Approved Nursing Diagnoses

North American Nursing Diagnosis Association (NANDA)
June 1990

Activity intolerance
Activity intolerance, potential
Adjustment, impaired
Airway clearance, ineffective
Anxiety
Aspiration, potential for
Body image disturbance
Body temperature, altered, potential
Bowel incontinence
Breastfeeding, effective
Breastfeeding, ineffective
Breathing pattern, ineffective
Cardiac output, decreased
Communication, impaired verbal
Constipation
Constipation, colonic
Constipation, perceived
Coping, defensive
Coping, family: potential for growth
Coping, ineffective family: compromised
Coping, ineffective family: disabling
Coping, ineffective individual
Decisional conflict (specify)
Denial, ineffective
Diarrhea
Disuse syndrome, potential for
Diversional activity deficit
Dysreflexia
Family processes, altered
Fatigue
Fear
Fluid volume deficit (1)
Fluid volume deficit (2)
Fluid volume deficit, potential
Fluid volume excess
Gas exchange, impaired
Grieving, anticipatory
Grieving, dysfunctional
Growth and development, altered
Health maintenance, altered
Health-seeking behaviors (specify)
Home maintenance management, impaired
Hopelessness
Hyperthermia
Hypothermia
Incontinence, functional
Incontinence, reflex
Incontinence, stress
Incontinence, total
Incontinence, urge
Infection, potential for

Injury, potential for
Knowledge deficit (specify)
Mobility, impaired physical
Noncompliance (specify)
Nutrition, altered: less than body requirements
Nutrition, altered: more than body requirements
Nutrition, altered: potential for more than body requirements
Oral mucous membrane, altered
Pain
Pain, chronic
Parental role conflict
Parenting, altered
Parenting, altered, potential
Personal identity disturbance
Poisoning, potential for
Post-trauma response
Powerlessness
Protection, altered
Rape-trauma syndrome
Rape-trauma syndrome: compound reaction
Rape-trauma syndrome: silent reaction
Role performance, altered
Self-care deficit, bathing/hygiene
Self-care deficit, dressing/grooming
Self-care deficit, feeding
Self-care deficit, toileting
Self-esteem disturbance
Self-esteem, chronic low
Self-esteem, situational low
Sensory/perceptual alterations (specify) (visual, auditory, kinesthetic, gustatory, tactile, olfactory)
Sexual dysfunction
Sexuality patterns, altered
Skin integrity, impaired
Skin integrity, impaired, potential
Sleep pattern disturbance
Social interaction, impaired
Social isolation
Spiritual distress (distress of the human spirit)
Suffocation, potential for
Swallowing, impaired
Thermoregulation, ineffective
Thought processes, altered
Tissue integrity, impaired
Tissue perfusion, altered (specify type) (renal, cerebral, cardiopulmonary, gastrointestinal, peripheral)
Trauma, potential for
Unilateral neglect
Urinary elimination, altered patterns
Urinary retention
Violence, potential for: self-directed or directed at others

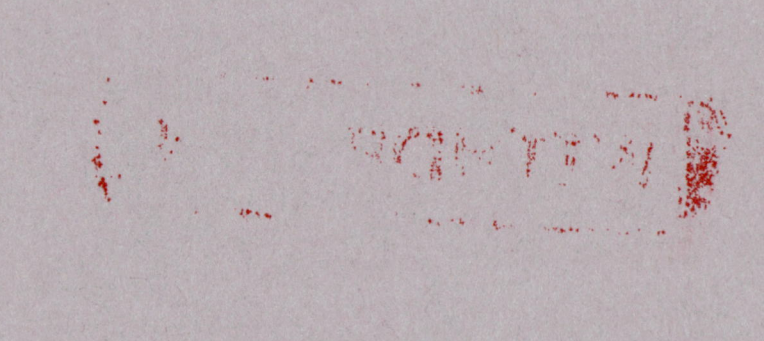

FUNDAMENTALS OF NURSING

Concepts, Process and Practice

FOURTH EDITION

FUNDAMENTALS OF NURSING

Concepts, Process and Practice

FOURTH EDITION

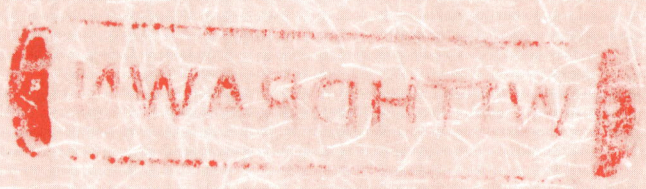

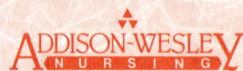

ADDISON-WESLEY
NURSING

A Division of The Benjamin/Cummings Publishing Company, Inc.
Redwood City, California • Menlo Park, California
Reading, Massachusetts • New York • Don Mills, Ontario • Wokingham, UK
Amsterdam • Bonn • Sydney • Tokyo • Madrid • San Juan

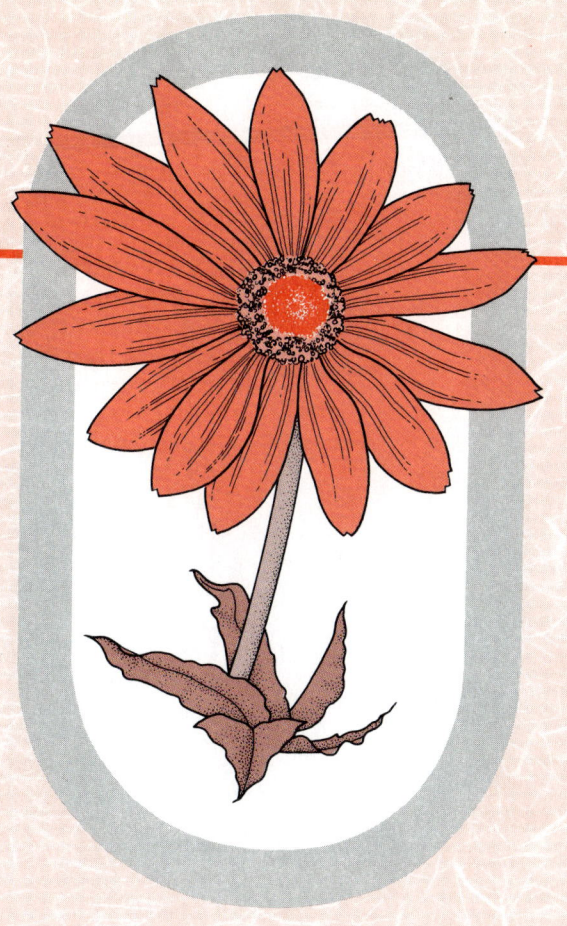

Barbara Kozier

RN, MN

Glenora Erb

RN, BSN

Rita Olivieri

RN, PHD

School of Nursing, Boston College, Chestnut Hill, Massachusetts

To Patti Cleary, sponsoring editor, and Wendy Earl, production editor, for their outstanding contributions to this book.

Sponsoring editor: *Patricia L. Cleary*
Production editor: *Wendy Earl*
Manuscript editor: *Antonio Padial*
Art editor: *Daniel J. Heller*
Photo editor: *Wendy Earl*
Interior designer: *Brenn Lea Pearson*
Insert designer: *Detta Penna*
Cover designer: *Rudy Zehntner/The Belmont Studio*
Text illustrator: *Jack P. Tandy*
Cover illustrator: *Joan Carol*
Insert illustrator: *Charles W. Hoffman*
Photographers: *Tom Ferentz, Judy Braginsky, Suzanne Arms Wimberley, Karen Stafford Rantzman, Tom Thompson, George B. Fry III*
Proofreader: *Jennifer Beachey*
Indexer: *Katherine Pitcoff*

Executive editor: *Debra S. Hunter*
Senior managing editor: *Glenda S. Epting*
Manufacturing supervisor: *Casimira Kostecki*

Compositor: *Graphic Typesetting Service*
Text and insert printer: *Rand McNally*
Cover printer: *Lehigh Press*

Photographic credits may be found on page 1448.

Library of Congress Cataloging-in-Publication Data
Kozier, Barbara.
    Fundamentals of nursing: concepts, process, and practice/ Barbara Kozier, Glenora Erb, Rita Olivieri.—4th ed.
        p.   cm.
    Includes bibliographical references and index.
    1. Nursing.   I. Erb, Glenora Lea.   II. Olivieri, Rita.
III. Title.
    [DNLM: 1. Nursing Care.   2. Nursing Process.   WY 100 K88fa]
RT41.K72   1991
610.73—dc20
DNLM/DLC   90-14491
for Library of Congress   CIP
ISBN 0-201-09202-6
5 6 7 8 9 10 -RN- 95 94 93 92

The authors and publisher thank the following institutions for their kind permission to photograph many of the clients who appear in this book:

Joseph M. Long Hospital, University of California, San Francisco, California
San Francisco General Hospital, San Francisco, California
Stanford University Medical Center, Palo Alto, California
Children's Memorial Hospital, Chicago, Illinois
El Camino Hospital, Mountain View, California
Mt. Sinai Hospital, Chicago, Illinois

In addition, the authors and publisher thank Patricia J. Larson, RN, DNSc, Mary Matejov, RN, and Patricia Wong, RN, and the 11 Long staff for their valuable assistance in providing client and nurse models; Karen Lou Kennedy, RN, FNP, for her images of decubitus ulcers; Eileen J. Plunkett, RN, for her collaboration on the physical assessment insert; and Tom Bauer of On•Gard Systems for providing the image of the On•Gard Recapper.

Care has been taken to confirm the accuracy of information presented in this book. The authors, editors, and the publisher, however, cannot accept any responsibility for errors or omissions or for consequences from application of the information in this book and make no warranty, express or implied, with respect to its contents.

The authors and publisher have exerted every effort to ensure that drug selections and dosages set forth in this text are in accord with current recommendations and practice at the time of publication. However, in view of ongoing research, changes in government regulations, and the constant flow of information relating to drug therapy and drug reactions, the reader is urged to check the package inserts of all drugs for any change in indications of dosage and for added warnings and precautions. This is particularly important when the recommended agent is a new and/or infrequently employed drug.

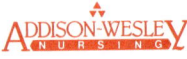

ADDISON-WESLEY
NURSING

A Division of the Benjamin/Cummings Publishing Company, Inc.
390 Bridge Parkway, Redwood City, California 94065

CONTRIBUTORS

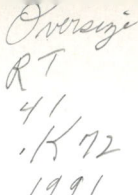

KATHLEEN KOERNIG BLAIS, RN, EDD
School of Nursing
Florida International University
Miami, FL
*Revised Chapter 31, Ethnic and Cultural Values.
Contributed three new care plans (sexuality, wound
care, and perioperative care). Reviewed all other care
plans*

PHYLLIS CARROLL, RN, MS
Saint Joseph College of Nursing
Joliet, IL
Contributed 13 nursing care plans

BONITA MORROW CAVANAUGH, RN, PHD
School of Nursing
University of Colorado
Denver, CO
Contributed two research notes

SARAH M. CIMINO, RN, MS
School of Nursing
Boston College
Chestnut Hill, MA
Revised Chapter 32, Spiritual and Religious Beliefs

JANICE DENEHY, RN, PHD
College of Nursing
The University of Iowa
Iowa City, IA
Contributed Chapter 28, Family Health

EDITH P. LEWIS, MN, FAAN
Former Editor of *Nursing Outlook*
*Contributed Appendix A, Significant Events in Nursing
History*

DIANA J. MASON, RNC, PHD
College of Nursing
Rutgers University
Newark, NJ
*Contributed information on power and political action
in Chapter 3, Changing Nursing Practice: Trends,
Research, and Politics*

RITA OLIVIERI, RN, PHD
School of Nursing
Boston College
Chestnut Hill, MA
*Revised Unit IV, The Nursing Process, and Unit VIII,
Promoting Health Through the Lifespan, Contributed
computer information in Chapter 3, Changing Nursing
Practice: Trends, Research, and Politics, and Chapter 17,
Documenting and Reporting*

ROSS A. STEWART, RPN, RN, MHSC
Department of Psychiatric Nursing
Douglas College
New Westminster, BC, Canada
Revised Chapter 30: Sexuality

SUSAN W. TALBOTT, RN, MA, MBA
Principal, Woman's Financial Center of Baltimore
Baltimore, MD
*Contributed information on power and political action
in Chapter 3, Changing Nursing Practice: Trends,
Research, and Politics*

HOLLY SKODOL WILSON, RN, PHD, FAAN
School of Nursing
University of California
San Francisco, CA
*Contributed nursing research material in Chapter 2,
Socialization and Roles of the Nurse, and Chapter 3,
Changing Nursing Practice: Trends, Research, and
Politics*

REVIEWERS

DEBBIE AMASON, BSN, MS
Department of Nursing
Cleveland State Community College
Cleveland, TN

KATHLEEN KOERNIG BLAIS, RN, EDD
School of Nursing
Florida International University
Miami, FL

DARLENE BOLTON, BSN, MSN, CRNP
School of Nursing
Troy State University
Troy, Alabama

JANIS C. CHILDS, RN, MSN, PNP
School of Nursing
University of Virginia
Charlottesville, VA

EMMA CLARK, RN, MSN
Department of Nursing
Nicolls State University
Thibodaus, LA

JUDY DAVY, BSN, MSH
Department of Nursing
Humboldt State University
Arcata, CA

PATRICIA A. DIEHL, RN, BSN, MA
School of Nursing
West Virginia University
Morgantown, WV

JEANNE C. DUFFY, CAES, MS
School of Nursing
Salem State College
Salem, MA

D. KAREN ENRIGHT, RN, PHD
Department of Nursing
Rhode Island College
Providence, RI

JOANNE M. FLANDERS, RN, MS
Department of Nursing
Midwestern State University
Wichita Falls, TX

MARY S. KOITHAN, BSN, MSN
Department of Nursing
University of Nevada, Las Vegas
Las Vegas, NV

LILY LEE, RN, BS, MSN, ADVANCED
CERTIFICATE IN EDUCATION
Department of Nursing
Illinois Central College
East Peoria, IL

RUTH LUDWICK, RNC, MSN
School of Nursing
Kent State University
Kent, OH

KATHLEEN MULRYAN, RN, BSN, MSN
Nursing Programs
La Guardia Community College
Long Island City, NY

JOYCE MURRAY, RN, BSN
Nursing Programs
Weber State University
Ogden, UT

IVY M. NELSON, RN, EdD
Director, Division of Nursing
University of the District
of Columbia
Washington, D.C.

MICHELE PORADZISZ, RN, BSN, MS
Department of Nursing
De Paul University
Chicago, IL

JANICE RUMFELT, RNC, BSN, MSN
School of Nursing
Southern Illinois University
Edwardsville, IL

JULIE G. SEBASTIAN, RN, MSN
College of Nursing
University of Kentucky
Lexington, KY

LINA K. SIMS, RNCS, BSN, MSN
St. Joseph's College of Nursing
Joliet, IL

HILARY STRAUB, BSN, MSED, PHD
Department of Nursing
Boise State University
Boise, ID

ANITA L. THORNE, BSNE, MA
College of Nursing
Arizona State University
Tempe, AZ

STEVEN RENE TOUSSAINT,
RN, MSN, OCN
School of Nursing
Linfield College
Portland, OR

ANN F. TULLY, RN, MSN
Department of Nursing
Highland Community College
Freeport, IL

DORCAS D. WILLIAMS,
RN, BA, BSN, MSN
College of Nursing
Chicago State University
Chicago, IL

LOLA WILMES, RN, BSNE, MSN
Department of Nurse Science
Oklahoma State University
Oklahoma City, OK

EMILY C. ZABROCKI, RN, PHD
Department of Nursing Education
Joliet Junior College
Joliet, IL

PREFACE

The complete, mature, or excellent nurse ... is the one who remains compassionate and sensitive to patients, who has thoroughly mastered nursing's technical skills, but who uses— and has the opportunity to use—her emotional and technical responses in a unique design that suits the peculiar needs of the person she serves and the situation in which she finds herself.

Virginia Henderson
"Excellence in Nursing"
American Journal of Nursing,
October, 1969

*N*ursing is a remarkably challenging and gratifying endeavor, synthesizing the mastery of technical procedure with the abililty to care for people in need. This powerful integration of broad knowledge, technical expertise, and humanistic caring defines contemporary nursing practice to a large degree.

It is an extraordinarily exciting time to become a nurse, a time of rapid technological innovation, of pioneering nursing research and literature, of ever-greater appreciation for human universality as well as diversity, and of significant gains toward achieving professional recognition.

With this edition, *Fundamentals of Nursing* continues its tradition of providing a solid foundation on which students can build their technical and interpersonal expertise. Because nursing is a dynamic art and science, every chapter has been meticulously revised and updated to incorporate the latest nursing research and technology and to reflect the increasing autonomy and accountability of nurses. The fourth edition also puts to advantage many valuable suggestions from reviewers and nurses using the text.

NEW FEATURES

Three New Chapters

- Socialization and Roles of the Nurse
- Theories and Conceptual Frameworks
- Changing Nursing Practice

Very Special Learning Aids

- Safety alert logos ⚠ indicating when safety precautions are essential.
- Blood and body fluid alert logos 🩸 to reinforce awareness of CDC body fluid precautions.
- A full-color section on physical health assessment.
- A full-color section on the nursing process.
- A full-color section showing common skin disorders, including decubitus ulcers.

Increased Application of Nursing Process

- Assessment interview boxes, designed in question format to help students obtain nursing history data and conduct interviews.
- Expanded lists of nursing diagnoses with contributing factors and tables showing assessment data clusters and related nursing diagnoses. The focus is on applying nursing diagnoses rather than on providing detailed information about each diagnosis, which is readily available from other sources.
- Expanded lists of outcome criteria in the planning sections.

Increased Emphasis on Wellness
See Chapter 5, Health and Illness, and Unit 8, Promoting Health Through the Life Span, Chapters 23–28. Wellness diagnoses are also included.

Focus on the Elderly
Eighteen boxes showing normal physical changes (in Chapter 19, Assessing Health Status) and an entire chapter (Chapter 27, Late Adulthood) devoted to promoting the health of the elderly.

Increased Application of Nursing Research
In each chapter, a box summarizing a related research study and explaining its clinical application. Each chapter then concludes with a list of related research.

Clinical Guidelines Boxes In many chapters, instant-access summaries of clinical dos and don'ts.

Teaching Boxes Quick-reference displays that focus on the client's learning needs.

ORGANIZATION

This edition has been organized into eleven units plus six appendixes, a glossary, and an index. The steps of the nursing process are a major organizational element in most chapters. Units and chapters are organized so that they can be used independently or in any sequence.

Unit 1, Contemporary Nursing Practice, introduces the student to the nursing profession and its role within the health care system. The first chapter includes information about contemporary nursing, such as definitions of nursing, historical perspectives, concepts of professionalism, and nurse practice standards. Chapter 4, Theories and Conceptual Frameworks, includes theories about nursing, selected theoretical views of human beings, theories about caring, and other theories that affect nursing practice. Information that influences the future of nursing, including trends, research, and political activism, has been integrated into Chapter 3, Changing Nursing Practice.

Unit 2, Health Perceptions and Management, focuses on concepts of health, health beliefs, wellness, well-being, illness, and disease. Current health trends, health care systems, and problems are included. Future challenges and implications for nursing are addressed. A discussion of the rights of clients is now included in Chapter 6, Health Care Delivery Systems.

Unit 3, Professional Accountability and Advocacy, highlights essential ethical and legal aspects of nursing practice. The acquisition of personal and professional values, nursing codes of ethics, and ethical issues and dilemmas are introduced. Also included are the many facets of the law affecting nursing, such as nurse-practice acts, contractual arrangements in nursing, areas of potential liability in nursing, and informed consent.

Unit 4, The Nursing Process, provides an in-depth discussion of the process as a whole, devoting separate chapters to each of the five components. This unit introduces the knowledge and abilities required (a) to assess the client's health status, (b) to cluster and analyze data and formulate nursing diagnoses, (c) to establish client goals and outcome criteria and select appropriate nursing interventions (that is, develop a nursing care plan), (d) to implement nursing interventions effectively, and (e) to perform ongoing evaluation of goal achievement and the effectiveness of nursing

interventions. Throughout these chapters, the discussion follows one client, building a nursing care plan. The unit, therefore, lays the groundwork for application of the process throughout the remainder of the text.

Unit 5, Interactive Processes, focuses on the skills needed to establish and maintain a helping relationship, to implement a teaching plan, and to exchange essential information about the client through recording and reporting. Group interaction has been streamlined and integrated with Chapter 15, Helping and Communicating. It focuses on types of health care groups, features of effective groups, and assessment and evaluation of group dynamics.

Unit 6, Assessing Health, explains clinical health assessment. It begins with the assessment of vital signs and continues with the general survey and a head-to-toe approach for assessing overall health status. A table comparing the body systems approach to functional health patterns is included for nurses who use a functional health pattern approach.

Unit 7, Protecting Health, describes current practices regarding the transfer of microorganisms and offers specific guidelines that nurses should follow to protect themselves and their clients from microbial infections.

Unit 8, Promoting Health through the Life Span, focuses on the nurse's role in providing health education to clients and fostering healthful behaviors in clients from infancy through late adulthood. Separate chapters are devoted to the concept of health promotion, theoretical views of growth and development, the older adult, and family health. Each stage of development includes physical, psychosocial, cognitive, moral, and spiritual development. Pertinent health education topics, such as colic in the infant and elder abuse, are included for each stage.

Unit 9, Supporting Psychosocial Health Patterns, discusses both psychosocial and biophysical concepts that help the student gain an understanding of human differences and responses. Specific chapters address self-concept and role relationships, sexuality, ethnic and cultural values, spiritual and religious beliefs, stress tolerance and coping, and the grieving process.

Unit 10, Supporting Physiologic Health Patterns, contains chapters on physiologic needs and nursing activities to help clients meet these needs. Like Unit 9, it uses the nursing process as a unifying thread and in addition, includes common techniques the nurse performs in daily practice.

Unit 11, Implementing Special Nursing Measures, introduces the student to underlying basic principles of commonly performed procedures, such as administering medications, providing wound care, caring for clients before and after surgery, and assisting clients during special diagnostic and therapeutic procedures. Current guidelines from the Centers for Disease Control have been integrated.

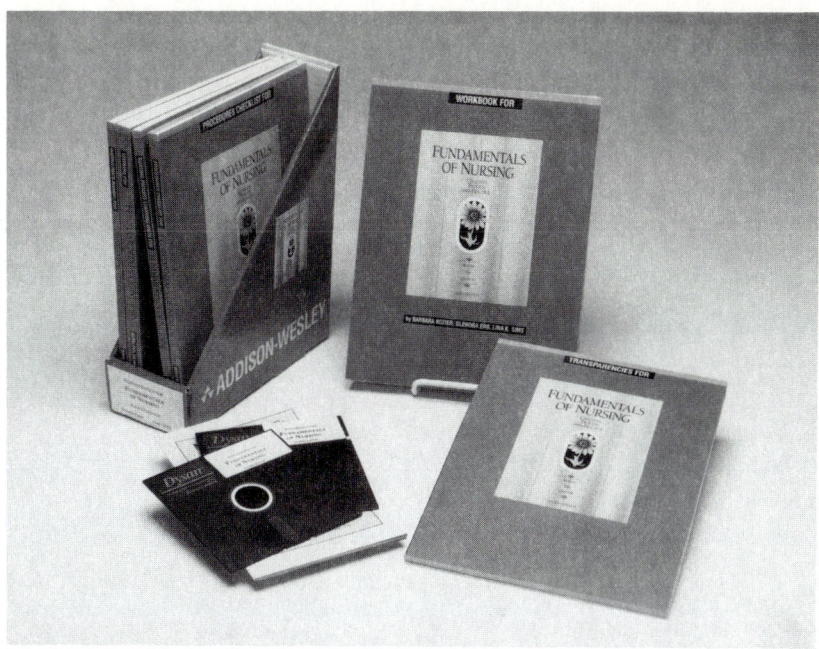

The comprehensive new supplement package contains six items to help instructors and students make the best use of this edition.

PEDAGOGICAL FEATURES

Procedures   Procedures have been streamlined to facilitate learning, with key rationales shown in italics. In addition, the Guide to Required Nursing Actions on page *xxx* lists nursing actions common to all procedures.

Nursing Care Plans   The number of nursing care plans has increased to 17, and all have been updated to reflect current NANDA terminology.

Enhanced Visual Appeal   Numerous illustrations, with color added to many of the line drawings, highlight focal points. Full-color guides to the nursing process, physical assessment, and skin disorders are included.

Appendixes, Glossary, and Index   To meet the student's need for quick reference materials, the authors have included six appendices on (a) significant events in nursing history; (b) nursing organizations; (c) NANDA-approved nursing diagnostic categories: *Taxonomy I Revised;* (d) root words, prefixes, and suffixes; (e) *Canada's Food Guide* (1985); and (f) weight and volume equivalents. A glossary and a comprehensive index end the book.

Inside Front and Back Cover Information
The Universal Precautions from the Centers for Disease Control, a complete list of the latest NANDA diagnoses, and a table of standard international (SI) units appear on the inside covers for easy accessibility.

SUPPLEMENTAL TEACHING/LEARNING PACKAGE

To help instructors make the best use of this new edition, the authors have developed a comprehensive new supplements package with the following components:

Workbook for Fundamentals of Nursing   This workbook, written by Lina K. Sims, challenges students to apply and extend knowledge as they complete inventive learning exercises. Each chapter contains learning objectives, questions in a variety of formats, self-assessment sections, and additional learning activities.

Fundamentals Resource Center (New)   This resource center is a special assortment of helpful tools for today's nurse educator. Free to adopters, this collection of valuable resources includes the following:

- *Nursing Process Learning Units,* by Judith M. Wilkinson, reinforce and help students to apply content in Unit 4, *The Nursing Process.* Each of six learning units provides a pretest, exercises in a variety of formats, a post-test, and answers to all three. Complete rationales are provided for correct and incorrect answers. These units are ideal for independent study.

- *Procedures Checklists* provide a tool to evaluate how well students perform each step of a given procedure.

- *Instructor's Manual,* by Lina K. Sims, provides chapter-by-chapter overviews, with objectives, key terms, discussion questions, classroom and clinical activities, recommended audiovisual aids, and teaching strategies.

- A *Test Bank* provides 1000 test items covering many cognitive levels. All questions are presented in NCLEX format.

The two following items are also available:

- A *Transparency Kit* includes 40 two-color transparencies to support classroom presentations.
- *Delta Testing Software* is a computerized version of the Test Bank for the IBM PC and Apple computers.

Just as nursing is influenced by forces from within and from without, this book continues to be shaped by comments from instructors and students who use it. The acceptance of the preceding editions has been most gratifying, and the authors continue to welcome suggestions for ways to make this book even more helpful to students.

Barbara Kozier
Glenora Erb
Rita Olivieri

ACKNOWLEDGMENTS

We would like to extend our warmest appreciation and sincere thanks to the many persons who participated in the development and production of this book:

- The contributors who provided content in their areas of expertise: Kathleen Blais, Phyllis Carroll, Bonita Cavanaugh, Sarah Cimino, Janice Denehy, Barbara Germino, Edith Lewis, Diana Mason, Rita Olivieri, Ross Stewart, Susan Talbott, and Holly Skodol Wilson.

- The nursing students and teachers who used previous editions of *Fundamentals* and who sent us many helpful suggestions for this edition.

- All reviewers, who provided so many valuable comments.

- Patti Cleary, the sponsoring editor, whose stimulating new ideas and commitment to excellence have greatly helped in the preparation of this manuscript. In addition, her enthusiasm, sense of what is needed, and competence have benefited every aspect of this project. Her input in so many areas has been invaluable.

- Wendy Earl, the production editor, whose sensitive and understanding nature, flexibility in manipulating schedules, and meticulous attention to detail has been indispensable to the authors. Her creative input into the book design and selection of photographs was also greatly appreciated.

- Armando Parcés Enríquez, for his editorial support and enthusiasm in the initial stages of this project.

- Antonio Padial and Sarah Carolina, who as copy editors provided many helpful suggestions on style and syntax.

- Debra Hunter, executive editor, and Glenda Epting, senior managing editor, for their continuing support.

- Daniel Heller, whose attention to detail in organizing and managing the art program for this text has been greatly appreciated.

- Brenn Lea Pearson, designer, for producing a contemporary design concept for the interior of this edition that resulted in a streamlined, visually appealing book.

- Dorthy Lee, editorial assistant, for her gracious help whenever it was needed.

- Jennifer Beachey, for her careful attention to detail when reading the galleys.

- Katherine Pitcoff, for her meticulous reading of the pages to create a comprehensive index.

- Lina K. Sims, for her dedicated and creative efforts in developing a new workbook for this edition.

- Photographers Tom Ferentz, Judy Braginsky, and Suzanne Arms Wimberley—new to this edition—for their creative, sensitive, and realistic photographs.

- Illustrator Jack Tandy of St. Louis, who provided the new line drawings that are, as usual, models of clarity.

- The typists, Allankah Goldy and Mary Tobin, who were so accommodating to the schedule and whose skills and flexibility enabled us to meet many deadlines.

- Joan Andrews, Andrew Stefanelli, and Linda Edge at the Registered Nurses's Association of British Columbia for their willing assistance in acquiring many reference materials for the manuscript.

- Finally, our understanding families and friends who once again were patient and supportive throughout yet another writing schedule.

BRIEF CONTENTS

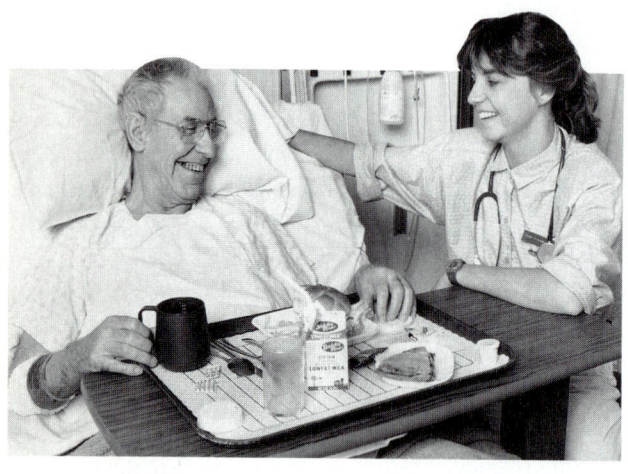

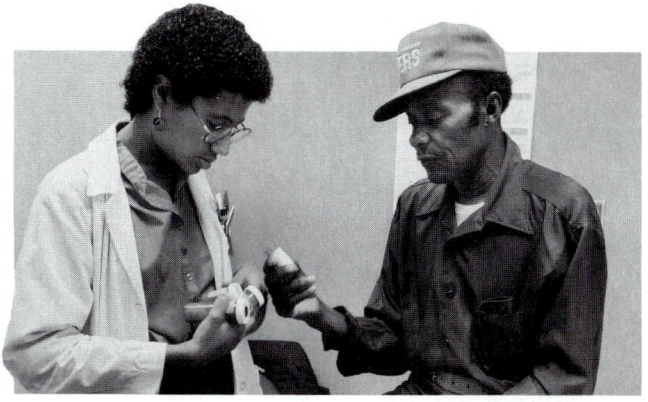

DETAILED CONTENTS

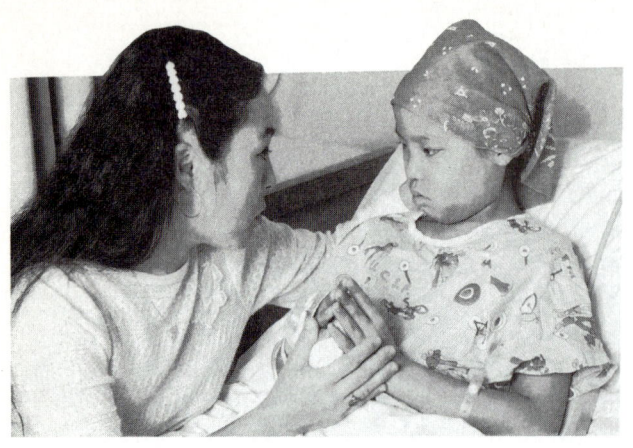

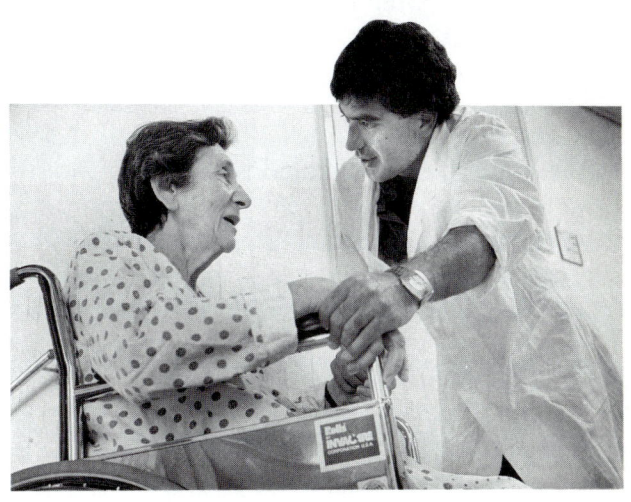

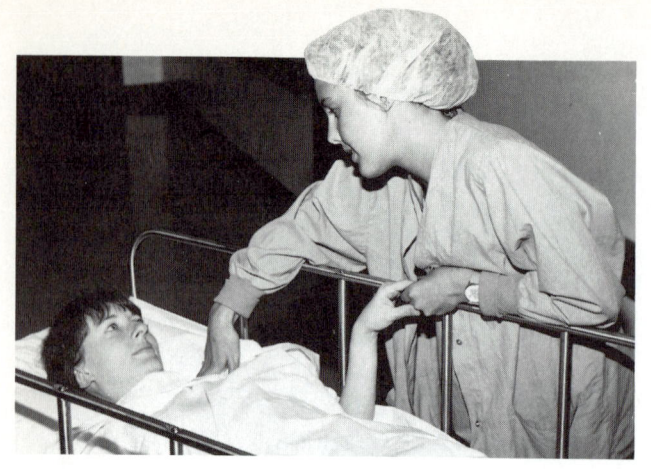

UNIT

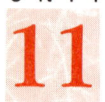

***IMPLEMENTING SPECIAL NURSING
MEASURES***   *1247*

CLINICAL SKILLS AND PROCEDURES

SUMMARY OF SPECIAL FEATURES

ASSESSMENT INTERVIEWS/GUIDELINES

CLIENT TEACHING

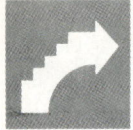

CLINICAL GUIDELINES

RESEARCH NOTES

NURSING CARE PLANS

The following logos are used throughout the text:

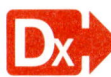 **Nursing Diagnoses**

This logo directs the reader to a list of relevant diagnoses for a particular client problem. Diagnoses are expressed in two-part format; they include problem statements as well as etiologies.

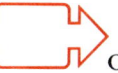 **Outcome Criteria**

This logo directs the reader to a list of outcome criteria that relate directly to the diagnoses stated earlier.

 Blood and Body Fluid Precautions

This logo draws attention to the need for blood and body fluid precautions. These precautions are intended to protect the nurse and others from infection. See the CDC Guidelines on the inside front cover, and check with your instructor regarding agency protocol to determine which precautionary measures to implement.

 Safety Precautions

This logo highlights nursing actions that are of particular significance for maintaining client and nurse safety. If you require clarification, consult your instructor or check agency protocol to ensure safe practice.

GUIDE TO REQUIRED NURSING ACTIONS

Specific nursing actions have been omitted from each procedure to avoid repetition. These actions, which underlie safe, competent nursing, are:

- Wash the hands before gathering any clean or sterile supplies, before implementing a procedure, and after contact with a client to avoid transmission of microorganisms to clients and others.

- Implement appropriate blood and body fluid precautions (see inside front cover). The authors suggest wearing gloves for most procedures that involve direct contact with any body fluid, even though blood may not be present in the body fluid and gloving may not always be necessary.

- Identify the client appropriately, e.g., by reading the client's wrist band.

- Explain the procedure to the client and, in some instances, to support persons, adjusting your explanation to their needs. Explaining what you plan to do reassures people by letting them know what to expect. Explanations are provided in some procedures.

- Provide privacy for the client when any aspect of the procedure could be embarrassing to the client or others and as an indication of respect even when the client is not conscious.

- Elevate the client's bed to a working level and lower the near side rail before starting a procedure. These actions help the nurse maintain good body mechanics.

- Following a procedure, lower the bed and raise the near side rail for clients requiring these precautions. These actions are taken for the client's safety.

- Ensure that the client is comfortable following the procedure.

- Dispose of used and unused supplies according to agency practice. This step includes cleaning and/or disinfecting equipment as necessary.

CONTEMPORARY NURSING PRACTICE

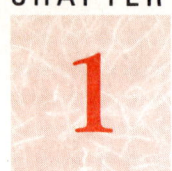

CHAPTER

1

Introduction to Nursing

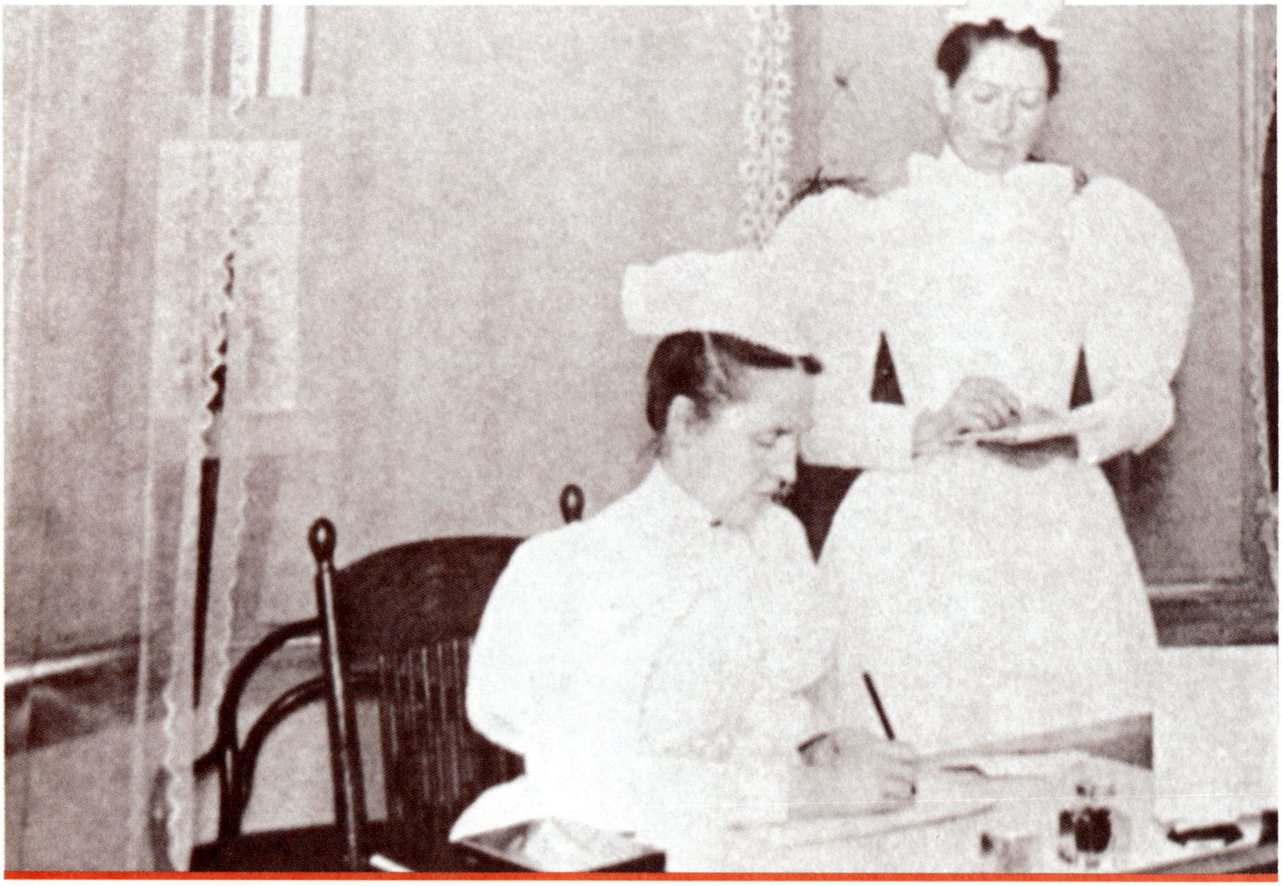

CONTENTS

- Identify the essential aspects of nursing.
- Explain the professional growth within nursing.
- Identify the functions that Styles cites as necessary for the preservation and development of a profession.
- Identify the critical attributes of professionalism in nursing as identified by Miller.
- Identify essential concepts in the historical development of nursing.
- Explain the significance of nurse practice acts.
- Describe the settings for nursing practice.
- Describe the importance of standards of nursing practice.
- Explain career mobility and expanded roles.
- Describe the various educational programs in nursing.
- Explain the functions of the national nurses' associations.

AN EMERGING DEFINITION OF NURSING

Nursing today is far different from nursing as it was practiced 50 years ago, and it takes a vivid imagination to envision how the nursing profession will change in the next 50 years in an ever-changing world. To comprehend present-day nursing and at the same time prepare for nursing in tomorrow's world, one must understand not only past events but also contemporary nursing practice and the sociologic factors affecting it.

Florence Nightingale defined nursing over 100 years ago as "the act of utilizing the environment of the patient to assist him in his recovery" (Nightingale 1860). Nightingale considered a clean, well-ventilated, and quiet environment essential for recovery. Often considered the first nurse theorist, Nightingale raised the status of nursing through education. Nurses were no longer untrained housekeepers but people trained in the care of the sick.

Virginia Henderson was one of the first modern nurses to define nursing. In 1960, she wrote, "The unique function of the nurse is to assist the individual, sick or well, in the performance of those activities contributing to health or its recovery (or to peaceful death) that he would perform unaided if he had the necessary strength, will, or knowledge, and to do this in such a way as to help him gain independence as rapidly as possible" (Henderson 1966, p. 3). Like Nightingale, Henderson described nursing in relation to the client and the client's environment. Unlike Nightingale, Henderson saw the nurse as concerned with both well and ill individuals, acknowledged that nurses interact with clients even when recovery may not be feasible, and mentioned the teaching and advocacy roles of the nurse.

In the latter half of the twentieth century, a number of nurse theorists developed their own views of nursing. A **nurse theorist** is a person who seeks to define basic principles of nursing practice systematically. Certain themes are common to many of these definitions: that nursing is caring, adaptive, individualized, holistic, family- and community-interrelated; that it involves teaching and direct/indirect services; and that it is a science as well as an art concerned with health promotion, health maintenance, health restoration, and the care of the dying. See Table 1–1 for definitions of nursing by selected nurse theorists.

Professional nursing associations have also examined nursing and developed their definitions of nursing. The American Nurses' Association (ANA) describes nursing practice as "direct, goal oriented, and adaptable to the needs of the individual, the family, and community during health and illness" (ANA 1973, p. 2). In 1980, the ANA published this definition of nursing: "Nursing is the diagnosis and treatment of human responses to actual or potential health problems" (ANA 1980, p. 9). In its 1987 House of Delegates, the ANA adopted a statement on the scope of nursing practice: "There is one scope of clinical nursing practice. The core, or essence, of that practice is the nursing diagnosis and treatment of human responses to health and to illness" (ANA 1987a, p. 76). The new statement further describes the differences between professional and technical nurses: The "depth and breadth to which the individual nurse engages in the total scope of the clinical practice of nursing are defined by the knowledge base of the nurse, the role of the nurse, and the nature of the client population within a practice environment" (ANA 1987a, p. 76). The Canadian Nurses' Association (CNA) published a definition in 1984 that serves as the professional standard for nurses in Canada.

"Nursing" or "the practice of nursing" means the identification and treatment of human responses to actual or potential health problems and includes the practice of and supervision of functions and services that, directly or indirectly, in collaboration with a client or providers of health care other than nurses, have as their objectives the promotion of health, prevention of illness, alleviation of suffering, restoration of health and optimum development of health potential and includes all aspects of the nursing process (CNA Connection 1984, p. 8).

AN EVOLVING PROFESSION

The profession of nursing has evolved over centuries. The traditional nursing role was one of humanistic caring, nurturing, comforting, and supporting. To these must be added

TABLE 1-1 *Definitions and Descriptions of Nursing*

Nursing Theorist and Theory	Definition/Description
Faye Abdellah (1960): Twenty-one nursing problems	Service to individuals and families; therefore, to society. An art and science that molds the attitudes, intellectual competencies, and technical skills of the individual nurse into the desire and ability to help people, sick or well, cope with their health needs. May be carried out under general or specific medical direction.
Virginia Henderson (1960): Fourteen basic needs	The unique function of the nurse: to assist clients, sick or well, in the performance of those activities contributing to health, its recovery, or peaceful death that clients would perform unaided if they had the necessary strength, will, or knowledge. Also, to do so in such a way as to help clients gain independence as rapidly as possible.
Dorothy E. Johnson (1980): Behavioral system theory	An external regulatory force that acts to preserve the organization and integration of the client's behavior at an optimal level under those conditions in which the behavior constitutes a threat to physical or social health or in which illness is found.
Imogene King (1971, 1981): Goal attainment theory	A helping profession that assists individuals and groups in society to attain, maintain, and restore health. If this is not possible, nurses help individuals die with dignity. Nursing is perceiving, thinking, relating, judging, and acting vis-a-vis the behavior of individuals who come to a nursing situation. A nursing situation is the immediate environment, spatial and temporal reality, in which nurse and client establish a relationship to cope with health states and adjust to changes in activities of daily living if the situation demands adjustment. It is an interpersonal process of action, reaction, interaction, and transaction whereby nurse and client share information about their perceptions in the nursing situation.
Madeleine Leininger (1984): Transcultural care theory	A learned humanistic art and science that focuses on personalized (individual and group) care behaviors, functions, and processes directed toward promoting and maintaining health behaviors or recovery from illness. Behaviors have physical, psychocultural, and social significance or meaning for those being assisted generally by a professional nurse or one with similar role competencies.
Myra Levine (1973): Four conservation principles	A human interaction; a discipline rooted in the organic dependency of the individual on relationships with other human beings. A subculture reflecting ideas and values unique to nurses, even though the values mirror the social template that created them.
Bette Neuman (1982): Systems theory	A unique profession in that it is concerned with all of the variables affecting an individual's response to stressors, which are intra-, inter-, and extrapersonal in nature. The concern of nursing is to prevent stress invasion, or, following stress invasion, to protect the client's basic structure and obtain or maintain a maximum level of wellness. The nurse helps the client, through primary, secondary, and tertiary prevention modes, to adjust to environmental stressors and maintain client system stability.
Dorothea Orem (1985): Self-care theory	A helping or assisting service to persons who are wholly or partly dependent—infants, children, and adults—when they, their parents, guardians, or other adults responsible for their care are no longer able to give or supervise their care. A creative effort of one human being to help another human being. Nursing is deliberate action, a function of the practical intelligence of nurses, and action to bring about humanely desirable conditions in persons and their environments. It is distinguished from other human services and other forms of care by its focus on human beings.
Hildegard Peplau (1952): Psychodynamic nursing	A therapeutic, interpersonal process. It functions cooperatively with other human processes that make health possible for people in communities. An educative instrument, a maturing force that aims to promote forward movement of the personality in the direction of creative, constructive, productive, personal, and community living.
Martha Rogers (1970): Unitary human beings, an energy field	A humanistic science dedicated to compassionate concern with maintaining and promoting health, preventing illness, and caring for and rehabilitating the sick and disabled. Nursing seeks to promote symphonic interaction between the environment and the person, to strengthen the coherence and integrity of the human beings, and to direct and redirect patterns of interaction between the person and the environment for the realization of maximum health potential.
Sister Callista Roy (1976, 1984): Adaptation theory	A theoretical system of knowledge that prescribes a process of analysis and action related to the care of the ill or potentially ill person. As a science, nursing is a developing system of knowledge about persons used to observe, classify, and relate the processes by which persons positively affect their health status. As a practice discipline, nursing's scientific body of knowledge is used to provide an essential service to people, that is, to promote ability to affect health positively.

specific characteristics of true professionalism, including education, a code of ethics, mastery of a craft, an informed membership involved in the organized profession, and accountability for actions (Flaherty 1979, p. 61).

Historical Perspective

As an activity that provides help to the ill, to children, and to babies, nursing has existed since the earliest times. Before the early Christian period (A.D. 1–500), caring for the sick was a function women performed in their homes. Later, monastic orders provided nursing functions as part of their activities. The first nursing order, the Augustinian Sisters, was established in the Middle Ages. This was probably the first organized group to provide purely nursing services to people.

Prior to the Protestant Reformation in the 16th century, hospital facilities were organized chiefly by the Roman Catholic Church. With the Reformation, beginning in 1517, came a decline in people's interest in and support of the church and religion. This change introduced an era known in nursing history as the "dark period." Hospitals were unsanitary places, dark and foreboding. Nursing was provided by women who were frequently described as drunk, heartless, and immoral. They were expected to carry out the housework of the hospital, wash the laundry, and do all the cleaning for very little reward. No training was required of nurses, and it was not unusual for a nurse to work from 12 to 40 consecutive hours. This period of decline lasted until the middle of the 19th century.

The era of reform in nursing is marked by the work of the British nurse, Florence Nightingale, during the Crimean War (1854–56). Nightingale's efforts made nursing a respectable vocation once again. However, Nightingale's reform activities did not stop at respectability. Besides crusading for cleanliness and comfort in hospitals, Nightingale also worked toward educating the populace regarding health measures in an effort to stave off the widespread diseases resulting from poor conditions in the cities. Nightingale believed in prevention and in nursing the whole person, calling upon nurses to make sure that patients always had fresh air, good water, proper medication, quiet, mobility, and knowledge of how to care for themselves in the future. Many of Nightingale's ideas are now standards of client care. Education of nurses was a major goal of this reformer. Among her many other accomplishments was the establishment of the Nightingale School of Nurses at St. Thomas' Hospital, London, in 1860. This school is credited with providing the first planned educational program for nurses. She also assisted in establishing the first organized home nursing services.

In North America, establishment of nursing and health services was slow before the American Revolution (1775–83). One notable organization was the Nurse Society of Philadelphia, which gave women minimal instruction in obstetrics to enable them to provide maternity nursing services in home settings.

The late 1800s was a time of rapid reform of nursing services in the United States and Canada. Schools of nursing with planned educational programs were started. A number of their graduates became the early leaders in the profession.

Isabel Hampton Robb had been a young school-teacher in Canada. She decided to change her profession and entered the Bellevue Hospital Training School in New York. After graduation, she nursed in Rome for two years, and then she became superintendent of the Illinois Training School at 26 years of age. Three years later she went to Baltimore to organize a new school in connection with Johns Hopkins Hospital. Among her many accomplishments was a nursing textbook, which became the standard text for nursing schools in America.

Mary Adelaide Nutting, also from Canada, was in the first class at Johns Hopkins. After graduation, she established a course of training for students prior to ward experience at Johns Hopkins. Later, she reduced the nursing students' hours from 12 to 8 and lengthened the nurses training to three years.

Mary Agnes Snively graduated from Bellevue and returned to Canada to take charge of the nurses' training at Toronto General Hospital. She is credited largely with the direction of Canadian nursing education and was the first president of the Canadian Nurses' Association.

Two American graduates of the New York Hospital, Lillian D. Wald and Mary Brewster, were the first to offer trained nursing services to the poor in the New York slums. Their home among the poor on the upper floor of a tenement is now famous as a center of public health nursing (the Henry Street Settlement). Soon after, school nursing was established as an adjunct to visiting nursing. Again, Wald was involved, along with Lina L. Rogers.

Linda Richards, who graduated in 1873 from the New England Hospital for Women and Children Training School for Nurses in Boston, is cited by many historians as America's first trained nurse. She is credited with reforming nursing in 12 major hospitals, some of which were specialized mental hospitals. She initiated training schools for students in mental health nursing. Her programs included a period of training in general hospitals. She also founded the first training school for nurses in Japan.

Some, however, dispute that Richards was the first trained nurse. Evidence in a series of reports of Women's Hospital of Philadelphia suggests that Harriet Newton Phillips was the first trained nurse to receive a certificate from that hospital in 1864 (Large 1976, p. 50). Phillips is also considered the first trained nurse in America to do community nursing, to do missionary service, and to take postgraduate training.

America's first trained black nurse was Mary Mahoney. She trained at the same hospital as Linda Richards and graduated in 1879.

The need for concerted action by nurses was first felt in England during the late 1800s. In 1894, the Matrons' Council of Great Britain and Ireland was organized, followed by the American Society of Superintendents of Training Schools for Nurses of the United States and Canada. Alumnae associations joined to form the Nurses' Associated Alumnae of the United States and Canada in 1897. From these North American organizations current national groups were founded. The Society of Superintendents divided nationally and ultimately became the Canadian National Association of Trained Nurses in 1908 (now the Canadian Nurses' Association) and the National League of Nursing Education in 1912. The Nurses' Associated Alumnae became the American Nurses' Association in 1911. See the section on nursing organizations later in this chapter. In 1908, the National Association of Colored Graduate Nurses was founded by a group of nurses who felt such an association could further not only the nursing cause but their own interests.

After World War I, the Frontier Nursing Service (FNS) was established by a notable pioneer nurse, Mary Breckinridge. In 1918, she worked with the American Committee for Devastated France, distributing food, clothing, and supplies to rural villages in France and taking care of sick children. In 1921, Breckinridge returned to the United States with plans to provide health care to the people of rural America. She initially prepared herself by taking courses at Teachers College in New York (where she met Mary Adelaide Nutting and gained her approval) and midwifery training in London and by developing prominent social contacts for fundraising. In 1925, Breckinridge and two other nurses began the FNS in Leslie County, Kentucky. Within this organization, Breckinridge began one of the first midwifery training schools in the United States.

The general trend from the beginning of formal organization of nursing of the late 1800s to the end of World War I was rapid expansion in the establishment of hospitals, with nursing schools dependent on them for support. Hospitals in turn depended on the schools to carry the chief nursing load. During the war, greater numbers of young women were accepted for entrance, and less consideration was given to selection requirements. Most schools by this time had adopted 3-year programs, but the 8-hour day originally proposed with those programs was less quickly adopted.

By 1920, the hospital system of educating nurses was increasingly criticized. In addition, the effectiveness of the nurse as a teacher of nurses was being questioned. Thus, a special postbasic course was offered at Teachers College, Columbia University, New York, to prepare nurses as teachers. Preparations for a postbasic public health nursing program were also made, in response to an influenza epidemic and the development of broader aims by the medical profession, which now included teaching the principles of healthful living to individuals, families, and community groups.

During the early 1920s, the Rockefeller Survey (Committee for the Study of Nursing Education) recommended that nursing schools be independent of hospitals and on a col-

lege level. As a result, two university schools of nursing were set up, one at Yale University, New Haven, Connecticut, the other at Western Reserve University, Cleveland, Ohio. The purpose of these experimental schools was to prove the feasibility of planning both classroom instruction and ward practice in accordance with the educational needs of the students. Emphasis was placed on the social welfare and health aspects of nursing. Both schools demonstrated the value of university standards in the nursing field.

Another far-reaching result of the Rockefeller Survey was a proposal by the National League of Nursing Education to undertake a comprehensive study of nursing education (1926–34) that would lead to the grading of nursing schools. It was believed that grading would establish standards for education in these schools. This was the beginning of the accreditation function now carried out by the National League for Nursing. See the section on nursing organizations later in this chapter.

During this period, the concept of the clinical nurse specialist arose. In 1933, the need for "experts in the nursing art and specialists in the clinical branches they represent" was recognized. This concept, currently seen by many as a new role in nursing, was discussed by nursing leaders in the 1930s and 1940s. In the early 1940s, it was thought that more emphasis needed to be placed on the clinical specialties in the advanced professional curricula of colleges and universities. Most advanced nursing curricula were preparing specialists in nursing school administration, teaching, and supervision, in public health, and in hospital administration and were not emphasizing clinical specialties. These specialties gained prominence in the postwar society. Nurses returning from overseas were required to work in clinical areas not familiar to them. One such area was psychiatric nursing, which helped individuals to readjust to civilian life. By 1946, many nursing programs in the United States were providing more clinical content. Today the clinical nurse specialist is a graduate of a master's or doctoral program in nursing with a major in a clinical specialty. These nurses are responsible for increasing their own clinical knowledge and competence and for enhancing the quality of nursing care and the quality of the organizational climate for learning and research (McPhail 1971, p. 16–18).

From its early days to the present, nursing has undergone change in every area. Rapid strides have been made in nursing education programs and in a wide variety of hospital and community nursing services. Throughout these changes, nursing has continued to provide a stable helping service to people. Appendix A outlines significant events in nursing history from the first century through the 1980s.

Growth of Professionalism

There are a number of ways to differentiate a profession from an occupation. A **profession** is a calling that requires special knowledge, skill, and preparation. Medicine and law have consistently been recognized as learned professions.

The terms *vocation* and *occupation* are often used synonymously. A **vocation** is the work that a person regularly performs or the work that especially suits him or her. An **occupation** is an activity in which one engages, e.g., a business. Thus, an occupation does not necessarily hold a special interest for the person and may be temporary, whereas a vocation often denotes employment in an area of interest on a regular basis. In this chapter, the more commonly used term *occupation* will be used to denote nonprofessions.

A profession is generally distinguished from other kinds of occupations by (a) its requirement of prolonged, specialized training to acquire a body of knowledge pertinent to the role to be performed and (b) an orientation of the individual toward service, either to a community or to an organization. The standards of education and practice for the profession are determined by the members of the profession, rather than by outsiders. The education of the professional involves a complete socialization process, more far-reaching in its social and attitudinal aspects and its technical features than is usually required in other kinds of occupations. In 1915, Abraham Flexner stated that professions are organized primarily for the achievement of social ends and secondarily for the assertion of rights and the protection of special interests (Flexner 1915, p. 901).

Styles (1983) writes that nursing organizations must perform the following five functions for the preservation and development of the profession:

1. Professional definition and regulation through the setting and enforcing of standards of education and practice for the generalist and the specialist. Regulation is largely achieved in the United States and Canada through the licensure of individual nurses, certification, and accreditation. See the section on credentialing of nurses in Chapter 8. Regulation is also achieved through the adoption of codes of ethics and norms of conduct (Styles 1983, p. 570).

2. Development of the knowledge base for practice in its broadest and narrowest components. Major contributions to the development of nursing knowledge have been made by various theorists. The primary purpose of nursing theories is to generate nursing knowledge. The challenge for nurses in the future is to generate questions and formulate hypotheses from these published theories and then test the hypotheses through nursing research. Since only research can determine the usefulness of a theory, research makes a major contribution to the development of nursing knowledge. Another significant contribution to nursing knowledge is the work of the North American Nursing Diagnosis Association (NANDA) (see Chapter 11). This group is generating and expanding a taxonomy of nursing diagnoses. Research is required to determine the validity and reliability of these diagnoses.

3. Transmission of values, norms, knowledge, and skill to neophytes and members of the profession for applica-

tion in practice. This function is largely performed through the education of nurses and the socialization processes. Socialization is the development in the individual of those qualities (skills, beliefs, habits, requirements) necessary to belong to and function in a group. See Chapter 2.

4. Communication and advocacy of the values and contributions of the field to several publics and constituencies. This function requires that nursing organizations speak for nurses from a position of broad agreement. It is essential for nurses to participate actively in the formulation of health legislation and policy.

5. Attendance to the social and general welfare of their members. This function is carried out by the professional nursing organizations of the country. Professional associations give their members social and moral support to perform their roles as professionals and to cope with their professional problems. Association journals, for example, disseminate updated knowledge, new ideas, and professional concerns. By participating in the collective bargaining process, nurses can improve their economic and working conditions.

In 1970, Moore and Rosenblum identified six elements of a profession. A profession should (a) have a systematic theory, (b) exert authority, (c) command prestige, (d) have a code of ethics, (e) have a professional culture, and (f) be the major source of income of those who practice it (Moore and Rosenblum 1970).

Miller states that the critical attributes of professionalism in nursing are the following:

- Gaining a body of knowledge in a university setting and a science orientation at the graduate level in nursing

- Attaining competencies derived from the theoretical base wherein the "diagnosis and the treatment of human responses to actual or potential health problems" (ANA 1980) can be accomplished

- Delineating and specifying the skills and competencies that are the boundaries of expertise (Miller 1985, p. 25)

The growth of professionalism in nursing can be viewed in relation to specialized education, knowledge base, ethics, and autonomy.

Specialized Education   Specialized education is an important aspect of professional status. Historically, nurses were educated in hospitals. In modern times, the trend has been toward nursing education programs in colleges and universities (see the discussion of the education of nurses later in this chapter).

People are the theoretical focus and concern of nursing, and the education of nurses should reflect this fact. Many nursing educators believe that the undergraduate nursing curriculum should include 2 years of liberal arts education. The ANA's position paper on education for nurses (1965, p.

107) states: "Education for those who work in nursing should take place within the general education system." In 1983, the National League for Nursing (NLN) voted at its convention to retain the baccalaureate degree as academic preparation for the professional nurse (Lewis 1983, p. 246).

In the United States today, there are five levels of entry into registered nursing: hospital diploma, associate degree, baccalaureate degree, master's degree, and doctoral degree (DeYoung 1985, p. 101). Programs for entry at the master's and doctoral levels are designed specifically for nonnurse college graduates.

Body of Knowledge

As a profession, nursing is establishing a well-defined body of knowledge and expertise. A number of nursing conceptual frameworks (discussed in Chapter 4) contribute to the knowledge base of nursing and give direction to nursing research and nursing education.

Increasing research in nursing is contributing to this body of knowledge. In the 1940s, nursing research was at a very early stage of development. In the 1950s, increased federal funding and professional support helped to establish centers for nursing research. In 1952, *Nursing Research,* the first journal to report findings of nursing studies, was founded. Since that time, more nurses with doctorates are carrying out nursing research.

Early research focused on the needs and resources of nursing and nursing education. In the 1960s, studies were often related to the nature and veracity of the knowledge base underlying nursing practice (Gortner 1980, p. 205). During the 1970s and 1980s, research was largely practice-related, and nursing's involvement in research continues to grow.

The ANA Commission on Nursing Research (1981b) identified the following as priorities for nursing research:

1. Promoting health and preventing illness
2. Decreasing the negative impact of health problems on coping abilities, productivity, and satisfaction
3. Developing strategies that provide effective nursing care to high-risk vulnerable groups
4. Developing cost-efficient delivery systems of nursing care

The establishment of the National Center for Nursing Research in 1986 has meant additional federal support for professional growth. See Chapter 3 for additional information about research.

Ethics

Nurses have traditionally placed a high value on the worth and dignity of others. The nursing profession requires integrity of its members; that is, a member is expected to do what is considered right regardless of the personal cost. Nurses must respect the professional judgment of others and must develop nursing standards and establish mechanisms for identifying and dealing with unethical behavior.

Ethical codes change as the needs and values of society change. Nursing has developed its own codes of ethics and in most instances has set up means to monitor the professional behavior of its members. See Chapter 7 for additional information on ethics.

Autonomy

A profession is autonomous if it regulates itself and sets standards for its members. Providing autonomy is one of the purposes of a professional association. If nursing is to have professional status, it must function autonomously in the formation of policy and in the control of its activity. To be autonomous, a professional group must be granted legal authority to define the scope of its practice, describe its particular functions and roles, and determine its goals and responsibilities in delivery of its services. The amount of autonomy a professional group possesses depends on its effectiveness at governance. **Governance** is the establishment and maintenance of social, political, and economic arrangements by which practitioners control their practice, their self-discipline, their working conditions, and their professional affairs. Nurses, therefore, must work within their professional organizations.

To practitioners of nursing, autonomy means independence at work, responsibility, and accountability for one's actions.

The ANA statement on the scope of practice describes the accountability of professional and technical nurses:

> Professional nurses develop nursing policies, procedures, and protocols and set standards for nursing care for all client populations in all practice settings. . . . Technical nurses use policies, procedures, and protocols developed by professional nurses in implementing an individual's plan of care. Technical nurses are accountable for practicing within these guidelines. (ANA 1987b, p. 77)

Autonomy is more easily achieved and maintained from a position of authority. Therefore, many nurses seek administrative positions rather than expanded clinical competence as a means to assure their autonomy in the workplace.

Professional Behaviors of Nurses

Miller states that the degree to which a nurse behaves as a professional is reflected in the following five behaviors. The professional:

1. Assesses, plans, implements, and evaluates theory, research, and practice in nursing. These behaviors are reflected in the entire nursing process. See also Chapters 10 through 14.
2. Accepts, promotes, and maintains the interdependence of theory, research, and practice. These three elements make nursing a profession and not a task-centered activity (Miller 1985, p. 26).
3. Communicates and disseminates theoretical knowledge, practical knowledge, and research findings to the nurs-

ing community. Professionalism must be demonstrated by supporting, counseling, and assisting other nurses (Miller 1985, p. 26).

4. Upholds the service orientation of nursing in the eyes of the public. This orientation differentiates nursing from an occupation pursued primarily for profit. Many consider altruism the hallmark of a profession. (Altruism is selfless concern for others.) Nursing has a tradition of service to others. This service, however, must be guided by certain rules, policies, or code of ethics (Miller 1985, p. 26). The nursing code of ethics is formulated by national nursing associations. In addition, society is protected by licensure and accreditation of nurses. These self-regulatory provisions give nurses the autonomy to function in the public's best interests rather than in the best interests of an institution or other profession.

5. Preserves and promotes the professional organization as the major referent. Operation under the umbrella of professional organization differentiates a profession from an occupation (Miller 1985, p. 26). In nursing, the American Nurses' Association in the United States and the Canadian Nurses' Association in Canada perform the self-regulatory functions.

NURSING PRACTICE

Nurses practice in an ever-increasing variety of ways and settings. The actual focus of practice is determined largely by the setting, the needs of the clients, the nurse practice acts of the area, and the standards of the professional organization.

Recipients of Nursing

The recipients of nursing are sometimes called *consumers,* sometimes *patients,* and sometimes *clients.* A **consumer** is an individual, a group of people, or a community that uses a service or commodity. A family that uses electricity in their home is a consumer of electricity. People who use health care products or services are consumers of health care.

A **patient** is a person who is waiting for or undergoing medical treatment and care. The word *patient* comes from a Latin word meaning to suffer or to bear. Traditionally, the person receiving health care has been called a patient. Usually, people become patients when they seek assistance because of illness or for surgery. Some nurses believe that the word *patient* implies passive acceptance of the decisions and care of health professionals. Additionally, with the emphasis on health promotion and prevention of illness, many recipients of nursing care are not ill. Moreover, nurses interact with family members and significant others in addition to the persons actually receiving nursing care.

For these reasons, nurses are increasingly referring to recipients of health care as clients.

A **client** is a person who engages the advice or services of another who is qualified to provide this service. The term *client* presents the receivers of health care less as passive recipients and more as collaborators in the care, i.e., as persons who are also responsible for their health. Thus, the health status of a client is the responsibility of the individual in collaboration with health professionals. In this book, *client* is the preferred term, although *consumer* and *patient* are used in some instances.

Focus of Nursing

Nursing involves an interrelationship of many people concerned with a client's responses to potential or actual health problems. Today, there is an emphasis, on the whole person; people are seen not merely as physical beings but as biopsychosocial beings. Nursing practice involves a complex of knowledge and skills applied to the whole client. Nurses are also involved with support persons and the community as a whole. For this reason, nurses must be aware of how the support persons and community affect the client's well-being and consider the well-being of these support persons and the community.

Nursing practice involves four areas related to health (health is discussed in Chapter 5):

1. Health promotion. Health promotion means helping people develop resources to maintain or enhance their well-being. The goal of health promotion is to move people toward their own optimum level of health and well-being or wellness (Black and McDowell 1984, p. 19). An example of a nursing action that promotes health is explaining the benefits of an exercise program to a client. Health promotion is discussed in more detail in Chapter 23.

2. Health maintenance. Health maintenance nursing activities are those actions that help clients to maintain their health status. An elderly person in a long-term care facility can be taught and encouraged to exercise to maintain muscle strength and mobility.

3. Health restoration. Health restoration means helping people to improve health following health problems or illness. Examples of activities that help restore health are teaching a client to protect an incision and to change a surgical dressing or assisting handicapped individuals to attain the highest level of physical strength of which they are capable.

4. Care of the dying. This area of nursing practice involves comforting and caring for people of all ages while they are dying. Nurses carrying out these activities work in homes, hospitals, and extended care facilities. Some agencies, called hospices, are specifically designed for this purpose.

Settings for Nursing

In the past, the acute care hospital was the only practice setting open to most nurses. Today, however, there are employment opportunities not only in acute and long-term chronic or rehabilitation hospitals but also in clients' homes, community agencies, ambulatory clinics or health maintenance organizations (HMOs), and nursing practice centers, for example. Table 1–2 shows areas of registered practice in the United States.

Nurses have different degrees of nursing autonomy and nursing responsibility in the various settings. Today, nurses have a variety of career choices and can pursue any number of interests. They may specialize, for example, in intensive care nursing or respiratory nursing. In addition to providing direct care, they teach clients and support persons, serve as nursing advocates and agents of change, and help determine health policies affecting consumers in the community

and in hospitals. For additional information regarding settings, see Chapter 6.

Models for Delivery of Nursing

Common configurations for the delivery of nursing care include the case method, the functional method, team nursing, primary nursing, and the case management system.

Case Method   The case method, also referred to as total care, is one of the earliest models developed. This method is client-centered. One nurse is assigned to and is responsible for the comprehensive care of a group of clients during an 8- or 12-hour shift. For each client, the nurse assesses needs, makes nursing plans, formulates diagnoses, implements care, and evaluates the effectiveness of care. In this method, a client has consistent contact with one nurse during a shift but may have different nurses on other shifts. The case method, considered the precursor of primary nursing, continues to be used in a variety of practice settings, e.g., intensive care nursing. With the shortage of nursing personnel during World War II, the case method could no longer be the chief mode of care for clients. To meet staff shortages, managers hired personnel with less educational preparation than the professional nurse and developed on-the-job training programs for auxiliary helpers. The total care method became unfeasible in such situations, and the functional method was developed in response.

Functional Method   This system of assignment, which evolved from concepts of scientific management used in the field of business administration, focuses on the jobs to be completed. In this task-oriented approach, personnel with less preparation than the professional nurse fulfill less complex care requirements. It is based on a production and efficiency model that gives authority and responsibility to the person assigning the work, e.g., the head nurse. Clearly defined job descriptions, procedures, policies, and lines of communication are required. The functional approach to nursing is economical and efficient and permits centralized direction and control. Its disadvantages are fragmentation of care (the client receives care from several different categories of nursing personnel) and the possibility that nonquantifiable aspects of care, such as meeting the client's emotional needs, may be overlooked.

Team Nursing   In the early 1950s, Eleanor Lambertson (1953) and her colleagues proposed a system of team nursing to overcome the fragmentation of care resulting from the task-oriented functional approach and to meet increasing demands for professional nurses created by advances in technologic aspects of care. **Team nursing** is the delivery of individualized nursing care to clients by a nursing team led by a professional nurse. A nursing team consists of registered nurses, licensed practical nurses, and often nurses' aides. This team is responsible for providing

TABLE 1–2   *Areas of Registered Nurse Employment*

Practice Setting	United States 1986 (percentage*)	Canada 1988 (percentage*)
Hospitals	68.1	73.0
Nursing homes/ homes for the aged	7.7	6.9
Community health, public health (U.S.) and physicians' offices (Canada)	6.8†	9.9
Family practice units (Canada)	—	2.5
Ambulatory care (U.S.)	6.6	—
Nursing education (U.S.)	2.7	—
Educational institutions (Canada)	—	2.6
Schools	2.9	—
Occupational health	1.5	—
Other, e.g., self-employed, insurance claims reviewers	3.7	3.9
Not stated	—	0.9

*Rounded to the first decimal
†These figures do not reflect the shift to home health care.

Sources: American Nurses' Association, *Facts about nursing 86–87.* (Kansas City, Mo.: ANA, 1987), p. 101 and Statistics Canada, *Registered nurse management data,* Pub. no. 613–990–8552 (Ottawa: Statistics Canada, 1988).

coordinated nursing care to a group of clients during an 8- or 12-hour shift. Compared to the functional system, team nursing emphasizes humanistic values and responds to the needs of both clients and employees. Individualized client care on a personal level rather than task-oriented care on an impersonal level is emphasized. Employees are stimulated to learn and develop new skills by the professional nurse leader, who instructs them, supervises them, and provides assignments that offer the potential for growth.

Basic to team nursing are the team conference, nursing care plan, and leadership skills. The conference, led by the professional nurse team leader, includes all personnel assigned to the team. Discussing the needs of clients, establishing goals, individualizing the plan of care, instructing personnel, and following up are all under the direction of the team leader. In essence, the team leader has a management role that requires a high degree of competence in coordination and leadership.

Although the team nursing approach has worked effectively in many health care agencies, certain weaknesses have been observed in some settings. The client may still perceive care as fragmented if the team leader does not establish a satisfactory relationship with the client. Teams may not have the appropriate health care personnel, and team members may not have the expertise to meet the needs of a particular client population. Ideally, several professional nurses should be team members. Often, there is only one professional nurse, who must assume the role of team leader. When there are no professional nurses assigned to the unit, technical nurses, who are not educationally prepared to fulfill the leadership role required of a team leader, are assigned to this role. To manage effectively, the leader may revert to using a functional mode of delivering care.

Primary Nursing
Primary nursing was introduced at the Loeb Center for Nursing and Rehabilitation, the Bronx, New York, under the leadership of Lydia Hall (1963). **Primary nursing** is a system in which one nurse is responsible for total care of a number of clients 24 hours a day, 7 days a week. It is a method of providing comprehensive, individualized, and consistent care.

Primary nursing uses the nurse's nursing knowledge and management skills. The primary nurse assesses and prioritizes each client's needs, identifies nursing diagnoses, develops a plan of care with the client, and evaluates the effectiveness of care. While associates provide some care, the primary nurse coordinates it and communicates information about the client's health to other nurses and other health professionals. Primary nursing encompasses all aspects of the professional role, including teaching, advocacy, decision making, and continuity of care. The primary nurse is the first-line manager of the client's care with all its inherent accountabilities and responsibilities.

Case Management System
Case management is a more recent nursing care delivery system in which *case*

managers are responsible for a case load of clients throughout their hospitalization. These managers may be aligned with case loads in a variety of ways, for instance (a) with specific physicians and their patients, (b) with patients geographically within a unit or units, and (c) by diagnosis. The case management system maintains the philosophy of primary nursing and requires a graduate of a bachelor's or master's program to implement high-level professional practice.

Nurse Practice Acts

Nurse practice acts, or acts for professional nursing practice, regulate the practice of nursing in the United States and Canada. Each state in the United States and each province in Canada has its own act. Although nurse practice acts differ in various jurisdictions, they all have a common purpose: to protect the public. Nurse practice acts are a formalized contract between society and the profession. They serve a public purpose and also meet the needs of the profession. The public is granted a mechanism to ensure minimum standards for entry into the profession and to distinguish the unqualified. The profession achieves partial implementation of its goal of maintaining standards in practice through appropriate entry credentialing (Snyder and Labar 1984, p. 2). During the past 10 years, many states have revised their nurse practice acts to permit expanded nursing roles. For additional information, see Chapter 8.

Standards of Nursing Practice

Establishing and implementing standards of practice are major functions of a professional organization. Nursing practice standards provide exact criteria against which clients, nurses, and employers can evaluate care for effectiveness and excellence.

In the ANA publication *Standards of Nursing Practice,* the association comments on this responsibility of the nursing profession to society:

> Nursing's concern for the quality of its services constitutes the heart of its responsibility to the public. The more expertise required to perform the service, the greater society's dependence upon those who carry it out. Nursing must control its practice in order to guarantee the quality of its service to the public. Behind that guarantee are the standards of the profession, which are directed toward assurance that service of a good quality will be provided. This is essential both for the protection of the public and for the profession itself. A profession which does not maintain the confidence of the public will soon cease to be a social force (ANA 1973, p. 1).

The profession's responsibilities inherent in establishing and implementing standards of practice include (a) to establish, maintain, and improve standards, (b) to hold members accountable for using standards, (c) to educate the public to appreciate the standards, (d) to protect the

TABLE 1–3   American Nurses' Association Standards of Nursing Practice

Standard	Rationale	Standard	Rationale
1. The collection of data about the health status of the client/patient is systematic and continuous. The data are accessible, communicated, and recorded.	Comprehensive care requires complete and ongoing collection of data about the client/patient to determine the nursing care and needs of the client/patient. All health status data about the client/patient must be available for all members of the health care team.	5. Nursing actions provide for client/patient participation in health promotion, maintenance, and restoration.	The client/patient and family are continually involved in nursing care.
2. Nursing diagnoses are derived from health status data.	The health status of the client/patient is the basis for determining the nursing care needs. The data are analyzed and compared to norms when possible.	6. The nursing actions assist the client/patient to maximize health capabilities.	Nursing actions are designed to promote, maintain, and restore health.
3. The plan of nursing care includes goals derived from the nursing diagnoses.	The determination of the results to be achieved is an essential part of planning care.	7. The client/patient's progress or lack of progress toward goal achievement is determined by the client/patient and the nurse.	The quality of nursing care depends upon comprehensive and intelligent determination of nursing's impact upon the health status of the client/patient. The client/patient is an essential part of this determination.
4. The plan of nursing care includes priorities and the prescribed nursing approaches or measures to achieve the goals derived from the nursing diagnoses.	Nursing actions are planned to promote, maintain, and restore the client/patient's well-being.	8. The client/patient's progress or lack of progress toward goal achievement directs reassessment, reordering of priorities, new goal setting, and revision of the plan of nursing care.	The nursing process remains the same, but the input of new information may dictate new or revised approaches.

Source: From American Nurses' Association, Standards of nursing practice (Kansas City, Mo.: ANA, 1973). Reprinted with permission.

public from individuals who have not attained the standards or willfully do not follow them, and (e) to protect individual members of the profession from each other (Phaneuf and Lang 1985, p. 2).

Nursing standards clearly reflect the specific functions and activities that nurses provide, as opposed to the functions of other health workers. The ANA's Standards of Nursing Practice are set forth in Table 1–3, and those of the CNA are summarized in Table 1–4. These standards apply to the practice of all registered nurses.

When standards of professional practice are implemented, they serve as yardsticks for the measurements used in licensure, certification, accreditation, quality assurance, peer review, and public policy (Phaneuf and Lang 1985, p. 7). Licensure, certification, and accreditation are discussed in Chapter 8. Quality assurance and peer review are discussed in Chapter 14.

TABLE 1–4   Canadian Nurses' Association Standards for Nursing Practice

I.	Nursing practice requires that a conceptual model(s) for nursing be the basis for that practice.
II.	Nursing practice requires the effective use of the nursing process.
III.	Nursing practice requires that the helping relationship be the nature of the client-nurse interaction.
IV.	Nursing practice requires nurses to fulfill professional responsibilities.

Source: Canadian Nurses' Association, February 1987. A definition of nursing practice: Standards for nursing practice. Ottawa, Ontario: CNA Pub. #ISBN 0-919 108-51-2. Reprinted with permission.

Career Mobility

The public image of the nurse is that of a hospital staff nurse who has been educated in a hospital school. Many laypeople are unaware of the variety of roles and educational backgrounds of nurses. Two kinds of mobility are open to the nurse: vertical and horizontal. Vertical mobility means advancing upward within a hierarchy, for example, from staff nurse to head nurse. Horizontal mobility refers to ability to change practice setting, such as from a nursing home to a community health agency.

Recognizing that nurses require encouragement, motivation, and recognition, some settings provide clinical ladder models for career development. Traditionally, a nurse's clinical competence was rewarded by moving the nurse away from client care into administrative roles. Clinical ladders provide nurses with recognition of their clinical competence, at the same time permitting them to continue clinical nursing practice.

Expanded Nursing Roles

A role is a pattern of behavior expected of individuals in specific social situations. An **expanded role** is one that a nurse assumes by virtue of education and experience. The nurse who assumes an expanded role has increased responsibilities and, usually, greater autonomy. Nurses are assuming expanded roles in both hospitals and community settings.

Nurse Practitioner   The role of the nurse practitioner is an extension of the nurse's basic caregiving role; it prepares nurses for an expanded role in the provision of primary care. Nurse practitioners have advanced educational preparation; often they have a certificate or a master's degree in nursing.

Nurse practitioners may be generalists, e.g., family nurse practitioners, or specialists, e.g., geriatric nurse practitioners. Nurse practitioners in a community may be employed in health maintenance organizations, health centers, schools, and physicians' offices. They are usually skilled at making nursing assessments, performing physical assessments, counseling, teaching, and treating (in concert with the physician) minor, self-limiting illnesses or stable, long-term illness. Nurse practitioners in hospitals are often employed in specialty areas, e.g., geriatric nursing.

Nurse Specialist   The nurse specialist has advanced knowledge and skills in a particular area of nursing. An educational prerequisite is a master's degree in nursing. The ANA's title of "certified specialist" (C.S.) is reserved for these three programs: clinical specialist in medical-surgical nursing, clinical specialist in adult psychiatric and mental health nursing, and clinical specialist in child and adolescent psychiatric and mental health nursing. By January 1988, 12,993 nurses had been certified as nurse specialists (*Amer-*

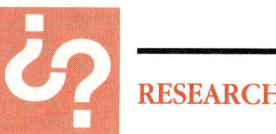

RESEARCH NOTE

A Tool to Help Nurses Build Career Plans?

Hefferin and Kleinknecht developed a Nursing Career Preference Inventory (NCPI) to assist nurses in determining which of four primary nursing practice areas—clinical, administration, research, or education—most reflect personal work activity interests or preferences, and in turn which of fourteen hospital nursing role positions (e.g., director of nursing service, clinical nurse specialist, community health nurse, and staff nurse) most often encompass the preferred work activity patterns. The authors invited registered nurses in six Veteran's Administration (VA) patient care facilities to identify their nursing positions and to list the types of tasks or functions they performed in their work roles. From these data fourteen nursing positions were identified as common to all participating facilities. The most common activities or tasks for each position were also determined. The NCPI was then tested in VA health facilities and non-VA community hospital settings across the country. Results indicated significant correlations between the work activity responses of both groups in the identified positions.

Implications: The NCPI may be used by career counselors to introduce new and experienced nurses to the type of work functions associated with a broad range of hospital-based nursing positions, and to help nurses plan their professional career goals.

Hefferin, E. A., and Kleinknecht, M. K. January/February 1986. Development of the nursing career preference inventory. *Nursing Research* 35:44–48.

ican Nurse September 1988). These nurses practice in hospitals or communities. In the hospital, such nurses give direct client care, advise other nurses, and coordinate nursing given by others. The clinical nurse specialist is a role model and is expected to keep abreast of new developments in the field.

Nurse Clinician   The term *nurse clinician* was first used by Frances Reiter in 1966. Such nurses provide bedside or direct care in a specialty area. They may or may not have advanced educational preparation.

Nurse Generalist   The nurse generalist certification programs conducted by the ANA issue certificates in seven areas: maternal-child health, child and adolescent, high-risk perinatal, medical-surgical, psychiatric and mental health, community health, and gerontologic. Through January 1,

1988, 29,888 nurses had been certified by the ANA (*American Nurse* September 1988). Their certification designation is R.N., C. (Registered Nurse, Certified).

EDUCATION FOR NURSES

The nurse's function today is so complex that a nursing student requires knowledge in the biologic, physical, and social sciences, in addition to nursing theory and practice. It is not possible for nurses to acquire a safe level of skill through empiric (experience and observation) means alone. They require specific knowledge and skills that can be gained only through an organized nursing curriculum.

The traditional focus of nursing education has been on teaching the skills required in hospitals. However, considerable evidence shows that the need for community and home services is increasing and that using these services overcomes some of the negative aspects of hospitalization, such as separation from family. As a result, nursing curricula now focus more broadly on health as well as illness and community as well as hospital, in addition to appropriate knowledge from the biologic, social, and physical sciences.

State laws in the United States and provincial laws in Canada recognize two types of nurses: the licensed practical (vocational) nurse (LPN or LVN) and the registered nurse (RN). Various types of programs exist to prepare nurses to enter practice.

Licensed Practical Nursing

Approved practical or vocational nursing programs are provided by high schools, community colleges, vocational schools, hospitals, and a variety of health agencies. These programs usually last 1 year and provide both classroom and clinical experiences. At the end of the program, the graduate takes National Council Licensing Examination (NCLEX) examinations to obtain a license as a practical or vocational nurse. Licensed practical nurses work in structured care settings, such as hospitals and long-term care agencies. Their skills are basically those required for bedside nursing under the guidance of a registered nurse, who has the knowledge and skills to make more sophisticated nursing judgments. In some areas of the United States, LPN programs are being expanded to the associate degree level.

Registered Nursing

In the United States, most basic education for registered nurses is provided in three types of programs: diploma, associate degree, and baccalaureate programs. In Canada, the 2-year diploma, 3-year (or more) diploma, and baccalaureate programs prepare registered nurses. Figures 1–1 and 1–2 indicate the numbers of graduates from these registered nursing programs.

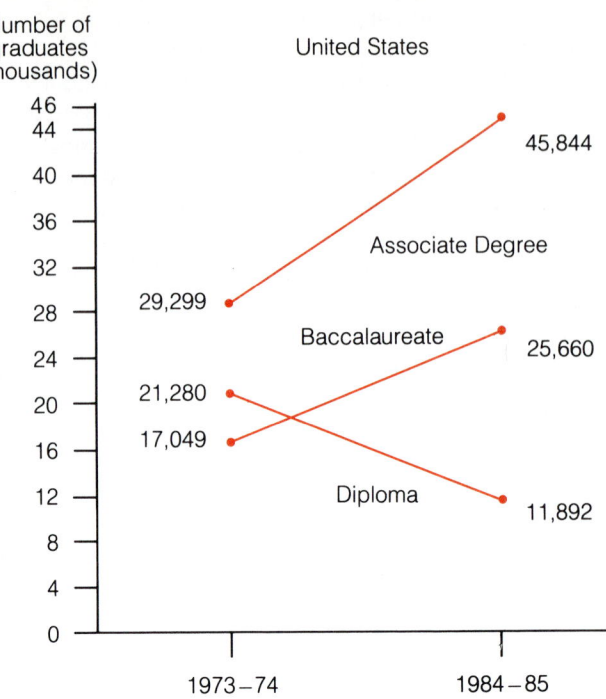

Figure 1–1 Number of graduates from registered nursing programs in the United States from 1973–74 to 1984–85. *Source:* American Nurses' Association, *Facts about nursing 86–87* (Kansas City, Mo.: ANA, 1987), p. 42.

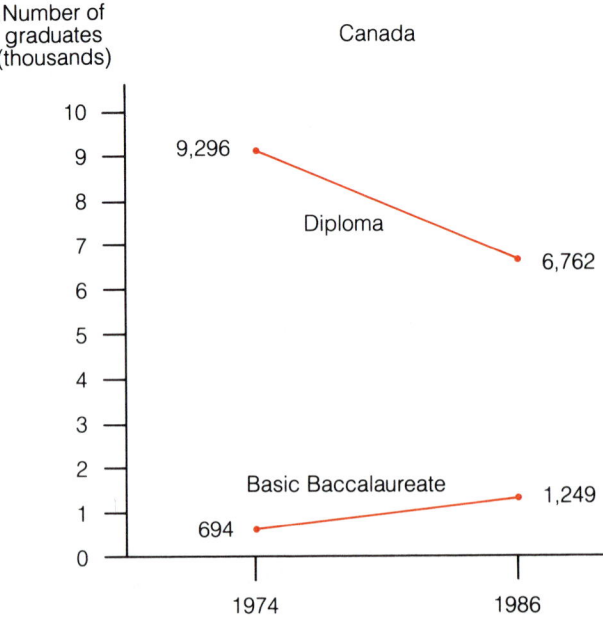

Figure 1–2 Number of graduates from registered nursing programs in Canada from 1974 to 1986. (Diploma refers to collegiate and hospital programs.) *Source:* Statistics Canada, *Nursing in Canada 1986* (Ottawa: Statistics Canada, 1988), pp. 33, 36.

Diploma Nursing education originated in hospital-based programs. First developed by Florence Nightingale (circa 1860), these programs were operated by hospitals as "training" schools for nurses, to ensure a source of qualified nurses. Today's diploma nursing programs have changed markedly from the original Nightingale model, becoming hospital-based educational programs that provide a rich clinical experience for nursing students. These programs may last 2 or more years and are often associated with colleges or universities. A significant number of nurses practicing today are graduates of diploma programs. Though the number of diploma nursing programs has declined since the ANA resolution in 1965, these programs are still providing one avenue for students desiring an education in nursing.

Associate Degree Associate degree programs in nursing were suggested in 1951 by Mildred L. Montag (1980) as a solution to the acute shortage of nurses that came about because of World War II. Associate degree programs are offered in the United States in junior colleges as well as in colleges and universities. The graduating student receives an associate degree in nursing (ADN), or an associate of arts (AA), associate of science (AS), or associate in applied science (AAS) degree with a major in nursing. In Canada, associate degrees are not offered, but similar programs confer a diploma upon graduation.

Although ADN programs relieved the post–World War II nursing shortage, the utilization of ADN graduates in hospital practice did not fulfill Montag's original intent; ADN and BSN graduates are often used interchangeably. This creates a discrepancy between the competence expected of new graduates and their actual competence. In an effort to resolve this discrepancy, differentiated competency statements were developed during two projects sponsored by the Midwest Alliance in Nursing and funded by the W. K. Kellogg Foundation (Primm 1986, pp. 135–37). Because ADN and BSN prepared nurses currently function under the same practice acts, "these differentiated statements provide a basis for discussion of collaborative ADN and BSN nursing practice" (Primm 1986, p. 136). A new organization, the National Organization of ADN Educators, has been formed recently to address issues in modern ADN education.

Baccalaureate Degree Although baccalaureate nursing education programs were established in universities in both the United States and Canada in the early 1900s, it was not until the 1960s that the number of students enrolled in these programs increased markedly. The 1965 ANA position paper provided considerable impetus to move nursing education out of hospitals and into the general education system.

Most baccalaureate programs also admit registered nurses who have diplomas or associate degrees. Some programs have special curricula to meet the needs of these students. Some universities also offer nursing students the oppor-tunity to pursue a self-paced or independent study program. Many accept transfer credits from other accredited colleges and universities and offer students the opportunity to take challenge examinations when they believe they have the knowledge or skills taught in a course.

Another impetus toward baccalaureate education for all nurses was a resolution of the ANA, passed in 1978, stating that the minimum educational preparation for entry into professional nursing practice by 1985 be a baccalaureate degree (BSN). The 1978 delegates also endorsed a resolution that diploma and associate degree graduates who are licensed to practice before 1985 not be affected. In 1984, the ANA House of Delegates adopted a different time frame for this change. The goal was to implement the requirement of a BSN for entry into professional nursing practice in 5% of states by 1986, 15% by 1988, 50% by 1992, and 100% by 1995 (Hood 1985, p. 592). In 1985, the ANA House of Delegates proposed that two and only two categories of nursing be established. See Chapter 3, Nursing Education.

In Canada in 1982, the Board of Directors of the CNA endorsed the recommendations of the Committee on Entry to Practice that the baccalaureate degree be the minimum entry level for professional nursing practice by the year 2000. Although many nurses recognize the move toward a baccalaureate degree as a requirement for entry into professional nursing practice, the issue of titling and licensure has yet to be resolved by individual state or provincial legislation. In addition, there are nurses who believe that the appropriate entry level for nursing should be at the master's or doctoral level.

Graduate Programs

Education at the graduate level requires critical thinking. Most graduate programs are conducted by departments within the graduate school of a university, and the applicant must first meet requirements established by the graduate school. Although all graduate schools have somewhat different requirements, common requirements for admission to graduate programs in nursing include the following (DeYoung 1985, p. 120):

- The applicant must be a registered nurse.
- The applicant must hold a baccalaureate degree in nursing from an approved college or university and have had an acceptable upper division major in nursing at the baccalaureate level.
- The applicant must give evidence of scholastic ability (usually a minimum grade point average of 2.7 to 3.0 on a 4.0 scale).
- The applicant must demonstrate satisfactory achievement on a qualifying examination.

Master's Programs Master's programs generally take from 1½ to 2 years to complete. Degrees granted are the

Master of Arts (MA), Master in Nursing (MN), Master of Science in Nursing (MSN), and Master of Science (MS).

Master's degree programs may focus on an area of advanced clinical practice, e.g., psychiatric mental health nursing, or on areas such as administration or nursing management.

The number of nurses obtaining master's degrees has increased. In 1988, 20,182 students were pursuing master's study, as compared to 5085 who obtained master's degrees in 1983 (Poteet and Hodges 1990, p. 145; ANA 1985, p. 155).

Doctoral Programs   Doctoral programs in nursing, which award the degrees of doctor of philosophy (PhD), doctor of nursing science (DNS or DNSc), or nursing doctorate (ND), began in the 1960s in the United States. These programs further prepare the nurse for advanced clinical practice, administration, education, and research. Before 1960, nurses acquired doctoral degrees in such related fields as psychology, sociology, physiology, and education.

The number of doctoral programs in nursing has greatly increased in the past decade. Between 1977 and 1987, the number of doctoral programs increased 156% from 18 to 46 (Lenz 1990, p. 114).

Content and approach vary among doctoral programs. One may focus on usual clinical areas, such as medical-surgical nursing, while others emphasize such nontraditional areas as transcultural nursing. Some programs emphasize theory development, but all emphasize research (DeYoung 1985, p. 119). In 1988, 2077 nurses were pursuing doctoral degrees (Poteet and Hodges 1990, p. 145).

Ladder Programs

The ladder concept fosters progression of an individual from one educational level to another. The nurse who wishes to progress "up the ladder" can often obtain credit for experience and/or courses at an earlier level. Although associate degree programs were not originally designed to lead to further education, many universities now grant academic credit toward a baccalaureate degree for the years spent in the associate degree program.

Often, baccalaureate programs emphasize independent learning and self-pacing. External degree programs, such as the New York State Regents Program and the California Statewide Nursing Program, provide alternatives to traditional university programs to allow for this independent, self-paced learning.

Continuing Education

The term *continuing education* refers to formalized experiences designed to enlarge the knowledge or skills of practitioners. Compared to advanced education programs, which result in an academic degree, continuing education courses tend to be more specific and shorter. Participants may receive certificates of completion or specialization.

Continuing education is the responsibility of each practicing nurse. Constant updating and growth are essential to keep abreast of scientific and technologic change and changes within the nursing profession. A variety of educational and health care institutions conduct continuing education programs. They are usually designed to meet one or more of the following needs: (a) to keep nurses abreast of new techniques and knowledge, (b) to help nurses attain expertise in a specialized area of practice, such as intensive care nursing, and (c) to provide nurses with information essential to nursing practice, for example, knowledge about the legal aspects of nursing

Some state laws now require nurses to obtain a certain number of continuing education credits to renew their licenses. In these states, required continuing education (CE) contact hours vary from 15 to 30 hours for every 2-year relicensure period. All, some, or none of these hours may be acquired through home study. Some home study courses are offered through professional journals. A few regions also require a certain number of hours of practice, either independently or in lieu of study hours, before license renewal.

In-Service Education

An in-service education program is administered by an employer; it is designed to upgrade the knowledge or skills of employees. For example, an employer might offer an in-service program to inform nurses about a new piece of equipment, about specific isolation practices, or about methods of implementing a nurse theorist's conceptual framework for nursing.

NURSING ORGANIZATIONS

One way nurses can demonstrate professional commitment is active involvement in a nursing organization. There are two types of organizations: professional and nonprofessional. "A professional organization is an organization of practitioners who judge one another as professionally competent and who have banded together to perform social functions which they cannot perform in their separate capacities as individuals" (Merton 1958, p. 50). Two examples of professional organizations are the American Nurses' Association (ANA), the professional organization for RN's in the United States, and the Canadian Nurses' Association (CNA) in Canada. The National League for Nursing (NLN) is an example of a nonprofessional nursing organization; nurses at various levels and nonnurses can join. Nursing organizations are established at local, national, and international levels. Selected nursing organizations, discussed below, are placed in alphabetical order. See also Appendix B for other nursing organizations in North America.

American Academy of Nursing (AAN)

The AAN was established in 1970 by the American Nurses' Association. Its purpose is to recognize those nurses who have made significant contributions to their profession. The first members were chosen by the Board of Directors of the ANA in 1973. The members are now chosen by current members. Nurses elected to the Academy may use the title of Fellow of the American Academy of Nursing (FAAN). The Academy is now separate from the ANA.

American Nurses' Association (ANA)

The ANA is the national professional organization for nursing in the United States. It was founded in 1896 as the Nurses Associated Alumnae of the United States and Canada. In 1911, the name was changed to the American Nurses' Association. It was a charter member of the International Council of Nurses along with Great Britain and Germany in 1899. The purposes of the ANA are to foster high standards of nursing practice and to promote the educational and professional advancement of nurses so that all people may have better nursing care. The ANA is composed of the nurses' associations from the 50 states, Guam, the Virgin Islands, Puerto Rico, and the District of Columbia. These state associations are in turn divided into regional and local chapters.

In 1982, the organization became a federation of state nurses' associations. Individuals can no longer belong to the ANA, but they participate by joining their state nurses' associations. Each state nurses' association is entitled to representation as a member of the federation. The number of seats allocated to each state's delegation depends on the number of members in each state organization. The official journal of the ANA is the *American Journal of Nursing,* and the *American Nurse* is the official newspaper. The functions of the ANA are shown in the accompanying box.

Canadian Nurses' Association (CNA)

The Canadian Nurses' Association (CNA) is the national nursing association of Canada. Nurses do not join the CNA independently but obtain membership by paying a fee to the provincial chapters. In November 1985, the Ordre des infirmières et infirmiers du Quebec (the Quebec Nurses' Association) withdrew from the CNA.

The CNA has developed national standards and a code of ethics, and it offers support to all provincial associations. Through the National Testing Services, the CNA prepares licensure examinations. These examinations are available to all provinces and territories and provide a national standard for licensure of registered nurses. Through the Canadian Nurses' Foundation, research grants, fellowships, and scholarships are offered to Canadian nurses. The official journal of the CNA, *Canadian Nurse,* is published monthly and sent to each nurse member.

Functions of the American Nurses' Association (ANA)

- Establish standards of nursing practice, nursing education, and nursing services
- Establish a code of ethical conduct for nurses
- Ensure a system of credentialing in nursing
- Initiate and influence legislation, governmental programs, national health policy, and international health policy
- Support systematic study, evaluation, and research in nursing
- Serve as the central agency for the collection, analysis, and dissemination of information relevant to nursing
- Promote and protect the economic and general welfare of nurses
- Provide leadership in national and international nursing
- Provide for the professional development of nurses
- Conduct an affirmative action program
- Ensure a collective bargaining program for nurses
- Provide services to constituent state nurses' associations
- Maintain communication with members through official publications
- Assume an active role as consumer advocate
- Represent and speak for the nursing profession with allied health groups, national and international organizations, governmental bodies, and the public

Source: American Nurses' Association. Bylaws, as revised July 1, 1982. Kansas City, Mo.: ANA, 1982. Used by permission.

International Council of Nurses (ICN)

The ICN was established in 1899. Nurses from both the United States and Canada were among the founding members. The council is a federation of national nurses' associations such as the ANA and CNA. In 1990, 101 national associations from different countries were affiliated with the ICN.

The purpose of the ICN is "to provide a medium through which the interests, needs, and concerns of member national nurses' associations can be addressed to the advantage of the public and nurses" (ICN 1973). The work of the ICN is based on four objectives (Quinn 1981):

1. To promote the development of strong nursing associations.

2. To assist national nursing associations to improve the standards of nursing and the competence of nurses.

3. To assist national nursing associations to improve the status of nurses.

4. To serve as an authoritative voice of nurses and nursing internationally.

International Honor Society: Sigma Theta Tau

Sigma Theta Tau, the international honor society in nursing, was founded in 1922 and is headquartered in Indianapolis, Indiana. The greek letters stand for the Greek words *storga, tharos,* and *tima,* meaning love, courage, and honor. The society is a member of the association of college honor societies. The society's purpose is professional rather than social. Membership is attained through academic achievement. Students in baccalaureate programs in nursing and nurses in master's, doctoral, and postdoctoral programs are eligible to be selected for membership.

The official journal of Sigma Theta Tau, *Image: Journal of Nursing Scholarship,* is published quarterly. The journal publishes scholarly articles of interest to nurses. The society also publishes *Reflections,* a quarterly newsletter that provides information about the organization and its various chapters.

National League for Nursing (NLN)

The National League for Nursing, formed in 1952, is an organization of both individuals and agencies. Its objective is to foster the development and improvement of all nursing services and nursing education. People who are not nurses but have an interest in nursing services, for example, hospital administrators, can be members of the league. This feature of the NLN—involving nonnurse members, consumers, and nurses from all levels of practice—is unique.

The purposes of the NLN are to strengthen and support nursing services, to promote research for widening the knowledge base of nursing education and practice, to maintain responsiveness to its membership, to promote public understanding and support of nursing, and to explore new avenues for promoting nursing, such as alternative health care settings (NLN 1983). The NLN has traditionally offered a wide range of services, including continuing education workshops and seminars, consultation, and educational aid. In terms of schools of nursing, the NLN offers two major services: (a) voluntary accreditation for educational programs in nursing, and (b) testing services, including preentrance testing for potential students, achievement testing throughout the program, and state board examinations for licensure. The NLN also conducts yearly surveys of nursing schools, newly registered nurses, and post-basic graduates. These surveys serve as a primary source of research data about nursing education in the United States. The official

journal of the NLN up to 1979 was *Nursing Outlook;* as of 1980, the official magazine became *Nursing and Health Care.*

National Student Nurses' Association (NSNA)

The National Student Nurses' Association (NSNA) is the official preprofessional organization for nursing students. It was formed in 1953 and incorporated in 1959. Originally, the NSNA functioned under the aegis of the ANA and NLN; however, in 1968 it became an autonomous body, although it communicates with the NLN and the ANA. To qualify for membership in the NSNA, a student must be enrolled in a state-approved nursing education program. The official magazine of the NSNA is the newsletter *Imprint.*

In Canada, nursing students have a similar organization, the Canadian University Student Nurses' Association. The provincial student nurses' associations also have programs related to the needs of nursing students and concerns within the health field in general.

World Health Organization (WHO)

The World Health Organization (WHO) is one of the special agencies of the United Nations. It is an intergovernmental agency, formed in 1948, whose primary aim is to bring all people in the world to the highest possible level of health. As of 1990, 166 countries were members of WHO. Its major activities are to provide assistance to countries to improve health standards, education, and training.

Nurses make an essential contribution to the activities of WHO. American and Canadian nurses are frequently asked to go to countries that require assistance in nursing education and public health. About 300 nurses currently work for WHO in countries other than their own.

Special Interest Organizations

A number of nursing organizations in the United States and Canada are involved with special interests of the nurses.

Alumni Associations The major purpose of alumni associations is to foster the high ideals of the nursing program from which the nurses graduated. Alumni associations offer an opportunity for nurses to socialize, participate in educational programs, and raise funds for nursing students.

Clinical Specialty Organizations During the past 15 years, many specialty organizations have formed to meet the needs of groups of nurses. The clinical areas for which specialty organizations have formed include critical care, nurse anesthesia, urology, and orthopedics. One of the major purposes of many of these organizations is the continuing education of its members. Many groups also have certification mechanisms that recognize achievement in their specialized area of practice.

Red Cross   The American Red Cross and the Canadian Red Cross are two of about 120 Red Cross, Red Crescent, Sun Societies, and Red Lion organizations around the world. The original Red Cross organization was founded by Henri Dunant in 1859. He organized a group of volunteers who worked to help the injured on the battlefield of Solferino in Italy. His work was nonpartisan, and both sides were helped by his group.

Nurses in the American Red Cross pioneered public health nursing in the United States. By 1930, however, most states had their own public health nursing services. At that time, the Red Cross extended its functions in the United States and Canada by establishing home nursing courses, organizing volunteers to assist in hospitals and nursing homes, and organizing disaster nursing and a blood donation program. Nursing students can volunteer their services with the Red Cross in many of these activities.

CHAPTER HIGHLIGHTS

▶ Florence Nightingale may be thought of as nursing's first nurse theorist, since she emphasized such independent nursing functions as preventive health care, humanistic care, comfort, and support of the client.

▶ There are many definitions and descriptions of nursing, but the essence of nursing is caring for and caring about people as holistic beings in matters related to health promotion, health maintenance, health restoration, and dying.

▶ A desired goal of nursing is professionalism, which necessitates a unique body of knowledge including specific skills and competencies, autonomous regulation, and formulation of a code of ethics.

▶ Although the majority of nurses today are employed in hospital settings, more nurses are working in other areas, such as home health care and community clinics.

▶ Nurse practice acts vary among states and provinces, and nurses must be aware of the act governing their practice.

▶ Standards of nursing practice provide criteria against which the effectiveness of nursing care can be evaluated.

▶ The career mobility of nurses increases with their education.

▶ Nurses are fulfilling expanded nursing roles, for instance, those of the nurse practitioner, the nurse specialist, the nurse clinician, and the nurse generalist, which allow greater independence and autonomy.

▶ Educational programs for nurses must reflect the health care demands and needs of a changing society, accommodate changes in the health care delivery system, and adhere to professional standards yet be responsible to concerns about rising costs of health care.

▶ Flexibility in nursing curricula and innovation in implementing curricula are needed to upgrade the educational achievement of nursing graduates from programs below the baccalaureate degree level.

▶ Both professional and nonprofessional nursing organizations and associations fulfill essential functions for the nursing profession and for individual nurses.

▶ Participation in the activities of nursing associations enhances the growth of involved individuals and helps nurses collectively influence policies affecting nursing practice.

READINGS AND REFERENCES

SUGGESTED READINGS

Diers, D. January 1990. Learning the art and craft of Nursing. *American Journal of Nursing* 90:65–66.

Diers writes about the *art* of nursing, which is described in part as self-discipline. The tool of the nurse in this context is the intellect. Diers describes the discipline of nursing as the constant attention to difference and unpredictability.

McBride, A. B. September/October 1985. Orchestrating a career. *Nursing Outlook* 33:244–47.

A career in nursing—as in any other field—advances through several stages. Understanding this process can smooth the way.

Mechanic, H. F. November/December 1988. Redefining the expanded role. *Nursing Outlook* 36:280–84.

In this article, Mechanic illustrates how nursing is changing. For example, some skills that were formerly associated with the expanded role are now part of the "common practice" of nursing. She emphasizes that redefining the expanded role is important so that nursing will continue to contribute to primary health care.

Zwolski, K. Winter 1989. Professional nursing in a technical system. *Image: Journal of Nursing Scholarship* 21:238–42.

Zwolski, discusses four principles that describe a technical system: (a) technique is distinguishable from technology; (b) a technique cannot produce the philosophy that directs it; (c) technology at its incomplete and imperfect stages creates new problems; and (d) technology produces fragmentation. The author points out that the more technical the health care system becomes, the greater the need for professionally prepared nurses.

RELATED RESEARCH

Baer, E. D. January/February 1987. "A cooperative venture" in pursuit of professional status: A research journal for nursing. *Nursing Research* 36:18–25.

———. May/June 1989. Nursing's divided loyalties: An historical case study. *Nursing Research* 38:166–71.

Fenton, M. V. March/April 1987. Development of a scale of humanistic nursing behaviors. *Nursing Research* 36:82–87.

Hefferin, E. A, and Kleinknecht, M. K. January/February 1986. Development of the nursing career preference inventory. *Nursing Research* 35:44–48.

Reverby, S. January/February 1987. A caring dilemma: Womanhood and nursing in historical perspective. *Nursing Research* 36:5–11.

Schank. M. J., and Weis, D. January/February 1989. A study of values of baccalaureate nursing students and graduate nurses from a secular and a nonsecular program. *Journal of Professional Nursing* 5:17–22.

SELECTED REFERENCES

American Journal of Nursing. February 1985. ANA gears up new drive for entry-level change: Despite opposition, some SNAs see success soon. *American Journal of Nursing* 85:194, 200–201.

American Nurse. September 1988.

American Nurses' Association. December 1965. American Nurses' Association first position on education for nursing. *American Journal of Nursing* 65:106–11.

———. 1973. *Standards of nursing practice.* Kansas City, Mo.: ANA.

———. April 1979. Credentialing in nursing: A new approach. Report of the Committee for the Study of Credentials in Nursing. *American Journal of Nursing* 79:674–83.

———. 1980. *Nursing: A social policy statement.* Kansas City, Mo.: ANA.

———. 1981a. *Facts about nursing 80–81.* New York: American Journal of Nursing Co.

———. 1981b. *The Nursing practice act: Suggested state legislation.* Kansas City, Mo.: ANA.

———. November/December 1982. Bylaws. *American Nurse* 14:15.

———. 1985. *Facts about nursing 84–85.* Kansas City, Mo.: ANA.

———. 1987a. *Facts about nursing 86–87.* Kansas City, Mo.: ANA.

———. 1987b. *Proceedings of the 1987 House of Delegates.* Kansas City, Mo.: ANA.

Balasco, E. M. January/February 1990. The nurse in relationship. *Journal of Professional Nursing* 6:4.

Barritt, E. R. 1973. Florence Nightingale's values and modern nursing education. *Nursing Forum* 12:6–47.

Baumgart, A. J., and Larsen, J. 1988. *Canadian nursing faces the future.* St. Louis: C. V. Mosby Co.

Black, A., and McDowell, I. April 1984. Healthstyles: Moving beyond disease prevention. *Canadian Nurse* 80:18–20.

Canadian Nurses' Association. 1982. *Credentialing in Nursing: Policy Statement and Background Paper.* Ottawa: CNA

———. April 1984. CNA Connection: Canada health act. *Canadian Nurse* 80:8–9.

———. 1987. *A definition of nursing practice: Standards for nursing practice.* Ottawa CNA.

Chamings, P. A., and Teevan, J. February 1979. Comparison of expected competencies of baccalaureate- and associate-degree graduates in nursing. *Image: Journal of Nursing Scholarship* 11:16–21.

Chaska, N. J., editor. 1990. *The nursing profession: Turning points.* St. Louis: C. V. Mosby Co.

CNA Connection. April 1984. Canada health act. CNA appears before commons committee. *Canadian Nurse* 80:8–9.

DeYoung, L. 1985. *Dynamics of nursing.* 5th ed. St. Louis: C. V. Mosby Co.

Ellis, J. R., and Hartley, C. L. 1988. *Nursing in today's world: Challenges, issues and trends.* 3d ed. Philadelphia: J. B. Lippincott Co.

Flaherty, M. J. 1979. The characteristics and scope of professional nursing. *Journal for Nursing Leadership and Management* 1:61, 63, 69.

Flexner, A. 1915. Is social work a profession? *School Society* 1:901.

Hall, L. November 1963. A center for nursing. *Nursing Outlook* 11:805–6.

Henderson, V. 1966. *The nature of nursing: A definition and its implications for practice, research, and education.* New York: Macmillan Co.

———. April 1990. Excellence in nursing. *American Journal of Nursing* 90:76–7.

Holleran, C. November/December 1989, I.C.N.: Still vital at 90. *International Nursing Review* 36:158.

Hood, G. May 1985. At issue: Titling and licensure. *American Journal of Nursing* 85:592, 594.

International Council of Nurses 1973. *Constitution and regulations.* Geneva: ICN.

King, I. M. 1971. *Toward a theory for nursing: General concepts of human behavior.* New York: John Wiley and Sons.

———. 1981. *A theory for nursing: Systems, concepts, process.* New York: John Wiley and Sons.

Kinney, C. D. May/June 1985. A reexamination of nursing role conceptions. *Nursing Research* 34:170–76.

Lambertson, E. 1953. *Nursing team organization and functioning.* New York: Teachers College Press.

Large, J. T. October 1976. Harriet Newton Phillips, the first trained nurse in America. *Image: Journal of Nursing Scholarship* 8:49–51.

Leddy, S., and Pepper, J. M. 1989. *Conceptual bases of professional nursing.* 2d ed.. Philadelphia: J. B. Lippincott Co.

Leininger, M. 1989. *Care: The essence of nursing and health.* 2d ed. Thorofare, N.J.: Charles B. Slack.

Lenz, E. R. 1990. Doctoral education: Present views, future trends. In Chaska, N. L., editor. *The nursing profession: Turning points.* St. Louis: C. V. Mosby Co.

Levesque, V. D. June 1985. Specialization and certification: A review of CNA's activities. *Canadian Nurse* 81:26–28.

Lewis, E. P. September/October 1983. News outlook: The issue that won't go away. A report on the 1983 NLN convention. *Nursing Outlook* 31:246–47.

———. September/October 1985. Taking care of business: The ANA House of Delegates. *Nursing Outlook* 33:239–43.

McPhail, J. October 1971. Reasonable expectations for the nurse clinician. *Journal of Nursing Administration* 1:16–18.

Merton, R. K. January 1958. The function of the professional organization. *American Journal of Nursing* 58:50–54.

Miller, B. K. April 1985. Just what is a profession? *Nursing Success Today* 2:21–27.

Montag, M. L. April 1980. Looking back: Associate degree education in perspective. *Nursing Outlook* 28:248–50.

Moore, W. E., and Rosenbaum, G. W. 1970. *The professions: Roles and rules.* New York: The Russell Sage Foundation.

National Commission on Nursing: Summary report and recommendations. July 1983. American Hospital Association. Chicago: The Hospital Research and Educational Trust, and American Hospital Supply Corporation.

National League for Nursing. March/April 1975. 1974 Annual Report. *NLN News* 23:3.

———. 1978a. *Characteristics of graduate education in nursing leading to the master's degree.* New York: NLN.

———. 1978b. *Competencies of the associate degree nurse on entry into practice.* New York: NLN.

———. 1978c. *Roles and competencies of graduates of diploma programs in nursing.* New York: NLN.

———. 1979. *Characteristics of baccalaureate education in Nursing.* New York: NLN

———. 1983. *NLN mission and goals, 1983–85.* New York: NLN.

———. 1989. *Nursing Student Census 1989* NLN Pub. no. 19–2291. New York: NLN.

National Student Nurses' Association. 1985. *Getting the pieces to fit 85/86. A handbook for state associations and school chapters.* New York: NSNA.

Neuman, B. 1982. *The Neuman systems model: Application to nursing education and practice.* New York: Appleton-Century-Crofts.

New federal nursing panel tackles the shortage. June 1990. *American Journal of Nursing* 90:118, 122.

Nightingale, F. 1860. *Notes on nursing: What it is, and what it is not.* London: Harrison. Reprinted in Bishop, F. L. A., and Goldie, S. 1962. *A bio-bibliography of Florence Nightingale.* London: Dawsons of Pall Mall.

O'Malley, J.; Loveridge, C. E.; and Cummings, S. H. February 1989. The new nursing organization. *Nursing Management* 20:29–32.

Orem, D. E. 1985. *Nursing: Concepts of practice.* 3d ed. New York: McGraw-Hill.

Palmer, I. S. June 1981. Florence Nightingale and international origins of modern nursing. *Image: Journal of Nursing Scholarship* 8:28–31.

Phaneuf, M. C., and Lang, M. 1985. *Issues in professional nursing practice 7: Standards of nursing practice.* Kansas City, Mo.: American Nurses' Association.

Pletsch, P. K. December 1981. Mary Breckinridge: A pioneer who made her mark. *American Journal of Nursing* 81:2188–90.

Poteet G. W., and Hodges, L. E. 1990. How to choose a graduate program. In McClosky, J. C., and Grace, H. K. *Current issues in nursing.* 3d ed. St. Louis: C. V. Mosby Co.

Poulin, M. A. 1985. *Issues in professional nursing practice 5, Configurations of nursing practice.* Kansas City, Mo.: American Nurses' Association.

Primm, P. L. May/June 1986. Entry into practice: Competency statements for BSNs and ADNs. *Nursing Outlook* 34:135–37.

Quinn, S. 1981. What about me? Caring for the careers. Geneva: International Council of Nurses.

Reiter, F. February 1966. The nurse-clinician. *American Journal of Nursing* 66:274–80.

Riehl, J. P., and Roy, C. 1980. *Conceptual models for nursing practice.* 2d ed. New York: Appleton-Century-Crofts.

Rogers, M. E. 1970. *An introduction to the theoretical basis of nursing.* Philadelphia: F. A. Davis Co.

———. 1980. Nursing: A science of unitary man. In Riehl, J. P., and Roy, C. *Conceptual models for nursing practice.* 2d ed. New York: Appleton-Century-Crofts.

Roy, C. 1984. *Introduction to nursing: An adaptation model.* 2d ed. Englewood Cliffs, N.J.: Prentice-Hall.

Segal, E. T. June 1985. Is nursing a profession? Yes no. *Nursing 85* 15:40–43.

Shortage is international problem. March 1990. *American Nurse* 22:5.

Snyder, M. E., and LaBar, C. 1984. *Issues in professional nursing practice 1. Nursing: Legal authority to practice.* Kansas City, Mo.: American Nurses' Association.

Statistics Canada. 1988. *Registered nurse management data.* Ottawa: Statistics Canada.

Stewart, I. April 1933. Postgraduate education—new and old. *American Journal of Nursing* 33:363.

Stull, M. K., May/June 1986. Entry skills for BSNs. *Nursing Outlook* 34:138, 153.

Styles, M. M. January 1978. Dialogue across the decades. *Nursing Outlook* 26:28–32.

———. November 1983. The anatomy of a profession. *Heart and Lung* 12:570–75.

Sultz, H. A.; Henry, O. M.; Bullough, B.; Buck, G. M.; and Kinyor, L. J. September/October 1983. Nurse practitioners: A decade of change. Part 3. *Nursing Outlook* 31:266–69.

Young, W. B. 1987. *Introduction to nursing concepts.* Norwalk, Conn.: Appleton & Lange.

Socialization and Roles of the Nurse

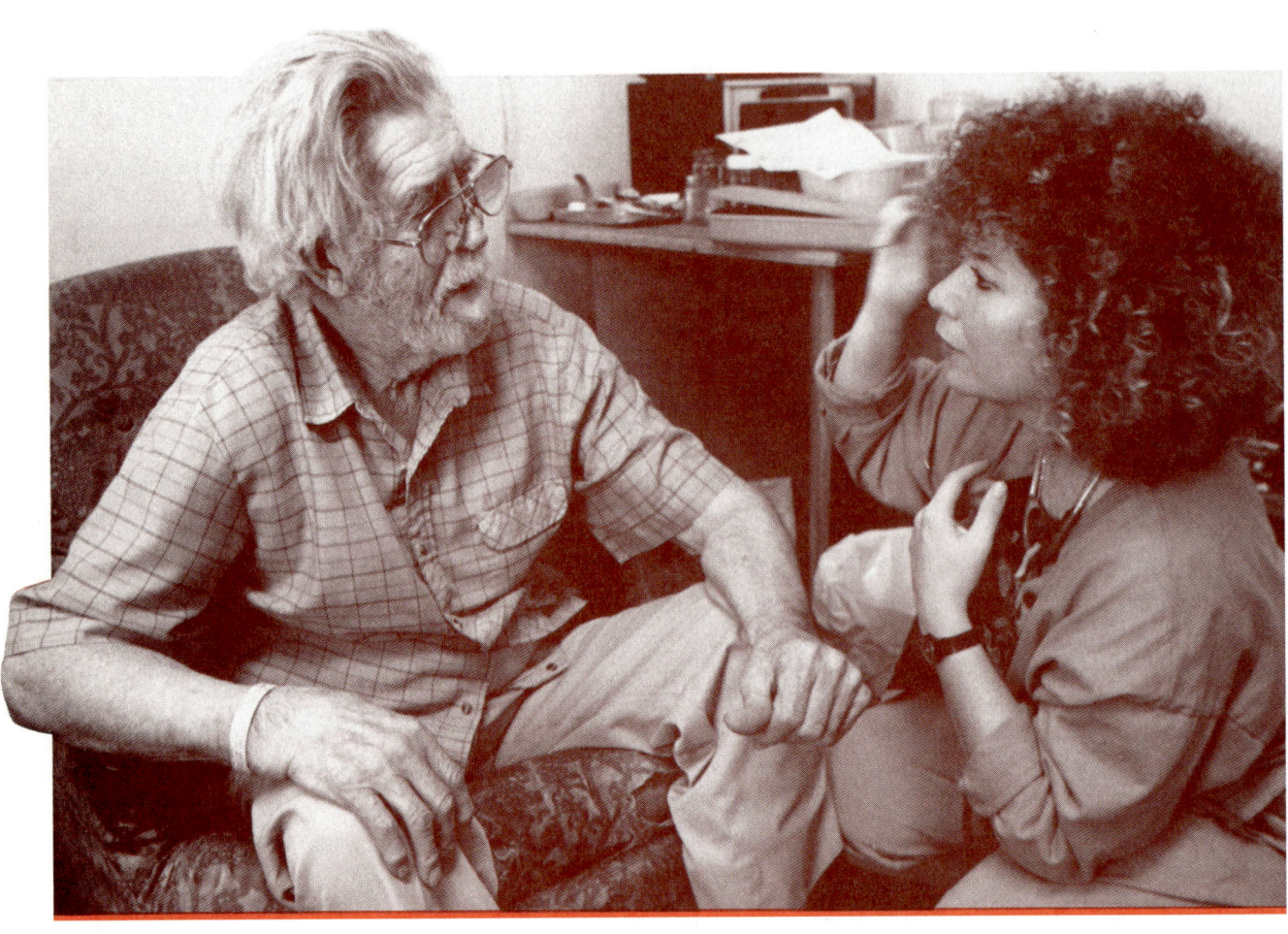

CONTENTS

OBJECTIVES

▶ Differentiate primary, secondary, and anticipatory socialization.

▶ Identify four critical values of professional nursing.

▶ Describe the process of professional socialization.

▶ Compare the socialization models of Simpson, Davis, Hinshaw, and Dreyfus.

▶ Compare Dalton's and Kramer's models of career development.

▶ Discuss essential aspects of the nurse's roles.

TYPES AND CHARACTERISTICS OF SOCIALIZATION

Socialization can be defined as the process by which people learn to become members of society (Berger and Berger 1975) or as the process by which people learn the social rules defining relationships into which they will enter (Tepperman and Richardson 1986). In short, socialization makes people skilled at following the rules for living. Although socialization goes on throughout life, the changes are most dramatic in childhood. By the time children begin school, they have learned to follow the rules given by people in authority (primarily adults), to cooperate with others, especially peers, to accept certain responsibilities, and to carry out assigned tasks at home.

The rules and roles learned in socialization are compatible with the values learned in acculturation. **Acculturation** is the process by which members of a society learn its culture and norms (Tepperman and Richardson 1986). The learning of cultural values is largely an unstructured and unconscious process. For example, young children are unaware that they are learning to speak the society's language. Related to acculturation and socialization is **assimilation,** the process by which adult members of foreign cultural groups learn the values and behaviors of a culture into which they have immigrated.

Sociologists have categorized socialization into primary and secondary phases. **Primary socialization** is early socialization that occurs from birth to adolescence. It is the process during which "children learn language, symbols, mores, norms, and values and develop a diverse set of cognitive skills that enable them to cope with the wide range of interactions they will experience during their lifetime" (Shaffir and Turowetz, 1987, p. 136). Because children have less power than adults and are unaware of alternatives, early primary socialization is largely imposed. However, socialization can also be *reciprocal.* Mutual learning usually occurs between peers but may also occur between children and parents or between students and teachers. Children influence parents and teachers in many ways, especially in situations where there is mutual respect, when the adult's exercise of power is not excessive, and when affection is high. Children may, for example, influence parents in their involvement in sports, leisure, personal care, politics, and attitudes toward handicapped persons, drugs, sexuality, and minority groups. Socialization therefore is usually considered a two-way process.

Secondary, or **adult, socialization** is the ongoing process of learning to adjust to new situations. Secondary socialization differs from primary socialization in that adults bring to new situations an accumulation of previous learning experiences and certain preconceptions about each new role. In secondary socialization, new values and appropriate behavior are developed for adult positions and group memberships. Every time a person enters a new group or assumes a new role (for example, becomes a nursing student, starts a new job, gets married, becomes a parent or grandparent), that person undergoes a period of formal or informal preparation or socialization for this new role. Even when an adult learns about a new set of beliefs through another person or exchanges ideas in a new social setting, the person is becoming socialized. Socialization is therefore an ongoing series of processes that continues throughout the life cycle. It is an adaptive process in which people learn about new and varied ways to look at the world. Characteristics of socialization are summarized in the accompanying box.

Anticipatory socialization is the process by which people prepare themselves for roles to which they aspire but which they do not yet occupy (Lundy and Warme 1986). In anticipatory socialization, there is some conscious motivation on the part of the person to acquire the skills and values of a given role. The person imagines what the new experience will be like. An example is the child who receives a nurse's or doctor's kit and enacts the role of nurse or doctor during play.

Resocialization entails learning a different way of looking at the world and is the process of changing behavior in rather dramatic ways. This becomes necessary whenever a person starts a new job, joins a club, changes marital status, or immigrates to another country, for example. Resocialization may or may not be a matter of free choice. For example, families generally choose to relocate for school or work. In other cases, however, resocialization is brought about by social changes beyond a person's control, as when the nature of a job is completely altered by technology.

Characteristics of Socialization

- It is a lifelong process by which a person learns the ways of a group or society in order to become a functioning participant.

- It is a reciprocal learning process brought about by interaction with other people.

- It involves all of a person's interactions with various agents of socialization—family, teachers, peers, media. Interactions may be conscious or unconscious, formal or informal.

- It is a universal process that varies according to a person's social class, ethnic origin, sex, and religion.

- It is a process that produces attitudes, values, knowledge, and skills required to participate effectively as an individual or a group member.

- It establishes boundaries of behavior.

- It develops a social self or awareness of others and their expectations.

- It is basic to group continuity and stability.

The most extreme form of resocialization occurs in institutions that control every aspect of a person's existence. Examples of such institutions are boarding schools, mental hospitals, prisons, and the armed services. Extreme socialization is aimed at stripping individuals of their own identity and replacing it with a new one. New recruits or members are issued uniforms or special clothing, their hair length may be regulated, and they are pressured to conform in thinking and behavior. They learn rituals, routines, and modes of presenting themselves, among other patterns of social behavior. Sometimes a formal period of orientation is offered to facilitate resocialization. For example, "boot camp" is provided in military training, and orientation weeks are commonly held at universities to introduce the informal side of university life.

In some situations, resocialization can create conflict with earlier experiences. Thus, conflict may be experienced by a worker promoted to supervisor or a staff nurse promoted to charge nurse. As a worker or staff nurse, the person may have felt loyal to workers and opposed to management, but as a supervisor or charge nurse the nurse must feel loyal to management. The structure and rules associated with specific roles and relationships, i.e., worker/supervisor or staff nurse/charge nurse, create conflict. People usually resolve conflict through resocialization and accomplish the transition even though it may not always be smooth.

SOCIALIZATION FOR PROFESSIONAL NURSING PRACTICE

Professional (or occupational) socialization is a very important part of adult socialization. People's work identities can be one of the most important parts of their social identities, since they are often judged by the ways in which they do their jobs and by how successful they are at achieving their goals. Watson (1981, p. 19) defines **professional socialization** as "the process whereby the values and norms of the profession are internalized into one's own behavior and concept of self; it is the process whereby the knowledge, skills, and attitudes characteristic of a profession are acquired." Hinshaw (1986, p. 20) defines socialization as "the process of learning new roles and the adaptation to them, and as such, continual processes by which individuals become members of a social group." She points out that from the perspective of professional nursing, the adult socialization/resocialization process focuses on the provision of values and behaviors basic to the delivery of quality client care. Standards for this process are derived from the norms of service professions and guide the specific role of professional nurses. Styles (1978, p. 29) in her analysis of the socialization process referred to this phenomenon simply as "the development of a professional soul."

Obviously, each person enters a nursing education program with many personal values that reflect the person's culture. Some of these values influence the person's choice of nursing as a profession. Most students enter nursing with a service orientation in which they foresee themselves doing things that will help the *sick* recover. However, the professional educational concept of the nurse is one who does the following (Hinshaw 1977, p. 5):

- Defines clients in terms of health and promoting and maintaining health
- Views the relationship between the nurse and clients as a therapeutic and analytic process
- Learns technical mastery of procedures and tools from the aspect of principles guiding their use
- Uses critical inquiry and creativity processes to manipulate knowledge in relation to the client's concerns
- Accepts responsibility and accountability for client care decisions

The socialization process therefore involves changes in knowledge, skills, attitudes, and values—changes that are often associated with strong emotional reactions and conflict.

Critical Values of Professional Nursing

It is within the nursing educational program that professional values are developed, clarified, and internalized. Specific professional nursing values are stated in nursing codes of ethics (see Chapter 7), in standards of nursing practice (see Chapter 1), and in the legal system itself (see Chapter 8). Watson (1981, pp. 20–21) outlines four values critical for the profession of nursing:

1. A strong commitment to the service that nursing provides for the public
2. Belief in the dignity and worth of each person
3. A commitment to education
4. Autonomy

The first value, a strong commitment to the service that nursing provides for the public, is considered essential. Nursing is a helping, humanistic service directed to the health needs of individuals, families, and communities. The nurse's role is therefore focused on *health* and *care*. Nurses, being responsible for assessing and promoting the health status of all humans, need to value their contribution to the health and well-being of people. Since "care and caring is the central core and essence of nursing" (Watson 1979), nurses also need to value the caring aspect of nursing.

The second value—the dignity and worth of each person—is based on Judeo-Christian philosophy of the sacredness of human life and the worth of the individual. Because nursing is a person-oriented profession, a basic value of the worth of each person regardless of nationality, race, creed, color, age, sex, politics, social class, and health status is basic to nursing. Applied to nursing practice this value means that the nurse always acts in the best interest of the client.

Commitment to education, the third value, reflects the lifelong value of learning in North American society. In terms of professional nursing, continuous education is needed for graduates to maintain and expand their level of competencies to meet professional criteria, to anticipate the role of the nurse in the future, and to expand the body of professional knowledge. Nurses need to question nursing knowledge and practice critically, to contribute to nursing's theoretical base, and to test theories in nursing practice.

The fourth value—autonomy, or the right of self-determination as a profession—is "the one where the greatest emphasis should be placed at this time" (Watson 1981, p. 21). Watson points out that "nurses must have freedom to use their knowledge and skills for human betterment and the authority and ability to see that nursing service is delivered safely and effectively." A future challenge for nurses is to become more assertive in promoting nursing care and to develop the ability for independent behavior.

Process of Socialization

Several models have been developed to explain the initial process of socialization into professional roles. The models described here include those of Simpson, Davis, Hinshaw, and Dreyfus. Each model outlines a sequential set of phases or "chain of events" beginning at the role of a lay person and ending at the role of a professional. Table 2–1 summarizes each model.

Ida Harper Simpson   Simpson (1967) outlines three distinct phases of professional socialization. In the first phase, the person concentrates on becoming proficient in specific work tasks. In the second phase, the person becomes attached to significant others in the work or reference group. In the third and final phase, the person internalizes the values of the professional group and adopts the prescribed behaviors.

Fred Davis   Davis (1966) describes a six-stage doctrinal conversion process among nursing students.

Stage 1: Initial innocence   When students enter a professional program, they have an image of what they expect to become and how they should act or behave. Nursing students usually enter a nursing program with a service orientation and expect to look after sick people. However, educational experiences often differ from what the students expect. For example, initial learning experiences for students often focus on the development of a relationship with healthy clients rather than on tasks performed for sick clients. During this phase students may express disappointment and frustration at experiences provided and may question their value.

Stage 2: Labeled recognition of incongruity   In this phase students begin to identify, articulate, and share their concerns. They learn that they are not alone in their value incongruencies: peers share the same concerns. Some students question whether to continue in the program.

Stages 3 and 4: "Psyching out" and role simulation   At this point, the basic cognitive framework for the internalization of professional nursing values begins to take shape. Students begin to identify the behaviors they are expected to demonstrate and through role modeling begin to practice the behaviors. In Davis's terms, this process becomes a matter of "psyching out" the faculty. The more effectively the role simulation is done, the more authentic the person believes the behavior to be, and it becomes part of the person. However, students may feel they are "playing a game" and are being "untrue to oneself," resulting in feelings of guilt and estrangement.

Stage 5: Provisional internalization   In stage five, students vacillate between commitment to their former image

TABLE 2–1   *Models of Socialization into Professional Roles*

Simpson (1967) Model	Davis (1966) Doctrinal Conversion Model	Hinshaw (1986) Model	Dreyfus (1980) Model
Stage 1 Proficiency in specific work tasks	*Stage 1* Initial innocence	*Phase I* Transition of anticipatory role expectations to role expectations of societal group	*Stage 1* Novice
Stage 2 Attachment to significant others in the work environment	*Stage 2* Labeled recognition of incongruity		*Stage 2* Advanced beginner
	Stage 3 "Psyching out" and role simulation		*Stage 3* Competent
Stage 3 Internalization of the values of the professional group and adoption of the behaviors it prescribes	*Stage 4* Increasing role simulation	*Phase II* Attachment to significant others/Labeling incongruencies	*Stage 4* Proficient
	Stage 5 Provisional internalization	*Phase III* Internalization of role values/behaviors	*Stage 5* Expert
	Stage 6 Stable internalization		

of nursing and performance of new behaviors attached to the professional image. Factors that increase the students' use of the new professional image are an increasing ability to use professional language and an increasing identification with professional role models, e.g., nursing faculty.

Stage 6: Stable internalization   During stage six, the student's behavior reflects the educationally and professionally approved model. However, preparation of the student for the work setting is only the initial process in socialization. New values and behaviors continue to be formed in the work setting.

Ada Sue Hinshaw   Hinshaw (1986) provides a three-phase general model of socialization that is an adaptation of Simpson's model.

Phase I: Transition of anticipatory role expectations to role expectations of societal group   During the first phase, individuals change their images of the role from anticipated concepts to the expectations of the persons who are setting the standards for them. Hinshaw states that (a) adults entering a profession have already learned a number of roles and values that help them to evaluate new roles and (b) these individuals are actively involved in the socialization process, having chosen to learn the new role expectations and enter the socialization process.

Phase II: Attachment to significant others/Label incongruencies   This phase has two components: (a) learners attach themselves to significant others in the system, and at the same time (b) they label situations that are incongruent between their anticipated roles and those presented by the significant others. In the initial professional socialization, significant others are usually a group of faculty; in the work setting, they are selected colleagues or immediate supervisors. Hinshaw emphasizes the importance of appropriate role models in both educational programs and work settings. At this stage, individuals are able to verbalize the expected role behaviors are not what they anticipated. It is a stage that often involves strong emotional reactions to conflicting sets of expectations. Successful resolution of conflicts depends on the existence of role models who demonstrate appropriate behaviors and who show how conflicting systems of standards and values can be integrated.

Phase III: Internalization of role values/behaviors   In this final phase the student internalizes the values and standards of the new role. The degree to which values and standards are internalized and the extent to which incongruencies in role expectations are resolved is variable. Kelman (1961) defines three levels of value orientation. Individuals may demonstrate one or a blend of three levels:

1. *Compliance.* The person demonstrates the expected behavior to get positive reactions from others but has not internalized the values. Compliance behavior can be dismissed when it no longer elicits positive responses.

2. *Identification.* The person selectively adopts specific role behaviors that are acceptable to that person. The person may accept only expected behaviors rather than values. Identification behavior usually changes as role models change.

3. *Internalization.* The person believes in and accepts the standards of the new role. The standards are a part of the person's own value system.

Stuart and Hubert Dreyfus   The Dreyfus model of skill acquisition is based on a study of chess players and airline pilots (Dreyfus and Dreyfus 1980). Benner (1984) has applied this model to nursing and discusses implications for teaching and learning. Five levels of proficiency are described: novice, advanced beginner, competent, proficient, and expert.

Stage 1: Novice   A novice may be a nursing student or any nurse entering a clinical setting where that person has no experience. Behavior of the novice is extremely limited, inflexible, and governed by rules. Because novices have no experience for the situations they face, their performance must be guided by rules. To help the novice enter situations and gain experience, context-free, objective, measurable attributes or procedures such as weight, temperature, and blood pressure measurement are often taught.

Stage 2: Advanced beginner   The advanced beginner can demonstrate marginally acceptable performance. The beginner has had experience with enough real situations to be aware of the meaningful "aspects" of a situation. "Aspects" require prior experience in real situations to be recognized. An example is recognition of the client's readiness to learn about how to manage a therapeutic regimen.

Stage 3: Competent   Competence is manifested by the nurse who has been on the job in a similar situation for 2 or 3 years. It develops when the nurse consciously and deliberately plans nursing care and coordinates multiple complex care demands. The nurse at this stage demonstrates organizational ability but lacks the speed and flexibility of the proficient nurse. The competent nurse knows which aspects of care are to be considered most important and which ones can be ignored. For example, the competent nurse will ensure that intravenous infusions are running, that clients will receive required medications, and that a client's urgent physical complaints and needs are dealt with before proceeding with other needs.

Stage 4: Proficient   The proficient nurse perceives situations as wholes rather than in terms of aspects. The nurse focuses on long-term goals and is oriented toward managing the nursing care of a client rather than performing specific tasks. This holistic understanding improves the decision making of the proficient nurse. Maxims are used as guides but can be applied only after a deep understanding of the situation is acquired. Maxims provide direction to what must be taken into consideration. For example, a nurse weaning a client from a respirator assesses the client's vital signs to discover any significant finding, but even then the nurse is aware that elevated readings may indicate anxiety. The decision whether to medicate to calm the client down is weighed against the knowledge that the medication may impair breathing. The nurse makes the decision according to the demands of the situation and the lessons of past experience. To the competent or novice performer, maxims appear as unintelligible nuances of a situation; they can mean one thing at one time and another thing at a different time.

Stage 5: Expert   The expert performer no longer relies on rules, guidelines, or maxims to connect an understanding of the situation to an appropriate action. The expert nurse intuitively grasps each situation and focuses on the accurate area of the problem without wasteful consideration of large ranges of unnecessary alternative diagnoses and solutions. The expert nurse may be inclined to say that a certain action was taken because "it felt right." Expert nurses have highly developed perceptual acuity or recognitional ability and their performance is fluid, flexible, and highly proficient. However, the nurse's highly skilled analytic ability is used in situations with which the nurse has had no previous experience.

Resocialization in the Employment Setting

When the new graduate enters the work setting, further socialization occurs. In the work setting, the nurse is faced with the need to put the values of the profession into operation in primarily bureaucratic settings that may not be supportive of professional career development (Leddy and Pepper 1989, p. 67). Various models of career stages have been developed. Two models by Dalton, Thompson, and Price (1977) and Kramer (1974) are summarized in Table 2–2.

ROLES OF THE PROFESSIONAL NURSE

The following nurse roles are ways of describing the nurse's activities in practice. Each role is described as a separate entity for the sake of clarity. However, the roles are not in actuality exclusive of one another. In practice, several roles often coincide. For example, the nurse may be acting as a client advocate while also caring, communicating, teaching or counseling, and acting as a change agent and a leader.

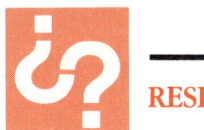

RESEARCH NOTE

How Similar Are the Nursing Role Identities of Students and Faculty Members?

In this study, the authors sought to determine the relationship between nursing role identities of students and faculty members in the baccalaureate nursing program at Fairleigh Dickinson University in Rutherford N.J. The participants in the study included 309 students and 23 full-time faculty members. With the exception of the department chairperson, all of the faculty members had clinical responsibilities. Most of the faculty were members of professional organizations (83%), belonged to the nursing honor society (74%), and had recently participated in workshops (95%). To measure the congruence between the student nurses' perceptions and faculty members' opinions of the professional nursing role, Crocker and Brodie's 59-item Nurses Professional Orientation Scale (NPOS) was used.

Results indicated the following: (a) the further students had advanced in the program, the more closely their responses correlated with those of the faculty; (b) during the first year, when students begin taking nursing courses, students started to substitute a professional view of nursing for a traditional view; (c) the congruency of scores of students who had completed their sophomore year and who had taken their first clinical nursing course were significantly higher than those of entering freshman; (d) there was a statistically significant higher relationship between students' congruency scores and the following variables: previous work experience as a nurses' aide, post–high school education before enrollment, high verbal scores on scholastic aptitude tests (SATs), high grade point averages, and high scores on the state board examination; and (e) the congruency scores of graduating seniors did not change between the time of the first survey and the time of the second, one year later, indicating that they had developed realistic role identities during the program.

Implications: Professional socialization is a complex process, and students need time to assimilate their professional identities. These authors suggest, therefore, that programs should offer both nursing courses and clinical experience under faculty guidance early on. To serve as effective role models, furthermore, faculty members should be expert clinicians as well as educators and have clinical responsibilities.

Source: B. J. Cohen and C. P. Jordet, Nursing schools: Students' beacon to professionalism? *Nursing and Health Care,* January 1988, 9:38–41.

TABLE 2–2   *Models of Career Development*

Dalton, Thompson, and Price Model	Kramer Model
Stage I Performs fairly routine duties under the direction of a mentor	*Stage I* Skill and routine mastery or development of technical expertise
Stage II Works independently as a competent colleague	*Stage II* Social integration; peer recognition of competence and acceptance into the group as the major concerns
Stage III Takes responsibility for influencing, guiding, directing, and developing others	*Stage III* Moral outrage at incongruities between conceptions of *bureaucratic* role associated with rules and regulations, *professional* role committed to continued learning, and *service* role concerned with the client as a person
Stage IV Influences the direction of the organization or a segment of it; has one of three roles: manager, internal entrepreneur, or idea innovator	*Stage IV* Conflict resolution by surrendering behaviors and/or values or by learning to use both the values and behaviors of the professional and bureaucratic system in a politically astute manner

Sources: G. W. Dalton, P. H. Thompson, and R. L. Price, The four stages of professional careers—A new look at performance by professionals, *Organ Dynamics,* Summer 1977 :19–42; and M. Kramer, *Reality check: Why nurses leave nursing* (St. Louis: C. V. Mosby Co., 1974).

Carer

The caring/comforting role of the nurse has traditionally included those activities that preserve the dignity of the individual and those often referred to as the "mothering actions" in nursing. However, caring involves knowledge and sensitivity to what matters and what is important to clients. (See caring theories in Chapter 4, page 71.) The caring role is difficult to define specifically. It is the role of human relations. The chief goal of the nurse in this role is to convey understanding about what is important and to provide support. The nurse supports the client by attitudes and actions that show concern for client welfare and acceptance of the client as a person, not merely a mechanical being.

Benner and Wrubel (1989, p. 4) state that "caring is central to effective nursing practice.... Nursing can never be reduced to mere technique and scientific knowledge because humor, anger, 'tough love,' administering medications, and even client teaching have different effects in a caring context than a noncaring one." Caring is central to most nursing interventions and an essential attribute of the expert nurse.

Communicator/Helper

Effective communication is an essential element of all helping professions, including nursing. Communication shapes relationships between nurses and clients, nurses and support persons, and nurses and colleagues. It plays a role in every action the nurse undertakes. The communication process, listening and responding skills, and ways to establish helping relationships are discussed in detail in Chapter 15.

Communication facilitates all nursing actions. The nurse communicates to other health care personnel the nursing interventions planned and implemented for each client. Planned nursing interventions are written on the client's care plan. Once the interventions are implemented, the nurse documents them on the client's record. Assessment findings, procedures implemented, and the client's responses are recorded. Pertinent information is communicated verbally by nurses at change of shift reports, when client's are transferred to another unit, at client rounds, and when clients are discharged to another health care agency. This type of communication needs to be concise, clear, and relevant. See Chapter 17 for details of reporting and recording.

Teacher

Teaching refers to activities by which the teacher helps the student to learn. It is an interactive process between a teacher and one or more learners in which specific learning objectives or desired behavior changes are achieved (Redman 1988, pp. 9 and 15). The focus of the behavior change is usually the acquiring of new knowledge or technical skills. The teaching process has four components—assessing, planning, implementing, and evaluating—which can be viewed as parallel to the parts of the nursing process. In the assessment phase, the nurse determines the client's learning needs and readiness to learn. During planning, specific learning goals and teaching strategies are set. During implementation, teaching strategies are enacted, and, during evaluation, learning is measured. See Chapter 16 for detailed information about the teaching/learning process.

Many factors have increased the need for health teaching by nurses. Today, there is a new emphasis on health promotion and health maintenance rather than on treatment alone; as a result, people desire and require more knowledge. Shortened hospital stays mean that the clients must be prepared to manage convalescence at home. The increase in long-term illnesses and disabilities often requires that both the client and the family understand the illness and its treatment.

Counselor

Counseling is the process of helping a client to recognize and cope with stressful psychologic or social problems, to develop improved interpersonal relationships, and to promote personal growth. It involves providing emotional, intellectual, and psychologic support. In contrast to the psychotherapist, who counsels individuals with identified problems, the nurse counsels primarily healthy individuals with normal adjustment difficulties. The focus is on helping the person develop new attitudes, feelings, and behaviors rather than on promoting intellectual growth. The client is encouraged to look at alternative behaviors, recognize the choices, and develop a sense of control.

Counseling can be provided on a one-to-one basis or in groups. Often nurses lead group counseling sessions. For example, on the individual level, the nurse counsels clients who need to decrease activity levels, stop smoking, lose weight, accept changes in body image, or cope with impending death. At the group level, the nurse may be a leader, member, or resource person in any self-help group in which the nurse may assume the role of structuring activities and fostering a climate conducive to group interaction and productive work.

Obviously, counseling requires therapeutic communication skills. In addition, the nurse must be a skilled leader, able to analyze a situation, synthesize information and experiences, and evaluate the progress and productivity of the individual or group. The nurse must also be willing to model and teach desired behaviors, to be sincere when dealing with people, and to demonstrate interest and caring in the welfare of others. The nurse-leader needs an inventive mind, a flexible attitude, and a sense of humor to deal with the varied experiences of people. Essential to leadership abilities is self-awareness, self-assurance, and self-understanding.

Client Advocate

An **advocate** pleads the cause of another or argues or pleads for a cause or proposal. Advocacy involves concern for and defined actions in behalf of another person or organization to bring about a change. A **client advocate** is an advocate of clients' rights. According to Disparti (1988, p. 140), advocacy involves promoting what is best for the client, ensuring that the client's needs are met, and protecting the client's rights. Some nurses believe client advocacy is an essential nursing function. Others believe that a client advocate need not be a nurse. All, however, recognize that many clients need an advocate to protect their rights and to help them speak up for themselves.

Some people believe that the client advocate should be accountable to the client and be the client's representative. The client advocate should be able to call in qualified consultants, participate actively in hospital committees monitoring the quality of client care, present complaints directly to the hospital director and hospital executive committee, delay discharges, and participate at the client's request and direction in discussions of the client's case (Annas 1975, pp. 209, 211). An advocate can represent a client by presenting the client's point of view and by interpreting and explaining the client's rights.

According to Kohnke, the actions of an advocate are (a) to inform clients about their rights in a particular situation and make sure they have all the necessary information to make an informed decision and (b) to support clients in their decisions. Support can involve actions or nonactions (Kohnke 1980, p. 2039). Kohnke further points out the difficulty of advocacy. It involves accepting and respecting the client's right to make a decision even if in the nurse's professional opinion that decision is wrong. In this role, nurses do not make decisions for clients; clients must make their own decisions freely. For example, Mr. Rae makes a decision not to have further chemotherapy for his malignancy after being fully informed about the treatment, the options, and the possible consequences. The client advocate informs Mr. Rae of his right to make this decision and supports him in his decision.

Underlying client advocacy are the following beliefs:

- Individuals have the right to select values they deem necessary to sustain their lives.
- Individuals have the right to exercise their judgment of the best course of action to achieve the chosen values.
- Individuals have the right to dispose of values in a way they choose without coercion by others (Donahue 1985, p. 1037).

Guidelines characteristic of responsible advocacy are outlined in the accompanying box.

Change Agent

A **change agent** is a person or group who initiates changes or who assists others in making modifications in themselves or in the system (Kemp 1986). Brooten, Hayman, and Naylor (1978) describe a *change agent* as a professional who relies on a systematic body of knowledge about change to guide the change process. Types, theories, and the process of change are discussed in Chapter 16.

The promotion of change is an essential component of nursing care. By using the nursing process, the nurse helps the client to propose, implement, and maintain changes (e.g., knowledge, skill, feelings, attitudes) that promote the client's health. Principles and strategies to promote change are integrated into all phases of the nursing process. During the assessment phase, the nurse establishes trust and identifies the client's health status and motivation for change. In the diagnosis phase, problems are specified. In the planning phase, objectives or goals for change are mutually established. In the implementation phase, the change strategies are implemented and maintained. In the evaluation phase, a judgment is made about whether the change process has been successful. For information about enhancing behavior change, see Chapter 23; for information about teaching and learning, see Chapter 16. On a larger scale, the nurse can be instrumental in promoting change at the institutional, professional, or societal levels.

An effective change agent must be a highly skilled communicator who is able to establish good interpersonal relationships. In addition, change agents must be self-aware and aware of others' attitudes about change and be able to handle disagreements and disappointments (Lancaster and Lancaster 1982, p. 21).

Lancaster and Lancaster describe the functions of a change agent in assisting a group as the following: (a) defining the problem; (b) listing all alternatives and positive and negative consequences; (c) determining the most suitable alternative for the situation and time; (d) organizing a plan to implement the change; (e) providing continuing support and direction; and (f) helping to develop an evaluation format (1982, p. 21).

When assuming the role of change agent, nurses must recognize that they serve as an important link between various components of the change project or people participating in the change project. The change agent should hold a variety of expectations and expect the final outcome to be different from the original plan. It is also important for the change agent to be accessible to all people involved in the change process. The change agent should be honest and straightforward about goals and problems.

A key element is trust. The change agent must trust the participants in the change and they in turn must trust the change agent. One of the greatest risks of change is that the system can become disrupted, even nonfunctional. For example, changing the method of nurse assignments could result in gaps and missed care for some clients. Close observation of the situation during the change process is important to avoid this problem.

A change agent may be formally or informally designated by the system. A *formally designated change agent* is one who has the role and responsibility for change, such as a clinical nurse specialist expected to make changes beneficial to specified clients. This person has the power to plan and implement change. An *informally designated change agent* does not have the authority to make change by virtue of a position but does have the leadership skills and respect of others and therefore can serve an important function in the change process.

Change agents may also be internal or external. An *internal change agent* is a person who is part of the situation or system, e.g., a charge nurse on a hospital unit or a nurse employed on a surgical unit. Internal change agents are familiar with the situation and the organization. However, they may have vested interests in the present system as well as biases. An *external change agent* comes to the situation from the "outside," e.g., a nurse from another state or another hospital. External change agents are able to view the problem and the situation objectively and usually have no biases; however, they are unfamiliar with the situation and the problems. There are advantages and disadvantages to both positions, and it is important for any change agent to be aware of these in each situation.

Change agents who are successful have effective leadership skills. That is, they can influence people in order to attain specified goals. A change agent should be oriented toward changing the group or individual rather than the agency (Kemp 1986).

Mauksch and Miller (1981) list three key characteristics of a change agent:

1. The ability to take risks. This involves the ability to calculate potential risks associated with the change and then to decide whether the risks are worth taking.

2. A commitment to the efficacy of the change. The change agent should investigate the change and be convinced of its value and effectiveness.

3. Comprehensive knowledge of nursing that combines research findings and basic science data; competence in nursing practice, interpersonal relations, and communication skills.

Leader

The leadership role can be applied at many different levels: individual, family, groups of clients, professional colleagues, or the larger society. At the client level, **nursing leadership** is defined as a process of interpersonal influence through which a client is assisted in the establishment and achievement of goals toward improved well-being (Leddy and Pepper 1989, p. 336). On a larger scale, leadership can be defined as translating innovative ideas into action or as influencing individuals or groups to take an active part in the process of achieving agreed-upon goals (Epstein 1982, p. 2). The purposes of leadership vary according to the level of application and include (a) improving health status of individuals or families, (b) increasing the effectiveness and level of satisfaction among professional colleagues who provide care, and (c) improving the attitudes of citizens and legislators toward the nursing profession and their expectations of it (Leddy and Pepper 1989, p. 336).

Leadership Style Three leadership styles have been described: autocratic, democratic, and laissez-faire. The three are often blended in a selective combination to fit the situation, the needs of the leader, and the needs of the group, rather than being implemented continuously in pure form. More recent leadership styles include participative (diffused) leadership and situational leadership.

In **autocratic leadership,** the leader makes the decisions for the group. This style is likened to dictatorship and presupposes that the group is incapable of making its own decisions. The leader determines policies and gives orders and directions to the members. Autocratic leadership generally has negative connotations and often makes group members dissatisfied. It may, however, be a necessary style of leadership when urgent decision making is required or when group members do not wish to participate in making a decision.

In **democratic leadership,** the leader participates as a facilitator, encouraging group discussion and decision making. This supportive style increases group productivity and satisfaction. It presupposes that group members are capable of making decisions, are motivated to do so, and value independence. Democratic leadership generally has positive connotations but requires time for consultation and collaboration. It may not always be the most effective method if an urgent decision is required or if members lack skills and information to make decisions.

In **laissez-faire leadership,** the leader participates minimally and often only on request of the members. This style is described as a "hands-off" approach. It recognizes the group's need for autonomy and self-regulation. It is most effective after a group has made a decision, is committed to it, and has the expertise to implement it. The leader acts as a resource person and consultant.

Participative leadership is an approach to group leadership in which functions are distributed. Inherent in this concept is the recognition that the leadership function is not held irrevocably by one person but rather is distributed among the group members. To clarify this concept, Francis and Young (1979, p. 63) distinguish the role of group manager (the formal head of the group) from that of group leader. Managers have special responsibilities and functions that are recognized by the organization and are vital to the group's performance as an energizing and creative force. However, group leadership is a broad function. Different members assume leadership in their areas of strength to suit the tasks at hand.

Participative leaders are guided by the following principles (Richards 1987, p. 114):

- Leadership is not concentrated but diffused throughout the group.
- Formal or designated leadership is situational, and other members may perform functions equal in importance to or more important than those of the formal leader.
- The more members who function as leader, the better, because the act of leadership develops initiative, creativity, and responsibility.
- Leadership is a set of learned behaviors.

Situational leadership theory encourages managers to combine certain profiles of leader task behavior, leader relationship behavior, and follower maturity levels into four options of leadership style (Teasley 1987, p. 112):

1. High task–low relationship
2. High task–high relationship
3. Low task–high relationship
4. Low task–low relationship

Task behavior refers to leadership activities that direct followers by setting goals and defining role expectations. The leader tells how, what, when, and where something must be done. For example, a nurse would use this style when teaching a client about a prescribed medication (e.g., insulin) and informing the client about the drug name, dosage, administration method, number of times to take the drug, any side effects to report, and so on.

Relationship behavior is concerned with communications between the leader and follower. It involves mutual listening, supporting, informing, and facilitating so that people see various sides of mutual problems and get to know one another through general conversation and a social atmosphere. For example, a vice president of nursing may hold regular coffee or lunch sessions with nursing coordinators or supervisory staff.

Follower maturity level refers to the follower's state of job and psychologic functioning (high to low) for specific activities in particular situations. This involves assessment of job maturity and psychologic maturity. Assessment of *job maturity* requires a description of the person's education, experience, and capability of performing a particular function. Assessment of *psychologic maturity* requires a description of the person's motivation to perform and willingness to accept responsibility for a specific assignment.

To choose the best leadership style for a specific follower on a particular occasion, the leader must first assess the follower's maturity level and match it with the appropriate style. The leader must be competent in performing all four styles listed above.

A high task–low relationship leadership style may be used when the followers have a low job maturity level. For example, a leader helps nursing staff adopt a new computer system with which they are unfamiliar. A high task–high relationship leadership style may be used when the staff, now more familiar with the system, is revealing consistent errors or problems with the system. Here, the leader empathizes with the followers, works with them, and reteaches them. A low task–high relationship style would be necessary in situations that create frustration and call for participation and communication. Low task–low relationship leadership styles are used when a follower has a high job maturity level, i.e., is proficient, interested, and motivated. In this situation, the leader may delegate certain activities and be available as a consultant. A situational leadership style can improve job performance, help followers develop professionally, and promote competence in the leader.

Effective Leadership Effective leadership is a learned process requiring an understanding of the needs and goals that motivate people, the knowledge to apply the leadership skills, and the interpersonal skills to influence others. Much has been written about effective leadership and style; some descriptive statements are listed in the accompanying box.

Manager

There is often confusion between management and leadership, because in much of the literature, leadership is associated with group interaction within an organizational setting. **Management** is defined as "the use of delegated authority within the formal organization to organize, direct, or control responsible subordinates . . . so that all service contributions are coordinated to attain a goal" (Yura, Ozimek, and Walsh 1981, p. 5). Leadership, by contrast, may or may not require delegated authority within a formal organization.

The nurse manages the nursing care of individuals, families, and communities. The nurse-manager also delegates

nursing activities to ancillary workers and other nurses, and supervises and evaluates their performance. Managing requires knowledge about organizational structure and dynamics, authority and accountability, leadership, change theory, advocacy, delegation, and supervision and evaluation.

Nurses function in various types of organizations. Some are *autocratic,* with one person having primary knowledge and power while other persons are subordinate. Some are *bureaucratic,* with control through policy, structured jobs, and compartmentalized actions. Others *decentralize* control and emphasize self-direction and self-discipline of members. Still others can be viewed as components of *systems* that interact interdependently and adapt dynamically to change. This organization is particularly useful for the nurse who manages the care of individuals, families, and communities. On a larger scale, the nurse-manager must work in the organizational framework of the employing agency.

Authority is the right to act and command. It is an integral component of managing. Authority is conveyed through leadership actions; it is determined largely by the situation, and it is always associated with responsibility and accountability.

Accountability means being responsible for one's actions and accepting the consequences of one's behavior. Accountability can be viewed within a hierarchical systems framework, starting at the individual level, through the institutional/professional level, and then to the societal level (Sullivan and Decker 1988, p. 5). At the individual or client level, accountability is reflected in the nurse's ethical decision-making processes, competence, commitment, and integrity. At the institutional level, it is reflected in the statement of philosophy and objectives of the nursing department and nursing audits. At the professional level, it is reflected in standards of practice developed by national or provincial nursing associations. At the societal level, it is reflected in legislated nurse practice acts.

Delegation is the sharing of responsibility and authority with others and holding them accountable for performance (Sullivan and Decker 1988, p. 251). Because it is often impossible to provide all of the nursing care needed by a group of clients, the nurse as a delegator must assign aspects of the client's care to other nursing personnel. Delegation is a major tool in making the most efficient use of time. Delegation is a high-level implementation skill. The nurse as a delegator must have the following information: (a) needs of the client and family, (b) goals of the client, (c) nursing activity that can help the client meet the goals, and (d) skills and knowledge of various nursing personnel.

The nurse-delegator must also determine how many nursing personnel are needed. This information may be indicated on the client's records. Other sources of this information are the client, the charge nurse, other nursing personnel, and the nurse-delegator's own judgment. Nurses may require assistance to give clients care quickly in certain situations. Assistance may also be necessary to ensure the client's safety; for example, a nurse administering an intramuscular injection to a 3-year-old might need help to prevent injury to the child. If in doubt, nurses should always obtain aid to safeguard the client.

After establishing that assistance is required, the nurse-delegator must identify what type of help is needed, e.g., lifting or holding; how long help is required; when it is required; and what assistance is available. The nurse must arrange for assistance, usually by asking the appropriate person on the unit, before commencing the nursing activity. Delegation does not mean that a nurse-delegator never gets involved in direct client care. Often the nurse-delegator performs nursing activities appropriate to personal knowledge and skills. An important aspect of delegation is the development of the potential of nursing personnel. By knowing the backgrounds, experiences, knowledge, skills, and strengths of each person, a nurse can delegate responsibilities that help develop their competence.

Nursing personnel to whom aspects of care have been delegated need to be supervised and evaluated. The amount of supervision required is highly variable, depending on the knowledge and skills of each person. The nurse-delegator contributes to this evaluation process as the person who assigns the activity and observes the performance. Because individual motivation varies, the nurse-delegator needs to realize that not all persons perform equally. Thus, the nurse should evaluate assigned personnel according to standards of performance stated in job descriptions rather than by comparing one person to another. It is essential, too, for the nurse-delegator to realize that people require ongoing feedback about the care they give. Feedback should be given in an objective manner and include both positive and negative input.

Researcher

The majority of researchers in nursing are prepared at the doctoral and postdoctoral level, although an increasing number of clinicians with master's degrees are beginning to participate in research activity as part of their nursing role. However, "if nursing is to emerge in society as a socially significant, credible, scientific, and learned profession with a commitment to high-quality patient care, then research (for all nurses) is a necessity" (Starzomski 1983). It may be unrealistic to expect each nurse to conduct a study in the clinical setting. Many constraints in clinical settings must be reckoned with before research can become a legitimate and comfortable activity. However, if nursing is to develop as a research-based practice, it is not unreasonable to expect the nurse in the clinical area to (a) have some awareness of the process and language of research, (b) be sensitive to issues related to protecting the rights of human subjects, (c) participate in the identification of significant researchable problems, and (d) be a discriminating consumer of research findings.

Nursing students must learn these investigative functions early in their careers to establish the connection that "knowing how we know is fundamental to doing what we do" (Wilson 1985, p. viii). Bridging the research-practice gap, that is, bringing research into the clinical practice arena, is a key strategy in uniting the scholarly, scientific, and caring aspects of nursing in the future. Table 2–3 summarizes this position in the ANA's *Guidelines for the Investigative Function of Nurses* (1981), which specifies the generally expected research competence of nurses with associate, bachelor's, master's, and doctoral degrees.

TABLE 2–3 *Investigative Functions of a Nurse at Various Educational Levels*

Associate Degree in Nursing

1. Demonstrates awareness of the value or relevance of research in nursing
2. Assists in identifying problem areas in nursing practice
3. Assists in collecting data within an established, structured format

Baccalaureate in Nursing

1. Reads, interprets, and evaluates research for applicability to nursing practice
2. Identifies nursing problems that need to be investigated and participates in the implementation of scientific studies

3. Uses nursing practice as a means of gathering data to refine and extend practice
4. Applies established findings of nursing and other health-related research to nursing practice
5. Shares research findings with colleagues

Master's Degree in Nursing

1. Analyzes and reformulates nursing practice problems so that scientific knowledge and scientific methods can be used to find solutions
2. Enhances the quality and clinical relevance of nursing research by providing expertise in clinical problems

and by providing knowledge about the way in which these clinical services are delivered

3. Facilitates investigations of problems in clinical settings through such activities as contributing to a climate supportive of investigative activities, collaborating with others in investigations, and enhancing nursing's access to clients and data
4. Conducts investigations for the purpose of monitoring the quality of the practice of nursing in a clinical setting
5. Assists others to apply scientific knowledge in nursing practice

TABLE 2-3 *(continued)*

Doctoral Degree in Nursing or a Related Discipline	3. Develops methods to monitor the quality of the practice of nursing in a clinical setting and to evaluate contributions of nursing activities to the well-being of clients	empiric research and analytic processes
1. Provides leadership for the integration of scientific knowledge with other sources of knowledge for the advancement of practice	*Graduate of a Research-Oriented Doctoral Program*	2. Uses analytic and empiric methods to discover ways to modify or extend existing scientific knowledge so that it is relevant to nursing
2. Conducts investigations to evaluate the contribution of nursing activities to the well-being of clients	1. Develops theoretical explanations of phenomena relevant to nursing by	3. Develops methods for scientific inquiry of phenomena relevant to nursing

Source: American Nurses' Association, Commission on Nursing Research, *Guidelines for the investigative function of nurses* (Kansas City, Mo.: ANA, 1981). Reprinted with permission.

CHAPTER HIGHLIGHTS

▶ Socialization is a lifelong process by which people become functioning participants of a society or a group. It is a reciprocal learning process brought about by interaction with other people and establishes boundaries of behavior.

▶ Primary socialization occurs from birth to adolescence and is largely imposed by authority figures.

▶ Secondary socialization is the ongoing process of learning to adjust to new situations.

▶ Anticipatory socialization prepares people for the roles to which they aspire but do not yet occupy.

▶ Resocialization is the process of adapting to a very different social situation and may or may not be a matter of free choice. The most extreme form occurs in institutions that control every aspect of a person's existence.

▶ Professional socialization is the process whereby the values and norms of the profession are internalized into one's own behavior and concept of self. Knowledge, skills, and attitudes characteristic of the profession are acquired.

▶ Socialization for professional nursing requires the development of critical values, including a strong commitment to the service that nursing provides to the public, a belief in the dignity and worth of each person, a commitment to education, and autonomy.

▶ Various models of the socialization process have been developed. Such models may serve as guidelines to establish the phase and extent of an individual's socialization.

▶ In nursing practice, the nurse functions in a variety of roles that are not exclusive of one another; in reality, they often occur together. The roles serve to clarify the nurse's activities and include carer, communicator/helper, teacher, counselor, client advocate, change agent, leader, manager, and researcher.

READINGS AND REFERENCES

SUGGESTED READINGS

Benner, P. 1984. *From novice to expert: Excellence and power in clinical nursing practice.* Menlo Park, Calif.: Addison-Wesley Publishing Co.
This book is a major contribution to nursing. It provides a lucid description of nursing practice as it is rendered by expert nurses. It provides profound implications for nurses in administration, education, and practice.

Kirk, R. February 1987. Being a proactive leader. *Journal of Nursing Administration* 17:6–8.
Although all nurses are managers, management is not leadership. This management consultant advocates proactive leadership rather than reactive leadership. Proactive leaders stimulate creativity, constantly seek out new opportunities for quality and productivity, and inspire others to cooperate in the planning

and implementation of these opportunities. Seven ways to develop this style of leadership are discussed.

Kramer, M. 1974. *Reality shock: Why nurses leave nursing.* St. Louis: C. V. Mosby Co.

Kramer describes a postgraduate resocialization model for the resolution of value and role conflict between the generalized knowledge and skills acquired in an educational program and the specific behaviors required for the work setting. Four stages are outlined: skill and routine mastery, social integration, moral outrage, and conflict resolution.

Robinson, M. B. 1985. Patient advocacy and the nurse: Is there a conflict of interest? *Nursing Forum* 22:58–63.

Robinson explains that a patient advocate must be able to relate to patients and staff at all levels and must have certain qualities: self-motivation, objectivity, empathy, tact, flexibility, tenacity, a sense of humor, and the ability to cope with stress and pressure. The nurse who becomes a patient advocate should be aware of the possible conflicts of interest and the restrictions of the role. Robinson points out that most hospitals do not have written policies to protect the nurse in the advocacy role.

Trandel-Korenchuk, D., and Trandel-Korenchuck, K. April 1983. Nursing advocacy of patients' rights: Myth or reality. Part 2. *Nurse Practitioner* 8:37, 40–42.

The authors discuss communication in the physician-nurse relationship. Evident in communication patterns are authoritarianism (physician), acceptance of dependence (nurse), and communication control (physician). The authors relate problems in nurse-to-nurse relationships to the problems in women's relationships. It is proposed that nurses will be better able to meet medicine and hospital bureaucracy on equal ground if nursing attains unity and influence.

Wierda, L. 1989. BSN students find a way to lessen the severity of reality shock. *Nursing Forum* 22:11–14.

Fear of "reality shock" influenced a group of BSN students to develop different variations in their clinical experience. The most successful and well-liked alternative was a module consisting of two students and three clients. Students said they felt more independent and liked having another person, other than the clinical instructor or staff nurses, with whom they could discuss their problems.

RELATED RESEARCH

Cohen, B. J., and Jordet, C. P. January 1988. Nursing schools: Students' beacon to professionalism? *Nursing and Health Care* 9:38–41.

Dobbs, K. K. April 1988. The senior preceptorship as a method for anticipatory socialization of baccalaureate nursing students. *Journal of Nursing Education* 27:167–71.

Furnham, A. 1988. Values and vocational choice: A study of value differences in medical, nursing and psychology students. *Social Science and Medicine* 26:613–18.

Green, G. J. July/August 1988. Relationships between role models and role perceptions of new graduate nurses. *Nursing Research* 37:245–48.

Irurita, V. September/November 1988. A study of nurse leadership. *Australian Journal of Advanced Nursing* 6:43–52.

Langston, R. A. 1990. Comparative effects of baccalaureate and associate degree educational programs on the professional socialization of nursing students. In Chaska, N. L. *The nursing profession: Turning points.* pp. 53–58. St. Louis: C. V. Mosby Co.

SELECTED REFERENCES

American Nurses' Association. Commission of Nursing Research. 1981. *ANA guidelines for investigative function of nurses.* Kansas City, Mo.: ANA.

Annas, G. J. 1975. The rights of hospital patients: The basic ACLU guide to a hospital patient's rights: New York: Avon Books.

Batra, C. January 1990. Socializing nurses for nursing entrepreneurship roles. *Nursing Health Care* 11:34–37.

Benner, P. 1984. *From novice to expert: Excellence and power in clinical nursing practice.* Menlo Park, Calif.: Addison-Wesley Publishing Co.

Benner, P., and Wrubel, J. 1989. *The primacy of caring: Stress and coping in health and illness.* Redwood City, Calif.: Addison-Wesley Nursing.

Berger, P., and Berger, B. 1975. *Sociology: A biographical approach.* 2d ed. New York: Basic Books.

Brooten, D. A.; Hayman, L.; and Naylor, M. 1978. *Leadership for change: A guide for the frustrated nurse.* Philadelphia: J. B. Lippincott, Co.

Cohen, B. J., and Jordet, C. P. January 1988. Nursing schools: Students' beacon to professionalism? *Nursing and Health Care* 9:38–41.

Dalton, G. W.; Thompson, P. H.; and Price, R. L. Summer 1977. The four stages of professional careers—A new look at performance by professionals. *Organ Dynamics* pp. 19–42.

Davis, F. September 1966. Professional socialization as subjective experience: The process of doctrinal conversion among student nurses. Sixth World Congress of Sociology Paper. Evian, France.

Disparti, J. 1988. Nutrition and self care. In Caliandro, G., and Judkins, B. L. *Primary nursing practice.* Glenview Ill.: Scott, Foresman & Co.

Donahue, M. P. 1985. Viewpoints. Euthanasia: An ethical uncertainty. In McCloskey, J. C., and Grace, H. K. *Current issues in nursing.* 2d ed. Boston: Blackwell Scientific Publications.

Dreyfus, S. E., and Dreyfus, H. L. February 1980. A five-stage model of the mental activities involved in directed skill acquisition. Unpublished report supported by the Air Force Office of Scientific Research (AFSC), USAF (Contract F49620–79–C–0063), University of California at Berkeley.

Epstein, C. 1982. *The nurse leader: Philosophy and practice.* Reston: Reston Publishing.

Francis, D., and Young, D. 1979. Improving work groups: A practical manual for team building. San Diego, Calif.: University Associates.

Hinshaw, A. S. November 1977. *Socialization and resocialization of nurses for professional nursing practice.* National League for Nursing Pub. no. 15–1659. New York: National League for Nursing.

———. 1986. Socialization and resocialization of nurses for professional nursing practice. In Hein, E. C., and Nicholson, M. J., editors. *Contemporary leadership behavior: Selected readings.* 2d ed. Boston: Little, Brown and Co.

Hollie, M. L., Blatchley, M. E. Winter 1989. Teaching leadership with role theory. *Nursing Connections* 2:53–61.

Kelman, H. 1961. Process of opinion changes. *Public Opinion Quarterly* 25:57.

Kemp, V. H. 1986. An overview of change and leadership. In Hein, E. C., and Nicholson, M. J., editors. *Contemporary leadership behavior: Selected readings.* 2d ed. Boston: Little, Brown and Co.

Kohnke, M. F. November 1980. The nurse as advocate. *American Journal of Nursing* 80:2038–40.

Kozier, B., and Erb, G. 1988. *Concepts and issues in nursing practice.* Redwood City, Calif.: Addison-Wesley Nursing.

Kramer, M. 1974. *Reality shock: Why nurses leave nursing.* St. Louis: C. V. Mosby Co.

Lancaster, J., and Lancaster, W. 1982. *Concepts for advanced nursing practice: The nurse as change agent.* St. Louis: C. V. Mosby Co.

Leddy, S., and Pepper, J. M. 1989. *Conceptual bases of professional nursing.* 2d ed. Philadelphia: J. B. Lippincott Co.

Lundy, K. L. P., and Warme, B. D. 1986. *Sociology: A window on the world.* Toronto: Methuen Publications.

Mauksch, I. G., and Miller, M. H. 1981. *Implementing change in nursing.* St. Louis: C. V. Mosby Co.

Redman, B. K. 1988. *The process of patient education.* 6th ed. St. Louis: C. V. Mosby Co.

Richards, M. B. November 1987. Developing "participative leaders." *Nursing Management* 18:113–15.

Shaffir, W. B., and Turowetz, A. 1987. Socialization and the self. In Rosenberg, M. M.; Shaffir, W. B.; Turowetz, A.; and Weinfeld, M., editors. *An introduction to sociology.* 2d ed. Toronto: Methuen Publications.

Simpson, I. H. Winter 1967. Patterns of socialization into professions: The case of student nurses. *Sociological Inquiry* 37:47–54.

Starzomski, R. September 1983. The place of research in nursing. *Canadian Nurse* 79:34–35.

Styles, M. M. June 1978. Why Publish? *Image: Journal of Nursing Scholarship* 10:28–32.

———. 1982. *On nursing: Toward a new endowment.* St. Louis: C. V. Mosby Co.

Sullivan, E. J., and Decker, P. J. 1988. *Effective management in nursing.* 2d ed. Redwood City, Calif.: Addison-Wesley Nursing.

Teasley, D. November 1987. Situational leadership for nurses. *Nursing Management* 18:112–3.

Tepperman, L., and Richardson, R. J., editors. 1986. *The social world: An introduction to sociology.* Toronto: McGraw-Hill Ryerson Ltd.

Watson, I. Summer 1981. Socialization of the nursing student in a professional nursing education programme. *Nursing Papers* 13:19–24.

Watson, J. 1979. *Nursing—The philosophy and science of caring.* Boston: Little, Brown and Co.

Wilson, H. S. 1985. *Research in Nursing.* Menlo Park, Calif.: Addison-Wesley Publishing Co.

———. 1989. *Research in Nursing.* Redwood City, Calif.: Addison-Wesley Nursing.

Yura, H.; Ozimek, D.; and Walsh, M. B. 1981. *Nursing leadership: Theory and process.* New York: Appleton-Century-Crofts.

Zusman, J. November/December 1982. Want some good advice? Think twice about being a patient advocate. *Nursing Life* 6:46–50.

Changing Nursing Practice:
Trends, Research, and Politics

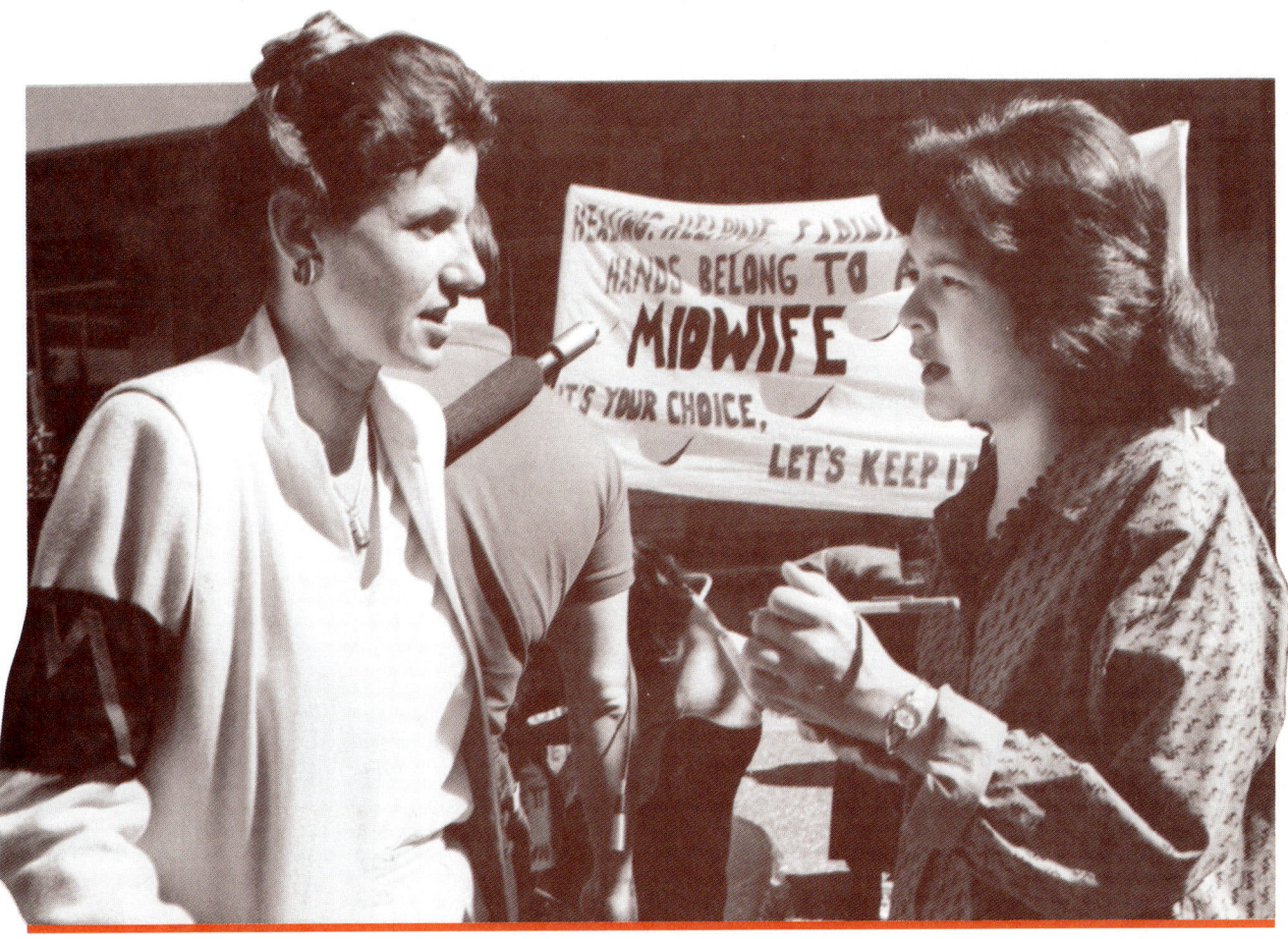

CONTENTS

▶ Describe Bennis, Benne, and Chin's strategies for change.

▶ Describe the change process.

▶ Identify the factors influencing nursing practice.

▶ Explain how nursing education affects nursing practice.

▶ Describe the role of nursing research as it influences current and future nursing practice.

▶ Describe the role of the nurse in protecting the rights of clients.

▶ Identify the attitudes and behaviors necessary to overcome powerlessness.

▶ Explain the various sources of power.

▶ Describe why nurses should be politically active.

▶ Explain the guiding principles for political action.

CHANGE

Change is all around us. It is a dynamic process and a normal part of people's lives. It is a means by which people grow, develop, and adapt. Change is also an integral aspect of nursing. To be effective and influential in today's world, nurses need to understand change theory and apply its precepts in the workplace, in government and professional organizations, and in the community. Planning and implementing change are professional responsibilities as well as largely unrealized power sources that are vital to the practice of nursing. Some synonyms for change are *alter, transform, modify, convert,* and *vary.* All these terms suggest that a fundamental difference or substitution is the outcome of change.

Brooten, Hayman, and Naylor (1978) define **change** as "the process which leads to alteration in individual or institutional patterns of behavior." Mauksch and Miller define change as "the process by which alterations occur in the function and structure of society." Further, they define **planned change** as a "deliberative and collaborative process including a change agent and a client system," this system being "an individual, group of people, an agency, an organization, or a social institution" (1981, p. 9). For further information about change, see Chapter 16.

A nurse can use a number of strategies to implement change. The three categories that follow are described by Bennis, Benne, and Chin (1985):

1. *Power-coercive.* Power-coercive strategies are based on the use of power as a result of legitimate authority or of economic influence. These strategies are particularly valuable when there is a lack of general agreement about a change. The use of this type of strategy may produce considerable resistance to the change and so should not be used without considering the subsequent consequences. A hospital administrator might demonstrate this strategy by establishing a policy that nurses on night shift can take only 15 minutes for a meal break. The administrator has the obvious power to make this decision.

2. *Empiric-rational.* This category of strategies uses knowledge as the basis for change. It assumes that people act in a rational manner. It is also assumed that the change agent has knowledge and has the power to persuade others to accept a change that is desirable for them. An example of this strategy is for a clinical nurse specialist to introduce a new method for recording intravenous infusions that is faster and more accurate than other methods of recordkeeping.

3. *Normative-reeducative.* This category of strategies is based on the assumption that people's actions are guided by sociocultural norms and values. Information is considered to be insufficient to change people's behavior. Therefore, the change must be brought about through skilled interpersonal communication. The change agent collaborates with the others involved in the change process. Normative-reeducative strategies foster personal growth and problem-solving. An example of normative-reeducative change strategy is having a well-known athlete talk to teenagers about the dangers associated with taking drugs. It is hoped that this person's influence will be greater than the peer pressure toward experimentation.

Taking a slightly different approach, Schaller (1972) outlined four general strategies for change: coercion, co-optation, conflict, and cooperation.

Coercion is the application of power to force a change. The individual or group that selects this strategy must gain power before introducing change.

Co-optation means bringing people or a person resisting the change into the prochange group. This may involve making promises of a certain position or money or some type of "buy-off." Co-optation can have the advantage of establishing a group with more diverse points of view; however, the disadvantage is that members may not agree with the promises given in exchange for support.

Conflict or confrontation strategy may clarify issues in the change process, but it may also have a divisive effect and may stimulate resistance that can impede the change (Brooten 1984).

The *cooperative* strategy is widely used in health care institutions. A climate for cooperative change is encouraged by an open exchange of information, opinions, and feelings (Mauksch and Miller 1981). In addition, it requires skills in communication and interpersonal relations. The need for the change must also be based on knowledge and fact.

Steps in the Change Process

The following steps are a model of planned change. The model outlines the actions one must take to plan and control change and make it serve a specific purpose (Spradley 1980).

1. Identify symptoms that indicate something needs changing.
2. Diagnose the problem by reviewing the symptoms and gathering additional data.
3. Explore alternative solutions in terms of their risks, benefits, driving and restraining forces, advantages, disadvantages, and probable outcomes. (An effective technique often used by change agents is brainstorming.)
4. Select one course of action from among the identified alternatives.
5. Plan the steps in the change process:
   a. Write measurable objectives.
   b. Determine a timetable.
   c. Plan a budget.
   d. Recruit individuals to carry out each aspect of the plan.
   e. Ensure ability of the change agents to work with the client system.
   f. Evaluate resources (driving forces) and resistance (restraining forces) and plan strategies to manage both.
   g. Design a plan to evaluate the outcomes of the change effort.
   h. Identify measures to refreeze or establish the change within the client system.
6. Implement the change. (Pilot testing a new idea affords one the opportunity to evaluate it on a small scale and to "sell" it to the larger client system.)
7. Evaluate the outcome(s) on the basis of the measurable objectives and make appropriate adjustments.
8. Refreeze the client system so that the changes are seen as standard operating procedures and the system is once again stable.

Examples of Change

It is exciting to realize how effective nurses can be when they determine the need for change and plan strategies to bring it about. The following examples outline changes initiated by nurses who have identified a need to "do something" in each of four spheres of influence: the workplace, organizations, government, and the community.

The Workplace   At each of three shift meetings Mrs. Hawkins, Head Nurse, listened to nurses complain about

problems with getting clients' laboratory work done and reported to the unit in a timely manner. She conferred with other head nurses and with the attending and resident physicians on her unit. It appeared that similar complaints were widespread.

At the next head nurse meeting, Mrs. Hawkins described the problem. The group appointed a task force, with Mrs. Hawkins as Chair, and asked it to present a plan to solve the problem at the next meeting. After gathering more data, the task force invited representatives from the attending and resident staff and the laboratory director to meet with them to review the data, consider alternative solutions, and select a plan to solve the problem.

By the next head nurse meeting, a preliminary plan to alter the system of laboratory reporting had been devised, and all concerned were working cooperatively to implement the plan.

The Professional Organization   Nurses on the Education Committee of a district nurses' association recognized the need to make a public policy statement concerning the care of clients with AIDS. Since the Board of Directors had recently expressed interest in promulgating such policy statements, the committee sensed the timing was right and that the board would welcome its draft despite the controversial subject matter.

Members of the committee researched and drafted a statement. The full committee offered a critique and selected an articulate spokesperson to present the statement to the association president and seek support before asking to have the statement presented to the board. Once the president had approved the statement, it was placed on the agenda for the next board meeting.

After making minor additions, the board approved it for distribution to the lay and nursing press and asked the Education Committee to suggest a nurse to present the statement at a local hearing of the City Council Health Committee.

The Government   While the pressure to contain health care costs escalated through the first half of the 1980s, a coalition representing the shared interests of the ANA, the NLN, and the American Association of Colleges of Nursing (AACN) mounted a campaign to convince Congress of the cost-effectiveness of a center for nursing research within the National Institutes of Health (NIH). Despite incredible odds, including a presidential veto and opposition from the American Medical Association, the American Association of Medical Colleges, and the NIH administrations, the proposal was passed by Congress in the fall of 1985. The success of this effort demonstrates the effectiveness of carefully planned change including the collaboration of nursing organizations. It also illustrates the clout organized nurses can wield on any level and in any sphere.

The Community   Every nurse plays several roles besides that of registered nurse. Each resides in a community, and many are parents. Some serve on school boards, belong to the League of Women Voters, or participate in religious, club, or scouting activities. There are numerous opportunities for nurses to contribute to the health and welfare of the communities in which they live. A group of nursing students recognized a health problem within their community and developed a plan to intervene. Many of the students were parents of children in local elementary schools where a high percentage of children were being sent home daily with head lice. Because of previously enacted budget cuts, the district's school nurses were each responsible for between three and five schools. The students volunteered to work with the district nurses to provide screening and health teaching at each of the elementary schools, thereby helping to resolve the community's problem.

All nurses are affected by change; nobody can avoid it. Knowledgeable nurses make rational plans to deal with both opportunities to initiate and guide needed change as well as to respond to change that affects them in the workplace, government, organizations, and the community. To recognize these opportunities for change and respond to the factors that influence nursing from without, it is helpful to consider the history of nursing, current trends in nursing, and present political, social, technological, and economic issues.

FACTORS INFLUENCING NURSING PRACTICE

To understand nursing as it is practiced today and as it will be practiced tomorrow requires not only a historical perspective of nursing's evolution but also an understanding of some of the social forces currently influencing this profession. These forces usually affect the entire health care system, and nursing, as a major component of that system, cannot avoid the effects. See Chapter 1 for the historical development of nursing.

Economics   Greater financial support provided through public and private health insurance programs has increased the demand for nursing care. Health services such as emergency room care, mental health counseling, and preventive physical examinations are increasingly being used by people who could not afford them in the past. Federal governments recognized this need and markedly increased their budgets for health care in the 1970s and early 1980s. This increase in expenditure is accompanied by increased employment opportunities for those who provide health services.

Costs of health care have also increased during this period as well. In response to these increasing costs, the Medicare payment system to hospitals was revised in 1982, establishing fees according to diagnostic related groups (DRGs). With the implementation of this legislation, more clients in hospitals are more acutely ill than before, and clients once considered sufficiently ill to be hospitalized are now treated at home.

These changes present challenges to nurses. Currently, the health care industry is shifting its emphasis from inpatients to outpatients with preadmission testing, posthospitalization rehabilitation, home health care, health maintenance, and physical fitness (Powell 1984, p. 33). Nurses need to identify how their knowledge and skills can fit into these settings. Rogers (1985, p. 10) suggests that before long a large majority of nurses will not work in hospitals. This change in the area of employment has implications for nursing education, nursing research, and nursing practice.

Nursing Shortage   In the U.S.A., 58% of hospitals report an acute shortage of registered nurses, particularly in areas such as intensive care, emergency, and operating rooms. A similar shortage also exists in Canada. This shortage is thought to be the result of many factors, e.g., a decline in student enrollment and an increase in the number of nurses leaving nursing (Graham and Sheppard 1990, p. 440–41).

The declining interest in nursing is a multifaceted problem. Students have wider career choices than in previous years. Inglehart (1987) points out that nurses' salaries and benefits do not reflect their levels of education, experience, or performance. In addition, weekend and shift work appears unattractive to many prospective students. Another factor considered to affect recruitment is nursing's public image. The public often has difficulty differentiating the "generic" nurse from other nursing personnel, such as nursing assistants and support personnel. This inability to identify and explain nursing and how it affects society is also reflected in recruitment.

Nursing associations, government agencies, employers, and nursing educators have studied the problem. The major organizations on the Tri-Council for Nursing have plans regarding the nursing shortage. The American Medical Association has recommended the preparation of a new class of health care worker, the registered care technologist (RCT) to answer the nursing shortage. Nursing groups have called the creation of such a technologist unnecessary and costly. Moreover, nursing groups believe that it will further fragment client care (DeBack 1990, p. 122). Some employer hospitals are testing strategies to change the role of the hospital nurse and to improve the practice environment. In addition, some nursing schools, in order to attract more students to nursing, have designed new models for nursing education, flexible scheduling of courses, and alternative fiscal support for students.

Consumer Demands   Consumers of nursing services (the public) have become an increasingly effective force in changing nursing practice. On the whole, people are better educated and have more knowledge about health and illness than in the past. Consumers also have become more aware of others' needs for care. The ethical and moral issues raised by poverty and neglect have made people more vocal about the needs of minority groups and the poor.

The public's concepts of health and nursing have also changed. Most now believe that health is a right of all people, not just a privilege of the rich. The media emphasize the message that individuals must assume responsibility for their own health by obtaining a physical examination regularly, checking for the seven danger signals of cancer, and maintaining their mental well-being by balancing work and recreation. Interest in health and nursing services is therefore greater than ever. Furthermore, many people now want more than freedom from disease—they want energy, vitality, and a feeling of wellness.

Increasingly, the consumer has become an active participant in making decisions about health and nursing care. Planning committees concerned with providing nursing services to a community usually have active consumer membership. Recognizing the legitimacy of public input, many state and provincial nursing associations and regulatory agencies have consumer representatives on their governing boards.

Family Structure

The need for and provision of nursing services are being influenced by new family structures. An increasing number of people are living away from the extended family and the nuclear family, and the family breadwinner is no longer necessarily the husband. An extended family consists of parents, children, grandparents, and sometimes aunts and uncles; a nuclear family consists only of parents and their children.

Today, many single men and women rear children, and in many two-parent families both parents work. It is also common for young parents to live at great distances from their own parents. These young families need support services such as day-care centers. Many such families do not have grandparents or other relatives readily available to help in times of illness or to offer advice about childbearing and child health. These parents usually get this advice from physicians and nurses as well as others. Similarly, grandparents who live alone and far from other members of the family require homemaker and visiting nurse services when they are ill because they cannot receive this care from younger members of the family.

Adolescent mothers also need specialized nursing services. These young mothers have the normal needs of teenagers as well as those of new mothers. In 1960, 13.9% of all births were to teenage mothers; this percentage has increased steadily despite the fact that an increasing number of women are choosing to delay motherhood. Many teenage mothers are raising their children alone. This type of single-parent family is especially vulnerable because motherhood compounds the difficulties of adolescence.

Science and Technology

Advances in science and technology affect nursing practice. For example, widespread immunization for poliomyelitis decreased the morbidity of that disease and the need for specialized nursing care. As physicians expand their knowledge base and technical skills, nurses acquire complementary knowledge and skills as they adapt to meet the new needs of clients.

In some settings, technologic advances have required that nurses become highly specialized. Nurses frequently have to use sophisticated computerized equipment to monitor or treat clients. As technologies change, nursing education changes, and nurses require increasing education to provide effective, safe nursing practice.

Advances in technology are exemplified by the many machines now used to help clients maintain life. There seems to be no end to the discoveries and the knowledge explosion of the twentieth century. With this knowledge explosion has come the charge that medical services—and some health professionals—have become dehumanized. Yet an increasing understanding of the psychologic, emotional, and spiritual aspects of care has developed to balance the technologic advances. As science and technology create methods of treating disease, it is the responsibility of all health professionals, and nurses in particular, to remember that clients are human beings requiring warmth, care, and acknowledgment of self-worth. Often equipment is frightening to clients and their support persons. Medical vocabulary appears mysterious and is frequently misunderstood. The nurse who deals with clients daily is in an ideal situation to humanize technology as much as possible. To humanize highly technical care, nurses can offer explanations, communicate their support, and recognize the clients' needs to understand and to be supported. This is the "high touch" aspect of a "high tech" environment.

Problems created by technologic change present new challenges to nurses. For example, some industries are hazardous to employees because of dangerous equipment or harmful chemical residues. Trauma (injury) and disease are frequently the direct result of advanced technology; the classic example is automobile accidents, which are among the top five causes of death in North America. In addition, our society frequently creates high levels of stress, which does not promote health.

Legislation

Legislation about nursing practice and health matters affects both the public and nursing. Legislation related to nursing is discussed in Chapter 8. Changes in legislation relating to health also affect nursing. For example, relaxation of laws governing abortions has been associated with reduced maternal morbidity from self-induced abortions.

Legislation regarding the Medicare payment system according to DRGs has had an enormous influence on nursing practice in hospitals and communities. Many clients leave hospitals sooner than they did in the past. As a result, more clients in hospitals are seriously ill, and more clients at home require more complex nursing care than in the past. Although this trend has contributed to a shortage of nurses in acute care settings, it has opened new opportunities for nurses in home health care.

Demography

Demography is the study of population, including statistics about distribution by age and place of residence, mortality (death), and morbidity (incidence of disease). From demographic data, needs of the population for nursing services can be assessed. For example:

- The total population in North America has increased since 1900. The proportion of elderly people has also increased, creating an increased need for nursing services for this group.
- The population is shifting from rural to urban settings. This shift signals increased needs for nursing related to problems caused by pollution and by the effects on the environment of concentrations of people. Thus, most nursing services are now provided in urban settings.
- Mortality and morbidity studies reveal the presence of "risk factors." Many of these "risk factors," e.g., smoking, are major causes of death and disease that can be prevented through changes in life-style. The nurse's role in assessing risk factors and helping clients to make healthy life-style changes is discussed in Chapter 23.

The Women's Movement

The women's movement has brought public attention to human rights. Persons are seeking equality in all areas, particularly educational, political, economic, and social equality. Because the majority of nurses are women, this movement has altered the perspectives of nurses about economic and educational needs. As a result, nurses are increasingly asserting themselves as professional people who have a right to equality with men in health professions, and nurses are demanding more autonomy in client care.

Collective Bargaining

More nurses are using collective bargaining to deal with their concerns. The ANA has participated in collective bargaining for more than 40 years through its economic and general welfare programs on behalf of nurses. Today, some nurses are joining other labor organizations that represent them at the bargaining table. In both the United States and Canada, nurses have gone on strike over certain demands and concerns. Often these concerns go beyond economic reward to issues about safe care for clients. Increasingly, nurses are becoming aware of the strength of organized, large numbers. DeCrosta (1985, p. 20) believes that nurses will increasingly look to unions as they attempt to resist staff cuts and perceived dilution of the quality of nursing care.

Nursing Associations

Professional nursing associations have provided leadership that affects many areas of nursing. Voluntary accreditation of nursing education programs by the NLN and by mandatory accreditation licensing boards in each state have also influenced nursing. Many programs have steadily improved to meet the standards for accreditation over the years. As a result, nurse graduates are better prepared to meet the demands of society.

In 1979, the ANA published findings of a committee on credentialing, which recommended the establishment of a center for credentialing in nursing (ANA 1979, p. 682). **Credentialing** is the process of determining and maintaining competence in nursing. The credentialing of expanded nursing roles, such as that of the nurse practitioner, is carried out by the ANA and certain nursing specialty organizations, such as the American Association of Critical-Care Nurses.

To influence health care policy-making, a group of professional nurses organized formally to take political action in the nursing and health care arenas. Nurses for Political Action (NPA) was formed in 1971 and became an arm of the ANA in 1974, when its name changed to Nurses Coalition for Action in Politics (N-CAP). In 1986, the name was changed to ANA-PAC. Through this group, nurses have lobbied actively for legislation affecting health care. A number of nursing leaders hold positions of authority in government. Attaining such positions is essential if nurses hope to exert ongoing political influence.

The drive for increased autonomy comes from the nursing profession itself. During the past 20 years, the increased autonomy of nurses has been evidenced by their function in specialty care units, such as intensive care units, and in their expanded roles, such as that of the nurse practitioner. Many states have rewritten their nurse practice acts to reflect such changes in nursing practice.

NURSING EDUCATION

Although current scientific, social, and economic influences may affect the utilization of nursing services, they do not determine nursing practice. Nursing is controlled from within the profession itself. The future of nursing lies not with the leaders of the past or present but rather with today's and tomorrow's nursing students. In recognition of this reality, the nursing profession is particularly interested in the educational preparation of nurses for the future.

Technical and Professional Levels of Practice

In 1985, the ANA House of Delegates proposed that two levels of nurses be delineated: technical and professional. The technical nurse is to be prepared in an associate degree program, and the professional nurse is to be prepared in a baccalaureate degree program. This proposal, if implemented by the state nursing associations, has many implications. One implication concerns "grandfathering" to protect those nurses already licensed to practice. Because at present both technical and professional nurses are licensed as registered nurses, there is substantial agreement about grandfathering those already licensed. However, even with a grandfather clause in place, many nurses fear that they will not be protected from discrimination when they compete with recent graduates for jobs.

Titling and Licensure

The designations *registered nurse* (RN) and *licensed practical* or *vocational nurse* (LPN, LVN) have been used since licensure laws were first enacted. In its 1985 proposal, the ANA endorsed that the professional nurse with a baccalaureate degree be licensed under the legal title *registered nurse* (RN) and that the technical nurse with an associate degree be licensed under the legal title *associate nurse* (AN). As a professional organization, however, the ANA cannot legislate these changes. It is the responsibility of each state to define the legal boundaries of nursing practice and to designate the titles to be used by those practitioners who meet the individual state's criteria for licensure. Thus, if this proposal is to be accepted nationally, each state will need to implement its own changes. Such changes have major implications for diploma nurses and LPNs, because their status is not discussed in the proposal. In addition, this proposal means that new standardized examinations must be developed to test the two levels of competence.

Economic Constraints

Stevens (1985, p. 124) states that "what is best for nursing may not coincide with what is best for society at large," and that "one can no longer assume that the *best* for society—at any price—is a feasible goal." Recognizing that no discipline has ever achieved professional status outside of the traditional academic institutions, Stevens (1985, pp. 125–26) points out that 4-year baccalaureate programs are more costly than 2-year programs, BSN graduates require higher salaries, and the financial resources of the health care industry are shrinking. For these reasons, the nursing profession must substantiate to the general public the claim that the BSN nurse can deliver qualitatively different care from that provided by the ADN nurse. The 2-year associate degree program, however, can potentially effect cost savings that can offset the high cost of educating and hiring the BSN nurse. How the two roles can be redesigned to best complement each other is a question that needs to be answered. The 1987 ANA statement on the scope of practice (see Chapter 1) begins to answer this question and calls for further differentiation between the professional and technical practice of nursing (ANA 1987, pp. 76–79).

Types of Educational Preparation

In the future, more nurses will be needed in home and community settings as a result of the prospective payment system in hospitals. What education will best prepare nurses to meet these needs? Because of nurses' greater autonomy in these areas, some nurse educators think that a baccalaureate degree is a minimum requirement. Others believe that ADN nurses can implement plans of care that are developed by a BSN primary nurse.

Given the expanding knowledge and technologic bases of nursing, it may be expected that curricula will have to be scrutinized to remove extraneous content and to ensure appropriate clinical experiences that relate to the theoretical content presented. Some educators are calling for inclusion of computer courses in nursing programs as society becomes more computer dependent. Before the implementation of the Medicare prospective payment system, many nurses had little knowledge of health care and nursing care economics. Perlich (1986, p. 6) advocates that nursing school curricula be changed to reflect such realities as cost containment and accountability of productivity so that future nurses are educated in their role in both influencing and implementing policies in this area.

The National Commission on Nursing Implementation Project (NCNIP 1987) recommended in its *Timeline for Transition into the Future System for Two Categories of Nurses* a time frame for systematic transition of the present system of nursing education into a future system of education of technical and professional nursing. See Figure 3–1. According to the paper's recommendations, the educational preparation of the professional and technical nurse will differ from the current preparation. Professional nurses will be prepared in liberal arts and nursing education. They will have baccalaureate or higher degrees with majors in nursing. Technical nurses will be prepared in general education

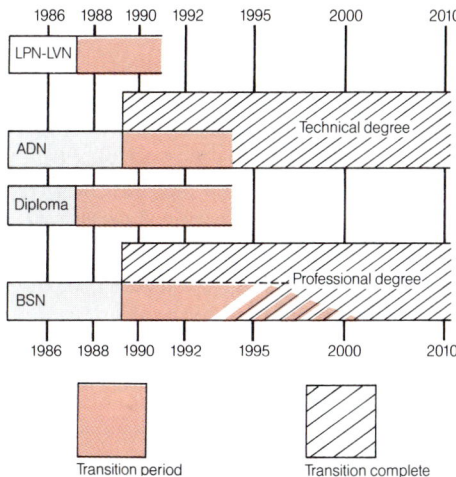

Figure 3–1 Timeline for transition into the future: nursing education system for two categories of nurse.
Source: National Commission on Nursing Implementation Project. (Milwaukee: NCNIP, 1987). Reprinted with permission.

courses and natural and behavioral sciences as well as nursing. They will be graduates of associate degree programs in nursing.

Post-RN Baccalaureate and Master's Degree Programs

The thrust to make the baccalaureate degree the minimum entry level for professional nursing practice has significantly increased the need for post-RN baccalaureate programs. Providing programs to meet these needs and demands is a challenge for universities, especially since the profile of returning nursing students indicates that most are married women in their 30s and 40s who have dependent children and hold either full-time or part-time jobs (Dugas 1985, p. 18). Universities must be flexible in planning and providing such programs for these adult learners. Some universities now offer courses in off-campus sites for post-RN baccalaureate and MSN students and use distance delivery techniques such as teleconferencing and shipments of basic reference materials to remote areas (Kerr 1985, p. 30).

Specialization

Basic nursing education programs are designed to develop nurses as generalists, not specialists in any aspect of nursing. Traditionally, educators and employers have perpetuated the idea that nurses should be generalists who can rotate among services and shifts with minimal preparation. Yet, with the technological advances affecting nursing practice over the past 10 years, the market demand for nurses with specialized knowledge and skills has grown significantly.

A **specialty** is a defined area of clinical practice that has a narrow, in-depth focus. Some clinical specialties are occupational health nursing, emergency and operating room nursing, enterostomal therapy nursing, intravenous therapy nursing, infection control nursing, nephrology nursing, neurology nursing, midwifery, critical care nursing, oncology nursing, and palliative care nursing.

There is a bewildering array of educational programs to prepare specialists. Aims, length, and content of the programs differ. Once prepared, the specialists are employed in a wide number of capacities and have a variety of job titles. There is a need for the national association to establish priorities for specialty development, program standards, credentialing mechanisms, and an accompanying need for employers to provide appropriate economic rewards for the performance of specialty services.

NURSING RESEARCH

Nursing research is more than just scientific investigations conducted by a person educated and credentialed as a nurse. It refers instead to research directed toward building a body of nursing knowledge about "human responses to actual or potential health problems" (ANA 1980, p. 9) and to the effects of nursing action on such human responses. The human responses of people may be reactions of individuals, groups, or families to actual health problems (e.g., the burden a family experiences when they must care for an elderly relative with senile dementia); and concerns of individuals and groups about potential health problems (such as accident prevention or stress management in an industrial setting). The purpose of nursing research is to improve health care while reflecting the traditional nursing perspective. In this perspective, the client is seen as a whole person, with physiologic, psychologic, social, cultural, and economic components.

In addition to reflecting concern for the whole person, a nursing perspective implies 24-hour-a-day responsibility. Thus, this perspective encompasses all of the factors in a client's environment, such as fatigue, noise, sensory deprivation, nutrition, and positioning, that might influence coping patterns. Diers (1979) enumerates three distinguishing properties of nursing research:

1. The final focus of nursing research must be on a difference that matters in improving client care.
2. Nursing research has the potential for contributing to theory development and the body of scientific nursing knowledge.

TABLE 3–1 *Examples of Nursing Studies*

Baker et al. (1983) reported on the use of therapeutic touch by nurses to increase the range of motion of joints and to decrease pain in persons with arthritis.

Baker et al. (1984) studied the effects of types of thermometer and length of time inserted on oral temperature measurements of afebrile subjects.

Dufault (1983) used observation, interviews, and case studies to conduct a descriptive, longitudinal field study that identified themes and patterns of hope in elderly cancer patients.

Fehring (1983) compared the effects of a particular relaxation technique with the effects of the same technique augmented with biofeedback on the symptoms of psychologic stress among healthy college students.

Itano et al. (1983) conducted a study in which they correlated factors such as locus of control, self-esteem, anxiety, client's understanding of the illness, client's perception of the severity of the nurse's care and concern plus several demographic factors to compliance to therapy among clients with cancer.

Norbeck and Sheiner (1982) used a social support scale to identify sources of social support related to single-parent functioning.

3. A research problem is a nursing research problem when nurses have access to and control over phenomena being studied.

The examples in Table 3–1 suggest the diversity of subjects, topics, and settings of actual nursing studies. The sample of contemporary nursing studies in this table only begins to show the diversity of fascinating and ultimately valuable research projects being conducted in the field of nursing.

Findings from nursing studies are being incorporated into textbooks such as this one. Clinical journals such as the *American Journal of Nursing, Heart and Lung,* and *Gerontological Nursing* are increasingly publishing the results of studies about nursing practice. Nursing journals such as *Advances in Nursing Science, Image: Journal of Nursing Scholarship,* the *Journal of Research in Nursing and Health, Nursing Research,* the *Western Journal of Nursing Research,* and the *International Journal of Nursing Studies* have editorial policies that stress science, research, and nursing scholarship and publish current research studies.

The *Cumulative Index to Nursing and Allied Health Literature,* the *International Nursing Index,* and the *Cumulative Medical Index* are excellent resources for locating research published on a topic or problem of interest. Computerized literature searches, such as Medline and MEDLARS, are available through many school libraries. They, too, help the student or researcher find relevant study reports. Since 1983, research on a variety of topics has been collected in yet another valuable resource, the *Annual Review of Nursing Research.*

It is unrealistic to expect each nurse to conduct a study in the clinical setting. Many constraints in clinical settings must be reckoned with before research can become a legitimate and comfortable activity. However, if nursing is to develop as a research-based practice, it is not unreasonable to expect that nurses (a) have some awareness of the process and language of research, (b) be sensitive to issues related to protecting the rights of human subjects, (c) participate in the identification of significant researchable problems, and (d) be discriminating consumers of research findings.

Bridging the research-practice gap, that is, bringing research into the clinical practice arena, is a key strategy in uniting the scholarly, scientific, and caring aspects of nursing in the future. Table 2–3 in Chapter 2 summarizes this position in the ANA's *Guidelines for the Investigative Function of Nurses* (1981a). The steps in the research process are listed in the accompanying box.

In February 1981, the Canadian Nurses' Association published a statement on research in nursing:

The Canadian Nurses' Association believes systematic investigation of the needs of individuals, groups and society forms an essential component of total health care. Research in nursing is needed to improve the quality of nursing care and to contribute to the efficiency and effectiveness of health care and the quality of life of Canadians. . . .

More research is needed to analyze and evaluate the skills and strategies nurses can use in giving nursing care:

- assisting individuals and families in developing constructive and healthy lifestyles,
- facilitating the maintenance of health, the prevention of illness and the restoration of health,
- supporting individuals and families through periods of crises,
- improving the quality of community settings,
- teaching individuals and families how nursing services can be used more effectively and appropriately. (CNA 1981)

Steps in the Research Process

1. Stating a research question or problem
2. Defining the purpose of a study
3. Reviewing related literature
4. Formulating hypotheses and defining variables
5. Selecting the research design
6. Selecting the population, sample, and setting
7. Conducting a pilot study
8. Collecting the data
9. Analyzing the data
10. Communicating conclusions and implications

Protecting the Rights of Human Subjects

Because nursing research usually focuses on humans, a major nursing responsibility is to be aware of and advocate clients' rights. All clients must be informed about the consequences of consenting to serve as research subjects. The client needs to be able to assess whether an appropriate balance exists between the risks of participating in a study and the potential benefits, either to the client or to the development of knowledge.

Research ethics not only protect the rights of human subjects but also encompass a broader list of characteristics. Most of these characteristics are reflected in the ANA's *Human Rights Guidelines for Nursing in Clinical and Other Research.* These guidelines are based on historic documents, such as the Nuremberg Code and the Declaration of Helsinki, and United States federal regulations, all of which set standards governing the conduct of research involving human subjects. The ANA Guidelines are presented in Table 3–2.

TABLE 3–2 *American Nurses' Association Human Rights Guidelines for Nurses in Clinical and Other Research*

The guidelines in this table attempt to specify several important entities: (1) the type of activities involved, (2) the rights to be protected, (3) the persons to be safeguarded, and (4) the mechanisms necessary to ensure that protection is adequate.

Guideline 1: Employment in Settings Where Research Is Conducted

Conditions of employment in settings in which clinical or other research is in progress need to be spelled out in detail for all potential workers. . . . Anyone employed in work that carries the potential of risk to others needs to be advised as to the types of risks involved, the ways of recognizing when risk is present, and the proper actions to take to counteract harmful effects and unnecessary danger.

Guideline 2: Nurses' Responsibilities for Vigilant Protection of Human Subjects' Rights

In all instances the prospective subject must be given all relevant information prior to participation in activities that go beyond established and accepted procedures necessary to meet the subject's personal needs. . . . Nurses must be increasingly vigilant in their concern for subjects and patients who by reason of their situation and/or illness are not able to protect themselves effectively from externally imposed threat or injury. They must be sensitive to the tendency toward exploitation of "captive" populations such as students, patients, and inmates in institutions and prisons. All proposals to be used need to be discussed with the prospective subject and with any worker who is expected to participate as a subject or data collector or both. Special mechanisms must be developed to safeguard the confidentiality of information and protect human dignity.

Guideline 3: Scope of Application

The persons to whom these human rights guidelines apply include all individuals involved in research activities and include the following groups: patients, donors of organs and tissue, informants, normal volunteers including students, and vulnerable populations that are "captive" audiences, such as the mentally disordered, mentally retarded, and prisoners.

Guideline 4: Nurses' Responsibility to Support the Accrual of Knowledge

Just as nurses have an obligation to protect the human rights of patients, so do they also have an obligation to support the accrual of knowledge that broadens the scientific underpinnings of nursing practice and the delivery of nursing services.

Guideline 5: Informed Consent

To safeguard the basic rights of self-determination, nurses must obtain consent from the prospective subject or the subject's legal representative to participate in research of unusual clinical activities. The subject needs to receive:

- A description of any benefit to the subject or the development of new knowledge that might be expected
- An offer to discuss or answer any questions about the study
- A clear statement to the subject that the subject is free to discontinue participation at any time the subject wishes to do so
- Full freedom from direct or indirect coercion and deception

Guideline 6: Representation on Human Subjects Committee

There is increasing public support for systematic accountability to ensure that individual rights are not denied to human subjects who participate in research studies. In most instances, the protective mechanism takes place through a committee judged competent to review studies and other investigative activities that involve human subjects. The profession of nursing has an obligation to publicly support the inclusion of nurses as regular members of institutional review committees of this kind.

Source: Adapted and summarized with permission from the American Nurses' Association, *Human rights guidelines for nurses in clinical and other research* (ANA Publication No. D-46 5M 7/75, 1975). Also found in ANA, *Guidelines in nursing research* (Kansas City, Mo.: ANA, 1975).

The Nurse's Role in Protecting Subjects' Rights

All nurses who practice in settings where research is being conducted with human subjects or who participate in such research as data collectors or collaborators play an important role in safeguarding the following rights:

Right Not to Be Harmed The Department of Health and Human Services defines **risk of harm** to a research subject as exposure to the possibility of injury going beyond everyday situations. The risk can be physical, emotional, legal, financial, or social. For instance, withholding standard care from a client in labor for the purpose of studying the course of natural childbirth clearly poses a potential physical danger. Risks can be less overt and involve psychologic factors, such as exposure to stress or anxiety, or social factors, such as loss of confidentiality, loss of privacy, and the like.

Right to Full Disclosure Even though it may be possible to collect data about a client as part of everyday care without the client's particular knowledge or consent, to do so is considered unethical. **Full disclosure** is a basic right. It means that deception, either by withholding information about a client's participation in a study or by giving the client false or misleading information about what participating in the study will involve, will not occur.

Right of Self-Determination

Many clients in dependent positions, such as people in nursing homes, feel pressured to participate in studies. They feel that they must please those doctors and nurses who are responsible for their treatment and care. The right of **self-determination** means that subjects should feel free from constraints, coercion, or any undue influence to participate in a study. Masked inducements, for instance, suggesting that they might become famous by making an important contribution to science or get special attention by taking part in the study, must be strictly avoided. Nurses must be assertive in advocating this essential right as well.

Right of Privacy and Confidentiality

Privacy enables a client to participate without worrying about later embarrassment. The anonymity of a study is ensured if even the investigator cannot link a specific subject to the information reported. **Confidentiality** means that any information a subject relates will not be made public or available to others. Investigators must inform research subjects about the measures that provide for these rights. Such measures may include using pseudonyms, code numbers, or reporting only aggregate or group data in published research.

Nurses who participate in scientific investigations that involve human subjects are in a key position to serve as advocates for research subjects. All of the study topics in Table 3–3 involve human subjects at risk.

TRENDS IN NURSING

A **trend** is a general direction or a prevailing tendency or inclination. Several trends are apparent in the nursing profession today. Some trends in nursing are subtle and emerge slowly, while others are obvious and seem to surface quickly. Not all trends complement one another; some may seem divergent, if not in conflict. Over time, some aspects of nursing become prevailing trends, while others may be modified by social forces or disappear altogether. A number of trends are apparent today: the broadening focus of nursing practice, the increasingly scientific basis of nursing practice (including nursing research), the increasing use of technology, and a heightened awareness of the need for "high touch" skills.

Broadening Focus

The focus of nursing has broadened from the care of the ill person to the care of people in illness and health, and from care of only the patient to care of the client, the family or

TABLE 3–3 *Research Studies with Ethical Issues at Stake*

---

1. A nurse who had worked for 6 years on a unit for nonviable clients was concerned about the tendency for nurses to avoid certain clients. She decided to conduct a study of how nurses care for nonviable clients.
2. In a study of unprofessional behavior, several nurse informants revealed some very personal and damaging information about themselves, but this was only a pilot study and they had not signed a consent form.
3. In a study of care of mentally retarded children, the researcher found that there were some glaring deficiencies in the care of these children. For example, children were often left in uncomfortable positions for hours at a time, were rarely offered fluids, and received diaper changes infrequently.

---

support persons, and, in some instances, the community. In the past, nursing, like medicine, was oriented toward disease and illness. Today, there is increasing recognition of people's need for health care as distinct from illness care and of the nurse's independent functions in this area.

A holistic philosophy is evident in modern nursing care. Today's nurse deals with clients as emotional and social as well as physical beings. Care is directed not toward a particular health problem but toward the response of the total person, the health of the whole person. The broadened focus of care requires an integration of skills and concepts.

Another aspect of the broader nursing focus is the movement of nursing practice into the community. In a sense, this is a return to the beginnings of nursing, e.g., before it became a recognized occupation. Throughout much of this century, however, nurses worked only in institutions; increasingly, nursing services are provided in the community, often in homes and in clinics. These nursing activities not only assist those who are ill but also help those who are healthy to maintain or enhance their health.

Scientific Basis

In the past, nursing largely was either intuitive or relied on experience or observation rather than on research. Through trial and error, the individual nurses discovered which measures would assist the client, and many nurses became highly skilled in providing care through experience. The past 20 years have brought an increased emphasis on nursing research and on the use of scientific data at the bedside.

Technology

Technology or mechanization is being applied in the health field extensively. Certain areas of a hospital, e.g., intensive care units and coronary care units, are more technologic than others. Nurses find themselves in the midst of this rapidly changing, increasingly technologic environment in hospitals and in clients' homes. Many feel they need more education to obtain the knowledge and skills necessary to use the new technology. Indicators of increasing technology are (a) the proliferation of technologic equipment in hospitals and homes, (b) the increasing costs of home and self-care equipment, and (c) the use of computers in many areas of health care.

A good example is the computer, which was relatively new 10 years ago. Today, computers are used on most campuses and in many hospitals and health agencies to keep client records, record and analyze vital signs, regulate medications, diagnose and treat, and analyze laboratory data. Nurses need to be flexible and ready to learn how to operate increasingly complex equipment.

Computers in Nursing

By the turn of the century, most nurses will use computers in many aspects of their professional practice. Already, "user-friendly" machines are of great help to the nurse in assessing, diagnosing, planning, implementing, and evaluating nursing care. The nurse educator and the nurse manager have also discovered the usefulness of computers in managing staffing, budgeting, producing grade reports, writing papers, and improving productivity. In fact, computer skills and knowledge will soon be expected and perhaps required for a great many positions. Those who ignore this technologic revolution may be left behind.

The nurse is clearly the manager of client care. Hospital information flows to and through nursing departments. Nurses who allow computer systems to design their practice may find themselves both frustrated and victimized. Instead, they must take an active role in the design, development, and implementation of any such systems. Those professional nurses who understand the conceptual framework of computer applications will find computers to be an extraordinarily useful tool in their professional practice.

In the past, hospital computer applications have been administrative. Tasks such as patient billing, maintaining financial records, and long-term planning are necessary aspects of the business side of the hospital. As computers get smaller, less costly, more powerful, and easier to use, they will be used increasingly in other areas of the health care system as well. Today, it is common to find a microcomputer system or computer terminal in the nurse's station. It is likely that such machines will become a more integral part of the nurse's activities during the next decade.

Using the computer to plan care

Automated client care systems allow "on-line" (i.e., directly connected to the computer) use of standardized nursing care plans (see Figure 3–2). After analyzing the assessment database and identifying the client's nursing diagnoses, nurses are able to create a care plan easily, customize it for each client, type in additions as needed, evaluate and update information at any time, and retrieve data appropriate to each specific nursing diagnosis. Specific ways in which an automated client care plan can facilitate the role of the nurse include the following:

1. Entry of nursing assessments is simplified; e.g., the nurse can touch a computer screen display of possibilities.
2. Laboratory data can be ordered by entering a request at a computer workstation.
3. Laboratory results can be retrieved in a shorter time with less paperwork.
4. The system facilitates complete and legible medication orders.
5. The system promotes consistent doctor's orders (verbal orders are not accepted).
6. The nursing implications of a doctor's order can be sent to the nurse. Client preparation needs for a particular test can be listed automatically in the client's nursing care plan.
7. The use of nursing diagnosis is facilitated; a common format can be used.
8. Current information can be updated easily. Discontinued medication orders can be detected easily, making all information timely, legible, and complete.

Using the computer as a consultant

The term *expert system* will no doubt become familiar to those in the health care professions over the next decade. An expert system is a computer-based model (using some of the principles of an exciting area of computer science called artificial intelligence) that strives to simulate the way human experts in a particular discipline gather data and make decisions. The human expert, for example, a clinical nurse specialist, is an important part of the design of these systems. In effect, the clinical nurse specialist is fulfilling a consulting role through the computer.

COMMES (Creighton On-Line Multiple Modular Expert Systems) is an artificial intelligence system that can simulate a consultation with a professional nurse. To do so, the system must have a current knowledge base and be able to mimic professional decision-making skills while avoiding the risk of providing incorrect or inappropriate data (Ryan 1985). Some expert systems are, in many ways, merely computer data bases that allow retrieval of data in various ways. It is quite likely that in the near future, expert systems will not only contain the information of a human considered an expert in a particular field but also, like that human expert, be able to analyze logically and make decisions. In this way, the "system" can begin to provide assistance in educational settings, hospital settings, and emergency settings and facilitate client care of consistent quality.

Using the computer as a research tool

Nursing research is also made easier by the computer's ability to access information in client records. Many hospitals main-

| Client name : | Martha Johnson | | Rm number | 403 |

Client name : Martha Johnson   **Rm number** 403

Admission date : 05/25/91

Sex : F   **Religion :** Catholic

Age : 58   **Date of birth :** 03/13/33

Admitting physician : Dr. Raymond Atkins

Medical diagnosis : Diabetes

Primary nurse : Judy Foster, R.N.

Allergies : Penicillin   **Diet :** 1500 c ADA

Risk factors : Hearing aid   **Vital signs :** T.I.D.

Nursing diagnosis : Impairment of skin integrity related to pruritus.

Long-term goals : Client will experience improved skin integrity within 48 hours.

Short-term goals	Nursing interventions	Evaluation
Given the prescribed care, client will experience decreased itching sensation	1. Infrequent baths. 2. Use cool water. 3. Soap substitute. 4. Blot skin dry. DO NOT RUB! 5. Lubricate skin with lotion after bath.	
Client will understand and implement health teaching.	1. Explain phenomenon of itching. 2. Teach avoidance of excessive warmth. 3. Teach need for increased humidity.	

Figure 3–2   Computer-generated nursing care plan.

tain extensive computerized records. If access to these data is permitted, the nurse researcher can gather information that may be important in a particular study or project. For example, a researcher interested in determining what interventions were most successful in caring for clients with the nursing diagnosis "impairment of skin integrity" can retrieve the care plans containing this information from the computer-based record. In addition, other key variables, such as the client's age, background, and sex, can be obtained and used to facilitate the analysis of the research problem.

Collecting these data manually (if they were available at all) would take a long time.

Using the computer for administrative tasks

The particular needs of the nursing administrator or manager can often be met by a hospital's computer system. The director of nurses or the division head of client services in a hospital needs data related to staffing, nurse scheduling, budgeting, and the evaluation of client services. If the appropriate information is stored in a computer-based

TABLE 3–4 *Selected Computer Applications Available in Health Education*

Computer Program	What It Does	Audience
Calculate with Care	Tutorial for mathematics	Beginning students
NURSESTAR	Review of nursing	RN students
TESTSTAR	Test construction	Nursing faculty
Build Medical Vocabulary	Tutorial/drill	Beginning students
Cardiac Arrest Simulation	Tutorial and simulation	Nurses and physicians
Hemodynamic Management	Clinical simulation	Critical care RNs
Clinical Nursing	Computer simulation	Advanced nursing students
Drug Interactions	Database of interactions	Nursing students
Nasogastric Suction	Client care simulations	Nursing students
Chest Suction	Client care simulations	Nursing students
Sugar	Hyperglycemia	Nursing students
Pre-lab Testing	30 pre-lab nursing test	Beginning students
Dosages and Solutions	Medication dosage math	Beginning students
Health History	Taking health histories	Beginning students
Genetic History	Basic human genetics	Nurses
Genetic Training	Basic human genetics	Nurses
Drug Therapy	Tutorial	Nursing students
CPR Certification	CPR exam	Nurses, students
Gross Anatomy	Tutorials	Nursing students
Automated Nurse Staffing	Staffing application	Administrators

information system, the manager can generate reports on the acuity levels of clients on each unit. These can be used to devise a formula for determining both the appropriate skill levels and the number of nurses required per shift and per floor. In addition, the scheduling of personnel is often made difficult by changing shifts, different skill levels, vacations, weekends, legal coverage requirements, and so on. Computer-based scheduling models can save much time and provide options that can be difficult to discover if the information is handled manually.

Using the computer for education   In the educational setting, the computer is becoming increasingly important, both as a teaching tool and as a resource for improving faculty and student productivity. It is likely that the use of the computer in these ways will increase dramatically over the next few years as these machines become easier to use. Table 3–4 shows some educational applications that are currently available. Although brief, the list in the table illustrates the variety of computer applications available in health education.

It is quite likely that the microcomputer will become even more pervasive as a resource for educators and students. Additional computer applications programs in nursing and health care will be developed, machines will become easier to use, and professional and academic organizations will begin to require graduates to have some familiarity with them.

The nurse's role in developing computer systems
Nurses can play many roles to integrate the computer into

their environment. One method is to become more comfortable with, knowledgeable about, and an advocate of the use of microcomputers. In addition (and perhaps more importantly), nurses need to become involved with the planning, design, and implementation of any computer systems that affect their profession. In most cases, health care applications are designed by persons or groups with computer expertise, who often lack skill in and knowledge of the application area in which they plan to put the computer to use. Sometimes, these developers seek out the active participation of those who will use the implemented system every day. Many times, no such attempt is made. It is essential that nurses demand involvement in the design of any systems that will eventually affect them and/or their clients. Otherwise, they run the risk of having to work with a computer system designed by someone unfamiliar with their needs. The likelihood of such systems being successful without this involvement is remote.

"High Touch"

The increasing use of technology in hospitals and homes has created an increasing need to humanize care. Nursing has traditionally been a caring and humanizing profession. Today more than ever, there is an expressed need for this "high touch" (DeCrosta 1985, p. 19). Indicators of this trend are (a) the increasing number of professional articles about balancing caring and technical skills, (b) many studies regarding caring as an aspect of nursing, and (c) increasing recognition in nursing of the needs of clients in technologic environments.

PROFESSIONAL CHANGE THROUGH POWER AND POLITICAL ACTION

Nurses are increasingly more knowledgeable about and capable of influencing the development of health care policy and the delivery of client care. Unless nurses develop their individual and collective political skills and use them to be advocates for the health of society and to promote the profession, client care and the nursing profession itself will be jeopardized.

In the past, nurses have often perceived themselves as powerless to influence nursing and bring about change. However, the sense of powerlessness is increasingly being recognized and overcome, and nurses are using power and political action to improve nursing and working conditions. Attitudes and behaviors necessary to overcome powerlessness are shown in the accompanying box.

Power

Patterns of behavior in groups are greatly influenced by the force of power. **Power** can be defined as the *capacity* to modify the conduct of others in a desired manner, while avoiding having one's own conduct modified in undesired ways by others (Stevens 1980, p. 208). Power is the ability to do or act, to deliver goods and services on one's own terms, or to be in control or command over others (Ferguson 1985, p. 89).

Many people have a negative concept of power, likening it to control, domination, and even coercion of others by muscle and clout. However, power can be viewed as a vital, positive force that moves people toward the attainment of individual or group goals. The overall purpose of power is to encourage cooperation and collaboration in accomplishing a task.

Often the terms *power, influence,* and *authority* are used interchangeably, but they need to be differentiated. **Power** is the source of influence, whereas **influence** is the result of proper use of power. **Authority** is the official or legitimized right to use a given amount or type of power, i.e., the right to act and the right to command (Claus and Bailey 1977, p. 21). Authority may be either delegated or acquired. Power theorists describe a variety of sources of a person's power. Understanding these sources of power is prerequisite to formulating a plan for developing one's own power and to recognizing it in others.

- *Legitimate* (or positional) *power* is derived from one's formal position or title in an organization. It is associated with the authority that the position gives its holder to make and enforce decisions. The title "Vice President for Nursing" implies that the holder has power by virtue of the position, regardless of who holds that position or how effective that person is.

Attitudes and Behaviors Necessary to Overcome Powerlessness

- Power is a positive force in nursing.
- There must be a commitment to continuing education in nursing.
- Professional nursing is a career and not just a job.
- Nursing is intrinsically valuable to society.
- Nurses must be actively involved in the women's movement because the advancement of nursing is tied directly to the advancement of all women's rights.
- Cohesiveness is developed among members of the nursing profession.
- Present nurse leaders are willing to empower the nurse leaders of the future by becoming mentors.
- Nurses support their leaders and regard them as advocates for nursing.
- Nurses are involved politically.
- The nurse's role is defined more clearly to the public.

Source: C. J. Huston and B. Marquis, Ten attitudes and behaviors necessary to overcome powerlessness, *Nursing Connections,* Summer 1988, 1:39–47. Reprinted by permission. Division of Nursing, The Washington Hospital Center, Washington, D.C., publisher.

- *Reward power* is derived from the perception of one's ability to bestow rewards or favors on others.
- *Coercive power,* by contrast, arises from the perception of one's ability to threaten, harm, or punish others.
- *Information power* is associated with persons who are perceived to control key information.

Reward, coercive, and information power all relate to the degree to which an individual can control the distribution of resources.

- *Referent* (charismatic, or personal) *power* is power derived from an individual's own vision, sense of self, and ability to communicate these so that others regard the person with admiration and are motivated to follow.
- *Connection power* is derived from the perception that one has important contacts or relationships with others. These connections can be an aspect of both formal and informal networks.
- *Expert* (or knowledge) *power* is power derived from one's expertise, talents, and skills. One can include in this category Benner's (1984) vision of power in caring; i.e., the positive power the nurse brings to the nurse-client relationship. This power enables the nurse to transform the client's life through advocacy and other means of caring.

Politics

What is politics? For many people the word *politics* evokes images of "crooked deals" hatched by men in "smoke-filled rooms," Watergate, the Iran-Contra dealings, bribes, and powerbrokers. More positive examples of political action are legislative initiatives to meet consumer needs and campaigns to elect nurse legislators. Although the words *crafty* and *unscrupulous* are sometimes included in the definition of *political,* a more positive definition is "having practical wisdom." Others describe politics as a means to an end, a process by which one can influence the decisions of others and thus exert control over events (Stevens 1980).

Politics can also be defined as "influencing the allocation of scarce resources" (Talbott and Vance 1981, p. 592). Defined in this way, the word denotes more than action in the governmental arena; it is also applicable to every sphere of life where resources are limited and more than one person or group competes for them (Ehrat 1983). The allocation of scarce resources involves everyone in some way. Consider the following examples:

- A student applying for a college loan or competing with other students for a fair share of a teacher's time and attention

- A patient advocate competing for hospital education funds to do more preoperative teaching

- A citizen lobbying against the school board's proposal to divide one RN's time between two large schools

- A member of a professional association seeking association action on a practice issue, such as care of clients with acquired immune deficiency syndrome (AIDS)

Despite nurses' experience with the political realities affecting the allocation of scarce resources, many nurses still harbor negative images of anything associated with the word *politics.* For example, it is not unusual to hear a colleague say, "I like her; she does not play politics." Although this remark is meant as a compliment, apolitical nurses in today's world hinder not only themselves and their colleagues but also the profession. For example, the nursing school dean, the head nurse, and the nurse researcher must all be politically skilled if they are to influence who gets how much of such scarce resources as funds for nursing education or nursing salaries, space for classrooms or offices, or release time to conduct research.

Why are nurses reluctant to engage in politics? Why do many view political activity as outside the realm of the professional nurse's role and responsibility? There are a number of reasons why nurses, and many women, have avoided becoming involved in political action. Among these are the following:

- There has been minimal recognition of the social activism of many of the profession's early leaders or of the efforts of nurses working together to effect legislative changes on issues relating to nursing and health.

- Prior to the contemporary wave of activism in women's rights, politics was considered an aggressive, men-only endeavor. Even though more women and nurses are becoming involved in governmental politics, many nurses have difficulty viewing the larger world of politics as an appropriate arena in which to participate. Women are socialized differently than men; for this reason, few women exert much influence on the male-dominated world of business and the professions.

- The fact that relatively few nurses know and appreciate their rich heritage also contributes to their discomfort with politics. Nurses who have been leaders and social activists, such as Lavinia Dock, Lillian Wald, Harriet Tubman, and Margaret Sanger, were all skilled politicians. Each was able to make significant contributions to the profession and society because of her political skills. Maybe they had read the wise words of the founder of modern nursing, Florence Nightingale:

> When I entered into service here, I determined that, happen what would, I *never* would intrigue among the Committee. Now I perceive that I do all my business by intrigue. I propose in private to A, B, or C the resolution I think A, B, or C most capable of carrying in Committee, and then leave it to them, and I always win (Huxley 1975, p. 53).

- Associated with the lack of appreciation of nursing history is the sparse education of nursing students, at the undergraduate and graduate level, on how to be politically astute. There is a critical need for students to have the opportunity to work with faculty and other preceptors who are skilled in the art of influencing governmental, organizational, workplace, and community politics.

Thus, a conscious effort needs to be made to educate nurses and nursing students about effective political action. Clearly, for such education to be effective, nurses must examine who they are as women and men and the values that they have been socialized to hold in relation to team play, power, and competition (Vance et al. 1985). This effort can be facilitated by learning more about how nursing leaders historically have used their political skills to bring about change, not only in the profession and health care but also in the values and actions of society as a whole.

Opportunities for Political Action

Government Most people think of political action in relationship to local, state, or federal government. By voting, responsible citizens convey their opinions to elected and appointed officials on matters of concern. Many women first learn about political action through the educational efforts of the League of Women Voters. Other organizations—including the ANA, CNA, NLN, and NSSA—publish articles on legislative matters and encourage nurses to take action in behalf of health care consumers and the nursing profession. Nursing lobbyists at the state and national level work to influence the development of health policy and legislation, but their success depends on the active support of nurses who back up these paid lobbyists by doing personal lobbying among their own elected officials.

Workplace   Since most nurses work in hospitals and too few nurses derive professional satisfaction from working in these bureaucratic institutions, it seems logical that nurses would work together to change the nature of their workplace. Evidence that hospitals can be rewarding places for delivering quality health care to clients is documented in the American Academy of Nursing's (1983) study of hospitals with a fine record of attracting and retaining professional nurses.

The politics of client care impinges on the practice of every nurse. For example, as the prospective payment system became the norm, hospital stays were cut more drastically in an effort to reduce health care costs (Shaffer 1984, p. 48). The need for nurses to be "faster and smarter" in delivering client care and client education will increase. Nurses are already feeling the pressure to prepare clients for discharge days earlier than before. How can nurses ensure that the quality of nursing care is maintained under the new system? One way is for nurses to collaborate with each other and other providers to eliminate nonnursing tasks, such as answering the telephone, emptying the garbage, and transporting nonacute clients. Developing a demonstration project that compares cost and quality of care issues under different hospital unit structures can provide the necessary data and generate support from other providers and administrators for changing the role of staff nurses. This sort of "proactive" planning can empower nurses to take charge of nursing practice in ways that benefit clients and health professionals while conserving scarce resources such as money, time, and supplies.

Organizations   Powerful and influential professional associations, such as the ANA and CNA and their affiliated state/province and district associations, provide a collective voice for promoting nursing and quality health care. As such, they exert influence on the individual nurse as well as in the spheres of government, the workplace, the community, and the profession. Associations monitor and influence laws and regulations affecting nursing and health care. Their role in workplace matters ranges from studying practice issues to acting as the collective bargaining agent for nurses. Additionally, the professional nursing organization is often a visible presence in the community because it presents the nursing perspective on health care issues.

Community   The community in which the nurse lives and works can include the local neighborhood, the corporate world, the nation, and the international community. The community encompasses the workplace, professional organizations, and government. Many nurses, including Lillian Wald, founder of the Henry Street Settlement and mod-

ern public health nursing, view the community as more than a practice setting. Nurses who live in the community where they work can understand and influence the complex interplay among individuals and groups that compete for scarce resources.

Many communities depend on nurses to help with a wide variety of health and social policy decisions, such as environmental pollution and the feminization of poverty (Archer 1985). For example, a nurse who serves as an elected member of the community school board can influence decisions that affect the health and health care of students, such as the hiring of nurses for the school system. Nurses' opinions on matters of the public health are frequently sought, and the enterprising nurse looks for opportunities to promote a positive image of nursing while serving the community (Frost 1985). The nurse also identifies ways in which fellow citizens can support both consumer health and nursing agendas.

Guiding Principles for Political Action

The following list of "commandments" is designed to help newcomers to political activism consider some ideas to enhance their effectiveness.

1. *Look at the big picture.* Step back and take a look at the larger environment in which you live, work, and study. In the governmental sphere especially, nurses are too often described as concerned only with nursing issues rather than with a broad variety of consumer and health care issues.

   Nurses will not enjoy credibility as health experts unless they become more sensitive to the concerns of others and employ their expertise in all spheres. In the workplace, nurses often focus their attention on their own unit, neglecting to view their position and unit in relationship to the larger organization.

   Astute nurses are aware of the environmental factors that impinge on their work setting. For example, the advent of the prospective payment system has had a major effect on nursing practice and raised many issues regarding the quality of client care. Nurses who make an effort to "take off the blinders" will see and understand the complex forces that affect their practice, the status of the nursing profession, and the nature of health care delivery.

2. *Do your homework.* Homework is not something that ends with graduation. Nurses must take stock of their goals and clarify their personal and professional positions on issues. Taking stock requires setting time aside for reflection. Nurses who use the nursing process as a basis for planning client care can use the same problem-solving approach in their own behalf. For example, developing a strategy to convince the head nurse to support the development of a formal continuing education program for staff nurses requires research and

planning and will be most successful if it is based on an understanding of change theory.

3. *Nothing ventured, nothing gained.* Nurses have always been risk takers. Margaret Sanger risked being jailed for promoting birth control. Lavinia Dock and her colleagues chained themselves to the White House fence to call attention to their belief that women should have the vote. Clara Maas lost her life while participating in research on malaria. If you have a dream, an idea, a vision of what might be—make it a reality.

4. *Get a toe in the door.* Incremental changes or actions may have a better chance of success than a major project. Resistance to change is more easily overcome if change is tested by a pilot project. For example, a nursing director is more apt to agree to the introduction of primary nursing on one unit rather than to an overall change in the nursing system of the whole hospital.

5. *"Quid pro quo."* "Something for something." "Scratch my back, and I'll scratch yours." Everything and everybody has a price." Many nurses are offended by the implications of these aphorisms, believing that they represent a cynical view of human and organizational relationships. Others, however, concede that they represent a realistic view of life. Consider how you relate to your friends and colleagues: Don't you often find yourself making trade-offs?

    When assessing your position within your school of nursing, the clinical area, or among your peers, review your friendships, connections, and pragmatic relationships. Frequently men say, "He owes me one," implying the person has received a favor and will reciprocate. Women and nurses, however, rarely use those words. In fact, they seem uncomfortable with the idea of being "in debt" or owing a favor despite the fact that they participate in give-and-take situations every day. It is important to develop an ease in professional and personal relationships so that one feels connected and supported rather than isolated and resentful.

6. *Walk a mile in another's moccasins.* Nurses learn to evaluate clients, to assess "where they are coming from." But how often do they make similar inquiries of peers,

supervisors, or friends? The politically astute nurse who wants to get ahead identifies the goals the head nurse has for the unit and finds ways to support those efforts and get help in meeting personal development goals. Identifying another's agenda can help one plan a win-win situation in which the staff nurse or student meets her or his own needs as well as those of the teacher or head nurse.

7. *Strike while the iron is hot.* Any plan for change must include a timetable that identifies the best time for a particular action. Few people would approach the head nurse to discuss the work schedule while a client is in cardiac arrest, but a surprising number of people give little thought to what might be an opportune time to discuss such a topic. Sometimes an eagerness to take action precludes some important questions: "Is this the best time to do this? Will it be received better now or later?"

8. *Read between the lines.* Some people reveal a lot by the information they choose not to share. Just as nurses listen with a "third ear" to their clients, politically astute nurses attend to colleagues, their bosses, and the work environment for cues that help them achieve some measure of control and influence.

9. *Half a loaf is better than none.* It is human nature to want it all, but the reality is that the world is far from perfect. People often need to learn to share the wealth and settle for less than they would like. One way to adjust to this reality is to develop an ability to identify alternative solutions or outcomes. Rather than setting one's heart on a particular goal, it is prudent to outline acceptable alternatives.

10. *Rome was not built in a day.* Because most nurses work in bureaucratic organizations, they need to accept the fact that change does not occur rapidly. Even in a small, flexible organization, change is often slow because the nature of the change process demands that one proceed only after careful deliberation. While political skills are gained only through practice, nurses who ponder and act on the principles that underlie political action gain the ability to view their efforts in perspective.

CHAPTER HIGHLIGHTS

▶ To be effective and influential in current and future health care delivery systems, nurses need to understand and apply change theory.

▶ Nurses have been effective in promoting change in the workplace, through professional organizations, in the legislative arena, and in the community.

▶ Nursing practice is influenced by economics, consumer demand, family structure, science and technology, legislation, demographic and social changes, and the nursing associations.

▶ Nursing education focuses on preparing today's nurs-

▶

ing students to fulfill current and future expectations and roles.

▶ Nursing research is having an increasing impact on nursing practice.

▶ All nurses practicing in settings where research is conducted have a role in safeguarding their clients' rights.

▶ Apparent trends in nursing today are: the broadening focus of nursing practice, the increasingly scientific basis of nursing practice, the increasing use of tech-nology in nursing, and a heightened awareness of the need for "high touch" skills.

▶ The use of the computer in nursing and health care is expanding and demands that nurses take an active role in developing computer application systems.

▶ Nurses are actively participating in political processes to promote change within the profession and to be influential in policy-making regarding health issues.

READINGS AND REFERENCES

SUGGESTED READINGS

Cahill, C. A., and Palmer, M. H. 1989. Individual professionalism: Part of the solution to the nursing shortage crisis. *Nursing Forum* 24:27–31.

The authors point out that nursing is currently faced with a number of problems, including who is to control nursing practice and its scope. The authors quote Styles: "If nursing is to become a profession, each nurse must be required to exhibit the characteristics of 'professionhood'" (1982, p. 119). The article further states that nurses must attain an understanding and mastery of their role.

Lynaugh, J. E., and Fagin, C. M. Winter 1988. Nursing comes of age. *Image: Journal of Nursing Scholarship* 20:184–90.

The authors base their article on two "realities": (a) nursing is made up of individuals from heterogeneous class, ethnic, and racial backgrounds, and (b) nursing care is undervalued in our society. Nursing practice in relation to the economic system, the women's issue, and oppression are reviewed. The concept of profession versus occupation is also discussed. The authors conclude that nursing has made considerable progress during the last century.

Orlando, I. J., and Dugan, A. B. February 1989. Independent and dependent paths: The fundamental issue for the nursing profession. *Nursing and Health Care* 10:76–80.

Orlando and Dugan address the dilemma of dependent versus independent nursing function. They write that the distinct function of nursing must be stated. In addition, the product of professional nursing practice must be identified.

RELATED RESEARCH

An examination of the relationship between Medicare prospective payment and the nursing shortage. November/December 1988. *Nursing Economics* 6:317–18.

Heiskanen, T. A. November 1988. Nursing staff's perceptions of work in acute and long-term care hospitals. *Journal of Advanced Nursing* 13:716–25.

Keefe, M. R.; Pepper, G.; and Stoner, M. November 1988. Toward research-based nursing practice: The Denver Collaborative Research Network. *Applied Nursing Research* 1:109–15.

Moody, L. E.; Wilson, M. E.; and Smyth, K. November/December 1988. Analysis of a decade of nursing practice research 1977–1986. *Nursing Research* 37:374–79.

SELECTED REFERENCES

Aiken, L. H. March 1988. Solutions to the nursing shortage bear repeating. *American Nurse* 20:4.

American Academy of Nursing. 1983. *Magnet hospitals: Attraction and retention of professional nurses.* Kansas City, Mo.: American Nurses' Association.

American Nurses' Association. April 1979. Credentialing in nursing: A new approach. Report of the Committee for the Study of Credentials in Nursing. *American Journal of Nursing* 79:674–83.

———. 1980. *Nursing: A social policy statement.* Kansas City, Mo.: ANA.

———. 1981. *The nursing practice act: Suggested state legislation.* Kansas City, Mo.: ANA.

———. Commission on Nursing Research. 1981a. *ANA guidelines for investigative functions of nurses.* Kansas City, Mo.: ANA.

———. Commission on Nursing Research. 1981b. *Priorities for the 1980s.* Kansas City, Mo.: ANA.

———. 1987. *Proceedings of the 1987 House of Delegates.* Kansas City, Mo.: ANA.

Archer, S. E. 1985. Politics and the community. In Mason, D. J., and Talbott, S. W., editors. *The political action handbook for nurses.* Menlo Park, Calif.: Addison-Wesley Publishing Co.

Baker, N., Carter, M. A., and Harrison, O. A. 1983. An experimental trial of therapeutic touch in the treatment of arthritis. *Western Journal of Nursing Research* 5:56.

———. April 1984. The effect of type of thermometer and length of time inserted on oral temperature measurements of afebrile subjects. *Nursing Research* 33:109–11.

Benner, P. 1984. *From novice to expert: Excellence and power in clinical nursing practice.* Menlo Park, Calif.: Addison-Wesley Publishing Co.

Bennis, W. G., Benne, K. D., Chin, R., editors. 1985. *The planning of change.* 4th ed. New York: Holt, Rinehart & Winston.

Brooten, D. A. 1984. *Managerial leadership in nursing.* Philadelphia: J. B. Lippincott Co.

Brooten, D. A., Hayman, L., and Naylor, M. 1978. *Leadership for change: A guide for the frustrated nurse.* Philadelphia: J. B. Lippincott Co.

Canadian Nurses' Association. February 1981. *CNA Position Statements.* Ottawa: CNA.

Claus, K. E., and Bailey, J. T. 1977. *Power and influence in health care: A new approach to leadership.* St. Louis: C. V. Mosby Co.

DeBack, V. 1990. Debate: Entry into practice: Will the 1985 proposal ever happen? In McCloskey, J. C., Grace, H. K., editors. *Current Issues in Nursing*. 3d ed. St. Louis: C. V. Mosby Co.

DeCrosta, T. May/June 1985. Megatrends in nursing: Ten new directions that are changing your profession. *Nursing Life* 5:17–21.

Diers, D. 1979. *Research in nursing practice*. Philadelphia, J. B. Lippincott Co.

Dufault, K. 1983. Process of hope in elderly cancer patients. *Western Journal of Nursing Research* 5:72.

Dugas, B. W. May 1985. Baccalaureate for entry to practice: A challenge that universities must meet. *Canadian Nurse* 81:17–19.

Ehrat, K. September 1983. A model for politically astute planning and decision making. *Journal of Nursing Administration* 13:29–34.

Fagin, C. M., and Maraldo, P. J. Sept. 1988. Feminism and the nursing shortage . . . do women have a choice? *Nursing and Health Care* 9:364–67.

Fehring, R. J. 1983. Effects of biofeedback relaxation on the psychological stress symptoms of college students. *Nursing Research* 32:362–66.

Ferguson, V. D. 1985. Power in nursing. In Mason, D. J., and Talbott, S. W., editors. *The political action handbook for nurses*. Menlo Park, Calif.: Addison-Wesley Publishing Co.

Frost, A. D. 1985. Working together: Local community action. In Mason, D. J., and Talbott, S. W., editors. *The political action handbook for nurses*. Menlo Park, Calif.: Addison-Wesley.

Graham, N. O., and Sheppard, C. 1990. Realities in retention and recruitment. In Chaska, N. L., editor. *The nursing profession: Turning points*. St. Louis: C. V. Mosby Co.

Huston, C. J., and Marquis, B. Summer 1988. Ten attitudes and behaviors necessary to overcome powerlessness. *Nursing Connections* 1:39–47.

Huxley, E. 1975. *Florence Nightingale*. New York: G. P. Putnam's Sons.

Inglehart, J. K. September 1987. Problems facing the nursing profession. *New England Journal of Medicine* 317:646–51.

Itano, J., Tanabe, P., Lum, J. L. J., Lamkin, L., Rizzo, E., Wieland, M., Sato, P., Winter, 1983. Compliance of cancer patients to therapy. *Western Journal of Nursing Research* 5:15–25.

Kerr, J. May 1985. Taking the campus to the student. *Canadian Nurse* 81:30–31.

Kramer, M. June 1990. Trends to watch at the magnet hospitals. *Nursing 90* 20:67–8, 70, 73–4.

Mason, D. J., and Talbott, S. W., editors. 1985. *The political action handbook for nurses: Changing the workplace, government, organizations, and community*. Menlo Park, Calif.: Addison-Wesley Publishing Co.

Mauksch, I. G., and Miller, M. H. 1981. *Implementing change in nursing*. St. Louis: C. V. Mosby Co.

Monheim, B. J. January/February 1989. Encouraging the growth of computer applications in nursing. *Computers in Nursing* 7:35, 34.

National Commission on Nursing Implementation Project. 1987. Timeline for transition into the future: Nursing education system for two categories of nurse. Milwaukee: National Commission on Nursing Implementation Project.

Norbeck, J. S., and Sheiner, M. 1982. Sources of social support related to single-parent functioning. *Research in Nursing and Health* 5:3–12.

Nyberg, J. May 1990. The effects of care and economics on nursing practice. *Journal of Nursing Administration* 20:13–18.

Perlich, L. J. M. March 1986. Catalyzing educational change . . . Issues of health care economics. *Journal of Nursing Administration* 16:6.

Pillar, B., Jacox, A. K., Redman, B. K. January/February 1990. Technology, its assessment, and nursing. *Nursing Outlook* 38:16–9.

Powell, D. J. January/February 1984. Nurses—"High touch" entrepreneurs. *Nursing Economics* 2:33–36.

Rogers, M. E. 1985. High touch in a high-tech future. Paper presented at the National League for Nursing convention, San Antonio, Texas.

Ryan, S. A. March/April 1985. An expert system for nursing practice: Clinical decision support. *Computers in Nursing* 3:77–84.

Schaller, L. 1972. *The change agent*. New York: Abingdon Press.

Sinclair, V. G. March/April 1990. Potential effects of decision support systems on the role of the nurse. *Computers in Nursing* 8:60–5.

Spradley, B. W. 1980. Making change creatively. *Journal of Nursing Administration* 10:32–37.

Stevens, B. J. November 1980. Power and politics for the nurse executive. *Nursing and Health Care* 1:208–10.

Stevens, K. R. May/June 1985. Does the 1985 education proposal make economic sense? *Nursing Outlook* 33:124–27.

Styles, M. M. 1982. *On nursing: Toward a new endowment*. St. Louis: C. V. Mosby Co.

Talbott, S. W., and Vance, C. 1981. Involving nursing in a feminist group—NOW. *Nursing Outlook* 29:592–95.

Tanner, C. A., Lindeman, C. A. 1989. *Using nursing research*. NLN Publ. #15-22-32-1-513.

Vance, C., Talbott, S. W., McBride, A. B., and Mason, D. J. November/December 1985. An uneasy alliance: Nursing and the women's movement. *Nursing Outlook* 33:281–85.

Theories and Conceptual Frameworks

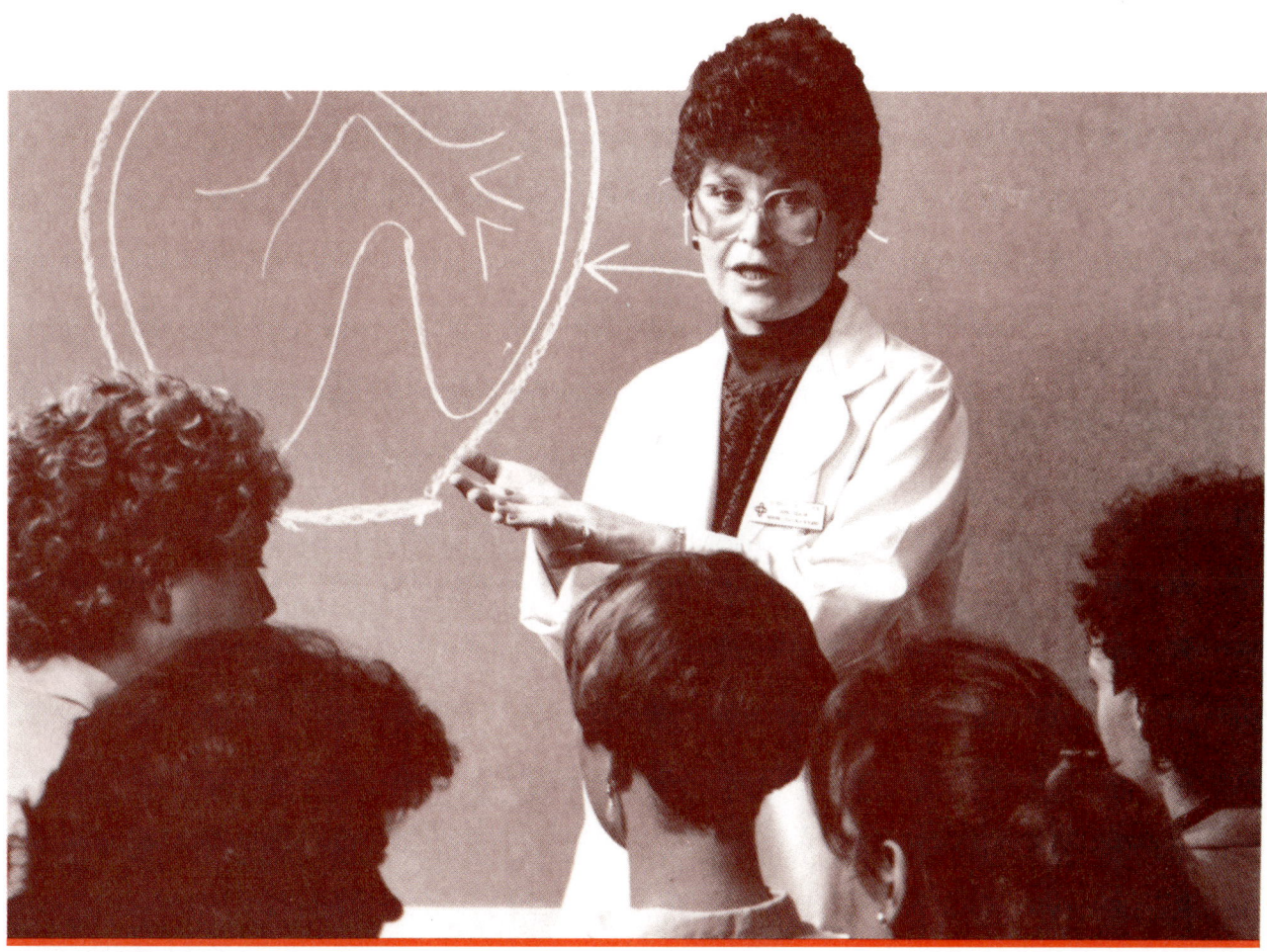

CONTENTS

OBJECTIVES

▶ Explain the purposes of nursing theories.

▶ Identify the concepts that form the metaparadigm of nursing.

▶ Differentiate a theory from a conceptual framework.

▶ Identify three essential elements of a theory.

▶ Identify three essential components and seven major units of a conceptual model of nursing. ▶

▶ Describe the relationship of the nursing process to conceptual models of nursing.

▶ Describe the relationship of nursing theory to nursing research.

▶ Compare selected conceptual models for nursing.

▶ Explain the relationship of holism to nursing.

▶ Identify selected characteristics of basic human needs and factors influencing priority of needs.

▶ Discuss various constructs of caring.

▶ Describe general systems theory.

▶ Describe various approaches to problem solving.

▶ Identify three phases of the decision-making process.

▶ Explain the relationship of perception theory to the nursing process.

NURSING THEORIES AND CONCEPTUAL FRAMEWORKS

Theory development is considered by many nurses to be one of the most crucial tasks facing the profession today. Historically, knowledge used by nurses has been derived from the physical and behavioral sciences. As an increasingly emerging profession, nursing is now deeply involved in identifying its own unique knowledge base—that is, the body of knowledge essential to nursing practice—or a so-called nursing science. Identification of this knowledge base requires the development and recognition of concepts and theories specific to nursing.

Theory development gained momentum in the 1960s and has progressed markedly since then through the work of several nurse theorists and the participation of nurses in theory conferences and in research to refine or validate the theories. Three approaches may be used to develop nursing theory:

1. Borrowing conceptual frameworks from other disciplines and applying them to nursing problems. The problem with this approach is that many theories are not easily applied to nursing practice.

2. Using an inductive approach; that is, looking at various aspects of nursing in nursing practice settings to discover theories and concepts that explain phenomena important to nurses.

3. Using a deductive approach; that is, looking for the compatibility or fit of a general theory of nursing with various aspects of nursing.

Nursing theories serve several essential purposes. Nursing theory (King 1978):

■ Generates knowledge that facilitates improved practice

■ Organizes information into logical systems

■ Discovers knowledge gaps in the specific field of study

■ Provides a rationale for collecting reliable and valid data about the health status of clients, which are essential for effective decision making and implementation

■ Provides a measure to evaluate the effectiveness of nursing care

■ Develops an organized way of studying nursing

■ Guides nursing research to expand knowledge

Conceptual frameworks and models offer ways of looking at (conceptualizing) a discipline (e.g., nursing) in clear, explicit terms that can be communicated to others. Although most nurses have a clear idea of what nursing is, its uniqueness needs to be clearly stated to other health care workers and the public. Professionalism and a desire for collegial status with other health professionals have made the need for conceptual frameworks of nursing to be explicit. If nurses are to be considered health professionals, they must communicate exactly what makes their place in the interdisciplinary team unique and important.

Before conceptual frameworks are discussed, the terms *concept, model, framework, conceptual model* or *framework,* and *theory* must be clarified. A **concept** is an abstract idea or mental image of phenomena or reality. Many concepts apply to nursing: concepts about human beings, health, helping relationships, and communication. The concepts that influence nursing most significantly and determine its practice include: the *person* receiving nursing care, the *environment* in which the person exists, *health* at the time of interaction with the nurse, and *nursing actions*. Together these concepts form the **metaparadigm of nursing.** The metaparadigm is the most global perspective of any discipline, its encapsulating unit or framework. It singles out the phenomena with which the discipline deals in a unique manner. Most disciplines have a single metaparadigm, but several conceptual models provide different views of the metaparadigm concepts.

A **model** is a pattern of something to be made, an abstract outline or architectural sketch of a genuine article, or an approximation or simplification of reality. A toy model, such as a toy car, illustrates the definition simply. The model is not actually a car, but its parts represent the features of a real car. A model can also show the features of a discipline. Nursing models include only those concepts that the model builder considers relevant and that aid understanding by others.

A **framework** is a basic structure supporting anything. A **conceptual framework** is a set of concepts and statements that integrate the concepts into a meaningful configuration (Fawcett 1984, p. 2). Conceptual frameworks, however, are not made up only of concepts. They are also made up of **propositions,** statements that express the relationships between concepts. Each nurse theorist's conceptual framework proposes a different view of the metaparadigm concepts.

A conceptual model gives clear and explicit direction to the three areas of nursing: practice, education, and research. (Some nurses add a fourth field of nursing, administration; however, many consider administration a component of each of the three areas.) All conceptual models are frames of reference (conceptual and theoretical), but not all frames of reference are models in that some are not specific enough to give clear direction to practice, education, and research.

A **theory,** like a conceptual model, is made up of concepts and propositions; however, a theory accounts for phenomena with much greater specificity. The primary purpose of a theory, as opposed to a conceptual framework, is to generate knowledge in a field. A conceptual framework, by contrast, provides a guide for nursing practice, education, and research. Numerous definitions of theory exist in the literature. Most definitions include three elements:

1. A set of well-defined constructs or concepts. For example, the constructs in Imogene King's (1981) theory of goal attainment include perception, communication, interaction, transaction, self, role, growth and development, stress, time, and space.

2. A set of propositions that specify the relationships among the constructs. For example, here are a few examples of the eight propositions King developed to describe the relationship among the concepts in her theory of goal attainment (Austin and Champion 1983):
   a. If perceptual accuracy is present in nurse-client interactions, transactions (goal attainment) will occur.
   b. If role expectations and role performance as perceived by the nurse and client are congruent, transactions will occur.
   c. If transactions are made in nurse-client interactions, growth and development will be enhanced.

3. Hypotheses that test the relationships between the constructs and propositions. Because theory is abstract, it cannot be applied to practice. Instead, hypotheses derived from the theory are tested. For example, here are some testable hypotheses derived from King's goal-attainment theory (King 1981):
   a. Perceptual accuracy in nurse-client interactions increases mutual goal setting.
   b. Communication increases mutual goal setting between nurses and clients and leads to satisfaction.
   c. Goal attainment decreases stress and anxiety in nursing situations.

In summary, the major distinction between a theory and a conceptual model is the level of abstraction. A conceptual model is an abstract system of related concepts. A theory is based on a conceptual model but is more limited in scope.

It contains more concrete concepts with definitions and detailed explanations of the premises or hypotheses linking them together.

As there are varying opinions on the nature and structure of nursing, theories continue to be developed. Each theory bears the name of the person or group who developed it and reflects the beliefs of the developer. Some well-known theories are Virginia Henderson's (1966) complementary-supplementary model; Dorothy E. Johnson's (1966, 1980) behavioral systems model; Imogene King's (1971, 1978, 1981, 1987) systems interaction model; Madeleine Leininger's (1984) transcultural care theory; Myra Levine's (1973) conservation theory; Betty Neuman's (1982) health care systems model; Dorothea E. Orem's (1971, 1980, 1985) self-care model; Martha Roger's (1970, 1980) life process theory; and Sister Callista Roy's (1976, 1984) adaptation model. Each nursing education program is based on a conceptual framework selected or developed by the program's faculty to guide student learning and to provide a nursing model for graduates.

Components of Nursing Models

Conceptual models have three components: assumptions, a value system, and major units.

Assumptions

Assumptions are statements of facts (premises) or suppositions that people accept as the underlying theoretical foundation for conceptualizations about nursing. Assumptions are derived from scientific theory or practice or both, and either have been or can be verified. Some nursing models draw assumptions from adaptation theories; others from general systems theories. Most models also draw assumptions from practice.

Assumptions differ greatly from model to model, since they are drawn from different premises. For example, assumptions about human beings (the client) vary considerably: Henderson views the client as a being with 14 fundamental needs; Roy, as a being with four modes of adaptation; Johnson, as a being with eight behavioral subsystems; and Orem, as an agent with six universal self-care requisites.

Value System

The beliefs underlying a profession are its value system. Generally, these beliefs are similar from model to model. Some of them are the following:

- Nurses have a unique function even though they share certain functions with other health professionals.

- Nursing is a service directed toward meeting the needs of well or ill persons or groups (families and communities) rather than directed toward specific aspects of disease or illness.

- Nursing uses a systematic process (see Chapter 9) to operationalize its conceptual model.

■ Nursing involves a series of interpersonal relationships. The nurse-client relationship (helping relationship) is of major importance. See Chapter 15.

Margretta Styles believes that the nursing profession must have a common ideology, just as nations have their pledges of allegiance, societies their oaths, and religions their creeds. Styles proposes a series of beliefs about the nature and purpose of nursing, as outlined in the accompanying box.

Major Units   Seven major units of nursing models are constructed from the assumptions and values: (a) Goal of nursing, (b) client (patient), (c) role of the nurse, (d) source of difficulty of the client, (e) intervention focus, (f) modes of intervention, and (g) consequences of nursing activity. A summary of these units in the major conceptual models is given in Table 4–1 on page 62.

Goal of nursing   The goal is the end or aim of nursing, what nursing is trying to achieve. This goal has to agree with the goals common to all health professionals—to improve health, to maintain health, to prevent health problems, to restore health, etc. However, each health discipline has a goal distinct enough to justify the presence of that discipline on the health team. Specific nursing goals vary from model to model, depending on its assumptions about people. Goals need to be broad enough (a) to indicate what end the nursing profession is working toward, (b) to indicate what to teach future practitioners, and (c) to apply to nursing practice in all practice settings (community, hospital, home, health center, etc.). Before the 20th century, Florence Nightingale believed the goal of nursing was to make the patient as comfortable as possible and to put the patient in the best possible condition for nature to act and for the physician's treatment to take effect. For current goals of nursing, see Table 4–1.

Client   The client unit refers not only to the intended recipient(s) of nursing service but also to conceptions about that person or group. Most models indicate that the client is a biopsychosocial being, but they differ in exactly how the client is conceptualized as such. Henderson views the client as a whole, complete, independent being who has 14 fundamental needs, while Johnson views the client as a behavioral system composed of eight subsystems. See Table 4–1 for further information.

Role of the nurse   The role of the nurse must be wanted, needed, and accepted by society just as the physician's curative role or the lawyer's defending role is wanted and accepted. Many nurses consider their role to be one of "caring"; however, caring is a vague concept that is difficult to operationalize. In Orem's self-care model, the role of the nurse is to provide assistance to influence the client's devel-

---

Declaration of Belief about the Nature and Purpose of Nursing

I. I believe in nursing as an *occupational force for social good,* a force that, in the *totality of its concern* for all human health states and for mankind's responses to health and environment, provides a distinct, unique, and vital perspective, value orientation, and service.

II. I believe in nursing as a *professional discipline,* requiring a sound education and research base grounded in its own science and in the variety of academic and professional disciplines with which it relates.

III. I believe in nursing as a *clinical practice,* employing particular physiological, psychosocial, physical, and technological means for human amelioration, sustenance, and comfort.

IV. I believe in nursing as a *humanistic field,* in which the fullness, self-respect, self-determination, and humanity of the nurse engage the fullness, self-respect, self-determination, and humanity of the client.

V. I believe that nursing's *maximum contribution* for social betterment is dependent on:
   A. The well-developed *expertise* of the nurse;
   B. The *understanding, appreciation,* and *acknowledgment* of that expertise by the public;
   C. The organizational, legal, economic, and political *arrangements* that enable the full and proper expression of nursing values and expertise;
   D. The ability of the profession to maintain *unity* within diversity.

VI. I believe in *myself* and in my nursing *colleagues:*
   A. In our *responsibility* to develop and dedicate our minds, bodies, and souls to the profession that we esteem and the people whom we serve;
   B. In our *right* to be fulfilled, to be recognized, and to be rewarded as highly valued members of society.

Source: Margretta M. Styles, *On nursing: Toward a new endowment* (St. Louis: C. V. Mosby Co., 1982), p. 61. Used by permission.

---

opment in achieving an optimal level of self-care; in Roy's adaptation model, the nurse's role is to promote the client's adaptive behaviors by manipulating stimuli. See Table 4–1 for additional information.

Source of difficulty The source of difficulty resides with the client, not the nurse. In other words, it is the probable origin or cause of any client problems amenable to nursing intervention. Clients in health care agencies have health problems that may be subcategorized as medical, psychologic, dietary, nursing, etc. The physician deals with medical problems, the psychologist or psychiatrist with psychologic problems, the dietitian with dietary problems, and the nurse with nursing problems. The source of difficulty is an explicit statement of the nursing problem. For example, in Henderson's model, the origin of the client's problem is lack of strength, will, or knowledge; in Johnson's model, it is functional or structural stress. Table 4–1 lists the sources of difficulty identified by other theorists.

Intervention focus Another unit of each model is the target or focus of nursing intervention. The universally accepted intervention focus for the physician is the client's pathology. In Orem's self-care model, the intervention focus for nurses is a deficit in the client's ability to maintain self-care; in Roy's adaptation model, it is the stimuli the client is having difficulty adapting to. See Table 4–1 for additional information.

Modes of intervention The modes of intervention unit clarifies the means at the nurse's disposal when intervening. It is closely allied to the intervention focus and spells out specific ways in which the nurse helps the client. For example, in Roy's adaptation model the intervention focus is stimuli and the mode of intervention is manipulation of the stimuli. In contrast, Florence Nightingale believed the mode of intervention was manipulation of the environment. This was done by providing warmth, fresh air, light, food, and sanitation. See Table 4–1 for other intervention modes.

Consequences The last unit states the expected consequences of nursing actions. It reflects the nursing goal and the concept of the client. See Table 4–1 for the consequences identified by specific models.

One Model Versus Several Models

Many nurses believe that there are advantages to having a single, universal model for nursing for these reasons:

- It would further the development of nursing as a profession.

- It would give all nurses a common framework, enhancing communication and research.

- It would promote understanding about the nurse's role in nontraditional nursing settings, such as independent nurse practitioner practice, self-help clinics, and health maintenance organizations (HMOs), since many people believe nurses provide care for only sick persons.

In contrast, advocates of several different conceptual models point out the following:

- Most disciplines have several conceptual models, which allow members to explore phenomena in different ways and from different viewpoints.

- Several models increase an understanding of the nature of nursing and its scope.

- Several models foster development of the full scope and potential of the discipline.

It is possible that in the 21st century many more models for nursing will be developed or that existing ones will be refined in accordance with societal needs and with their tested usefulness.

Relationship to the Nursing Process

Conceptual models for nursing are abstractions that are operationalized or made real by the use of the nursing process. See Chapters 9–14 for detailed information on the nursing process. This systematic process, similar to the scientific or problem-solving process, consists of five steps:

1. *Assessing.* The specific data collected about a client's health needs relate directly to the second unit of the conceptual model for nursing, the client. For example, if the client is seen as having 14 fundamental needs, data are collected about these 14 needs.

2. *Diagnosing.* In this step, the assessment data are analyzed to identify actual, potential, and possible nursing diagnoses. The client's actual or potential health problems are outlined or written as a nursing diagnostic statement in accordance with the nursing model used.

3. *Planning.* Planning also relates directly to the conceptual nursing model. Goals for resolution of client problems, nursing interventions aimed at achieving those goals, and outcome criteria by which the nurse can evaluate whether or not the goals are met are established in accordance with the modes of intervention outlined in the conceptual model.

4. *Implementing.* Implementing the planned interventions draws on scientific knowledge that is not part of the nursing model. The nursing model instructs the nurse what to do and directly influences what nursing interventions are planned, but it does not tell the nurse how to do it.

5. *Evaluating.* Evaluating is a continuous nursing function. How is the client adjusting and reacting? What does the client see as needs? How does the client see these needs changing? Has the client achieved the desired consequences? The answers to these questions help the nurse evaluate the effectiveness of the total nursing process and the nursing model.

(continued on page 66)

TABLE 4–1 *Summary of Major Units from Selected Conceptual Models for Nursing**

Theorist	Goal of Nursing	Client	Role of the Nurse
Virginia Henderson (1966): complementary-supplementary model	Independence in the satisfaction of human beings' 14 fundamental needs	A whole, complete and independent being who has 14 fundamental needs to breathe, eat and drink, eliminate, move and maintain posture, sleep and rest, dress and undress, maintain body temperature, keep clean, avoid danger, communicate, worship, work, play, and learn	A complementary-supplementary role to maintain or restore independence in the satisfaction of clients' 14 fundamental needs
Dorothy Johnson (1980): behavioral systems model	Behavioral system equilibrium and dynamic stability	A behavioral system composed of seven subsystems: affiliative, achievement, dependence, aggressive, eliminative, ingestive, and sexual	A regulator and controller of behavioral system stability and equilibrium
Imogene King (1971, 1978, 1981, 1987): systems interaction model	Attainment, maintenance, or restoration of health to allow clients to achieve maximum potential for daily living and function in social roles	Three interacting systems: individuals (personal systems), groups (interpersonal systems), and society, (social systems); the personal system is a unified, complex, whole self who perceives, thinks, desires, imagines, decides, identifies goals, and selects means to achieve them	An interaction process
Myra Levine (1973): conservation model	Promotion of wholeness	Holistic being: an open system of systems that in its wholeness expresses the organization of all its parts; the person retains personal integrity through adaptive capability; the life process of the system is unceasing change that has direction, purpose, and meaning	Therapeutic, i.e., to influence adaptation favorably or move client toward renewed social well-being; or supportive, i.e., to maintain the status quo
Betty Neuman (1982): health care systems model	Attainment and maintenance of client system equilibrium	Open system consisting of a basic structure or central core of survival factors surrounded by concentric rings that are bounded by lines of resistance, a normal line of defense, and a flexible line of defense. The total person is a composite of physiologic, psychologic, sociocultural, and developmental variables	To identify intrapersonal, interpersonal, and extrapersonal stressors and assist the individual to respond to stressors

*The models are listed in alphabetical order.

TABLE 4 – 1 (*continued*)

Source of Client Difficulty	Intervention Focus	Modes of Intervention	Consequences of Nursing Activity
Lack of strength, will, or knowledge	The deficit that is the source of client difficulty	Actions to replace, complete, substitute, add, reinforce, or increase strength, will, or knowledge	1. Increased independence in satisfaction of the client's 14 fundamental needs, or 2. Peaceful death
Functional or structural stress; inadequate development or stimulation of the system or its parts; breakdown in regulatory system; exposure to noxious influences; lack of environmental input	1. The mechanisms of control and regulation 2. The functional requirements	Imposing external regulatory control mechanisms; changing structural units; fulfilling functional requirements; helping to regulate subsystem balance	Efficient and effective client behavior
Stressors in the internal and external environment	Perception of client difficulty and goal setting through communication	Interaction process in which both client and nurse perceive and communicate, thus creating action; actions result in reactions, and, if there is no disturbance, goals may be set, means to achieve them explored and agreed upon, and transactions made	Goal attainment
Altered relationship with the internal and external environment	Enhancing patterns of adaptive response	Four conservation principles: actions to conserve energy, structural integrity, personal integrity, and social integrity	Adaptive responses that retain wholeness
Intrapersonal, interpersonal, and extrapersonal stressors in the internal and external environments	Strengthening normal and flexible lines of defense and reducing stress factors	Primary intervention, i.e., strengthening the person's flexible line of defense; secondary prevention, i.e., strengthening internal lines of resistance; and tertiary prevention, i.e., maintaining the person's existing energy resources	Reconstitution, i.e., movement from a variance of wellness to the desired level of wellness and client system stability

Theorist	Goal of Nursing	Client	Role of the Nurse
Dorothea Orem (1971, 1980, 1985): self-care model	Achievement of optimal client self-care so that clients can achieve and maintain an optimal health state	A unity who can be viewed as functioning biologically, symbolically, and socially and who initiates and performs self-care activities on own behalf in maintaining life, health, and well-being; self-care activities deal with air, water, food, elimination, activity and rest, solitude and social interaction, hazards to life and well-being, and being normal (the tendency to conform to the norm)	To provide assistance to influence clients' development in achieving an optimal level of self-care
Rosemarie Parse (1987): human-living-health model	Transforming or changing health patterns	An open being, more than and different from the sum of its parts, in mutual simultaneous interchange with the environment, who chooses from options (value priorities) and bears responsibility for choices	Guided by three principles: meaning, rhythmicity, and cotranscendence; exploration of personal meanings of lived experiences (meaningful moments); helping clients to illuminate different rhythms; presenting energizing ways of becoming or reaching beyond what *is* toward the possible; helping clients to experience a shift in everyday rhythms.
Martha Rogers (1970, 1980): science of unitary human beings	Achievement of maximum health potential	A unified whole possessing integrity and manifesting characteristics that are more than and different from the sum of its parts; an organized patterned energy field that continually exchanges matter and energy with the environmental energy field, resulting in continuous repatterning. The human being has the capacity for abstraction and imagery, language and thought, and sensation and emotion	To help clients develop patterns of living that accommodate environmental changes rather than conflict with them
Sister Callista Roy (1976, 1981, 1984): adaptation model	Adaptation in each of the four adaptive modes in situations of health and illness	A biopsychosocial being who is in constant interaction with the environment and who has four modes of adaptation, based on: physiologic needs, self-concept (physical self, moral-ethical self, self-consistency, self-ideal and expectancy, and self-esteem), role function, and interdependence relations	To promote clients' adaptive behaviors by manipulating focal, contextual, and residual stimuli

Source of Client Difficulty	Intervention Focus	Modes of Intervention	Consequences of Nursing Activity
Any interference with self-care, by a person, object, condition, event, circumstance, or any combination of interferences	Inability to maintain self-care (a deficit in the self-care agency)	Five general ways of assisting: acting for or doing for, guiding, supporting, providing a developmental environment, and teaching	Achievement of the client's optimal level of self-care
Patterns of relating and values at a given moment	Provision of attentive listening (true presence) or empathetic sounding board for clients to express and therefore uncover the meaning of thoughts, feelings, values, and changing views	Illuminating meaning by explicating what is happening through language; synchronizing rhythms by *dwelling with* the flow of connecting-separating; mobilizing transcendence by moving toward possibles in transforming	Changed health patterns
Unharmonious person-environment interactions that are determined by social values	Coordinating environmental field and human field rhythmicities	Actions to promote harmonious interaction between the client and environment, to strengthen the integrity of the human field, and to direct and redirect patterning of the human and environmental fields	Maximum health potential, unity, and increasing complexity of organization
Coping activity that is inadequate to maintain integrity in the face of a need deficit or excess	The focal, contextual, and residual stimuli	Manipulation of the stimuli by increasing, decreasing, and/or maintaining them	Adaptive responses to stimuli by the client

Relationship of Nursing Theory to Research

Because the primary purpose of nursing theory is to generate scientific knowledge, nursing theory and nursing research are closely related. Scientific knowledge is derived from testing hypotheses generated by theories for nursing. Research determines the utility of those hypotheses, and research findings may be developed into theories for nursing. In the research process, comparisons are made between the observed outcomes of research and the relationship predicted by the hypotheses.

Several approaches can be used to test or develop theory:

- *Inductive*. Research is first conducted, and the findings are used to develop a theory. In this inductive method, a theory is developed from multiple data. The following premise and conclusion illustrate the inductive method: If X (e.g., low self-esteem) is true of persons A1, A2, . . . , A100, and if the persons are all members of the same class (e.g., rape victims) then X is true of all members of that class.

- *Deductive*. A theory is devised, hypotheses generated, and then research is conducted. For example, in deductive research a premise (hypothesis) is first proposed, e.g., All rape victims have low self-esteem. Among many others, Mary, Joan, Ellen, and Judy are rape victims, and their level of self-esteem is tested. Because it is low, it is concluded that the hypothesis is valid.

- *Combined*. Both inductive and deductive methods are used.

SELECTED THEORETICAL VIEWS OF HUMAN BEINGS

The nurse's view of human beings influences the focus of nursing interventions. Although most nurses agree that humans are biopsychosocial beings, they differ in how they view human beings as recipients of nursing services. Nursing theorists have developed these viewpoints from systems, adaptation, and interactive theories. The conceptualizations of the client according to selected nursing theorists are summarized in Table 4–1, earlier.

The Person as a System

The human being is an *open system* in constant interaction with a changing environment (Roy 1980, p. 180). Systems theory is discussed later in this chapter. In other words, the individual engages in a dynamic interchange with the environment, and this interchange is an essential factor of the system's viability, reproductive ability or continuity, and ability to change. Constant input (stimuli) into the system and feedback to it maintain the system in a state of dynamic equilibrium. This premise directs the nurse to look at envi-

ronmental factors influencing the system and to provide nursing interventions that help the client maintain and achieve a state of dynamic equilibrium.

Human beings interact with the environment by adjusting themselves to it or adjusting it to themselves (Neuman 1980, p. 122). This premise directs the nurse to look at ways the client handles changing situations. Does the client withdraw from the environment, alter the environment, or alter self?

Humans are open systems with many interrelated subsystems. Because humans are biopsychosocial beings, their biologic, psychologic, social, and spiritual components can be regarded as systems with hierarchic subsystems. (See Systems theory later in this chapter.)

The *biologic system* can be subdivided into the neurologic, musculoskeletal, respiratory, circulatory, gastrointestinal, and urinary subsystems, among others. Each subsystem can in turn be subdivided. For example, the urinary system consists of the kidneys, the ureters, and the bladder; the circulatory system consists of the heart and the blood vessels; the neurologic system consists of the brain, the spinal cord, and the nerves. The biologic system can also be subdivided into categories of needs or functional health patterns or activities of daily living, such as nutrition and hydration, sleep/rest, activity/exercise, elimination, etc.

The *psychologic and social systems* consist of subsystems that include thinking, feeling, and interaction patterns. Names of the psychologic and social subsystems vary considerably according to the individual nursing theorist and model. For example, Johnson (1980, p. 228), who describes the human system in terms of behaviors, lists the following psychologic subsystems: affiliative, dependency, aggressive/protective, and achievement. Orem (1980, p. 316) categorizes the psychologic and social systems as conditions of being alone or with people, situations that threaten the well-being of the individual, and the tendency to conform to the norm. (See Table 4–1.)

According to King (1976, p. 51) the primary concerns of nursing are human behavior, social interactions, and social movements. Therefore, she includes three dynamic interacting systems in her concept of person: individuals (*personal systems*), groups (*interpersonal systems*), and society (*social systems*). Each of these systems has a set of related concepts that King sees as relevant for understanding human beings.

The Person as an Adaptive System

Adaptation is a process of change allowing the individual to respond to environmental changes yet retain personal integrity or wholeness (Levine 1969, p. 95). In this sense, **environment** means all the conditions, circumstances, and influences surrounding and affecting the development of an organism or group of organisms. It refers to both the internal and external environments. Roy states that the person, as an adaptive system, functions as a totality. **Adaptive behavior** is the behavior of the whole person. Roy identifies two major internal processor subsystems of the adaptive system: the regulator and the cognator (Roy and Roberts 1981, p. 43). The individual uses these subsystems to adapt to or cope with internal and external environmental stimuli. The regulator mechanism has neural, endocrine, and perception-psychomotor components. The cognator mechanism encompasses psychosocial pathways and apparatus for perceptual/information processing, learning, judgment, and emotion. These two mechanisms are linked by the process of perception.

Concept of Holism

Nurses are concerned with the individual as a whole, complete, or holistic person, not as an assembly of parts and processes. The terms **holistic** and **holism** are derived from the Greek word meaning "whole." The term *holism* itself was coined by Jan Smuts, a South African statesman, in his book *Holism and Evolution* (1926). In holistic theory, all living organisms are seen as interacting, unified wholes that are more than the mere sums of their parts. Viewed in this light, any disturbance in one part is a disturbance of the whole system; in other words, the disturbance affects the whole being.

When applied to humans and health, the concept of holism emphasizes the fact that "nurses must keep the self-identity of the 'whole' person in mind and must strive to understand simultaneously the relationship of the 'part' of the individual under concern to the totality of that individual's interactions and the relationship of the whole to its parts" (Krieger 1981, p. 4). Therefore, when studying one part of an individual, the nurse must consider how that part relates to all others. The nurse must also consider the interaction and relationship of the individual to the external environment and to others. For example, a nurse helps a man who is recuperating from a heart attack to consider his life-style and other contributing factors so that he can improve his health in the future. The nurse asks the client why he thinks the attack happened, what stresses he feels in his life, whether he smokes, what his eating habits are, and how much exercise he normally gets. Using the holistic approach, the nurse considers all contributing factors so that the client can prevent a recurrence.

Holistic health involves the total person: the whole of the person's being and the overall quality of life-style. It includes physical fitness, primary prevention of negative physical and emotional states, stress management, sensitivity to the environment, self-awareness, and spiritual insight (Smith 1984, p. 5). Many holistic health care centers have been established across North America. They help clients to take responsibility for their health, to seek alternative, healthy, self-fulfilling behaviors, and to mobilize inner healing capacities.

Human Needs

Although each individual has unique characteristics, certain needs are common to all people. Nursing theorists define *need* in various ways. Orlando defines a need as "a requirement of the person which, if supplied, receives or diminishes his immediate distress or improves his immediate sense of adequacy or well-being." (Orlando 1961, p. 5). King defines need as "a state of energy exchange within and external to the organism which leads to behavioral responses to situations, events, and persons" (King 1971, p. 80). Roy defines a need as "a requirement within the individual which stimulates a response to maintain integrity" (Roy 1980, p. 184). For the purposes of this book, a **need** is something that is desirable, useful, or necessary.

The humanist Abraham Maslow developed his theory of human needs in the 1940s. To Maslow, needs motivate the behavior of the individual. His model of human needs includes both physiologic and psychologic needs, which he ranks according to how critical to survival they are. Maslow believes that the needs at one level must be met before the needs on the next level can be met. Thus, the physiologic needs must be met before the safety needs are met. Maslow's five categories or levels of needs, in hierarchical order, are physiologic needs, safety and security needs, love and belonging needs, self-esteem needs, and the need for self-actualization (1970, p. 37). See Figure 4–1.

Throughout life, people strive to meet their needs at each level; however, the dominant needs *within one level* may vary at different times of life. Maslow sees humans as beings who continue to grow and develop from conception until death. Once a need is completely met, Maslow believes, the individual is no longer aware of it. Needs can be completely met, partially met, or not met at all. An individual usually persists in behavior to meet a need until it is met.

Maslow also states that an individual who apparently meets all needs still looks further to self-actualization. Maslow discusses two additional needs: the need to know and the need to understand. He believes that these needs are always present and permit people to meet the other needs more efficiently.

Maslow includes air, food, water, shelter, rest and sleep, activity, and temperature maintenance as the basic physiologic needs. A person who is starving or deprived of fluid for an extended time will center all activities around meeting that need. After the physiologic needs are met, the need to feel safe in one's environment emerges. This need for safety has both physical and psychologic aspects; the person needs to *be* safe and to *feel* safe, both in the physical environment and in relationships.

The third level of needs (for love, affection, and belonging) emerges after the needs for safety are met. According to Maslow, the need for love encompasses both giving and receiving. Belonging needs include attaining a place in a group, e.g., having a family and the feeling of belonging. The need for esteem is at the fourth level. The individual

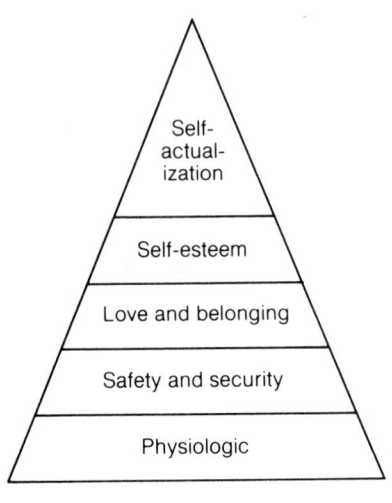

Maslow's hierarchy of needs

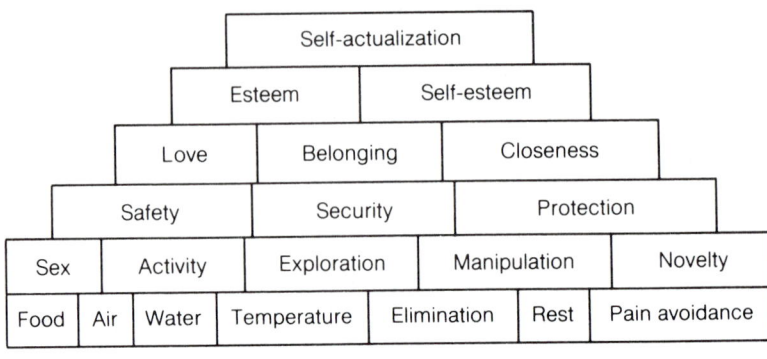

Maslow's hierarchy of needs, as adapted by Kalish

Figure 4–1 Maslow's needs. *Source:* From *The Psychology of Human Behavior,* 5th ed., by R. A. Kalish. Copyright © 1966, 1970, 1973, 1977, 1983 by Wadsworth, Inc. Reprinted by permission of Brooks/Cole Publishing Company, Monterey, Calif. 93940.

needs both *self-esteem* (i.e., feelings of independence, competence, and self-respect) and *esteem from others,* i.e., recognition, respect, and appreciation.

When the need for esteem is satisfied, the individual strives for **self-actualization.** Self-actualized persons have realized their full potential. Such a person has the ability to connect the past and the future to the present while living fully in the present, is inner-directed, and is autonomous in contrast to being other-directed.

To be inner-directed means that the individual is guided by a few basic values and principles, whatever the situation. To be autonomous is to be free from parental and social pressures and to apply these values or principles to behavior in a manner that appears appropriate to the individual. The other-directed individual is influenced by outside pressures, accepts guidance and direction from others, and adheres to this guidance to gain approval.

Not all people become fully self-actualized, and Maslow does not believe that intelligence is required for self-actualization. However, if all the "lower" needs are met, an individual may aspire to become self-fulfilled or self-actualized. Maslow sees self-actualization as a product of maturity that comes about through relating to people in autonomous and time-competent ways.

The fully self-actualized person may not always be happy, successful, or well adjusted. Maslow views many of the subjects he believes to be self-actualized as prideful, vain, and possessing doubts and fears. However, they are able to deal positively with their fears, doubts, and failures. See the accompanying box for the major characteristics of a self-actualized person.

In later research, Maslow identified the growth needs, in contrast to the deficiency needs. He calls the growth needs **Being values (metaneeds,** B-values). These "being values" resemble needs because, when metaneeds are not met, the person has a "sickness of the soul," or *metapathology* (Maslow 1971, p. 43). Maslow believes that for some people being values give meaning to life. There are 14 "being values:" truth, goodness, beauty, wholeness, aliveness, uniqueness, perfection, completion, justice, simplicity, richness, effortlessness, playfulness, and self-sufficiency. These needs are not ranked (Goble 1970, pp. 47–48).

Richard Kalish (1977, p. 32) has adapted Maslow's hierarchy and suggests an additional category of needs between the physiologic needs and the safety and security needs. This category includes sex, activity, exploration, manipulation, and novelty. See Figure 4–1. Kalish emphasizes that children need to explore and manipulate their environments to achieve optimal growth and development. He notes that adults, too, often seek novel adventures or stimulating experiences before considering their safety or security needs. Maslow, by contrast, includes the pursuit of knowledge and aesthetic needs in the category of self-actualization needs.

Halbert Dunn's (1958) model presents a series of needs

Characteristics of Basic Needs   All people have the same basic needs; however, each person's needs are modified by that person's culture. A person's perception of a need varies according to learning and the standards of the culture. For example, professional achievement may be important in one culture or subculture and unimportant in another.

- People meet their own needs relative to their own priorities. For example, during a drought, a mother might give up her share of water and die so that her child might have sufficient water to live.
- Although basic needs generally must be met, some needs can be deferred. An example is the need for independence, which an ill person can defer until well.
- Failure to meet needs results in one or more homeostatic imbalances, which can eventually result in illness.
- A need can make itself felt by either external or internal stimuli. An example is the need for food. A person may experience hunger as a result of thinking about food (internal stimulation) or as a result of seeing a beautiful cake (external stimulation).
- A person who perceives a need can respond in several ways to meet it. The choice of response is largely a result of learned experiences and the values of the culture. For example, the professional woman who comes home from work feeling tired may meet the need for relaxation by having a cocktail. This response reflects her experience and culture.
- Needs are interrelated. Some needs cannot be met unless related needs are also met. The need for hydration can be seriously altered if the need for elimination of urine is not also met. Likewise, the need for security can be markedly altered if the need for oxygen is threatened by a respiratory obstruction.

Needs can be satisfied in healthy and unhealthy ways. Individuals can succeed in their profession as a way of meeting the needs for belonging and self-esteem. Ways of meeting basic needs are considered healthy when they are not harmful to others or to self, conform to the individual's sociocultural values, and are within the law. Conversely, unhealthy behavior has one or more of the following characteristics: It may be harmful to others or to self, does not conform to the individual's sociocultural values, or is not within the law. Maslow found that people who satisfy their basic needs are healthier, happier, and more effective than those whose needs are frustrated (Goble 1970, p. 50).

Factors Affecting Needs Satisfaction   Gauging whether physiologic needs are met is largely an objective judgment by the nurse, although it may be subjective for the client. For example, the nurse can judge whether an

that the individual must meet to achieve a state of maximum functioning or high-level wellness. Dunn's basic needs are survival, communication, fellowship, growth, imagination, love, balance, environment, communication with the universe, philosophy of living, dignity, freedom, and space. At any specific time, different needs assume a greater relative importance to the individual.

Jourard (1963) believes that people rank their needs according to their relative importance in their lives. He adds the needs for health (physical and mental), freedom, challenge, cognitive clarity, and varied experience to Maslow's list.

individual's need for food has been met by weighing that person, using calipers to measure body fat, or reviewing the results of laboratory tests that analyze the metabolic processes of the body. Gauging whether psychologic needs have been met, however, is largely a subjective judgment. If a person believes a psychologic need (e.g., for love) is not satisfied, then for that person it is not met, regardless of external appearances. Several factors affect people's abilities to satisfy their needs. Four of these are illness, significant relationships, self-concept, and development stage.

Illness frequently interferes with people's abilities to meet their own needs. Nurses help ill clients to meet their physiologic needs on a number of levels. The man recovering from abdominal surgery probably requires oxygen, intravenous fluids, assistance in moving, and reassurance immediately after surgery. Enacting each of these interventions helps to meet a different need. As he recovers, his requirements for nursing help will decrease. As his physiologic needs are met, the client attends to needs at the next level (e.g., safety needs, according to Maslow) and so on. Ailing people often direct all their energies to meeting physiologic (survival) needs and may not identify needs at higher levels until later.

A second variable affecting needs satisfaction is *significant relationships*. Often these relationships are with family and support persons. Nurses also frequently establish significant relationships with clients because they are present at critical times in people's lives. Through these relationships, nurses can help clients become aware of their needs and establish healthy ways of meeting them.

A person's *self-concept* affects not only the ability to meet basic needs but also the awareness of whether or not these needs are satisfied. People who feel good about themselves are more likely to change, to recognize needs, and to establish healthy ways of meeting those needs. Those with a poor self-concept are less likely to meet these needs independently and may require more assistance from the nurse. Self-concept is discussed with greater depth in Chapter 29.

A fourth variable is an individual's *developmental stage*. According to Erikson's model of psychosocial human development (see Table 24–5), if an individual satisfactorily achieves the development task of learning to trust, then the basic needs of feeling safe and secure are readily resolved. The person who has already learned to trust others transfers those feelings to the health personnel caring for the person. As another example, if the developmental tasks of establishing identity and intimacy have been achieved, the individual has an increased sense of belonging and being loved at a time of illness.

Assigning Priorities to Needs

Although Maslow's needs are presented in a hierarchy, sometimes clients and nurses must adjust the priority of the needs. People are continually changing and growing; thus, their needs do not stay constant but also continually change. Depending upon the situation, the nurse may be able to help a client meet several needs at once, partially meet one need and then go on to another, or deal with one need at a time. Needs related to life-threatening situations, e.g., a suffocating client's need for air, always assume first priority.

In many situations, one need does not stand out as priority one. In these cases, the client and nurse consider several factors, such as the client's health, the client's and support persons' perceptions about health and areas of need, and the client's sociocultural background. A person may not perceive a specific need. If so, the nurse may allocate it a low priority, often deferring action until the person is ready. For example, a man who smokes heavily might not see the need to stop.

Socioeconomic and cultural backgrounds affect how people rank their needs. For example, a man may place his need to return to work ahead of his need to learn exercises. A woman may perceive that getting her husband's breakfast is more important than resting in bed. See Chapter 31 for more information about cultural influences.

Applications in Nursing

A knowledge of human needs helps nurses in several ways. First, it helps nurses understand themselves so that they can meet personal needs outside of the client situation. Second, by understanding human needs, nurses can understand people's behavior better. Recognizing the causes of certain behavior helps nurses be less judgmental and more objective. In addition, understanding the reason for behavior helps nurses respond therapeutically rather than emotionally. For example, by repeatedly turning on his signal light, a man may be reflecting a need for safety (he feels frightened), a need for belonging or affect, or a need for esteem. The nurse can discuss his feelings to determine what his need is and thus how to respond. If the client is turning on his light because he is frightened, the nurse can employ a variety of methods to reassure him, including explaining about the hospital, answering his call promptly, anticipating some of his needs, and telling him when the nurse will return and returning at that time.

Third, knowledge of basic needs can provide a framework for, and be applied in, the nursing process at the individual and family levels. Human needs can serve as a framework for assessing, assigning priorities to problems, and planning nursing interventions. A client's unmet need for blood can be of high priority and calls for immediate nursing action, whereas the same client's self-esteem needs are of lower priority during that emergency.

Fourth, nurses can apply their knowledge of human needs to relieve distress. To meet or help a client meet unmet needs and thereby alleviate distress, the nurse requires a knowledge not only of needs but also of the situations that bring about these unmet needs and the manner in which the client conveys the need.

Fifth, the nurse can use a knowledge of human needs to help people develop and grow. Sometimes people are unaware or only partially aware of their own needs. Nurses can often help clients move toward self-actualization by helping them to find meaning in their illness experience. To encourage the client's growth toward self-actualization nurses can help them to (a) understand what is happening to them, (b) maintain some control over events affecting them, (c) maintain their identities and self-respect, (d) accept inevitable outcomes, and (e) feel good about themselves.

THEORIES ABOUT CARING

Humanistic Theory

Humanism is a concern for human attributes, for those characteristics that are considered human. Some of these attributes are universal, that is, they occur in all cultures. Examples of humanistic behaviors are empathy, compassion, sympathy toward other people, and respect for life.

Humanism has received increased attention in nursing in response to the technologic advances that have affected nursing practice. Humanism in nursing refers to an attitude and an approach to the client and support persons recognizing them as human beings with human needs, rather than as "the appendectomy in Room 192" or "the catheterization in bed 6A."

North American societies are multiethnic (i.e., they comprise diverse ethnic groups). They are person-centered in their humanism and embody human rights concepts. This means that individuals are seen as autonomous and have certain rights and freedoms; in fact, each person has the right to be treated as an individual. By contrast, in certain societies, the tribe or the family, not the person, is the primary unit endowed with values and rights. Other characteristics of American humanism—though not necessarily unique to it—are belief in helping the poor and the suffering and respect for the ways and values of others, even if these differ from one's own.

The nurse who takes a humanistic approach to nursing practice takes into account all that is known about a client—thoughts, feelings, values, experiences, likes, desires, behavior, and body (La Monica 1985, p. 2). This humanistic approach, the traditional "caring" aspect of nursing, is characterized by understanding and action. Understanding requires the ability to listen to another and perceive that person's feelings. Action requires the ability to respond to another with genuineness and warmth to promote optimal well being (Slevin and Harter 1987, p. 24). The caring aspect of nursing is a core construct upon which the nurse builds the knowledge and skill of professional practice.

Caring Constructs

The terms *nursing care* and *caring* have been used by nurses for more than a century. Leininger (1984, p. 3) states: "Care is the essence and the central, unifying, and dominant domain to characterize nursing: it is an essential human need for the full development, health maintenance, and survival of human beings in all world cultures...yet care has not received the same degree of attention by professionals and the public as cure." In an address to the 75th Annual Registered Nurses' Association of Nova Scotia, Benner (1984, p. 3) made this statement: "Caring is often frankly curative because it facilitates healing." Leininger (1984, p. 6) says that there can be no curing without caring, but there may be caring without curing.

Definitions and a clear understanding of the terms *care* and *caring* have been lacking. Systematic research is needed to describe caring behaviors, values, and practices in nursing so that this knowledge can be incorporated into nursing education and practice areas. Some definitions of care and caring are provided in Table 4–2.

TABLE 4–2 *Definitions and Descriptions of Care and Caring*

Delores Gaut	There is no clear-cut rule for the use of *caring* in common language, but the family of meanings is related to the notion of caring in three senses: (a) attention to or concern about; (b) responsibility for or providing for; and (c) regard or fondness for.
	The term *caring* in both lay and scholarly literature is found in discussions of: (a) certain feelings or dispositions within a person; (b) the doing of certain activities that seem to identify that person as a caring individual; or (c) a combination of both attitudes and actions in which caring about the other disposes the one to carry out activities for the other.
	Caring is intentional activity.*
Madeleine Leininger	*Care* in a generic sense refers to those assistive, supportive, or facilitative acts toward or for another individual or group with evident or anticipated needs to ameliorate or improve a human condition or lifeway.
	Caring refers to the direct (or indirect) nurturant and skillful activities, processes, and decisions related to assisting people in such a manner that reflects behavioral attributes that are empathetic, supportive, compassionate, protective, succorant, educational, dependent upon the needs, problems, values, and goals of the individual or group being assisted.

TABLE 4–2 *Definitions and Descriptions of Care and Caring* (*continued*)

Madeline Leininger (continued)	*Professional caring* embodies the cognitive and deliberate goals, processes, and acts of professional persons or groups providing assistance to others, and expressing attitudes and actions of concern for them, in order to support their well-being, alleviate undue discomforts, and meet obvious or anticipated needs.
	Scientific caring refers to those judgments and acts of helping others based on tested or verified knowledge.
	Humanistic caring refers to the creative, intuitive, or cognitive helping process for individuals or groups based upon philosophic, phenomenologic, and objective and subjective experiential feelings and acts of assisting others.[†]
M. Mayeroff	We sometimes speak as if caring did not require knowledge, as if caring for someone, for example, were simply a matter of good intentions or warm regard. . . . To care for someone, I must know many things. I must know, for example, who the other is, what his powers and limitations are, what his needs are, and what is conducive to his growth; I must know how to respond to his needs and what my own powers and limitations are.
	Caring is an important means for self-growth. To help another person grow is at least to help him to care for something or someone apart from himself, and it involves encouraging and assisting him to find and create of his own in which he is able to care. Also, it is to help that other person to come to care for himself, and by becoming responsive to his own needs, to care and to become responsible for his own life.[‡]
Jean Watson	Human caring in nursing is not just an emotion, concern, attitude, or benevolent desire. Caring connotes a personal response. Human caring involves values, a will and a commitment to care, knowledge, caring actions, and consequences. All of human caring is related to intersubjective human responses to health-illness conditions; a knowledge of health-illness; environmental-personal interactions; a knowledge of the nurse caring process; self-knowledge; [and] knowledge of one's power and transaction limitations.
	The ideal and value of caring is a starting point, a stance, an attitude, which has to become a will, an intention, a commitment, and a conscious judgment that manifests itself in concrete acts. The most abstract characteristic of a caring person is that he or she is somehow responsive to a person as a unique individual, perceives the other's feelings, and sets apart one person from another from the ordinary. The uncaring person is by contrast insensitive to another person as a unique individual, [not] perceptive of the other's feelings, and does not necessarily distinguish one person from another in any significant way.[§]

Sources:
[*]D. Gaut, A theoretic description of caring as action, in M. Leininger, *Care: The essence of nursing and health* (Thorofare, N.J.: Charles B. Slack, 1984), pp. 27–28.
[†]M. Leininger, *Care: The essence of nursing and health* (Thorofare, N.J.: Charles B. Slack, 1984), pp. 4, 46.
[‡]M. Mayeroff, *On caring* (New York: Harper and Row, 1971), P. 13.
[§]J. Watson, *Nursing: Human science and human care—A theory of nursing* (National League for Nursing, 1988), pp. 29, 31, 32, 34.

In her transcultural care theory, Leininger (1984, pp. 5–6) points out that human caring, although a universal phenomenon, varies among cultures in its expressions, processes, and patterns; it is largely culturally derived. These differences in caring values and behaviors lead to differences in the expectations of those seeking care. For example, cultures that perceive illness primarily as a personal and internal body experience—caused by physical, genetic, and intrabody stresses—tend to use more medications and physical techniques than cultures that view illness as an extrapersonal experience.

Leininger identifies many caring and nursing care constructs. Examples are comfort, compassion, concern, coping behaviors, empathy, enabling, involvement, health acts (consultative, instructive, maintenance), love, nurturance, presence, sharing, tenderness, touching, and trust. Each of these constructs has many subdescriptions. Leininger believes the goal of health care personnel should be to work toward an understanding of care and the health of different cultures so that each culture's care, values, beliefs, and life-styles will be the basis for providing culture-specific care.

Watson (1979, pp. 10–208; 1988, p. 75) identifies ten caring factors in nursing:

1. Forming a humanistic-altruistic system of values. This factor relates to satisfaction through giving and extending the sense of self. Although the values are learned early in life, they can be greatly influenced by educators.

2. Instilling faith and hope. Feelings of faith and hope promote wellness by helping the client to adopt health-seeking behaviors. By developing an effective nurse-client relationship, the nurse facilitates feelings of optimism, hope, and trust.

3. Cultivating sensitivity to one's self and others. Nurses who are able to recognize and express their feelings are better able to allow others to express theirs.

4. Developing a helping-trust (human care) relationship. This kind of relationship involves effective communication, empathy, and nonpossessive warmth. It promotes and accepts the expression of positive and negative feelings.

5. Expressing positive and negative feelings. Sharing feelings of sorrow, love, and pain is a risk-taking experience. The nurse must be prepared for negative feelings.

6. Using a creative problem-solving caring process. Caring linked to the nursing process contributes to a creative problem-solving approach to nursing care.

7. Promoting interpersonal teaching-learning. This factor separates caring from curing and shifts responsibility for wellness to the client.

8. Providing a supportive, protective, or corrective mental, physical, sociocultural, and spiritual environment. Because the client can experience change in any aspect of the internal and external environments, the nurse must assess and facilitate the client's abilities to cope with mental, emotional, and physical changes.

9. Assisting with gratification of human needs. Caring is conveyed by recognizing and attending to the physical, emotional, social, and spiritual needs of the client.

10. Being sensitive to existential-phenomenologic-spiritual forces. Phenomenology describes data of the immediate situation that help people understand the phenomena in question. The **phenomenal field** is the individual's frame of reference; this field can be known only to the person. Existential psychology is a science of human existence that employs the method of phenomenologic analysis. Persons possess three spheres of being: mind, body, and soul (Watson 1988, p. 54). Allowing for expression of these forces leads to a better understanding of self and others.

Benner and Wrubel examine the relationship among caring, stress and coping, and health and claim that caring is primary. To Benner and Wrubel, **caring** means that persons, events, projects, and things matter to people (1989, p. 1). They state that caring is *primary* for any health care practice and view it as central to human expertise, to curing, and to healing. Caring is primary in three ways:

1. "Since caring sets up what matters to a person, it also sets up what counts as stressful, and what options are available for coping."

2. It is an enabling condition of connection and concern. When there is caring and concern, people find ways to cope. "Coping based on caring may not abolish loss and pain but it allows for the possibility of joy and the satisfactions of attachment."

3. "It sets up the possibility of giving and receiving help. A caring relationship sets up the conditions of trust that enable the one cared for to accept the help offered and to *feel* cared for" (Benner and Wrubel 1989, pp. 1–4).

The Power of Caring

Benner (1984, pp. 209–15) identifies six different qualities of power associated with caring:

1. *Transformative power.* With this power, the nurse can help clients to regain a sense of control and to participate actively in situations they thought were beyond their control. For example, clients often need help to realize that they have a choice and can abandon whatever role they wish.

2. *Integrative caring.* Caring can also reintegrate individuals into their own social world. For example, when prolonged or permanent disability is inevitable, the nurse can help clients to continue with meaningful life activities despite their limitations.

3. *Advocacy power.* Clients and families frequently need the nurse to act on their behalf. They may be confused by medical jargon, or their understanding may be hampered by anxiety or fear. The nurse can interpret necessary information to the client and to the physician. Advocacy removes obstacles; it is a standing alongside and enabling of the client.

4. *Healing power.* To establish a healing relationship and climate, the nurse (a) mobilizes hope within the self, the staff, and the client; (b) finds an interpretation or understanding of the situation (e.g., illness, pain, fear, or other stressful emotion) that is acceptable and clarifying to the client; and (c) helps the client find social, emotional, and spiritual support. A healing relationship helps the client to mobilize internal and external resources by bringing hope, confidence, and trust.

5. *Participative/affirmative power.* By participating, a nurse finds meanings in specific events. The nurse may experience pain but may also experience strength and affirmation. A detached, avoiding approach usually offers only frail protection and develops no positive inner resources.

6. *Problem solving.* Caring is the prerequisite for creative problem solving. The most difficult problems require perceptual ability as well as conceptual reasoning, and perception requires involvement and attentiveness. Caring provides a sensitivity to cues that allows persons to search for solutions and even makes it possible to recognize solutions when they are not directly sought.

OTHER THEORIES THAT AFFECT NURSING PRACTICE

Many other theories integrated throughout this book have a potential impact on nursing practice. These include theories about health and wellness in Chapter 5, change theory in Chapter 16, stress and adaptation theory in Chapter 33, and growth and development theories in Chapter 24. This section includes the following theories: general systems theory, problem-solving and decision-making theory, and perception theory.

General Systems Theory

General systems theory explains the breaking of whole things into parts and the working together of those parts in systems. The theory explains the relationship between wholes and parts, a description of concepts about them, and predictions about how the parts will behave and react. This theory is relevant in the nursing process as it is applied to the individual, family, and community.

The basic concepts of systems theory were proposed in the 1950s. One of its major proponents, Ludwig von Bertalanffy (1969) introduced systems theory as a universal theory that could be applied to many fields of study. Systems theory is being used increasingly by nurses as a way of understanding not only biologic systems but also systems in families, communities, and nursing and health care. General systems theory provides a way of examining interrelationships and deriving principles.

A **system** is a set of interacting identifiable parts or components. A system can be an individual, a family, or a community. The fundamental components of a system are matter, energy, and communication. Without any one of these, a system does not exist. The individual or the human system has matter (the body), energy (chemical or thermal), and communication (e.g., the nervous system). The **boundary** of a system, such as the skin in the human system, is a real or imaginary line that differentiates one system from another system or a system from its environment.

Systems may be complex and therefore are often studied as *subsystems*. Each subsystem belongs to a higher system. In the individual or human system, the subsystems (or lower level systems) are the organ systems, such as the respiratory system and the digestive system; the *suprasystems* are the family systems. See Figure 4–2 for a hierarchy of the human system.

Because all the parts of a system are interrelated, the whole system responds to changes in one of its parts. This interrelatedness is the basis for nursing's holistic view of the client. For example, a tumor of the liver affects the whole individual, that is, the person may be nauseated, tired, anxious, and so on. A psychologic problem such as stress or anxiety may also manifest itself by physiologic symptoms such as sleeplessness, nausea, or changes in cardiac function.

There are two general types of systems: closed and open. A **closed system** does not exchange energy, matter, or information with its environment; it receives no input from the environment and gives no output to the environment. An example of a closed system is a chemical reaction that takes place in a test tube. In reality, no closed systems exist. In an **open system,** energy, matter, and information move into and out of the system through the system boundary. All living systems, such as plants, animals, people, families, and communities, are open systems, since their survival depends on a continuous exchange of energy. They are, therefore, in a constant state of change.

For its functioning, an open system depends on the quality and quantity of its input, output, and feedback. **Input** consists of information, material, or energy that enters the system. After the input is absorbed by the system, it is processed in a way useful to the system. This process of transformation is called **throughput.** For example, in the digestive system, food is input; it is digested (throughput) so that it can be used by the body. **Output** from a system is energy, matter, or information given out by the system as a result of its processes. Output from the digestive system is feces and caloric energy.

Feedback is a process that enables a system to regulate itself by redirecting the output of a system to determine the input of the same system, thus forming a feedback loop. See Figure 4–3. Numerous examples of this feedback mechanism are found within individual, family, and community systems. In the individual, for example, the autonomic nervous system relies on a feedback system to balance the effects of the sympathetic and parasympathetic centers, which reg-

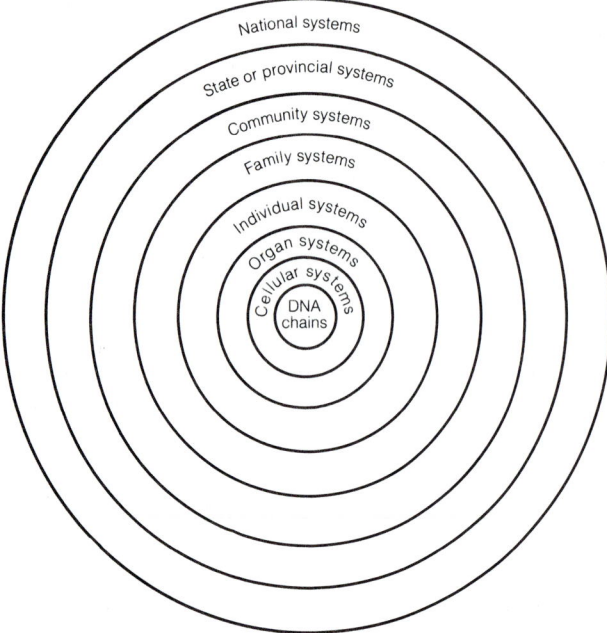

National systems

State or provincial systems

Community systems

Family systems

Individual systems

Organ systems

Cellular systems

DNA chains

Figure 4–2 A common system hierarchy.

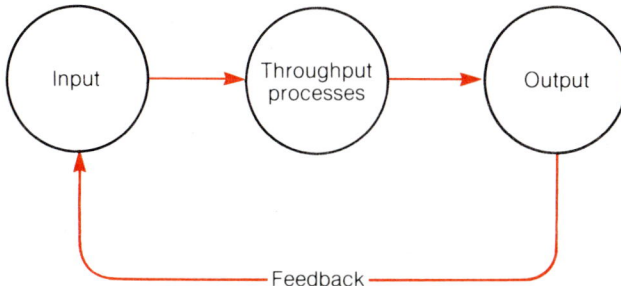

Figure 4–3 An open system with a feedback mechanism.

ulate, among other processes, heart and respiratory rates. In the family system, parents provide feedback to children to regulate behavior. In the community, laws, rules, and regulations regulate the behavior of citizens.

To survive, open systems must maintain a special balance often referred to as *dynamic equilibrium, homeostasis,* or *homeodynamics.* In the human being, examples of this balance include maintenance of normal body temperature, regardless of variations in environmental temperature from freezing to 85 F, and regulation of heart and respiratory rate within normal limits, in spite of varying degrees of physical exertion from watching television to running a marathon.

The nursing process has some of the characteristics of an open system: it is open, flexible, and dynamic; it is planned and goal directed; it interacts with the environment; and it emphasizes feedback. The nursing process can be viewed as a system with input, throughput, output, and feedback. Input (data) from the client and nurse is then transformed by the processes of analyzing, planning, and implementing, all of which are throughput. The output (client's response) is then evaluated.

Problem-Solving and Decision-Making Theory

Problem solving and decision making are used in applying the nursing process. Although these two terms are often used interchangeably, they are separate processes that are related in some situations. Solving a problem may require making a number of decisions, and making a decision may involve solving a number of problems. In addition, not all decisions involve problem solving. In many nursing situations, however, decision making is an aspect of problem solving.

Problem-Solving Methods   There are various approaches to problem solving. Four of the most commonly used are trial and error, intuition, experimentation, and the scientific method.

Trial-and-error problem solving   One way to solve problems is to try a number of approaches until a solution is found. However, the reason one solution works is not known when alternatives are not considered systematically. Trial-and-error methods in nursing care can be dangerous because the client might suffer harm if an approach is inappropriate.

Intuitive problem solving   Intuition as a problem-solving method has not been considered either sound or legitimate. Rather, it has been viewed as a form of guessing and, as such, an inappropriate basis for nursing decisions. However, according to recent investigations, intuition appears to be an essential and legitimate aspect of clinical judgment acquired through knowledge and experience (Benner and Tanner 1987). **Intuitive judgment** in nursing is developed through clinical experience with similar types of situations. In other words, expertise in a specialty area, such as cardiovascular nursing, is developed by continuous and meaningful exposure to clients who have experienced cardiovascular problems.

Intuition is based on experience and knowledge. The nurse must first have the knowledge base necessary to practice in

RESEARCH NOTE

Is Intuition Used In Nursing?

Intuition is the ability to recognize and understand something immediately without using analysis. People say, "I had a feeling that this was the appropriate choice." This statement describes intuition. In this study, the researchers wanted to determine if nurses use intuition while providing nursing care. They discovered that nurses do use intuition very effectively. They also found that nurses (a) recognized that the clients' signs and symptoms were falling into a particular pattern; (b) were able to draw on their experience to recognize how a particular client's symptoms were similar to those of other clients that they had cared for; (c) were able to identify quickly the most important pieces of information about the client to consider; and (d) anticipated that certain events would occur.

Implications: The researchers of this project suggest that although experience plays a very important role in improving this skill, some of these techniques can be taught. This teaching is most effective when students are given a complete description of all the factors surrounding the client's situation. In addition, experienced nurses should work with students and let them know whether their intuitions were correct or incorrect.

Source: P. Benner and C. Tanner. Clinical judgment: How expert nurses use intuition, *American Journal of Nursing,* January 1987, 87:23–31.

the clinical area, then use that knowledge in clinical practice. Clinical experience allows the nurse to recognize cues and patterns and begin to make correct decisions.

The intuitive method of problem solving is gaining recognition as part of nursing practice. It is not a valid method of decision making for novices or students, however, because they usually lack the knowledge base on which to make a valid judgment.

Experimentation Experimentation is more controlled than trial and error. It is based on knowledge and research, and it is therefore a more valid method than trial-and-error or intuitive problem solving. Examples of experimentation are pilot projects or limited trials in an effort to solve a problem. For example, a nurse caring for a client with intractable pain may try one specific nursing intervention for 3 days to reduce the pain. If the pain is not reduced, the nurse may then implement a second plan for another 3 days. Many research projects designed and implemented by nurse researchers are done to determine the most effective nursing interventions and ultimately improve nursing care.

Scientific method The **scientific method** is a logical, systematic approach to solving problems. The classic scientific method is most useful in a laboratory where the scientist is working in a controlled situation. The steps of the scientific method are outlined in Table 4–3.

Although the scientific method has certain applications in nursing, there are differences between the scientist's laboratory setting and the nurse's practice setting. Three of these differences are as follows:

1. The nurse's time frame is often shorter than the scientist's. The scientist may take months or even years to carry out a study, whereas a nurse, for example, must give immediate help to a client in pain.

2. The nurse's environment makes complete scientific control impossible, whereas the scientist strives to establish precise scientific controls in experiments. For example, a home care nurse striving to help regulate a client's diabetes through diet and insulin injections can outline a regimen and teach the client to administer insulin but has no control over whether the client will follow instructions later.

3. The nurse deals with multiple, complex problems, especially since most clients have more than one problem when they are ill. The scientist often isolates and studies a single aspect of a problem.

The scientific method, therefore, must be adapted for nursing practice. The nurse requires a problem-solving system that is scientific, systematic, yet flexible enough to deal with the complex situations in the health care system.

Modified scientific method (problem-solving process) Health professionals require a modified approach of the scientific method for solving problems. This modified scientific problem-solving method is used in the nursing process as well as the medical process. Like the scientific process, it has seven steps. See Table 4–3 for a comparison of the problem-solving process, the nursing process, and the scientific method.

Decision-Making Process **Decision making** is a process of choosing a particular and best action to meet a desired goal. Three conditions must prevail: freedom, rationality, and voluntary (Schaefer 1974, p. 1852). Freedom means that the individual makes the decision without pressure from others and has the authority to make the decision. Rationality, in the context of decision making, means that the best or optimal decision is made and that it is con-

TABLE 4–3 *Comparison of Steps in the Problem-Solving Process, the Nursing Process, and the Scientific Method*

Problem-Solving Process	Nursing Process	Scientific Method
1. Encounter the problem	1. Assessing	1. Recognize and define the problem
2. Collect data		2. Collect data from observation and experimentation
3. Analyze information and identify exact nature of the problem	2. Diagnosing	3. Formulate hypothesis (an assumption made to test the logic of a proposition)
4. Determine a plan of action	3. Planning	4. Select plan to test the hypothesis
5. Carry out the plan	4. Implementing	5. Test the hypothesis
6. Evaluate the plan and its outcomes	5. Evaluating	6. Interpret test results (evaluate whether the hypothesis is correct)
7. Terminate or modify the plan		7. Conclude or modify hypothesis

sistent with the decision maker's values and preferences. Rationality involves both deliberation and judgment. Voluntarity is making a choice voluntarily.

Decision making involves two types of reasoning: inductive and deductive. In **inductive reasoning,** generalizations are formed from a set of facts or observations. When viewed together, certain bits of information suggest a particular interpretation. For example, the nurse who observes that a client has dry skin, poor turgor, sunken eyes, and dark amber urine may make the generalization that the client is dehydrated. **Deductive reasoning,** by contrast, is reasoning from the general to the specific. The nurse starts with a conceptual framework—for example, Maslow's hierarchy of needs or a self-care framework—and makes descriptive interpretations of the client's condition in relation to that framework. For example, the nurse who uses the needs framework might categorize data and define the client's problems in terms of elimination, nutrition, or protection needs.

Several authors have described the decision-making process. For the purposes of this text, a three-phase decision-making process is chosen: deliberation, judgment, and discrimination (choice).

Deliberation   During this initial phase, the nurse considers all the available data. The data are categorized and any gaps, inconsistencies, or conflicts are identified. At this time, solutions are considered, including all alternative actions and their consequences.

Judgment   During the judgment phase of the decision-making process, each course of action is analyzed in terms of (a) effectiveness related to the goal of the action and (b) efficiency of the action. Included in the analysis are the risk factors involved.

Discrimination (choice)   The third phase in the decision-making process is choosing one alternative action and the consequences. Insufficient deliberation and judgment can lead to poor choices, and inadequate consideration of the consequences can also lead to poor choices. However, thorough deliberation and judgment can lead to an effective choice of action.

Decision-making, like the nursing process, is cyclical. Assessing, the gathering of data about a client, is similar to the deliberation phase of the decision-making process (see Table 4–4). The analyzing stage of the nursing process is parallel to the judgment phase of decision-making. Planning, in the nursing process, is like the discrimination (choice) phase. Intervention involves continuous collection of data, analyses of the data, and nursing judgments regarding the effectiveness of the intervention. Any change in data may change the plan and the intervention. All three phases of decision-making apply to this stage of the nursing process. During evaluation, the nurse continues to gather data, reassess the effectiveness of the intervention, and make

TABLE 4–4   *A Comparison of the Steps of the Nursing Process and Decision Making*

Nursing Process Steps	Decision-Making Phases
1. Assessing	Deliberation
2. Diagnosing	Judgment, discrimination
3. Planning	Discrimination
4. Implementing	Deliberation, judgment, discrimination
5. Evaluating	Deliberation, judgment, discrimination

decisions about it. In effect, the nurse also evaluates the effectiveness of the decision-making process itself.

Perception Theory

Perception is a major means by which people gain information about themselves, their needs, and the environment. **Perception** is the process of selecting, organizing, and interpreting sensory stimuli into a meaningful and coherent picture of the world. When looking around, a person sees a whole range of different objects, forms, and colors. People also see depth; all objects appear three-dimensional. Why does the world look the way it does to a person? A superficial answer is that things look the way they do because that is the way they are; they mirror reality.

Perception, however, is more complex than a response to sensory stimuli. It is also the interpretation of the sensation in the light of previous learning. Perception is a person's conscious awareness of reality and is based on an individual's knowledge and past experiences.

People tend to see what they want to see. What people anticipate as a result of past experience can become so firmly embedded into their thinking that people can be "blinded" to reality. Differences in people's perceptual fields are evident when, for example, witnesses to an accident give different reports of the same event. Often, there are as many different reports as witnesses. Observers are prone to make inferences from fragments of information, and the inferences are influenced by what the observer expects to perceive.

Three main factors influence people's perceptual fields: (a) the persons' needs, (b) their values or beliefs, and (c) their self-concept. For example, hungry shoppers perceive themselves as needing more food than those who are not hungry; people who value another's property perceive the taking of an apple from a neighbor's tree as theft, while others perceive it as all right as long as they are not seen. Persons who have a low self-concept, i.e., think of themselves as weak, will selectively ignore stimuli that refute it.

An understanding of perceptual theory is essential for the nurse who wishes to communicate with clients and acquire and interpret data about them. Analysis of data is an inductive process. To share information accurately with a client, the nurse must perceive what the client intends to be perceived.

To enhance the ability to collect data and the accuracy of inferences made about the client, nurses must continually strive to increase their observational or perceptual field. This can be achieved by the following:

1. Using all senses—sight, smell hearing, touch, and taste—when collecting data.

2. Not focusing attention on only particular events or aspects of a stimulus.

3. Resisting the expectation that certain types of stimulation or responses will occur.

4. Asking for feedback about the client's perceptions, sharing and comparing perceptions, and reaching a common understanding. When eliciting feedback, the nurse can say, "I don't understand" or nonverbally indicate a question with a raised eyebrow or other gesture.

5. Being aware of their own values, beliefs, and biases, which may affect how nurses interpret what they see and hear. Nurses need to overcome the tendency to attend only to a person's positive attributes (that is, those that are similar to the nurse's own values) or to attend overly to negative attributes (that is, those in conflict with the nurse's values).

CHAPTER HIGHLIGHTS

▶ Three directions have been used to develop nursing theories: borrowing from conceptual frameworks in other disciplines, using an inductive approach, and using a deductive approach.

▶ A conceptual framework is a way of looking at a discipline in clear, explicit terms that can be communicated to others.

▶ Concepts that influence nursing most significantly include the person, the environment, health, and nursing actions. Together these concepts form the metaparadigm of nursing.

▶ A conceptual model gives clear and explicit directions to the three areas of nursing: practice, education, and research.

▶ A theory is made up of concepts, propositions, and hypotheses. Whereas a conceptual framework provides guidelines, a theory serves to generate knowledge in a field.

▶ A number of models have been developed by nurse theorists, including Henderson, Johnson, King, Levine, Neuman, Orem, Parse, Rogers, and Roy.

▶ The three basic components of nursing models are assumptions, a value system, and major units. The seven major units of nursing models (constructed from the assumptions and values) are goal of nursing, client, role of the nurse, source of difficulty of the client, intervention focus, modes of intervention, and consequences of nursing activity.

▶ Conceptual models for nursing are operationalized by the nursing process. This process consists of five steps:

assessing, diagnosing, planning, implementing, and evaluating.

▶ Much research must be conducted before the usefulness of a conceptual model for nursing can be realized.

▶ Nursing involves viewing the individual holistically.

▶ How nurses view human beings influences how they assess and intervene.

▶ Humans can be viewed as open systems with many interrelated subsystems.

▶ Maslow defined a hierarchy of human needs, from physiologic (survival) needs to self-actualization.

▶ People vary in how they rank their needs at any given moment.

▶ Needs satisfaction can be altered by illness, significant relationships, self-concept, and developmental levels.

▶ A knowledge of human needs helps nurses understand behavior, can provide a framework for applying parts of the nursing process, and can help nurses relieve distress and help people develop and grow.

▶ Definitions and a clear understanding of the terms *care* and *caring* are being developed. The major theorists involved to date are Leininger, Watson, and Benner.

▶ Many theories, other than nursing theories, also have an impact on nursing practice. Included are theories about health and wellness, change theory, stress and adaptation theory, growth and development theories, general systems theory, problem-solving and decision-making theory, and perception theory.

READINGS AND REFERENCES

SUGGESTED READINGS

Storch, J. L. January 1986. In defense of nursing theory. *Canadian Nurse* 82:16–20.

Storch suggests that nursing theory may be the key to meeting the changing needs of health consumers. She discusses how theory can make a significant difference in the quality of client care.

RELATED RESEARCH

Baer, E. D., and Lowery, B. J. September/October 1987. Patient and situational factors that affect nursing students' like or dislike of caring for patients. *Nursing Research* 36:298–302.

Benner, P., and Tanner, C. January 1987. Clinical judgment: How expert nurses use intuition. *American Journal of Nursing* 87:23–31.

Slevin, A. P., and Harter, M. O. November/December 1987. The teaching of caring: A survey report. *Nurse Educator* 12:23–26.

SELECTED REFERENCES

Andres, H. A., and Roy, C. 1986. *Essentials of the Roy Adaptation Model*. Norwalk, Conn.: Appleton-Century-Crofts.

Austin, J. K., and Champion, V. L., 1983. King's theory for nursing: Explication and evaluation. In Chinn, P. L., editor. *Advances in nursing theory development*. Rockville, Md.: Aspen Systems Corporation.

Benner, P. 1984. *From novice to expert: Excellence and power in clinical nursing practice*. Menlo Park, Calif.: Addison-Wesley Publishing Co.

Benner, P., and Tanner, C. January 1987. How expert nurses use intuition. *American Journal of Nursing* 87:23–31.

Benner, P. and Wrubel, J. 1989. *The primacy of caring: Stress and coping in health and illness*. Menlo Park, Calif.: Addison-Wesley Publishing Co.

Canadian Nurses' Association. 1984. *A definition of nursing practice: Standards for nursing practice*. Ottawa: Canadian Nurses' Association.

DeYoung, L. 1985. *Dynamics of nursing*. 5th ed. St. Louis: C. V. Mosby Co.

Dunn, H. H. November 1958. What high level wellness means. *Canadian Journal of Public Health* 50:447–57.

Fawcett, J. 1984. *Analysis and evaluation of conceptual models of nursing*. Philadelphia: F. A. Davis Co.

Gaut, D. 1984. A theoretic description of caring as action. In Leininger, M. pp. 27–28. *Care: The essence of nursing and health*. Thorofare, N.J.: Charles B. Slack.

George, J. B., editor. 1985 *Nursing theories: The base for professional nursing practice*. 2d ed. Englewood Cliffs, N.J.: Prentice-Hall.

Goble, F. G. 1970. *The third force: The psychology of Abraham Maslow*. Richmond Hill, Ontario: Simon and Schuster.

Henderson, V. 1966. *The nature of nursing: A definition and its implications for practice, research, and education*. New York: Macmillan Co.

———. October 1969. Excellence in nursing. *American Journal of Nursing* 69:2133–37.

Johnson, D. E. 1980. The behavioral system model for nursing. In Riehl, J. P., and Roy, C., editors. pp. 207–16. *Conceptual models for nursing practice*. 2d ed. New York: Appleton-Century-Crofts.

Jourard, S. 1963. *Personality adjustment*. 2d ed. New York: Macmillan Co.

King I. M. 1971. *Toward a theory for nursing: General concepts of human behavior*. New York: John Wiley and Sons.

———. 1978. The "why" of theory development. In *Theory development: What, why, how?* New York: National League for Nursing.

———. 1981. *A theory for nursing: Systems, concepts, process*. New York: John Wiley and Sons.

———. 1987. King's theory of goal attainment. In Parse, R. R., editor. *Nursing science: Major paradigms, theories, and critiques*. Philadelphia: W. B. Saunders Co.

Krieger, D. 1981. *Foundations for holistic health nursing practices: The Renaissance nurse*. Philadelphia: J. B. Lippincott Co.

La Monica, E. L. 1985. *The humanistic nursing process*. Monterey, Calif.: Wadsworth Health Sciences.

Leddy, S., and Pepper, J. M. 1989. *Conceptual bases of professional nursing*. 2d ed. Philadelphia: J. B. Lippincott Co.

Leininger, M. 1984. *Care: The essence of nursing and health*. Thorofare, N.J.: Charles B. Slack.

Levine, M. E. January 1969. The pursuit of wholeness. *American Journal of Nursing* 69:93–98.

———. 1973. *Introduction to clinical nursing*. 2d ed. Philadelphia: F. A. Davis Co.

Malinski, V. M. 1986. Explorations on Martha Rogers' science of unitary human beings. Norwalk, Conn.: Appleton-Century-Crofts.

Mariner-Tomey, A. 1989. *Nursing theorists and their work*. 2d ed. St. Louis: C. V. Mosby Co.

Maslow, A. H. 1968. *Toward a psychology of being*. 2d ed. New York: Van Nostrand Reinhold Co.

———. 1970. *Motivation and personality*. 2d ed. New York: Harper and Row.

———. 1971. *The farther reaches of human nature*. New York: Penguin Books.

Mayeroff, M. 1971. *On caring*. New York: Harper and Row.

Mitchell, G. J., Pilkington, B. Summer 1990. Theoretical approaches in nursing practice: A comparison of Roy and Parse. *Nursing Science Quarterly* 3:81–7.

Neuman, B. 1974. The Betty Neuman health-care systems model: A total person approach to patient problems. In Riehl, J. P., and Roy, C., editors. *Conceptual models for nursing practice*. New York: Appleton-Century-Crofts.

———. 1980. The Betty Neuman health-care systems model: A total person approach to patient problems. In Riehl, J. P., and Roy, C., editors. *Conceptual models for nursing practice*. 2d ed. New York: Appleton-Century-Crofts.

———. 1982. *The Neuman systems model: Applications to nursing education and practice*. New York: Appleton-Century-Crofts.

Newman, M. A. Spring 1990. Newman's theory of health as praxis. *Nursing Science Quarterly* 3:37–41.

Orem, D. E. 1971. *Nursing: Concepts of practice*. New York: McGraw-Hill.

———. 1980. *Nursing: Concepts of practice*. 2d ed. New York: McGraw-Hill.

———. 1985. *Nursing: Concepts of practice*. 3d ed. New York: McGraw-Hill.

Orlando, I. J. 1961. *The dynamic nurse-patient relationship: Function, process and principles.* New York: G. P. Putnam's Sons.

Parse, R. R. 1987. *Nursing science: Major paradigms, theories, and critiques.* Philadelphia: W. B. Saunders Co.

Ray, M. A. Spring 1990. Critical reflective analysis of Parse's and Newman's research. *Nursing Science Quarterly* 3:44–6.

Rogers, M. E. 1970. *An introduction to the theoretical basis of nursing.* Philadelphia: F. A. Davis Co.

———. 1980. Nursing: A science of unitary man. In Riehl, J. P., and Roy, C., editors. *Conceptual models for nursing practice.* 2d ed. New York: Appleton-Century-Crofts.

———. 1986. Science of unitary human beings. In Malinski, V. M. pp. 3–8. *Exploration on Martha Rogers' science of unitary human beings.* Norwalk, Conn.: Appleton-Century-Crofts.

Roy, C. 1976. *Introduction to nursing: An adaptation model.* Englewood Cliffs, N. J.: Prentice-Hall.

———. 1980. The Roy adaptation model. In Riehl, J. P., and Roy, C., editors. *Conceptual models for nursing practice.* 2d ed. New York: Appleton-Century-Crofts.

———. 1984. *Introduction to nursing: An adaptation model.* 2d ed. Englewood Cliffs, N. J.: Prentice-Hall.

———. 1987. Roy's adaptation model. In Parse, R. pp. 35–45. *Nursing science: Major paradigms, theories, and critiques.* Philadelphia: W. B. Saunders Co.

Roy, C., and Roberts, S. L. 1981. *Theory construction in nursing: An adaptation model.* Englewood Cliffs, N. J.: Prentice-Hall.

Schaefer, J. October 1974. The interrelatedness of decision making and the nursing process. *American Journal of Nursing* 74:1852–55.

Slevin, A., and Harter, M. November/December 1987. The Teaching of Caring: A Survey Report. *Nurse Educator.* 12:23–26.

Smith, M. P. August 1984. The new frontier. *RNABC* (Registered Nurses Association of British Columbia) *News* 16:5.

Smuts, J. 1926. *Holism and evolution.* New York: Macmillan Co.

Styles, M. M. 1982. *On nursing: Toward a new endowment.* St. Louis: C. V. Mosby Co.

von Bertalanffy, L. 1969. *General system theory.* New York: George Braziller.

Watson, J. 1979. *Nursing: The philosophy and science of caring.* Boston: Little, Brown and Co.

———. 1988. *Nursing: Human science and human care.* A theory of nursing. National League for Nursing Pub. no. 15–2236. New York: National League for Nursing.

HEALTH PERCEPTIONS AND MANAGEMENT

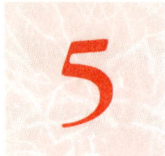

CHAPTER

5 Health and Illness

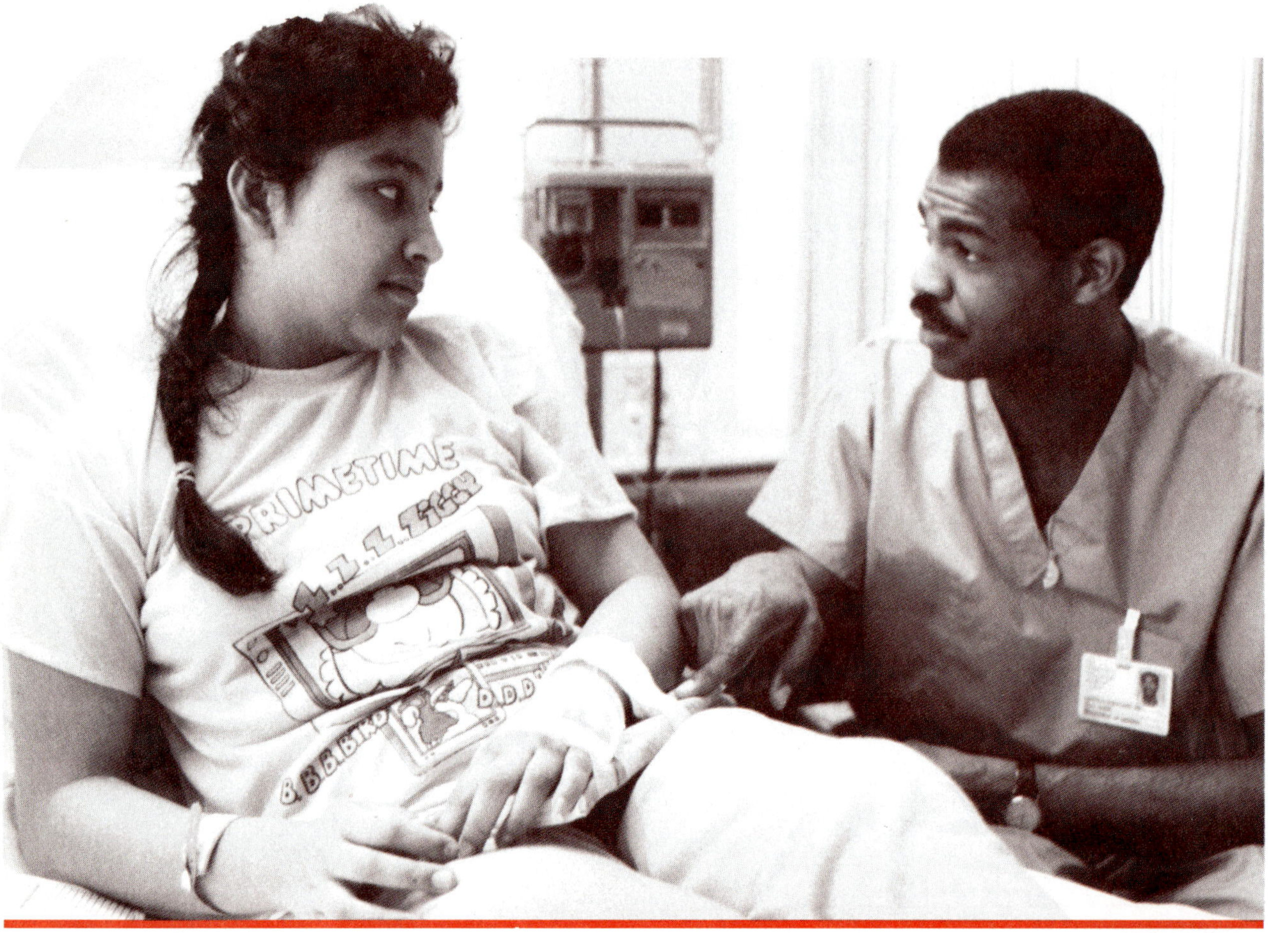

CONTENTS

OBJECTIVES

- Differentiate health, wellness, well-being, sickness, illness, and disease.
- Identify factors that influence a person's concept of health.
- Describe how individual perceptions affect a person's health behavior.
- Describe factors affecting compliance.
- Identify nursing interventions to improve compliance.
- Describe Suchman's five stages of illness.

of an individual for the effective performance of his roles and tasks" (Parsons 1972, p. 107). An emphasis in this definition is the capacity of the individual rather than a commitment to roles and tasks.

It is assumed in this model that sickness is the inability to perform one's work. A problem with this model is the assumption that a person's most important role is the work role. People usually fulfill several roles, e.g., mother, daughter, friend, and certain individuals may consider nonwork roles paramount in their lives.

Adaptive Model

Adaptive Model The focus of the adaptive model is adaptation. This model is derived from the writings of Dubos (1978), who views health as a creative process. Individuals are actively and continually adapting to their environments. In Dubos's view, the individuals must have sufficient knowledge to make informed choices about their health and also the income and resources to act on choices. Dubos believes that complete well-being is unobtainable, thus contradicting the 1947 WHO definition.

In the adaptive model, disease is a failure in adaptation. The aim of treatment is to restore the ability of the person to adapt, i.e., to cope. According to this model, extreme good health is flexible adaptation to the environment and interaction with the environment to maximum advantage (Smith 1981, p. 45). The focus of this model is stability, although there is also an element of growth and change.

Murry and Zentner indicate this growth and change in their definition of health: "a state of well-being in which the person is able to use purposeful, adaptive responses and processes, physically, mentally, emotionally, spiritually, and socially, in response to internal and external stimuli (stressors) in order to maintain relative stability and comfort and to strive for personal objectives and cultural goals" (Murray and Zentner 1985, pp. 4–5).

Eudaemonistic Model

Eudaemonistic Model The eudaemonistic model incorporates the most comprehensive view of health (Smith 1981, p. 44). Health is seen as a condition of actualization or realization of a person's potential. Actualization is the apex of the fully developed personality. (Maslow presents this concept of health. See Chapter 4). In this model, the highest aspiration of people is fulfillment and complete development, i.e., actualization. In the words of Dubos (1978, p. 74), health is primarily a "measure of each person's ability to do what he wants to do and become what he wants to become." It is the same as high-level wellness (see the next section). Illness, in this model, is a condition that prevents self-actualization.

Pender includes stabilizing and actualizing tendencies in her definition of health: "Health is the actualization of inherent and acquired human potential through satisfying relationships with others while adjustments are made as needed to maintain structural integrity and harmony with the environment" (1987, p. 27).

RESEARCH NOTE

How Do Adults Define Health?

Do health care professionals and the consumers of health care share the same views about health? In order to make health promotion activities more effective, it is important to know the public's view of health. The purpose of a study done by Colantonio (1988) was to investigate the concept of health in an adult population. One hundred men and women were asked to respond in an interview to the question "What does being healthy mean to you?" Based on the responses, seven categories were identified. The approximate response frequencies for each category are as follows:

Being fit (36%):	"able to work," "able to take care of oneself"
Feeling well (16%):	"fresh," "feeling happy"
Not being ill (23%):	"not spending time at the doctor's"
Good health behaviors (12%):	"eating well," "not drinking too much"
Looking well (10%):	"good complexion," "not overweight"
Environment (4%):	"clean air," "having enough money"
Other (10%):	no response

The findings of this study indicate that the most common concept of health refers to feeling fit. This means being able to fulfill those activities of daily living that are both necessary and desirable and being in a positive emotional and physical state. The role of good health habits is considered an important factor in the maintenance of this positive state. Further statistical analysis reveals that there are no significant differences in the perceptions of health concepts between men and women or between younger and older age groups.

Implications: These findings suggest that providers of health care services should be aware that the consumer's concept of health may vary from that of the health care professional.

The results of the study also suggest that (a) health promotion communication should be delivered in positive terms; (b) the information provided may not have to vary for males and females or for different age groups; and (c) indicators of health status may be more useful if they are based on the degree of fitness rather than the degree of illness.

Source: A. Colantonio, Lay concepts of health, *Health Values,* September/October 1988, 12:3–7.

Personal Definitions of Health

Health is a highly individual perception. Meanings and descriptions of health vary considerably. An individual's personal definition of health may not agree with that of health professionals. The following factors influence an individual's definition of health.

- *Developmental status.* The idea of health is frequently related to a person's level of development. The ability to conceptualize a state of health and the ability to respond to changes in health are related directly to age. The nurse's knowledge of an individual's developmental status (see Chapter 24) can facilitate assessment of the appropriateness of the person's behavior and help anticipate future behaviors.

- *Social and cultural influences.* Culture and social interactions also influence a person's notion of health. Each culture has ideas about health, and often these are transmitted from parents to children. For example, in some traditional Chinese families health is defined as a flow of energy (yin and yang). Yin is dark, cold, wet, negative, and female; yang is light, warm, dry, positive, and male. An imbalance of yin and yang results in disease.

- *Previous experiences.* Experiences with health and illness also affect people's perceptions of health. Some people may consider a pain or dysfunction normal because they have experienced it once or often before. Knowledge gained from these past experiences helps determine people's definitions of health.

- *Expectations of self.* Some people expect to be functioning at a high level physically and psychosocially all the time when they are healthy. They perceive any change in that level of functioning, therefore, as illness. Others expect variations in their level of functioning, and their definitions of health accommodate those variations.

- *Perception of self.* Another factor is how the individual perceives the self generally. These perceptions relate to such aspects of self as esteem, body image, needs, roles, and ability. When there is any threat or perceived threat to these views of self, the individual usually feels some anxiety and may need to reassess health and to redefine health itself. For example, a 75-year-old man who can no longer move large objects as he was accustomed to do may need to examine and redefine his concept of health in view of his age and abilities.

Nurses should be aware of their own personal definitions of health and should appreciate that other people have their own individual definitions as well. The person's definition of health influences behavior related to health and illness. By understanding clients' perceptions of health and illness, nurses can provide more meaningful assistance to help clients regain or attain a state of health. To facilitate development of a personal definition of health, see the accompanying box.

Developing a Personal Definition of Health

The following questions can help nurses develop a personal definition of health.

- Is a person more than a biophysiologic system?
- Is health more than the absence of disease symptoms?
- Is health solely the result of the interaction between host, agent, and environment?
- Is health the ability of an individual to perform work?
- Is health the ability of an individual to adapt to the environment?
- Is health a condition of a person's actualization?
- Is health a state or a process?
- Is health the effective functioning of self-care activities?
- Is health static or changing?
- Are health and wellness the same?
- Are disease and illness different?
- Are there levels of health?
- Are health and illness separate entities or points along a continuum?
- Is health socially determined?
- How do you rate your health and why?

Illness, Sickness, and Disease

Illness is a highly personal state in which the person feels unhealthy or ill. Illness may or may not be related to disease. An individual could have a disease, for example, a growth in the stomach, and not feel ill. Parsons defines illness as "a state of disturbance in the normal functioning of the total human individual, including both the state of the organism as a biological system, and of his person and social adjustments" (Parsons 1972, p. 107).

Sickness is a status or social entity that is usually associated with disease or illness but can occur independently of them (Twaddle 1977, p. 97). When a person is defined as sick, several dependent behaviors are accepted that otherwise might be considered unacceptable. Bauman (1965, p. 206) found that people use three distinct criteria to determine whether they are ill:

1. The presence of symptoms, such as elevated temperature or pain

2. Their perceptions of how they feel; for example, good, bad, sick

3. Their ability to carry out daily activities, such as a job or schoolwork

Disease is a medical term that can be described as an alteration in body functions resulting in a reduction of capacities or a shortening of the normal life span (Twaddle 1977, p. 97). Disease may further be described as *acute* or *chronic, communicable, congenital, degenerative, functional, malignant, psychosomatic,* or *idiopathic.* Intervention by physicians has the goal of eliminating or ameliorating disease processes. Primitive people thought disease was caused by "forces" or spirits. Later, this belief was replaced by the single-causation theory. Increasingly, a number of factors are considered to interact in causing disease and determining the individual's response to treatment.

The causation of disease is called its **etiology.** A description of the etiology of a disease includes the identification of all causal factors that act together to bring about the particular disease. For example, the tubercle bacillus is designated as the biologic agent of tuberculosis. However, other etiologic factors, such as age, nutritional status, and even occupation, are involved in the development of tuberculosis and influence the course of infection. Although there are many diseases for which the cause is unknown (e.g., diabetes, many types of cancer, multiple sclerosis) common causes of disease include the following:

- Genetic or familial predisposition
- Environmental abnormalities during critical periods of gestation (e.g., chemicals, viruses)
- Biologic agents, such as viruses, bacteria, rickettsia, fungi, protozoa, and helminths (worms)
- Physical agents, such as temperature extremes, radiation, and electricity.
- Chemical agents, such as alcohol, strong acids and bases, many drugs, heavy metals, and industrial poisons
- Faulty chemistry in the production of antibodies resulting in hypersensitivities or allergies
- Faulty chemical or metabolic processes, e.g., excessive or inadequate production of body secretions such as hormones and enzymes
- Continued, unabated stress

Risk factors are situations, habits, or other phenomena that increase a person's vulnerability to illness or injury. Risk factors can be categorized into five interrelated areas: genetic makeup, age, physiologic factors, life-style, and environment: Examples of each follow:

- *Genetic makeup.* A person with a family history of diabetes mellitus or cancer is at risk of developing the disease later in life.
- *Age.* The risk of birth defects and complications of pregnancy increases after age 35; the risk of communicable disease is higher in school-age children; and the risk of cardiovascular disease increases with age for both sexes.
- *Physiologic factors.* Pregnancy places the fetus and mother

at increased risk of disease; obesity increases the risk of heart disease.

- *Life-style or health habits.* Overeating increases the risk of heart disease; smoking increases the risk of lung cancer; poor nutrition leads to several deficiencies; promiscuity increases the risk of sexually transmitted disease; excessive use of alcohol increases the risk of accident, liver disease, and disability; unabated stress increases the risk of accidents and illness; and certain activities such as skiing or mountain climbing increase the risk of injury.
- *Environment.* Exposure to specific hazards, such as asbestos, rubber, and plastic, increases the risk of certain kinds of cancer; unclean, overcrowded living conditions predispose people to infections and other communicable diseases; air, water, and noise pollution all increase susceptibility to illness.

All of these risks present challenges to health care workers, especially nurses, in terms of prevention. Measures to enhance health include maintaining ideal body weight; eating regular meals with few snacks; elimination of cigarette smoking; moderation of alcohol consumption; safety measures, such as using seat belts, to prevent accidents and injuries; and periodic screening for such health problems as cancer. See "Three Levels of Preventive Care" in Chapter 23.

In 1974, Marc Lalonde, Canadian minister of national health and welfare, introduced the **health field concept.** In this view, all causes of death and disease have four contributing elements: (a) human biologic factors, such as genetic makeup and age; (b) behavioral factors or unhealthy life-styles; (c) environmental hazards; and (d) inadequacies in the health care system (Canadian Department of National Health and Welfare 1974, pp. 31—34). Using these four elements as a framework, a group of United States experts devised a method to assess the relative contributions of each of these elements to the ten leading causes of death in 1976. The results indicated that approximately 50% of deaths were due to unhealthy behavior or life-style; 20% to human biologic factors; 20% to environmental factors; and 10% to inadequacies in health care (U.S. DHEW 1979, p. 9). These results have implications for nursing; the most important is that a substantial number of deaths could be avoided by efforts directed at health promotion and illness prevention. The leading causes of death in the United States in 1986 are shown in Table 5–2 on page 88.

Traditionally, medical practitioners have dealt with disease at a subsystem level. Subsystems are those aspects of the body subsumed in the larger system of the whole body. (See systems theory in Chapter 4.) A subsystem may be a cell, an organ, or an organ system. Only recently have medical practitioners started looking at the person as an entity, or whole. Nurses, by contrast, have traditionally viewed the person as an entity, taking a holistic view of people. Nursing practice today is based on the multiple-causation theory of health problems. Unemployment, pollution, life-style, and

TABLE 5–2 *Leading Causes of Death in the United States in 1986*

Cause	Deaths per 100,000 Residents
Diseases of the heart	317.5
Malignant neoplasms	194.7
Cerebrovascular diseases	62.1
Accidents	39.5
Chronic obstructive pulmonary disease	31.8
Pneumonia and influenza	29.0
Diabetes mellitus	15.4
Suicide	12.8
Chronic liver disease and cirrhosis	10.9
Atherosclerosis	9.4
Homicide	9.0

Source: U.S. Center for Health Statistics, U.S. Bureau of the Census, *Monthly vital statistics report,* vol. 37, no. 6 supplement, in *Statistical abstract of the United States,* 109th ed. (Washington D.C.:U.S Government Printing Office, 1989), p. 79, Table 118.

ronment. Hettler proposes six dimensions of wellness (see Figure 5–2). The *physical dimension* encourages regular physical activity, cardiovascular flexibility and strength, knowledge about food and nutrition, medical self-care, and appropriate use of the medical system. It discourages excessive use of tobacco, drugs, and alcohol.

The *emotional dimension* focuses on the degree to which a person feels positive about the self and enthusiastic about life. It emphasizes awareness and acceptance of one's feelings, the capacity to manage one's feelings, the ability to cope effectively with stress, the ability to maintain satisfying relationships with others, and the assessment and acceptance of one's limitations. The *social dimension* focuses on the interdependence with others and nature, development of harmony in the family, and contribution to the welfare of the human and environmental community. The *intellectual dimension* encourages stimulating and creative mental activities and the use of available community resources to expand one's knowledge and increase the potential for sharing with others. The *occupational dimension* focuses on preparation for work that will produce personal satisfaction and enrichment of life. The *spiritual dimension* involves seeking meaning and purpose in human life.

stressful events, while not disease, may all contribute to illness. These can be considered suprasystem problems, i.e., problems stemming from systems in which the individual is a subsystem. See Figure 5–1. Thus, the concept of illness must include all aspects of the total person as well as the biologic and genetic factors that contribute to disease. Illness, then, is influenced by a person's family, social network, environment, and culture (Kneisl and Ames 1986, p. 18).

Wellness and Well-Being

Wellness Some people believe *wellness* and *health* are synonymous, while others believe they differ. Wellness is similar to actualization as defined in the eudaemonistic model of health. In 1959, Dunn differentiated good health from wellness: "Good health can exist as a relatively passive state of freedom from illness in which the individual is at peace with his environment—a condition of relative homeostasis. Wellness is an integrated method of functioning which is oriented toward maximizing the potential of which the individual is capable, within the environment where he is functioning" (Dunn 1959b, p. 4).

Wellness can also be defined as an "active process of becoming aware of and making choices toward a higher level of well-being" (Hettler, 1979). These choices are influenced by the individual's self-concept, culture, and envi-

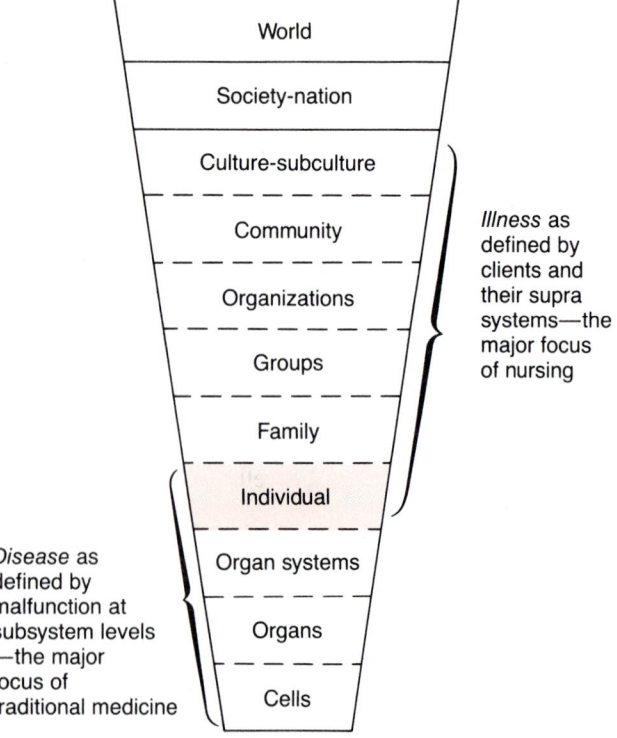

Figure 5–1 A systems hierarchy differentiating illness from disease and nursing from traditional medicine.
Source: Knopke, H. J., and Diekelmann, N. L., editors, *Approaches to teaching primary health care* (St. Louis: C. V. Mosby Co., 1981). St. Louis, Mosby © 1981. Used with permission.

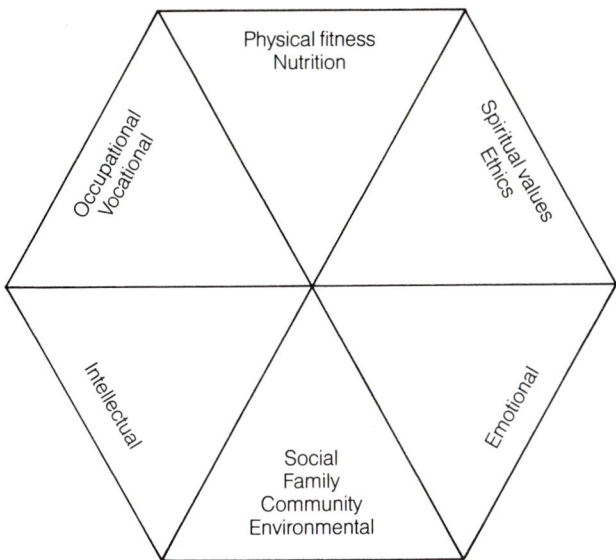

Figure 5–2 Six dimensions of wellness. *Source:* Bill Hettler, M.D., *Six dimensions of wellness* (Stevens Point, Wis.: National Wellness Institute, Inc., South Hall, 1319 Fremont Street, Stevens Point, WI 54481 (715) 346-2172). Used by permission.

Clark's concept of wellness includes both health and illness. She describes wellness (1986, p. 3) as a process of moving toward greater awareness of oneself and the environment; it is unique to the individual and purposeful in direction. Wellness, health, and illness are dynamic patterns, changing with time and social patterns. Therefore, they must be continuously reevaluated. Ill persons can experience wellness if they have joy in living or a purpose and appreciation of life. The wellness process can be pursued to prevent illness, to assist in rehabilitation, to enhance the quality of life, or to maximize one's potential (Murray and Zentner 1989, p. 570).

In his book about high-level wellness in the individual, Dunn (1973) explores the concept of wellness as it relates to family, community, environment, and society. He believes that family wellness enhances wellness in individuals. In a well family that offers trust, love, and support, the individual does not have to expend energy to meet basic needs and can move forward on the wellness continuum. By providing effective sanitation and safe water, disposing of sewage safely, and preserving beauty and wildlife, the community enhances both family and individual wellness. Environmental wellness is related to the premise that humans must be at peace with and guard the environment. Societal wellness is significant because the status of the larger social group affects the status of smaller groups. Dunn believes that social wellness must be considered on a worldwide basis.

Well-Being   **Well-being** is a subjective perception of balance, harmony, and vitality (Leddy and Pepper 1989, p. 207). According to Leddy and Pepper, well-being occurs in levels. At the highest levels, a person feels satisfaction and a sense of contributing; such persons might place their state of well-being at the top of a plus-3 scale. At the lowest levels, people see themselves as ill and may place their state of well-being at the bottom of a minus-3 scale. Leddy and Pepper also state that well-being is a state that can be described objectively and therefore can be measured. In contrast, health, which encompasses "well-being, illness, disease and nondisease is an evolving potential that cannot be quantified" (Leddy and Pepper 1989, p. 208).

The Health-Illness Continuum

Health and illness can be considered either as points along one continuum, as related but separate entities, or as separate entities. (A **continuum** is a grid or graduated scale.)

Dunn describes a health grid in which a health axis and an environmental axis intersect. The resulting quadrants represent degrees of health and wellness. See Figure 5–3. This grid is intended to demonstrate the interaction of the environment with the continuum from well-being to illness. Jahoda conceptualizes health and illness along separate but coexisting continua (see Figure 5–4 on page 90). The double continuum reflects the fact that people exhibit health and illness in varying degrees at the same time (Jahoda 1958, p. 75). This approach allows one to view a person's strengths (health) and illnesses at the same time.

The concept of wellness is related to health promotion (see Chapter 23), which places emphasis on the whole person and self-responsibility for health. Ryan and Travis (1981) incorporate this idea in their health-illness continuum ranging from high-level wellness to premature death. They

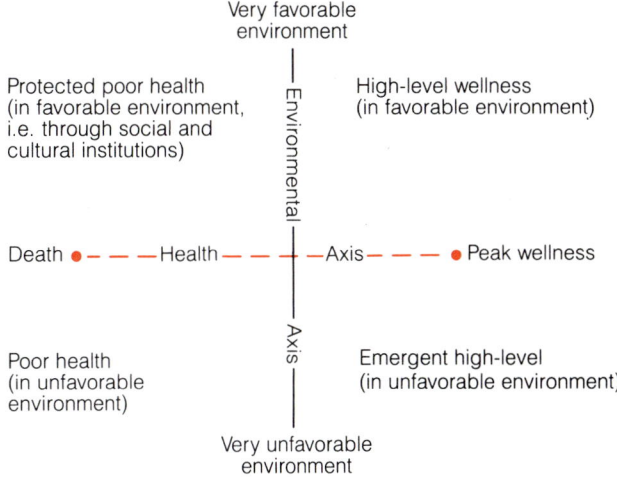

Figure 5–3 Dunn's health grid: its axes and quadrants. *Source:* H. L. Dunn, High-level wellness for man and society, *American Journal of Public Health,* June 1959, 49:788. Reprinted with permission.

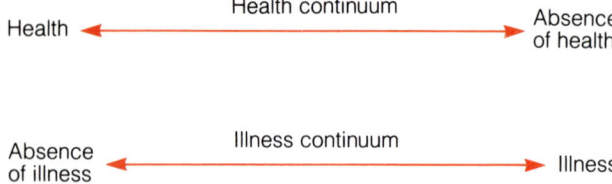

Figure 5–4 Jahoda's coexisting health and illness continua.

include a treatment model and a wellness model. See Figure 5–5.

HEALTH STATUS, BELIEFS, AND BEHAVIORS

The **health status** (state) of an individual is the health of that person at a given time. In its general meaning, the term may refer to anxiety, depression, or acute illness and thus describes the individual's problem in general. *Health status* can also describe such specifics as pulse rate and body temperature. The **health beliefs** of an individual are those concepts about health that an individual believes true. Such beliefs may or may not be founded on fact. Some of these are influenced by culture, such as the "hot-cold" system of some Hispanic Americans. In this system, health is viewed as a balance of hot and cold qualities within a person. Citrus fruits and some fowl are considered cold foods, and meats and bread are hot foods. In this context, hot and cold do not denote temperature or spiciness but innate qualities of the food. For example, a fever is said to be caused by an excess of hot foods. Another example of a culturally related health belief is the belief that health and illness are closely associated with the amount and quality of blood in the body. For example, among some Southern whites and blacks, "high blood," caused by too much blood in the body, causes headaches and dizziness (Mitchell and Loustau 1981, pp. 41–42). For additional information about ethnic views of health and illness, see Chapter 31.

Health behaviors are the actions people take to understand their health state, maintain an optimal state of health, prevent illness and injury, and reach their maximum physical and mental potential. Behaviors such as eating wisely, exercising, paying attention to signs of illness, following treatment advice, and avoiding known health hazards such as smoking are all examples. The ability to relax, emotional maturity, productivity, and self-expression also affect one's health (McCann/Flynn and Heffron 1988, pp. 37–38).

Individual health behaviors may or may not be recommended by health care professionals. For example, an individual who believes that drinking several bottles of beer each day keeps the intestines free of infection may refuse to accept advice against this practice, even in life-threatening situations.

Health behavior is intended to prevent illness or disease or to provide for early detection of disease. Nurses preparing a plan of care with an individual need to consider the person's health beliefs before they attempt to change health behaviors. Otherwise, the individual may reject the nurses' suggestions and become angry because of intrusion into personal habits.

Variables Affecting Health Status

Multiple variables influence a person's health status. Some of these are internal factors, such as the person's genetic makeup, and others are external, such as the person's culture and physical environment.

Genetic Makeup Genetic makeup influences biologic characteristics, innate temperament, activity level, and intellectual potential. It has been related to susceptibility to specific disease, such as diabetes and breast cancer.

Race Disease distribution is associated with race. For example, blacks have a higher incidence of sickle-cell anemia and hypertension than the general population, and native American Indians have a higher rate of diabetes.

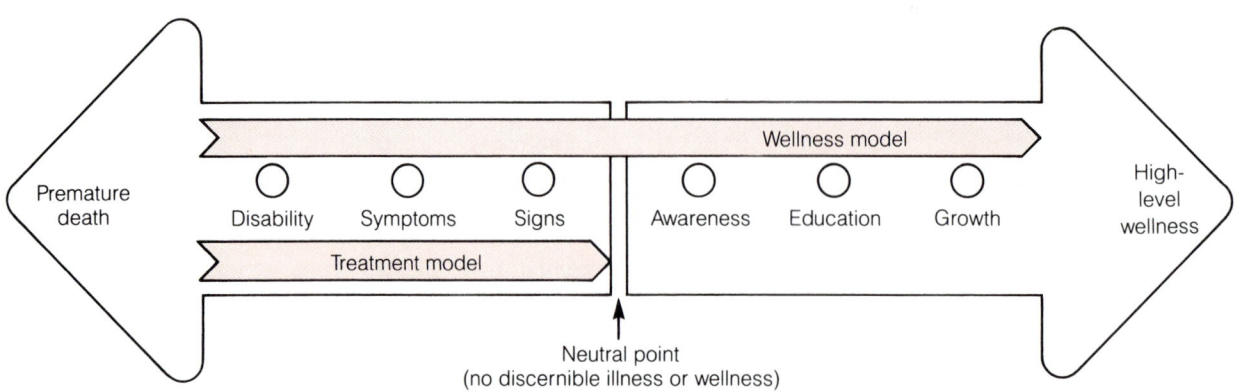

Figure 5–5 Health-illness continuum. *Source:* R. S. Ryan and J. W. Travis, *Wellness workbook for health professionals* (Berkeley, Calif.: Ten Speed Press, 1981). Used by permission.

Sex   Certain acquired and genetic diseases are more common in one sex than in the other. Disorders more common among females are osteoporosis; autoimmune disease, such as rheumatoid arthritis and systemic lupus erythematosus; anorexia nervosa and bulimia; gallbladder disease; obesity; and thyroid disease. Those more common among males are stomach ulcers, abdominal hernias, respiratory diseases, arteriosclerotic heart disease, hemorrhoids, and tuberculosis. Obviously, diseases that affect reproductive organs, such as testicular or uterine tumors, are sex dependent.

Age and Developmental Level   Distribution of disease varies with age. For example, arteriosclerotic heart disease is common in middle-aged males but occurs infrequently in younger persons; such communicable diseases as whooping cough and measles are common in children but are rare in older persons, who have acquired immunity to them. Developmental level is also a significant factor. Capabilities for responding to disease are less during the first few years of life and again near the end of life. Infants lack physiologic and psychologic maturity. Declining physical and sensory-perceptual abilities in older persons limit their ability to respond to environmental hazards and stressors.

Mind-Body Relationship   Mind-body relationships—i.e., how emotional responses to stress affect body function and what emotional reactions occur in response to body conditions—also influence health. Emotional distress may increase susceptibility to organic disease or precipitate it. Emotional distress may influence the immune system through central nervous system and endocrine alterations. Alterations in the immune system are related to the incidence of infections, cancer, and autoimmune diseases. Increasing attention is being given to the mind's ability to direct the body's functioning. Relaxation, meditation, and biofeedback techniques are gaining wider recognition by individuals and health care professionals.

Life-Style   A person's life-style includes patterns of eating; exercise; use of tobacco, drugs, and alcohol; and methods of coping with stress. Overeating, getting insufficient exercise, and being overweight are closely related to the incidence of heart disease, arteriosclerosis, diabetes, and hypertension. Excessive sugar intake increases the risk of dental caries. Abuse of drugs and alcohol is physically and mentally debilitating. Excessive use of tobacco is clearly implicated in lung cancer, emphysema, and cardiovascular diseases.

Physical Environment   The physical environment, including housing and sanitation facilities also affects health. Air, food, and water pollutants are often directly or indirectly related to various types of cancer. Extreme fluctuations in environmental temperature cause temporary disruptions in a person's internal environment, and the person in such an environment must expend more energy to restore physiologic stability. Persons with minimal physical coping responses are more susceptible to the effects of hypothermia and hyperthermia. Seasonal variations also affect health and the incidence of certain illnesses. For example, drownings and insect bites occur more frequently in the summer, whereas allergic reactions occur more frequently when pollen and related allergens are present.

Standards of Living   An individual's standard of living (reflecting occupation, income, and education) is related to health, morbidity, and mortality. Hygiene, food habits, and the propensity to seek health care advice and follow health regimens vary among high- and low-income groups. For example, preventing illness may not have as high a priority among the poor as generating and maintaining an income; even when it is a priority, the poor may not be able to afford regular medical examinations, housing, or nutritious foods that promote health. Occupational roles, also predispose people to certain illnesses. For instance, some industrial workers may be exposed to carcinogenic agents. More affluent people may fulfill stressful social or occupational roles that predispose them to stress-related diseases. Such roles may also encourage overeating or social use of drugs or alcohol.

Cultural Beliefs   How a person perceives, experiences, and copes with health and illness is partly determined by cultural beliefs. Some people may perceive home remedies or tribal health customs as superior and more dependable than the health care practices of North American society. Cultural rules, values, and beliefs give people a sense of being stable and able to predict outcomes. The challenging of old beliefs and values by second-generation ethnic groups may give rise to conflict, instability, and insecurity, in turn contributing to illness.

Family   In addition to transmitting genetic predispositions, the family passes on patterns of daily living and life-styles to offspring. Physical or emotional abuse may cause long-term health problems. Emotional health depends on a social environment that is free of excessive tension and does not isolate the person from others. A climate of open communication, sharing, and love fosters the fulfillment of the person's optimum potential.

Self-Concept   How a person feels about the self (the self concept) affects how that person perceives and handles situations. Such attitudes can affect health practices and the times when treatment is sought. A sense of extreme hopelessness, despair, or fear may cause disease and even death. An example is the anorexic woman who deprives herself of needed nutrients because she believes she is too fat even through she is well below an acceptable weight level.

Support Network and Job Satisfaction   Having a support network (family, friends, or a confidant) and job satisfaction helps people avoid illness (Grasser and Craft 1984, p. 210). Support people also help the person confirm that illness exists. Persons with inadequate support networks sometimes allow themselves to become increasingly ill before confirming the illness and seeking therapy. Support people also provide the stimulus for an ill person to become well again. Job satisfaction positively influences both the individual's self-concept and mind-body relationship.

Geography   Geography determines climate, and climate affects health. For instance, malaria and malaria-related conditions, e.g., sickle-cell hemoglobin, occur more frequently in tropical than temperate climates (Overfield 1985, p. 84). Multiple sclerosis is more prevalent in northern and central Europe, southern Canada, and the northern United States, for example, than in Asia, Africa, Mexico, and Alaska (Overfield 1985, p. 127).

Factors Influencing Health Behavior

Some factors affecting health status also affect health behavior; cultural and family influences are two examples. However, people can usually control their health behaviors and can choose healthy or unhealthy activities. In contrast, people have little or no choice over their genetic makeup, age, sex, physical environments, culture, or area of residence. This section outlines the factors that affect a person's health beliefs and behavior.

Health Belief Model   In the 1950s, Rosenstock (1974) proposed a **health belief model** (HBM) intended to predict which individuals would or would not use such preventive measures as screening for early detection of cancer. Becker (1974) modified the health belief model to include these components: *individual perceptions, modifying factors,* and *variables likely to affect initiating action.*

The health belief model is based on motivational theory. Rosenstock assumed that good health is an objective common to all people. Becker added "positive health motivation" as a consideration. See Figure 5–6.

Individual Perceptions   Individual perceptions include the following:

- *Perceived susceptibility.* A family history of a certain disorder, such as diabetes or heart disease, may make the individual feel at high risk.

- *Perceived seriousness.* The question here is: In the perception of the individual, does the illness cause death or have serious consequences? Growing concern about the spread of AIDS (acquired immune deficiency syndrome) reflects the general public's perception of the seriousness of this illness.

- *Perceived threat.* According to Becker, perceived susceptibility and perceived seriousness combine to determine the total perceived threat of an illness to a specific individual. For example, a person who perceives that many individuals in the community have AIDS may not necessarily perceive a threat of the disease; if the person is a

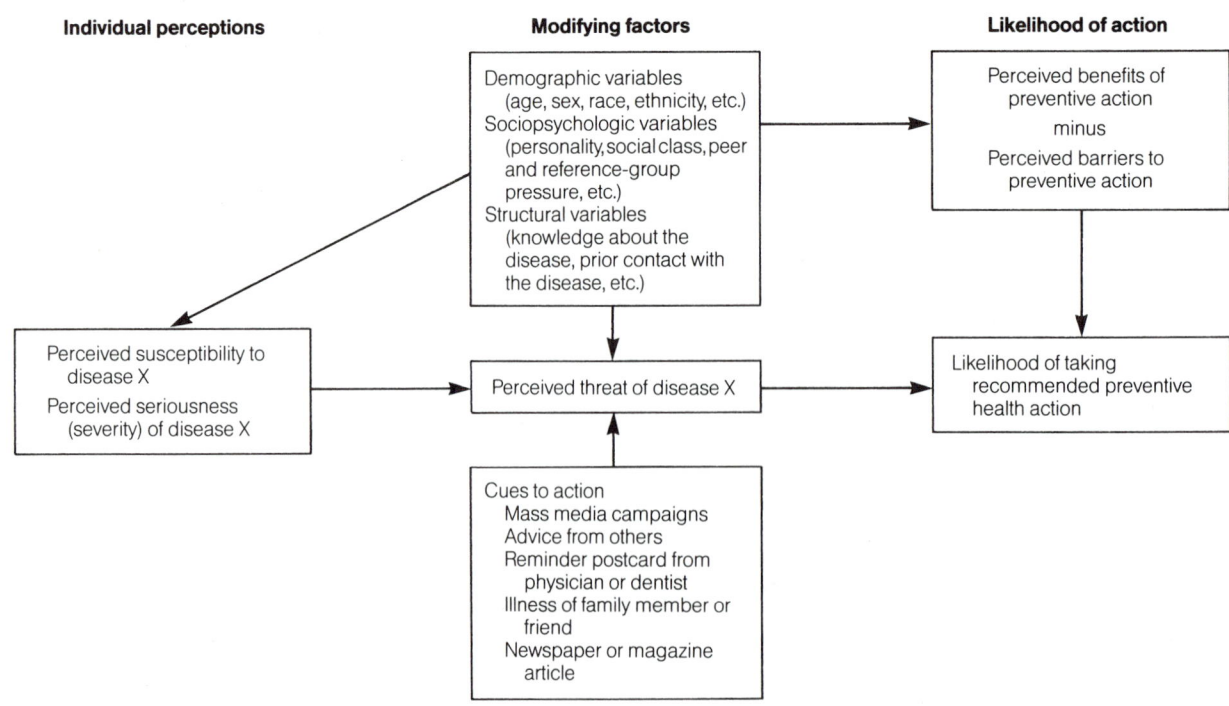

Figure 5–6   The health belief model.   *Source:*   From Becker, M. H., Haefner, D. P., Kasi, S. V. et al. Selected psychosocial models and correlates of individual health-related behaviors. *Medical Care* 1977. 15:27–46. Used with permission.

drug addict or a homosexual, however, the perceived threat of illness is likely to increase because of the combined susceptibility and seriousness.

Modifying Factors

Factors that modify a person's perceptions include the following:

- *Demographic variables* such as age, sex, race, ethnicity, etc. An infant, for example, does not perceive the importance of a healthy diet; an adolescent may perceive peer approval as more important than family approval and participate as a consequence in hazardous activities or adopt unhealthy eating and sleeping patterns; some ethnic groups consider it inappropriate to seek medical advice unless one is seriously ill.

- *Sociopsychologic variables.* Social pressure or influence from peers or other reference groups (e.g., self-help or vocational groups) may encourage preventive health behaviors even when individual motivation is low. Expectations of others may motivate people, for example, to obtain immunizations for their children, not to drive an automobile after drinking alcohol, to attend dental clinics, and to perform techniques such as breast self-examination for the early detection of cancer.

- *Structural variables* presumed to influence preventive behavior are knowledge about the target disease and prior contact with it. Becker found higher compliance rates with prescribed treatments among mothers whose children had frequent ear infections and occurrences of asthma.

- *Cues to action.* Cues can be either internal or external. Internal cues include feelings of fatigue, uncomfortable symptoms, or thoughts about the condition of an ill person who is close. External cues are listed in Figure 5–6.

Likelihood of Action

The likelihood of a person taking recommended preventive health action depends on the perceived benefits of the action minus the perceived barriers to the action.

- *Perceived benefits of preventive action.* Examples include refraining from smoking to prevent lung cancer and to increase ventilatory capacity; eating nutritious foods and avoiding snacks to maintain slenderness.

- *Perceived barriers to action* can include cost, inconvenience, unpleasantness, and life-style changes.

Pender (1975) adds two further considerations: The importance of health as perceived by the individual and perceived control.

1. *The importance of health to the person.* Behavior indicating that health is perceived as something of value includes providing special foods and vitamins to keep children well, having regular dental checkups, and participating in screening tests for cervical cancer, breast cancer, and cardiovascular disorders.

2. *Perceived control.* People who perceive that they have control over their own health are more likely to use preventive services than people who feel powerless. Control over health can relate to such behaviors as not smoking, maintaining an appropriate weight, using seat belts, or obtaining immunizations for influenza.

Nurses play a major role in helping clients implement healthy behaviors. Nurses help clients monitor health, supply anticipatory guidance, and impart knowledge about health. Nurses can also reduce barriers to action, e.g., by minimizing inconvenience or discomfort, and can support preventive actions. For additional information about nursing activities that promote health and instruments to assess perceptions of health control, see Chapter 23.

Health Care Compliance

Compliance is the extent to which a person's behavior coincides with health practitioners' advice. Clients' compliance with health care advice is of concern to all health professionals. Yoos reports that 86% of studies of compliance report noncompliance in more than 30% of clients (Yoos 1981, p. 27). Compliance can be complete, partial, or nonexistent.

Whether a person complies to a therapeutic regimen depends on many variables, among them age, education, costs, the complexity of the regimen and its convenience, the individual's value of health, and the inconvenience of the illness itself. In 1974, Becker published a sick role model to explain how people react to illness and to predict whether they will comply with health care advice (Becker 1974). See Figure 5–7. Becker's model indicates that compliance is related to (a) the client's motivation to become well, (b) the value the client places on reducing the threat of illness, and (c) the client's belief that compliance will reduce that threat. Modifying and enabling factors of people's behavior include age, cost, duration, attitudes of health care personnel, interaction with health care personnel, previous health care experiences, and sources of advice.

Researchers have investigated why some people comply with therapeutic regimens and others do not and how to help clients comply with therapeutic regimens. The first step is identifying noncompliance. The nurse can ask the client if the regimen is being followed. If the client is not complying, the nurse needs to find out why and intervene to assist the client in complying. To enhance compliance, nurses can do the following:

- *Demonstrate caring.* The nurse can do so by showing sincere concern about the client's problems and decisions and at the same time accepting the client's right to a course of action. For example, a nurse might tell a client who is not taking his heart medication, "I can appreciate how you feel about this, but I am very concerned about your heart."

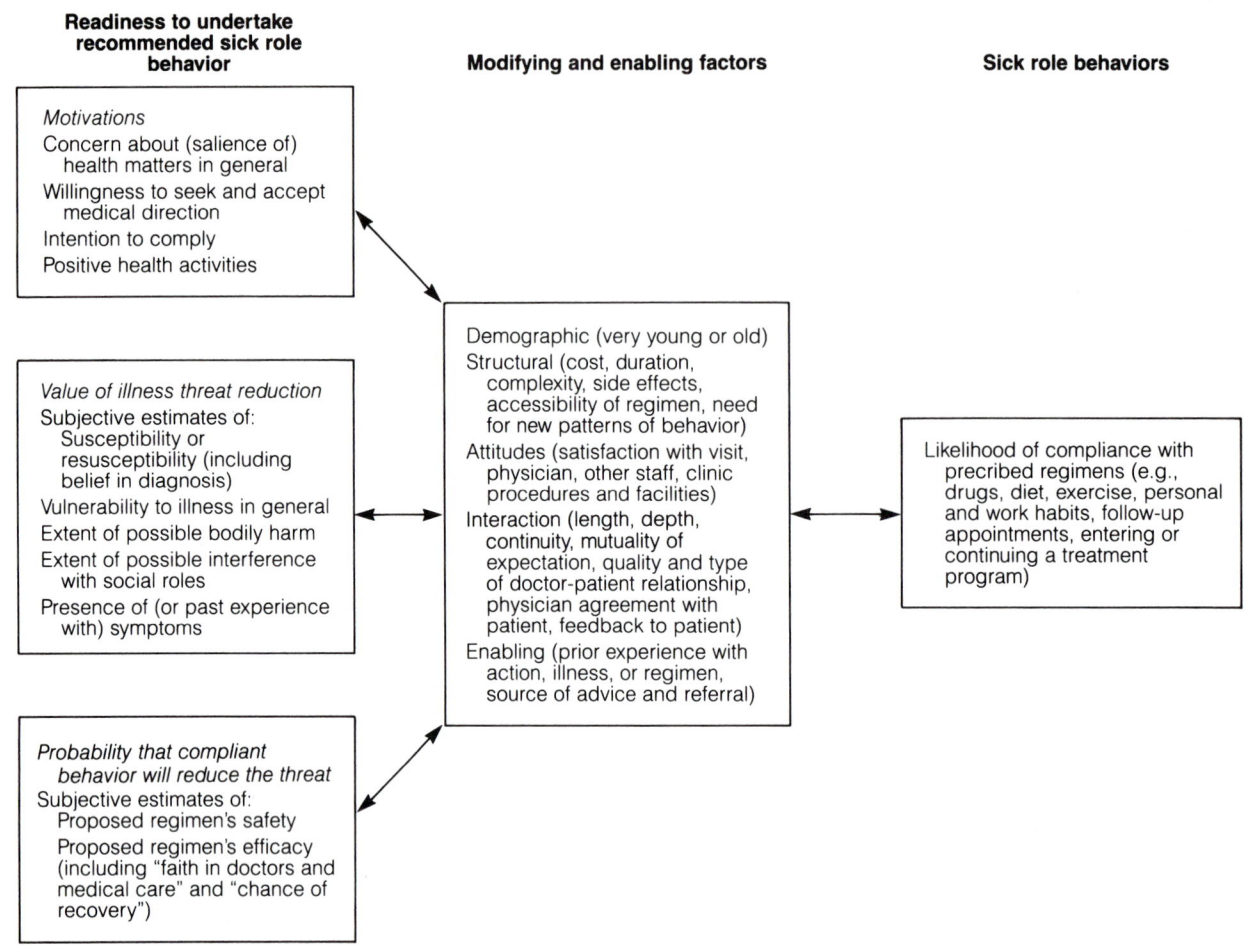

Readiness to undertake recommended sick role behavior

Motivations
Concern about (salience of) health matters in general
Willingness to seek and accept medical direction
Intention to comply
Positive health activities

Value of illness threat reduction
Subjective estimates of:
Susceptibility or resusceptibility (including belief in diagnosis)
Vulnerability to illness in general
Extent of possible bodily harm
Extent of possible interference with social roles
Presence of (or past experience with) symptoms

Probability that compliant behavior will reduce the threat
Subjective estimates of:
Proposed regimen's safety
Proposed regimen's efficacy (including "faith in doctors and medical care" and "chance of recovery")

Modifying and enabling factors

Demographic (very young or old)
Structural (cost, duration, complexity, side effects, accessibility of regimen, need for new patterns of behavior)
Attitudes (satisfaction with visit, physician, other staff, clinic procedures and facilities)
Interaction (length, depth, continuity, mutuality of expectation, quality and type of doctor-patient relationship, physician agreement with patient, feedback to patient)
Enabling (prior experience with action, illness, or regimen, source of advice and referral)

Sick role behaviors

Likelihood of compliance with precribed regimens (e.g., drugs, diet, exercise, personal and work habits, follow-up appointments, entering or continuing a treatment program)

Figure 5–7 Sick role model. *Source:* Modified from M. H. Becker, The health belief model and sick role behavior, in M. H. Becker, editor, *The health belief model and personal health behavior* (Thorofare, N.J.: Charles B. Slack, 1974). Reprinted with permission.

- *Encourage healthy behaviors through positive reinforcement.* If the man who is not taking his heart medication is walking every day, the nurse might say, "You are really doing well with your walking."

- *Establish why the client is not following the regimen.* Where indicated, the nurse can provide information, correct misconceptions, attempt to decrease expense, or suggest counseling if psychologic problems are interfering with compliance.

- *Use aids to reinforce teaching.* For instance, the nurse can leave pamphlets for the client to read later or make a "pill calendar," a paper with the date and number of pills to be taken.

- *Establish a therapeutic relationship of freedom, mutual understanding, and mutual responsibility with the client and support persons.* By providing knowledge, skills, and information, the nurse gives clients control over their health and establishes a cooperative relationship, which results in greater compliance (MacElveen-Hoehn 1983, p. 535).

ILLNESS BEHAVIORS

Various scientists have described the stages of illness. By knowing these stages and the illness behaviors that accompany them, nurses can better understand their clients' behavior and determine ways to assist them. **Illness behavior** is "any activity undertaken by a person who feels ill, to define the state of his health and to discover a suitable remedy" (Igun 1979, p. 445). How people behave when they are ill is affected by many variables, such as age, sex, occupation, socioeconomic status, religion, ethnic origin, psychologic stability, personality, education and modes of coping. Suchman (1972, p. 145) describes five stages of illness:

Symptom Experience Stage   The symptom experience stage is the transition stage during which people come to believe something is wrong. Either a significant person mentions that they look unwell, or people experience some symptoms, which can appear insidiously. The symptom experience stage has three aspects:

- The physical experience of symptoms (e.g., pain or elevated temperature)
- The cognitive aspect (the interpretation of the symptoms in terms that have some meaning to the person)
- The emotional response (e.g., fear or anxiety)

During this stage, unwell persons usually consult others close to them about their symptoms or feelings. People validate with their spouses or support persons that the symptoms are real. At this stage, sick persons sometimes try home remedies, such as laxatives or cough medicines.

Assumption of the Sick Role

The second stage signals acceptance of the illness. At this time, individuals decide that their symptoms or concerns are sufficiently severe to suggest that they are sick. Some people seek professional help quickly; others continue self-treatment, often following the suggestions of family and friends.

In this stage, sick people are usually afraid, but they now accept that they are ill even though they may not be able to accept the possible reasons. In conferring with people close to them, sick people seek not only advice but also support for the decision to give up some activities and, for example, stay home from work.

At the end of this stage, sick people experience one of two outcomes. They may find that the symptoms have changed and that they feel better. If family members support the perceptions of such persons, they are no longer considered or consider themselves sick. Then the recovered persons resume normal obligations, such as returning to work or attending a school concert.

If, however, the symptoms persist or increase and if lack of improvement is validated by the family or significant others, then sick people know they should seek some treatment. The choice of a treatment plan is often affected by the known available alternatives and previous experience.

Medical Care Contact Stage

Sick people seek the advice of a health professional either on their own initiative or at the urging of significant others. When people go for professional advice they are really asking for three types of information:

- Validation of real illness
- Explanation of the symptoms in understandable terms
- Reassurance that they will be all right or prediction of what the outcome will be

If the health professional does not validate illness, people have two recourses: to return to normal activities or to seek other advice. If the symptoms disappear, people often per-ceive that they really are not ill. If symptoms continue, people usually return to the health professional or go to a second person for care. People who are repeatedly told that they are not ill may seek out quasi-practitioners as a last resort to alleviate the perceived symptoms. Some people will go from health professional to health professional until they find someone who provides a diagnosis that fits their own perceptions.

Most people also want an understandable explanation of their symptoms. When symptoms are not explained, people may assume the health professional does not believe them or perhaps that they are imagining the symptoms. Overly technical explanations, however, often confuse and frighten people.

People often experience anxiety about seeking help with health problems. Even minor symptoms can be construed as serious. Therefore, clients need reassurance that they will be cured. Even when this reassurance cannot be given, most people want to know the likely outcome.

Dependent Patient Role Stage

When a health professional has validated that the person is ill, the individual becomes a client, dependent on the professional for help. During this stage, sick people may or may not be reluctant to accept a professional's recommendations. They may vacillate about what is best for them and alternately accept and reject the professional's suggestions. People vary greatly in the degree of ease with which they can give up their independence, particularly in relation to life and death. Role obligations—such as those of wage earner, father, mother, student, baseball team member, or choir member—complicate the decision to give up independence.

It is also common for the client and the health professional to hold different notions of the nature of the illness, unless complete and open communication exists. During this stage, a nurse can often provide information that may allay some fears and/or provide data that support the person. Misconceptions can result from limited information, which clients interpret in the light of their experiences. For example, a woman may be told by a physician that there is a small encapsulated growth in the right groin and that surgical removal is advised. If the woman's mother died after being told she had a growth in her breast, that person may assume that she also will die.

Most people accept their dependence on the physician, although they retain varying degrees of control over their own lives. For example, some people request precise information about their diseases, their treatment, and the cost of treatment, and they delay the decision to accept treatment until they have all this information. Others prefer that the physician proceed with treatment and do not request additional information.

During this period, sick people often become more passive and accepting. They require a predictable environment in which people are genuinely concerned about them. In addition to being concerned about themselves, some sick people regress to an earlier behavioral stage in their development. As a result, they may have fewer coping mechanisms (physical and emotional adaptive or defensive abilities). Frequently reactions are related to previous experiences and to misconceptions about what will happen.

People have varying dependence needs. For some, illness may meet dependence needs that have never been met and thus provide satisfaction. Other people have minimal dependence needs and do everything possible to return to independent functioning. A few may even try to maintain independence to the detriment of their recovery.

Recovery or Rehabilitation Stage
During the fifth stage, the client learns to give up the sick role and return to former roles and functions. For people with acute illnesses, the time as an ill person is generally short, and recovery is usually rapid. Thus, most find it relatively easy to return to their former life-styles. People who have long-term illnesses and who must make adjustments in life-style may find recovery more difficult. Recovery is particularly difficult for people who have to relearn skills such as walking or talking.

During this stage, readiness for social functioning may not coincide with physical readiness. People may be physically able to go out to dinner but find that functioning socially is still too stressful or they may find that they have the *desire* to perform activities but not the strength. Nurses can help clients function with increasing independence by planning with them those functions they can accomplish by themselves and those with which they need assistance. It is also important for nurses to convey an attitude of hope and to support the client's return to health.

Sick Role Behavior

Sick role behavior is "the activity undertaken by those who consider themselves ill, for the purpose of getting well" (Igun 1979, p. 455). Parsons (1972, pp. 436–37) describes four aspects of the sick role:

1. Clients are not held responsible for their condition.
2. Clients are excused from certain social roles and tasks.
3. Clients are obliged to try to get well as quickly as possible.
4. Clients or their families are obliged to seek competent help.

Many North Americans believe that illness, though undesirable, is beyond a person's control and that individuals are not responsible for incurring an illness. Some subcultures view illness as punishment from God, and therefore consider the infirm responsible for their illnesses, because of their sins. This folk belief persists to some degree in American society. A client may say something like, "What have I done to deserve this?" This remark reflects a sense that illness is a punishment. Today, because of the recog-

nition that life-style contributes to illness and disease, some people—for example, the cardiac client who smokes or the overweight person who develops diabetes—are being held increasingly responsible for developing some illnesses.

Nurses can help clients by providing factual information and by not judging the client. It is important to encourage behaviors that promote health and not to reinforce behaviors that may have helped bring about an illness.

The sick person is usually excused from some normal duties. Social pressures on the sick and people's expectations of the sick usually depend on the prognosis and the severity of the illness. People who are severely ill and whose prognosis is poor or uncertain are permitted more dependence than people who are less seriously ill. People who are not seriously ill and whose prognosis is good are more likely to be encouraged to fulfill personal and social responsibilities. The person with a cold may still be expected to give a scheduled speech or to take an examination. People who are chronically ill may be permanently exempted from some duties or activities by society.

Some people may express feelings of guilt because they are unable to fulfill their normal responsibilities. Nurses can express support to clients who cannot fulfill their perceived roles and help them substitute other appropriate activities, when desirable. For example, a young father who cannot play ball with his son may be able to help his son build a model airplane, thereby fulfilling the father's role in another way.

Another aspect of the sick role is the obligation of the person to get well as quickly as possible. The sick role is a dependent one, at least in some respects. The person who fears dependence may be threatened by assuming a sick role and having to seek help. This individual might ignore advice despite the most serious consequences. Some people, however, find dependence gratifying. Some clients find dependence so satisfying that they perpetuate the sick role and do not try to get well or continue to complain of symptoms even after they are physically well. Some people in the dependent stage also find it satisfying to control others through excessive demands. With exceptions, people usually try to get well as quickly as possible.

Nurses can help clients assume a dependence appropriate to their developmental status and health. Part of the nurse's function is to reinforce both dependence and increasing independence at the appropriate times. For example, a man who is acutely ill may have to be shaved by the nurse; however, once he is stronger the nurse can assist him by providing shaving supplies and later complimenting him on his appearance.

An essential aspect of the sick role is seeking competent help. This presupposes that competent help is available to the client. It should also be recognized that the client's notion of competent help may be different from the general population's. For example, a man with a whiplash injury may become dissatisfied with his physician's treatment because of his slow recovery and may go to a healer who uses hypnotism. Or a domineering, talkative woman may reject advice to see a therapist and decide instead to join a cult of young people, considering the members of the cult competent help.

Nurses need to encourage some people to obtain competent help from health professionals. Nurses who are aware of the health facilities available in a community can assist people to obtain care. People may require considerable support before seeking assistance because, for example, they fear the health problem might be serious or they believe competent help might not be available. A nurse's function in these instances is to provide accurate information about available health facilities while recognizing clients' beliefs and their right to hold them.

Effects of Hospitalizaton

Normal patterns of behavior generally change with illness; with hospitalization, the change can be even greater. Hospitalization usually disrupts a person's privacy, autonomy, life-style, roles, and finances.

Loss of Privacy
When a client enters a hospital or nursing facility, the loss of privacy is instantly obvious. **Privacy** has been described as a comfortable feeling reflecting a deserved degree of social retreat. Its dimensions and duration are controlled by the individual seeking the privacy. It is a personal internal state that cannot be imposed from without (Schuster 1976, p. 245).

People need varying degrees of privacy and establish boundaries for privacy; when these boundaries are crossed, they feel invaded. Hospital personnel sometimes show little concern for clients' privacy. Clients are asked to provide information that often they consider private; they may share a room with strangers; and their health is frequently discussed with many health professionals.

The boundaries of privacy are highly individual. The adult who lives alone may be used to privacy while eating, sleeping, and reading. A child from a large family may be accustomed to sharing these activities with others. It is important for nurses to ascertain what privacy means to the individual and try to support accustomed practices whenever possible. See also the discussion of Territoriality in Chapter 15, page 253.

Altered Autonomy
Autonomy is the state of being independent and self-directed without outside control. People vary in their sense of autonomy; some are accustomed to functioning independently in most of their life activities, while others are more accustomed to direction from others. An example of the former is a writer who lives alone and works independently. By contrast, a wife in a patriarchal home may be accustomed to having decisions made by her husband and receiving direction from him.

Hospitalized people frequently give up much of their autonomy. Decisions about meals, hygienic practices, and sleeping are frequently made for them. This loss of individuality is often difficult to accept, and the client may feel dehumanized into "just a piece of machinery." Nurses have a major responsibility to humanize care by learning about the client as a person and by individualizing nursing care plans.

Altered Life-Style
Hospitalization marks a change in life-style. Many hospitals determine when people wake up and when they sleep. The woman who normally rises at 8:00 A.M. and the man who usually works until 11:00 P.M. must change their habits. Food in a hospital is usually mass produced, and individual differences in taste are not always accommodated. Occasionally hospitals have relatively large populations from a particular culture and make special food arrangements, for example, a Chinese menu for traditional Chinese clients or Kosher foods for traditional Jewish clients. However, individual preferences are not always met.

Nurses can help clients adapt to life in a hospital in several ways:

■ Providing explanations about hospital routines

■ Making arrangements wherever possible to accommodate the client's life-style, such as providing a bath in the evening rather than in the morning

■ Encouraging other health professionals to become aware of the person's life-style and to support healthy aspects of that life-style

■ Reinforcing desirable changes in practices with a view to making them a permanent part of the client's lifestyle

Economic Burden
Hospitalization often places a genuine financial burden on clients and their families. Even though many people have health insurance, it may not reimburse all costs; in addition, many lose wages while they are hospitalized. Nurses can be aware of these costs and provide care that is as economical as is safely possible; for instance, they can use only the minimum supplies necessary for safe care. In some agencies, nurses may initiate referrals to the social service department to assist clients in making arrangements to address the financial burdens imposed by hospitalization. When this is not an independent nursing function, the nurse should consult with the client's physician to obtain such a referral.

Effects of Illness on Family Members

A person's illness affects not only the person who is ill but also the family or significant others. The kind of effect and its extent depend chiefly on three factors: (a) which member of the family is ill, (b) how serious and long the illness is, and (c) what cultural and social customs that family follows.

The changes that can occur in the family include the following:

■ Role changes

- Task reassignments
- Increased stress due to anxiety about the outcome of the illness for the client and conflict about unaccustomed responsibilities
- Financial problems
- Loneliness as a result of separation and pending loss
- Change in social customs

Each member of the family is affected differently depending upon which member of the family is ill, because each plays a different role in the family and supports the family in different ways. Parents of young children, for example, have greater family responsibilities than parents of grown children.

The degree of change that family members experience is often related to their dependence on the sick person. For example, when a child is ill, there are few changes other than added responsibilities directly related to the child's illness. When the mother is ill, however, many changes are often necessary because other family members must assume her functions.

Sick Elderly Persons   When an elderly person is ill, a son or daughter often assumes the role of parent to the elderly person, providing housing, meals, and assistance with daily needs over a prolonged time. In other words, the parent-child roles are frequently reversed. This role reversal may be only temporary and may end when the illness ends, or it may become permanent.

The whole family, particularly the spouse of the sick person, experiences stress and concern about the outcome of the illness. Usually, the sick person's spouse feels a pending loss or separation most keenly. After a marriage of 50 or 60 years, elderly people may find it difficult to envisage what life will be like without a husband or wife. Younger persons in the family may deal with serious illness in an elderly person by stating, "He has led a good life" or "She had so much pain the past years." In this way, the young prepare themselves for that person's death. This same reasoning is rarely applied to a child or younger adult who is ill.

When an elderly person is ill, adult sons and daughters may face conflicting responsibilities. A daughter who lives some distance away needs to maintain her job and look after her own family, but at the same time her parents need her in another city. How often should she visit? How should she fulfill her responsibilities? These questions pose problems for many families today who live far apart.

The financial problems of the sick elderly can be a major problem for a family as well as a community. Because illness in this age group tends to be chronic, the costs of illness are often considerable. The greatest change in life-style is that the family must now allot time for hospital visits to the elderly relative.

Sick Parents   When the sick person is a parent, the degree to which the family experiences change is related to the responsibilities the individual has and the number and age of dependents in the person's care. For example, when a father is ill for a long time, his roles are usually taken over by other members of the family, frequently the mother. Such tasks as doing chores in the house or attending a child's basketball games, for example, are either reassigned or not performed at all. Anxiety of family members about the outcome of a parent's illness is usually high, especially if the parent is a wage earner. The implications to the family of prolonged illness or death are great in almost all areas of living because of the needs of the dependents.

Prolonged illness of the mother can have equally serious consequences. Often the children do not understand why their mother is in the hospital, and they may feel lonely and unwanted. Sometimes the mother's functions are taken over by grandparents or by aunts and uncles as well as by the father. When a young mother has a serious illness of unknown outcome, the father and family face worrisome problems of how to manage over a long period of time. Most arrangements have financial implications and involve role changes for the father and children. In this situation, the father must become both father and mother and give up many of his normal social activities. The children may also need to assume more housekeeping functions.

Sick Children   Because a child is dependent on parents for so many daily needs, both sick children and their families may need to make fewer role adjustments than sick adults and their families. Task reassignments are also generally minimal. Sometimes a younger sibling takes over a paper route for a sick brother or sister, and other members of the family share the sick child's chores.

However, all members of the family experience anxiety if the outcome of the child's illness is in doubt. A permanent disability has implications for schooling, earning a living, and future needs. Financial responsibility for chronic illness or a disability often can be a serious problem for young parents. Other children may feel neglected if an unusual amount of attention is given to the ill child. Husband and wife may also expend most of their energies visiting the hospital and have little time for each other. If extended, this situation can place great stress on a marriage.

When a child is admitted to the hospital, parents and siblings may experience some sense of loss; however, children usually continue with their daily activities, and there frequently is minimal disruption in the home.

CURRENT HEALTH TRENDS

The health of North Americans is steadily improving. Probable reasons for this improvement include the following:

- Earlier preventive efforts based on new knowledge obtained through research.

- Improvements in sanitation, housing, nutrition, and immunization essential to disease prevention.
- Individual measures to promote health and prevent disease. For example, increasing attention is being paid to exercise, nutrition, environmental health, and occupational health.

Trends

Evidence of current health status and changes in the last few decades are measured in various ways. Measurements are made of the type of health behavior people practice; longevity (life expectancy); mortality rates and causes; morbidity rates and causes; and the amount and kind of health services used.

The following facts and statistics are derived from *Statistical Abstract of the United States,* 109th ed. (U.S. Bureau of the Census 1989) unless otherwise indicated.

Health Behaviors   The number of cigarette smokers in America has declined since 1964, when the Surgeon General's first *Report on Smoking and Health* was released. The sharp rise in smoking among teenage females that occurred in the 1970s has been curbed. However, the ratio of male to female smokers was about equal in 1983, whereas in 1965 male smokers outnumbered female smokers by 150%. In addition, among people who smoke, the percent who smoke 25 or more cigarettes per day has been increasing (U.S. DHHS 1985, p. 17).

Dietary practices, especially those related to the consumption of saturated fats, have had notable effects on the health of people. Over the past 20 years, the mean serum cholesterol level of adults aged 20 to 74 years has declined for every age group for both men and women. High serum cholesterol levels are associated with heart attacks and strokes. Another indicator of positive health behavior relates to hypertension control. The proportion of people with hypertension who kept their blood pressure below the level of 160/95 mm Hg nearly doubled from 1960–1962 to 1976–1980. This is thought to be due in part to adherence to prescribed medication regimens (U.S. DHHS 1985, p. 18). See also Tables 5–3 and 5–4.

Longevity   In 1950, life expectancy at birth for males was 65.6 years and for females 71.1 years. By 1987, it had reached 71.5 years for males and 78.3 years for females, an increase of 5 to 7 years. Differences, however, exist between white and black people; the life expectancy for blacks is 4 to 6 years less. In 1987, life expectancy for black males was only 65.4 years and for black females 73.8 years.

Mortality   The infant **mortality** (death) rate has declined by over 50% since 1960. In 1986, the rate fell to 10.4 per 1000 live births from 26.0 per 1000 in 1960. This decline is attributed largely to advances in medical science related to newborn treatment, improved socioeconomic conditions, and increased availability of maternal and infant care services. Infant mortality rates, however, are still relatively high for certain groups; rates are higher for black babies and babies of unmarried mothers, teenage mothers, and mothers over 35 years of age.

The major causes of death in infants during the first 6 days of life are immaturity (low birth weights) and birth-associated events, such as lack of oxygen. Among infants 1 year and younger, the three most important causes of death are congenital malformations, sudden infant death syndrome, and respiratory distress syndrome.

Major causes of death in the general population were shown earlier in Table 5–2. By age group, accidents are the leading cause for people up to age 35 years. Suicide is another major cause for people over age 15, and malignant neoplasms become a significant factor after age 25 years. From the years of 35 to 55 years, major causes of death are (in

TABLE 5–3   *Health Behaviors of People Over 18 Years (1985)*

Behavior	Percentage of Population
Current smokers	30.1
Have 5 or more alcoholic drinks per day	37.5
Obese (30% or more above desirable weight)	13.0
Less physically active than contemporaries	16.4
Never eat breakfast	24.3
Snack every day	39.0
Sleep 6 hours or less	22.0

Source: U.S. National Center for Health Statistics, U.S. Bureau of the Census, *Health promotion and disease prevention,* United States 1985 series 10, no. 163, In *Statistical abstract of the United States,* 109th ed. (Washington D.C.: U.S. Government Printing Office, 1989), p. 118, Table 190.

TABLE 5–4   *Percentage of Women Who Performed or Obtained Breast Self-Exam and Pap Smear in 1985*

Knew how to do it	87.0
Did at least 12 times per year	37.3
Had breast exam within past year	50.3
Had Pap smear within past year	45.6

Source: U.S. Bureau of the Census, *Statistical Abstract of the United States,* 109th ed. (Washington D.C.:U.S. Government Printing Office, 1989), p. 117, Table 189.

descending order); malignant neoplasms, diseases of the heart, and accidents. Over age 55 years, malignant neoplasms remain a major cause, but at age 65, heart disease becomes the primary cause. After age 65 years cerebrovascular disease becomes prominent as a major cause of death.

Morbidity   **Morbidity** means illness; the morbidity rate is the ratio of sick to well people in a population. Morbidity statistics are more difficult to obtain than mortality statistics. Two ways to measure the illness of children is to determine (a) absenteeism from school and (b) changes in average heights and weights, since growth is characteristic of healthy, well-fed children. The number of school days lost because of acute illnesses was about the same in the early 1980s as it was in the early 1960s. Influenza outbreaks account for one-third of all absences from school. Little change occurred in the heights and weights of boys and girls 6 to 17 years of age from 1960 onward. A growing concern about the physical and mental health of children today is the growing divorce rate. Increasing numbers of children are involved in divorce.

The health of adults can be measured by considering the days of work lost, bed-disability days, and restricted-activity days. The rates of absenteeism from work declined for both men and women since the mid 1970s, but women had higher absenteeism rates than men. The rate of restricted-activity days increased since the late 1960s, and there has been a slight increase in bed-disability days. Because this increase correlates with increased physician utilization, the increase may reflect earlier detection of illness and better health management. Many people may be limiting their activities at the onset of illness to prevent more serious health consequences (U.S. DHHS 1985, p. 7).

In midlife and later life, illness, disability, and impairment pose more problems. Of the three leading causes of death in later life—heart disease, cancer, and stroke—the rate of death from strokes declined 60% and the rate of death from heart disease 36% from 1960 to 1982. However, rates of death from cancer increased about 11%. Respiratory cancer was a major factor in the increased cancer death rates.

Implications for Nursing

As nurses assume an increasingly more visible role in providing health care services, it is helpful to consider the trends and behaviors noted above and to structure nursing services to ensure:

- Increased prenatal maternal and infant care services to reduce factors contributing to low birth weight, such as inadequate nutrition, smoking, and alcohol consumption. Services are especially required for black mothers, teenage mothers, mothers over 35 years of age, and the babies of these mothers.

- Early identification of problems that deprive the fetus of oxygen during labor and delivery, or prompt management of such problems when they do occur.

- Instruction in accident prevention to people of all ages.

- Maintenance of immunization programs to prevent infectious diseases.

- Promotion of measures to ensure optimal childhood development.

- Increased emphasis on supportive emotional care for children of divorced parents.

- Instruction to young adults about motor vehicle safety.

- Improved screening programs to assist in the early identification of disease.

- Improvement in life-styles to help individuals avoid major risk factors responsible for disease.

- Improvement in the health of adolescents and young adults; their physical, psychologic, and social attitudes; and their health habits to prevent later susceptibility to chronic diseases.

- Education to help youths acquire skills and information to prevent pregnancy, alcohol and drug abuse, and sexually transmitted diseases.

- Concerted efforts to reduce respiratory cancer rates by assisting people, especially women between 54 and 64 years of age and teenagers, to stop smoking.

- Increased assistance to help the elderly population with self-care and home management.

- Guidance to help all people acquire early treatment for illness and comply with therapy.

- Attention to occupational and environmental hazards.

CHAPTER HIGHLIGHTS

▶ The perspective from which health is viewed has changed; instead of absence of disease, health has come to mean a high level of wellness or the fulfillment of one's maximum potential for physical, psychosocial, and spiritual functioning.

▶ Models developed to explain health include the clinical, ecologic, role performance, adaptive, and eudaemonistic models.

▶ Because notions of health are highly individual, the

▶

nurse must determine each client's perception of health in order to provide meaningful assistance. Nurses too should be aware of their own personal definitions of health.

▶ Each person's concept of health is molded by social and cultural influences, previous experiences, expectations of self, and perceptions of self.

▶ Illness, sickness, and disease all have different meanings. Illness and sickness are usually associated with disease but may occur independently of it.

▶ The single-causation theory of disease is being replaced by a multiple-causation theory. For many diseases, the cause is still unknown.

▶ Five categories of risk factors that predispose individuals to illness and disease are genetic, age, physiologic, life-style, and environment.

▶ Marc Lalonde's *health field concept* views all causes of death and disease as having four contributing elements: human biologic factors, unhealthy lifestyles, environmental hazards, and inadequacies in the health care system.

▶ Wellness is an active, six-dimensional process of becoming aware of and making choices toward a higher level of well-being.

▶ The health status of a person is affected by many internal and external variables over which the person has varying degrees of control.

▶ Whether or not people choose to implement health behaviors depends on such factors as the importance of health to the person, perceived control, a perceived threat of a particular disease, perceived familial susceptibility, perceived seriousness of an illness, perceived benefits of preventive actions, and perceived value of early detection.

▶ Whether or not people take action to improve their health often depends on the cost, inconvenience, and unpleasantness involved and on the degree of life-style change necessary.

▶ People realize they are ill when certain symptoms indicate that something is wrong; they accept that they are ill when significant others or a health care professional verifies the illness.

▶ Increasingly, persons are being held responsible for some illnesses but are excused from certain roles and tasks during the illness; they are obliged, however, to get well as quickly as possible and to seek competent help.

▶ Nurses need to be aware that the illness of one member of a family affects all other members.

▶ Nurses need to be aware of a hospitalized client's life-style, roles, economic situation, and need for privacy and autonomy, and provide care accordingly.

▶ People have the right and ability to make judgements about complying with health regimens after obtaining complete information.

▶ Health trends indicate that nurses need to assume a major role in helping people make life-style and environmental changes that will prevent accidents, disease, and occupational hazards.

READINGS AND REFERENCES

SUGGESTED READINGS

Collins, H. L. May 1989. How well do nurses nurture themselves? *RN* 52:39–41.
  This author reports the results of a poll about whether nurses take their own health as seriously as they take their clients'. Diet, exercise, rest and relaxation, and preventive medicine practices are surveyed.

Hogsteal, M. O., and Kashka, M. January/February 1989. Staying healthy after 85. *Geriatric Nursing* 10: 16–18.
  These researchers interviewed 302 individuals 85 years or older about longevity patterns in their families, their lifelong health practices, and their major health care problems and needs. Eleven factors they believed contributed most to their long life are provided. Included are exercise, religion, and a positive attitude.

RELATED RESEARCH

Allen, J. D. 1987. Identification of health risks in a young adult population. *Journal of Community Health Nursing* 4:223–33.

Eiser, C., and Eiser, J.R. December 1987. Implementing a "life-skills" approach to drug education: A preliminary evaluation. *Health Education Research* 2:319–27.

Lichtenstein, R. L., and Thomas, J. W. Winter 1987. A comparison of self-reported measures of perceived health and functional health in an elderly population. *Journal of Community Health* 12:213–30.

Williams, R. O. September/October 1988. Factors affecting the practice of breast self-exam in older women. *Oncology Nursing Forum* 15:611–16.

Woods, N. F. October 1988. Being healthy: Women's images. *Advances in Nursing Science* 11:36–46.

SELECTED REFERENCES

Ames, S. A., et al. 1981. A systems approach to curricula in primary health care nursing. In Knopke, H. J., and Diekelmann, N. L., editors. *Approaches to teaching primary health care*. St. Louis: C. V. Mosby Co.

Bauman, B. 1965. Diversities in conceptions of health and physical fitness. In Skipper, J. K., Jr. and Leonard, R. C., editors. *Social interaction and patient care*. Philadelphia: J. B. Lippincott Co.

Becker, M. H., editor. 1974. *The health belief model and personal health behavior*. Thorofare, N. J.: Charles B. Slack.

Brown, N. Spring 1983. The relationship among health beliefs, health values, and health promotion activity. *Western Journal of Nursing Research* 5:155–63.

Canadian Department of National Health and Welfare. 1974. *A new perspective on the health of Canadians: A working document*. Ottawa: Department of National Health and Welfare.

Clark. C. C. 1986. *Wellness nursing*. New York: Springer Publishing Co.

Colantonio, A. September/October 1988. Lay concepts of health. *Health Values* 12:3–7.

Dubos, R. 1978. Health and creative adaptation. *Human Nature* 74(1):entire issue.

Dunn, H. L. June 1959a. High-level wellness in man and society. *American Journal of Public Health* 49:786.

———. November 1959b. What high-level wellness means. *Canadian Journal of Public Health* 50:447.

———. 1973. *High-level wellness*. Arlington, Va.: R. W. Beatty Co.

Grasser, C., and Craft, B. J. G. June 1984. The patient's approach to wellness. *Nursing Clinics of North America* 19:207–18.

Hegyvary, S. T. January/February 1990. Redefining community: As the center of our health care model. *Journal of Professional Nursing* 6:7.

Hettler, B. 1979. *Six dimensions of wellness*. Stevens Point, Wis.: National Wellness Institute, Inc.

Horgan, P. A. December 1987. Health status perceptions affect health-related behavior. *Journal of Gerontological Nursing* 13:30–33, 34–35.

Igun, U. A. 1979. Stages in health-seeking: A descriptive model. *Social Science and Medicine* 13A:445—56.

Jahoda, M. 1958. *Current concepts of positive mental health*. New York: Basic Books.

Kneisl, C. R., and Ames, S. W. 1986. *Adult health nursing: A biopsychosocial approach*. Menlo Park, Calif.: Addison-Wesley Publishing Co.

Leddy, S., and Pepper, J. M. 1989. *Conceptual bases of professional nursing*. 2d ed. Philadelphia: J. B. Lippincott Co.

MacElveen-Hoehn, P. 1983. The cooperation model for care in health and illness. pp. 515–39. In Chaska, N. L., editor. *The nursing profession: A time to speak*. New York: McGraw-Hill.

McCann/Flynn, J. B., and Heffron, P. B. 1988. *Nursing: From concept to practice*. 2d ed. East Norwalk, CT: Appleton & Lange.

Minister of Supply and Services. 1985. *Mortality, Vol. 3, 1983*. Cat. 84-206, ISSIV 0225-7394. Ottawa: Minister of Supply and Services.

Mitchell, P. H., and Loustau, A. 1981. *Concepts basic to nursing*. 3d ed. New York: McGraw-Hill.

Moll, J. A. January 1982. High-level wellness and the nurse. *Topics in Clinical Nursing* 3:61–67.

Muhlenkamp, A. F., and Broerman, N. A. May 1988. Health beliefs, health value, and positive health behaviors. *Western Journal of Nursing Research* 10:637–46.

Murray, R. B., and Zentner, J. P. 1985. *Nursing concepts for health promotion*. 3d ed. Englewood Cliffs, N.J.: Prentice-Hall.

Overfield, T. 1985. *Biologic variation in health and illness: Race, age, and sex differences*. Menlo Park, Calif.: Addison-Wesley Publishing Co.

Parsons, T. 1972. Definitions of health and illness in the light of American values and social structure. In Jaco, E. G., editor. *Patients, physicians and illness*. 2d ed. New York: Free Press.

Payne, L. September 1983. Health: A basic concept in nursing theory. *Journal of Advanced Nursing* 8:393–95.

Pender, N. J. June 1975. A conceptual model for preventive health behavior. *Nursing Outlook* 23:385–90.

———. 1987. *Health promotion in nursing practice*. 2d ed. East Norwalk, Conn.: Appleton & Lange.

President's Commission on Health Needs of the Nation. 1953. *Building American's health*. Vol. 2 Washington, D.C.: U.S. Government Printing Office.

Redeker, N. S. Spring 1988. Health beliefs and adherence in chronic illness. *Image: Journal of Nursing Scholarship* 20:31–35.

Reynolds, C. L. July 1988. The measurement of health in nursing. *Advances in Nursing Science* 10:23–31.

Rosenstock, I. M. 1974. Historical origins of the health belief model. In Becker, M. H., editor. *The health belief model and personal health behavior*. Thorofare, N.J.: Charles B. Slack

Rosenstock, I. M.; Strecher, V. J.; and Becker, M. H. Summer 1988. Social learning theory and the health belief model. *Health Education Quarterly* 15:175–83.

Ryan, R. S., and Travis, J. W. 1981. *Wellness workbook for health professionals*. Berkeley, Calif.: Ten Speed Press.

Schuster, E. A. October 1976. Privacy: The patient and hospitalization. *Social Science Medicine* 10:245.

Smith, J. A. April 1981. The idea of health: A philosophical inquiry. *Advanced Nursing Science* 3:43–50.

Soeken, K. L., Bausell, R. B., Winklestein, M. et al. December 1989. Preventive behavior: Attitudes and compliance of nursing students. *Journal of Advanced Nursing* 14:1026–33.

Suchman, E. A. 1972. Stages of illness and medical care. In Jaco, E. G., editor. *Patients, physicians and illness*. 2d ed. New York: Free Press.

Tatro, S., and Gleit, C. J. March 1983. A wellness model for nursing: Promoting high-level wellness in any setting through independent nursing functions. *Nursing Leadership* 6:5–9.

Twaddle, A. C. 1977. *A sociology of health*. St. Louis: C. V. Mosby Co.

U.S. Bureau of the Census. 1989. *Statistical abstract of the United States*. 109th ed. Washington, D.C.: U.S. Government Printing Office.

U.S. Department of Health and Human Services. December 1985. *Health United States 1985*. Pub. no. (PHS) 86-1232. Hyattsville, Md.: Public Health Service.

Wallston, B. S.; Wallston, K. A.; Kaplan, G. D.; and Maides, S. A. 1976. Development and validation of the health locus of control scale. *Journal of Consulting and Clinical Psychology* 44:580–85.

World Health Organization. 1947. *Constitution of the World Health Organization: Chronicle of the World Health Organization 1*. Geneva: WHO.

Yoos, L. September/October 1981. Compliance: Philosophical and ethical considerations. *Nurse Practitioner* 6:27, 29–30, 34.

Health Care Delivery Systems

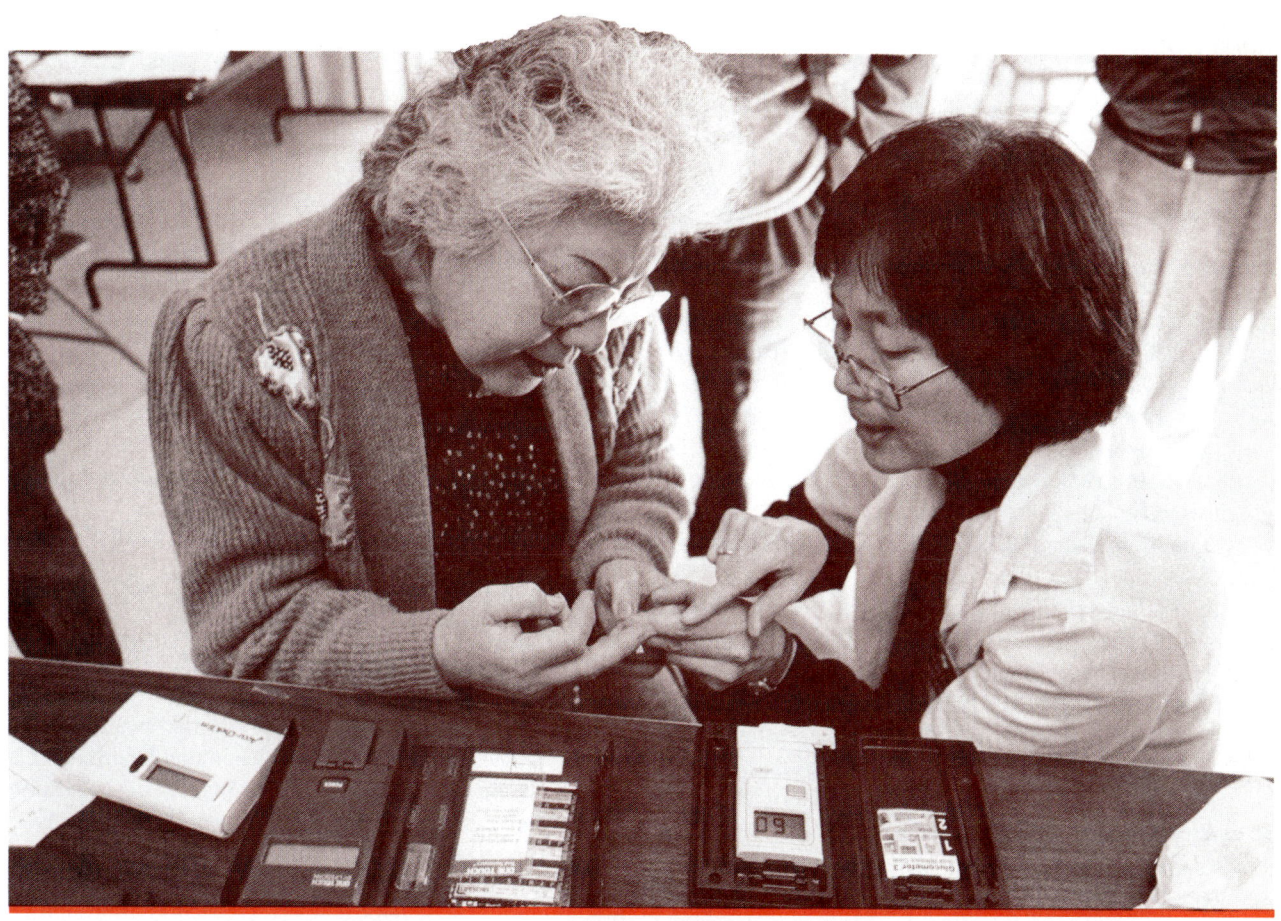

CONTENTS

OBJECTIVES

▶ Describe ways in which consumers are influencing changes in health care delivery.

▶ Relate demographic influences to health care delivery.

▶ Describe the effects of specific social changes on health care delivery.

▶ Explain the effects of poverty and unemployment on health care delivery.

▶ Describe effects of the prospective payment system on health care delivery services.

▶ Explain how political decisions affect health care delivery.

▶ Compare various systems of payment for health care services.

▶ Describe the functions and purposes of various health care delivery systems.

▶ Identify the roles of various health care personnel.

▶ Outline the essentials of the Patient's Bill of Rights established by the American Hospital Association.

▶ Explain contemporary problems in the health care system.

▶ Discuss specific health care priorities and the requirements for promoting health and improving health care delivery services in the future.

▶ Describe the implications for nursing of changes in health care delivery systems.

HEALTH CARE SYSTEM

A **health care system** is the totality of services offered by all health disciplines. Traditionally, the health care delivery system in North America provides two general types of services: illness care services (restorative) and health care services (preventive). Illness care services help the ill or injured. Health care services promote better health and help prevent disease and accidents. Although most facilities within the system—for example, hospitals, clinics, and physicians' offices—provide both types of services, illness care services predominate. In recent years, however, there has been increased awareness of the need to promote health and to prevent disease. Considerable emphasis has been placed on the role of the nurse in these areas.

In the past, health care facilities have been influenced largely by the needs of the people providing the service. For example, hospitals have developed in relation to medical and technologic advances and generally reflect the needs of physicians. Also, the public viewed health care facilities as sources of help primarily for the ill or injured. As a result, preventive health care facilities have been slower to develop. This delay can be attributed in great part to three factors:

1. Physicians are largely oriented to illness in their practice.

2. Consumers have been more aware of treatment of illness than of prevention and health promotion.

3. The nurse's role as the chief provider of preventive health care and health promotion has been slow to evolve, and frequently the treatment of illness takes precedence over preventive health care activities.

In recent years, however, many people have become more conscious of their health, and comprehensive health care, including health promotion and disease prevention services, are receiving increased attention. In the future, increased efforts by nurses, all health professionals, and governments can be instrumental in helping people gain a greater awareness of health as a way of life. Greater empha-

sis must be given to the ill effects of smoking, excessive consumption of alcohol, taking illicit drugs, and overuse of prescribed and over-the-counter medications, rather than treatment of the consequences of these activities. Measures to prevent disease or reduce risks must also be emphasized. Examples are immunizing children; reducing the incidence of road accidents, particularly among adolescents; and preventing accidents in the home, especially among children and older people.

FACTORS INFLUENCING HEALTH CARE SERVICES

People in this society generally believe that health care is a right of everyone. This does not mean that health itself is a right; people can work toward being healthy, but the health care system cannot provide health for all people. However, society can strive to provide health care for all people. The question is not whether all people should have health care but how it can be provided.

Change within the health care system has accelerated during the past decade. This change and future changes are a result of many influences in society.

Health Care Consumer Comprehensive, holistic, and humanistic health care is being emphasized today. People want comprehensive care. They want to have their health care needs met at one time at one agency rather than to seek help for an abdominal pain at one place, for a tooth problem at another place, and for an emotional problem at yet another. Holistic health practitioners emphasize the effects of one problem on the person as biopsychosocial whole. Consumers, therefore, expect health care that reflects this view of the total person and the person's roles and functions.

In the past few decades, many North Americans have come to expect more of the health care system than disease prevention or cure. Consumers today are more aware and knowledgeable about the effects of life-style on health. As a result, they desire more information and services related to health promotion and illness prevention. Although the diagnosis and treatment of illness are still a necessity, the focus of health care has changed. Traditionally, health care was viewed as synonymous with professional and medical care. Now health care professionals are increasingly viewed as a supplementary resource for individuals carrying out their own health maintenance and health promotion activities. As a result, a wide range of health promotion programs have arisen. Some are provided through the traditional health care agencies, but many are developing in community facilities along with physical fitness centers. The media, too, reflect this change. It is not rare for characters in movies, for instance, to exhibit positive health behaviors, such as exercising and not smoking. In Canada, alcohol and tobacco advertisements have been restricted.

Mutual Support and Self-Help Groups

In North America today, there are more than 500 mutual support or **self-help groups** that focus on nearly every major health problem or life crisis people experience. Such groups arose largely because people felt their needs were not being met by the existing health care system. Alcoholics Anonymous, which formed in 1935, served as the model for many of these groups. The National Self-Help Clearinghouse provides information on current support groups and guidelines about how to start a self-help group. Groups vary in effectiveness, but most provide education to encourage self-care as well as social and emotional support. Before referring clients to specific groups, the nurse needs to assess the group's effectiveness and availability to the client.

Women's Movement

The women's movement has been instrumental in changing health care practices. Examples are the provision of childbirth services in more relaxed hospital settings or the home, and the provision of overnight facilities for parents in children's hospitals. The literature on the health concerns of women and research into women's unique health experiences are growing.

Family Characteristics

The characteristics of the North American family have changed considerably in the last few decades. There is a marked increase in single-parent families because of divorce and increased acceptance of children born out of wedlock. Most single-parent families are headed by women. Serious illness or hospitalization can create major financial and home management difficulties for single-parent families. See Chapter 28 for additional information on family health.

Increasing Population

Statistics reflect an increase in the total population and indicate the need for increased health services. See Figure 6–1. In both the United States and Canada, there has been tremendous population growth.

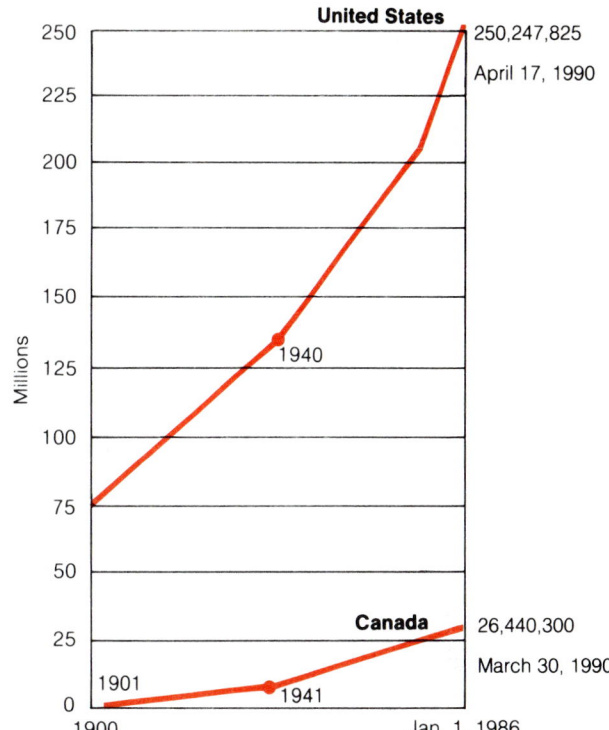

Figure 6–1 Increases in population in the United States, 1900–1987, and in Canada, 1901–1986. *Source:* U.S. Department of Commerce, Bureau of the Census, *Population profile of the United States,* April 17, 1990, 1980 Series P, no. 363 (Washington, D.C.: U.S. Government Printing Office, June 1981), p. 9; Statistics Canada, *The Daily: Quarterly Demographic Statistics for Canada, Provinces and Territories,* March 30, 1990; and Statistics Canada, *Census of Canada* Ottawa: Minister of Supplies and Services, 1981), p. 6.

The impact of the growing elderly population on the health care system is a major social issue. About 30 cents of each health care dollar in the United States are allocated to this group, which now exceeds 28 million and constitutes almost 12% of the population (U.S. Department of Commerce 1984).

By the year 2000, it is estimated that the elderly will number approximately 35 million, constituting 13.1% of the population (U.S. Bureau of the Census 1989, p. 25). In Canada, a similar increase in the number of older people is anticipated: from 1.9 million in 1976 (Statistics Canada 1980, p. 10) to 3.2 million by the year 2000. By the year 2031, 21% of the population will be over age 65 (Statistics Canada 1981). Since only 5% of older people are institutionalized because of health problems, substantial home management and nursing support services are required to assist those in their homes and communities.

The frail aged population over age 85 is the second fastest growing population in North America, exceeded only by the baby boom generation now between 40 and 55. More research into the health and economic conditions of this population is needed.

Because people over 65 are becoming an increasingly large part of the population, their health needs deserve special concern. Long-term illnesses are most prevalent in this group, and these illnesses frequently make special housing, treatment services, and financial support necessary. The elderly need to feel they are still part of a community even though they are approaching the end of their lives. Feelings of being useful, wanted, and productive citizens are essential to their health. Special programs are being designed in communities so that the talents and skills of this group will be used and not lost to society. These programs—e.g., partial employment—are designed especially for the elderly person.

Environmental Change
Air and water pollution from industrial waste is a notable change in this century. Many cities publish a daily air quality index so that persons with respiratory disease will know whether the outside air is safe to breathe. Tragic industrial and nuclear leaks are also of concern.

Many work environments also pose health hazards for employees. Coal miners and textile workers are prone to lung disease. Increasingly, the public is demanding smokeless air in work settings. Many corporations and cities have already banned smoking in certain work areas.

Cultural Diversity
The health care system of North America reflects largely Western, white values and does not adequately accommodate the values of the many different cultural groups living in this country. Language barriers and inequities in income and education hinder access of minority ethnic groups to health care. The more sophisticated and impersonal health services become, the less accessible they are to ethnic groups, who often have a strong family tradition, and prefer personalized care from someone who understands them and their families. Many such people look on the modern health care system with distrust. See Chapter 31 for more information about cultural diversity.

Economic Influences
The health care delivery system is very much affected by a country's total economic status. Inflation and the economic recession of the early 1980s brought increasing concern about escalating health care costs. The United States spends $1 billion a day on health care, and costs are still rising. Medical care costs have increased more than 400% since 1965. They increased an average of 12.6% annually between 1970 and 1984 and about 7.5% in 1986 (Dougherty 1988, p. 16). In Canada, health care expenditures have increased at a similar rate. Some reasons for this sizable increase are advanced techniques and technology, inflation, increased utilization of health services, and the system of payment for hospitals and physicians.

Prospective payment system (PPS)
Efforts to curtail health care costs in the United States were made in 1983, when Congress passed legislation putting the **prospective payment system** into effect. This legislation limits the amount paid to hospitals that are reimbursed by Medicare. Reimbursement is made according to a classification system known as **diagnostic related groups (DRGs).** The system has categories that establish pretreatment diagnosis billing categories.

Under this system, the hospital is paid a predetermined amount for clients with a specific diagnosis. For example, a hospital that admits a client with a diagnosis of uncomplicated asthma is reimbursed a specified amount, such as $1300, regardless of the cost of services, the length of the stay, or the acuity or complexity of the client's illness. In the past, Medicare reimbursed hospitals according to the reasonable cost of services provided to its clients. The hospital billed retrospectively, after the services were rendered. In contrast, prospective payment or billing is formulated before the client is even admitted to the hospital; thus, the record of admission, rather than the record of treatment, now governs payment. DRG rates are set in advance of the prospective year during which they apply and are considered fixed except for major, uncontrollable occurrences. The prospective rates are paid by clients and/ or third parties.

This legislation has had a tremendous impact on health care delivery in the United States, since the providers of care, rather than Medicare or other third-party payers, run the risk of monetary losses. If a hospital's cost per case exceeds the defined limit, it incurs a loss; if the cost is less than the defined limit, it receives a surplus. Thus, PPS offers financial incentives for withholding unnecessary tests or procedures and avoiding prolonged hospital stays.

Notable effects of the DRG system to date are earlier discharge of clients, a decline in admissions, and a reduction of services and staff, especially nurse's aides and LPN/LVN staff. With the decline in admissions, most clients now admitted are seriously ill and have multiple health problems. Many hospitals are now employing only registered nurses (RNs), believing that RNs can provide the broadest range of nursing care. The earlier discharge of clients has given rise to home care agencies that provide needed home nursing care.

To protect clients from DRG abuses, Medicare introduced state peer review organizations (PROs). Made up of physicians and other health care professionals, PROs are intended to monitor the hospitals and ensure high-quality care under DRGs. PROs have developed screening guidelines that govern whether admissions or procedures should occur and are used to review records, render payment decisions, and handle difficulties.

The implication of DRGs for nursing education, practice, and research are many. The Health Care Financing Administration (HCFA) funds research to study alternative systems for classifying severity of illness through nursing diagnosis (Caterinicchio 1984, p. 130) and to shed light on the relationship between DRGs, nursing resource utilization, and nursing costs (ANA 1985).

Unemployment and poverty   Unemployment and poverty, whether the result of recessions, new microchip technology, or inadequate education and technical skills, affect which health services are offered and used. Because the unemployed do not receive employment-based health insurance, they do not use health care services to the same extent as the general population. Even though some government aid is available, eligibility for government insurance programs and benefits varies considerably from state to state. Canada's economic problems are similar to those of the United States; however, the overall effects are not always as apparent because Canada has a smaller population. The National Health Care program in Canada ensures medical care and hospitalization for the poor and unemployed.

Political Influences   Health care is affected by political decisions. For example, political decisions affect health insurance programs, health care funding, allocation of resources (people, money, and equipment), and laws governing the duties of health care workers and the rights of clients, e.g., of women to have abortions. The attitude of people in government health ministries largely determines whether the focus of health care delivery is primary care, secondary care, or tertiary care. *Political activity by nurses (see Chapter 3) is essential.*

FINANCING HEALTH CARE SERVICES

Funding for personal health care can come from a variety of sources: Governments (social insurance), the client, and health insurance are the major sources.

Social Insurance

Federal funding is largely through the social insurance programs Medicare and Medicaid in the United States, and the National Medical Care Insurance program in Canada. A nationally funded program to cover the health costs of all United States citizens has been discussed for the past 20 years.

United States   In the United States, the 1965 **Medicare** amendments (Title 18) to the Social Security Act provided a national and state health insurance program for the aged. By the mid 1970s, virtually everyone over 65 years was protected by hospital insurance under Part A, which also includes posthospital extended care and home health benefits. Medicaid was established the same year under Title 19 of the Social Security Act. **Medicaid** is a federal public assistance program paid out of general taxes to people who require financial assistance, i.e., low-income groups.

In 1972, Congress directed the Department of Health, Education, and Welfare to create professional standards review organizations (PSROs) to monitor the appropriateness of hospital use under the Medicare and Medicaid programs. In 1974, the National Health Planning and Resources Development Act established health systems agencies (HSAs) throughout the United States for comprehensive health planning. In 1978, the Rural Health Clinics Act provided for the development of health care in medically underserved rural areas. This act opened the door for nurse practitioners to provide primary care.

In addition, disabled or blind persons may be eligible for special payments called **Supplemental Security Income** (SSI) benefits. These benefits are also available to people not eligible for Social Security, and payments are not restricted to health care costs. Clients often use this money to purchase medicines or to cover costs of extended health care.

Canada   The Canadian National Hospital Insurance program was started in 1958, and the National Medical Care Insurance Program (Medicare) began in 1968. Through these programs, every Canadian can obtain health insurance. Not all hospital and medical services are covered by provincial hospital insurance or Medicare plans; there are slight differences between provinces. The Canada Health Act was passed in 1984 by Parliament to provide federal government reimbursement to provincial governments for health services they provide. This act replaced two acts: the Hospital Insurance and Diagnostic Services Act and the Medical Care Act. The new act penalizes provinces that permit extra billing of clients by physicians by a levy of a dollar-for-dollar assessment. The act also creates incentives for home care, community health clinics, and health promotion.

Voluntary Insurance

Health care costs are also covered by private insurance plans. The costs of these insurance plans, such as Blue Shield and Blue Cross, are borne by the individual or shared by the employer and the employee. One type of voluntary health insurance is the prepaid group plan offered by HMOs. Prepaid group plans provide for services required by the participants 24 hours a day. By advance payment, the individual takes out insurance against any health requirements in the future. These plans place heavy emphasis on promotion of health and prevention of disease and injury among participants.

Workmen's Compensation

Workers who are injured on the job may collect workmen's compensation payments during their recovery. In some instances, all health care costs are paid by workmen's compensation. Employer companies contribute to a workmen's compensation fund to make money available when accidents occur.

Charitable Resources

Charitable resources for medical payments are supported by donations from individuals or groups and by bequests. Charitable donations are still made by some philanthropic organizations to assist the poor and to support innovations. On the whole, however, charitable donations as a means of paying for health care are declining in importance.

HEALTH CARE AGENCIES

Official Agencies

Government (official) agencies are established at the local, state (provincial), and federal levels. Health agencies at the state, county, or city level vary according to the need of the area. Their funds, generally from taxes, are administered by elected or appointed officials. Local health departments (county, bicounty, or tricounty) traditionally have responsibility for developing programs to meet the health needs of the people, providing the necessary staff and facilities to carry out these programs, continually evaluating the effectiveness of the programs, and monitoring changing needs. State health organizations are responsible for assisting the local health departments. In some remote areas, state departments also provide direct services to people.

The Public Health Service (PHS) of the United States Department of Health and Human Services is an official agency at the federal level. Its functions include conducting research and providing training in the health field, providing assistance to communities in planning and developing health facilities, and assisting states and local communities through financing and provision of trained personnel. Also at the national level in the United States are research institutions such as the National Institutes of Health (NIH). The National Institute on Drug Abuse, the National Institute on Alcohol Abuse and Alcoholism, and the National Institute of Mental Health work with federal, regional, and state agencies. The Centers for Disease Control (CDC) in Atlanta, Georgia, administer a broad program related to surveillance of diseases. By means of laboratory and epidemiologic investigations, data are made available to appropriate authorities. The CDC also publishes recommendations about the prevention and control of infections and administers a national health program. The federal government also administers a number of Veterans Administration (VA) hospitals in the United States.

The Canadian Department of Health and Welfare (CDHW) administers such federal programs as native health in the north and health care in the territories. However, provincial governments generally have responsibility for administering health services to the people of each province.

Agencies Providing Health Care

Health care agencies can be viewed as giving primary, secondary, and tertiary care.

Primary Care

Primary care agencies are the point of entry into the health care system, i.e., the point at which initial health care is given. Primary care includes health maintenance, health promotion, and disease prevention activities. Aydelotte writes, "The major purposes of primary care centers will be to provide: (1) entry into the system; (2) emergency care; (3) health maintenance; (4) long-term and chronic care; (5) treatment of temporary malfunctioning that does not require hospitalization" (Aydelotte 1983, p. 812). It is in this area that increased services are expected to reduce health care costs and improve health. Settings for primary care are various health centers in the community, homes, schools, physicians' offices, and industry and business. Primary care is frequently inadequate in rural and economically depressed areas, due to lack of physicians. Emergency departments of hospitals are often crowded and overtaxed, in many instances with nonemergency health problems.

Ambulatory care centers are being used more frequently in many communities. They usually have diagnostic and treatment facilities and may or may not be attached to or associated with an acute care hospital. They provide medical, nursing, laboratory, and radiologic services. Some ambulatory care centers provide services to people who require minor surgical procedures that can be performed outside the hospital. After surgery, the client returns home the same day. These centers have two advantages: They permit the client to live at home while obtaining needed health care, and they free costly hospital beds for seriously ill clients. Nurses in ambulatory care centers frequently function as nurse practitioners or clinical nurse specialists, e.g., in gastroenterology or urology.

The term *ambulatory care center* has replaced the term *clinic* in many places. The term *clinic* can refer to a department in a hospital or a group practice of physicians. Traditionally, a hospital clinic was called an outpatient clinic, serving only outpatients, as opposed to those admitted to the hospital (inpatients). The role of the nurse in a clinic may be similar to that of a nurse practitioner or a nurse in a physician's office.

The *physician's office* is a traditional primary care setting in North America. The majority of physicians either have their own offices or work with several other physicians in a group practice. People usually go to a physician because they consider themselves ill, because a relative thinks the client is ill, or because the client needs medical advice.

Nurses employed in physicians' offices have a variety of roles. Some nurses carry out the traditional functions of registering the client, preparing the client for an examination or treatment, and providing information. Other nurses function as nurse practitioners and have the responsibility of providing primary care to clients in stable health.

The *industrial clinic* is gaining importance as a setting for primary care. Employee health has long been recognized as important to productivity. Today, an increasing number of companies are recognizing the value of healthy employees and encouraging healthy life-styles. Some companies provide exercise facilities, while others provide healthy snacks, such as fruit, instead of coffee. More businesses are prohibiting smoking in the work setting.

Community health nurses in the occupational setting have a variety of roles. Worker safety has been a traditional concern of occupational nurses. Today, nursing functions include health education, screening for such health problems as hypertension and obesity, counseling, and initial care after accidents.

A **health maintenance organization (HMO)** is a group health care agency that provides basic and supplemental health maintenance and treatment services to voluntary enrollees. The enrollees prepay a fixed periodic fee that is set without regard to the amount or kind of services received. The basic idea of the HMO arose in the 1930s, when prepaid health care experiments were sponsored by unions, cooperatives, corporations, municipalities, and other organized groups. HMOs did not become popular, however, until after the passage, in 1973, of the Health Maintenance Organization Act. In 1984, 11 million people were served by HMOs (Curtin and Zurlage 1984, p. 34).

To be federally qualified, an HMO company must meet certain requirements. It must offer physicians' services, hospital and outpatient services, emergency services, short-term mental health services, treatment and referral for drug and alcohol problems, laboratory and radiologic services, preventive dental services for children under 12, and preventive health services. By encouraging preventive health care and by offering ambulatory services, HMOs have reduced the cost of health insurance to the consumer.

A client of an HMO signs a contract to pay a specified amount to the HMO for unlimited care. The plan stresses wellness; the better the health of the person, the less the client needs HMO services and the greater the agency's profit. Because of the emphasis on health promotion and prevention of illness, nurses who work in HMOs focus on these aspects of care, frequently as nurse practitioners, client educators, and consultants.

Although not in every community, HMOs have been established across the United States. The largest HMO, the Kaiser-Permanente Medical Care Program, serves clients in California, Oregon, Hawaii, Ohio, and Colorado. A person with private health insurance can obtain services in most hospitals, but the clients of an HMO must use its facilities.

The **preferred provider organization (PPO)** has emerged as another alternative health delivery system. It consists of a group of physicians or a hospital that provides companies with health services at a discounted rate. Hospitals, physicians, and insurance companies are the major sponsors of PPOs. PPOs were first established in 1980 in the United States. Physicians can belong to one or several PPOs, and the client can choose among the physicians belonging to that PPO.

Individual practice associations (IPA) are somewhat like HMOs and PPOs. The IPA provides practice in offices, just as the providers belonging to a PPO do. The difference is that clients pay a fixed prospective payment to the IPA, and the IPA pays the provider. In some instances, the health care provider bills the IPA for services; in others, the provider receives a fixed fee for services given. At the end of the fiscal year, any surplus money is divided among the providers; any loss is assumed by the IPA.

Crisis centers provide emergency services. The clients are often people experiencing life crises. These centers may operate out of a hospital or in the community and usually provide 24-hour telephone service. Some also provide direct counseling to people at the center or in their homes. The primary purpose of a crisis center is to help people cope with an immediate crisis and then provide guidance and support for long-term therapy.

Nurses working in crisis centers need well-developed communication and counseling skills. The nurse must immediately identify the person's problem, offer assistance to help the person cope, and perhaps later provide guidance about resources for long-term support.

Secondary Care   **Secondary care** focuses on preventing complications of disease conditions. It has traditionally been the province of hospitals; however, other agencies now increasingly provide this level of service. Secondary care centers of the future will focus on the treatment of temporary dysfunctions that require hospitalization but not highly skilled services and high-risk interventions, the evaluation of long-term illness that requires hospitalization to determine any needed change in treatment, and the provision of counseling and therapy that cannot be provided in a primary care center (Aydelotte 1983, p. 813). Agencies that provide secondary care include hospitals, home health agencies, and ambulatory care centers.

Hospitals traditionally have provided restorative care to the ill and injured. They vary in size from the 12-bed rural hospital to the 1500-bed metropolitan hospital with a 50-bed day surgery center. Hospitals can be classified according to their ownership or control as governmental (public) and nongovernmental (private). Governmental hospitals are either federal, state, city, or county hospitals in the United States and federal or provincial hospitals in Canada. In both countries, governments have traditionally provided hospital facilities for veterans, merchant mariners, and individuals with long-term illness.

Although hospitals are chiefly viewed as institutions that provide care, they have other functions, such as providing resources for health-related research and teaching.

Hospitals also are classified by the services they provide. General hospitals admit clients requiring a variety of services, such as medical, surgical, obstetric, pediatric, and psychiatric services. Other hospitals offer only specialty services, such as psychiatric or pediatric care.

Hospitals can be further described as acute or chronic. An acute hospital provides assistance to clients who are acutely ill or whose illness and need for hospitalization are relatively short-term, for example, 2 days. Long-term hospitals provide health services for longer periods, sometimes for years or the remainder of the client's life.

Hospitals in the United States are undergoing massive change. In the past, hospitals were virtually the sole providers of secondary care; however, ambulatory care centers and HMOs have forced hospitals to reorganize and adopt different practices. Some hospitals have merged or sold out to large multihospital for-profit corporations, e.g., Humana, Inc., and Hospital Corporation of America. Other hospitals are providing innovative services, such as fitness classes, day care for elderly people, and nutrition classes. Some hospitals have even established alternative birth centers (ABCs) to attract new families.

In the United States today, all but the most seriously ill are treated outside of a hospital. Because so many of these are elderly, some general hospitals are becoming acute care hospitals solely for the elderly. Because of the increasing acuity of illness among clients, general hospitals are becoming intensive care centers.

Tertiary Care

Tertiary care is also called rehabilitation or long-term care. It is largely provided through home health care, long-term care facilities, rehabilitation centers, and hospices. **Home health care agencies** are rapidly becoming major tertiary care providers. Home care is one aspect of comprehensive health care. Its purposes include promoting, maintaining, and restoring health, specifically maximizing independent functioning and minimizing the disabling effects of illness, including terminal illness. Services appropriate to the needs of clients and their families are planned, coordinated, and delivered by providers organized for the delivery of home health care through the use of contractual arrangements, employed staff, or a combination of the two (Warhola 1980).

Home care services are appropriate when an individual or family does not need full-time care, observation, or the special facilities of an institution such as a hospital or nursing home, yet does need care that family members or others cannot provide without assistance or teaching. Home care may or may not be associated with a hospitalization. It may precede or follow institutional care in a hospital or long-term care facility, or it may be provided along with ambulatory care (Lundberg 1984). Self-care and care given by health professionals and allied health personnel in the home account for the majority of health care provided in this country today. The time a person spends in a hospital receiving care for acute conditions is generally a very small percentage of the person's life. The need for home care services is increasing as the population of the United States ages and the incidence of chronic illness increases correspondingly (Lundberg 1984).

The nature of home care services has broadened to include both acute, short-term care as well as long-term monitoring of problems associated with chronic illness. Comprehensive home care includes both direct and indirect services.

Direct services involve direct contact between a caregiver and a client for the purposes of administering treatment or nursing care measures, assessment, teaching, counseling, or planning care. Direct services provided may be complex technical procedures, such as intravenous chemotherapy for cancer and respiratory therapy. Such services are becoming more widely available at home. Symptom management, teaching for self-care, monitoring adaptation to long-term illness, family counseling, physical and occupational therapy, and nutritional counseling are direct services provided by a variety of home care agencies. Such basic nursing care measures as bathing, skin care, assistance with ambulation, toileting, feeding, dressing changes, catheter care, and administration of medications have long been and continue to be direct service components of home care. Home care nursing also includes such direct services as providing ongoing assessment, anticipation and planning for problems or crises before they occur, helping clients think through problems and their options for dealing with them, managing symptoms, teaching, counseling, and assisting individuals and families to meet their health care goals.

Indirect services in home care include those measures taken to provide or facilitate direct services in nursing practice (McCorkle and Germino 1984). Consulting with other professionals and allied health personnel about client problems and needs, coordinating care within the home care agency, coordinating community resources and referrals outside the agency, supervising allied health workers providing services, and evaluating the effectiveness of care provided are all examples of indirect services currently provided by home care nurses. In addition, nurses involved in home care may be liaisons with acute care facilities and serve as facilitators and contact persons for clients and families who need access to special health care resources.

Long-Term Care Facilities

There are a wide variety of **long-term care facilities.** Traditionally, they were all called nursing homes. Long-term care facilities now include skilled nursing facilities for extended care, intermediate care, and personal care for those who are chronically ill or are no longer able to care for themselves without assistance.

Because long term illness occurs most often in the elderly, many long-term care facilities have programs that are oriented to the needs of this age group. Nursing homes are intended for people who require not only personal services (such as assistance in bathing and dressing, and meal preparation) but also some regular nursing care and occasional medical attention. However, the type of care provided varies considerably. Some admit and retain only residents who can dress themselves and are ambulatory. Other long-term care facilities provide bed care for clients who are more incapacitated. Nursing homes can, in effect, become the clients' home, and consequently the people who live there are frequently referred to as residents rather than patients or clients.

In 1987, the Congress of the United States passed the Omnibus Budget Reconciliation Act (OBRA) to bring a measure of quality assurance to the nursing home industry. There was growing concern whether minimal essential standards were being met in many nursing home facilities. One of the provisions of OBRA that concerns nursing is the requirement for nurse's aide training. Specific requirements include the following:

- A training program of 75 hours in length for nurse's aides
- Competency evaluation of newly trained nurse's aides
- Competency evaluation of nurse's aides already providing care
- A registry for nurse's aides

For nursing, implications of this OBRA 1987 provision include the following (Kelly 1989, p. 792):

1. Concern about which state agency is to be responsible for implementing the requirements. If the state agency is other than a board of nursing, the nursing community could have less than the desired control over nursing functions to be delegated by licensed nurses to nurse's aides. Legally, a licensed registered or practical nurse is accountable for acts delegated.

2. The 75-hour training requirement may not be sufficient to prepare aides to carry out routine care for nursing home clients who have complex problems.

3. The evaluation requirement necessitates job analysis and the development of standard criteria at the state level.

4. The establishment of a registry system for nurse's aides implies the establishment of a discipline function and a process to identify those at risk to the public. Licensed nurses, therefore, will need to be alerted to their responsibilities in monitoring for the three problems cited by OBRA as calling for the investigation of care provided by aides: (a) neglect of residents, (b) abuse of residents, and (c) misappropriation of resident property.

Rehabilitation Centers

Rehabilitation centers usually are independent community centers or special units in hospitals. However, rehabilitation ideally starts the moment a client enters the health care system. Thus, nurses are involved in rehabilitation whether they are employed on pediatric, psychiatric, or surgical units of hospitals or in the community. Today, the concept of rehabilitation is applied to all illness (physical and mental), to injury, and to chemical addiction. Rehabilitation affects every age group and

segment of society. **Rehabilitation** is a process of restoring people to useful function in physical, mental, social, economic, and vocational areas of their lives. Rehabilitation, then, is a process of restoring people to their previous level of health (i.e., to their previous capabilities) or to the level that is possible for them. Rehabilitation, as distinct from maintenance, is an active concept and can be considered largely an educational function.

Hospice Services

Traditionally, a **hospice** was a place where travelers could rest. Recently, the term has come to mean a health care facility for the dying. The hospice movement subsumes a variety of services given to the terminally ill, their families, and support persons. The movement sprang initially from dissatisfaction with the preoccupation of health personnel with technologic care and insufficient emphasis on caring and psychologic support. In the 1970s, the movement gained momentum. It derived impetus from new attitudes toward death and from the work of such people as Elisabeth Kübler-Ross, whose books challenged prevailing attitudes, and Cicely Saunders, founder of St. Christopher's Hospice in London, England. Saunders believed that the physical and social environments of dying people are as important as medical interventions on their behalf.

In recent years, hospices have provided a variety of services to terminally ill clients and their families; indeed, hospices have inspired a social movement. Basic to the movement is a humanistic belief in the individuality of people and their needs. Hospice programs are institution and community based. Some supply services in the home, either directly or through community resources. Reimbursement for these services is variable, often voluntary.

Hospices are a haven for the dying because they emphasize the needs of the individual and help clients and their families plan for death. The central concept of the hospice movement, as distinct from the acute care model, is not saving life but improving or maintaining the quality of life until death. Important in this care are **palliative measures** for relief rather than cure. Comfort and relief from pain are frequently the most important needs of the dying. Hospice care addresses the needs of the mind and the spirit as well: It is truly holistic.

PROVIDERS OF HEALTH CARE

The providers of health care, also referred to as the **health care team,** are health personnel from different disciplines who coordinate their skills to assist a client and/or support persons. The choice of personnel for a particular client depends on the needs of the client. In the present system of health care in North America, health teams commonly include nurses, physicians, pharmacists, dietitians, physiotherapists, respiratory therapists, occupational therapists, paramedical technologists, social workers, and chaplains.

Nurse The role of the nurse varies with the needs of the situation. The advent of expanded nursing roles has established new dimensions for nursing practice. In the past, nursing was thought to comprise three types of skills: psychomotor, affective, and cognitive. While these skills remain important, the role of the nurse is seen more broadly today because of the acceptance of the nursing process as a framework for nursing practice and the recognition of other nursing roles, e.g., manager and counselor.

Psychomotor skills are the traditional skills of nurses. These skills involve the use of the hands. For example, manipulating equipment or repositioning a client is a psychomotor skill. **Affective skills** include the ability to incorporate cultural, attitudinal, and emotional elements into nursing. The nurse uses affective skills to individualize care. Caring and communicating activities require affective skills. **Cognitive skills** include the ability to think, recall knowledge, apply knowledge, and evaluate. Cognitive skills are required in all aspects of the nursing process.

A number of nursing personnel often participate actively on a health team. Sometimes nurses find it necessary to provide some services normally given by other members of the team, especially in settings where all the health services required by a client are not available 24 hours a day. For example, a nurse might assist a client who has had a cerebrovascular accident (stroke) by giving remedial exercises to restore function of the left arm.

Physician A **physician** is a person who is licensed to practice medicine in a particular jurisdiction. The physician has successfully completed a course of medical studies. In a hospital setting, the physician is responsible for medical diagnosis and for determining the therapy required by a person who has a disease or injury. The traditional role of the physician is the treatment of disease and trauma (injury). However, many physicians, especially family practice physicians, are now including health promotion and disease prevention in their practice. In a community setting, the physician is often involved in diagnosis and therapy. Some physicians are specialists in surgery and are referred to as surgeons. An example is a neurosurgeon or an orthopedic surgeon. Some physicians extend their roles by employing a **physician's assistant** who is educated to perform certain tasks and authorized to practice under the direction of the physician.

Pharmacist A **pharmacist** is a person who prepares and dispenses pharmaceuticals in hospital and community settings. The role of the pharmacist in monitoring and evaluating the actions and effects of medications on clients is becoming increasingly prominent. Pharmacists are also actively involved in preparing individual dosages for clients in hospitals that employ the unit dose system. In some settings, pharmacists prepare medications for intravenous therapy. A **clinical pharmacist** is a specialist who guides physicians in prescribing medications. A **pharmacy assis-**

tant is also recognized in some states. This member of the health team administers medications to clients or works in the pharmacy under the direction of the pharmacist.

Dietitian or Nutritionist When dietary and nutritional services are required, the dietitian or nutritionist may be a member of a health team. A **dietitian** is a person who has special knowledge about the diets required to maintain health and to treat disease. Dietitians in hospitals generally are concerned with therapeutic diets, may design special diets to meet the nutritional needs of individual clients, and supervise the preparation of the meals to ensure that clients receive the proper diet.

A **nutritionist** is a person who has special knowledge about nutrition and food. The nutritionist in a community setting recommends healthy diets and gives broad advisory services about the purchase and preparation of foods. Community nutritionists often function at the preventive level. They promote health and prevent disease, for example, by advising families about balanced diets for growing children and pregnant women.

Physiotherapist (Physical Therapist) The physiotherapist assists clients with musculoskeletal problems. **Physiotherapists** treat the body by means of heat, water, exercise, massage, and electric current. They provide physical therapy in response to a physician's order. The physiotherapist's functions include assessing clients' mobility and strength, providing therapeutic measures (e.g., exercises and heat applications to improve mobility and strength), and teaching new skills (e.g., how to walk with an artificial leg). Most physiotherapists provide their services in hospitals; however, independent practitioners establish offices in communities and serve clients either at the office or in the home.

Respiratory Therapist A **respiratory therapist** is skilled in therapeutic measures used in the care of clients with respiratory problems. These therapists are knowledgeable about oxygen therapy devices, intermittent positive pressure breathing respirators, artificial mechanical ventilators, and accessory devices used in inhalation therapy.

Occupational Therapist An **occupational therapist** assists clients with some impairment of function to gain the skills to perform activities of daily living. For example, a man with severe arthritis in his arms and hands might be taught how to adjust his kitchen utensils so that he can continue to cook. The therapist also teaches skills that are therapeutic and at the same time provide some satisfaction. For example, weaving is a recreational activity but also exercises the arthritic man's arm and hands.

Paramedical Technologists Laboratory technologists, radiologic technologists, and nuclear medicine technologists are just three kinds of paramedical technologists in an expanding field of medical technology. **Paramedical** means having some connection with medicine. Laboratory technologists examine specimens such as urine, feces, blood, and discharges from wounds to provide exact information that facilitates the medical diagnosis and the prescription of a therapeutic regimen. The radiologic technologist assists with a wide variety of x-ray film procedures, from simple chest radiography to more complex fluoroscopy. The nuclear medicine technologist uses radioactive substances to provide diagnostic information, for example, about a client's liver, and can administer therapeutic doses of radioactive materials as part of a therapeutic regimen. These technologists have highly specialized skills and knowledge important to client care.

Social Worker   A **social worker** counsels clients and support persons about social problems, such as finances, marital difficulties, and adoption of children. It is not unusual for health problems to produce problems in living. For example, an elderly woman who lives alone and has a stroke resulting in impaired walking may find it impossible to continue to live in her third-floor apartment. Finding a more suitable living arrangement can be the responsibility of the social worker if the client has no support network in place. The current trend toward shorter acute care hospitalizations has lead to an increased need for rehabilitative services in skilled nursing facilities or in the home. For this reason, social workers, who usually make the placement arrangements, are playing an increasingly important role in the health care team.

Chaplains   Hospital **chaplains** serve as part of the health care team by attending to the spiritual needs of clients. In most facilities, local clergy volunteer their services on a regular or "on-call" basis. Hospitals affiliated with specific religions, as well as many large medical centers, have full-time chaplains on staff. They usually offer regularly scheduled religious services. The nurse is often instrumental in identifying the client's desire to see a chaplain, either by responding promptly to the client's request or by informing the client of the chaplain's services.

RIGHTS TO HEALTH CARE

The movement for clients' rights in health care arose in the late 1960s. At that time, the broad goals of the movement were to improve the quality of health care and to make the health care system more responsive to clients' needs. Today, clients are also seeking more self-determination and control over their own bodies when they are ill. Informed consent, confidentiality, and the right of the client to refuse treatment are all aspects of this self-determination. The need for clients' rights is largely the result of two circumstances: the vulnerability of the client because of illness and the complexity of the relationships in the health care setting.

When people are ill, they are frequently unable to assert their rights as they would if they were healthy. Asserting rights requires energy and an underlying awareness of one's rights in the situation.

The complexity and variety of health care relationships also increase the need for clients' rights. In this day of specialization, a client is often helped by a variety of health professionals. The client becomes one person among many health professionals. Thus, the client's needs or priorities, for example, can become lost in the communications among health professionals.

A new pattern of health care relationships is emerging as a result of several forces in society, including a more knowledgeable consumer and recognition of the role of life-style in disease. Today, the goals of health include the return or autonomy and independence to the client and the acceptance of good health as a responsibility of the care provider, the client, and society. These goals cannot be met unless clients accept active responsibility for their health and health care and unless clients and care providers have mutual respect.

Annas and Healey (1974, p. 26) list four rights that are assertable in a health care facility: (a) the right to the whole truth, (b) the right to privacy and personal dignity, (c) the right to retain self-determination by participating in decisions regarding one's health, and (d) the right of complete access to medical records, both during and after the hospital stay.

A Patient's Bill of Rights

In 1973, the American Hospital Association published "A Patient's Bill of Rights" in an effort to promote the rights of hospitalized clients. See Table 6–1. Frequently clients do not know their rights, although many hospitals today give clients upon admission a statement of their rights while in hospital.

The nursing implications of the Patient's Bill of Rights are

1. *The patient has a right to considerate and respectful care.* The client has a right to an explanation about what will happen, why, and when. Clients also have the right to participate in planning their care. Considerate and respectful care also includes respect for the dignity of each person. Nurses can convey respect by listening carefully to clients and their support persons and reporting their concerns to the appropriate people.

2. *The patient has the right to obtain from his physician complete current information concerning his diagnosis, treatment, and prognosis, in terms the patient can be reasonably expected to understand.* The responsibility for divulging this information belongs to the physician. If a client asks a nurse for this information, the nurse should relay the questions to the physician and document the client's questions and the nurse's actions on the client's record.

TABLE 6-1 *A Patient's Bill of Rights*

1. The patient has the right to considerate and respectful care.

2. The patient has the right to obtain from his physician complete current information concerning his diagnosis, treatment, and prognosis, in terms the patient can be reasonably expected to understand. When it is not medically advisable to give such information to the patient, the information should be made available to an appropriate person in his behalf. He has the right to know by name the physician responsible for coordinating his care.

3. The patient has the right to receive from his physician information necessary to give informed consent prior to the start of any procedure and/or treatment. Except in emergencies, such information for informed consent should include but not necessarily be limited to the specific procedure and/or treatment, the medically significant risks involved, and the probable duration of incapacitation. Where medically significant alternatives for care or treatment exist, or when the patient requests information concerning medical alternatives, the patient has the right to such information. The patient also has the right to know the name of the person responsible for the procedures and/or treatment.

4. The patient has the right to refuse treatment to the extent permitted by law and to be informed of the medical consequences of his action.

5. The patient has the right to every consideration of his privacy concerning his own medical care program. Case discussion, consultation, examination, and treatment are confidential and should be conducted discreetly. Those not directly involved in this care must have the permission of the patient to be present.

6. The patient has the right to expect that all communications and records pertaining to his care should be treated as confidential.

7. The patient has the right to expect that within its capacity a hospital must make reasonable response to the request of a patient for services. The hospital must provide evaluation, service, and/or referral as indicated by the urgency of the case. When medically permissible, a patient may be transferred to another facility only after he has received complete information and explanation concerning the needs for and alternatives to such a transfer. The institution to which the patient is transferred must first have accepted the patient for transfer.

8. The patient has the right to obtain information as to any relationship of his hospital to other health care and educational institutions insofar as his care is concerned. The patient has the right to obtain information as to the existence of any professional relationships among individuals, by name, who are treating him.

9. The patient has the right to be advised if the hospital proposes to engage in or perform human experimentation affecting his care or treatment. The patient has the right to refuse to participate in such research projects.

10. The patient has the right to expect reasonable continuity of care. He has the right to know in advance what appointment times and physicians are available and where. The patient has the right to expect that the hospital will provide a mechanism whereby he is informed by his physician or a delegate of the physician of the patient's continuing health.

11. The patient has the right to examine and receive an explanation of his bill regardless of source of payment.

12. The patient has the right to know what hospital rules and regulations apply to his conduct as a patient.

Source: American Hospital Association. 1973. A patient's bill of rights, *Nursing Outlook,* February 1973, 21:82, and January 1976, 24:29. Reprinted with the permission of the American Hospital Association.

Many people believe that even when ill, clients still have a right to the whole truth, i.e., complete information about their health care. Nurses should explain independent nursing actions truthfully and completely. Because these activities are solely in the nurse's domain, the nurse has sole responsibility for explaining them. However, dependent nursing functions, i.e., those nursing activities ordered by the physician, should be explained only after the nurse completely understands the physician's and client's positions. See Chapter 13 for information about independent and dependent nursing actions. Usually, a physician has no objection to a client understanding the ordered treatments; however, occasionally a physician does not wish a client to be fully informed, e.g., about a medication for a malignancy before the client has been informed of the diagnosis. Although the client has a right to be fully informed, not all jurisdictions accept the Patient's Bill of Rights as law. Therefore nurses should inform the physician about the client's questions, discuss the matter thoroughly, and document the client's questions.

3. *The patient has the right to receive from his physician information necessary to give informed consent prior to the start of any procedures and/or treatment.* The client has the right to give or withhold informed consent. Obtaining informed consent is the physician's responsibility. The nurse's role in obtaining informed consent is discussed in Chapter 8, page 153.

An important nursing strategy is to "coordinate the medical, technical, and nursing activities on behalf of the patient's well-being into a meaningful process that the patient and family can utilize in the shared decision process" (Bandman and Bandman 1990, p. 95). It has been found that in many instances treatments are refused because of conflicting information. Therefore, when nurses and other health professionals collaborate and encourage the client's participation, the client feels more secure and more comfortable about making decisions regarding care.

4. *The patient has the right to refuse treatment to the extent permitted by law and to be informed of the medical consequences of his action.* Clients have the right to self-determination. Just as they have the right to informed consent, they also have the right to refuse a treatment. An adult client who is conscious and medically competent has the right to refuse any medical or surgical procedure (Annas 1975, p. 79). When the client refuses treatment, no person has to impose the treatment. The clients still have the right to the best possible care within the limitations they impose. In regard to a parent's refusal to allow treatment of a child, Annas states: "It is only in extreme cases involving the potential of death or permanent disability to the child that courts are likely to overrule a parent's refusal of treatment for a child" (Annas 1975, p. 87).

5. *The patient has the right to every consideration of his privacy concerning his own medical care program.* People vary in what they consider an invasion of privacy and a threat to dignity. Therefore only the client can decide whether to permit any invasion of privacy. Although a client who signs a consent form for an examination or treatment may be giving up certain aspects of privacy in the course of the examination or treatment, the invasion of the client's privacy must be kept to the minimum. For example, a client who consents to a physical examination is expected to disrobe; however, the nurse can provide some degree of privacy by supplying an appropriate gown, drapes, and a room or enclosed area. Also, by consenting to the examination, the client does not also agree to the presence of people other than those directly involved in the examination.

The right to privacy is closely linked to the individual's personal dignity. Individuals "on exhibit" can feel demeaned and embarrassed. The experience of being viewed by a group of health professionals, e.g., nursing students, can live in a person's memory for many years as a distasteful incident. Nurses must ensure that the client fully understands and consents to the presence of health personnel not directly involved in treatment.

The right to privacy is the second item in the ANA Code (ANA 1976, p. 2). In addition, clients have a right to be examined and seen by only the people directly concerned with their care. Physicians normally have responsibility for obtaining consent if, for example, a medical student needs to examine the client. Clients have a right to privacy even after death. Privacy also means not intruding into the client's private life and

disclosing confidential information. Nurses can be held legally liable for taking any action without consent that would offend a reasonable person's sensibilities (Good Intentions Gone Awry 1986, p. 55). Ways of intruding into a client's private life include eavesdropping on a conversation, searching a client's clothes or handbag, taking photographs of an unconscious client, or asking questions that have no relation to the client's health. See Chapter 8 for additional information regarding the invasion of privacy.

6. *The patient has the right to expect that all communications and records pertaining to his care should be treated as confidential.* Privacy is closely related to confidentiality. Only clients have the power to let people not directly involved in their care view their medical records. Only the client has the right to provide information to support persons or others. Confidentiality is also included in the ANA ethical code. See Chapter 7.

Another aspect of confidentiality is related to computers. Although computers have facilitated health care in a number of ways, any person who knows an access code can view confidential client information. Therefore, nurses and all health professionals must guard the confidentiality of client records and not give computer codes to unauthorized people.

7. *The patient has the right to expect that within its capacity a hospital must make a reasonable response to the request of a patient for services.*

8. *The patient has a right to obtain information as to any relationship of his hospital to other health care and educational institutions insofar as his care is concerned.* Rights 8 and 9 are largely related to hospital administration. However, nurses are becoming increasingly involved in such matters as budget as it relates to client care. Clients who believe their care is inadequate should communicate this fact to the appropriate person in the hospital. Every health agency should have a procedure for handling client grievances. One trend in health care is client advocacy, a function assumed by nurses in some settings.

9. *The patient has the right to be advised if the hospital proposes to engage in or perform human experimentation affecting his care or treatment.* Clients also have a right to consent or refuse to participate in any research or experimentation. Both the ANA and the CNA have published guidelines for nurses who participate in research.

10. *The patient has the right to expect reasonable continuity of care.* Clients have a right to know what health care they will need after they are discharged from a hospital. It is often the nurse's responsibility to teach follow-up care and to make appropriate referrals to other health agencies. Discharge planning is discussed in Chapter 12.

11. *The patient has the right to examine and receive an explanation of his bill regardless of the source of payment.* Nurses often record billable items such as dressings, medications, and the like. In some settings, it may be the nurse's responsibility to explain a bill to a client, although this task is often carried out by someone in the hospital's business office.

12. *The patient has the right to know what hospital rules and regulations apply to his conduct as a patient.* Some agencies provide pamphlets that list rules, such as those governing visiting hours, and explain services, such as cafeteria and telephone service. Often nurses clarify information and answer a client's questions about hospital rules. Nurses also explain rules associated with special procedures, such as those that apply when oxygen is in use or when a client has an infection.

Another right not mentioned specifically in the AHA Patient's Bill of Rights is the right of access to medical records. Although in some jurisdictions clients have the right of access to their health records, agency practices vary widely in this regard. Some hospitals, e.g., military hospitals, permit clients to keep records at the bedside. At the other extreme, some agencies release records to clients only if they have a subpeona. A number of state legislatures have passed laws requiring health agencies to establish reasonable policies by which clients are permitted access to their records. Laws about access to records have changed in recent years, and it is generally recognized that only clients can grant others access to their records or permit the release or transfer of their records.

PROBLEMS IN THE HEALTH CARE SYSTEM

Although the health care system is changing, problems still exist. Many of the problems stem, at least partially, from the enormous changes in health care during the past 30 years. Major advances in medicine and technology have meant better care for many. With this improved care, however, have come such problems as fragmentation of care and high costs.

Other problems have always existed with health care delivery systems and are present today. Some of these are unmet needs of low-income people and the special needs of the homeless and the elderly. Another problem is uneven national distribution of health care services; limited resources are available in rural and inner-city areas, whereas more services are available in more prosperous urban and suburban areas. The consumer is becoming more aware of these problems and is exerting increasing pressure to have them corrected, but corrections are gradual and must accommodate to economic and political realities.

Fragmentation of Care

Highly specialized techniques and new knowledge emerging during the past 30 years of research mean that an increasing number of health care personnel provide specialized services. They may be highly specialized technicians or technologists who have relatively narrow but exacting jobs, such as respiratory technologists, biomedical electronic technologists, and nuclear medicine technologists. Increased specialization is evident also among physicians. In 1982, about 83% of all physicians classified themselves as being in a specialty (Jonas 1986, p. 128). All this specialization means fragmentation of care and, often, increased cost of care. To clients, it may mean receiving care from 5 to 30 people during their hospital experience. This seemingly endless stream of personnel is often confusing and frightening. The individual feels like a cog in the wheel and asks, "Who really cares about me?" and "Who is really responsible?" The increasing number of health workers creates problems with the smooth flow of information and plans to help the client. Again, the person wonders, "Will someone forget to order my medication?" The concept of total care is more difficult to implement when so many people are involved.

Increased Cost of Services

The problem of financing health-illness services is increasingly severe. There are six major reasons for increased costs:

1. Existing equipment and facilities are continually becoming obsolete as research uncovers new and better methods in health-illness care.

2. Additional space and sophisticated equipment are required to provide the newest diagnostic and treatment methods.

3. Inflation increases all costs.

4. The total population has grown, and the demand for services has increased.

5. People increasingly recognize that health is a right of *all* people, hence larger numbers of people are seeking assistance in health matters.

6. The relative number of people who provide health-illness services has increased.

Health Care for the Homeless

The number of homeless people in towns and cities continues to grow. Estimates vary widely, but advocates of the homeless estimate this number at 2 million to 3 million in the United States. Reasons for this increase include the following (Lindsay 1989, p. 78):

- Rising cost of housing

- Reduction in federal subsidies for low-income housing

- Economic recessions of the late 1970s and early 1980s

resulting in continued low or minimum wages, plant closures, and unemployment
- Alcohol and drug abuse
- Deinstitutionalization of mental health facilities and a change in the laws governing commitment of the mentally ill. About 30 to 40% of the homeless are mentally ill.

The homeless differ from those who are poor; they are alone, lack some type of permanent residence, and are disaffiliated from family and friends. Because of the conditions in which homeless people live (in shelters, on the streets, in parks, in tents, under scrap material covers, under viaducts, in all-night movie theaters, in transportation terminals, or in cars), their health problems are often exacerbated and sometimes become chronic. Major health problems of the homeless include the following (Lindsay 1989, p. 79):

- Chronic health problems such as diabetes, hypertension, and drug and alcohol abuse
- Risk of communicable diseases such as tuberculosis, scabies, lice, and AIDS
- Hypothermia in the winter
- Malnutrition
- Dental problems
- Peripheral vascular problems
- Traumatic injuries and risk of assault
- Children at risk of abuse, neglect, and missing immunizations, making them vulnerable to disease

The 1987 Report of the Panel on Health Goals for Ontario has suggested several basics to good health (Spasoff 1987): "peace; an adequate income; adequate housing and food; a valued role to play in family, work, and community; a safe environment; and a healthy lifestyle." These basics, however, are beyond the reach of the homeless population, many of whom are multiply handicapped by physical, mental, social, and emotional problems. Several factors contribute to poor health among the homeless (see the accompanying box).

One of the most critical contributors to poor health of the homeless is the lack of access to health care services, even though most of the homeless live in the cities that have an abundance of health services. In the United States, the majority of homeless people have no benefits such as Medicard, Aid for Families with Dependent Children, veteran's benefits, and private health insurance. In Canada—even with its national health insurance system—many homeless have lost their hospital insurance number and other forms of identification and lack other resources such as money and a home address to obtain new identification. Homeless people without proper identification find it humiliating to be turned away when they seek health care.

Because the life-style of the homeless is usually outside the experience of health care providers, it is difficult for them to understand and appreciate the health care needs of this group. In addition, many health care providers find

---

Factors Contributing to Poor Health of the Homeless

- Poor physical environment resulting in increased susceptibility to infections
- Inadequate rest and privacy
- Improper nutrition
- Poor access to facilities for personal hygiene
- Exposure to the elements
- Lack of social support
- Few personal resources
- Questionable personal safety (physical assault is a constant threat)
- Inadequate health care
- Poor compliance with treatment plans

---

it distasteful to deal with the homeless because of their poor hygiene, unkempt appearance, body odors, and sometimes offensive remarks and behavior. Those who have had experience with the homeless have learned that traditional approaches and routine health care instructions are not appropriate for this group of people. For example, Judd and Forgues (1989, p. 19) state that simple treatment instructions such as "get plenty of rest," "drink clear fluids," and "soak your wound in salt and water three times a day" may be impossible for homeless persons to carry out, given their meager resources (e.g., no bed, no money, and no hygienic facilities). Experienced health professionals have learned, too, that the homeless want to be healthy and that they will, with support, benefit from health care services.

Health care workers can help in providing health care to the homeless in these ways (Judd and Forgues 1989, p. 19):

- Valuing the right of the homeless to receive the same health care as others in the society
- Establishing nursing care services in shelters and on the streets

In 1983, the Robert Wood Johnson Foundation (RWJ) and the Pew Memorial Trust announced the Health Care for the Homeless Program (The RWJ/Pew homeless program initiative), in which they would provide funds for four-year demonstration projects providing health care to the homeless. Several cities in the United States have successfully applied for funding and have demonstrated that the homeless can be reached and that health care can be provided to them. In Canada, one approach to helping the homeless was started in Toronto in 1985 by Dilin Baker, who originated a service called Street Health. Street Health is owned and operated by street people who are members of the board of directors and who work in the clinics. This type of service enables nurses to establish contact, gain trust, act as resource persons, attend to minor wounds and conditions, listen to and act on their concerns, teach illness management to shelter workers, help the homeless secure identification, and through the office provide an address for these people to receive mail. The ultimate goal of Street Health is to lead the homeless to existing health services.

Special Needs of the Elderly

Because people over 65 are becoming an increasingly large group in the population, their health needs deserve special concern. Long-term illnesses and disability are most prevalent in this group, and with these illnesses frequently come special needs for housing, treatment services, and financial support.

The health of the elderly is also associated with social deprivation. For instance, problems such as hypothermia, incontinence, and depression have been linked to inadequate heating and housing and feelings of rejection (Tinker 1983, p. 61).

Uneven Distribution of Health Services

Serious problems in the distribution in health services exist in both the United States and Canada. Two facets of this problem are (a) uneven distribution and (b) increased specialization. Uneven distribution is evidenced by the relatively higher number of nurses per population in the New England states and lowest number in Louisiana and Oklahoma. Physicians are also unevenly distributed: Mississippi has the lowest number of physicians per 100,000 (120), whereas Massachusetts has the highest (Jonas 1986, pp. 61, 103).

CHALLENGES FOR THE FUTURE

Health for All

In 1977, the World Health Organization launched the movement known as Achieving Health for All. The goal of this movement was—and still is today—for all persons to obtain a level of health by the year 2000 that will permit them to lead socially and economically productive lives.

Achieving the goal of equal access to appropriate health care for all people in the future requires the efforts of all people and a focus on the following (O'Neill 1983, pp. 117–18):

1. Establishment of community-based health systems in which primary health care is the major function. Such systems would need to be backed up by hospital services and other specialty services. Health and welfare centers of the future need to be planned together and cover all aspects of health. Such centers should be places that the local people can approach whatever their health requirement.

2. Redistribution of health and specialty services to overcome regional inequities. Currently, health care services and professionals are concentrated in the more prosperous urban areas. In rural and low-income areas, such as declining inner city areas, there is a notable lack of services.

3. Emphasis on self-reliance and participation by the individual and community members in health matters. This will require a changed emphasis by health workers on home and community care rather than institutional care. More research will be needed about the cost-effectiveness of home and community services, self-care, and self-help approaches.

4. Increased emphasis on provision of services to specific target groups, such as children and adolescents, the elderly, the disabled, the dying, single mothers, the mentally ill, and working mothers. A whole array of services that now exist need expansion. Examples are health education for children, home help, and child care for working women.

5. Increased involvement of existing health organizations and groups. Many existing health and social groups, e.g., AA, groups for the elderly, and paraplegic associations, can use their specialized talents to bring about change.

6. Expanded education of health professionals—medical practitioners, nurses, nurse-midwives—in community and health care as well as traditional hospital and acute care. Graduating physicians and nurses will need to think and practice in terms of health rather than disease, apply techniques of prevention and health promotion in addition to those of cure and rehabilitation, focus practice on the family and community and not the individual sick person, and work as members of a health team that invites the active participation of the consumer. Clients are now beginning to play a critical, active role rather than their traditional, uncritical role of passively accepting everything the health professional says and does.

7. Expansion of traditional roles and change in the current hierarchical health profession. As O'Neill (1983, p. 72) says: "Health professionals have before them a dramatic new role in addition to the exercise of their clinical skills: that of health leaders, educators, guides, and generators of simpler and more socially acceptable technologies. To fulfill this role they will require a combination of sagacity, scientific and technical knowledge, social understanding, managerial acumen and, above all, political persuasiveness."

8. New focus by government on health rather than cure and on the roles that transportation, housing, and industry can play in bringing about a healthy society.

Future Health Care Environment

O'Malley, Loveridge, and Cummings (1989) state that the changing health care environment challenges nurses to redesign nursing care delivery systems. Several future changes in the health care environment are outlined in the accompanying box.

Aydelotte (1987, p. 118) predicts a health care system divided into four branches:

1. Health promotion, health education, self-help, and health evaluation

2. Chronic disease management

3. Trauma and severe illnesses

4. Care of the frail elderly, the physically limited elderly, and the dying

Within each of these branches at least four classes of nursing roles are needed (Aydelotte 1987, p. 119):

1. Provider of direct services

2. Researcher and developer, who will develop new knowledge, educational programs, technology, media, *telematics* (new information technologies), and the like

3. Case manager in the health promotion and maintenance branch, who will emphasize prevention rather than remedy

4. Executives to administer groups of nurses in the units, who will secure resources; allocate resources; develop policy; and distribute, evaluate, and revise services

Nurses will provide these services through four different arrangements (Aydelotte 1987, p. 119):

Future Changes in the Health Care Environment

- The elderly will be the fastest growing segment of the population, because the baby boomers are entering middle age; therefore, the number who are young and who provide services to this group will be relatively small.

- Hospitals will restructure their organizations and redirect their goals toward a health-maintenance versus illness-based culture.

- Health promotion services, child-rearing services, and weight reduction programs will increasingly be provided by the same organizations that offer long-term care and physical rehabilitation.

- The organizational design of the health care service will be decentralized and information-based rather than centralized and bureaucratic.

- The service focus will become consumer-focused and information-based rather than treatment focused and highly technologic.

Source: J. O'Malley, C. E. Loveridge, and S. H. Cummings, The new nursing organization, *Nursing Management,* February 1989, 20:29–32.

---

1. Professional corporations headed by nurses, which will contract with specific groups or other organizations to provide nursing services such as school nursing, home health care, or intensive care

2. Nurse specialty practice groups, which will provide special services such as counseling, health maintenance, and certain technological services on a contractual basis with individuals or groups

3. Practice on an individual basis, which will provide highly specialized nursing service on a one-to-one basis or consultation with other health care professionals (this service will also be arranged by contracts).

4. Employment in profit and nonprofit health care systems primarily oriented toward acute care

Implications for Nursing

The changes and future trends in the health care system have many implications for nursing practice. Aydelotte (1987, pp. 118–20; 1983, pp. 814–15) describes the following strategies:

- The nature of the profession needs to be clarified and understood. The knowledge of nursing should be exclusive, and the education of nurses should be on a professional level. The title "nurse" should be more highly restricted to only one class, i.e., the *professional,* and not include support personnel.

- Individuals entering nursing must meet high standards of intelligence and motivation, especially motivation to public service. The nursing profession must be concerned with building a nucleus of true professionals.

- The nursing education system needs to be remodeled, so that it will be much more extensive and sound. Such a remodeling should include more depth in the sciences, an understanding of economics, emphasis on legal and ethical issues, an introduction to management and business, an increased understanding of information technology, and greater clinical application.

- Preparation in self-governance and self-management is needed for the professional of the future. Ways to develop clinical nursing judgment need to be explored and made available to students.

- Nursing's relationship with the public and the power elite must change. Political action should extend beyond the legislative arena into every aspect of community affairs. Nursing leaders need to make a concerted effort to become college and university presidents and vice presidents, leaders in business and community affairs, heads of corporations, and chairpersons of boards. Increased leadership skills for functioning in corporate structures will be needed.

- The costs of nursing services will need to be established. Currently, nursing costs are often disguised as hospital room costs or payments to nonnurse supervisors. Thus, a system of reimbursement that pays directly to nursing services obtained by contracts needs to be developed. To develop such a system, nurses will need to learn the management of contracts and business, attach a value to services, and, at the same time, ensure the maintenance or quality of care provided.

■ Nursing strategies need to be designed to meet the health promotion and health maintenance needs of people, especially the elderly, low-income persons, rural residents, the chronically ill, the unemployed, pregnant women, working women, children, and adolescents. The nurse's role in primary care needs to be expanded in hospitals, homes, and industry, and the public and government need to be convinced that such services would coordinate care, decrease fragmentation, and be cost-efficient. Nurses will need to develop the following:
   a. Improved assessment and evaluation skills
   b. Increased skills in communication, e.g., a second language or computer skills
   c. Increased knowledge and acceptance of cultural diversity
   d. Increased acceptance of change
   e. Increased use of technology in teaching clients

Humanizing Health Care

Although the goal of any health care delivery system is intrinsically human, the system is perceived as increasingly dehumanizing. Dehumanization is associated with vulnerability, powerlessness, and loss of identity in large, faceless institutions. The blame usually falls on society in general, technologic change, the rat race, or bureaucratic red tape.

Howard and Strauss (1975, p. 73) discuss four ways nurses and other health care professionals can humanize care:

1. Value the concept of inherent worth, which reflects notions of equality among people. Health systems now recognize the inherent worth of persons by trying to prolong life, reduce pain, and restore social functioning. Clients themselves emphasize that they should be treated with dignity and respect even if discriminated against in the larger society. The concept of inherent worth needs to apply to *all* professional/client interactions and must be reflected in institutional policy.

2. Recognize that each person is a unique individual, even though all humans have some commonalities, and avoid stereotyping or treating clients in a routine, uniform way. Remember that at any given moment, the sum of a person's past and present experience influences the person's feelings, attitudes, and actions.

3. Recognize that although humans do not have infinite freedom of action, most people have considerable control and choice over their destinies and need to be given the freedom to consider all options available to them. Clients are restricted by such factors as illness, ignorance, and financial constraints. Practitioners are restricted by institutional commitments, colleague pressures, scarce resources for therapy, and cost considerations. Sharing decision making and responsibility (a) reflects the ideology that all clients, regardless of education, have a right to participate as much as possible in decisions about their care and (b) makes the client and provider partners and therefore, in a way, equals. To share in decision making, the client must be informed about prognoses, alternative therapies, and the rationales behind them.

   The client's level of education will influence the client's desire and capacity to accept shared responsibility for care. In addition, some clients may be too sick, anxious, or irrational to analyze facts and to make appropriate decisions.

4. Convey empathy and positive affect. *Empathy* is the ability to identify and sympathize with others. Clients expect health care professionals to show sympathy and concern. Otherwise, clients feel depersonalized and dehumanized. For example, in the words of one client, "He should know how much my leg hurts and what it means to me." The dilemma of the practitioner is that too much empathy can be emotionally draining. In some instances, it may also be impossible to put oneself in the client's shoes. For example, an able-bodied nurse who cares for paraplegics knows that these clients are well aware the nurse has two legs and cannot possibly identify with them as well as another paraplegic. Thus, a balance between too little and too much empathy is necessary. The means of achieving this balance needs research.

   Positive affect is the conveying of genuine feelings of warmth to the client. Positive feelings appear to be necessary for continued human-to-human contact.

CHAPTER HIGHLIGHTS

▶ Consumer attitudes—their view of health care as a right and their demand for comprehensive, holistic, and humanistic health care—are noticeably influencing health care delivery.

▶ Consumers are demanding greater emphasis on health promotion and illness prevention rather than on treatment of disease.

▶ The idea that health is the responsibility of each individual in society is gaining greater acceptance.

▶

- Social changes, such as the women's movement, the rise in single-parent families and in women working outside the home, cultural diversity, and the growing elderly population, are influencing the type and quantity of health care services needed.

- Health care services are currently financed through social insurance, such as Medicaid and Medicare in the United States and the National Medical and Hospital Insurance programs in Canada; direct client payments; voluntary insurance plans, such as Blue Cross and Blue Shield; and charitable donations.

- The prospective payment system (PPS) was introduced in the United States to curtail the escalating costs of health care.

- Because of fewer hospital admissions, earlier discharges, and staff reductions—the results of PPS—the need for home health care has increased.

- Government health care agencies, established at the local, state (provincial), and federal levels, are supported by revenues obtained through taxes.

- Agencies providing health care can be viewed as giving primary, secondary, and tertiary care.

- *Primary care* agencies focus on health maintenance, health promotion, and disease prevention.

- *Secondary care agencies,* such as hospitals and ambulatory care clinics, focus on the treatment of illness and the prevention of complications of disease conditions.

- *Tertiary care agencies* provide long-term care and rehabilitation services and focus on restoring the client to optimum functioning after physical or mental illness.

- Several alternative health care delivery systems, such as health maintenance organizations, preferred provider organizations, and individual practice associations, have arisen in the past decade to encourage preventive health care and to reduce the cost of health care to the consumer.

- A variety of hospice services meets the special needs of the terminally ill in settings other than acute care agencies; caring and psychologic support are emphasized.

- Health care services are provided by a variety of health care personnel in a variety of settings.

- Problems in the health care system include fragmentation of care, increased costs, and health care for the homeless, elderly, and low-income groups.

- The unemployed and poverty-stricken have unique health care needs that require increasing attention.

- Future challenges in health care delivery are to promote health as a way of life, to prevent ill health, and to provide community care for all.

- In the future, nurses will need to be prepared to practice in primary care settings and to develop the skills to work in these settings. They will also need to learn the management of contracts and business.

READINGS AND REFERENCES

SUGGESTED READINGS

Curtin, L. L. March 1980. Is there a right to health care? *American Journal of Nursing* 80:462–65.

In this thought-provoking article, Curtin discusses "human rights" as related to health care and presents these in relation to "human wants." Curtin suggests that reasonable health guidelines should be developed and that the intrusion of government in the health of people should be limited.

Davis, G. C. November/December 1988. Nursing values and health care policy. *Nursing Outlook* 36:289–92.

Davis describes the relationship between society's and nursing's values and how these relate to public policy. Five nursing beliefs are described, and some suggestions for influencing health policy conclude the article.

Dimond, M. March/April 1989. Health care and the aging population. *Nursing Outlook* 37:76–77.

Dimond relates the increasing number of aging people in the population to the problems in the present health care delivery system. Dimond then explains some of the challenges facing health care providers given the limited financial resources. Long-term care as a health care deficiency and the problem of aging as a women's problem are described.

Grassi, L. C. 1989. Nurses' assessment of DRGs on quality patient care. *Nursing Forum* 24:32–34.

Grassi describes a survey of how several nurses perceive the impact of DRGs on client care. The survey revealed that the nurses had specific concerns about the quality of health care for their clients.

RELATED RESEARCH

Beachy, W. November 1988. Multicompetent health professionals: Needs, combinations, and curriculum development. *Journal of Allied Health* 17:319–29.

Bremer, A. 1989. A description of community health nursing practice with the community-based elderly. *Journal of Community Health Nursing* 6:173–84.

Cameron, E.; Badger, F.; and Evers, H. May 1989. District nursing, the disabled and the elderly: Who are the black patients? *Journal of Advanced Nursing* 14:376–82.

Wilson, S. L.; Rudman, S. V.; and Snyder, J. R. May/June 1989. Health educators in HMOs: A study of utilization and effectiveness. *Health Values* 13:9–14.

SELECTED REFERENCES

American Nurses' Association. 1976, 1985. *Code for nurses with interpretative statements.* Kansas City, Mo.: ANA.

American Nurses' Association. Center for Research. June 1985. *DRGs and nursing care.* Kansas City, Mo.: ANA.

American Hospital Association. January 1976. A patient's bill of rights. *Nursing Outlook* 24:29 (also February 1973, *Nursing Outlook* 21:82).

Annas, G. J. 1975. *The rights of hospital patients: The basic ACLU guide to a hospital patients' rights.* New York: Avon Books.

Annas, G. J., and Healey, J. May/June 1974. The patient rights advocate. *Journal of Nursing Administration* 4:25–31.

Aydelotte, M. K. 1983. The future health care delivery system in the United States. In Chaska, N. L. *The nursing profession: A time to speak.* New York: McGraw-Hill.

———. May/June 1987. Nursing's preferred future. *Nursing Outlook* 35:114–20.

Bandman, E. L., and Bandman, B. 1990. *Nursing ethics in the lifespan.* 2d ed. Norwalk, CT.: Appleton and Lange.

Bentley, J. D., and Butler, P. 1980. Case mix reimbursements: Measures, applications, experiments. *Hospital Financial Management* 3:14.

Brecht, M. C. January/February 1990. Nursing's role in assuring access to care. *Nursing Outlook* 38:6–7.

Caterinicchio, R. P., editor. 1984. *DRGs: What they are and how to survive them—A sourcebook for professional nursing.* Thorofare, N.J.: Charles B. Slack.

Curtin, L. L., and Zurlage, C. 1984. *DRGs: The reorganization of health.* Chicago: S-N Publications.

Davis, C. K. 1983. The federal role in changing health care financing. *Nursing Economics* 1:10–11.

Deines, E. October 1985. Coping with PPS and DRGs: The levels of care approach. *Nursing Management* 16:43–44, 46–48, 52.

Dimond, M. March/April 1989. Health care and the aging population. *Nursing Outlook* 37:76–77.

Dougherty, C. J. 1988. *American health care: Realities, rights, and reforms.* New York: Oxford University Press.

Good intentions gone awry. March/April 1986. *Nursing Life* 6:55–56.

Griffith, H. September/October 1983. Competition in health care. *Nursing Outlook* 31:262–65.

———. May 1985. Who will become the preferred provider? *American Journal of Nursing* 85:538–42.

Griffith-Kenney, J. 1986. *Contemporary women's health: A nursing advocacy approach.* Menlo Park, Calif.: Addison-Wesley Publishing Co.

Hamilton, C. L., and Wilson, C. N. January 1989. The new Medicare Catastrophic Coverage Act: Will it affect nursing? *Nursing and Health Care* 10:30–34.

Hamilton, J. January/February 1986. Consumer alert: DRGs—Are hospitals saving money at your expense? *American Health* 41–45.

Howard, J., and Strauss, A., editors. 1975. *Humanizing health care.* New York: John Wiley and Sons.

Jonas, S. 1986. *Health care delivery in the United States.* 3d ed. New York: Springer Publishing Co.

Judd, V., and Forgues, C. November 1989. Canada's homeless: Breaking down the barriers to health care. *Canadian Nurse* 85:18–19.

Kelly, M. September 1989. The Omnibus Budget Reconciliation Act of 1987: A policy analysis. *Nursing Clinics of North America* 24:791–94.

Lindsay, A. M. March/April 1989. Health care for the homeless. *Nursing Outlook* 37:78–81.

Lundberg, C. J. 1984. Home health care: A logical extension of hospital services. *Topics in Health Care Financing* 11:22–33.

McCorkle, R., and Germino, B. 1984. What nurses need to know about home care. *Oncology Nursing Forum* 11:63–69.

McManis, G. L. February 10, 1989. AIDS crisis: A catalyst for needed changes. *Modern Health Care* 19:30.

Micheletti, J. A., and Shlala, T. J. October 1985. PROs and PPS: Nursing's role in utilization management. *Nursing Management* 16:37–42.

Morris, E. M., and Fonseca, J. D. 1984. Home care today: An interview. *American Journal of Nursing* 84:340–42.

Omachonu, V. K., and Nanda, R. April 1989. Measuring productivity: Outcome vs. output. *Nursing Management* 20:35–38, 40.

O' Malley, J.; Loveridge, C. E.; and Cummings, S. H. February 1989. The new nursing organization. *Nursing Management* 20:29–32.

O'Neill, P. 1983. *Health crisis 2000.* London: William Heinemann.

Porter-O'Grady, T. October 1985. Strategic planning: Nursing practice in the PPS. *Nursing Management* 16:53–56.

Pryga, E., and Bachofer, H. June 24, 1983. *Hospice care under Medicare.* Working paper. Chicago: Office of Public Policy Analysis, American Hospital Association. Cited in Amenta, M. O. September/October 1984. Hospice U.S.A. 1984: Steady and holding. *Oncology Nursing Forum* 11:68–74.

RNABC News. January/February 1990. Health in the 1990's. *RNABC News* 22:11–13.

Smith, C. E. January 1985. DRGs: Making them work for you. *Nursing 85* 15:34–41.

Spasoff, R. 1987. *Health for all: Report of the Panel on Health Goals for Ontario.* Toronto: Ontario Ministry of Health.

Statistics Canada. 1980. *Perspectives Canada III.* Ottawa: Minister of Supply and Services.

———. 1981. *Canada year book 1980–81.* Ottawa: Statistics Canada.

Thatcher, R. M. September 1989. Community support: Promoting health and self-care. *Nursing Clinics of North America* 24:725–31.

Tinker, A. 1983. *The Elderly in Modern Society.* 2d ed. London: Longman.

U.S. Bureau of the Census. 1980. *Statistical abstract of the United States.* 101st ed. Washington, D.C.: U.S. Government Printing Office.

U.S. Department of Commerce. July 1, 1984. *Statistics on elderly population.* Washington, D.C.: Bureau of the Census.

U.S. Department of Health and Human Services. August 1985a. *Charting the nation's health trends since 1960.* Pub. no. (PHS) 85-1251. Hyattsville, Md.: Public Health Service.

———. December 1985b. *Health United States.* Pub. no. (PHS) 86-1232. Hyattsville, Md.: Public Health Service.

U.S. Department of Health, Education, and Welfare. 1979. *Healthy people: The surgeon general's report on health promotion and disease prevention.* Pub. no. 79-55071. Washington, D.C.: U.S. Government Printing Office.

Walker, A. 1987. Demand and supply of health care services. In Economics Council of Canada, *Aging with limited health resources: Proceedings of a colloquium on health care, May 1986.* Ottawa: Minister of Supplies and Services.

Warhola, C. 1980. *Planning for home health services: A resource book.* Pub. no. (HRA) 80-14017. Washington, D.C.: Public Health Service, Department of Health and Human Services.

Weinstein, S. M. 1984. Specialty teams in home care. *American Journal of Nursing* 84:342–45.

Zarle, N. C. September 1989. Continuity of care: Balancing care of elders between health care settings. *Nursing Clinics of North America* 24:697–705.

PROFESSIONAL ACCOUNTABILITY AND ADVOCACY

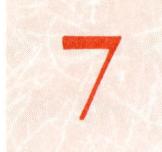
Ethical Aspects of Nursing Practice

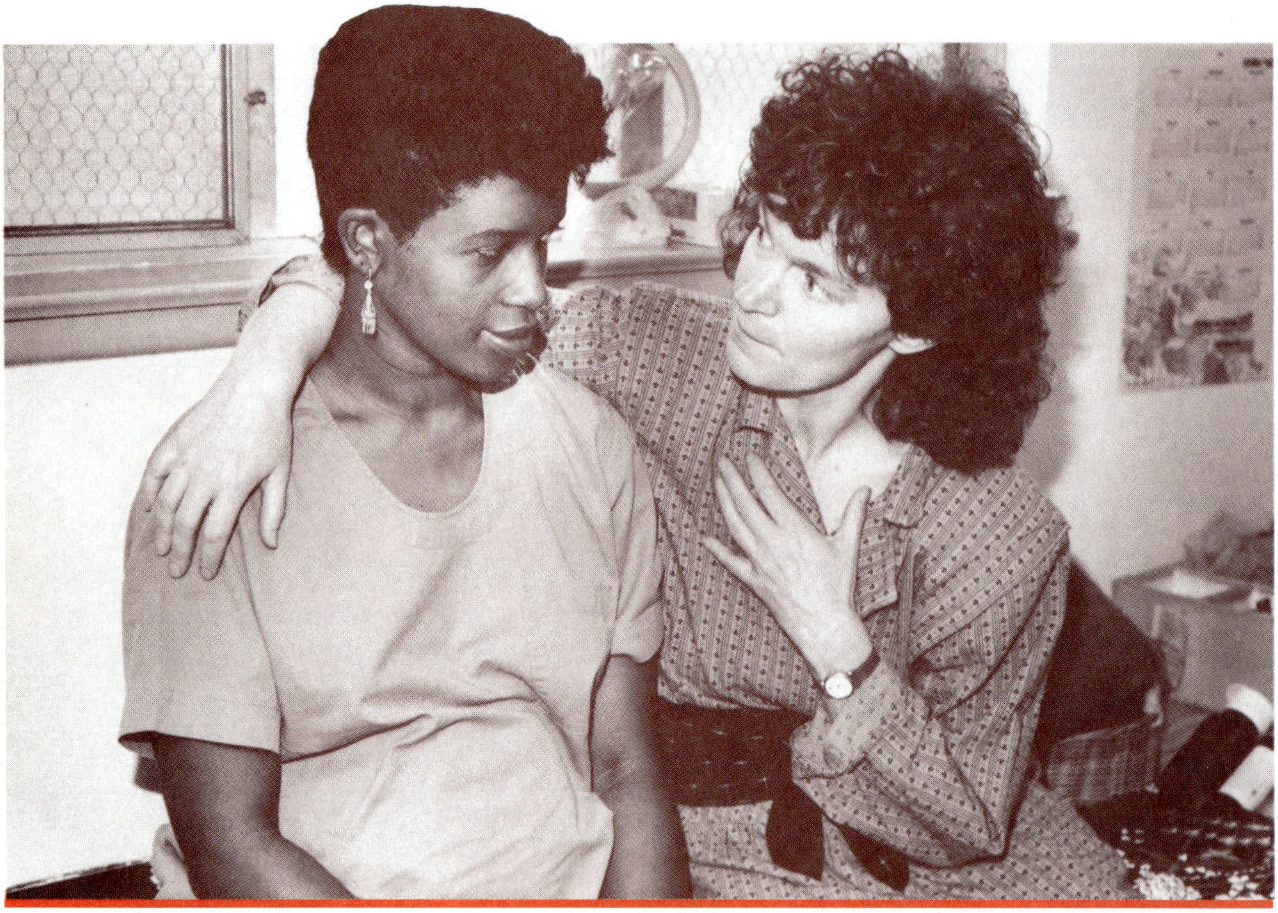

CONTENTS

OBJECTIVES

▶ Identify various ways in which values, beliefs, and attitudes are learned.

▶ Describe four methods of transmitting values.

▶ Explain Rath's values clarification process.

▶ Describe reasons for identifying clients' values.

▶ State three elements of a moral dilemma.

▶ Identify professional values incorporated in nursing codes.

▶ Describe the purposes of codes of ethics.

▶ Discuss the types of ethical issues encountered by nurses.

▶ Discuss the process for resolving ethical dilemmas.

VALUES, BELIEFS, ATTITUDES, AND ETHICS DEFINED

Nurses are becoming increasingly aware of the values, beliefs, and attitudes of clients and their support persons and of the ethics involved in nursing practice. Values, beliefs, and attitudes differ from one another but are often interconnected.

A **value** can be defined as something of worth, a belief held dear by a person. A value is an affective disposition toward a person, object, or idea (Steele and Harmon 1983, p. 1). According to Simon et al. (1978), "values are a set of personal beliefs and attitudes about the truth, beauty, worth of any thought, object, or behavior. They are action oriented and give direction and meaning to one's life." Values develop from associations with people, the environment and self; they are derived from life experiences (Steele and Harmon 1983, p. 1). Values form a basis for behavior; a person's real values are shown by consistent patterns of behavior. Once one is aware of one's values, the values become an internal control for behavior. "Values are significant in choice making" (Salladay and McDonnell 1989, p. 544).

Values common to many people are peace, truth, and freedom, for example. Values exist in some relationship to one another within a person. A **value system** is the organization of a person's values along a continuum of relative importance. Values underlie people's purposive behavior. **Purposive behavior** refers to actions that are performed "on purpose" with the intention of reaching some goal or bringing about a certain result (Muldary 1983, p. 200). Purposive behavior, then, is based on a person's decisions or choices, and these decisions or choices are based on underlying values.

There are two types of values: intrinsic and extrinsic. An **intrinsic value** relates to the maintenance of life, e.g., food and water have intrinsic value. An **extrinsic value** originates outside the individual and is not necessary for the maintenance of life, e.g., health, holism, and humanism (Steele and Harmon 1983, p. 2).

Values can be either positive or negative. A positive value is a view of what is desirable or how something *should be*. For example, some nurses value a holistic approach to nursing. Negative values, by contrast, are views of what is undesirable or how something *should not be*. For example, talking unkindly about clients is considered by many nurses to be undesirable. Therefore, being unkind is a negative value.

A **belief** (opinion) is something accepted as true by a judgment of probability rather than actuality. It is a special type of attitude whose cognitive (intellectual) component is based more on faith than on fact. People hold beliefs that may be true or that can, with reliable evidence, be proved true. Family traditions and folklore are beliefs passed from one generation to another.

Beliefs may or may not involve values. For example, a client may believe that all nurses are honest. The client has accepted that a relationship exists between "nurse" and "honesty," nurse being the object and honesty the value. The client considers this relationship self-evident. A belief of this type is sometimes called a value judgment.

An **attitude** is a feeling tone directed toward a person, object, or idea. Attitudes have behavioral, cognitive, and affective components. The behavioral component of an attitude is exemplified by the tendency of the person to take action. It reflects the inclination of the individual to act as a result of his or her attitude. For example, a nurse who dislikes a peer's behavior toward a client is inclined to think, "If she speaks that way to Mr. B again, I am going to. . . ." This is the inclination to act, a part of one's attitude toward the peer. The cognitive component of an attitude includes the beliefs and factual information associated with the attitude, e.g., nursing is a high-stress occupation. The affective component may be the central component of an attitude. It is the feelings that are associated with the belief, knowledge, and the target of the attitude. Feelings vary greatly among people; for example, one client may feel very strongly about the sound from a television in the next room, whereas another client dismisses it as unimportant. The affective component of one's attitudes is usually rooted in a person's values (Muldary 1983, p. 210).

Attitudes are made up of many beliefs (Steele and Harmon 1983, p. 3). For example, a child may learn such attitudes as cooperation and kindness from parents and in turn exhibit these in behavior. According to values clarification theory, a belief or attitude can become a value only if the belief satisfies seven criteria. See the section on values later in this chapter.

Ethics are the rules or principles that govern right conduct. The word *ethics* is derived from the Greek *ethos,* meaning custom or character. An ethic is "what ought to be." The term *bioethics* is being used increasingly in the health field. **Bioethics** is the ethics concerning life.

In nursing, ethical practice refers to a nurse's moral behavior and decisions regarding ethical dilemmas (Ketefian 1989, p. 509).

Morality is a word often used interchangeably with ethics. "Morality concerns behavior which involves judgments, actions, and attitudes based on rationally conceived and effectively established norms" (Steele and Harmon 1983, p. 49). In other words, **morality** denotes what is right and wrong in conduct, character, or attitude and what individuals must do to live together in society. The way a person perceives the requirements for living together and responds to them is **moral behavior.**

Some authors use the term **moral reasoning** to refer to the cognitive and developmental process of reasoning about moral choice. Moral judgment and moral development are terms often used synonymously for moral reasoning (Ketefian 1989, p. 509). People learn moral reasoning during their **socialization,** the process by which individuals learn the knowledge, skills, and dispositions of their social group or society. Lawrence Kohlberg sees six stages in the moral development of individuals. See Chapter

24 for Kohlberg's theory and other theories of moral development as proposed by Kegan and Gilligan. Also see Table 7–1 for a summary of moral development.

VALUES

Each person, e.g., nurse, client, and physician, has a personal set of values. A **value set** is the group of values a person holds. Individuals incorporate personal values into their lives as a result of observing the behavior and attitudes of parents and teachers and interacting with their cultural, religious, and social environments. Personal values also reflect experiences and a person's intelligence.

Professional values are a reflection and expansion of personal values (Fromer 1981, p. 15). These values are acquired as a nurse is socialized into the nursing profession.

Acquisition of Values

Raths, Harmin, and Simon (1978) identified seven criteria that must be met for beliefs, attitudes, activities, or feelings to become values:

TABLE 7–1   *Summary of Moral Development*

Developmental Stage	Moral Development	Examples of Values Developed
Infant (0 to 1 years)	The infant is generally considered not to have values but perceives emotions and the behavior of others. A mother's or caregiver's behavior toward the infant can reflect her or his values.	Parents who communicate love to their infants and convey pleasure in the infant's pleasure teach the infant the values of love and caring.
Toddler (1 to 3 years)	The toddler learns values largely through copying others; i.e., through modeling. Toddlers don't understand the meaning behind a value.	By showing appreciation and saying thank you when others give gifts and when the toddler starts to give the parents toys, objects, or food, parents teach toddlers that "giving" makes others feel good and, in turn, makes one feel good about oneself.
Preschooler (4 to 5 years)	The preschooler learns the right and wrong of singular acts but does not possess a concept of right and wrong.	By pointing out to her son that taking a toy away from a sister or friend is wrong and makes the other person feel as badly as he would if the same happened to him, a mother teaches the child to consider other person's feelings and to treat everyone as you want to be treated.
School-aged child (6 to 12 years)	People with diverse values have contact with school-aged children. Parents who provide alternatives in situations help the school-aged child solve problems, make decisions, and learn the value of self-determination.	Parents who help and encourage a child with a school project teach the child the value of industry and completing projects once started.
Adolescent (12 to 18 years)	Adolescents encounter a multitude of new values. Adolescents learn to identify some of their own significant values. Parents continue to be a major source of values.	Parents who recognize that adolescents and other people have the right to their own tastes and preferences convey to the adolescent the value of respect for others.
Early adulthood	Most young adults can identify many of their own values. Although these may be tested through experience, the young adult establishes these as part of self. Some values may differ from those of the parents.	By moving away from home and through widening experiences, a young adult develops values associated with health, e.g., becomes a vegetarian and exercises daily.
Middle adulthood	Middle-aged adults who are secure and satisfied with their values will experience pleasure and a sense of serenity with each day. People who are dissatisfied and insecure may discard held values.	A man who values youth and helping others spends much of his time with scouts.
Late adulthood	Older adults may see their values challenged in a changing society. Older adults often learn to appreciate differing values of others but at the same time keep their own values.	A woman accepts that her grandson is living with his girlfriend, although she feels that people of the opposite sex should marry before doing so.

1. Having been freely chosen without outside pressure
2. Having been chosen from among alternatives
3. Having been chosen after reflection
4. Having been prized and cherished
5. Having been affirmed to others
6. Having been incorporated into actual behavior
7. Having been repeated in one's life (1978, p. 47)

A value must meet the above criteria, i.e., it is a belief put into practice (Thompson and Thompson 1985, p. 78). Values are also hierarchical, i.e., each person has an individual hierarchy of values, ranging from the most important value to the least important value. For information about health beliefs and values, see Chapter 5.

Values Transmission

Each person has a relatively small number of values. The origin of these values can be traced to culture, society, institutions, and personality. In addition, these few values guide virtually all aspects of behavior. Values are learned and are greatly influenced by a person's sociocultural environment. For example, Puerto Ricans often value treatment by a folk healer over treatment by a physician. For additional information about cultural and ethnic values relative to health and illness, see Chapter 31.

Values are learned throughout life; however, many values are learned in early childhood. Acquiring values is usually a gradual process of which the individual is unaware. People do not always realize they have a specific set of values or that they base the decisions they make on values. Values are transmitted in a variety of ways. Four approaches are modeling, laissez-faire, moralizing, and responsible choice (Simon et al. 1978, pp. 15–18).

Modeling
Modeling is a process by which a person engages in ideal behavior to serve as an example to be imitated by other persons (Johnson 1972, p. 189). There are two steps in modeling: (a) one person must engage in the ideal behavior, and (b) the second person must imitate the first person's behavior.

Parents are important models. Young children often want to be like their parents and will copy their parents' behavior. Through modeling, they behave in a manner that they perceive represents ideal values. However, modeling also can transmit socially unacceptable values. For example, a man who repeatedly hits his wife during an argument is modeling a socially unacceptable way to resolve a disagreement.

Laissez-faire
In this approach, people are left alone "to do their own thing." For example, a child is left free to have new experiences and to form his or her own values without parental guidance. The problem with this approach is that children can become confused when the adults around them do not support any behavior. For young people or people being socialized into roles, e.g., the nursing role, a laissez-faire approach to learning values can result in conflict and frustration.

Moralizing
Moralizing is a direct method of inculcating values in another person. In some religions, moralizing is the basis of indoctrination into the religion: people are told what is "right" and what is "wrong." People who learn their values through moralizing can have difficulty making responsible choices later in life because they have no experience doing so. Moralizing is a rigid approach to transmitting values: Alternatives are not provided, and the individual has no choice if he or she wishes to do or believe what is "right."

Responsible Choice
Values are also transmitted through responsible choice. The individual does not have free choice but is given limited choices. An example is the teenager who is allowed to use the family car only if it is returned by ten o'clock. The teenager has two choices that control behavior: not to use the car or to use it and return it on time. It is questionable, however, whether the teenager in this situation learns any values on which to base future behavior.

Values are also taught, usually by parents and by teachers in school and in religious organizations. For example, a parent will explain to a toddler that he or she should ask for a cookie before taking one, or a father will explain to a son how to be considerate on his first date. People also learn values through experience. For example, a young boy who drinks alcohol and then has an accident with the family car can learn from that experience to value safety and concern for others as well as himself when he drives. Additional information about teaching strategies may be found in Chapter 16.

Personal and Professional Values

The nurse enters the profession of nursing with values that guide personal actions. Through the process of socialization into the profession, the nurse may choose additional values. Personal and professional values are closely related and often can be the same. Hall (1973, pp. 23–32) identifies two primary values that are related to and must be in harmony with each other.

1. Self-value, or the idea that one is of worth to others
2. The idea that others are of equal worth

These primary values are not only vital as personal values in North American society but also vital as professional values, since nursing is based on relationships with clients, colleagues, and others.

Nurses' personal values influence client-nurse interactions and the practice of nursing. Steele and Harmon (1983, p. 7) believe that nurses can enact their professional roles with minimal discomfort when their personal and professional values are reasonably congruent. Thompson and Thompson (1985, p. 81) agree that nurses who are comfortable with their professional roles probably experience greater satisfaction and possibly provide better care for clients but question the latter point. A nurse who is comfortable with her or his role may not necessarily practice in an ethical manner. For example, the nurse who is comfortable in her or his role may decide not to "make waves" or may fail to take a stand against a decision that goes against her or his sense of ethics.

Personal Values
Most people derive some values from the society or subgroup of society in which they live. Values developed by society ensure its continued functioning and enable people to live harmoniously together. Examples of societal values common to Western civilization are shown in the accompanying box. A person may internalize

---

Universal Moral Values Basic to Clinical Nursing Practice

- Respect for persons
- Autonomy (self-determination)
- Beneficence (doing good)
- Nonmaleficence (avoiding harm)
- Veracity (truth telling)
- Confidentiality (respecting privileged information)
- Fidelity (keeping promises)
- Justice (treating people fairly)

Source: American Nurses' Association, *Code for Nurses with Interpretive Statements* (Kansas City, Mo.: American Nurses' Association, 1985).

Selected Societal and Personal Values

Societal Values	Personal Values
■ Human life	■ Family unity
■ Individual rights	■ Self-worth
■ Individual autonomy	■ Worth of others
■ Liberty	■ Independence
■ Democracy	■ Religion
■ Equal opportunity	■ Honesty
■ Power	■ Fairness
■ Health	■ Love
■ Wealth	■ Sense of humor
■ Youth	■ Safety
■ Vigor	■ Peace
■ Intelligence	■ Financial security
■ Imagination	■ Material things
■ Education	■ Money
■ Technology	■ Property of self
■ Conformity	■ Property of others
■ Friendship	■ Leisure time
■ Courage	■ Work
■ Compassion	■ Travel
■ Family	■ Plants
	■ Animals
	■ Physical activity
	■ Intellectual activity
	■ Artistic activity
	■ Neatness

---

some or all of these values and perceive them as personal values. In addition to internalizing societal values, people have values that are important to them as individuals. Purtilo (1978, p. 71) points out that most people find fulfillment only if they can integrate both societal and personal values into a satisfactory life-style. People need societal values to feel like an accepted part of the society and humankind, and they need personal values to individualize themselves.

Professional Values
Because nursing is a profession based on caring, professional values relate to both competence and compassion. Universal moral values are shown in the box above. Nurses develop these values during socialization into the profession and from professional codes of ethics, discussed later in this chapter.

Values Clarification

Values clarification is a process by which individuals find their own answers (values) to situations. It is not the transmission of "correct" values or rules, but a process of identifying and developing individual values. The principle of values clarification is that no one set of values is right for everyone.

The process of values clarification was formulated by Louis Raths in 1966, who built on the thinking of John Dewey. Raths was chiefly concerned with the process of valuing, not the content of the values. Valuing is composed of seven processes, which can be placed in three groups (Simon et al. 1978, p. 19):

Prizing one's beliefs and behaviors

1. Prizing and cherishing
2. Publicly affirming beliefs and behaviors when appropriate

Choosing one's beliefs and behaviors

3. Choosing from alternatives

4. Choosing according to consequences

5. Choosing freely

Acting on one's beliefs

6. Acting

7. Acting with a pattern, consistency, and repetition

A belief, attitude, or feeling becomes a value when all seven steps have been satisfied. The individual applies each of the seven steps to an emerging or already formed belief, behavior pattern, or attitude.

By using these seven steps in values clarification, nurses can clarify their own values and enhance their personal growth. These steps also can be applied to client situations; the nurse can help clients identify conflict areas, examine and choose from alternatives, set goals, and act (Coletta 1978, p. 2057).

Steele and Harmon (1983, p. 77) point out that nurses must exhibit ethical behavior to clients whether or not the nurse and client hold the same values. Nurses should, therefore, be "value-neutral"; that is, they should not believe that their own values are right and that a client's values are right or wrong. This attitude permits a nurse to establish an effective relationship with clients who have differing values.

Prizing and Cherishing

Prizing or cherishing is a continuous process in which the individual asks, "Do I cherish or prize my position or belief?" Unprized beliefs may still influence behavior, but they cannot be considered values.

Publicly Affirming When Appropriate

Public affirmation or appropriate sharing is an indication of the quality of a value. Individuals who feel strongly about an issue may publicly stand up and share the value with others. For example, nurses who value the autonomy of clients may refuse to obtain a signed consent form from a client without first explaining the procedure to the client. Thus the nurses are affirming to others their autonomy.

Choosing from Alternatives

For a belief to be a value, it must be chosen from among other alternatives. Individuals must consider the other options before they commit themselves to one choice.

Choosing After Consideration of Consequences

The individual must be able to consider the consequences of a choice, i.e., the significance of the decision. The person may reject or confirm the choice because of or in spite of the consequences. For example, a nurse may refuse to give a client a medication that the nurse believes may harm the client. The nurse considers the consequences of this behavior in terms of client and of self. The nurse is concerned for the client's welfare, but the refusal could result in disciplinary action. After considering all the alternatives, the nurse may confirm the choice of not giving the medication or select another course of action, e.g., dis-

cussing the medication with a physician before making a decision. If an individual's behavior is not the consequence of considering the results of action, it cannot be considered to reflect a value.

Choosing Freely

A value must be chosen freely. Some beliefs are not freely chosen by the individual but are accepted from parents or others without much thought and without choice. These beliefs are not values. Behavior determined by fear or coercion, for example, does not reflect values.

Acting

A value involves action. Therefore, a value must be incorporated into behavior. If it is not, it is not a value but a belief or an attitude.

Acting with a Pattern, Consistency, and Repetition

Behavior must be consistent over a period of time to reflect a value. The behavior is repeated in many aspects of life. For example, a nurse who values health will eat a healthful diet and get enough sleep.

It is important for nurses (a) to examine their own values and clarify them, (b) to recognize the differences in the values of clients and to accept them, and (c) to recognize the differences in the values of peers, other health care professionals, and health care organizations. Nurses need to recognize how such differences can affect them. Often, values represent an ideal; when that ideal is not achievable, some adaptation or compromise has to be made. Awareness of one's own values is a first step. The next step is to learn how to make the best possible compromise of values that circumstances allow. See "Resolving Ethical Dilemmas," later in this chapter.

Advantages of Values Clarification

Clarification of values has the following advantages (Steele and Harmon 1983, pp. vii, 13; Thompson and Thompson 1985, p. 78):

■ It is a process of discovery that brings to conscious awareness the values that guide one's actions.

■ It fosters the making of choices. It is not synonymous with ethical decision-making, however.

■ It leads to human growth because it fosters awareness, empathy, and insight.

■ It serves as a guide for assessing client values and provides direction for nursing interventions.

■ It gives insight into the source of a particular value. This awareness allows the individual to retain or change the value.

Identifying Personal Values

Nurses need to know in particular what values they hold about life, health, illness, and death. To explore personal values, the nurse can begin by answering questions such as

(Thompson and Thompson 1985, pp. 77–80): "What ten things do I like to do?" "What ten things do I like about myself?" "What ten things do I dislike about myself?" An awareness of things nurses dislike can lead to thoughts about what they may like to change. After initial exercises, nurses may then list ten values that guide their daily interactions or activities. By comparing their lists with a trusted friend or in a group that fosters trust and mutual respect, nurses can see similarities and differences with others. Resulting discussion often reveals reasons for the items listed. An example of a strategy called values voting is illustrated in the accompanying box. Another strategy for gaining awareness of personal values is to consider individual attitudes to such issues as abortion, unwanted pregnancy, euthanasia, sex-role stereotypes, and sexuality.

Examples of some questions and issues adapted from Corey et al. (1984, pp. 57–94) follow. When considering these issues, ask yourself: "Can I accept this or live with this?" "Why does this bother me?" "What would I do or want done in this situation?"

Values Clarification Strategy: Values Voting

This exercise, adapted from Uustal (1978, p. 2060) and Bernal (1985, p. 174), demonstrates that there are many facets to every issue. How do you determine your position? What factors influence your thoughts and feelings? How will your choice be reflected in your behavior? Talk with some colleagues. Do they feel similarly or differently?

Where do you stand on the following issues? Indicate your responses in the following manner:

SA	strongly agree	D	disagree
A	agree	SD	strongly disagree
U	undecided		

Do you believe:

1. ____ Clients have the right to participate in all decisions related to their health care.
2. ____ Clients have a right to refuse extraordinary treatment that is life-sustaining.
3. ____ Refusing life-sustaining treatments is a form of suicide.
4. ____ Clients have a right *not* to be interfered with in a rational act of suicide.
5. ____ Health professionals have a responsibility to assist a client in an act of rational suicide that does not cause injury to others.
6. ____ Comfort measures should always be provided.
7. ____ Health professionals should always do their best to sustain a person's life.

---

1. *Sexuality.* What are your attitudes toward?
   a. Teenage sex
   b. Casual sex
   c. Sex as an expression of love and commitment
   d. Group sex

2. *Right to die and the choice of suicide.* See the Values Clarification Strategy box.

3. *Abortion.* Indicate whether you agree or disagree with the following statements.
   a. A woman should have the right to choose abortion.
   b. Abortion at any point during gestation is murder.
   c. Abortion is wrong.
   d. Abortion should be performed if the woman's health is endangered.
   e. A mentally handicapped woman should be encouraged to have an abortion.
   f. Abortion should not be performed after 20 weeks' gestation, when a living infant can be borne.
   g. Abortion should be encouraged when parents have genetically transmissible diseases.

4. *Health.* Various definitions of health were proposed in Chapter 5. The nurse who defines and values health as physiologic, emotional, social, cultural, and spiritual well-being does not give the same nursing care as the nurse who defines health as the absence of illness. Remember that values are what the nurse actually puts into practice. Consider whether you agree or disagree with the following:
   a. To be most effective in nursing practice, the nurse must be a role model of health.
   b. An obese nurse can effectively instruct an obese client about nutrition and exercise.
   c. A nurse who smokes can effectively help a client to stop smoking.
   d. The nurse who has been pregnant and delivered an infant is most effective in helping a client through this experience.

5. *Health care.* Aroskar (1982, p. 24) lists four mind-sets about health care that can influence ethical nursing practice. These views are shown in Table 7–2.

Identifying Client Values

People's values change from time to time as their situation in life changes. State of health greatly influences a person's values. For example, a client with failing eyesight will probably place a high value on the ability to see; a client with failing neuromuscular ability will value the ability to stand or walk; and a client with chronic pain will value comfort. Normally, people take such things for granted. Nurses, therefore, need to identify the major values, beliefs, and behaviors of clients as they influence and relate to a particular health problem.

Reasons for identifying a client's value system include the following: (a) helping a client discover a new and mean-

TABLE 7-2 *Mind-Sets About Health Care and Effects on the Nurse*

Health Care Mind-Set	Effects on the Nurse
The medical cure of disease	The nurse is considered primarily accountable to the physician. Medical values dominate.
A commodity to be sold to others	The nurse's major accountability is to the institution. Concerns for the client may conflict with this view.
The client's right to relief from pain and other debilitating conditions	The nurse's obligation is to the clients and their needs as defined by the clients themselves. By supporting the client's autonomy, the nurse abdicates responsibility; needs as defined by the client supersede the nurse's knowledge and experience.
The promotion, maintenance, and restoration of health within a cooperative community	All participants' values are considered in decision making. Both clients and providers have rights and responsibilities.

Source: M. A. Aroskar, Are nurses' mind-sets compatible with ethical nursing practice? Adapted from *Topics in Clinical Nursing,* April 1982, 4:24, with permission of Aspen Publishers, Inc. Copyright © April 1982.

ingful value system following injury or illness; (b) providing information about the client's responses to injury or illness; (c) helping the client explore alternative goals and intervention strategies when valued goals cannot be realized; (d) and planning nursing interventions that support the client's cultural and health care beliefs.

There are several ways of learning a client's values (Purtilo 1978, p. 75):

- Converse with the clients about their jobs, families, pets, hobbies, past achievements, goals, or material possessions.

- Listen to the client's family and friends. Friends or family members often provide clues through casual remarks, such as "I'll tell you something; he used to be a great concert pianist."

- Review the client's health records, which can reveal personal values.

Values clarification can be a useful tool to help clients whose unclear or conflicting values are detrimental to their health. Behaviors that may indicate the need for values clarification are listed in the accompanying box.

To help clients clarify their values, the nurse needs to help the clients think about what is and what is not important to them. It is helpful to ask the following questions, each associated with one of the seven steps in values clarification:

1. *List alternatives.* Make sure that the client is aware of all alternative actions and has thought about the consequences of each. Ask: "Are you considering other courses of action?"

2. *Examine possible consequences of choices.* Ask: "What do you think you will gain by doing that?" "What benefits do you foresee from doing that?"

3. *Choose freely.* To determine whether the client chose freely, ask: "Did you have any say in that decision?" "Did you have a choice?"

4. *Feel good about the choice.* To determine how the client feels about a decision or action, ask: "How do you feel about that decision (or action)?" Because some clients may not feel satisfied with their decision and feel badly about a bad choice, a more sensitive question may be: "Some people feel good after a decision is made; others feel bad. How do you feel?"

5. *Affirm the choice.* Ask: "What will you say to others (family, friends) about this?"

6. *Act on the choice.* To determine whether the client is prepared to act on the decision, ask: "Will it be difficult to tell your wife about this?"

7. *Act with a pattern.* Help the client determine whether he or she consistently behaves in a pattern. Ask: "How many times have you done that before?" or "Would you act that way again?"

When implementing these seven steps, the nurse assists the client to think each question through, never imposing personal values. The nurse never offers an opinion, e.g., "It

---

Behaviors That May Indicate Unclear Values

Behavior	Example
Ignoring a health professional's advice	A client with heart disease who values hard work ignores advice to exercise regularly
Inconsistent communication or behavior	A pregnant woman says she wants a healthy baby but continues to drink alcohol and smoke tobacco
Numerous admissions to a health agency for the same problem	A middle-aged, obese woman repeatedly seeks help for back pain but does not lose weight
Confusion or uncertainty about which course of action to take	A woman wants to obtain a job to meet financial obligations but also wants to stay at home to care for an ailing husband

would be better to do it this way," or offers a judgment, e.g., "That's not the right thing to do." The nurse offers an opinion only when the client asks the nurse for it and then only with care.

Value Conflicts

A **value conflict** occurs when two or more values are incongruent. For example, a nurse may value life yet be expected to collaborate with a physician in disconnecting a client from a life support system. Incongruent values may not present a problem until some action must be taken, as in the example above. There is now a value conflict that may confuse the nurse and make it difficult to make a decision.

An ethical or moral **dilemma** is "a situation involving a choice between equally satisfactory or unsatisfactory alternatives or a difficult problem that seems to have no satisfactory solution" (Thompson and Thompson 1985, p. 94). In a moral dilemma there is no right or wrong. For example, a nurse is alone at night on a hospital unit and two clients experience cardiac arrest at almost the same time. What does the nurse do? It may be possible to save one client, but not both. Moral dilemmas are arising with increasing frequency in nursing.

According to Thompson and Thompson (1985, p. 94), for a situation to be a moral dilemma, it must fulfill three criteria:

1. *Awareness of different options.* The individual must be aware of the different options that are open. The awareness may be cognitive, or it may be a feeling that something is wrong.

2. *Moral nature of the dilemma.* Is the dilemma the nurse faces a moral issue? Not all situations that appear confusing to nurses are moral dilemmas, e.g., a conflict between two nurses about how to proceed with specific client care may not be a moral dilemma but simply a differing interpretation of facts or even differing assessments. For example, one nurse may believe that a client's respirations indicate the need for oxygen, while another nurse may believe that the administration of morphine sulfate, as ordered by the physician, will suppress the Hering-Breuer reflex and ease respirations. Both nurses may in fact be right.

3. *Two or more options with true choice.* For a situation to be a moral dilemma, one must have a choice between two or more actions.

For example, a physician tells a client that when he performed the surgery he did all he could. The nurse present at the conversation knows that a resident physician performed the surgery because the client's surgeon could not be reached. The nurse's choices are (a) to tell the client his physician did not perform the surgery, (b) say nothing, (c) report the discussion to the charge nurse, or (d) discuss the conversation with the physician. The nurse in this example has free choice.

ETHICS

Since ethics govern right conduct, they deal with what "should" or "ought to" be done. Ethics are not unlike the law in that each deals with rules of conduct that reflect underlying principles of right and wrong and codes of morality. Ethics are designed to protect the rights of human beings. In nursing, ethics provide professional standards for nursing activities; these standards protect both the nurse and the client.

Although *ethics* and *morals* are often used interchangeably, Jameton differentiates the two. Ethics refers to publicly stated and formal sets of rules or values, while morals are values or principles to which one is personally committed (Jameton 1984, p. 5).

Nursing Codes of Ethics

A **code of ethics** provides a means by which professional standards of practice are established, maintained, and improved. It is essential to a profession. Codes of ethics are formal guidelines for professional action. They are shared by the persons within the profession and should be generally compatible with a professional member's personal values.

A code of ethics gives the members of the profession a frame of reference for judgments in complex nursing situations. No two situations are identical, and nurses are frequently in situations that require judgment about which course of action to take. A code of ethics serves as a guide in many of these situations. It identifies the values and beliefs behind ethical standards (Thompson and Thompson 1985, p. 12).

Codes of ethics are frequently a mixture of creeds and commandments. Benjamin and Curtis (1981) describe a **creed** as an affirmation of professional regard for high ideals of conduct and as a commitment of members of a profession to honor them. An example of a creed is the opening statement of the 1973 *Code for Nurses* of the International Council of Nurses (ICN): "The fundamental responsibility of the nurse is fourfold: to promote health, to prevent illness, to restore health and to alleviate suffering." See Table 7–3. As **commandments,** codes of professional ethics provide prescriptions designed to regulate conduct in more specific situations (Benjamin and Curtis 1981, p. 6). An example of a commandment is this statement in the ICN *Code for Nurses:* "The Nurse holds in confidence personal information and uses judgment in sharing this information."

International, national, state, and provincial nursing associations have established codes of ethics. If a nurse violates

TABLE 7-3 International Council of Nurses Code for Nurses

The fundamental responsibility of the nurse is fourfold: to promote health, to prevent illness, to restore health, and to alleviate suffering.

The need for nursing is universal. Inherent in nursing is respect for life, dignity, and rights of man. It is unrestricted by considerations of nationality, race, creed, color, age, sex, politics or social status.

Nurses render health services to the individual, the family and the community and coordinate their services with those of related groups.

Nurses and People

The nurse's primary responsibility is to those people who require nursing care.

The nurse, in providing care, promotes an environment in which the values, customs and spiritual beliefs of the individual are respected.

The nurse holds in confidence personal information and uses judgment in sharing this information.

Nurses and Practice

The nurse carries responsibility for nursing practice and for maintaining competence by continual learning. The nurse maintains the highest standards of nursing care possible within the reality of a specific situation.

The nurse uses judgment in relation to individual competence when accepting and delegating responsibilities.

The nurse when acting in a professional capacity should at all times maintain standards of personal conduct which reflect credit upon the profession.

Nurses and Society

The nurse shares with other citizens the responsibility for initiating and supporting action to meet the health and social needs of the public.

Nurses and Coworkers

The nurse sustains a cooperative relationship with coworkers in nursing and other fields. The nurse takes appropriate action to safeguard the individual when his care is endangered by a coworker or any other person.

Nurses and the Profession

The nurse plays the major role in determining and implementing desirable standards of nursing practice and nursing education.

The nurse is active in developing a core of professional knowledge.

The nurse, acting through the professional organization, participates in establishing and maintaining equitable social and economic working conditions in nursing.

Source: International Council of Nurses, *ICN code for nurses: Ethical concepts applied to nursing* (Geneva, Switzerland: Imprimeries Populaires, 1973). Reprinted with permission of the ICN.

the code, the association may expel the nurse from membership. Increasingly, professional nursing associations are taking an active part in improving and enforcing standards.

Purposes of ethical nursing codes are as follows:

1. Providing a basis for regulating the relationship between the nurse, the client, coworkers, society, and the profession.

2. Providing a standard basis for excluding the unscrupulous nursing practitioner and for defending a practitioner who is unjustly accused.

3. Serving as a basis for professional curricula and for orienting the new graduate to professional nursing practice.

4. Assisting the public in understanding professional nursing conduct.

In 1953, the International Council of Nurses (ICN) developed and adopted their first code of ethics. This code was revised in 1965 and again in 1973. See Table 7-3. The code should be considered together with the relevant data in each situation; thus it provides assistance in setting prior-

ities and in taking action. For the nurse practitioner, the code specifically provides assistance in making judgments and in developing attitudes appropriate to nursing.

The American Nurses' Association (ANA) first adopted a code of ethics in 1950, which was revised in 1968, 1976, and 1985. See Table 7-4. This code is designed to provide guidance for nurses by stating principles of ethical concern. In 1988, the ANA published *Ethics in Nursing,* which addresses a wide range of nursing situations that involve ethical action. Nurses have a responsibility to be familiar with the code that governs their nursing practice.

In 1980, the Canadian Nurses' Association adopted a code of ethics. It was revised in 1985. See Table 7-5.

Ethical Issues in Nursing

A discussion of all the ethical issues facing nurses today cannot be complete because of the large number of dilemmas currently encountered in nursing practice. Davis (1989, p. 571) attributes the increase in international discussion

TABLE 7–4   *American Nurses' Association Code for Nurses*

1. The nurse provides services with respect for human dignity and the uniqueness of the client unrestricted by considerations of social or economic status, personal attributes, or the nature of health problems.

2. The nurse safeguards the client's right to privacy by judiciously protecting information of a confidential nature.

3. The nurse acts to safeguard the client and the public when health care and safety are affected by the incompetent, unethical, or illegal practice of any person.

4. The nurse assumes responsibility and accountability for individual nursing judgments and actions.

5. The nurse maintains competence in nursing.

6. The nurse exercises informed judgment and uses individual competence and qualifications as criteria in seeking consultation, accepting responsibilities, and delegating nursing activities to others.

7. The nurse participates in activities that contribute to the ongoing development of the profession's body of knowledge.

8. The nurse participates in the profession's efforts to implement and improve standards of nursing.

9. The nurse participates in the profession's effort to establish and maintain conditions of employment conducive to high quality nursing care.

10. The nurse participates in the profession's effort to protect the public from misinformation and misrepresentation and to maintain the integrity of nursing.

11. The nurse collaborates with members of the health professions and other citizens in promoting community and national efforts to meet the health needs of the public.

Source: American Nurses' Association, *Code for nurses* (Kansas City, Mo.: American Nurses' Association, 1985). Reprinted with permission.

of nursing ethics to the following: (a) more ethical dilemmas in the health care field have been identified; (b) the general public, policy makers, and health professionals are more aware of these dilemmas; and (c) communication technology has increased our knowledge of how others, including people in other parts of the world, deal with ethical dilemmas.

The changing scope of nursing practice has led to an increasing incidence of conflicts between clients' needs and expectations and nurses' professional values. Some of these areas of conflict are AIDS, abortions, withholding food and fluid, and confidentiality.

Acquired Immune Deficiency Syndrome (AIDS)

AIDS has had a profound impact upon the whole of society, including the nursing profession. Because of its association with homosexual and bisexual behavior, prostitution, illicit intravenous drug use, and inevitable physical decline and death, it bears enormous social stigma and elicits fear in nurses and all health care personnel. Some nurses have value systems that are incongruent with caring for clients who have AIDS or who test HIV seropositive, yet the profession expects the nurses to care for such clients. Nurses have a responsibility to the clients. There is a moral obligation for a nurse to care for an HIV-infected person (ANA 1988b, p. 8). According to the ANA's *Nursing and the Human Immunodeficiency Virus: A Guide for Nursing's Response to AIDS,* the moral obligation to care for an HIV-infected client cannot be set aside *unless* the risk exceeds the responsibility. The ANA has published a statement regarding risk versus responsibility in providing nursing care to clients who have infectious diseases such as AIDS, Hansen's disease, and typhoid fever.

"Not only must nursing care be readily available to individuals afflicted with communicable or infectious diseases, but nurses must also be advised on the risks and the responsibilities they face in providing care to those individuals. Accepting personal risk which exceeds the limits of duty is not morally obligatory; it is a moral option" (ANA 1988b, p. 31).

In addressing the issue of risk to nurses versus their responsibility to clients, the ANA presents four fundamental criteria to differentiate the nurse's moral duty from the moral option to care for a client:

1. The patient is at significant risk of harm, loss, or damage if the nurse does not assist.

2. The nurse's intervention or care is directly relevant to preventing harm.

3. The nurse's care will probably prevent harm, loss, or damage to the patient.

4. The benefit the patient will gain outweighs any harm the nurse might incur and does not present more than minimal risk to the health care provider (ANA 1988b, p. 32).

When all four of these criteria are met, the nurse is obliged to give care. In most instances, therefore, it is morally obligatory to care for a client with AIDS (ANA 1988b, p. 32).

Abortion

Abortion is a highly publicized issue about which many people, including nurses, feel very strongly. If a nurse cannot be "value-neutral" (Steele and Harmon 1983, p. 77), another nurse should support and care for a client having an abortion.

In most states and provinces, there are provisions in the law known as *conscience clauses.* These clauses permit

TABLE 7–5 *Canadian Nurses' Association Code of Ethics for Nursing**

Clients

I. A nurse is obliged to treat clients with respect for their individual needs and values.

II. Based upon respect for clients and regard for their right to control their own care, nursing care should reflect respect for the right of choice held by clients.

III. The nurse is obliged to hold confidential all information regarding a client learned in the health care setting.

IV. The nurse has an obligation to be guided by consideration for the dignity of clients.

V. The nurse is obligated to provide competent care to clients.

VI. The nurse is obliged to represent the ethics of nursing before colleagues and others.

VII. The nurse is obliged to advocate the client's interest.

VIII. In all professional settings, including education, research, and administration, the nurse retains a commitment to the welfare of clients. The nurse bears an obligation to act in such a fashion as will maintain trust in nurses and nursing.

Health Team

IX. Client care should represent a cooperative effort, drawing upon the expertise of nursing and other health professions. Acknowledging personal or professional limitations, the nurse recognizes the perspective and expertise of colleagues from other disciplines.

X. The nurse, as a member of the health care team, is obliged to take steps to ensure that the client receives competent and ethical care.

The Social Context of Nursing

XI. Conditions of employment should contribute to client care and to the professional satisfaction of nurses. Nurses are obliged to work toward securing and maintaining conditions of employment that satisfy these connected goals.

Responsibilities of the Profession

XII. Professional nurses' organizations recognize a responsibility to clarify, secure and sustain ethical nursing conduct. The fulfillment of these tasks requires that professional organizations remain responsive to the rights, needs and legitimate interests of clients and nurses.

*This represents only one element of the code—*values. Standards,* which provide more specific directions for conduct than values, and *limitations,* which describe exceptional circumstances in which a value or standard cannot receive its usual application, are provided with each value in the publication cited above.

Source: Canadian Nurses' Association, February 1985. *Code of ethics for nursing.* Ottawa, Ontario. Reprinted with permission.

individual physicians and nurses, as well as institutions, to refuse to assist in performing abortions if doing so violates their religious or moral principles. In these instances, the individual or institution can exercise the right to refuse without fear of reprisal.

Nurses, however, have no right to impose their values on a client. Nurses should, therefore, choose a type of nursing practice that does not conflict with personal values.

Withdrawing or Withholding Food and Fluid

Food and fluid are necessary to sustain health and life. It is generally accepted that providing food and fluid is part of nursing practice and, therefore, one of a nurse's moral duties. A nurse is morally obligated, however, to withhold feedings, when it is more harmful to administer than to withhold them (ANA 1988a, p. 2). A clinical example is the withholding of food or fluid preoperatively and postoperatively. In this instance, withholding food and fluid is clearly in the client's best interest despite any resulting discomfort. Ethical dilemmas can occur when it is not clear whether withholding the food or fluid is beneficial or harmful to the client. "It is morally as well as legally permissible for nurses to honor the refusal of food and fluid by competent patients

in their care" (ANA 1988a, p. 3). The *Code for Nurses* supports this statement through the nurse's role as a client advocate and through the principle of autonomy, i.e., the moral principle of respect for others. It is important that clients who refuse food and/or fluid understand their situations, the alternatives, and the associated harms and benefits. It is equally important that a nurse establish the client's competency to do this. If a client is not currently competent but has previously expressed a personal preference—e.g., through a living will made when the client was competent—the nurse should respect the client's values. In almost all instances, the giving of fluid and food must be in the client's best interests.

Confidentiality

"The nurse safeguards the clients' right to privacy by judiciously protecting information of a confidential nature" (ANA 1985b, p. 1). Confidentiality dilemmas can arise when clients and their support persons are breaking the law, when clients tell a nurse they have committed a crime, and when a health professional shares information about a client with others not directly involved with the clients' care.

Confidentiality is an aspect of respect for the individual. Nurses must explain to clients that it is often necessary to share pertinent information with others caring for the client. The nurse is not in violation of client trust if the client knows about this sharing (College of Nurses of Ontario 1985, p. 15). The nurse may also find that preventing harm to someone overrides the responsibility of confidentiality. For example, a postoperative client tells the nurse in confidence that he is taking amphetamines that a friend brings him while he is in hospital. The nurse tells the client that this information must be shared with the other health professionals because of the possible harmful effect to the client's health.

Termination of Life-Sustaining Treatment
The withdrawal of equipment from clients whose lives are being sustained by artificial means (e.g., ventilators) is a highly complex issue. The Hastings Center (1987, pp. 6–8) has prepared guidelines for the termination of life-sustaining treatment. These guidelines are governed by four values:

1. The client's well-being
2. Client autonomy
3. The integrity of the health professional
4. Justice or equity

A nursing decision in these situations should be based on the four values. If it is the client's wish to die, the nurse must establish the client's competency to make this decision. An agency ethics committee can provide a forum for discussion of this and similar situations.

Safeguarding Client Health and Safety
The *Code of Nurses* states that nurses act as client advocates "to safeguard the client and the public when health care and safety are affected by the incompetent, unethical or illegal practice of any person" (ANA 1985b, p. 1). Each agency should have an established process for reporting and handling practices that jeopardize the health and safety of clients. A nurse's first obligation is to protect a client; in some situations, therefore, it may be necessary to intervene before a client is harmed. For example, a client tells the nurse that he intends to walk out of the hospital even though he is receiving intravenous infusion, has been receiving oxygen, and has a newly sutured abdominal incision. The nurse's judgment is that the client will harm himself if he is permitted to leave his bed. The nurse should follow the agency practices regarding reporting the situation and restraining the client before he is harmed.

Accountability
Nurses are repeatedly faced with conflicting responsibilities. On the one hand, the nurse is frequently employed by and thus responsible to a health agency. On the other hand, the nurse is a professional person with professional ethics. In addition, the nurse is an individual with personal values.

Nurses should be able to identify priorities in their personal value systems. If the nurse perceives a conflict of values between the nurse and a client, the nurse should be able to respect the client's values and provide the necessary care. "The nurse provides services with respect for human dignity and the uniqueness of the client" (ANA 1985b, p. 1). If it is impossible for the nurse to do this, the nurse (or other nursing personnel) should arrange for someone else to carry out the client's care.

Resolving Ethical Dilemmas

To make ethical judgments, one must rely on rational thought, not emotions. Such judgments require conscious, cognitive skills necessary to perceive the client's needs and provide client care (Sigman 1986, p. 21). Every day, nurses make decisions that affect their clients, and these decisions are frequently based on ethics. See the accompanying Research Note.

A number of ethical theories and ethical decision-making models can guide nurses in making ethical decisions. Purtilo and Cassel suggest a four-step process: gather relevant data, identify the dilemma, decide what to do, and complete the action (Purtilo and Cassel 1981, pp. 27–29).

Thompson and Thompson (1981) propose a ten-step bioethical decision model to help nurses examine ethical issues and make a decision. See Table 7–6.

There are three primary ways to approach bioethical issues: teleology, deontology, and intuitionism. **Teleology** is a

RESEARCH NOTE

How Do Nurses Respond to Moral Dilemmas?

At times nurses confront fundamental moral dilemmas arising from their work. Swider, McElmurry, and Yarling examined this and related questions in their study of decisions reported by 775 senior baccalaureate nursing students from 16 midwestern colleges and universities presented with an ethical dilemma in nursing practice. Loyalties to clients, institutions, and physicians were addressed and analyzed. Most of the first decisions out of the chain of decisions to follow were institution-centered. The study revealed, however, that an overall sense of confusion prevails.

Implications: In clinical areas nurses must explore seriously the choices they make in order to practice maturely.

Swider, S. M.; McElmurry, B. J.; and Yarling, R. R. March/April 1985. Ethical decision making in a bureaucratic context by senior nursing students. *Nursing Research* 34:108–12.

TABLE 7–6 *A Bioethical Decision Model*

Step One	Review the situation to determine health problems, decision needed, ethical components, and key individuals
Step Two	Gather additional information to clarify situation
Step Three	Identify the ethical issues in the situation
Step Four	Define personal and professional moral positions
Step Five	Identify moral positions of key individuals involved
Step Six	Identify value conflicts, if any
Step Seven	Determine who should make the decision
Step Eight	Identify range of actions with anticipated outcomes
Step Nine	Decide on a course of action and carry it out
Step Ten	Evaluate/review results of decision/action

Source: J. B. Thompson and H. O. Thompson, *Ethics in nursing.* (New York: Macmillan, 1981). Used by permission.

doctrine that explains phenomena by results; a person who takes a teleologic approach to ethics is concerned with the consequences of ethical decisions. This approach is often summarized in the notion "the end justifies the means." The terms *teleology* and *utilitarianism* are sometimes used interchangeably; however, utilitarianism is also considered a type of teleology, summarized in the ideas "the end justifies the means" and "the greatest good for the greatest number." Many people in medical research support this approach to the ethics of medical problems. For example, Dr. Brown, a surgeon who has had no experience with a particular type of surgery, goes ahead and operates anyway. Although the surgeon recognizes that the surgery may not be successful largely because of his lack of experience, the knowledge he believes he will gain justifies his actions.

Deontology is the theory or study of moral obligation. A simplification of the deontologic approach is that the morality of an ethical decision is completely separate from its consequences. For instance, a nurse might believe it is necessary to tell the truth no matter who is hurt.

The difference in these approaches is shown by applying them to an ethical issue, abortion. A person who takes a teleologic approach to the ethical issue of abortion might consider that saving the mother's life (the end) justifies the abortion (the means). One taking a deontologic approach to abortion might consider any termination of life as morally bad and therefore would not harm the fetus regardless of the consequences. The approach does not determine the decision, e.g., a person taking a teleologic approach might consider that saving the life of the fetus justifies the death

of the mother. The approach, however, guides the steps in the making of ethical decisions.

The third approach to ethical issues is **intuitionism,** summarized as the notion that people inherently know what is right or wrong; it is not a matter of rational thought or of learning. For example, a nurse inherently knows it is wrong to strike a client—this does not need to be taught.

According to Fromer, the four most important principles in a deontologic approach are autonomy, nonmaleficence, beneficence, and justice. **Autonomy** is personal liberty of action; it implies independence, self-reliance, freedom of choice, and the ability to make decisions (Fromer 1986, pp. 82–83).

Nonmaleficence means the duty to do no harm. This principle is the basis of most codes of nursing ethics. Although this would seem to be a simple principle to follow in nursing practice, in reality it is complex. Harm can mean deliberate harm, risk of harm, and harm that occurs during beneficial actions (Fromer 1986, p. 83). In nursing, intentional harm is always unacceptable. However, the risk of harm is not so clear. A client may be at risk of harm during a nursing intervention that is intended to be helpful. For example, a client may react adversely to a medication. Sometimes, the degree to which a risk is morally permissible can be a conflict.

Beneficence means "doing good." Nurses are obligated to "do good," that is, to implement actions that benefit clients and their support persons. However, in an increasingly technologic health care system, "doing good" can also pose a risk of doing harm. For example, a nurse may advise a client about an exercise program to improve general health but should not do so if the client is at risk of a heart attack.

Justice, the fourth principle, is often referred to as fairness. Nurses frequently face decisions in which a sense of justice should prevail. For example, a nurse is alone on a hospital unit, and one client arrives to be admitted at the same time another client requires a medication for pain. Instead of running from one client to the other, the nurse should weigh the facts in the situation and then act based on the principle of justice.

In resolving ethical problems, nurses need to be aware of (a) the ethical theory with which they are most comfortable and (b) their own hierarchy of principles or values in that theory.

Although codes of ethics offer general guidelines for decision making, more specific guidelines are necessary in many cases to resolve the everyday ethical dilemmas encountered by nurses in practice settings. Suggested guidelines for the nurse to resolve these dilemmas are as follows:

1. Establish a sound database.

2. Identify the conflicts presented by the situation.

3. Outline alternative actions to the proposed course of action.

4. Outline the outcomes or consequences of the alternative actions.

5. Determine ownership of the problem and the appropriate decision maker.

6. Define the nurse's obligations.

Establishing the Database

To establish a sound database, the nurse needs to gather as much information as possible about the situation. Aroskar (1980, p. 660) suggests that nurses get answers to the following questions:

1. What persons are involved and what is their involvement in the situation?

2. What is the proposed action?

3. What is the intent of the proposed action?

4. What are the possible consequences of the proposed action?

For example, Mrs. Green, a 67-year-old woman, is hospitalized with multiple fractures and lacerations caused by an automobile accident. Her husband, also in the accident, is admitted to the same hospital and dies. Mrs. Green, who was the driver of the automobile, constantly questions the primary nurse about her husband. The surgeon, Dr. Mario Gonzales, however, has told the nurse not to tell the client about the death of her husband. The nurse is not provided with any reason for such a direction and expresses concern to the charge nurse, who says the surgeon's orders must be followed.

In this example, the database includes

Persons involved: Client (concerned about husband's welfare), husband (deceased), surgeon, charge nurse, and primary nurse.

Proposed action: Withhold information about the husband's death.

Intention of proposed action: Unknown; possibly to protect Mrs. Green from psychologic trauma, overwhelming guilt feelings, and consequent deterioration of her physical condition.

Consequences of proposed action: If information is withheld, the client may become increasingly anxious and angry and may refuse to cooperate with necessary care, delaying recovery.

Identifying Conflicts

A conflict is a clash between opposing elements or ideas. The conflicts for the primary nurse in the example are

- Need to be honest with Mrs. Green without being disloyal to the surgeon and the charge nurse

- Need to be loyal to the surgeon and charge nurse without being dishonest to Mrs. Green

- Conflict about the effects on Mrs. Green's health if she is informed or if she is not informed.

Outlining Courses of Action and Outcomes

Alternative courses of action to the proposed action for Mrs. Green and their outcomes might include:

- Follow the surgeon's and charge nurse's advice and do as the surgeon suggests. The outcomes for the nurse would be (a) approval from the charge nurse and surgeon, (b) risk of being seen as nonassertive, (c) violation of own value to be truthful to Mrs. Green, (d) possible benefit to Mrs. Green's health, and (e) possible detriment to her health.

- Discuss the situation further with the charge nurse and surgeon, pointing out Mrs. Green's rights to autonomy and information. The outcomes might be: (a) the surgeon may acknowledge the client's right to be informed and may then inform the client, (b) the surgeon may state that the client's rights have no legal basis and may adhere to the action originally proposed, based on a judgment about the effects of information on Mrs. Green.

Determining Ownership

In some ethical dilemmas, nurses do not make decisions about their own actions but assist clients to make a decision. For example, if a client states he does not want to have an operation, the question of ownership arises. In this example, it is obvious that the client owns the problem and that it is his right to choose this course of action. Associated with ownership, however, is knowledge about the probability and the risk of consequences attending various courses of action. Therefore, the nurse does not abandon the client with this decision. The nurse has the professional knowledge and expertise to ensure that the client makes an informed decision. Thus the client needs information from the professional's frame of reference about the consequences of decisions.

A series of questions that evolve from decision-making theories can help nurses determine who owns a certain problem (Davis and Aroskar 1983, p. 218):

1. Who should be involved in making the decision and why?

2. For whom is the decision being made?

3. What criteria (social, economic, psychologic, physiologic, or legal) should be used in deciding who makes the decision?

4. What degree of consent is needed by the subject (client and other)?

5. What, if any, moral principles (rights, values) are enhanced or negated by the proposed action?

In the example of Mrs. Green, the surgeon obviously believes the decision is his to make for Mrs. Green, and the charge nurse agrees. However, the criteria used to decide who the decision maker should be are not clear. If the criteria were spelled out, perhaps the conflict about the effects on Mrs. Green's health of knowing or not knowing about her husband's death could be resolved. Is it psychologically advantageous for Mrs. Green to know or not to know? Is it physically advantageous? What will the social and economic effects be?

Value systems also influence the decision about problem ownership. The value of Mrs. Green's right to information about her husband will be enhanced if she is told, negated if not. Her right to autonomy will also be affected.

This example shows that there are no clearly defined right or wrong answers to ethical dilemmas. If there were, they would not be ethical dilemmas. To resolve the ethical dilemma about Mrs. Green, it may be necessary for the involved health professionals to confer and clearly establish approaches that will be in Mrs. Green's best interests. Once an approach is agreed on, the nurses and physician can devise consistent continuing methods of support for Mrs. Green. That approach may dictate actions by the nurse that conflict with her or his own value system. However, the action chosen for Mrs. Green's best interest takes precedence.

Defining the Nurse's Obligations When nurses are determining an ethical course of action, Moser and Cox (1980, p. 43) advise them to list their nursing obligations, to assess the conflicts that will arise if all obligations are met, and to determine the alternatives from which the nurse can choose. Examples of obligations are

- To maximize the client's well-being
- To balance the client's need for autonomy and family members' responsibilities for the client's well-being
- To support each family member and enhance the family support system
- To carry out hospital policies
- To protect other clients' well-being
- To protect the nurse's own standards of care

CHAPTER HIGHLIGHTS

▶ Values give direction and meaning to life and guide a person's behavior.

▶ Every individual has a personal set of values influenced by societal standards, parents, teachers, culture, religion, and other life experiences.

▶ Values are freely chosen, prized and cherished, affirmed to others, and consistently incorporated into behavior.

▶ Nurses enter nursing practice with personal sets of values and through socialization acquire additional professional values that influence and guide their actions.

▶ Nursing is a profession based on caring; its professional values relate to both competence and compassion.

▶ Clarification of personal values is important for nurses to identify values that guide one's actions and to facilitate the making of choices.

▶ Values often represent an ideal that is not always achievable; compromises are thus necessary in the practice situation.

▶ Value conflicts do not present problems for the nurse until some action must be taken.

▶ Moral dilemmas are situations in which there is no right or wrong choice; the individual must choose between two equally undesirable alternatives.

▶ Professional standards for nursing activities are founded in ethics and designed to protect the rights of clients and nurses.

▶ Ethical issues in nursing may arise because of conflicts between personal values and professional responsibilities or between people involved in client care.

▶ To resolve an ethical dilemma, a nurse must establish a sound database, identify value conflicts, outline courses of action and outcomes, determine who owns the problem, and define the nurse's obligations.

READINGS AND REFERENCES

SUGGESTED READINGS

Muyskens, J. L. July/August 1984. No easy choice resolving everyday ethical dilemmas. *Nursing Life* 4:28–32.
    Should a nurse ever force clients to accept treatment, lie to them about their condition, or reveal their confidences? Muyskens advises nurses to assess their priorities when the answer is neither black nor white.

Omery, A. June 1989. Values, moral reasoning, and ethics. *Nursing Clinics of North America* 24:499–508.

Omery writes that nurses are facing increasing numbers of moral/ethical dilemmas in professional practice. Values are explained, and moral values as a special kind of values are discussed. In addition, moral reasoning is described using Kohlberg's and Gilligan's models. Ethics is differentiated from values. Omery explains that values and moral reasoning reflect the "is." Moral reasoning is the mental process that nurses use to come to a decision of right or wrong in a moral dilemma. Values are motivational preferences or dispositions. Ethics, according to Omery, is the "ought."

Sheehan, J. July 1985. Ethical considerations in nursing practice. *Journal of Advanced Nursing* 10:331–36.

Some ethical implications for nursing practice are considered in relation to three issues: competence, honesty, and obedience. Sheehan discusses factors that contribute to conformity, obedience, and authoritarianism and suggests respect for other people as a guiding principle for ethically acceptable conduct.

Yarling, R. R., and McElmurry, B. J. January 1986. The moral foundation of nursing. *Advances in Nursing Science* 8:63–73.

The authors argue that the major predicament facing nurses in their professional practice is their lack of freedom to act morally. It is suggested that two changes are necessary: the emergence of a strong sense of professional autonomy and a change in the locus of accountability from other health professionals to the client. Yarling and McElmurry provide the reader with a historical perspective and present-day realities. They state that nurses have a moral instinct founded on conscience but seldom act on their consciences when their actions are in opposition to the power structure that controls their professional and economic destiny. The authors urge that nursing ethics should be viewed as reform ethics.

RELATED RESEARCH

Crisham, P. March/April 1981. Measuring moral judgment in nursing dilemmas. *Nursing Research* 30:104–110.

Ketefian, S. May/June 1981. Moral reasoning and moral behavior among selected groups of practicing nurses. *Nursing Research* 30:171–176.

Ketefian, S. July/August 1985. Professional and bureaucratic role conceptions and moral behavior among nurses. *Nursing Research* 34:248–253.

SELECTED REFERENCES

American Nurses' Association. 1976, 1985a. *Code for nurses with interpretive statements.* Kansas City, Mo.: ANA.

———. 1985b. *Ethical dilemmas confronting nurses.* Kansas City, Mo.: ANA Committee on Ethics.

———. 1988a. *Ethics in nursing: Position statements and guidelines.* Kansas City, Mo.: ANA.

———. 1988b. *Nursing and the human immunodeficiency virus: A guide for nursing's response to AIDS.* Kansas City, Mo.: ANA

Aroskar, M. A. April 1980. Anatomy of an ethical dilemma. *American Journal of Nursing* 80:658–63.

———. April 1982. Are nurses' mind-sets compatible with ethical nursing practice? *Topics in Clinical Nursing* 4:24–26.

Bandman, E. L., and Bandman, B. 1990. *Nursing ethics through the life span.* 2d ed. Norwalk, Conn.: Appleton & Lange.

Benjamin, M., and Curtis, J. 1981. *Ethics in nursing.* New York: Oxford University Press.

Bernal, E. W. April 1985. Values clarification: A critique. *Journal of Nursing Education* 24:174–75.

Chinn, P. L., editor. 1986. *Ethical issues in nursing.* Rockville, Md: Aspen Publishers.

Coletta, S. S. December 1978. Values clarification in nursing: Why? *American Journal of Nursing* 78:2057.

College of Nurses of Ontario. 1985. *Guidelines for ethical behavior in nursing.* Toronto: The College of Nurses.

Corey, G.; Corey, M. S.; and Callahan, P. 1984. *Issues and ethics in the helping professions.* 2d ed. Monterey, Calif.: Brooks/Cole Publishing Co.

Curtin, L., and Flaherty, M. J. 1982. *Nursing ethics: Theories and pragmatics.* Bowie, Md.: Brady Communications Co.

Davis, A. J. June 1989. New developments in international nursing ethics. *Nursing Clinics of North America* 24:571–77.

———. May 1990. Professional obligations, personal values in conflict. *American Nurse* 22:7.

Davis, A. J., and Aroskar, M. A. 1978. *Ethical dilemmas and nursing practice.* New York: Appleton-Century-Crofts.

Fenner, K. M. 1980. *Ethics and law in nursing professional perspectives.* New York: D. Van Nostrand Co.

Fowler, M. D. M. January 1988. Ethical guidelines. *Heart and Lung* 17:103–4.

———. March 1988. Acquired immunodeficiency syndrome and refusal to provide care. *Heart and Lung* 17:213–15.

Fromer, M. J. 1981. *Ethical issues in health care.* St. Louis: C. V. Mosby.

———. 1986. Solving ethical dilemmas in nursing practice. In Chinn, P. L., editor. *Ethical issues in nursing.* Rockville, Md.: Aspen Publishers.

Fry, S. T. July 1989. Toward a theory of nursing ethics. *Advances in Nursing Science* 9–22.

Grady, C. February, 1989. Acquired immunodeficiency syndrome: The impact on professional nursing practice. *Cancer Nursing* 12:1–9.

———. June 1989. Ethical issues in providing nursing care to human immunodeficiency virus-infected populations. *Nursing Clinics of North America* 24:523–34.

Hall, B. P. 1973. *Value clarification as a learning process.* New York: Paulist Press.

The Hastings Center. 1987. Termination of life-sustaining treatment and care of the dying.

International Council of Nurses. 1973. *ICN code for nurses: Ethical concepts applied to nursing.* Geneva: Imprimeries Populaires.

Jameton, A. 1984. *Nursing practice: The ethical issues.* Englewood Cliffs, N.J.: Prentice-Hall.

Jarczewski, P. H. May/June 1990. What is an ethical decision? Ethics for contemporary nursing practice. *Advancing Clinical Care* 5:28.

Johnson, D. W. 1972. *Reaching out: Interpersonal effectiveness and self-actualization.* Englewood Cliffs, N.J.: Prentice-Hall.

Ketefian, S. June 1989. Moral reasoning and ethical practice in nursing. *Nursing Clinics of North America* 24:509–21.

Lund, M. March/April 1990. Conflict in ethics: Is giving pain relief always right? *Geriatric Nursing* 11:83–4.

Moser, D., and Cox, J. M., editors. May 1980. Perspectives: Resolving an ethical dilemma. *Nursing 80* 10:39–43.

Muldary, T. W. 1983. *Interpersonal relations for health professionals: A social skills approach.* New York: Macmillan Co.

Murphy, C. P. 1985. *Ethical dilemmas in nursing practice.* Pub. no. NP-68D. Kansas City, Mo.: American Nurses' Association.

Murphy, P. June 1989. The role of the nurse on hospital ethics committees. *Nursing Clinics of North America* 24:551–56.

Purtilo, R. 1978. *Health professional/patient interaction.* 2d ed. Philadelphia: W. B. Saunders Co.

Purtilo, R. B., and Cassel, C. K. 1981. *Ethical dimensions in the health professions.* Philadelphia: W. B. Saunders Co.

Raths, L. E.; Harmin, M.; and Simon, S. B. 1978. *Values and teaching.* 2d ed. Columbus, Ohio: Charles E. Merrill Books.

Salladay, S. A., McDonnell, Sr. M. M. June 1989. Spiritual care, ethical choices, and patient advocacy. *Nursing Clinics of North America* 24:543–49.

Sheehan, J. July 1985. Ethical considerations in nursing practice: Competence, honesty, and obedience. *Journal of Advanced Nursing* 10:331–36.

Sigman, P. 1986. Ethical choice in nursing. In Chinn, P. L. (editor). *Ethical issues in nursing.* Rockville, Md.: Aspen Publishers.

Simon, S. B.; Howe, L. W.; and Kirschenbaum, H. 1978. *Values clarification: A handbook of practical strategies for teachers and students.* Rev. ed. New York: Hart Publishing Co.

Steele, S. M. May 1986. AIDS: Clarifying values to close in on ethical questions. *Nursing and Health Care* 7:247–8.

Steele, S. M., and Harmon, V. M. 1983. *Values clarification in nursing.* 2d ed. Norwalk, Conn.: Appleton-Century-Crofts.

Swider, S. M.; McElmurry, B. J.; and Yarling, R. R. March/April 1985. Ethical decision making in a bureaucratic context by senior nursing students. *Nursing Research* 34:108–12.

Thompson, J. B., and Thompson, H. O. 1981. *Ethics in nursing.* New York: Macmillan Co.

———. 1985. *Bioethical decision making for nurses.* Norwalk, Conn.: Appleton-Century-Crofts.

Twomey, J. G. Jr. April 1989. Analysis of the claim to distinct nursing ethics: Normative and nonnormative approaches. *Advances in Nursing Science* 11:25–32.

Uustal, D. B. December 1978. Values clarification: Application to practice. *American Journal of Nursing* 78:2058–63.

Van Hooft, S. February 1990. Moral education for nursing decisions. *Journal of Advanced Nursing* 15:210–15.

CHAPTER

8

Legal Aspects of Nursing Practice

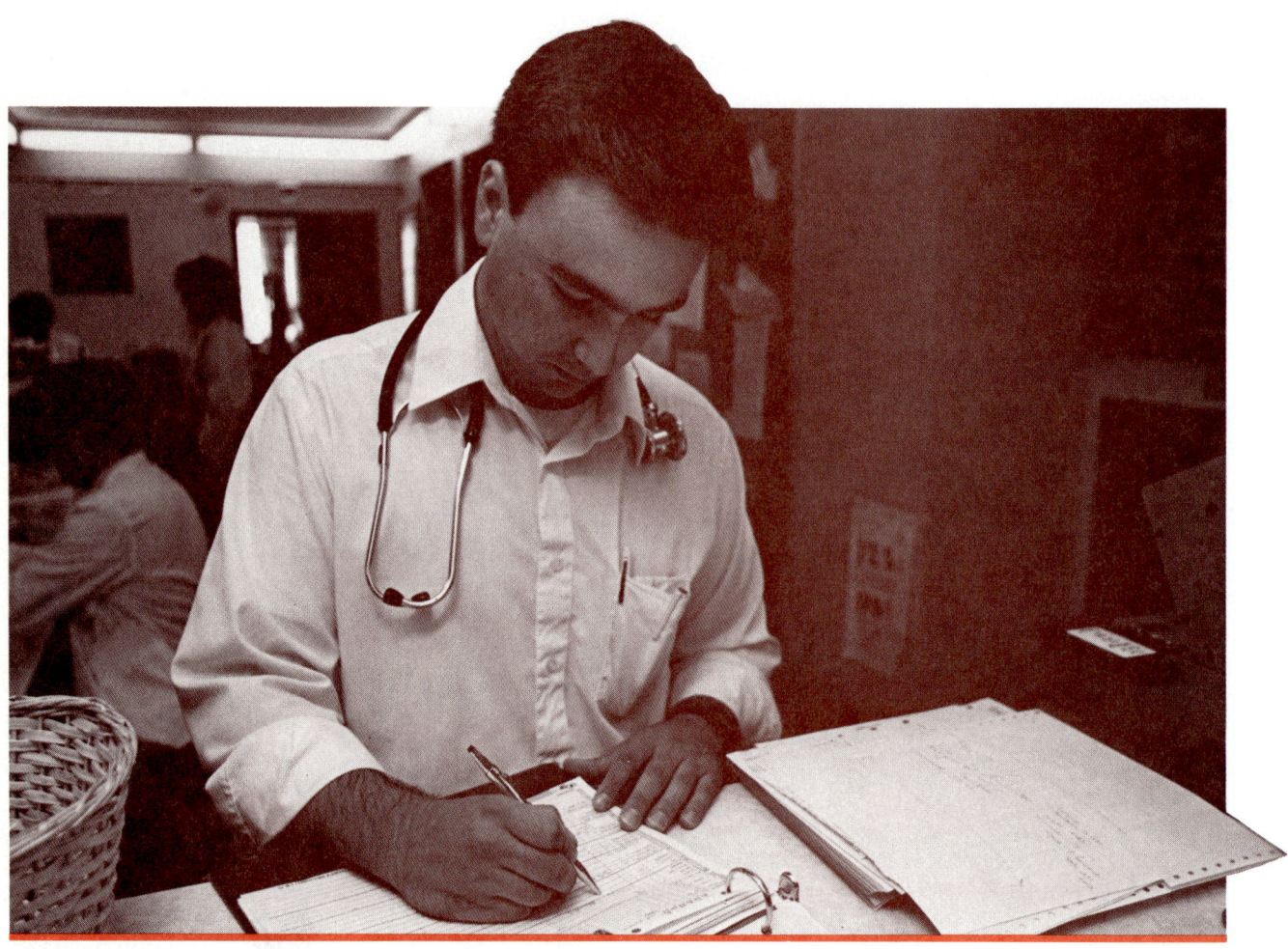

CONTENTS

OBJECTIVES

- ▶ Describe general legal concepts as they apply to nursing.
- ▶ Explain how nurse practice acts legally help the nurse practitioner.
- ▶ Differentiate mandatory from permissive licensure.
- ▶ Describe ways standards of care, agency policies, and nurse practice acts affect the scope of nursing practice.
- ▶ Identify ways nursing students can minimize chances of liability.
- ▶ Identify essential types and elements of contracts.
- ▶ Identify rights and obligations associated with the nurse's legal roles.
- ▶ Describe collective bargaining with reference to nursing.
- ▶ Identify areas of potential liability for nurses.
- ▶ Differentiate crimes from torts and give examples in nursing.
- ▶ Describe the purpose and essential elements of informed consent.
- ▶ List information that needs to be included in an incident report.
- ▶ Describe actions a nurse should take when a client is injured.
- ▶ Explain the positive and negative aspects of living wills.
- ▶ Describe the purpose of professional liability insurance.

GENERAL LEGAL CONCEPTS

Nursing practice is governed by many legal concepts. It is important for nurses to know the basics of legal concepts because nurses are accountable for their professional judgments and actions. Accountability is an essential concept of professional nursing practice and the law. Knowledge of laws that regulate and affect nursing practice is needed for two reasons:

1. To ensure that the nurse's decisions and actions are consistent with current legal principles
2. To protect the nurse from liability

Law can be defined as "a system of principles and processes by which people, who live in a society, attempt to control human conduct in an effort to minimize the use of force as a means of resolving conflicting interests" (Rhodes and Miller 1984, p. 1).

Functions of the Law in Nursing

The law serves a number of functions in nursing:

- ■ It provides a framework for establishing which nursing actions in the care of clients are legal.
- ■ It differentiates the nurse's responsibilities from those of other health professionals.
- ■ It helps to establish the boundaries of independent nursing action.
- ■ It assists in maintaining a standard of nursing practice by making nurses accountable under the law.

Sources of Law

The legal systems in both the United States and Canada have their origins in the English common law system. Three primary sources of law are constitutions, statutes, and decisions of courts (common law).

Constitutions   The Constitution of the United States and the Constitution of Canada are the supreme laws of each country. They establish the general organization of the federal governments, grant certain powers to them, and place limits on what federal and state or provincial governments may do. Constitutions create legal rights and responsibilities and are the foundation for a system of justice. The rights created, however, do not relate directly to the nurse-client relationship.

Constitutions have due process and equal protection clauses. The due process clause applies to state or provincial and local agencies, including public hospitals, and to actions that deprive a person of life, liberty, or property. **Due process** has two primary elements:

1. The rules being applied must be reasonable and not vague.
2. Fair procedures must be followed when enforcing the rules.

Equal protection means that like persons must be dealt with in like fashion.

Legislation (Statutes)   Laws enacted by any legislative body are called **statutory laws.** When there is a conflict between federal and state or provincial laws, federal law supersedes. Likewise, state or provincial laws supersede local laws.

The regulation of nursing is a function of state or provincial law. State or provincial legislatures pass statutes that define and regulate nursing, i.e., nurse practice acts. These acts, however, must be consistent with constitutional and federal provisions. Nurses practice acts, Good Samaritan laws, and adult or child abuse laws are examples of statutes that affect nurses.

Legislatures delegate responsibility and power to implement various laws to many administrative agencies who have the time and the expertise to address complex issues. State or provincial administrative agencies oversee the practice of the professions and regulate various aspects of commerce and public welfare. Examples pertinent to nurses are the state boards of nursing and provincial nursing associations, which implement and enforce nurse practice acts.

Common Law   The body of principles that evolves from court decisions is referred to as **common law,** or decisional laws. Although courts are called upon to interpret and apply constitutional or statutory law, they also are asked to resolve disputes between two parties. In such disputes, statutory and constitutional laws cannot support the case. Common law is continually being adapted and expanded. In deciding specific controversies, courts generally adhere to the doctrine of *stare decisis*—"to stand by things decided"—usually referred to as "following precedent." In other words, in a current case, the court applies the same rules and principles as applied in similar cases decided previously and arrives at the same ruling. Courts may depart from precedent when slight differences are noted between cases or when it is thought that a particular common-law rule no longer applies to the needs of society.

Types of Laws

Laws govern the relationship of private individuals with government and with each other.

Public law refers to the body of law that deals with relationships between individuals and the government and governmental agencies. An important segment of public law is **criminal law,** which deals with actions against the safety and welfare of the public. Examples are homicide, manslaughter, and theft. Crimes are classified as felonies or misdemeanors in the United States or as indictable offenses or summary conviction offenses in Canada. See the discussion of crimes and torts later in this chapter. Public law also includes numerous regulations designed to enhance societal objectives. Private individuals and organizations are required to follow specified courses of action in their activities. Noncompliance with these regulations can lead to criminal penalties.

Private law, or civil law, is the body of law that deals with relationships between private individuals. It is categorized as contract law and tort law. **Contract law** involves the enforcement of agreements among private individuals or the payment of compensation for failure to fulfill the agreements. **Tort law** defines and enforces duties and rights among private individuals that are not based on contractual agreements. The word *tort* comes from the Latin word *tortus,* meaning twisted. Loosely translated, it means "wrong" or "bad." Some examples of tort laws applicable to nurses are negligence and malpractice, invasion of privacy, and assault and battery. See Figure 8–1 and also Table 8–1 for selected categories of law affecting nurses.

Principles of Law

The system of law rests on four simple principles that are often cloaked in complex terminology (Fenner 1980, p. 84):

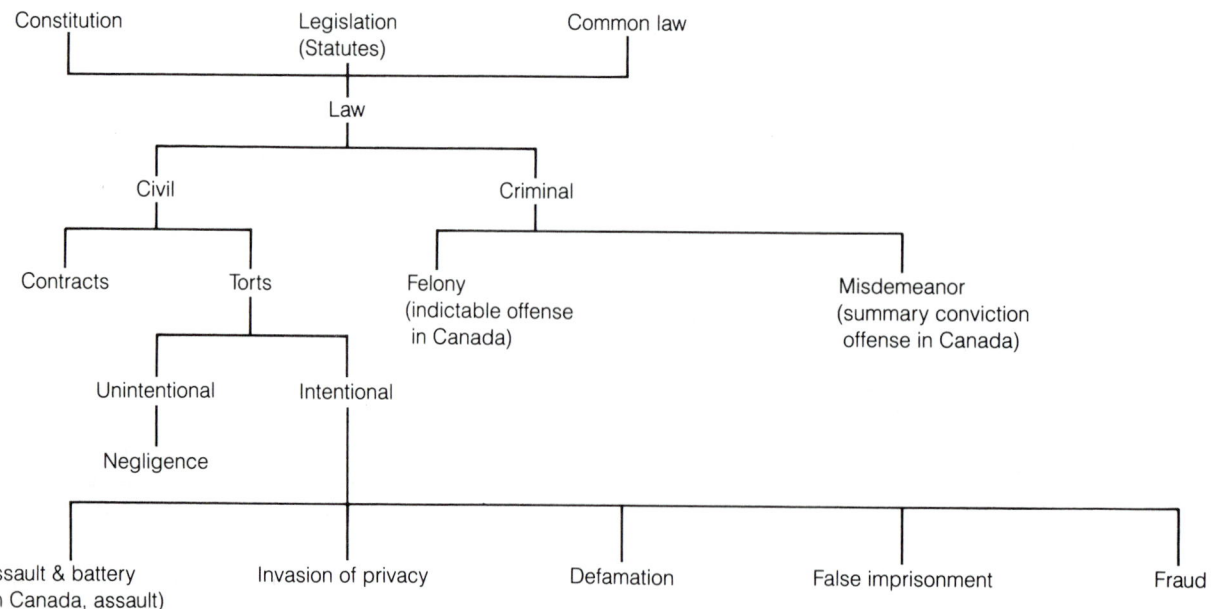

Figure 8–1   Categories of law pertinent to nurses.

TABLE 8–1 *Selected Categories of Laws Affecting Nurses*

Category	Examples
Constitutional	Due process
	Equal protection
Statutory (legislative)	Nurse practice acts
	Good Samaritan acts
	Child and adult abuse laws
	Living wills
Criminal (public)	Homicide, manslaughter
	Theft
	Arson
	Active euthanasia
	Rape
	Illegal possession of controlled drugs
Contracts (private/civil)	Nurse and client
	Nurse and employer
	Nurse and insurance
	Client and agency
Torts (private/civil)	Negligence
	Libel and slander
	Invasion of privacy
	Assault and battery
	False imprisonment

Source: American Nurses' Association. *Standards of Nursing Practice.* Kansas City, Mo.: ANA, 1973. Used by permission.

1. *Law is based on a concern for justice and fairness.* The law seeks to protect the rights of one party from the transgressions of another by setting guidelines for conduct and mechanisms to enforce those guidelines.

2. *Law is characterized by change.* Social and technologic changes occur rapidly and often without predictions of problems to follow. In response to these changes, the legal system also must change. Often the legal system reacts rather than acts. For example, after technologic devices such as respirators were developed to prolong life, it became necessary for the law to change its guidelines about indications of death—from cessation of heart function to absence of electric currents from the brain for at least 24 hours.

3. *Actions are judged on the basis of a universal standard of what a similarly educated, reasonable, and prudent person would have done under similar circumstances.* All nurses are expected to function the same way that another nurse with similar education and experience would function. This rule of reasonable and prudent conduct is the basis for evaluating a person's actions, e.g., for judging whether or not actions were negligent (see the discussion of negligence and malpractice later in this chapter).

4. *Each individual has rights and responsibilities.* **Rights** are privileges or fundamental powers that individuals possess unless they are revoked by law or given up voluntarily; **responsibilities** are the obligations associated with these rights. Failure to meet one's responsibilities can endanger one's rights. For example, a registered nurse has the right to practice nursing within the constraints of the law (nurse practice acts). If the nurse fails to observe these constraints (e.g., prescribes medications or conducts a surgical procedure), the behavior is considered irresponsible, and the right to practice can be revoked.

Kinds of Legal Actions

There are two kinds of legal actions: civil or private actions and criminal actions. **Civil actions** deal with the relationships between individuals in society; for example, a man may file a suit against a person who he believes cheated him. Civil actions that are of concern to nurses include the torts and contracts listed in Table 8–1. Other civil actions that might be of concern to nurses include those relating to wills and the estates of deceased persons. These cases are known as **probate proceedings. Criminal actions** deal with disputes between an individual and the society as a whole; for example, if a man shoots a person, society brings him to trial.

The Civil Judicial Process

The judicial process primarily functions to settle disputes peacefully and in accordance with the law. A lawsuit has strict procedural rules. There are generally five steps:

1. A document called a **complaint** is filed by a person referred to as the **plaintiff,** who claims that the person's legal rights have been infringed upon by one or more persons, referred to as **defendants.**

2. A written response, called an **answer,** is made by the defendants.

3. Both parties engage in pretrial activities, referred to as **discovery,** in an effort to gain all the facts of the situation.

4. In the **trial** of the case, all the relevant facts are presented to a jury or a judge.

5. The judge renders a **decision,** or the jury renders a **verdict.** If the outcome is not acceptable to one of the parties, an appeal can be made for another trial.

During a trial, a plaintiff must offer evidence of the defendant's wrongdoing. This duty of proving an assertion is called the **burden of proof.** An additional aspect of this burden of proof is that the plaintiff must have a greater amount of convincing evidence than the defendant if the plaintiff is to prevail.

Nurses as Expert Witnesses

When called into court as a witness, the nurse has a duty to assist justice as far as possible. An **expert witness** is one who, by education or experience, possesses knowledge and skill needed to understand the matter about which the person is to testify (Rhodes and Miller 1983, p. 18). Such a witness is usually called to help a judge or jury understand evidence pertaining to the extent of damage and the standard of care.

Privileged Communication

A **privileged communication** is information given to a professional person who is forbidden by law from disclosing the information in a court without the consent of the person who provided it.

Legislation regarding privileged communications is highly complicated. A nurse would be unwise to encourage disclosures or advise a client about the subject. The privileged communication law is for the benefit of the client; a nurse who is given confidential information should be prepared to answer questions fully and honestly if required to testify in a court of law. Many states with statutes granting privileged communications between the client and various health care providers do not extend the privilege to nurse-client communication.

The matter of privileged communications is referred to in the ANA's *Code for Nurses* (1976). It advises the nurse to seek legal counsel in regard to a privileged communication and to become familiar with the rights and privileges of the client and the nurse.

In Canada, confidentiality of information is incorporated as an ethic in the legislation on nursing practice. Failure to maintain confidentiality can result in disciplinary action against the nurse.

LEGAL ASPECTS OF NURSING

Nurse Practice Acts

Each state in the United States has nurse practice acts, and each province in Canada has a nurse practice act or an act for professional nursing practice. Nurse practice acts protect the nurse's professional capacity and legally control nursing practice through licensing. Nurse practice acts legally define and describe the scope of nursing practice, which the law seeks to regulate, thereby protecting the public as well. Because of the number of acts there are many definitions and descriptions of nursing. In 1981, the ANA described nursing practice as including but not limited to "administration, teaching, counseling, supervision, delegation, and evaluation of practice and execution of the medical regimen, including the administration of medications and treatments prescribed by any person authorized by state law to prescribe" (ANA 1981, p. 6).

Many states have an additional clause that pertains to actions that may be performed only by certain nurses with education beyond the minimum required for licensure under the act. For example, many of the clauses address the practice of nurse-midwives or nurse-anesthetists. Some address the nurse-practitioner role. These clauses conflict with the ANA policy, which advises against legal regulation of advanced or specialty nursing practice. The ANA's position is that it is the function of the professional association, not the law, to establish the scope and desirable qualifications required for each specialized area of practice (Snyder and Labar 1984, p. 7).

Credentialing

Credentialing is the process of determining and maintaining competence in nursing practice. The credentialing process is one way in which the nursing profession maintains standards of practice and is accountable for the educational preparation of members. Credentialing includes licensure, registration, certification, and accreditation.

The ANA enumerated the principles of credentialing; these principles reflect the belief that credentialing exists primarily to protect and benefit the public. See Table 8–2.

Licensure and Registration   **Licenses** are legal permits granted by a government agency to individuals to engage in the practice of a profession and to use a particular title. A particular jurisdiction or area is covered by the license. For a profession or occupation to obtain the right to license its members, it generally must meet three criteria:

1. There is a need to protect the public's safety or welfare.
2. The occupation is clearly delineated as a separate, distinct area of work.
3. There is an organization suitable in ability to assume the obligations of the licensing process.

In the United States, nurses are issued a license by the state board of nursing or by an administrative governmental agency that is empowered by government to grant licenses. Licenses are issued to registered nurses who have (a) successfully completed a course of studies in a school of nursing accredited by the state board, (b) passed the national qualifying examinations with a score that is acceptable to the board, and (c) paid the required fee. A state board may also grant a license to a nurse who holds an active practicing license in another state, through a process of endorsement, without the candidate having to rewrite examinations. The candidate, however, must have attained a passing score on

TABLE 8–2 *Principles of Credentialing*

1. In addition to benefiting and protecting the public, credentialing also benefits those who are credentialed.

2. The legitimate interests of the involved occupation or institution and of the general public should be reflected in each credentialing mechanism.

3. Accountability should be an essential component of any credentialing process.

4. A system of checks and balances within the credentialing system should assure equitable treatment for all parties involved.

5. Periodic assessments with the potential for sanction are essential components of an effective credentialing mechanism.

6. Objective standards and criteria and persons competent in their use are essential to the credentialing process.

7. Representation in credentialing systems of the community of interests directly affected by credentialing mechanisms should assure consideration of the legitimate concerns of each group.

8. Professional identity and responsibility should evolve from the credentialing process.

9. An effective system of role delineation is fundamental to any credentialing mechanism for individuals.

10. An effective system of program identification is fundamental to any credentialing mechanism for institutions.

11. Coordination of credentialing mechanisms should lead to efficiency and cost effectiveness and avoid duplication.

12. Geographic, including interstate, mobility should be improved by the credentialing of the individual.

13. Widely accepted definitions and terminology are basic to an effective credentialing system.

14. Communications and understanding between health care providers and society should be facilitated through the credentialing process.

Source: Report of the Committee for the Study of Credentialing in Nursing, American Nurses' Association. *American Journal of Nursing* April 1979, 79:674. Used by permission.

the national examinations that is equal to, or above, that considered acceptable in the state in which the nurse wishes to practice.

In Canada, nurses are not licensed except in the province of Quebec. They are, however, registered by their provincial nursing association and by the College of Nurses of Ontario. Nurses in the United States are also registered but must in addition be granted a license to practice. **Registration** is the listing of an individual's name and other information on the official roster of a governmental or nongovernmental agency. Nurses who are registered are permitted

to use the title "Registered Nurse." To be registered, the nurse must have completed a basic course of nursing studies in a program approved by the registering body and have passed the national qualifying examinations with an acceptable grade. Canada has a national comprehensive registered nurse examination, offered in both French and English. All state boards of nursing consider the same score an acceptable passing grade. Nurses from other provinces in Canada and from other countries may be granted registration by endorsement provided they meet the requirements of the registering body. Both licensure and registration must be renewed on an annual basis (in some states every 2 years) to be valid.

There are two types of licensure/registration: mandatory and permissive. Under mandatory licensure/registration, anyone who practices nursing must be licensed or, in Canada, registered. The only exceptions are: (a) practice in an emergency, (b) practice by nursing students as part of their education, and (c) practice by nurses employed by the federal government (nurses who practice in Veterans Administration hospitals and in public health must be currently licensed in some jurisdiction but not necessarily where the facility is located). Under permissive licensure/registration, the title RN is reserved for licensed or, in Canada, registered practitioners, but the practice of nursing is not prohibited to others who are not licensed or registered.

Registration is mandatory in most provinces of Canada. In the United States, nursing licensure is mandatory in all states. There is a strong movement underway in Canada to make registration mandatory in all provinces.

In each state and province there is a mechanism by which licenses (or registration in Canada) can be revoked for just cause, e.g., incompetent nursing practice; professional misconduct; conviction of a crime such as using illegal drugs or selling drugs illegally; obtaining a license through deception, falsifying school records, or hiding a criminal history; and, in some areas, aiding in a criminal abortion. In each situation, all the facts are generally reviewed by a committee at a hearing. Nurses are entitled to be represented by legal counsel at such a hearing. If the nurse's license is revoked as a result of the hearing, an appeal can be made to a court, or, in some states, an agency is designated to review the decision before any court action is initiated.

Certification **Certification** is the voluntary practice of validating that an individual nurse has met minimum standards of nursing competence in specialty areas, such as maternal-child health, pediatrics, mental health, gerontology, and school nursing. Certification programs are conducted by the ANA and by specialty nursing organizations. A certification program has not yet been established in Canada, but the CNA is currently considering the establishment of a certification program for nurses in specialized fields of nursing.

Accreditation/Approval of Basic Nursing Education Programs

Accreditation is a process by which a voluntary organization (e.g., the NLN) or governmental agency (e.g., the state board of nursing) appraises and grants accredited status to institutions and/or programs or services that meet predetermined structure, process, and outcome criteria (ANA 1979). Minimum standards for basic nursing education programs are established in each state of the United States and in each province in Canada. State accreditation or provincial approval is granted to schools of nursing meeting the minimum criteria. NLN accreditation is concerned with optimum, rather than minimum, standards. In other words, accreditation by the NLN certifies that an educational program not only meets minimum standards but also is considered "good" by national standards. It is not a legal requirement as is state or provincial accreditation.

Standards of Practice

Another way the nursing profession attempts to ensure that its practitioners are competent and safe to practice is through the establishment of standards of practice (see Chapter 1). These standards are often used to evaluate the quality of care provided by nurses. In addition to this basic set of standards, which are applicable in any practice setting, the ANA has developed standards of nursing practice for specific areas such as maternal-child, medical-surgical, geriatric, psychiatric, and community health nursing.

CONTRACTUAL ARRANGEMENTS IN NURSING

A contract is the basis of the relationship between a nurse and an employer—for example, a nurse and a hospital or a nurse and a physician. A **contract** is an agreement between two or more competent persons, upon sufficient consideration (remuneration), to do or not to do some lawful act. A contract may be written or oral; however, a written contract cannot be changed legally by an oral agreement. If two people wish to change some aspect of a written contract, the change must be written into the contract, because one party cannot hold the other to an oral agreement that differs from the written one.

A contract is considered to be *expressed* when the two parties discuss and agree orally or in writing to its terms, e.g., that a nurse will work at a hospital for a stated length of time and under stated conditions. An *implied* contract is one in which there has been no discussion between the parties, but the law considers that a contract exists. In the contractual relationship between nurse and client, clients have the right to expect that nurses caring for them have the competence to meet their needs. This *implies* that the nurse has a responsibility to remain competent. The nurse

has the associated right to expect the client to provide accurate information as required.

Contract law requires that four elements be met to make a contract valid (Fenner 1980, p. 94):

1. The act contracted for must be legal. The nurse's employment must be legal, and the duties to be performed and services provided must be within the law. For example, the nurse cannot be required to provide services that are not permitted in the nurse practice act.

2. The parties to the contract must be of legal age (majority) and competent (free of mental impairment) to enter a binding agreement.

3. There must be mutual agreement about the service to be contracted for. A contract becomes invalid, for example, if the nurse does not accept an offer of hire.

4. There must be compensation (or promise of it) for the service to be provided.

These four elements are also required for contracts made by clients (with nurses, other health professionals, or health care institutions) to be valid. For example, the activity contracted for between a client and a hospital is health care, which is legal. Clients who are minors are not usually admitted for care without consent from their parents or legal guardians. The parties agree to the terms of the contract when the client gives informed consent for care and the hospital offers care. The client promises to reimburse the hospital for its services through insurance coverage or other means.

Legal Roles of Nurses

Nurses have three separate, interdependent legal roles, each with rights and associated responsibilities:

1. *Provider of service.* The nurse is expected to provide safe and competent care so that harm (physical, psychologic, or material) to the recipient of the service is prevented. Implicit in this role are several legal concepts: liability, standard of care, and contractual obligations.

   Liability is the quality or state of being legally responsible to account for one's obligations and actions and to make financial restitution for wrongful acts. A primary nurse or team leader, for example, has an obligation to practice and direct the practice of others under supervision so that harm or injury to the client is prevented and standards of care are maintained. Even when a nurse is directed by a physician, the responsibility for nursing activity is the nurse's. When a nurse is requested to carry out an activity that the nurse believes will be injurious to the client, the nurse's responsibility is to refuse to carry out the order and report this to the nurse in charge.

   The **standards of care** by which a nurse acts or fails to act are legally defined by nurse practice acts and by the rule of reasonable and prudent action—what a reasonable and prudent professional with similar preparation and experience would do in similar circumstances. A nurse, for example, would be acting illegally in diagnosing a medical condition or treating a client for a tumor because these functions are within the scope of the physician's practice, and nurses are constrained from engaging in them. **Contractual obligations** refer to the nurse's duty of care, that is, duty to render care, established by the presence of an expressed or implied contract discussed earlier.

2. *Employee or contractor for service.* A nurse who is employed by a hospital works as an agent of the hospital, and the nurse's contract with clients is an implied one. However, a nurse who is employed directly by a client, for example, a private nurse, may have a written contract with that client in which the nurse agrees to provide professional services for a certain fee. If the client is dying, the nurse can be protected by a written contract that allows collection of the fee from the client's estate. A nurse might be prevented from carrying out the terms of the contract because of illness or death. However, personal inconvenience and personal problems, such as the nurse's car failure, are not legitimate reasons for failing to fulfill a contract.

   Contractual relationships vary among practice settings. An independent nurse practitioner is a contractor for service, whose contractual relationship with the client is an independent one. The nurse employed by a hospital functions within an employer-employee relationship, in which the nurse represents and acts for the hospital and therefore must function within the policies of the employing agency. This type of legal relationship creates the ancient legal doctrine known as **respondeat superior** ("let the master answer"). In other words, the master (employer) assumes responsibility for the conduct of the servant (employee) and can also be held responsible for malpractice by the employee. By virtue of the employee role, therefore, the nurse's conduct is the hospital's responsibility.

   This doctrine does not imply that the nurse cannot be held liable as an individual. Nor does it imply that the doctrine will prevail if the employee's actions are extraordinarily inappropriate, i.e., beyond those expected or foreseen by the employer. For example, if the nurse hits a client in the face, the employer could disclaim responsibility, since this behavior is beyond the bounds of expected behavior. Criminal acts, such as assisting with criminal abortions or taking tranquilizers from a client's supply for personal use, would also be considered extraordinarily inappropriate behavior. Nurses can be held liable for failure to act as well. For example, if a nurse sees another nurse hitting a client and fails to do anything to protect the client, the observer may also be considered negligent.

   The nurse in the role of employee or contractor for service has obligations to the employer, the client, and other personnel. The nursing care provided must be within the limitations and terms specified. The nurse has an obligation to contract only for those responsibilities that the nurse is competent to discharge. As an employee, the nurse is expected to uphold the good name of the employer and therefore should not criticize the employer unjustifiably. The employer, in turn, is obligated to provide adequate working conditions, e.g., a safe, functional employment setting.

   The nurse is expected to respect the rights and responsibilities of other health care participants. For example, although the nurse has responsibility to explain nursing activities to a client, the nurse does not have the right to comment on medical practice in a way that disturbs the client or causes problems for the physician. At the same time, the nurse has the right to expect reasonable and prudent conduct from other health care providers.

3. *Citizen.* The rights and responsibilities of the nurse in the role of citizen are the same as those of any individual under the legal system. Rights of citizenship protect clients from harm and ensure consideration for their personal property rights, rights to privacy, confidentiality, and other rights discussed later in this chapter and in Chapter 6. These same rights apply to nurses. For example, nurses have the right to physical safety and need not perform functions that are considered to pose an unreasonable risk.

Nurses move in and out of these roles when carrying out professional and personal responsibilities. An understanding of these roles and the rights and responsibilities associated with them promotes legally responsible conduct and practice by nurses. See Table 8–3 for examples of the responsibilities and rights associated with each role.

Collective Bargaining

Collective bargaining is a formalized decision-making process between management and labor representatives concerning salaries, work environment, and conditions of employment (Crawford et al. 1985, p. 155). Through a written agreement, both employer and employees legally commit themselves to observe the terms and conditions of employment. Collective bargaining is a controversial issue among nurses. Some nurses argue against collective bargaining on the grounds that it is contrary to the nature of professionalism, it is not necessary, it fosters discord, and it undermines the nurse-administrator's role (McClelland 1983, p. 36). Others argue that collective bargaining is necessary to obtain control of nursing practice and economic security.

The collective bargaining process involves the recognition of a certified bargaining agent for the employees. This agent can be a union, a trade association, or a professional organization. The agent represents the employees in negotiating a contract with management.

TABLE 8–3 *Nurses' Legal Roles, Rights, and Responsibilities*

Role	Responsibilities	Rights
Provider of service	To provide safe and competent care commensurate with the nurse's preparation, experience, and circumstances	Right to adequate and qualified assistance as necessary
	To inform clients of the consequences of various alternatives and outcomes of care	Right to reasonable and prudent conduct from clients, e.g., provision of accurate information as required
	To provide adequate supervision and evaluation of subordinates for whom the nurse is responsible	
	To remain competent	
Employee or contractor for service	To fulfill the obligations of contracted service with the employer	Right to adequate working conditions, e.g., safe equipment and facilities
		Right to compensation for services rendered
	To respect the rights and responsibilities of other health care participants	Right to reasonable and prudent conduct by other health care givers
Citizen	To protect the rights of the recipients of care	Right to respect by others of the nurse's own rights and responsibilities

When collective bargaining breaks down because an agreement cannot be reached, the employees usually call a strike. A **strike** is an organized work stoppage by a group of employees to express a grievance, enforce a demand for changes in conditions of employment or solve a dispute with management (Crawford et al. 1985, p. 162).

Because nursing practice is a service to people (often ill people), striking presents a moral dilemma to many nurses. Actions taken by nurses can affect the safety of people. When faced with a strike, each nurse must make an individual decision to cross or not to cross a picket line. Nursing students may also be faced with decisions about crossing picket lines in the event of a strike at a clinical agency used for learning experiences. The ANA supports striking as a means of achieving economic and general welfare.

Collective bargaining is more than the negotiation of salary terms and hours of work; it is a continuous process in which day-to-day working problems and relationships can be handled in an orderly and democratic manner. Day-to-day difficulties or grievances are handled through the grievance procedure, a formal plan established in the contract that outlines the channels for handling and settling grievances through progressively higher levels of administration. A **grievance** is any dispute, difference, controversy, or disagreement arising out of the terms and conditions of employment. Grievances fall into four main categories outlined in Table 8–4.

TABLE 8–4 *Categories and Examples of Grievances*

Category	Examples
Contract violations	Shift or weekend work is assigned inequitably.
	A nurse is dismissed without cause.
Violations of federal and state law	A female nurse is paid less than a male nurse for the same work.
	Appropriate payment is not given for overtime work.
	Minority group nurses are not promoted.
Management responsibilities	Appropriate locker room facilities are not provided.
	Safe client care is jeopardized by inadequate staffing.
Violation of agency rules	Performance evaluations are conducted only at termination of employment, but the contract requires annual evaluations.
	A vacation period is assigned without the nurse's agreement, as required in personnel policies.

Source: American Nurses' Association, *The grievance procedure* (Kansas City, Mo.: ANA, 1985), pp. 2–4. Used by permission.

AREAS OF POTENTIAL LIABILITY IN NURSING

Crimes and Torts

A **crime** is an act committed in violation of public (criminal) law and punishable by a fine and/or imprisonment. A crime does *not* have to be intended in order to be a crime. For example, a nurse may accidentally give a client an additional and lethal dose of a narcotic to relieve discomfort.

Crimes are classified as either felonies (or in Canada, indictable offenses) or misdemeanors (or in Canada, summary conviction offenses). A **felony** is a crime of a serious nature, such as murder, punishable by a term in prison. In some areas, second-degree murder is called **manslaughter.** A nurse who accidentally gives an additional and lethal dose of a narcotic can be accused of manslaughter. Other examples of felonies are arson and armed robbery.

Crimes are punished through criminal action by the state or province against an individual. A **misdemeanor** is an offense of a less serious nature and is usually punishable by a fine or short-term jail sentence, or both. A nurse who slaps a client's face could be charged with a misdemeanor.

A **tort** is a civil wrong committed against a person or a person's property. Torts are usually litigated in court by civil action between individuals. In other words, the person or persons claimed to be responsible for the tort are sued for damages. Tort liability almost always is based on fault, i.e., something was done incorrectly (an unreasonable act of commission) or something that should have been done was not done (act of omission).

Torts may be classified as intentional or unintentional. Intentional torts include fraud, invasion of privacy, libel and slander, assault and battery, and false imprisonment. **Fraud** is the false presentation of some fact with the intention that it will be acted upon by another person. For example, it is fraud for a nurse applying to a hospital for employment to fail to list two past employers for deceptive reasons when asked to list the previous five employers.

The right to privacy is the right of individuals to withhold themselves and their lives from public scrutiny. Invasion of privacy is a direct wrong of a personal nature. It injures the feelings of the person and does not take into account the effect of revealed information on the standing of the person in the community. The right to privacy can also be described as the right to be left alone. Liability can result if the nurse breaches confidentiality by passing along confidential client information to others or intrudes into the client's private domain.

In this context, there is a delicate balance between the need of a number of people to contribute to the diagnosis and treatment of a client and the client's right to confidentiality. In most situations, necessary discussion about a client's medical condition is considered appropriate, but unnecessary discussions and gossip are considered a breach of confidentiality. Necessary discussion involves only those engaged in the client's care.

Most jurisdictions of the country have a variety of statutes that impose a duty to report certain confidential client information. Four major categories are (a) vital statistics: e.g., births and deaths, (b) infections and communicable diseases, e.g., diphtheria, syphilis, and typhoid fever, (c) child or elder abuse, and (d) violent incidents, e.g., gunshot wounds and knife wounds.

Both libel and slander are wrongful actions that come under the heading of defamation. **Defamation** is communication that is false, or made with a careless disregard for the truth, and results in injury to the reputation of a person. **Libel** is defamation by means of print, writing, or pictures. **Slander** is defamation by the spoken word, stating unprivileged (not legally protected) or false words by which a reputation is damaged. A nurse has a qualified privilege to make statements that could be considered invasions of a client's privacy, both orally and in writing, but only as a part of nursing practice and only to a physician or another health team member caring directly for the client.

In the United States, the terms *assault* and *battery* are often heard together, but each has its own meaning. **Assault** can be described as an attempt or threat to touch another person unjustifiably. Assault precedes battery; it is the act that causes the person to believe a battery is about to occur. For example, the person who threatens someone by making a menacing gesture with a club or a closed fist is guilty of assault. In nursing, a client may perceive that a nurse is *about* to administer an injection without the client's consent.

Battery is the willful touching of a person (or the person's clothes or even something the person is carrying), which may or may not cause harm. To be actionable at law, however, the touching must be wrong in some way, e.g., done without permission, embarrassing, or causing injury. For example, the nurse who administers a hypodermic injection to a client or ambulates a client without the client's consent could be held liable for battery. Liability applies even though the physician ordered the medication or the activity and even if the client benefits from the nurse's action.

In Canada, the term *battery* is not used. Instead assault is classified into three categories: assault with intention to injure (for example, threatening someone by making a menacing gesture with a knife), assault causing bodily injury, and sexual assault. **False imprisonment** is unjustifiable detention that deprives a person of personal liberty for any length of time. For example, a nurse who locks a client in a room unjustifiably is guilty of false imprisonment. False imprisonment accompanied by forceful restraint or threat of restraint is assault (Creighton 1986, p. 197).

Although nurses may suggest under certain circumstances that a client remain in the room or in bed, the client must not be detained against the client's will. The client has a right to insist upon leaving even though it may be detri-

TABLE 8–5 *Comparison of Intentional and Unintentional Torts*

Intentional	Unintentional (Negligence)
1. They involve the commission of a prohibited act.	1. They can result from either an act of commission or an act of omission.
2. The act in question is willful and deliberate (intentional).	2. The wrong results from failure to use due care.
3. They involve certain specific types of conduct listed as "wrong."	3. They are not spelled out in an all-inclusive list.

mental to health. In this instance, the client can leave by signing an AWA (absence without authority) form.

Negligence and malpractice are examples of unintentional torts that may occur in health care settings. **Negligence** is "the omission to do something that a reasonable person, guided by those ordinary considerations which ordinarily regulate human affairs, would do, or doing something which a reasonable and prudent person would not do" (Creighton 1986, p. 141). **Malpractice** is that part of the law of negligence applied to the professional person: It is, in effect, any professional misconduct or unreasonable lack of professional skill. A nurse could be liable for malpractice if the nurse injured a client while performing a procedure differently from the way other nurses would have done it.

Nurses are responsible for their own actions whether they are independent practitioners or employees of a health agency. The descriptions of negligence and malpractice do not mention good intentions; it is not pertinent that the nurse did not intend to be negligent. If a nurse administers an incorrect medication, even in good faith, the fact that the nurse failed to read the label correctly indicates malpractice if all of the elements of negligence are met.

Another significant aspect of negligence and malpractice is that both omissions and commissions are included. That is, a person can be negligent by forgetting to give a medication as well as by giving the wrong medication. See Table 8–5 for a summary of the differences between intentional and unintentional torts.

Potential Malpractice Situations in Nursing

If a nurse wishes to avoid charges of malpractice, it is helpful to recognize those nursing situations in which negligent actions are most likely to occur and to take measures to prevent them. The most common situation is the *medica-*

tion error. Because of the large number of medications on the market today and the variety of methods of administration, these errors may be on the increase. Nursing errors include failing to read the medication label, misreading or incorrectly calculating the dosage, failing to identify the client correctly, preparing the wrong concentration, or administering a medication by the wrong route (e.g., intravenously instead of orally). Some medication errors are very serious and can result in death. For example, administering dicumarol to a client recently returned from surgery could cause the client to have a hemorrhage. Nurses always need to check medications very carefully. Even after checking, the nurse is wise to recheck the medication order and the medication before administering it if the client states, for example, that the client "did not have a green pill before."

Sponges or other small items can be left inside a client during an operation because the nurse either failed to count them before the surgeon closed the incision or counted them incorrectly. In either case, the nurse responsible for the *sponge count* can be held liable for malpractice.

A relatively frequent malpractice action attributed to nurses is *burning a client.* Burns may be caused by hot water bottles, heating pads, and solutions that are too hot for application. Elderly, comatose, or diabetic people are particularly vulnerable to burns due to their decreased sensitivity. Hot objects can burn these people before they notice it. A nurse may also be held negligent for leaving a client without taking precautions (giving warnings or providing protections), for example, when using a steam vaporizer.

Clients often fall accidentally, sometimes with resultant injury. Some falls can be prevented by elevating the side rails on the cribs, beds, and stretchers of babies and small children, and of adults when necessary. If a nurse leaves the rails down or leaves a baby unattended on a bath table, that nurse is guilty of malpractice if the *client falls* and is injured as a direct result of not placing the siderails up or leaving the child unattended. Most hospitals and nursing homes have policies regarding the use of safety devices such as side rails and restraints. The nurse needs to be familiar with these policies and to take indicated precautions to prevent accidents.

In some instances, nurses are found guilty of malpractice by ignoring a client's complaints. This type of malpractice is termed *failure to observe and take appropriate action.* The nurse who does not report a client's complaint of acute abdominal pain is negligent and may be found guilty of malpractice for ensuing appendix rupture and death. By failing to take the blood pressure and pulse and to check the dressing of a client who has just had a kidney removed, a nurse omits important assessments. If the client hemorrhages and dies, the nurse may be held responsible for the death as a result of this malpractice.

Incorrectly identifying clients is a problem, particularly in busy hospital units. Nurses have prepared the wrong client for an operation with unfortunate results such as a healthy gallbladder being removed from the wrong person.

Cases of *mistaken identity* are costly to the client and render the nurse liable for malpractice.

Client property, such as jewelry, money, and dentures, is a constant concern to hospital personnel. Today, agencies are taking less responsibility for property and are generally requesting clients to sign a waiver on admission relieving the hospital and its employees of any responsibility for property. There are, however, situations in which the client cannot sign a waiver, and the nursing staff must follow prescribed policies for safeguarding the client's property. In hospital units, dentures are often a major problem; they can be lost in bedding or left on a meal tray. Nurses are expected to take reasonable precautions to safeguard a client's property, and they can be held liable for its *loss or damage* if they do not exercise reasonable care.

Reporting Crimes, Torts, and Unsafe Practices

Nurses may need to report nursing colleagues or other health professionals for practices that endanger the health and safety of clients. For instance, alcohol and drug use, theft from a client or agency, and unsafe nursing practice should be reported. Reporting a colleague is not easy. The person reporting may feel disloyal, incur the disapproval of others, or endanger chances for promotion. When reporting an incident or series of incidents, the nurse must be careful to describe observed behavior only and not make inferences as to what might be happening. The accompanying box outlines guidelines for reporting a crime, tort, or unsafe practice. In cases of substance abuse, states such as California have established voluntary programs that allow nurses to receive help in resolving their problems without losing their licenses to practice.

Guidelines for Reporting a Crime, Tort, or Unsafe Practice

- Write a clear description of the situation you believe you should report.
- Make sure that your statements are accurate.
- Make sure you are credible.
- Obtain support from at least one trustworthy person before filing the report.
- Report the matter starting at the lowest possible level in the agency hierarchy.
- Assume responsibility for reporting the individual by being open about it. Sign your name to the letter.
- See the problem through once you have reported it.

Source: D. M. Price and P. Murphy, How—and when—to blow the whistle on unsafe practices, *Nursing Life,* January/February 1983, 3:50–54.

SELECTED LEGAL FACETS OF NURSING PRACTICE

Informed Consent

Informed consent is an agreement by a client to accept a course of treatment or a procedure after complete information, including the risks of treatment and facts relating to it, has been provided by the physician. Informed consent, then, is an exchange between a client and a physician. Usually the client signs a form provided by the agency. The form is a record of the informed consent, not the informed consent itself.

Obtaining informed consent is the responsibility of a physician. Although this responsibility is delegated to nurses in some agencies, the practice is highly undesirable. The nurse's responsibility is often to witness the giving of informed consent. This involves the following:

- Witnessing the exchange between the client and the physician
- Witnessing the client's signature
- Establishing that the client really did understand, i.e., was really informed

If a nurse witnesses only the client's signature and not the exchange between the client and the physician, the nurse should write "witnessing signature only" on the form (Northrop 1988, p. 218). If the nurse finds that the client really does not understand the physician's explanation, then it is important that the physician be notified.

Northrop (1988, p. 218) describes three major elements of informed consent:

1. The consent must be given voluntarily.
2. The consent must be given by an individual with the capacity and competence to understand.
3. The client must be given enough information to be the ultimate decision maker.

To give informed consent voluntarily, the client must not feel coerced. Sometimes fear of disapproval by a health professional can be the motivation for giving consent; such consent is not voluntarily given.

To give informed consent, the client must receive sufficient information to make a decision; otherwise, the client's right to decide has been usurped. Information needs to include benefits, risks, and alternative procedures. It is also important that the client understand. Technical words and language barriers can inhibit understanding. If a client cannot read, the consent form must be read to the client before it is signed. If the client does not speak the same language as the health professional who is providing the information, an interpreter must be acquired.

If given sufficient information, the client can make decisions regarding health. To do so, the client must be competent and an adult. A competent adult is a person over 18 years of age who is conscious and oriented. A person under 18 years who is considered "an emancipated minor," i.e., self-supporting or married, can also give consent. A client who is confused, disoriented, or sedated is not considered functionally competent at that time.

There are three groups of people who cannot provide consent. The *first* is minors. In most areas, consent must be given by a parent or guardian before minors can obtain treatment. The same is true of an adult who has the mental capacity of a child if a guardian has been appointed. In some states, however, minors are allowed to give consent for such procedures as blood donations, treatment for drug dependency and sexually transmitted disease, and procedures for obstetric care. The *second* group is persons who are unconscious or injured in such a way that they are unable to give consent. In these situations, consent is usually obtained from the closest adult relative if existing statutes permit. In an emergency, if consent cannot be obtained from the client or a relative, then the law generally agrees that consent is assumed. The *third* group is mentally ill persons who have been judged to be incompetent. State and provincial mental health acts or similar statutes generally provide definitions of mental illness and specify the rights of the mentally ill under the law as well as the rights of the staff caring for such clients.

Recordkeeping

The client's medical record is a legal document and can be produced in court as evidence. Often the record is used to remind a witness of events surrounding a lawsuit, since it usually takes several months or years for the suit to go to trial. The effectiveness of a witness's testimony can depend on the accuracy of such records. Nurses, therefore, need to keep accurate and complete records of nursing care provided to clients. Failure to keep proper records can constitute negligence and be the basis for tort liability. Insufficient or inaccurate assessments and documentation can hinder proper diagnosis and treatment and result in injury to the client. Types of records and essential facts about recording are discussed in Chapter 17.

Controlled Substances

United States and Canadian laws regulate the distribution and use of controlled substances such as narcotics, depressants, stimulants, and hallucinogens. Misuse of controlled substances leads to criminal penalties. Controlled substances are kept in securely locked drawers or cupboards, and only authorized personnel have access to them. See Chapter 45 for the legal aspects of drug administration.

The Incident Report

An incident report is an agency record of an accident or incident. This report is used to make all the facts about an accident available to agency personnel, to contribute to statistical data about accidents or incidents, and to help health

---

Information to Include in an Incident Report

- Identify the client by name, initials, and hospital or identification number.
- Give the date, time, and place of the incident.
- Describe the facts of the incident. Avoid any conclusions or blame. Describe the incident as you saw it even if your impressions differ from those of others.
- Identify all witnesses to the incident.
- Identify any equipment by number and any medication by name and number.
- Document any circumstance surrounding the incident, e.g., another client (Mrs. Losas) was experiencing cardiac arrest.

---

personnel prevent future accidents. All accidents are usually reported on incident forms. Some agencies also report other incidents, e.g., the occurrence of client infection or the loss of personal effects. The box above lists the information to be included in an incident report. The report should be completed as soon as possible, always within 24 hours of the incident.

Incident reports are often viewed by an agency committee, which decides whether to investigate the incident further. The nurse may be required upon further investigation to answer such questions as: Why do you believe the acci-

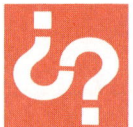

RESEARCH NOTE

When Do Incidents Occur in a Health Care Facility?

A study of all incident reports in five special-care homes of various resident capacities in Saskatchewan revealed that (a) the incidents per client day increased inversely with the size of the facility, (b) all facilities reported fewer incidents on the 2300 to 0700 hour shift, (c) in two facilities the evening shift had more incidents than the day shift, (d) in one facility there were more incidents during the day shift than the evening shift, and (e) falls accounted for the largest percentage of incidents.

Implications: In practice, nurses can help prevent accidents to clients by being alert to when and why accidents are likely to occur.

Source: V. Wasiatu, Reporting incidents: How many is too many? *Dimensions in Health Service,* September 1982, 59:16–18.

dent occurred? How could it have been prevented? Should any equipment be adjusted? Nurses who believe they may be dismissed or that suit may be brought should obtain legal advice. Even if the agency clears the nurse of responsibility, the client or the client's family may file suit. The plaintiff, however, bears the burden of proof that the accident occurred because reasonable care was not taken. Even if the accepted standard of care was not given, the plaintiff must prove that the accident was the direct result of unacceptable standards of care and that the accident caused physical, emotional, or financial injury.

When an accident occurs, the nurse should first assess the client and intervene to prevent injury. If a client is injured, nurses must take steps to protect the client, themselves, and their employer. Most agencies have policies regarding accidents. It is important to follow these policies and not to assume one is negligent. Although this may be the case, accidents do happen even when every precaution has been taken to prevent them.

Wills

A **will** is a declaration by a person about how the person's property is to be disposed of after death. In order for a will to be valid the following conditions must be met:

- The person making the will must be of sound mind, that is, able to understand and retain mentally the general nature and extent of the person's property, the relationship of the beneficiaries and of relatives to whom none of the estate will be left, and the disposition being made of the property. A person, therefore, who is seriously ill and unable to carry out usual roles may be still able to direct preparation of a will.

- The person must not be unduly influenced by anyone else. Sometimes a client may be persuaded by someone who is close at that particular time to make that person a beneficiary. Clients sometimes are persuaded to leave their estates to persons looking after them rather than to their relatives. Frequently, the relatives contest the will in such situations and take the matter to court, claiming undue influence.

Nurses may be requested from time to time to witness a will, although most agencies have policies that nurses not do so. In most states and provinces, a will must be signed in the presence of two witnesses. In some situations, a mark can suffice if the person making the will cannot write a signature. If a nurse is a witness to a will, the nurse should note on the client's chart the fact that a will was made and the nurse's perception of the physical and mental condition of the client. This record provides the nurse with accurate information if the nurse is called as a witness later. The record may also be helpful if the will is contested. If a nurse does not wish to act as a witness—for example, if in the nurse's opinion undue influence has been brought on the client—then it is the nurse's right to refuse to act in this capacity.

Euthanasia and the Right to Die (Living Wills)

Euthanasia is the act of painlessly putting to death persons suffering from incurable or distressing disease. It is commonly referred to as mercy killing. Regardless of compassion and good intentions or moral convictions, euthanasia is *legally wrong* in both Canada and the United States and can lead to criminal charges of homicide or to a civil lawsuit for withholding treatment or providing an unacceptable standard of care. Because advanced technology has enabled the medical profession to sustain life almost indefinitely, people are increasingly considering the meaning of quality of life. For some people, the withholding of artificial life-support measures or even the withdrawal of life support is a desired and acceptable practice for clients who are terminally ill or who are incurably disabled and believed unable to live their lives with some happiness and meaning.

Voluntary euthanasia refers to situations in which the dying individual desires some control over the time and manner of death. All forms of euthanasia are illegal except in states where right-to-die statutes and living wills exist. Right-to-die statutes legally recognize the client's right to refuse treatment.

Living wills (an individual's signed request to be allowed to die when life can be supported only mechanically or by heroic measures) and right-to-die statutes have received increasing attention in recent years. Most nurses agree that people have a right not to participate in medical treatment or to refuse treatment once it has started. When a person is being maintained on life-sustaining machines, however, a conflict may arise between a physician's ability to prolong life physiologically and the individual's right to die with dignity. Living wills grew out of this conflict. California was the first state to enact legislation, the California Natural Death Act of 1976, that gives legal recognition to a person's desire to control his or her right to die. Since then, 37 other states and the District of Columbia have enacted similar laws (Bellocq 1988, p. 313). Some oppose these laws, contending there is no need for such laws, the laws exclude family from the decision, and the laws hasten death. For a sample living will, see Figure 8–2.

Nurses need to familiarize themselves with statutes that authorize living wills in the state where they are employed. Where statutes do exist, policy and procedures are usually detailed specifically. They may include the need to obtain a court order, a medical opinion, the agreement of an ethics or medical committee, family confirmation, or some combination of these. The statutes usually grant civil and criminal immunity to those who carry out living-will requests.

No-Code and Slow-Code Orders

Physicians may order "no code" or "slow code" for clients who are in a stage of terminal, irreversible illness or expected death. **No code** means no effort is to be made to resuscitate

To My Family, My Physician, My Lawyer And All Others Whom It May Concern

Death is as much a reality as birth, growth, and aging—it is the one certainty of life. In anticipation of decisions that may have to be made about my own dying and as an expression of my right to refuse treatment, I_____, being of sound mind, make this statement of my wishes and instructions concerning treatment.

(print name)

By means of this document, which I intend to be legally binding, I direct my physician and other care providers, my family, and any surrogate designated by me or appointed by a court, to carry out my wishes. If I become unable, by reason of physical or mental incapacity, to make decisions about my medical care, let this document provide the guidance and authority needed to make any and all such decisions.

If I am permanently unconscious or there is no reasonable expectation of my recovery from a seriously incapacitating or lethal illness or condition, I do not wish to be kept alive by artificial means. I request that I be given all care necessary to keep me comfortable and free of pain, even if pain-relieving medications may hasten my death, and I direct that no life-sustaining treatment be provided except as I or my surrogate specifically authorize.

This request may appear to place a heavy responsibility upon you, but by making this decision according to my strong convictions, I intend to ease that burden. I am acting after careful consideration and with understanding of the consequences of your carrying out my wishes. *List optional specific provisions in the space below. (See other side)*

Figure 8–2 A sample living will. *Source:* For more information and a complete document, contact: Concern for Dying, or The Society for the Right to Die, 250 W. 57th Street, New York, NY 10107. Reproduced with permission.

the client. No-code orders may also be written as *"no heroics"* or *DNR* (do not resuscitate or do not make resuscitative efforts). **Slow code** means "half-hearted" resuscitation measures are to be initiated and implemented. "Slow-code" orders are frequently not written orders, but are conveyed in an informal manner (i.e., the physician issuing the order does *not* want it to be written as a verbal or telephone order) and are *not* legally acceptable. The legality of no-code and slow-code orders is not well established in most settings. New York state has a law that permits adults and minors (through a parent or guardian) to consent to a DNR order. It applies only to CPR, not to the withholding or withdrawing of other medical treatment. The statute also permits a competent adult to designate a surrogate to direct

that CPR be withheld if the individual becomes incompetent (Bellocq 1988, p. 313).

The American Heart Association (AHA) has issued "Standards and Guidelines for Cardiopulmonary Resuscitation and Emergency Cardiac Care" outlining the medicolegal considerations and offering recommendations about DNR orders for physicians (AHA 1986, p. 2880). Although these standards, like those of any professional organization, are not legally binding, they are persuasive to a judge and jury. They indicate that CPR is intended to prevent *unexpected* death and that its intent is not to continue life when death is *expected*. The implications of the AHA no-code standards mean that the nurse must:

- Ensure that the DNR order is written on the client's order sheet and progress notes. Verbal orders can be easily misunderstood and disclaimed.

- If the physician refuses to write such an order, follow agency policies and procedures. Some agencies have established formal protocols for nurses to follow. Because such procedures are usually carefully reviewed by legal counsel, they can minimize the risk of legal liability substantially.

- If the agency does not have a well-established procedure, seek a legal opinion through the agency attorney or state or provincial nursing association.

- If none of the above steps provides the nurse with sufficient guidelines, the nurse must make a personal decision based on moral values and sense of humanity. Even when there are appropriate guidelines, the guidelines may conflict with the nurse's personal ethics. Thus, DNR orders may create an ethical dilemma as well as a legal dilemma for the nurse.

Abortions

Abortion laws provide specific guidelines for nurses about what is legally permissible. In 1973, when the *Roe vs. Wade* and *Doe vs. Bolton* cases were decided, the Supreme Court of the United States held that the constitutional rights of privacy give a woman the right to control her own body to the extent that she can abort her fetus in the early stages of pregnancy. The state, however, has a legitimate interest in controlling abortion during later stages of pregnancy. The results of the Supreme Court rulings are:

1. It is not legally permissible for the state to restrict or regulate abortions during the first trimester (first 3 months) of pregnancy except to require that the abortion be performed by a licensed physician.

2. During the second trimester of pregnancy (4 to 6 months), the mother's privacy rights must yield to *reasonable* restrictions designed to protect the health and safety of the mother. Restrictions include that the facility in which the abortion is performed be licensed.

3. During the third trimester of pregnancy, the state has the right to prohibit abortion. The rationale for this ruling is that by this stage of pregnancy the state's interest in protecting the viable but unborn child outweighs the woman's right to privacy.

Since these rulings, many states have enacted statutes. In addition, the Supreme Court no longer requires that the parents of a pregnant minor consent to abortion, nor that the father of the woman's child (whether he is her husband or not) consent; however, there are opportunities to appeal these waivers.

In 1989 the Supreme Courts' decision in *Webster vs. Reproductive Health Services* upheld a Missouri law banning the use of public funds or facilities for performing or assisting with abortions. The ANA's statement in 1989 includes "abortion is largely a symptom of social failure." The ANA supports equal access to care, freedom of choice, and right to privacy (ANA 1989).

Many statutes also include conscience clauses, upheld by the Supreme Court, designed to protect nurses and hospitals. These clauses give hospitals the right to deny admission to abortion clients and give health care personnel, including nurses, the right to refuse to participate in abortions. When these rights are exercised, the statutes also protect the agency and employee from discrimination or retaliation.

The abortion issue is before the Parliament of Canada at time of writing. It is proposed that abortion be a matter between a woman and her physician. Currently, abortion may be indicated only if a woman's physical, mental, or emotional health is in danger. Abortion that does not fit these criteria is considered a criminal offense.

Death and Related Issues

Legal issues surrounding death include the death certificate, labeling of the deceased, autopsy, organ donation, and inquest. By law, a death certificate must be made out when a person dies. It is usually signed by the attending physician and filed with a local health or other government office. The family is usually given a copy to use for legal matters, such as insurance claims.

Nurses have a duty to handle the deceased with dignity and label the corpse appropriately. Mishandling can cause emotional distress to survivors. Mislabeling can create legal problems if the body is inappropriately identified and prepared incorrectly for burial or a funeral. Usually, the deceased's wrist identification tag is left on, and another tag is tied to the client's ankles, in case one of the tags becomes detached. Tags tied to the ankles are preferred, since any tissue damage they cause will be concealed by bed linen or clothing. A third tag is attached to the shroud. All identification tags should include the client's name, hospital number, and physician's name.

An **autopsy** or **postmortem examination** is an examination of the body after death. It is performed only in certain cases. The law describes under what circumstances an autopsy must be performed, e.g., when death is sudden or when it occurs within 48 hours of admission to a hospital. The organs and tissues of the body are examined to establish the exact cause of death, to learn more about a disease, and to assist in the accumulation of statistical data.

It is the responsibility of the physician or, in some instances, of a designated person in the hospital to obtain consent for autopsy. Consent must be given by the decedent (before death) or by the next of kin. Laws in many states and provinces prioritize the family members who can provide consent as follows: surviving spouse, adult children, parents, siblings. After autopsy, hospitals cannot retain any tissues or organs without the permission of the person who consented to the autopsy.

Organ Donation   Under the Uniform Anatomical Gift Act in the United States or the Human Tissue Act in Canada, any person 18 years or older and of sound mind may make a gift of all or any part of the body for the following purposes: for medical or dental education, research, advancement of medical or dental science, therapy, or transplantation (Annas et al. 1981, p. 227). The donation can be made by a provision in a will or by signing a cardlike form in the presence of two witnesses. This card is usually carried at all times by the person who signed it. In most states and provinces, the gift can be revoked either by destroying the card or by an oral revocation in the presence of two witnesses. Nurses may serve as witnesses for persons consenting to donate organs. In some states (e.g., California) health care workers are required to ask survivors for consent to donate the deceased's organs.

Inquest   An **inquest** is a legal inquiry into the cause or manner of a death. When a death is the result of an accident, for example, an inquest is held into the circumstances of the accident to determine any blame. The inquest is conducted under the jurisdiction of a coroner or medical examiner. A **coroner** is a public official, not necessarily a physician, appointed or elected to inquire into the causes of death, when appropriate. A **medical examiner** is a physician who usually has advanced education in pathology or forensic medicine. Agency policy dictates who is responsible for reporting deaths to the coroner or medical examiner.

LEGAL PROTECTIONS FOR NURSES

Good Samaritan Acts

Good Samaritan acts are laws designed to protect health care providers who provide assistance at the scene of an emergency against claims of malpractice unless it can be shown that there was a gross departure from the normal standard of care or willful wrongdoing on their part. Gross negligence usually involves further injury or harm to the person. For example, an injured child left on the side of the road may be struck by an automobile when the nurse leaves to obtain help.

In the United States, most state statutes do not require citizens to render aid to people in distress. Such assistance is considered more of an *ethical* than a *legal* duty. A few states, however, have enacted legislation that requires people educated in health care to stop and aid the injured. To encourage citizens to be good Samaritans, most states have now enacted legislation releasing the good Samaritan from legal liability for injuries caused under such circumstances, even if the injuries resulted from negligence of the person offering emergency aid.

In Canada, some provinces specify in traffic acts that it is the responsibility of people to give aid at the scene of an accident. Alberta is the only province that exempts physicians and nurses from liability unless gross negligence is proved. However, lawsuits against good Samaritans are rarely successful.

It is generally believed that a person who renders help in an emergency, at the level of helping that would be provided by any reasonably prudent person under similar circumstances, cannot be held liable. The same reasoning applies to nurses, who may be the people best prepared to help at the scene of an accident. If the level of care a nurse provides is of the caliber that would have been provided by any other nurse, then the nurse will not be held liable.

Professional Liability Insurance

Because of the increase in the number of malpractice lawsuits against health professionals, nurses are advised in many areas to carry their own liability insurance. Most hospitals have liability insurance that covers all employees, including all nurses. However, some smaller facilities, such as "walk-in" clinics, may not. Thus the nurse should always check with the employer at the time of hiring to see what coverage the facility provides. A physician or a hospital can be sued because of the negligent conduct of a nurse, and the nurse can also be sued and held liable for negligence or malpractice. Because hospitals have been known to countersue nurses when they have been found negligent and the hospital was required to pay, nurses are advised to provide their own insurance coverage and not rely on hospital-provided insurance.

Liability insurance coverage usually defrays all costs of defending a nurse, including the costs of retaining an attorney. The insurance also covers all costs incurred by the nurse up to the face value of the policy, including a settlement made out of court. In return, the insurance company may have the right to make the decisions about the claim and the settlement.

Nursing faculty and nursing students are also vulnerable to lawsuits. In hospital nursing education programs, in-structors and students are often specifically covered for liability by the hospital. An instructor, however, can still be sued by a hospital in cases of negligence and malpractice.

Students and teachers of nursing employed by community colleges and universities are less likely to be covered by the insurance carried by hospitals and health agencies. It is advisable for these people to check with their school about the coverage that applies to them. Increasingly, instructors are carrying their own malpractice insurance in both the United States and Canada. In the United States, insurance can be obtained through the ANA or private insurance companies; in Canada, it can usually be obtained through provincial nurses' associations. Nursing students in the United States can also obtain insurance through the National Student Nurses Association. In some states, hospitals do not allow nursing students to provide nursing care without liability insurance.

LEGAL RESPONSIBILITIES IN NURSING PRACTICE

Carrying Out Physician's Orders

Nurses are expected to know basic information about procedures and medications ordered by the physician. It is the nurse's responsibility to seek clarification of ambiguous or seemingly erroneous orders from the prescribing physician. Clarification from any other source is unacceptable and regarded as a departure from competent nursing practice.

If the order is neither ambiguous nor apparently erroneous, the nurse is responsible for carrying it out. For example, if the physician orders oxygen to be administered at 4 liters per minute, the nurse must administer oxygen at that rate, and not at 2 or 6 liters per minute. If the orders state that the client is not to have solid food after a bowel resection, the nurse must ensure that no solid food is given to the client. Nurses also have a responsibility to check for changes in orders from previous shifts of duty.

Becker (1983, pp. 21–23) outlines four orders that nurses must question to protect themselves legally:

1. Question any order a client questions. For example, if a client who has been receiving an intramuscular injection tells the nurse that the doctor changed the order from an injectable to an oral medication, the nurse should recheck the order before giving the medication.

2. Question any order if the client's condition has changed. The nurse is considered responsible for notifying the physician of any significant changes in the client's condition, whether the physician requests notification or not. For example, if a client who is receiving an intravenous infusion suddenly develops a rapid pulse, chest pain, and a cough, the nurse must notify the physician immediately and question continuance of the ordered rate of infusion. If a client who is receiving morphine

for pain develops severely depressed respirations, the nurse must withhold the medication and notify the physician.

3. Question and record verbal orders to avoid miscommunications. In addition to recording the time, the date, the physician's name, and the orders, the nurse documents the circumstances that occasioned the call to the physician, reads the orders back to the physician, and documents that the physician confirmed the orders as the nurse read them back.

4. Question standing orders, especially if the nurse is inexperienced. *Standing orders* give the nurse added responsibility to exercise appropriate judgment when implementing them. The nurse is delegated the authority to, for example, adjust the amount of a medication or other substances and make decisions about when a medication is needed. Nurses need to take the same precautions when implementing these orders as when implementing any other orders. In addition, the nurse who does not feel confident about exercising discretionary judgment should request specific guidelines from the physician or assistance from a more experienced nurse. In some states, standing orders are not allowed except in intensive care or coronary care units.

Implementing Delegated and Independent Nursing Interventions

Nurses implementing care need to take the following precautions (Grane 1983, pp. 17–20; Rhodes and Miller 1984, pp. 153–60):

- Know their job description. This enables nurses to function within the scope of the description and know what is and what is not expected. Job descriptions vary from agency to agency.
- Follow the policies and procedures of the agency in which they are working.
- Always identify clients, particularly before initiating major interventions, e.g., surgical or other invasive procedures, or when administering blood transfusions.
- Make sure the correct medications are given in the correct dose, by the right route, at the scheduled time, and to the right client. See Chapter 45 for more detailed information about the administration of medications.
- Perform procedures appropriately. Negligent incidents during procedures generally relate to equipment failure, improper technique, and improper performance of the procedure. For instance, the nurse must know how to safeguard the client in the event that a respirator or other equipment fails.
- Promptly and accurately document all assessments and care given. Records must show that the nurse provided and supervised the client's care daily.

- Report all incidents involving clients. Prompt reports enable those responsible to attend to the client's well-being, to analyze why the incident occurred, and to prevent recurrences.
- Build and maintain good rapport with clients. Keeping clients informed about diagnostic and treatment plans, giving feedback on their progress, and showing concern for the outcome of their care prevent a sense of powerlessness and a build-up of hostility in the client.
- Maintain clinical competence in their area of practice. For students, this demands study and practice before caring for clients. For graduate nurses, it means continued study, including maintaining and updating clinical knowledge and skills.
- Know their own strengths and weaknesses. For example, nurses who recognize that they have difficulty calculating medication dosages should always ask someone to check the calculations before proceeding.
- When delegating nursing responsibilities, make sure that the person who is delegated a task understands what to do and that the person has the required knowledge and skill. The delegating nurse can be held liable for harm caused by the person to whom the care was delegated.
- Be alert when implementing nursing interventions and give each task their full attention and skill.

Ways nurses can protect themselves legally are summarized in the accompanying Clinical Guidelines box.

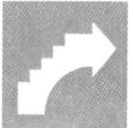

CLINICAL GUIDELINES
Legal Precautions for Nurses

- Function within the scope of your education, job description, and area nurse practice act.
- Follow the procedures and policies of the employing agency.
- Observe and monitor the client accurately.
- Communicate and record significant changes in the client's condition to the physician.
- Check any orders that a client questions.
- Identify clients before initiating any interventions.
- Protect clients from falls and preventable injuries.
- Document all nursing assessments and interventions accurately.
- Ask for assistance and supervision in situations for which you feel inadequately prepared.
- Delegate tasks to persons with the knowledge and skill to carry them out.
- Build and maintain good rapport with clients.

LEGAL RESPONSIBILITIES OF STUDENTS

Nursing students are responsible for their own actions and liable for their own acts of negligence committed during the course of clinical experiences. When they perform duties that are within the scope of professional nursing, such as administering an injection, they are legally held to the same standard of skill and competence as a registered professional nurse (Rhodes and Miller 1984, p. 163). Lower standards are *not* applied to the actions of nursing students.

In cases arising from negligent acts by nursing students, the student has traditionally been treated as an employee of the hospital, which was held liable under the doctrine of *respondeat superior.* Today, associate degree and baccalaureate nursing students are not usually considered employees of the agencies in which they receive clinical experience, since these nursing programs contract with agencies to provide clinical experiences for students. In future cases of negligence involving such students, the hospital or agency (e.g., public health agency) and the educational institution will be held potentially liable for negligent actions by students (Rhodes and Miller 1984, p. 164).

Students in clinical situations must be assigned activity within their capabilities and be given reasonable guidance and supervision. Nursing instructors are responsible for assigning students to the care of clients and for providing reasonable supervision. Failure to provide reasonable supervison and/or the assignment of a client to a student who is not prepared and competent can be a basis for liability.

To fulfill responsibilities to clients and to minimize chances for liability, nursing students need to

- Make sure they are prepared to carry out the necessary care for assigned clients.

- Ask for additional help or supervision in situations for which they feel inadequately prepared.

- Comply with the policies of the agency in which they obtain their clinical experience.

- Comply with the policies and definitions of responsibility supplied by the school of nursing.

Students who work as part-time or temporary nursing assistants or aides must also remember that *legally* they can perform only those tasks that appear in the job description of a nurse's aide or assistant. Even though a student may have received instruction and acquired competence in administering injections or suctioning a tracheostomy tube, the student cannot legally perform these tasks while employed as an aide or assistant.

CHAPTER HIGHLIGHTS

▶ Accountability is an essential concept of professional nursing practice under the law.

▶ Nurses need to understand laws that regulate and affect nursing practice to ensure that the nurses' actions are consistent with current legal principles and to protect the nurse from liability.

▶ Nurse practice acts legally define and describe the scope of nursing practice that the law seeks to regulate.

▶ Competence in nursing practice is determined and maintained by various credentialing methods, such as licensure, registration, certification, and accreditation, which protect the public's welfare and safety.

▶ Standards of practice published by national and state or provincial nursing associations and agency policies, procedures, and job descriptions further delineate the scope of a nurse's practice.

▶ The nurse has specific legal obligations and responsibilities to clients and employers. As a citizen, the nurse has the rights and responsibilities shared by all individuals in the society.

▶ Collective bargaining is one way nurses can improve their working conditions and economic welfare.

▶ Nurses can be held liable for intentional torts, such as fraud, invasion of privacy, defamation, assault and battery, and false imprisonment; and for unintentional torts, or negligence.

▶ Negligence or malpractice of nurses can be established when (a) the nurse (defendant) owed a duty to the client, (b) the nurse failed to carry out that duty, (c) the client (plaintiff) was injured, and (d) the client's injury was caused by the nurse's failure to carry out that duty.

▶ The nurse is responsible for ensuring that the physician obtains informed consents from clients (or from the closest relative in emergencies or from parents or guardians when the client is a minor) before treatment regimens and procedures begin.

▶ Informed consent implies that (a) the consent was given voluntarily; (b) the client was of age and had the capacity and competence to understand; and (c) the client was given enough information on which to make an informed decision.

▶ When a client is accidentally injured or involved in an unusual situation, the nurse's first responsibility is to

▶

take steps to protect the client and then to notify appropriate agency personnel.

- ▶ Living wills are receiving increasing attention; because statutes that authorize living wills vary, nurses need to familiarize themselves with their specifications.

- ▶ The legality of no-code and slow-code orders is not well established; nurses are advised to follow the state law for no-code orders.

- ▶ Nurses must be knowledgeable about their responsibilities in regard to legal issues surrounding death: death certificate, labeling of the deceased, autopsy, organ donation, and inquest.

- ▶ Good Samaritan acts protect health professionals from claims of malpractice when they offer assistance at the scene of an emergency, provided there is no willful wrongdoing or gross departure from normal standards of care.

- ▶ Practicing nurses who are not covered by liability insurance in their employing agency can obtain liability insurance through professional nursing associations.

- ▶ Nursing students need to make sure they are prepared to provide the necessary care to assigned clients and to ask for help or supervision in situations for which they feel inadequately prepared.

READINGS AND REFERENCES

SUGGESTED READINGS

Arbeiter, J. S. October 1988. Are you merely a witness to the patient's consent? *RN* 51:53–57.

Arbeiter writes about the approaches of two panelists to the issue of informed consent. According to one panelist, about 99% of the responsibility for obtaining informed consent is the physician's. The issue of when a client is not fully informed is discussed. A questionnaire regarding witnessing a consent is also described. The alternatives open to a nurse who refuses to witness an informed consent are also described.

Baer, O. J. May/June 1985. Protecting your patient's privacy. *Nursing Life* 5:50–53.

Baer discusses clients' rights to privacy under the law. Such problems as responding to a family's questions, responding to media inquiries, and discussing clients with others are addressed. The author reviews reporting guidelines and discusses how court decisions affect clients' right to privacy. Baer recommends that nurses secure professional liability insurance and then make sure it is never needed.

Klimon, E. L. March/April 1985. Do you swear to tell the truth? *Nursing Economics* 3:98–102.

Klimon describes what may happen when a health professional must testify at a malpractice suit. Klimon tells nurses how to prepare for a deposition; gives advice on appearance, demeanor, and enunciation; and prepares the reader for the personal and professional information that one may need to provide. Points addressed include identifying exhibits, understanding the question, and keeping answers brief. It is exceedingly important to tell the truth and not to qualify favorable facts.

Parsons, M. S. November/December 1986. 5 common legal risks: Could these stories have happened to you? *Nursing Life* 6:26–30. Parsons describes five common legal risks: falls, restraining a client, client teaching, equipment malfunction, and understaffing. An example of each circumstance is given, followed by guidelines to reduce the risk of liability.

Rabinow, J. February 1989. Where you stand in the eyes of the law. *Nursing 89* 19:34–42.

Rabinow explains that there may be 2000 nurses sued by 1989. She describes a number of nursing and legal trends, such as expanding nursing responsibilities and their legal implications. The legal process is diagrammed in the article, and incident reports are discussed.

RELATED RESEARCH

Wasiuta, V. September 1982. Reporting incidents: How many is too many? *Dimensions in Health Service* 59:16–18.

SELECTED REFERENCES

Alford, D. M. March 1987. A probate judge's view: Nurse attorneys. *Journal of Gerontological Nursing* 13:32–34.

Alford, D. September/October 1987. How to avoid being a nurse defendant. *Nursing Life* 7:22–23.

American Heart Association. June 6, 1986. Standards and guidelines for cardiopulmonary resuscitation and emergency cardiac care. *Journal of the American Medical Association*. 255:2841–3044.

American Nurses' Association. 1961. *Legal definition of nursing.* Kansas City, Mo.: ANA.

———. July 1973. ANA issues statement on diploma graduates. *American Journal of Nursing* 73:1135.

———. 1975. *Human rights guidelines for nurses in clinical and other research.* Publication no. D-46 5M 7/75. Kansas City, Mo.: ANA.

———. 1976. *The code for nurses.* Kansas City, Mo.: ANA.

———. April 1979. Credentialing in nursing. A new approach. Report of the Committee for the study of Credentialing in Nursing. *American Journal of Nursing* 79:674–83.

———. 1981. The nursing practice act: Suggested state legislation. Kansas City, Mo.: ANA.

———. 1985. *The grievance procedure.* Kansas City, Mo.: ANA.

American Nurses' Association Cabinet on Economic and General Welfare. 1985. *The nature and scope of ANA's economic and general welfare program.* Kansas City, Mo.: ANA.

———. 1987. Credentialing in nursing: Contemporary developments and trends. Kansas City, Mo.: ANA.

Annas, G. J.; Glantz, L. H.; and Katz, B. F. 1981. *The right of doctors, nurses and allied health professionals.* New York: Avon Books.

Arbeiter, J. S. October 1988. Are you merely a witness to the patient's consent? *RN* 51:53–57.

Baer, O. J. May/June 1985. Protecting your patient's privacy. *Nursing Life* 5:50–53.

Barbash, J. 1980. Collective bargaining: Contemporary American experience—A commentary. In Sommers, G. H., editor. *Collective bargaining: Contemporary American experience.* Madison, Wis.: Industrial Relations Research Association.

Becker, M. January/February 1983. Five orders you must question to protect yourself legally. *Nursing Life* 3:21–23.

Bellocq, J. A. September/October 1988. Legal and ethical issues: Changing attitudes about death. *Journal of Professional Nursing* 4:313.

Brill, J. M. April 1990. Informed consent may entail risk. *American Nurse* 22:42.

Cournoyer, C. P. March/April 1985. Protecting yourself legally after a patient's injured. *Nursing Life* 5:18–22.

Crawford, M.; Fisher, M.; and Kilbane, N. February 1983. Law for the nurse manager. Incident reports subject to discovery? *Nursing Management* 14:55, 57.

———. 1985. Collective bargaining in nursing. In DeYoung, L. *Dynamics of nursing.* 5th ed. St. Louis: C. V. Mosby Co.

Creighton, H. November 1982. Board of nursing has authority to establish standards for programs . . . only associate and baccalaureate degree graduates could sit for examinations. *Nursing Management* 18:26, 28, 30, 32.

———. November 1985. Law for the nurse manager. Relatives sue for putting patient on life support. *Nursing Management* 16:56, 60.

———. 1986. *Law every nurse should know.* 5th ed. Philadelphia: W. B. Saunders Co.

Curtin, L. L. October 1982. Informed consent: Rights, responsibilities, and roles. *Nursing Management* 13:7–8.

Cushing, M. August 1985. Incident reports: For your eyes only? *American Journal of Nursing* 85:873–74.

———. February 1986. How courts look at nurse practice acts. *American Journal of Nursing* 86:131.

Davis, A. January/February 1985. Informed consent: How much information is enough? *Nursing Outlook* 33:40–42.

Doe v. Bolton, 410 U.S. 179 (1973); Roe v. Wade, 410 U.S. 113 (1973).

Ellstrom, K., Bella, L. D. May 1990. Understanding your role during a code. *Nursing 90* 20:36–44.

Facts to know about living wills. January/February 1984. *Nursing Life* 4:26–27.

Fenner, K. 1980. *Ethics and the law in nursing.* New York: D. Van Nostrand Co.

Fiesta, J. 1983, 1988. *The law and liability: A guide for nurses.* 2d ed. New York: John Wiley and Sons.

Flanagen, L. 1983. *Collective bargaining and the nursing profession.* Kansas City, Mo.: American Nurses' Association.

Grane, N. B. January/February 1983. How to reduce your risk of a lawsuit. *Nursing Life* 3:17–20.

Kemerer, A. A. March/April 1989. Nurse practice acts. *A D Nurse* 4:29–33.

Labor-Management Relations Act. 1947. Section 8(d).

Lacombe, D. C. June 1990. Avoiding a malpractice nightmare. *Nursing 90* 20:42–3.

Lewis, E. P. September/October 1985. Taking care of business: The ANA house of delegates. *Nursing Outlook* 33:239–43.

McClelland, J. Q. November 1983. Professionalism and collective bargaining: A new reality for nurses and management. *Journal of Nursing Administration* 13:36–38.

Mackert, M. E., and Hemelt, M. D. September/October 1985. Avoiding legal risks in the E.D. *Nursing Life* 5:26–29.

Marks, D. T. March 1987. Legal implications of increased autonomy. *Journal of Gerontological Nursing* 13:26, 28–31.

Moylan, L. B. June 1988. Implications of the National Labor Relations Act. *Nursing Management* 19:80.

Murchison, I.; Nichols, T. S.; and Janson, R. 1982. *Legal accountability in the nursing process.* 2d ed. St. Louis: C. V. Mosby Co.

Nichols, B. 1986. Legal and professional responsibilities in the regulation of nursing practice. *Issues* 7:1–3.

Northrop, C. 1988. Legal aspects of nursing. In McCann Flynn, J. B., and Heffron, P. B. *Nursing: From concept to practice.* 2d ed. East Norwalk, Conn: Appleton & Lange.

———. January 1985. The ins and outs of informed consent. *Nursing 85* 15:21.

———. March/April 1988. Nursing practice and the legal presumption of competency. (Legal Outlook). *Nursing Outlook* 36:112.

Numerof, R. E., and Abrams, M. N. Spring 1984. Collective bargaining among nurses: Current issues and future prospects. *Health Care Management Review* 9:61–67.

Nursing education and students' rights: Legalities . . . when charged with academic dishonesty. August 1983. *Regan Report on Nursing Law* 24:4.

A *Nursing Life* poll report on ethics. March/April 1983. Do you make your patient live . . . or let him die? *Nursing Life* 3:54–55.

Oberst, M. November/December 1985. Another look at informed consent. *Nursing Outlook* 33:294–95.

Orr, M. L. March 1987. Enabling professional nursing practice in New York State. *Journal of the New York State Nurses' Association* 18:30–38.

Ozimek, D. February 1982. Rights and responsibilities of students and faculty. *Imprint* 29:50–51.

Parsons, M. S. November/December 1986. 5 common legal risks: Could these stories have happened to you? *Nursing Life* 6:26–30.

Pettengill, M. M. September/October 1985. Multilateral collective bargaining and the health care industry: Implications for nursing. *Journal of Professional Nursing* 1:275–82.

Price, D. M., and Murphy, P. January/February 1983. How—and when—to blow the whistle on unsafe practices. *Nursing Life* 3:50–54.

Rhodes, A. M., and Miller, R. D. 1984. *Nursing and the Law.* 4th ed. Rockville, Md.: Aspen Systems Corporation.

Rudy, E. B. June 1985. The living will: Are you informed? *Focus on Critical Care* 12:51–57.

Smith, G. R. July/August 1985. Unionization for nurses: An issue for the 1980s. *Journal of Professional Nursing* 1:192–201.

Snyder, M. E., and LaBar, C. 1984. *Issues in professional nursing practice 1. Nursing: Legal authority for practice.* Kansas City, Mo.: American Nurses' Association.

Snyder, R., Westerfield, J. June 1990. Should nurses pronounce death? *Nursing 90* 20:41.

Tobin, B. K. September/October 1986. Living wills: The spectrum of new possibilities. *Nursing Life* 6:44–45.

U.S. Department of Labor. 1979. *Impact of the 1974 health care amendments to the NLRA on collective bargaining in the health care industry.* Washington, D.C.: U.S. Government Printing Office.

Williams, R. M. March/April 1984. Collective bargaining and political lobbying: Tools to accomplish professional nursing goals. *Michigan Nurse* 57:1.

The Nursing Process

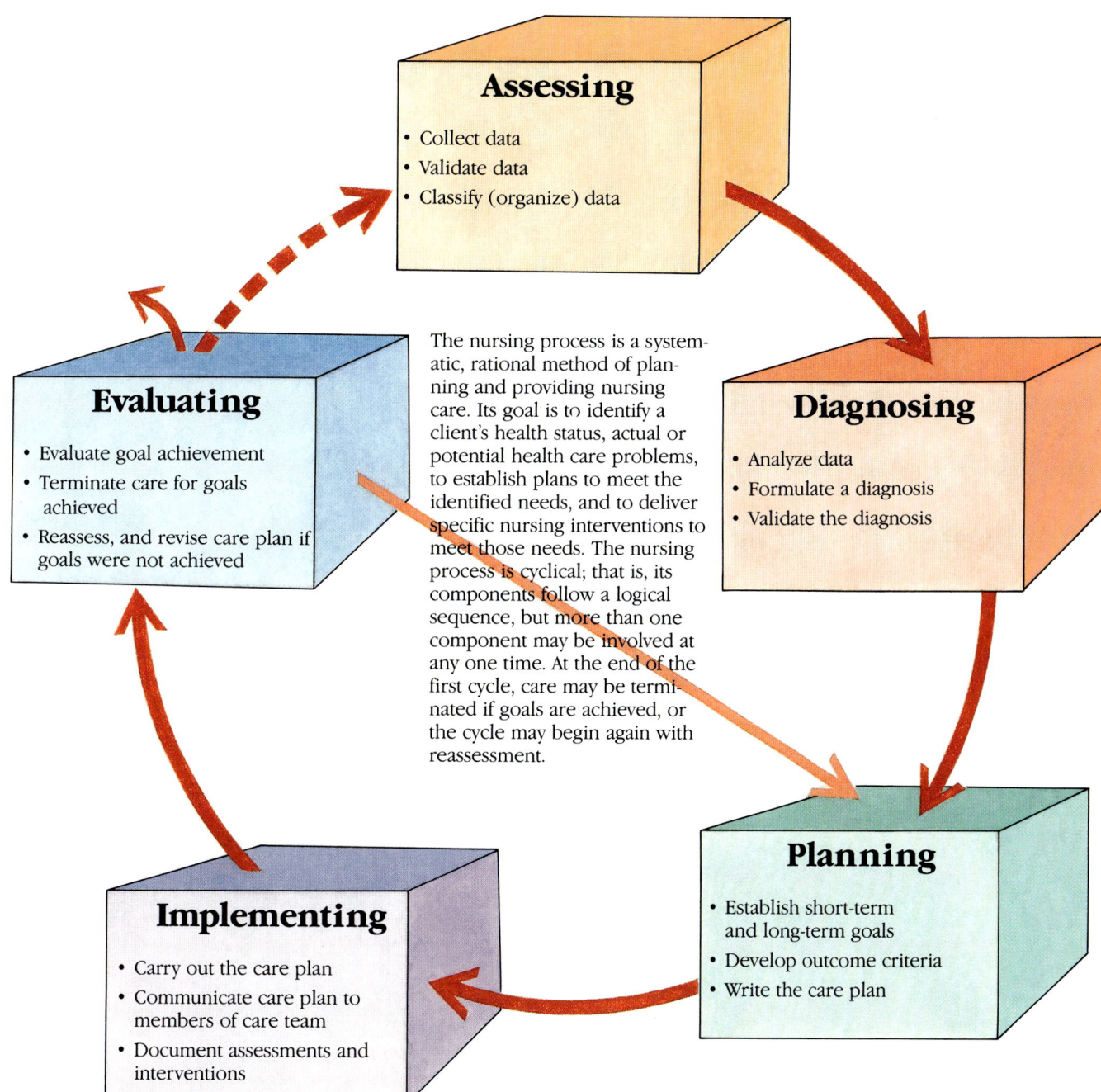

Assessing

- Collect data
- Validate data
- Classify (organize) data

The nursing process is a systematic, rational method of planning and providing nursing care. Its goal is to identify a client's health status, actual or potential health care problems, to establish plans to meet the identified needs, and to deliver specific nursing interventions to meet those needs. The nursing process is cyclical; that is, its components follow a logical sequence, but more than one component may be involved at any one time. At the end of the first cycle, care may be terminated if goals are achieved, or the cycle may begin again with reassessment.

Diagnosing

- Analyze data
- Formulate a diagnosis
- Validate the diagnosis

Evaluating

- Evaluate goal achievement
- Terminate care for goals achieved
- Reassess, and revise care plan if goals were not achieved

Planning

- Establish short-term and long-term goals
- Develop outcome criteria
- Write the care plan

Implementing

- Carry out the care plan
- Communicate care plan to members of care team
- Document assessments and interventions

The nursing process in practice . . .

Luisa Westley, a 28-year-old married attorney, was admitted to the hospital with an elevated temperature, a nonproductive cough, and rapid, labored respirations. In taking a nursing history, Mary Medina, RN, finds that Ms. Westley has had a "chest cold" for two weeks, and has been experiencing shortness of breath upon exertion. Yesterday she developed an elevated temperature and began to experience "pain" in her "lungs."

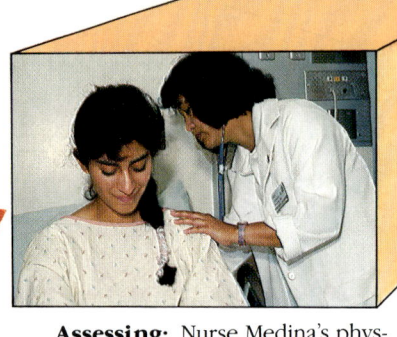

Assessing: Nurse Medina's physical assessment reveals that Ms. Westley's vital signs are: Temperature, 39.4 C (103 F); pulse, 92 BPM; respirations, 28; and blood pressure, 122/80 mm Hg. Nurse Medina observes that Ms. Westley's skin is dry, her cheeks are flushed, and she is experiencing chills. Auscultation reveals inspiratory crackles with diminished breath sounds in the right lung.

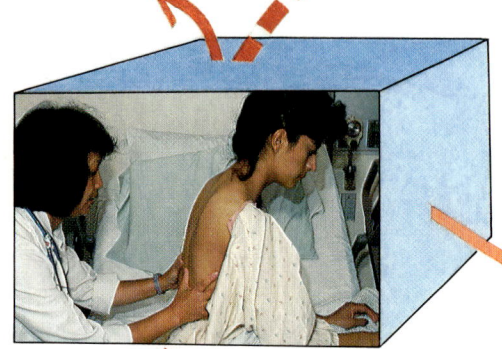

Evaluating: Upon assessment of respiratory excursion, Nurse Medina detects failure of the client to achieve maximum ventilation. She and Ms. Westley reevaluate the care plan and modify it to increase coughing and deep breathing exercises to q2h.

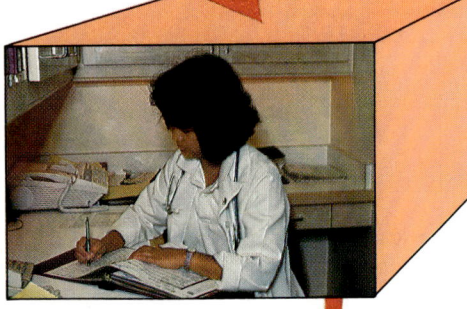

Diagnosing: After analysis, Nurse Medina formulates a nursing diagnosis:
Ineffective airway clearance
related to thick sputum obstructing airways.

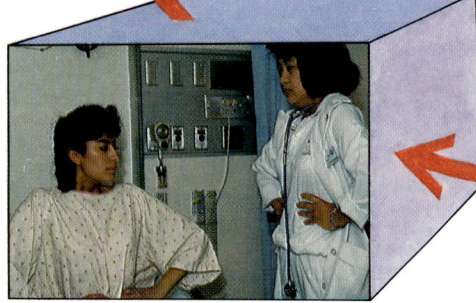

Implementing: Ms. Westley agrees to practice deep breathing exercises q3h during the day. In addition, she understands the need to increase her fluid intake and to plan her morning activities to accommodate postural drainage.

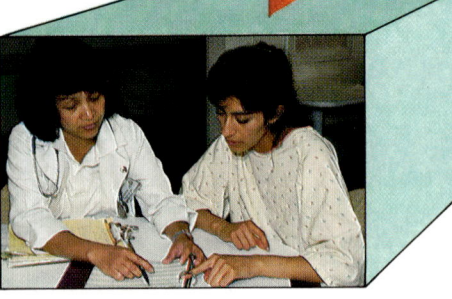

Planning: Nurse Medina and Ms. Westley collaborate to establish goals (e.g., restore effective breathing pattern and lung ventilation); set outcome criteria (e.g., have a symmetrical respiratory excursion of at least 4 cm and so on); and develop a care plan that includes, but is not limited to, coughing and deep breathing exercises q3h, fluid intake of 3000 mL daily, and daily postural drainage.

THE NURSING PROCESS

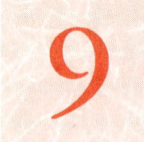
Introduction to the Nursing Process

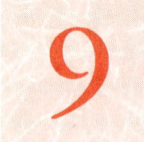

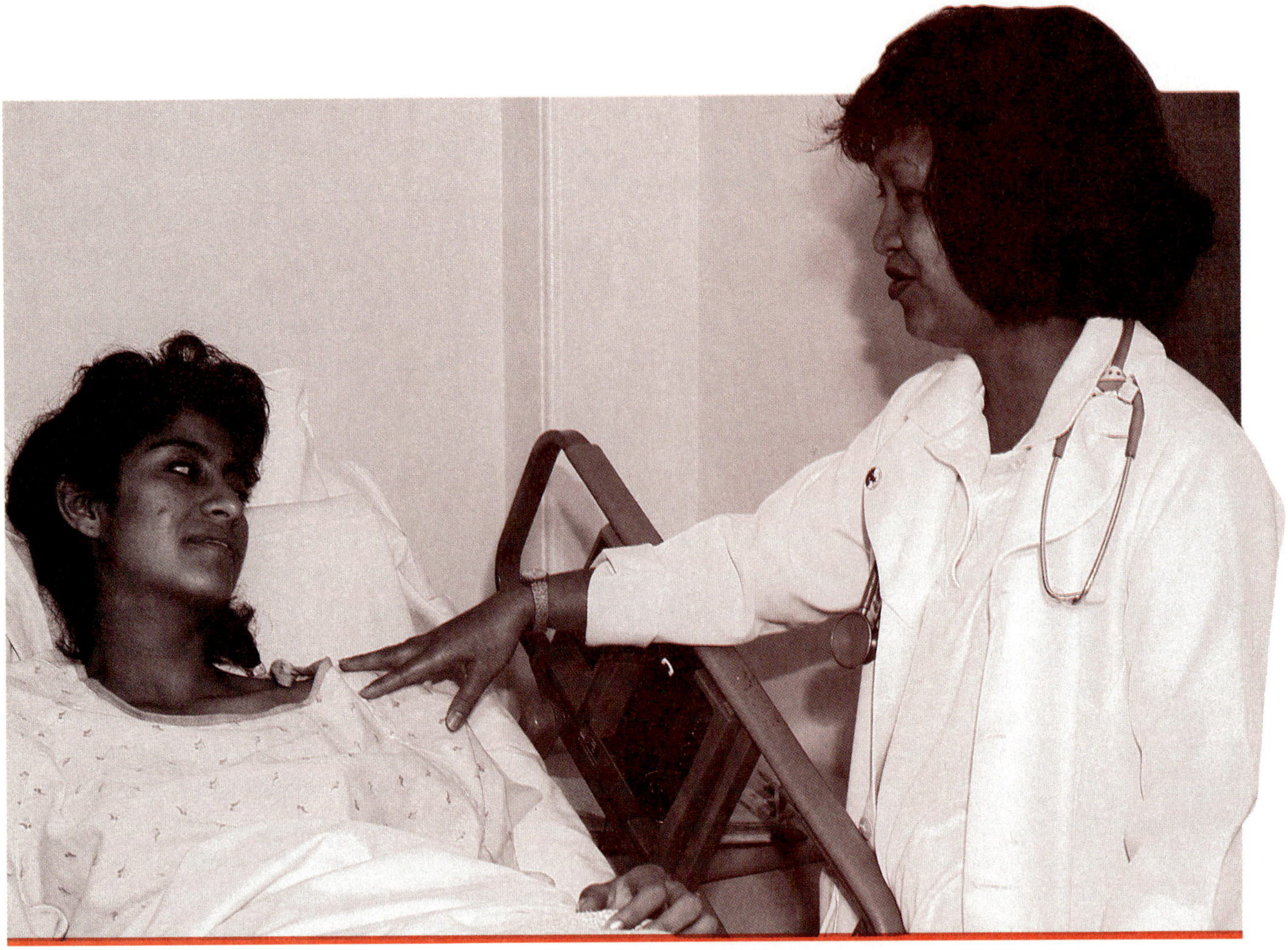

OBJECTIVES

▶ Describe the components of the nursing process.

▶ Identify the contribution of selected nurses to the development of the nursing process.

▶ Identify nursing activities involved in each component of the nursing process.

▶ Identify essential characteristics of the nursing process.

▶ List benefits of the nursing process to the client.

▶ List benefits of the nursing process to the nurse.

▶ Describe how the nursing process is a framework for accountability and responsibility.

HISTORICAL PERSPECTIVE OF THE NURSING PROCESS

Before the nursing process was developed, nurses tended to provide care that was based on medical orders written by physicians and focused on specific disease conditions rather than on the person being cared for. Nursing practice that was provided independently of the physician was often guided by intuition and experience rather than a scientific method.

The term **nursing process** and the framework it implies are relatively new. In 1955, Hall originated the term *nursing process*. Since then, various nurses have described the process of nursing in different ways. Wiedenbach (1963) described three steps in nursing: observation, ministration of help, and validation. Later, Knowles (1967, pp. 248–72) suggested "five Ds" necessary for the practice of nursing: discover, delve, decide, do, and discriminate. During the first two stages, the nurse collects data about the client. During the third stage (decide), the nurse determines a plan of action; and during the fourth stage (do), the nurse implements the plan. In the fifth stage (discriminate), the nurse assesses the client's reaction to the nursing actions.

In 1967, the Western Interstate Commission on Higher Education identified a nursing process with five steps: perception, communication, interpretation, intervention, and evaluation. WICHE defined the nursing process as "the interrelationship between a patient and a nurse in a given setting; it incorporates the behaviors of patient and nurse and the resulting interaction" (WICHE 1967). Also in 1967, the nursing faculty of the Catholic University of America proposed four components of the nursing process: assessment, planning, intervention, and evaluation.

The use of the nursing process in clinical practice gained additional legitimacy in 1973 when the American Nurses' Association (ANA) published *Standards of Nursing Practice,* which describes the five steps of the nursing process; assessing, diagnosing, planning, intervention, and evaluation (ANA 1973). See Table 1-3, page 12. Subsequently, a number of states revised their nurse practice acts to reflect these aspects of nursing.

As the nursing process developed both theoretically and clinically, the term **nursing diagnosis** gained considerable recognition in the nursing literature. The concept of a nursing diagnosis, as it evolved in the 1950s and 1960s, applied to the identification of client problems or needs. The term was not easily accepted, although many nursing authors regarded the nursing diagnosis as basic to professional nursing (Durand and Prince 1966; Rothberg 1967). Nearly a decade later, Bloch defined the terms that were crucial in nursing and found that the term diagnosis—in relation to nursing practice—was still quite controversial (Bloch 1974, pp. 689–94).

In 1973, Gebbie and Lavin at St. Louis University School of Nursing helped to form the first national conference on the classification of nursing diagnoses. The participants at this conference defined the nursing diagnosis as the "conclusion or judgment which occurs as a result of nursing assessment" (Gebbie and Lavin 1975, p. 70). Subsequently, conferences have been held every two years and have gained support and interest. In 1982, the conference group accepted the name North American Nursing Diagnosis Association (NANDA), thus recognizing the participation and contributions of Canadian nurses. This group has currently established and accepted about 100 diagnostic categories (NANDA 1990).

In 1980, ANA declared that "nursing is the diagnosis and treatment of human responses to actual or potential health problems" (ANA 1980). Clearly, the ANA saw diagnosis as a nursing function even though it was not unusual for some people to believe diagnosis was the prerogative of the physician. In 1982, the National Council of State Boards of Nursing defined and described the five-step nursing process in terms of nursing behaviors: assessing, analyzing, planning, implementing, and evaluating (National Council of State Boards of Nursing 1982). Table 9–1 lists some of the nurses and groups who contributed to the development of the nursing process and nursing diagnosis movements.

TABLE 9–1 *Evolution of the Nursing Process*

Nurse	Selected Contributions	Nurse	Selected Contributions
Peplau, H. 1952	Identified four phases in an interpersonal relationship: orientation, identification, exploitation, and resolution. The phases are sequential and focus on interpersonal therapeutic interaction (George 1985, pp. 60–65).		nursing care and directing the family and the nursing auxiliary as they give nursing care. These were considered to promote the quality of professional practice (Kreuter 1957, p. 302).
Hall, L. 1955	Originated the term *nursing process* (George 1985, p. 116).	Johnson, D. E. 1959	Saw the nursing process as assessing situations, arriving at decisions, implementing a course of action designed to resolve nursing problems, and evaluating (Johnson 1959, p. 200).
Kreuter, F. R. 1957	Described steps in a nursing process as coordinating, planning, and evaluating		

TABLE 9–1 *Evolution of the Nursing Process* (continued)

Nurse	Selected Contributions	Nurse	Selected Contributions
Orlando, I. J. 1961	Saw the nursing process as interactive (Orlando, 1961, p. 29). Stated that the process included three phases: client's behavior, reaction of the nurse, and nursing actions (George 1985, pp. 162–68).	Catholic University of America 1967	Proposed four components of the nursing process: assessment, planning, intervention, and evaluation (Yura and Walsh 1988, p. 22).
Henderson, V. 1965	Stated that the nursing process was the same as the steps of the scientific method (Henderson 1965, pp. 3–10; Henderson 1980, p. 907).	Orem, D. 1971	Stated that there were three steps in nursing care: (a) initial and continuing determination of need for nursing care; (b) designing nursing actions for the client that will contribute to the client's achievement of health goals; and (c) the initiating, conducting, and control of assisting actions (Orem 1985, p. 224).
Wiedenbach, E. 1963, 1970	Introduced a three-step nursing process model: identify help needed, minister help, validate that help was given.		
Heidgerken, L. 1965	Described steps of professional nursing care as evaluating behavior and situations; recognizing physical symptoms; diagnosing, planning, and meeting nursing needs; and coordinating the client's regimen through all stages of care (Heidgerken 1965, p. 95).	ANA Standards of Nursing Practice 1973	Referred to a five step process: assessing, diagnosing, planning, intervention, and evaluation.
		Bloch, D. 1974	Suggested a five-step nursing process that was similar to the four-step model: collection of data, definition of problem, planning of intervention, implementation of the intervention, and evaluation of the intervention (Bloch 1974, p. 693).
McCain, R. A. 1965	Was the first to use the term *assessment* in an article published in 1965. Used the functional abilities of the client as the framework for assessment. Collected and recorded objective and subjective data in assessment (McCain 1965, pp. 82–84).		
		Gebbie, K., and Lavin, M. A. 1975	Initiated first national conference on the classification of nursing diagnoses in 1973, which led to the use of a five-step nursing process model: assessment, nursing diagnosis, planning, intervention, and evaluation.
Knowles, L. 1967	Introduced a process model called the "five Ds"; discover, delve, decide, do, and discriminate. Stated that nurses collected data about the client's health during the first two stages.	Roy, Sr. C. 1976	Used six-step nursing process: assessment of client behaviors, assessment of influencing factors, problem identification, goal setting, intervention, selection of approaches, and evaluation. Advocated the use of the term *nursing diagnosis* (Roy 1976, pp. 23–38).
WICHE (Western Interstate Commission on Higher Education) 1967	Listed the steps of the nursing process as perception and communication; interpretation; intervention; and discrimination.		

COMPONENTS OF THE NURSING PROCESS

A **process** is a series of planned actions or operations directed toward a particular result. The **nursing process** is a systematic, rational method of planning and providing nursing care. Its goal is to identify a client's health status, actual or potential health care problems, to establish plans to meet the identified needs, and to deliver specific nursing interventions to meet those needs. The nursing process is cyclical; that is, the components of the nursing process follow a logical sequence, but more than one component may be involved at any one time. See Figure 9–1.

To carry out the nursing process most effectively and individualize approaches to each person's particular needs, the nurse must collaborate with the client. An individual, a family, or a community may be considered a client. If the client is unable to take part in the planning and decision-

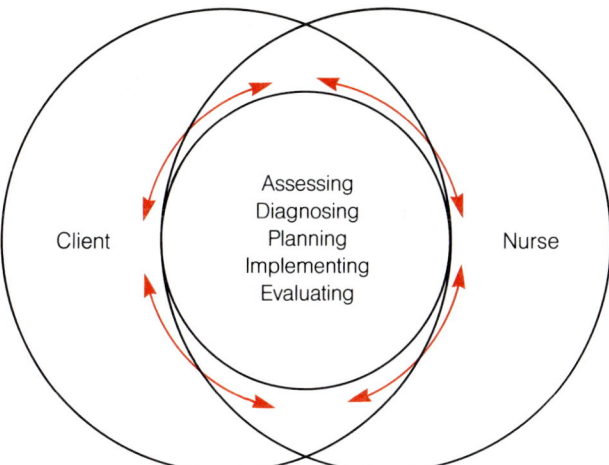

Figure 9–1 The interrelationship of the client, the nurse, and the nursing process.

making process, a family member may be asked to participate on the client's behalf. Application of the nursing process requires that the nurse have a variety of skills, including interpersonal, technical, and intellectual. Interpersonal skills include communicating; listening; conveying interest, compassion, knowledge, and information; developing trust and obtaining data in a manner that enhances the individuality of the client, promotes the integrity of the family, and contributes to the viability of the community. Technical skills are manifested in the use of equipment and the performance of procedures. Intellectual skills required by a nurse include problem solving, critical thinking, and making nursing judgments. Decision making is involved in every component of the nursing process (Yura and Walsh 1988, p. 108).

The nursing process consists of a series of four or five components or steps. The four-step process is assessing, planning, implementing, and evaluating. In this system, diagnosing is included in the assessing phase. The five-step nursing process is assessing, diagnosing, planning, implementing, and evaluating. Some authorities believe the five-component nursing process gives greater prominence to diagnosing than the four-component process.

Both the four- and five-step nursing processes provide an organizational structure for achieving the goals of the process. In both nursing processes, interaction between the client and the nurse is essential, as illustrated in Figure 9-1.

Nursing theorists may use different terms to describe these steps. In spite of these differences, the activities of the nurse using the process are similar. To avoid misunderstanding, nurses should be familiar with alternate terms that describe steps in the process. For example, *nursing diagnosis* may be called *analysis,* and *implementation (implementing)* may be called *intervention or intervening.*

An overview of the five-step nursing process used in this book follows. See also Tables 9–2 and 9–3. Each of the five

TABLE 9–2 *Overview of the Purposes and Activities of the Nursing Process*

Component and Purpose(s)	Activities
Assessing To establish a database	Obtain health history
	Perform physical assessment
	Review records, e.g., laboratory records, other health care records
	Interview support persons
	Review literature
	Validate assessment data
Diagnosing To identify the client's health care needs and to prepare diagnositc statements	Organize data
	Compare data against standards
	Cluster or group data (generate tentative hypotheses)
	Identify gaps and inconsistencies
	Determine the client's health problems, risks, and strengths
	Formulate nursing diagnoses statements
Planning To identify the client's goals and appropriate nursing interventions	Set priorities in collaboration with client
	Write evaluation goals and outcome criteria in collaboration with client
	Select nursing strategies
	Consult other health personnel
	Write nursing orders
	Write nursing care plan
Implementing To carry out planned nursing interventions to help the client attain goals	Reassess client
	Update database
	Review and revise care plan
	Perform or delegate planned nursing interventions
Evaluating To determine the extent to which goals of nursing care have been achieved	Collect data about the client's response
	Compare the client's response to evaluation (outcome) criteria
	Analyze the reasons for the outcomes
	Modify the care plan

TABLE 9–3 *Selected Knowledge and Abilities Needed for the Nursing Process*

Component	Knowledge	Abilities
Assessing	Biopsychosocial and spiritual systems of humans Developmental needs of humans Health Illness Pathophysiology Family system Culture and values of self and client Environment	Observe systematically Communicate effectively Establish a helping relationship Obtain a health history Perform a nursing physical assessment
Diagnosing	Nursing diagnosis categories that nurses can identify and treat Etiologic factors of nursing diagnoses Signs or characteristics of nursing diagnoses Risk factors associated with potential nursing diagnoses Normal measurement standards Individual coping mechanisms	Differentiate cues* and inferences† Think critically Reason inductively and deductively Organize data Identify cue patterns and relationships Generate and test tentative hypotheses Make a nursing diagnosis
Planning	Client's strengths and weaknesses Values and beliefs of the client Scope of nursing practice Resources available to implement nursing interventions Roles of other health care personnel	Problem solve Make decisions Write client goals that relate to the nursing diagnosis in collaboration with client Set priorities Write measurable outcome criteria that relate to the goals Select and create nursing strategies that are safe and appropriate to meet client goals Write nursing orders Elicit the cooperation and participation of the client and other health care personnel
Implementing	Physical hazards and safety Asepsis Procedures Use of equipment Organization Management Learning Change theory Advocacy Client rights Client's developmental level	Observe systematically Communicate effectively Maintain a helping relationship Perform psychomotor techniques Teach self-care Convey caring Act as a client advocate Counsel clients Delegate Supervise and evaluate the work of others Implement medical orders
Evaluating	Client goals and outcome criteria Client responses to nursing intervention	Obtain relevant data to compare with outcome criteria Draw conclusions about goal attainment Relate nursing actions to outcome criteria Reassess the nursing care plan

*Cue: A fact that one acquires through the use of the five senses
†Inference: The nurse's judgment or interpretation of a cue

components of the nursing process is discussed in depth in subsequent chapters of this unit.

1. **Assessing** is collecting, verifying, and organizing data about a client's health status. Data about the physical, emotional, developmental, social, cultural, intellectual, and spiritual aspects of the client are obtained from a variety of sources and are the basis for actions and decisions taken in subsequent phases. Skills of observation, communication, interviewing, and physical assessment are essential to perform this phase of the nursing process.

2. **Diagnosing** is a process which results in a diagnostic statement or nursing diagnosis. **Nursing diagnosis** is a statement of a client's potential or actual alteration of health status. Implicit in the diagnosis is a statement of the client's response that nurses are licensed and able to treat. In this phase, the nurse sorts and clusters the data and asks, "What are the actual and potential health problems for which the client needs nursing assistance?" and "What factors contributed to this problem?" Responses to those questions establish the nursing diagnoses. The process used to establish a nursing diagnosis is analyzing. **Analyzing** is breaking down a whole into component parts, e.g., identifying the various systems (component parts) of the body. An **actual health problem** is a problem that currently exists. A **potential health problem** is the presence of risk factors that predispose persons and families to a health problem.

3. **Planning** involves a series of steps in which the nurse and the client set priorities, write goals or expected outcomes, and establish a written care plan designed to resolve or minimize the identified problems of the client and to coordinate the care provided by all health team members. In collaboration with the client, the nurse develops specific interventions for each nursing diagnosis.

4. **Implementing** is putting the nursing care plan into action. During the implementation phase, the nurse continues to collect data, carries out the prescribed nursing activities or delegates the care to an appropriate person, and validates the nursing care plan. Continued data collection is essential not only to keep track of changes in the client's condition but also to obtain evidence for the evaluation of goal achievement in the next phase. To validate the care plan, the nurse determines (a) whether the client's priorities are being considered, (b) whether planned nursing actions are realistic and help the client achieve the desired outcome or goal, and (c) whether the plan is individualized to meet the particular needs of the client.

5. **Evaluating** is assessing the client's response to nursing interventions and then comparing the response to predetermined standards. These standards are often referred to as **outcome criteria.** The nurse determines the extent to which the goals or predetermined outcomes of care have been achieved, partially achieved, or not met. If goals have not been met, reassessment of the care plan is needed. Reassessment may involve changes in any or all of the previous phases of the nursing process.

The nursing process is an adaptation of problem-solving techniques and systems theory. It can be viewed as parallel to but separate from the medical process. Table 9–4 lists the two processes for comparison. The focus of the medical process is examining, diagnosing, planning, treating or curing disease processes, and evaluating the effectiveness of the treatment. The focus of the nursing process is gathering data, diagnosing (analyzing), planning, implementing, and evaluating the degree to which the client's goals have been met.

Both processes begin with data gathering and analysis and base action (intervention or treatment) on a problem statement (nursing diagnosis or medical diagnosis). Both processes include an evaluative component. Where the focus of the medical process is on the disease process, however, the nursing process is directed toward a client' *response* to illness.

The nurse can be highly creative when using the nursing process. Nurses are not bound by standard responses but may apply problem-solving skills, creativity, critical thinking, and their own knowledge and skills to assist clients. The nursing process is universally applicable. It can be applied in a variety of situations. It can be used with individuals of all ages, groups, and communities.

The five steps of the nursing process are not discrete entities but overlapping, continuing subprocesses. For example, assessing, the first step of the nursing process, may also be carried out during implementing and evaluating. Each step must be continually updated as the situation changes. Just as a client's health is never static but constantly changing, the nursing process, because it is responsive to the client's health, is also dynamic.

Each step or phase of the nursing process affects the others; they are closely interrelated. For example, if an inadequate database is used during assessment, the nursing diagnoses will be incomplete or incorrect; this will be reflected in the planning, implementing, and evaluating phases. Incomplete or incorrect assessment necessarily means equivocal evaluation because the nurse will have incomplete or incorrect criteria against which to evaluate changes in the client and the effectiveness of intervention.

The nursing process individualizes the approach to each client. In the assessment phase, data are collected to determine the habits, routines, and needs of the client. This data about the normal health patterns of the client allows the nurse to write a care plan that incorporates these prior routines whenever possible. The nursing process is also interpersonal. To assure the delivery of quality nursing care, the nurse and client must share concerns and problems and participate in continuous evaluation of the care plan. The success of the nursing process depends on open and meaningful communication and the development of

TABLE 9–4 *Comparison of the Nursing Process and the Medical Process*

Nursing Process	Medical Process	Nursing Process	Medical Process

1. Assessing
   Collection of data from:
   a. Nursing history
   b. Health examination
   c. Review of records
   d. Consultation with other team members
   e. Review of literature
	1. Assessing
	   Collection of data from:
	   a. Medical history
	   b. Physical examination
	   c. Diagnostic tests
	   d. Review of literature
		b. Implementation
		   c. Postimplementation strategies: update database, review and revise care plan
			b. Medical therapy
			   c. Referrals

2. Diagnosing
   a. Analysis and synthesis of data
   b. Identification of the health problems
   c. Formulation of nursing diagnosis
	2. Medical diagnosis*
	   a. Organization of data
	   b. Analysis and interpretation of the data
	   c. Formulation of a diagnosis
		5. Evaluating
		   a. Collection of data about the client's response
		   b. Comparison of the data to the established objectives and goals
		   c. Determination of the effectiveness of the nursing plan
		   d. Analysis of variables affecting the outcomes
		   e. Modification of the care plan
			5. Evaluating
			   a. Establishment of the effectiveness of the medical therapy in terms of the goals
			   b. Analysis of variables
			   c. Revision of the plan of therapy as necessary

3. Planning
   a. Establishment of priorities
   b. Establishment of goals
   c. Development of objectives
   d. Written nursing care plan
   e. Delegation of nursing activities
	3. Medical planning
	   a. Establishment of priorities
	   b. Establishment of goals for therapy
	   c. Written plan of therapy		

4. Implementing
   a. Preimplementation interventions
	4. Therapy
	   a. Physician's orders		

*Medical diagnosis has four or five phases:
1. Suspected diagnosis following the patient's initial complaint
2. Tentative diagnosis following the medical history
3. Provisional diagnosis following the physical examination
4. Definitive diagnosis following diagnostic tests
5. Anatomic diagnosis following a postmortem

---

rapport between the client and the nurse. See the accompanying box for a summary of the characteristics of the nursing process.

BENEFITS OF THE NURSING PROCESS

The nursing process is important to both the client and the nurse. The following benefits have been described (Atkinson and Murray 1986, pp. 5–7).

Benefits for the Client

- Quality client care. The nursing care is planned to meet the unique needs of the individual, family, or community. Continuous evaluation and reassessment of the client's changing needs ensure an appropriate level of care.

- Continuity of care. The written care plan is accessible to all persons involved in the client's care and prevents the client from having to repeat information and preferences to each caregiver.

- Participation by the clients in their health care. The process can help clients to develop skills related to their health care and to become more committed to the goals of care.

Benefits for the Nurse

- Consistent and systematic nursing education. The National League for Nursing (NLN), which administers a voluntary accreditation of nursing education programs, requires graduates to be competent in the use of the nursing process (NLN 1978). In addition, licensure examinations for nurses in the United States are organized around nursing process activities.

- Job satisfaction. Well-written care plans give nurses confidence that nursing interventions are based on correct identification of the client's problems, thus preventing uncoordinated, trial-and-error nursing. Plans also can instill a sense of pride when the goals of care are accomplished.

- Professional growth. By evaluating the effectiveness of the nursing interventions, the nurse learns which inter-

Characteristics of the Nursing Process

- The system is open, flexible, and dynamic.
- It individualizes the approach to each client's particular needs.
- It is planned.
- It is goal directed.
- It is flexible to meet the unique needs of client, family, or community.
- It permits creativity for the nurse and client in devising ways to solve the stated health problem.
- It is interpersonal. It requires the nurse to communicate directly and consistently with clients to meet their needs.
- It is cyclical. Since all steps are interrelated, there is no absolute beginning or end.
- It emphasizes feedback, which leads either to reassessment of the problem or to revision of the care plan.
- It is universally applicable. The nursing process is used as a framework for nursing care in all types of health care settings, with clients of all age groups.

ventions are effective and which ones can be adapted to meet the needs of other clients. This process enhances the skill and expertise of the nurse. In addition, the shared knowledge and experience gained in collaborating with colleagues when formulating a care plan enhance the nurse's knowledge.

- Avoidance of legal action (Philpott 1985, p. 79). When every step of the nursing process is used in delivering nursing care, the nurses are carrying out their legal obligations to the client. Failure to conduct a complete nursing assessment or failure to document data appropriately can have adverse legal consequences. (See also Chapter 8.)
- Meeting professional nursing standards. The criteria in *Standards of Nursing Practice* developed by the American Nurses' Association are based on the steps or phases of the nursing process (ANA 1973). A portion of the Canadian Nurses' Association *Standards for Nursing Practice* (1980) also includes standards related to the nursing process. See Table 1–4 in Chapter 1. Learning and implementing the nursing process when providing client care is a basic requirement for professional nursing competence. The nursing process, therefore, is a framework for nurses' accountability. It holds the nurse both accountable and responsible for assessing, diagnosing, planning, implementing, and evaluating client care.
- Meeting standards of accredited hospitals. In the United States, the Joint Commission on Accreditation of Health

Organizations (JCAHO) requires that nursing process be utilized and a written plan of care be available for each hospitalized patient. The registered nurse is responsible for the initial nursing assessment (JCAHO 1989, pp. 133–143).

A FRAMEWORK FOR ACCOUNTABILITY

Accountability is the condition of being answerable and responsible to someone for specific behaviors that are part of the nurse's professional role. The nursing process provides a framework for accountability and responsibility in nursing and maximizes accountability and responsibility for standards of care (Law 1983, p. 34). Nurses are accountable to the client (public), to their professional statutory nursing body, to colleagues, to the employing agency, and to themselves. The nursing process provides a framework for accountability in all areas. The professional nurse is accountable for activities in all five phases of the nursing process.

Assessing　The nurse is accountable for collecting information, encouraging client participation, and for judging the validity of the collected data. When assessing, the nurse is accountable for gaps in data or conflicting data, inaccurate data, and biased data.

Diagnosing　During the second phase, nurses are accountable for the judgments made about the client's health problems, i.e., the diagnostic statements. Is the health problem recognized by the client or only by the nurse? Did the nurse consider the client's values, beliefs, and cultural practices when determining the health problems? When making judgments, nurses are accountable for considering a broad spectrum of client sociocultural backgrounds.

Planning　Accountability at the planning stage involves determining priorities, establishing client goals, predicting outcomes, and planning nursing activities. These are all incorporated into a written nursing care plan available to all involved nurses. In this phase, nurses are also accountable for ensuring that the *clients'* priorities are considered as well as the nurse's.

Implementing　Nurses are accountable for all their actions in delivering nursing care. These actions may be performed directly or in collaboration with others, or they may be delegated to another. Even though a nurse delegates an activity to another person, the nurse is still accountable for the delegated action as well as for the act of delegating. The nurse should be able to give reasoned answers as to why the activity was delegated, why the person was chosen to perform the activity, and how the delegated action was carried out. Nursing actions must be charted after being carried out, thereby providing a written record.

Evaluating   By establishing the degree to which the objectives have been attained, the nurse is accountable for the success or failure of the nursing actions. The nurse must be able to explain why a client goal was not met and what phase or phases of the nursing process require changing and why.

The nursing process provides the framework for nurses to help clients with their health needs and to produce a record of the actions and their effectiveness. The nursing process makes nurses responsible primarily to the client. An implicit part of applying the nursing process is having the knowledge and skills to make the required decisions and to implement the required nursing actions. Therefore, nurses are also accountable to themselves for having the knowledge and skills to use the nursing process in a specific situation.

CHAPTER HIGHLIGHTS

▶ The nursing process is a systematic, rational method of planning and providing nursing care. The nursing process is also cyclical, because all steps are interrelated.

▶ The goals of the nursing process are to identify a client's actual or potential health care needs (assessment and diagnosis), to establish plans to meet the identified needs, and to deliver and evaluate specific nursing interventions to meet those needs.

▶ The basic components of the nursing process are assessing, diagnosing, planning, implementing, and evaluating.

▶ Specific nursing activities and responsibilities are associated with each component of the nursing process.

▶ The nursing process can be applied to individuals, families, and communities.

▶ Assessing is collecting, verifying, and organizing data about a client's status.

▶ Diagnosing is the process of making a clinical judgment (nursing diagnosis) about a client's potential or actual health problem that nurses are licensed and able to treat.

▶ Planning involves setting priorities, writing goals, and establishing a written plan for nursing interventions designed to prevent, resolve, or identify problems or potential problems.

▶ Implementing is carrying out or delegating the nursing interventions. It incorporates all of the activities performed or supervised by the nurse to promote health, prevent complications, treat present problems, and facilitate the client's coping with chronic alterations in health status.

▶ Evaluating involves the nurse and the client in determining whether the client goals or predetermined outcomes of care have been met, identifying factors that facilitated or inhibited goal achievement, and modifying or terminating the care plan accordingly.

▶ The nursing process is goal oriented. It facilitates the communication of client goals and individualizes care to facilitate goal achievement.

▶ The nursing process provides a framework for nurses' accountability and responsibility.

READINGS AND REFERENCES

SUGGESTED READINGS

Bodnar, B., and Pedersen, S. 1986. The nursing process. In Edelman, C., and Mandle, C., editors. pp. 44–71. *Health promotion throughout the life span*. St. Louis: C. V. Mosby Co.
    The authors present the nursing process in a wellness perspective. Theorists who contributed to a health focus for nursing are discussed. An example of an assessment tool for use with healthy clients is included. A modified definition of the nursing process to include wellness is presented, and the need for health-oriented nursing diagnoses is discussed.
Capers, C. F., and Kelly, R. May 1987. Neuman nursing process: A model of holistic care. *Holistic Nursing Practice* 1: 19–26.
    The authors describe the implementation of the three-phase method of the Neuman prescribed nursing process: the diagnosis phase, the goals phase, and the outcome phase. A unique aspect of this model is the detailed comparison of the perceptions of the nurse and the client. The authors provide a sample database detailing five client variables—psychologic, physiologic, developmental, sociocultural, and spiritual. Examples of nursing diagnoses, outcomes, and approaches are also presented.

RELATED RESEARCH

Moss, A. R. September 1988. Determinants of patient care: Nursing process or nursing attitudes? *Journal of Advanced Nursing* 13: 615–620.

SELECTED REFERENCES

Alfaro, R. 1990. *Applying Nursing Diagnosis and Nursing Process: A Step-by-Step Guide.* 2nd ed. Philadelphia: J. B. Lippincott Co.

American Nurses' Association. 1973. *Standards of nursing practice.* Kansas City, Mo.: ANA.

————. 1980. *Nursing: A social policy statement.* Publication no. NP-63. Kansas City, Mo.: ANA.

Atkinson, L. D., and Murray, M. E. 1990. *Understanding the nursing process.* 4th ed. Elmsford, NY.: Pergamon Press, Inc.

Bloch, D. November 1974. Some crucial terms in nursing: What do they really mean? *Nursing Outlook* 22:689–94.

Canadian Nurses' Association. February 1987. *A definition of nursing practice: Standards for nursing practice.* Ottawa: CNA.

Durand, M., and Prince, P. 1966. Nursing diagnosis: Process and decision. *Nursing Forum.* 5(4):50–64.

Gebbie, K., and Lavin, M. 1975. *Classification of nursing diagnosis.* St. Louis: C. V. Mosby Co.

George, J. B., editor. 1985. *Nursing theories: The base for professional nursing.* 2d ed. Englewood Cliffs, N.J.: Prentice-Hall.

Gordon, M. 1987. *Nursing diagnosis: Process and application.* 2d ed. New York: McGraw-Hill.

Griffith, J. W., and Christensen, P. J. 1986. *Nursing process: Application of theories, frameworks, and models.* 2d ed. St. Louis: C. V. Mosby Co.

Hall, L. June 1955. Quality of nursing care. *Public health news.* Newark, N.J.: State Department of Health.

Hannah, K. J.; Reimer, M.; Mills, W. C.; and Letourneau, S., editors. 1987. *Clinical judgment and decision making: The future with nursing diagnosis.* New York: John Wiley and Sons.

Heidgerken, L. E. 1965. *Teaching and learning in schools of nursing: Principles and methods.* 3d ed. Philadelphia: J. B. Lippincott.

Henderson, V. January/February 1965. The nature of nursing. *International Nursing Review* 12:23–30.

————. May 22, 1980. Nursing: Yesterday and tomorrow. *Nursing Times* 76:905–7.

Iyer, P.; Taptich, B.; and Bernocchi-Losey, D. 1991. *Nursing process and nursing diagnosis.* 2nd ed. Philadelphia: W. B. Saunders Co.

Johnson, D. E. April 1959. A philosophy of nursing. *Nursing Outlook* 7:198–200.

Joint Commission on Accreditation of Health Organizations. 1989. *Accreditation manual for hospitals.* Chicago: Joint Commission on Accreditation of Health Organizations, Nursing Services.

Knowles, L. 1967. *Decision-making in nursing: A necessity for doing:* ANA Clinical Sessions, 1966. New York: Appleton-Century-Crofts.

Kreuter, F. R. May 1957. What is good nursing care? *Nursing Outlook* 5:302–304.

La Monica, E. L. 1985. *The humanistic nursing process.* Monterey, Calif.: Wadsworth Health Sciences.

Law, G. M. October 5–11, 1983. Accountability in nursing: Providing a framework . . . the nursing process and accountability are inextricably linked. Part 2. *Nursing Times* 79:34–36.

McCain, R. F. April 1965. Nursing by assessment—Not intuition. *American Journal of Nursing* 65:82–84.

McCann-Flynn, J. B., and Heffron, P. B. 1988. *Nursing: From concept to practice.* 2d ed. Norwalk, Conn.: Appleton & Lange.

National Council of State Boards of Nursing. 1982. *Test plan for the National Council licensure examination for registered nurses.* Chicago: National Council of State Boards of Nursing.

National League for Nursing. 1978. *Competencies of the associate degree nurse on entry into practice.* Publication no. 23-1731C. New York: National League for Nursing.

North American Nursing Diagnosis Association. Summer 1988. New diagnosis accepted. *Nursing Diagnosis Newsletter,* 15:1–3.

Orem, D. 1971. *Nursing: Concepts of practice.* New York: McGraw-Hill.

————. 1985. *Nursing: Concepts of practice.* 3d ed. New York: McGraw-Hill.

Orlando, I. 1961. *The dynamic nurse-patient relationship.* New York: G. P. Putnam's Sons.

Peplau, H. E. 1952. *Interpersonal relations in nursing.* New York: G. P. Putnam's Sons.

Philpott, M. 1985. *Legal liability and the nursing process.* Toronto: W. B. Saunders Co., Canada.

Rothberg, J. May 1967. Why nursing diagnosis? *American Journal of Nursing.* 67:1040–42.

Roy, C. 1976. *Introduction to nursing: An adaptation model.* Englewood Cliffs, N.J.: Prentice-Hall.

Western Interstate Commission on Higher Education. 1967. *Defining clinical content.* Graduate Nursing Programs, Medical and Surgical Nursing. Boulder, Colo.: Western Interstate Commission on Higher Education.

Wiedenbach, E. November 1963. The helping art of nursing. *American Journal of Nursing.* 63:54.

————. May 1970. Nurses' wisdom in nursing theory. *American Journal of Nursing.* 70:1057–62.

Yura, H., and Walsh, M. B. 1988. The nursing process: Assessing, planning, implementing, evaluating. 5th ed. Norwalk, Conn.: Appleton & Lange.

10

Assessing

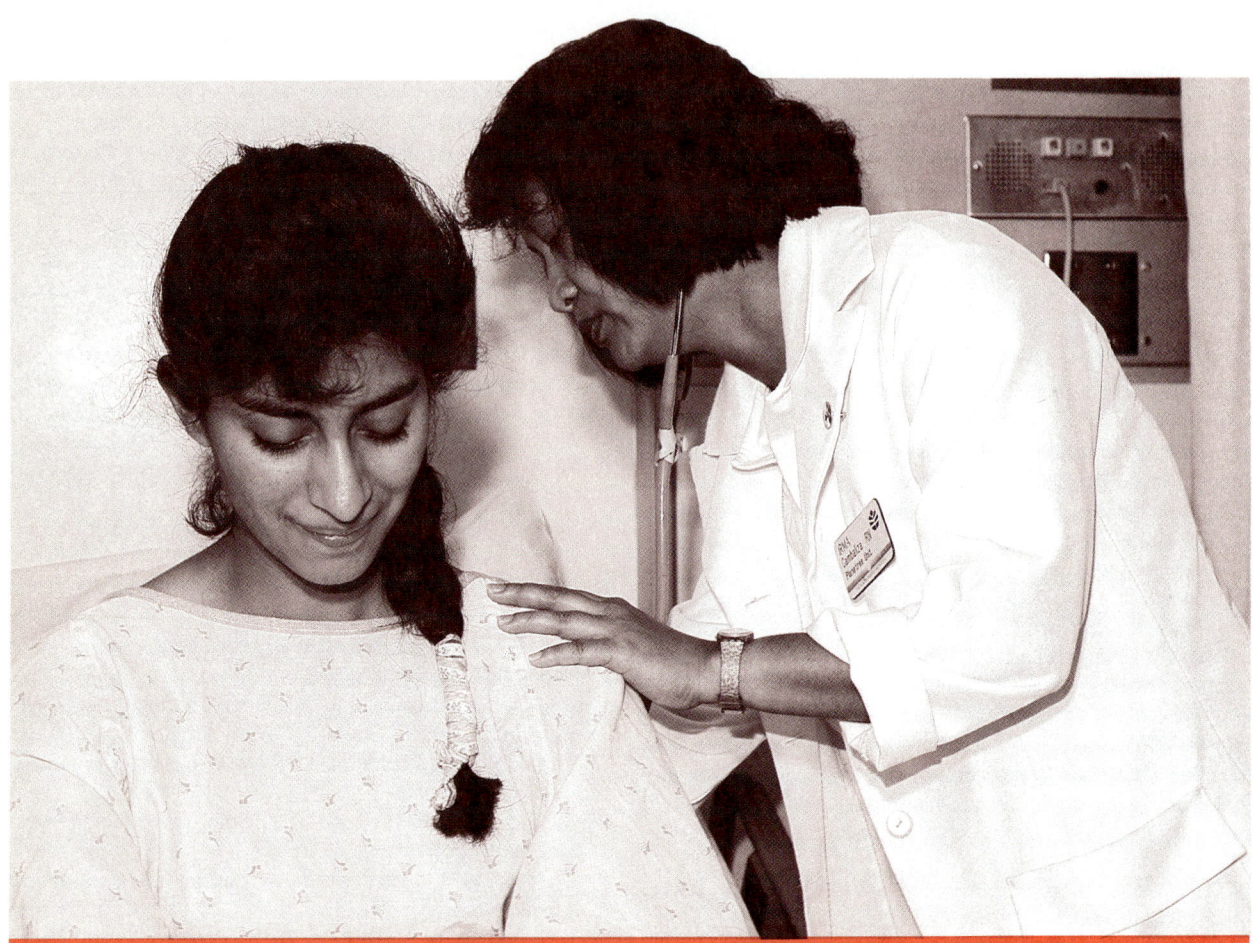

CONTENTS

OBJECTIVES

▶ Identify the purpose of assessing.

▶ Differentiate objective and subjective data and variable and constant data.

▶ Identify three methods of data collection.

▶ Identify the purposes of each method of data collection and give examples of how each is useful.

▶ Compare directive and indirective approaches to interviewing.

▶ Compare closed and open-ended questions, providing examples and listing advantages and disadvantages of each.

▶ Describe important aspects of the interview setting.

▶ Explain common health areas the nurse assesses.

▶

▸ Contrast various frameworks used for nursing assessment.

▸ Describe the importance of assessing to nursing diagnosis.

▸ Describe the importance of reassessing during other phases of the nursing process.

PURPOSE OF ASSESSING

Assessing is the first phase of the nursing process. It involves data collection and validation and is necessary before a nursing diagnosis can be made. "Assessment is part of each activity the nurse does for and with the patient" (Atkinson and Murray 1986, p. 11). In effect, assessing is a continuous process carried out during all phases of the nursing process. It may be used during the diagnosis phase to validate a diagnosis. During the planning and implementing stages, data collection may be used before writing a nursing intervention or in obtaining information about a client's response to the nursing strategies. In the evaluation phase, assessment is done to determine the outcomes of the nursing strategies and to evaluate goal achievement. All phases of the nursing process depend on the accurate and complete collection of **data** (information).

In *Nursing: A Social Policy Statement* (ANA 1980, p. 9), the American Nurses' Association states that nursing is "the diagnosis and treatment of human responses to actual or potential health problems." Thus the focus of assessment is to establish a database about a client's *response* to health concerns or illness in order to determine the client's nursing care needs. Clients' responses include areas of daily living, health, and biophysical, emotional, socioeconomic, cultural, and religious concerns. In contrast to other health professionals, the nurse is concerned with human needs that affect the total person rather than one problem or segment of need fulfillment (Yura and Walsh 1988, p. 110).

A **database** (baseline data) is all the information about a client; it includes the nursing health history and physical assessment, the physician's history and physical examination, results of laboratory and diagnostic tests, and material contributed by other health personnel. **Data collection** is the process of gathering information about a client's health status. It must be both systematic and continuous. Systematic data collection can largely prevent the omission of significant data, and continuous data collection maintains the currency of the data, reflecting a client's changing health.

Assessing involves active participation by both the client and the nurse. The client may be one or more individuals, a family, or even a community. Both the nurse and the client enter the relationship with specific knowledge and previous experiences that influence their perceptions and interpretations (see the discussion of perception theory in Chapter 4). It is important for nurses to be aware that their interpretations or assumptions may not be fact. For example, a nurse seeing a man holding his arm to his chest might assume that he is experiencing chest pain when in fact he has a painful hand. Another example of mistaking interpretation for fact is assuming that a client who states that her husband died three weeks ago feels sadness when in fact the death was a great relief.

The acceptance of assumptions as fact is called **premature closure.** To build an accurate database and avoid premature closure, nurses must validate assumptions regarding the client's physical or emotional behavior. In the first of the previous two examples, the nurse should question the client as to why he is holding his arm to his chest. The response of the client may validate the assumptions of the nurse or lead to further questioning. In the second example, the nurse should ask the client how she feels about her husband's death. Failure to validate or verify leads to the acceptance of assumptions as fact, and an inaccurate or incomplete nursing assessment. If the nursing process is to be a successful framework for nursing care, the information gathered during the assessment phase must be complete, factual, and accurate. To collect data accurately, nurses need to be aware of their own biases, values, and beliefs and separate fact from inference.

TYPES OF DATA

Data can be objective or subjective. **Objective data** are detectable by an observer or can be tested against an accepted standard. They can be seen, heard, felt, or smelled. For example, a discoloration of the skin, a blood pressure reading, the act of crying, or a hand tremor are objective data. **Subjective data** are apparent only to the person affected and can be described or verified only by that person. Itching, pain, and feeling worried are examples of subjective data. Subjective data are collected during the nursing health history and include the client's perception of personal health status and life situation. Information supplied by family members, significant others, or other health professionals is also considered subjective, if it is based on opinion rather than fact.

Objective data are sometimes called **signs** or **overt data,** and subjective data are sometimes called **symptoms** or **covert data.** Data can also be described as **variable** or **constant.** Blood pressure is variable in that it changes from day to day or even hour to hour and needs updating. Constant data, for example, a date of birth, are unchanging.

Client data should include past history as well as current problems. For example, a history of an allergic reaction to penicillin is a vital piece of historical data. Past surgical procedures and chronic diseases are also examples of historical data. Current data relate to present circumstances, such as pain, nausea, vision changes, and sleep patterns.

Data are recorded in a factual manner and not interpreted by the nurse. For example, the nurse records the client's breakfast intake (objective data) as "coffee 240 ml, juice 120 ml, 1 egg, and 1 slice of toast," rather than as "appetite good" (a judgment). A judgment or a conclusion such as "appetite good" or "normal appetite" may have different meanings for different people. To increase accuracy, the nurse records subjective data in the client's own words. Restating in other words what someone says increases the chance of changing the original meaning.

A common error in assessing is to offer opinions, generalizations, and interpretations as data. For example, a nurse may describe a client as "uncooperative" rather than record the specific behavior (e.g., refusing to take a deep breath and to cough after surgery). A specific description of the behavior is more useful than an interpretation because the causes of specific behavior can be explored. Perhaps the client refuses to cough because she is afraid of rupturing a suture line, or perhaps she experiences severe pain upon coughing. "I do not want to cough; it hurts too much" is a noninterpretive reporting of the problem. Another common error is obtaining incomplete information, i.e., leaving out information about pain because the client does not mention it and the nurse did not ask.

Clients can generalize or be nonspecific. They may describe the reason for their hospitalization as a "weak spell" or as "chest pain." It is important for the nurse to elicit specific information from the client. For example, the documentation of the chest pain needs to include how the client described it, where it was felt, what activity preceded it, when it occurred, whether it was a new experience and how it was relieved. The nurse should briefly summarize the information collected, using correct medical terms.

SOURCES OF DATA

Sources of data are *primary* or *secondary*. The client is the primary source of data. Secondary or indirect sources are significant others, other health personnel, records and reports, and relevant literature.

Client   The chief source of data is usually the client unless the client is too ill, young, or confused to communicate clearly. The client can usually provide subjective data that no one else can offer. However, a stoic client may understate symptoms, while another person may exaggerate.

Significant Others   Significant others or support persons know the client well and often can provide data.

They may supplement information or verify information provided by the client. They might convey information about the stresses the client was experiencing before the illness, family attitudes to illness and health, and the client's home environment.

Significant others are an important source of data, particularly when the client is very young, unconscious, or confused. In some cases—when the client is an abused child, for example—the person giving information may wish to remain anonymous.

Health Personnel   Health personnel are often sources of information about a client's health. Nurses, social workers, physicians, and physiotherapists, for example, may have information from either previous or current contact with the client. A physician who knows the client's home setting may provide valuable data about the family and environmental stressors.

Medical Records   Medical records are often a source of a client's present and past health and illness patterns. These records can provide nurses with information about a client's coping behaviors, health practices, previous illnesses and allergies. A **coping behavior** is behavior learned by a person in response to stress; it may be an adaptive mechanism or a task-oriented behavior. For additional information about coping see Chapter 33. Medical records also contain data regarding the client's occupation, religion, marital status, and reports from other hospital personnel, e.g., dietitians, social workers, and physicians.

The appropriateness of the information in medical records to the present situation must always be considered. For example, if the most recent medical record is 10 years old, it is likely that the client's health practices and coping behaviors have changed. Stressors in an individual's life often change, e.g., an alcoholic husband leaves home, a sick infant is now healthy.

Other Records and Reports   Other records and reports can also provide pertinent health information. Laboratory tests are frequently ordered as part of the physician's initial examination to aid in a medical diagnosis. Laboratory tests are also used to monitor medical treatment, e.g., determination of blood glucose level to monitor the administration of oral hypoglycemic medications. In some cases, nurses can use the same laboratory test to monitor the effectiveness of nursing measures, such as teaching about diet and taking medications.

Any laboratory data about a client must be compared to established norms for that particular test and for the client's age, sex, and so on. Laboratory tests vary among agencies, and norms can therefore be different.

In most settings, laboratory tests are ordered by physicians and independent nurse practitioners, although this practice varies greatly. In some agencies, protocols are written that direct nurses to order and/or carry out specific tests, e.g., urinalysis and routine blood tests, by following prescribed guidelines. For instance, a nurse may order and carry out a throat culture for a client with a temperature of 38.8 C (102 F), a sore throat, and white patches on the tonsils.

Other records and reports—for example, a social agency's report on a client's living conditions or a home health care agency's report on a client's coping at home—can also be helpful to the nurse conducting an assessment.

Literature   The review of nursing and related literature, such as professional journals and reference texts, can provide additional information for the database. A literature review includes but is not limited to the following information:

- Standards or norms against which to compare findings, e.g., height and weight tables, normal developmental tasks for an age group
- Cultural and social health practices
- Spiritual beliefs
- Additional required assessment data
- Nursing interventions and evaluation criteria relative to a client's health problems
- Information about medical diagnoses, treatment, and prognoses

METHODS OF DATA COLLECTION

The major methods of collecting data are observing, interviewing, and examining. Although these nursing activities are often carried out during the implementing and evaluating phases of the nursing process, they are the main nursing activities during the assessing phase. During assessment, observation occurs whenever the nurse is in contact with the client or support persons. The primary interviewing process during the assessment phase is the nursing health history. Examining during the assessment phase is the major method used in the physical health assessment. Consulting, another nursing activity, is discussed in Chapter 12, page 218.

Observing

To **observe** is to gather data by using the five senses. Although nurses observe mainly through sight, all of the senses are engaged during careful observations. Observation has two aspects: (a) noticing the stimuli and (b) selecting, organizing, and interpreting the data, i.e., perceiving them. A nurse who observes that a client's face is flushed must relate that observation to, for example, body temperature, activity, environmental temperature, and blood pressure. Because observation involves selecting, organizing, and interpreting data, there is a possibility of error. For example, a nurse might not notice certain signs simply because they are unexpected in a certain client or situation

or because they do not conform to preconceptions about a client's illness. Another source of error is faulty organization and misinterpretation of data. A nurse may interpret a client's wish not to talk as depression when in fact the client is very tired.

Observation is a conscious, deliberate skill that is developed only through effort and with an organized approach. Nurses often need to focus on specific stimuli in a clinical situation; otherwise they are overwhelmed by a multitude of stimuli. Observing, therefore, involves discriminating among stimuli, that is, separating stimuli in a meaningful manner. For example, nurses caring for newborns learn to ignore the usual sounds of machines in the nursery but respond quickly to an infant's cry or movement.

The experienced nurse is often able to attend to an intervention, e.g., giving a bed bath or monitoring an IV infusion and at the same time make important observations, e.g., a change in respiratory status or the sudden flushing of a client's face. This simultaneous observation and task completion often needs to be learned by the beginning student.

Nursing observations must be organized so that nothing significant is missed. Most nurses develop an individual sequence for observing events. For example, a nurse walks into a client's room and observes the following:

1. Clinical signs of client distress, e.g., pallor or flushing, labored breathing, and behavior indicating pain or emotional distress
2. Threats to the client's safety, real or anticipated, e.g., a lowered side rail
3. The presence and functioning of associated equipment, e.g., intravenous equipment and oxygen
4. The immediate environment, including the people in it

Interviewing

An **interview** is a planned communication or a conversation with a purpose. Some possible purposes are to gather data, to give information, to identify problems of mutual concern, to evaluate change, to teach, to provide support, and to provide counseling or therapy. Interviewing can be viewed as a process that is applied in most phases of the nursing process. One example of the interview is the nursing health history, which is the primary tool for data collection during the assessment phase of the nursing process. (See Nursing Health History later in this chapter.)

There are two approaches to interviewing: directive and nondirective. The **direct interview** is highly structured and elicits specific information. The nurse establishes the purpose of the interview and controls the interview, at least at the outset, by asking closed questions (see the next section) that call for a specific amount of data. The client responds to questions but may not have an opportunity to ask questions or discuss concerns. Directive interviews are frequently used to gather and to give information in a limited amount of time. During a **nondirective,** or rapport building **interview,** the nurse allows the client to control the purpose, subject matter, and pacing. **Rapport** is an understanding between two or more people. The nurse encourages communication by using open-ended questions (see the next section) and empathetic responses. Nondirective interviewing is used for problem solving, counseling, and performance appraisal (Stewart and Cash 1988, p. 7).

A combination of directive and nondirective approaches is usually appropriate during the information gathering interview. The goals of the information gathering interview are to collect data and to begin to establish rapport. The nurse begins by using open ended questions to determine areas of concern for the client. If, for example, a client expresses worry about surgery, the nurse pauses to explore the client's worry and to provide support. Simply to note the worry, without dealing with it, can leave the impression that the nurse does not care about the client's concerns or dismisses them as unimportant. As the interview evolves, the nurse may use closed questions to obtain needed data and to complete the nursing health history. Griffin and Christensen (1986, p. 62) suggest using as little authority or structure as possible to obtain the data needed within the allotted time frame.

Kinds of Interview Questions

Although there are many ways to categorize questions, in this book they are classified as open-ended or closed, and neutral or leading. The type a nurse chooses depends on the needs of the client at the time. For example, the nurse asks closed questions in an emergency or other acute situation when information must be obtained quickly. **Closed questions,** used in the directive interview, are restrictive and generally require only short answers giving specific information. Thus the amount of information gained is generally limited. Closed questions often begin with "when," "where," "who," "what," "do (did, does)," "is (are, was)" and sometimes "how." Examples of closed questions are: "What medication did you take?" "Are you having pain now? Show me where it is." "How long has it been since you had your last physical examination?" "What is your occupation?" "How old are you?" "When did you fall?" "What were you doing before the fall?" The highly stressed person and the person who has difficulty communicating will find closed questions easier to answer than open questions.

Open-ended questions, associated with the non-directive interview, are ones that lead or invite clients to explore (elaborate, clarify, or illustrate) their thoughts or feelings. They allow clients the freedom to talk about what they wish. They also place responsibility on clients to explore and to understand themselves, in contrast to receiving advice from another. An **open-ended** question is broad, specifies only the topic to be discussed, and invites answers longer than one or two words. Such questions give the client the freedom to divulge only information he or she is ready to disclose. The response may also convey attitudes and beliefs the client holds. The chief disadvantage of the open-ended question is that the client may spend time conveying irrel-

evant information. However the open-ended question is useful at the beginning of an interview or to change topics.

Examples of open-ended questions and suggestions are: "How have you been feeling lately?" "What brought you to the hospital?" "How do you feel about coming to the hospital?" "How did you feel in that situation?" "What do you think she meant by that remark?" "Would you describe more about how you relate to your child?" "What would you like to talk about today?" These questions or statements require more than a "yes" or "no" or other short response, such as "yesterday" or "I don't know." They encourage clients to discover what their thoughts and feelings truly are. Such questions usually begin with "what" or "how."

The nurse often finds it necessary to use a combination of directive and indirective techniques throughout an interview to accomplish the goals of the interview and obtain needed information. See Table 10-1 for advantages and disadvantages of open and closed questions.

A client can answer a **neutral question** without direction or pressure from the nurse. Examples are: "How do you feel about that?" "Why do you think you had the operation?" A **leading question** directs the client's answer. Examples are: "You're stressed about surgery tomorrow aren't you?" "You don't think this illness is fair?" "You will take your medicine, won't you?" The leading question does not give the client an opportunity to decide if the answer is true or not. The interviewer suggests the expected answer by the way the question is asked. Leading questions create problems if the client, in an effort to please the nurse, gives inaccurate responses.

Planning the Interview and Setting

It is important to plan an interview before beginning it. The nurse reviews what information is already available such as a postoperative record, information about the current illness, or literature about the client's health problem. The nurse also reviews the data collection form to make sure that the data to be collected are really needed and will serve some purpose related to the client's care. If a form is not available, most nurses prepare an interview guide to remember areas of information and determine what questions to ask. The guide includes a list of topics and subtopics rather than a series of questions.

Each interview and its setting is influenced by time, place, and seating arrangement. In all instances, the client should be made to feel comfortable and unhurried.

Time Interviews with hospitalized clients need to be scheduled for a time when the client is physically comfortable and free of pain, and when interruptions by friends, family, and other health professionals are absent or minimal. Interviews with clients in their homes should be scheduled at a time selected by the client.

Place The place of the interview must have adequate privacy to promote communication. A well-lighted, well-ventilated, moderate-sized room that is relatively free of

TABLE 10–1   *Selected Advantages and Disadvantages of Open and Closed Questions*

Open Questions		Closed Questions	
Advantages	**Disadvantages**	**Advantages**	**Disadvantages**
1. They let the interviewee do the talking.	1. They take more time.	1. Questions and answers can be controlled more effectively.	1. They may provide too little information and require follow-up questions.
2. The interviewer is able to listen and observe.	2. Only brief answers may be given.	2. They require less effort from the interviewee.	2. They may not reveal how the interviewee feels.
3. They are easy to answer and nonthreatening.	3. Valuable information may be withheld.	3. They may be less threatening, since they do not require explanations or justifications.	3. They do not allow the interviewee to volunteer possibly valuable information.
4. They reveal what the interviewee thinks is important.	4. They often elicit more information than necessary.	4. They take less time.	4. They may inhibit communication and convey lack of interest by the interviewee.
5. They may reveal the interviewee's lack of information, misunderstanding of words, frame of reference, prejudices, or stereotypes.	5. Responses are difficult to document and require skill in recording.	5. Information can be asked for before the information is volunteered.	5. The interviewer may dominate the interview with questions.
6. They can provide information the interviewer may not ask for.	6. The interviewer requires skill in controlling an open-ended interview.	6. Responses are easily documented.	
7. They can reveal the interviewee's degree of feeling about an issue.	7. Responses require psychologic insight and sensitivity from the interviewer.	7. They are easy to use and can be handled by unskilled interviewers.	
8. They can convey interest and trust because of the freedom they provide.			

Table constructed, with permission, from material on pp. 80–85 of Stewart, Charles J., and William B. Cash, Jr., *Interviewing: Principles and practices,* 4th ed. © 1985 Wm. C. Brown Publishers, Dubuque, Iowa. All rights reserved.

noise, movements, and interruptions encourages communication. Constant interruptions, such as telephone calls, the noise of traffic outside a window, or people moving about in or near the location can disrupt thought patterns, concentration, and moods and may convey the impression that the nurse is too busy or uninterested. In addition, a place where others cannot overhear or, if possible, see the client is desirable. Most people are inhibited when answering personal questions in the hearing of others and expressing strong feelings in the sight of others.

Seating arrangement   Seating arrangement can help or hinder the interview. A seating arrangement with the nurse behind a desk and the client seated across creates a formal setting that suggests a business meeting between a superior and a subordinate. In contrast, a seating arrangement in which the parties sit on two chairs placed at right angles to a desk or table or a few feet apart with no table between creates a less formal atmosphere, and the nurse and client tend to feel on equal terms. In groups, a horseshoe or circular chair arrangement can avoid a superior or head-of-the-table position.

When interviewing a client in bed, the nurse can sit at a 45° angle to the bed. This position is less formal than sitting behind a table in the room or standing at the foot of the bed. During an initial admission interview, a client may feel less confronted if there is an overbed table between the client and the nurse (Davis 1984, p. 66). Sitting on a client's bed hems the client in and makes staring difficult to avoid.

Distance   The distance between the interviewer and interviewee is also important. The distance should be neither too small nor too great. Most people feel uncomfortable when talking to someone who is too close or too far away. Most people feel comfortable 3 to 4 ft apart during an interview. A distance of 5 to 6 ft encourages a client to talk longer (Davis 1984, p. 66). For additional information, see the discussion of personal space in Chapter 15.

Height also affects communication. By standing and looking down at a client, the nurse may intimidate the client. Status is associated with greater space and the freedom to move about (Davis 1984, p. 68). Therefore, the client may perceive the nurse who stands during an interview as having greater status.

Stages of an Interview   An interview has three major stages: the opening or introduction, the body or development, and the closing.

The opening   The opening can be the most important part of the interview since what is said and done at that time sets the tone for the remainder of the interview. An inadequate opening can be misleading and create problems during and following the interview. The opening is a two-step process: establishing rapport and orienting the interviewee (Stewart and Cash 1988, p. 39). Either step can come first depending on the situation, the relationship between the two parties, or the interviewer's choice. The rapport and orientation stages may occur at the same time since they are often indistinguishable.

Establishing rapport is a process of creating good will and trust. It can begin with a greeting—"Good morning, John"—or a self-introduction—"Good morning. I'm Becky James, a nursing student"—accompanied by non-verbal gestures such as a smile, a handshake, and a friendly manner. Next the rapport stage is developed by asking questions about the person and proceeding with some small talk about the weather, sports, families, and the like. The nurse must be careful not to overdo this stage since too much superficial talk can arouse anxiety about what is to follow and may appear insincere.

The orientation step consists of explaining the purpose and nature of the interview, e.g., what information is needed, how long it will take, and what is expected of the client. For instance, the nurse might state that the client has the right not to provide data or might tell the client how the information will be used.

The following is an example of an interview introduction:

Step 1—Establish rapport

Nurse: Hello, Ms. Goodwin, I'm Ms. Fellows. I'm a nursing student, and I'll be assisting with your care here.
Client: Hi. Are you a student from the college?
Nurse: Yes, I'm in my final year. Are you familiar with the campus?
Client: Oh! yes! I'm an avid football fan. My nephew graduated in 1985 and I often attend football games with him.
Nurse: That's great! Sounds like fun.
Client: Yes, I enjoy it very much.

Step 2—Orientation

Nurse: May I sit down with you here for about 10 minutes to talk about how I can help you while you're here?
Client: All right. What do you want to know?
Nurse: Well, to plan your care after your operation, I'd like to get some information about your normal daily activities and what you expect here in the hospital. I'd like to make notes while we talk to get the important points and have them available to the other staff who will also look after you.
Client: OK. That's all right with me.

Nurse: If there is anything you don't want to talk about, please feel free to do so, and if there is anything you would rather I didn't write down, just tell me. Is this a good time for you?
Client: Sure, that will be fine.

The body   In the body of the interview, the client communicates what he or she thinks, feels, knows, and perceives in response to questions from the nurse. Transition from the opening stage to this stage can often be facilitated by the use of an open-ended question that is related to the stated purpose, is easy to answer, and does not embarrass or place stress on the person. For example: "What brought you to the hospital today?"

Effective development of the interview demands that the nurse use communication techniques that make both parties feel comfortable and serve the purpose of the interview. See communication techniques in Chapter 15. Brief guidelines for communicating during an interview are outlined in the accompanying box.

The closing   The interview is usually terminated by the nurse, although in some cases the client terminates it. Nurses normally terminate interviews when they have obtained the information they need. Clients terminate interviews when they decide not to give any more information or are unable to offer more information for some other reason—fatigue, for example. The closing is important in maintaining the rapport and trust established during the interview and in facilitating future interactions. The following ways are commonly used to close an interview (Stewart and Cash 1988, pp. 50–52):

1. Signal that the interview is coming to an end by offering to answer questions: "Do you have any questions?" "I would be glad to answer any questions you have." Be sure to allow time for the person to answer, or the offer will be regarded as insincere.

2. Declare completion of the purpose or task by saying "Well, that's about all I need to know for now" or "Well, those are all the questions I have for now." Preceding a remark with the word *well* generally signals that the end of the interaction is near.

3. State appreciation or satisfaction about what was accomplished: "I really enjoyed meeting you, and I think we accomplished a great deal." "Those are all the questions I have. Thank you for your time and help." "The questions you have answered will be helpful in planning your nursing care."

4. Express concern for the person's welfare and future: "Take care of yourself. I'll see you on Thursday." "I hope all goes well for you. If you run into additional problems, be sure to get in touch with me."

5. Plan for the next meeting, if there is to be one. Include the day, time, place, topic, and purpose: "Let's get together

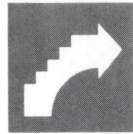

■ Listen attentively, using all your senses, and speak slowly and clearly.

■ Use language the client understands and clarify points that are not understood, for instance, by asking the person to describe what a word means to him or her.

■ Plan questions to follow a logical sequence.

■ Ask only one question at a time. Double questions limit the client to one choice and may confuse both the nurse and the client.

■ Allow the client the opportunity to look at things the way they appear to him or her and not the way they appear to the nurse or someone else.

■ Do not impose your own values on the client.

■ Avoid using personal examples, such as saying, "If I were you . . ."

■ Nonverbally convey respect, concern, interest, and acceptance.

■ Use and accept silence to help the client search for more thoughts or to organize them.

■ Use eye contact and be calm, unhurried and sympathetic.

Source: Adapted from A. Benjamin, *The helping interview,* 3d. ed. (Boston: Houghton-Mifflin Co., 1981), pp. 20–55.

again here on the fifteenth at 9:00 A.M. to see how you are managing then."

6. Reveal what will happen next. For example: "Ms. Goodwin, I will be responsible for giving you care three mornings per week while you are here. I will be in to see you each Monday, Tuesday, and Wednesday between eight o'clock and noon. At those times, we can adjust your care if we need to."

7. Signal that the time is up if a time limit was agreed upon or explain why the interview must close at that time: "Well, I see our time is up; did it ever go quickly today." Or: "I'm sorry, but we're going to have to end our discussion; I have another appointment in 10 minutes."

8. Provide a summary to verify accuracy and agreement. Summarizing serves several purposes: it helps to terminate the interview, it reassures the client that the nurse has listened, it checks the accuracy of the nurse's perceptions, it clears the way for new ideas, and it helps the client to note progress and forward direction (Brammer 1985, p. 74). Sometimes clients may spontaneously offer a summary; at other times the nurse must initiate it or ask the client to do so. "Let's look at what has happened in this interview. What do you think has been accomplished?" Summaries are particularly helpful for clients who are anxious or who have difficulty staying with the topic. "Well, it seems to me that you are especially worried about your hospitalization and chest pain because your father died of a heart attack 5 years ago, your wife has multiple sclerosis and depends on you for support and care, and you don't want to ask for too much help from your children. Is that correct? . . . We'll do the best we can to help you with these concerns. I'll discuss this with you again tomorrow, and we'll decide what plans need to be made to help you."

Examining

Nurses perform physical assessments to obtain the objective data needed to complete the assessment phase of the nursing process. A complete database of both subjective and objective data allows the nurse to formulate nursing diagnoses, develop client goals, and intervene to promote health and prevent disease. Developing the skills needed for physical assessment requires knowledge, practice, and time. However, the student nurse often begins to develop assessment skills by describing the general appearance of the client, assessing skin, range of motion, and mobility often during morning care, and by monitoring vital signs.

The physical assessment is carried out systematically. It may be organized according to the examiner's preference, in a head-to-toe approach or as a body systems approach. Usually, the nurse records a general impression about the client's overall appearance and health status, e.g., age, body size, mental and nutritional status, speech, and behavior. Then, measurements such as vital signs, height, and weight are taken. The nurse conducting a physical examination using the head-to-toe (**cephalocaudal**) approach begins the assessment at the head, progresses to the neck, thorax, abdomen, and extremities and ends at the toes. The nurse using a body systems approach investigates each system individually, i.e., the respiratory system, the circulatory system, the nervous system, and so on. During the physical assessment, the nurse assesses all body parts and determines anthropometric measurements. (An **anthropometric measurement** is a measurement of the size and composition of the body.) These techniques are discussed in detail in Chapters 18, 19, and 39. Instead of giving a complete examination, the nurse may focus on a specific problem area noted from the nursing assessment, such as the inability to urinate. On occasion, the nurse may find it necessary to resolve a client complaint or problem prior to completing the examination, e.g., if the client appears short of breath. Alternatively, the nurse may perform a screening examination. A **screening examination,** also called a review of systems, is a brief review of essential functioning of various body parts or systems. An example of a screening examination is the nursing admission assessment form shown in Figure 10–1. Data obtained from this examination
(continued on page 186)

Welcome to UCSF! Your nurses will be planning your hospital care with you to meet your individual needs. We would appreciate your help in answering the following questions. This information will help us learn about your general health and your condition, and assist us in planning for your discharge. The information is confidential. You do not have to answer any questions, or complete the form unless you want to. Thank you!

Please complete both sides of this page, and return it to the person who gave it to you. A relative or friend may ask you the questions and/or write your answers for you.

GENERAL INFORMATION:

What language do you find it easiest to read & write? English __✓__ ; Other_____

What is (or was) your occupation? *cattle rancher and farmer*

What is the highest level of school you have completed (circle one): Grammar school (High School) College

Other_____

HEALTH PERCEPTION/HEALTH MAINTENANCE:

What has caused this hospitalization? *no energy and shortness of breath*

Do you:	NO	YES	If yes, please explain:
Follow a special diet		✓	Type of diet *no sugar - I have diabetes*
Smoke	✓		Packs per day _____
Use alcohol	✓		Drinks per day *none*
Take drugs or medicines which are not prescribed for you	✓		_____
Get up at night to go to the bath-room			How often? _____

Have you experienced any problems with the following within the past year:

	NO	YES	Comments/additional information:
Weight loss		✓	Amount: *5 lbs*
Weight gain	✓		Amount: _____
Change in appetite or thirst	✓		
Eating or swallowing	✓		Do you wear dentures? ___No ___Yes
Changes in bowel habit	✓		Do you use laxatives? ___No___ Yes; name _____ frequency_____
Urinating		✓	*go too often*
Energy for daily activities		✓	*can't do my daily chores anymore*
Falling			
Sleeping	✓		Do you use anything to help you sleep? ___No ✓ Yes; name _____
Difficulty hearing		✓	Do you use a hearing aid? ✓ No ___ Yes;
Difficulty seeing	✓		Do you wear glasses? ___No ✓ Yes Contact lenses? ✓ No ___ Yes
Changes in memory	✓		
Shortness of breath		✓	
Muscle weakness			
Pain or discomfort	✓		Describe the pain and what you do to relieve it: _____

__ALLERGIES:__ ✓ No Known Allergies ____ Allergic to:_____

MEDICATIONS

NAME	DOSE	FREQUENCY	LAST TAKEN	PURPOSE OF MEDICATION/WHY TAKING IT	WITH PT YES	NO
Tolinase	250 mg	every day	7/22	diabetes		
Lasix	20 mg	every day	7/22	for bad heart valve		
Slow K	20 mEq.	every day	7/22	to replace potassium		
NTG 1/150	2	when necessary	2 months ago	angina		

602-02 R. 2/89

UCSF
The Medical Center
at the University of California, San Francisco
San Francisco, California 94143

NURSING ADMISSION ASSESSMENT   8

Figure 10–1   Nursing Admission Assessment

Source   (Courtesy of the Department of Nursing, The Medical Center at the University of California, San Francisco.)

DISCHARGE PLANNING ASSESSMENT:

1. Where do you live? City _Portola Valley_ State _California_ County_____
2. Where do you plan to stay after hospitalization? _✓_ Home _____ Other_____
3. Do you live alone? _____ yes _✓_ no...With whom do you live? _wife and 6 of my 13 children_
4. In what areas do you need assistance? _____ transportation; _____ personal care; _✓_ preparation of meals; _✓_ shopping
   other_____
5. If you need help in any of the above areas, who can assist you _wife_
6. Have you received help from any community agency? _✓_ No _____ Yes... _____ home health agency; _____ Meals on Wheels;
   _____ visiting nurse; _____ homemaker; _____ other..._____
7. Is there any other information about yourself which you feel would assist us in planning your care while in the hospital or after you go
   home?_____
   _____

Completed by _____ _Joe Smith_ _____ Date _7/23/90_ If someone other than patient completed this form, what
is your relationship to the patient?_____

Thank you for your assistance. The nurse will complete the rest of the form.

FUNCTIONAL ASSESSMENT: Document the patient's level of functioning prior to this episode of illness.

ACTIVITY	INDEP	NEED ASSIST	UNABLE TO DO	EXPLAIN
1. Bath/shower	✓			
2. Dressing	✓			
3. Toileting	✓			
4. Moving to/from bed/chair	✓			*moves slowly since hip operation*
5. Walking				
6. Eating	✓			
7. Meal preparation	wife			
8. Household chores	wife			

If patient is not independent in any of the above areas, consider the need to initiate a nursing diagnosis and/or refer patient to: 1) PT; 2) Nutritionist; 3)Social Worker; 4)CNS; 5) Home Care liaison nurse or other appropriate resource.

ORIENTED TO UNIT:

	YES		YES
Phone	✓	Meal times/menu	✓
Bed controls	✓	Care of valuables	✓
TV	✓	Visiting hours	✓
Call light	✓	Smoking	✓
Dentures	✓	Belongings sheet completed	✓

EQUIPMENT NEEDED IN:

	Hospital	Home
Crutches	-----	-----
Walker/cane	-----	-----
Wheelchair	-----	-----
Highrise toilet seat	-----	-----
Oxygen	-----	-----
Other _____		

HIGH RISK FOR FALLS ASSESSMENT :
(Circle those that apply)

65 or older	__1__
Mental status limitations	__5__
History of falls	__5__
Mobility limitations	__4__
Elimination needs	__2__
Medications	__1__
TOTAL SCORE	_____

INITIATE NURSING CARE PROBLEM FOR SCORE OF 6 OR MORE

Disposition of meds brought to hospital:_____None brought to hospital; _X_ Meds located:_____
Completed by: _Mary Jones RN_ DATE _7/23/90_ TIME _1530_

PHYSICAL ASSESSMENT (To be completed by the registered nurse.)

GENERAL APPEARANCE: ☑ Ambulatory ☑ Alert ☑ Responds appropriately to interview _Pleasant but not talkative_

COGNITIVE SCREEN: *Complete screen if patient meets one of the following criteria:: 1) over 65 years of age; 2) report or shows evidence of short–term memory deficit and/ or confusion or 3) diagnosis of central nervous system dysfunction.*

INTRODUCTION TO PATIENT: *"I would like to ask you a few questions. Some you will find very easy and others may be very hard. Just do your best."*

(Maximum score)

Memory:
(4 points)
_4_ *(score)*

Please repeat these words after me and remember them. I will ask for them later: TABLE, LION, ORANGE, GLOVE *(1 point for each word on first repetition)*

Orientation:
(10 points)
_10_ *(score)*

What is your full name? *(0 point)* What day of the week is this? *(1 point)*
What month is this? *(1 point)* What is today's date? *(1 point)*
What year is this? *(2 points)* What city are we in? *(2 points)*
What place is this? (need to say UC Hospital) *(2 points)* What time is it? (within an hour) *(1 point)*

Attention:
(10 points)
_10_ *(score)*

Count backward from 20 to 1. *(Stop the patient after 10 answers.)*

_4_ *(score)*

Repeat the four words I told you earlier and asked you to remember. *(1 point for each word remembered)*

_28_ TOTAL SCORE

PHYSICAL ASSESSMENT (Continued)

COGNITIVE SCREEN: (continued)

If the patient scores 19 or less out of 28, take one of the following actions: 1) implement nursing actions for care of patients with altered thought processes and/or for falls prevention; and/or 2) call the Gerontology CNS, Psychiatric Liaison CNS, Neurology/ Neurosurgery CNS, head nurse or nursing supervisor to discuss the need for further evaluation or action.

SKIN INTEGRITY:
☑ No areas of erythema   ☑ Skin intact

Pink, intact, good turgor

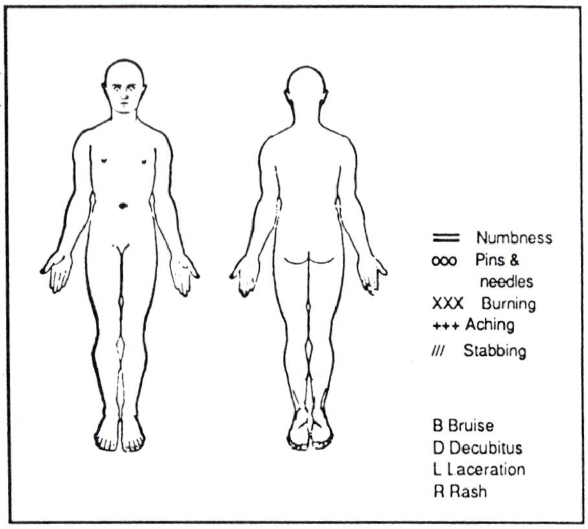

PRESSURE SORE RISK ASSESSMENT SCORING SCALE:
TOTAL SCORE ___19___ *(Circle #'s, then total; If ≤ 14, initiate a nursing diagnosis.)*

Phys. Cond.	Ment. Cond.	Activity	Mobility	Incontin.
④ Good	④ Alert	④ Ambulat.	4 Full	④ Not
3 Fair	3 Apathetic/ Withdrawn	3 Walk/help	③ Sl. Limit.	3 Occassional
2 Poor	2 Confused	2 Chair	2 V. Limited	2 Usually/urine
1 Very bad	1 Stuporous/ unresponsive	1 Bed	1 Immobile	1 Urine & stool

Legend (body diagram):
- ═══ Numbness
- ∞∞ Pins & needles
- XXX Burning
- +++ Aching
- /// Stabbing
- B Bruise
- D Decubitus
- L Laceration
- R Rash

HEENT: (trach; eyes; cranial facial abnormalities)
☑ No abnormalities noted ☑ Wears glasses *for reading only*

PULMONARY: (Breath sounds; cough or sputum; chest symmetry; respiratory effort)
☑ Lungs clear to auscultation   ☑ No respiratory distress *Equal expansion. Rales in bases bilaterally which do clear with coughing. No sputum.*

CARDIOVASCULAR: (pulses 4+=bounding, 3+=v. strong, 2+=normal, 1+=weak/thready, 0=unable to palpate;

Pulse	R	L
Radial	2+	2+
Fem.	3+	4+
Pop.	2+	0
D.P	2+	0

☑ Apical pulse regular ☑ Skin warm & dry ☑ No peripheral edema
Loud murmur in aortic area.
Ⓛ limb cooler than Ⓡ

GASTRO–INTESTINAL: (Urgency; frequency; burning; vaginal discharge)
Abdomen: ☑ soft; ☑ non–tender ☑ Bowel sounds active, within normal limits *Last BM 7/22 a.m.*

GENITOURINARY/GYNECOLOGICAL:
☑ No abnormalities reported; Is there any possiblility you might be pregnant? ☐YES ☐NO
↑ frequency c̄ Lasix noted by client

MUSCULO–SKELETAL: (atrophy; swelling/edema; ROM; prosthetic devices)
☑ Moves all extremeties

NEUROLOGICAL: (gait/balance; LOC; speech disorders)
☐ See neuro assessment sheet ☑ Able to maintain balance ☑ Gait steady *Slight limp*

Signature *Mary Jones RN*   Date *7/23/90*

Figure 10–1   (continued)

184

ADMISSION NURSING NOTE:

Admitted to: _525 W_ From: _home_ Time: _1500_ Weight: _95.3 kg_

Admitted for cardiac catheterization and probable aortic valve replacement. Has hx (6 mos.) of angina. Over past year client has noted marked decrease in energy and episodes of SOB on exertion.
T 36.5, P 80R, R 16, BP 124/80 · Ht. 171 cm Wt. 95.3 kg
States he has "always been healthy" since he "eats a good diet, and doesn't drink or smoke" but lately is "too weak to do day to day work on the farm". Says "my son Tom" is most helpful even for talking things over." "I am usually too busy to worry about things." Hopes his family can visit frequently. Requested to see a hospital chaplain and location of chapel.

Signature _Mary Jones_ Date _7/23/90_

DISCHARGE NURSING NOTE:

Discharged to:_____ Home _____ Other _____ DATE_____ TIME_____

_____ Ambulatory _____Wheelchair _____Ambulance _____Other_____

Person Accepting Responsibility for Patient: _____Self _____Other_____

Status of admitting problem and/or other active problems: _____

_____

_____

_____

Resources to be used post–hospitalization:_____

_____

_____

Medication Instruction: ☐ See Patient Teaching Record; If no patient teaching record... ☐ instructed by pharmacist; ☐ instructed by nurse... ☐ Information given/discussed;☐ appropriate feedback/independent;☐ needs reinforcement...Plan: _____

_____

_____

_____

_____

Signature   Date

Past Medical History (Optional)	Past Surgical History (Optional)
	Ⓛ hip replacement 18 months ago
	S̄ complications

UNIT SPECIFIC INFORMATION/Other:

_____

_____

_____

_____

_____

■ *Health-perception–health-management pattern.* Describes client's perceived pattern of health and well-being and how health is managed

■ *Nutritional-metabolic pattern.* Describes pattern of food and fluid consumption relative to metabolic need and pattern indicators of local nutrient supply

■ *Elimination pattern.* Describes patterns of excretory function (bowel, bladder, and skin)

■ *Activity-exercise pattern.* Describes pattern of exercise, activity, leisure, and recreation

■ *Cognitive-perceptual pattern.* Describes sensory-perceptual and cognitive pattern

■ *Sleep-rest pattern.* Describes patterns of sleep, rest, and relaxation

■ *Self-perception–self-concept pattern.* Describes self-concept pattern and perceptions of self (e.g., body comfort, body image, feeling state)

■ *Role-relationship pattern.* Describes pattern of role-engagements and relationships

■ *Sexuality-reproductive pattern.* Describes client's patterns of satisfaction and dissatisfaction with sexuality; describes reproductive patterns

■ *Coping–stress-tolerance pattern.* Describes general coping pattern and effectiveness of the pattern in terms of stress tolerance

■ *Value-belief pattern.* Describes patterns of values, beliefs (including spiritual), or goals that guide choices or decisions

Source: M. Gordon, *Nursing diagnosis: Process and application,* 2d ed. (New York: McGraw-Hill, 1987), p. 93. Copyrighted by Mosby-Year Book, Inc. St. Louis

are measured against norms or standards, such as ideal height and weight standards or norms for body temperature or blood pressure levels.

To conduct the examination, the nurse uses techniques of inspection, auscultation, palpation, and percussion. These techniques are discussed in Chapter 19.

STRUCTURING DATA COLLECTION

To obtain data systematically the nurse needs to use an organized assessment framework or structure. This systematic method of collecting desired data about the client is referred to as a **nursing health history** or, more recently, **a nursing assessment.** The purpose of the nursing assessment is to gather as much information as possible about the client in order to identify problems for nursing interventions (Yura and Walsh 1988, p. 116). The data collected during the nursing health history between the nurse and client largely constitute a *subjective assessment.* The nurse obtains information about the client, the client's health, responses to illness, sociocultural factors, health beliefs and practices, coping patterns, and day-to-day activities. Details about the nursing assessment are discussed in Chapter 19.

There are many nursing models and frameworks that guide data collection through structured assessment tools. An example is Newman's tool, an assessment/intervention tool

TABLE 10–2 *Areas of Data Collection Delineated by Dorothea Orem and Sister Callista Roy*

Orem (1985)	Roy (1984)
Universal self-care requisites	Adaptive modes
1. The maintenance of a sufficient intake of air	1. Physiologic needs
2. The maintenance of a sufficient intake of water	a. Exercise and rest
3. The maintenance of a sufficient intake of food	b. Nutrition
	c. Elimination
4. The provision of care associated with elimination processes and excrements	d. Fluid and electrolytes
	e. Oxygen and circulation
	f. Regulation: temperature
5. The maintenance of a balance between activity and rest	g. Regulation: the senses
	h. Regulation: endocrine system
6. The maintenance of a balance between solitude and social interaction	2. Self-concept
	a. Physical self
7. The prevention of hazards to human life, human functioning, and human well-being	b. Moral-ethical self
	c. Self-consistency
	d. Self-ideal and expectancy
	e. Self-esteem
8. The promotion of human functioning and development within social groups in accord with human potential, known human limitations, and human desire to be normal. (Normalcy is used in the sense of that which is essentially human and that which is in accord with the genetic and constitutional characteristics and the talents of individuals.)	3. Role function
	4. Interdependence

that has seven categories: intake summary, stressors as perceived by the client, stressors as perceived by the caregiver, intrapersonal factors, interpersonal factors, extrapersonal factors, and formulation of the problem (Cross 1985, pp. 271–72).

Abdellah (1961) and Henderson (1966) developed earlier frameworks used or adapted in many settings. More recently, Gordon (1987) established a framework of 11 functional health patterns. See the box on page 186. Gordon uses the word *pattern* to signify a sequence of behavior. The nurse collects data about dysfunctional as well as functional behavior. Thus, using Gordon's framework to analyze data, nurses are able to discern emerging patterns.

Roy (1984) outlines the data to be collected according to the Roy Adaptation model and classifies observable behavior into four categories: physiologic, self-concept, role function, and interdependence. Orem (1985) delineates eight universal self-care requisites of humans. See Table 10–2.

Other frameworks and models from other disciplines are also helpful for data collection. Some are Maslow's hierarchy of needs (see Chapter 4). Piaget's assessment of cognitive development (see Chapter 24). Selye's stress theory (see Chapter 33). These frameworks are narrower than the model required in nursing; therefore, the nurse usually needs to combine these with other approaches to obtain a complete history. Figure 10–1 is an example of an eclectic nursing admission assessment form that reflects Gordon's and other frameworks.

CHAPTER HIGHLIGHTS

▶ Assessment is the collection, verification, and documentation of subjective and objective data about a client's health status.

▶ Assessing involves active participation by the client and the nurse.

▶ The nursing assessment must be complete and accurate, since nursing diagnosis and interventions are based on this information.

▶ Observation is a conscious, deliberate skill.

▶ The observations of the nurse must be validated; interpretations of client's behavior must not be used as fact.

▶ Subjective data are the client's personal perceptions often gathered during the nursing health history.

▶ Objective data are detectable by an observer; an example is data collected during the physical examination.

▶ The nurse often uses a combination of directive and nondirective interviewing approaches to obtain the nursing health history.

▶ Skills required for data collection are communicating, interviewing, observing, and examining.

READINGS AND REFERENCES

SUGGESTED READINGS

Brown, M. D. May 1988. Functional assessment of the elderly. *Journal of Gerontological Nursing* 14:13–17.
  With advanced age, the cumulative effects of age and disease have a significant impact on the functional reserve of all organ systems. Comprehensive functional assessment of the elderly is therefore essential. Brown describes the functional assessment protocol used in one geriatric clinical setting.
Guzzetta, C. E., Bunton, S. D.; Prinkey, L. A.; Sherer, A.; and Seifert, P. April 1988. Unitary person assessment tool: Easing problems with nursing diagnoses. *Focus on Critical Care* 15:12–24.
  The authors discuss an assessment tool developed to facilitate the use of nursing diagnoses in the critical care setting. The NANDA nursing diagnosis *Taxonomy I, Revised* and the unitary person framework were analyzed by the authors, a tool was developed based on this analysis, and the tool was refined for clinical practice. The complete tool is presented and offered as an example for nurses to adapt to other clinical settings.

RELATED RESEARCH

Lenihan, A. A. July/August 1988. Identification of self-care behaviors in the elderly: A nursing assessment tool. *Journal of Professional Nursing* 4:285–288.
Loveridge, C. E. and Heinkeken, J. May 1988. Confirming interactions. *Journal of Gerontological Nursing* 14:27–30, 38–39.

SELECTED REFERENCES

Abdellah, F. G., et al. 1961. *Patient-centered approaches to nursing.* New York: Macmillan Co.
American Nurses' Association. 1980. *Nursing: A social policy statement.* Kansas City, Mo: ANA.
Atkinson, L. D., Murray, M. E. 1986. *Understanding the nursing process.* 3d ed. New York: Macmillan Co.
Barker, P. November/December 1987. Assembling the pieces: Assessment is like a jigsaw puzzle. *Nursing Times* 83:67–68.

Brigdon, P., Todd, M. January 1990. In search of the perfect assessment. *Professional Nurse* 5:181–84.

Carnevali, D. L. 1983. *Nursing care planning: Diagnosis and management.* 3d ed. Philadelphia: J. B. Lippincott Co.

Cross, J. R. Betty Newman. In George, J. B., editor, 1985. pp. 258–86. *Nursing theories: A base for professional practice.* 2d ed. Englewood Cliffs, NJ: Prentice-Hall.

Gordon, M. 1987. *Nursing diagnosis: Process and application.* 2d ed. New York: McGraw-Hill.

Griffith, J. W., Christensen, P. J. 1986. *Nursing Process: Application of theories, frameworks, and models.* 2d ed. St. Louis: C. V. Mosby.

Hanna, D. V., Wyman, N. B. November 1987. Assessment + diagnosis = care planning: A tool for coordination. *Nursing Management* 18:106–9.

Henderson, V. 1966. *The nature of nursing.* New York: Macmillan.

La Monica, E. L. 1985. *The humanistic nursing process.* Monterey, Calif.: Wadsworth Health Sciences.

Merry, J. A. January 1988. Take your assessment all the way down to the toes. *RN* 51:60–63.

Orem, D. E. 1985. *Nursing: Concepts of practice.* 3d ed. New York: McGraw-Hill.

Roy, Sr. C. 1984. *Introduction to nursing: An adaptation model.* 2d ed. Englewood Cliffs, N.J.: Prentice-Hall.

Schamel, K. October 1987. How to assess the patient on long-term care. *RN* 50:65–68.

Schare, B. L., Gilman, B.; Adams, G.; and Albright, J. C. February 1988. Health assessment skill utilization by sophomore nursing students. *Western Journal of Nursing Research* 10:55–65.

Sherwood, M. J.; Szczech, P. C.; Glasgow, G. M.; and Munoz, C. C. 1988. *Determining diagnosis through assessment.* Baltimore: Williams & Wilkins.

Yura, H., and Walsh, M. B. 1988. *The nursing process: Assessing, planning, implementing, evaluating.* 5th ed. Norwalk, Conn.: Appleton & Lange.

Diagnosing

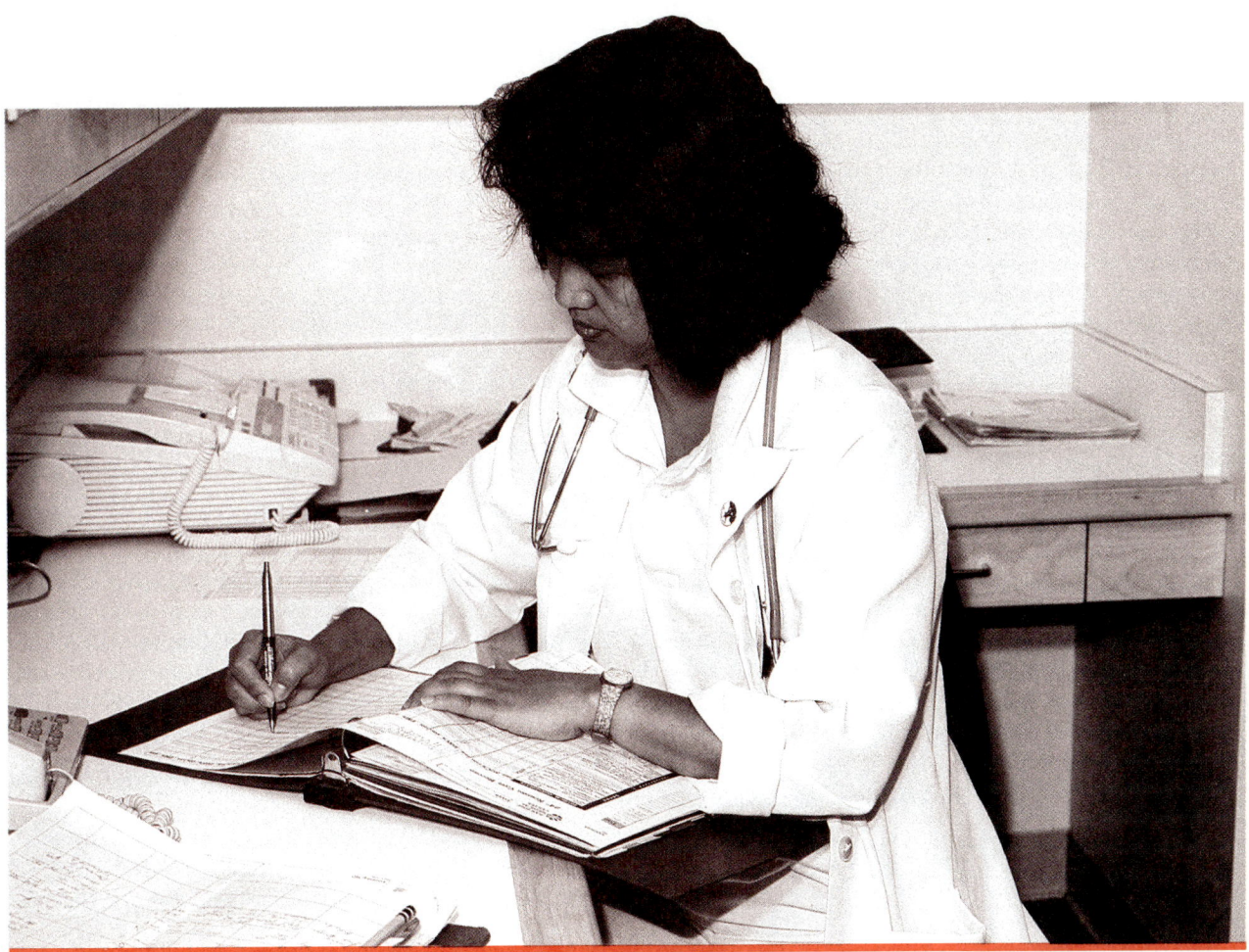

CONTENTS

OBJECTIVES

▶ Define the term *nursing diagnosis*.
▶ Compare medical and nursing diagnoses.
▶ Identify basic steps in the diagnostic process.
▶ Describe the PES format for writing nursing diagnoses.

▶ Describe the characteristics of a nursing diagnosis.

▶ List common errors in writing diagnostic statements.

▶ Describe the evolution of the nursing diagnoses movement.

▶ List advantages of a taxonomy of nursing diagnoses.

▶ Identify the challenges of the profession related to nursing diagnoses.

NURSING DIAGNOSIS

Definitions

Nursing diagnosis emerged in the 1970s and provided the profession with an appropriate focus on the content and the diagnostic categories that were in the domain of nursing. The term *diagnosis*, according to the dictionary, is derived from the Greek word *diagignoskein,* which means "to distinguish." Definitions include (a) the art of identifying a disease from its signs and symptoms, (b) a statement or conclusion concerning the nature of some phenomenon, and (c) analysis of the course or nature of a condition, situation, or problem. Although the first definition pertains to physicians, diagnosis is not restricted to one particular profession and must be qualified by a professional designation. In fact, anyone who makes a statement or conclusion about the nature of a condition or problem is diagnosing.

The term *nursing diagnosis* refers to both the process of making a diagnosis and to the clinical judgment reached and expressed in a category name or label (Gordon 1987b, p. 7). Several definitions of nursing diagnosis have been stated since the early 1950s. Each has a different emphasis, but all have many similarities. The earliest definition of nursing diagnosis was formulated by Abdellah (1957, p. 4), who stated that it was the "determination of the nature and extent of nursing problems presented by the individual patients or families receiving nursing care."

In 1973, the First National Conference on the Classification of Nursing Diagnosis accepted this definition: A **nursing diagnosis** "is the judgment or conclusion [that] occurs as a result of nursing assessment" (Gebbie and Lavin 1975). To Gordon (1976, p. 1299), *nursing diagnoses,* or clinical diagnoses made by professional nurses, describe a combination of signs and symptoms that indicate actual or potential health problems that nurses by virtue of their education and experience are able, licensed, and accountable to treat. To Edel (1982, p. 6), a *nursing diagnosis* is the statement of a potential or actual altered health status of a client, which is derived from nursing assessment and which requires intervention from the domain of nursing. Edel's definition emphasizes that the entity to be diagnosed is *health status,* which avoids the negative connotation of problem and allows for positive diagnoses of clients. (**Health status** is the health of a person at a given time.) The strengths and the problems of the person are considered. To Shoemaker (1984, p. 109), a *nursing diagnosis* is a clinical judgment about an individual family or community that is derived through a deliberate, systematic process of data collection and analysis. The diagnosis is the basis for prescriptions of definitive therapy for which the nurse is accountable. It is expressed concisely and includes the etiology (when known) of the condition.

In March 1990, the Ninth Conference on the Classification of Nursing Diagnoses in Orlando, Florida accepted the working definition of nursing diagnosis shown in the accompanying box.

Implied in these definitions are the following characteristics:

■ Professional nurses (registered nurses) are the persons responsible for making nursing diagnoses. Even though other nursing personnel may contribute data to the process of diagnosing and may implement specified nursing care, the formulation of a diagnostic statement lies within the realm of the professional nurse.

■ A **health problem** is any condition or situation in which a client requires help to promote, maintain, or regain a state of health or to achieve a peaceful death. It does not always refer to an undesirable state but does refer to a situation for which the client needs nursing assistance.

■ Nursing diagnoses describe (a) **actual health problems** (deviations from health), (b) **potential health problems** (risk factors that predispose persons and families to health problems), and (c) areas of enriched personal growth. Examples of actual health problems are **Ineffective airway clearance, A fluid volume deficit,** and **Knowledge deficit.** Examples of potential health problems are **Potential for infection,** and **Potential for injury.** Examples of areas of enriched personal growth

---

1990 NANDA Definition of Nursing Diagnosis

"Nursing diagnosis is a clinical judgment about individual, family, or community responses to actual and potential health problems/life processes. Nursing diagnoses provide the basis for selection of nursing interventions to achieve outcomes for which the nurse is accountable."

Ninth Conference on the Classification of Nursing Diagnoses, March 17–21, 1990, Orlando, Florida.

are self-development, health maintenance management, and parenting.

- The domain of nursing diagnosis includes only those health states that nurses are able and licensed to treat. For example, nurses are not educated to diagnose or treat diseases such as diabetes mellitus; this task is defined legally as within the practice of medicine. Yet they can diagnose a **Knowledge deficit, Ineffective individual coping, Altered nutrition,** and **Potential for injury,** all of which may accompany diabetes mellitus. These problems are within the nurse's capabilities and the scope of the nurse's licensing laws; thus, the nurse is responsible and accountable for the treatment provided for these nursing diagnoses.

- A nursing diagnosis is a judgment made only after a thorough, systematic process of data collection.

Differentiating Nursing Diagnosis from Medical Diagnosis

To clarify the domain of nursing and make it distinct from the medical profession, nurses had to define the characteristics of a nursing diagnosis. This was accomplished most definitively by Shoemaker (1984). She surveyed 111 experts in the field to determine the essential characteristics of a nursing diagnosis. These findings describe and define a nursing diagnosis and also allow for differentiation from medical diagnoses. For a summary, see Table 11–1. A medical diagnosis describes a specific pathophysiologic response that is fairly uniform from one client to the other. In contrast, a nursing diagnosis describes a client's response to an illness or a potential health problem; this response varies among individuals. Nursing diagnoses are oriented to the individual and change as the client's responses change. For example, two clients with a medical diagnosis of rheumatoid arthritis can have quite similar disease processes but very different responses. A 70-year-old woman may respond with acceptance, viewing her condition as part of the aging process, whereas a 20-year-old woman may respond with anger and hostility because of the changes this condition will make in her personal identity, body image, role performance, and self-esteem.

Medical diagnoses are described in concise phrases of two or three words according to a universally accepted taxonomy (system of classification). For nursing diagnoses, however, the format is a two-part statement that includes the **etiology** (cause or source) when known. Some nursing diagnoses are long and complex. It is doubtful that nursing diagnoses will ever be as condensed as medical diagnoses. A nursing diagnosis may be complementary to a medical diagnosis but is separate and distinct. A client who has one or more medical diagnoses and medical orders may also have one or more nursing diagnoses and nursing orders. These diagnoses and orders are complementary rather than contradictory.

TABLE 11–1 *Comparison of Nursing and Medical Diagnoses*

Nursing Diagnosis	Medical Diagnosis
Describes an individual's response to a disease process condition or situation	Describes a specific disease process
Is oriented to the individual	Is oriented to pathology
Changes as the client's responses change	Remains constant throughout the duration of illness
Guides independent nursing activities: planning, intervening and evaluating	Guides medical management, some of which may be carried out by the nurse
Is complementary to the medical diagnosis	Is complementary to the nursing diagnosis
Has no universally accepted classification system; such systems are in the process of development	Has a well-developed classification system accepted by the medical profession
Consists of a two-part statement with etiology when known	Consists of two or three words

A nursing diagnosis is a statement of a nursing judgment, and refers to a condition that nurses are licensed to treat. In contrast, a medical diagnosis is made and treated by a physician. Nursing diagnoses refer to physical, sociocultural, psychologic, and spiritual conditions, whereas medical diagnoses refer to disease.

Nursing diagnoses relate to the nurse's **independent functions,** i.e., the areas of health care that are unique to nursing and are separate and distinct from the care included in medical management. Even though the nurse is obligated to carry out medical orders, i.e. **dependent functions,** the nurse is also obligated to diagnose and prescribe within the limits of nurse practice acts.

Some of the advantages of using nursing diagnoses are outlined in the box on the following page.

THE DIAGNOSTIC PROCESS

Diagnosis is a process of analysis and synthesis. **Analysis** is the separation into components, i.e., breaking down the whole into its parts. **Synthesis** is the opposite, i.e., putting together the parts into the whole.

The cognitive skills required for analysis and synthesis are objectivity, critical thinking, decision making, and inductive and deductive reasoning (Risner 1986a, p. 126). Deductive and inductive reasoning and decision making are discussed in Chapter 4, page 77. To be **objective** is to be without bias; i.e., the values and beliefs of the nurse do not affect how data are viewed and analyzed. To be objective, nurses must be aware of their own values and beliefs. **Critical thinking** is a cognitive process during which data are reviewed and explanations considered before an opinion is formed. In this process, nurses use all the subjective and objective data acquired and validated during the assessment phase as well as their knowledge to develop a nursing diagnostic statement.

The diagnostic process is used continuously by most nurses working in hospitals, ambulatory care settings, clients' homes, and long-term care facilities. An experienced nurse may enter a client's room and immediately observe significant data about the client. The nurse is able to do this because of knowledge, skill, and expertise in the practice setting. The outcome of the diagnostic process, the statement of the nursing diagnosis, is recorded in the care plan. This conclusion or statement provides nurse colleagues with a common language and direction for individualized interventions.

Although experienced practitioners are able to perform these mental processes automatically, the novice needs guidelines to understand and formulate diagnoses. The diagnostic process has the following steps:

1. Data processing—interpreting collected data

2. Determining the client's health problems, health risks, and strengths

3. Formulating nursing diagnoses

Data Processing

Data processing, the first aspect of analyzing, is the act of interpreting collected data. It involves the following steps:

1. Organize data
2. Compare data against standards (identify significant cues)
3. Cluster data (generate tentative hypotheses)
4. Identify gaps and inconsistencies

These activities occur continuously rather than sequentially.

Organizing the Data   Once the data are collected, they need to be organized into a usable framework for the nurse and others who may need access to them. As discussed in Chapter 10, theoretical frameworks and conceptual models often guide the format of the assessment tool, thus facilitating the organization of data. The nurse may choose one or more nursing models and develop skill by using them consistently. For further information on nursing models, see Chapter 4.

To illustrate data organization, the client example (Joe Smith) given in Chapter 10 will be used (see Figure 10–1 on page 182). A summary of the nursing assessment data for this client using a functional health pattern assessment format is shown in the accompanying box.

Comparing Data against Standards   The nurse compares the client's data to a wide range of standards, such as normal health patterns, normal vital signs, laboratory values, basic food groups, growth, and development. The nurse also uses personal knowledge—e.g., of physiology, psychology, and sociology—as well as past experience when comparing the data.

A **standard** or **norm** is a generally accepted rule, model, pattern, or measure. To be used in comparing, however, a standard must be both relevant and reliable. To be relevant, it must be of the same class as the data to which it is compared. Just as oranges cannot be the standard used to judge apples, the ideal breakfast for a teenager cannot be used as a standard for the breakfast of a person over 65 years of age. To be reliable, the standard must be based on data from a sufficiently large sample. For example, to determine the average interests of 12-year-olds, one must survey a large number of teenagers, not just three.

Standards used for comparison include the Daily Food Guides (Chapter 39), Erickson's stages of development, and the Metropolitan Life Insurance charts for normal ranges of height and weight. When comparing data against standards, the nurse must know the client's view of "normal," which may differ from that of the nurse. For example, a client may think it is perfectly normal to bathe once a week whereas the nurse may believe once a day is normal. What is considered normal varies according to the client's expectations, culture, values, socioeconomic status, and knowledge. It is important to gather and record useful and specific data. Thus, if the client states, "My urinary elimination is normal," the nurse should ask for clarification: "Can you explain what you mean by normal?" The nurse compares the client data against standards and norms in order to identify significant and relevant cues. A **cue** is a piece of information or data that influences decisions (Gordon 1987b, p. 182). Cues are acquired through the use of the five senses (taste, touch, smell, hearing, and sight). Gordon (1987b, p. 191) suggests the following guidelines to assist in determining significant cues.

1. *Cues that point to change in a client's health status or pattern.* These may be positive or negative. For example the client states: "I have recently experienced shortness of breath while climbing stairs" or "I have not smoked for three months."

2. *Cues that vary from norms of the client population.* The client's pattern may fit within cultural norms but vary from norms of the general society. The client may consider a pattern—for example, eating very small meals and having a poor appetite—to be normal. This pattern,

however, may not be productive and may require further exploration.

3. *Cues that indicate a developmental delay.* Changes in health patterns occur as the person grows and develops. By age 9 months, the infant is usually able to sit alone without support, stand while holding on, and turn the wrists to examine objects (James and Mott 1988, p. 96). The infant who has not accomplished these tasks needs further assessment for possible developmental delays. To identify significant cues, the nurse must be aware of normal patterns and changes.

The nurse must always consider the client's interpretation of the situation. Making diagnostic decisions without eliciting the perceptions of the client or family may lead to missed diagnoses or misdiagnoses. The client's perceptions are an important aspect of the decision-making process.

Clustering Data

Clustering or grouping data is a process of determining the relatedness of facts and finding patterns in the facts. This is the beginning of synthesis. Data are examined to determine whether any patterns are present, whether the data represent isolated incidents, and whether the data are significant. The process of data clustering is influenced by the nurse's background of scientific knowledge, past nursing experiences, and concept of nursing. Together, these factors are a mental reference file of facts and principles the nurse uses to verify the significance of the data. The nurse may cluster data inductively by combining data from different assessment areas to form a pattern, or the nurse may begin with a framework, such as Gordon's functional health patterns, and cluster the subjective and objective data into the appropriate categories. The latter is a deductive approach to data clustering, or pattern formation.

To relate and group data, the nurse must consider nursing diagnostic categories or areas of nursing responsibility. Gordon (1987b, p. 20) states that clustering information involves a search in the nurse's memory stores for previously learned meaningful groups of clinical cues that are associated with a diagnostic category. Gordon believes that clustering occurs in conjunction with data collection and interpretation, as evidenced in remarks or thoughts such as, "I'm getting a picture of" or "This cue doesn't fit the picture." The novice nurse does not have the knowledge base or the clinical experience that facilitates the recognition of cues related to diagnostic categories. Thus, the novice must take careful assessment notes, search data for abnormal cues, and use textbook resources for comparing the client's cues with the defining characteristics and etiologic factors of the accepted nursing diagnoses. (A list of accepted nursing diagnostic categories is shown on the inside front cover.) After comparing the client cues against available resources, the novice can group data into clusters.

Data clustering involves making inferences. An **inference** is the nurse's judgment or interpretation of cues.

Inferences are made throughout the diagnostic process. During data clustering, the nurse interprets the possible meaning of the cues and labels the cue clusters with tentative diagnostic hypotheses. Data clustering or grouping for Mr. Joe Smith is illustrated in Table 11–2. The data are clustered according to nursing diagnostic categories.

Identifying Gaps and Inconsistencies in Data

Gaps are missing information needed to determine a data pattern. For example, during the assessment phase, the nurse needs data about a client's definition of health to interpret his statement "I am sick all the time." Data may be completely missing or incomplete. For example, information about a 15-month-old child's mobility may not specify whether the child crawls or walks. This information is essential for establishing the child's developmental stage.

Inconsistencies are conflicting data. Possible sources of conflicting data include: measurement error, expectations, and conflicting or unreliable reports (Gordon, 1987b, p. 259). For example, if the client reports a history of high blood pressure but the nurse obtains a low reading, the nurse should check the equipment and procedure for possible error. In another situation, a nurse may learn from the nursing history that the client reports not seeing a doctor in 15 years, yet during the physical health examination he states, "My doctor takes my blood pressure every week." All inconsistencies must be clarified before a valid pattern can be established.

Determining the Client's Health Problems, Health Risks, and Strengths

After data are processed, the nurse and the client can together identify strengths and problems. This is primarily a decision-making process.

Health Problems and Risks

During data processing, the nurse groups data according to categories and labels the clusters with tentative diagnoses. However, for health problems (existing or potential) to have a successful outcome, the client must accept the existence of the problem. The nurse, by contrast, determines whether the client needs help dealing with the problem. The nurse and the client can then make any of the following judgments (Yura and Walsh 1988, pp. 126–129):

1. No problem exists, and the client's health status is confirmed.

2. No problem exists, but there is a potential problem.

3. A problem exists, but the client is coping effectively.

4. A problem exists, and the client needs help in handling it.

5. A problem exists, but the client cannot deal with it at this time.

6. A problem requires further study and diagnosis.

TABLE 11–2 *Formulating Nursing Diagnoses for Mr. Joe Smith*

Diagnostic Category	Data Clustering/ Grouping Data	Determining Strengths and Health Problems	Formulating Nursing Diagnostic Statements
Activity intolerance	Shortness of breath Lacks energy to do daily chores Does not smoke	Does not smoke (strength) Activity intolerance (problem)	**Activity intolerance** related to shortness of breath and lack of energy secondary to decreased strength of cardiac contraction
Ineffective airway clearance	Rales in bases of both lungs relieved by coughing	Able to expel secretions by coughing (strength) Secretions in lung bases (problem)	**Potential ineffective airway clearance** postoperatively related to chest incision
Potential for injury	Left hip replacement Movement slightly limited Joint stiffness Slight limp	Carries out daily activities independently (strength) Movement slightly limited (problem)	**Potential for injury** (trauma) related to joint stiffness and limp from hip replacement surgery
Altered nutrition	Is diabetic Takes tolazamide (Tolinase) daily "No sugar" in diet "Eats a good diet" Overweight for height Weight loss of 5 pounds in past year	Controls diabetes with Tolinase and "no sugar" (strength) Weight loss of 5 pounds in past year (strength) Overweight (problem)	**Altered nutrition: more than body requirements** related to imbalance of intake versus activity expenditure
Knowledge deficit	Takes furosemide (Lasix) daily Takes Slow K daily Urinates frequently	Complies with medical regime (strength) Does not relate urinary frequency to diuretic (problem)	**Knowledge deficit:** side-effects of diuretic therapy
Altered peripheral tissue perfusion	Vital signs normal Heart rhythm regular Loud heart murmur (aortic area) Femoral pulses stronger than normal Absent pulses (popliteal, dorsalis pedis, posterior tibial) in left leg Left leg cooler than right leg Integument pink and intact	Vital signs within normal range (strength) Skin intact and of good color (strength) Impaired circulation in left leg (problem)	**Altered peripheral tissue perfusion** (left leg) related to impaired arterial circulation
Fear	Hospitalized for cardiac catheterization and possible aortic valve replacement States family "scared" about illness Wants to see chaplain Wants family to visit Perceives son Tom as helpful Says is usually too busy to worry about things	Perceives family as supportive (strength) Says family anxious about illness. Did not indicate own feelings (problem)	**Fear** related to cardiac catheterization, possible surgery, and its outcome
Pain	History of angina (6 months) Takes nitroglycerin for angina	Has not needed nitroglycerin for 2 months (strength)	**Potential (angina)** related to excessive activity or stress

7. A problem is not presently incapacitating but will be at a later date.

8. A problem places heavy demands on the client's ability to cope.

9. A problem is critical to the client.

10. The problem is long term and permanent.

See Table 11–2 for examples of Mr. Joe Smith's problems.

Strengths At this stage, the nurse and client also establish the client's strengths, resources, and abilities to cope. Generally, people have a clearer perception of their problems or weaknesses than of their strengths and assets, which are often taken for granted. By taking an inventory of strengths, the client can develop a more well-rounded self-concept and self-image. Strengths can be an aid to mobilizing health and regenerative processes.

A client's strengths might be that his weight is within the normal range for his age and height, thus enabling him to cope better with surgery. In another instance, a client's strengths might be that she is allergy-free and a nonsmoker. The same client's resources could be a supportive family and an ability to cope. Coping is a learned pattern or response that helps an individual deal with crises and stressful events. Nurses must remember, however, that because of the magnitude of an event, the number of stressful events occurring at one time, or the unfamiliarity of the situation, a client may be unable to cope and require assistance of the nurse.

A client's strengths can be found in the nursing assessment record (health, home life, education, recreation, exercise, work, family and friends, religious beliefs, and sense of humor, for example), the health examination, and the client's records. See Table 11–2 for examples of Mr. Joe Smith's strengths.

FORMULATING NURSING DIAGNOSES

At this final stage, the nurse formulates causal relationships between the health problems and the factors related to them. These factors may be, for example, environmental, sociologic, psychologic, physiologic, or spiritual. More than one factor may be related to one health problem. It is also important to determine at this time that the problem can be resolved by independent nursing interventions. If it cannot, the nurse should refer the client to the appropriate health team member. By including the causal factors in diagnostic statements, the nurse can tailor a plan of care for the client. For example, the diagnosis **Impaired physical mobility** tells the nurse the problem but does not suggest the direction the nursing intervention should take, whereas **Impaired physical mobility related to neuromuscular impairment** suggests a direction for plans and interventions to deal with the problem. Obviously, the causative factor *neuromuscular impairment* suggests a different direction than the factor *fear of falling* would.

Nurses can refer to a list of accepted nursing diagnoses, shown on the inside front cover, to select a diagnostic category. The causal factors are obtained from the data. If no causal factor appears in the data, the nurse may wish to make a tentative diagnosis based on scientific nursing knowledge and experience. The nurse should then review the database for inconsistencies and gaps and the analysis/synthesis for error. Once the causal relationships have been established, the nurse is ready to write the diagnostic statements.

Prior to writing the diagnostic statement in the care plan, the beginning diagnostician reviews the following checkpoints (Gordon 1987b, p. 257):

1. Do I understand client data, and have I verified any questionable data? Have I been careful and objective regarding my observations?

2. Have I recognized diagnostic cues accurately?

3. Have I processed data and reports accurately? Did I test data with standards and compare data from different sources to ensure accuracy?

4. Have I considered several tentative diagnoses to explain the cues, and ruled out incorrect ones?

5. Have I reviewed all the *major* and *minor* defining characteristics for the tentative diagnostic statements? See *Nursing Diagnosis Format* below. Have I accurately assessed the client for these signs and symptoms?

6. Do I have adequate cues to support the formulation of the nursing diagnoses?

See Table 11–2 for Mr. Joe Smith's nursing diagnostic statements.

Nursing Diagnosis Format

There are three essential components of nursing diagnostic statements; they are referred to as the **PES format** (Gordon 1976, p. 1299). Nurses need to consider these components when developing new diagnostic categories and writing diagnoses for specific clients. The components are:

1. *The terms describing the problem (P).* This component, referred to as the *diagnostic category label* or *title,* is a description of the client's (individual, family, community) health problem (actual or potential) for which nursing therapy is given. The state of the client is described clearly and concisely in a few words. See the inside back cover for a list of nursing diagnostic categories adopted by the Ninth National Conference on Classification of Nursing Diagnoses in 1990. To be clinically useful, category labels need to be specific. When the word *specify* follows a category label in the list on the inside back-cover, the nurse states the area in which the problem occurs. For example, a knowledge deficit may be in the area of medication prescription, dietary adjustments, or disease process and therapy.

2. *The etiology of the problem (E)* or contributing factors.

This component identifies one or more probable causes of the health problem and gives direction to the required nursing therapy. Etiology may include behaviors of the client, environmental factors, or interactions of the two. For example, the probable causes of alteration in health maintenance include perceptual or cognitive impairment, lack of gross or fine motor skills, lack of material resources, and ineffective individual coping. See Table 11–3. Several authors have identified etiologies for many diagnoses (Carpenito 1989, Gordon 1987a, Kim and McFarland 1989). Differentiating among possible causes in the nursing diagnosis is essential because each may require different nursing therapies.

3. *The defining characteristics or cluster of signs and symptoms (S).* The defining characteristics provide information necessary to arrive at the diagnostic category label (component 1). Each nursing diagnostic category is associated with signs and symptoms that occur as a clinical entity. *Major* signs and symptoms are those that must be present to make a valid diagnosis. *Minor* characteristics may or may not be present. Nursing diagnostic categories are similar to medical diagnostic categories. For example, the medical diagnostic category myocardial infarction (heart attack) is associated with a standard set of signs and symptoms that are universally understood and accepted. Likewise, the nursing diagnostic category **Altered health maintenance** is associated with a standard cluster of signs and symptoms. See Table 11–3. For most nursing diagnoses the list of defining characteristics is still being developed and refined. Partial listings have been published to assist nurses in developing and validating nursing diagnoses.

Writing a Diagnostic Statement

A nursing diagnostic statement (nursing diagnosis) is a clear statement about a client's actual or potential health problem that is within the scope of independent nursing intervention. It is the outcome of the diagnostic process: the second phase in the nursing process.

Nurses may write diagnoses as either two-part or three-part statements. The two-part nursing diagnostic statement includes

1. Problem (P)—Statement of the client's response
2. Etiology (E)—Factors contributing to or probable causes of the responses

The two parts are joined by the words *related to* or *associated with* rather than *due to*. The phrase *due to* implies a cause-and-effect relationship; one clause causes or is responsible for the other clause. By contrast, the phrases *related to* and *associated with* merely imply a relationship. The phrase *related to* is most commonly used. If one part of the diagnostic statement changes, the other part may change as well. Legal hazards are thus avoided. Here are some examples of nursing diagnoses containing two parts:

- **Ineffective breathing pattern** (problem) related to *pain* (etiology)
- **Disturbance in self-esteem** (problem) related to *altered body image* (*loss of arm*)(etiology)
- **Grieving** (problem) related to *anticipated loss* (etiology) secondary to *husband's illness* (etiology)

A three-part nursing diagnosis statement includes

1. Problem (P)—Statement of the client's response

TABLE 11–3 *Components of a Nursing Diagnostic Category*

Diagnosis	Definition	Etiology	Defining Characteristics
Altered health maintenance	Inability to identify, manage, and/or seek out help to maintain health	Lack of or significant alteration in communication skills (written, verbal, and/or gestural)	Demonstrated lack of knowledge regarding basic health practices
		Lack of ability to make deliberate and thoughtful judgments	Demonstrated lack of adaptive behaviors to internal or external environmental changes
		Perceptual or cognitive impairment	Reported or observed inability to take the responsibility for meeting basic health practices in any or all functional pattern areas
		Complete or partial lack of gross and/or fine motor skills	
		Ineffective individual coping; dysfunctional grieving	History of lack of health-seeking behavior
		Lack of material resources	Expressed interest in improving health behaviors
		Unachieved developmental tasks	Reported or observed lack of equipment, financial, and/or other resources
		Ineffective family coping: disabling spiritual distress	Reported or observed impairment of personal support system

Source: M. J. Kim, G. K. McFarland, and A. M. McLane, editors, *Pocket guide to nursing diagnoses,* 3d ed. St. Louis: C. V. Mosby Co., 1989), pp. 29–30. Used by permission.

2. Etiology (E)—Factors contributing to or probable causes of the response

3. Signs and symptoms (S)—Defining characteristics manifested by the client

The three-part diagnostic statement includes the problem, the etiology, and the observed signs and symptoms (PES). Actual nursing diagnoses can be documented by using the three-part statement (using *related to* and *manifested by*), since the signs and symptoms have been identified. Several alternatives for writing the PES format have been suggested (Carpenito 1987, Guzzetta 1988).

1. Nurses learning to write diagnoses may find it helpful to list the signs and symptoms before (even though the S is last) or after the two-part diagnostic statement in a care plan format. The defining characteristics may include both objective and subjective data.

2. Signs and symptoms may be written after the diagnostic statement joined by the words *manifested by* or *evidenced by*.

Here are some examples of three-part statements:

- **Disturbance in self-esteem** (problem) related to *altered body image (loss of arm)* (etiology) manifested by *crying and hostility* (signs and symptoms)

- **Anticipatory grieving** (problem) related to *husband's terminal illness* (etiology) manifested by *anorexia and withdrawn behavior* (signs and symptoms)

- **Altered family processes** (problem) related to *mother's hospitalization* (etiology) as manifested by son's *unmet physical and emotional needs* (signs and symptoms)

Potential nursing diagnoses are used when a client's responses can be predicted or when health promotion can contribute to well-being. Predictable responses are based on a client's health history, known complications of a disease process, or the nurse's experience. For example, a client who has smoked two packages of cigarettes per day for 40 years may have a potential postoperative nursing diagnosis of **Potential for ineffective airway clearance** (P) related to *smoking* (E).

Possible nursing diagnoses are used when evidence about a response is unclear or when the related factors are unknown. The nurse writes the possible nursing diagnosis and collects more data either to support or refute the possible response. For example, an elderly widow who lives alone is admitted to hospital. The nurse notices that she has no visitors and is pleased with attention and conversation from the nursing staff. Until more data are collected, the nurse may write a possible nursing diagnosis of **Social isolation** related to *unknown etiology*. Characteristics of a diagnostic statement are summarized in the accompanying box.

Common Diagnostic Errors

Clear, concise, client-centered nursing diagnoses can be written by following the guidelines presented in Table 11–4. Some common errors in writing diagnostic statements are

1. Writing the client's response as a need instead of a problem

2. Using judgmental statements

3. Placing the etiology before the client's response

4. Using statements that provide no specific direction for planning independent nursing interventions

5. Using medical rather than nursing terminology

6. Starting the diagnosis with a nursing intervention

7. Using a single symptom as the client's response

The accuracy of nursing diagnostic statements also depends on a complete database and appropriate data processing. If data are omitted, a diagnosis can be missed. If data are not processed properly, e.g., are not clustered appropriately, a diagnosis can be made prematurely or incorrectly, or be missed. Gordon (1987b, p. 286) categorizes diagnostic errors as (a) errors of omission, i.e., failure to diagnose a problem and (b) errors of commission, i.e., diagnosing a problem when no problem exists. Both errors can occur during data collection, data interpretation, and data clustering.

To avoid such errors during assessment, the nurse needs to ensure that relevant data are not missed and that large quantities of irrelevant data are not obtained. The nurse can prevent data omissions by using an organized assessment plan, striving for accuracy, and drawing on personal knowledge. Collecting irrelevant data can be avoided if the nurse asks appropriate questions. An overload of irrelevant data hinders the nurse's capacity to process information.

Data interpretation errors occur when the meaning of cues is misinterpreted. The nurse can avoid inaccurate interpretation of cues by determining how the client perceives the health problem, its probable cause, and actions taken to remedy it. For example, the nurse observes that a client repeatedly gets out of bed after the physician has ordered complete bed rest. The nurse may interpret this behavior as noncompliance. However, the client may be experiencing diarrhea and may be embarrassed to use the bedpan or may be refusing to accept a dependent sick role. Obviously, inaccurate interpretation of cues leads to diagnostic errors. Another source of diagnostic errors in data interpretation is overgeneralization from one isolated observation of client behavior. For example, one episode of angry behavior does not mean that the client is hostile.

A diagnosis may be made prematurely, before all relevant data have been considered or collected. For example, a nurse, learning of a client's history of angina and his pre-

---

Characteristics of a Diagnostic Statement

- A diagnostic statement is clear and concise.
- It is specific and client centered.
- It relates to one client problem.
- It is accurate.
- It is based on reliable and relevant assessment data.

TABLE 11-4 *Guidelines for Writing a Nursing Diagnostic Statement*

Guideline	Correct Statement	Incorrect and/or Ambiguous Statement
1. State in terms of a problem, not a need	**Actual fluid volume deficit** (problem) related to fever	**Fluid replacement** (need) related to fever
2. State so that it is legally advisable	**Impaired skin integrity** related to immobility (legally acceptable)	**Impaired skin integrity** related to improper positioning (implies legal liability)
3. Use nonjudgmental statements	**Spiritual distress** related to inability to attend church services secondary to immobility (nonjudgmental)	**Spiritual distress** related to strict rules necessitating church attendance (judgmental)
4. Make sure that both elements of the statement do *not* say the same thing	**Potential impaired skin integrity** related to immobility	**Impaired skin integrity** related to ulceration of sacral area (response and probable cause are the same)
5. Make sure that the client's response precedes the contributing or causal factor	**Noncompliance with diet** (response) related to lack of knowledge (contributing factor)	**Knowledge deficit** (contributing factor) related to noncompliance with diet (response)
6. Use statements that provide guidance for planning independent nursing interventions	**Social isolation** related to loss of speech (loss of speech provides direction for planning alternative communication methods)	**Social isolation** related to laryngectomy (the nurse can do nothing about the laryngectomy)
7. Word diagnosis specifically and precisely to provide direction for planning nursing intervention	**Altered oral mucous membrane** related to decreased salivation secondary to radiation of neck (specific)	**Altered oral mucous membrane** related to noxious agent (vague)
8. Use nursing terminology rather than medical terminology to describe the client's response	**Potential ineffective airway clearance** (nursing terminology)	**Potential pneumonia** (medical terminology)
9. Use nursing terminology rather than medical terminology to describe the probable cause of the client's response	**Potential ineffective airway clearance** related to accumulation of secretions in lungs (nursing terminology)	**Potential ineffective airway clearance** related to emphysema (medical terminology)
10. Do not start the nursing diagnosis with a nursing intervention	**Altered nutrition: less than body requirements** related to inadequate intake of protein (directs but does not state nursing intervention)	Provide high-protein diet because of **Potential altered nutrition** (starts with nursing intervention)
11. Avoid using a symptom such as nausea as the client's response. A symptom does not reflect a pattern and requires additional data collection	Insufficient data for a diagnosis	**Nausea** related to medication

scription for nitroglycerin, may write this diagnostic statement: **Pain (anginal).** Additional data, however, reveal that angina has not been a problem since the client had cardiac bypass surgery a year ago and that pain is therefore not a current problem.

Incorrect clustering of data also leads to diagnostic errors. For example, by clustering "urinary frequency" and "has diabetes," the nurse could erroneously begin a diagnostic statement for Mr. Joe Smith with **Altered urinary elimination pattern.** However, clustering other data such as "takes furosemide (Lasix, a diuretic) daily," "shortness of breath," "no energy," and "aortic valve insufficiency," changes

the diagnostic focus from a urinary problem to **Activity intolerance** or **Decreased cardiac output.**

THE NURSING DIAGNOSIS MOVEMENT

The identification and development of nursing diagnoses began formally in 1973 when the National Conference Group for the Generation and Classification of Nursing Diagnoses was formed. This group originated through the efforts of two faculty members of Saint Louis University, Kristine Gebbie and Mary Ann Lavin, who perceived a need to identify their roles in an ambulatory care setting. The First National Conference held to identify nursing diagnoses was sponsored by the Saint Louis University School of Nursing and Allied Health Professions in 1973. Since that time, national conferences have been held in 1975, 1978, 1980, 1982, 1984, 1986, 1988, and 1990. The proceedings of the conferences have been published (Gebbie and Lavin 1975; Gebbie 1976; Kim and Moritz 1982; Kim, MacFarland, and McLane 1984; Hurley 1986; McLane 1987). Through the efforts of these groups, much progress has been made in defining, classifying, and describing nursing diagnoses. International recognition was shown by the First Canadian Conference, held in Toronto in 1977, and the International Nursing Conference held in May 1987 in Calgary, Alberta, Canada. In 1982, the conference group accepted the name North American Nursing Diagnosis Association (NANDA), thus recognizing the participation and contributions of nurses in the United

States and Canada. The purpose of NANDA is to "define, refine and promote a taxonomy of nursing diagnostic terminology of general use to professional nurses" (NANDA 1982). The members of NANDA include staff nurses, clinical specialists, faculty, directors of nursing, deans, theorists, and researchers. In 1988, NANDA and the American Nurses' Association established a collaborative working agreement to "pursue development of the taxonomy" (Gordon 1988). The system developed by NANDA is recognized as the diagnostic classification system for the nursing profession. The group has currently approved approximately 100 nursing diagnostic categories or labels for clinical use and testing. See the list on the inside back cover.

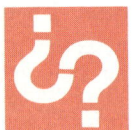

RESEARCH NOTE

Are Nursing Diagnoses Actually Used?

The researchers in this project were interested in determining if the list of nursing diagnoses that was prepared by the North American Nursing Diagnosis Association were actually being used. In particular, they were interested in their use in diagnosing the needs of the elderly.

To examine this, they gathered data from elderly residents in a large long-term care facility in Iowa and compared their findings with the results of four other studies that were done in similar settings.

They discovered that the following nursing diagnoses were used with more than 10% of the patients in these facilities:

- Impaired physical mobility
- Altered thought process
- Impaired skin integrity
- Pain
- Constipation
- Altered nutrition: less than body requirements

These findings indicated that the listings that were developed by NANDA to describe nursing diagnoses were being used and that they were useful in actual practice.

Implications: Studies such as this one bring credibility to NANDA'S efforts to establish professional standards and descriptions of the diagnoses that nurses will use in a variety of health care settings.

M. Hardy, M. Maas, and J. Akins, The prevalence of nursing diagnoses among elderly and long-term care residents: A descriptive study. In R. M. Carroll-Johnson, editor, *Classification of nursing diagnoses, Proceedings of the Eighth Conference* (Philadelphia, J. B. Lippincott, 1989).

Approval of Nursing Diagnosis Categories

Nursing diagnosis categories approved by NANDA are recognized by the nursing profession as areas of concern in education, practice, and research. Kritek (1986, p. 36) states that nursing diagnoses should be generated and classified simultaneously. Each process enhances and challenges the other. Professional nurses wishing to submit a nursing diagnosis to NANDA do so through a review process developed by the Diagnosis Review Committee (DRC). In the first step of the review process, the DRC reviews the proposed diagnosis, requests critiques from a task force of appropriate clinical experts, and then makes recommendations to the NANDA Board of Directors. The diagnoses accepted by the board are then presented to the members of NANDA at the biennial meeting for approval. Finally, the diagnosis is either accepted or rejected by the membership through a mail ballot. Diagnoses accepted by the membership are then included in the approved NANDA taxonomy. These diagnoses or categories are considered diagnoses to be tested and used in clinical practice. The categories are tentative and will be modified and/or refined as necessary, according to clinical research data. At present these labels are considered the standard for use in the United States and Canada and represent a professional focus for independent nursing practice.

Taxonomy of Nursing Diagnoses

A **taxonomy** is a classification system of groups, classes, or sets. A taxonomy may be natural or artificial and hierarchic or nonhierarchic (Rasch 1987). Animals and plants, for example, are classified in a taxonomy that is hierarchic, which means that the groups are increasingly inclusive and thus more general. The genus contains one or more species; the family, one or more genera; and so on. One example of a nonhierarchic taxonomy is a telephone book in which numbers are arranged alphabetically by last name or by category (e.g., florists, plumbers, and so on). A taxonomy is natural when the characteristics of the groupings are considered basic or fundamental to them. The classification of people according to gender is an example of a natural division.

The first taxonomy of nursing diagnoses was done in 1973, at the First National Conference on the Classification of Nursing Diagnoses. Following the approval of the 31 diagnostic categories, the diagnoses were then grouped alphabetically (Gebbie and Lavin, 1975). The nonhierarchic alphabetical ordering (see inside front cover) was considered unscientific by some, and a hierarchic structure was sought.

NANDA's Taxonomy I, Revised

In 1978, the Nurse Theorist Group of NANDA proposed the utilization of the "nine patterns of unitary man" as an organizing principle. This proposal was accepted by NANDA in 1982. An initial taxonomic tree was generated. One of the major reasons for classifying and coding nursing diagnosis is to facilitate computer storage and access of information.

In 1984 NANDA renamed the "patterns of unitary man" as "human response patterns." See the box below. In 1986, NANDA accepted the system as *Taxonomy I* (McLane, 1987). In 1988, some refinements and revisions were made after the acceptance of new diagnoses, and the new taxonomy was called *Taxonomy I, Revised*. All nursing diagnoses, once accepted, now become subcategories of these nine human response patterns. For example, the human response pattern *Feeling* includes:

- Anxiety
- Pain or chronic pain
- Grieving (anticipatory, dysfunctional)
- Fear
- Potential for violence (self-directed or directed at others)
- Post-trauma response
- Rape-trauma syndrome (compound reaction, silent reaction)

The taxonomy is numerically coded and organized from the most abstract (Level I) to the most concrete (Level IV or V). Each of the nine human response patterns constitute Level I concepts, which are the most abstract. Level II concepts refer to alterations in the human response patterns, and subsequent levels refer to more specific responses. See

Appendix C for the coding of all nine human response patterns and their related nursing diagnoses.

Translating Taxonomy I Revised into ICD Code

To prepare the taxonomy for possible inclusion into the World Health Organization's 10th revision of the *International Classification of Diseases* (ICD 10), the NANDA Taxonomy Committee, in liaison with the American Nurses' Association, made further revisions to conform to the ICD framework (Fitzpatrick et al. 1989, pp. 493–495).

These revisions approved by the NANDA board include:

1. Arranging the nine human response patterns in alphabetical order: choosing, communicating, exchanging, feeling, knowing, moving, perceiving, relating, and valuing.

2. Decreasing the levels of abstraction from four, five, or six levels to only two levels.

3. Modifying the diagnostic coding to meet ICD criteria. A four character code is used: an alphabetical character (Y) is placed first, followed by three numerical characters. For example Y27.1 is the code for **Skin integrity, impaired.**

The box below indicates the proposed ICD-10 version of the first (previously fifth) human response pattern: *Choosing*. Note that there are some changes in wording from previously accepted NANDA diagnostic labels; e.g., the word "ineffective" is changed to "impaired."

Human Response Patterns

1. Exchanging: mutual giving and receiving.
2. Communicating: sending messages
3. Relating: establishing bonds
4. Valuing: assigning relative worth
5. Choosing: selection of alternatives
6. Moving: activity
7. Perceiving: reception of information
8. Knowing: meaning associated with information
9. Feeling: subjective awareness of information

Proposed ICD-10 Version of the First Human Response Pattern

Human Response Pattern: Choosing

Y100	Family coping, impaired*
Y00.0	Compromised
Y00.1	Disabled
Y01	[Health-seeking behavior]†
Y01.0–9	Health-seeking behaviors (specify)
Y02	Individual coping, impaired*
Y02.0	Adjustment, impaired
Y02.1	Conflict: decisional
Y02.2	Coping: defensive
Y02.3	Denial, impaired*
Y02.4	Noncompliance

---

*Denotes change in wording from previously accepted NANDA diagnostic label.
†Item in brackets is not an accepted diagnosis.

Source: J. J. Fitzpatrick, M. E. Kerr, V. K. Saba, L. M. Hoskins, M. L. Hurley, W. C. Mills, B. C. Rottkamp, J. J. Warren, and L. J. Carpenito, Nursing diagnosis: Translating nursing diagnosis into ICD code, *American Journal of Nursing* April 1989, 89:494.

Advantages of a Nursing Diagnosis Taxonomy

■ *Nursing diagnosis promotes professional accountability and autonomy by defining and describing the independent area of nursing practice.* It provides a standardized terminology for categorizing clusters of signs and symptoms for specific conditions. These category names, such as **Knowledge deficit** or **Self-care deficit** focus the nursing interventions needed to achieve the desired outcomes (Maas and Hardy 1988, p. 13).

■ *Nursing diagnoses provide an effective vehicle for communication among nurses and other health care professionals.* Because a nursing diagnosis consolidates a great deal of information into concise statements and includes assessment parameters, it provides a shorthand method of communication. A nurse who knows that a client has a certain nursing diagnosis knows about that client's problem, the causal or contributing factors, and the necessary nursing actions.

■ *Nursing diagnoses provide an organizing principle for the building of meaningful research.* A valid nursing diagnosis taxonomy would more clearly define the scope of nursing practice. This ability to access such client data in relation to their nursing diagnoses would provide a framework for testing the validity of nursing interventions and also provide feedback for further development of nursing's unique body of knowledge. In addition, the organization of data in this manner would facilitate retrieval and analysis by computer-based information systems.

Challenges for the Future

The evolution of nursing diagnostic categories is in its early developmental stages, and the list of diagnoses is not to be considered a comprehensive guide for nursing practice.

Although some nurses feel constrained and frustrated with the existing list of diagnoses, it is well to remember that disciplines with well-established taxonomies, such as medicine, have taken many decades to develop. Each NANDA publication emphasizes that the existing list is not at all definitive. McLane (1987, p. 469) states that this taxonomy "is an investment by NANDA which can be . . . tested, refined, revised and expanded. A major task of all nurses is to locate diagnoses that are neglected, to test and develop them, and to present them for inclusion in future listings."

A relationship between the nursing diagnosis taxonomy and theoretical frameworks for nursing is yet to be demonstrated. The diagnostic focus of proposed conceptual frameworks for nursing depends on the concepts outlined in the nursing theory. For this reason, such frameworks do not necessarily fit the taxonomy of nursing diagnoses. This point is illustrated in Table 11–5, which gives examples of the diagnostic focus of two nursing theories. Dialogue between nursing practitioners and theorists is essential for continued development in this area.

The taxonomy needs to be tested for reliability and validity. Although it has been approved and accepted by participants at the national NANDA conferences, the usefulness of each diagnostic category must still be validated by appropriate research. **Validation** is the determination that the diagnosis accurately reflects the problem of the client, that the methods used for data gathering were valid, and that the conclusion or diagnosis is justified by the data.

There is some concern that the use of nursing diagnoses may lead to stereotyping by the nurse and lessen the client's role in the decision-making process. Nurses must ensure that the client's perception of the problem is the focus of care. They need to be aware of the problems involved in professional labeling and make every effort to provide individualized client care. Henderson (1987, p. 15) suggests the use of client questionnaires to maintain a consistent approach.

A weakness of the present nursing diagnoses taxonomy is the lack of focus on health promotion and health edu-

TABLE 11–5 *Variations of Diagnostic Focus and Contributing Factors in Selected Conceptual Frameworks for Nursing*

Nursing Theory	Diagnostic Focus	Contributing Factors (Etiology)
Orem's self-care agency theory	Actual or potential deficit between the powers of self-care agency and the demands placed on it in relation to three self-care categories: 1. Universal 2. Developmental 3. Health deviation	Lack of knowledge, skills, interest, or motivation; disease process; or type of therapy
Roy's adaptation theory	Actual maladaptation problems or potential adaptation problems in relation to four modes: 1. Physiologic 2. Self-concept 3. Role function 4. Interdependence	Coping activity that is inadequate to maintain integrity in the face of a need deficit or excess

cation. Nationally and internationally there is now an emphasis on consumer education and activities to promote a healthy life-style. However, the present taxonomy of nursing diagnoses is mainly focused on client problems. Assessing the strengths of the client and promoting wellness activities are also important nursing functions and should be more visible in the nursing diagnoses taxonomy. See examples of wellness diagnoses in Chapter 23.

The development of *Taxonomy I, Revised* based on the nine human response patterns is receiving some criticism. Porter (1986, p. 136) points out that the human response patterns provide a theoretical or conceptual framework for the diagnostic categories rather than a true taxonomic structure that is based on principles of classification. Modifications therefore may need to be made to *Taxonomy I, Revised,* or an alternative taxonomy may have to be developed.

One of the major purposes of nursing diagnoses is to establish a method of validating independent nursing functions that would define nursing's unique role. A major task that is yet to be considered is the development of nursing interventions specific to each nursing diagnosis. Nurses will be accountable for these prescribed interventions. To date, a taxonomy of accepted clinical nursing interventions does not exist. However, lists of independent nursing functions are being developed. See Chapter 13 for further information.

CHAPTER HIGHLIGHTS

▶ A nursing diagnosis is a statement of an actual or potential health problem amenable to independent nursing intervention.

▶ The diagnostic process is one of analysis and synthesis.

▶ The cognitive skills for analysis/synthesis are objectivity, critical thinking, decision making, and deductive and inductive reasoning.

▶ The three phases of the diagnostic process are data processing; determination of the client's health problems, health risks, and strengths; and formulation of nursing diagnoses.

▶ A nursing diagnostic statement should be clear, concise, client-centered, related to one problem, and based on reliable and relevant assessment data.

▶ A nursing diagnostic statement may have two or three parts: A two-part statement includes (a) the client's response and (b) factors contributing to the response or probable causes of the response. A three-part statement includes the defining characteristics of the problem as well.

▶ Nursing diagnoses provide direction for planning independent nursing interventions.

▶ A valid nursing diagnoses taxonomy would define the independent scope of practice, facilitate nursing research, and clarify communication among nurses and other health professionals.

▶ The development of a taxonomy of nursing diagnoses is an ongoing process.

READINGS AND REFERENCES

SUGGESTED READINGS

Gordon, M. December 1987. Implementation of nursing diagnoses: An overview. *Nursing Clinics of North America* 22:875–879.
  Gordon discusses some of the forces fueling the diagnosis movement including professional policy and practice changes and the usefulness of diagnosis to communicate and demonstrate nursing's productivity and effectiveness. The history of the North American effort to identify and classify nursing diagnosis is also outlined briefly.

Hutcherson, A. H. July/August 1989. Care plan hints. *Advanced Clinical Care* 4:8–10.
  Examples illustrate the use of defining characteristics. These examples help explain the relationship of the various components of the care plan and the nursing process.

Rasch, R. F. R. Fall 1987. The nature of taxonomy. *Image: Journal of Nursing Scholarship* 19:147–149.
  Rasch discusses the general characteristics of a taxonomy and the approaches that can be used to develop a taxonomy. The history of the NANDA taxonomy is reviewed and critiqued, and

the problems in the development of *Taxonomy I* are presented.

Tribulski, J. December 1988. Nursing diagnosis: Waste of time or valued tool? *RN* 51:30–34.
  Tribulski uses a case study to demonstrate the importance and practical use of nursing diagnosis. The common complaints related to using nursing diagnosis are presented and challenged, and guidelines are offered for writing diagnoses and developing a plan of care.

RELATED RESEARCH

Brunckhorst, L.; Placzek, L.; Payne, J.; McInerney, J.; and Parzuchowski, J. February 1989. Who's using nursing diagnoses? *American Journal of Nursing* 89:267–268.

Fredette, S. L., and O'Neill, E. S. 1987. Can theory improve diagnosis? An examination of the relationship between didactic content and the ability to diagnose in clinical practice. In AM McLane, editor. pp. 423–435. *Classification of nursing diagnoses: Proceedings of the seventh national conference.* St. Louis: C. V. Mosby, 1987.

Hardy, M., Maas, M., and Akins, J. 1989. The prevalence of nursing diagnoses among the elderly and long-term care residents: A descriptive study. In R. M. Carroll-Johnson, editor. *Classification of nursing diagnoses, Proceedings of the eighth national conference*. Philadelphia: J. B. Lippincott Co., 1989.

Holden, G. W., and Klingner, A. M. January 1988. Learning from experience: Differences in how novice vs. expert nurses diagnose why an infant is crying. *Journal of Nursing Education* 27:23–29.

Johnson, C. F., and Hales, L. W. January/February 1989. Nursing diagnosis anyone? Do staff nurses use nursing diagnoses effectively? *Journal of Continuing Education in Nursing* 20:30–35.

Levin, R. F.; Krainovitch, B. C.; Bahrenburg, E.; and Mitchell, C. A. Spring 1989. Diagnostic content validity of nursing diagnoses. *Image: Journal of Nursing Scholarship* 21:40–44.

SELECTED REFERENCES

Abdellah, F. G. June 1957. Methods of identifying covert aspects of nursing. A key to improved clinical teaching. *Nursing Research* 57:4–23.

Alfaro, R. 1990. *Applying Nursing Process and Diagnosis: A step-by-step guide*. 2nd ed. Philadelphia: J. B. Lippincott Co.

Baretich, D. M., and Anderson, L. B. September 1987. Diagnostics. Should we diagnose strengths? No—stick to the problem. *American Journal of Nursing* 87:1211–1212.

Carpenito, L. J. 1991. *Nursing diagnosis: Application to clinical practice*. 4th ed. Philadelphia: J. B. Lippincott Co.

———. 1991. *Handbook of Nursing Diagnosis*. Philadelphia: J. B. Lippincott Co.

Derdiarian, A. March 1988. A valid profession needs valid diagnoses. *Nursing and Health Care*. 9:136–140.

Edel, M. 1982. The nature of nursing diagnosis. In Carlson, J. H., Craft, C. A., and McGuire, A. D. *Nursing diagnosis*. Philadelphia: W. B. Saunders Co.

Gebbie, K. M. 1976. *Classification of nursing diagnoses: Summary of the second national conference*. St. Louis: C. V. Mosby Co.

Gebbie, K. M., and Lavin, M. A., editors. 1975. *Classification of nursing diagnoses*: Proceedings of the First National Conference. St. Louis: C. V. Mosby Co.

Gordon, M. August 1976. Nursing diagnosis and the diagnostic process. *American Journal of Nursing*. 76:1298–300.

———. 1987a. *Manual of nursing diagnosis*. New York: McGraw Hill.

———. 1987b. *Nursing diagnosis: Process and application. 2d. ed.* New York: McGraw-Hill.

———. December 1987c. Implementation of nursing diagnoses. An overview. *Nursing Clinics of North America*. 22:875–879.

———. Summer 1988. President's column. North American Nursing Diagnosis Association. *Nursing Diagnosis Newsletter*. 15:4–5.

Griffith, J. W., and Christensen, P. J., editors. 1986. *Nursing process: Application of theories, frameworks, and models*. 2d ed. St. Louis: C. V. Mosby Co.

Guzzetta, C. 1988. Nursing diagnosis. In McCann Flynn, J. B., and Burroughs Heffron, P. *Nursing: From concept to practice*. 2d ed. Norwalk, Conn: Appleton & Lange.

Guzzetta, C.; Bunton, S.; Prinkey, L.; Sherer, A.; and Seifert, P. 1989. *Clinical assessment tools for use with nursing diagnosis*. St. Louis: C. V. Mosby Co.

Hannah, K. J.; Reimer, M.; Mills, W. C.; and Letourneau, S., editors. 1987. *Clinical judgment and decision making: The future with nursing diagnosis*. New York: John Wiley and Sons.

Henderson, V. May 1987. Nursing process—A critique. *Holistic Nursing Practice* 1:7–18.

Hurley, M. E., editor. 1986. *Classification of nursing diagnoses. Proceedings of the sixth conference. North American Nursing Diagnosis Association*. St. Louis: C. V. Mosby Co.

James, S., and Mott, S. 1988. *Child Health Nursing*. Menlo Park, Calif. Addison-Wesley Publishing Co.

Kim, M. J., McFarland, G. K., and McLane, A. M. 1989. *Pocket guide to nursing diagnoses,* 3d ed. St. Louis: C. V. Mosby Co.

Kim, M. J., McFarland, G. K., and McLane, A. M., editors. 1984. *Classification of nursing diagnoses: Proceedings of the Fifth National Conference*. St. Louis: C. V. Mosby Co.

Kim, M. J., and Moritz, D. A., editors. 1982. *Classification of nursing diagnosis: Proceedings of the Third and Fourth National Conferences*. New York: McGraw-Hill.

Kritek, P. P. 1986. Development of a taxonomic structure for nursing diagnoses: A review and an update. In Hurley, M. E., editor. *Classification of nursing diagnoses. Proceedings of the sixth conference. North American Nursing Diagnosis Association*. St. Louis: C. V. Mosby Co.

Lederer, J. R.; Marculescu, G.; Mocnik, B.; and Seaby, N. 1990. *Care planning pocket guide: A nursing diagnosis approach*. 3d ed. Redwood City, Calif.: Addison-Wesley Nursing.

Maas, M., and Hardy, M. March 1988. Focus: Nursing diagnosis. A challenge for the future. *Journal of Gerontological Nursing* 14:8–13.

McLane, A. M., editor. 1987. *Classification of nursing diagnoses: Proceedings of the Seventh Conference*. St. Louis, C. V. Mosby Co. North American Nursing Diagnosis Association. 1982 Bylaws. St. Louis, Mo.

———. Summer 1988. NANDA approved nursing diagnostic categories for clinical use and testing. *Nursing Diagnoses Newsletter* 15:1–3.

Popkess-Vawter, S., and Pinnell, N. September 1987. Diagnostics. Should we diagnose strengths? Yes: Accentuate the positive. *American Journal of Nursing*. 87:1211, 1216.

Porter, E. J. Winter 1986. Critical analysis of NANDA nursing diagnosis taxonomy I. *Image: Journal of Nursing Scholarship* 18:136–139.

Rasch, R. F. R. Fall 1987. The nature of taxonomy. *Image: Journal of Nursing Scholarship*. 19:147–149.

Risner, P. B. Analysis and Synthesis. 1986a. In Griffith, J. W., and Christensen, P. J., editors. pp. 124–150. *Nursing process: Application of theories, frameworks, and models*. St. Louis: C. V. Mosby Co.

———. 1986b. Nursing diagnosis. In Griffith, J. W., and Christensen, P. J., editors. pp. 151–168. *Nursing process: Application of theories, frameworks, and models*. St. Louis: C. V. Mosby Co.

Roy, C. 1984. *Introduction to nursing: An adaptation model*. Englewood Cliffs, N. J.: Prentice-Hall.

Shoemaker, J. 1984. *Essential features of nursing diagnoses*. In Kim, M. J., McFarland, G. K., and McLane, A. M., editors. pp. 104–115. *Classification of nursing diagnoses: Proceedings of the Fifth National Conference*. St. Louis: . V. Mosby Co.

Turkoski, B. May/June 1988. Nursing diagnosis in print, 1950–1985. *Nursing Outlook* 36:142–144.

Woolley, N. January 1990. Nursing diagnosis: Exploring the factors which may influence the reasoning process. *Journal of Advanced Nursing* 15:110–7.

Yura, H., and Walsh, M. B. 1988. *The nursing process: Assessing, planning, implementing, evaluating*. 5th ed. Norwalk, Conn. Appleton & Lange.

Planning

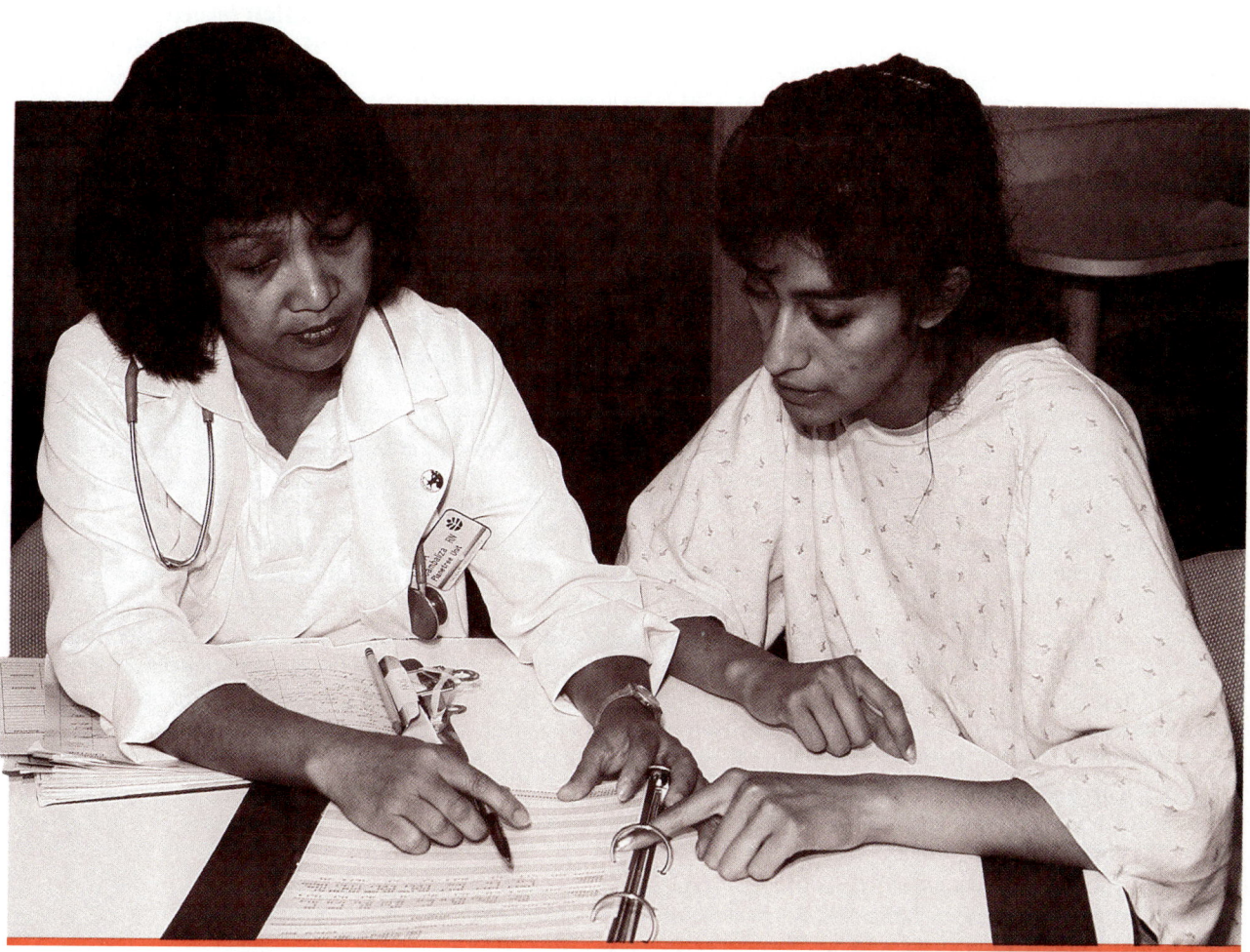

OBJECTIVES

▶ Describe the essential aspects of the planning phase of the nursing process.

▶ Identify four components of planning.

▶ Identify criteria that help the nurse and client set priorities.

▶ State the purposes of establishing client goals.

▶ Describe the relationship of goals to the nursing diagnoses.

▶ Differentiate between goals and outcome criteria.

▶ Identify guidelines for writing goals and outcome criteria.

▶ Describe three aspects of planning nursing strategies.

▶ Identify major purposes of a written care plan.

DEFINITION AND PROCESS

In general, planning is designing or arranging the parts of something to achieve an end or goal. In nursing, planning is the third step of the nursing process. In this context, **planning** is the process of designing the nursing strategies or interventions required to prevent, reduce, or eliminate those client health problems identified and validated during the diagnostic phase. The following people can be involved in planning nursing strategies: one or more nurses; the client, family members, support persons, and/or caregivers; and sometimes members of other health professions. Although the planning process is basically the responsibility of the nurse, input from the client and support persons is essential if a plan is to be effective. It is no longer sufficient that nurses plan *for* the client; whenever possible, the client must participate actively.

For a client in a home setting, the home health care nurse needs to involve the client, if the client's health permits, as well as the client's support persons and/or the caregiver. With the nurse's guidance, these people can implement the plan of care; thus, its effectiveness depends largely on them. They can also provide information about problems previously unknown to the nurse. For example, Mrs. Robson is a 59-year-old woman with impaired physical mobility because of paralysis of her right side. Her 60-year-old husband cares for her at home. One of the client's health problems is **Bathing/hygiene self-care deficit** related to impaired physical mobility of the right side. Mrs. Robson is developing skin irritations of the groin and inner thighs. One of the alternative nursing strategies could be: "Demonstrate for the husband how to lift Mrs. Robson onto a seat in the bathtub," where thorough washing can be carried out. However, Mr. Robson explains that he is unable to lift or exert himself because of heart disease. It is then necessary to consider alternative ways of washing Mrs. Robson's perineal area or other ways for her to move into the tub. The nurse may have remained unaware of the husband's heart condition had Mr. Robson not been involved in developing nursing strategies to deal with the problem.

When a client is admitted to the hospital or long-term care setting, it is important for the nurse to know if the person required care at home prior to admission. If care was necessary, input from the family and other caregivers assists the nursing staff in continuing to implement appropriate interventions and thus provide the client optimum continuity of care.

For example, Mrs. Chapman, a 45-year-old client admitted with a medical diagnosis of metastatic cancer, has nursing diagnoses of **Fluid volume deficit** related to nausea and vomiting, and **Potential bathing/hygiene self-care deficit** related to fatigue. For the past several months, the client's husband and sons have been assisting her with activities of daily living (ADLs). Mr. Chapman explained to the nurse that his wife's daily routine consists of getting up prior to breakfast, sponging herself in the bathroom, and getting dressed in comfortable clothes such as a jogging suit. Other routines include measures to control pain and nausea and to maintain bowel regularity.

Discussing Mrs. Chapman's activities and care in the home gives the nurse valuable information. With the assistance of her husband and sons, Mrs. Chapman has developed routine measures that assist in her daily care. The primary nurse uses this information to develop goals and nursing strategies, and to provide continuity in the client's care as much as possible.

Planning is a deliberative, systematic process that is critical to the attainment of quality nursing care. It is a process in which decision making and problem solving are carried out. The planning process uses (a) data obtained during assessing and (b) the diagnostic statements that present the client's health problems (potential and actual). Accurate nursing diagnoses provide direction for determining client goals and developing a plan of care.

COMPONENTS OF PLANNING

The six components of planning are:

1. Setting priorities
2. Establishing client goals and outcome criteria
3. Planning nursing strategies
4. Writing nursing orders
5. Writing the nursing care plan
6. Consulting

Setting Priorities

Priority setting is the process of establishing a preferential order for nursing strategies. To set priorities, the nurse and the client first order the nursing diagnoses preferentially, i.e., they decide which deserves attention first, which second, and so on. Diagnoses can be grouped as having high, medium, or low priority. This priority setting, however, does not mean that all the high-priority diagnoses must be resolved before any others are considered. A high-priority diagnosis may be dealt with partially, and then a diagnosis of lesser priority may be dealt with. In addition, the nurse may address more than one diagnosis at a time. Because client problems are usually multiple, this is often the case. See Table 12–1 for the assignment of priorities to the diagnostic statements for Mr. Joe Smith.

Setting priorities is made easier by using a framework such as a nursing model or theory. One frequently used framework is Maslow's hierarchy of needs. See Figure 4–1 on page 68. Maslow's physiologic needs, such as air, food, and water, are basic to life and receive higher priority than the need for security or activity.

Life-threatening problems, such as loss of respiratory or cardiac functioning, have the highest priority. Health-threatening problems, either actual or potential, such as acute illness and decreased coping ability, may result in delayed development or impaired functioning. Health-threatening problems usually have medium priority. Growth needs, such as self-esteem, are not necessary for sustaining life. Thus, when the nurse plans care for a client with unmet physiologic needs and unmet growth needs, the basic or physiologic needs are the first priority.

The importance of the client's involvement in setting priorities cannot be overemphasized. Although a nurse may believe she or he knows a client, the client's values may be different than the nurse supposes, and the client may set priorities differently. For example, one nursing diagnosis may relate to smoking and another to nutrition. The nurse may give the smoking problem a higher priority than the problem of obesity, but the client may see the problem of obesity as more important. When there is such a difference of opinion, the client and nurse should discuss it openly or resolve the conflict. However, in a life-threatening situation, the nurse needs to take the initiative.

The priorities assigned to problems should not remain fixed. Nursing priorities must change as a client's health problems and therapy change.

TABLE 12–1 *Assigning Priorities to Diagnostic Statements for Mr. Joe Smith (before cardiac catheterization)*

Diagnostic Statement List	Priority Rating	Rationale
Activity intolerance related to shortness of breath and lack of energy secondary to decreased strength of cardiac contractions	Medium priority	Lack of energy is the client's stated major concern. Too much activity can create excessive cardiac demands, resulting in further decreased cardiac output with lowered blood pressure and inadequate circulation. However, because Mr. Smith is able to handle basic activities of daily living, strategies to deal with this diagnostic statement can be deferred until after cardiac catheterization and/or cardiac surgery.
Potential ineffective airway clearance postoperatively related to chest incision	Low priority	Until surgery is performed, ineffective airway clearance is not likely since he is currently able to clear his airways by coughing.
Potential for injury (trauma) related to joint stiffness and limp from hip replacement surgery	High priority	The client is independent and moves slowly to accommodate his limitations. However, new surroundings and a sedative given before cardiac catheterization increase his risk of injury.
Knowledge deficit: side effects of diuretic therapy	Medium priority	Although the client complies with his medical regime, he does not seem to understand the side-effects of the prescribed diuretic, e.g., its relation to increased urination.
Altered peripheral tissue perfusion (left leg) related to impaired arterial circulation	High priority	Decreased circulation and tissue perfusion to the client's left leg can result in damage to the tissues of the limb.
Fear related to cardiac catheterization, possible heart surgery, and its outcome	High priority	Extreme fear could impair his coping capacity.
Potential pain (angina) related to excessive activity or stress	Medium priority	Angina has not been a problem for 2 months, but it could recur with the stress of hospitalization and planned treatments.

Client's Health Values and Beliefs
Values concerning health may be very important to the nurse but not to the client. For example, a client may see attendance at school or being home for the children as more urgent than a health problem.

Client's Priorities
Offering the client the opportunity to set own priorities allows client participation in care planning and enhances cooperation between the nurse and client. Sometimes, however, the client's perception of what is important conflicts with the nurse's knowledge of potential future problems or complications. For example, an elderly female may not regard ambulation or turning and repositioning every 2 hours as important, preferring to be undisturbed. The nurse, however, aware of the potential complications of prolonged bed rest (e.g., muscle weakness and decubitus ulcers), needs to inform the client and implement necessary interventions to prevent such debilitating effects.

Resources Available to the Nurse and Client
If money, equipment, or personnel are scarce, then a health problem may be given a lower priority than usual. Nurses in a home setting, for example, do not have the resources of a hospital; therefore, if the resources needed for specific nursing strategies are not available, the solution of that problem might need to be postponed, or the client may need referral.

Client resources, such as finances or coping abilities, may also influence the setting of priorities. For example, a client who is unemployed may defer dental treatment; a client whose husband is terminally ill and dependent on her may consider nutritional guidance directed toward weight loss as too much to handle.

Time Needed for the Nursing Strategies
Each client feels comfortable with a certain pace of action. Some clients may want to discuss the problem with family members or think about it overnight. Others may want "to get on with it." The nurse must allow adequate time for the necessary nursing strategies resulting from the nursing diagnosis.

Urgency of the Health Problem
Life-threatening situations require that the nurse establish priorities quickly. This also applies to situations that affect the integrity of the client, i.e., that could have a negative or destructive effect on the client. Such health problems as drug abuse and radical alteration of self-concept due to amputation can be destructive not only to the individual but also to the family. These health problems should receive high priority.

Medical Treatment Plan
The priorities for treating health problems must be congruent with treatment by other health professionals. For example, a high priority for the client might be to become ambulatory; however, if the physician's therapeutic regimen calls for extended bed rest, then ambulation must assume a lower priority in the nursing strategy plan. In such a case, however, the nurse can provide or teach exercises to facilitate ambulation later, provided the client's health permits. The diagnostic statement related to ambulation is not ignored; it is merely deferred.

Establishing Client Goals and Outcome Criteria

Goals
A **client goal** is a desired outcome or change in client behavior in the direction of health. Goal attainment reflects the resolution of the client concern or health problem that is specified in the nursing diagnosis. The nursing diagnosis guides the type of goal statement: goals may reflect health restoration, health maintenance, or health promotion (Christensen 1986, p. 173).

In the past, nursing goals were often written to direct care. For example, a nursing goal might have been stated as follows: "Increase the client's exercise," or "Teach client about diabetic diet." From these nursing goals, specific nursing activities were derived, such as ambulating the client at specified intervals, offering instruction about needed dietary adjustments, and ensuring that the correct diet was provided. Recently, however, nurses have begun to state goals in terms of desired *client behavior,* not in terms of nursing activities. The term *outcome* means the result of an activity rather than the activity itself.

The concept of goals varies in nursing literature. In nursing education, goals are often referred to as objectives. In nursing process literature, some nurses separate goals from objectives; others use the terms synonymously. Still others use the term *outcomes* or *outcome criteria* synonymously with objectives. In this book, the terms *goal* and *outcome criteria* are differentiated, whereas *outcome criteria* and *behavioral objectives* are used synonymously. Goals are broadly stated and require further specification. Outcome criteria are specific and measurable.

A *client goal,* then, is a broad statement about the expected or desired change in the status of the client after he or she receives nursing interventions. Since goals are broad indicators of performance, the use of such verbs as *increase, decrease, maintain, improve, develop,* and *restore* is appropriate. See examples of client goals in the accompanying box.

The purpose of client goals is to:

1. Provide direction for planning nursing interventions that will achieve the anticipated changes in the client.
2. Provide direction for establishing evaluation criteria to measure the effectiveness of the interventions.

Relationship of goals to the nursing diagnosis
Client goals are derived from the first clause of the nursing diagnosis, i.e., from the identified client response. For example, if the first clause of the nursing diagnosis or problem (P) is **Feeding self-care deficit,** the goal might be stated as follows: "Client will demonstrate increased ability

to feed self." See establishing goals from nursing diagnosis in the box below. More specific client outcomes (criteria) are then set from this goal; these criteria form the basis of evaluation. For example, if the goal is "The client will demonstrate increased ability to feed self," two criteria might be, "Will drink from a glass through a straw" and "Will feed self using utensils with sponge-wrapped handles." See the section on outcome criteria next in this chapter.

Long-term and short-term goals   Goals may be short term or long term. A short-term goal might be, "Client will raise right arm to shoulder height by Friday." In the same context, a long-term goal might be, "Client will regain full use of right arm in 6 weeks." Because a great deal of the nurse's time is focused on the immediate needs of the client, most goals are short term. In addition, the nurse is better able to evaluate the client's progress or lack of it with short-term goals.

Long-term goals are often used for clients living at home and having chronic health problems or clients in nursing homes, extended care facilities, and rehabilitation centers. Short-term goals are useful (a) for clients who require health care for only a short time and (b) for persons who are frustrated by long-term goals that seem difficult to attain and who need the satisfaction of achieving a short-term goal.

Outcome Criteria   Outcome criteria or objectives are needed to add specificity to the broad goal statements. A **criterion** is a standard or model that can be used in judging. **Outcome criteria** are statements that describe specific, observable, and measurable responses of the client. They determine whether the stated goals have been achieved and are therefore essential to the evaluation phase of the nursing process.

Outcome criteria serve four purposes:

1. They provide direction for nursing interventions.
2. They provide a time span for planned activities.
3. They serve as criteria for evaluation of progress toward goal achievement.
4. They enable the client and nurse to determine when the problem has been resolved.

Relationship of outcome criteria to client goals
Outcome criteria are derived from and relate to the client goals. Client goals, as described previously, are derived from the first clause of the nursing diagnosis. For example, if the nursing diagnosis is **Potential impaired skin integrity** related to imposed bed rest, and the client goal is, "Maintain intact skin, particularly over bony prominences," the outcome criteria might be as follows. The client:

- Demonstrates correct technique for positioning and turning, and the use of pillows to prevent pressure, within two days.
- Discusses two methods for reducing pressure over bony prominences, within two days.
- Has an absence of redness or irritation to skin when discharged from the hospital.

Generally, three to six outcome criteria are needed for each goal. Some nurses consider outcome criteria to be part of goals and add criteria directly to the goal statement, as follows: "Client's hydration status will be maintained (goal) as evidenced by (outcome criteria): (a) fluid intake of at least 2500 ml daily, (b) urinary output in balance with fluid intake, (c) normal skin turgor, (d) moist mucous membranes." Other nurses find this method cumbersome and separate the goal statement from the criteria statements.

Whichever method is used, the process of developing outcome criteria is the same. The nurse needs to ask two questions:

1. How will the client look or behave if the desired goal is achieved?
2. What must the client do and how well must the client do it before the goal is attained?

Characteristics of well-stated outcome criteria are shown in the accompanying box.

Components of outcome criteria   Outcome criteria generally have all or some of the following four components:

1. *Subject.* The subject, a noun, is the client, any part of the client, or some attribute of the client, such as the client's pulse or urinary output. Often, the subject is omitted in nursing care plan goals; it is assumed that the subject is the client unless indicated otherwise.
2. *Verb.* The verb denotes an action the client is to perform, e.g., what the client is to do, learn, or experience. Verbs that denote directly observable behaviors, such as *administer, demonstrate, show, walk, drink, tell, list, state,* etc., are used.
3. *Conditions or modifiers.* Conditions or modifiers may be added to the verb to explain the circumstances under which the behavior is to be performed. They explain what, where, when, or how. For example:

   Walks *with the help of a walker* (how)

   After attending two group diabetes classes, lists signs and symptoms of diabetes (when)

   When at home, maintains weight at existing level (where)

   Discusses *four food groups and recommended daily servings* (what)

Characteristics of Well-Stated Outcome Criteria

- Each outcome criterion relates to the established goal.
- The outcome stated in the criterion is possible to achieve.
- Each criterion is a statement of *one* specific outcome.
- Each criterion is as specific and concrete as possible, to facilitate measurement.
- Each criterion is appraisable or measurable, i.e., the outcome can be seen, heard, felt, or measured by another person.

Conditions need not be included if the standard of performance clearly indicates what is expected.

4. *Criterion of desired performance.* The criterion indicates the standard by which a performance is evaluated or the level at which the client will perform the specified behavior. These criteria may specify time or speed, accuracy, distance, and quality. To establish a time-achievement criterion, the nurse needs to ask "how long?" To establish an accuracy criterion, the nurse asks "how well?" Similarly, the nurse asks "how far?" and "what is the expected standard?" to establish distance and quality criteria, respectively. Examples are:

Weighs 75 kg *by April* (time)

Lists *five out of six* signs of diabetes (accuracy)

Walks *one block per day* (time and distance)

Administers insulin *using aseptic technique* (quality)

See Table 12–2 for other examples of outcome criteria.

TABLE 12–2   *Components of Outcome Criteria*

Subject	Verb	Conditions/Modifiers	Desired Performance Standard
Client	drinks	2500 ml of fluid	daily (time)
Client	administers	correct insulin dose	using aseptic technique (quality standard)
Client	lists	three hazards of smoking (after reading literature)	(accuracy indicated by number of hazards)
Client	recalls	five symptoms of diabetes before discharge	(accuracy indicated by number of symptoms)
Client	walks	the length of the hall without a walker	by date of discharge (time)
Client's ankle	measures	less than 10 inches in circumference	in 48 hours (time)
Client	carries out	leg ROM exercises as taught	every 8 hours (time)
Client	identifies	foods high in salt from a prepared list	before discharge (time)
Client	states	the purposes of his medications	before discharge (time)

Guidelines for Writing Goals and Outcome Criteria

The following guidelines can help nurses write goals and outcome criteria:

1. Write goals and outcome criteria in terms of client behavior. Begin each goal and outcome criteria with "the client." This helps to focus on what the client will be able to do when the outcome criteria are achieved. Outcome criteria should focus on what the client will accomplish, *not what the nurse will do*. For example, a postoperative client may have the following goal (and outcome criteria): The client will maintain clear, open airways (goal) and manifest normal breath sounds (e.g., no wheezing or rales), normal rate of respirations, and absence of dyspnea and cyanosis (outcome criteria).

   Avoid statements that start with *enable, facilitate, allow, let, permit,* or similar verbs followed by the word *client* (Carnevali 1983, p. 191). These verbs indicate what the nurse hopes to accomplish, not what the client will do. For example, the statement "assist the client to deep breathe and cough every two hours" is a nursing action, not an observable behavior.

2. Make sure the goal statement is appropriate for the nursing diagnoses and that the outcome criteria are appropriate for the goal. Validate the outcomes. If the outcomes are accomplished, will the goal be achieved? Validate the goal statement. If the goal is accomplished, will the client's nursing diagnosis be resolved?

3. Make sure that the outcome criteria are realistic for the client's capabilities, internal and external limitations, and designated time span, if it is indicated. *Internal limitations* refer to the person's physical and mental health status and coping mechanisms. *External limitations* refer to finances, equipment, family support, social services, and time. For example, the goal "The client will walk with crutches on level surfaces and on stairs" may be unrealistic for an elderly woman with a heavy leg cast. "The client will walk with crutches from bed to bathroom with assistance" may be more realistic. The goal "Measures insulin accurately" may be unrealistic for a client who has poor vision due to cataracts.

4. Make sure the client considers the goals important and values them. Outcomes are value decisions (Gordon 1987, p. 309). Some outcomes, such as those for problems related to self-esteem, parenting, and communication, involve choices that are best made by the client or in collaboration with the client. Whenever possible, clients should be given information that will allow them to make informed choices with regard to goals.

   Some clients may know what they wish to accomplish with regard to their health problem. For instance, the client's goal may be "relief of pain." Other clients may not know all the outcome possibilities for their specific problem. The nurse must actively listen to the client to determine personal values, goals, and desired outcomes in relation to current health concerns. Then, discuss the nursing diagnosis and goals to determine if the client agrees with the stated problem and goals. Clients are usually motivated and expend the necessary energy to reach a goal if they consider it important.

5. Ensure that the goals and outcome criteria are compatible with the work and therapies of other professionals. The goal "Increase the client's activity tolerance" and the attending criterion "Will increase the time spent out of bed by 15 minutes each day" are not compatible with a physician's prescribed therapy of bed rest for 3 days.

6. Make sure that each *goal* is derived from only one nursing diagnosis. For example, the goal "The client will increase the amount of nutrients ingested and show progress in the ability to feed self" is derived from two nursing diagnoses: **Feeding self-care deficit** related to neuromuscular impairment and **Altered nutrition: less than body requirements** related to anorexia. Keeping the goal statement related to only one diagnosis ensures that outcome criteria and planned nursing interventions are clearly related to the diagnosis.

7. When writing *outcome criteria,* use observable, measurable terms; avoid words that are vague and require interpretation or judgment by the observer. For example, such phrases as "increase daily exercise," "increase participation in social activities," and "improve knowledge of nutrition" can mean different things to different people. If used in criteria, these phrases can lead to disagreements about whether the criterion was met. These phrases may be suitable for a broad client goal but are not sufficiently clear and specific for use in outcome criteria used to evaluate the client's response. Examples of client goals and outcome criteria associated with the diagnostic statements for Mr. Joe Smith are shown in Table 12–3 on page 212. Note that the diagnostic statements have been reordered according to established priorities.

Planning Nursing Strategies

Nursing strategies or interventions are nursing actions chosen to treat a specific nursing diagnosis in order to achieve client goals. The specific strategies chosen for actual nursing diagnoses should focus on eliminating or reducing the cause of the nursing diagnosis, which is the second clause of the diagnostic statement. When nurses determine strategies for *potential* nursing diagnosis, the interventions should focus on measures to reduce the client's contributing factors, i.e., signs and symptoms.

The correct identification of the etiology during the nursing assessment provides the framework for choosing successful nursing interventions. For example, **Activity intolerance** may have several etiologies—pain, weakness, sedentary life-style, anxiety, or cardiac arrhythmias. The interventions will vary depending on the cause of the problem.

TABLE 12–3 *Goals and Outcome Criteria for Mr. Joe Smith (before cardiac catheterization)*

Diagnostic Statement*	Client Goals	Outcome Criteria
1. **Fear** related to cardiac cathet-erization, possible heart sur-gery, and its outcome	Experience increased emo-tional comfort and feelings of control	Verbalizes specific concerns.
		Communicates thoughts clearly and logically.
		Facial expressions, voice tone, and body posture corre-spond to verbal expressions of increased emotional com-fort or feelings of control
		After instruction, describes the cardiac catheterization procedure and what is expected of him before and after the procedure
2. **Altered peripheral tissue perfusion (left leg)** related to impaired arterial circulation	Improve circulation to left leg and foot	Skin intact, pink, and moist
		Skin temperature warm (as other foot)
		Left dorsalis pedis, posterior tibial, and popliteal pulses palpable and of same strength as corresponding right pulses
		Verbalizes factors that improve and inhibit peripheral circulation
		Capillary refill of left toenails within 1 to 3 seconds
3. **Potential for injury (trauma)** related to joint stiff-ness and limp from hip replacement surgery	Prevent injury	Moves in and out of bed and ambulates without falling or injuring self
4. **Activity intolerance** related to shortness of breath and lack of energy secondary to de-creased strength of cardiac con-traction	Avoid performance of activ-ities causing shortness of breath and excessive car-diac workload	Rests after meals
		No shortness of breath during activities
		Pulse and blood pressure remain stable at 80 beats per minute and 124/80 mm Hg

*Note new order of diagnostic statements to reflect highest priorities.

Selecting nursing strategies is a decision-making process. Planning nursing strategies involves generating a number of alternative nursing actions likely to solve the client's problem, considering the consequences of each alternative action, and choosing one or more nursing strategies.

Generating Alternative Nursing Strategies The client and nurse can use several methods of generating alternative nursing strategies at this stage: brainstorming, hypothesizing, and extrapolating.

Brainstorming is a technique used by more than one person, usually a group of people. In this process, one per-son's idea elicits an idea from another, and so forth. The ideas should not be evaluated while they are being gener-ated. An idea is expressed, developed by another, modified by another, and so on, until a solution acceptable to all is established. The results of this process are often creative solutions.

Hypothesizing is a technique of predicting which actions will solve a problem or meet a goal. Hypothesized alter-natives are the result of knowledge and experience, and

each of the proposed alternatives is likely to be effective. Hypothesizing is *not* guessing because the alternatives have been tried successfully in the past.

Extrapolating is inferring facts or data from known facts or data. In this technique, the individual suggests an action because everything that is known about the problem sug-gests the action will be effective. For example, Mrs. Redden says, "I am unable to sleep at night." Mrs. Redden knows that Miss Hollis in the next bed has a glass of warm milk at 10:00 P.M. and sleeps well at night. Mrs. Redden extrapolates that the warm milk will help her sleep. Therefore, her sug-gested solution for her insomnia is to take a glass of warm milk at bedtime. If, however, Mrs. Redden knew that she was unable to sleep at night because of the side-effects of a medication, she or the nurse might suggest another solu-tion to the problem.

Often, the nurse and the client can establish a number of nursing strategies for each problem statement. Too many alternatives can be confusing. Usually three to five alter-native nursing strategies for each health problem are sat-isfactory. See Table 12–4.

TABLE 12-4 *Developing Alternative Nursing Strategies*

Diagnostic Statement	Client Goal	Alternative Nursing Strategies
Sleep pattern disturbance related to anxiety	Obtain 6 to 9 hours of sleep	Provide warm milk and a snack in the evening
		Provide more activity during daytime
		Encourage client to decrease activity 2 hours before bedtime
		Assess diet for stimulants, i.e., caffeine
		Provide soft music
		Encourage verbalization of worries

Considering the Consequences of Each Strategy

The next step is to consider the consequences of each action, including the risks. Often, each action will have more than one consequence. For example, the strategy "Provide accurate information" could result in the following client behaviors:

1. Increased anxiety
2. Decreased anxiety
3. Wish to talk with the physician
4. Desire to leave hospital
5. Relaxation

Establishing the consequences of each strategy requires nursing knowledge and experience. The nurse's experience may suggest that providing information before the client's bedtime may increase the client's worry and tension and that maintaining the usual rituals before sleep is more effective. Perhaps some alternative nursing actions should be implemented during the day to facilitate sleep at night, e.g., providing accurate information during the day and increasing daytime activity.

Choosing Nursing Strategies

After considering the consequences of the alternative nursing strategies, the nurse chooses one or more that are likely to be most effective. Although the nurse bases this decision on knowledge and experience, the client's input is very important. For example, a client may say: "I always have a sandwich and glass of milk before going to bed when I am home. I know I'll sleep if I can have that." Maintaining the client's routine may indeed help the client sleep, and this action might be the first choice as a nursing strategy.

The following criteria can help the nurse choose the best nursing strategy. The planned action must be:

1. Safe and appropriate for the individual's age, health, and so on.
2. Achievable with the resources available (e.g, in the previous example, sandwiches and milk must be available).
3. Congruent with the client's values and beliefs.
4. Congruent with other therapies (e.g., if the client is not permitted food, the strategy of an evening snack must be deferred until health permits).

RESEARCH NOTE

Selecting Nursing Activities for Hospitalized Clients

This study was conducted to investigate how important 50 selected nursing activities were to elderly hospitalized clients and their nurses and how much agreement there was between nurses and clients about their importance. The areas of nursing activities studied included: physical and psychosocial care, discharge planning, and the implementation of doctor's orders. A random sample of 50 pairs of nurses and their clients at a private southwestern hospital responded independently to a five-point questionnaire. The possible responses ranged from 1 (the intervention had no importance) to a 5 (the intervention was extremely important).

The results revealed that nurses and clients agreed that interventions related to physical activities and the implementing of doctor's orders were extremely important. Areas of disagreement included nursing interventions related to psychosocial care and discharge planning. The nurses perceived psychosocial care activities as of significant importance, whereas the clients did not. The clients, by contrast, perceived interventions related to discharge planning as very important, whereas the nurses saw them as less important.

Implications: The results of this study suggest that (a) nurses need to educate clients of their capability to manage psychosocial aspects of care and (b) nurses need to be aware of the importance of discharge planning activities to the elderly, who may have multiple health problems that need to be managed at home.

J. E. Johnson. Selecting nursing activities for hospitalized clients. *Journal of Gerontological Nursing,* October 1987, 13:29–33.

5. Based on nursing knowledge and experience or knowledge from relevant sciences. Example:

Client's Diagnosis

Potential impaired skin integrity related to immobility

Nursing Strategies

Assess skin integrity over bony prominences q2h.
Turn and change position q30 minutes.
Pad pressure points.
Use egg crate mattress on bed.

Rationale

Continuous pressure on a body area compresses tissue, obstructs blood flow to and from an area, and can result in damaged tissue.

6. Within established standards of care as determined by state laws, professional associations (American Nurses' Association, Canadian Nurses' Association), and the policies of the institution.

Each state has nurse practice acts that govern the scope of nursing practice. What nurses can do varies somewhat from state to state. Nurses should know the laws of the state where they practice and remain aware of current changes.

Many agencies have policies to guide nursing activities and the activities of other health professionals. Policies are usually intended to safeguard clients, e.g., rules for visiting hours, procedures to follow when a client has cardiac arrest, and so on. If a policy does not benefit clients, nurses have a responsibility to bring this to the attention of the appropriate people.

Writing Nursing Orders

Carnevali (1983, p. 222) says the term *nursing order* is preferable to the terms *approaches, activities, actions,* and *interventions* because *order* connotes a sense of accountability for the nurse who gives the order and for the nurse who carries it out. **Nursing orders** are the specific actions the nurse takes to help the client meet established health care goals.

The degree of detail included in the nursing orders depends to some degree on the health personnel who will carry out the order. It is advisable, however, to be exact in writing orders.

Nursing orders should include the following five components (Carnevali 1983, p. 222):

Date
Nursing orders are dated when they are written and reviewed regularly at intervals that depend on the individual's needs. If a client is acutely ill, in an intensive care unit, for example, the plan of care will be continually monitored and revised. In a community clinic, weekly or biweekly reviews may be indicated.

Action Verb
The verb starts the order and needs to be precise. For example, "Explain (to the client) the actions of insulin" is a more precise statement than "Teach (the client) about insulin." "Measure and record ankle circumference daily at 0900 hr" is more precise than "Assess edema of left ankle daily." Sometimes a modifier for the verb can make the nursing order more precise. For example, "Apply spiral bandage to left lower leg *firmly*" is more precise than "Apply spiral bandage to left leg." Two examples of imprecise verbs (Carnevali 1983, p. 223) are shown in the box below.

Content Area
The content is the where and the what of the order. In the above order, "spiral bandage" and "left leg" state the what and the where of the order. The nurse can also clarify in this example whether the foot or toes are to be left exposed.

Time Element
The time element answers when, how long, or how often the nursing action is to occur. Examples are: "Assist client with tub bath at 0700 daily"; "Immerse client's left arm in sterile saline soak for 1 hr"; or "Assist client to change position every 2 hr between 0700 and 2100 hr."

Signature
The signature of the nurse prescribing the order shows the nurse's accountability and has legal significance.

Nursing orders (plans) may be categorized as:

- Orders for nursing therapy of a problem
- Orders for collection of additional data to define a problem better or facilitate its management
- Orders for dissemination of information about the management of a problem

Orders for *nursing therapy* include those activities that maintain or restore the client's usual patterns, alleviate symptoms, and prevent additional problems. These make up the majority of orders.

Examples of Imprecise Action Verbs

Imprecise verbs	Suggested alternatives
Have the client	Ask the client if he will _____
	Request the client to _____
	Remind the client to _____
Reassure the client	Inform the client of _____
	Listen to the client _____
	Stay with the client _____

The *collection of additional data* is often necessary to define a nursing diagnosis better or to learn how to manage a problem. For example, if the nurse notices that a client appears withdrawn, worried, and tense, the nurse needs additional data from the client to clarify the contributing causes of this behavior. The nurse may write a tentative nursing diagnosis of **Anxiety** and then write nursing orders that guide interventions toward confirming the cause. For example, a nursing order may state, "Talk with client to determine cause of anxiety."

If the nurse needs information about *how to manage a problem,* data may be collected from many sources. One example is the order "RN to consult physician about method of cleaning ulcer." The nurse may consult with a pharmacist about the side-effects of a medication, a dietitian about the foods allowed on a certain diet, a physical therapist about appropriate exercise, and so on. See *Consulting* later in this chapter.

Nursing orders may specify the need to distribute information about continuing management of a problem to the client's support persons or other health team members. For example, a family member may need to learn how to help the client manage a long-term illness, or a visiting nurse association may need information about follow-up nursing care requirements for a client who is being discharged.

Writing the Nursing Care Plan

The **nursing care plan** is a written guide that organizes information about a client's health into a meaningful whole; it focuses on the actions nurses must take to address the client's identified nursing diagnoses and meet the stated goals. It is also referred to as the *client care plan,* since its focus is the client.

The nurse in charge (head nurse, primary nurse, or team leader) starts the care plan as soon as a client is admitted to the health care agency. It is constantly updated and revised throughout the client's stay, in response to changes in the client's condition and evaluations of goal achievement.

The purposes of a written care plan are:

1. To provide direction for *individualized care* of the client. The plan is organized according to each client's unique nursing care needs. Although many agencies have devised standardized care plans as guides for providing essential nursing care to specified groups of clients, such plans should be used in conjunction with a plan developed for each client. Standardized plans, developed and accepted by the nursing staff of the agency, ensure that the minimally acceptable standards of care are provided. These plans, however, do not ensure individualized care.

2. To provide for *continuity of care.* The written plan is a means of communicating and organizing the actions of a constantly changing nursing staff. The initial plan, updated to show nursing interventions and new assess-

ment data, is often conveyed to all nursing staff at change of shift reports, nursing rounds, and client care conferences.

3. To provide *direction about what needs to be documented* on the client's progress notes. The care plan specifically outlines which observations to make, what nursing actions to carry out, and what instructions the client or family members require. In this way, recording is facilitated.

4. To serve as a *guide for assigning staff* to care for the client. Certain aspects of the client's care may need to be delegated to someone who can make necessary judgments about the client's responses.

5. To serve as a *guide for reimbursement* from medical insurance companies, often called third-party reimbursement. The medical record is used by the insurance companies to determine what they will pay in relation to the hospital care received by the client. If nursing care has not been documented precisely in the care plan, the nurse has no way to prove that it was done, and the insurers will not pay for care that is not documented. Nursing care plans carefully written and implemented facilitate hospital reimbursement for the professional services the nurse provides.

Format   Although formats differ from agency to agency, the plan is generally organized into four columns or categories: (a) nursing diagnoses or problem list, (b) goals, (c) nursing strategies/interventions/nursing orders, and (d) outcome or evaluation criteria. Some agencies have a five-column plan that includes a column for assessment data before the nursing diagnoses column. Others use a three-column plan that subsumes the evaluation (outcome criteria) column under the goal column.

To help students learn to write care plans and apply their knowledge, educators often modify this plan by adding a column headed "Rationale" after the nursing intervention column. See Table 12–5 on page 216. A **rationale** is the scientific reason for selecting a specific nursing action. Students may also be required to cite supporting literature for this stated rationale.

Many agencies use a nursing Kardex or Rand system for organizing and storing nursing care plans. A nursing *Kardex* or Rand is a file of specially designed 6-by-11-inch index cards containing the care plan for a group of clients. Most Kardexes include not only space for the nursing diagnoses, goals, nursing actions, and evaluations but also:

- A concise profile of the client, with the client's name, medical diagnosis, religion, marital status, occupation, allergies, next of kin, and so on.

- Information about medications the client is receiving, parenteral therapy and other treatments, current operations, and planned laboratory and diagnostic studies. With

TABLE 12–5 *Nursing Orders with Rationale for Mr. Joe Smith*

Diagnostic Statement	Goals	Nursing Orders	Rationale	Outcome Criteria
1. **Fear** related to cardiac catheterization, possible heart surgery, and its outcome	Experience increased emotional comfort and feelings of control	Establish a trusting relationship with the client and family	Mistrust in health care providers increases fear	Verbalizes specific concerns
		Encourage client and family to express feelings and concerns	Expression of feelings often relieves tension and enables supportive feedback or correction of misinformation	Communicates thoughts clearly and logically Facial expressions, voice tone, and body posture correspond to verbal expressions of increased emotional comfort or feelings of control
		Discuss the cardiac catheterization procedure and what is expected of him before and after the procedure	Knowledge of the procedure and of what is expected of him will reduce fears of the unknown and feelings of powerlessness	After instruction, describes the cardiac catheterization procedure and what is expected of him before and after the procedure
		Encourage conversation with another client who has recuperated from similar surgery	Another client who has recuperated from heart surgery can provide more hope about the outcome of surgery than the nurse.	
2. **Altered peripheral tissue perfusion (left leg)** related to impaired arterial circulation	Improve circulation to left leg and foot	Consult with physician about exercise program, such as walking and range-of-motion exercises to hip, knee, and ankle	Walking and range-of-motion exercises increase peripheral circulation, but because the conditions causing impaired arterial circulation are unknown, the physician must prescribe them	Skin intact, pink, and moist Skin temperature warm (as other foot)
		Keep the extremity in a *dependent* position (i.e., lower than the heart)	A dependent position facilitates arterial blood flow by gravity	Left dorsalis, posterior tibial, and popliteal pulses palpable and of same strength as corresponding right pulses
		Use Doppler ultrasound stethoscope (DUS) to assess blood flow in left dorsal pedis, posterior tibial, and popliteal arteries q2h	The DUS detects and indicates movement of blood through arteries by a pulsating sound. When pulses are not palpable, the DUS can determine blood flow	Capillary refill of left toenail within 1 to 3 seconds

knowledge of the time and frequency of tests, treatments, and other activities, the nurse can coordinate all care for the client and organize the clinical assignment. Coordinating care is essential to preserve the client's energy.

Some health care agencies have adopted 8½-by-11-inch nursing care plan records that correspond to the standard chart size and require that the plan be written in ink so that it can be retained as part of the client's permanent legal record. In other agencies, problem-oriented medical records (POMR) are used; in this situation, the nursing care plan is documented in a SOAP format. See Chapter 17. In still other agencies, medical orders are not included on the nursing care plan.

TABLE 12—5 *(continued)*

Diagnostic Statement	Goals	Nursing Orders	Rationale	Outcome Criteria
		Instruct client to keep his leg warm, e.g., wear warm socks but discourage use of external heat sources	Warmth increases circulation; because decreased sensation is often associated with impaired perfusion, external heat may not be perceived and cause burning	
3. **Potential for injury (trauma)** related to joint stiffness and limp from hip replacement surgery	Prevent injury	Closely assess ambulation and transfers during first few days	Close supervision enables assessment of independence and safety in mobility	Moves in and out of bed and ambulates without falling or injuring self
		Keep bed at lowest level	Low level facilitates safer transfers into and out of bed	
		Encourage to request assistance to ambulate during the night	New surroundings can cause confusion in older people and be the cause of accidents	
		Closely attend or put side rails up when client is sedated	Sedation can alter perception and impair motor abilities	
4. **Activity intolerance** related to shortness of breath and lack of energy secondary to decreased strength of cardiac contraction	Avoid performance of activities causing shortness of breath and excessive cardiac workload	Organize client care and provide undisturbed rest periods	A balance of activity and rest is necessary to stabilize cardiac effort	Rests after meals No shortness of breath during activities
		Discuss energy conservation methods such as taking periodic rest periods	Implementing energy conservation methods reduces the cardiac workload and deleterious effects of reduced cardiac output	Pulse and blood pressure remain stable at 80 beats per minute and 124/80 mm Hg
		Tell the client to reduce the intensity, duration, and frequency of activity if he experiences chest pain, shortness of breath, dizziness, or abnormal pulse and blood pressure after activity	These signs indicate inadequate cardiac output	
		Monitor vital signs q2h and report decreasing blood pressure, increasing heart rate, or increasing respiratory rate	These signs are indicative of additional reduced cardiac output and cardiac failure	

Guidelines for Writing Nursing Care Plans

In addition to following the earlier suggestions for writing nursing orders, the nurse can use the following guidelines when writing nursing care plans:

1. Date and sign the plan. The date the plan is written is essential for evaluation, review, and future planning.

The signature of the nurse who is writing the plan demonstrates accountability to the client and to the nursing profession, since the effectiveness of nursing actions can be evaluated.

2. Use the category headings "Nursing Diagnoses," "Goals," "Nursing Orders/Interventions," and "Evaluation" and include a date for the evaluation of each goal.

3. Indicate that goals are met or revised by a signature or some other method specified by the agency.

4. List the nursing orders for each goal in order of priority. For example, the nursing orders for a client with a decubitus ulcer might include "Apply an occlusive dressing for 24 hours" and "Clean the ulcer with Betadine solution daily." The appropriate sequence is to clean the ulcer before applying the dressing, and the orders should be listed in that sequence. Another example of priority listing is to explore a client's feelings about administering injectable insulin before demonstrating how to do it.

5. Use standardized medical or English symbols and key words rather than complete sentences to communicate your ideas. For example, write "Turn and reposition q2h" rather than "Turn and reposition the client every two hours." Or write, "Clean decubitus ulcer c̄ H_2O_2 bid" rather than "Clean the client's decubitus ulcer with hydrogen peroxide twice a day, morning and evening."

6. Refer to procedure books or other sources of information rather than including all the steps on a written plan. For example, write: "See unit procedure book for tracheostomy care," or attach a standard nursing plan about such procedures as radiation-implantation care and preoperative or postoperative care. Using these adjuncts for commonalities of care among clients not only saves the nurse time but also focuses the care plan on the unique differences that individualize the care of clients.

7. Tailor the plan to the unique characteristics of the client by ensuring that the client's choices, such as preferences about the times of care and the methods used, are included. This reinforces the client's individuality and sense of control. For example, the written nursing order "Provide prune juice at breakfast rather than regular juice" indicates that the client was given the choice between beverages.

8. Ensure that the nursing plan incorporates *preventive* and health maintenance aspects as well as restorative. For example, carrying out the order "Provide active-assistance ROM exercises to affected limbs q2h" prevents joint contractures and maintains muscle strength and joint mobility.

9. Include collaborative and coordination activities in the plan. For example, the nurse may write orders to ask a nutritionist or physical therapist about specific aspects of the client's care.

10. Include plans for the client's discharge and home care needs. It is often necessary to consult and make arrangements with the community health nurse, social worker, and specific agencies that supply client information and needed equipment.

Consulting

Consulting is deliberating between two people. Nurses consult a variety of personnel, including other nurses, throughout the nursing process. Consulting implies that the nurse involved in the care seeks advice or clarification regarding client goals. Also, the nurse may serve as a resource to provide assistance in health- or client-related issues. Increasingly nurses consult with other nurses within the agency about a variety of specialized nursing practice areas. Nurses may also consult with other health care personnel including physicians, nutritionists, physical therapists, and social workers. Some agencies have a protocol to be followed by those consulting a health professional not presently involved in the client's care. For example, if a nurse wants to discuss a client's depression with an agency psychiatrist, the nurse may need to send a form to the psychiatrist requesting a consultation. However, many consultations are done on an informal basis. For example, the nurse may discuss a client's skin problem with the physician during the physician's rounds.

Nurses generally consult to verify findings, implement change, and obtain additional knowledge. Nurses frequently ask other nurses to verify assessment data, such as extremely low blood pressure or exceptionally fast pulse, when their findings are unexpected or they are uncertain about them. Sometimes nurses discuss a client's care plan with another nurse, often to make sure the best possible plan has been arranged, or to implement change in the plan. A second person's ideas can often generate new approaches to the client's care. Consultation to obtain knowledge is desirable. No nurse can know everything about nursing, and another nurse may have knowledge and experience about a particular problem.

The consulting process has seven steps: (1) identify the problem, (2) collect pertinent data about the client, (3) select the consultant, (4) communicate the problem and pertinent information, (5) discuss the recommendations with the consultant, and (6) include the recommendations in the client's nursing care plan.

Identify the Problem Before consulting another person, the nurse must have the problem clearly in mind, including circumstances surrounding the problem. For example, a nursing student is unsure how to place the dressings on a draining wound to catch all the drainage because the student did not see the previous dressing before the physician removed it. The problem is clearly described, i.e., how to place the dressing, and the circumstances include the site of the source of the drainage, the amount of drainage, and the present absence of a correct dressing.

Collect Pertinent Data About the Client When planning to consult a health professional who is unfamiliar with the client, collect all the data relevant to the problem, e.g., the client says, "I am afraid I am bleeding all the time," and the client is thin and at risk of developing pressure sores.

Select the Consultant

The nurse who has identified a problem regarding nursing care should consult a recognized health professional who has the skills or knowledge required—a nurse with special knowledge and skills. For example, if Mrs. Kinney has a malignancy and is experiencing acute pain in spite of analgesics, a logical consultant would be the oncology nurse specialist. This nurse is likely to have knowledge and experience to teach the nurse how to help Mrs. Kinney. As another example, a nurse might consult an enterostomal therapist about the best way to care for a client's stoma and incision.

Communicate the Problem and Pertinent Information

This information often varies with each client and each problem. However, it is important to convey information about the client's strengths and problems. Convey the information clearly and objectively so that the consultant does not become biased yet obtains a clear picture of the situation. Make sure the data provided are factual and not interpretive. For example, "Mrs. Marsh cries each time she moves" describes her behavior factually, but "Mrs. Marsh is seeking attention" or "Mrs. Marsh is acting like a child" interprets the crying judgmentally and conveys bias.

Discuss the Recommendations with the Consultant

The consultant may provide recommendations at the time the nurse describes the problem, or a later meeting may be necessary. For example, an oncology nursing consultant may give immediate recommendations regarding activity, positioning, timing of medication, or the consultant might prefer to obtain further data before making recommendations.

Include the Recommendations in the Client's Nursing Care Plan

Once recorded, the recommendations become part of the client's record and are available to all health professionals involved in the client's care. After implementing the recommendations, the nurse needs to evaluate their effectiveness and to record these. If they are not effective, it may be necessary to see the consultant again and make further adjustments in the client's nursing plan.

DISCHARGE PLANNING

Because the average client stay in acute care hospitals has become shorter due to cost-containment efforts, people are sometimes discharged still needing care. Such care is increasingly being delivered in the home. *Discharge planning,* the process of anticipating and planning for needs after discharge from a hospital or other facility, is becoming a crucial part of comprehensive health care and should be addressed in each client's care plan. Effective discharge planning begins with the admission of the person and continues with ongoing assessment of both client and family needs, until discharge. It involves a comprehensive assessment not only of physical care needs but also of the availability of family and friend caregivers, the home environment as described by the client and family, client and family resources, and community resources.

Some large hospitals have *discharge planners,* nurses whose primary responsibility is to assess anticipated needs after discharge. In most settings, however, staff, head nurses, and clinicians, with the help of social workers, are doing discharge planning. To facilitate collecting the assessment data needed for effective discharge planning, hospital staff may establish liaisons with community-based nurses who can visit the home before the client's discharge, thereby having the opportunity to anticipate needs and plan with the family in advance of discharge.

Effective two-way communication is obviously essential for the coordination of information and planning. The nurse can be effective in helping family members think through their typical day and week and process the changes they can anticipate when the ill person is at home. Thinking through "what-if" situations (e.g., What if the client falls? What if there is an emergency? What if the caregiver needs to go to the store or do other essential errands?) helps families to confront what is happening to them at their own pace and in their own style and to plan for anticipated problems, thereby experiencing a sense of control and confidence (McCorkle and Germino 1984). It also provides the nurse an opportunity to identify the learning needs of clients and families. These learning needs can be met by individualized teaching prior to discharge or, if necessary, after discharge by the home health nurse. (See Chapter 16.)

When possible, referrals and other actions should be initiated before the day of discharge so that preparations for the client's return home are complete when he or she arrives. In this way, the client's and family's anxiety about the return is kept to a minimum. Referrals of a hospitalized client for home care are often initiated and implemented by the nurses caring for that client, but signed physician's orders for care are required if care is to be reimbursed by third-party payment. The physician may order treatments, medications, adjunctive therapies (e.g., physical, occupational, or speech therapy), and skilled nursing care. See Figure 12–1 on page 220 for a sample home health referral form.

Patient Name: *Mr. Donald Phillips*

Medical Record Number: *5447652001*

INTER-AGENCY REFERRAL FORM
ALLIED HEALTH INFORMATION

(addressograph stamp)

Address Reply To:
STANFORD UNIVERSITY HOSPITAL
Patient Care Planning Program
300 Pasteur Drive
Stanford, CA 94305-5232

Medicare No. *0721569702*	Medi-Cal No.	From (Ward or Clinic) *4 SOUTH*	(415) 725- *4499*

Admission Date: *7/15/91*	Discharge Date: *8/1/91*	Medications Administered Day of Discharge:

Name and Address of Nearest ~~Relative or~~ Friend:
KAY JONES (neighbor)
14 MONTGOMERY ST., MENLO PARK, CA

COUMADIN 5mg @ 0900 hrs.

NURSING EVALUATION

	GOOD	FAIR	POOR
Vision	✓		
Hearing		✓	
Speech			✓
Bladder Control			✓
Bowel Control		✓	
Date of last BM	*7/31/91*		

PATIENT USES:	YES	NO	COMMENTS
Glasses	✓		
Hearing Aide	✓		
Dentures	✓		
Catheter *(condom)*	✓		Type: △'d.
Tubes		✓	Type: △'d.
Prosthesis		✓	Type:
Colostomy		✓	△'d.

MOBILITY		PERSONAL NEEDS	
	Walks		Call Bell
	Cane	A	Feeds Self
	Crutches		Eating Device
	Walker	A	Commode
A	Wheelchair		Bedpan
A	Bed/Chair	I	Urinal
	Bedfast	A	Bathing
		I	Wash Face
CODE:		A	Shave/Make-Up
I = Independent		I	Comb Hair
A = Assist		A	Brush Teeth/Dentures
D = Dependent			

PATIENT IS:	YES	Describe Atypical Behavior
Alert/Appropriate		
Confused		
Combative		
Noisy		
Withdrawn	✓	*DEPRESSED ABOUT DYSPHASIA*
Wanderer		

SKIN (describe), DRESSING CHANGES, or TREATMENTS:
SKIN DRY BUT INTACT. SLING APPLIED TO Ⓛ ARM

Myra Brown RN *7/31/91*
SIGNATURE · TITLE · DATE

PHYSICAL AND OCCUPATIONAL THERAPY:
ROM exercises to Ⓛ arm and Ⓛ leg daily. Quadriceps exercises to Ⓡ leg. *Larry Agnew, PT 7/31/91*
SIGNATURE · TITLE · DATE

DIET: *NO RESTRICTIONS*

TEACHING:
SIGNATURE · TITLE · DATE

SOCIAL (Current/future living arrangements; family composition, etc.)
AND OTHER PERTINENT INFORMATION:
THIS 86 YR OLD WIDOWER LIVES ALONE. HAS ONE DAUGHTER (IN NEW YORK CITY) WHO IS EXPLORING LONG TERM CARE FACILITIES IN THIS AREA. CLIENT'S ATTEMPTS TO VERBALIZE NEED TO BE ENCOURAGED. HE UNDERSTANDS SLOW, DISTINCT SPEECH. *Myra Brown* RN *7/31/91*
SIGNATURE · TITLE · DATE

REPLY TO BE COMPLETED WITHIN 4 WEEKS:

SIGNATURE · TITLE · DATE

Figure 12-1 Patient referral form. *Source:* Stanford University Hospital, Stanford, California.

CHAPTER HIGHLIGHTS

▶ Planning is the process of designing nursing strategies required to prevent, reduce, or eliminate a client's health problems.

▶ Planning can involve the nurse, the client, support persons, and caregivers.

▶ Nursing strategies are planned around a client's diagnostic statements and goals.

▶ Six components of planning are setting priorities, establishing client goals, planning nursing strategies, writing nursing orders, writing a nursing care plan, and consulting.

▶ Nursing diagnoses are assigned high, medium, and low priorities in consultation with the client, if health permits.

▶ Client goals are used to plan nursing strategies that will achieve anticipated changes in the client.

▶ Client goals are derived from the *first* clause of the nursing diagnosis.

▶ Outcome criteria describe specific and measurable client responses and help the nurse evaluate the effectiveness of the nursing intervention.

▶ Goal statements and outcome criteria are written in terms of the client's behavior.

▶ Nursing strategies are focused on the etiology or *second* clause of the nursing diagnosis.

▶ Nursing strategies can be generated by brainstorming, hypothesizing, and extrapolating.

▶ Establishing the consequences of each nursing strategy requires nursing knowledge and experience.

▶ Nursing orders are the specific actions taken by the nurse to help the client meet established health care goals.

▶ The nursing care plan provides direction for individualized care of the client.

▶ The nurse consults with other nurses or health professionals to verify information, implement changes, or obtain additional knowledge to aid in client goals.

▶ Shorter acute care hospitalizations necessitate careful discharge planning.

READINGS AND REFERENCES

SUGGESTED READINGS

McElroy, D., and Herbelin, K. February 1988. Writing a better patient care plan. *Nursing 88* 18:50–51.

The authors present the basic reasons for writing a good care plan: assuring quality nursing care, documenting in case of lawsuits, and validating care for reimbursement purposes. The purpose and parts of the care plan are reviewed, and a sample care plan is presented for examination.

RELATED RESEARCH

Aasen, N. June 1987. Interventions to facilitate personal control: The nursing home experience. *Journal of Gerontological Nursing* 13:20–28.

Brett, J. L. L. November/December 1987. Use of nursing practice research findings. *Nursing Research* 36:344–49.

Johnson, J. E. October 1987. Selecting nursing activities for hospitalized clients. *Journal of Gerontological Nursing* 13:29–33, 44–45.

McCorkle, R. and Germino, B. 1984. What nurses need to know about home care. *Oncology Nursing Forum* 11(6):63–69.

Petrucci, K. E.; McCormick, K. A.; and Scheve, A. A. S. November 1987. Documenting patient care needs: Do nurses do it? *Journal of Gerontological Nursing* 13:34–38, 46–48.

SELECTED REFERENCES

Atkinson, L. D., and Murray, M. E. 1986. *Understanding the nursing process.* 3d ed. New York: Macmillan Co.

Breyerman, K. L. Summer 1988. Consultation roles of the clinical nurse specialist: A case study. *Clinical Nurse Specialist* 2:91–95.

Bulechek, G. M., and McCloskey, J. C. May 1987. Nursing interventions: What they are and how to choose them. *Holistic Nursing Practice* 1:36–44.

Carnevali, D. L. 1983. *Nursing care planning: Diagnosis and management.* 3d ed. Philadelphia: J. B. Lippincott Co.

Christensen, P. J. 1986. Planning: Priorities, goals and objectives. In Griffith, J. W., and Christensen, P. J., editors. pp. 169–182. *Nursing Process: Application of theories, frameworks, and models.* St. Louis: C. V. Mosby Co.

Gordon, M. 1987. *Nursing diagnosis: Process and application.* 2d ed. New York: McGraw-Hill.

Griffith, J. W., and Christensen, P. J. 1986. *Nursing Process: Application of theories, frameworks, and models.* 2d ed. St. Louis: C. V. Mosby Co.

Hanna, D. V., and Wyman, N. B. November 1987. Assessment + diagnosis = care planning: A tool for coordination. *Nursing Management* 18:106–9.

La Monica, E. L. 1985. *The humanistic nursing process.* Monterey, Calif.: Wadsworth Health Sciences.

Lederer, J. R.; Marculescu, G. L.; Mocnik, B.; and Seaby, N. 1990. *Care planning pocket guide: A nursing diagnosis approach.* 3d ed. Redwood City, Calif.: Addison-Wesley Nursing.

MacLeod, E., and MacTavish, M. Spring 1988. Solving the nursing care plan dilemma: Nursing diagnosis makes the difference. *Journal of Nursing Staff Development.* 4:70–73.

Yura, H., and Walsh, M. B. 1988. *The nursing process: Assessing, planning, implementing, evaluating* 5th ed. Norwalk, Conn.: Appleton & Lange.

Implementing

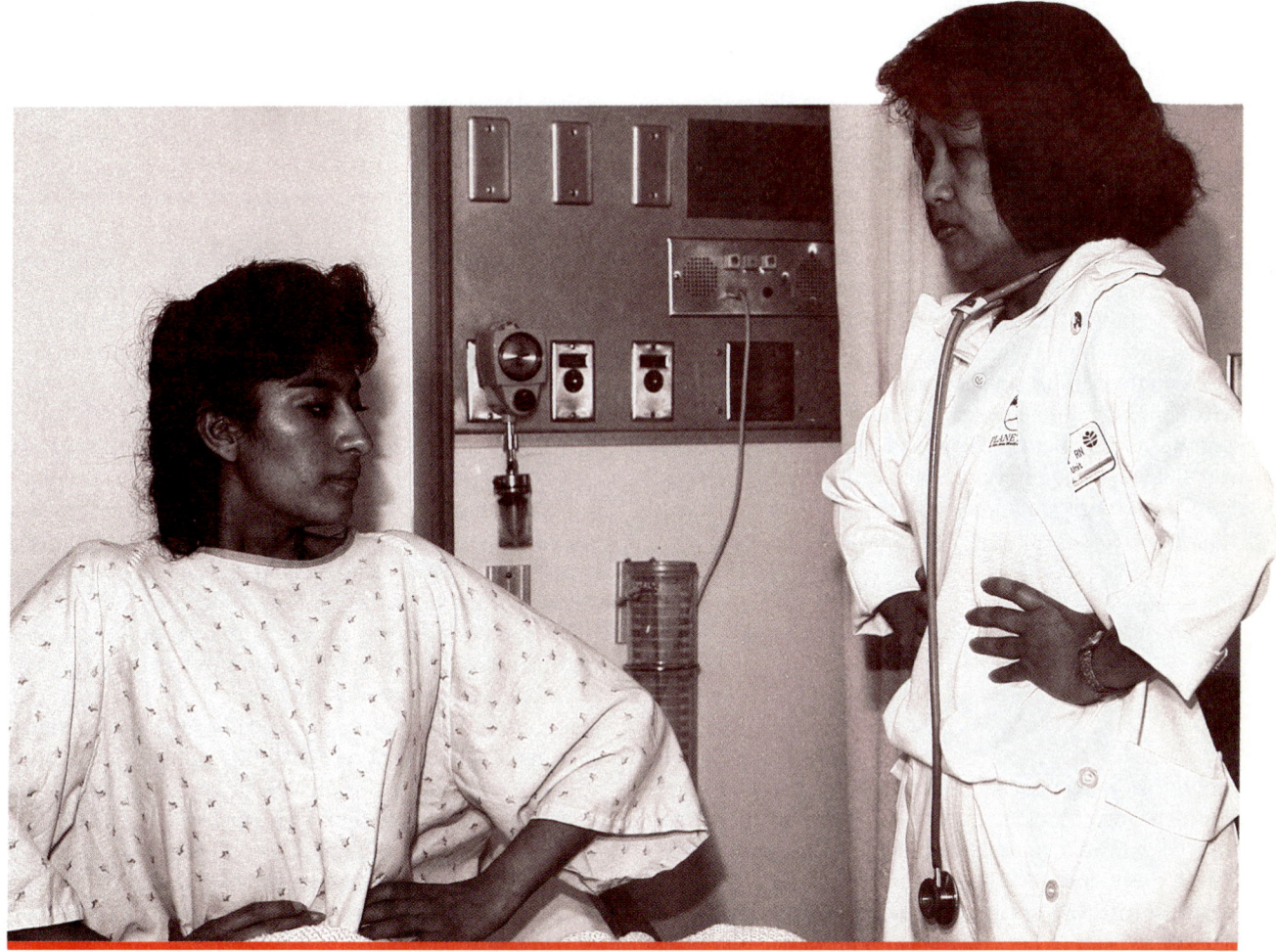

CONTENTS

OBJECTIVES

▶ Differentiate independent, dependent, and collaborative nursing actions.

▶ Compare protocols and standing orders.

▶ Identify five essential aspects of implementing nursing strategies.

▶ Describe two processes that continuously operate throughout the implementing phase.

▶ Describe three categories of skills used to implement nursing strategies.

▶ Identify four cognitive skills nurses use when implementing nursing strategies.

▶ Differentiate critical and creative thinking.

▶ Identify essential guidelines for implementing nursing strategies.

IMPLEMENTING DEFINED

Implementing, also called intervening, is putting the nursing strategies listed in the nursing care plan into action; it is the nursing action taken to attain the desired outcome or the client's goals. According to Marriner (1983), implementing involves carrying out nursing orders *and* physician's orders. Within the context of the nursing process, Bulechek and McCloskey (1985, p. 8) define nursing intervention (implementation) as "an autonomous action based on scientific rationale that is executed to benefit the client in a predicted way related to the nursing diagnosis and stated goals." By this definition, nursing interventions *do not* include those strategies resulting from a physician's order.

The client is always the primary participant in implementing the nursing care plan, although the nurse may act on the client's behalf, e.g., referring the client to a community health nurse for home care. The client's degree of participation often depends on the client's health status. For example, because an unconscious man is unable to participate in his care, he needs to have care given to him. By contrast, an ambulatory client may require very little care from the nurse and carry out health care activities independently. The nurse or nurses, other health professionals, support persons, and/or caregivers can all be involved in implementing nursing.

TYPES OF NURSING ACTIONS

The terms *independent, dependent,* and *collaborative* (interdependent) are often used to describe nursing actions. An action, in this context, is an activity appropriate to a person's role. It is also called a nursing strategy. An **independent nursing action** is an activity that the nurse initiates as a result of the nurse's own knowledge and skills. Mundinger prefers the term *autonomous nursing practice* to *independent nursing practice.* She states, "Knowing why, when, and how to position clients and doing it skillfully makes the function an autonomous therapy" (Mundinger 1980, p. 4). In this instance, the nurse determines that the client requires certain nursing interventions, either carries these out or delegates them to other nursing personnel, and is accountable for the decision and the actions. To be **accountable** is to be answerable. An example of an independent action is planning and providing special mouth care to a man after assessing his mouth. Independent nursing actions are receiving increasing attention from nurses today.

Bulechek and McCloskey (1987) have identified a taxonomy of independent nursing interventions. A **taxonomy** is a set of classifications that are ordered and arranged on the basis of a single principle or consistent set of principles

(Bloom 1956, p. 10). See Table 13–1 for a beginning taxonomy of nursing interventions.

Dependent nursing actions are those activities carried out on the order of the physician, under the physician's supervision, or according to specified routines. An example of a dependent action is giving an antibiotic by injection to a client as a result of a physician's written order. The dependent activity in nursing practice is usually directly related to the client's disease, and its importance should not be minimized. In addition to the task of carrying out the physician's order, the nurse who performs a dependent nursing action also conducts the appropriate nursing activities associated with the order. In the example above, for instance, the nurse would also monitor the client for signs of improvement, worsening infection, or toxic effects of the antibiotic.

Collaborative nursing actions are those activities performed either jointly with another member of the health care team or as a result of a joint decision by the nurse and another health care team member. Collaborative nursing activities sometimes illustrate the overlapping responsibilities of health personnel and reflect the collegial relationship between health professionals. For example, a nurse and a respiratory therapist together may decide on a schedule of breathing exercises for a woman. The therapist may initially teach the exercises to the client, and the nurse reinforces the learned behavior and assists the client in the therapist's absence.

A social policy statement by the American Nurses' Association (ANA) describes collaboration as "true partnership, in which the power on both sides is valued by both, with recognition and acceptance of separate and combined spheres of activity and responsibility, mutual safeguarding of legitimate interests of each party, and a commonality of goals that is recognized by both parties" (ANA 1980, p. 7). To achieve effective collaborative nursing practice, nurses must have clinical competence, feel confident of their knowledge and skills, and assume responsibility for their own actions.

The amount of time that the nurse spends in an independent versus a collaborative or dependent role will vary according to the clinical area, type of institution, and specific position of the nurse. Guzzetta (1987, p. 634) estimates that the critical care nurse spends only about 10% of the day functioning in the independent nursing role. In other settings, e.g., home health care, nurses may find that they function independently 50% of the time. Clinical nurse specialists may work independently 100% of the time. Often, so many activities are integrated into a clinical day that it is difficult for many nurses to assess how much of their time is spent in an independent practice role.

Protocols and Standing Orders

A **protocol** is a written plan specifying the procedure to be followed in a particular situation. For example, agencies

TABLE 13–1 *Beginning Taxonomy of Nursing Interventions*

Most Abstract			Most Concrete
Level 1	Level 2	Level 3	Level Nth
Stress management	Relaxation training Cognitive reappraisal Music therapy		Nursing orders
Life-style alteration	Self-modification Patient contracting Counseling Nutritional counseling Sexual counseling Reminiscence therapy Role supplementation Patient teaching Values clarification Support groups Exercise programs Group psychotherapy Assertiveness training		
Acute care management	Preparatory sensory information Crisis intervention Preoperative teaching Surveillance Presence		
Self-care assistance	Ambulation Bathing Bladder training Bowel training Feeding Oral hygiene Positioning Skin care		
Communication	Active listening Advocacy Cultural brokerage Truth telling Discharge planning		

Source: Reprinted from *Holistic Nursing Practice,* Vol. 1, No. 3, p. 38, with permission of Aspen Publishers, Inc., © May 1987.

often have protocols regarding a client's admission and discharge. Nurse practitioners in a community clinic often have protocols about which clients to refer to the physician and which clients to treat directly. Nurses in a home setting usually have protocols about the procedure to follow when a client dies. Nurses in hospitals often have protocols regarding the steps to follow when a postoperative client returns to the unit.

A **standing order** is a written document about policies, rules, regulations, or orders regarding client care. Standing orders give nurses the authority to carry out specific actions under certain circumstances, often when a physician is not immediately available. In a hospital critical care unit, a common example is the administration of emergency antiar-

rhythmic medications when a client's cardiac monitoring pattern changes.

In a home care setting, a physician may write a standing order for the administration of epinephrine for a client who becomes excessively dyspneic.

PROCESS OF IMPLEMENTING

The process of implementing normally includes reassessing the client, validating the nursing care plan, determining the need for nursing assistance, implementing the nursing strategies, and communicating the nursing actions. Reassessing the client and validating the nursing care plan are subprocesses that operate continuously throughout the implementing phase.

Reassessing the Client

As was mentioned in Chapter 10, assessing or reassessing is carried out throughout the nursing process, i.e., during assessing, implementing, and evaluating—in fact, whenever the nurse has contact with the client. While providing care, nurses must continue to collect data about changes (subtle or acute) in the client's level of wellness, i.e., health problems as well as reactions, feelings, and strengths.

Following an extensive assessment during the first phase of the nursing process, reassessing in later phases usually focuses on more specific needs or responses of the client, i.e., fluid intake, pain, pulse rate, and urine output. Through this mechanism, nurses are able to determine whether planned nursing strategies are currently appropriate for the client.

It should never be assumed that once nursing strategies are established or ordered they must be implemented without assessing the client first. For example, Mr. Raymond Ball's nursing diagnosis is: **Constipation** related to prolonged bed rest, decreased fluid intake, and a soft, low-fiber diet. Before administering an enema to Mr. Ball, the nurse establishes that he had a large bowel movement that morning. Therefore, the enema is not needed. However, encouraging Mr. Ball to take fluids and to exercise in bed as his health permits are still appropriate nursing interventions.

New data may, in the nurse's judgment, indicate a need to change the priorities of care or the nursing strategies. For example, a nurse is turning a client, Mr. Dolan, from a supine to left lateral position according to the turning schedule. The nurse observes a reddened area on Mr. Dolan's left hip even though he has not lain on that side for several hours. The nurse decides not to position Mr. Dolan on his left side but turns him to his right side and records the reddened area and the change of nursing strategy. As a further example, a nurse begins to teach a client who has diabetes, Miss Eves, how to give herself insulin injections. Shortly after beginning the teaching, the nurse realizes that Miss Eves is not concentrating on the lesson. Subsequent discussion reveals that she is worried about her eyesight and fears she is going blind. The nurse ends the lesson because the client's level of stress is interfering with her learning and makes arrangement for a physician to examine the client's eyes. The nurse also provides supportive communication to alleviate the client's stress and revises the nursing care plan appropriately.

Validating the Nursing Care Plan

A nursing care plan cannot be fixed; it must be a flexible tool. When new data are collected, they should be compared with the database. Sometimes, the new data are incongruent with baseline data. The nurse must judge the value of the new data and determine whether the nursing care plan is still valid. When a client's health status changes, i.e., when physical or psychosocial responses change, the nursing care plan needs to be adjusted.

If the data regarding the client's health status are unchanged, the nurse proceeds with the implementing process. For information on modifying or changing the nursing care plan, see Chapter 14, page 234.

Determining the Need for Assistance

When implementing some nursing strategies, the nurse may require assistance for one of the following reasons: The nurse is unable to implement the nursing strategies safely alone (e.g., turning an obese client in bed) and to reduce stress upon a client (e.g., turning a person who has acute pain when moved). In addition, nurses should obtain assistance if they lack the knowledge or skills to implement a particular nursing activity. For example, a nurse who is not familiar with a particular model of oxygen mask needs assistance the first time it is applied.

Implementing Nursing Strategies

Nursing strategies are implemented to help the client meet his or her health goals.

There are four primary areas of nursing practice: health promotion, health maintenance, health restoration, and care of the dying. Nursing actions in each of these areas can be independent, dependent, or collaborative.

Six important considerations for implementing nursing strategies are

1. The client's individuality. Individualized actions are needed, while care is taken not to violate the scientific basis of the activity. For example, a client may prefer to have an oral medication after meals rather than before. However, this might not be justified if the medication will not act in the stomach in the presence of food.

2. The client's need for involvement. Some clients want to be totally involved in their care, while others prefer little involvement. The amount of desired involvement is often related to the client's energy, severity of illness; number of stressors, fear, understanding of the illness, and understanding of the intervention.

3. Prevention of complications. When changing a sterile dressing, for example, the nurse must observe sterile technique to prevent the complication of infection.

4. Preservation of the body's defenses. For example, when turning a client, the nurse protects the client's skin from abrasions, which could permit microorganisms to enter the body and establish an infection.

5. Provision of comfort and support to the client.

6. Accurate and careful implementation of all nursing activ-

ities. The nurse takes care to administer the correct dosage of a medication by the ordered route, for example.

Communicating Nursing Actions

Nursing actions are communicated in writing and often verbally *after* they have been carried out. Nursing actions must not be recorded in advance because the nurse may determine upon reassessing the client that the action should not or cannot be implemented. For example, a nurse is authorized to inject 10 mg of morphine sulfate subcutaneously to a client, but the nurse finds that the client's respiratory rate is 4 breaths per minute. This finding contraindicates the administration of morphine (a respiratory depressant). The nurse withholds the morphine and reports the client's respiratory rate to the nurse in charge and/or physician. A nurse might also find that a planned nursing action cannot be implemented, e.g., the client objects; the client is too weak to ambulate; the nurse encounters an obstruction when inserting a rectal tube. Nursing activities, therefore, are always recorded after they are completed, when the nurse can accurately record exactly what occurred.

In some instances, it is important to record a nursing action immediately after it is implemented. This is particularly true of medications, treatments, etc., because recorded data about a client must be up to date, accurate, and available to other nurses and health care professionals. Immediate recording helps safeguard the client, for example, from receiving a second dose of medication.

The nurse may record such nursing actions as mouth care every 2 hours or turning a client at the end of a shift; in the meantime, the nurse maintains a personal record of these interventions so that they can be accurately recorded later. The method of documentation will be guided by the policies of the health care agency. Many agencies have special forms for this type of recording. See Chapter 17 for additional information regarding recording.

Nursing actions are often communicated verbally as well as in writing. When a client's health is changing rapidly, the charge nurse and/or the physician may want to be kept up to date with verbal reports. Verbal reports are given to another nurse or other health professionals. Nurses also give verbal reports regarding clients at a change of shift and upon a client's discharge to another unit or health agency. Some hospitals use tape recorders to facilitate change of shift reports. For additional information about evaluating the client's response, see Chapter 14; for information on recording and reporting, see Chapter 17.

IMPLEMENTING SKILLS

Three skills are needed to implement nursing actions: cognitive, interpersonal, and technical skills.

The necessary **cognitive** (intellectual) skills for implementing are problem solving, decision making, critical thinking, and creativity. They are crucial to safe, intelligent nursing care. Problem solving and decision making are discussed in Chapter 4.

Critical thinking is a pattern of thinking based on knowledge, experience, and the abilities to conceptualize and analyze relationships. To conceptualize means to form a concept. A **concept** is an abstract idea generalized from particular instances. Critical thinking involves organizing information, picking out relevant information, relating, conceptualizing, and making judgments. Critical thinking enables nurses to make decisions quickly without bias.

Critical thinking, like problem solving, is directed thinking in contrast to associative thinking. **Directed thinking** has a goal and is purposeful. A person uses this type of thinking when trying to form a judgment. For example, when determining whether a client would be wise to sit up in a chair for meals, a nurse uses directed thinking. In this example, the goal is a decision about the client, and the data involve relevant information about the client's health and health problems. **Associative thinking,** by contrast, has very little direction and often involves random thoughts. An example is daydreaming.

The ability to think critically is learned. It requires knowledge or experience, and mature, healthy nervous systems. As people grow and develop, they attempt to deal with new experiences largely through trial and error. As a result, individuals build up a repertoire of thinking skills. With increasing knowledge and experience, individuals enlarge their repertoire, test and modify their skills, and learn to think critically.

Creativity, often called creative thinking, is also a form of directed thinking. **Creative thinking** is establishing new relationships and new concepts, solving problems innovatively. When thinking creatively, the individual cannot always weigh alternatives or establish the logic behind all actions. For nurses, planning nursing strategies and changing nursing actions provide opportunities for creative thinking. Creative thinking helps nurses change a nursing activity efficiently.

Interpersonal skills are all the activities people use when communicating directly with one another. They may be verbal and nonverbal. The effectiveness of a nursing action often depends largely on the nurse's ability to communicate with others. Even when giving a medication to a client, the nurse needs to understand the client and in turn to be understood. A nurse who is delegating a nursing action also needs to be understood.

Interpersonal skills are necessary for all nursing activities: caring, comforting, referring, counseling, and supporting are just a few. They include conveying knowledge, attitudes, feelings, interest, and appreciation of the client's cultural values and life-style. Before nurses can be highly skilled in interpersonal relations, they must have self-awareness and sensitivity to others. See Chapter 15 for more detailed explanations on interpersonal skills.

Technical skills are "hands-on" skills such as manipulating equipment, giving injections and bandaging, moving, lifting, and repositioning clients. These tasks are also called procedures or psychomotor skills. The term *psychomotor* includes the interpersonal component, e.g., the communication need of the client. Technical skills require considerable knowledge on the part of the nurse, including the principles behind the steps of the procedure, knowledge about equipment and supplies, and in some instances knowledge about when the procedure is required. Knowledge of the principles underlying the procedure is of particular importance because it enables the nurse to adapt a procedure to the individual client safely. For example, if a female client cannot turn on her left side for an enema, the nurse can adjust the client's position and still administer the enema effectively if the nurse understands the position of the rectum and large intestine in the body and the flow of fluids by gravity.

When the nurse carries out procedures requiring technical skills, it is important that the nurse make significant assessments of the client *before, during,* and *after* the procedure. Before nurses initiate any procedure, they must relate their own knowledge and competence to the needs of the client. Sometimes assistance is necessary to prevent undue stress on the client and to ensure that the procedure is both safe and effective. It is equally important to evaluate the effectiveness of the procedure.

Technical skills require knowledge and, frequently, manual dexterity. The number of technical skills expected of a nurse has increased greatly in recent years. Because of the trend toward increased use of technology, especially in acute care hospitals, humanizing health care has become a recognized need for clients. See Chapter 6, page 120.

IMPLEMENTING ACTIVITIES

To implement nursing care, the nurse generally performs the following activities: caring, communicating, helping, teaching, counseling, acting as a client advocate and change agent, leading, and managing. These activities are associated with nursing roles (see Chapter 2) and include (a) assigning and delegating care to other nursing personnel and (b) supervising and evaluating the nursing activities of others.

The task of learning what the nurse should do may at times seem overwhelming to the student. Guidelines for implementing nursing strategies, shown in the accompanying box, serve as a blueprint.

Guidelines For Implementing Nursing Strategies

- Nursing actions are based on scientific knowledge and nursing research. The nurse must be aware of the scientific rationale for all interventions and any possible side effects or complications of the activities.

- Nursing actions resulting from a physician's order must be understood by the nurse. The nurse is responsible for intelligent implementation of these orders. This requires a knowledge of the activity, procedure, or medication; its purpose in the client's plan of care; and any contraindications (e.g., allergies) or changes in the client's condition that may be applicable. If the nurse has any question regarding prescribed nursing actions, the nurse-manager or supervisor and/or physician must be consulted.

- Nursing actions are adapted to the individual. A client's beliefs, values, age, health status, and environment are factors that can affect a nursing action.

- Nursing actions should always be safe. Nurses and clients need to take precautions to prevent injury. For example, when changing a sterile dressing, the nurse practices sterile technique to prevent infection; when turning a client, the nurse protects the client's skin from abrasions, which could also lead to infection.

- Nursing actions often require teaching, supportive, and comfort components. These independent nursing activities can often enhance the effectiveness of a specific nursing action.

- Nursing actions should always be holistic. The nurse must always view the client as a whole and consider the client's responses in that light.

- Nursing actions should respect the dignity of the client and enhance the client's self-esteem. Providing privacy and encouraging clients to make their own decisions are ways of respecting dignity and enhancing self-esteem.

- The client's active participation in implementing nursing actions should be encouraged as health permits. Active participation enhances the client's sense of independence and control. Clients vary in the degree of participation they desire. Some clients want total involvement in their care, while others prefer little involvement. The amount of involvement desired is often related to the severity of the illness and the number of stressors, as well as the client's energy, fear, understanding of the illness, and understanding of the intervention.

CHAPTER HIGHLIGHTS

▶ Implementing is putting planned nursing strategies into action.

▶ Reassessing and validating the nursing care plan occur continuously during the implementing phase.

▶ Cognitive, interpersonal, and technical skills are used to implement nursing strategies.

▶ Cognitive skills include problem solving, decision making, critical thinking, and creativity.

▶ Creative thinking helps the nurse and the client to establish innovative nursing actions.

▶ Implementing activities are communicating, caring, teaching, counseling, leading, managing, and acting as a client advocate and change agent.

▶ Caring and communicating are essential for all nursing activities and for establishing relationships.

▶ The implementing phase of the nursing process is terminated with the documentation of the nursing activities.

▶ All nursing activities, all assessment data, and all client responses to the nursing activities require documentation.

▶ Nurses are accountable for all their nursing actions.

READINGS AND REFERENCES

SUGGESTED READINGS

Bulechek, G. M. and McCloskey, J. C. May 1987. Nursing interventions: What they are and how to choose them. *Holistic Nursing Practice* 1:36–44.
    The authors discuss the role and development of independent nursing interventions and offer a beginning list or ordering of the levels of nursing interventions. Five guidelines for choosing nursing interventions for diagnosis are presented, and problems related to implementation and evaluation are discussed.

Walker, L. June 1986. Nursing diagnoses and interventions: new tools to define nursing's unique role. *Nursing and Health Care* 7:323–326.
    The author examines and supports the nursing diagnosis movement as a means of providing coherent communication among nurses. She questions, however, whether nursing diagnoses can be useful without specific nursing interventions that relate to them. She suggests that the nursing profession develop a taxonomy of nursing interventions.

RELATED RESEARCH

Becker, H., and Sands, D. May 1988. The relationship of empathy to clinical experience among male and female nursing students. *Journal of Nursing Education* 27:198–203.

Gropper-Katz, E. I. August 1987. Reality orientation research. *Journal of Gerontological Nursing* 13:13–18.

SELECTED REFERENCES

Alfaro, R. 1986. *Application of nursing process: A step by step guide.* Philadelphia: J. B. Lippincott Co.

American Nurses' Association. 1980. *Nursing: A social policy statement.* Kansas City, Mo.: A.N.A. Pub. no. NP–63 35M 12/80.

Bloom, B. S. (editor) 1956. *Taxonomy of Educational Objectives.* New York: David McKay Company.

Bulechek, G. M. and McCloskey, J. C. 1985. *Nursing interventions: Treatments for nursing diagnoses.* Philadelphia: W. B. Saunders.

DeYoung, L. 1985. *Dynamics of nursing.* 5th ed. St. Louis: C. V. Mosby.

Flynn, J. B., and Heffron, P. B. 1988. *Nursing: From concept to practice.* 2d ed. San Mateo: Appleton & Lange.

Guzzetta, C. E. November 1987. Nursing diagnoses in nursing education: Effect on the profession. Part 1. *Heart and Lung.* 16:629–35.

La Monica, E. L. 1985. *The humanistic nursing process.* Belmont, Calif.: Wadsworth Health Sciences.

Leddy, S., and Pepper, J. M. 1989. *Conceptual bases of professional nursing.* 2d ed. Philadelphia: J. B. Lippincott Co.

Marriner, A. 1983. *The nursing process: A scientific approach to nursing care.* 2d ed. St. Louis: C. V. Mosby Co.

Moss, A. R. September 1988. Determinants of patient care: Nursing process or nursing attitudes? *Journal of Advanced Nursing* 13:615–20.

Mundinger, M. O. 1980. *Autonomy in nursing.* Germantown, Md.: Aspen Systems Corporation.

Paterson, J. G. 1988. *Humanistic nursing.* New York: National League for Nursing N.L.N. Pub. no. 41–2218:3–129.

Peplau, H. E. 1987. Interpersonal constructs for nursing practice. *Nurse Education Today* 7:201–8.

Yura, H., and Walsh, M. B. 1988. *The nursing process: Assessing, planning, implementing, evaluating.* 5th ed. Norwalk, Conn.: Appleton & Lange.

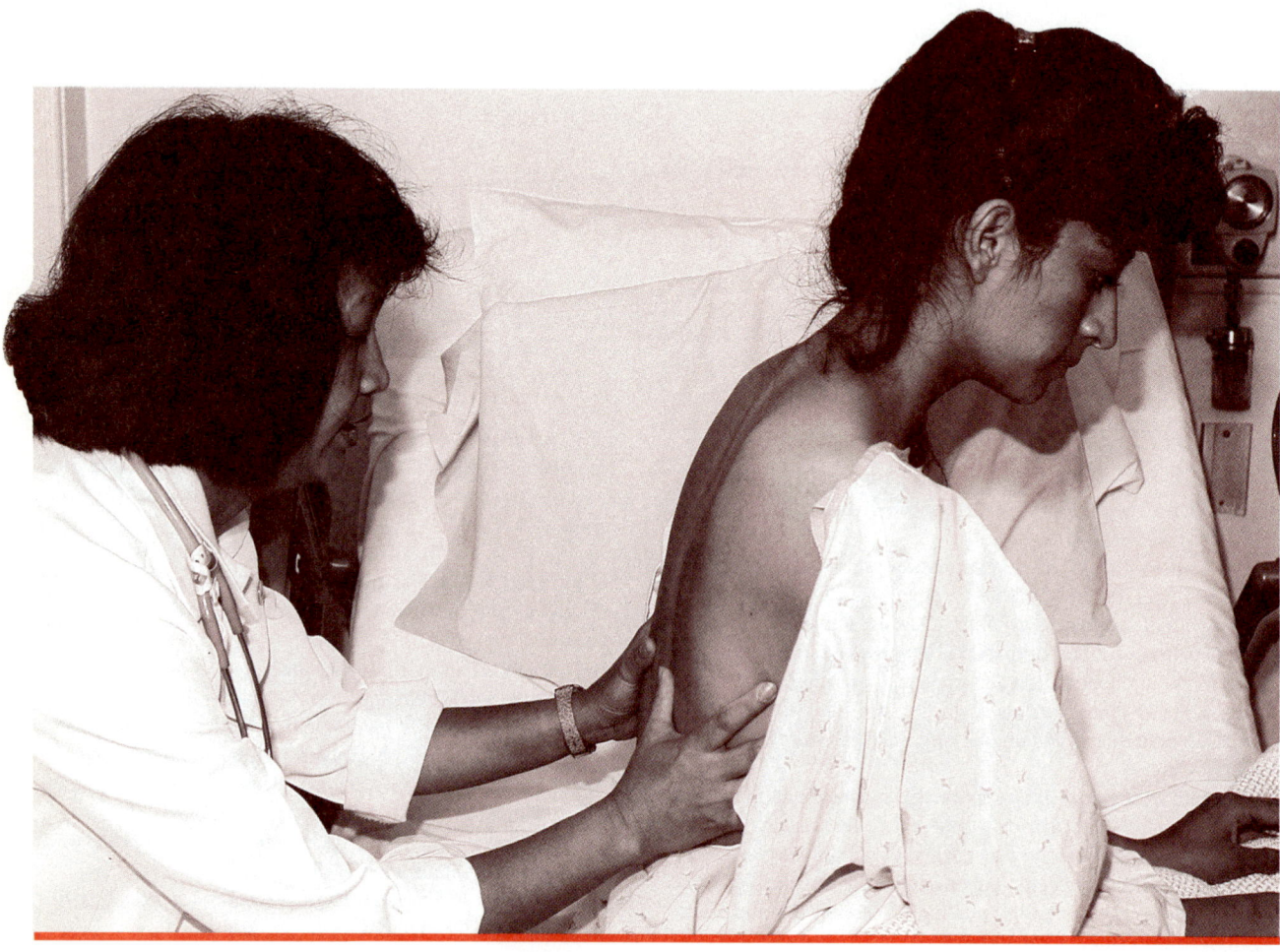

CONTENTS

OBJECTIVES

▶ Describe six components of the
  evaluation process.

▶ Describe the steps involved in reexamining the client's care plan both
  when goals are met and when they
  are not met.

▶ Differentiate quality assessment from
  quality assurance.

▶ Describe three approaches to quality evaluation.

▶ Identify essential steps in developing tools to evaluate quality care.

▶ Identify various methods used to
  evaluate nursing care.

DEFINITION OF EVALUATION

To evaluate is to judge or to appraise. In the context of the nursing process, evaluation is the fifth and last phase. Here, to **evaluate** means to identify whether or to what degree the client's goals have been met. Evaluation is an exceedingly important aspect of the nursing process because conclusions drawn from the evaluation determine whether the nursing interventions can be terminated or must be reviewed or changed.

Evaluating is a concurrent and a terminal process: It is concurrent in that the nurse normally evaluates during the implementing phase of the process. How is the client reacting to this nursing action? Is the reaction expected or unexpected? At this stage, the nurse may change a nursing action to help the client meet the planned goals. It is a terminal process because after completing the nursing activity, the nurse evaluates whether the client's goals have been met. Often the time frame (if stated) in the outcome criteria is used.

Evaluating is a purposeful and organized activity. Through evaluating, nurses accept responsibility for their actions, indicate interest in the results of the nursing actions, and demonstrate a desire not to perpetuate ineffective actions but to adopt more effective ones.

PROCESS OF EVALUATING

The evaluation process has six components:

1. Identifying the **outcome criteria** (standards for measuring success) that will be used to measure achievement of the goals
2. Collecting data related to the identified criteria
3. Comparing the data collected with the identified criteria and judging whether the goals have been attained
4. Relating nursing actions to client outcomes
5. Reexamining the client's care plan
6. Modifying the care plan

Identifying Outcome Criteria

The identification of outcome criteria used to evaluate the client's response to nursing care is discussed in Chapter 12. See Table 12–3 on page 212. Criteria serve two purposes: They establish the kind of evaluative data that need to be collected, and they provide a standard against which the data are judged. For example, the goal "Client's urinary elimination pattern will be maintained" does not tell the nurse what data to collect while caring for the client. When these criteria are added, however, any nurse caring for the client knows what data to collect:

■ Daily fluid intake will be not less than 2500 ml.

■ Urinary output will be in balance with fluid intake. Residual urine will be less than 100 ml.

Criteria that are clearly stated, precise, and measurable guide the next step of the evaluation process: data collection.

Collecting Data

Data are collected so that conclusions can be drawn about whether goals have been reached. The nurse collects data in relation to the specified criteria, either by observation, direct communication, and purposeful listening or from reports of other health professionals.

Collection of both objective and subjective data may be necessary. Objective, measurable data are preferred for evaluation purposes; for example, "Respirations increased from 12 to 16 breaths per minute, and pulse rate increased from 70 to 90 beats per minute after client walked around the corridor." However, the nurse often needs to collect subjective data and some objective data that require interpretation. Examples of objective data requiring interpretation are the degree of tissue turgor of a dehydrated client or the degree of restlessness of a client with pain. Examples of subjective data include complaints of nausea or pain by the client.

When objective data require interpretation, the nurse may obtain the views of one or more other nurses to substantiate changes. When subjective data are required, the nurse must rely upon either (a) the client's statements (e.g., "My pain is worse now than it was after breakfast") or (b) objective indicators of the subjective data, even though these indicators may require interpretation (e.g., decreased restlessness, decreased pulse and respiratory rates, and relaxed facial muscles as indicators of pain relief). Data collected must be recorded concisely and accurately to facilitate the third part of the evaluating process. Flowsheets and problem-oriented medical records in the SOAP format (discussed in Chapter 17) are recording aids.

Judging Goal Achievement

If the first two parts of the evaluation process have been carried out effectively, determining whether a goal has been achieved is relatively simple. Both the nurse and the client play active roles in this. The data collected are compared with established criteria. Did the client drink 3000 ml of fluid in 24 hours? Did the client walk unassisted the specified distance per day? There are three possible outcomes of evaluation:

1. The goal was met; i.e., the client responded as expected.
2. The goal was partially met; i.e., a short-term goal was achieved, but the long-term goal was not; or, some, but not all, of the outcome criteria were attained.
3. The goal was not met.

See Table 14–1 on page 232 for evaluation examples of Mr. Joe Smith's outcome criteria.

TABLE 14-1 *Evaluating Goal Achievement for Mr. Joe Smith*

Assessment Data	Diagnostic Statement	Goal
Hospitalized for cardiac catheterization and possible aortic valve replacement States family scared about illness Wants to see chaplain Wants family to visit Perceives son Tom as helpful Says is usually too busy to worry about things	**Fear** related to cardiac catheterization, possible heart surgery, and its outcome	Experience increased emotional comfort and feelings of control
Vital signs normal Heart rhythm regular Loud heart murmur (aortic area) Femoral pulses stronger than normal Absent pulses (popliteal, dorsalis pedis, posterior tibial) in left leg Left leg cooler than right leg Integument pink and intact	**Altered peripheral tissue perfusion (left leg)** related to impaired arterial circulation	Improve circulation to left leg and foot
Left hip replacement Movement slightly limited Joint stiffness Slight limp	**Potential for injury(trauma)** related to joint stiffness and limp from hip replacement surgery	Prevent injury
Shortness of breath Lacks energy to do daily chores Does not smoke	**Activity intolerance** related to shortness of breath and lack of energy secondary to decreased strength of cardiac contraction	Avoid performance of activities causing shortness of breath and excessive cardiac workload

TABLE 14 – 1 *(continued)*

Nursing Orders	Outcome Criteria	Evaluation
Establish a trusting relationship with the client and family Encourage client and family to express feelings and concerns Discuss what the cardiac catheterization procedure entails and what is expected of him before and after the procedure Encourage conversation with another client who has recuperated from similar surgery	Verbalizes specific concerns Communicates thoughts clearly and logically Facial expressions, voice tone, and body posture correspond to verbal expressions of increased emotional comfort or feelings of control After instruction, describes the cardiac catheterization procedure and what is expected of him before and after the procedure	*Goal met* Verbalized concerns: "I'm worried about how my wife will support the family especially if anything bad happens during surgery." Asked questions about cardiac catheterization and surgery Nonverbal and verbal communication are congruent Described what to expect and what is expected of him before and after the cardiac catheterization procedure, e.g., "I know I will be taking a pill to help me relax before the procedure."
Consult with physician about exercise program, such as walking and range-of-motion exercises to hip, knee, and ankle Keep the extremity in a dependent position (i.e., lower than the heart) Use Doppler ultrasound stethoscope (DUS) to assess blood flow in left dorsalis pedis, posterior tibial, and popliteal arteries q2h Instruct client to keep his legs warm, e.g., by wearing warm socks, but discourage use of external heat	Demonstrates intact, pink, and moist skin Exhibits warm skin temperature (as other foot) Demonstrates palpable left dorsalis pedis, posterior tibial, and popliteal pulses of same strength as corresponding right pulses Verbalizes factors that improve and inhibit peripheral circulation Demonstrates capillary refill of left toenails within 1 to 3 seconds	*Goal partially met* Skin of left foot and ankle intact but pale Skin temperature still cooler in left than right foot Left popliteal pulse palpable but weak Left dorsalis pedis and posterior tibial pulses not palpable Blood flow evident only by DUS Capillary refill in left toenails within 7 seconds
Closely assess ambulation and transfers during first few days Keep bed at lowest level Encourage client to request assistance to ambulate during the night Closely attend client or put side rails up when client is sedated	Moves in and out of bed and ambulates without falling or injuring self	*Goal met* Ambulated and moved in and out of bed safely
Organize client care and provide undisturbed rest periods Discuss energy conservation methods, such as taking periodic rests Tell the client to reduce the intensity, duration, and frequency of activity if he experiences chest pain, shortness of breath, dizziness, or abnormal pulse and blood pressure after activity Monitor vital signs q2h and report decreasing blood pressure, increasing heart rate, or increasing respiratory rate	Rests after meals No shortness of breath during activities Shows stable pulse rate and blood pressure at 80 bpm and 124/80 mm Hg	*Goal met* Rested after meals and activities Experienced no shortness of breath while performing ADLs Pulse rate and blood pressure remained stable at 80 bpm and 124/80 mm Hg

Relating Nursing Actions to Client Outcomes

The fourth aspect of the evaluating process is determining whether the nursing actions had any relation to the outcomes. It should never be assumed that a nursing action was the cause of or the only factor in meeting, partially meeting, or not meeting a goal. For example, Mrs. Sophi Ringdale was obese and needed to lose 14 kg (30 lb). When the nurse and client drew up a care plan, one outcome criterion was "Lose 1.4 kg (3 lb) by 4/7/91." A nursing strategy in the care plan was "Explain how to plan and prepare a 900-calorie diet." On 4/7/91, the client weighed herself and had lost 1.8kg (4 lb). The goal had been met, in fact, exceeded. It is easy to assume that the nursing strategy was highly effective. However, it is important to collect more data before drawing that conclusion. Upon questioning the client, the nurse could find any of the following: (a) the client planned a 900-calorie diet and prepared and ate the food; (b) the client planned a 900-calorie diet but did not prepare the correct food; (c) the client did not understand how to plan a 900-calorie diet, so she did not bother with it. If the first possibility is found to be true, the nurse can safely judge that the nursing strategy "Explain how to plan and prepare a 900-calorie diet" was effective in helping the client lose weight. However, if the nurse learns that either the second or third possibility actually happened, then it must be assumed that the nursing strategy did not affect the outcome. The next step for the nurse is to collect data about what the client actually did to lose weight. It is important to establish the relationship (or lack thereof) of the nursing actions to the outcomes.

Reexamining the Client's Care Plan

Evaluating goal achievement provides the feedback necessary to determine if the care plan was effective in resolving, reducing, or preventing the client's problems. It is then necessary for the nurse to reexamine all aspects of the care plan, whether or not the goals have been met. Reexamining is a process of reassessing and replanning. See Table 14–1, earlier, for an example of evaluating goal achievement for Mr. Joe Smith.

When Goals Are Met
If a goal or goals have been met, one of the following decisions may be made:

- The nurse may decide that the problem stated in the diagnosis no longer exists. In this instance, the nurse must document that the goal was met and that the care planned to meet this goal is discontinued.
- The nurse may decide that the problem still exists even though the goal was met. For example, if the criterion is "Client will ingest 3000 ml of fluid daily," and the goal is "Client's state of hydration will be maintained," nursing interventions need to continue even though the goal and criterion have been met.

When Goals Are Not Met
When goals are not met or only partially met, the nurse needs to reexamine the client's database, nursing diagnoses statements, goal statements, and nursing strategies.

Database   An incomplete or incorrect database influences all subsequent steps of the nursing process and care plan. In some instances, new data may invalidate the database, necessitating new nursing diagnoses, new goals, and new nursing actions.

Diagnostic statements   If the database is incomplete, new diagnostic statements are required. If the database is complete, the nurse needs to analyze whether the problem was identified correctly and whether the nursing diagnoses are relevant to that database.

Goal statements   If the nursing diagnostic statement is inaccurate and requires correcting, it is obvious that the goal statement needs revision. If the nursing diagnostic statement is appropriate, the nurse then checks that the goal statements are realistic and attainable. Unrealistic, unattainable goals require correction. The nurse should also determine whether priorities have changed and whether the client and nurse still agree on the priorities. For example, a priority for the nurse may be to increase the client's fluid intake, but a priority for the client may be to decrease intake because of nausea.

Nursing strategies   Last, the nurse investigates whether the nursing strategies are related to the goals and whether the best nursing strategies were selected. Even when the diagnoses and goals are appropriate, the nursing strategies selected may not have been the best ones to achieve the goal. Before selecting new strategies, the nurse should check whether the ordered nursing actions have been carried out. Other personnel may not have carried them out, either because the orders were unclear or because the orders were unreasonable in terms of such external constraints such as money, staff, and equipment.

Modifying the Care Plan

When it is determined that the care plan needs revising, the nurse follows five steps:

1. Change the data in the assessment column to reflect the more recent findings. The new data should be dated and

flagged in some way to indicate they are new. Follow agency practice: Some nurses use ink of a different color; others put a colored tab at the edge of the paper.

2. Revise the nursing diagnoses to reflect the new data. The new nursing diagnoses are also dated.

3. Revise the client's priorities, goals, and outcome criteria to reflect the new nursing diagnoses. These are also dated.

4. Establish new nursing strategies to correspond to the new nursing diagnoses. New nursing strategies may reflect increased or decreased need of the client for nursing care, scheduling changes, and rearrangement of nursing activities to group similar activities or to permit longer rest or activity periods for the client. For example, the nurse might assist Mr. Carter to walk after a rest period and before a meal so that he can ambulate when he is rested and sit up for the meal if his health permits.

5. Change the outcome criteria to reflect the other changes in the plan. These changes should project the desired level of wellness indicted by the client. Criteria that apply to outdated nursing diagnoses should be deleted. See Table 14-2 on pages 236-237.

EVALUATING THE QUALITY OF NURSING CARE

Over the past 30 years, there has been considerable work on the evaluation of the quality of nursing care to determine what good care is, whether the care nurses give is appropriate and effective, and whether the quality of care provided is good. Evaluating the quality of nursing care is an essential part of professional accountability. Other terms used for this measurement are quality assessment and quality assurance. **Quality assessment** is an examination of services only; **quality assurance** implies that efforts are made to evaluate *and* ensure quality health care.

Historical Perspective

Evaluation of the quality of care is not a new concept. Florence Nightingale's *Notes on Hospitals,* published in 1859, included an evaluation of medical and nursing care. Since that time, evaluation has progressed through a number of stages. Initially, it focused on the environment, e.g., whether equipment was available at the time it was needed. Later, organizational standards in agencies were developed. For example, the ratio of nurses to clients was studied and evaluated in terms of clients' needs. Since 1952, the Joint Commission on Accreditation of Hospitals (JCAH), a voluntary organization, has surveyed hospitals. Objective criteria were applied to evaluate a client's record after discharge from the hospital. This was called a **retrospective audit. (Ret-**rospective** means relating to a past event, and **audit** means an examination or review of records.) A **nursing audit** is a review of clients' charts to evaluate nursing competence or performance.

In 1972 and 1973, the JCAH revised its standards to include the requirement that hospitals be subjected to medical and nursing audits before receiving accreditation. The maximum length of accreditation is three years, with reports submitted periodically to determine the institution's progress toward the recommendations submitted by the surveyors at the last visit.

In 1972, the United States government enacted legislation to control health care costs and evaluate the quality of health care services received by Medicare and Medicaid patients. Since that time a national and statewide system of professional review organizations (PROs) has been developed (Gordon 1987). The purposes of the PROs include developing standards and monitoring the quality of, cost of, and access to care. Hospitals are required to contract with a PRO for utilization review. The objective of these procedures is to ensure that the care given under federal programs was necessary and that the appropriate facilities were chosen to provide the care. Once problems are identified, an education process may be suggested to facilitate the correction of unacceptable staff practices, or penalties may be imposed on noncompliant care providers.

The PRO's are based on the concept of peer review. A **peer review** is an encounter between two persons equal in education, abilities, and qualifications, during which one person critically reviews the practices that the other has documented in a client's record. These evaluative processes may be **concurrent audits,** that is, reviews of present practices.

Approaches to Quality Evaluation

Three aspects of care—structure, process, and outcome—can be evaluated. Standards of care for each type of evaluation have been developed based on nursing and health-related research and expert opinion.

The Structure in Which Client Care Takes Place
Structure evaluation focuses on the organization of the client care system, for instance, administrative and financial procedures that direct the provision of care, staffing patterns, management styles, availability of equipment, and physical facilities. Information about these support structures can be obtained easily. All of these factors indirectly influence care. For example, the hospital administration determines the number of nursing positions that the hospital can afford. Quality care cannot be delivered without adequate staff and resources. However, adequate staffing patterns and adequate facilities do not ensure quality care.

TABLE 14–2 *Modified Care Plan for Mr. Joe Smith after Cardiac Surgery (selected examples only)*

Assessment Data	Diagnostic Statement	Goal
Rales in bases of both lungs relieved by coughing before surgery Painful chest incision	**Potential ineffective airway clearance** related to chest incision	Maintain a clear airway
Aortic valve replacement (7/15) Heart rhythm regular at rest Pulse: 80 beats per minute (bpm) BP: 110/80 mm Hg	**Potential decreased cardiac output** related to physical exertion and/or shock	Maintain cardiac output and blood volume
Left dorsalis pedis pulse and posterior tibial artery not palpable Skin of left extremity cool and pale	**Altered tissue perfusion** related to impaired arterial circulation	Improve arterial circulation
Aortic valve replacement	**Potential activity intolerance** related to reduced strength of cardiac contraction	Increase activity tolerance

TABLE 14 – 2 *(continued)*

Nursing Orders	Rationale	Outcome Criteria
Administer analgesics q4h during first 48 hours	Pain relief makes coughing less uncomfortable and more effective	Normal breath sounds auscultated in all areas of both lungs
Splint incision with pillows or hands during coughing	Splinting minimizes pain	
Turn q2h during first 48 hours	Turning prevents the accumulation of secretions in one lung area	
Assist with deep breathing and coughing (DB & C) exercises q2h	DB & C exercises help to move and expel secretions	
Assess vital signs q1h for first 24 hours, q2h if stable for next 48 hours, and q4h thereafter if stable	A lowered blood pressure and rapid pulse indicate lowered blood volume or inadequate cardiac output	Stable vital signs
Assess apical pulse and heart rhythm, not radial pulse		Pulse: 80–100 bpm
Report an increase in resting pulse rate above 110 bpm and a BP below 100 mm Hg		BP: not less than 110/80 mm Hg
		Respirations not more than 15 breaths per minute
Keep client's legs warm (especially left leg) with blankets or socks	Warmth increases circulation	Left posterior tibial and dorsalis pedis pulses palpable and of same strength as corresponding right pulses
Assess blood flow in left dorsalis pedis artery and posterior tibial artery q2h using DUS	The DUS detects and indicates movement of blood through the arteries	Skin warm, intact, pink
Keep left leg in dependent position	A dependent position facilitates arterial blood flow by gravity	Capillary refill of left toenails within 1 to 3 seconds
Consult physician about a schedule for increasing activity	A gradual increase in activity helps the heart muscle and new valve accommodate increased demands	After activity, heart rate remains below 110 bpm and within 6 bpm of resting pulse after 3 minutes
Monitor and later show the client how to monitor his response to increased activity by:	Pulse rate monitoring provides awareness of activities that do not overly exert the heart	
1. Taking a resting pulse before activity 2. Taking pulse immediately after activity 3. Taking pulse 3 minutes after activity 4. Noting rate decreases, rates about 110, rates not within 6 bpm of resting pulse after 3 minutes		
Monitor blood pressure after activity	A drop in blood pressure indicates a reduction in cardiac output	
Starting on 7/19, discuss factors contributing to increased cardiac workload, such as stress, excessive weight, overactivity, large meals	Knowledge of factors contributing to increased cardiac workload may facilitate necessary life-style changes, such as eating smaller meals, losing weight, and altering activity patterns	
Starting on 7/19, discuss the effects of reduced cardiac output such as shortness of breath, pain, fatigue, edema	Knowledge of the effects of reduced cardiac output may motivate him to avoid excessive activity	

The Process of Care   The focus of process evaluation is the activities of the nurse i.e., the performance of the caregiver in relation to the client's needs. This approach may be the most effective in determining the quality of care provided. The care given by the nurse is evaluated by talking with the client, auditing the client's record, and observing the nursing activities. Evaluators may seek answers to questions such as these: Are medications recorded properly? Was client teaching documented? Is the care plan complete? This type of evaluation is time consuming and requires the judgment of expert practitioners. The American Nurses' Association (ANA) *Standards of Practice* (1973) are process standards that provide the nursing profession with a framework for the delivery and evaluation of care.

Outcomes of the Care   The focus of outcome evaluation is the client's health status, welfare, and satisfaction, or the results of care in terms of changes in the client. Its advantage is that outcomes may be easily observed, especially in relation to medical care, which focuses on disease entities. In nursing, however, outcomes are more difficult to determine, since nursing takes a holistic view of the client. Defining emotional, social, and behavioral outcomes is more complex than defining medical outcomes. In addition, client outcomes cannot be wholly attributed to nursing care. The client's own physical and psychologic mechanisms and contributions by family and other health professionals collectively produce outcomes. Outcome evaluation can focus on the client's change in behavior toward goal achievement prior to discharge (concurrent audit), or the client's record may be reviewed after discharge for evidence of goal attainment (retrospective audit).

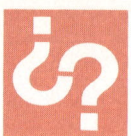

RESEARCH NOTE

What Nursing Care Behaviors Predict Client Satisfaction?

The purpose of this study was to (a) determine how satisfied hospitalized clients were with nursing care behaviors and (b) predict which nursing behaviors were associated with client satisfaction. Client satisfaction was based on how closely the care the client received (actual) approached the care the client would have liked to receive (ideal). A patient satisfaction instrument (PSI) measured three nursing care variables: trust, patient education, and professional technical aspects. The subjects included 24 women and 26 men with a mean age of 60.36 years. Some nursing care behaviors associated with client satisfaction included being friendly, spending time talking to the client, following through with directions, explaining the diagnosis, and showing the client how to carry out physicians' orders. The subjects were least satisfied with the amount and type of information the nurse gave them.

Implications: This study suggests (a) that placing an emphasis on meeting the emotional and psychologic needs of clients and (b) providing more information to clients about themselves and their situation would increase client satisfaction. Clients need more information to take an active part in health care decisions.

M. M. M. Bader, Nursing care behaviors that predict patient satisfaction, *Journal of Nursing Quality Assurance*, May 1988, 2:11–17.

Tools and Methods for Measuring Quality Care

Measuring the quality of care is a complex task. Development of tools involves four steps (Wright 1984, pp. 457–61):

1. Defining and clarifying the nature of nursing.

2. Deciding what approach to take (structure, process, outcome).

3. Developing standards and criteria. **Standards** are optimum levels of care against which actual performance is compared. **Criteria** are predetermined indicators of measures of health care, the presence, absence, and completeness of which indicate the quality of services (Meisenheimer 1985, p. 333, 338). Here is an example of a standard and its criteria:

   Standard IV: Each client has a written nursing care plan.

   Criteria: The nursing care plan is initiated within 8 hours of admission. It is based on information from the nursing health history and physical assessment. Goals are mutually set with the client and family, and the nursing care plan is evaluated and modified according to the client's needs.

4. Testing the criteria. Criteria must be valid and reliable. A **valid criterion** measures what it is intended to. A **reliable criterion** produces consistent results when used by the same person over time or by a different person.

Several established tools are available for measuring the quality of care. Some are process tools, some are outcome tools, and others are process-outcome tools. Each tool consists of standards and criteria. Developing effective quality care evaluation tools is a challenge for the nursing profession. Much work is continuing even on established tools.

Methods of using these tools also vary. Some evaluate by retrospective audits of nursing records using nursing audit committees. Others evaluate using a concurrent audit process, i.e., direct observation of the nurse or nurses providing the nursing care by educated observers or by peers. Data may also be obtained by questioning and observing clients, questioning the family, and observing the client's environment and the general environment. The time period for measurement also varies. Some tools are designed for use over a 2-hour period; some are designed to evaluate the whole process of care given to the client from admission to discharge.

Scoring systems differ among tools. Levels of care may be rated as *excellent, good, incomplete, poor,* and *unsafe.* Some tools require only simple *yes* or *no* responses. Nurses' performances may be rated on a scale of 5 (best nurse) to 1 (worst nurse).

CHAPTER HIGHLIGHTS

▶ Evaluation determines whether or to what degree the client goals have been met.

▶ Evaluating is both a concurrent and terminal process.

▶ Evaluating is purposeful and organized.

▶ Identifying outcome criteria is the first aspect of evaluating.

▶ Outcome criteria determine the evaluative data that must be collected to judge whether the goals have been met.

▶ Outcome criteria must be measurable and precise.

▶ Reexamining the client care plan is a process of reassessing and replanning.

▶ Evaluating the quality of nursing care is an essential aspect of professional accountability.

READING AND REFERENCES

SUGGESTED READINGS

Porter, A. L. September 1988. Assuring quality through staff nurse performance. *Nursing Clinics of North America* 23:649–655.

The author describes the importance of a quality nursing staff to ensure quality patient care. The nurse must have the basic educational and personal credentials and then demonstrate quality performance as determined by preestablished standards. Clinical standards and performance appraisal methods must be clearly stated and effectively designed. Continuing education is suggested as a method to assist the nursing staff to refine and improve ineffective behaviors.

Smeltzer, C. H. August, 1988. Evaluating a successful quality assurance program: The process. *Journal of Nursing Quality Assurance* 2:1–9.

For a quality assurance program to benefit the nursing profession, it must be understood by all departments, implemented in a timely and appropriate manner, and include an ongoing evaluation component to determine effectiveness. Smeltzer presents and examines criteria for a successful quality assurance program that will provide a systematic method for evaluation of quality professional practice.

RELATED RESEARCH

Bader, M. M. M. May 1988. Nursing care behaviors that predict patient satisfaction. *Journal of Nursing Quality Assurance* 2:11–17.

Fink, A., Siu, A. L., and Brook, R. H. October 9, 1987. Assuring the quality of health care for older persons: an expert panel's priorities. *Journal of the American Medical Association* 258:1905–8.

Smeltzer, C. H., Hinshaw, A. S., and Feltman, B. May 1987. The benefits of staff nurse involvement in monitoring the quality of patient care. *Journal of Nursing Quality Assurance* 1:1–7.

SELECTED REFERENCES

Bachrach, M. K.; Ballesteros, P.; and Black, A. N. Winter, 1988. Using patient outcomes to define nursing practice. *Nursing Administration Quarterly* 12:45–51.

Gordon, M. 1987. *Nursing diagnosis: Process and application.* 2d ed. New York: McGraw Hill.

Joint Commission on Accreditation of Health Organizations. 1989. *Accreditation Manual for Hospitals.* Chicago: Joint Commission on Accreditation of Health Organizations, Nursing Services.

Latreille, D. D.; Roth, M. J.; and Burgoyne, J. A. January 1988. Quality assurance. *Journal of Psychosocial Nursing and Mental Health Services* 26:28–31, 36, 38.

Lieske, A. 1985. Standards: The basis of a quality assurance program. In Meisenheimer, C., editor. *Quality assurance: A complete guide to effective programs.* Rockville, Md.: Aspen Systems Corporation.

Marker, C. G. S. May 1987. The Marker Umbrella model for quality assurance: Monitoring and evaluating professional practice. *Journal of Nursing Quality Assurance* 1:52–63.

Meisenheimer, C. 1985. *Quality assurance: A complete guide to effective programs.* Rockville, Md.: Aspen Systems Corporation.

O'Brien, B. November 1988. QA: A commitment to excellence. *Nursing Management* 19:33–34, 38–40.

Patterson, C. H. September 1988. Standards of patient care: The Joint

Commission focus on nursing quality assurance. *Nursing Clinics of North America* 23:625–638.

Porter, A. L. September 1988. Assuring quality through staff nurse performance. *Nursing Clinics of North America* 23:649–655.

Rinke, L. 1987. *Outcome measures in home care.* Vol. 1. New York: National League for Nursing (Pub. no. 21-2194).

Rinke, L., and Wilson, A. 1987. *Outcome measures in home care.* Vol. 2. New York: National League for Nursing (Pub. no 21-2195).

Westfall, U. E. February 1987. Standards of practice: Nursing values made visible. *Journal of Nursing Quality Assurance* 1:21–30.

Whittaker, A. and McCanless, L. February 1988. Nursing peer review: Monitoring the appropriateness and outcome of nursing care. *Journal of Nursing Quality Assurance* 2:24–31.

Wright, D. September 1984. An introduction to the evaluation of nursing care: A review of the literature. *Journal of Advanced Nursing* 9:457–67.

Yura, H., and Walsh, M. B. 1988. *The nursing process: Assessing, planning, implementing, evaluating.* 5th ed. Norwalk, Conn.: Appleton & Lange.

INTERACTIVE PROCESSES

Helping and Communicating

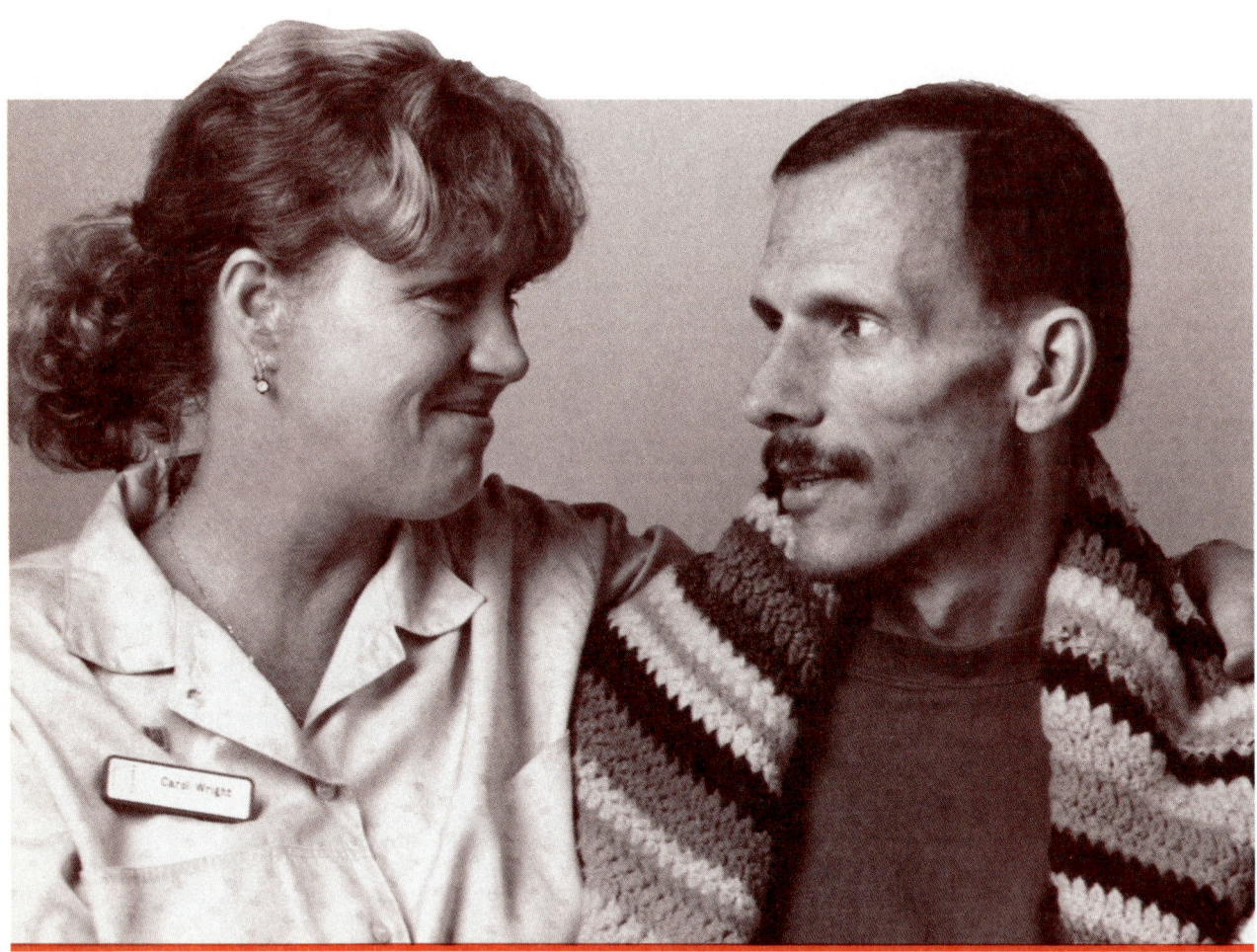

CONTENTS

OBJECTIVES

▸ Describe four phases of the helping relationship.

▸ Describe essential aspects of communication and the communication process.

▸ Explain the four elements of the communication process outlined in this chapter.

▸ Identify ways in which selected factors influence the communication process.

▸ Differentiate verbal and nonverbal communication.

▸ Give guidelines for assessing problems in communication.

▸ List examples of nursing diagnoses pertaining to communication.

▸ Describe strategies for planning to resolve communication problems.

▸ Describe effective and ineffective methods used by nurses when communicating with clients.

▸ List outcome criteria that can be used to evaluate whether or not communication problems have been resolved.

▸ Identify features of effective groups.

THE HELPING RELATIONSHIP

Nurse-client relationships are referred to by some as *interpersonal relationships,* by others as *therapeutic relationships* and by still others as *helping relationships.* Helping is a growth-facilitating process in which one person assists another to solve problems and to face crises in the direction the assisted person chooses (Brammer 1988, p. 5). Several terms are used to describe the persons involved in a helping relationship: *helper* and *helpee; giver* and *receiver;* and *counselor* and *client.* For purposes of consistency, in this text the term *nurse* or *helper* will refer to the person who gives the help, and the term *client* will denote the person receiving the help. However, we recognize that various people in all walks of life act as helpers and receivers of help.

Imogene King (1981) uses the terms *nurse/client interaction* rather than *interpersonal relationship.* According to King (1981, p. 60), "The process of *interactions* between two or more individuals represents a sequence of verbal and nonverbal behaviors that are goal directed." In King's theory, *interpersonal relationships* are a subconcept of the *interaction.* She points out that in many nurse practice settings, such as critical care, where the nurse only has time to attend to physiologic variables that are life-threatening, interpersonal relationships cannot be established. In the interactive process, two individuals mutually identify goals and the means to achieve them. When they agree on the means to implement the goals, they move toward transactions. *Transaction* is defined as goal attainment (King 1981, p. 61).

Phases of the Helping Relationship

This relationship process can be described in terms of four sequential phases, each of which is characterized by identifiable tasks and skills. Progression through the stages must occur in succession, as each builds on the one before. Nurses can identify the progress of a relationship by understanding these phases: preinteraction phase, introductory phase, working (maintaining) phase, and termination phase. Table 15–1 on page 244 summarizes the tasks and skills required for each phase.

Preinteraction Phase   The **preinteraction phase** is similar to the planning stage before an interview. In most situations, the nurse has information about the client before the first face-to-face meeting. Such information may include the client's name, address, age, medical history, and/or social history. Planning for the initial visit may generate some anxious feelings in the nurse. By recognizing these feelings and identifying specific information to be discussed, positive outcomes will evolve.

Introductory Phase   The **introductory phase** is also referred to as the *orientation phase* or the *prehelping phase.* This phase is important, since the tone for the rest of the relationship phases is set during this phase. Three stages of this introductory phase are (a) opening the relationship, (b) clarifying the problem, and (c) structuring and formulating the contract (Brammer 1988, p. 51). Other important tasks of the introductory phase include getting to know each other and developing a degree of trust.

During the initial parts of the introductory phase, the client may display some resistive behaviors and some testing behaviors. *Resistive behaviors* are those that inhibit involvement, cooperation, or change. Three major reasons for their occurrence are (a) difficulty in acknowledging the need for help and thus a dependent role, (b) fear of exposing and facing feelings, and (c) anxiety about the discomfort involved in changing problem-causing behavior patterns. *Testing behaviors* are those that examine the nurse's interest and sincerity. For example, a client may refuse to talk to test whether the nurse will stay with her for the prescribed period of time.

TABLE 15–1 *Tasks and Skills for Each Phase of the Helping Relationship*

Phase	Tasks	Skills
Preinteraction phase	The nurse reviews pertinent knowledge, considers potential areas of concern, and develops plans for interaction.	Recognizing limitations and seeking assistance as required.
Introductory phase 1. Opening the relationship	Both client and nurse identify each other by name. When the nurse initiates the relationship, it is important to explain the nurse's role to give the client an idea of what to expect. When the client initiates the relationship, the nurse needs to help the client express concerns and reasons for seeking help. Vague, open-ended questions, such as "What's on your mind today?" are helpful at this stage.	A relaxed attending attitude to put the client at ease. It is not easy for all clients to receive help.
2. Clarifying the problem	Because the client initially may not see the problem clearly, the nurse's major task is to help clarify the problem.	Attentive listening, paraphrasing, clarifying, and other effective communication techniques discussed in this chapter. A common error at this stage is to ask too many questions of the client.
3. Structuring and formulating the contract (obligations to be met by both the nurse and client)	Nurse and client develop a degree of trust and verbally agree about: (a) location, frequency, and length of meetings, (b) overall purpose of the relationship, (c) how confidential material will be handled, (d) tasks to be accomplished, and (e) duration and indications for termination of the relationship.	Communication skills listed above and ability to overcome resistive and/or testing behaviors if they occur.
Working phase	Nurse and client accomplish the tasks outlined in the introductory phase, enhance trust and rapport, and develop caring.	
1. Responding and exploring	The nurse assists the client to explore thoughts, feelings, and actions. The client explores feelings and actions associated with problems (self-exploration or self-disclosure).	Listening and attending skills and four responding skills: first-level empathy, respect, genuineness, and concreteness.
2. Integrative understanding and dynamic self-understanding	The nurse acquires integrative understanding about the client. The client develops the skill of listening and gains insight into personal behavior.	In addition to those of the first stage, skills required by the nurse are advanced-level empathy, self-disclosure, and confrontation. Skills required by the client are nondefensive listening and dynamic self-understanding.
3. Facilitating and taking action	The nurse plans programs within the client's capabilities and considers long- and short-term goals. The client needs to learn to take risks (i.e., accept that either failure or success may be the outcome). The nurse needs to reinforce successes and help the client recognize failures realistically.	Decision-making and goal-setting skills. In addition: For the client: risk-taking. For the nurse: reinforcement skills.
Termination phase	Nurse and client accept feelings of loss. The client accepts the end of the relationship without feelings of anxiety or dependence.	For the nurse: summarizing skills. For the client: abilities to handle problems independently.

By the end of the introductory phase, the client begins to develop trust in the nurse. Both participants also begin to view each other as unique individuals. Characteristics of trusting individuals include (a) a feeling of comfort with growth in self-awareness, (b) an ability to share this awareness with others, (c) acceptance of others as they are without needing to change them, (d) openness to new experiences, (e) consistency between words and actions, (f) openness and honesty about motives, (g) willingness to confide, offer information and opinions, and (h) ability to delay gratification (Thomas 1970, p. 118; and Kaul and Schmidt 1971, p. 542).

Working Phase   During the **working phase** the nurse and the client begin to view each other as unique individuals. They begin to appreciate this uniqueness and care about each other. *Caring* is sharing deep and genuine concern about the welfare of another person. Once caring develops, the potential for empathy increases. The working phase has three successive stages: (a) responding and exploring, (b) integrative understanding and dynamic self-understanding, and (c) facilitating and taking action (Egan 1975, pp. 34–40).

Stage 1: Responding and exploring   In addition to listening and attending skills, the nurse requires four skills for this first stage.

1. *First-level empathy.* Nurses must communicate (respond) in ways that indicate they have listened to what was said and understand how the client feels. The nurse responds to content or feelings or both, as appropriate. The nurse's nonverbal behaviors are also important. In a study of five nurses and five clients, Hardin and Halaris (1983, p. 15) found that nonverbal communication and specific nonverbal behaviors may be linked to empathy. They observed the engaging and defensive nonverbal behaviors of clients and nurses and compared nurses whom the clients rated as either highly empathetic or not empathetic. Nonverbal engaging behaviors included direct gaze, slight smile, laugh, forward torso, gestures, head nods, and leg position. Defensive behaviors included cross arms and crossed legs. Their findings indicated that *high-empathy nurses* employed moderate head nodding, a steady gaze, moderate gesturing, and little activity or body movement. The *low-empathy nurse* used frequent head nodding and gesturing, laughed more than the high-empathy nurse, and displayed more eye movement, leg movement, and torso movement.

2. *Respect.* The nurse must show respect for the clients, willingness to be available, and desire to work with the client.

3. *Genuineness.* Personal statements can be helpful in solidifying the rapport between the nurse and the client. The nurse might offer such comments as "I recall when I was in (a similar situation), and I felt angry about being put down." Egan (1982, p. 128) states that the helper "must be spontaneous, open. He can't hide behind the role of counselor. He must be a human being to the human being before him." Egan refers to this quality as *genuineness* and outlines five behaviors that are components of it. See the accompanying box. Nurses need to exercise caution when making references about themselves. These statements must be used with discretion. The extreme of matching each of the client's problems with a better story of the nurse's own is of little value to the client.

4. *Concreteness.* The nurse must assist the client to be concrete and specific rather than to speak in generalities.

Behaviors/Components of Genuineness

- The genuine helper does not take refuge in or overemphasize the role of counselor.
- The genuine person is spontaneous.
- The genuine person is nondefensive.
- The genuine person displays few discrepancies—that is, the person is consistent and does not think or feel one thing but say another.
- The genuine person is capable of deep self-disclosure (self-sharing) when it is appropriate.

Source: G. Egan, *The skilled helper. Model, skills, and methods for effective helping,* 2d ed. (Monterey, Calif.: Brooks/Cole Publishing Co., 1982), pp. 127–31.

When the client says, "I'm stupid and clumsy," the nurse narrows the topic to the specific by pointing out, "You tripped on the scatter rug."

During this first stage of the working phase, the intensity of interaction increases, and feelings such as anger, shame, or self-consciousness may be expressed. If the nurse is skilled in this stage and if the client is willing to pursue self-exploration, the outcome is a beginning understanding on the part of the client about behavior and feelings.

Stage 2: Integrative understanding and dynamic self-understanding   In this second stage, clients achieve an objective understanding of themselves and their world (dynamic self-understanding). This ultimately enables clients to change and to take action. More self-exploration occurs, and more information is produced. As a result of this process, isolated pieces of information can now be integrated into larger contexts that reveal behavior patterns or themes.

For this stage, the nurse needs the following three skills in addition to those of the first stage:

1. *Advanced-level empathy.* The nurse responds in ways that indicate an understanding not only of what is said but also of what is hinted at or implied nonverbally. Isolated statements become connected.

2. *Self-disclosure.* The nurse willingly but discreetly shares personal experiences.

3. *Confrontation.* The nurse points out discrepancies between thoughts, feelings, and actions that inhibit the client's self-understanding or exploration of specific areas. This is done empathetically, not judgmentally.

Stage 3: Facilitating and taking action   Ultimately the client must make decisions and take action to become more effective. The responsibility for action belongs to the client. The nurse, however, collaborates in these decisions, provides support, and may offer options or information.

Termination Phase   This phase of the relationship is often expected to be difficult and filled with ambivalence. However, if the previous phases have evolved effectively, the client generally has a positive outlook and feels able to handle problems independently. However, because caring attitudes have developed, it is natural to expect some feelings of loss, and each person needs to develop a way of saying good-bye.

Many methods can be used to terminate relationships. Summarizing or reviewing the process can produce a sense of accomplishment. This may include sharing reminiscences of how things were at the beginning of the relationship, compared to now. It is also helpful for both the nurse and the client to express their feelings about termination openly and honestly. Thus termination discussions need to start in advance of the termination interview. This allows time for the client to adjust to independence. In some situations referrals are necessary, or it is appropriate to offer an occasional standby meeting to give support as needed.

Developing Helping Relationships

Whatever the practice setting, the nurse establishes some sort of helping relationship in which mutual goals are set with the client, or with support persons if the client is unable to participate. Although *special* training in counseling techniques is advantageous, there are many ways of helping clients that do not require special training. Shanken and Shanken (1976, pp. 24–27) have outlined 11 of these:

1. *Listen actively.* (See the discussion of attentive listening, later in this chapter.)

2. *Help to identify what the person is feeling.* Often clients who are troubled are unable to identify or to label their feelings and consequently have difficulty working them out or talking about them. Responses by the nurse such as "You seem angry about taking orders from your boss" or "You sound as if you've been lonely since your wife died" can help clients recognize what they are feeling and talk about it.

3. *Put yourself in the other person's shoes.* The ability to do this is referred to as **empathy.** According to Egan (1975, p. 76), empathy involves the ability to discriminate what the other's world is like and to communicate to the other this understanding in a way that shows the other that the helper has picked up both the client's *feelings* and the *behavior* and *experience* underlying these feelings.

4. *Be honest.* In effective relationships nurses honestly recognize any lack of knowledge by saying, "I don't know the answer to that right now"; openly discuss their own discomfort by saying, for example, "I feel uncomfortable about this discussion"; and admit tact-fully that problems do exist, for instance, when a client says "I'm a mess, aren't I?"

5. *Do not tell a person not to feel.* Feelings expressed by clients often make nurses uncomfortable. Common examples are a client's expressions of anger or worry or a client's crying. When a nurse feels this discomfort, common responses are "Don't worry about it, everything will be fine" or "Please don't cry." Such responses inhibit the client's expression of feelings. Unless feelings are extremely inappropriate, it is best to encourage the client to ventilate (voice) them. Ventilation allows the client to express feelings in words and examine them objectively. Indirectly, such an attitude conveys this message: "Your feelings are not that awful, since I am not bothered by them."

6. *Do not tell a person what to feel.* Statements that indicate to clients how they should feel, rather than how they actually do feel, in essence deny clients' true feelings and suggest that they are inappropriate. Examples are: "You shouldn't complain about pain; many others have gone through this same experience stoically" and "You should be glad that you are alive and not worry about the loss of your arm."

7. *Do not make excuses for the other person.* When a person reacts with an intense feeling such as anger or grief and seems to have lost control of behavior to the astonishment or discomfort of others, a common error is to explain the behavior by offering excuses. Examples are: "Well, Mr. Brown, you're upset about not finishing your lunch, but the dietician and I gave you too much" and "I guess you've had a tough session in physical therapy." These responses discourage and divert the person from discussing feelings of anger or inadequacy. The nurse has made assumptions about the reasons for the client's behavior and therefore inhibits exploration of what the client is really experiencing and feeling.

8. *Be genuine.* See the discussion of this topic earlier in this chapter.

9. *Use your ingenuity.* There are always many courses of action to consider in handling problems. Whatever course is chosen needs to further achievement of the client's goals, be compatible with the client's value system, and offer the probability of success. The client needs to choose the ways to achieve goals; however, the nurse can assist in identifying options. For example, a client has asked for help because he is depressed and anxious about retirement. The nurse knows he loves animals, young children, and story telling. In this case, the nurse might direct his thoughts toward acquiring a puppy, writing children's stories, and volunteering at the public library.

10. *Know your role and your limitations.* Every person has unique strengths and problems. When the nurse feels

unable to handle some problems, the client should be informed and referred to the appropriate health professional.

COMMUNICATION IN NURSING

The term **communication** has various meanings, depending on the context in which it is used. To some, communication is the interchange of information between two or more people; in other words, the exchange of ideas or thoughts. This kind of communication uses methods such as talking and listening or writing and reading. However, painting, dancing, and story telling are also methods of communication. Thoughts are conveyed to others not only by spoken or written words but also by gestures or body actions.

Communication may have a more personal connotation than the interchange of ideas or thoughts. It can be a transmission of feelings, or a more personal and social interaction between people. In this context, communication often is synonymous with relating. Frequently one member of a couple comments that the other is not communicating. Some teenagers complain about a generation gap—being unable to communicate with understanding or feeling to a parent or authority figure. Sometimes a nurse is said to be efficient but lacking in something called *bedside manner.* For the purpose of this text, *communication* is any means of exchanging information or feelings between two or more people. It is a basic component of human relationships.

The intent of any communication is to elicit a response. Thus, communication is a process. It includes all the techniques by which an individual affects another. It has two main purposes: to influence others and to obtain information. Communication can be described as helpful or unhelpful. The former encourages a sharing of information, thoughts, or feelings between two or more people. The latter hinders or blocks the transfer of information and feelings.

Communication is a significant aspect of nursing practice. Nurses who communicate effectively are better able to initiate change that promotes health, establish a trusting relationship with a client and support persons, and prevent legal problems associated with nursing practice. Effective communication is essential for the establishment of the nurse-client relationship.

Nursing practice involves three kinds of communication: social, structured, and therapeutic. **Social communication** is unplanned communication, often carried out in an informal setting and usually at a leisurely pace. It is usually satisfying to all parties participating. **Structured communication** refers to definite planned content (Sundeen, Stuart, Rankin, and Cohen 1989, p. 129). An example of structured communication is teaching a client to give an injection or discussing postoperative care with a person anticipating surgery. **Therapeutic communication** is also used by nurses. It is defined by Ruesch as a process that helps "overcome temporary stress, to get along with other people, to adjust to the unalterable, and to overcome psychological blocks which stand in the way of self-realization" (1961, p. 7). Therapeutic communication is used by nurses in many settings and in many circumstances, for example, to support the anxious preoperative client or to help the person who has cancer accept and cope with this diagnosis. Structured communication is discussed in Chapter 16.

MODES OF COMMUNICATION

Communication is generally carried out in two different modes: verbal and nonverbal. **Verbal communication** uses the spoken or written word; **nonverbal communication** uses other forms, such as gestures or facial expressions. Although both kinds of communication occur concurrently, the majority of communication (some say 80 to 90%) is nonverbal. This may be surprising to those who associate communication with only verbal expression. Learning about nonverbal communication is thus an important consideration for nurses in developing effective communication patterns and relationships with clients.

Verbal Communication

Verbal communication is largely conscious, because people choose the words they use. The words used vary among individuals according to culture, socioeconomic background, age, and education. As a result, countless possibilities exist in the way ideas are exchanged. An abundance of words can be used to form messages. In addition, a wide variety of feelings can be conveyed when talking. The intonation of the voice can express animation, enthusiasm, sadness, annoyance, or amusement. The number of different intonations heard when people say "hello"or "good morning" illustrates the variety that is possible. The pacing or rhythm of a person's communication is another variable. Monotonous rhythms or very rapid rhythms can be products of lack of energy or interest, anxiety, or fear.

When choosing words to say or to write, nurses need to consider several criteria of effective communication. These include (a) simplicity, (b) clarity, (c) timing and relevance, (d) adaptability, and (e) credibility.

Simplicity   The best teachers can state complex ideas in simple words. The same holds true for persons communicating everyday concerns. Simplicity includes the use of commonly understood words, brevity, and completeness. Many people have a tendency to overcommunicate. Their messages are wordy, contain too many extraneous explanations, or use words that are highly academic, technical, or slangy. In the world of nursing, many complex technical terms become natural to nurses. However, these terms can often be misunderstood even by informed laypeople. Words such as *vasoconstriction* or *cholecystectomy* are meaningful to the speaker and easy to use but are ill-advised when communicating with clients. Nurses need to learn to select simple words intentionally even though effort is required to do so. For example, instead of saying to a client, "The nurse will be catheterizing you tomorrow for a urine specimen," it is better to say "Tomorrow we need a sample of urine and we will collect it by putting a tube into your bladder." The latter statement is likely to produce a response from the client about why it is needed and whether it will hurt or be uncomfortable. The former statement may simply make the client wonder what the nurse means.

Another aspect of simplicity is brevity. Most people have heard others give lengthy explanations of events, to which they respond, "Get to the point." By using short sentences and avoiding unnecessary material, the speaker or writer can achieve brevity. Brevity is of particular importance in writing, e.g., nurse's notes (see Chapter 17). Reports or memos need to be concise and should be condensed into a single paragraph or page, if possible.

The opposite of overcommunicating is undercommunicating. Shortcuts for the sake of simplicity can lead to incomplete or unclear communication. For example, initials or abbreviations such as b.i.d. (twice a day) or ICU (intensive care unit) should be avoided unless the nurse is certain that the client will understand them. Because clarification is required, abbreviations can waste the listener's or reader's time. At the first use, names should be expressed in full; later they can be shortened when the nurse is sure that the client or reader knows the meanings.

Clarity

Clarity means saying exactly what is meant. It also is aligned with meaning what is said. The latter involves a blending of the speaker's behavior (nonverbal communication) with the words that are spoken. When the words and the behavior blend together or are unified, the communication is regarded as consistent or congruent.

The goal of clarity is to communicate so that people know the what, how, why (if necessary), when, who, and where of any specific event. Without knowing these facts, people are left to make assumptions. To ensure clarity in communication, the nurse also needs to speak slowly and enunciate words well. It may be helpful to repeat the message and to reduce distractions such as surrounding noises.

Some common pitfalls that can produce unclear communications are ambiguous statements, generalizations, and opinions. For example, "Men are stronger than women" is both a generalization and an opinion, and the term *stronger* is open to several interpretations. Another example is a nurse's statement to a client, "Mrs. Smith, you need to keep busy today." The specific actions Mrs. Smith is expected to

RESEARCH NOTE

The Words Clients Don't Understand

Some nurses think that today's clients are better informed than clients of years ago because they receive better health education and watch more television. However, in a research study of 100 randomly selected clients, Aina Apse found that many are bewildered by 41 commonly used clinical terms: Not one of the research subjects could correctly define all of the terms. The results ranged from one client who understood only 4% of the terms to another who understood 97%. Most of the clients understood between 51% and 75% of the terms.

The least understood terms included *N.P.O., ambulate,* and *impaction.* Surprisingly, 63% didn't understand the term *blood pressure;* and 29% didn't understand *malignant.* Some clients thought *dilate* means "smaller," *orally* means "every hour," *P.O.* means "afternoon."

Implications: This research demonstrates how important it is for the nurse to find out which terms a particular client understands and then to avoid using potentially confusing terms.

A. Apse, Avoiding terms of bewilderment, *Nursing 85,* December 1985, 15:42–43.

carry out and the reasons for them are open to many interpretations.

Timing and Relevance

No matter how clearly or simply words are stated or written, the timing needs to be appropriate to ensure that words are heard. Moreover, the messages need to relate to the person or to the person's interests and concerns. Consider the woman whose children are crying and whose doorbell is ringing while she is on the telephone with a salesperson. This is not the best time to make a sale, even if the woman is interested.

Nurses need to be aware of both relevance and timing when communicating with clients. This involves being sensitive to the client's needs and concerns. For example, if a female client is enmeshed in fear of cancer, she may not hear the nurse's explanations about the expected procedures before and after her gallbladder surgery. In this situation it is better for the nurse first to encourage her to express her concerns, and to then deal with those concerns. The necessary explanations can be provided at another time.

Another pitfall is to ask several questions at once. For example, a nurse enters a client's room and says in one breath, "Good morning, Mrs. Brody. How are you this morning? Did you sleep well last night? Your husband is coming to see you before your surgery, isn't he?" The client no doubt would feel bombarded and confused and wonder which question to answer first, if any. A related pattern of poor timing is to ask a question and then not wait for an answer before making another comment. To Mr. Ramirez the nurse says, "How is that swollen leg this morning? I'm getting your bath water now before the doctor comes."

Adaptability   Spoken messages need to be altered in accordance with behavioral cues from the receiver. This adjustment is referred to as *adaptability*. Moods and behavior may change minute by minute, hour by hour, or from day to day. In this sense the nurse needs to avoid routine or automatic speech. What the nurse says and how it is said must be individualized and carefully considered. This requires astute assessment and sensitivity on the part of the nurse. For example, a nurse who usually smiles, appears cheerful, and greets her client every afternoon with an enthusiastic "Hi, Mr. Brown!" notices that he is not smiling and appears distressed when she appears. In response to the client's cues, the nurse adapts her usual greeting and tones down her cheery manner. She may say "Hi" in a much softer and caring manner and express concern in her facial expression while she moves toward him.

Credibility   *Credibility* means worthiness of belief, trustworthiness, reliability. Credibility may be the most important criterion of effective communication. A nurse's credibility to clients depends in part on the opinion of others. If other health professionals and clients regard the nurse as trustworthy, then the client also is likely to.

To become credible, the nurse needs to be knowledgeable about the subject matter being discussed and to have accurate information. Nurses also need to convey confidence and certainty in what they are saying. This is often referred to as *positivism*. People tend to perceive confidence, which is dynamic and emphatic, as more credible than hesitance or uncertainty, which is less forceful and less active. However, the nurse should not sound overconfident or authoritarian. To avoid this perception by the client, the nurse states messages in a constructive way and focuses on being helpful to clients.

Reliability is developed by being consistent, dependable, and honest. People value the nurse who acknowledges limitations and can say, "I don't know the answer to that, but I'll find someone who does."

Nonverbal Communication

Nonverbal communication is sometimes called *body language*. It includes gestures, body movements, and physical appearance, including adornment. The majority of communication is nonverbal. Nonverbal communication often tells others more about what a person is feeling than what is actually said, because nonverbal behavior is controlled less consciously than verbal behavior. Nonverbal communication either reinforces or contradicts what is said verbally. For example, a nurse may say to a client, "I'd be happy to sit here and talk to you for a while," yet if she glances nervously at her watch every few seconds, the actions contradict the verbal message. The client is more likely to believe the nonverbal behavior, which conveys "I am very busy."

Observers cannot always be sure of the correct interpretation of the feelings expressed nonverbally. On the one hand, the same feeling can be expressed nonverbally in more than one way. For example, anger may be communicated by aggressive or excessive body motion, or it may be communicated by a frozen stillness. On the other hand, a variety of feelings, such as embarrassment, pleasure, or anger, can be expressed by a single nonverbal cue, such as blushing.

Observing and interpreting the client's nonverbal behavior are essential skills for nurses. Interpreting the observations requires validation with the client. The nurse's own nonverbal behavior is under constant scrutiny by clients. It is therefore necessary for nurses to gain awareness of their actions and to learn to convey understanding, respect, and acceptance to clients.

To observe nonverbal behavior efficiently requires a systematic approach. As part of an initial assessment, the nurse should observe the person's overall physical appearance, including adornments, posture, and gait, and then assesses specific parts of the body, such as the face and the hands for nonverbal cues. The person's overall appearance includes physical characteristics and manner of dress. Physical characteristics can denote the person's state of health. Skin color and texture, length of fingernails, weight, and deformities causing physical limitations are a few examples. The skin may appear dry, mottled, or pale. Weight may indicate malnourishment. Nails may be well manicured or extremely short. Whatever is observed, the nurse needs to exercise caution in interpretation. For example, pale skin may be normal for that person. Nails may be short because they were bitten nervously or because they were broken by hard manual labor.

Clothing and adornments are sometimes rich sources of information about a person. Choice of apparel is highly personal. Clothing may convey social and financial status, culture, religion, group association, and self-concept. Adornments such as jewelry, perfume, and cosmetics reveal additional information.

How a person dresses is often an indicator of how the person feels. People who are tired or ill may not have the energy or the desire to maintain their normal grooming. The nurse also needs to be alert to sudden changes in a person's dress. When a person known for immaculate grooming becomes lax about appearance, the nurse may suspect a loss of self-esteem or a physical illness. For clients in acute general hospital settings, a change in grooming habits or personal adornment often signals that the client is feeling better. A male client may request a shave, or a female client may request a mirror and her lipstick.

Posture and Gait   The ways people walk and carry themselves are often reliable indicators of self-concept, current mood, and health. Erect posture and an active, purposeful stride suggest a feeling of well-being. Slouched posture and a slow, shuffling gait suggest dejection or physical discomfort. Tense posture and a rapid, determined gait suggest anxiety or anger. Likewise, the sitting or lying postures of clients can communicate feelings.

Facial Expression   No part of the body is as expressive as the face. See Figure 15–1. Feelings of joy, sadness, fear, surprise, anger, and disgust can be conveyed by facial expressions. The muscles around the eyes and the mouth are particularly expressive. Although actors learn to control these muscles to convey emotions to audiences, facial expressions generally are not consciously controlled.

Clients are quick to notice the nurse's facial expression, particularly when they feel unsure or uncomfortable. The client who questions the nurse about a feared diagnostic result will watch the nurse to see whether the nurse maintains eye contact or looks away when answering. The client who has had disfiguring surgery will examine the nurse's face for signs of disgust. Nurses, like actors, need to be aware of their facial expressions and what they are communicating to others. Although it is impossible to control all facial expressions, the nurse must learn to control feelings such as fear and disgust in certain situations.

Many facial expressions convey a universal meaning. The smile conveys happiness. Contempt is conveyed by the mouth turned down, the head tilted back, and the eyes directed down the nose. No single expression can be interpreted accurately, however, without considering (a) other reinforcing physical cues, (b) the setting in which it occurs, and (c) the expression of others in the same setting.

Eye contact is another essential element of facial communication. Mutual eye contact acknowledges recognition of the other person and a willingness to maintain communication. Often a person initiates contact with another person with a glance, capturing the person's attention prior to communicating. A person who feels weak or defenseless often averts the eyes or avoids eye contact. The communication received may be too embarrassing or too dominating. Animals are known to succumb to dominance by averting first their eyes and then their presence.

Hand Movements and Gestures   Like faces, hands are expressive. They can communicate feelings at any given moment. An anxious person, for instance a man awaiting word about his daughter in surgery, may wring his hands or pick his nails; relaxed persons may interlock their fingers over their laps or allow their hands to fall over the ends of armrests. Hands also communicate by touch: slapping someone's face or caressing another's head communicates obvious feelings.

Hands are frequently involved in gestures. The handshake, the victory sign, the wave good-bye, the hand motion to ask a visitor to sit down are gestures that have relatively universal meanings. Some gestures, however, are culture-specific. European women walk together holding hands as a sign of friendship; in North American society, this gesture may be regarded as unacceptable. Even the same gesture can have different meanings in different cultures. The North American gesture meaning "shoo away" or "go away" means "come here" or "come back" in some Asian cultures.

Hands are also very expressive in illustrating or stylizing verbal communication. The French and Italians are noted for using their hands in this manner. When describing the shape and size of an object, a French person uses the hands to reinforce the verbal message.

For people with special communication problems, such as the deaf, the hands are invaluable in communication. Many deaf people learn sign language. Ill persons who are unable to reply verbally can similarly devise a unique communication system using the hands. The client may be able to raise an index finger once for "yes" and twice for "no." Other signals can often be devised by the client and the nurse to denote other meanings.

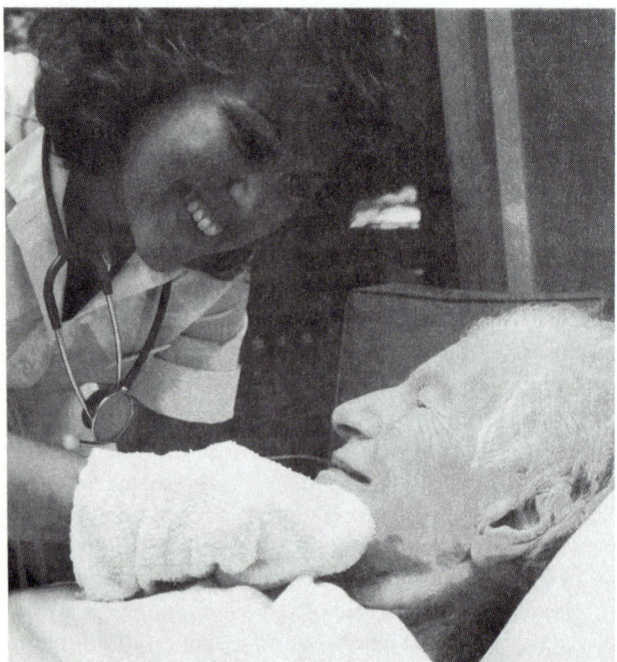

Figure 15–1   The nurse's facial expression communicates warmth and caring.

THE COMMUNICATION PROCESS

There are two major models of nurses' communication in nurse-client interaction: the therapeutic model and "interpersonally competent" model. The *therapeutic model* originated as part of the patient-centered approach to nursing that emphasized the nurse's responsibility to the total well-being of the client. This model focuses on the learning and practicing of a now well-accepted set of skills and abilities such as listening, responding empathetically, using non-evaluative language and nonverbal cues, and demonstrating behaviors that stress confirmation and acknowledgment. See the discussion of therapeutic responses, later in this chapter.

The *interpersonally competent model* was introduced by Kasch in 1984. This model assumes that communication is related to health outcomes. It defines effective communication as that which is interpersonally competent rather than that which is psychologically therapeutic. It is based upon two types of abilities. The first is *social cognitive competence*: the ability to interpret the message content in interactions from many perspectives and to make judgments about the effectiveness and appropriateness of potential responses. The second is *strategic message competence*: the ability to control and strategically use language and other behavioral capabilities to achieve objectives of the nursing process (Harrison et al 1989, p. 77).

Both models emphasize the necessity to learn and perform certain basic communication skills, but the interpersonally competent model stresses these skills as part of the strategic message competence. It adds to these basic skills analytic and interpretational skills in communicating (Harrison et al. 1989, p. 77). Interpretation involves perception, symbolization, memory, and thinking.

The purpose of a model is to break down the process of communication into its essential components so that it can be better understood. A communication model has two main parts: people and messages. In face-to-face communication there is a sender, a message, a receiver, and a response (feedback). See Figure 15–2. In its simplest form, communication is a two-way process involving the sending and the receiving of a message. Since the intent of communication is to elicit a response, the process is ongoing; the receiver of the message then becomes the sender of a response, and the original sender then becomes the receiver.

Sender

The sender, a person or group who wishes to convey a message to another, is sometimes called the *source-encoder.* This term suggests that the person or group sending the message must have an idea or reason for communicating (source) and must put the idea or feeling into a form that can be transmitted. **Encoding** involves the selection of specific signs or symbols (codes) to transmit the message, such as which language and words to use, how to arrange the words, and what tone of voice and gestures to use. For example, if the receiver speaks English, English words will usually be selected. If the message is "No, Johnny, you may not have any more cookies before dinner!" the tone of voice selected will be one of firmness, and a shake of the head

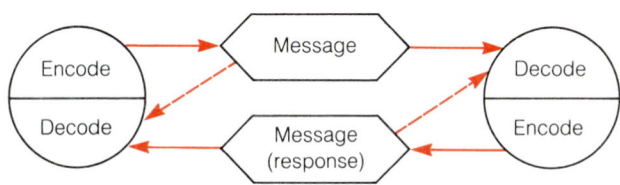

Figure 15–2 The communication process. The dashed arrows indicate internal feedback from the sender of the message (or response).

or a pointing index finger can reinforce it. The nurse must not only deal with dialects and foreign languages but also must cope with two language levels—the layperson's and the health professional's.

Message

The second component of the communication process is the message itself—what is actually said or written, the body language that accompanies the words, and how the message is transmitted. Various channels can be used to convey messages, and frequently combinations are used. It is important that the channel be appropriate for the message and make the intent of the message clear.

Talking face-to-face with a person may be more effective in some instances than telephoning or writing a message. Recording messages on tape or communicating by radio or television may be more appropriate for larger audiences. Written communication is often appropriate for long explanations or for a communication that needs to be preserved. The nonverbal channel of touch is often highly effective.

Receiver

The receiver, the third component of the communication process, is the listener, who must listen, observe, and attend. This person, sometimes called the *decoder,* must perceive what the sender intended (sensation) and then analyze the information received (interpretation). Perception involves use of all the senses to receive all verbal and nonverbal messages. To **decode** means to relate the message perceived to the receiver's storehouse of knowledge and experience and to sort out the meaning of the message. Whether the message is decoded accurately by the receiver, according to the sender's intent, depends largely on their similarities in knowledge and experience. For example, Johnny may perceive the message accurately—"No more cookies for me right now." However, if experience has taught him that he can help himself to the cookie jar without punishment, he will interpret the intent of the message differently.

Response

The fourth component of the communication process, the response, is the message that the receiver returns to the sender. It is also called **feedback.** Feedback can be either positive or negative. Nonverbal examples are a nod of the head or a yawn. Either way, feedback allows the sender to correct or reword a message. In the case of Johnny, the receiver may cry or move away from the cookie jar or say, "Well, Judy had three cookies and I only had two." The sender then knows the message was interpreted accurately. However, now the original sender becomes the receiver, who is required to decode and respond.

The receiver is not the sole source of feedback. Communicators constantly receive *internal feedback* from themselves. Internal feedback is often used for written messages. For example, after composing a letter, a person will read it silently or out loud to see how it sounds; or a person who makes a social blunder (*faux pas*) may instantly realize the mistake and say, "That isn't what I really meant" or "I didn't mean it that way."

Factors Influencing the Communication Process

In addition to factors such as a person's sociocultural background, language, age, and education, and the limitations and attributes of nonverbal communication, the following factors affect the communication process: ability of the communicator; perceptions; personal space; territoriality; roles and relationships; time; environment; attitudes; and emotions and self-esteem.

Ability of the Communicator

The person's abilities to speak, hear, see, and comprehend stimuli influence the communication process. People who are hard of hearing may require messages that are short, loud, and clear. Those who are unable to read will be unable to comprehend written information. Some, because of disease processes, are unable to see or to speak, and individual methods for communication need to be devised with them.

The receiver of a message also needs to be able to interpret the message. Mental faculties can be impaired for such reasons as brain damage or use of sedative drugs or alcohol. Even if a client is free of physical impairments, the nurse needs to determine how many stimuli the client is capable of receiving in a given time frame. Frequently the receiver is expected to assimilate too much information. The nurse may be talking too quickly or presenting too many ideas at once. This is of particular importance when offering health instruction.

Perceptions

Because each person has unique personality traits, values, and life experiences, each will perceive and interpret messages differently. For example, the nurse may draw the curtains around a crying woman and leave her alone. The woman may interpret this as "The nurse thinks that I will upset others in the room and that I shouldn't cry" or "The nurse doesn't like crying" or "The nurse respects my need to be alone." It is important in many situations to validate or correct the perceptions of the receiver.

Personal Space

Personal space is the distance people prefer in interactions with others. **Proxemics** is the study of distance between people in their interactions. Middle-class North Americans use definite distances in various interpersonal relationships, along with specific voice tones and body language. Communication thus alters in accordance with four distances, each with a close and a far phase, that have been described by Hall (1969, p. 45):

1. Intimate: Physical contact to 1½ feet
2. Personal: 1½–4 feet
3. Social: 4–12 feet
4. Public: 12 feet and beyond

Intimate distance communication is characterized by body contact, heightened sensations of body heat and smell, and vocalizations that are low. Vision is intense, restricted to a small body part, and may be distorted. Intimate distance is frequently used by nurses. Examples occur in cuddling a baby, touching the sightless client, positioning clients, observing an incision, and restraining a toddler for an injection. It is a natural protective instinct for people to maintain a certain amount of space immediately around them, and the amount varies with individuals. When someone who wants to communicate steps too close, the receiver automatically steps back a pace or two. In their therapeutic roles, nurses often are required to violate this personal space. However, it is important for them to be aware when this will occur and to forewarn the client. In many instances, the nurse can respect (not come as close as) a person's intimate distance. In other instances, the nurse may come within intimate distance to communicate warmth and caring.

Personal distance is less overwhelming than intimate distance. Voice tones are moderate, and body heat and smell are noticed less. Physical contact such as a handshake or touching a shoulder is possible. More of the person is perceived at a personal distance, so that nonverbal behaviors such as body stance or full facial expressions are seen with less distortion. Much communication between nurses and clients occurs at this distance. Examples occur when nurses are sitting with a client, giving medications, or establishing an intravenous infusion. Communication at a close personal distance can convey involvement by facilitating the sharing of thoughts and feelings. At the outer extreme of 4 ft, however, less involvement is conveyed. Bantering and some social conversations are usual at this distance.

Social distance is characterized by a clear visual perception of the whole person. Body heat and odor are imperceptible, eye contact is increased, and vocalizations are loud enough to be overheard by others. Communication is therefore more formal and is limited to seeing and hearing. The person is protected and out of reach for touch or personal sharing of thoughts or feelings. Social distance allows more activity and movement back and forth. It is expedient in communicating with several people at the same time or within a short time. Examples occur when nurses make rounds or wave a greeting to someone. Social distance is important in accomplishing the business of the day. However, it is frequently misused. For example, the nurse who stands in the doorway and asks a client "How are you today?" will receive a more noncommittal reply than the nurse who moves to personal distance to inquire.

Public distance requires loud, clear vocalizations with careful enunciation. Although the faces and forms of people are seen at public distance, individuality is lost. Instead, a general notion is perceived about a group of people or a community.

Territoriality

Territoriality is a concept of the space and things that an individual considers as belonging to the self. Territories marked off by people may be visible to others. For example, clients in a hospital often consider their territory as bounded by the curtains around the bed unit or by the walls of a private room. This human tendency to claim territory must be recognized by all health care workers. Clients often feel the need to defend their territory when it is invaded by others; for example, when a visitor removes a chair to use at another bed, the visitor has inadvertently violated the territoriality of the client whose chair was moved.

Roles and Relationships

The roles and the relationship between sender and receiver affect the communication process. Roles such as nursing student and instructor, client and physician, or parent and child will affect the content and responses in the communication process. Choice of words, sentence structure, and tone of voice vary considerably from role to role. In addition, the specific relationship between the communicators is significant. The nurse who meets with a client for the first time will communicate differently from the nurse who has previously developed a relationship with that client.

Time

The time factor in communication includes the events that precede and follow the interaction. The hospitalized client who is anticipating surgery or who has just received news that a spouse has lost a job will not be very receptive to information. A client who has had to wait for some time to express needs may respond quite differently from one who has endured no waiting period. The setting also influences communication. If the room lacks privacy or is hot, noisy, or crowded, the communication process can break down.

Nurses' use of time can facilitate or inhibit a client's communication. The nurse who tells a client "I'll be back in a moment" while delivering medications is likely to convey "I haven't time now" or "I've got work to do." This inhibits client communications. However, if this nurse says to the client, "Would you tell me now what your concern is about, and then when I've finished delivering medications I'll come back and help you with it," the communication process is facilitated.

Environment

People usually communicate most effectively in a comfortable environment. Temperature extremes, excessive noise, and a poorly ventilated environment can all interfere with communication. Also, lack of privacy may interfere with a client's communication about matters the client considers private. For example, a client who is worried about the ability of his wife to care for him after discharge from hospital may not wish to discuss this concern with a nurse within the hearing of other clients in the room. Environmental distraction can impair and distort communication.

Attitudes

Attitudes convey beliefs, thoughts, and feelings about people and events. They are communicated convincingly and rapidly to others. Attitudes such as caring, warmth, respect, and acceptance facilitate communication, whereas condescension, lack of interest, and coldness inhibit communication.

Caring and *warmth* convey a feeling of emotional closeness, in contrast to impersonal distance. Caring is more enduring and intense than warmth. It conveys deep and genuine concern for the person. Warmth, on the other hand, conveys friendliness and consideration, shown by acts of smiling and attention to physical comforts (Brammer 1988, p. 37). Caring involves giving feelings, thoughts, skill, and knowledge. It requires psychologic energy and poses the risk of gaining little in return, yet by caring, people usually reap the benefits of greater communication and understanding.

Respect is an attitude that emphasizes the other person's worth and individuality. It conveys that the person's hopes and feelings are special and unique even though similar to others in many ways. People have a need to be different from—and at the same time similar to—others. Being too different can be isolating and threatening. Respect is conveyed by listening open-mindedly to what the other person is saying, even if the nurse disagrees. Nurses can learn new ways of approaching situations when they conscientiously listen to another person's perspective.

Acceptance emphasizes neither approval nor disapproval. The nurse willingly receives the client's honest feelings and actions without judgment. An accepting attitude allows clients to express personal feelings freely and to be themselves. The nurse may need to restrict acceptance in situations where clients' actions are harmful to themselves or to others.

In contrast, *condescension* is an attitude that conveys superiority over the other person. Clients who feel helpless often perceive nurses to be in a superior position because of their knowledge and skill. In these instances, the nurse may convey condenscension by an air of superiority and intellectualism. One common condescending act by nurses is to call clients "honey" or "dear." This casts the nurse in the role of the superior mother and the client in the role of the inferior child. Another condescending act is patting an elderly client on the head.

Lack of interest also inhibits communication by saying "I'm not concerned" or "What you say is not important." The nurse conveys lack of interest by forgetting part of the client's conversation or not concentrating on it sufficiently to respond. Being tired near the end of a long day's work or in a hurry to complete tasks may contribute to giving the appearance of not being interested in client.

Coldness is the opposite of caring and warmth. Nurses convey this attitude to clients by appearing more interested in the technical and procedural aspects of nursing than in the concerns of the person receiving the therapy. For example, the nurse can convey coldness by appearing more concerned about the neatness of the client's bed than about the client's restlessness or more interested in the efficient functioning of a cardiac monitor than in the client's anxiety. A rigid body posture and aloof tone of voice also convey a nurse's lack of genuine concern for the client.

Emotions and Self-Esteem

Most people have experienced overwhelming joy or sorrow that is difficult to express in words. Anger may produce loud, profane vocalizations or controlled speechlessness. Fright may produce screams of terror or paralyzed silence.

Emotions also affect a person's ability to interpret messages. Large parts of a message may not be heard, or the message may be misinterpreted when the receiver is experiencing strong emotion. This situation occurs frequently in nursing. For example, the client feeling great fear may not remember all the preoperative instructions offered by a nurse.

Self-esteem also influences communication patterns. People whose self-esteem is high communicate honestly, with confidence, and with **congruence** (agreement or coinciding) between verbal and nonverbal messages. For example, a nurse explaining the importance or preoperative exercises would present a sincere and serious facial expression. Those with low self-esteem or under high stress tend to give double messages; that is, their verbal and nonverbal messages are incongruent (lack consistency). For example, while explaining about a client's colostomy to the client's family, a nurse laughs.

LANGUAGE DEVELOPMENT

The development of language, from the cry of the infant to the verbal fluency of the adult, is a complex process described in various theories of language development, a topic beyond

TABLE 15–2 *Language Development*

Stage	Normal Behavior
Newborn	At birth—cries as air passes over vocal cords. Within 2 to 3 weeks—cries become differentiated.
Infant	At 2 to 3 months—babbling begins. At 7 months—repeats sounds heard from environment. At 10 to 12 months—responds to a few familiar words; single words are pronounced. At 15 months—can say about four words.
Toddler	At 2 years—initially has over 50-word vocabulary; this increases progressively to about 800–1000 words by 3 years. Associates symbols with form, e.g., words, pictures. Grammatical errors are common.
Preschooler	At 4 years—vocabulary has grown to about 1600 words. Sentences are complete. By 5 to 6 years—most infantile pronunciations have disappeared.
School-age child	At 6 years—has command of most sentence structures. Speech is less egocentric. Vocabulary continues to increase; comprehension exceeds use. Slang and swear words become part of vocabulary. At 8 to 12 years—boasting commonly occurs.
Adolescent	Uses language of subgroup. Speech reflects consideration of hypotheses.
Adulthood	Has full speech skills. Language often reflects specialized education.

the scope of this book. Table 15–2 provides a brief summary of language development from birth through adolescence.

Phases of Development

The first sound of a newborn is the birth cry as air moves across the vocal cords. This is a reflexive response associated with the air pressure and the temperature changes of extrauterine life. Although infants are speechless for almost 1 year, they do communicate their needs. Within 2–3 weeks after birth, parents can describe notable differences in the cries of their infant. Smiling is noted in a number of infants as early as the second week of life. Soon after, some begin small, throaty, cooing sounds while feeding or bathing. Babies usually make these comfort sounds when they are contented, for example, when they are cuddled or when others talk to them.

Until the age of 10 months to 1 year the infant's sounds are not related to language and therefore are considered *prelinguistic*. This phase includes reflexive vocalization, babbling, and echolalia. **Reflexive vocalization** is a term for the nondescriptive sounds infants make in response to various stimuli and environmental conditions. These are the discomfort cries and the comfort coos.

Babbling begins when infants become aware that they are making noises. They spend more time making noises and will talk to themselves when alone. Babbling often occurs just after waking up or before going to sleep. By about 7 months, babbling includes some sounds infants have picked up from their environment. This is referred to as lalling: Infants are repeating sounds they have heard.

Echolalia is the repetition of sounds just spoken by another. This involves definite acoustic awareness. At this point there is no meaning associated with the infant's sounds, but they have learned to manipulate their tongue, lips, and throat and to imitate sounds spoken by others. Language and speech development proceed at a faster pace if the parent at this time repeats the baby's sounds. The baby in turn echoes the parent's sounds. The *first word* of the infant is a notable event for proud parents. By about 10 to 12 months of age children develop a *passive* understanding of the language. They will respond to a few familiar words, such as "no," and familiar names—their own and those of family members and household pets. Even when family members are not present, children will turn to look for them when their names are mentioned.

Active use of language follows. The first words that children use may be unrecognized by parents, since children often invent their own first words. True speech begins at 12 to 18 months of age, when the child correctly uses a conventional word or facsimile of the word. It is used with intent, and a response is anticipated; a child may bang a cup on the high chair and say "wawa" (water). This type of speech is referred to as **holophrastic speech** (one word expresses a whole sentence). By 2 years of age children learn to put words together. This period is considered the beginning of complete speech, the use of different word combinations in grammatical form.

The French psychologist Jean Piaget (1952) categorized the conversation of children from ages 4 to 11 into egocentric and socialized speech. **Egocentric speech** is self-centered, noncommunicative speech. Children talk merely to please themselves or to please anyone who happens to be there to hear. Although the conversation is not directed at anyone in particular, the talking is about the child's thoughts and activity of the moment. The child is thinking out loud.

In contrast to Piaget, the Russian psychologist Lev Vygotsky (1962, pp. 16–17) proposed that egocentric speech is a form of self-guidance and assists the child in problem-solving situations. He believes that egocentric speech is both goal oriented and communicative. It is the state between external speech and what he refers to as "silent inner speech" (Vygotsky 1962, p. 149). Egocentric or external speech goes underground and becomes internalized as thought processes.

Socialized speech refers to the exchange of thoughts with others. It includes questions, answers, commands, and criticism of others. In school-age children the use of egocentric speech gradually diminishes, and communicating thoughts to other people becomes predominant.

Semantics is the study of the meanings of words in a given language. Children learn the meanings of concrete words and their categories first; later, abstract words and their categories are understood. A child learns "chair" and "table" before learning the meaning of the category "furniture," or learns "apple" and "orange" before learning the category "fruit." Abstract words such as "quality" or "relation" are learned primarily after the preschool years.

Factors Influencing Language Development

Growth in language development is affected by a number of factors: intelligence, sex, bilingualism, status as a single child or twin, parental stimulation, and socioeconomic components.

Intelligence
Brighter children begin to talk earlier than those with lower intelligence. Vocabulary development of intelligent children occurs more rapidly, and they articulate better and use sentences that are longer and grammatically more correct. Mentally defective children show notable lags in vocabulary growth.

Sex
During the first year there is not much difference in the sounds produced by boys and girls. After this time girls tend to be superior in both the rate of vocabulary development and articulation. In later school years boys tend to equal girls in reading abilities and be superior in use of certain words. Females on the whole exceed males in grammatical word usage and spelling tests.

Bilingualism
Research has contradicted the belief that a child of a bilingual home is hindered in language development. Lambert and Tucker (1972) found that language development was not retarded in bilingual children over a 7-year period. The bilingual children also scored high on tests of creativity.

Status as a Single Child or Twin
Evidence suggests that twins and triplets exhibit certain aspects of retarded language development, particularly during the preschool years. It is thought that (a) twins may receive less verbal stimulation from parents, (b) they grow up so close together that they understand each other's speech patterns early, and (c) they lack the motivation to verbalize with others. The school years are often instrumental in resolving these problems.

Parental Stimulation   Vocabulary growth occurs at a more rapid pace in children who are spoken to more frequently by their parents. Less rapid growth has been noted in children who spend most of their time with other children and who watch a great deal of television. Vocabulary is enhanced in children who travel away from their homes and who have contact with several different adults.

Socioeconomic Components   The social and economic family setting in which the child is reared affects language development. Children whose parents are highly educated, e.g., lawyers and doctors, use many more words even by age 3 than children from families headed by unskilled workers. The caliber of conversation overheard by youngsters is an influencing factor in their choice of vocabulary and sentence structure.

Stimulating Children's Language Development

Nurses can be instrumental in assisting parents to become active stimulants in language development and helping children when they are hospitalized. The following interventions are suggested.

- *Improve the parental model.* Parents can be encouraged to provide the best possible instruction and to become good models.
- *Encourage verbal and nonverbal means of communications.* Children need different verbal experiences, such as rhyming games, reading aloud, and songs, with accompanying nonverbal gestures, such as smiling and laughing. See Figure 15–3.

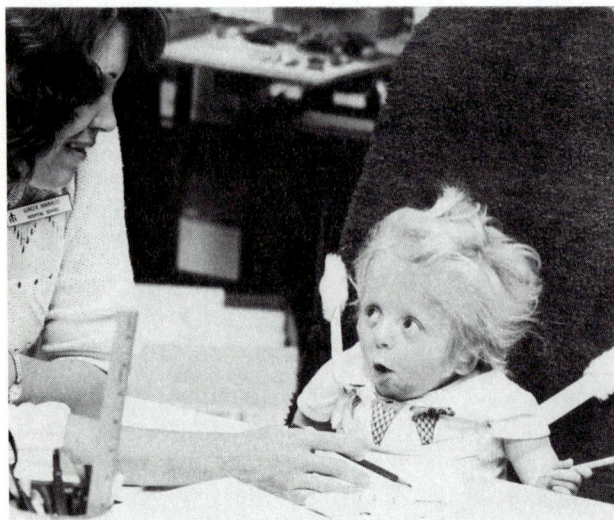

Figure 15–3   Development of a child's language is stimulated by reading together.

- *Provide experiences to talk about.* Children talk when they have something to talk about. Whenever possible, parents and/or nurses need to provide pets, toys, picture books, numbers, and colors that the child can experiment with and talk about.
- *Encourage listening.* Articulation skills of children can be enhanced by teaching them to pay attention and to listen to sounds.
- *Encourage speech as a substitute for action.* Children's ability to express themselves verbally can be enhanced when parents, rather than responding to physical action, direct them to say what they want. The child who tugs at a playmate's tricycle can be instructed by the parent to express a want verbally by the remark "Tell him what you want; perhaps he will let you have it."
- *Use exact terms.* Children learn to distinguish color, size, shape, position, and ownership of objects when exact terms are used. Parents can be encouraged to say, "Bring the big red ball from the playroom table," rather than "Bring that thing from over there—you know what I mean."

ASSESSING COMMUNICATION

When nurses assess the communication of clients, they need to include language development, nonverbal behavior, and communication style.

Language Development

The nurse assesses the following aspects of language development:

- The language skills presented by the client, compared to the language skills normally expected (see Table 15–2)
- Adequacy of the language skills in relation to the individual's need
- The chief method of communicating, e.g., words or gestures
- Obstacles to language development, such as deafness or absence of environmental stimuli
- Specific forms of language impairment, e.g., a school-age child's inability to write or lack of abstractions in the language of an adult
- Cultural influences on language development, e.g., the language used in the home or customs about when and how to speak

Nonverbal Behavior

In assessing nonverbal communication, the nurse considers the following:

- Gestures used by the individual.
- Posture and facial expressions employed.
- Use of touch as a means of communication. See the discussion of touch, later in this chapter.
- The interpersonal distance with which the person feels comfortable, e.g., whether the person assumes an intimate distance for most discussions.
- The grooming and appearance of the individual. These may affect the communication process, e.g., when dress is inconsistent with a setting or presents a stereotype that may evoke biases.

Style of Communication

A person's style of communication is often affected by such factors as health, culture, education, stress level, fatigue, and cognitive ability. In assessing communication style, the nurse considers the following:

- The vocabulary of the individual, particularly any changes from the vocabulary normally used. For example, a person who normally never swears may indicate increased stress or illness by an uncharacteristic use of profanity.
- The use of symbols and gestures to communicate. Some uses of symbols and gestures are culturally determined; for example, a Puerto Rican girl may be taught not to look an adult in the eyes, as a sign of respect and obedience; the gesture should not be interpreted as a sign of guilt.
- The presence of hostility, aggression, assertiveness, reticence, hesitance, anxiety, or loquaciousness (incessant verbalization) in the communication.
- Difficulties with verbal communication, such as slurring, stuttering, inability to pronounce a particular sound, lack of clarity in enunciation, inability to speak in sentences, loose association of ideas, flight of ideas, or the inability to find or name words or identify objects.
- Refusal or inability to speak.

DIAGNOSING COMMUNICATION PROBLEMS

Impaired verbal communication is the nursing diagnosis given to clients with communication problems. Impaired verbal communication is the "state in which an individual experiences, or could experience, a decreased ability to send or receive messages, i.e., has difficulty exchanging thoughts, ideas, or desires" (Carpenito 1989, p. 227). Contributing factors for impaired verbal communication follow.

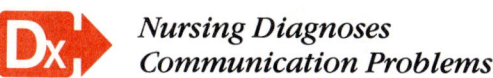

Nursing Diagnoses Communication Problems

Impaired verbal communication related to:

- Development or age-related stage(s)
- Anatomic deficit, such as cleft palate
- Cultural difference or inability to speak dominant language
- Physical conditions such as cerebrovascular accident or brain tumor, or surgery such as laryngectomy or tracheostomy.
- Psychologic conditions, such as extreme anger, severe anxiety or panic, moderate and severe depression, fear, shyness, loneliness, and unrealistic or inadequate self-concept
- Pharmacologic therapy, such as central nervous system depressant

Ineffective individual coping, Ineffective family coping, Anxiety, and **Fear** may be appropriate diagnoses for some clients. These definitions, defining characteristics, and contributing factors are discussed in Chapter 33.

PLANNING FOR EFFECTIVE COMMUNICATION

When problems in communication have been identified, the nurse and client set goals and begin planning ways to promote effective communication. The overall client goal for persons with impaired verbal communication is to reduce or resolve the impaired communication. Specific nursing interventions are planned from the stated etiology. Among these interventions are (a) developing listening skills, (b) becoming aware of how people respond and (c) developing a helping relationship. More specific interventions may include the following:

- Anticipate needs until effective communication is established.
- Discuss individual methods of dealing with the impairment.
- Keep communication simple, using visual, auditory, and kinesthetic modes for conveying information.
- Plan for alternate methods of communication, such as a typewriter, slate, or letter/picture board.
- Respond with simple, straightforward, honest statements to provide reality orientation and correct faulty perception.
- Use and assist clients to learn facilitative communication techniques, e.g., active listening skills. See the discussion of therapeutic and nontherapeutic communication skills later in this chapter.

- Help the client look at the effects of nonfacilitative communication techniques.
- Teach and encourage expression of feelings.
- Point out discrepancies in verbal and nonverbal behavior.
- Encourage the client to ask for feedback when communicating with others.
- Refer the client to appropriate resources such as speech therapy, group therapy, or individual or family counseling.

Examples of outcome criteria to evaluate the achievement of client goals and the effectiveness of nursing interventions follow.

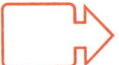

Outcome Criteria
Communication Problems

The client:

- Attends to appropriate communication input.
- Perceives input accurately.
- Gives clear, concise, understandable messages.
- Uses effective communication techniques, e.g., active listening, silence, reflecting, restating.
- Avoids the use of nonfacilitative techniques such as offering advice.
- Expresses congruent verbal and nonverbal behavior.
- Expresses feelings appropriately.
- Uses resources appropriately.
- Establishes a method of communication in which needs can be expressed.

IMPLEMENTING

Techniques for Therapeutic Communication

Therapeutic communication promotes understanding by both the sender and the receiver. A number of techniques can help establish a constructive relationship between the nurse and the client, although the use of the techniques is no guarantee of effective communication. So many factors are involved in communication that the nurse is ill-advised to rely on any one technique or even several techniques. Not all people feel comfortable with all techniques, and skill in using them appropriately is essential. The nurse must be comfortable with the technique used and convey sincerity to the client. A phony or false response is usually quickly identified by clients and hinders the development of an effective relationship.

Nurses can learn much by examining and becoming aware of their own reactions (feelings) and responses. Although it is difficult for nurses to see their own nonverbal communication other than by videotape feedback, much can be learned by reflecting on what was heard, what the nurse said, and when and how it was said. Methods such as role playing, process recordings, and audiotapes can be useful.

Nurses need to respond not only to the content of a client's verbal message but also to the feelings expressed. It is important to understand how the client views the situation and feels about it before responding. The content of the client's communication is the words or thoughts, as distinct from the feelings. Sometimes people can convey a thought in words while their emotions contradict the words; i.e., words and feelings are incongruent. For example, a client says, "I am glad he has left me; he was very cruel." However, the nurse observes that the client has tears in her eyes as she says this. To respond to the client's *words,* the nurse might simply rephrase, saying "You are pleased that he has left you." To respond to the client's *feelings,* the nurse would need to acknowledge the tears in the client's eyes, saying, for example, "You seem saddened by all this." Such a response helps the client to focus on her feelings. In some instances, the nurse may need to know more about the client and her resources for coping with these feelings.

Sometimes clients need time to deal with their feelings. Strong emotions are often draining. People usually need to deal with feelings before they can cope with other matters, such as learning new skills or planning for the future. This is most evident in hospitals when clients learn that they have a terminal illness. Some require hours, days, or even weeks before they are ready to start other tasks. Some need only time to themselves, others need someone to listen, others need assistance identifying and verbalizing feelings, and others need assistance making decisions about future courses of action.

Attentive Listening   It is essential, in therapeutic communication, that nurses listen and respond to clients purposefully and deliberately. Attentive listening is listening actively, using all the senses, as opposed to listening passively with just the ear. It is probably the most important technique in nursing. Attentive listening is an active process that requires energy and concentration. It involves paying attention to the total message, both verbal messages and nonverbal messages that can modify what is spoken, and noting whether these communications are congruent. Attentive listening means absorbing both the content and the feeling the person is conveying, without selectivity. The listener does not select or listen to solely what the listener wants to hear; the nurse does not focus on the nurse's own needs but rather on the client's needs. Attentive listening conveys an attitude of caring and interest, thereby encouraging the client to talk. In summary, attentive listening is a highly developed skill, but fortunately it can be learned with practice.

A nurse can convey attentiveness in listening to clients in various ways. Common responses are nodding the head, uttering "uh huh" or "mmm," repeating the words that the client has used, or saying "I see what you mean." Each nurse has characteristic ways of responding, and the nurse must take care not to sound insincere or phony.

Egan (1982, pp. 60–61) has outlined five specific ways to convey physical attending. He defines physical attending as the manner of being present to another or being with another. Listening, in his frame of reference, is what a person does while attending. The five actions of physical attending, which convey a "posture of involvement," follow:

1. *Face the other person squarely.* This position says, "I am available to you." Moving to the side lessens the degree of involvement.

2. *Maintain good eye contact.* Mutual eye contact, preferably at the same level, recognizes the other person and denotes a willingness to maintain communication. Eye contact neither glares at nor stares down another but is natural.

3. *Lean toward the other.* People move naturally toward one another when they want to say or hear something— by moving to the front of a class, by moving a chair nearer a friend, or by leaning across a table with arms propped in front. The nurse conveys involvement by leaning forward, closer to the client.

4. *Maintain an open posture.* The nondefensive position is one in which neither arms nor legs are crossed. It conveys that the person wishes to encourage the passage of communication, as the open door of a home or an office does.

5. *Remain relatively relaxed.* Total relaxation is not feasible when the nurse is listening with intensity, but the nurse can show relaxation by taking time in responding, allowing pauses as needed, balancing periods of tension with relaxation, and using gestures that are natural. See Figure 15–4.

These five attending postures need to be adapted to the specific needs of clients in a given situation. For example, leaning forward may not be appropriate at the beginning of an interview. It may be reserved until a closer relationship grows between the nurse and the client. The same applies to eye contact, which is generally uninterrupted when the communicators are very involved in the interaction.

Paraphrasing   **Paraphrasing,** also called *restating,* involves listening for the client's basic message and then repeating those thoughts and/or feelings in similar words. Usually fewer words are used. Paraphrasing conveys that the nurse has listened and understood the client's basic message. It may also offer clients a clearer idea of what they have said. The client's response to the paraphrase may tell the nurse whether the paraphrase was accurate or helpful. (It may be necessary for the nurse to ask for a response.)

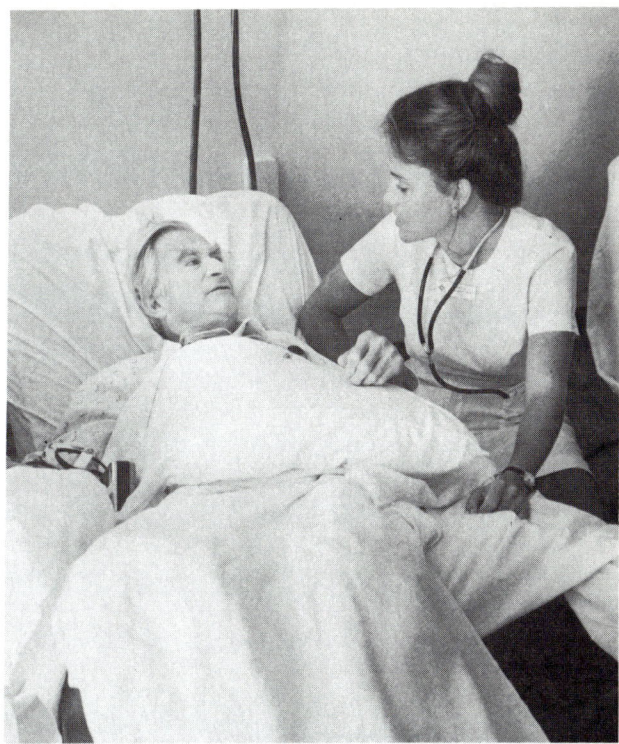

Figure 15–4 The nurse conveys attentive listening through a posture of involvement.

Client: I couldn't manage to eat any of my dinner last night— not even the dessert.

Nurse: You had difficulty eating yesterday.

Client: Yes, I was very upset after my family left.

Clarifying   *Clarifying* is a method of making the client's message more understandable. It is used when paraphrasing is difficult, when the communication has been rambling or garbled. To clarify the message the nurse can make a guess and restate the basic message or confess confusion and ask the client to repeat or restate the message (Davis 1984, p. 9). In the former situation, if the client says, "I didn't sleep at all last night," the nurse might say, "You didn't sleep at all last night." In the latter instance the nurse might say, "I'm puzzled" or "I'm not sure I understand that" and "Would you please say that again?" or "Would you tell me more?"

Nurses sometimes need to clarify their own messages to clients. The need to do so is generally discovered from the client's nonverbal feedback. Then the nurse might ask a question or say, "It seems to me I didn't make that clear" and repeat or rephrase the message. Sometimes only one word or phrase in a message needs clarifying.

Clarifying also includes *verifying what is implied.* In this instance, the client implies or hints at something without actually saying it. The nurse then tries to clarify the client's statement without interpreting it.

Client: There is no point in asking for a pain pill.

Nurse: Are you saying that no one gives you an analgesic when you have pain?

or

Nurse: Are you saying that your pills are not helping your pain?

Another clarifying technique is **perception checking,** or *consensual validation*. This verifies the accuracy of the nurse's listening skills by giving and receiving feedback about what was communicated. It involves paraphrasing what the nurse believes to have heard and asking the client for confirmation. It is important to allow the client to correct inaccurate perceptions. The advantage of frequent perception checking is that inaccurate perceptions are corrected before communications become confused and misunderstandings arise. Examples of perception checking are: "You sound annoyed with me—is that correct?" or "You seem to have some doubts about the decision you made, and I'd like to see if what I'm hearing is accurate."

Sometimes it is important for nurses to clarify reality when a client has misrepresented it. This assists the client to differentiate the real from the unreal.

Client: Someone took my magazine last night.

Nurse: Your magazine is here in your drawer.

Client: There is a dead mouse in that corner.

Nurse: It is a discarded washcloth, not a mouse.

It may also be necessary to clarify a sequence of events or a time period.

Client: I vomited this morning.

Nurse: Was that after breakfast?

Client: I feel that I have been asleep for weeks.

Nurse: You had your operation Monday, and today is Tuesday.

Using Open-Ended Questions and Statements
The use of *open-ended questions* is discussed in Chapter 10 (see "Interviewing" on page 177). Examples of *open-ended statements* are "I'd like to hear more about that" and "Tell me about . . ."

Focusing
Focusing is used when the client's communication is vague, when the client is rambling, or when the client seems to be talking about numerous things. Focusing can be compared to using a telephoto lens, which focuses sharply on a certain aspect of a view; similarly, the nurse assists or leads the client to focus on one specific aspect of a communication. It is important for the nurse to wait until the clients think they have talked about the main concerns before attempting to focus. The focus may be an idea or a feeling; however, a feeling is often emphasized, to help the client recognize an emotion disguised behind words.

Client: My wife says she will look after me, but I don't think she can, what with the children to take care of, and they're always after her about something—clothes, homework, what's for dinner that night.

Nurse: You are worried about how well she can manage.

Being Specific, Tentative, and Informative
When responding to another person's comments, it is helpful to make statements that are (a) specific rather than general, (b) tentative rather than absolute, and (c) informative rather than authoritarian. Examples are: "You scratched my arm" (specific statement); "You're as clumsy as an ox" (general statement); "You seemed unconcerned about Mary" (tentative statement); "You don't give a damn about Mary and you never will" (absolute statement); "I haven't finished yet" (informative statement); "Stop interrupting!" (authoritarian statement).

In being informative, the nurse needs to present facts or specific information simply and directly. If the nurse does not know some fact, this is also stated simply, together with a suggestion about where or how the information can be obtained.

Client: I don't know the visiting hours.

Nurse: The visiting hours are 9 A.M. to 9 P.M. each day.

Client: When will my doctor be in?

Nurse: I don't know. But Ms. Lu, the charge nurse, will be here in a few minutes, and she may know.

Another way to be informative is to make an observation. This indicates that the nurse has noticed a change of behavior but is not placing a value judgment on it. For example: "You have washed your hair" (neutral observation); "Your hair looks better now that you have washed it" (value judgment); "You are holding your arm carefully; is it painful?" (observation; verifying implication).

Using Touch
Certain forms of touching indicate affection. For example, cheek patting, hand patting, and putting an arm over the person's shoulder are valued forms of affection in North America. The "laying on of hands" is a common expression indicating curative and comforting actions. This expression is often attributed to individuals in the healing professions such as religion, medicine, and nursing. Tactile contacts vary considerably among individuals, families, and cultures. Some families have a great deal of tactile contact among members. Other families, even within the same culture, have minimal contact. Appropriate forms of touch can be helpful in reinforcing caring feelings by the nurse. See Figure 15–5. The use of touch alone often says much more than words for clients, such as for those who are terminally ill or who are unable to speak for whatever reason. It is important, however, for the nurse to be sensitive to the differences in attitudes and practices related to touch among individuals, including the nurse's own attitudes.

Using Silence In everyday conversations natural pauses or silences are often accepted without thought. The listener attentively waits until the talker resumes conversation. These natural pauses are generally used to recall a name or event or to put thoughts or feelings into the most accurate words possible. Pauses or silences that extend for several seconds or minutes, however, make some listeners extremely uncomfortable. The listener who interjects thoughts, questions, or explanations to reduce the discomfort in essence "puts words into the other person's mouth." The unfortunate result is that self-expression is blocked for the initial communicator.

When people are ill, communication about how they feel is often difficult for them. Many prefer to remain stoically silent until they are sure that the nurse is interested or trustworthy. Once communication is initiated, it may be expressed awkwardly, with many pauses. The nurse needs to learn to be silent in these situations and to wait patiently until the person is able to put thoughts and feelings into words.

Providing General Leads By providing a general lead, the nurse encourages the client to verbalize and at the same time choose the topic of conversation.

Client: I am sure glad yesterday is over.

Nurse: Perhaps you would like to talk about it.

or

Nurse: Would it help you to discuss your feelings?

Summarizing Summarizing the main points of a discussion is a useful technique near the end of an interview, after a significant discussion, or to review a health-teaching session. It clarifies for both the nurse and the client the relevant points discussed and often acts as an introduction to future care planning. For example, the nurse might say, "During the past half hour we have talked about. . . . Tomorrow afternoon we may explore this further" or "In a few days, I'll review what you have learned about the actions and effects of your insulin." A word of caution about summarizing: No new material should be added.

Nontherapeutic Responses

Nurses need to recognize nontherapeutic techniques that interfere with effective communication. These include failing to listen; unwarranted reassurance; judgmental responses; defensive responses; and probing, testing or challenging responses.

Failing to Listen Because listening is the most effective technique to facilitate communication, the opposite, failure to listen, is the primary inhibitor to communication. It says to the client, "I'm not interested" or "I'm bored" or "You are not important." It suggests that nurses need to be

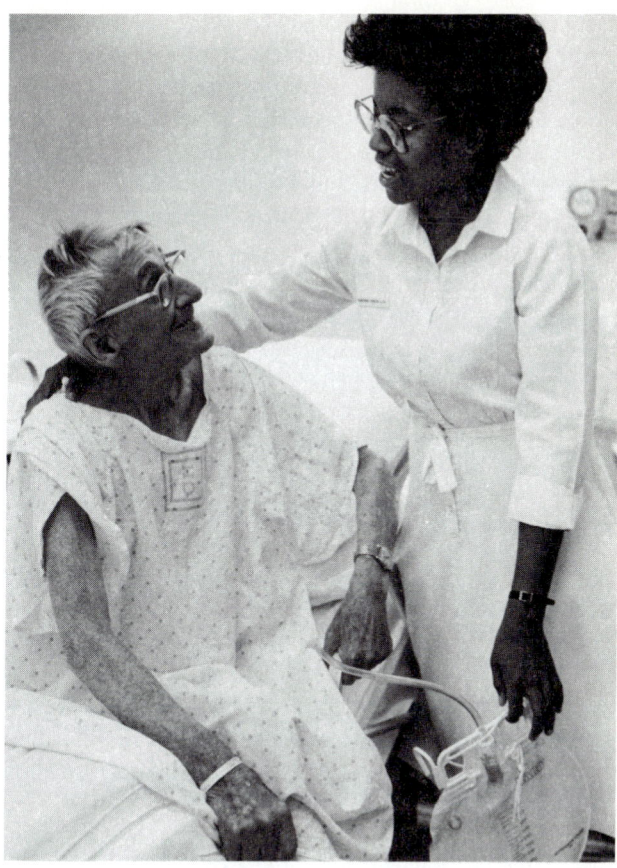

Figure 15–5 Appropriate forms of touch can communicate caring.

entertained, that the nurses' needs require attention, or that nurses prefer to discuss topics that concern themselves.

Unwarranted Reassurance Statements such as "You'll feel better soon," "I'm sure everything will turn out all right," "Don't worry," and "You're looking better each day" are futuristic and intended to provide hope for the client. However, they disregard the client's feelings of the moment and in many instances are said when there is no hope of improvement. The client who fears death, for example, needs to express these concerns rather than have them dismissed with false reassurance. The nurse who offers reassurance in this manner needs to examine her or his own feelings and recognize that this type of response is of more help to the nurse than to the client.

Judgmental Responses Passing judgment on the client implies that the client *must* think as the nurse thinks—the client's values must be the same as the nurse's—if the client is to be accepted. Approving or disapproving responses, such as "That's good (bad)," "You shouldn't do that," and "That's not good enough," tell clients they must measure up to the nurse's standards rather than to their own goals. Perhaps what the nurse considers "bad" the client considers "good."

Giving common advice, another nontherapeutic response, removes decision-making control from the client to the nurse. It suggests that the client is inferior and less wise than the nurse. Moreover, it fosters dependence, and often the advice is not followed. Note that *common,* not *expert,* advice is spoken of here. This differentiation is significant, since giving expert advice can be therapeutic. Brammer (1985, p. 7) writes:

> Advice can be helpful if it is given by trusted persons with expert opinions based on solid knowledge of a supporting field such as law, medicine, or child rearing. Sometimes . . . clients need a recommended course of action supported by wide experience and . . . facts.

Common advice, on the other hand, refers to matters dealing with individual choice. For example, a client asks, "Should I move from my home to a nursing home?" or "I'm separated from my wife. Do you think I should have sexual relations with another woman?" Offering advice such as "If I were you . . ." is unwise for the nurse. Clients need support to make their own decisions.

Stereotyping responses are judgmental, since they categorize clients and negate their uniqueness as individuals. *Stereotypes* are generalized and oversimplified beliefs we hold about various groups of people, which are based upon experiences too limited to be valid. The less one knows about a person, the more the tendency to stereotype. Examples of stereotyping statements are: "Two-year-olds are brats," "Women are complainers," and "Men don't cry." Communication between nurse and client can be inhibited, depending on how emotionally charged the stereotype is for the nurse. For example, if the nurse is not deeply committed to the "brat" theory, the communication pattern with a 2-year-old who is cooperative may be only temporarily affected. On the other hand, the nurse who has marked feelings about men who cry will probably ignore the individualism of a male client who expresses his grief in that manner.

Another common error is to offer meaningless stereotyped responses to clients.

Client: I'm sure having a lot of pain.

Nurse: Really? Most people don't have pain after this type of surgery.

Client: I don't have the energy I'd like to have.

Nurse: Rome wasn't built in a day.

Agreeing and disagreeing imply that the client is either right or wrong and that the nurse is in a position to judge this. They can deter clients from thinking through their position. Disagreement sometimes causes the client to defend a position.

Client: I don't think Dr. Broad is a very good doctor. He doesn't seem interested in his patients.

Nurse: Dr. Broad is head of the Department of Surgery and is an excellent surgeon.

Defensive Responses

Many clients offer opinions or comments about their care, directed toward the nurse, the nurse's colleagues, or the institution. Feeling threatened or attacked, the nurse may become defensive and prevent the client from expressing feelings. Following are two examples:

Client: The food here is lousy.

Nurse: It's a lot better here than in the county hospital. You should consider yourself lucky.

Client: Those night nurses must just sit around and talk all night. They didn't answer my light for over an hour.

Nurse: I'll have you know we literally run around on nights. You're not the only client, you know.

These responses prevent the client from expressing true concerns. The nurse is saying, "You have no right to complain." Defensive responses protect the nurse from admitting weaknesses in the health care services, including personal weaknesses.

Probing, Testing, and Challenging Responses

Probing, testing, and challenging are often considered hostile responses. **Probing** is asking for information chiefly out of curiosity rather than with the intent to assist the client. Usually probing is considered prying, and the client feels that privacy is not being respected. Often asking "why" is probing and can place the client in a defensive posture:

Client: I was speeding along the street and didn't see the stop sign.

Nurse: Why were you speeding?

Client: I didn't ask the doctor when he was here.

Nurse: Why didn't you?

Testing is questioning by nurses to make clients admit to something. With testing, the nurse usually asks a question that permits the client only limited answers. Testing often meets the nurse's need rather than the client's. Examples of testing questions are: "Who do you think you are?" This question forces clients to admit that their status in the health care agency is that of "only a client." Another testing question is "Do you think I am not busy?" which forces the client to admit that the nurse really *is* busy.

Challenging is giving a response that makes clients prove their statement or point of view. Usually clients' feelings are not considered, and they feel it necessary to defend a position. Challenging a client's perceptions rarely changes them; often it strengthens them, because the client feels forced to find proof to support the position.

Client: I felt nauseated after that red pill.

Nurse: Surely you don't think I gave you the wrong pill?

Client: I feel as if I am dying.

Nurse: How can you feel that way when your pulse is 60?

Client: I believe my husband doesn't love me.

Nurse: You can't say that; why, he visits you every day.

EVALUATING COMMUNICATION

Evaluation activities involve an appraisal of both client communication and nurse communication. To evaluate whether client goals have been achieved, the nurse obtains data in relation to the outcome criteria established. This is accomplished by actively listening to the client's style of verbal communication and observing the client's nonverbal communication with the nurse and others. Examples of evaluative statements indicating goal achievement are "The client expressed feelings of anger and fear about diagnosis and inability to speak," or "Using slateboard effectively to indicate needs × 1 week," or "The client stated, 'I listened more closely to my daughter yesterday and discovered how she feels about our divorce.'"

For nurses to evaluate the effectiveness of their own communications with clients, process recordings are frequently used. A **process recording** is a verbatim (word-for-word) account of a conversation. It can be taped or written, and it includes all verbal and nonverbal interactions.

One method of writing a process recording is to make three columns on a page. The first column lists what the client said and did, the second what the nurse said and did, and the third contains interpretive comments about the nurse's responses. See Table 15–3.

Once a process recording his been completed, it should be analyzed in terms of (a) the direction and development of the interaction (process), and (b) the content. The nurse's interaction can be analyzed for process according to a number of questions:

1. Was the client's verbal and nonverbal behavior really heard and seen?

2. Were any cues missed?

3. Were the nurse's verbal responses and behavior congruent?

4. Did the client respond to the nurse or independently of the nurse?

5. Did the communication process flow smoothly?

6. Were the nurse's responses consistent with what the nurse observed and heard? Or were they unrelated, exaggerated, or underresponsive?

7. Were the nurse's responses therapeutic or nontherapeutic? See the previous sections on responding therapeutically or nontherapeutically.

Each response can also be analyzed for content in terms of facilitating or inhibiting communication. See Table 15–3 for a sample analysis.

TABLE 15–3   *Sample Process Recording*

Mary Jane Adams, a nursing aide, reports to Irene Olsen, the staff nurse, that Sandra Barrett, the client in room 815, had finished only her orange juice when Ms. Adams collected the breakfast trays. Mrs. Barrett had been admitted two days earlier for diagnostic studies. Concerned about her client, Miss Olsen walks down the corridor to room 815, knocks, and enters. Mrs. Barrett turns away from the window, tears in her eyes, as Miss Olsen enters.

Client	Nurse	Comments
	Good morning, Mrs. Barrett.	Acknowledging.
Hello.		
	I understand you didn't eat your breakfast.	Making a specific statement, but ignoring the nonverbal.
I wasn't hungry.	Is something wrong?	Asking a closed-ended question that fails to facilitate exploration.
No. (Eyes fill with tears.)	You look sad; as if you're about to cry.	Giving feedback.
(Cries)	I'll sit here a while with you. (Sits down.)	Offering self.
(Continues to cry.)	(After a 30-second pause): Sometimes it's hard to share the things you're concerned about with someone you don't know well. I'd like to be able to help.	Empathizing. Supporting. Offering self.
(Angrily): You can help me by telling me the truth.		
	(Leans forward and maintains eye contact.)	Actively listening and demonstrating interest.

TABLE 15-3 *Sample Process Recording* (*continued*)

Client	Nurse	Comments
Everyone beats around the bush when I ask them what's wrong with me. The head nurse said, "What do *you* think is wrong?" That kind of put-off drives me up the wall!		
	You're angry because you're not getting any answers. It seems as if the staff knows something about your condition and they're keeping it from you.	Paraphrasing.
They all seem to be in cahoots. Nobody tells me anything. (Pause). (Softly): If the news was good, they wouldn't beat around the bush.		
	I'm wondering if you're worried that because people haven't answered your question it means that you have a serious illness?	Paraphrasing.
Good news is always easy to give.		
	Yes, people do seem to be able to deliver good news easier and faster. I also know that we don't have any news—good or bad—to give you because none of the laboratory or x-ray results are back yet. I know that doesn't help answer your questions, but I hope it relieves you a bit from worrying that there is some bad news that's being withheld.	Giving information. Supporting.
Well, when my father-in-law had surgery for a bleeding ulcer, the x-ray and laboratory results were available immediately.		
	When there's a question of emergency surgery being needed, then tests results are asked for immediately. Usually, though, it's preferable to wait for an accurate reading and a thorough written report.	Giving information.
Are you absolutely sure?		
	You don't sound convinced.	Acknowledging the implied.
Listen, I don't mean to give you a hard time. It's just that . . . it may not seem like an emergency to my doctor or the lab people, but it sure is to me. I can't stand not knowing. I don't know the results of the tests I had yesterday. I don't know how many more tests I have to have. Will I have to have surgery? When can I go home?		
	The problem you need help with now is finding out the answers to four questions: What are the results of yesterday's tests? Is your doctor considering any other tests for you, and if so what are they? Is surgery being planned? And when can you go home? Let's try to figure out how you can get the answers to these questions.	Summarizing. Encouraging problem solving.

▶

TABLE 15–3 *(continued)*

Client	Nurse	Comments
Well, I can't call my doctor on the phone. All his receptionist will do is take the message. And, anyway, I'm afraid that he'll be offended if he thinks I'm complaining about him. You won't tell him, will you?		
	No, not unless you and I decide together that it would be the best solution.	Encouraging collaboration.
I suppose I could try to forget about it and be patient, just like everyone tells me to.		
	You've tried that, but you're still worried, fearful, and angry. Let's think of some other possibilities.	Encouraging further exploration.
Maybe you could call his office for me! Since you're a nurse, they'll probably put your call right through.		
	So far there are three possible solutions—calling his office yourself, waiting until he comes to visit you later this afternoon, or having me call his office. Are there any other possible solutions that we haven't considered?	Focusing on solutions.
I can't think of any others.		
	Okay, then, which do you think would be best?	Demonstrating respect for the client.
I guess I'd feel better if you called his office. I just don't want him to think that I'm criticizing him.		
	You're concerned about what he might think of you because of this phone call. Let's discuss how I should handle the call and what I should say.	Paraphrasing. Encouraging collaboration and problem solving.

After a few minutes they develop a plan for calling Mrs. Barrett's physician, and Miss Olsen makes the call. The physician has decided to call both the laboratory and the X-ray department for the results of Mrs. Barrett's tests and promises to phone her as soon as he learns the results. They will discuss further possible tests and treatment plans that afternoon when he makes his hospital rounds. Mrs. Barrett asks Miss Olsen to stay with her while she receives the physician's telephone call about the test.

Courtesy of Carol Ren Kneisl, President and Educational Director, Nursing Transitions, Williamsville, New York.

GROUP INTERACTION

People are born into a group (i.e., the family) and interact with others at all stages of their lives in various groups: peer groups, work groups, recreational groups, religious groups, etc. A **group** is defined as two or more persons who have shared needs and goals, who take each other into account in their actions, and who thus are held together and set apart from others by virtue of their interactions. Groups exist to help people achieve goals that would be unattainable by individual effort alone. For example, groups can often solve problems more effectively than one person by pooling the ideas and expertise of several individuals; in addition, information can be disseminated to groups more quickly than to individuals. Moreover, groups often take greater risks than do individuals. Just as responsibilities for actions are shared by group members, so are the consequences of actions. The overall effectiveness of groups in attaining goals depends on many factors, discussed in this chapter.

Classifications of Groups

Groups are classified as either primary or secondary, according to their structure and type of interaction. A **primary group** is a small, intimate group in which the relationships among members are personal, spontaneous, sentimental, cooperative, and inclusive. Examples are the family, a play group of children, informal work groups, and friendship groups. Members of a primary group communicate with each other largely in face-to-face interactions and develop a strong sense of unity or "oneness." What belongs to one person is often seen as belonging to the group. For example, a success achieved by one member is shared by all and is seen as a success of the group.

Primary groups set standards of behavior for the members but also support and sustain each member under stresses he or she would otherwise not be able to withstand. Expectations are informally administered and involve primarily internal constraints imposed by the group itself. To its members, the primary group has a value in itself, not merely as a means to some other goal. The group has a sense of "we" and "our" to it, in contrast to "I" and "mine." Affective relationships are stressed.

The role of the primary group, particularly the family, in health care is increasingly recognized. It is to the primary group that people turn for help and support when they have health problems. Treatment and health care of individuals therefore are developing an expanded focus that includes the family.

A **secondary group** is generally larger, more impersonal, and less sentimental than a primary group. Examples are professional associations, task groups, ad hoc committees, political parties, and business groups. Members view these groups simply as means of getting things done. Interactions do not necessarily occur in face-to-face contact and do not require that the members know each other in any inclusive sense. Thus, there is little sentiment attached to such relationships. Expectations of members are formally administered through impersonal controls and external restraints imposed by designated enforcement officials. Once the goals of the group are achieved or change, the interaction is discontinued.

Groups may be also classified as formal, semiformal, or informal. The most common example of the *formal group* is the work organization. People become familiar with many different formal work groups during their lifetimes and spend a major part of their working hours in such groups. Formal groups usually exist to carry out a task or goal rather than to meet the needs of group members. Some examples of *semiformal groups* are churches, lodges, social clubs, PTAs, and some labor unions. Many of a person's social needs and ego needs are satisfied by membership in these groups.

All people, from childhood on, have membership in numerous *informal groups*. These groups provide much of a person's education and develop most cultural values. Five types of groups are representative of the numerous informal groups in existence.

1. *Friendship groups.* The first groups formed in life are friendship groups. They are often formed on the basis of common interests. Many arise out of semiformal group interactions or are formed spontaneously from work organization.

2. *Hobby groups.* Hobby groups bring together a wide variety of people from all walks of life. The differences in members' personalities and backgrounds are largely ignored in the interests of the hobby itself.

3. *Convenience groups.* Many examples of convenience groups are found both in and out of the work setting. Two examples are the car pool and the child-care group organized by mothers.

4. *Work groups.* Informal work groups can make or break an organization. Managers need to be sensitive to such groups and cultivate their cooperation and good will. Friendships often arise out of such groups between a new member and the first person who makes that member feel a welcome addition to the group.

5. *Self-protective groups.* Self-protective groups can be found anywhere but are particularly common in work organizations. They arise spontaneously out of a real or perceived threat. For example, a supervisor may approach a worker too strongly and find a group of workers organizing a united front against the threat. Such groups dissipate as soon as the threat has subsided.

Types of Health Care Groups

Much of a nurse's professional life is spent in a wide variety of groups, ranging from **dyads** (two-person groups) to large professional organizations. As a participant in a group, the nurse may be required to fulfill different roles: member or leader, teacher or learner, adviser or advisee, etc.

Common types of health care groups include task groups, teaching groups, self-help groups, self-awareness/growth groups, therapy groups, and work-related social support groups. There are similarities and differences among the characteristics of these various types of groups and the nurse's role.

Task Groups   The task group is one of the most common types of work-related groups to which nurses belong. Examples are health care planning committees, nursing service committees, nursing team meetings, nursing care conference groups, and hospital staff meetings. The focus of such groups is the completion of a specific task, and the format is defined at the outset by the leader and/or members. The methods used to perform the task vary according to the task to be performed.

The leader of a task group, usually called the *chairperson,* must be accepted by the members as an appropriate leader and therefore should be an expert in the area of task emphasis. The chairperson's role is to identify the specific task, clarify communication, and assist in expressing opinions and offering solutions. *Committee members* are generally selected in terms of their individual functional role and employment status, rather than in terms of their personal characteristics. Member participation is determined by the task. A target date for termination of the group is usually set in advance.

Teaching Groups   The major purpose of teaching groups is to impart information to the participants. Examples of teaching groups include group continuing education and client health care groups. Numerous subjects are often handled via the group teaching format: childbirth techniques, birth control methods, effective parenting, nutrition, management of chronic illness such as diabetes, exercise for middle-aged and older adults, and instructions to family members about follow-up care for discharged clients. A nurse who leads a group in which the primary purpose is to teach or learn must be skilled in the teaching-learning process discussed in Chapter 16.

Self-Help Groups   A self-help group is a small, voluntary organization composed of individuals who share a similar health, social, or daily living problem (Rollins 1987, p. 403). These groups are based on the helper-therapy principle: those who help are helped most. One of the central beliefs of the self-help movement is that persons who experience a particular social or health problem have an understanding of that condition which those without it do not.

The self-help group process can be classified as either behaviorally or cognitively oriented (Levy 1979). Behaviorally oriented processes include social reinforcement, self-control behaviors, modeling, and promoting change. Cognitively oriented processes include the provision of information and advice, demystifcation of troubling experiences, and discovering alternative perceptions of problems and methods of solutions. There are many self-help groups available for a range of problems (e.g., stillbirth, parenting, pregnant adolescents, divorce, drug abuse, cancer, menopause, mental illness, diabetes, AIDS, women's health, caregivers of elderly people, and grief). Alcoholics Anonymous was the first self-help group established. Positive aspects of self-help groups are outlined in the accompanying box.

There are three major reasons why people join self-help groups. First, individuals want to be self-reliant and as independent as possible from health and/or social services. Second, people like to give help as well as receive it—a value is placed on the idea of mutual aid. Third, members feel that they have power through collective action.

According to Katz (1970, p. 58), self-help groups have the following characteristics.

- They are similar to small autonomous groups and form along the lines of friendship networks.
- They are problem-centered and organized with reference to a specific problem or problems.
- Members of the group tend to be peers.
- The members of the group have common goals, and the group's goals are formed by the group.
- The action of the group is group action. According to Corbin (1983, p. 12), "this is one of the main reasons for joining a group rather than 'going it alone.'"

Positive Aspects of Self-Help Groups

- Members can experience almost instant kinship, since the essence of the group is the idea that "you are not alone."
- Members can talk about their feelings and listen to the concerns of others, knowing they all share this experience.
- The group atmosphere is generally one of acceptance, support, encouragement, and caring.
- Many members act as role models for newer members and can inspire them to attempt tasks they might consider impossible.
- The group provides the opportunity for people to help as well as to *be* helped—a critical component in restoring self esteem.

Source: V. J. Gilbey, Self-help, *Canadian Nurse,* April 1987, 83:25.

- A norm of the group is helping others. Riessman (1976, p. 42) lists three reasons why people who help others obtain special benefits: (a) the helper is less dependent; (b) in struggling with another's problems that are like one's own, helpers have an opportunity to view their own problems from a distance; and (c) the helper attains a feeling of social usefulness.
- Power and leadership are on a peer basis. Leaders evolve from the group over a period of time.

The program of a self-help group has several aspects: First, the members should gain confidence in their abilities to handle their problems. Second, a member's failure to deal with a problem should afford an opportunity for that person to learn how to deal with the failure. Third, peers, in self-help groups need to balance support with critical feedback. Peers in a self-help group are generally judgmental, critical, active, and supportive, whereas a therapist in an orthodox psychotherapy group is usually noncritical, nonjudgmental, and neutral. Fourth, peers in a self-help group serve as role models; therefore they act as reminders to the other members that "it can be done." Fifth, a self-help group helps the members assume a "wellness role" rather than a "sickness role" in which one is dependent and helpless. Finally, the emphasis in these groups is on self-control or will power. The locus of control is within, not external to, the member.

The major functions of the nurse's role in self-help groups include

1. Helping clients form such groups by identifying key people who can act as facilitators.
2. Sharing expertise with clients and helping them gain appropriate knowledge and skills.

3. Informing clients and support persons about existing self-help groups available to them. Some self-help groups are organized nationally, e.g., Alcoholics Anonymous (alcoholism), Weight Watchers (obesity), and United Ostomy Association (any ostomy). Community service organizations and social work agencies can usually provide the name of self-help groups.

4. Participating as a member of a self-help group when this is appropriate. For example, a nurse in a nursing home might participate in a self-help group of elderly clients, or a nurse could be a member of a self-help group in the larger community. The nurse's role is that of a resource person, i.e., being "on tap, but not on top."

5. Helping out in times of crisis. A self-help group may flounder after operating successfully for some time for several reasons. For example, group time may compete with other aspects of a member's social life, or people who are caregivers may not have the time or energy to take part in the activities designed to help them.

Involvement in a self-help group can supplement and complement any health worker's role. They can profit from learning of people's experiences and in turn offer more insightful counseling to future clients and their families.

Self-Awareness/Growth Groups

The purpose of self awareness/growth groups is to develop or use interpersonal strengths. The overall aim is to improve the perception of members or to improve the functioning of the group to which they return, whether job, family, or community. From the beginning broad goals are usually apparent, e.g., to study communication patterns, group process, or problem solving. Because the focus of these groups is interpersonal concerns around current situations, the work of the group is oriented to reality testing with a here-and-now emphasis. Members are responsible for correcting inefficient patterns of relating and communicating with each other. They learn group process through participation and involvement.

The leader of self awareness/growth groups is usually referred to as a *trainer* and the members as *trainees*. To maintain effective control of interpersonal tensions, the trainer must have sufficient preparation and skill to understand and facilitate group process and experience. When the trainees learn and implement similar skills, the trainer's superior role diminishes.

Selection criteria are variable. Members may merely express a desire to become more self-aware or to address specific personality characteristics. Members may or may not be interviewed and/or requested to complete a questionnaire regarding personal data and personality characteristics before entry. Effectiveness of these groups is facilitated when an agenda and structure are defined by all members and the leader. A target date for termination is usually set in advance.

Therapy Groups

Therapy groups are clearly defined to do the work of therapy. Members work toward self-understanding, more satisfactory ways of relating or handling stress, and changing patterns of behavior toward health. The focus of the group is member-centered. Depending on the leader's orientation, past experiences may be just as relevant as current concerns.

The leader of the group, referred to as a *therapist,* differs from the members in having superior skills in a specialized area such as group psychotherapy. The therapist never truly becomes a member but may at times take on a member role. The overall role of the therapist is to establish and facilitate group interaction between the therapist and individual members and among group members.

Members of the therapy group are referred to as clients or, in some settings, as patients. They are selected by health professionals after extensive selection interviews that consider the pattern of personalities, behaviors, needs, and identification of group therapy as the treatment of choice. Duration of therapy groups is not usually set. A termination date is usually mutually determined by the therapist and members.

Work-Related Social Support Groups

Many nurses experience some of the high levels of vocational stress, e.g., hospice, emergency, and critical care nurses. Social support groups can help reduce stress for such nurses if various types of support are provided to buffer the stress. Richman and Rosenfeld (1987, p. 205) delineate four types of social support (listed in order of importance) that effective support groups need to provide to buffer stress:

1. *Technical challenge.* Group members who know about the work of others can encourage and challenge members to be more creative and enthusiastic about their work and to achieve more. For example, a nurse may help another team member consider alternative strategies for intervention.

2. *Shared social reality.* Group members act as sounding boards and verify perceptions of the social context with other members who have similar priorities, values, and perspectives. For example, two nurses working with a difficult client can share similar feelings of frustration.

3. *Emotional challenge.* Group members provide emotional challenge to each other when they question whether others are doing their best to achieve goals and overcome obstacles. For example, a nurse who has difficulty explaining a hospice concept to a physician is encouraged by other members to question whether she blames the physician for her own inability to provide a clear explanation.

4. *Listening.* Group members share the joys of success and the frustration of failure through active listening without giving advice or making judgments. This type of social support is best given *outside* of the work-related support

group, since mere reflective listening is counterproductive for stress reduction. It is difficult for members to combine listening support with other types.

Features of Effective Groups

To be effective, a group must achieve three main functions:

1. Accomplish its goals
2. Maintain its **cohesion** (degree of group unity or oneness; sense of members being "we")
3. Develop and modify its structure to improve its effectiveness.

Characteristics of an effectively functioning group are shown in Table 15–4.

Assessing Group Dynamics

During recent years the terms *group dynamics* and *group process* have frequently appeared in literature and discussions among group workers, educators, and professional

TABLE 15–4 *Comparative Features of Effective and Ineffective Groups*

Factor	Effective Groups	Ineffective Groups
Atmosphere	Informal, comfortable, and relaxed. It is a working atmosphere in which people demonstrate their interest and involvement.	Obviously tense. Signs of boredom may appear.
Goal setting	Goals, tasks, and objectives are clarified, understood, and modified so that members of the group can commit themselves to cooperatively structured goals.	Unclear, misunderstood, or imposed goals may be accepted by members. The goals are competitively structured.
Leadership and member participation	Shift from time to time, depending on the circumstances. Different members assume leadership at various times, because of their knowledge or experience.	Delegated and based on authority. The chairperson may dominate the group, or the members may defer unduly. Member participation is unequal, with high-authority members dominating. One or more functions may not be emphasized.
Communication	Open and two-way. Ideas and feelings are encouraged, both about the problem and about the group's operation.	Closed or one-way. Only the production of ideas is encouraged. Feelings are ignored or taboo. Members may be tentative or reluctant to be open and may have "hidden agendas" (personal goals at cross-purposes with group goals).
Decision making	By consensus, although various decision-making procedures appropriate to the situation may be instituted.	By the highest authority in the group, with minimal involvement by members; or an inflexible style is imposed.
Cohesion	Facilitated through high levels of inclusion, trust, liking, and support.	Either ignored or used as a means of controlling members, thus promoting rigid conformity.
Conflict tolerance	High. The reasons for disagreements or conflicts are carefully examined, and the group seeks to resolve them. The group accepts unresolvable basic disagreements and lives with them.	Low. Attempts may be made to ignore, deny, avoid, suppress, or override controversy by premature group action.
Power	Determined by the members' abilities and the information they possess. Power is shared. The issue is how to get the job done.	Determined by position in the group. Obedience to authority is strong. The issue is who controls.
Problem solving	High. Constructive criticism is frequent, frank, relatively comfortable, and oriented toward removing an obstacle to problem solving.	Low. Criticism may be destructive, taking the form of either overt or covert personal attacks. It prevents the group from getting the job done.
Self-evaluation as a group	Frequent. All members participate in evaluation and decisions about how to improve the group's functioning.	Minimal. What little evaluation there is may be done by the highest authority in the group rather than by the membership as a whole.
Creativity	Encouraged. There is room within the group for members to become self-actualized and interpersonally effective.	Discouraged. People are afraid of appearing foolish if they put forth a creative thought.

Source: H. S. Wilson and C. R. Kneisl, *Psychiatric nursing,* 3d ed. (Menlo Park, Calif.: Addison-Wesley Publishing Co., 1988), p. 276. Used by permission.

organizations. **Group dynamics** (or **group process**) are forces in the group situation that determine the behavior of the group and its members. They are a way of looking at groups. Every group has its own unique dynamics and constantly changing patterns of forces, just as each individual has unique forces from within that shape the person's character. To study the dynamics of a group, several factors, in addition to group structure and organization, may be analyzed: (a) commitment, (b) leadership style, (c) decision-making methods, (d) member behaviors, (e) interaction patterns, (f) cohesiveness, and (g) power.

Commitment   The members of effective groups have a **commitment** (agreement, pledge, or obligation to do something) to the goals and output of the group. Because groups demand time and attention, members must give up some autonomy and self-interest. Inevitably conflicts arise between the interests of individual members and those of the group. However, members who are committed to the group feel close to each other and willingly put themselves out for the group. These are some indications of group commitment:

- Members feel a strong sense of belonging.
- Members enjoy each other.
- Members seek each other for counsel and support.
- Members support each other in difficulty.
- Members value the contributions of other members.
- Members are motivated by working in the group and want to do their tasks well.
- Members express good feelings openly and identify positive contributions.
- Members feel that the goals of the group are achievable and important.

Leadership Style   Leadership styles and characteristics of effective leaders are discussed in Chapter 2, page 30. To determine which group members carry out leadership functions, the following questions may be asked:

- Who starts the meeting or the work?
- Who contributes additional information to help the group carry out its functions?
- Who represents the group with other groups?
- Who encourages contributions from group members?
- Who provides support to members with difficult situations?
- Who clarifies thoughts expressed in discussions?
- Who keeps the discussions relevant?

Decision-Making Methods   Five methods of decision making have been identified:

1. *Individual or authority-rule decisions.* The designated leader of the group makes the decision, and group members or others involved in the decision are expected to abide by it. Authority-rule decisions may be made without discussion or consultation with the group or may be made after discussing the issue and eliciting the group's ideas and views. Decisions made without discussion are often advantageous for simple, routine matters. Those made after discussion are advantageous in that they use the resources of the group and gain the benefits of discussion. However, this type of decision making does not develop a commitment in members to implement the decision, and it fails to resolve controversies among members.

2. *Minority decision.* A few group members meet to discuss an issue and make a decision that is binding for all. This method of decision making is advantageous when the total group is unable to meet together because of time pressures. It is useful for routine decisions. Its limitations are similar to those of decision making by authority rule. Often, executive committees of large groups exercise minority control in decision making.

3. *Majority decisions.* More than half of those involved make the decision. This method is commonly used in large groups when complete member commitment is unnecessary. It is an effective method to close a discussion on issues that are not highly important for the group and when sufficient time is lacking for a decision by consensus.

4. *Consensus decisions.* Each group member expresses an opinion, and a decision is made by which members can abide, if not in whole, at least in part. This type of decision making takes a great deal of time and energy and therefore is not effective when time pressures are great or when an emergency is in progress. It is useful, however, when important and complex decisions requiring commitment from all members need to be made. This method has several advantages: (a) it produces creative, high-quality decisions, (b) it elicits commitment by all members and responsibility for implementing action, (c) it uses the resources of all members, and (d) it enhances the future decision-making ability of the group.

5. *Unanimous decisions.* Every group member agrees on the decision and can support the action to be taken. This method is commonly used for issues that are highly important to the group and require complete member commitment. Unanimous decisions are not practical for simple, routine matters or controversial issues, however.

Making sound decisions is essential to effective group functioning. Effective decisions are made when

- The group determines which decision method to adopt.
- The group listens to all the ideas of members.
- Members feel satisfied with their participation.
- The expertise of group members is well used.
- The problem-solving ability of the group is facilitated.
- The group atmosphere is positive.

- Time is used well; i.e., the discussion focuses on the decision to be made.
- Members feel committed to the decision and responsible for its implementation.

Member Behaviors   The degree of input by members into goal setting, decision making, problem solving, group evaluation, and so on is due in part to the group structure and leadership style, but members, too, have responsibilities for group behavior and participation. Effective member behaviors include the following:

- Offer facts, opinions, ideas, suggestions, and relevant information to help group discussion.
- Ask for facts, information, opinions, ideas, and feelings from other members, to help group discussion.
- Focus attention on the task to be done.
- Restate and summarize the major points discussed.
- Identify sources of difficulties the group has in working effectively and blocks to progress in accomplishing the group's goals.
- Stimulate a higher quality of work from the group.
- Examine the practicality and workability of ideas; evaluate alternative solutions, and apply them to real situations to see how they will work.
- Encourage everyone to participate, giving recognition for contributions, demonstrating acceptance and openness to the ideas of others.
- Persuade members to analyze their differences of opinion constructively, search for common elements in conflicts, and try to reconcile disagreements.
- Make sure that each group member understands what other members are saying.
- Listen and serve as an interested audience for other members; be receptive to others' ideas.

Interaction Patterns   Interaction patterns can be observed and ascertained by a **sociogram,** a diagram of the flow of verbal communication within a group during a specified period, e.g., 5 or 15 minutes. This diagram indicates who speaks to whom and who initiates the remarks. Ideally, the interaction patterns of a small group would indicate verbal interaction from all members of the group to all members of the group. See Figure 15–6. In reality, however, such an interaction pattern does not occur. See Figure 15–7. This second diagram illustrates that not all communication is a two-way process. The lines with arrowheads at each end indicate that the statement made by one person was responded to by the recipient; a short cross-line drawn near one of the arrowheads indicates who initiated the remark. One-way communication is indicated by lines with an arrowhead at only one end. Remarks made to the group as a whole are indicated by arrows drawn to only the middle

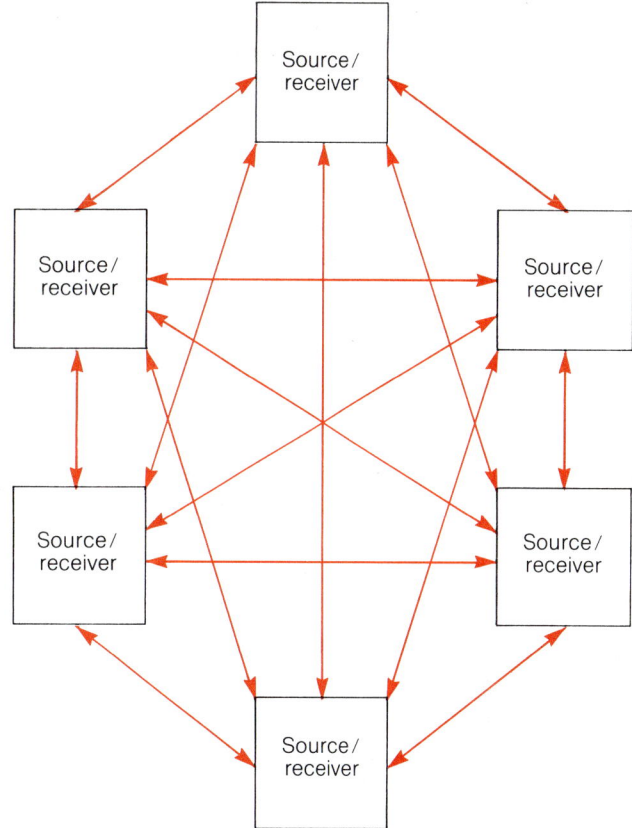

Figure 15–6   An ideal small-group interaction pattern. All members interact with all other members.

of the circle. By using a sociogram, nurses can analyze strengths and weaknesses in a group's interaction patterns. Used in conjunction with member behavior tools, this can offer considerable data about the group's dynamics.

Cohesiveness   Cohesive groups (those that cohere or "hang together") possess a certain group spirit, a sense of being "we," and a common purpose. Groups lacking in cohesiveness are unstable and prone to disintegration. Membership attitudes and behaviors and group properties that characterize high-cohesion groups include the following (Kneisl 1988, p. 284):

- Members like one another, are friendly, and enjoy interacting with one another.
- Members receive support on issues from one another.
- Members praise one another for accomplishments.
- Members share similar opinions and attitudes.
- Members are likely to influence one another and are willing to be influenced by other members.
- Members accept assigned tasks and roles readily and value group goals.
- Members trust one another.

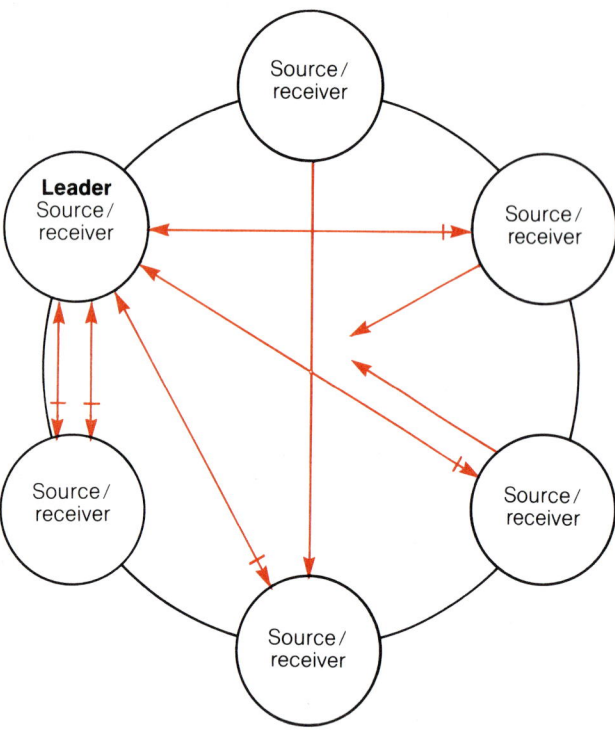

Figure 15–7 A sociogram indicating the flow of verbal communication within a group during a specific period. Note that five questions or comments calling for a response were directed at the leader.

■ Members are loyal to group and defend it against external criticism and attack.

■ Attendance risk taking, participation, and communication are high.

■ "We" is frequently heard in discussions, and group output and productivity are high.

■ Leadership is democratic.

■ Satisfaction with members and work of group is high.

Power Power can be viewed as a vital, positive force that moves people toward the attainment of individual or group goals. It is impossible to interact with others without influencing and being influenced by them; hence, group members are constantly adjusting to one another and modifying their behavior. The various types and sources of power are detailed in Chapter 3, page 51.

The unequal distribution of power within a group (i.e., a group in which certain members have much power and others have little) can adversely affect the task and maintenance functions of the group. Members who believe they have little influence in the group are less likely to feel committed to group goals and to participate in decision making.

Dissatisfaction with the group decreases its attractiveness and reduces its cohesion.

High-power people often are the most popular or have the most authority. However, neither circumstance is appropriate for high-quality decision making. High-quality decisions are the result of power based on expertise, competence, and relevant information, not on popularity or authority. To ensure rational and humane decision making and to avoid unquestioning obedience to authority, group members need to assess and critique suggestions from the authority person.

Group Self-Evaluation

Groups need to set up mechanisms for feedback of information to the members about their method of operation. Only when a group acquires information about itself can it make adjustments to improve its efficiency. Several mechanisms can be set up for group feedback and self-evaluation: use of a group-productivity observer, use of a group self-evaluation guide, general open discussion initiated by the group leader prior to the end of the meeting, or combinations of these.

Some groups establish a rotating position for a group-productivity observer, just as positions are established for a recorder; others acquire the assistance of an outsider specially trained in this area. The responsibility of this person is to observe the group during its discussions, rather than participate, and to provide feedback to the group about perceptions of the group's behavior. The observer notes the general atmosphere of the group, leadership techniques, orientation of the group, participation by members, and any factor considered to affect the productivity of the group. See Table 15–5 for a sample group self-evaluation guide that can be used by the observer.

The provision of feedback requires skill by the observer in presenting comments. It is helpful to present objective data first and then phrase comments in the form of tentative hypotheses, alternative solutions, or expressions of the observer's feelings. This allows group members the chance to reject a comment if they are not ready to handle it. The observer can be viewed as "in error." For example, the observer of the group meeting evaluated in Table 15–5 might comment:

Objective data: During the time we were trying to suggest solutions to problems, two of us seemed impatient to tear a new idea apart. Out of five suggestions made, four were immediately criticized. Right after that, suggestions for solutions lagged.

Alternative solution: I was wondering at the time whether more and better ideas might have emerged if we had withheld our critical comments until after most of the ideas about solutions were on the blackboard.

Open discussion needs to follow such comments.

TABLE 15—5 *Example of Group Self-Evaluation Guide*

Criteria	Comments
A. Group direction and orientation	
1. How much was achieved?	1. Only one-third of agenda covered. Too much time spent on irrelevant material
2. How clear are goals and purposes?	2. A few members not clear about purposes.
3. How clear is procedure to achieve goals?	3. No discussion about how to try to achieve task.
4. Was sufficient relevant information available?	4. Yes
B. Group motivation and unity	
5. What degree of interest is there in task?	5. A few do not think problem is important.
6. Was interest maintained throughout?	6. Interest lagged when one member made lengthy lecture.
7. Is group united in purpose?	7. Feelings of unity not evident in two members.
C. Group atmosphere	
8. Formal?	
9. Informal?	9. Yes
10. Permissive?	10. Yes
11. Inhibited?	
12. Cooperative?	12. Yes
13. Competitive?	
14. Friendly?	14. Yes
15. Hostile?	
D. Member contributions	
16. What is degree of participation by members?	16. All participated. Some monopolization by one member.
17. Were contributions relevant, factual, and problem-centered?	17. Most were.
18. Were members listening to what others said?	18. A few were not, at point of high interest in discussion.
19. How did special members serve group?	19.
a. Leader	a. Facilitated discussion. Could have handled dominating member better. Let group wander too much.
b. Recorder	b. Asked for clarification of some points. Assisted group to focus on issue.
c. Resource person	c. Provided essential clarifying information.
d. Others	d. Two members criticized four out of five ideas while they were being suggested. After that, fewer suggestions were offered.
20. How did majority of members feel about meeting?	
a. Poor	
b. Mediocre	20b. Yes
c. Okay	
d. Good	
e. Excellent	

Source: Adapted from David H. Jenkins, "Feedback and group self-evaluation" from the *Journal of Social Issues,* Vol. IV, No. 2, pp. 50–60. Reprinted by permission of The Society for the Psychological Study of Social Issues, Ann Arbor, MI.

CHAPTER HIGHLIGHTS

▶ The effective nurse-client relationship is a growth-facilitating process.

▶ Four phases of the helping relationship include the preinteraction phase, the introductory phase, the working phase, and the termination phase; each has a specific purpose or goal and requires specific skills of the nurse.

▶ Communication incorporates exchanging information between two or more people and is a basic component of human relationships and nurse-client relationships.

CHAPTER HIGHLIGHTS (continued)

▶ Communication is usually categorized as verbal or nonverbal.

▶ Verbal communication is effective when the criteria of simplicity, clarity, timing, relevance, adaptability, and credibility are met.

▶ Nonverbal communication often reveals more about a person's thoughts and feelings than verbal communication; it includes physical appearance, posture and gait, facial expressions, hand movements, and other gestures.

▶ When assessing nonverbal behaviors, the nurse needs to consider cultural influences and be aware that a variety of feelings can be expressed by a single nonverbal expression.

▶ When communication is effective, verbal and nonverbal expressions are congruent.

▶ Communication is a two-way process involving the sender of the message and the receiver of the message.

▶ Because the sender must encode the message and determine the appropriate channels for conveying it, and because the receiver must perceive the message, decode it, and then respond, the communication process includes four elements: sender, message, receiver, and feedback.

▶ Many factors influence the communication process: the ability of the communicator, perceptions, personal space (intimate, personal, social, and public distance), territoriality, roles and relationships, purposes, time and setting, attitudes, emotions, and self-esteem.

▶ The development of communication is a complex process; the nurse needs to be familiar with the phases of language development for assessment purposes.

▶ Factors that influence language development are intelligence, sex, bilingualism, single child versus twin status, parental stimulation, and socioeconomic components.

▶ There are three broad areas for assessing communication: language development, nonverbal behavior, and style of communication.

▶ Many techniques facilitate therapeutic communication: attentive listening; paraphrasing; clarifying; using open-ended questions and statements; focusing; being specific; using touch and silence; clarifying reality, time, or sequence; providing general leads; and summarizing.

▶ Techniques that inhibit communication include offering unvalidated reassurance, stating approval or dis-

approval, giving common (not expert) advice, stereotyping, and being defensive.

▶ Process recordings are frequently made by nurses to evaluate their own communication. With them, nurses can analyze both the process and the content of the communication.

▶ Most people's lives are spent interacting with other human beings in groups. A person's sense of being evolves through membership in groups that help achieve goals they set for themselves.

▶ Groups can be classified as primary or secondary, according to their structure or according to their type of interaction. In small, primary groups, relationships are spontaneous, personal, and sentimental. In larger, secondary groups, relationships are impersonal and less sentimental.

▶ Effective groups produce outstanding results, succeed in spite of difficulties, and have members who feel responsible for the output of the group. They accomplish their goals, maintain cohesion, and develop and modify their structure in ways that improve effectiveness.

▶ Regardless of setting or composition, several forces shape and modify the structure and functioning of groups. They include member commitment, leadership styles and roles, methods of decision making, member behaviors, interaction patterns, cohesiveness, and power and influence.

▶ Sound decision making that leads to well-conceived, well-understood, and well-accepted realistic actions toward the goals agreed on by the group is the hallmark of a group that functions effectively.

▶ Groups make decisions by consensus, selection of a group of experts, averaging members' opinions, majority vote, minority control, authority rule after discussion, and authority rule without discussion. Each method is appropriate at certain times.

▶ Power and influence in groups operate constantly and force members to adjust to one another and modify their behavior.

▶ Group self-evaluation is essential to improving the efficiency of a group.

▶ Nurses interact with groups of clients and colleagues in a wide variety of settings. To use groups rationally and effectively, nurses must understand the forces that underlie small group interactional processes and recognize their own patterns of participation.

READINGS AND REFERENCES

SUGGESTED READINGS

Bilderback, B. January 1989. Surviving the stages of peer consultation. *American Journal of Nursing* 89:113–14, 116.

This education specialist at St. Francis Hospital, Tulsa, Oklahoma, describes the stages of development of a *peer consultation group*. *Peer consultation* involves group collaboration to resolve clinical or organizational problems. After one year of struggling toward peer consultation, these group members learned to define problems succinctly for the group and ask the right (consultative) questions.

Peplau, H. E. July 1960. Talking with patients. *American Journal of Nursing* 60:964–66.

This classic article differentiates nursing communication with a client from that of a layperson. In this article, Peplau offers the beginning nursing student helpful suggestions for meaningful communication with clients.

Scott, A. L. August 1988. Human interaction and personal boundaries. *Journal of Psychosocial Nursing and Mental Health Services* 26:23–27.

Scott discusses the different meanings of *boundaries* and their major characteristics. The behaviors of people with open and closed boundaries are listed in a table. The development of an individual's boundaries is reviewed and the assessment of a client's boundaries discussed.

Seaman, L. May/June 1982. Affective nursing touch. *Geriatric Nursing* 3:162–64.

The need to be touched continues throughout life and may even be intensified by the sensory and personal losses that occur with aging. The author discusses why touch is important and implications for nursing touch, including appropriate ways of touching.

Travelbee, J. February 1963. What do we mean by rapport? *American Journal of Nursing* 63:70–72.

The basic ingredients of rapport are outlined in this classic article. Nurses are constantly reminded that they need to develop rapport with patients but often are unable to explain its meaning.

Truglio-Londrigam, M., and Hayes, P. M. November/December 1986. Carers learn to cope . . . families caring for elders at home. *Geriatric Nursing* 7:310–12.

Families caring for elders at home need information, know-how, and support from peers. In recognition of this need, these geriatric nurse practitioners and clinical nurse specialists started a support group using Orem's self-care model, adult learning theory, and systems theory. Group goals, planned content, group profile, and concerns are discussed.

RELATED RESEARCH

Appleby, F. M. March 1987. Professional support and the role of support groups. *Health Visitor* 60:77–78.

Banning, M. R. August 1987. The effects of activity-elicited humor and group structure on group cohesion and affective responses. *American Journal of Occupational Therapy* 41:510–14.

Chapman, G. E. March 1988. Reporting therapeutic discourse in a therapeutic community. *Journal of Advanced Nursing* 13:255–64.

Coeling, H. V. E., and Wilcox, J. R. November 1988. Understanding organizational culture: A key to management decision-making. *Journal of Nursing Administration* 18:16–24.

Edwards, E. M. J. September 1988. Group dynamics in psychotherapy. *Canadian Nurse* 84:59.

Forrest, D. Autumn 1983. Analysis of nurses' verbal communication with patients. *Nursing Papers* 15:48–56.

Harrison, T. M.; Pistolessi, T. V.; and Stephen, T. D. February 1989. Assessing nurses' communication: A cross-sectional study. *Western Journal of Nursing Research* 11:75–91.

Rosendahl, P. B., and Ross, V. October 1982. Does your behavior affect your patient's response? *Journal of Gerontological Nursing* 8:572–75.

Trojan, A. 1989. Benefits of self-help groups: A survey of 232 members from 65 disease-related groups. *Social Science and Medicine* 29(2):225–32.

Walton, J., and Youngkin, E. May/June 1987. The effect of a support group on self-esteem of women with premenstrual syndrome. *Journal of Obstetric, Gynecologic, and Neonatal Nursing* 16:174–78.

Wintersteen, R. T., and Young, L. July 1988. Effective collaboration with family support groups. *Psychosocial Rehabilitation Journal* 12:19–31.

SELECTED REFERENCES

Apse, A. December 1985. Avoiding terms of bewilderment. *Nursing 85* 15:42–43.

Bandler, R., and Grinder, J. 1975. *The structure of magic,* Volume 1. Palo Alto, Calif.: Science and Behavior Books.

Bee, H. 1985. *The developing child.* 4th ed. New York: Harper & Row.

Brammer, L. M. 1988. *The helping relationship: Process and skills.* 4th ed. Englewood Cliffs, N.J.: Prentice-Hall.

Brockopp, D. Y. July 1983. What is NLP? *American Journal of Nursing* 83:1012–14.

Carkhuff, R. R., and Anthony, W. A. 1979. *The skills of helping.* Amherst, Mass.: Human Resource Development Press.

Carpenito, L. J. 1989. *Nursing diagnosis. Application to clinical practice.* 3d ed. Philadelphia: J. B. Lippincott Co.

Clark, C. C. 1987. *The nurse as group leader.* 2d ed. New York: Springer Publishing Co.

Consider this . . . Social support groups. February 1988. *Journal of Nursing Administration* 18:3.

Corbin, D. E. May/June 1983. Self-help groups: What the health educator should know. *Health Values* 7:10–14.

Davis, A. J. 1984. *Listening and responding.* St. Louis: C. V. Mosby Co.

Dreher, B. B. 1987. *Communication skills for working with elders.* New York: Springer Publishing Co.

Egan, G. 1975. *The skilled helper: A model for systematic helping and interpersonal relating.* Monterey, Calif.: Brooks/Cole Publishing. Co.

————. 1982. *The skilled helper: Model, skills, and methods for effective helping.* 2d ed. Monterey, Calif.: Brooks/Cole Publishing Co.

Fisher, D. W. January 1985. Guidelines to effective group functioning. *Point of View* 22:6–8.

Harrison, T. M., Pistolessi, T. V., Stephen, T. M. February 1989. Assessing nurses' communication: A cross-sectional study. *Western Journal of Nursing Research* 11:75–91.

Gilbey, V. J. April 1987. Self-help. *Canadian Nurse* 83:23, 25.

Hall, E. T. 1969. *The hidden dimension.* Garden City, N.Y.: Doubleday and Co.

Hardin, S. B., and Halaris, A. L. January 1983. Nonverbal communication of patients and high- and low-empathy nurses. *Journal of Psychosocial Nursing and Mental Health Services* 21:15–20.

Hurst, J. B., and Keenan, M. January 1986. Do you have any other ideas for improvement? *Nursing Success Today* 3:1–29.

Kasch, C. R. 1984. Interpersonal competence and communication in the delivery of nursing care. *Advances in Nursing Science* 6(2):71–88.

Katz, A. H. January 1970. Self-help organizations and volunteer participation in social welfare. *Social Work* 15:57–60.

Kaul, T., and Schmidt, L. 1971. Dimensions of interviewer trustworthiness. *Journal of Counselling Psychology* 34:134–39.

Kim, M. J.; McFarland, G. K.; and McLane, A. M. 1989. *Pocket guide to nursing diagnoses.* 3d ed. St. Louis: C. V. Mosby Co.

King, I. M. 1981. *A theory for nursing. Systems, concepts, process.* New York: John Wiley and Sons.

Kneisl, C. R. 1988. Group process. In Wilson, H. S., and Kneisl, C. R., pp. 270–289. *Psychiatric nursing.* 3d ed. Menlo Park, Calif.: Addison-Wesley Publishing Co.

Knowles, R. D. July 1983. Building rapport. Through neuro-linguistic programming. *American Journal of Nursing* 83:1011–14.

Leonard, R. November 1985. Speak for yourself. *Nursing 85* 15:30–31.

Levy, L. 1979. Processes and activities in groups. In Lieberman M. A., and Borman, L. D., and Associates, editors. pp. 244–257. *Self-help groups for coping with crisis: Origins, members, process, and impact.* San Francisco: Jossey-Bass.

Morgan, B. S., and Barden, M. E. September 1985. Nurse-patient interaction in the home setting. *Public Health Nursing* 2:159–67.

NANDA approved nursing diagnostic categories for clinical use and testing. Summer 1988. *Nursing Diagnosis Newsletter* 15:1–3.

Northhouse, P. G., and Northhouse, L. L. 1985. *Health education. A handbook for health professionals.* Englewood Cliffs, N.J.: Prentice-Hall.

Orr, J. August 1987. In our own hands . . . self-help groups are a growing concern. *Nursing Times* 83:26–28.

Piaget, J. 1952. *The language and thought of the child.* London: Routledge and Kegan Paul.

Raudsepp, E. April 1990. Seven ways to cure communication breakdowns. *Nursing 90* 20:132, 134, 137–38.

Richman, J. M. February 1988. Social support groups. *Journal of Nursing Administration* 18:3, 19.

Richman, J. M., and Rosenfeld, L. B. Summer 1987. Stress reduction for hospice workers: A support group model. *Hospice Journal* 3:205–21.

Riessman, F. 1976. How does self-help work? *Social Policy* 7:41–45.

Rollins, J. A. November/December 1987. Self-help groups for parents. *Pediatric Nursing* 13:403–9.

Ruesch, J. 1961. Therapeutic Communication. New York: W. W. Norton and Co.

Salvage, J. June 21–27 1989. Take me to your leader . . . what makes a good nursing leader. *Nursing Times* 85:34–35.

Shanken, J., and Shanken, P. February 1976. How to be a helping person. *Journal of Psychiatric Nursing and Mental Health Services* 14:24–28.

Stewart, C. J., and Cash, W. B. 1988. *Interviewing principles and practices.* 5th ed. Dubuque, Iowa: Wm. C. Brown Publishers.

Sundeen, S. J.; Stuart, G. W.; Rankin, E. A. D.; and Cohen, S. A. 1989. *Nurse-client interaction.* 4th ed. St. Louis: C. V. Mosby Co.

Teasley, D. November 1987. Situational leadership for nurses. *Nursing Management* 18:112–13.

Thomas, E. J. 1984. *Designing interventions for the helping professions.* Beverly Hills, Calif.: Sage Publications.

Thomas, M. 1970. Trust in the nurse-patient relationship. In Carlson, Carolyn E. editor. *Behavioral concepts and nursing intervention.* Philadelphia: J. B. Lippincott Co.

Vygotsky, L. S. 1962. *Thought and language.* Cambridge, Mass.: MIT Press.

Wilkinson, R. April 1986. Communication: Learning from the market. *Nursing Management* 17:42J, 42L.

Wilson, M. 1985. *Group theory/process for nursing practice.* Bowie, Md.: Brady Communications Co.

Wold, J. E. November 1986. Group decision-making: Teaching the process—an introductory Guided Design project. *Journal of Nursing Education* 25:388–89.

Teaching, Learning, and Planned Change

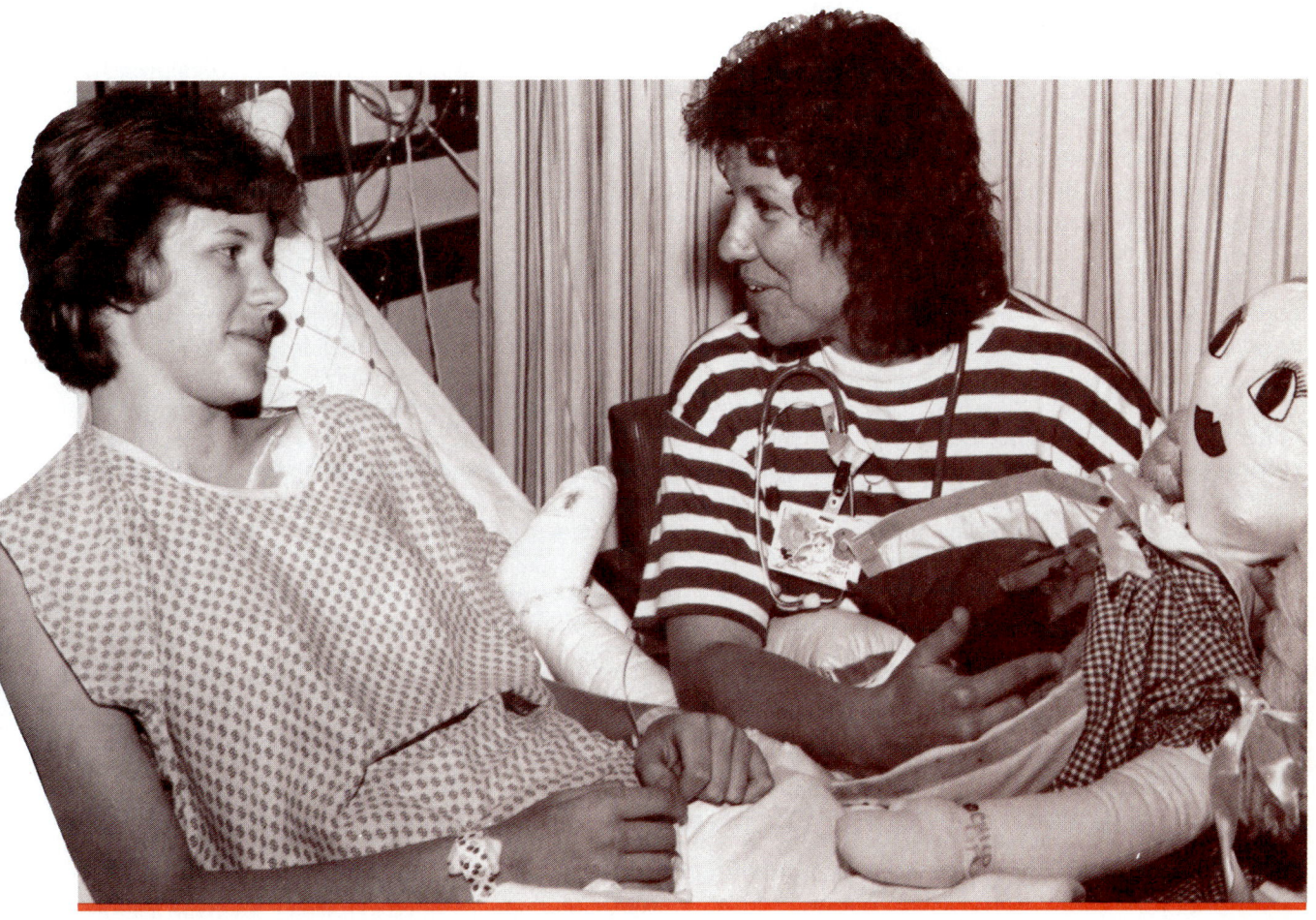

OBJECTIVES

▶ Explain how andragogy can guide client teaching.

▶ Describe types of change.

▶ Explain three theories of change.

- List factors that facilitate learning.
- Explain the three domains, or areas, of learning.
- Outline five principles of teaching.
- Describe the essential aspects of a teaching plan.
- Explain essential factors in assessing for learning.
- Identify eight guidelines that help plan teaching.

FACILITATING LEARNING

Education incorporates two processes: teaching and learning. However, these processes are not interdependent. Teaching can occur without any learning taking place, and learning can occur in the absence of teaching. Client education is a major aspect of nursing practice and an important independent nursing function. In 1972, the American Hospital Association passed the Patients' Bill of Rights mandating client education as a right of all clients. In addition, legislation relating to nursing frequently has included client teaching as a function of nursing, thereby making teaching a legal and professional responsibility (Phillips and Heckelman 1983, pp. 42–46).

Client education is multifaceted, involving promoting, protecting, and maintaining health. It involves teaching about reducing health risk factors, increasing a person's level of wellness, and providing information about specific protective health measures.

Clients have a variety of learning needs. A **learning need** is a need to change behavior or "a gap between the information an individual knows and the information necessary to perform a function or care for self" (Gessner 1989, p. 593). **Learning** is a change in human disposition or capability that persists over a period of time and that cannot be solely accounted for by growth. Learning is represented by a change in behavior. An important aspect of learning is the individual's desire to learn and to act on the learning. This is referred to as **compliance.** Compliance is best illustrated when the person recognizes and accepts the need to learn, willingly expends the energy required to learn, and then follows through with the appropriate behaviors that reflect the learning. For example, a man diagnosed as having diabetes willingly learns about the special diet he needs, and then plans and follows the learned diet.

Theories of Learning

Theories of learning have been developed to explain how and why people learn. Three main theoretical areas are behaviorism, cognitivism, and humanism.

Behaviorism was originally advanced by Edward Thorndike, who believed that transfer of knowledge could occur if the new situation closely resembled the old situation. To Thorndike, the term *understanding* was used in the context of building connections. One of his major contributions applicable to client teaching is that learning should be based on the learner's behavior.

Cognitivism depicts learning as a complex cognitive activity. Kurt Lewin's field theory, i.e., theories of motivation and perception, were considered precursors of the more recent cognitive theories. Lewin believed that learning involved four different types of changes: change in cognitive structure, change in motivation, change in one's sense of belonging to the group, and gain in voluntary muscle control.

Humanism or humanistic theories of learning assume that there is a natural tendency for people to learn and that learning flourishes in an encouraging environment. Implementing humanistic theory involves providing options for the client and the resources and equipment for learning.

More recently, in the 1970s and 1980s, theories of adult learning have been increasingly applied in client teaching. Malcolm Knowles coined the term *andragogy.*

Andragogy is "the art and science of helping adults learn" (Knowles 1980, p. 43) in contrast to *pedagogy,* the discipline concerned with helping children learn. Nurses can use the following andragogic concepts about learners as a guide for client teaching (Knowles 1984):

- As people mature, they move from dependence to independence.
- An adult's previous experiences can be used as a resource for learning.
- An adult's readiness to learn is often related to a developmental task or social role.
- An adult is more oriented to learning when the material is immediately useful, not useful sometime in the future.

Types of Change

Implicit in the definition of learning is **change.** There are many types of change; in fact, change can occur without effort on anyone's part. Change of this type is also referred to as "drift." It occurs as individuals and groups respond to the environment and is usually recognized retrospectively. For example, after the birth of a baby, changes may take place in the parents' life-style. They may go out socially less frequently and spend less money. They may become aware of this change only after a period of time, when they realize they have not been going to movies as they were accustomed.

There is also traditional change, which can be approached in five different ways. See Table 16–1. Traditional change is effective in some circumstances and is usually planned.

TABLE 16-1 *Traditional Change Strategies*

Strategy	Basis	Application in Nursing
Exposition and propagation	Ideas change the world, and ideas can be responsible for change.	Workshops, client teaching, advertising.
Elite corps	Knowledge is power; people with knowledge in power positions assure change by an elite corps.	The nurse assumes an elitist position in relation to clients and uses this position to convince the client to change.
Psychoanalytic insight	People in power require knowledge, insight, and awareness of psychologic factors operating in a situation. Psychologic insights provide power to effect change.	The nurse uses insights about the client when proposing change.
Scholarly consultation	Experts with special knowledge serve as outside consultants and propose solutions or change.	A nurse acts as a consultant to a client and/or family and uses knowledge to propose changes.
Circulation of ideas to the elite group	Circulating ideas about change to the power group can effect change.	A nurse conveys ideas about change to the nurse in charge, hoping this will result in the desired change.

However, most of these approaches have limitations: Anyone wanting to use these strategies to effect change has to be in a position of superior knowledge and power. Today, social scientists recognize that change is not a simple phenomenon but has far-reaching effects involving many people, usually an entire system, e.g., a family or a broader social group.

Other types of change have been described. *Developmental change* refers to the physiopsychosocial changes that occur during the life cycle. This type of change is normally gradual. An example of this is the decreasing physical capability of an elderly person. This kind of change is slow and generally permits the individual time to adapt. *Situational change* occurs without any control by a person or group. An example is the change that occurs as a result of a war or a hurricane. However, not all situational changes are negative; for example, Nurse Smith may be unexpectedly offered a position in a hospital that she has wanted for a long time.

Changes may also be considered covert or overt. A *covert* change is hidden or occurs without the individual's awareness. For example, a person can become increasingly deaf without being aware of this fact. *Overt* change is change about which a person is aware, for example, the development of abdominal pain or shortness of breath while walking up stairs. People who experience overt change may also experience anxiety. Overt change often necessitates behavioral changes that are at variance with the person's needs or goals. An example is a diagnosis of cancer and the subsequent need for therapy even though it interferes with the person's work and family life.

Change is frequently differentiated as unplanned or planned. **Unplanned change** is usually haphazard, and the results can be unpredictable. **Planned change,** by contrast, involves problem-solving and decision-making skills

as well as interpersonal competence (Welch 1979, p. 307). It is deliberate and carried out consciously. According to Lippitt (1973), planned change is an intended, purposive attempt by an individual, group, organization, or larger social system to influence the status quo of itself, another organism, or a situation. Planned change refers to "changes that are proposed to improve living, working or recreational conditions" (Mauksch and Miller 1981, p. 20). However, according to Bennis, Benne, and Chin (1985, p. 21), not all people want the stated benefits of change.

There are a number of theories of planned change. They all have in common an emphasis less on knowledge than on collaboration among the people involved. Four theories about change of particular value to nurses are those proposed by Lewin, Lippitt, Havelock, and Rogers. See Table 16-2 on page 280.

Kurt Lewin (1948) originated classical change theory. He saw change as having three basic stages: unfreezing, moving, and refreezing.

During the *unfreezing* stage, the motivation to establish some sort of change occurs. The individual becomes aware of the need for change. This stage is a cognitive process in which the person becomes aware of a problem or of a better method of accomplishing a task and hence of the need for change. Having identified this need, the individual must also identify restraining and driving forces. The restraining forces are those that inhibit change, and the driving forces are those that support change. For example, a charge nurse who wants nurses recognized for their nursing excellence may identify the new vice-president of nursing as a driving force but may see nurses on the unit who are resistant to change as restraining forces.

In the second stage, *moving,* the actual change is planned in detail and then started. Information about the problem is gathered from one or several sources. At this stage, it is

TABLE 16-2 *Theories of Change*

Lewin (1948)	Lippitt (1958)	Havelock (1973)	Rogers (1983)
1. Unfreezing	1. Diagnosing the problem	1. Building a relationship	1. *Knowledge.* The individual, called the decision-making unit, is introduced to change and begins to comprehend it.
2. Moving	2. Assessing the motivation and the capacity for change	2. Diagnosing the problem	2. *Persuasion:* The individual develops an attitude toward the change that may be favorable or unfavorable.
3. Refreezing	3. Assessing the change agent's motivation and resources	3. Acquiring relevant resources	3. *Decision.* The person makes a choice to adopt or not to adopt the change.
	4. Selecting progressive change objectives	4. Choosing the solution	4. *Implementation.* The person acts on the choice. At this time, alterations may take place.
	5. Choosing an appropriate role for the change agent	5. Gaining acceptance	5. *Confirmation.* The individual looks for confirmation that the choice was right. If the person encounters mixed messages, the choice may be changed.
	6. Maintaining the change once it has been initiated	6. Stabilization and generating self-renewal	
	7. Terminating the helping relationship		

Sources: K. Lewin, *Field theory in social science* (New York: Harper and Row, 1951); R. Havelock, *The change agent's guide to innovations in education* (Englewood Cliffs, N.J.: Educational Technology Publications, 1973); E. Rogers, *Diffusion of innovations,* 3d ed. (New York: Free Press, 1983). R. Lippitt, Jeanne Watson, and B. Westley: *The Dynamics of Planned Change.* (New York. Harcourt, Brace and World, Inc., 1958)

important that the people involved agree that the status quo is undesirable. In the above example, the charge nurse would help nurses to see the disadvantages of not recognizing clinical excellence and to view the problem from another perspective—i.e., how recognition can be accomplished. The charge nurse could also guide the nurses in their search for information about this problem.

The charge nurse, as a change agent, should provide an environment that is conducive to the change. Rewards may need to be provided to reinforce desired behaviors. An environment that fosters change should be supportive, non-threatening, and educational (Olson 1979).

In the third stage, *refreezing,* the changes are integrated and stabilized. According to Welch (1979), the individuals involved in the change integrate the idea into their own value system. Thus, in the above example the nurses on the unit would come to value recognition of clinical excellence and would integrate this idea into their own value systems.

Gordon Lippitt (1958) described planned change as having seven phases. See Table 16-2. For a detailed discussion of each of these seven stages, see Welch (1979).

Ronald Havelock (1973) modified Lewin's theory regarding planned change. See Table 16-2. In his theory, the emphasis is on planning the change process, which he believed takes the most time and involves the most significant changes (Welch 1979).

Everett Rogers (1983) viewed people's backgrounds and the environment as important in the process of change. He described change as a five-step process, which he called the *innovation-decision process* (Rogers 1983). See Table 16-2.

The individual who undergoes change can also reject the change at a later time. Rogers thus introduced the idea that an adopted change is not necessarily permanent but may be reversed in the future. Rogers emphasized that for successful change, the people involved must be interested in the change and committed to implementing it.

Acceptance of Change

Important aspects of planning change are establishing the likelihood of change being accepted and then identifying the criteria by which it can be identified. Acceptance of change often takes time, particularly when change does not fit into an individual's attitudinal frame of reference; in such a case, change may not occur at all. For example, to stop smoking may not be accepted as a desirable behavior change by an individual who values smoking and does not believe it is harmful. Optimally, this belief changes before the change in behavior is tried. Stages in the acceptance of change are shown in the accompanying box.

Resistance to Change

When a change agent encounters resistance, it is important to determine whether the resistance should be overcome. Sometimes the change is inadvisable, as when there are insufficient resources for making the change. Resistance to change is often greatest when the idea is not concurrent with existing trends, such as trying to change from primary nursing to functional nursing when primary nursing is currently popular. Also, resistance is usually great when the proposed change would alter a situation with which people are comfortable.

Reasons for Resistance

Resistance to change is not merely lack of acceptance but rather behavior intended to maintain the status quo—that is, to prevent the change. However, not all behavior that opposes change is resistance. Sometimes change is opposed for valid, logical reasons. According to New and Couillard (1981), people resist change for one or more of the following reasons: (a) threatened self-interest, (b) inaccurate perceptions, (c) objective disagreement with the change, (d) psychological reactance, and (e) low tolerance for change.

Threatened self-interest as a reason for resistance to change often involves people's perception that the personal costs will be greater than any gains. These costs may occur in time, money, or status, for example. Opposition to a change may be based on *incorrect perceptions* of the change itself. Incomplete or inaccurate information may cause apprehension about the change, resulting in resistance on the part of the people involved. *Objective disagreement* can also cause resistance to a change. In some instances, people may have information that leads them to believe the change will not attain stated objectives. Sometimes individuals have more experience or information than the change agent, and their resistance can result in reconsideration of a planned change and perhaps benefits for the people involved. *Psychologic reactance* is a reaction motivated by perceived loss of freedom to engage in particular behaviors. According to New and Couillard (1981), psychologic reactance is manifested when threatened or eliminated behaviors suddenly assume

greater importance than previously, and the person attempts to reestablish eliminated behaviors.

Some people have a *low tolerance* for change. Although they may intellectually understand the change, they are unable to accept it emotionally. This may be due to feelings of low self-esteem, fear of risk, or minimal tolerance for uncertainty.

Stages of Resistance

Stevens (1975) described six stages of resistance to change:

1. Undifferentiated resistance arises from various sources.
2. The sides for and against the change line up and develop their stands.
3. The two sides have direct conflicts. The resistance is either overcome or reduced.
4. The people for the change come into power.
5. The people against the change begin the stages of acceptance.
6. Few opponents are found and most people don't recall that they opposed the change.

Dealing with Resistance

Reinhard (1988) gives the following guidelines for dealing with resistance:

- Communicate with the people who oppose the change and identify the cause of their opposition.
- Clarify information and give accurate feedback.
- Be open to revisions in the plan, but be clear about areas that cannot be changed.
- Induce guilt in the people who oppose the change by, for example, explaining the consequences of their resistance on client care or on available money for care.
- Enhance psychological security and reduce threats to it. This can be done by emphasizing the positive aspects of the change.
- Encourage the people who are resisting to maintain face-to-face contact with supporters. Encourage both sides to empathize with the other: recognize valid objections, and relieve unnecessary fears.
- Maintain a climate of trust, support, and confidence.

PRINCIPLES OF LEARNING

Learning involves the entire person and can affect the person's life-style, methods of handling problems, attitudes, and knowledge. Learning requires energy and the ability to concentrate. To be effective client teachers, nurses must understand those factors that facilitate learning and those that inhibit it.

Factors Facilitating Learning

Motivation to learn is the desire to learn. It is a term that describes forces acting on or from within the person to initiate, direct, and maintain behavior and to explain differences in the intensity and direction of behavior (Redman 1988, p. 21). Such motivation is generally greatest when a person recognizes a need and believes the need will be met through learning. It is not enough for the need to be identified and verbalized by the nurse; it must be experienced by the client. Often the nurse's task is to help the client personally work through the problem and identify the need. Sometimes clients or families need help identifying relevant situational elements before they can see a need. For instance, clients with heart disease may need to know the effects of smoking and being overweight before they recognize the need to stop smoking or adopt a weight-reduction diet. Or adolescents may need to know the consequences of an untreated sexually transmitted disease before they see the need for treatment.

Readiness to learn is the behavior that reflects motivation at a specific time. Readiness sometimes comes with time, and the nurse's role is often to encourage its development (Redman 1988, p. 36).

Active involvement in the learning process makes learning more meaningful. For example, if the learner actively participates in planning and discussion, learning is faster and retention is better. See Figure 16–1. Passive learning, such as listening to a lecture or watching a film, does not foster optimal learning.

Once learners have succeeded in accomplishing a task or understanding a concept, they gain self-confidence in their ability to learn. This reduces their anxiety about failure and can motivate greater learning. Successful learners have increased confidence with which to accept failure. People learn best when they believe they are accepted and will not be judged. The person who expects to be judged as a "poor"

or "good" client will not learn as well as the person who feels no such threat.

Feedback is information relating a person's performance to a desired goal. It has to be meaningful to the learner. Feedback that accompanies practice of psychomotor skills helps the person to learn those skills. Support or desired behavior through praise, positively worded corrections, and suggestions of alternative methods are ways of providing positive feedback. Negative feedback such as ridicule, anger, or sarcasm can lead people to withdraw from learning. Such feedback, viewed as a type of punishment, may cause the client to avoid the teacher in order to avoid punishment.

Learning is facilitated by material that is logically organized and proceeds from the *simple to the complex*. Such organization enables the learner to comprehend new information, assimilate it with previous learning, and form new understandings. Of course, simple and complex are relative terms, depending on the level at which the person is learning. What is simple for one person may be complex for another.

Repetition of key concepts and facts facilitates retention of newly learned material. Practice of psychomotor skills improves performance of those skills and facilitates their transfer to another setting. When a person appreciates the relevance of specific material, learning is facilitated. For example, the man who understands the relevance to his health of a special diet is better able to learn about the diet than a person who sees no such connection.

People retain information and psychomotor skills best when the *time between learning and use is short*; the longer the time interval, the more is forgotten. For example, a woman who is taught how to administer her own insulin but is not permitted to do so until discharge from hospital is unlikely to remember much of what she learned. However, if she is allowed to give her own injections while in hospital, her learning will be enhanced.

An *optimal learning environment* has adequate lighting that is free from glare, a comfortable room temperature, and good ventilation. Most students know what it is like to try to learn in a hot, stuffy room; the subsequent drowsiness interferes with concentration. Noise can also distract the student and interfere with listening and thinking. For the best learning in a hospital setting, nurses should choose a time when there are no visitors present and interruptions are unlikely. Privacy is essential for some learning. For example; when a client is learning to irrigate a colostomy, the presence of others can be embarrassing and thus interfere with learning.

Factors Inhibiting Learning   A greatly *elevated anxiety* level can impede learning. Clients or families who are very worried may not hear spoken words or may retain only part of the communication. Extreme anxiety might be reduced by medications or by information that relieves uncertainty. By contrast, clients who appear disinterested

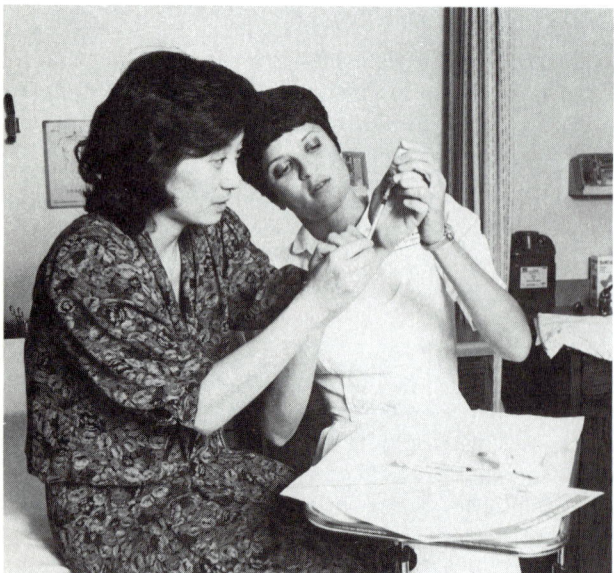

Figure 16–1 Learning is facilitated when the client is interested and actively involved.

and unconcerned may need to be told about potential problems, to increase their anxiety slightly and enhance their motivation to learn.

Learning can be inhibited by *physiologic events* such as a critical illness, pain, or impaired hearing. Because the client cannot concentrate and apply energy to learning, the learning itself is impaired. There are also *cultural barriers* to learning, such as language or values. Obviously the client who does not understand the nurse's language will learn little. Another impediment to learning is differing values held by the client and the health team. For example, a client who does not value being thin may have difficulty learning about a reducing diet.

Domains of Learning
Bloom (1956) has identified three domains, or areas of learning: cognitive, affective, and psychomotor. The *cognitive domain* includes intellectual skills such as thinking, knowing, and understanding. The *affective domain* includes feelings, emotions, interests, attitudes, and appreciations. The *psychomotor domain* includes motor skills such as giving an injection. Nurses should include each of these three domains in client teaching plans. For example, teaching a client how to irrigate a colostomy is the psychomotor domain. An important part of such a teaching plan is to teach the client why a specific amount of fluid is used and when the irrigation should be carried out; this is the cognitive domain. Helping the client accept the colostomy and maintain self-esteem is in the affective domain.

TEACHING

Teaching is a system of activities intended to produce learning. The teaching process is intentionally designed to produce specific learning. Teaching is considered one of the functions of nursing. In some states in the United States teaching is included in the legal definition of nursing, making it a required function under the law.

The teaching/learning process involves dynamic interaction between teacher and learner. Each participant in the process communicates information, emotions, perceptions, and attitudes to the other. The teaching process and the nursing process are very much alike. See Table 16–3.

Teaching also involves a type of communication for which there are specific goals. For example, clients who need to administer their own eye drops or to change an incision dressing share these goals with the nurse. Another aspect of teaching is the relationship between the teacher and the learner. It is essentially one of trust and respect. The learner trusts that the teacher has the knowledge and skill to teach, and the teacher respects the learner's ability to attain the recognized goals. Once a nurse starts to instruct a client and/or support persons, it is important that the teaching process continue until the participants reach the goals,

TABLE 16–3 *Comparison of the Teaching Process and the Nursing Process*

Step	Teaching Process	Nursing Process
1	Collect data; analyze client's learning strengths and deficits.	Collect data; analyze client's strengths and deficits.
2	Make educational diagnoses.	Making nursing diagnoses.
3	Prepare teaching plan.	Plan nursing intervention.
4	Implement teaching plan.	Implement nursing strategies.
5	Evaluate client learning (effectiveness of teaching plan)	Evaluate effectiveness of nursing interventions.

change the goals, or decide that the goals will not help meet the learning objectives.

The following five *principles of teaching* may be helpful to nursing students:

1. Teaching activities should help the learner meet individual learning objectives. These objectives should be mutually determined. If certain activities do not assist the learner, these need to be reassessed; perhaps other activities can replace them. For example, explanation alone may not be able to teach a client to handle a syringe. Actually handling the syringe may be more effective.

2. Rapport between teacher and learner is essential. A relationship that is both accepting and constructive will best assist learning.

3. The teacher who can use the client's previous learning in the present situation encourages the client and facilitates the learning of new skills. For example, a person who already knows how to cook can use this knowledge when learning about a special diet.

4. A teacher must be able to communicate clearly and concisely. The words the teacher uses need to have the same meaning to the learner as to the teacher. For example, a client who is taught not to put water on an area of the skin may think a wet washcloth is permissible for washing the area. In effect, the nurse needs to explain that no water or moisture should touch the area.

5. The teaching activities need to be oriented around the learning objectives. Thus information and skills not related to the learner's objectives need to be eliminated from the teaching process. If they remain, they may confuse the learner or be a distraction from effective learning.

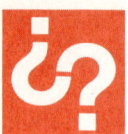

RESEARCH NOTE

Do Hospitalized Clients Understand Medical Terminology?

Byrne and Edeani found in their study that the more clients said they knew about medical terminology, the more they actually did know. In comparing the results of their study in 1980 with a similar study in 1961, knowledge of most medical terminology had increased significantly; however, there was no increase in knowledge of some terms such as *symptom* and *constipation*.

Implications: Despite an overall increase in clients' knowledge of medical terminology, nurses should not assume that all clients understand medical vocabulary.

T. J. Byrne and D. Edeani. Knowledge of medical terminology among hospital patients, *Nursing Research* May/June 1984, 33:178–81.

ASSESSING

Assessing for teaching essentially has two foci: the identification of the client's learning needs and the assessment of relevant data about the client.

Identifying Client Learning Needs

Smitherman (1981, pp. 125–28) describes three sources for identifying learning needs.

1. *The client.* Clients' learning needs may be identified by the clients themselves. A client aware of a learning need may ask pertinent questions or seek out the needed information in some other way.

2. *The client's behavior.* Learning needs are not always easily detected; frequently, consultation with the client is necessary to confirm or deny the existence of these needs. For example, a client who appears angry may be insecure or worried because the client does not understand what is happening; only after the discussion with the client can the nurse be sure that the client has a need for information.

3. *Health care professionals.* Anticipatory learning needs related to the client's health problem often are known by health professionals. For example, a client anticipating surgery will probably need to learn about deep breathing and leg exercises. Or a client receiving oxygen who is being discharged from hospital will need to know how to operate the oxygen equipment and the appropriate safety measures to employ while at home.

Relevant Client Data

Particular client data that need to be collected and examined include client readiness, client motivation, and personal characteristics such as socioeconomic factors, age, and health beliefs and practices.

Readiness   Clients who are ready to learn often behave differently from those who are not. A client who is ready may search out information, for instance, by asking questions, reading books or articles, talking to others, and generally showing interest. The person unready to learn is more likely to avoid the subject or situation and hope or believe that someone else will take care of the problem (Smitherman 1981, pp. 126–27). In addition, the unready client may change the subject when it is brought up by the nurse. For example, the nurse might say, "I was wondering about a good time to show you how to change your dressing," and the client responds, "What did you think of the ball game last night?" Furthermore, somatic symptoms (such as headaches, upset stomach, or gas pains experienced by clients having surgery) may make it difficult for clients to pay attention (Laird 1975, p. 1340).

Tyson (1984) points out that in assessing readiness there are two major factors: emotional and experiential. Emotional factors affecting readiness include anxiety. If the anxiety level of the client is high, perceptions are narrowed and thus interfere with learning. Experiential factors include occupational status, client capabilities, and educational level. In health, physical readiness is also important to consider. Clients may be too ill or weak to attend to learning.

Nurses can sometimes facilitate a client's readiness by tactfully calling attention to a learning need (for example, "Have you thought about learning to change your dressing?"). Two other ways to facilitate readiness are by giving the client information to read and by pointing out an opportunity to learn (for instance, "There is a baby bath demonstration at 3 P.M. today in the next room").

Motivation   As discussed earlier, motivation relates to whether the client wants to learn and is usually greatest when the client is ready, the learning need is recognized, and the content is meaningful to the client (Smitherman 1981, p. 127).

Assessment of motivation to learn is often part of a general health assessment or of a more specific problem assessment. A nurse assessing motivation and a client's present abilities must have a full understanding of the subject to be learned. For example, a man who has had diabetes for several years may already understand how to test his urine for sugar, but he may not know how to administer insulin hypodermically because he has always taken a medication by mouth.

Increasingly, tools are being developed to measure motivation to learn; for example, focus groups may be formed to help identify trends and knowledge held by a selected group of consumers. Another example is a questionnaire given to clients to elicit information about perceptions and expectations related to their illness.

Nurses can positively influence a client's motivation in three ways:

1. By relating the learning to something the client values and helping the client see the relevance of the learning
2. By helping the client to make the learning situation pleasant
3. By encouraging self-direction

To influence the externally motivated learner a nurse can use *positive reinforcement,* which involves rewarding the learner for achievements, e.g., giving praise, or reading a bedtime story to a child. Reinforcement is most effective when given immediately after the desired response. **Negative reinforcement,** or punishment for undesirable responses, is considered less motivating than positive reinforcement. However, negative reinforcement can be motivating if it is accompanied by encouragement and an explanation of how to correct the response (for instance: "I agree that looks right, but if you place the tube like this the urine should flow more readily").

Socioeconomic Factors

Many cultural groups have their own beliefs and practices, a number of them related to diet, health, illness, and life-style. It is therefore important to know how the practices and values held by client's impinge on their learning needs. Although a nurse may be inclined to assume that because a client belongs to a specific ethnic or cultural group the client will follow the norms of the group, this is not always the case. Thus, nurses should avoid stereotyping and should determine the relevant beliefs and values of each client. For example, although the diet of some Jews excludes pork, other Jews have no objection to eating pork.

Folk beliefs of certain groups in North America, e.g., low-income Hispanics, may also affect learning. Although the client may readily understand the health care information being taught, this learning may not be implemented in the home, where folk medical practices prevail. See Chapter 31 for additional information.

Economic factors can also affect a client's learning. For example, a client who cannot afford to obtain a new sterile syringe for each injection of insulin may find it difficult to learn to administer the insulin when the nurse teaches that a new syringe should be used each time.

Learning Style

Considerable research has been done on people's learning styles. It has been suggested that in terms of perception, people can be classified as either sensing types or intuitive types. Sensing people use their senses to perceive data, whereas intuitive people use their perception of meanings, relationships, and possibilities by way of insight to perceive data (Lawrence 1982, p. 7). For example, a sensing person will likely gather data by using sight or hearing when meeting another person, whereas an intuitive person will more likely be aware of meanings and relationships in the same situation.

In terms of judgement processes, people may be classified as thinking or feeling persons. A thinking person uses logical decision making to arrive at a conclusion, whereas a feeling person is more likely to arrive at conclusions using subjective personal values. Attitudes in the latter group tend to result from a preference for feeling; these people find interpersonal skills more interesting than technical skills (Lawrence 1982, p. 8). A nurse will best stress logic and knowledge when teaching a thinking person but should stress interpersonal skills when teaching a feeling person.

Age

Age provides information on the person's developmental status. Simple questions to school-age children and adolescents will elicit information on what they know. Observing children in play provides information about their motor and intellectual development as well as relationships with other children. For the elderly person, conversation and questioning may reveal slow recall or limited psychomotor skills and learning difficulties. For additional information, see "Special Teaching Strategies" later in this chapter.

Health Beliefs and Practices

A client's health beliefs and practices are important to consider in any teaching plan. The health belief model described in Chapter 5, page 92, provides a predictor of preventive health behavior. However, even if a nurse is convinced that a client's health beliefs should be changed, doing so may not be possible because so many factors are involved in a person's health beliefs.

Education

Clients' education will probably influence their present knowledge as well as the teaching method that is most effective. Although some research indicates that education does not always affect learning, the client's ability to read or write does affect the teaching style.

DIAGNOSING

Nursing diagnoses pertinent to a client's learning needs are all grouped under the diagnostic category of **Knowledge deficit.** It is extremely important that the nurse specify which exact deficits individual clients manifest. Examples include the following:

- **Knowledge deficit: low-calorie diet** related to newly ordered therapy
- **Knowledge deficit: diabetic diet** related to prescribed treatment
- **Knowledge deficit: preoperative care** related to impending surgical procedure

- **Knowledge deficit: medications** related to language differences
- **Knowledge deficit: home safety hazards** related to denial of declining health
- **Knowledge deficit: substance abuse** related to lack of motivation to acquire information

PLANNING

Developing a teaching plan is accomplished in a series of steps. Involving the client at this time promotes the formation of a meaningful plan and stimulates client motivation. The client who participates in the formulation of the teaching plan is more likely to achieve the desired outcomes.

Determining Teaching Priorities

The client's learning needs must be ranked according to priority. The client and the nurse should do this together, with the client's priorities always being considered. Once a client's priorities have been addressed, the client is generally more motivated to concentrate on other identified learning needs. For example, a man who wants to know all about diabetes mellitus may not be ready to learn how to give himself injections until his own knowledge needs are met. Nurses can also use theoretical frameworks to establish priorities, such as Maslow's hierarchy of needs. See Chapter 4.

Setting Learning Objectives

The terms *goals* and *objectives* are used interchangeably by some educators and distinguished by others. Used interchangeably, they can be considered as both immediate and long-term aims to be accomplished in a learning situation. However, goal is often the more general term, describing a general, long-range intended outcome of learning, whereas objective is used to mean a specific immediate, short-range intended outcome of a learning situation.

The setting of goals and objectives is done by the client (or support persons) and the nurse. Objectives relate to immediate client needs, such as perineal care after birth of a baby. Goals relate to long-term needs, such as an obese new mother's need to lose weight (in which case the goal may be a specific weight loss through diet and exercise).

The objectives for learning should be both specific and observable in terms of behavior. A specific objective might be "to take 60 mg furosemide (Lasix) upon identifying ankle edema." An objective needs to be stated in terms of client behavior, not nurse behavior: for example, "Will write his own diets as instructed" (client behavior), not "To teach the client about his diet" (nurse behavior). See Table 16–4 for a list of behavioral (observable) verbs and nonbehavioral verbs.

TABLE 16–4 *Selected Verbs for Objectives*

Behavioral Verbs	Nonbehavioral Verbs
Defines	Knows
Identifies	Understands
Chooses	Appreciates
Demonstrates	Feels
Differentiates	
Applies	
Compares	

Objectives should contain three types of information: performance, conditions, and criteria (Mager 1975, p. 21) *Performance,* or behavior, describes what the learner will be able to do after mastering the objective. The objective must reflect an observable activity. The performance may be visible, e.g., walking, or invisible, e.g., adding a column of figures. However, it is necessary to be able to deduce whether an unobservable activity has been mastered from some performance that represents the activity. Therefore, the performance of an objective might be written: "Writes the total for a column of figures in the indicated space" (observable), not "Adds a column of figures" (unobservable).

In some instances it is necessary to state the *conditions* under which a performance is to be carried out so that the objective is clear. For example, "Walks to the end of the hall and back without crutches" describes a performance clearly; "without crutches" is a condition of the objective. Nurses always need to determine the conditions in which an activity will be carried out. Then the objectives for the learning plan can reflect those conditions. For example, if Mr. Jones lives alone and must irrigate his own colostomy, then "Irrigates his colostomy *independently* as taught" is the correct objective.

Criteria state the standards of performance that are considered acceptable. Each objective should specify a standard against which the performance can be measured. Examples include speed, quality, and accuracy. Learners need to understand the criteria so that they can evaluate their performance validly.

Selecting Teaching Strategies

The method of teaching chosen by the nurse should be suited to the individual, to the material to be learned, and to the teacher. For example, the person who cannot read needs material presented in other ways; a discussion is usually not the best strategy for teaching to give an injection; and a teacher using group discussion for teaching should be a competent group leader. Some people are visually oriented and learn best through seeing; others learn best through hearing and having the skill explained. These attributes should be considered during the planning phase. If this fact is not identified until the teaching plan has been implemented, the plan may need revising. See Table 16–5 for selected teaching strategies.

Choosing Content

The content to be taught is determined by the objectives. For instance, "Identify appropriate sites for insulin injections" means the nurse must include content about the body sites suitable for insulin injections.

There are many sources for content information. Nurses will have some knowledge as a result of their own education. Pamphlets, books, and journals can also assist nurses and clients. In addition, clients can learn a great deal from peers. For example, the client who has recently had a colostomy often can learn a great deal from a person who has had a colostomy for several years. Self-help groups function on this premise.

Audiovisual aids (film strips, films, posters, line drawings) often are helpful for client learning. It is important, however, that the nurse review these aids before presenting them to clients, for sometimes they are out of date, or they differ in content from other materials (even minimal differences can be confusing to clients).

Ordering Learning Experiences

Some health agencies have developed teaching guides for lessons that nurses commonly give. The guides save nurses time in constructing their own guides. They also standardize content and assist staff in remembering it. Figure 16–2 on the next page shows one such guide. Whether the nurse is implementing a plan devised by another or developing an individualized teaching plan, some guidelines can help the nurse order the learning experience.

(continued on page 291)

TABLE 16–5 Selected Teaching Strategies

Strategy	Major Type of Learning	Characteristics
Explanation or description (e.g., lecture)	Cognitive	Teacher controls contents and pace. Feedback is determined by teacher. May be given to individual or group. Encourages retention of facts.
One-to-one discussion	Affective, cognitive	Encourages participation by learner. Permits reinforcement and repetition at learner's level. Permits introduction of sensitive subjects.
Answering questions	Cognitive	Teacher controls most of content and pace. Teacher must understand question and what it means to learner. Can be used with individuals and groups. Teacher sometimes needs to confirm whether question has been answered by asking learner, e.g., "Does that answer your question?"
Demonstration	Psychomotor	Often used with explanation. Can be used with individuals, small or large groups. Does not permit use of equipment by learners.
Group discussion	Affective, cognitive	Learner can obtain assistance from supportive group. Group members learn from one another.
Practice	Psychomotor	Allows repetition and immediate feedback. Permits "hands-on" experience.
Printed and audiovisual materials	Cognitive	Forms include books, pamphlets, films, programmed instruction, and computer learning. Learners can proceed at their own speed. Nurse can act as resource person, need not be present during learning.
Role playing	Affective, cognitive	Permits expression of attitudes, values, and emotions. Can assist in development of communication skills. Involves active participation by learner.
Modeling	Affective, psychomotor	Nurse sets example by attitude, psychomotor skill.

Teaching Plan

Home IV Antibiotic Administration

Equipment:
Alcohol swabs
Needles
IV tubing & add-a-line connector
IV antibiotics
Heparin lock solution
Metal/plastic disposal container

Goal	Behaviors	Comments about practice sessions
1. Applies the principles of sterile technique	1.1 Washes hands before initiating intermittent IV antibiotic infusion. 1.2 Stabilizes arm that holds heparin lock to prevent contamination (using Velcro apparatus). 1.3 Does not touch needle when removing cover sheath before hooking up line to heparin lock. 1.4 Wipes heparin lock plug with alcohol wipe before inserting needle. 1.5 Checks needle hub connection to prevent leaking and maintain a closed system. 1.6 Demonstrates ability to insert needle into stabilized heparin lock without contaminating either surface.	
2. Identifies signs and symptoms of IV site infiltration	2.1 Checks heparin lock site before each IV dose and observes for redness, swelling, tenderness, or leakage during or after each infusion. 2.2 Observes rate of infusion to	

Figure 16–2   Sample teaching plan for home use.   *Source:*   Courtesy of the Department of Nursing, University of British Columbia Health Sciences Centre Hospital.

	verify potency of infusion system.
3. Follows procedure to change heparin lock if IV site is interstitial	3.1 Stops infusion if signs and symptoms in 2.1 are observed.
	3.2 Discontinues antibiotic drip; caps needle using sterile technique.
	3.3 Reports to emergency department for a change of site.
4. Initiates infusion of IV antibiotic independently	4.1 Sets up IV flush solution (D_5W bag) and add-a-line tubing with IV antibiotic using sterile technique (see 1.1 – 1.6).

Priming the bulb chambers to prevent air emboli:

4.2 Ensures antibiotic mini-bag is elevated higher than flush bag.

4.3 Flushes IV tubing with flush D_5W solution.

4.4 Stabilizes arm holding heparin lock with Velcro apparatus.

4.5 Inserts needle into heparin lock using sterile technique, and begins to check the site for signs of infiltration (see 2.1 – 2.2). Tapes into place.

4.6 Proceeds to flush with D_5W solution by opening IV control ¼ way. If heparin lock site is clear and pain-free, switches open the IV antibiotic tubing line control knob.

4.7 Observes IV drip chamber, and adjusts to run for 15-20 mins.

4.8 When IV antibiotic mini-bag is empty, the IV flush bag

should automatically begin to drip.

4.9 Checks to confirm that medication is completely absorbed. Flushes tubing with D_5W solution. Closes control knob on IV tubing.

Terminates infusion of IV antibiotic

4.10 Removes needle from heparin lock plug using sterile technique; caps the needle.

5. Stores IV antibiotics appropriately to maintain sterile technique

5.1 Keeps IV antibiotic mini-bags refrigerated in separate plastic container with seal-tight lid.

5.2 Checks label on IV mini-bag for correct drug, dosage, and expiration date.

6. Handles and disposes of equipment to promote safety

6.1 Uses a new IV tubing and add-a-line q2 days.

6.2 Uses a new needle for each IV antibiotic dose following sterile technique.

6.3 Disposes of needles in a metal/plastic container.

7. Identifies support systems in the community

7.1 Knows when public health nurse will visit.

7.2 Knows telephone numbers of emergency department and physician.

7.3 Knows how to contact family members in case of problems with care.

8. Demonstrates emergency procedure if heparin lock becomes dislodged

8.1 Applies clean gauze to site.

8.2 Applies pressure to site.

8.3 Calls for assistance and reports to emergency department to replace IV heparin lock.

T. Savage
H. Lobo
M. Pringle
G. Gleason
2a
June 1991

Figure 16–2 Sample teaching plan (continued)

- Start with something the learner is concerned about, e.g., before learning how to administer insulin to himself, an adolescent wants to know how he can adjust his life-style and still play football.

- Begin with what the learner knows and proceed to the unknown. This gives the learner confidence. Sometimes a nurse does not know the client's knowledge or skill base and needs to elicit this information either by asking questions or by having the client fill out a form, such as a pretest.

- Any area of learning that is anxiety provoking should be taught first. A high level of anxiety can impair concentration in other areas. For example, a woman highly anxious about turning her husband in bed might not be able to learn about bathing him until she has successfully learned to turn him.

- Teach the basics first, then proceed to the variations or adjustments. It is very confusing to learners to have to consider every possible adjustment and variation before the basic concepts are understood. For example, when teaching a female client how to insert a retention catheter, it is best to teach the basic procedure before teaching any adjustments that might be needed if the catheter stops draining after insertion.

IMPLEMENTING

The nurse needs to be flexible in implementing any teaching plan, since the plan may need revising, e.g., because the client tires sooner than anticipated, the client is faced with too much information too quickly, the client's needs change, or external factors intervene. For instance, the nurse and the client, Mr. Brown, may have planned for him to learn to administer his own insulin at a particular time, but when the time comes the nurse finds that he wants additional information before actually giving himself the insulin. In this case, the nurse alters the teaching plan and discusses the desired information, provides written information, and defers teaching the psychomotor skill until the next day.

It is also important for nurses to use teaching techniques that enhance learning and to consider any barriers to learning. See Table 16–6 for barriers to learning. When implementing a teaching plan, the nurse may find the following eight guidelines helpful.

1. The optimal time for each session depends largely on the learner. Some people, for example, learn best at the beginning of the day, when they are most rested; others prefer late afternoon, when no other activities are scheduled.

2. The pace of each teaching session also affects learning. Nurses should be sensitive to any signs that the pace is too fast or too slow. A client who appears confused or does not comprehend material when questioned may be finding the pace too fast. When the client appears bored and loses interest, the pace may be too slow, the learning period may be too long, or the client may be tired.

3. An environment can detract from or assist learning; e.g., noise or interruptions usually interfere with concentration, whereas a comfortable environment promotes learning. Environmental characteristics that should be

TABLE 16–6 *Barriers to Learning*

Barrier	Explanation	Nursing Implications
Acute illness	Client requires all resources to cope with illness.	Defer teaching until client is less ill.
Pain	Pain decreases ability to concentrate.	Deal with pain before teaching.
Age	Vision, hearing, and motor control can be impaired in the elderly.	Allow for sensory and motor defects in teaching.
Prognosis	Client can be preoccupied with illness and unable to concentrate on new information.	Defer teaching to a better time.
Biorhythms	Mental and physical performances have a circadian rhythm.	Change time of teaching to suit client.
Emotion (e.g., anxiety, denial, depression)	Emotions require energy and distract from learning.	Deal with emotions first and possible misinformation.
Language and ethnic background	Client may not be fluent in the nurse's language.	Obtain services of an interpreter or nurse with appropriate language skills.
Iatrogenic barriers	The nurse may set up barriers by appearing condescending or hurried or ignoring client cues.	Establish a helping relationship and be sensitive to client's needs.

considered are: lighting, temperature, sound, ventilation, visibility, and a chair or support for the learner.

4. Teaching aids can foster learning. Posters and displays, for example, can help focus a learner's attention. To ensure the transfer of learning, the nurse should use the type of supplies or equipment that the client will eventually use.

5. Learning is more effective when the learners discover the content for themselves. Ways to increase learning include stimulating motivation and stimulating self-direction, e.g., by providing specific objectives, giving feedback, and helping the learner derive satisfaction from learning. Nurses can maximize learner satisfaction by setting realistic goals with the learner.

6. Repetition—e.g., summarizing content, rephrasing (using other words), and approaching the material from another point of view—reinforces learning. For instance, after discussing the kinds of foods that can be included in a diet, the nurse describes the foods again, but in the context of the three meals eaten during one day.

7. It is helpful to employ "organizers" to introduce material to be learned and to present it at a higher level of abstraction, generality, or inclusiveness (Rorden 1987, p. 120). Advanced organizers provide a means of relating unknown material to known material and generating logical relationships. For example: "You understand how urine flows down a catheter from the bladder. Now I will show you how to inject fluid so that it flows up the catheter into the bladder." The details that follow such an introduction are then seen within its framework, and the details have added meaning.

8. Using a layperson's vocabulary enhances communication. So often nurses use terms and abbreviations that have meaning to other health professionals but make little sense to clients. Even words such as *urine* or *feces* may be unfamiliar to clients, and abbreviations such as "RR" (recovery room) or "PAR" (postanesthesia room) are often misunderstood.

Special Teaching Strategies

There are a number of special teaching strategies that nurses can use: client contracting, group teaching, behavior modification, and various accelerated strategies.

Client Contracting

Client contracting involves establishing a contract with a client that specifies certain objectives and when they are to be met. The contract, drawn up and signed by the client and the nurse, specifies not only the learning objectives but also the responsibilities of the client and the nurse, and the teaching plan. The agreement allows for freedom, mutual respect, and mutual responsibility. For additional information about client contracting see Chapter 23 page 574.

Group Teaching

Group instruction is economical and it provides members with an opportunity to share with and learn from others. A small group allows for discussion in which everyone can participate. A large group often necessitates a lecture technique.

It is important that all members involved in group instruction have a need in common, e.g., prenatal health, preoperative instruction. It is also important that sociocultural factors be considered in the formation of a group. Whereas middle-class Americans may value sharing experiences with others, people from a culture such as Japan may consider it inappropriate to reveal their thoughts and feelings.

Behavior Modification

The behavior modification system for changing behavior has as its basic assumptions that human behaviors are learned and can be selectively strengthened, weakened, eliminated, or replaced and that a person's behavior is under conscious control. Under this system, desirable behavior is rewarded and undesirable behavior is ignored. The client's response is the key to behavior change. For example, clients trying to quit smoking are not criticized when they smoke, but they are praised or rewarded when they go without a cigarette for a certain period of time. For some people a learning contract is combined with behavior modification.

Some pertinent features of behavior modification are the following:

- Positive reinforcement—e.g., praise—is used.

- The client participates in the development of the learning plan.

- Undesirable behavior is ignored, not criticized.

- The expectation of the client and the nurse is that the task will be mastered, i.e., the behavior will change.

- Success is maximized through positive reinforcement; failure and the threat of failure are minimized.

Teaching Throughout the Life Span

Infants and Toddlers

The primary caregiver, i.e., the parent, is the best person to teach the infant or toddler. Infants learn by exploring their environment with their senses. An infant's routines normally should not be changed, unless they involve something that is making the infant ill. Predictable routines help infants feel secure. When teaching toddlers before surgery, the nurse should make sure they are able to hold the mask or the equipment with which they will come into contact later. Toddlers like to explore, e.g., handle equipment. They also need to be reassured that their parents have seen the room in which they will "wake up," because then the children know their parents will be able to find them.

Toddlers who reply "no" when they are being taught a new activity such as brushing their teeth are asserting their independence; this does not mean they will not learn. Better results will usually be produced if the nurse postpones the teaching to another time and repeats the lesson rather than arguing with the toddler.

Preschoolers   Most preschoolers want to learn. They have limited verbal abilities and like to explore, just as toddlers do. Most preschoolers like to practice procedures such as bandaging; such activity helps them deal with their fears.

Preschoolers like to ask questions, but the nurse's answers should be short and at a level that can be understood. Preschoolers like explanations, and they worry about such things as providing a blood specimen because the nurse "may take all my blood." The nurse should emphasize that treatment is not punishment.

School-Age Children   School-age children know more about their bodies than do preschoolers. Since their attention span is short, they learn best in brief stages. They usually like to handle objects and to draw pictures and color in books. Although their vocabulary is limited, they are learning new things. A school-age child's day is often filled with short projects.

School-age children love to ask why. They require explanations that meet their needs and that use words they understand. Children at this age should be encouraged to express their feelings, including fear about dying. School-age children love to do things the "right way," and any changes they consider as not "right" they often do not accept.

Adolescents   Adolescents may prefer to learn in the absence of their parents. Although they do have knowledge about their bodies, some of it may be incorrect. Adolescents learn best when they see immediate benefit to themselves. For example, an adolescent who understands that taking his medicine regularly will permit him to continue playing football is more likely to follow through than if he is told the medication will prevent heart problems when he is in his forties.

Young and Middle-Aged Adults   Young adults often take health for granted ("It won't happen to me"), and they may not be interested in learning about other people's problems. However, when young adults understand how something affects them, learning is facilitated. Young adults not living at home may find it unacceptable to be dependent on parents for health matters, and they may prefer a friend or the nurse to help them through a health problem.

Middle-aged adults are usually aware of the problems that can result from unhealthy life-styles. This is the period when changes in life-style are often indicated. Some middle-aged people change despite difficulty, and others still believe "it won't happen to me."

Elderly Adults   Healthy elderly adults can learn new techniques and procedures and usually desire to do so if it will mean their continued health and independence. Recent research has shown that there is no general decline in intelligence with age.

Teaching methods should be geared to the older person's memory. Those who, for example, have difficulty with recent memory should be taught by methods that take this into consideration. In addition, like people of other ages, elderly people must be motivated to learn. People who have always assumed responsibility for their own health will probably be better motivated to change life-style and learn skills designed to improve health than will people who have had others assume this responsibility. Also, elderly people who prefer dependence may find it difficult to learn health practices that promote independence.

Teaching methods should also consider the individual's past learning methods. Visualization using pictures may be preferable to discussion. The acuity of an elderly person's senses is an important consideration in this regard. The following physiologic changes commonly occur in old age (Kick 1989, pp. 682–84).

- Reaction time is longer, but a decrease in speed is often compensated by an increase in accuracy.
- High-pitched sound is often difficult to discriminate.
- Background noises such as a fan can interfere with hearing.
- Visual acuity is decreased.
- Color discrimination may be less acute, e.g., red, yellow, blue, and orange are less readily read on white paper.
- The senses of taste and smell and fine discrimination in touch, pressure, and temperature are less acute.
- Cerebral function can be compromised by decreases in oxygenation, cerebral blood flow, and hemoglobin.
- Recent memory recall may be more difficult than recall of events long past.

EVALUATING

Evaluating is an ongoing and terminal process in which the client, the nurse, and often the support persons determine what has been learned. Both short-term objectives and long-term goals need to be evaluated. Learning is measured against the predetermined objectives. Thus, the objectives serve not only to direct the teaching plan but also to provide criteria for evaluation. For example, the objective "Selects foods that are low in carbohydrates" can be evaluated by asking the client to name such foods or to select low-carbohydrate foods from a list.

The best method for evaluating depends on the type of learning. In cognitive learning, asking questions of the client is one way to determine what has been learned. The acquisition of psychomotor skills is best evaluated by observing the client carry out a procedure, such as changing a dressing or carrying out a urinary self-catheterization. Affective learning is more difficult to evaluate. Whether attitudes or values have been learned may be inferred by listening to the client's responses to questions and by the way the client speaks about relevant subjects and by observing the client's behavior. For example, has an obese client learned to value health sufficiently to follow a reducing diet? Do clients who state that they value health actually stop smoking?

Following evaluation, the nurse may find it necessary to modify or repeat the teaching plan if the objectives have not been met or have been met only partially. For the hospitalized client, follow-up teaching in the home may be needed.

It is important for nurses to evaluate their own teaching. This should include a consideration of all factors—the timing, the teaching strategies, the amount of information, whether it was helpful, etc. The nurse may find, for example, that the client was overwhelmed with too much information, was bored, or was motivated to learn more.

The following guidelines (Smitherman 1981, pp. 141–44) can assist nurses in the evaluative process:

- Forgetting is normal and should be anticipated. Nurses can suggest to clients that they write down information they might forget. Often, clients are provided printed instructions, because such information may be easily forgotten.

- Both the client and the teacher should evaluate the learning experience. The learner may tell the nurse what was helpful, interesting, etc. Questionnaires and videotapes of the learning sessions can also be helpful.

- Behavior change does not always take place immediately after learning. Often individuals will accept change intellectually first and then may change their behavior only periodically (e.g., Mrs. Green, who knows that she must lose weight, diets and exercises off and on). If the new behavior is to replace old behavior, it must emerge gradually; otherwise, the old behavior may prevail. Nurses can assist clients with behavior change by allowing for client vacillation and by providing encouragement.

DOCUMENTATION

Documentation of the teaching process is essential, for this provides a legal record that the teaching took place and communicates the teaching to other health professionals. According to Omdahl, client teaching has been identified as "the most underdocumented skilled service because most nurses in home care do not recognize the scope and depth of the teaching they do" and "tend to view much of their teaching as commonsense suggestions" (Omdahl 1987, p. 1033).

The record should include the client's achievements. A specific client teaching record or the nurse's notes can be used. The client's reaction to the teaching should also be included, and this reaction should be incorporated into further planning. Documentation of the responses of support persons are also important to include.

The record of the teaching process should include written teaching plans, nursing Kardexes (see Chapter 17, page 302), and planning sessions with other health team members. Documentation of the teaching/learning process serves several other functions as well: reference for client learning and support-person learning; reevaluation of the teaching plan; reinforcement of identified areas of learning need; and revision of the teaching strategies (Corkadel and McGlashan 1983, pp. 14–15).

CHAPTER HIGHLIGHTS

▸ Planned change requires problem-solving and decision-making skills and interpersonal competence.

▸ Nurses frequently act as formal or informal change agents in relation to clients, support systems, and communities.

▸ Resistance to change can have a number of causes, including threatened self-interest, inaccurate perceptions, objective disagreement, psychological reactance, and low tolerance for change.

▸ Nurses who assume a change agent role can implement change using a nursing process framework.

▸ Learning is represented by a change behavior.

▸ Bloom identified three learning domains: cognitive, affective, and psychomotor.

▸ A number of factors facilitate learning, including motivation, readiness, active involvement, and success at learning.

▸ Factors such as extreme anxiety, certain physiologic processes, and cultural barriers impede learning.

▸ Teaching is a system of activities intended to produce learning. Rapport between the teacher and the learner is essential for effective teaching.

▸ Assessment relative to the preparation of a teaching plan must include identification of the client's learning needs and relevant client data such as readiness to learn, motivation, socioeconomic factors, learning style, age, and health beliefs and practices.

- ▸ Readiness is an important aspect of assessment *prior* to teaching.

- ▸ Learning objectives guide the content of the teaching plan and are written in terms of client behavior.

- ▸ Teaching strategies should be suited to the client, the material to be learned, and the teacher.

- ▸ A teaching plan is a written plan and must be revised when the client's needs change or the teaching strategies prove ineffective.

- ▸ Evaluation of the teaching/learning process is an ongoing and terminal process.

- ▸ Documentation of client teaching is essential to communicate the teaching to other health professionals and to provide a record for legal purposes.

READINGS AND REFERENCES

SUGGESTED READINGS

Kick, E. September 1989. Patient teaching for elders. *Nursing Clinics of North America* 24:681–87.
  Kick introduces this article by briefly explaining two myths about the elderly: older people experience a decline in mental abilities, and older people cannot learn. An overview of four ways in which aging affects learning is provided. Kick discusses how older persons learn and concludes the article with information about instructional settings.

Robinson, Y. K. January 1986. Teaching adults: Some issues in adult education for health education. *Physiotherapy* 72:49–52.
  Discusses adults as learners, including a list of ten beliefs about an andragogical humanistic approach to adult learning. The author sees learning as a cooperative effort on the part of the teacher and the learner, and describes participatory and group learning as well as individual differences and cognitive style and change.

Tripp-Reimer, T. September 1989. Cross-cultural perspectives on patient teaching. *Nursing Clinics of North America* 24:613–19.
  Tripp-Reimer states at the beginning of this article that "individual health behavior largely is culturally patterned." The author maintains that nurses should carry out a cultural assessment and a cultural negotiation before establishing a teaching plan. The author also points out that nurses should establish rapport and assess the problem and readiness to learn. Throughout the article Tripp-Reimer describes the significance of considering cultural values.

Welch, L. B. June 1979. Planned change in nursing: The theory. *Nursing Clinics of North America* 14:307–21.
  Welch describes the theories of Lewin, Lippitt, Havelock, and Rogers. Welch maintains that planned change is an essential part of nursing intervention and important for quality client care.

RELATED RESEARCH

Brown, S. A. July/August 1988. Effects of educational interventions in diabetes care: A meta-analysis of findings. *Nursing Research* 37:223–29.

Feldman, M. J., and Ventura M. R. May/June 1984. Evaluating changes in using non-interval data. *Nursing Research* 33:182–84.

Streiff, L. D. Summer 1986. Can clients understand our instructions? *Image: Journal of Nursing Scholarship* 18:48–52.

Vessey, J. A. September/October 1988. Comparison of two teaching methods on children's knowledge of their internal bodies. *Nursing Research* 38:262–87.

SELECTED REFERENCES

Armstrong, M. L. September 1989. Orchestrating the process of patient education: Methods and approaches. *Nursing Clinics of North America* 24:597–604.

Bennis, W. G., Benne, K. D., Chin, R., editors 1985. *The planning of change.* 4th ed. New York: Holt, Rinehart & Winston.

Bloom, B. S., editor. 1956. *Taxonomy of educational objectives.* Book 1, *Cognitive domain.* New York: Longman, Inc.

Corkadel, L., and McGlashan, R. January/February 1983. A practical approach to patient teaching. *The Journal of Continuing Education in Nursing* 14:9–15.

Cross, K. P. 1988. *Adults as learners.* San Francisco: Jossey-Bass.

Fox, V. August 1986. Patient teaching: Understanding the needs of the adult learner. *AORN Journal* 44:234–42.

Gessner, B. A. September 1989. Adult education: The cornerstone of patient teaching. *Nursing Clinics of North America* 24:589–95.

Havelock, R. 1973. *The change agent's guide to innovations in education.* Englewood Cliffs, N.J.: Educational Technology Publications.

Johnson, E. A., and Jackson, J. E. September 1989. Teaching the home care client. *Nursing Clinics of North America* 24:687–93.

Kanter, F. H. and Goldstein, A. P., editors. *Helping people change: A textbook of methods.* New York: Pergamon Press.

Kick, E. September 1989. Patient teaching for elders. *Nursing Clinics of North America* 24:681–86.

Knowles, M. S. 1980. *The modern practice of adult education:* From pedagogy to andragogy. Chicago: Follett.

———. 1984. *Andragogy in action.* San Francisco: Jossey-Bass.

Laird, M. August 1975. Techniques for teaching pre- and post-operative patients. *American Journal of Nursing* 75:1338–40.

Lawrence, G. 1982. *People types and tiger stripes: A practical guide to learning styles.* Gainesville, Florida: Center for Applications of Psychological Type, Inc.

Lewin, K. 1951. *Field theory in social science.* New York: Harper and Row.

———. 1948. *Resolving Social Conflicts.* G.W. Lewin, ed. New York: Harper and Brothers.

Lippitt, G. L. 1973. *Visualizing change: Model building and the change process.* La Jolla, Calif.: University Associates

Lippitt, R., Hooyman, G., Sashkin, M., and Kaplan, J. 1978. *Resourcebook for planned change.* Ann Arbor, Mich.: Human Resource Development Associates of Ann Arbor, Inc.

Lippitt, R., Watson, J., and Westley, B. 1958. *The dynamics of planned change.* New York: Harcourt Brace and Co.

Mager, R. F. 1975. *Preparing instructional objectives.* 2d ed. Belmont, California: Fearon Publishers, Inc.

McGovern, W. N., and Rodgers, J. A. May 1986. Change theory. *American Journal of Nursing* 86:566–7.

Mauksch, I. G., and Miller, M. H. 1981. *Implementing change in nursing.* St. Louis: C. V. Mosby Co.

New, J. R., and Couillard, N. A. March 1981. Guidelines for introducing change. *Journal of Nursing Administration* 11:17–21.

Olson, E. M. June 1979. Strategies and techniques for the nurse change agent. *Nursing Clinics of North America* 14:323–36.

Omdahl, D. J. August 1987. Preventing home care denials. *American Journal of Nursing* 87:1031–33.

Phillips, J. A., and Hekelman, F. P. September/October 1983. The role of the nurse as a teacher: A position paper. *Nephrology Nurse* 5:42–46.

Redman, B. K. 1988. *The process of patient education.* 6th ed. St. Louis: C. V. Mosby Co.

Reinhard, S. C. 1988. Managing and initiating change. In Sullivan, E. J., and Decker, P. J. *Effective management in nursing* 2d ed. Redwood City, California: Addison-Wesley Publishing Co.

Rodgers, J. A. 1973. Theoretical considerations involved in the process of change. *Nursing Forum* 12:160.

Rogers, E. 1983. *Diffusion of innovations.* 3d ed. New York: Free Press.

Rorden, J. W. 1987. *Nurses as health teachers: A practical guide.* Philadelphia: W. B. Saunders Co.

Smith, C. E., editor. 1987. *Patient education: Nurses in partnership with other health professionals.* Orlando Florida: Grune & Stratton.

Smitherman, C. 1981. *Nursing actions for health promotion.* Philadelphia: F. A. Davis Co.

Stevens, B. February 1975. Effecting change. *Journal of Nursing Administration.* 5:23–25.

Thurlow, J. G. Spring 1990. Tools for patient education. *Gastroenterological Nursing* 12:286–88.

Tyson, J. 1984. Before we educate. *Diabetes Educator* (special issue) 10:23–24.

Ward, D. B. January 1986. Why patient teaching fails. *RN* 49:45–47.

Documenting and Reporting

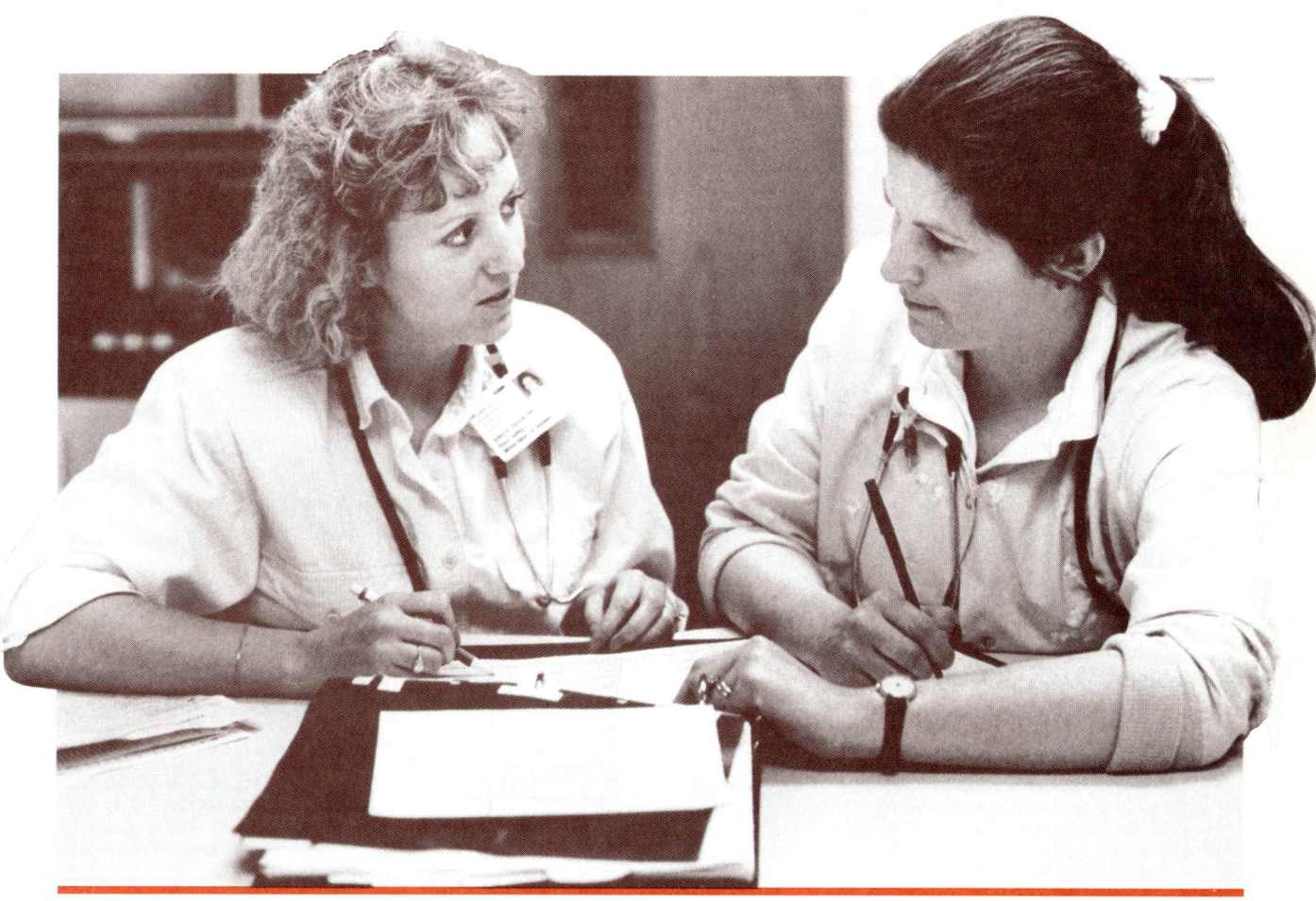

CONTENTS

OBJECTIVES

▶ Identify seven purposes of client records.

▶ Describe the components of source-oriented medical records and problem-oriented medical records (POMR).

▶ Describe three types of progress records.

▶ Differentiate between narrative, SOAP, focus charting, and charting by exception.

▶

▶ Identify measures used to ensure that recording meets legal standards.

▶ Identify abbreviations and symbols commonly used for charting.

▶ Identify measures used to maintain the confidentiality of client records.

▶ Describe the change-of-shift report.

▶ Identify essential guidelines for reporting client data.

▶ Compare the advantages and disadvantages of nursing care conferences and nursing care rounds.

IMPORTANCE OF COMMUNICATION AMONG HEALTH TEAM MEMBERS

Written and verbal communication among health team members is vital to the quality of client care. Generally, health team members communicate through discussions, reports, and records. A *discussion* is an informal oral consideration of a subject by two or more members of the health team, often leading to a decision. A *report* is an oral or written account by one member to others in the health team; for instance, nurses always report on clients at the end of a hospital work shift. A *record* is always written; it is a formal, legal documentation of a client's progress and treatment.

Accurate, complete communication serves several purposes:

■ It helps coordinate care given by several people.

■ It prevents the client from having to repeat information to each health team member.

■ It promotes accuracy in the provision of care and lessens the possibility of error.

■ It helps health personnel make the best use of their time by avoiding overlapping of activities.

PURPOSES OF CLIENT RECORDS

A client's **medical record,** or **chart,** is an account of the client's health history, current health status, treatment, and progress. It is a highly confidential, legal document by means of which physicians, nurses, social workers, and other health team members communicate about that client. When a client goes to a physician's office or enters a hospital, a record is usually started. Records are generally kept in folders, in binders, or on clipboards, and they are updated continually while clients attend the health care facility. When clients are discharged, their records are stored for future reference in the medical records department of the agency.

Although the forms of client records may vary considerably from place to place, nurses are universally required to make entries about clients' health, including, for example, all assessments and interventions. The process of making entries on client records is called **recording** (or **charting**).

Client records are kept for a number of purposes: communication, legal documentation, research, statistics, education, audit, and planning client care.

Communication   The record serves as the vehicle by which different members of the health team communicate with each other. Although these members also communicate verbally, the record is an efficient and effective method of sharing information. It also allows health team members on different shifts to convey meaningful data about the client to one another.

Legal Documentation   The client's record is a legal document and is admissible in court as evidence. In some jurisdictions, however, the record is considered inadmissible as evidence when the client objects, because information the client gives to the physician is confidential. A record is usually considered the property of the agency, although there is increasing belief that the client has a right to the information in the record upon request. Legal decisions have recognized this right (Creighton 1986, p. 104).

Research   The information contained in a record can be a valuable source of data for research. The treatment plans for a number of clients with the same illness can yield information helpful in treating a particular client. A record made years earlier may also assist members of the health team with a current problem. A client's memory of an illness may provide limited data, but a record of that illness will generally reveal additional and accurate data.

Statistics   Statistical information from client records can help an agency anticipate and plan for people's future needs. For example, the number of births or kinds of illnesses can be obtained from records. Some statistics, such as records of births and deaths, are required by law. They are filed with a government agency and become a part of the local, national, and international statistics.

Education   Students in health disciplines often use client records as educational tools. A record can frequently provide a comprehensive view of the client, the illness, and the kinds of assistance given. In this context, records are used by nursing students, medical students, dietitians, and other health team members.

Audit   The client's record is used to monitor the care the client is receiving and the competence of the people giving that care. During a nursing **audit,** for example, the nursing interventions are monitored and measured against established standards. Often the audit is a retrospective audit, in that the care has already been given.

A nursing audit carried out by other nurses is sometimes referred to as a *peer review*. Many agencies have audit committees that monitor the practice of individual nurses. Audits are also carried out by outside groups for approval and accreditation purposes.

Planning Client Care   The entire health team uses data from the client's record to plan care for that client. A physician, for example, may order a specific antibiotic after establishing that the client's temperature is steadily rising and that laboratory tests reveal the presence of a certain microorganism. Nurses use data from the history they took on the client's admission to establish an individual nursing care plan. The social worker's data about the client's home environment can assist the nurse in developing an appropriate discharge teaching plan. Data from the physical therapist help the nurse to implement specific physical exercises for the client.

TYPES OF RECORDS

Source-Oriented Medical Records

In the traditional client record, or **source-oriented medical record,** each person or department makes notations in a separate section or sections of the client's chart. For example, the admission department has an admission sheet; the physician has a doctor's order sheet, a doctor's history sheet, and progress notes; nurses use the nurse's notes; and other departments or personnel have their own records. In this type of record, information about a particular problem is distributed throughout the record. For example, if a client had left hemiplegia (paralysis of the left side of the body), data about this problem might be found in the doctor's history sheet, on the doctor's order sheet, in the nurse's notes, in the physical therapist's record, and in the social service record.

Source-oriented client records generally have five components:

- Admission sheet
- Physician's order sheet
- Medical history sheet
- Nurse's notes
- Special records and reports

The *admission sheet* is a part of the record in most agencies. It generally contains demographic data about the client such as name, address, date of birth, marital status, and admitting diagnosis.

The *physician's order sheet* is a written record of orders. The physician is expected to write the date of the order and sign each order (or sign for several orders written at once). Various agencies have different methods (e.g., using red "flags" on the front or extending out from the chart and/or placing the chart in a designated area of the nursing station) of indicating to the nurse or clerk that there is a new order. When the doctor phones in orders about a client, these are written on the physician's sheet by the recipient of the call and signed by that person, indicating a telephone order. Often the physician is expected to countersign the telephone order within 24 or 48 hours of the call. Before a nurse can accept a verbal order from a physician, however, agency policies and procedures must be checked. Usually, nursing students are not allowed to accept verbal orders.

The *medical history sheet* is a record of the client's health history, written by the physician. The physician may also use this sheet to record progress notes on the client and future plans, although most agencies have separate records for progress notes. At some facilities, the record of the client's admitting physical examination may also be on the history sheet, which is then usually called the *history and physical* sheet.

The *nurse's notes* are a record of the nursing assessments of the client, identified nursing diagnoses, interventions carried out, and evaluations of the effectiveness of the interventions. See Nurse's Notes later in this chapter.

Special records and reports also become part of the client's permanent record. These may include consultations from medical specialists, roentgenographic reports, laboratory findings, reports of surgery, anesthesia records, physical therapy records, occupational therapy records, and social service records. In addition, special flowsheets are often used to record certain data about the client. These include graphic records for vital signs, fluid intake and output, and medications. See page 305 later in this chapter for details.

Problem-Oriented Medical Records

In a **problem-oriented medical record (POMR** or **POR),** data about the client are recorded and arranged according to the problems the client has, rather than according to the source of the information. The record integrates all data about a problem, whether gathered by physicians, nurses, or others involved in the client's care. Plans for each active problem are drawn up, and progress notes are recorded for each problem. Unlike the traditional record, which separates the medical data on a problem from the nursing data and other data into different sections of the record, the POR coordinates the care given by all health team members and focuses on the client and his or her health problems.

The POR has four basic components:

- Defined database
- Problem list
- Initial list of orders or care plans
- Progress notes

Defined Database   The defined database consists of all information known about the client when the client first entered the health care agency. It includes the nursing assessment, the physician's history, and the physical health examination. To these are added social and family data from other sources, such as the social worker, and baseline laboratory and roentgenographic data. In most agencies, a standardized form is used to help team members obtain a complete database.

Problem List   The problem list is a list of problems that is carefully compiled once the databases have been collected and analyzed. Some problems are obvious on initial contact with the client; others are established as additional data are gathered. In this context, a problem is essentially a need that the client is unable to meet without assistance from members of the health care team.

The initial problem list is usually made either by the first health care worker to encounter the client or by the person who assumes primary responsibility for the client's care. Subsequent contributions are made by other members of the health team.

To be complete, the problem list should include socioeconomic, demographic, psychologic, and physiologic problems. The list is usually found at the front of the client's record. Each problem is labeled and numbered so that it can be identified throughout the record. This list has been likened to an index or table of contents. See Figure 17-1. Problems are usually categorized as active or inactive.

A problem that is potential rather than actual is generally entered on the progress notes rather than the problem list. Only when a problem actually becomes active is it added to the list.

Signs, symptoms, and abnormal diagnostic measures, if used, are considered temporary labels until diagnosis is established. With the development of nursing diagnoses, many nurses are now using the NANDA taxonomy of nursing diagnoses to state nursing problems. Problem statements should refer to one problem only, be written unambiguously (so that no interpretation is required) in behavioral terms, and should provide direction for client care.

When several problems have a common etiology or cause, two methods are used to relate the problems: sublisting and cross-referencing. A *sublist* is a group of all manifestations of a major problem that require separate management. Manifestations may be either behavioral or clinical indicators of the same problem. For example, consider the following segment of Figure 17-1:

No.	Client Problem
1	Several CVAs resulting in Rt hemiplegia and left-sided weakness
1A	Self-care deficit (hygiene, toileting, grooming, feeding)

1B	Impaired physical mobility
1C	Total incontinence
1D	Progressive dysphasia

The *cross-referencing method* lists all problems separately, using consecutive numbers. A "Related to" column to the right of the "Client Problem" column lists the number of the major problem to which the manifestations are related. For example, Figure 17-1 could also include the following:

No.	Client Problem	Related to
1	Multiple CVAs resulting in Rt hemiplegia and left-sided weakness	
2	Self-care deficit (hygiene, toileting, grooming, feeding)	#1
3	Impaired physical mobility	#1
4	Total incontinence	#1
5	Progressive dysphasia	#1

Major problems can also be cross-referenced to other major problems. An example of this would be the following:

No.	Client Problem	Related to
1	Cerebral vascular disease	#4
4	Essential hypertension	#1

"Redefinition" of problems is often necessary to reflect a change in the client's problem or to increase understanding of the problem. Redefining does *not* involve changing the stated nature of the problem; it involves changing the wording of the problem to reflect a change in its frequency or intensity, or increased knowledge. The problem retains the same number (e.g., see Figure 17-1):

No.	Client Problem
1C	Total incontinence Redefined Nov 10/92
1C	Nocturnal urinary incontinence

Initial List of Orders or Care Plans   The initial list of orders or care plans is made with reference to the active problems. Care plans or orders are generated by the person who lists the problems. Physicians write physician's orders or medical care plans; nurses write nursing orders or nursing care plans. The written plan in the record is listed under each problem in the progress notes (discussed next) and is not isolated as a separate list of orders.

Progress Notes   Progress notes in the POMR are made by all members of the health team involved in a client's care: nurse, occupational therapist, dietitian, physician, social

No.	Date Entered	Date Inactive	Client Problem	Related to
#1	Mar 9/91		Several CVAs resulting in Rt hemiplegia and left-sided weakness. Redefined Feb 7/92	
#1A	Mar 9/91		Self care deficit (hygiene, toileting, grooming, feeding)	
#1B	Mar 9/91		Impaired physical mobility. Redefined Feb 7/92	
#1C	Mar 9/91		Altered patterns of urinary elimination: total incontinence. Redefined Nov 10/92	
#1D	Mar 9/91		Progressive dysphasia	
#2	Mar 9/91		Altered bowel elimination constipation. Redefined Nov 10/91	
#3	Mar 9/91		History of depression	
#4	Mar 9/91		Essential hypertension	
#5	June 6/91	Nov 91	Pruritus	
#2	Nov 10/91		Potential for constipation	
#1C	Nov 10/92		Nocturnal urinary incontinence	
#1	Feb 7/92		Cerebral vascular disease (multiple CVAs) resulting in bilateral hemiplegia	
#1B	Feb 7/92		Needs major assist. to transfer/unable to walk	

Figure 17–1 A client's problem list using the sublisting method to relate problems. Note that problems 1, 1B, 1C, and 2 were redefined on the dates indicated and listed subsequently. *Source* Courtesy of the Nursing Department, University Hospital—UBC site, Vancouver, British Columbia.

worker, and others. All members of the health team add progress notes on the same type of sheet. Progress notes are numbered to correspond to the problems on the problem list. See Types of Progress Records later in this chapter.

Kardex and Nursing Care Plan

The **Kardex** is a widely used, concise method of organizing and recording data about a client, making information quickly accessible to all members of the health team. The system consists of a series of cards kept in a portable index file. The card for a particular client can be quickly turned up to reveal specific data. Often Kardex data are recorded in pencil so that they can be changed and kept up to date. The information on Kardexes may be organized into sections, for example:

- Pertinent information about the client, such as name, room number, age, religion, marital status, admission date, doctor's name, diagnosis, type of surgery and date, occupation, and next of kin
- List of medications, with the date of order and the times of administration for each
- List of intravenous fluids, with dates of infusions
- List of daily treatments and procedures, such as irrigations, dressing changes, postural drainage, or measurement of vital signs
- List of diagnostic procedures ordered, such as roentgenography or laboratory tests

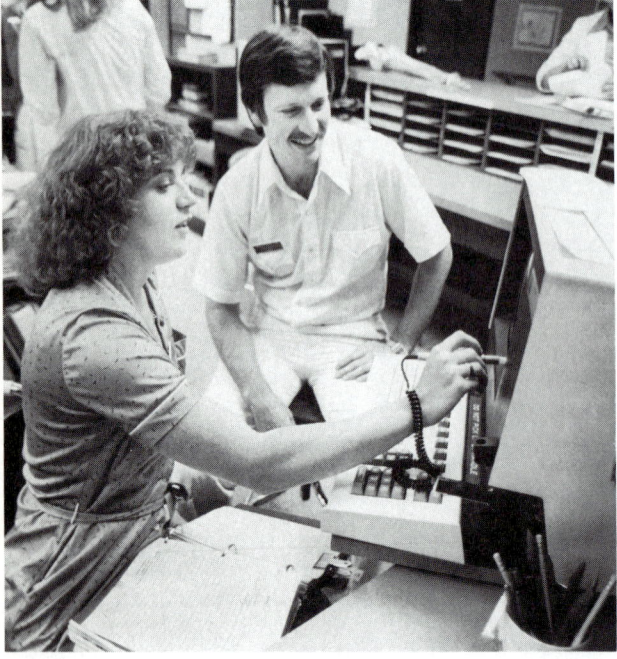

Figure 17–2 User-friendly computers offering light-pen input are used by many agencies.

- Allergies
- Specific data on how the client's physical needs are to be met, such as type of diet, assistance needed with feeding, elimination devices, activity, hygienic needs, and safety precautions (use of side rails, etc.)
- A problem list, stated goals, and a list of nursing approaches to meet the goals and relieve the problems.

Although much of the information on the Kardex may be recorded by the nurse in charge or a delegate (e.g., the ward clerk), any nurse who cares for the client plays a key role in initiating the record and keeping the data current. When caring for the client, a nurse has the best opportunity to assess and reassess with the client the accuracy of the information and the effectiveness of treatment.

Computer Records

In about 1968, a number of health institutions introduced computers. Initially, computers were installed primarily in hospital business offices. However, increasing numbers of computers are being used in health care planning and delivery as well as in laboratories and physicians' clinics. By the turn of the century, most nurses will use computers in many aspects of their practice. Already, "user friendly" machines, often operated with a light-pen and simple keyboard (see Figure 17–2), are of great help to the nurse in assessing, planning, implementing, recording, and evaluating nursing care. Computer skills and knowledge will soon be expected and perhaps required for a great many positions in nursing.

In the past, hospital computer applications have been administrative (e.g., tasks such as client billing, maintaining financial records, and long-term planning). As computers get smaller, less costly, more powerful, and easier to use, they are being used increasingly in other areas of the health care system as well. Today, it is common to find a microcomputer system or computer terminal in the nurse's station. It is likely that such machines will become a more integral part of the nurse's activities during the next decade. By using computerized systems, nursing staffs are able to create care plans easily, customize them for each client, type in additions as needed, evaluate and update information at any time, and retrieve data appropriate to a specific nursing diagnosis. Such systems can be programmed to provide work lists, as needed, directly from the computer. In this way, lists generated for treatments, procedures, and medications can always be kept up-to-date. Such an application eliminates the need for multiple flowsheets, since all of the same information is available both in the computer and on computer-printed update forms. To record nursing actions, the nurse either enters data directly into the computerized records or completes the computer-generated flowsheet in the client's chart.

A well-designed database system can make the entry and retrieval of information a relatively easy task for the nurses who use it. Figure 17–3 is an illustration of how a portion of a client's record might appear on the computer screen. The nurse enters the appropriate information into the form by typing it on the computer's keyboard. Changes can be made easily to update this record. Later, as the needs of the nurse dictate, information about a particular client, diagnosis, or physician can be recalled to the screen.

Specific ways in which an *automated client care plan* can facilitate the role of the nurse include the following:

1. Entry of nursing assessments is simplified; e.g., the nurse can touch a computer screen display of possibilities.

2. Laboratory data can be ordered by entering a request at a terminal in the nurse's station, and results can be retrieved over the same terminal in a shorter time with less paperwork.

3. The system facilitates complete and legible medication orders.

4. The nursing implications of a doctor's order can be sent to the nurse. Client preparation needs for a particular test can be listed automatically in the client's nursing care plan.

5. The use of nursing diagnosis is facilitated; a common format can be used.

6. Current information can be updated easily. Discontinued medication orders can be deleted easily, making all information timely, legible, and complete.

With access to a completely automated care plan, the nurse can prepare client discharge summaries that include information from the time of admission. These reports can include all current unresolved nursing diagnoses and the relevant interventions. Computer-generated reports can include relevant information for teaching the client, including instructions about the use of drugs, details of a required diet, activity restrictions, and the date of the next visit to the physician's office.

In addition to facilitating individualized client care, computerized records can also be beneficial to nurse-managers who may use stored data to generate reports on the acuity levels of clients on each unit. These can be used to devise a formula for determining both the appropriate skill levels and the number of nurses required per shift and per floor. The scheduling of personnel is often made difficult by changing shifts, different skill levels, vacations, weekends, legal coverage requirements, and so on. Computer-based scheduling models can save much time and provide options that can be difficult to discover if the information is handled manually.

Nurses are bound by their professional ethics to maintain a client's privacy. This means that information about a client cannot be disseminated outside of the realm of the caregivers. The use of computer-based information systems to store client data has increased the risk of an accidental or intentional violation of a client's rights. Just as computers are becoming easier to use, they are becoming easier to abuse. Clients have a right to privacy and confidentiality

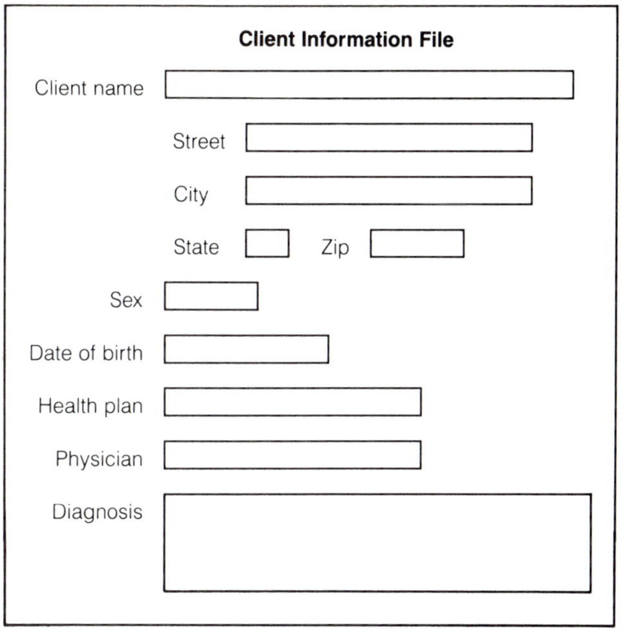

Figure 17–3 Segment of a client's database.

even where computer-based information systems are used. Nurses should not give their signature codes to anyone or let anyone without an access code use the computer.

In today's information age, health care providers tend to collect more data, share more databases, and access more client information than in earlier days. Client records are queried for insurance claims, during audits of the nursing (as well as some other) departments, and sometimes on the demand of the courts. There has not been a similar growth in the sophistication of the security systems (both manual and computerized) that are used to limit access to these data. Passwords limiting access to data can often be guessed; disgruntled employees may change, delete, or disseminate data; computer "enthusiasts" may deem it a challenge to "break into" a hospital's computer information system. Nurses must be aware of these problems and risks if they are to fulfill their responsibility to the client. The specific role of the nurse (or student, educator, researcher, manager) does not absolve that person from accountability for ensuring a client's right to privacy.

TYPES OF PROGRESS RECORDS

Three kinds of progress notes are generally recognized; nurse's, or narrative, notes; flowsheets; and discharge notes or referral summaries. These are used in both source-oriented and problem-oriented medical records.

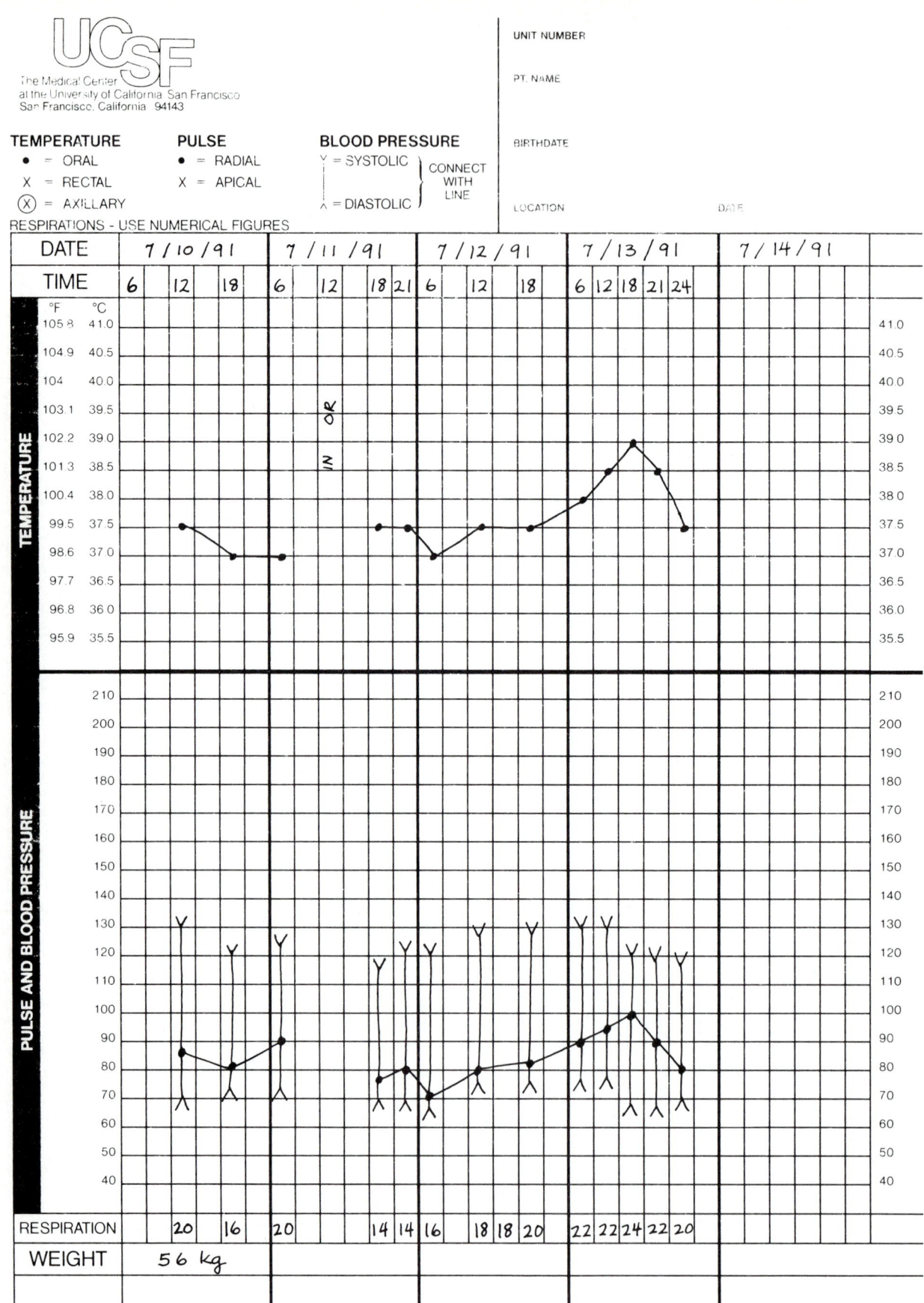

Figure 17–4 A clinical graph record. ***Source*** Courtesy of the Department of Nursing, The Medical Center at the University of California, San Francisco.

Nurse's Notes

Nurse's notes record the client's progress descriptively. In some hospitals, because of the prospective payment system based on diagnostic related groups (DRGs), discussed in Chapter 6, page 106, a note *must* be written every 24 hours. In general, the nurse's notes record the following kinds of information:

- Assessments of the client by various nursing personnel, e.g., pale or flushed skin color or dark or cloudy urine
- Independent nursing interventions, such as special skin care or health teaching, carried out on the nurse's initiative
- Dependent nursing interventions, such as medications or treatments ordered by a physician
- Evaluation of the effectiveness of each nursing intervention
- Measures carried out by the physician (e.g., shortening a postoperative drainage tube) that affect subsequent nursing measures
- Visits by members of the health team, such as a consulting physician, social worker, or chaplain

Nurse's notes and the manner of recording vary, depending on whether a source-oriented medical record or POR is used. See *Formats for Writing Progress Notes* later in this chapter.

Flowsheets

When specific client variables such as pulse, blood pressure, medications, and progress in learning a new skill need to be recorded accurately, narrative notes are often too long. Instead the **flowsheet,** a graphic record, is used as a quick way to reflect the client's condition. The time parameters for flowsheets can vary from minutes to months. In a hospital intensive care unit, a client's blood pressure may be monitored by the minute, whereas in an ambulatory clinic, a client's blood glucose level may be recorded once a month.

Flowsheets commonly used are the clinical record (also called the graphic chart or graphic observation record), the fluid intake and output record, the medication record, and daily nursing care records.

Clinical Record   The *clinical record* shown in Figure 17–4 indicates body temperature, pulse rate, respiratory rate, blood pressure readings, and weight.

Some agencies also show special medications (such as dicumarol), central venous pressure (CVP), 24-hour fluid intake and output, bowel movement, glucose and acetone in the urine, etc.

24-Hour Fluid Balance Record   A *24-hour fluid balance* record is shown in Figure 17–5. Before notations

EL CAMINO HOSPITAL

INTAKE AND OUTPUT RECORD

PATIENT LABEL

PATIENT NAME _____

PATIENT # _____

PHYSICIAN _____

INTAKE					OUTPUT				
TOTAL IV	INTRAVENOUS	TUBE FEED	ORAL	TIME	URINE	NG	EMESIS	BM	MISC.
				DATE:					
				6-2					
				2-10					
				10-6					
				24°					
				DATE:					
				6-2					
				2-10					
				10-6					
				24°					

Figure 17–5   A sample 24-hour fluid intake and output record.   ***Source***   Courtesy of El Camino Hospital, Mountain View, California.

are made on a 24-hour fluid balance record, the nurse records the amount of the client's fluid intake and output on a form kept at the client's bedside. The client and support persons should be taught to use this record. It documents intake and output for the duration of one shift only (8 or 12 hours). The totals for each shift are then recorded on the 24-hour fluid balance record. In the sample shown in Figure 17–5, the totals for each 8-hour shift (days, evenings, and nights) are recorded, and then the 24-hour totals are calculated.

All routes of fluid intake and all routes of fluid loss or output must be measured and recorded. Information about ways to measure and record specific amounts of fluid intake and output are described in Chapter 40.

Medication Record
Medication flow sheets usually include designated areas for the date of the medication order, the expiration date, the medication name and dose, the frequency of administration and route, and the nurse's signature. Some records also include a place to document the client's allergies.

Daily Nursing Care Record
In POMRs the daily nursing care is often recorded on a flowsheet. See Figure 17–6.

Discharge Note and Referral Summary

A discharge note and referral summary are completed when the client is being discharged and transferred to another institution or to a home setting where a visit by a public health nurse is required. See Figure 17–7 on page 309. Referral summaries usually include the following:

- Any active health problems
- Current medications
- Current treatments that are to be continued
- Eating and sleeping habits
- Self-care abilities
- Support networks
- Life-style patterns
- Religious preferences

This exchange of information ensures continuity of health care for the client. See also Figure 12–1 on page 220.

FORMATS FOR WRITING PROGRESS NOTES

Four methods used to write progress notes are narrative charting, the SOAP format, focus charting, and charting by exception.

Narrative Charting

Narrative charting is a description (narration) of information, and **chronologic charting** records data in sequence as time moves forward. Chronologic charting is commonly associated with source-oriented medical records. Figure 17–8 on page 310 is an example of narrative nurse's notes. The forms used for the nurse's notes may vary from place to place. Some agencies have separate columns for treatments, nursing observations, and comments. The major disadvantage of narrative charting is that it is difficult for a reader to find all the data about a specific problem without examining all of the recorded information. For this reason, specific flow records discussed earlier are often used for certain information.

SOAP Format

SOAP is an acronym for subjective data, objective data, assessment, and planning. The SOAP format originated with the POMR but is used increasingly in many different types of records. The acronyms SOAPIE and SOAPIER refer to formats that add implementation, evaluation, and revision. Many agencies use only the SOAP format. A more recent format is the **APIE** (assessment, plan, implementation, and evaluation), which condenses the client data into fewer statements (Groah and Reed 1983, p. 1184). In APIE, the assessment combines the subjective and objective data with the nursing diagnosis; the plan combines the nursing actions with the expected outcomes; and the implementation and evaluation are the same. See Figure 17–9 on page 310 for an example of a nurse's progress notes using the SOAP, SOAPIER, and APIE formats.

Subjective data report what the client perceives and the way the client expresses it. **Objective data** include measurements such as vital signs, observations made by health team members using their senses, laboratory and roentgenographic findings, and client responses to diagnostic and therapeutic measures such as medications. Examples of subjective and objective data are provided in Chapter 10.

In the **assessment stage,** the observer makes interpretations and draws conclusions from the subjective and objective data. Again, all team members have made assessments, using the knowledge in their possession. At this point, the nurse writes a nursing diagnostic statement in accordance with the guidelines discussed in Chapter 11. The *plan* is a plan for action based on the above data. The initial plan is written by the person who enters the problem into the record. All subsequent plans, considered revisions, also are entered into the progress notes. Plans may include termination of certain activities if the problem is resolved, initiation of new actions if the problem is unchanged, and activities being done to resolve a particular problem.

continued on page 311

NURSING CARE FLOW SHEET

IMPORTANT CONSIDERATIONS

1. The assigned R.N. is responsible for the documentation of all nursing care. Charting for acute care patients is completed on the Nurses' Notes at least every 24 hrs. Nurses' Notes are completed for long term care patients at least weekly.

2. The initialling of the flow sheet indicates that the required hourly observations of the patient's well-being by nursing staff members have been conducted (including functioning of all equipment, e.g. I.V. infusions).

3. Charting in the Nurses' Notes is necessary when the flow sheet does not adequately reflect the patient's status. $\boxed{NN}$ indicates documentation on Nurses' Notes.

4. Complete all boxes. Use a circle $\boxed{O}$ for areas that are not applicable.

5. Select the abbreviation that most accurately reflects the patient's condition. Place a tick $\boxed{\checkmark}$ e.g. eating well $\boxed{\checkmark}$ if the statement reflects the patient's condition.

6. Do not chart pedal pulses or dressings on this flow sheet.

IDENTIFYING INFORMATION

Date — Insert new date at 0730. This date is for the time frame 0730-0730.

Time Period — Maximum time period is 12 hours $\boxed{\begin{array}{c}0730\\1930\end{array}}$ Start a new column for shorter time periods that correspond to changes in patient status (e.g. pre-post op).

Initials — Assigned nurse inserts initials and completes the Nurses' Signature Record with a full legible signature.

INSTRUCTION FOR COMPLETION OF SUB-SYSTEMS

Urine — Insert $\boxed{QS}$ if patient voiding adequate amounts.
— Insert $\boxed{HNV}$ if patient has not voided.
— Insert amount if measuring urine (ml.)
— Insert $\boxed{FB}$ if recording amount on Fluid Balance Record.

Stool — Record number with $\boxed{0}$ $\boxed{1}$ $\boxed{SC}$ — Stool Chart.

Diet — Insert $\boxed{T}$ if patient is on a therapeutic diet. Chart in Nurses' Notes when therapeutic diet is initiated or changed.

Turns — Record frequency e.g. q2h etc.

Bedrails — Indicate if one $\boxed{x1}$ or, if both, $\boxed{x2}$ are raised.

Mobility — Record highest level of activity achieved. Indicate $\boxed{WC}$ under chair, if using wheelchair.

INSERT ONLY THESE ITEMS INTO BLANK SPACES

Blank spaces are provided for recording other routine nursing care not requiring Nurses' Notes.

1. Heparin Lock Intact.
2. I.V. Intact.
3. TPN Intact.
4. Telemetry Intact.
5. Holter Monitor Intact.
6. Urine Strained.
7. Catheter Care.
8. Calorie Count.

Use a $\boxed{\checkmark}$ if no problem observed. Chart in Nurses' Notes $\boxed{NN}$ where a problem exists.

9. Extremity Check: (CWMS)
colour/warmth, movement, sensation of area (identify) and side, e.g. CWMS rt. foot.

Use a $\boxed{\checkmark}$ if no problems observed. Document in Nurses' Notes $\boxed{NN}$ if problem observed.

10. Eye Patch Intact. ⎫
11. Eye Shield Intact. ⎬ (Identify side)
12. Tensor Bandage Intact (Identify side and area). ⎭

Use a $\boxed{\checkmark}$ if no problems observed. Document in Nurses' Notes $\boxed{NN}$ if problem observed.

13. Oral Intake.
14. Davol Drain.
15. Penrose Drain.
16. Heyer Drain.

Insert measured amount. Use the FLUID BALANCE RECORD if patient has an I.V. or a 24 hr. fluid balance is necessary.

17. Cardiac Activity Level.
18. Seizure Level.

Insert number that indicates assigned level. Indicate measurement in box.

19. Abdominal Girth. (Centimeter, Time)

Figure 17–6 A nursing care flowsheet used in conjunction with the problem-oriented record. *Source* Courtesy of the Nursing Department, University Hospital—UBC site, Vancouver, British Columbia.

UBC HEALTH SCIENCES CENTRE HOSPITAL

NURSING CARE FLOW SHEET

Legend:
I — Independent   T — Total Care
S — Supervised   NN — Refer to Nurses' Notes
Ⓐ — Assisted

			10/2							
	Date 9/									
	Time Period		0730 1930							
	Initials of nurse assigned to patient		BKE							
EXCRE-TORY CT – Catheter CM – Condom I – Incontinent		Urine	CT 750 ml							
		Stool (#)	1							
INGESTIVE N – Normal B – Blenderized MS – Mechanical Soft FF – Fluid CF – Clear Fluid P – Pureed NPO		Diet (T – Therapeutic)	NPO							
		Eating Poorly								
		Eating Well								
		Weight (kg.)								
PROTECTIVE	HYGIENE	Sponge Bath	✓							
		Tub Bath								
		Shower								
		Mouth Care	q 6h							
	SKIN INTEGRITY	Intact								
		Turns	q 2h							
	SAFETY P – Posey W – Wrist M – Mitts LT – Lap Tray LR – Lap Restraint	Restraint	M							
		Bed Rails Up (x1) (x2)	x 2							
REPARATIVE	MOBILITY AIDS C – Cane CR – Crutches W – Walker WC – Wheelchair	Bedrest (+D = Dangle)	✓ + D							
		B.R.P.								
		Chair								
		Walking								
	REST DURING NIGHT	Slept Poorly	✓							
		Slept Well								
	Catheter Care		x 1							
	I. V. Intact		✓							

KN 109-1-85 Rev 1

Figure 17–6   Nursing care flowsheet *(continued)*

THE UNIVERSITY OF BRITISH COLUMBIA
HEALTH SCIENCES CENTRE
EXTENDED CARE UNIT

NURSING SUMMARY

MISS ANN SMITH
Age 82 years BD: 1 Aug. 06
Admitted: March 5, 1991

DISCHARGE SUMMARY - June 10, 1991

Admitted March 5, 1991 from Victoria General Hospital in Victoria, B.C.

Problems

1. Multiple CVAs with bilateral hemiplegia resulting in need for assistance with ADLs and mobility/transfers--needs 2 person assist to transfer, needs maximum assist with ADLs; dressing, washing and bathing done by staff. She is concerned about her appearance.
2. Continent of urine if routinely toileted during the day--occasionally incontinent of urine at night.
3. Prone to constipation--has soft formed BM q 2-3 days when toileted--needs occasional glycerine suppository and receives Metamucil 15cc daily.
4. Essential hypertension--B.P. ranges from 150/90 to 184/108--monitored 2 days weekly (Tues & Fri.). Receives Nadolol 80 mg daily
5. Has a history of depression--has become lethargic, withdrawn and weepy at times. Minimal response to antidepressant drugs (Amitriptyline 25 mg ghs - was D/C May 19/81). Involved in numerous social groups and 1-1 interaction--responded well to both. Family visited frequently and very supportive.
6. Diet--minced--has occasional difficulty swallowing and tongue mobility due to dysarthria.
7. Progressive dysphasia--speech slurred--difficult to understand; very slow to respond; appreciates help from staff.

Next of Kin

Ray Smith--phone 123-4567 (brother)
Sue Brown--phone 261-0941 (niece)

Medical regime

Metamucil 15 cc daily
Nadolol 80 mg daily
Brandy 30 cc q h.s. prn

Allergies

--elastoplast--suffered period of general pruritis but was unable to relate to specific drugs or food--spontaneously resolved.

Safety Needs

Vision--good/able to read clock on wall and small print
Hearing--able to hear normal conversation
Mechanical aids--side rails and support in chair with pillows and belt restraints
--trunk balance poor
Orientation--well oriented to time, place, person despite deterioration in physical condition

Strengths and Resources

Miss Smith has a very supportive family. She is concerned about her appearance and feels comfortable letting staff know what her needs are.

Resident and family wish Miss Smith to move to LTC facility (X-E.C.U) in South Vancouver as it is much closer for family to visit--family visits 2-3 x weekly.

J. Doe, R.N.

June 10, 1991
Date

J. Doe, R.N.
Signature

Figure 17–7 A nursing discharge summary. ***Source*** Courtesy of the Nursing Department, University Hospital—UBC site, Vancouver, British Columbia.

NURSING NOTES

Date	Time	
2/13/91	1400	Passive ROM exercises provided for R arm and leg. Active assistive exercises to L arm and leg. Has scratch marks on L and R forearms. States, "My skin on my back and arms has been itchy for a week." Rash not evident. No previous history of pruritis. Is allergic to elastoplast but has not been in contact. Dr. J. Wong notified. ———————— Tom Ritchie, R.N.
	1430	Applied calamine lotion to back and arms. Incontinent of urine. Is restless. ——— Tom Ritchie, R.N.

Figure 17–8 An example of narrative nurse's notes.

SOAP Format

2/13/91 #5 Generalized pruritus

1400 S —"My skin is itchy on may back and arms and it's been like this for a week."

O —Skin appears clear—no rash or irritations noted. Marks where client has scratched noted on left and right forearms. Allergic to elastoplast but has not been in contact.
No previous history of pruritus.

A —Potential for infection related to scratching secondary to pruritus

P —Instructed to not scratch skin
—Applied calamine lotion to back and arms at 1430 hrs.
—Cut fingernails
—Assess further to determine if recurrence associated with specific drugs or foods
—Refer to physician and pharmacist for assessment
　　　　　　Tom Ritchie, R.N.

SOAPIER Format

2/13/91 #5 Generalized pruritus

1400 S —"My skin is itchy on back and arms and it's been like this for a week."

O —Skin appears clear—no rash or irritation noted. Marks where client has scratched noted on left and right forearms. Allergic to elastoplast but has not been in contact.
No previous history of pruritus.

A —Potential for infection

P —Instruct not to scratch skin
—Apply calamine lotion as necessary
—Cut nails to avoid scratches
—Assess further to determine if recurrence associated with specific drugs or foods
—Refer to physicians and pharmacist for assessment

I —Instructed not to scratch skin
Applied calamine lotion to back and arms at 1430 hrs.
Assisted to cut fingernails
Notified physician and pharmacist of problem

1600 E —States "I'm still itchy. That lotion didn't help."

R —Remove calamine lotion and apply hydrocortisone ungt. as ordered.
　　　　　　Tom Ritchie, R.N.

APIE Format

2/13/91 #5 Generalized pruritus

1400 A —Potential for infection (scratching) States "My skin is itchy on my back and arms and it's been like this for a week." Skin appears clear

—No rash or irritations noted. Marks where client has scratched noted on left and right forearms. Allergic to elastoplast but has not been in contact. No previous history of pruritus.

P —Instruct not to scratch skin
—Apply calamine lotion as necessary
—Cut nails to avoid scratches
—Assess further to determine if recurrence associated with specific drugs or foods
—Refer to doctor and pharmacist for assessment

I —Instructed not to scratch skin
Applied calamine lotion to back and arms at 1430 hrs.
Assisted to cut fingernails
Notified physician and pharmacist of problem

E —States "I'm still itchy. that lotion didn't help."
　　　　　　Tom Ritchie, R.N.

Figure 17–9 Examples of nursing progress notes using the SOAP, SOAPIER, and APIE formats.

Implementation, or *intervention,* is documentation of activities in the plan that were actually done for the client. These entries specify which plans were actually carried out. *Evaluation* is documentation of the client's response to the plan, stated in terms of client behavior (e.g., what the client did or said). The question asked at this stage is "Does the client's behavior indicate that the plan was unsuccessful in lessening or alleviating the identified problem?" *Revision,* or *reassessment,* refers to changes that must be made in the initial or original plan. From the evaluation notes and decision, one may determine that the client's condition may have improved or deteriorated. New data may now be available.

Focus Charting

Focus charting uses key words that describe what is happening to the client. Unlike problem-oriented charting, focus charting is *not* limited to clinical problems. The term "focus" was developed to encourage nurses to view the client's status from a positive perspective rather than the negative one that "problem" suggested. The term "focus" has a broad definition. It can denote (Lampe 1985, p. 43)

- A current client concern or behavior (e.g., decreased fluid intake)
- A significant change in the client status or behavior (e.g., sudden loss of sensation in one extremity)
- A significant event in the client's therapy (e.g., return from surgery)

In sum, a nursing focus outlines the occasions for and the activities of the *nursing care* the client is receiving. A focus is *not* a medical diagnosis, but it sometimes describes what is happening to the client as a result of the medical diagnoses. For example, some of the foci for a client with a medical diagnosis of myocardial infarction may include admission information, chest pain, anxiety about medical diagnosis, and education about cardiac medications.

The focus charting system uses three columns in the nurse's notes:

Date/Hour	Focus	Notes
2/11/91 0900	Neuro status	DATA. Unresponsive to verbal stimuli; responsive to painful stimuli. Pupils pinpoint and equal. Dr. Ward visited. ACTION. Neuro assessment and vital signs q2h. RESPONSE. See flowsheets.

Compared with a narrative documentation, this list facilitates (a) more rapid scanning to find the desired entries and (b) better communication. In the nurse's notes column, the SOAP format is replaced by DAR (data, action, response). *Data* include client behaviors, client status, and nursing observations. *Action* includes plans for action and immediate nursing actions. *Response* includes the client response

to nursing and/or medical care. This system is therefore compatible with use of the nursing process: data equates with assessment, action with planning and implementation, and response with evaluation.

Focus charting relies on an adequate database or assessment forms and the use of flowsheets such as vital signs records, neurologic checklists, intake and output flowsheets, and hygiene checklists. Agencies that use focus charting often provide a simple assessment checklist of key words that pertain to the special needs of clients in specific nursing units. For each key word, the checklist shows both normal and abnormal characteristics. Those applicable to the client can be circled. Normal characteristics may be underlined.

Charting by Exception

Charting by exception (CBE), developed in 1983 by staff nurses at St. Luke's Hospital in Milwaukee, is a documentation system in which only significant findings or exceptions to norms are recorded. CBE incorporates three key components (Burke and Murphy 1988, p. 7):

1. Unique *flowsheets* that highlight significant findings and define assessment parameters and findings. These include the nursing/physician order flowsheet, the graphic record, the patient teaching record, and the patient discharge note.

2. Documentation by reference to *Standards of Nursing Practice,* which eliminates much of the repetitive charting of routine care. The *standards* must therefore be specific in describing actual nursing practice and apply to every nurse regardless of clinical area. Unit-specific standards may also be developed. Examples of standards related to hygiene patterns include: "The nurse shall ensure that the client has a complete linen change every three days and as needed," and "The nurse shall ensure that the client is offered oral care t.i.d." Documentation of care according to these specified standards involves only a check mark in the routine standards box on the graphic record. If all standards are not implemented, an asterisk with reference to the nurse's notes is made. All exceptions to the standards are clearly outlined in narrative form on the nurse's notes.

3. Bedside accessibility of documentation forms. In the CBE system, all flowsheets are kept at the client's bedside to allow immediate recording and to eliminate the need for transcribing data from the nurse's worksheet to the permanent record.

GUIDELINES ABOUT RECORDING

Because the client's record is a legal document and may be used to provide evidence in court, many factors are considered in recording. Health care personnel not only maintain the confidentiality of the client's record but also meet legal standards in the process of recording. Some of these factors are restricted access, use of ink, signature, errors, blanks, accuracy, appropriateness, completeness, use of standard terminology, and brevity.

For *each* notation, documentation of the *date* and *time* is essential not only for legal reasons but also for safe care. For example, the time at which a narcotic was administered to a client needs to be determined before the next one can safely be given. Time can be recorded in the conventional manner (i.e., 9:00 A.M. or 3:20 P.M.) or according to the 24-hour clock (military clock), which avoids confusion about whether a time was A.M. or P.M. See Figure 17–10.

Restricted Access

The client's record is protected legally as a private record of the client's care. Thus, access to the record is restricted to health workers involved in giving care to the client. Insurance companies, for example, have no legal right to demand access to medical records, even though they may be determining compensation to the client. On the other hand, a client who is making a claim for compensation may ask to have the medical history used as evidence. In this instance, the client must sign an authorization for review, copying, or release of information from the record. This form clearly indicates what information is to be released and to whom. In no instance may a nurse allow access to a client's record by family members or any person other than a caregiver.

For purposes of education and research, most agencies allow student and graduate health professionals access to client records. The records are used in client conferences, clinics, rounds, and written papers or client studies. The student or graduate is bound by a strict ethical code to hold all information in confidence. Some agencies code medical records when they are filed, so that the names of clients are removed. This allows records to be used without identifying individuals. When this is not the practice, it is the responsibility of the student or health care professional to protect the client's privacy by *not* using a name or any statements in the notations that would identify the client. Many agencies also require documentation from the student or health professional wishing to use medical records of discharged clients. A permission note from the student's instructor will confirm the person's status as a student at a particular school.

Use of Ink

All entries on the client's record are made in dark-colored ink so that the record is permanent and changes can be identified. Dark-colored ink is generally required because it reproduces well on microfilm and in duplication processes. Entries need to be legible. Hand printing or easily understood handwriting is permissible.

Signature

Each recording on the nursing notes is signed by the nurse making it. The signature includes the *name* and *title,* for example, "Susan J. Green, RN." The following title abbreviations are often used, but nurses are advised to check the practice in their agencies.

RN registered nurse

LVN licensed vocational nurse

LPN licensed practical nurse

NA nursing assistant

NS nursing student

SN student nurse

Errors

When an error is made in charting, a line is drawn through it, and the word "error" is written above it, with the nurse's initials or name (depending on agency policy). Errors should not be erased or blotted out, so that there is no doubt about the nursing care given or the charting error made.

Sample Recording

Date: Dec 10/91	Time: 0100

error A.J.R.

Pulse ~~180 beats/minute~~ 108 beats/minute

_____ Abby J. Roberts, NS

If the nature of the error is not clear, many attorneys feel it is helpful and legally acceptable to indicate what the error was, in order to protect the client and the nurse. An example might be, "Charted for wrong client." The policy of the agency, however, needs to be checked.

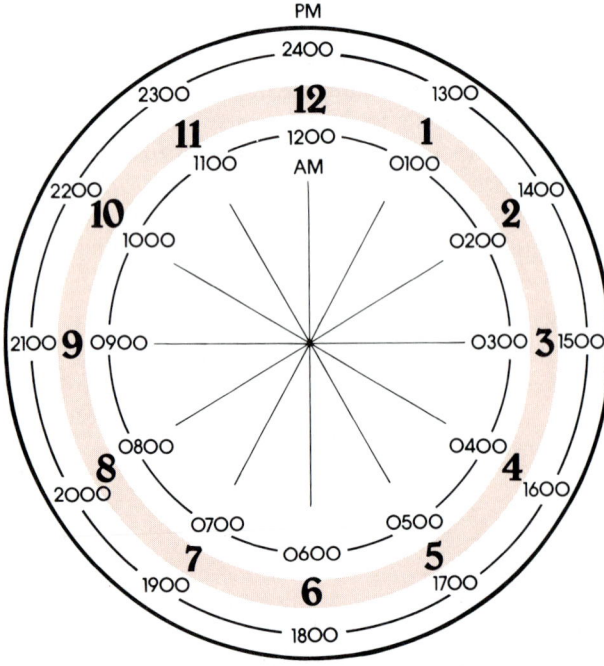

Figure 17–10 The 24-hour clock.

Blanks   If a blank appears in a notation, a line is drawn through the blank space so that no additional information can be recorded at any other time or by any other person, and it is signed.

Sample Recording

Date: Nov 7/91	Time: 0730

Urine appears cloudy, light brown with dark flecks. No odor. ——— Lin I. Ma, NS C/o burning pain in pubic region prior to voiding. ——————— Lin I. Ma, NS

Accuracy   It is essential that notations on records be accurate and correct. Accurate notations consist of facts or exact observations, rather than opinions or interpretations of an observation. It is more accurate, for example, to write that the client "refused medication" (fact) than to write that the client "was uncooperative" (opinion); to write that a client "was crying" (observation) is preferable to noting that the client "was depressed" (interpretation). Opinions or interpretations may or may not be accurate. Similarly, when a client expresses worry about the diagnosis or problem, this should be quoted directly on the record: "Stated: 'I'm worried about my leg.'" Nurses should record what they hear as well as what they observe.

Correct spelling is essential for accuracy in recording. If unsure how to spell a word, the nurse looks it up in a dictionary. Most agency units have one available for this purpose. Two decidedly different medications may have similar spellings—for example, digitoxin and digoxin.

Appropriateness   Only information that pertains to the client's health problems and care is recorded. Any other personal information that the client conveys to the nurse is inappropriate for the record. If irrelevant information is recorded, it can be considered an invasion of the client's privacy and/or libelous. A client's disclosure that she was a prostitute and has smoked marijuana, for example, *would not* be recorded on the client's medical record unless it had a direct bearing on the client's health problem.

Completeness   Not all data that a nurse obtains about a client can be recorded. However, the information that is recorded needs to be complete and helpful to the client, physicians, other nurses, and participating health care workers. Incomplete records could be used as evidence in court to show that the client did not receive the quality of care considered to meet generally accepted standards. For example, if a diabetic client's record does not indicate that insulin was given and that the urine was tested, the record could be used as evidence of negligence on the part of the nurse responsible for providing care. Of course, other examples and evidence would be needed to support a finding of negligence by the nurse. However, the client's record can be used to indicate the kind of care given. A complete

notation for a client who has vomited, for example, includes the time, the amount, the color, the odor of the vomit, and any other data about the client (e.g., pain).

Sample Recording

Date: Aug 12/91	Time: 1410

Vomited approx 500 ml of black liquid with foul fecal odor. C/o cramplike pain in epigastric region immediately prior to vomiting. ——————— Nancy R. Long, NS

The following guide may assist nurses in selecting essential and complete information to record about clients. Note that the emphasis is on facts that denote a change in the client's health status or behavior or that indicate a deviation from what is usually expected. Essential information includes the following:

1. Any behavior changes, for example
   - Indications of strong emotions, such as anxiety or fear
   - Marked changes in mood
   - A change in level of consciousness, such as stupor
   - Regression in relationships with family or friends
2. Any changes in physical function, such as
   - Loss of balance
   - Loss of strength
   - Difficulty hearing or seeing
3. Any physical sign or symptom that
   - Is severe, such as severe pain
   - Tends to recur or persist
   - Is not normal, such as elevated body temperature
   - Gets worse, such as gradual weight loss
   - Indicates a complication, such as inability to void following surgery
   - Is not relieved by prescribed measures, such as continued failure to defecate or to sleep
   - Indicates faulty health habits, such as lice on the scalp
   - Is a known danger signal, such as a lump in the breast
4. Any nursing interventions provided, such as
   - Medications administered
   - Therapies
   - Activities of daily living, if agency policy dictates
   - Teaching clients self-care
5. Visits by a physician or other members of the health team

In a legal battle, incomplete medical records may present difficulties that cannot be overcome. Courts take a dim view of evidence based on recall unsupported by written documentation, especially when a great deal of time has elapsed between the events and the trial. A plaintiff's attorney will never lose an opportunity to point out to the jury that an important event went unrecorded by the providers of care. Some courts have held that lack of exactitude in documentation implies lack of attention. In extreme cases, lack of

TABLE 17–1 *Commonly Used Abbreviations*

Abbreviation	Term	Abbreviation	Term
abd	abdomen	dc (disc)	discontinue
ABO	the main blood group system	drsg	dressing
ac	before meals (*ante cibum*)	Dx	diagnosis
ADL	activities of daily living	ECG (EKG)	electrocardiogram
ad lib	as desired (*ad libitum*)	F	Fahrenheit
adm	admitted or admission	fld	fluid
A.M.	morning (*ante meridiem*)	GI	gastrointestinal
amb	ambulatory	GP	general practitioner
amt	amount	gtt	drops (*guttae*)
approx	approximately (about)	h (hr)	hour (*hora*)
bid	twice daily (*bis in die*)	H_2O	water
BM (bm)	bowel movement	hs	at bedtime (*hora somni*)
BP	blood pressure	I & O	intake and output
BR	bed rest	IV	intravenous
BRP	bathroom privileges	Lab	laboratory
c̄ (C)	with	liq	liquid
C	Celsius (centigrade)	LMP	last menstrual period
CBC	complete blood count	lt (L)	left
CBR	complete bed rest	meds	medications
Cl	client	ml (mL)	milliliter
c/o	complains of	mod	moderate
DAT	diet as tolerated	neg	negative

documentation could be considered evidence of negligence (Cushing 1982).

Use of Standard Terminology   The nurse needs to use only commonly accepted *abbreviations, symbols,* and *terms* that are specified by the agency. Then, if the record is used in court as evidence, other professionals responsible for interpreting the data can do so correctly. Many abbreviations are standard and used universally; others are used only in certain geographic areas. Some agencies supply a list of the abbreviations they accept. When in doubt about whether to use an abbreviation, the nurse writes the term out in full, until certain about the abbreviation. Table 17–1 lists some commonly used abbreviations (except those used for medications, which are described in Chapter 45). Table 17–2 indicates commonly accepted symbols.

Medical terminology is generally made up of root words, prefixes, and suffixes. A root word may be derived from Latin or Greek. A prefix is a sequence of letters that comes before the word and often describes a variation of the normal. A suffix is a sequence of letters that occurs at the end

TABLE 17–2 *Commonly Used Symbols*

Symbol	Term	Symbol	Number
>	greater than	ō	0
<	less than	ss̄	½
=	equal to	ī	1
↑	increased	īī	2
↓	decreased	īīī	3
♀	female	īv̄	4
♂	male	v̄	5
°	degree	v̄ī	6
#	number; fracture	v̄īī	7
ʒ	dram	v̄īīī	8
℥	ounce	īx̄	9
×	times	x̄	10
@	at		

TABLE 17–1 *Commonly Used Abbreviations* (*continued*)

Abbreviation	Term	Abbreviation	Term
nil (ō)	none	qd	every day (*quaque die*)
no. (#)	number	qh (q1h)	every hour (*quaque hora*)
NPO (NBM)	nothing by mouth (*per ora*)	q2h, q3h, etc	every two hours, three hours, etc
NS (N/S)	normal saline	qhs	every night at bedtime (*quaque hora somni*)
O₂	oxygen	qid	four times a day (*quater in die*)
od	daily (*omni die*)	req	requisition
OD	right eye (*oculus dexter*); overdose	Rt (rt, R)	right
OOB	out of bed	S (s̄)	without (*sine*)
os	mouth	SI	seriously ill
OS	left eye (*oculus sinister*)	spec	specimen
pc	after meals (*post cibum*)	stat	at once, immediately (*statim*)
PE (PX)	physical examination	tid	three times a day (*ter in die*)
per	by or through	TL	team leader
P.M.	afternoon (*post meridiem*)	TLC	tender loving care
po	by mouth (*per os*)	TPR	temperature, pulse, respirations
postop	postoperative(ly)	Tr.	tincture
preop	preoperative(ly)	VO	verbal order
prep	preparation	VS (vs)	vital signs
prn	when necessary (*pro re nata*)	WNL	within normal limits
pt	patient	wt	weight
q	every (*quaque*)		

of the word; it often describes a condition of or act performed on the root word. Root words, suffixes, and prefixes are provided in Appendix D. Further terms are given in the glossary at the end of the book.

Brevity   Recordings need to be brief as well as complete, to save time in communication. The client's name and the word *client* are omitted. For example, the nurse may write "Perspiring profusely. Respirations shallow, wet, 28/min." Each thought or sentence is terminated with a period.

REPORTING

Reports can be either oral or written. The purpose of reporting, in general, is to communicate specific information to a person or group of people. A report should be concise. A good report includes pertinent information, but not extraneous detail. Two common types of reports are the change of shift report and the incident report. The incident report is discussed in Chapter 8 on page 154.

A *change-of-shift report* is an oral report usually given by the on-duty charge nurse to all nursing personnel coming on duty. Variations occur, however. In units where primary nursing is employed, the report may be given from one RN to another; in units where team nursing is practiced, the report may be given from one team leader to another. Change-of-shift reports may be given either in a face-to-face exchange or by audiotape recording. The face-to-face report allows the listener to ask questions during the report, although if given to all on-coming nurses it can be time-consuming. On-coming nurses, for example, are required to listen to the report on all clients, including many not under their care. The tape-recorded report is often briefer and less time-consuming. Some agencies or units combine these methods of giving the change-of-shift report, following the taped report or a brief report to all oncoming staff with a more extensive individual report given by the nurse going off duty to the nurse who will be providing client care during the coming shift. This more detailed report is often given at the bedside, and clients as well as nurses may participate in the exchange of information.

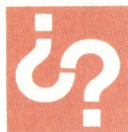

RESEARCH NOTE

Is There Congruence Between Intershift Reports and Client's Actual Conditions?

After listening to 57 intershift reports (face-to-face and taped) on adult medical-surgical units of an 800-bed metropolitan hospital, distributed over day, evening, and night shifts, this investigator verified the reports by checking each client. Predetermined pertinent items were analyzed for congruence, incongruence, omissions, and omissions resulting from incongruence between the stated conditions of clients during the intershift reports and the actual conditions of the clients. No attempt to determine the cause of discrepancies was made; only their occurrence was noted.

The overall congruence was 70%, with 70% congruence for the day shift, 72% for the evening shift, and 68% for the night shift. The omission rate was 11.8%; the most common omissions were in the category of intake and output. The overall incongruence was 12.4%; the most common instances were in the category of intravenous infusion sites. The rate of omissions resulting in incongruence was 6%. It is suggested that overload may be an important variable in determining the occurrence of omissions and incongruencies.

Implications: The results of this study indicate that nurses cannot assume that what is stated during the intershift report is congruent with the conditions of the clients immediately following the report.

Richard, J. A. Spring 1988. Congruence between intershift report and patients' actual conditions. *Image: Journal of Nursing Scholarship* 20:4–6.

The following guidelines can help nurses prepare and present reports about clients (Hesse 1983, Smith 1986):

- Follow a particular order when reporting about a series of clients. For example, follow room numbers in a hospital or times of appointments in a community clinic.

- Identify the client by name, room number, and bed designation. For example, Ms. Jessie Jones, 702, Bed D. This enables the listeners, especially float nurses or those returning from days off or vacation, to relate subsequent information immediately to this client's case.

- Depending on the type of unit, provide the reason for admission, that is, the client's medical diagnosis or original complaint. This information may not be necessary in long-term geriatric units or newborn nurseries; in acute-care settings, however, it is often necessary because of multiple tests, consultations, and transfers.

- Include diagnostic tests and/or results and other therapies performed in the past 24 hours, such as blood transfusions, surgery, initiation of intravenous therapy, narcotics administered, blood gas levels, and group therapy data.

- Note any significant changes in the client's condition. Oncoming nurses must know about changes for the worse to monitor the client's condition appropriately. Significant improvements toward goal attainment should also be noted so that the nurse can provide positive feedback to the client.

- When reporting about changes, present the pertinent information in this order: assessment, nursing diagnoses (if appropriate), planning, intervention, and evaluation. For example, "Mr. Ronald Oakes said he had an aching pain in his left calf at 1400 hours. Inspection revealed no other signs. Calf pain is related to altered blood circulation. Rest and elevation of his legs on a footstool for 30 minutes provided relief."

- Provide exact information, such as "Ms. Jessie Jones received Demerol 100 mg intramuscularly at 2000 hours (8 P.M.)," not "Ms. Jessie Jones received some Demerol during the evening."

- Do not include unremarkable measurements such as normal temperature, pulse, and blood pressure unless a desired change is involved. For example, a normal body temperature for a client who has had an elevated temperature should be reported.

- Report the client's emotional responses that need attention before other interventions can be implemented. For example, a client who has just learned his biopsy results revealed malignancy and who is now scheduled for a laryngectomy needs time to discuss his feelings before the nurse commences preoperative teaching.

Nursing students may want to practice giving report in clinical post-care conferences or by taping themselves giving a simulated report of the current status of their assigned clients.

CONFERRING

To **confer** is to consult another person or persons for advice, information, ideas, or instructions. Nurses confer with colleagues and other health professionals about some aspect of client care or to elicit or validate data needed to plan nursing care. Two ways nurses share information are through the nursing care conference and nursing care rounds.

A **nursing care conference** is a meeting of a group of nurses to discuss possible solutions to certain problems of a client, such as inability to cope with an event or lack of progress toward goal attainment. Examples: a middle-aged woman is so distressed about her body image after mastectomy that she is not perceiving her husband's love and not performing her arm exercises; an adolescent boy with severe diabetes is not following his diet but is eating chocolate bars and milk shakes that he has enticed his friends to bring into the hospital for him. The nursing care conference allows each nurse an opportunity to offer an opinion about possible solutions to the problem. Other health practitioners or nurse-clinicians may be invited to attend the conference to offer their expertise; for example, a nurse-clinician may discuss the emotional problems of a severely burned child and his responses, or a dietitian may discuss dietary problems.

Nursing care conferences are most effective when there is a climate of respect—i.e., nonjudgmental acceptance of others even though their values, opinions, and beliefs may seem different. The nurse needs to accept and respect each person's contributions, listening with an open mind to what others are saying even when the nurse disagrees. Everyone can learn new ways of approaching situations when they conscientiously listen to another perspective.

Nursing care rounds are procedures in which a group of nurses visit all or selected clients at each client's bedside to

- Obtain information that will help plan nursing care
- Provide clients the opportunity to discuss their care
- Evaluate the nursing care the client has received

During rounds, the nurse assigned to the client provides a brief summary of the client's nursing needs and the interventions being implemented. The advantage of nursing rounds for the clients is that they can participate in the discussions; the advantage for the nurses is that they can see the client being discussed. To facilitate client participation in nursing care rounds, nurses need to use terms that the client can understand. Medical terminology excludes the client from discussion.

CHAPTER HIGHLIGHTS

- Health team members must communicate among themselves effectively to provide coordinated, high-quality care.

- When there is accurate communication, all health team members become informed about client needs, and overlapping of activities is avoided.

- Written records ensure transmission of information to all health workers caring for the client; are a source of research, educational, and statistical data; and allow the audit of client care standards.

- Client records are admissible as evidence in a court of law.

- The problem-oriented medical record (POMR or POR) (Weed system) is increasingly recognized as a method that provides a client-centered problem-solving approach to care.

- The POR has four basic components: a defined database, a complete problem list, an initial plan for each identified problem, and progress notes.

- Progress notes follow the systematic SOAP format and include narrative notes, flowsheets, and discharge notes.

- Traditional client records are source-oriented records, in that each category of health worker keeps separate records.

- Traditional records generally have six parts: admission sheet, face sheet, physician's order sheet, medical history sheet, nurses' notes, and other special records such as the laboratory records.

- The Kardex record is widely used for quick access to current data about clients.

- Computerized information systems are being used increasingly in health care agencies.

- Record entries should be brief, accurate, legible, chronologic, made on consecutive lines, and appropriately signed.

- Record entries are made after nursing interventions and usually when the client is admitted or transferred.

- Because the record is a legal document, nurses sign their full legal names and use standard terms and abbreviations.

- Erasures on the client record are not permitted.

- Reports about clients need to be concise and pertinent and must include significant changes in the client's condition and therapy.

- Two ways in which nurses share information needed to plan nursing care are the nursing care conference and nursing rounds.

READINGS AND REFERENCES

SUGGESTED READINGS

Buckley-Womack, C., and Gidney, B. October 1987. A new dimension in documentation: The PIE method. *Journal of Neuroscience Nursing* 19:256–60.

The authors report the results of a pilot program to implement the problem identification, intervention, and evaluation method of documentation (PIE). This method incorporates the care plan into the progress notes, eliminating the need for a traditional care plan. The authors report that since this method was first put into use, the quality of documentation has improved and the time spent on charting has decreased.

Cohen, M. R. July 1987. Play it safe: Don't use these abbreviations. *Nursing 87* 17:46–47.

Even though some abbreviations may be approved for use by staff, Cohen maintains that some abbreviations should never be used because they are so easily misunderstood. Alternatives are provided.

Harkins, B. December 1986. Keep your eye on the patient's problems. *RN* 49:30–32.

Harkins advocates a problem-oriented charting system because it specifically lists the client's problems and the interventions used to solve them. A step-by-step guide for using this system is provided, with many examples specific to a postoperative client.

King, I. M. April 1984. Effectiveness of nursing care: Use of a goal-oriented nursing record in end stage renal disease. *The American Association of Nephrology Nurses and Technicians Journal* 1:11–17, 60.

King's theory of goal attainment provides the basis for this goal-oriented nursing record (GONR). The GONR system, a modification of the problem-oriented medical record designed for physicians, was designed for nurses to gather data in a systematic way, to record data, to identify nursing problems, make a nursing diagnosis, construct a goal list, write orders for nursing care, and report the effectiveness of nursing care through goal attainment. In this article, King discusses the seven elements of GONR: database, problem list, goal list, nursing orders, flowsheets, progress notes, and discharge summary and applies them to a client with end-stage renal disease (ESRD).

McKiel, R. E., and Rogers, C. A. March/April 1986. The chart critique: A learning activity for nursing students. *Nurse Educator* 11:23–24. This article describes the chart critique, a written assignment designed to help students develop skill in using a client's chart as one resource for identifying actual and potential problems and planning nursing care. The chart critique questionnaire is provided.

Rutkowski, B. October 1985. How DRGs are changing your charting. *Nursing 85* 15:49–51.

Because of DRGs, peer review organizations and hospital administrators are looking at nursing notes more thoroughly than ever before. Nursing notes therefore must be more concise, specific, and complete. The SOAP format is discussed as one way to meet the current need.

SELECTED REFERENCES

Afferbach, D. January 1986. A flow sheet that saves time and trouble. *RN* 49:42–44.

Allison, S., and Kinloch, K. December 1981. Four steps to quality assurance: Problem-oriented recording. Part 2. *The Canadian Nurse* 77:36–40.

Andreoli, K., and Musser, L. A. January/February 1985. Computers in nursing care: The state of the art. *Nursing Outlook* 33:16–21.

Bailey-Allen, A. M. January/February 1986. Avoid legal pitfalls in charting. *Orthopedic Nursing* 5:21–23.

———. April 1988. More about charting with a jury in mind. *Nursing 88* 18:50–58.

Blount, M.; Green, S. S.; Hamory, A.; Kinney, A. B.; and Sanborn, C. W. September 1978. Documenting with the problem-oriented record system. *American Journal of Nursing* 78:1539–42.

Buckley-Womack, C., and Gidney, B. October 1987. A new dimension in documentation: The PIE method. *Journal of Neuroscience Nursing* 19:256–60.

Burke, L. J., and Murphy, J. 1988. *Charting by exception: A cost-effective, quality approach.* New York: John Wiley and Sons.

Costello, S., and Summers, B. Y. June 1985. Documenting patient care: Getting it all together. *Nursing Management* 16:31–34.

Creighton, H. 1986. *Law every nurse should know.* 5th ed. Philadelphia: W. B. Saunders Co.

Cushing, M. December 1982. The legal side: Gaps in documentation. *American Journal of Nursing* 82:1899–1900.

Fairless, P. R. September 1986. Nine ways a computer can make your work easier. *Nursing 86* 16:54–56.

Groah, L., and Reed, E. A. May 1983. Your responsibility in documenting care. *Association of Operating Room Nurses Journal* 37:1174, 1176–77, 1180–85.

Gruber, M., Gruber, J. M. Spring 1990. Nursing malpractice: The importance of documentation, or saved by the pen! *Gastroenterological Nursing* 12:255–9.

Hesse, G. February 1983. A better shift report means better nursing care. *Nursing 83* 13:65. Canadian edition 13:17.

Kilpack, V., and Dobson-Brassard, S. October 1987. Intershift report: Oral communication using the nursing process. *Journal of Neuroscience Nursing* 19:266–70.

Laing, M. December 1981. Flow sheets: Meeting the charting challenge. *The Canadian Nurse* 77:40–42.

Lampe, S. S. 1984. *Focus Charting.* Minneapolis, Minn.: Creative Nursing Management.

———. July 1985. Focus charting: Streamlining documentation. *Nursing Management* 16:43–46.

Memorial Hospital of Burlington County, Mt. Holly, N.J. September/October 1985. Cut documentation time by 50%. *Nursing Life* 5:30–32.

Murphy, J., Burke, L. J. May 1990. Charting by exception: A more efficient way to document. *Nursing 90* 20:65, 68–69.

Philpott, M. August 1986. Twenty rules for good charting. *Nursing 86* 10:63.

Rich, P. L. July 1985. With this flow sheet less is more. *Nursing 85* 15:25–29.

Rocerto, L. R., and Maleski, C. M. July/August 1984. All about rights to medical records. *Nursing Life* 4:50–51.

Rutkowski, B. October 1985. How DRGs are changing your charting. *Nursing 85* 15:49–51.

Simpson, K. June 1985. Using Kardex cards to improve the quality of patient care. *The Canadian Nurse* 81:37–40.

Sklar, C. L. May 1984. The patient's record, an invaluable communication tool. *The Canadian Nurse* 80:50–52.

Smith, C. E. February 1986. Upgrade your shift reports with the three R's. *Nursing 86* 16:63–64.

Svanda, C. December 1986. Key words show what's important . . . focus charting. *RN* 49:32–33.

Vaughan-Wrobel, B. D., and Henderson, B. S. 1982. *The problem-oriented system in nursing.* 2d ed. St. Louis: C. V. Mosby Co.

Weed, L. L. 1971. *Medical records, medical education and patient care: The problem-oriented record as a basic tool.* Cleveland: Case Western Reserve University Press.

Assessing Vital Signs

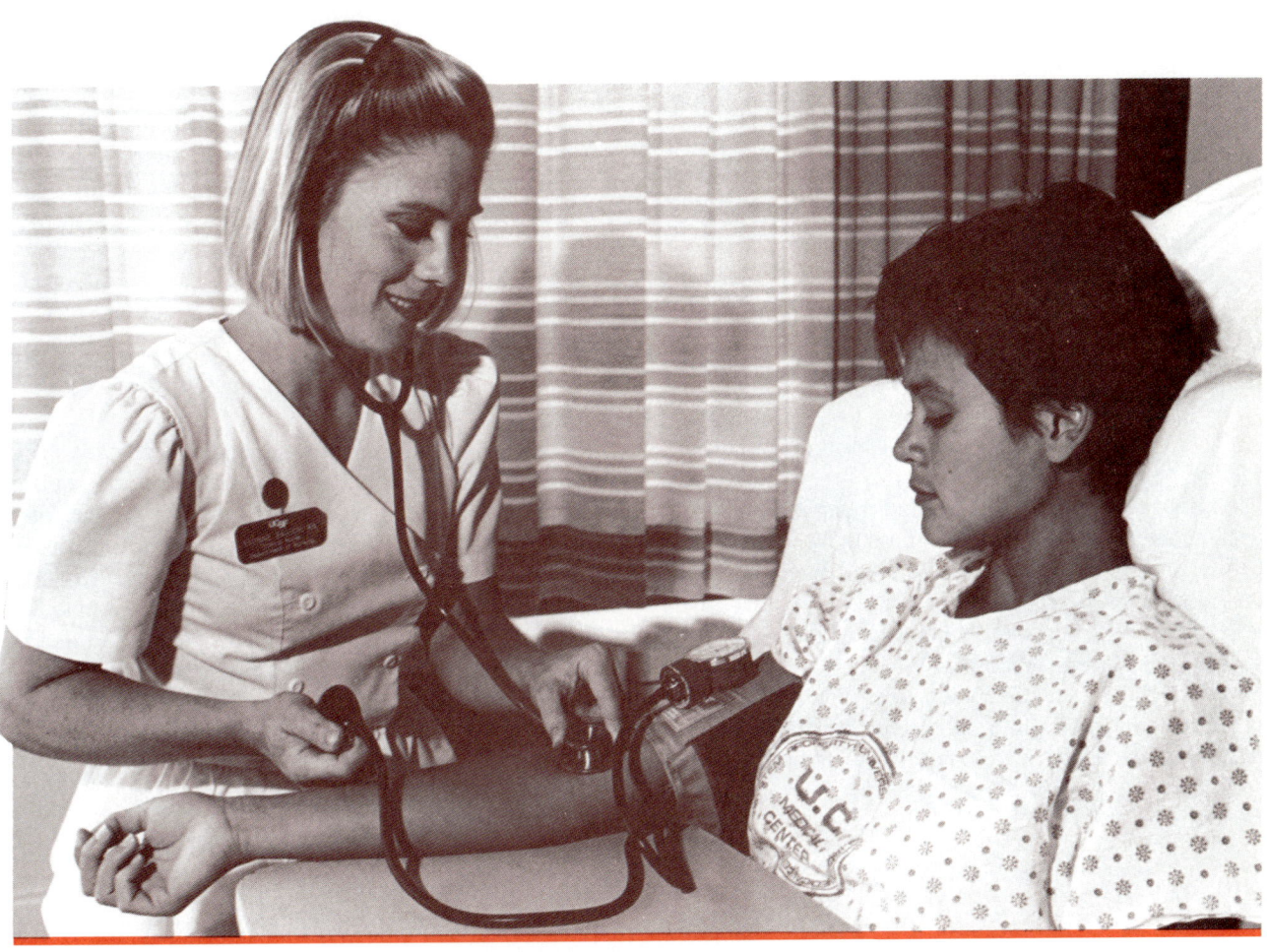

CONTENTS

OBJECTIVES

- Define terms and abbreviations used when measuring body temperature, pulse, respirations, and blood pressure.
- Describe five factors influencing the body's heat production.
- Identify four ways in which the body loses heat.
- Describe the body's temperature-regulating system.
- Compare oral, rectal, and axillary methods of measuring body temperature.

- Identify situations in which specific methods for measuring body temperature are indicated or contraindicated.
- Identify recommended intervals required to obtain accurate temperature readings for each method and for different types of equipment.
- Describe selected alterations of body temperature and appropriate nursing care for these alterations.
- Identify nine pulse sites commonly used to assess the pulse and state the reasons for their use.

- List the characteristics that should be included when assessing pulses.
- Explain how to measure the apical pulse and apical-radial pulse.
- Describe the mechanics of breathing and the mechanisms that control respirations.
- Identify the characteristics that should be included in a respiratory assessment.
- Differentiate systolic from diastolic blood pressure.
- Describe various methods and sites used to measure blood pressure.

VITAL SIGNS

The **vital** or **cardinal signs** are body temperature, pulse, respirations, and blood pressure. These signs, which should be looked at in total, are used to monitor the functions of the body. The signs reflect changes in function that otherwise might not be observed. Monitoring a client's vital signs should not be an automatic or routine procedure; it should be a thoughtful, scientific assessment. Vital signs, which should be evaluated with reference to the client's present and prior health status, are compared to accepted normal standards.

When and how often to assess a specific client's vital signs are chiefly nursing judgments depending on the client's health status. Some agencies have policies about taking clients' vital signs, and physicians may specifically order assessment of a vital sign, e.g., "Blood pressure q2h." Ordered assessments, however, should be considered the minimum; nurses should measure clients' vital signs more often if their health status requires it. Examples of times to assess vital signs are listed in the accompanying box.

BODY TEMPERATURE

Body temperature is the balance between the heat produced by the body and the heat lost from the body. There are two kinds of body temperature: core temperature and surface temperature. **Core temperature** is the temperature of the deep tissues of the body, e.g., cranium, thorax, abdominal cavity, and pelvic cavity. It remains relatively constant (37 C, 98.6 F). The **surface temperature** is the temperature of the skin, the subcutaneous tissue, and fat. It, by contrast, rises and falls in response to the environment.

The normal core body temperature is not an exact point on a scale but a range of temperatures. When measured orally, the average body temperature of an adult is between 36.7 C (98 F) and 37 C (98.6 F). See Figure 18–1 for the normal ranges of body temperature.

The body continually produces heat as a by-product of metabolism. Carbohydrates, fats, and proteins are used to synthesize large quantities of adenosine triphosphate (ATP), which in turn is used as a source of energy by body cells. However, about 50% of the energy in food becomes heat rather than ATP, and further heat is produced as the food

---

Times to Assess Vital Signs

- Upon admission to a health care agency to obtain baseline data
- When a client has a change in health status or reports symptoms such as chest pain or feeling hot or faint
- According to a nursing or medical order
- Before and after surgery or an invasive diagnostic procedure
- Before and after the administration of a medication that could affect the respiratory or cardiovascular systems; for example, before giving a digitalis preparation
- Before and after any nursing intervention that could affect the vital signs, e.g., ambulating a client who has been on bed rest

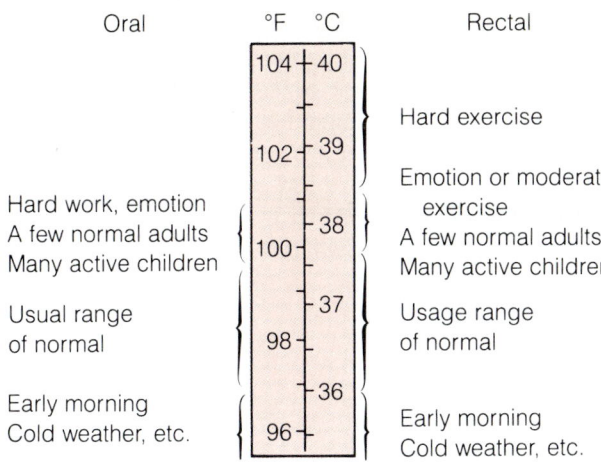

Oral	°F	°C	Rectal
	104 — 40		
			Hard exercise
	102 — 39		
			Emotion or moderate
Hard work, emotion	— 38		exercise
A few normal adults	100 —		A few normal adults
Many active children			Many active children
	— 37		
Usual range	98 —		Usage range
of normal			of normal
	— 36		
Early morning			
Cold weather, etc.	96 —		Early morning
			Cold weather, etc.

Figure 18–1 Estimated ranges of body temperatures in normal persons. *Source:* E. F. DuBois, *Fever and the regulation of body temperature* (Springfield, Ill.: Charles C. Thomas, 1948). Courtesy of Charles C. Thomas, Publisher, Springfield, Illinois.

is changed to ATP (Guyton 1986, p. 844). When the amount of heat produced by the body exactly equals the amount of heat lost, the person is in **heat balance.** See Figure 18–2.

A number of factors affect the body's heat production. The most important are these five:

1. *Basal metabolic rate (BMR).* The **basal metabolic rate** (**BMR**) is the rate of energy utilization in the body required to maintain essential activities such as breathing. BMRs vary with sex and age. After the age of 2 years, a female's BMR is usually about 5 to 10% less than a male's of the same age and size. Metabolic rates decrease with age. In general, the younger the person, the higher the BMR (Marieb 1989, p. 844).

2. *Muscle activity.* Muscle activity, including shivering, can greatly increase metabolic rate. For example, maximum muscle exercise can increase heat production to about 50 times normal (Guyton 1986, p. 845).

3. *Thyroxine output.* Increased thyroxine output increases the rate of cellular metabolism throughout the body. This effect is called **chemical thermogenesis,** the stimulation of heat production in the body through increased cellular metabolism.

4. *Epinephrine, norepinephrine, and sympathetic stimulation.* These hormones immediately increase the rate of cellular metabolism in many body tissues. Epinephrine and norepinephrine directly affect liver and muscle cells, thereby increasing cellular activity. Of more importance is sympathetic stimulation of brown fat. When the cells of this fat are stimulated, they produce a large amount of heat.

5. *Increased temperature of body cells (fever).* Fever increases the cellular metabolic rate. Chemical reactions increase an average of about 120% for every 10 C rise in temperature (Guyton 1986, p. 846). This means that for every 1 C (0.9 F) rise in temperature, there are about 12% more chemical reactions taking place. Although this mechanism is mediated somewhat by the body's temperature control system (see later in this chapter), the presence of fever acts to increase the body's temperature further.

Heat is lost from the body through radiation, conduction, convection, and vaporization. Sweating, panting, lowering the environmental temperature, and wearing light clothing all promote heat loss. **Radiation** is the transfer of heat from the surface of one object to the surface of another without contact between the two objects. For example, radiation accounts for 60% of the heat lost by a nude person standing in a room at normal room temperature (Guyton 1986, p. 850). Most heat loss through radiation is in the form of infrared rays.

Conduction is the transfer of heat from one molecule to another. Again, a temperature gradient is implied. The heat transfers to a molecule of lower temperature. Conductive transfer cannot take place without contact between the molecules and normally accounts for minimal heat loss

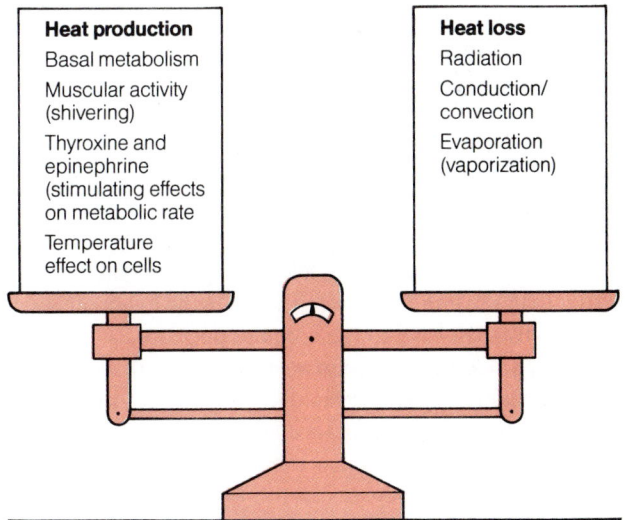

Heat production	Heat loss
Basal metabolism	Radiation
Muscular activity (shivering)	Conduction/ convection
Thyroxine and epinephrine (stimulating effects on metabolic rate	Evaporation (vaporization)
Temperature effect on cells	

Figure 18–2 As long as heat production and heat loss are properly balanced, body temperature remains constant. Factors contributing to heat production (and temperature rise) are shown on the left side of the scale; those contributing to heat loss (and temperature fall) are shown on the right side of the scale. Adapted from E. N. Marieb, *Human anatomy and physiology* (Redwood City, Calif.: Benjamin/Cummings, 1989). Adapted with permission.

except, for example, when a body is immersed in ice water. The amount of heat transferred depends on the temperature difference and the amount and duration of contact.

Convection is the dispersion of heat by air currents. There is usually a small amount of warm air adjacent to the body. This warm air rises and is replaced by cooler air, and so people always lose a small amount of heat through convection. **Vaporization** (evaporation) is continuous evaporation of moisture from the respiratory tract and from the mucosa of the mouth and from the skin. This continuous and unnoticed water loss is called insensible water loss, and the accompanying heat loss is called **insensible heat loss.** Insensible heat loss accounts for about 10% of basal heat production. When the body temperature increases, vaporization accounts for greater heat loss.

Regulation of Body Temperature

The system that regulates body temperature has three main parts: sensors in the shell and in the core, an integrator in the hypothalamus, and an effector system that adjusts the production and loss of heat. Most *sensors* or *sensory receptors* are in the skin, which is a major part of the shell. There are fewer receptors in the tongue, respiratory tract, and viscera. The skin has receptors of both cold and warmth; however, far more receptors detect cold than warmth (Guyton 1986, p. 854). Therefore, skin sensors detect cold more efficiently than warmth.

When the skin becomes chilled over the entire body, three physiologic processes to increase the body temperature take place:

1. Shivering increases heat production.
2. Sweating is inhibited to decrease heat loss.
3. Vasoconstriction decreases heat loss.

The receptors in the body's core, i.e., in the abdominal viscera, in the spinal cord, and in or around the large veins, respond only to the body's core temperature, not to the body's surface temperature. They also detect mainly cold rather than warmth. Thermoreceptors in the hypothalamus are likewise sensitive to the core temperature.

The **hypothalamic integrator,** the center that controls the core temperature, is located in the preoptic area of the hypothalamus. Some sensors are sensitive to heat, and some are sensitive to cold. Neurons transmit signals in response to signals from the sensors in the body shell. When the sensors in the hypothalamus detect heat, they send out signals intended to reduce the temperature, i.e., decrease heat production and increase heat loss. When the cold sensors are stimulated, signals are sent out to increase heat production and decrease heat loss.

The signals from the cold-sensitive receptors of the hypothalamus initiate *effectors* such as vasoconstriction, shivering, and the release of epinephrine, which increases cellular metabolism and hence heat production. Stimuli also

suppress the release of thyroxine by the thyroid gland. When the warmth-sensitive receptors in the hypothalamus are stimulated, the effector system sends out signals that initiate sweating and peripheral vasodilation. Another part of the effector system is the somatic nervous system. When this system is stimulated the person consciously makes appropriate adjustments, such as putting on additional clothing in response to cold or turning on a fan in response to heat.

Factors Affecting Body Temperature

Nurses should be aware of the factors that can affect a client's body temperature so that they can recognize normal temperature variations and understand the significance of body temperature measurements that deviate from normal. See Table 18–1 for a summary of the normal values of the vital signs at various ages. Among the factors that affect body temperature are the following:

1. *Age.* The infant is greatly influenced by the temperature of the environment and must be protected from extreme changes. Children's temperatures continue to be more labile than those of adults until puberty. Studies by Kolanowski and Gunter indicate that many elderly people, particularly those over 75 years, are at risk of hypothermia (temperatures below 36 C, or 96.8 F) for a variety of reasons, such as lack of central heating, inadequate diet, loss of subcutaneous fat, lack of activity, and reduced thermoregulatory efficiency. Elderly people are also particularly sensitive to extremes in the environmental temperature due to decreased thermoregulatory controls (Kolanowski and Gunter 1981, p. 362).

2. *Diurnal variations.* Body temperatures normally change throughout the day, varying as much as 2.0 C (1.8 F) between the early morning and the late afternoon. The point of highest body temperature is usually reached between 2000 and 2400 hours (8:00 P.M. and midnight), and the lowest point is reached during sleep between 0400 and 0600 hours (4:00 and 6:00 A.M.) See Figure 18–3.

3. *Exercise.* Hard work or strenuous exercise can increase body temperature to as high as 38.3 to 40 C (101 to 104 F) measured rectally.

4. *Hormones.* In women, progesterone secretion at the time of ovulation raises body temperature by about 0.35 C (0.5 F) above basal temperature (Olds, London, and Ladewig 1988, p. 136). Just before this time, as ovulation approaches, the production of estrogen increases and at its peak may decrease basal temperature slightly. Thyroxine, norepinephrine, and epinephrine also affect body temperature.

5. *Stress.* Stimulation of the sympathetic nervous system can increase the production of epinephrine and norepinephrine, thereby increasing metabolic activity and

TABLE 18–1 *Variations in Vital Signs by Age*

Age	Average Temperature	Pulse rate at Rest/Min		Respiratory Rate/Min	Mean Blood Pressure
		Average	Range		
Newborn	36.1–37.7C 97.0–100.0 F (axilla)	125	70–190	30–80	78 systolic 42 diastolic by flush technique: 30–60
1 year	37.7 C 99.7 F	120	80–160	20–40	96 systolic 65 diastolic
2 years	37.2 C 98.9 F	110	80–130	20–30	100 systolic 63 diastolic
4 years		100	80–120	20–30	97 systolic 64 diastolic
6 years	37.0 C 98.6 F (oral)	100	75–115	20–25	98 systolic 65 diastolic
8 years		90	70–110		106 systolic 70 diastolic
10 years		90	70–110	17–22	110 systolic 72 diastolic
12 years		Male: 85 Female: 90	65–105 70–110	17–22	116 systolic 74 diastolic
14 years		Male: 80 Female: 85	60–100 65–105		120 systolic 76 diastollic
16 years		Male: 75 Female: 80	55–95 60–100	15–20	123 systolic 76 diastolic
18 years		Male: 70 Female: 75	50–90 55–95	15–20	126 systolic 79 diastolic
Adult		Same as 18 years		15–20	120 systolic 80 diastolic
Elderly (over 70 years)	36.0 C 96.8 F	Same as 18 years		15–20	Diastolic pressure may increase

Sources: Pulse rates: R. E. Behrman and V. C. Vaughan, III, editors, *Nelson textbook of pediatrics,* 12th ed. (Philadelphia: W. B. Saunders, 1983), p. 1100. G. H. Lowrey, *Growth and development of children,* 7th ed. Chicago: Year Book, 1978) p. 450. For newborn and 1 year ages, National Heart, Lung, and Blood Institute, Task Force on Blood Pressure Control in Children: Report of the Task Force on Blood Pressure Control in Children, *Pediatrics* (May) 1977, 39(Suppl):819–20.

heat production. Nurses may anticipate that a highly stressed or anxious client could have an elevated body temperature for that reason.

6. *Environment.* Extremes in environmental temperatures can affect a person's temperature regulatory systems. The limits of extreme heat that a person can tolerate vary according to humidity. If the air is completely dry and if sufficient convection air currents are flowing to promote rapid evaporation from the body, a person can withstand several hours of air temperature at 150 F with no apparent ill effects (Guyton 1986, p. 859). If, however,

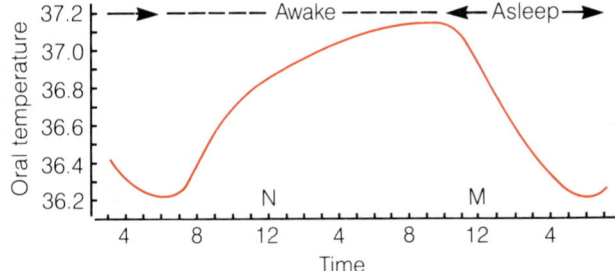

Figure 18–3 Range of oral temperature during 24 hours for a healthy young adult.

the air is 100% humidified or if the body is in water, the body temperature begins to rise whenever the environmental temperature rises above approximately 94 F. If the person is performing very heavy work, this critical temperature level may be as low as 85 to 90 F (Guyton 1986, p. 859).

Alterations in Body Temperature

Pyrexia   A body temperature above the usual range is called **pyrexia, hyperthermia,** or (in lay terms) **fever.** A very high fever, e.g., 41 C (105.8 F) is called **hyperpyrexia.** See Figure 18–4.

Four common types of fevers are intermittent, remittent, relapsing, and constant. During an **intermittent fever,** the body temperature alternates at regular intervals between periods of fever and periods of normal temperatures. During a **remittent fever,** a wide range of temperature fluctuations occurs over the 24-hour period, all of which are *above* normal. In a **relapsing fever,** short febrile periods of a few days are interspersed with periods of 1 or 2 days of normal temperature. During a **constant fever,** the body temperature fluctuates minimally but always remains elevated.

The clinical signs of fever vary with the onset, course, and abatement stages of the fever (see the accompanying box). These signs occur as a result of changes in the *set-*

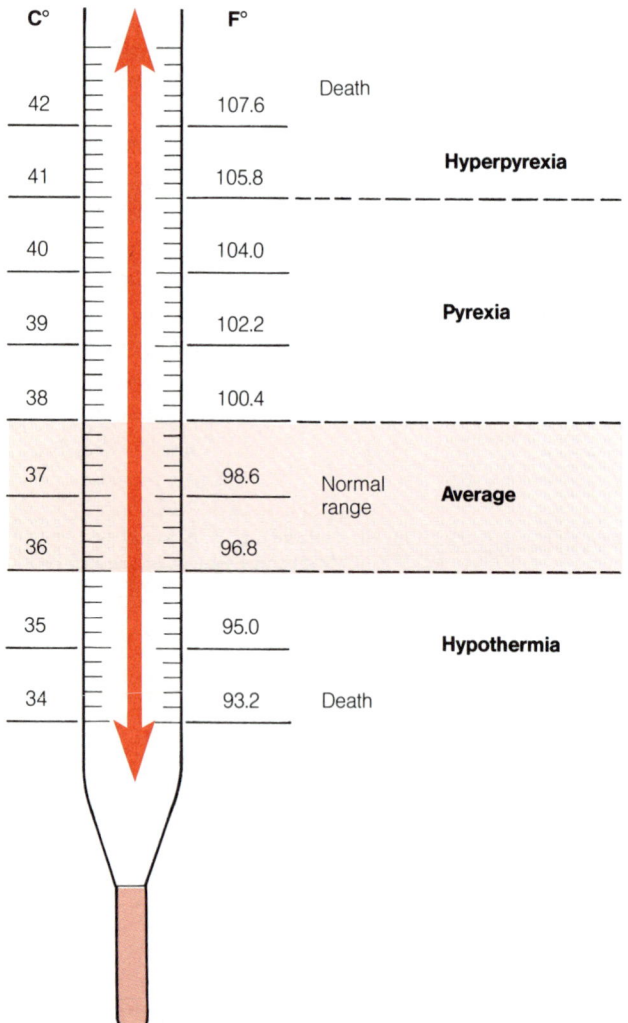

Figure 18–4   Terms used to describe alterations in body temperature (oral measurements).

Clinical Signs of Fever

Onset (cold or chill stage)

- Increased heart rate
- Increased respiratory rate and depth
- Shivering due to increased skeletal muscle tension and contractions
- Pallid, cold skin due to vasoconstriction
- Cyanotic nail beds due to vasoconstriction
- Complaints of feeling cold
- "Gooseflesh" appearance of the skin due to contraction of the arrector pili muscles
- Cessation of sweating
- Rise in body temperature

Course

- Absence of chills
- Skin that feels warm
- Feelings of being neither hot nor cold
- Increased pulse and respiratory rates
- Increased thirst
- Mild to severe dehydration
- Simple drowsiness, restlessness, or delirium and convulsions due to irritation of the nerve cells
- Herpetic lesions of the mouth
- Loss of appetite with prolonged fever
- Malaise, weakness, and aching muscles due to protein catabolism

Defervescence (fever abatement)

- Skin that appears flushed and feels warm
- Sweating
- Decreased shivering
- Possible dehydration

point of the temperature control mechanism regulated by the hypothalamus. Normally, the core temperature of the body is maintained at about 37 C (98.6 F), since the mechanisms of heat production and heat loss are continually being adjusted. Whenever the core temperature rises above 37 C, the rate of heat loss is greater than heat production, resulting in a fall in temperature toward the set-point level. Conversely, when the core temperature falls below 37 C, the rate of heat production is greater than heat loss, resulting in a rise in temperature toward the set-point.

In *pyrexic* conditions, however, the set-point of the hypothalamic thermostat changes suddenly from the normal level to a higher than normal value (e.g., 39.5 C) as a result of the effects of tissue destruction, pyrogenic substances, or dehydration on the hypothalamus. Although the set-point changes rapidly, the core body temperature, i.e., the blood temperature, reaches this new set-point only after several hours. During this interval, the usual heat production responses that cause elevation of the body temperature occur: chills, feeling of coldness, cold skin due to vasoconstriction, and shivering.

When the core temperature reaches the new set-point, the person feels neither cold nor hot and no longer experiences chills. Depending on the degree of temperature elevation, various other signs (shown in the box on page 326) may occur at this stage. Very high temperatures, such as 41–42 C (106–108 F), damage the parenchyma of cells throughout the body, particularly in the brain, where destruction of neuronal cells is irreversible. Damage to the liver, kidneys, and other body organs can be great enough to disrupt functioning and eventually cause death.

When the cause of the high temperature is suddenly removed, the set-point of the hypothalamic thermostat is suddenly reduced to a lower value, perhaps even back to the original normal level. In this instance, the hypothalamus now attempts to lower the temperature to 37 C, and the usual heat loss responses causing a reduction of the body temperature occur: excessive sweating and a hot, flushed skin due to sudden vasodilation. This sudden change of events is known as the **crisis** or the **flush** or the *defervescent stage* of a pyrexic condition. A more gradual return of the body temperature to normal is referred to as resolution of pyrexia by **lysis.**

Nursing interventions for a client who has a fever are designed to support the body's normal physiologic processes, provide comfort, and prevent complications. During the course of fever, the nurse needs to monitor the client's vital signs closely.

Nursing measures during the chill phase are designed to help the client decrease heat loss. At this time, the body's physiologic processes are attempting to raise the core temperature to the new set-point temperature. During the flush or crisis phase, the body processes are attempting to lower the core temperature to the reduced or normal temperature set-point. At this time, nursing measures are designed

Nursing Interventions for Clients with Fever

- Monitor vital signs.
- Assess skin color and temperature.
- Monitor white blood cell count, hematocrit value, and other pertinent laboratory records.
- Remove excess blankets when the client feels warm, but provide extra warmth when the client feels chilled.
- Provide adequate food and fluids (e.g., 2500–3000 ml per day) to meet the increased metabolic demands and prevent dehydration, if health permits. Clients who sweat profusely can become dehydrated.
- Measure intake and output.
- Maintain prescribed intravenous fluids.
- Reduce physical activity to limit heat production, especially during the flush stage.
- Administer antipyretics (drugs that reduce the level of fever) as ordered.
- Provide oral hygiene to keep the mucous membranes moist. They can become dry and cracked as a result of excessive fluid loss.
- Provide a tepid sponge bath to increase heat loss through conduction.
- Provide cool circulating air by using a fan to increase heat loss through convection.
- Provide dry clothing and bed linens to increase heat loss through conduction.

to increase heat loss and decrease heat production. Nursing interventions for a client with fever are shown in the box above.

Hypothermia   **Hypothermia** is a core body temperature below the lower limit of normal. The ability of the hypothalamus to regulate temperature is greatly impaired when the body temperature falls below 34.5 C (94 F), and death usually occurs when the temperature falls below 34 C (93.2 F). With severe hypothermia, the rate of heat production in each cell is reduced substantially. Sleepiness and even coma are likely to develop, which depress the activity of heat control mechanisms further and prevent shivering. Thus, the three physiologic mechanisms of hypothermia are (a) excessive heat loss, (b) inadequate heat production to counteract the heat loss, and (c) impaired hypothalamic thermoregulation.

The major clinical signs of hypothermia include the following:

- Decreased body temperature
- Severe shivering (initially)
- Feelings of cold and chills
- Pale, cool, waxy skin
- Hypotension
- Decreased urinary output
- Lack of muscle coordination
- Disorientation
- Drowsiness progressing to coma

Hypothermia may be accidental or induced. *Accidental hypothermia* can occur as a result of exposure to a cold environment, i.e., below 16 C (60.8 F) or from immersion in cold water. In elderly people, the problem can be compounded by a decreased metabolic rate and the use of sedatives, which depress the metabolic rate further. Management includes removing the client from the cold and rewarming the client's body. Methods of rewarming include the application of blankets for mild hypothermia and the application of a hyperthermia blanket (an electronically controlled blanket that provides a specified temperature) and warm intravenous fluids when the client has severe hypothermia. Wet clothing, which increases heat loss because of the high conductivity of water, should be replaced with dry clothing. In a person wearing wet clothes, the rate of heat loss increases as much as 20-fold (Guyton 1986, p. 852). Because rapid rewarming can cause vasodilation and subsequent additional heat loss, the client should be monitored closely, usually in an intensive care unit.

Induced hypothermia is the deliberate lowering of the body temperature to decrease the need for oxygen by the body tissues. Induced hypothermia can involve the whole body or a body part. It is sometimes indicated prior to surgery, e.g., cardiac and brain surgery.

Assessing Body Temperature

There are a number of methods of measuring body temperature. The three most common are oral, rectal, and axillary. Each of the sites has advantages and disadvantages. See Table 18–2. Since body heat is produced in the body's core

TABLE 18–2 *Advantages and Disadvantages of Three Sites for Body Temperature Measurement*

Site	Advantages	Disadvantages
Oral	Most accessible and convenient	Mercury-in-glass thermometers can be broken if bitten, thereby injuring the client. Therefore, it is contraindicated for infants, children under 6 years, and clients who are confused or who have convulsive disorders. Inaccurate if client has just eaten very hot or cold food or fluid or smoked.
		Inaccurate if client breathes through the mouth, therefore contraindicated for clients who have nasal surgery.
		Could injure the mouth following oral surgery.
Rectal	Most reliable measurement	Inconvenient and more unpleasant for clients; difficult for client who cannot turn to the side.
		Could injure the rectum following rectal surgery.
		Placement of the thermometer at different sites within the rectum yields different temperatures, yet placement at the same site each time is difficult.
		A rectal thermometer does not respond to changes in arterial temperatures as quickly as an oral thermometer, a fact that may be potentially dangerous for febrile clients, since misleading information may be acquired.
		Presence of stool may interfere with thermometer placement. If the stool is soft, the thermometer may be embedded in stool rather than against the wall of the rectum. If the stool is impacted, the depth of thermometer insertion may be insufficient.
		In newborns and infants, insertion of the rectal thermometer has resulted in ulcerations and rectal perforations. *Many agencies advise against using rectal thermometers on neonates.*
Axillary	Safest and most noninvasive	The thermometer must be left in place a long time to obtain an accurate measurement.

and because heat dissipates as it moves to the surface of the body, the surface of the body is cooler than the core. Among the common ways to assess temperature, the most accurate method (i.e., that best measures the core, rather than the surface, temperature) is the rectal method. In a resting adult, rectal temperature is slightly higher than the temperature of the arterial blood, about the same as the temperature of the liver, and slightly lower than that of the brain. When measured in the axilla or orally (by mouth), the temperature is about 0.65 C (1 F) less than the rectal temperature.

The body temperature is usually measured *orally*. This method reflects changing body temperature more quickly than the rectal method (Blainey 1974, p. 1861). Traditionally, the oral method was not used for clients receiving oxygen, since the accuracy of the measurement was considered questionable. Recent evidence, however, suggests that oral readings are accurate in clients receiving oxygen by nasal cannula, aerosol mask, Venturi mask, and nasal prongs (Graas 1974, p. 1863; Hasler and Cohen 1982, p. 265). Before taking a temperature orally, nurses should wait 30 minutes if a client has been taking cold or hot food or fluids or smoking to ensure that the temperature of the mouth is not affected by the temperature of the food, fluid, or warm smoke (Erickson 1980, p. 164).

Rectal temperature readings are considered to be the most accurate. In some agencies, taking temperatures rectally is contraindicated for clients with myocardial infarction. It is believed that inserting a rectal thermometer can produce vagal stimulation, which in turn can cause myocardial damage. Recent research, however, indicates that the rectal method has no deleterious effects on the heart (Creative Care Unit 1977, p. 997).

Although the *axillary* temperature was considered less accurate than the rectal or oral method, studies now indicate that there is no clinically important difference in accuracy between axillary and rectal temperatures (Axillary temps safer 1978, p. 1081; Eoff and Joyce 1981, p. 1011; Schiffman 1982, p. 274). The axilla is therefore the preferred site for temperature measurements in children, not only because it is easily accessible but also because there is less likelihood of rectal perforation and subsequent peritonitis (Axillary temps safer 1978, p. 1081; Eoff and Joyce 1981, p. 1010). Clients for whom the axillary method of temperature assessment is appropriate include newborns and infants, toddlers and preschoolers, clients with oral inflammation or wired jaws, clients recovering from oral surgery, clients who are breathing through their mouths (e.g., following nasal surgery), irrational clients, and clients for whom oral and rectal temperatures are contraindicated.

Types of Thermometers

Traditionally, body temperatures have been measured using *mercury-in-glass thermometers*. Oral thermometers may have long slender tips, short rounded tips, or pear-shaped tips. See Figure 18–5. The rounded thermometer can be used at the rectal as well

CENTIGRADE

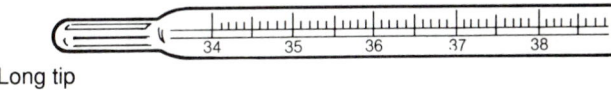

Long tip

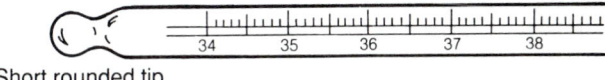

Short rounded tip

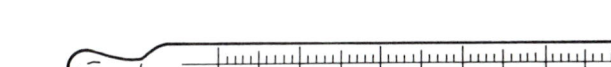

Pear-shaped tip

Figure 18–5 Three types of thermometer tips.

as other sites. In some agencies, thermometers may be color coded; for example, blue-colored thermometers may be used for rectal temperatures and silver-colored ones for oral and axillary temperatures. *Disposable thermometers* are also manufactured; these are used only once.

Electronic thermometers offer another method of assessing body temperatures. They can provide a reading in only 2 to 60 seconds, depending on the model. The equipment consists of a battery-operated portable electronic unit, a probe that the nurse attaches to the unit, and a probe cover, which is usually disposable. See Figure 18–6. Some models

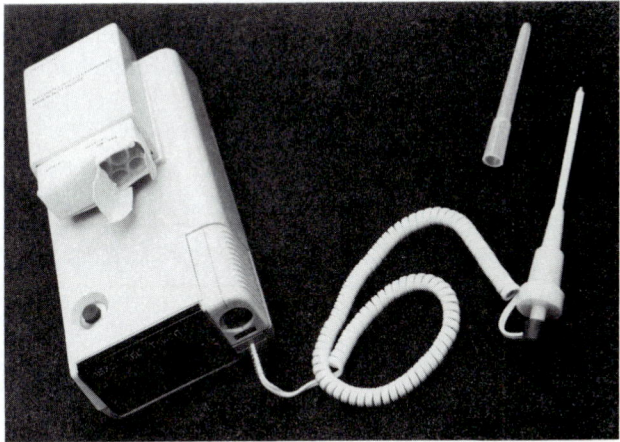

Figure 18–6 An electronic thermometer. Note the probe and the probe cover beside it.

have a different circuit for each method of measurement, and the nurse needs to make sure that the correct circuit is switched on before taking the temperature.

Chemical disposable thermometers are also used to measure body temperatures. They come in individual cases and are discarded after use. One type has small chemical dots at one end that respond to body heat by changing color, thereby providing a reading of the body temperature. The thermometer comes in a plastic case. To activate the chemicals, nurses hold the thermometer with the handle toward themselves, move the handle up and down, and then pull the plastic straight off the thermometer. The thermometer is inserted under the client's tongue, in the same way as a glass thermometer, and left in place for the time recommended by the manufacturer (e.g., 45 seconds). After it is removed, the dots are observed for a change in color. To read the temperature, the nurse notes the highest reading among the dots that have changed color. See Figure 18–7. The chemical thermometer is discarded after use.

Temperature-sensitive tape may also be used to obtain a general indication of body surface temperature. When applied to the skin, usually of the forehead or abdomen, the tape responds by changing color. The skin area should be dry. After the length of time specified by the manufacturer (e.g., 15 seconds), a color appears on the tape. The tape is removed and discarded after the color has been compared to the scale provided by the manufacturer. This method is particularly useful at home and for infants whose temperatures are to be monitored for any reason.

Temperature Scales

The body temperature is measured in degrees on two scales: Celsius and Fahrenheit. A common type of thermometer is a glass tube with a column of mercury inside it. Heat expands the mercury, thus expanding the column along the tube, where it can be measured against marked calibrations. The Celsius scale normally extends from 34.0 to 42.0 C. The Fahrenheit scale usually extends from 94 to 108 F. See Figure 18–8. Body temperatures rarely extend beyond these scales.

Sometimes a nurse needs to convert a Celsius reading to Fahrenheit, or vice versa. To convert from Fahrenheit to

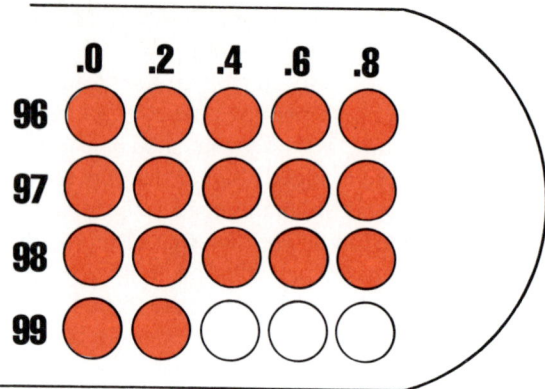

Figure 18–7 A chemical thermometer showing a reading of 99.2 F.

Celsius, deduct 32 from the Fahrenheit reading and then multiply by the fraction 5/9; that is:

$$C = (\text{Fahrenheit temperature} - 32) \times 5/9$$

For example, when the Fahrenheit reading is 100:

$$
\begin{aligned}
C &= (100 - 32) \times 5/9 \\
&= (68) \times 5/9 \\
&= 37.7
\end{aligned}
$$

To convert from Celsius to Fahrenheit, multiply the Celsius reading by the fraction 9/5 and then add 32; that is:

$$F = (\text{Celsius temperature} \times 9/5) + 32$$

For example, when the Celsius reading is 40:

$$
\begin{aligned}
F &= (40 \times 9/5) + 32 \\
&= (72) + 32 \\
&= 104
\end{aligned}
$$

Procedure 18–1 explains how to measure body temperature.

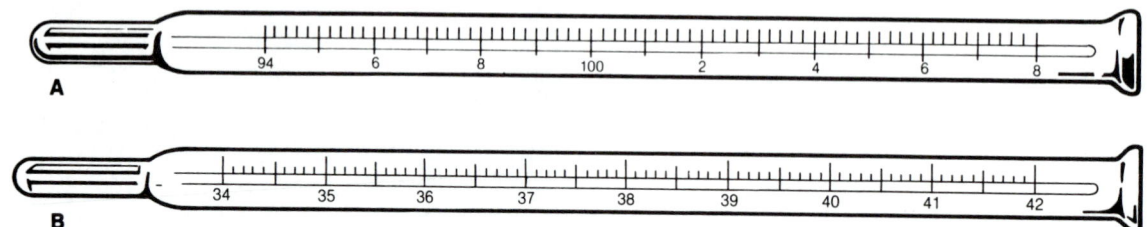

Figure 18–8 Thermometers. The upper one shows the Fahrenheit scale; the lower one, the Celsius (centigrade) scale.

PROCEDURE 18–1*

ASSESSING BODY TEMPERATURE USING A MERCURY THERMOMETER

Equipment ☑

Oral, rectal, or axillary thermometer

Towel if the axillary site is being used

Lubricant if the rectal site is being used

Disposable gloves

Intervention

1. **Assess the client.**

■ Note signs of hypothermia or hyperthermia (other than body temperature) (see page 326).

2. **Prepare the client.**

■ Ascertain which method of taking the temperature is appropriate.

For an oral temperature:

■ Determine the time the client last took hot or cold food or fluids or smoked. *To obtain an accurate oral temperature reading, it is recommended that you allow at least 15 minutes to elapse between a client's intake or smoking and the measurement* (Blainey 1974, p. 1861).

For a rectal temperature:

■ Assist the client to assume a lateral position. A newborn may be placed in a lateral or prone position (Axillary temps safer in infants 1978, p. 1081).

■ Provide privacy before folding the bedclothes back to expose the buttocks. *Privacy is essential, since exposure of the buttocks embarrasses most people.*

For an axillary temperature:

■ Expose the client's axilla. If the axilla is moist, dry it with the towel, using a patting motion. *Friction created by rubbing can raise the temperature of the axilla.*

3. **Prepare the equipment.**

■ Remove the thermometer from its package, and check the temperature reading on the thermometer.

■ Shake down the mercury (if necessary) by holding the thermometer between the thumb and forefinger at the end farthest from the bulb. Snap the wrist downward.

■ Repeat until the mercury is below 35 C (95 F).

4. **Take the temperature.**

For an oral temperature:

■ Place the thermometer or probe at the base of the tongue to the right or left of the frenulum (posterior sublingual pocket). See Figure 18–9. *The thermometer needs to reflect the core temperature of the blood in the larger blood vessels of the posterior pocket.*

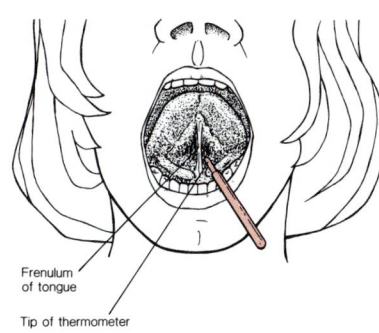

Frenulum of tongue

Tip of thermometer

Figure 18–9 The tip of an oral thermometer is placed beside the frenulum.

■ Ask the client to close the lips, not the teeth, around the thermometer. *A client who bites the thermometer can break it and injure the mouth.*

■ Leave the thermometer in place a sufficient time for the temperature

to register or for the length of time recommended by the agency. The recommended time is 2 minutes (Baker et al 1984, p. 111) or 3 minutes (Graves and Markarian 1980, p. 323). If an electronic oral thermometer is used, the client holds the thermometer under the tongue 10–20 seconds or until it completes registering.

For a rectal temperature:

■ Place some lubricant on a piece of tissue. Then apply lubricant to the thermometer about 2.5 cm (1 in) above the bulb. *The lubricant facilitates insertion of the thermometer without irritating the mucous membrane.*

■ Don a disposable glove on the dominant hand. With your nondominant hand, raise the client's upper buttock to expose the anus.

■ Ask the client to take a deep breath, and insert the thermometer into the anus anywhere from 1.5–4 cm (0.5–1.5 in.), depending on the age and size of the client (for example, 1.5 cm [0.5 in.] for an infant, 2.5 cm [0.9 in.] for a child, and 3.7 cm [1.4 in.] for an adult). *Taking a deep breath often relaxes the external sphincter muscle, thus easing insertion.*

■ Do not *force* insertion of the thermometer. *Inability to insert the thermometer into a newborn could indicate the rectum is not patent.*

■ Hold the thermometer in place for 2 minutes (Nichols 1972, p. 1093) or for the length of time recommended by the agency. For neonates hold the thermometer in place for 5 minutes (Schiffman 1982, p. 276). *The thermometer may become displaced inside or outside of the anus if not held in place.*

---

*See the *Guide to Required Nursing Actions* on page xxx for preliminary steps required for all procedures in this text.

For an axillary temperature:

■ Place the thermometer in the client's axilla. See Figure 18–10.

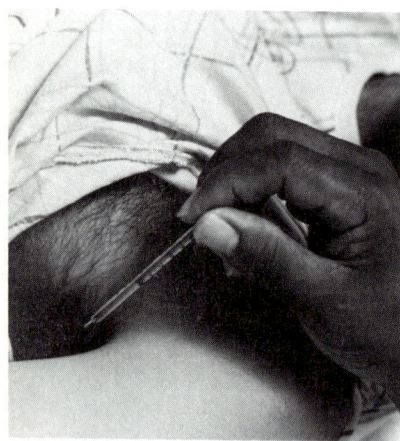

Figure 18–10 The bulb of the thermometer is placed in the center of the axilla.

■ Assist the client to place the arm tightly across the chest to keep the thermometer in place.

■ Leave the thermometer in place for 9 minutes (Nichols et al 1966, p. 310). For infants and children, leave the thermometer in place 5 minutes (Eoff and Joyce 1981, p. 1011).

■ Remain with the client and hold the thermometer in place if the client is irrational or very young.

5. **Remove the thermometer.**

■ Remove the plastic sheath, or wipe the thermometer with a tissue. Start at the end held by you, and wipe in a rotating manner toward the bulb. *The thermometer is wiped from the area of least contamination to that of greatest contamination.*

■ Discard the tissue in a receptacle used for contaminated items.

6. **Read the temperature.**

■ Hold the thermometer at eye level, and rotate it until the mercury column is clearly visible. The upper end of the mercury column registers the client's body temperature. On the Fahrenheit thermometer, each long line reflects 1 degree and each short line 0.2 degree. On the centigrade thermometer, each long line reflects 0.5 degree and each short line 0.1 degree.

7. **Clean and shake down the thermometer.**

■ Wash the thermometer in tepid, soapy water. Organic material such as mucus must be removed before the thermometer is stored. *Organic materials on the thermometer can harbor microorganisms.*

■ Rinse it in *cold* water, dry it, and store it dry. *Cold water is used because hot water expands the mercury and may break the thermometer.*

■ Shake down the thermometer and return it to its container or discard it. Some agencies also have special equipment for spinning down the mercury levels.

■ If the thermometer is to be disinfected before storage, use isopropyl alcohol 70%.

■ Return an electronic thermometer to the battery base for recharging.

8. **Document the temperature.**

■ Record the temperature to the nearest indicated tenth (for example, 98.4 F, 37.1 C) on a flowsheet or in a notebook. *Recording the temperature immediately ensures it is not forgotten.*

Variation: Using an Electronic Thermometer

■ Remove the electronic unit from the battery charging area.

■ Remove the temperature probe from the unit. If the probe is not attached, attach it to the appropriate circuit (oral, rectal, or axillary) in models that have separate circuits for each.

■ Place a disposable cover securely on the probe.

■ Warm up the machine by switching it on if removal of the probe does not automatically prepare the machine for functioning.

■ Take the temperature as indicated above in step 4.

■ Listen for a sound indicating that the maximum measurement has been reached and read the temperature on the dial or readout.

■ Remove the thermometer.

■ Remove and discard the probe cover.

Identifying Clients at Risk for Altered Body Temperature

The nursing assessment should include identifying individuals at risk for alterations in body temperature, as well as the clinical signs of specific conditions and the defining characteristics of possible nursing diagnoses. See the accompanying box.

Relationship of Vital Signs to Nursing Diagnoses

Abnormalities in specific measurements of vital signs are the defining characteristics of several NANDA nursing diagnostic categories in addition to the diagnostic categories discussed below. See Table 18–3.

There are currently four accepted NANDA diagnostic categories concerning body temperature that reflect clients' actual and potential health problems. These are **Potential altered body temperature, Hyperthermia, Hypothermia,** and **Ineffective thermoregulation. Potential altered body temperature** is the state in which an individual is at risk for failure to maintain body temperature within normal range (Kim, McFarland, and McLane 1989, p. 7) due to internal factors such as the effects of disease and/or injury to the individual. Although modifying the causative factors is a medical responsibility (i.e., the physician orders measures to modify the internal factor causing the alteration in body temperature), the nurse is responsible

---

Clients at Risk for Hypothermia and Hyperthermia

People at risk for **hypothermia:**

- People who participate in cold-weather sports, e.g., skiing and mountain climbing
- Infants and children whose thermoregulatory systems are immature
- Elderly people who have insufficient food, clothing, or fuel
- People who have neurologic deficits and are unable to identify or respond to cold
- Alcoholics who have extreme heat loss secondary to vasodilation
- "Street people" who lack adequate clothing and shelter

People at risk for **hyperthermia:**

- People who have an infection
- Debilitated clients who are vulnerable to infection
- People with disease processes of the central nervous system that may impair thermoregulation
- People who have head trauma causing increased intracranial pressure
- Neonates who have ineffective thermoregulation

TABLE 18–3 *Variations in Vital Signs Associated With NANDA Diagnoses*

Diagnostic Category	Variations in Vital Sign(s)	Diagnostic Category	Variations in Vital Sign(s)
Activity intolerance	Abnormal heart rate or blood pressure response to activity	**Fear**	Cardiovascular excitation
Ineffective airway clearance	Changes in rate or depth of respiration Tachypnea	**Fluid volume excess**	Change in respiratory pattern Blood pressure changes
Anxiety	Cardiovascular excitation	**Pain**	Blood pressure and pulse rate changes Increased or decreased respiratory rate
Ineffective breathing pattern	Tachypnea Respiratory depth changes	**Altered tissue perfusion**	Diminished arterial pulsations Blood pressure changes in extremities
Decreased cardiac output	Arrhythmias Decreased peripheral pulses		
Ineffective individual coping	High blood pressure		
Dysreflexia	Paroxysmal hypertension Bradycardia or tachycardia		

for maintaining comfort, hydration, and nutrition appropriate for the individual client (Carpenito 1989, p. 147).

The remaining three nursing diagnoses reflect changes in body temperature in response to external factors such as the environment. **Hyperthermia** is the state in which body temperature is elevated above the individual's normal range, i.e., greater than 37.8 C (100 F) orally or 38 C (100.5 F) rectally. **Hypothermia** is the state in which body temperature is reduced below the individual's normal range but not below a rectal temperature of 35.6 C (96 F) in adults and children and 36.4 C (97.5 F) in newborns (Kim, McFarland, and McLane 1989, p. 33). **Ineffective thermoregulation** exists when the client's temperature fluctuates between hyperthermia and hypothermia (Kim, McFarland, and McLane 1989, p. 64). The major nursing responsibility to clients with any of these three diagnoses related to external factors is modifying or controlling the causative factor or factors. Both hyperthermia and hypothermia, if not treated promptly, can result in medical emergencies; therefore, the nursing focus is often on prevention of these conditions in clients known to be at risk. The diagnoses are often recorded on the nursing care plan as **Potential hyperthermia** or **Potential hypothermia** (Carpenito 1989, p. 150). Examples of nursing diagnoses and contributing factors for clients with various alterations in body temperature follow. Examples of assessment data clusters and related nursing diagnoses are shown in Table 18–4.

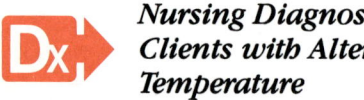

Nursing Diagnoses
Clients with Altered Body
Temperature

Potential altered body temperature related to:

- Illness or trauma affecting temperature regulation
- Medication causing vasoconstriction, vasodilation, altered metabolic state, or sedation
- Inactivity or vigorous activity

Hyperthermia related to:

- Exposure to excessively hot environment
- Increased metabolic rate
- Dehydration

Hypothermia related to:

- Exposure to excessively cool environment
- Debilitating illness or trauma
- Lack of adequate clothing and shelter

Ineffective thermoregulation related to:

- Decreased basal metabolism secondary to aging
- Trauma or illness

TABLE 18–4 *Examples of Assessment Data Clusters and Related Nursing Diagnoses*

Data Cluster	Nursing Diagnosis
Tommy Jones, aged 3, was admitted to hospital with pyrexia of unknown origin. T, 39.8 C (104 F), P, 118; and R, 24. Skin is dry, flushed, and warm to touch. Mother reports he has been vomiting, has not been able to tolerate food or fluids for 48 hours, has become increasingly listless, and has had all required immunizations.	**Hyperthermia** related to illness not yet diagnosed and to dehydration.
Mickey Finn, aged 71, was brought to a homeless shelter by two other street people. T, 35.8 C (96.7 F), P, 122; and R, 20 and shallow; skin is pale and cool; nail beds are cyanotic. Friends state he is an alcoholic who sleeps under a viaduct but has little warm clothing or bedding for this cold winter climate.	**Hypothermia** related to exposure to cold environment and consumption of alcohol.

PULSE

The **pulse** is a wave of blood created by contraction of the left ventricle of the heart. The heart is a pulsatile pump, and the blood enters the arteries with each heartbeat, causing pressure pulses or pulse waves (Guyton 1986, p. 225). Generally, the pulse wave represents the stroke volume output and the compliance of the arteries. **Stroke volume output** is the amount of blood that enters the arteries with each ventricular contraction. Normally the heart empties about 70% of its volume with each contraction, i.e., about 70 ml of blood in a healthy adult (Guyton 1986, p. 155). **Compliance** of the arteries is the distensibility of the arteries, i.e., their ability to contract and expand. When a person's arteries lose their distensibility, as can happen in old age, greater pressure is required to pump the blood into the arteries.

When an adult is resting, the heart pumps 4 to 6 liters of blood each minute. This volume is called the **cardiac output**. The cardiac output (CO) is the result of the stroke volume (SV) times the heart rate (HR) per minute:

$$CO = SV \times HR$$

In a healthy person, the pulse reflects the heartbeat, i.e., the pulse rate is the same as the rate of the ventricular contractions of the heart. However, in some types of cardiovascular disease the heartbeat and pulse rates can differ. For example, a client's heart may produce very weak or small pulse waves that are not detectable in a peripheral pulse. In these instances, the nurse should assess the heartbeat *and* the peripheral pulse. See the section on assessing the apical pulse, later in this chapter. A **peripheral pulse** is a pulse located in the periphery of the body, e.g., in the foot, hand, or neck. The **apical pulse,** in contrast, is a central pulse; i.e., it is located at the apex of the heart.

The pulse rate is regulated by the autonomic nervous system (ANS). Impulses pass through the parasympathetic branch to the sinoatrial node (SA node), which is the pacemaker of the heart. These impulses decrease the heart rate. When body demands indicate a need for an increased heart rate, the impulses of the parasympathetic system are inhibited and the impulses of the sympathetic system increase.

Factors Affecting Pulse Rate

The rate of the pulse is expressed in beats per minute. A pulse rate varies according to a number of factors. The nurse should consider each of the following factors when assessing a client's pulse:

- *Age.* As age increases, the pulse rate gradually decreases. See Table 18–1 for specific variations in pulse rates from birth to adulthood.

- *Sex.* After puberty, the average male's pulse rate is slightly lower than the female's.

- *Exercise.* The pulse rate normally increases with activity. The rate of increase in the professional athlete is often less than in the average person because of greater cardiac size, strength, and efficiency.

- *Fever.* The pulse rate increases (a) in response to the lowered blood pressure that results from peripheral vasodilation associated with elevated body temperature and (b) because of the increased metabolic rate.

- *Medications.* Some medications decrease the pulse rate, and others increase it. For example, cardiotonics (e.g., digitalis preparations) decrease the heart rate, whereas epinephrine increases it.

- *Hemorrhage.* Loss of blood from the vascular system (hemorrhage) normally increases pulse rate. The loss of a small amount of blood, e.g., 500 ml, as after a blood donation, results in a temporary adjustment of the heart rate as the body compensates for the lost blood volume. An adult has about 5 liters of blood in the system and can usually lose up to 10% without adverse effects.

- *Stress.* In response to stress, sympathetic nervous stimulation increases the overall activity of the heart. Stress increases the rate as well as the force of the heartbeat. Emotions such as fear and anxiety as well as the perception of severe pain stimulate the sympathetic system.

- *Position changes.* When a person assumes a sitting or

standing position, blood usually pools in dependent vessels of the venous system. Pooling results in a transient decrease in the venous blood return to the heart and a subsequent reduction in blood pressure. These changes are primarily mediated through the sympathetic nervous system, increasing cardiac rate, force of the ventricular contractions, and tone of the veins and arteries.

Pulse Sites

Nine of the sites where a pulse is commonly taken (see Figure 18–11) are the following:

1. *Temporal,* where the temporal artery passes over the

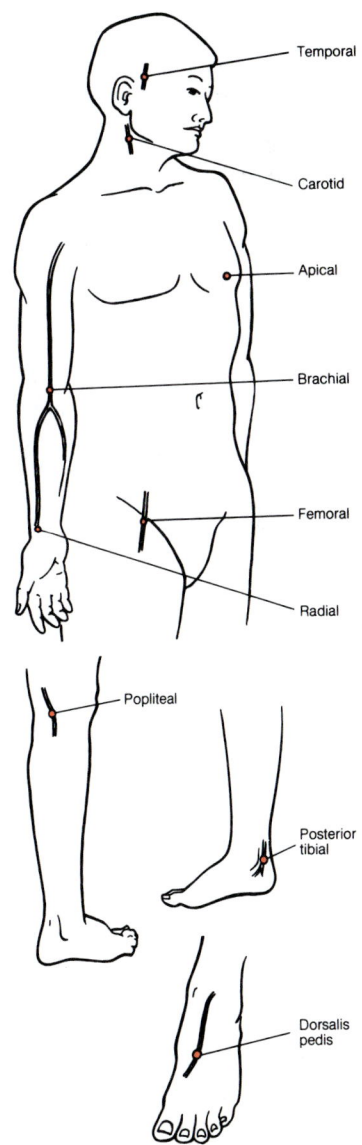

Figure 18–11 Nine sites commonly used for assessing a pulse.

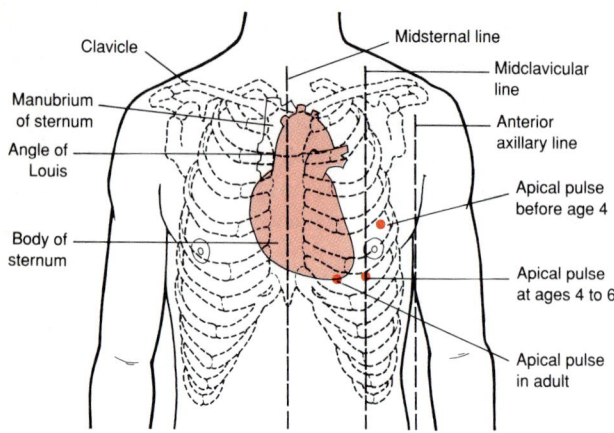

Clavicle
Manubrium of sternum
Angle of Louis
Body of sternum

Midsternal line
Midclavicular line
Anterior axillary line
Apical pulse before age 4
Apical pulse at ages 4 to 6
Apical pulse in adult

Figure 18–12 Location of the apical pulse for a child under 4 years, a child 4 to 6 years, and an adult.

temporal bone of the head. The site is superior (above) and lateral to (away from the midline of) the eye.

2. *Carotid,* at the side of the neck below the lobe of the ear, where the carotid artery runs between the trachea and the sternocleidomastoid muscle.

3. *Apical,* at the apex of the heart. In an adult this is located on the left side of the chest, no more than 8 cm (3 in) to the left of the sternum (breastbone) and under the fourth, fifth, or sixth intercostal space (area between the ribs). For a child 7 to 9 years of age, the apical pulse is located between the fourth and fifth intercostal spaces. Before 4 years of age it is left of the midclavicular line (MCL); between 4 and 6 years it is at the MCL. See Figure 18–12.

4. *Brachial,* at the inner aspect of the biceps muscle of the arm (especially in infants) or medially in the antecubital space (elbow crease).

5. *Radial,* where the radial artery runs along the radial bone, on the thumb side of the inner aspect of the wrist.

6. *Femoral,* where the femoral artery passes alongside the inguinal ligament.

7. *Popliteal,* where the popliteal artery passes behind the knee. This point is difficult to find, but it can be palpated if the client flexes the knee slightly. See also Figure 18–24, later in this chapter.

8. *Posterior tibial,* on the medial surface of the ankle where the posterior tibial artery passes behind the medial malleolus.

9. *Pedal (dorsalis pedis),* where the dorsalis pedis artery passes over the bones of the foot. This artery can be palpated by feeling the dorsum (upper surface) of the foot on an imaginary line drawn from the middle of the ankle to the space between the big and second toes.

The reasons for use of each site are given in Table 18–5. The radial site is most commonly used. It is easily found in most people and readily accessible.

TABLE 18–5 *Reasons for Using Specific Pulse Sites*

Pulse Site	Reasons for Use
Radial	Readily accessible and routinely used
Temporal	Used when radial pulse is not accessible
Carotid	Used for infants
	Used in cases of cardiac arrest
	Used to determine circulation to the brain
Apical	Routinely used for infants and children up to 3 years of age
	Used to determine discrepancies with radial pulse
	Used in conjunction with some medications
Brachial	Used to measure blood pressure
	Used during cardiac arrest for infants
Femoral	Used in cases of cardiac arrest
	Used for infants and children
	Used to determine circulation to a leg
Popliteal	Used to determine circulation to the lower leg
	Used to determine leg blood pressure
Posterial tibial	Used to determine circulation to the foot
Pedal	Used to determine circulation to the foot

Assessing the Pulse

A pulse is commonly assessed by palpation (feeling) or auscultation (hearing). The middle three fingertips are used for palpating all pulse sites except the apex of the heart. A stethoscope is used for assessing apical pulses and fetal heart tones. Increasingly, a Doppler ultrasound stethoscope (DUS; see Figure 18–13) is being used for pulses that are difficult to assess. The DUS headset has earpieces similar to standard stethoscope earpieces, but it has a long cord attached to a volume-controlled audio unit and an ultrasound transducer. The DUS detects movement of red blood cells through a blood vessel. In contrast to the conventional stethoscope, it excludes environmental sounds. The DUS can detect blood flow if the blood cells are moving faster than 6 cm per second and at a depth of about 5 cm (Hudson 1983, p. 55). It cannot detect blood flow in deep vessels or in those underlying bone, such as the vessels in the abdomen, thorax, or skull. The DUS is battery operated, and batteries must be replaced about every 6 months.

The cardiac monitoring machine is another device for assessing the apical pulse. It indicates the rate on a screen or readout graph.

A pulse is normally palpated by applying moderate pres-

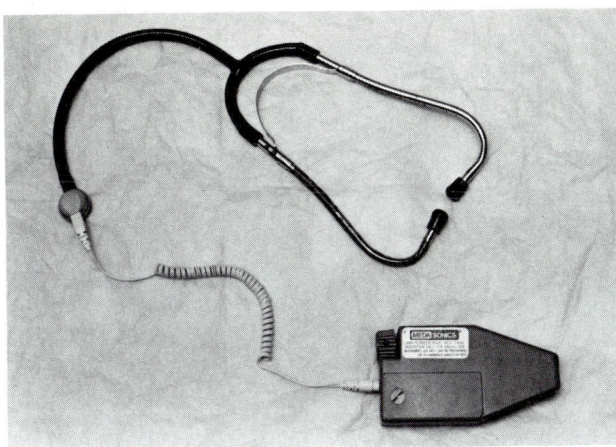

Figure 18–13 An ultrasound (Doppler) stethoscope.

sure with the three middle fingers of the hand. The pads on the most distal aspects of the finger are the most sensitive areas for detecting a pulse. With excessive pressure, one can obliterate a pulse, whereas with too little pressure, one may not be able to detect it. Before the nurse assesses the *resting* pulse, the client should assume a comfortable position. The nurse should also be aware of the following:

- Any medication that could affect the heart rate.

- Whether the client has been physically active. If so, wait 10 to 15 minutes until the client has rested and the pulse has slowed to its usual rate.

- Any baseline data about the normal heart rate for the client. For example, a physically fit athlete may have a heart rate below 60 beats per minute.

- Whether the client should assume a particular position, e.g., sitting. In some clients, the rate changes with the position because of changes in blood flow volume and autonomic nervous system activity.

When assessing the pulse, the nurse collects the following data: the rate, rhythm, volume, arterial wall elasticity, and presence or absence of bilateral equality. The *normal pulse rates* are shown in Table 18–1 on page 325. An excessively fast heart rate, e.g., over 100 beats per minute in an adult, is referred to as **tachycardia.** A heart rate in an adult of 60 beats per minute or less is called **bradycardia.** If a client has either tachycardia or bradycardia, the apical pulse should be assessed.

The **pulse rhythm** is the pattern of the beats and the intervals between the beats. Equal time elapses between beats of a normal pulse. A pulse with an irregular rhythm is referred to as a **dysrhythmia** or **arrhythmia.** It may consist of random, irregular beats or a predictable pattern of irregular beats. When a dysrhythmia is detected, the apical pulse should be assessed. An electrocardiogram (ECG or EKG) is necessary to define the dysrhythmia further.

Pulse volume, also called the pulse strength or amplitude, refers to the force of blood with each beat. Usually, pulse volume is the same with each beat. It can range from

absent to bounding. A normal pulse can be felt with moderate pressure of the fingers and can be obliterated with greater pressure. A forceful or full blood volume that is obliterated only with difficulty is called a *full* or *bounding* pulse. A pulse that is readily obliterated with pressure from the fingers is referred to as *weak, feeble,* or *thready.* A pulse volume is usually measured on a scale of 0 to 3. See Table 18–6.

The **elasticity of the arterial wall** reflects its expansibility or its deformities. A healthy, normal artery feels straight, smooth, soft, and pliable. Elderly people often have inelastic arteries that feel twisted (tortuous) and irregular upon palpation. The elasticity of the arteries may not affect the pulse rate, rhythm, or volume, but it does reflect the status of the client's vascular system.

When assessing a peripheral pulse to determine the adequacy of blood flow to a particular area of the body, the nurse should also assess the corresponding pulse on the other side of the body. The second assessment gives the nurse data with which to compare the pulses. For example, when assessing the blood flow to the right foot, the nurse assesses the right dorsalis pedis pulse and then the left dorsalis pedis pulse. If the client's right and left pulses are the same, the client's dorsalis pedis pulses are *bilaterally equal.*

TABLE 18–6 *Scale for Measuring Pulse Volume*

Scale	Description of Pulse
0	Absent, not discernible
1	Thready or weak, difficult to feel
2	Normal, detected readily, obliterated by strong pressure
3	Bounding, difficult to obliterate

Peripheral Pulse Assessment

A peripheral pulse, usually the radial pulse, is assessed by palpation for all individuals *except:*

- Newborns and children up to 2 or 3 years. Apical pulses are assessed in these clients.

- Very obese or elderly clients, whose radial pulse may be difficult to palpate. Doppler equipment may be used for these clients, or the apical pulse is assessed.

- Individuals with a heart disease, who require apical pulse assessment.

- Individuals in whom the circulation to a specific body part must be assessed; e.g., following leg surgery the pedal (dorsalis pedis) pulse is assessed.

Procedure 18–2 on the following page provides guidelines for assessing peripheral pulses.

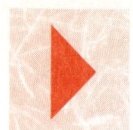

ASSESSING A PERIPHERAL PULSE

Equipment ☑

Watch with a second hand or indicator

If using Doppler ultrasound stethoscope, the transducer in the DUS probe, a stethoscope headset, and transmission gel. See Figure 18–13, earlier.

Intervention

1. **Assess the client.**

■ Ascertain the client's emotional status and activity level. *Emotion and activity, e.g., anxiety and exercise, can increase the pulse rate.*

■ Assess the color and warmth of a foot if taking a pedal pulse. *Color and warmth reflect the adequacy of the blood supply to the area.*

■ Assess the client for facial pallor and any cyanosis of the lips and nail beds. *These can reflect the adequacy of generalized blood flow.*

2. **Prepare the client.**

■ Select the pulse point. Normally, the radial pulse is taken, unless it cannot be exposed or circulation to another body area is to be assessed.

■ Assist the client to a comfortable resting position. When the radial pulse is assessed, the arm can rest alongside the client with the palm facing downward. Or, the forearm can rest at a 90° angle across the chest with the palm downward. For the client who can sit, the forearm can rest across the thigh with the palm of the hand facing downward or inward.

3. **Palpate and count the pulse.**

■ Place two or three middle fingertips lightly and squarely over the pulse point. See Figure 18–14.

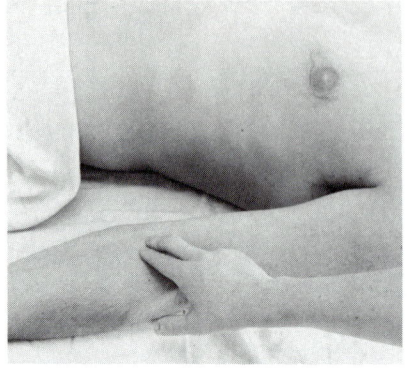
A

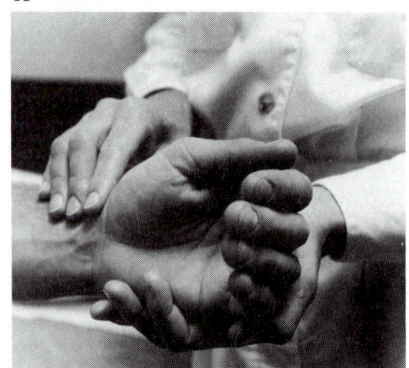
B

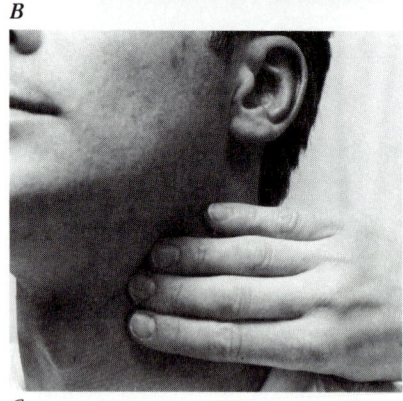
C

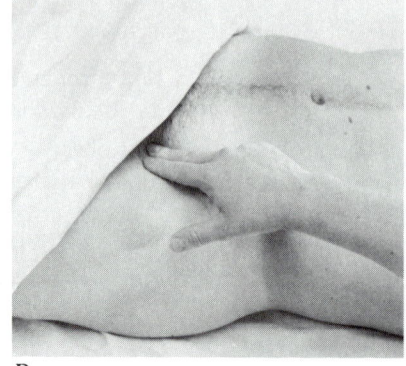
D

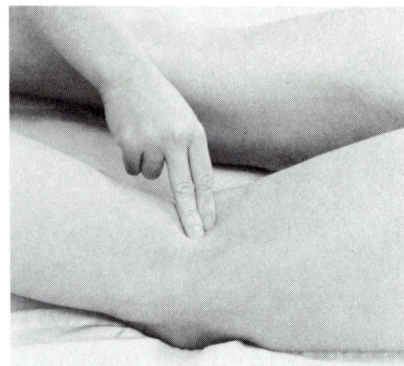
E

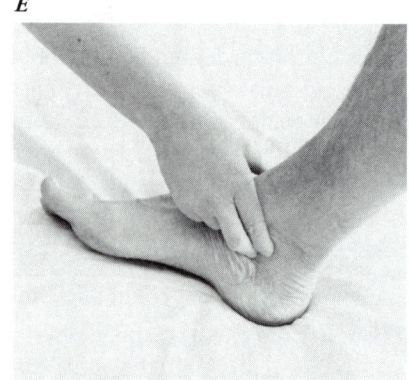
F

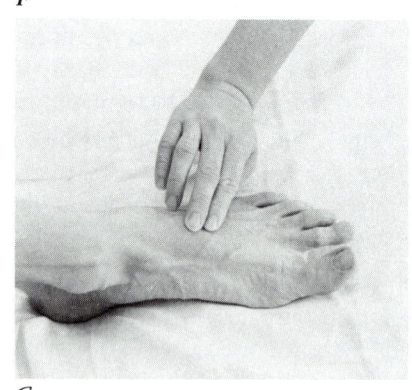
G

Figure 18–14 Assessing the pulses: *A,* brachial; *B,* radial; *C,* carotid; *D,* femoral; *E,* popliteal; *F,* posterior tibial; and *G,* pedal.

Using the thumb is contraindicated because the thumb has a pulse that the nurse could mistake for the client's pulse.

■ Count the pulse for 30 seconds and multiply by 2 if the pulse is regular. If it is irregular, count for 1 minute. If taking a client's pulse for the first time or when obtaining baseline data, count the pulse for a full minute. *An irregular pulse requires a full minute's count for a correct assessment.*

4. Assess the pulse rhythm and volume.

■ Assess the pulse rhythm by noting the pattern of intervals between the beats. A normal pulse has equal time periods between beats. If this is an initial assessment, assess for 1 minute.

■ Assess the pulse volume. A normal pulse can be felt with moderate pressure, and the pressure is equal with each beat. A forceful pulse volume is full; an easily obliterated pulse is weak.

5. Assess the arterial wall.

■ Compress the artery firmly and run a finger distal to the heart along the artery. See Figure 18–15. A normal arterial wall is smooth and straight.

6. Document and report pertinent assessment data.

■ Document the pulse rate, rhythm, and volume, and the condition of the arterial wall. See sample recording below.

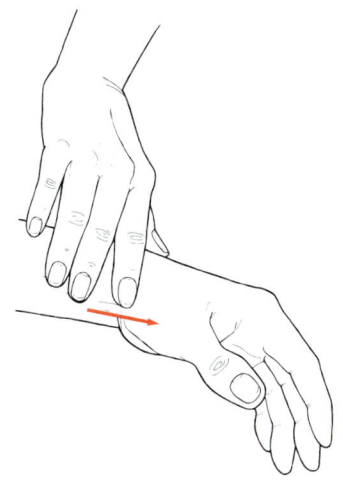

Figure 18–15 Assessing status of the arterial wall.

■ Report to the nurse in charge pertinent data such as (a) pale skin color and cool skin temperature, (b) a pulse rate faster or slower than normal for the client, (c) a full, bounding or weak pulse volume, (d) an irregular pulse rhythm, and (e) a tortuous arterial wall.

Sample Recording

Date 5/8/91	Time: 0900

Pale and listless. Pulse 116, weak and thready. Arterial wall feels soft and pliable. Reported above to Ms. N. McNamara.
———————— Sally M. Sahara, NS

Variation: Using a DUS

■ Plug the stethoscope headset into one of the two output jacks located next to the volume control. DUS units have jacks for two headpieces and accessory loudspeakers so that another person can listen to the signals.

■ Apply transmission gel either to the probe (a device resembling a small transistor radio), at the narrow end of the plastic case housing the transducer, or to the client's skin. *Ultrasound beams do not travel well through air. The gel makes an airtight seal, which promotes optimal ultrasound wave transmission.*

■ Press the "on" button.

■ Hold the probe at a 45° angle against the skin over the pulse site. Use a light pressure, and keep the probe in contact with the skin. *Too much pressure can stop the blood flow and obliterate the signal.*

■ Distinguish between artery and vein sounds. The artery sound (signal) is distinctively pulsating and has a pumping quality. The venous sound is like the wind, is intermittent, and varies with respirations. *Both artery and vein sounds are heard simultaneously through the DUS, since major arteries and veins are situated close together throughout the body.*

■ If you have difficulty hearing arterial sounds, reposition the probe.

■ After assessing the pulse, remove all the gel from the probe to prevent damage to its surface. Clean the transducer with aqueous solutions. *Alcohol or other disinfectants may damage the face of the transducer.* Remove all gel from the client (Hudson 1983, p. 56).

Apical Pulse Assessment

Assessment of the apical pulse is indicated for clients whose peripheral pulse is irregular as well as for clients with known cardiovascular, pulmonary, and renal diseases. It is commonly assessed prior to administering medications that affect heart rate. The apical site is also used to assess the pulse for newborns, infants, and children up to 2–3 years old. Procedure 18–3 presents guidelines for assessing the apical pulse.

Apical-Radial Pulse Assessment

An **apical-radial pulse** may need to be assessed for clients with certain cardiovascular disorders. Normally, the apical and radial rates are identical. An apical pulse rate greater than a radial pulse rate can indicate that the thrust of the blood from the heart is too feeble for the wave to be felt at the peripheral pulse site, or it can indicate that vascular disease is preventing impulses from being transmitted. Any discrepancy between the two pulse rates needs to be reported promptly. In no instance is the radial pulse greater than the apical pulse.

An apical-radial pulse can be taken by two nurses or one nurse, although the two-nurse technique may be more accurate. In the two-nurse technique, one nurse counts the radial pulse at exactly the same time as the other nurse counts the apical beat. The nurse who is assessing the radial pulse often holds the watch and indicates when they should start counting. In the one-nurse technique, the nurse first assesses the apical pulse for 60 seconds and then assesses the radial pulse for 60 seconds.

PROCEDURE 18–3

ASSESSING AN APICAL PULSE

Equipment ☑

Watch with a second hand or indicator

Stethoscope with a bell-shaped or flat-disc diaphragm. See Figure 18–16.

Antiseptic wipes

If using ultrasound, a DUS, probe (transducer), and transmission gel.

Intervention

1. **Assess the client.**

- Assess the client for skin pallor and cyanosis of the lips or nail beds and for dyspnea and restlessness. *Pallor and/or cyanosis and dyspnea can reflect circulatory problems.*

- Assess the emotional status of the client. *Emotions such as anxiety can affect the cardiac rate.*

2. **Position the client appropriately.**

- Assist an adult or young child to a comfortable supine position with the head of the bed elevated or to

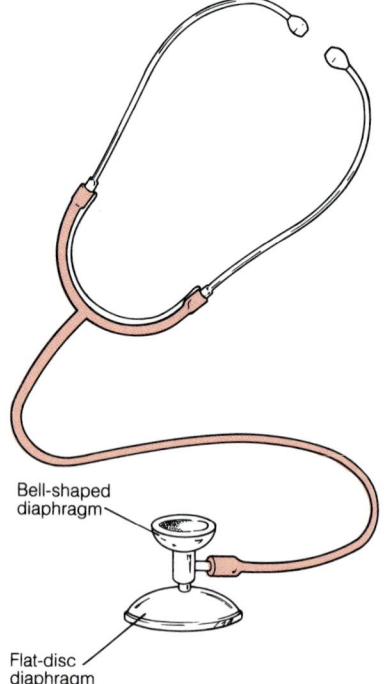

Figure 18–16 A stethoscope with both bell-shaped and flat-disc diaphragms.

Bell-shaped diaphragm

Flat-disc diaphragm

a sitting position on a chair, the edge of the bed, or the examination table.

- Place a baby in a supine position, and offer a pacifier if the baby is crying or restless. *Crying and physical activity increase the pulse rate.* For this reason, the nurse also takes the apical pulse rate of infants and small children before assessing body temperature.

- Expose the area of the chest over the apex of the heart.

3. **Locate the apical impulse.**

- This is the point over the apex of the heart where the apical pulse can be most clearly heard. It is also referred to as the point of maximal impulse (PMI). In 50% of the adult population, the apical impulse can be palpated (Malasanos et al. 1990, p. 337).

- Palpate the angle of Louis (the angle between the manubrium and the body of the sternum). It is palpated just below the suprasternal notch and is felt as a prominence. See Figure 18–12, earlier.

■ Place your index finger just to the left of the client's sternum and palpate the second intercostal space.

■ Place your middle or next finger in the third intercostal space and continue palpating downward until you locate apical impulse, usually about the fifth intercostal space, if the client is an adult or a child 7 years or older. If the client is a young child, palpate downward to the fourth intercostal space. *The apex of the heart is normally located in the fifth intercostal space, in individuals who are 7 years of age and over; it is in the fourth intercostal space in young children and one or two spaces above the adult apex during infancy* (Malasanos et al. 1990, p. 627).

■ Palpate the apical impulse. For an adult move your index finger laterally along the fifth intercostal space to the MCL. Normally, the apical impulse is palpable at or just medial to the MCL. For a young child move your finger along the fourth intercostal space to a position between the MCL and the anterior axillary line. See Figure 18–12, earlier.

4. Auscultate and count the heartbeats.

■ Use antiseptic wipes to clean the earpieces and diaphragm of the stethoscope if their cleanliness is in doubt. The diaphragm needs to be cleaned and disinfected if soiled with body substances.

■ Warm the diaphragm of the stethoscope by holding it in the palm of the hand for a moment. *The metal of the diaphragm is usually cold and can startle the client when placed immediately on the chest.*

■ Insert the earpieces of the stethoscope into your ears. The earpieces may be straight or bent. If they are bent, place them in the direction of the ear canals, slightly forward, to facilitate hearing.

■ Place the diaphragm of the stethoscope over the apical impulse and listen for the normal S_1 and S_2 heart sounds, which are heard as "lub dub." Each lub dub is counted as one heartbeat. *The heartbeat is normally loudest over the apex of the heart. The two heart sounds are produced by closure of the valves of the heart.* The S_1 heart sound, heard as lub, occurs when the atrioventricular valves close after the ventricles have been sufficiently filled. The S_2 heart sound, heard as dub, occurs when the semilunar valves close after the ventricles empty.

■ Count the heartbeats for 30 seconds and multiply by 2 if the rhythm is regular; count the beats for 60 seconds if the rhythm is irregular or if the apical impulse is being taken on an infant or child. *A 60-second count provides a more accurate assessment of an irregular pulse than a 30-second count.*

5. Assess the rhythm and the strength of the heartbeat.

■ Assess the rhythm of the heartbeat by noting the pattern of intervals between the beats. A normal pulse has equal time periods between beats.

■ Assess the strength (volume) of the heartbeat. Normally, the heartbeats are equal in strength and can be described as strong or weak.

6. Document and report pertinent assessment data.

■ Record the pulse site, rate, rhythm, and volume. See sample recording below.

■ Report to the nurse in charge pertinent data such as pallor, cyanosis, dyspnea, tachycardia, bradycardia, irregular rhythm, and reduced strength of the heartbeat.

Sample Recording

Date 1/26/91	Time: 0900

Apical pulse 56. Beats strong and equal. Digitoxin withheld. Notified Ms. S. Santos, RN. ——————Thomas A. Jones, NS

RESPIRATIONS

Respiration is the act of breathing; it includes the intake of oxygen and the output of carbon dioxide. Reference is often made to **external respiration** and **internal respiration.** The former refers to the interchange of oxygen and carbon dioxide between the alveoli of the lungs and the pulmonary blood. Internal respiration, by contrast, takes place throughout the body; it is the interchange of these same gases between the circulating blood and the cells of the body tissues.

The term **inhalation** or **inspiration** refers to the intake of air into the lungs. **Exhalation** or **expiration** refers to breathing out or the movement of gases from the lungs to the atmosphere. **Ventilation** is another word that is used to refer to the movement of air in and out of the lungs. **Hyperventilation** refers to very deep, rapid respirations; **hypoventilation** refers to very shallow respirations.

There are basically two types of breathing that nurses observe, **costal** (thoracic) breathing and **diaphragmatic** (abdominal) breathing. Costal breathing involves chiefly the external intercostal muscles and other accessory muscles, such as the sternocleidomastoid muscles. It can be observed by the movement of the chest upward and outward. By contrast, diaphragmatic breathing chiefly involves the contraction and relaxation of the diaphragm, and it is observed by the movement of the abdomen, which occurs as a result of the diaphragm's contraction and downward movement.

Mechanics and Control of Breathing

Respiration includes the intake of oxygen and the output of carbon dioxide. During *inhalation* the following processes normally occur (see Figure 18–17): The diaphragm contracts (flattens), the ribs move upward and outward, and the sternum moves outward, thus enlarging the thorax and permitting the lungs to expand. During *exhalation* (see Figure 18–18), the diaphragm relaxes (its curvature increases), the ribs move downward and inward, and the sternum moves inward, thus decreasing the size of the thorax as the lungs are compressed. Breathing is normally carried out automatically and effortlessly. Normal breathing is called **eupnea.** An inspiration normally lasts 1 to 1.5 seconds, and an expiration lasts 2 to 3 seconds.

Respiration is controlled by (a) respiratory centers in the medulla oblongata and the pons of the brain and (b) by chemoreceptors located centrally in the medulla and peripherally in the carotid and aortic bodies. These centers and receptors respond to changes in the concentrations of oxygen (O_2), carbon dioxide (CO_2) and hydrogen (H^+) in the arterial blood. See "Regulation of Respiration" in Chapter 41, page 1095, for details.

Assessing Respirations

Resting respirations should be assessed when the client is at rest because exercise affects respirations, increasing their rate and depth. Anxiety is likely to affect respiratory rate and depth as well. Respirations may also need to be assessed after exercise to identify the client's tolerance to activity. Before assessing a client's respirations, a nurse should be aware of

- The client's normal breathing pattern
- The influence of the client's health problems on respirations
- Any medications or therapies that might affect respirations
- The relationship of the client's respirations to cardiovascular function

The rate, depth, rhythm, and special characteristics of respirations should be assessed.

The *respiratory rate* is normally described in breaths per minute. A healthy adult normally takes between 15 and 20 breaths per minute. For the respiratory rates for different age groups, see Table 18–1. Several factors influence respiratory rate; some are listed in Table 18–7.

The *depth* of a person's respirations can be established by watching the movement of the chest. Respiratory depth is generally described as normal, deep, or shallow. *Deep respirations* are those in which a large volume of air is inhaled and exhaled, inflating most of the lungs. *Shallow respirations* involve the exchange of a small volume of air and often the minimal use of lung tissue. During a normal inspiration and expiration, an adult takes in about 500 ml of air. This volume is called the **tidal volume.**

Vital capacity is the total of the tidal volume plus the inspiratory reserve volume plus the expiratory reserve volume. The capacity of the lungs varies with sex, age, stature, physical development, and body position. Men generally have a greater lung capacity than women of the same age. Variance by age is obvious: Babies have less vital capacity than children, children less than adolescents, and adolescents 18 to 19 years old less than adults. However, elderly people usually have less vital capacity than young adults. Stature affects lung volume: Tall, thin people usually have a greater vital capacity than obese people. The athlete in top condition usually has a vital capacity that is above normal. See Chapter 41, page 1091, for detailed information about respiratory volumes.

Body position also affects the amount of air that can be inhaled. People in a supine position experience two physiologic processes that suppress respiration: an increase in the volume of the intrathoracic blood and compression of the chest. Consequently, clients in a supine position have poorer lung aeration, which can predispose them to the stasis of fluids and subsequent infection. Certain medications also affect the respiratory depth. For example, such

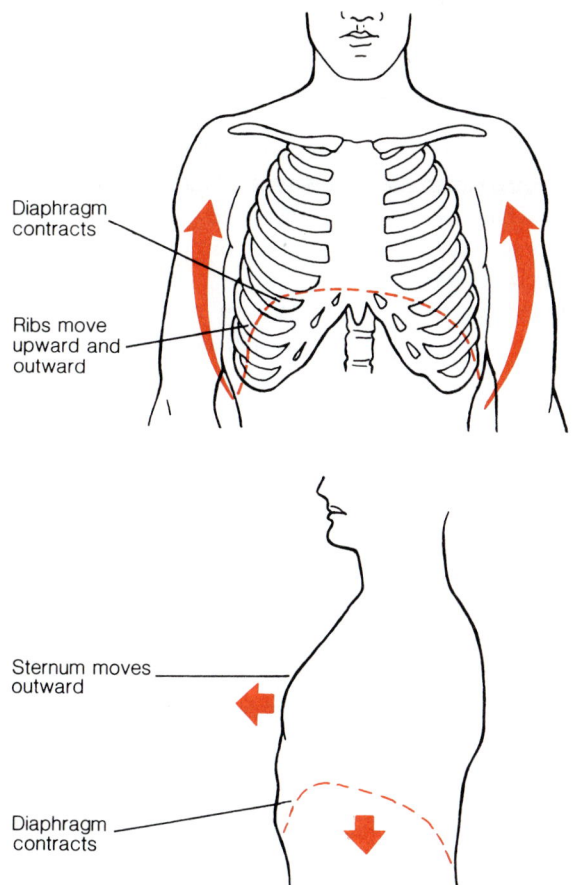

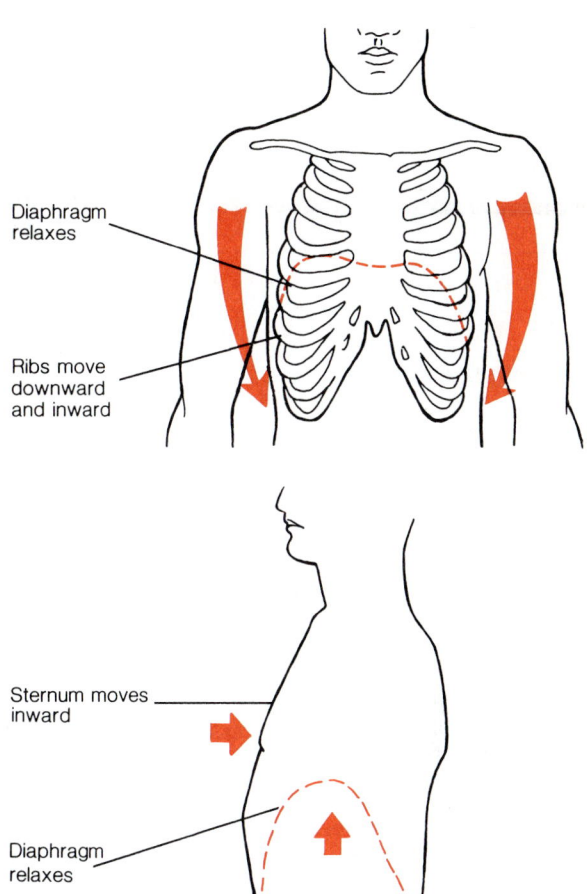

Figure 18–17 Respiratory inhalation: anterior and lateral views.

Figure 18–18 Respiratory exhalation: anterior and lateral views.

barbiturates as secobarbital sodium, when taken in large doses, depress the respiratory centers in the brain, thereby depressing the respiratory rate and depth.

Respiratory rhythm or **pattern** refers to the regularity of the expirations and the inspirations. Normally, respirations are evenly spaced. Respiratory rhythm can be described as *regular* or *irregular.* An infant's respiratory rhythm may be less regular than an adult's. Some disease conditions affect a person's respiratory rhythm. See Chapter 41, page 1098 for details about abnormal respiratory rhythms.

Respiratory quality or **character** refers to those aspects of breathing that are different from normal, effortless breathing. Two of these are the amount of effort a client must exert to breathe and the sound of breathing. Usually, breathing does not require noticeable effort; some clients, however, breathe only with decided effort.

The sound of breathing is also significant. Normal breathing is silent, but a number of abnormal sounds such as a wheeze are obvious to the nurse's ear. Many sounds occur as a result of the presence of fluid in the lungs and are most

TABLE 18–7 *Major Factors Influencing Respiratory Rate*

Factor	Influence
Exercise: increases metabolism	Increase
Stress: readies the body for "fight or flight"	Increase
Environment: increased temperature	Increase
Increased altitude: lower oxygen concentration	Increase
Certain medications, e.g., narcotic, analgesic	Decrease

clearly heard with a stethoscope. See Chapter 19, pages 401–403, for auscultation and percussion methods used to assess lung sounds. For details about altered breathing patterns and terms used to describe normal and abnormal patterns and sounds, see Chapter 41, pages 1097–1100. Procedure 18–4 provides guidelines for assessing respirations.

ASSESSING RESPIRATIONS

Equipment ☑

Watch with a second hand or indicator

Intervention

1. Assess the client.

■ Assess
  a. Skin and mucous membrane color, e.g., for cyanosis and/or pallor
  b. Position assumed for breathing, e.g., whether the client is orthopneic.
  c. Any change that might indicate cerebral anoxia (decreased oxygen to the brain), e.g., anxious behavior, irritability, restlessness, drowsiness, or loss of consciousness.
  d. Specific chest movements, such as intercostal retractions (indrawing between the ribs) and substernal or suprasternal retractions (indrawing below or above the sternum) if severe respiratory disease is present.

■ Determine the client's activity schedule so as to choose a suitable time to monitor the respirations. *A client who has been exercising will need to rest for a few minutes to permit the accelerated respiratory rate to return to normal. An infant or child who is crying will have an abnormal respiratory rate and will need quieting before the accurate assessment of the respirations can be made.*

2. Observe or palpate and count the respiratory rate.

■ Place a hand against the client's chest to feel the client's chest movements, or place the client's arm across the chest and observe the chest movements, while supposedly taking the radial pulse.

■ Count the respiratory rate for 30 seconds if the respirations are regular. Count for 60 seconds if they are irregular. An inhalation and an exhalation count as one respiration.

3. Observe the depth, rhythm, and character of respirations.

■ Observe the respirations for depth by watching the movement of the chest. During deep respirations a large volume of air is exchanged; during shallow respirations a small volume is exchanged.

■ Observe the respirations for regular or irregular rhythm. Normally, respirations are evenly spaced.

■ Observe the character of respirations—the sound they produce and the effort they require. Normally, respirations are silent and effortless.

4. Document and report pertinent assessment data.

■ Document the respiratory rate, depth, rhythm, and character on the appropriate record. See sample below.

■ Report to the nurse in charge:
  a. a respiratory rate significantly above or below the normal range,
  b. an irregular respiratory rhythm,
  c. an inadequate respiratory depth,
  d. an abnormal character of breathing—orthopnea, wheezing, stridor, rales, or rhonchi, and
  e. any complaints of dyspnea.

Sample Recording

Date 6/20/91	Time: 0900

R 38 and shallow. Dyspneic when talking. P 122. BP 94/60. Dr. Woo notified. ————————————John P. Brown, NS

BLOOD PRESSURE

Arterial blood pressure is a measure of the pressure exerted by the blood as it pulsates through the arteries. Because the blood moves in waves, there are two blood pressure measures: the **systolic pressure,** which is the pressure of the blood as a result of contraction of the ventricles, i.e., the pressure of the height of the blood wave; and the **diastolic pressure,** which is the pressure when the ventricles are at rest. Diastolic pressure, then, is the lower pressure, present at all times within the arteries. The difference between the diastolic and the systolic pressures is called the **pulse pressure.**

The average blood pressure of a healthy adult is 120/80 mm Hg. A number of conditions are reflected by changes in blood pressure. The most common is **hypertension,** an abnormally high blood pressure over 140 mm Hg systolic and/or 90 mm Hg diastolic when these are confirmed during a minimum of two consecutive visits by a client. See Table 18–8 for classifications of hypertension and recommendations for follow-up care. **Hypotension,** or an abnormally low blood pressure, is a systolic pressure below 100 mm Hg.

TABLE 18−8 *Classification of Hypertension in Adults 18 Years or Older and Recommended Follow-Up*

Blood Pressure Findings	Follow-Up
Diastolic Blood Pressure	
< 85 Normal	Recheck within 2 years.
85–90 High-normal	Recheck within 1 year.
90–104 Mild hypertension	Confirm within 2 months.
105–114 Moderate hypertension	Evaluate or refer promptly to source of care within 2 weeks.
> 115 Severe hypertension	Refer immediately to source of care.
Systolic Blood Pressure When Diastolic Is Less than 90	
< 140 Normal	Recheck within 2 years.
140–159 Borderline isolated systolic hypertension	Confirm within 2 months.
> 160 Isolated systolic hypertension	If below 200, confirm within 2 months. If above 200, refer promptly for care within 2 weeks.

Source: U.S. Department of Health and Human Services, Public Health Service, National Institutes of Health. May 1988. *The 1988 Report of the Joint National Committee on Detection, Evaluation, and Treatment of High Blood Pressure.* NIH Pub. no. 88–1088, pp. 3 and 6.

Because blood pressure can vary considerably among individuals, it is important for the nurse to know a specific client's baseline blood pressure. For example, if a client's usual blood pressure is 180/100 mm Hg and it is assessed following surgery to be 120/80 mm Hg, this drop in pressure must be reported to the charge nurse or physician. A number of conditions influence blood pressure. Some of these are listed in Table 18–9.

Physiology of Arterial Blood Pressure

The arterial blood pressure is the result of the cardiac output times the resistance the blood encounters while it flows, i.e., the peripheral vascular resistance. A person's blood pressure is directly affected by the *volume* of blood in the systemic circulation. The human body normally has about 5 liters of blood. Of this 5 liters, about 80 to 90% is in the systemic circulation and 10 to 20% is in the pulmonary circulation. Blood flows in the vascular system along a *pressure gradient*. The pressure of the blood in the aorta, for example, is higher than the pressure in the arterioles, and in the arterioles it is higher than in the capillaries. See Figure 18–19.

Cardiac output increases with fever and exercise, and the systolic pressure may increase as a result. However, cardiac output can be decreased as a result of heart disease, and the systolic pressure may then be low. *Peripheral resistance* can increase blood pressure. The diastolic pressure especially is affected. Some factors that create resistance in the

TABLE 18−9 *Selected Conditions Affecting Blood Pressure*

Condition	Effect	Cause
Fever	Increase	Increases metabolic rate
Stress	Increase	Increases cardiac output
Arteriosclerosis	Increase	Decreases artery compliance
Obesity	Increase	Increases peripheral resistance
Hemorrhage	Decrease	Decreases blood volume
Low hematocrit	Decrease	Decreases blood viscosity
External heat	Decrease	Increases vasodilation and thus decreases peripheral vascular resistance
Exposure to cold	Increase	Causes vasoconstriction and thus increases peripheral vascular resistance

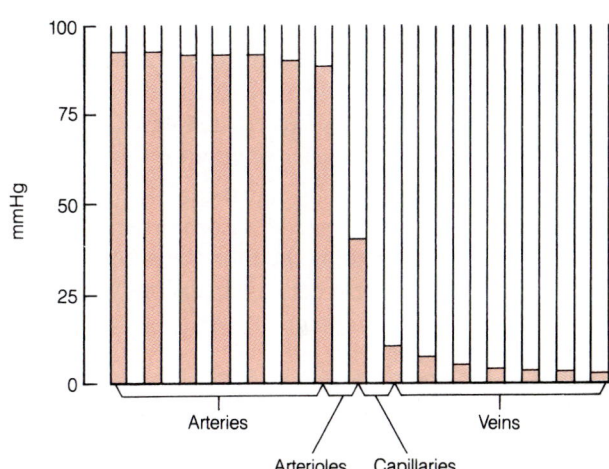

Figure 18−19 The mean blood pressure in the different parts of the vascular system. *Source:* Adapted from R. L. Vick, *Contemporary medical physiology* (Menlo Park, Calif.: Addison-Wesley Publishing Co., 1984), p. 198.

arterial system are the size of the arterioles and capillaries, the compliance of the arteries, and the viscosity of the blood.

The *size* of the arterioles and the capillaries determines in great part the peripheral resistance to the blood in the body. A **lumen** is a channel within a tube: the smaller the lumen of a vessel, the greater the resistance. Normally, the arterioles are in a state of partial constriction. Increased vasoconstriction raises the blood pressure, whereas decreased vasoconstriction lowers the blood pressure.

The arteries contain smooth muscles that permit them to contract, thus decreasing their **compliance** (distensibility). Arteries normally relax and contract somewhat during systole and retract during diastole. The arteries account for most of the peripheral resistance. The major factor reducing arterial compliance is pathologic change affecting the arterial walls. The elastic and muscular tissues of the arteries are replaced with fibrous tissue; thus, the arteries lose much of their compliance. The condition, most common in middle-aged and elderly adults, is known as **arteriosclerosis.**

Viscosity is a physical property that results from friction of molecules in a fluid. In a viscous (or "thick") fluid, there is a great deal of friction among the molecules as they slide by each other. The blood pressure is higher when the blood is highly viscous, i.e., when the proportion of red blood cells to the blood plasma is high. This ratio is referred to as the **hematocrit.** The viscosity increases markedly when the hematocrit is more than 60 to 65%.

Factors Affecting Blood Pressure

Among the factors influencing blood pressure are age, exercise, stress, race, obesity, sex, medications, and diurnal variations:

- *Age.* In older adults, the diastolic pressure often increases as a result of the reduced compliance of the arteries.
- *Exercise.* Physical activity increases both the cardiac output and hence the blood pressure; thus, a rest of 20 to 30 minutes following exercise is indicated before the blood pressure can be reliably assessed unless the blood pressure is being assessed during or after exercise.
- *Stress.* Stimulation of the sympathetic nervous system increases cardiac output and vasoconstriction of the arterioles, thus increasing the blood pressure reading; however, severe pain can decrease blood pressure greatly and cause shock by inhibiting the vasomotor center and producing vasodilation.
- *Race.* Black males over 35 years have higher blood pressures than white males of the same age.
- *Obesity.* Pressure is consistently higher in some overweight and obese people than in people of normal weight (Overfield 1985, p. 46).
- *Sex.* After puberty, females usually have lower blood pressures than males of the same age; this difference is thought

to be due to hormonal variations. After menopause, women generally have higher blood pressures than before.

- *Medications.* Many medications may increase or decrease the blood pressure; nurses should be aware of the specific medications a client is receiving and consider their possible impact when interpreting blood pressure readings.
- *Diurnal variations.* Pressure is usually lowest early in the morning, when the metabolic rate is lowest, then rises throughout the day and peaks in the late afternoon or early evening.
- *Disease process.* Any condition affecting the cardiac output, blood viscosity, and/or compliance of the arteries has a direct effect on the blood pressure. See the discussion in the previous section.

Assessing Blood Pressure

Equipment   Blood pressure is measured with a **blood pressure cuff**, a **sphygmomanometer,** and a **stethoscope.** The blood pressure cuff consists of a rubber bag that can be inflated with air. It is called the **bladder.** See Figure 18–20. It is usually covered with cloth and has two tubes attached to it. One tube connects to a rubber bulb that inflates the bladder. When turned counterclockwise, a small valve on the side of this bulb releases the air in the bladder. When the valve is tightened (turned clockwise),

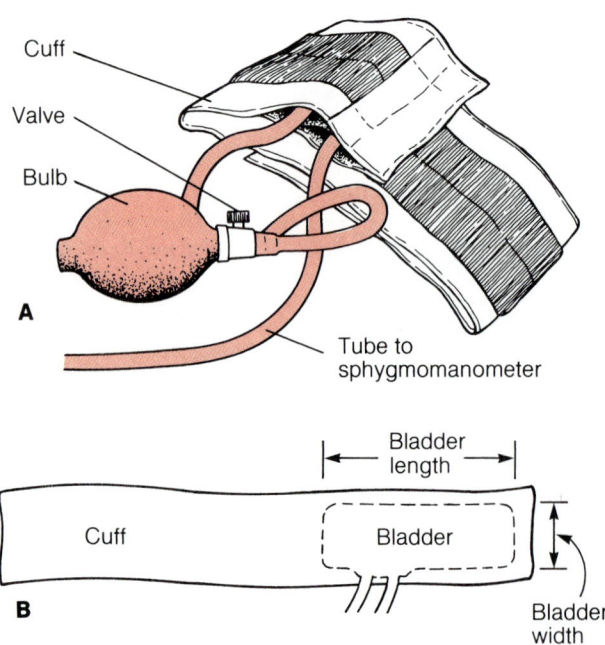

Figure 18–20   A, A blood pressure cuff and bulb; B, the bladder inside the cuff.

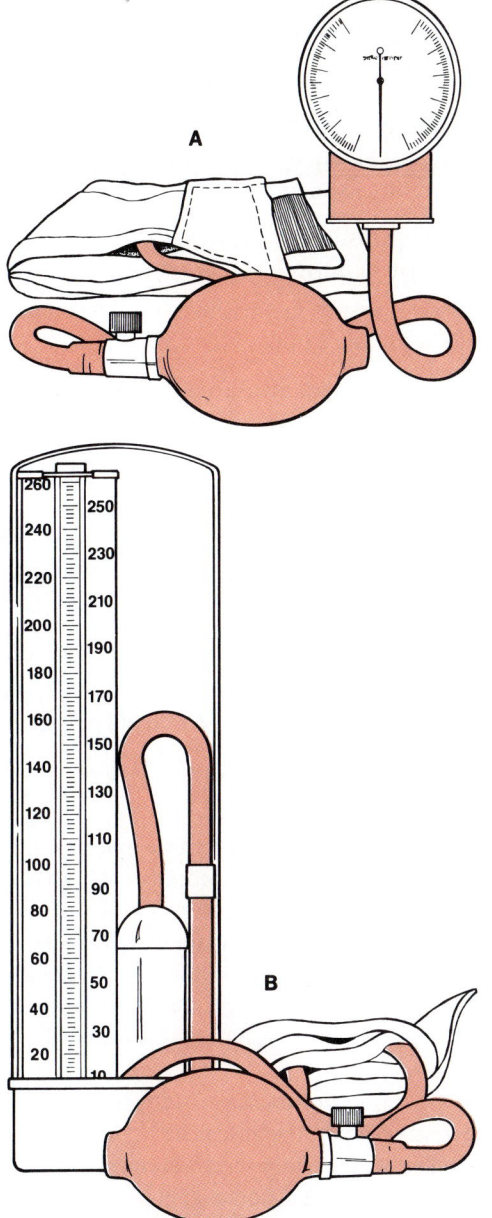

Adult Size	Arm Circumference (cm)	Cuff Size (cm)
Child (small)	<22	9 x 18
Adult (regular)	22-33	12 x 23
Adult (large)	33-41	15 x 33
Adult (thigh)	>41	18 x 36

Source: American Heart Association, *Recommendations for human blood pressure determination by sphygmomanometers,* Pub no. 701005 (American Heart Association, 1987) p. 10.

Figure 18-21 Blood pressure equipment: *A,* an aneroid manometer and cuff; *B,* a mercury manometer and cuff.

air pumped into the bladder remains there. The other tube is attached to a sphygmomanometer.

The sphygmomanometer indicates the pressure of the air within the bladder. There are two types of sphygmomanometers: **aneroid** and **mercury.** See Figure 18-21. The aneroid sphygmomanometer is a calibrated dial with a needle that points to the calibrations. The mercury sphygmomanometer is a calibrated cylinder filled with mercury. The pressure is indicated at the point to which the **meniscus** of the mercury (the crescent-shaped top surface of the col-

umn) rises. It is important to view the meniscus at eye level to avoid distortions in the reading.

Some agencies use electronic sphygmomanometers, which eliminate the need to listen to the sounds of the client's systolic and diastolic blood pressures through a stethoscope. With some electronic sphygmomanometers, as the pressure in the cuff is lowered, a light flashes to indicate the systolic and diastolic pressures.

Ultrasound (Doppler) stethoscopes are also used to assess blood pressure. See Figure 18-13, earlier. These are of particular value when blood pressure sounds are difficult to hear, e.g., in infants, obese clients, and clients in shock. Transmission gel is applied to a transducer probe, which is placed over the pulse point, and the blood pressure is measured. A systolic blood pressure assessed with a Doppler stethoscope is recorded with a large D, e.g., 85D. Systolic pressure may be the only blood pressure obtainable with some ultrasound models.

Blood pressure cuffs come in various sizes, since the bladder must be the correct width and length for the client's arm. If the bladder is too narrow, the blood pressure reading will be erroneously elevated; if it is too wide, the reading will be erroneously low. The width should be 40% of the circumference, or 20% wider than the diameter of the midpoint of the limb on which it is used (American Heart Association 1987, p. 4). The bladder dimensions by arm circumference are shown in Table 18-10; the arm circumference, not the age of the client, should always be used to determine bladder size. The nurse can also determine whether the width of a blood pressure cuff is appropriate: Lay the cuff lengthwise at the midpoint of the upper arm, and hold the outermost side of the bladder edge laterally on the arm. With the other hand, wrap the width of the cuff

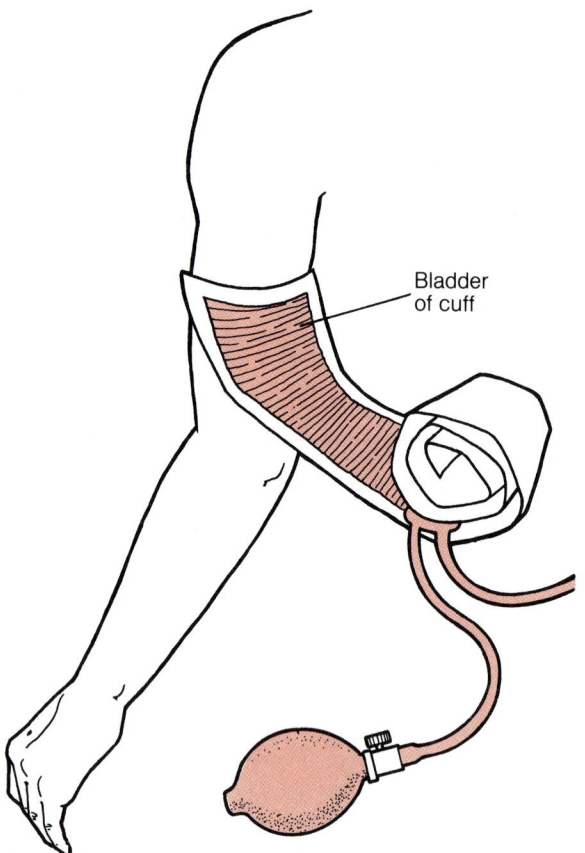

Figure 18–22 Determining that the bladder of a blood pressure cuff is 40% of the arm circumference or 20% wider than the diameter of the midpoint of the limb.

around the arm, and ensure that the width is 40% of the arm circumference. See Figure 18–22.

The length of the bladder also affects the accuracy of measurement. The bladder should be sufficiently long almost to encircle the limb and to cover at least two-thirds of its circumference.

Blood pressure cuffs are made of nondistensible material so that an even pressure is exerted around the limb. Most cuffs are held in place by hooks, snaps, or Velcro. Others have a cloth bandage that is long enough to encircle the limb several times; this type is closed by tucking the end of the bandage into one of the bandage folds.

Sites   The blood pressure is usually assessed in the client's arm using the brachial artery and a standard stethoscope. If the arm is very large or grossly misshapen and the conventional cuff cannot be properly applied, leg or forearm measurements can be taken. To obtain a *leg blood pressure,* a standard-sized cuff is applied over the lower leg with the distal border of the cuff at the malleoli. Blood pressure sounds are auscultated over the posterior tibial or dorsalis pedis arteries. To obtain a *thigh blood pressure,* an appro-

priate-sized cuff is applied to the thigh, and the pulsations of the blood are auscultated over the popliteal artery. To obtain a *forearm blood pressure* an appropriate-sized cuff is applied to the forearm 13 cm (5 in) from the elbow. Blood pressure sounds then can be heard over the radial artery.

Assessing the blood pressure on a client's thigh is usually indicated in these situations:

- The blood pressure cannot be measured on either arm, e.g., because of burns or other trauma.
- The blood pressure in one thigh is to be compared with the blood pressure in the other thigh.

Blood pressure is *not* measured on a client's arm or thigh in the following situations:

- The shoulder, arm, or hand (or the hip, knee, or ankle) is injured or diseased.
- There is a cast or bulky bandage on any part of the limb.
- The client has had breast or axilla (or hip) surgery on that side.
- The client has an intravenous infusion or a blood transfusion running.
- The client has an arteriovenous fistula (e.g., for renal dialysis).

Methods   Blood pressure can be assessed directly or indirectly. *Direct (invasive monitoring) measurement* involves the insertion of a catheter into the brachial, radial, or femoral artery. Arterial pressure is represented as wavelike forms displayed on an oscilloscope. Generally, physicians insert the catheters, and nurses monitor the pressure readings. With proper placement, this pressure reading is highly accurate.

There are three *noninvasive indirect methods* of measuring blood pressure: the auscultatory, palpatory, and flush methods. The *auscultatory method* is most commonly used in hospitals, clinics, and homes. Required equipment is a sphygmomanometer, cuff, and a stethoscope. External pressure is applied to a superficial artery, and the nurse reads the pressure from the sphygmomanometer when the blood flow is first heard through a stethoscope. When carried out correctly, the auscultatory method is relatively accurate.

When taking a blood pressure using a stethoscope, the nurse identifies five phases in the series of sounds called **Korotkoff's sounds.** First, the nurse pumps the cuff up to about 30 mm Hg above the point where the last sound is heard; that is the point when the blood flow in the artery is stopped. Then the pressure is released slowly (2 to 3 mm Hg per sound), while the nurse observes the pressure readings on the manometer and relates them to the sounds heard through the stethoscope. Five phases occur (American Heart Association 1980, p. 11):

Phase 1   The period initiated by the first faint clear tapping sounds. These sounds gradually become more intense.

To ensure that they are not extraneous sounds, the nurse should identify at least two consecutive tapping sounds.

Phase 2 The period during which the sounds have a swishing quality.

Phase 3 The period during which the sounds are crisper and more intense.

Phase 4 The period during which the sounds become muffled and have a soft, blowing quality.

Phase 5 The point where the sounds disappear.

The American Heart Association (AHA) recommends that the systolic pressure be considered the point where the first tapping sound is heard (phase 1). In adults, the diastolic pressure is the point where the sounds become inaudible (phase 5). In children, however, the AHA recommends that diastolic pressure be considered to be the onset of phase 4, where the sounds become muffled. In agencies where the fourth phase is considered the diastolic pressure of adults, three measures are recommended (systolic pressure, diastolic pressure, and phase 5). These may be referred to as systolic, first diastolic, and second diastolic pressures. The phase 5 (second diastolic pressure) reading may be zero; that is, the muffled sounds are heard even when there is no air pressure in the blood pressure cuff. In some instances, muffled sounds are never heard, in which case a dash is inserted where the reading would normally be recorded.

The *palpatory method* is sometimes used when Korotkoff's sounds cannot be heard and electronic equipment to amplify the sounds is not available, or when an auscultatory gap occurs. An **auscultatory gap,** which occurs particularly in hypertensive clients, is the temporary disappearance of sounds normally heard over the brachial artery when the cuff pressure is high and the reappearance of the sounds at a lower level. This temporary disappearance of sounds occurs in the latter part of phase 1 and phase 2 and may cover a range of 40 mm Hg. Instead of listening for the blood flow sounds, the nurse palpates the pulsations of the artery as the pressure in the cuff is released. The systolic pressure is read from the sphygmomanometer when the first pulsation is felt. A single whiplike vibration, felt in addition to the pulsations, identifies the point at which the pressure in the cuff nears the diastolic pressure (Enselberg 1961, p. 273). This vibration is no longer felt when the cuff pressure is below the diastolic pressure. To palpate the diastolic pressure, the nurse applies light to moderate pressure over the pulse point.

The *flush method* for determining blood pressure is another method used when Korotkoff's sounds cannot be heard by auscultation and electronic equipment is not available. The measurement is determined by a change in skin color when blood flow to an extremity resumes, i.e., when the extremity is no longer extremely pale but becomes reddened (vascular flush). The cuff is applied to the client's arm and the limb is wrapped in a bandage distally to proximally to force venous blood out of and restrict arterial flow into the extremity. The cuff is then inflated and the bandage is removed. The cuff pressure is released, and the nurse reads the pressure from the sphygmomanometer when the extremity flushes. This reading is the **mean blood pressure,** the midway point between the systolic and diastolic pressures. Procedure 18–5 gives guidelines for assessing blood pressure.

PROCEDURE 18–5

ASSESSING BLOOD PRESSURE (ARM)

Equipment ☑

Stethoscope or DUS (see Figure 18–13, earlier)

Blood pressure cuff of the appropriate size (newborn, infant, child, small adult, adult, large adult, thigh)

Sphygmomanometer

Intervention

1. **Assess the client.**

- Make sure the client has not smoked or ingested caffeine within 30 minutes prior to measurement (U.S. Department of Health 1988, p. 5).

- Make sure that the bladder of the cuff encircles at least two-thirds of the arm and that the width of the cuff is appropriate.

- Assess the client for any other signs of altered blood pressure. Signs of hypertension include frequent nosebleeds, irritability, and ringing in the ears. Signs of hypotension include increased pulse rate, cold clammy skin, dizziness.

2. **Position the client appropriately.**

- Position the client in a sitting position unless otherwise specified. The arm should be slightly flexed with the palm of the hand facing up and the forearm supported at heart level. Readings in any other position should be specified. *The blood pressure is normally similar in sitting, standing, and lying positions, but it can vary significantly by position in certain persons and may need to be measured in all three positions. There is an increase in the blood pressure when the arm is below heart level and a decrease when it is above heart level.*

■ Expose the upper arm.

3. Wrap the deflated cuff evenly around the upper arm.

■ Apply the center of the bladder directly over the medial aspect of the arm. *The bladder inside the cuff must be directly over the artery to be compressed if the reading is to be accurate.*

■ For an adult blood pressure, place the lower border of the cuff about 2.5 cm (1 in.) above the antecubital space. The lower edge can be nearer the antecubital space of an infant.

4. If this is the client's initial examination, perform a preliminary palpatory determination of systolic pressure. The initial estimate tells the nurse the maximal pressure to which the manometer needs to be elevated in subsequent determinations. It also prevents underestimation of the systolic pressure or overestimation of the diastolic pressure should an auscultatory gap occur.

■ Palpate the brachial artery with the fingertips. The brachial artery is normally found medially in the antecubital space. See Figure 18−23.

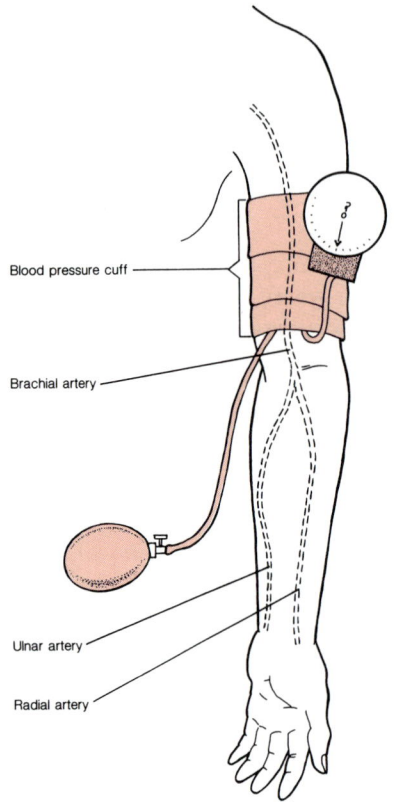

Blood pressure cuff

Brachial artery

Ulnar artery

Radial artery

Figure 18−23 Location of the brachial artery.

■ Close the valve on the pump by turning the knob clockwise.

■ Pump up the cuff until you no longer feel the brachial pulse. *At that pressure the blood cannot flow through the artery.*

■ Note the pressure on the sphygmomanometer at which the pulse is no longer felt. *This gives an estimate of the maximum pressure required to measure the systolic pressure.*

■ Release the pressure completely in the cuff and wait 1−2 minutes before further measurements are made. *A waiting period gives the blood trapped in the veins time to be released.*

5. Position the stethoscope appropriately.

■ Insert the ear attachments of the stethoscope in your ears so that they tilt slightly forward. *Sounds are heard more clearly when the ear attachments follow the direction of the ear canal.*

■ Ensure that the stethoscope hangs freely from the ears to the diaphragm. *Rubbing the stethoscope against an object can obliterate the sounds of the blood within an artery.*

■ Place the diaphragm of the stethoscope over the brachial pulse. Use the bell-shaped diaphragm of the stethoscope (see Figure 18−16, earlier). *Since the blood pressure is a low-frequency sound, it is best heard with the bell-shaped diaphragm.* Hold the diaphragm with the thumb and index finger.

6. Auscultate the blood pressure.

■ Pump up the cuff until the sphygmomanometer registers about 30 mm Hg above the point where the brachial pulse disappears.

■ Release the valve on the cuff carefully so that the pressure decreases at the rate of 2 to 3 mm Hg per second. *If the rate is faster or slower, an error in measurement may occur.*

■ As the pressure falls, identify the manometer reading at each of the five phases.

■ Deflate the cuff rapidly and completely.

■ Wait 1 to 2 minutes before making further determinations. *This permits blood trapped in the veins to be released.*

■ Repeat the above steps once or twice as necessary to confirm the accuracy of the reading.

7. Remove the cuff from the client's arm.

8. If this is the client's initial examination, repeat the procedure on the client's other arm.

- There should be a difference of no more than 10 mm Hg between the arms.

- The arm found to have the higher pressure should be used for subsequent examinations.

9. Document and report pertinent assessment data.

- Document the blood pressure according to agency policy. See sample that follows. Record two pressures in the form "130/80" where "130" is the systolic (phase 1) and "80" is the diastolic (phase 5) pressure. Record three pressures in the form "130/110/90," where "130" is the systolic, "110" is the first diastolic (phase 4), and "90" is the second diastolic (phase 5) pressure. Use the abbreviations *RA* for right arm and *LA* for left arm. Record a difference of greater than 10 mm Hg in the arms.

- Report any significant change in the client's blood pressure to the nurse in charge. Also report findings such as:
  a. Systolic blood pressure (of an adult) above 140 mm Hg

  b. Diastolic blood pressure (of an adult) above 90 mm Hg
  c. Systolic blood pressure (of an adult) below 100 mm Hg

Sample Recording

Date 8/14/91	Time: 1300

BP 130/90 in RA in bed-sitting position. P 115. R-20. Color pale. Ruth P. O'Shea, SN

Variation: Taking a Thigh Blood Pressure

- Help the client to assume a prone position. If the client cannot assume this position, measure the blood pressure while the client is in a supine position with the knee slightly flexed. *Slight flexing of the knee will facilitate placing the stethoscope on the popliteal space.*

- Expose the thigh, taking care not to expose the client unduly.

- Wrap the cuff evenly around the midthigh with the compression bladder over the posterior aspect of the thigh. *The bladder must be directly over the artery if the reading is to be accurate.*

- If this is the client's initial examination, perform a preliminary palpatory determination of systolic pressure by palpating the popliteal artery. See Figure 18–24. The systolic pressure in the popliteal artery is usually 10 to 40 mm Hg higher

than that in the brachial artery because of use of a larger bladder; the diastolic pressure is usually the same.

- Auscultate the pressure as above.

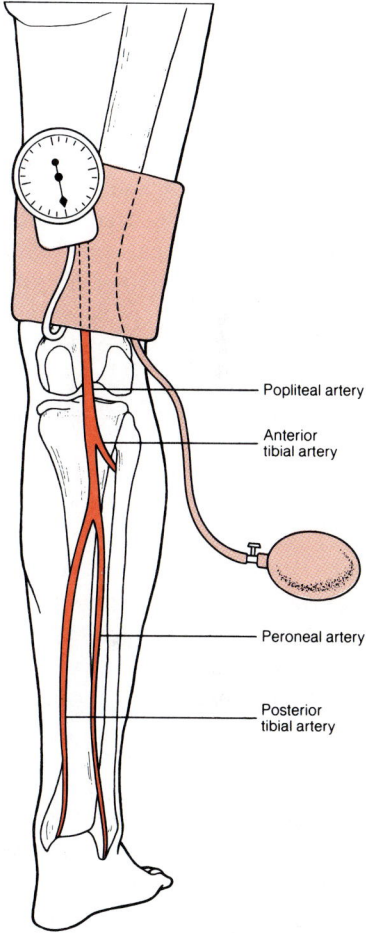

Figure 18–24 Location of the popliteal artery.

Common Errors in Assessing Blood Pressure

The importance of the accuracy of blood pressure assessments cannot be overemphasized. Many judgments about a client's health are made on the basis of blood pressure. It is an important indicator of the client's condition and is used extensively as a basis for nursing interventions. Mitchell and Van Meter found a mean difference of 7 mm Hg or less for recordings of systolic, diastolic phase 4, and diastolic phase 5 pressures as taken by nursing personnel and the investigators. There was also a difference of greater than 10 mm Hg in 37 to 46% of the readings. Nursing personnel consistently recorded higher readings than the investigators (Mitchell and Van Meter 1971, p. 352). Two possible reasons for the blood pressure errors are haste on the part of the nurse and subconscious bias. For example, a nurse may be influenced by the client's previous blood pressure measurements or diagnosis and "hear" a value consonant with the practitioner's expectations. An example of such a bias is "digit preference," a predilection for pressures ending with zero, e.g., 130 systolic, 70 diastolic, more often than would be expected (AHA 1980, p. 21). Some reasons for erroneous blood pressure readings are given in Table 18–11.

TABLE 18–11 Sources of Error in Blood Pressure Assessment

Error	Effect
Bladder cuff too narrow	Erroneously high
Bladder cuff too wide	Erroneously low
Arm unsupported	Erroneously high
Insufficient rest before the assessment	Erroneously high
Repeating assessment too quickly	Erroneously high systolic or low diastolic readings
Cuff wrapped too loosely or unevenly	Erroneously high
Deflating cuff too quickly	Erroneously low systolic and high diastolic readings
Deflating cuff too slowly	Erroneously high
Failure to use the same arm consistently	Inconsistent measurements
Arm above level of the heart	Erroneously low
Assessing immediately after a meal or while client smokes or has pain	Erroneously high
Failure to identify auscultatory gap	Erroneously low

CHAPTER HIGHLIGHTS

▶ Vital signs reflect changes in body function that otherwise might not be observed.

▶ Various sites and methods can be used to assess vital signs. The nurse selects the site and method that is safe for the client and that will provide the most accurate measurement possible.

▶ The most accurate values are obtained when the client is at rest and comfortable.

▶ Changes in one vital sign can trigger changes in other vital signs.

▶ Vital signs are assessed when a client is admitted to a health care agency to establish baseline data and when there is a change or possibility of a change in the client's condition.

▶ Data obtained from measurements of vital signs are used to plan and implement appropriate nursing interventions.

▶ Measurements of vital signs are also used to evaluate a client's response to nursing interventions or prescribed medical therapy.

▶ Knowledge of the normal ranges of vital signs and of the factors that regulate and influence vital signs helps the nurse interpret the measurements that deviate from normal.

▶ Body temperature is the balance between heat produced by the body and heat lost from the body.

▶ Heat is produced by the body's metabolic processes, which can be accelerated by muscle activity, thyroxine output, stimulation of the sympathetic nervous system, and fever.

▶ Heat is lost from the body by radiation, conduction, convection, and vaporization.

▶ Knowledge of factors affecting heat production and heat loss helps the nurse to implement appropriate interventions when the client has a fever or hypothermia.

▶ The system that regulates body temperature has three parts: sensory receptors, primarily in the skin; the hypothalamic integrator, which controls the core temperature; and an effector system, which initiates responses that either prevent heat loss and increase heat production (e.g., peripheral vasodilation, shivering, and release of epinephrine, which increases metabolism) or increase heat loss through sweating and peripheral vasodilation.

▶ Factors affecting body temperature include age, diurnal variations, exercise, hormones, stress, and environmental temperatures.

▶ Pyrexia (fever) is a common sign of disease. Four common types of fever are intermittent, remittent, relapsing, and constant. Clinical signs of fever vary during the onset, course, and abatement stages.

▶ During a fever, the set-point of the hypothalamic thermostat changes suddenly from the normal level to a higher than normal level, but several hours elapse before the core temperature reaches the new set-point.

▶ Hypothermia involves three mechanisms: excessive heat loss, inadequate heat production by body cells, and increasing impairment of hypothalamic thermoregulation.

▶ Body temperature can be measured orally, rectally, or by axilla. The nurse selects the most appropriate site according to the client's age and condition.

▶ An important nursing function is to identify clients at risk for altered body temperature.

▶ Four NANDA nursing diagnoses are associated with body temperature: **Potential altered body temperature, Hyperthermia, Hypothermia,** and **Ineffective thermoregulation.** Each has specific defining characteristics and contributing factors.

▶ Pulse rate and volume reflect the stroke volume output, the compliance of the client's arteries, and the adequacy of blood flow.

▶ Normally, a peripheral pulse reflects the client's heartbeat, but it may differ from the heartbeat in clients with certain cardiovascular diseases; in these instances, the nurse takes an apical pulse and compares it to the peripheral pulse.

▶ Many factors affect a person's pulse rate: age, sex, exercise, presence of fever, certain medications, hemorrhage, stress, and (in some situations) position changes.

▶ Although the radial pulse is the site most commonly used, eight other sites may be used in certain situations.

▶ Respirations are normally quiet, effortless, and automatic and are assessed by observing respiratory rate, depth, rhythm, and sound.

▶ Blood pressure reflects cardiac output and peripheral vascular resistance; peripheral vascular resistance varies according to the size of the arterioles and capillaries, compliance of the arteries, and blood viscosity.

READINGS AND REFERENCES

SUGGESTED READINGS

Birdsall, C. July 1985. How do you interpret pulses? *American Journal of Nursing* 85:785–86.

Using a question-and-answer format, Birdsall lists the pulses that should be recorded, discusses what an absent pulse means, and describes the different types of pulses, e.g., pulsus alternans, paradoxical pulse.

Davis, C., and Lentz, M. J. April 1989. Circadian rhythms: Charting oral temperatures to spot abnormalities. *Journal of Gerontological Nursing* 15:34–39.

This article describes a research study of body temperature measurements of a group of elderly people. A normal daily variation in body temperature was found. The researchers also found that normal oral temperature was lower in elderly people than in younger people and that elderly people may be more prone to hypothermia in the early morning hours, when their body temperatures are normally lower. Bathing may cause the body temperature to drop up to 1 C. When analyzing temperature data, the nurse must consider the time of day as well as any symptoms of infection.

Gurevich, I. December 1985. Fever: When to worry about it. *RN* 48:14, 17, 19.

Gurevich describes the basic physiology of fever and reviews the many causes of fever, including surgery, drug hypersensitivity, central nervous system disease, and factitious problems. The author also describes the significance of different types of fevers and points out that most fevers are self-limiting and best left untreated. However, in certain cases treatment is called for (e.g., clients with temperatures of 106 F or above or those with cardiac or respiratory diseases). Methods of treatment include administering aspirin or acetaminophen and applying cooling blankets.

RELATED RESEARCH

Graves, R. D., and Markarian, M. F. September/October 1980. Three-minute intervals when using an oral mercury-in-glass thermometer without J-temperature sheaths. *Nursing Research* 29:323–24.

Hahn, W. K.; Brooks, J. A.; and Hite, R. February 1989. Blood pressure norms for healthy young adults: Relation to sex, age, and reported parental hypertension. *Research in Nursing and Health* 12:53–56.

Henneman, E. A., and Henneman, P. L. May 1989. Intricacies of blood pressure measurement: Reexamining the rituals. *Heart and Lung* 18:263–73.

Mason, D. J. September/October 1988. Circadian rhythms of body temperature and activation and the well-being of older women. *Nursing Research* 37:276–81.

Rebenson-Piano, M.; Holm, K.; Foreman, M. D.; and Kirchhoff, K. T. January/February 1989. An evaluation of two indirect methods of blood pressure measurement in ill patients. *Nursing Research* 38:42–45.

White, H. E.; Thurston, N. E.; Blackmore, K. A.; et al. October 1987. Body temperature in elderly surgical patients. *Research in Nursing and Health* 10:317–21.

SELECTED REFERENCES

American Heart Association. 1987. *Recommendations for human blood pressure determination by sphygmomanometers.* Pub No. 701005. American Heart Association.

Axillary temps safer in infants. June 1978. (Medical Highlights.) *American Journal of Nursing* 78:1081.

Baker, N. C.; Cerone, S. B.; Gaze, N.; and Knapp, T. R. March/April 1984. The effect of thermometer and length of time inserted on oral temperature measurements of afebrile subjects. *Nursing Research* 33:109–11.

Birdsall, C. July 1985. How do you interpret pulses? *American Journal of Nursing* 85:785–86.

Blainey, C. G. October 1974. Site selection in taking body temperature. *American Journal of Nursing* 74:1859–61.

Boylan, A., and Brown, P. February 13–19, 1985a. Student observations: More than "doing the obs" . . . the significance of pulse and blood pressure measurement. *Nursing Times* 81:24–25.

———. February 13–19, 1985b. Student observations: The pulse and blood pressure. *Nursing Times* 81:26–29.

———. March 13–19, 1985c. Student observations: Respiration. *Nursing Times* 81:35–38.

———. April 17–23, 1985d. Student observations: Temperature. *Nursing Times* 81:36–40.

Carpenito, L. J. 1989. *Nursing diagnosis: Application to clinical practice.* 3d ed. Philadelphia: J. B. Lippincott Co.

Creative Care Unit. June 1977. Turnabout: Rectal temperatures for postcoronary patients. *American Journal of Nursing* 77:997.

Enselberg, C. D. 1961. Measurement of diastolic blood pressure by palpation. *New England Journal of Medicine* 265:272–74.

Eoff, M. J., and Joyce, B. May 1981. Temperature measurement in children. *American Journal of Nursing* 81:1010–11.

Erickson, R. May/June 1980. Oral temperature differences in relation to thermometer and technique. *Nursing Research* 29:157–64.

Graas, S. October 1974. Thermometer sites and oxygen. *American Journal of Nursing* 74:1862–63.

Graves, R. D., and Markarian, M. F. September/October 1980. Three-minute intervals when using an oral mercury-in-glass thermometer without J-temperature sheaths. *Nursing Research* 29:323–24.

Guyton, A. C. 1986. *Textbook of medical physiology.* 7th ed. Philadelphia: W. B. Saunders Co.

Hasler, M. E., and Cohen, J. A. September/October 1982. The effect of oxygen administration on temperature assessment. *Nursing Research* 31:265–68.

Hill, M. N. May 1980. Hypertension: What can go wrong when you measure blood pressure. *American Journal of Nursing* 80:942–45.

Hudson, B. May 1983. Sharpen your vascular skills with the Doppler ultrasound stethoscope. *Nursing 83* 13:55–57.

Kennedy, W. C., Jr. May 1990. Vital signs: reading the essentials. *Journal of Emergency Medical Services* 15:26–30, 34, 36–39.

Kim, M. J.; McFarland, G. K.; and McLane, A. M. 1989. *Pocket guide to nursing diagnoses.* 3d ed. St. Louis: C. V. Mosby Co.

Kolanowski, A., and Gunther, L. September/October 1981. Hypothermia in the elderly. *Geriatric Nursing* 2:362–65.

Malasanos, L.; Barkauskas, V.; Moss, M.; and Stoltenberg-Allen, K. 1990. *Health Assessment.* 4th ed. St. Louis: C. V. Mosby Co.

Marieb, E. N. 1989. *Human anatomy and physiology.* Redwood City, Calif.: Benjamin/Cummings.

Mitchell, P. W., and Van Meter, M. J. July/August 1971. Reproducibility of blood pressure recorded on patients' records by nursing personnel. *Nursing Research* 20:348–52.

NANDA approved nursing diagnostic categories for clinical use and testing. Summer 1988. *Nursing Diagnosis Newsletter* 15:1–3.

Nichols, G. A.; Ruskin, M. M.; Glor, B. A. K.; and Kelly, W. H. Fall 1966. Oral, axillary, and rectal determinations and relationships. *Nursing Research* 15:307–16.

Nichols, G. A. June 1972. Taking adult temperatures: Rectal measurement. *American Journal of Nursing* 72:1092–93.

Nichols, G. A., and Kucha, D. H. June 1972. Taking adult temperatures: Oral measurement. *American Journal of Nursing* 72:1090–92.

Olds, S. B.; London, M. L.; and Ladewig, P. A. 1988. *Maternal-newborn nursing: A family-centered approach.* 3d ed. Menlo Park, Calif.: Addison-Wesley Publishing Co.

Overfield, T. 1985. *Biologic variation in health and illness.* Menlo Park, Calif.: Addison-Wesley Publishing Co.

Schiffman, R. F. September/October 1982. Temperature monitoring in the neonate: A comparison of axillary and rectal temperatures. *Nursing Research* 31:274–77.

U. S. Department of Health and Human Services, Public Health Service National Institutes of Health. May 1988. *The 1988 Report of the Joint National Committee on Detection, Evaluation, and Treatment of High Blood Pressure.* NIH Pub. no. 88–1088.

Physical Assessment

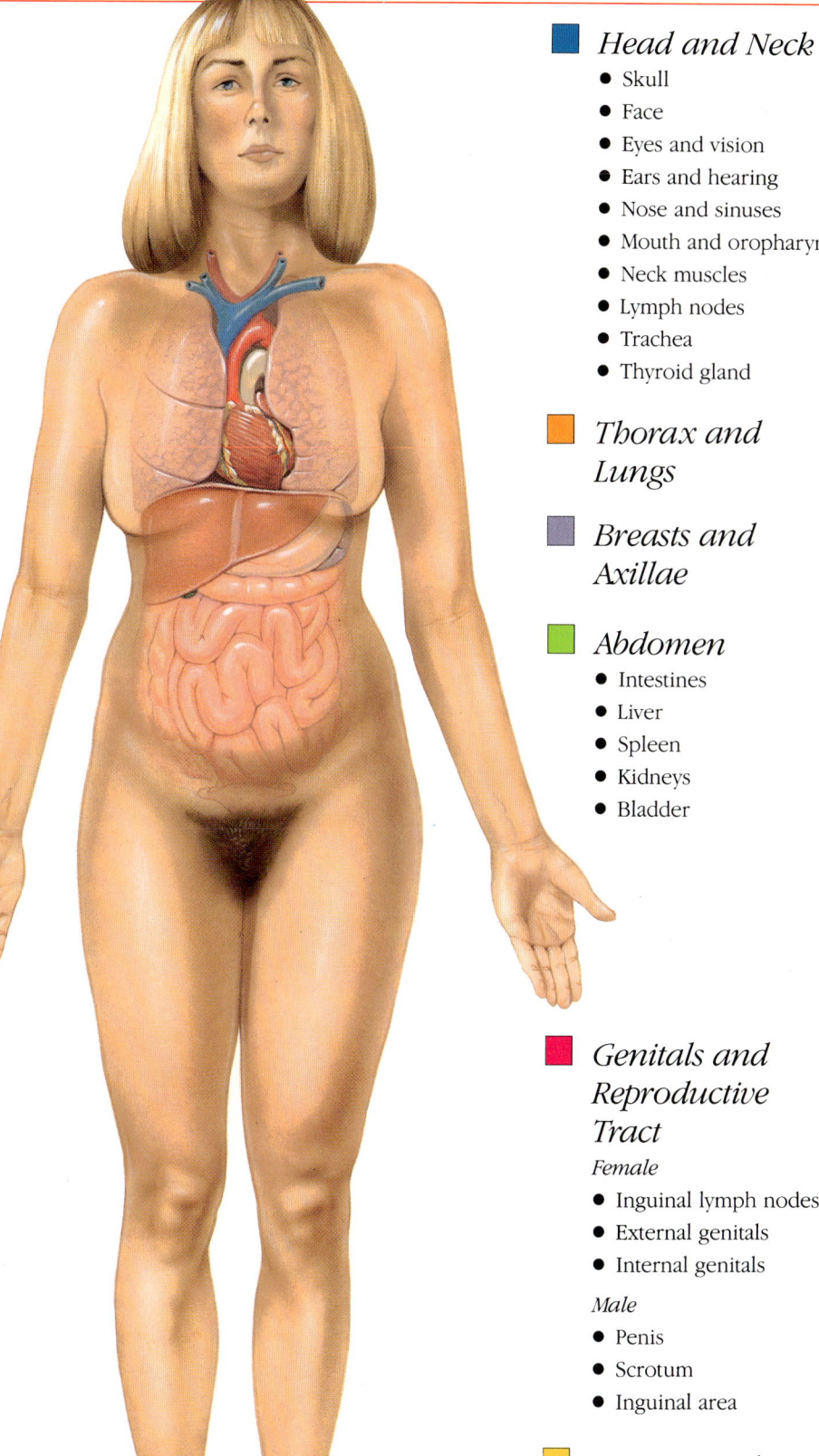

Integument
- Skin
- Hair
- Nails

Neurologic System
- Level of consciousness
- Mental status
- Cranial nerves
- Reflexes
- Motor function
- Sensory function

Cardiovascular System
- Heart
- Peripheral vascular system

Musculoskeletal System
- Muscles
- Bones
- Joints

Head and Neck
- Skull
- Face
- Eyes and vision
- Ears and hearing
- Nose and sinuses
- Mouth and oropharynx
- Neck muscles
- Lymph nodes
- Trachea
- Thyroid gland

Thorax and Lungs

Breasts and Axillae

Abdomen
- Intestines
- Liver
- Spleen
- Kidneys
- Bladder

Genitals and Reproductive Tract
Female
- Inguinal lymph nodes
- External genitals
- Internal genitals

Male
- Penis
- Scrotum
- Inguinal area

Rectum and Anus

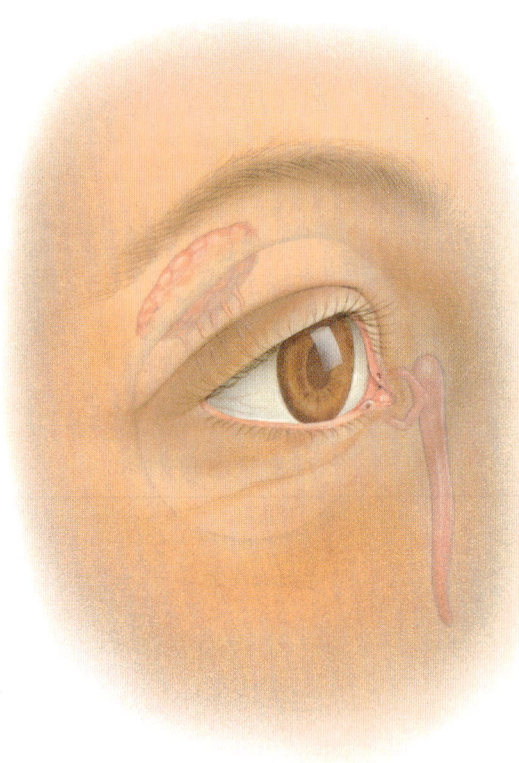

Eyes and Vision

- Inspect the external eye structures.
  - Eyebrows for hair distribution and alignment, skin quality, and movement
  - Eyelashes for evenness of distribution and direction of curl
  - Eyelids for surface characteristics, position, and movement
  - Palpebral and bulbar conjunctiva for color, texture, and lesions
  - Lacrimal apparatus for edema or tenderness
  - Cornea for clarity and texture
  - Anterior chamber for transparency and depth
  - Pupils for color, size, and equality
- Test visual acuity.
- Test peripheral visual fields.
- Test extraocular movements.
- Using an opthalmoscope, inspect the internal eye structures.
  - Red reflex through the pupil
  - Optic disc and cup for color, size, and shape
  - Retinal blood vessels for size, color, pattern, and arteriovenous crossings
  - Retinal background for color and surface characteristics
  - Macula and fovea centralis for color and surface characteristics

Ears and Hearing

- Inspect the auricles for color, texture, symmetry of size, position, and angle.
- Palpate the auricles for texture, elasticity, and areas of tenderness.
- Using an otoscope, inspect the external ear canals for cerumen, inflammation, scaling, foreign bodies, or other lesions.
- Using an otoscope, inspect each internal ear.
  - Tympanic membrane for color and gloss
  - Appearance of the annulus, pars flaccida, pars tensa, malleus, umbo, and light reflex
- Test hearing acuity.
  - Gross hearing acuity by response to voice tones
  - Tuning fork tests (Weber, Rinne, Schwabach tests)

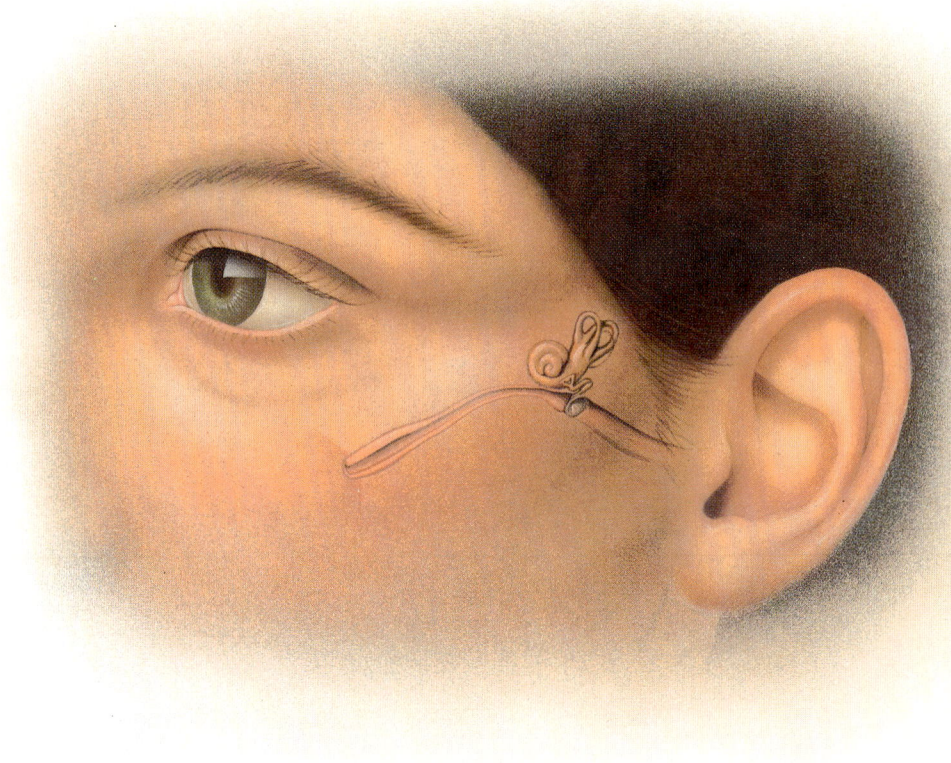

Nose and Sinuses

- Inspect the mucosa for redness, swelling, growths, discharge, and nasal polyps.
- Inspect the nasal septum for deviation.
- Palpate the external nose for tenderness.
- Palpate the maxillary and frontal sinuses for tenderness.
- Transilluminate the maxillary and frontal sinuses for the presence of air or fluid.

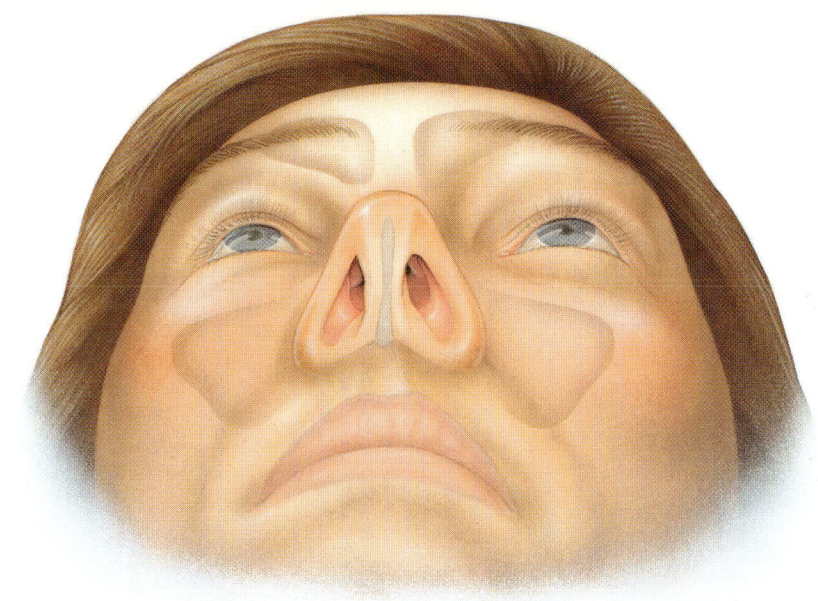

Neck

- Inspect the neck muscles for swellings or masses.
- Assess neck movement and strength of muscles.
- Palpate for enlarged lymph nodes.

- Palpate trachea for position.
- Inspect and palpate thyroid gland for symmetry and masses.

Mouth and Oropharynx

Mouth

- Inspect the lips for symmetry of contour, color, and texture.
- Using gloves, inspect the inner mucosa and the buccal mucosa for color, moisture, texture, and lesions; palpate the mucosa.
- Inspect the teeth for color, presence of fillings, dental caries, partial or complete dentures, and tartar.
- Inspect the gums for bleeding, color, retraction, edema, and lesions; palpate the gums to determine firmness and texture.
- Inspect the tongue for color, size, texture, position, mobility, and coating.
- Palpate the tongue and floor of the mouth for tenderness, nodules, lumps, or excoriated areas.

- Examine the hard and soft palates for color, shape, texture, and the presence of bony prominences.
- Observe the uvula for position and mobility.
- Inspect the salivary gland openings for swelling or redness.

Oropharynx

- Inspect the palatine arches for redness, lesions, and plaques.
- Inspect the tonsils for color, discharge, and size.
- Inspect the oropharynx for edema, inflammation, lesions, or exudate.
- Assess the gag reflex.

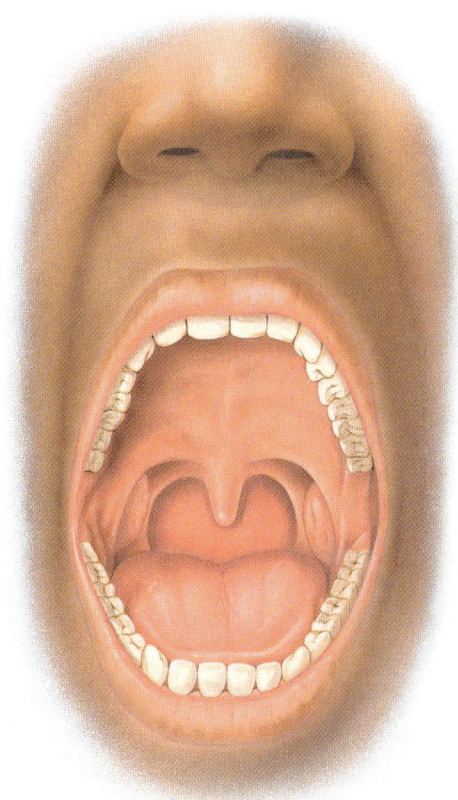

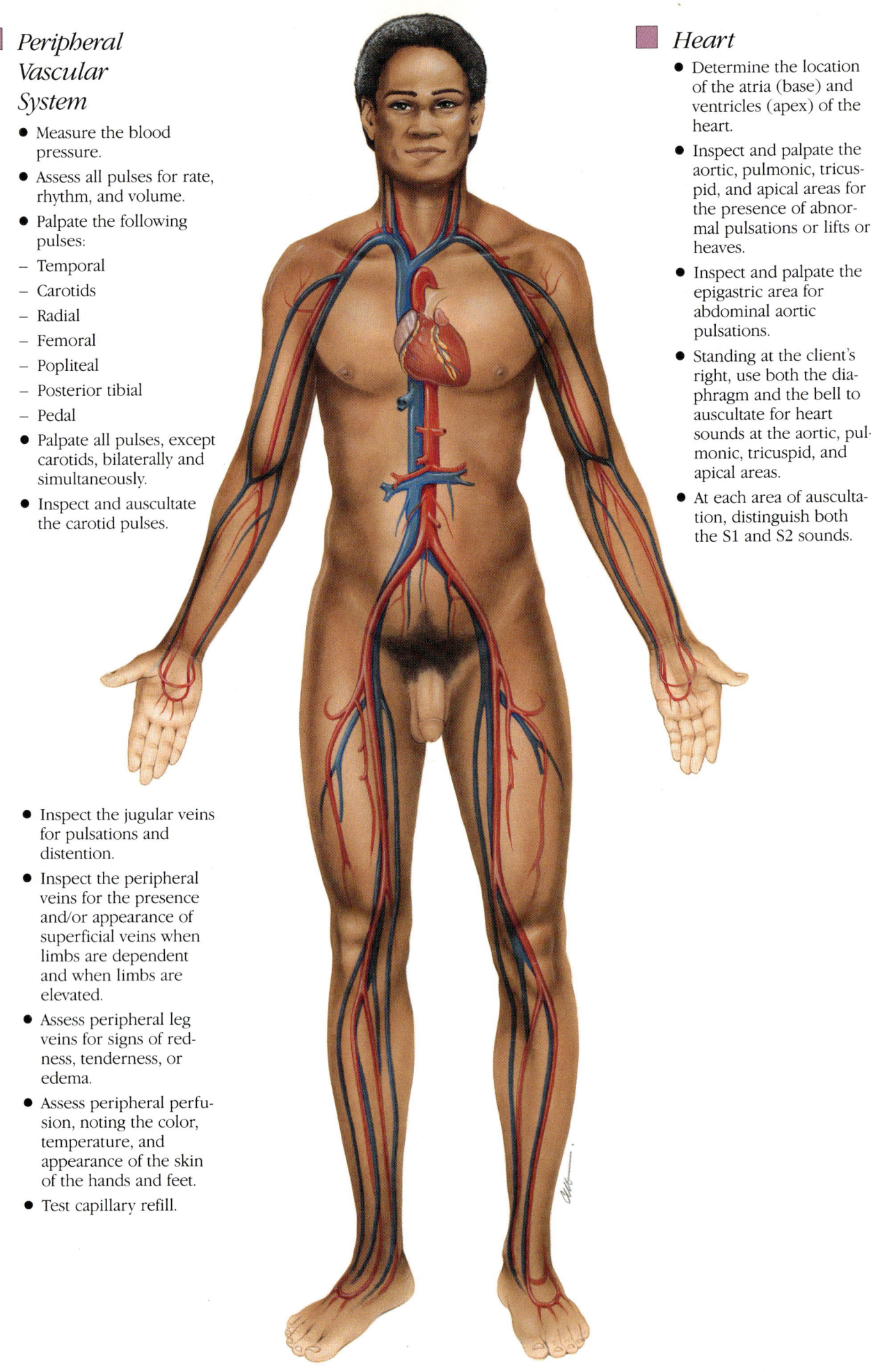

Peripheral Vascular System

- Measure the blood pressure.
- Assess all pulses for rate, rhythm, and volume.
- Palpate the following pulses:
  - Temporal
  - Carotids
  - Radial
  - Femoral
  - Popliteal
  - Posterior tibial
  - Pedal
- Palpate all pulses, except carotids, bilaterally and simultaneously.
- Inspect and auscultate the carotid pulses.

- Inspect the jugular veins for pulsations and distention.
- Inspect the peripheral veins for the presence and/or appearance of superficial veins when limbs are dependent and when limbs are elevated.
- Assess peripheral leg veins for signs of redness, tenderness, or edema.
- Assess peripheral perfusion, noting the color, temperature, and appearance of the skin of the hands and feet.
- Test capillary refill.

Heart

- Determine the location of the atria (base) and ventricles (apex) of the heart.
- Inspect and palpate the aortic, pulmonic, tricuspid, and apical areas for the presence of abnormal pulsations or lifts or heaves.
- Inspect and palpate the epigastric area for abdominal aortic pulsations.
- Standing at the client's right, use both the diaphragm and the bell to auscultate for heart sounds at the aortic, pulmonic, tricuspid, and apical areas.
- At each area of auscultation, distinguish both the S1 and S2 sounds.

Musculoskeletal System

- Observe body posture standing and sitting.
- Observe muscles and tendons for contractures.
- Inspect the muscles for size bilaterally.
- Palpate muscles at rest to determine tonicity.
- Test muscle strength.
- Observe muscles for fasciculations and tremors.
- Inspect each joint for swelling.
- Palpate each joint for tenderness, smoothness of movement, swelling, crepitation, and the presence of nodules.
- Determine the range of motion of the body joints bilaterally.

Neurologic System

- Assess level of consciousness.
- Assess mental status.
  - Assess for aphasias and related language deficits
  - Determine orientation to time, place, and person
  - Assess attitude and affect
  - Evaluate attention span and calculation
  - Listen for lapses in memory
  - Test judgment
  - Assess abstract reasoning
- Assess cranial nerve function.
- Test deep tendon reflexes.
  - Biceps
  - Triceps
  - Brachioradialis
  - Patellar
  - Achilles
  - Plantar (Babinski)

- Test motor function.
  - Conduct gross motor and balance tests
  - Conduct fine motor tests for the upper and lower extremities
- Assess sensory function.
  - Assess light touch sensation and tactile location
  - Assess pain sensation
  - Test temperature sensation
  - Test vibratory sense
  - Test for kinesthetic sensation
  - Test tactile discrimination

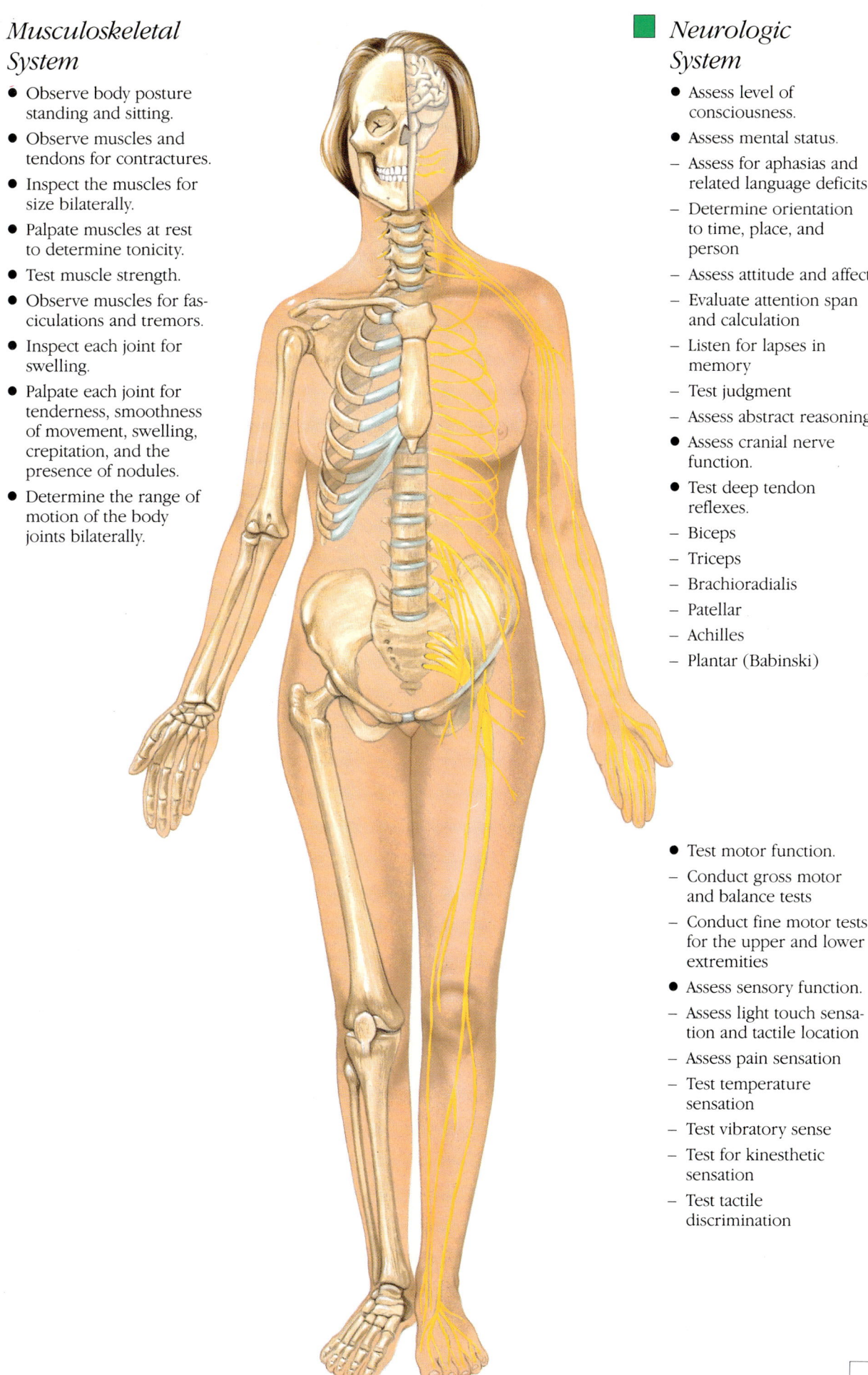

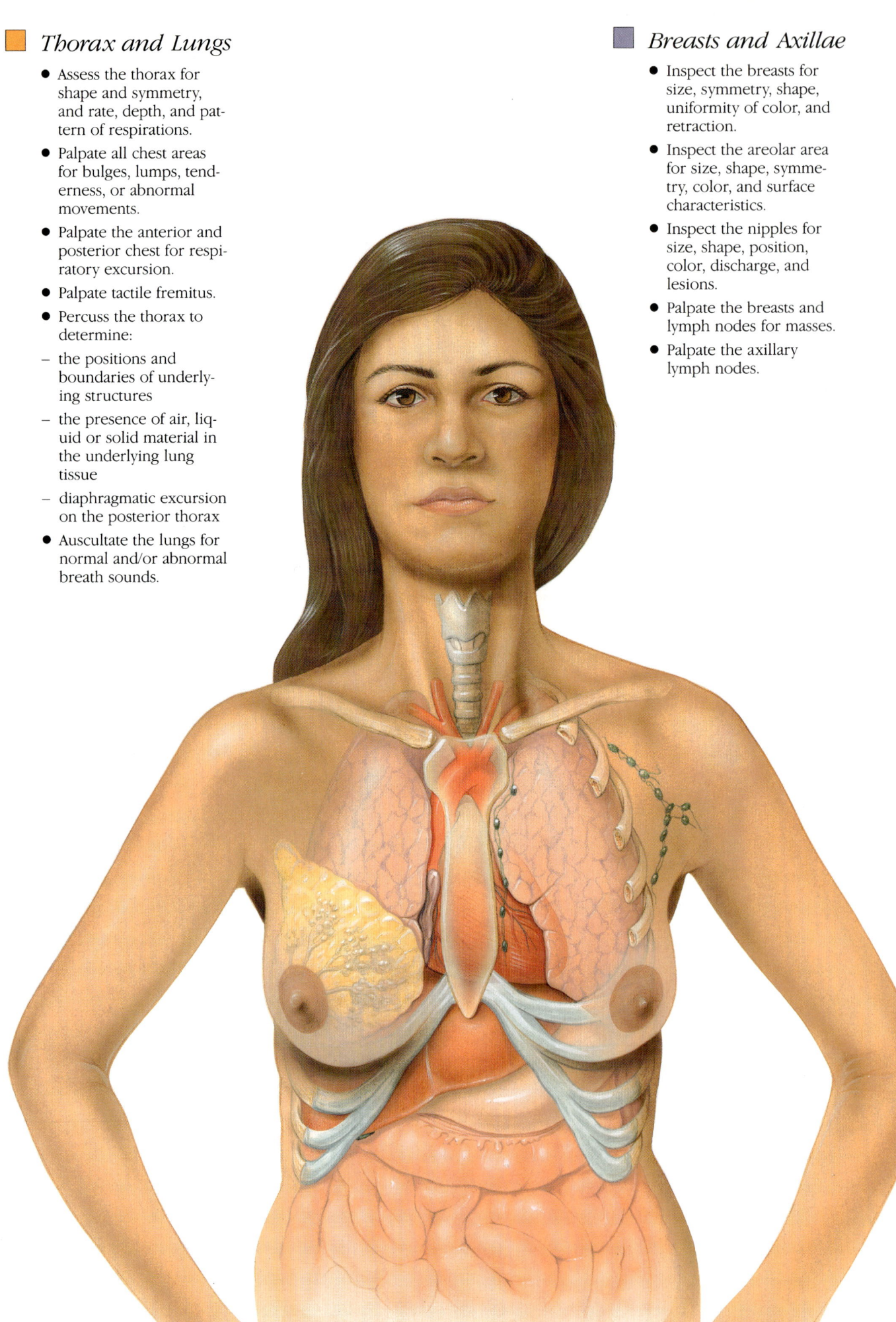

Thorax and Lungs

- Assess the thorax for shape and symmetry, and rate, depth, and pattern of respirations.
- Palpate all chest areas for bulges, lumps, tenderness, or abnormal movements.
- Palpate the anterior and posterior chest for respiratory excursion.
- Palpate tactile fremitus.
- Percuss the thorax to determine:
  - the positions and boundaries of underlying structures
  - the presence of air, liquid or solid material in the underlying lung tissue
  - diaphragmatic excursion on the posterior thorax
- Auscultate the lungs for normal and/or abnormal breath sounds.

Breasts and Axillae

- Inspect the breasts for size, symmetry, shape, uniformity of color, and retraction.
- Inspect the areolar area for size, shape, symmetry, color, and surface characteristics.
- Inspect the nipples for size, shape, position, color, discharge, and lesions.
- Palpate the breasts and lymph nodes for masses.
- Palpate the axillary lymph nodes.

Female Genitals and Reproductive Tract

- Inspect the amount, distribution, and characteristics of pubic hair.
- Inspect the pubic skin for parasites, inflammation, swelling, and lesions.
- Palpate the inguinal lymph nodes for enlargement and tenderness.
- Using gloves, inspect the clitoris, urethral orifice, and vaginal orifice for lesions, discharge, and inflammation.
  - Palpate Bartholin's glands
  - Assess the integrity of the pelvic musculature
- Insert a vaginal speculum and examine the internal genitals.
  - Inspect the cervix for shape of the os, color, size, and position
  - Obtain a specimen for a Papanicolaou smear
  - Inspect the vaginal walls for color, texture, and secretions

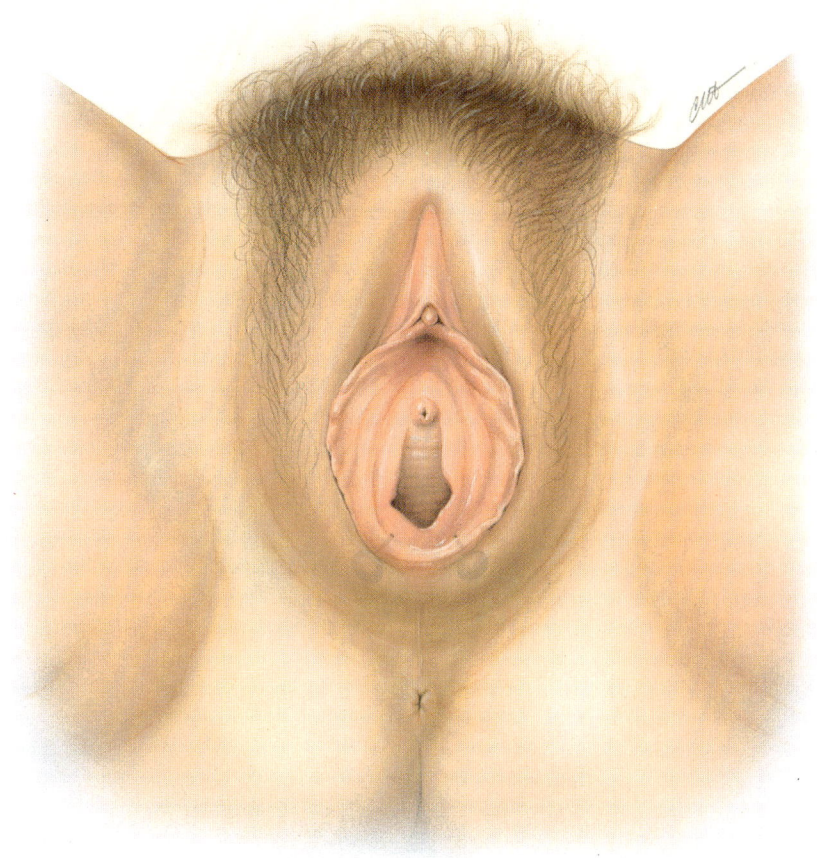

Male Genitals and Reproductive Tract

- Observe the amount, distribution, and characteristics of pubic hair.
- Using gloves, inspect the penile shaft, glans, and urethral meatus for lesions, nodules, swelling, inflammation, and discharge.
- Observe the color and position of the urethral meatus.
- Inspect the scrotum for appearance, general size, and symmetry.
- Palpate the scrotum, testicles, epididymis, and spermatic cord for swelling, irregularities, and tenderness.
- Inspect the inguinal areas for hernias.
- Palpate for inguinal and femoral hernias.

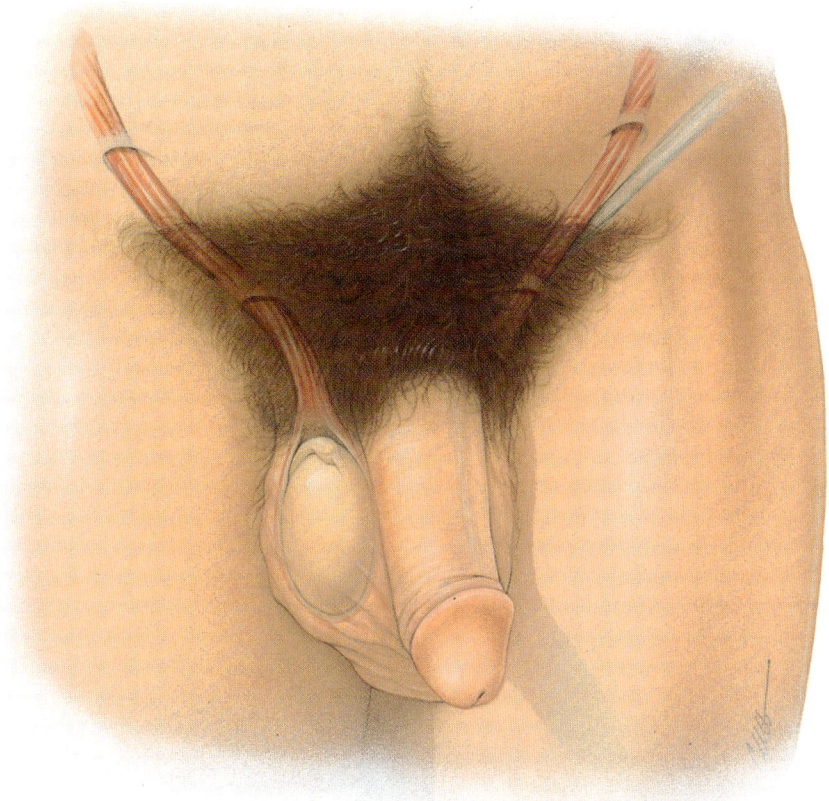

Abdomen

- Inspect the abdomen for skin integrity, contour, and symmetry.
- Observe any movements associated with respiration, peristalsis, or aortic pulsations.
- Auscultate the abdomen for bowel sounds, vascular sounds, and any peritoneal friction rubs.
- Percuss the abdomen for tympany and dullness.
- Percuss the abdomen to determine liver and spleen size.
- Percuss the abdomen to detect areas of tenderness over the liver and kidney.
- Percuss the abdomen to define the outline of a distended bladder.
- Palpate the liver, spleen and kidneys to determine position and size.
- Palpate the abdomen to detect tenderness, presence of masses, and distention.

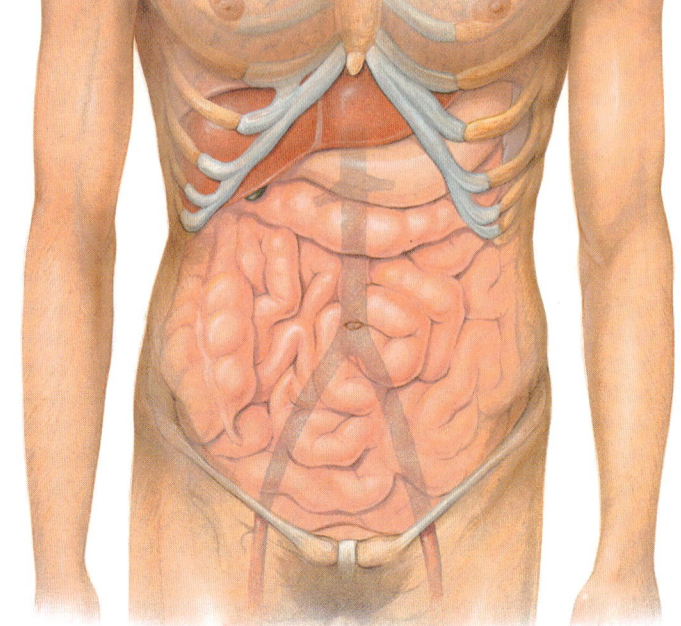

Rectum and Anus

- Using gloves, spread the buttocks with both hands and inspect the anus and surrounding tissue for skin lesions, fissures, ulcers, protruding hemorrhoids, fistula openings, and rectal prolapse.
- Ask the client to bear down and note any bulges, rectal prolapse, polyps, internal hemorrhoids, or rectal fissures.
- Using a gloved, lubricated index finger, palpate for nodules, masses, and tenderness.
- Ask the client to tighten the anal sphincter and note the tone.
- In the male, palpate the prostate gland.
- In the female, palpate the cervix of the uterus.

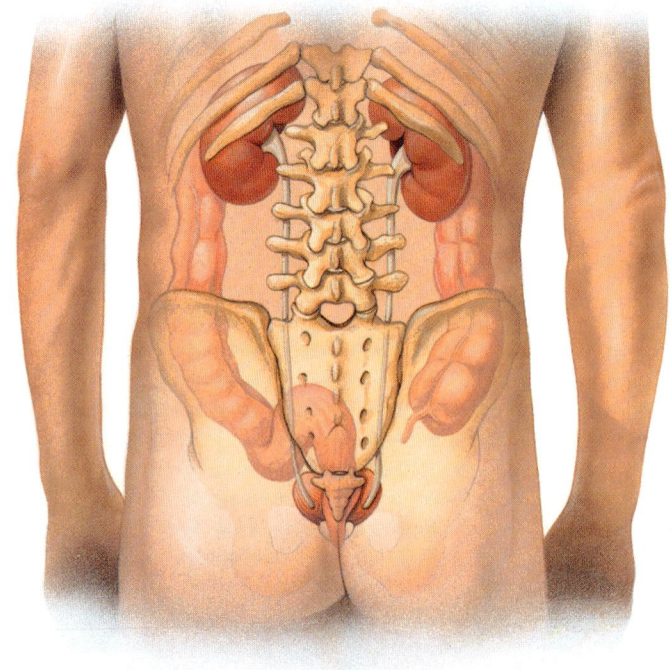

Assessing Health Status

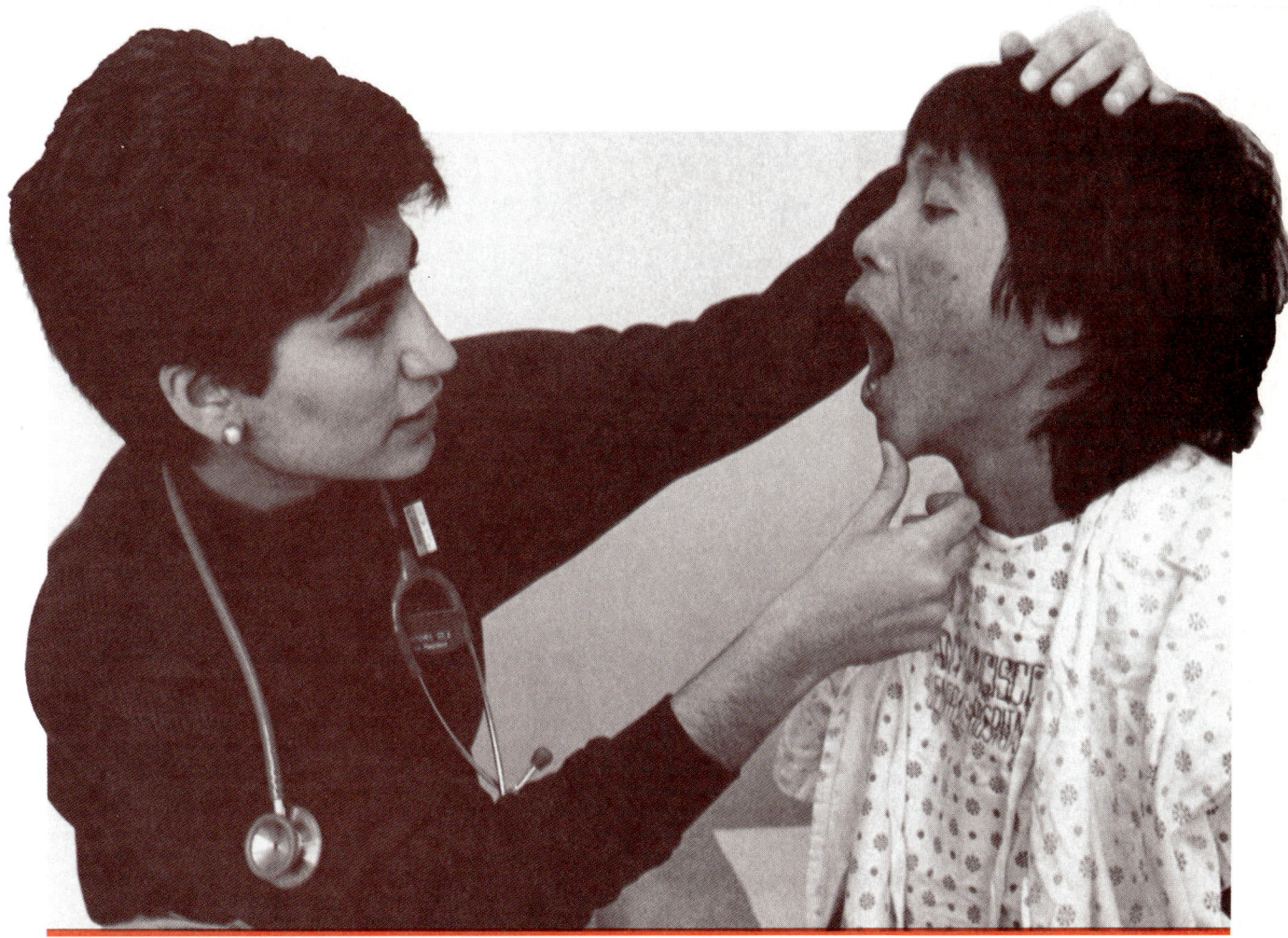

CONTENTS

CONTENTS *(continued)*

OBJECTIVES

▶ Define terms associated with health assessment.

▶ Identify purposes of physical health assessment.

▶ Compare and contrast the four modes of physical assessment.

▶ Explain the significance of selected physical findings.

▶ Identify expected outcomes of health assessment.

▶ Identify the various steps in selected assessment procedures.

▶ Describe suggested sequencing to conduct a physical health assessment in an orderly fashion.

NURSING HEALTH HISTORY

The nursing health history interview is the first part of the assessment of the client's health status and is usually carried out before the physical examination. This is a structured interview designed to collect specific health data and to obtain a detailed health record of the client. Its purposes are

- To elicit information about all the variables that may affect the client's health status
- To obtain data that help the nurse understand and appreciate the client's life experiences
- To initiate a nonjudgmental, trusting interpersonal relationship with the client

Data obtained are then used in collaboration with the client to develop nursing diagnoses and subsequent plans for individualized care. Skill in interviewing is essential when obtaining a health history (see Chapter 10, page 177).

Detailed nursing histories are discussed in each chapter in Units 9 and 10, Supporting Psychosocial and Physiologic Health Patterns. Many health history forms are designed as checklists that the client fills out independently. The nurse then reviews the information with the client and clarifies or amplifies the data as needed. Components of the nursing history include (a) biographic data, (b) chief complaint or reason for visit, (c) history of present illness (current health status), (d) past history, (e) family history of illness, (f) review of systems, (g) life-style, (h) social data, (i) psychologic data, and (j) patterns of health care.

Biographic Data

Biographic data obtained include the client's name, address, age, sex, race, marital status, occupation, religious orientation, health care financing, and usual source of medical care.

Chief Complaint or Reason for Visit

The chief complaint (CC) is the answer given to the question "What is troubling you?" or "What brought you to the hospital or clinic?" and should be recorded in the client's own words. If the client states, "I have heart trouble," or "I have cancer," the nurse should encourage the client to elaborate by discussing specific symptoms and their duration. Further investigation may produce a chief complaint, e.g., "I've had chest pain for the past two hours," or "I've lost 45 pounds in the past month."

History of Present Illness

The history of present illness (HPI) is a sequentially developed, four-part elaboration of the chief complaint (Block and Nolan 1986, p. 11): (a) usual health status, (b) chronologic story; (c) relevant family history, and (d) disability assessment. To obtain a description of the client's *usual health status,* ask the client, "How would you describe your health up until this time?" Answers such as "terrible" or "good" need to be clarified further. For example, ask the client, "What do you mean by terrible (or good)?"

The *chronologic story* is a narrative section where the client's chief complaint is documented in the proper sequence of events. The chronologic story includes these items:

- When the symptoms started
- Whether the onset of symptoms was sudden or gradual
- If available, specific dates when the problem was experienced
- How often the problem occurs
- Exact location of the distress
- Character of the complaint (e.g., intensity of pain or quality of sputum, emesis, or discharge)
- Amount of discharge, mucus, blood, stool, or urine or the size of a lesion
- Activity in which the client was involved when the problem occurred
- Phenomena or symptoms associated with the chief complaint
- Factors that aggravate or alleviate the problem

In the third part of the HPI, the *relevant family history,* the nurse asks the client about related problems of family members. If the client's chief complaint is chest pain, for example, the nurse may ask the client whether there is any family history of heart disease. If so, the specific problem of each affected family member is documented.

In the last part of the HPI, the *disability assessment,* the nurse explores how the problem has interfered with the client's daily life in terms of work or school and family resources and relationships. This part of the HPI provides the nurse with information about the severity of the problem from the client's perspective.

Past History

Included in the past history are all previous immunizations and experiences with illness, including the following:

- *Childhood illnesses,* such as chickenpox, mumps, measles, rubella (German measles), rubeola (red measles), streptococcal infections, scarlet fever, rheumatic fever, and other significant illnesses
- *Childhood immunizations* and the date of the last tetanus shot
- *Allergies* to drugs, animals, insects, or other environmental agents and the type of reaction that occurs
- *Accidents and injuries:* how, when, and where the incident occurred, type of injury, treatment received, and any complications
- *Hospitalization* for serious illnesses: reasons for the hospitalization, dates, location of the hospital, name of the physician, surgery performed, course of recovery, and any complications
- *Medications:* all currently used prescription and over-the-counter medications, such as aspirin, nasal spray, vitamins, or laxatives

Family History of Illness

The family history reveals risk factors for certain diseases. This information should include the ages of siblings, parents, and grandparents and their current state of health or (if they are deceased) the cause of death. Particular attention should be given to disorders such as heart disease, cancer, diabetes, hypertension, obesity, allergies, arthritis, tuberculosis, jaundice, bleeding, ulcers, migraine, and alcoholism.

Review of Systems (ROS)

The ROS is a review of all health problems by body system. Its purpose is to prevent the omission of data related to the present illness and to discover any other problems that might have been missed. It is a review of the past and present status of each system. Generally, a head-to-toe approach is used, and agency checklists are often available. A head-to-toe approach is also used in the physical examination, but the data obtained in this part of the history focus on *subjective data* given by the client. An example of a client checklist for the review of systems is shown in the box on page 358. The client is asked to circle or underline any symptoms experienced. The nurse then explores in depth with the client any symptoms that have not previously been mentioned. An alternative frame of reference for the ROS is the *functional health pattern* approach. See Table 19–1 on page 359 for comparative outlines.

Assessment of specific functional health patterns are shown throughout this book. See assessment interviews in each chapter in Units 7, 9, and 10.

Life-Style

Investigation of the client's life-style provides data about factors that can be used for planning health promotion, maintenance, and restoration. The nurse obtains data about personal habits, diet, sleep/rest patterns, activities of daily living, and recreation/hobbies.

- *Personal habits.* The nurse documents the frequency of all substance abuse, including the use of tobacco, alcohol, coffee, cola, tea, and illicit or recreational drugs. The type of tobacco (cigarette, cigar, or pipe) and the number of packs or smokes per day should be described. The nurse also notes the number of years the client has smoked. The type of alcohol (e.g., beer, wine, or hard liquor), number of bottles or glasses per day, and pattern of drinking (morning, evenings, or weekends) should also be specified. The same descriptive data apply to the consumption of coffee, tea, and cola. When asking about the use of illicit or recreational drugs, the nurse focuses on drugs used extensively in the past, frequency and duration of use, and the good and bad effects.
- *Diet.* Dietary data may include the description of a typical diet on a normal day or of any prescribed special diet,

- *General health.* Weight loss, weakness, feelings of fatigue, mood changes, night sweats, or bleeding tendencies?

- *Skin.* Skin diseases such as eczema, psoriasis, acne; change in pigmentation; tendency toward bruising; excessive dryness or moisture; jaundice; itching, rashes, hives; change in color or size of moles; or open sores that are slow to heal?

- *Hair.* Itchy scalp, loss of hair, excessive body hair? Do you wear a wig?

- *Nails.* Color changes, biting, clubbing, splitting?

- *Head.* Frequent or severe headaches, fainting, dizziness, fall or accident resulting in unconsciousness?

- *Eyes.* Difficulty seeing, eye infection, eye pain, excessive tearing, double vision, blurring, sensitivity to light, cataracts, itching, spots in front of eyes? Do you wear glasses (for near or far vision) or contact lenses? When was your last eye examination?

- *Ears.* Any infection, loss of hearing, pain, discharge, ringing in the ears? Do you wear a hearing aid?

- *Nose.* Frequent colds, nosebleeds, allergies, pain, tenderness, postnasal drip?

- *Mouth and throat.* Sore gums; bleeding gums; sores, lumps or white spots on mouth lips or tongue; toothaches, cavities, difficulty swallowing; voice change or hoarseness? Do you wear dentures (upper, lower, partial)? When was your last dental appointment?

- *Neck.* Pain, swelling, stiffness, limited movement, swollen glands?

- *Breasts.* Nipple discharge, scaling or cracks around nipples, dimples, lumps, pattern of breast self-examination? When did you last have a mammogram?

- *Respiratory system.* Chest pain; cough; shortness of breath; wheezing; coughing up blood; lung disease such as tuberculosis, emphysema, asthma, bronchitis? Have you ever had a chest x ray? When? Results?

- *Cardiovascular system.* Heart disease, palpitations, heart murmur, high blood pressure, anemia, varicose veins, leg swelling or ulcer?

- *Gastrointestinal system.* Nausea, vomiting, loss of appetite, indigestion, heartburn, bright blood in stools, tarry-black stools, diarrhea, constipation, abdominal pain, excessive gas, hemorrhoids, rectal pain, colostomy, ileostomy?

- *Genitourinary system.* Frequency, dribbling, urgency, urination at night, difficulty starting stream, blood in urine, incontinence, pain or burning upon urination, urinary tract infection, ureterostomy, sexually transmitted disease such as gonorrhea ("clap" or "morning drip") or syphilis ("bad blood")? *Females:* Age of menarche, last menstrual period (LMP), duration, amount of flow, regularity of cycle? Any problem with painful menstruation, bleeding between periods, pain during intercourse, vaginal discharge, vaginal itching, vaginal infection? *Males:* Penile discharge, swelling, masses or lesions, difficulty in sexual functioning?

- *Musculoskeletal system.* Muscular pain, swelling, or weakness; joint swelling, soreness, or stiffness; leg cramps; bone defects?

- *Neurologic system.* Difficulty walking; unconsciousness; seizures; tremors; paralysis; numbness, tingling, or burning sensations in any body part; weakness on one side of body; speech problems; loss of memory; disorientation; forgetfulness; unclear thinking; changes in emotional state?

- *Endocrine system.* History of goiter; heat or cold intolerance; diabetes; excessive thirst; excessive eating?

number of meals and snacks per day, who cooks and shops for food, ethnically distinct food patterns, methods used for food preparation, and food likes, dislikes, and allergies. A detailed nutritional history form is provided in Chapter 39, page 1009.

- *Sleep/rest patterns.* Sleep and rest clearly affect the total well-being of the client. The nurse notes the usual daily sleep/wake times, difficulties sleeping, and remedies used for difficulties. A detailed sleep/rest history is provided in Chapter 37, page 948.

- *Activities of daily living (ADLs).* The nurse collects data about the client's perception of any difficulties experienced in the basic activities of eating, grooming, dressing, elimination, and locomotion.

- *Recreation/hobbies.* The client's exercise activity and tolerance, hobbies and other interests, vacations, and time spent with family and friends are discussed.

Social Data

Social assessment includes family relationships and friendships, ethnic affiliation, educational history, occupational history, economic status, and home and neighborhood conditions.

TABLE 19–1 *Comparison of Data Obtained by Functional Health Patterns Framework and Body Systems Framework*

Functional Health Pattern	Body Systems
Health perception and health management	All body systems.
Nutrition and metabolism	Integumentary system (skin, hair, nails); gastrointestinal system, including mouth and throat; endocrine system, with specific reference to the thyroid gland and pancreas for diabetes.
Elimination	Lower gastrointestinal system (anus and rectum); musculoskeletal system, with specific reference to altered mobility and bone defects; neurologic system, with specific reference to problems influencing bowel or bladder control; genitourinary system; integumentary system, with specific reference to impaired perineal skin integrity from incontinence.
Activity/exercise	Cardiovascular, respiratory, musculoskeletal, and neurologic systems.
Cognitive/perceptual	Neurologic system, with specific reference to sensory deficits, altered thought processes, level of consciousness, and orientation.
Sleep and rest	All body systems may affect sleep/rest patterns; sleep disorders may affect various body systems.
Self-perception (self-concept)	Any body system alteration may threaten body image or self-concept.
Role/relationship	Any body system alteration that changes life-style or activities of daily living may alter usual roles and relationships.
Sexuality and reproduction	Reproductive system (breasts, external genitals, internal genitals).
Coping and stress tolerance	Effects of stress may be manifested in the cardiovascular, respiratory, gastrointestinal, integumentary, and endocrine systems.
Values and beliefs	Not applicable.

Family Relationships/Friendships   Because of the many different types of "family" arrangements and relationships in society today (e.g., single parents, unmarried couples, homosexual couples), the nurse must obtain such data with care. The nurse needs to keep in mind the purposes of eliciting such data, which are to determine (a) whether the client has a support system in times of stress, (b) what effect the client's illness has on the family, and (c) whether any "family" problems are affecting the client. The nurse may ask these questions: "Do you live alone? Who helps you in times of need? What person would you like us to contact in case of an emergency? What person do you feel close to in your family? What effect has your illness on family members or friends? Are the other members of your family healthy?" If problems are suspected, the nurse may need to explore the quality of support relationships. To explore specific relationships, the nurse may ask, for example, "How would you describe your father? How would your father describe you?" Open-ended statements, such as "Tell me more about it," also encourage elaboration by the client. See also the discussion of family assessment in Chapter 28, page 688.

Ethnic Affiliation   Data about ethnic affiliation help the nurse understand the client's customs and beliefs. Ethnic data may be obtained by indirect assessment of the client's language, manner of dress, and food preferences or by direct questions such as these: "What country are you and your parents and grandparents from? Do you identify with a particular ethnic group? What cultural practices should we know about that may affect your health care and recovery?" See also the detailed ethnic/cultural assessment guide in Chapter 31, page 765.

Educational History   Data about the client's highest level of education attained and any past difficulties with learning can help the nurse make appropriate adjustments in plans for client teaching.

Occupational History   The occupational history should focus on all jobs the client has held, the client's current employment status, the number of days missed from work because of illness, any history of accidents on the job, any occupational hazards with a potential for future disease or accident, the client's need to change jobs because of past illness, the employment status of both spouses or partners and the way child care is handled, and the client's overall satisfaction with the work.

Economic Status   Financial status is another sensitive area of inquiry that is best handled initially by an open-ended question, e.g., "How would you describe your financial status?" The nurse obtains information about how the client is paying for medical care (including what kind of medical and hospitalization coverage the client has), whether the client feels the family income is sufficient to meet the family's basic needs, and whether the client's illness presents financial concerns.

Home and Neighborhood Conditions

Information about the client's home environment reveals conditions that may or may not be conducive to health. Much of these data may already be surmised from economic, employment, and financial data. The client's physical and mental status and age are especially important in the nurse's review of home safety measures and adjustments in physical facilities that may be required to help the client manage a physical disability, activity intolerance, and activities of daily living. The nurse also inquires about the availability of neighborhood and community services to meet the client's needs.

Psychologic Data

The general survey of appearance and behavior (a component of the physical assessment) reveals much information about the client's emotional state. When a further psychologic assessment is indicated, the nurse notes the client's major stressors, usual coping pattern, communication style, self-concept, and mood.

- *Major stressors.* Determine major stressors the client has experienced in the past year and the client's perception of them.
- *Usual coping pattern.* Ask what the client normally does to cope with a serious problem or a high level of stress. See the section on assessing client coping in Chapter 33, page 806.
- *Communication style.* Observe the client's nonverbal communication and ability to verbalize appropriate emotion. Nonverbal communication—e.g., eye movements, gestures, use of touch, and posture—and the client's interactions with support persons can reveal anxiety, suspicion, withdrawal, anger, or other feelings. Note particularly the congruence of nonverbal behavior and verbal expression. Examples of incongruent expression are being overly cheerful in response to bad news, laughing while discussing a serious topic, or crying when talking about a pleasant topic.
- *Self-concept.* See questions in Chapter 29.
- *Mood.* The nurse may need to ask about mood if the client appears underactive (flat or unresponsive). Ask if the client sleeps well at night, gets discouraged, feels down, or cries frequently. The client's answers help the nurse determine whether the client is depressed. The nurse can then ask other questions to probe the depth of a depression. For example, a nurse may ask whether the client ever feels

life is not worth living or whether things are getting too bad for the client to cope. Affirmative answers to these questions warrant other questions: "Have you ever thought of killing yourself or tried to kill yourself?" "How did you do it or how did you plan to do it?" By gradually leading up to questions of suicide, the nurse can gauge the depth of depression.

Patterns of Health Care

The nurse needs to note all health care resources the client is currently using and has used in the past. These include the family physician, specialists (e.g., ophthalmologist or gynecologist), dentist, folk practitioners (e.g., herbalist or curandero), health clinic, or health center. In addition, the nurse should determine whether the client considers the care being provided adequate and whether access to health care is a problem.

PHYSICAL HEALTH EXAMINATION

A complete health assessment is generally conducted from the head to the toes; however, the procedure can vary in many ways according to the age of the individual, the severity of the illness, the preferences of the nurse, and the agen-

TABLE 19–2 *Examples of Nursing Assessments Addressing Specific Client Situations*

Situation	Physical Assessment
Client complains of abdominal pain.	Inspect, palpate, and auscultate the abdomen; assess vital signs.
Client is admitted with a head injury.	Assess level of consciousness using Glasgow Coma Scale; assess pupils for reaction to light and accommodation; assess vital signs.
The nurse administers a cardiotonic drug to a client.	Assess apical pulse and compare with baseline data.
The nurse administers postural drainage.	Auscultate lungs before and after the procedure.
The client has just had a cast applied to the lower leg.	Assess peripheral perfusion of toes, capillary blanch test, pedal pulse if able, and vital signs.
The client's fluid intake is minimal.	Assess tissue turgor, fluid intake and output, and vital signs.

cy's priorities and procedures. Regardless of what procedure is used, the client's energy and time need to be considered. The health assessment is therefore conducted in a systematic and efficient manner that requires the fewest position changes for the client.

Frequently, nurses assess a specific body area instead of the entire body. These specific assessments are made in relation to client complaints, the nurse's own observation of problems, the client's presenting problem, nursing interventions provided, and medical therapies. Examples of these situations and assessments are provided in Table 19–2. For clients *without* specific complaints or problems, an abbreviated physical health assessment may be provided. See guidelines in Table 19–3.

These are some of the purposes of the physical health examination:

1. To obtain baseline data about the client's functional abilities
2. To supplement, confirm, or refute data obtained in the nursing history
3. To obtain data that will help the nurse establish nursing diagnoses and plan the client's care
4. To evaluate the physiologic outcomes of health care and thus the progress of a client's health problem
5. To screen for the presence of cancer (see the American Cancer Society's guidelines shown on page 362)

TABLE 19–3 *Abbreviated Physical Health Assessment for Clients Without Specific Complaints or Problems*

Body Area or System	Essential Examination Techniques
General survey	Assess all aspects: appearance and behavior, height and weight, vital signs.
Skin	Inspect all skin areas exposed throughout the examination. Check skin turgor if dehydration is suspected.
Hair	Cursory inspection only.
Nails	Cursory inspection only.
Head (skull)	Cursory inspection only.
Face	Cursory inspection only.
Eyes	Cursory inspection of external eye structures only. May conduct visual acuity tests for near and far vision.
Ears	Cursory inspection only.
Nose and sinuses	No examination necessary.
Mouth	Inspect status of lips, mucous membranes, teeth, gingiva, tongue, palates, uvula, and opening of the salivary glands.
Oropharynx	Inspect oropharynx and tonsils and elicit gag reflex.
Neck	Inspect for abnormal lumps or masses. Palpate lymph nodes and observe movement of thyroid gland during swallowing.
Thorax and lungs	Inspect respirations and shape and symmetry of thorax. Palpate for respiratory excursion. Auscultate for adventitious breath sounds.
Heart	Inspect precordium for lifts or heaves. Auscultate heart rate and rhythm and identify S1 and S2 heart sounds.
Peripheral vascular	Assess blood pressure. Inspect, palpate, and auscultate carotid arteries. Test capillary refill of large toe nails.
Breasts/axillae	Inspect breasts. Palpate breasts annually in females beginning at age 40.
Abdomen	Perform light and deep palpation of abdomen. Palpate liver for enlargement.
Musculoskeletal	No examination necessary.
Neurologic	No examination necessary. May assess reflexes.
Female genitals and reproductive tract	Palpate inguinal area for lymph node enlargement and presence of hernias. Inspect external genitalia. See cancer screening guidelines for pelvic examination and Papanicolaou smears.
Male genitals	Inspect external genitals and assess the presence of any hernias. Palpate scrotum.
Rectum and anus	Inspect external structures. Perform digital rectal examination annually in persons beginning at age 40 years.

client should also be told that appropriate draping will be provided so that the body will not be unnecessarily exposed.

Most clients should empty their bladders before the examination. Doing so helps them feel more relaxed and facilitates palpation of the abdomen and pubic area. Since an empty rectum facilitates rectal examination, the client should be encouraged to defecate before a complete physical examination. If a urinalysis is required, the urine should be collected in a container for that purpose. Clients must often assume special positions during the health examination. See Table 19–4.

Dorsal and Horizontal Recumbent and Supine Positions

The appropriate drapes for a client in these positions usually include (a) a hospital gown or bath towel for the chest and (b) a bath blanket or sheet to cover the remainder of the body from the waist to the toes. The bath towel is placed across the chest, and the bath blanket or sheet is placed diagonally over the person. If the client's perineal area is to be examined, opposite corners of the sheet are wrapped around the feet to cover the legs. The corner between the client's legs can be raised to expose the perineum at the appropriate time. See Figure 19–1.

Sitting Position

This position is frequently assumed during examinations of the chest, neck, and head. The client requires a gown.

Lithotomy Position

The lithotomy position is frequently used for examinations of the vagina and sometimes for urinary catheterizations in women.

The drapes usually used are (a) a gown for the upper body (optional), (b) a rectangular sheet or a fenestrated sheet, and (c) socks for the clients' feet (optional). The socks are put on the client before the feet are placed in the

Preparation of the Client

Most people need an explanation about the physical health examination. The nurse should explain when and where the examination will take place, why it is necessary, who will conduct it, and what will happen during the examination. Children need explanations that address their concerns (e.g., that most examinations are not painful, how the child can assist, whether a parent can accompany the child, and that a nurse will be there to help). Special circumstances—for instance, the need to go to a different room or assume a special position—should be explained. The

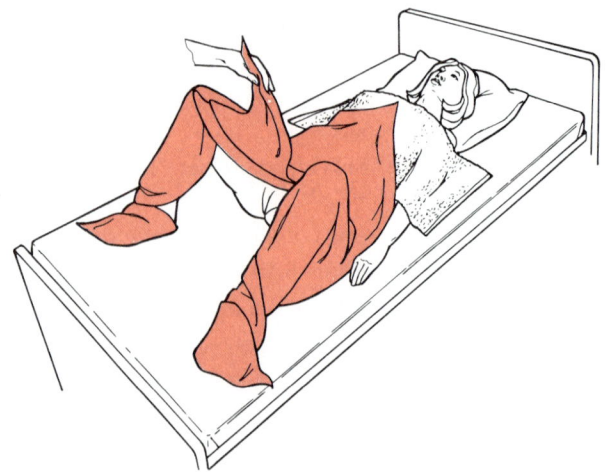

Figure 19–1 A client draped in a dorsal recumbent position.

Position	Description	Areas Examined	Cautions
Dorsal recumbent	Back-lying position with knees flexed and hips externally rotated; small pillow under the head	Head and neck, axillae, anterior thorax, lungs, breasts, heart, abdomen, extremities, peripheral pulses, vital signs, and vagina	May be difficult for clients who have cardiopulmonary problems to assume
Horizontal recumbent	Back-lying position with legs extended; small pillow under the head	Head, neck, axillae, anterior thorax, lungs, breasts, heart, extremities, peripheral pulses	Not used for abdominal assessment because of the increased tension of abdominal muscles
Dorsal (supine)	Back-lying position without a pillow	As for horizontal recumbent	Tolerated poorly by clients with cardiovascular and respiratory problems
Sitting	A seated position, back unsupported and legs hanging freely	Head, neck, posterior and anterior thorax, lungs, breasts, axillae, heart, vital signs, upper and lower extremities, reflexes	Elderly and weak clients may require support
Lithotomy	Back-lying position with feet supported in stirrups; the hips should be in line with the edge of the table	Female genitals, rectum, and female genital reproductive tract	May be difficult and tiring for elderly people
Genupectoral	Kneeling position with torso at a 90° angle to hips	Rectum	Uncomfortable position, tolerated poorly by clients who have respiratory problems
Sims's	Side-lying position with lowermost arm behind the body and uppermost leg flexed (See Chapter 36)	Rectum, vagina	Difficult for the elderly and people with limited joint movement
Prone	Face-lying position, with or without a small pillow	Posterior thorax, hip movement	Often not tolerated by the elderly and people with cardiovascular and respiratory problems.

stirrups. The sheet is placed diagonally on the client so that the top part covers the client's chest and abdomen. The side corners are wrapped around the client's legs and feet. If the client is wearing socks, the drape need not cover the feet, but it should overlap the socks. See Figure 19−2. The corner between the client's legs is lifted to expose the perineal area. A fenestrated drape is placed the same way as a rectangular sheet but with the opening directly over the area to be examined.

Genupectoral (Knee-Chest) Position

In this kneeling position, the head is turned to one side and the arms are held above the head. Special tables, provided in many agencies, support clients in this position.

The drapes required are (a) a hospital gown to cover the upper body, (b) socks to cover the feet and lower legs (optional), and (c) a fenestrated drape to cover the client's back, buttocks, and thighs. The hole in the drape exposes

(continued on page 364)

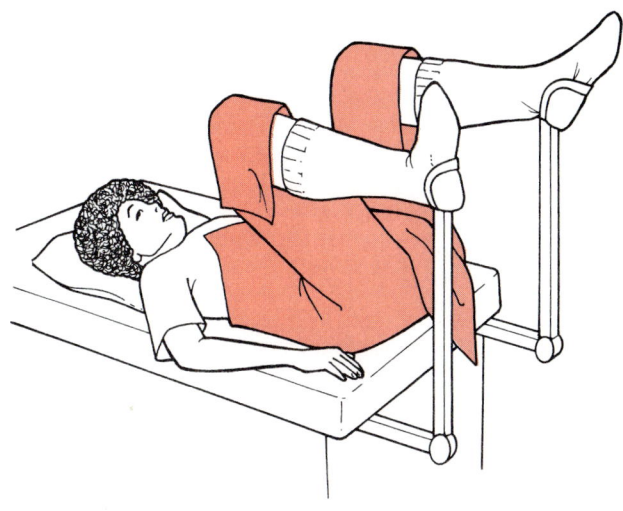

Figure 19−2 A client draped in the lithotomy position.

only the area to be examined. See Figure 19–3. A rectangular drape can be used instead. The two lateral corners are tucked around the client's thighs. The corner between the thighs can then be lifted up to expose the area to be examined, e.g., the anus. See Figure 19–4.

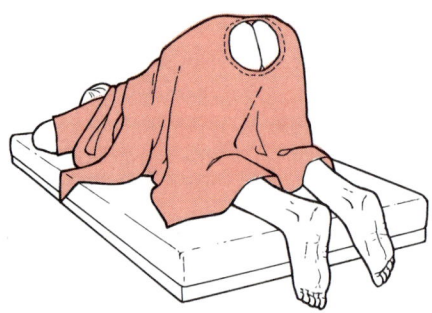

Figure 19–3 A fenestrated drape exposes only the anal area of a client in the genupectoral position.

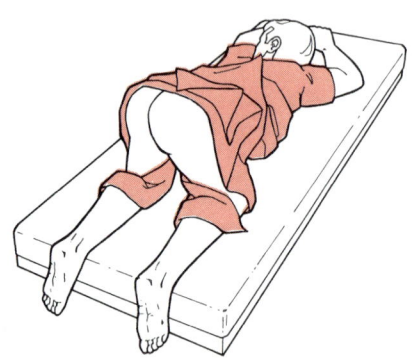

Figure 19–4 A client draped in the genupectoral position.

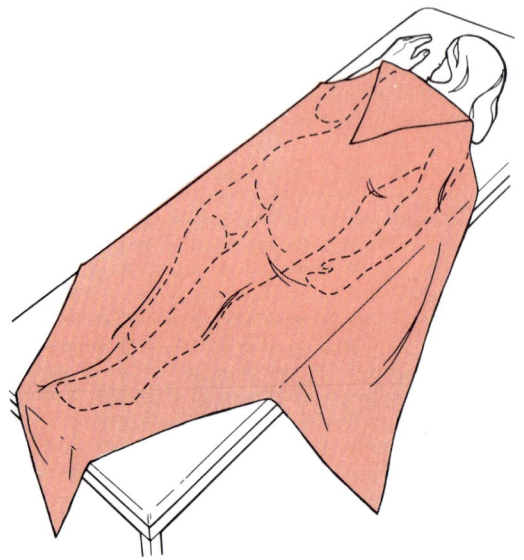

Figure 19–5 A client draped in Sims's position.

Sims's Position

In Sims's position, the lower arm is behind the client, and the upper arm is flexed at both the shoulder and the elbow. Both legs are also flexed, the upper one more so at the hip and the knee than the lower one.

The drape is usually one rectangular sheet, placed diagonally on the client. See Figure 19–5. At the time of examination, the corner is folded back to expose the area. Because this position can be difficult for some clients to assume, particularly the elderly and the obese, it is normally not assumed until immediately before the examination. For additional information, see Chapter 36, page 911.

Prone Position

A client in the prone position usually turns the head to the side. See Figure 36–16 on page 909. A sheet to cover the client is required.

Methods of Examining

Four primary techniques are used in the physical examination: inspection, palpation, percussion, and auscultation. These are discussed throughout this chapter as they apply to each body system.

Inspection

Inspection is the visual examination, i.e., assessing using the sense of sight. The nurse inspects with the naked eye and with a lighted instrument such as an otoscope (used to view the ear). Some authors consider the use of the senses of hearing and smell as part of inspection (Malasanos, Barkauskas, and Stoltenberg-Allen 1990, p. 138). Nurses frequently use this technique to assess color, rashes, scars, body shape, facial expressions that may reflect emotions, and body structures, e.g., the inner eye. Inspection is an active process, not a passive one. The nurse must know what to look for and where. Inspection should be systematic, so that nothing is missed. Lighting must be sufficient; either natural or artificial light can be used.

Palpation

Palpation is the examination of the body using the sense of touch. The pads of the fingers are used because their concentration of nerve endings makes them highly sensitive to tactile discrimination. Palpation is used to determine

- Texture, e.g., of the hair
- Temperature, e.g., of a skin area
- Vibration, e.g., of a joint
- Position, size, consistency, and mobility of organs or masses
- Distention, e.g., of the urinary bladder
- Presence and rate of peripheral pulses
- Tenderness or pain

There are two types of palpation: light and deep. *Light* (superficial) palpation should always precede *deep* palpation, because heavy pressure on the fingertips can dull the sense of touch. For *light palpation,* the nurse extends dominant hand fingers parallel to the skin surface and presses gently downward while moving the hand in a circular fash-

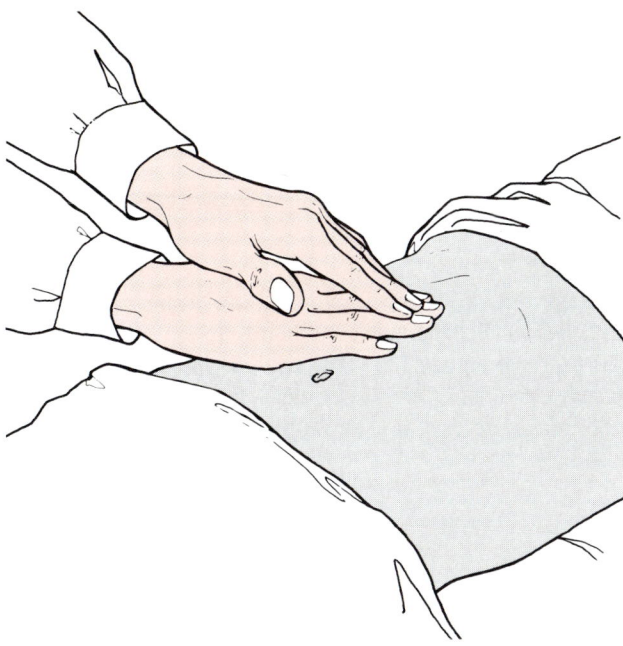

Figure 19–6 The position of the hands for deep bimanual palpation.

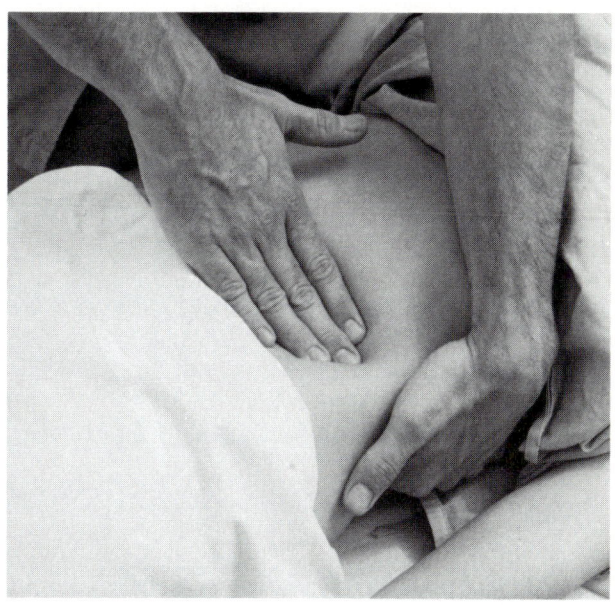

Figure 19–7 Deep palpation using one hand under the body for support while the upper hand palpates the organ.

ion. If it is necessary to determine the details of a mass, the nurse presses lightly several times rather than holding the pressure.

Deep palpation is done with two hands (bimanually) or one hand. In deep bimanual palpation, the nurse extends the dominant hand as for light palpation, then places the fingerpads of the nondominant hand on the dorsal surfaces of the distal interphalangeal joint of the middle three fingers of the dominant hand. See Figure 19–6. Pressure is applied by the top hand while the lower hand remains relaxed to perceive the tactile sensations. For deep palpation using one hand, the fingerpads of the dominant hand press over the area to be palpated. Often the other hand is used to support a mass or organ from below. See Figure 19–7. Deep palpation is a technique used more commonly by nurse practitioners and clinical specialists than by nurses in general practice.

The effectiveness of palpation depends largely on the client's relaxation. Nurses can assist a client to relax by (a) gowning and/or draping the client appropriately; (b) positioning the client comfortably; (c) ensuring that their own hands are warm before beginning, e.g., running them under warm water if they are cold; and (d) commencing palpation with areas that are not painful. During palpation, the nurse should be sensitive to the client's verbal and facial expressions indicating discomfort.

Percussion   **Percussion** is an assessment method in which the body surface is struck to elicit sounds that can be heard or vibrations that can be felt. There are two types of percussion: direct, or immediate, percussion and indirect, or mediate, percussion. In *direct percussion,* the nurse

strikes the area to be percussed directly with the pads of two, three, or four fingers or with the pad of the middle finger. The strikes are rapid, and the movement is from the wrist. This technique is not generally used to percuss the thorax but is useful in percussing an adult's sinuses. The second type, *indirect percussion,* is the striking of an object (e.g., a finger) held against the body area to be examined. In this technique, the middle finger of the nondominant hand, referred to as the **pleximeter,** is placed firmly on the client's skin. Only the distal phalanx and joint of this finger should be in contact with the skin. Using the tip of the flexed middle finger of the other hand, called the **plexor,** the nurse strikes the pleximeter, usually at the distal interphalangeal joint. Some nurses may find a point between the distal and proximal joints to be a more comfortable pleximeter point. See Figure 19–8 on page 366. The striking motion should come from the wrist; the forearm remains stationary. The angle between the plexor and the pleximeter should be 90 degrees, and the blows must be firm, rapid, and short to obtain a clear sound.

Percussion is used to determine the size and shape of internal organs by establishing their borders. It indicates whether tissue is fluid-filled, air-filled, or solid. Percussion elicits five types of sound: flatness, dullness, resonance, hyperresonance, and tympany. **Flatness** is an extremely dull sound produced by very dense tissue such as muscle or bone. **Dullness** is a thudlike sound produced by dense tissue such as the liver, spleen, or heart. **Resonance** is a hollow sound such as that produced by lungs filled with air. **Hyperresonance** is not produced in the normal body. It is described as booming and can be heard over an emphysematous lung. **Tympany** is a musical or drumlike sound

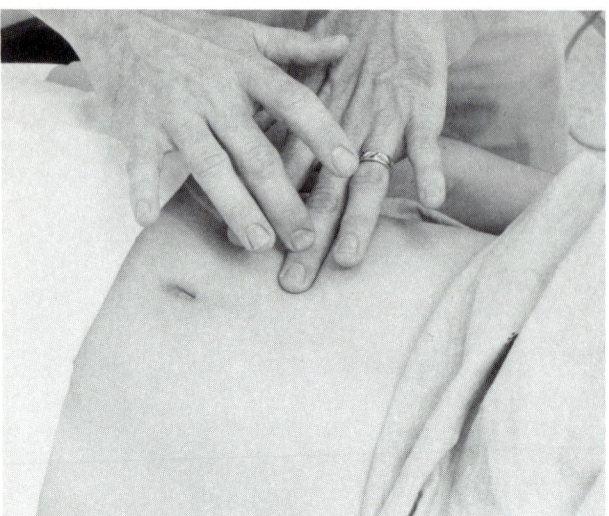

Figure 19–8 The position of the fingers for percussion. Only the middle finger of the nondominant hand is firmly in contact with the client's skin.

produced from an air-filled stomach. On a continuum, flatness reflects the most dense tissue (least amount of air) and tympany the least dense tissue (the most amount of air). A percussion sound is described according to its intensity, pitch, duration, and quality. See Table 19–13 on page 401.

Auscultation **Auscultation** is the process of listening to sounds produced within the body. Auscultation may be direct or indirect. *Direct auscultation* is the use of the unaided ear, e.g., to listen to a respiration wheeze or the grating of a moving joint. *Indirect auscultation* is the use of a stethoscope, which amplifies the sounds and conveys them to the nurse's ears. A stethoscope is used primarily to listen to sounds from within the body, e.g., bowel sounds or valve sounds of the heart.

The stethoscope should be 30 to 25 cm (12 to 14 in) long, with an internal diameter of about 0.3 cm (⅛ in). It should have both a flat-disc and a bell-shaped diaphragm. See Figure 18–16. The flat-disc diaphragm best transmits high-pitched sounds, e.g., bronchial sounds, and the bell-shaped diaphragm best transmits low-pitched sounds, such as some heart sounds. The earpieces of the stethoscope should fit comfortably into the nurse's ears. The diaphragm of the stethoscope is placed firmly but lightly against the client's skin. If a client is very hairy, it may be necessary to dampen the hairs with a moist cloth so that they will lie flat against the skin and not cause scratching sounds.

Auscultated sounds are described according to their pitch, intensity, duration, and quality. The **pitch** is the frequency of the vibrations (the number of vibrations per second). Low-pitched sounds, e.g., some heart sounds, have fewer vibrations per second than high-pitched sounds, such as bronchial sounds. The **intensity** (amplitude) refers to the loudness or softness of a sound. Some body sounds are loud, e.g., bronchial sounds heard over the trachea, while others are soft, e.g., normal breath sounds heard in the lungs. The **duration** of a sound is its length (long or short). The **quality** of sound is a subjective description of a sound, e.g., whistling, gurgling, or snapping.

Instrumentation

Illustrations of various equipment are shown throughout the chapter. Equipment is frequently set up on trays ready for use. See Figure 19–9. All equipment required for the health examination should be clean, in good working order, and readily accessible. See Table 19–5.

GENERAL SURVEY

The nurse assesses many components of the general survey while taking the health history. Other data obtained as part of the general survey include appearance and behavior, vital signs, and height and weight.

Appearance and Behavior

The general appearance and behavior of an individual must be assessed in terms of culture, educational level, socioeconomic status, and current circumstances. An individual who has recently experienced a personal loss may appropriately appear depressed. Points to consider when observing the client's general appearance include the following:

■ *Age, sex and race.* This information is useful in interpreting findings that suggest increased risk for known conditions.

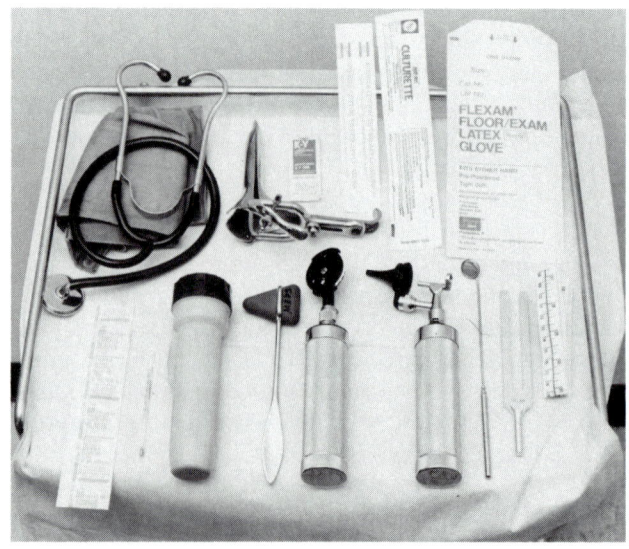

Figure 19–9 Equipment on a tray ready for a health examination.

- *Body build, height, and weight in relation to the client's age, life-style, and health.* Note whether the client is excessively thin, obese, or muscular.
- *Posture and gait.* Note whether the client (a) is relaxed or tense, (b) has an erect, slouched, or bent posture, and (c) has coordinated or uncoordinated movements or tremors.
- *Hygiene and grooming.* Relate findings to the person's activities prior to the assessment.
- *Dress.* Note whether dress is appropriate to age, life-style, climate, socioeconomic status, culture, and current circumstances.
- *Body and breath odor.* Note these in relation to activity level.

- *Signs of distress.* Posture, behavior, and facial expression (e.g., wincing or labored breathing) can reflect distress.
- *Obvious signs.* Note obvious signs of health or illness.
- *Attitude.* Attitude is reflected in appearance, speech, and behavior; note whether the client is cooperative, withdrawn, negative, or hostile.
- *Affect* (the emotional state as it appears to others) and *mood* (the emotional state as described by the individual). Assess whether client's responses are appropriate or inappropriate to the circumstances.
- *Speech.* Listen for quantity (amount of speech and the pace of talking), quality (loudness, clarity, and inflection), and organization (coherence of thought, overgeneralization, and vagueness).

TABLE 19–5 *Equipment and Supplies Used for a Health Examination*

Instruments and Supplies	Purpose
Flashlight or penlight	To assist viewing of the pharynx and cervix or to determine the reactions of the pupils of the eye
Head mirror	To direct light to a specific body area, e.g., the pharynx
Laryngeal or dental mirror	To observe the pharynx and oral cavity
Nasal speculum	To permit visualization of the lower and middle turbinates; usually a penlight is used for illumination
Neurologic hammer	To test reflexes; often has a soft brush and needle in the handle that come out when it is unscrewed
Ophthalmoscope	A lighted instrument to visualize the interior of the eye
Otoscope	A lighted instrument to visualize the eardrum and external auditory canal (a nasal speculum may be attached to the otoscope to inspect the nasal cavities)
Percussion (reflex) hammer	An instrument with a rubber head to test reflexes
Smells (1 or 2 vials)	To test the sense of smell
Sphygmomanometer and cuff	To measure the blood pressure
Stethoscope	To auscultate body sounds, e.g., blood pressure, chest, bowel sounds
Thermometer	To measure body temperature
Tuning fork	A two-pronged metal instrument used to test hearing acuity and vibratory sense
Vaginal speculum (various sizes)	To assess the cervix and the vagina
Ayre spatula	To obtain a cervical scrape
Assorted containers and slides	For specimens
Cotton applicators	To obtain specimens
Disposable pads	To absorb liquid
Drapes	To cover the client
Gauze dressings	To cover wounds
Gloves (sterile and unsterile)	To protect the nurse
Lubricant	To ease insertion of instruments, e.g., vaginal speculum
Sterile safety pins	To test sensory function
Tongue blades (depressors)	To depress the tongue during assessment of the mouth and pharynx

■ *Thought processes.* Listen for relevance and organization of the thoughts.

Mental status and the *level of consciousness* or state of awareness are often determined at the beginning of the physical examination. Ask the client to state name, the day or date, present location, and the reason for hospitalization or for seeking assistance. Record the client's ability to provide this information. For clients who are unable to speak, describe their specific responses to verbal and physical stimuli. See Neurologic Assessment later in this chapter.

Vital Signs

Vital signs are measured (a) to establish baseline data against which to compare future measurements and (b) to detect actual and future health problems. See Chapter 18 for measurements of temperature, pulse, respirations, and blood pressure.

Height and Weight

In adults, the ratio of weight to height provides a general measure of health. In infants and growing children, these measurements are an index of normal or abnormal growth and are essential in calculating body surface area to determine safe dosages of medications. By asking clients about

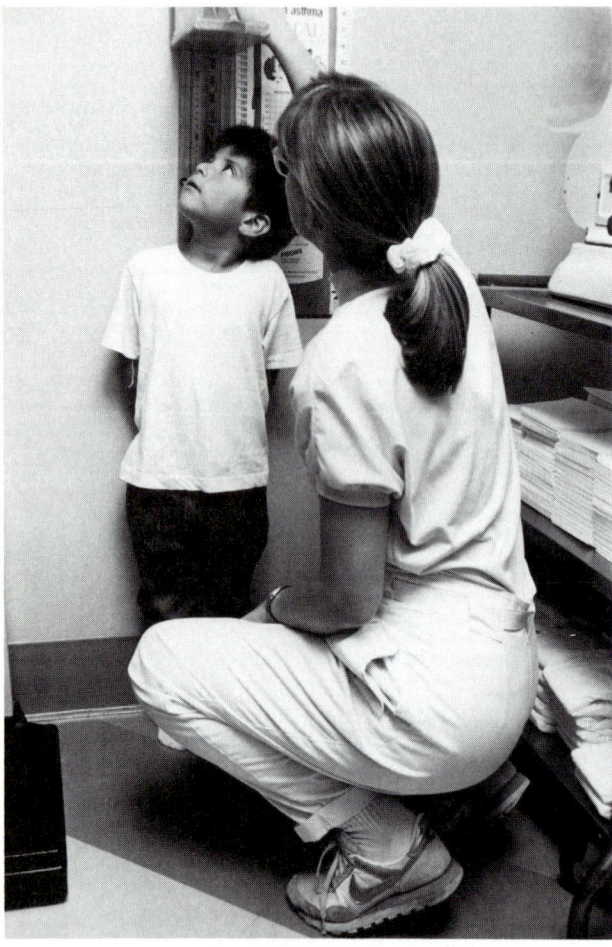

Figure 19–10   Measuring the height of a child.

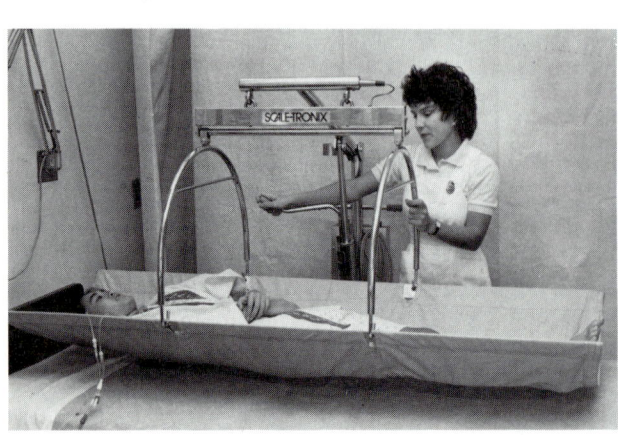

Figure 19–11   A bed scale.

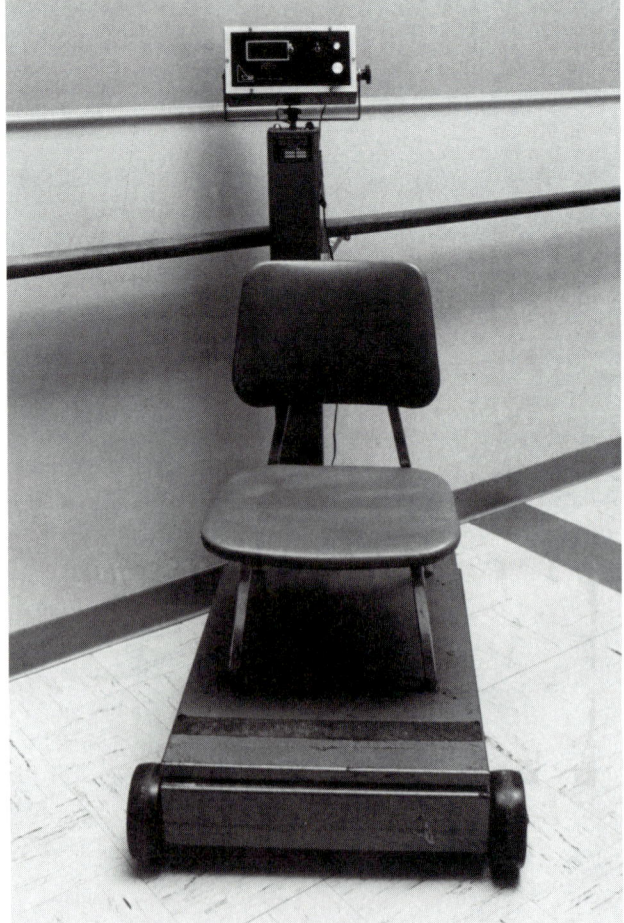

Figure 19–12   A chair scale.

their height and weight before actually measuring them, the nurse obtains some idea of the person's self-image. Excessive discrepancies between the client's responses and the measurements may provide clues to actual or potential problems in self-concept. It is also important that the nurse and client be aware of any weight gains or losses over a specific time period.

Height is measured with a measuring stick attached to weight scales or to a wall. See Figure 19–10. The client removes the shoes and stands erect with heels together, buttocks and head against the measuring stick, and eyes looking straight ahead. The nurse raises the L-shaped sliding arm on the weight scale until it rests on top of the client's head or places a small flat object, such as a ruler or book, on the client's head. The edge of the ruler should abut the measuring guide. More accurate results can be obtained with a right-angled instrument.

Weight is usually measured when a client is admitted to a health agency and often regularly, e.g., each morning before breakfast. When accuracy is essential, the nurse should use the same scale each time (since every scale weighs differently), take the measurements at the same time each day, and make sure the client wears the same kind of clothing and no shoes. The client stands on a platform, and the weight is read from a digital display panel or a balancing arm. Clients who cannot stand are weighed on bed and chair scales. See Figures 19–11 and 19–12. The bed scales have canvas straps or a stretcherlike apparatus. A machine lifts the client above the bed, and the weight is reflected either on a digital display panel or on a balance arm like that of a standing scale.

Standardized charts reflect average heights and weights of children and adults. See Table 19–6. To date, most of these charts are based on Caucasian standards. Studies indicate that black children tend to be taller and heavier at all ages than whites (Robson, Larkin, Bursick, and Perri 1975, pp. 1017–18). It is important to remember that standardized charts reflect average heights and weights and provide only general guidelines for assessing growth, development, and nutritional status.

INTEGUMENT

The integument includes the skin, hair, and nails. The examination begins with a generalized inspection using a good source of lighting, preferably indirect natural daylight.

TABLE 19–6 *1983 Metropolitan Height and Weight Tables, Men and Women, Ages 25 to 59*

	Men				Women		
	Weight (lb)*				Weight (lb)*		
Height	Small Frame	Medium Frame	Large Frame	Height	Small Frame	Medium Frame	Large Frame
5' 2"	128–134	131–141	138–150	4'10"	102–111	109–121	118–131
5' 3"	130–136	133–143	140–153	4'11"	103–113	111–123	120–134
5' 4"	132–138	135–145	142–156	5' 0"	104–115	113–126	122–137
5' 5"	134–140	137–148	144–160	5' 1"	106–118	115–129	125–140
5' 6"	136–142	139–151	146–164	5' 2"	108–121	118–132	128–143
5' 7"	138–145	142–154	149–168	5' 3"	111–124	121–135	131–147
5' 8"	140–148	145–157	152–172	5' 4"	114–127	124–138	134–151
5' 9"	142–151	148–160	155–176	5' 5"	117–130	127–141	137–155
5'10"	144–154	151–163	158–180	5' 6"	120–133	130–144	140–159
5'11"	146–157	154–166	161–184	5' 7"	123–136	133–147	143–163
6' 0"	149–160	157–170	164–188	5' 8"	126–139	136–150	146–167
6' 1"	152–164	160–174	168–192	5' 9"	129–142	139–153	149–170
6' 2"	155–168	164–178	172–197	5'10"	132–145	142–156	152–173
6' 3"	158–172	167–182	176–202	5'11"	135–148	145–159	155–176
6' 4"	162–176	171–187	181–207	6' 0"	138–151	148–162	158–179

*Weights at ages 25–59 based on lowest mortality. Weight in indoor clothing weighing 5 lb for men, 3 lb for women; height in shoes with 1" heels

Source of basic data: 1979 Build Study, Society of Actuaries and Association of Life Insurance Medical Directors of America, 1980. Courtesy Metropolitan Life Insurance Company.

Skin

Assessment of the skin involves inspection and palpation. In some instances, the nurse may also need to use the olfactory sense to detect unusual skin odors; these are usually most evident in the skinfolds or in the axillae. Pungent body odor is frequently related to poor hygiene, **hyperhidrosis** (excessive perspiration), or **bromhidrosis** (foul-smelling perspiration). The entire skin surface may be assessed at one time or as each aspect of the body is assessed.

Skin Inspection

The skin is inspected for color, uniformity of color, and the presence of edema, injury, or skin lesions. *Skin color* varies over the body; therefore, the skin color should be assessed in areas that have not been exposed to the sun. Normal skin pigmentation varies from light to deep brown, from ruddy pink to light pink, or from yellow overtones to olive. Abnormal findings include **pallor** (absence of normal skin color, reflected in a whitish gray tinge resulting from decreased blood flow to the peripheral blood vessels or from decreased hemoglobin in the blood), **cyanosis** (a bluish tinge to the skin, caused by decreased oxyhemoglobin binding in the blood or by decreased oxygenation of the blood), and **jaundice** (a yellow or green hue to the skin occurring when tissue bilirubin is increased).

Pallor may be difficult to determine in clients with dark skin. It is usually characterized by the absence of underlying red tones in the skin and may be most readily seen in the buccal mucosa. In brown-skinned clients, pallor may appear as a yellowish brown tinge; in black-skinned clients, the skin may appear ashen gray. Pallor in people with light skins may also be evident in the face, the conjunctiva of the eyes, and the nails. *Cyanosis* is most evident in the nail beds, lips, and buccal mucosa. In dark-skinned clients, close inspection of the palpebral conjunctiva and palms and soles may also show evidence of cyanosis. *Jaundice* may first be evident in the sclera of the eyes and then in the mucous membranes and the skin. Nurses should take care not to confuse jaundice with the normal yellow pigmentation in the sclera of a dark-skinned or black client. In these clients, the best place to inspect is the part of the sclera that is observable when the eye is open. If jaundice is suspected, the posterior part of the hard palate should also be inspected for a yellowish color tone.

Uniformity of skin color is also assessed. Generally, the color of the skin is uniform over the body except in areas exposed to the sun. Dark-skinned clients have areas of lighter pigmentation, such as the palms, lips, and nail beds. Localized areas of hyperpigmentation (increased pigmentation) and hypopigmentation (decreased pigmentation) may also occur as a result of changes in the distribution of melanin or in the function of the melanocytes in the epidermis. An example of hyperpigmentation in a defined area is a birthmark; an example of hypopigmentation is vitiligo. **Vitiligo,** seen as patches of hypopigmented skin, is caused by the destruction of melanocytes in the area. **Albinism** is the complete or partial lack of melanin in the skin, hair, and eyes. Other localized color changes may indicate a problem such as edema or a localized infection. **Edema** is the presence of excess interstitial fluid. An area of edema appears swollen, shiny, and taut and tends to blanch skin color. The location, color, temperature, and shape of edematous skin and the degree to which it remains indented or pitted when pressed by a finger should be assessed. See the accompanying box for a scale describing degrees of edema. Edema is most often an indication of impaired venous circulation and in some cases reflects cardiac dysfunction or vein abnormalities.

Numerous *skin lesions* may be observed; the color section following page 402 illustrates selected lesions. The nurse who observes any lesions is responsible for describing them accurately as follows:

- *Type or structure.* Skin lesions are classified as primary (those that appear initially in response to some change in the external or internal environment of the skin) and secondary (those that do not appear initially but result from modifications such as chronicity, trauma, or infection of the primary lesion). For example, a vesicle (primary lesion) may rupture and cause an erosion (secondary lesion). Table 19–7 lists some common lesions. In some instances, lesions may need to be palpated to determine their texture and actual shape.

- *Color.* There may be no discoloration, one discrete color (e.g., red, brown, or black), or several colors, as with **ecchymosis** (a bruise), in which colors are initially dark red or blue and fade to a yellow color. When color changes are limited to the edges of a lesion, they are described as *circumscribed;* when spread over a large area, they are described as *diffuse.*

- *Distribution.* Distribution is described according to the location of the lesions on the body and symmetry or asymmetry of findings in comparable body areas.

- *Configuration.* Configuration refers to the arrangement of lesions in relation to each other. Configurations of lesions may be annular (arranged in a circle); clustered together or grouped; linear (arranged in a line); arc- or bow-shaped; merged together, or indiscrete; follow the course of cutaneous nerves; or meshed in the form of a network.

Scale for Describing Edema

- 1+ Barely detectable
- 2+ Indentation of less than 5 mm
- 3+ Indentation of 5 to 10 mm
- 4+ Indentation of more than 10 mm

TABLE 19–7 *Skin Lesions*

Type of Lesion	Description	Examples
Primary		
Macule	A flat, circumscribed area of color with no elevation of its surface; 1 mm to 1 cm	Freckles, flat nevi (moles)
Patch	Same as macula, but larger than 1 cm	Port wine birthmark
Papule	A circumscribed, solid elevation of skin; less than 1 cm	Warts, acne, pimples
Plaque	Same as papule, but larger than 1 cm	Eczema
Nodule	A solid mass that extends deeper into the dermis than does a papule	Pigmented nevi
Tumor	A solid mass larger than a nodule	Epitheliomas
Vesicle	A circumscribed elevation containing serous fluid or blood; less than 1 cm	Blister, chickenpox
Bulla	A larger fluid-filled vesicle	Blister, second-degree burns
Pustule	A vesicle or bulla filled with pus	Acne vulgaris, impetigo
Wheal	A relatively reddened, elevated, localized collection of edema fluid; irregular in shape	Mosquito bites, hives
Telangiectasia	Dilated capillary; fine red lines	Seen chiefly in pregnancy and cirrhosis of the liver
Petechiae	Pinpoint red spots	May indicate a problem in blood-clotting mechanisms
Secondary		
Scale	Thickened epidermal cells that flake off	Dandruff, psoriasis
Crust	Dried serum or pus on the skin surface	Impetigo, scab on abrasion
Fissure	A linear crack	Athlete's foot
Erosion	Loss of all or part of the epidermis	Chickenpox and smallpox following rupture
Excoriation	Linear or hollowed out crusted area exposing dermis	Scratch, abrasion
Atrophy	A decrease in the volume of epidermis	Striae, aged skin
Scar	A formation of connective tissue	Healed wound
Ulcer	An excavation extending into the dermis or below	Stasis ulcer

Skin Palpation   The skin is palpated to determine changes in temperature, moisture, texture, and turgor. Palpation is usually carried out immediately following inspection of each body part to amplify the findings noted during inspection. Skin temperature should always be assessed when there is concern about the blood circulation to a body part. Normally, a person's skin temperature is relatively uniform over the body. When skin temperature is higher or lower in one area, the nurse should palpate the corresponding area on the other side of the body to gain comparative data. Localized areas of skin *hyperthermia* may be noticed where a burn or infection is present; localized areas of skin *hypothermia* may occur in extremities afflicted by arteriosclerosis. Generalized skin hyperthermia (involving all of the skin) may occur when there is a fever; generalized hypothermia occurs when the client is in shock. *Moisture* of the skin may be observed visually as well as by palpation. Moisture refers both to wetness and to oiliness. The skinfolds and axillae are normally moist. The moisture varies according to environmental temperature and humidity, muscular activity, and body temperature. Skin is often dry when environmental temperature and humidity are low, and often

The Elderly: Physical Changes of the Skin

- Aging changes of the skin occur as a result of many factors: enzymatic changes in connective and epithelial tissues, heredity, inadequate nutrition from vascular changes, and endocrine changes. Aging changes in white skin occur at an earlier age than in black skin.

- The skin loses its elasticity, and it wrinkles. Wrinkles first appear on the skin of the face and neck, which are abundant in collagen and elastic fibers.

- The skin appears yellow-white (like parchment), thin, and translucent because of loss of dermis and subcutaneous fat. Atrophy of the epidermal structures results from degeneration of collagen and elastin.

- The skin is dry and flaky because sebaceous and sweat glands are less active. Dry skin is more prominent over the extremities, where circulation is not as efficient.

- The skin takes longer to return to its natural shape after being pinched between the nurse's thumb and finger. Since there is loss of skin turgor over the extremities, the skin of the forehead is recommended for the pinch-fold test for dehydration.

- Flat tan to brown-colored macules, referred to as *senile lentigines* or *melanotic freckles,* are normally often apparent on the back of the hand and other skin areas that are exposed to the sun. These macules may be as large as 1 to 2 centimeters. They occur because cells lose their ability to spread out melanin.

- Warty lesions (*seborrheic keratosis*) with irregularly shaped borders and a scaly surface often occur on the face, shoulders, and trunk. These benign lesions begin as yellowish to tan and progress to a dark brown or black.

- Some skin areas may lack pigment, appearing whiter than surrounding skin areas. This phenomenon, referred to as *vitiligo,* tends to increase with age and is thought to be the result of an autoimmune response.

- Cutaneous tags (*acrochordons*) are most commonly seen in the neck and axillary regions. These skin lesions vary in size and are soft, often flesh colored, and pedicled.

- Visible, bright red, fine dilated blood vessels (*telangiectasias*) commonly occur as a result of the thinning of the dermis and the loss of support for the blood vessel walls.

- Pink to slightly red lesions with indistinct borders (*actinic keratoses*) may appear at about age 50, often on the face, ears, backs of the hands, and arms. They often become malignant.

moist when they are elevated. The elderly commonly have dry skin. Excessive oiliness, especially on the face, neck, and upper trunk, may occur during adolescence. Although there is some variation in the *texture* of normal skin, it is usually smooth, soft, and flexible. Skin can become dry and rough as a result of certain diseases, such as hypothyroidism (insufficient thyroid activity). The thickness of the skin varies widely. The skin is thicker in areas that are exposed to pressure, friction, or other types of irritation, such as the soles of the feet and the palms of the hands.

Turgor means fullness or elasticity. Skin or tissue turgor refers to the normal skin fullness, or the capacity of the skin and underlying tissue to return to their prior condition after being lifted and pinched. If skin turgor is poor (e.g., in a dehydrated client), the skin returns to its original shape slowly, remaining pinched or tented after it is released. Loss of skin turgor is often related to advanced age, when the skin becomes lax and wrinkled. See the accompanying box for physical changes of the skin in older adults.

Hair

Assessment of an individual's hair includes inspection of the hair, consideration of developmental changes, and determination of the individual's hair care practices and the factors influencing them. Much of the information about hair can be obtained by questioning the client. See the assessment interview in Chapter 22, page 537.

Normal hair is resilient and evenly distributed. People with severe protein deficiency (kwashiorkor) have faded hair colors that appear reddish or bleached and coarse, dry hair texture. Some therapies for cancer cause **alopecia** (hair loss), and some disease conditions affect the coarseness of hair.

Hair is assessed for

- The evenness of growth over the scalp and, in particular, any patchy loss of hair

- Texture, i.e., whether it is coarse or silky

- Oiliness, i.e., whether it is dry or greasy

- Thickness or thinness

The Elderly: Physical Changes of the Hair

- The age at which the scalp hair grays is influenced largely by genetic factors.

- There is loss of scalp, pubic, and axillary hair.

- In women, the hair of the eyebrows and some facial hair become coarse.

- Hairs of the eyebrows, ears, and nostrils become bristlelike and coarse.

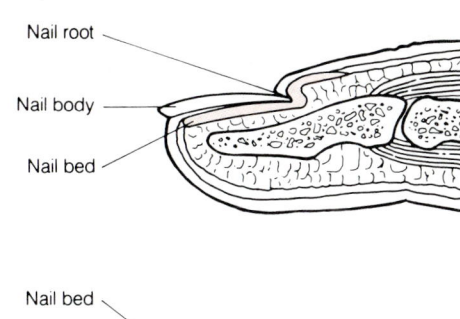

Nail root

Nail body

Nail bed

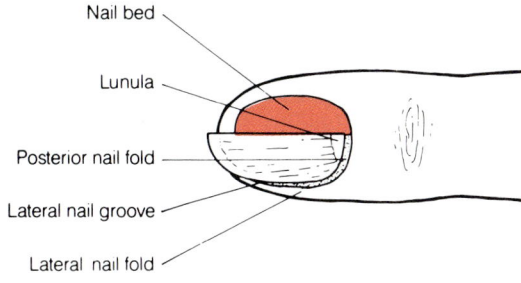

Nail bed

Lunula

Posterior nail fold

Lateral nail groove

Lateral nail fold

Figure 19–13   The parts of a nail.

- Presence of infections or infestations on the scalp, including flaking, sores, lice, nits (louse eggs), and ringworm
- Presence on the body (**hirsutism** is the presence of unusually dark, thick hair on the body. It has little significance in men but should be noted in children and women, since it may be associated with endocrine problems.)

See the box on page 372 for a description of hair changes in the elderly.

Nails

Parts of the nail are shown in Figure 19–13. Nails are inspected for nail plate shape, angle between the nail and the nail bed, nail texture, nail bed color, and the intactness of the tissues around the nails. The nail plate is normally colorless and a convex curve. The angle between the nail and the nail bed is normally 160°. See Figure 19–14. One nail abnormality is the spoon shape. Here, the nail curves upward from the nail bed. See Figure 19–15. This condition is called **koilonychia** and may be seen in clients with iron deficiency anemia. **Clubbing** is a condition in which the angle between the nail and the nail bed is 180° or greater. It may be caused by long-term oxygen lack and is seen in the elderly. See Figure 19–16.

Nail texture is normally smooth. Excessively thick nails can appear in the elderly or in the presence of poor circulation; excessively thin nails or the presence of grooves or furrows can reflect prolonged iron-deficiency anemia. *Beau's lines* are horizontal depressions in the nail that can result from injury or severe illness. See Figure 19–17.

The nail bed is highly vascular, a characteristic that accounts for its pink color in Caucasians. In blacks, brown or black pigmentation in longitudinal streaks or along the edge of the nail bed may normally be present. A bluish or purplish

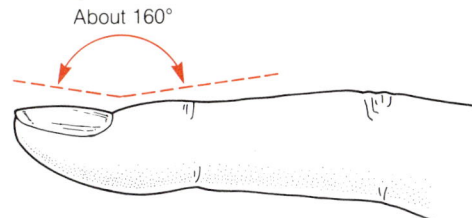

About 160°

Figure 19–14   A normal nail, showing the convex shape and the nail plate angle of about 160°.

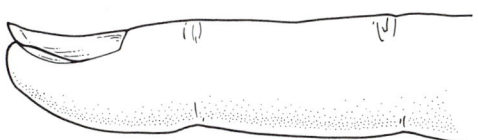

Figure 19–15   A spoon-shaped nail.

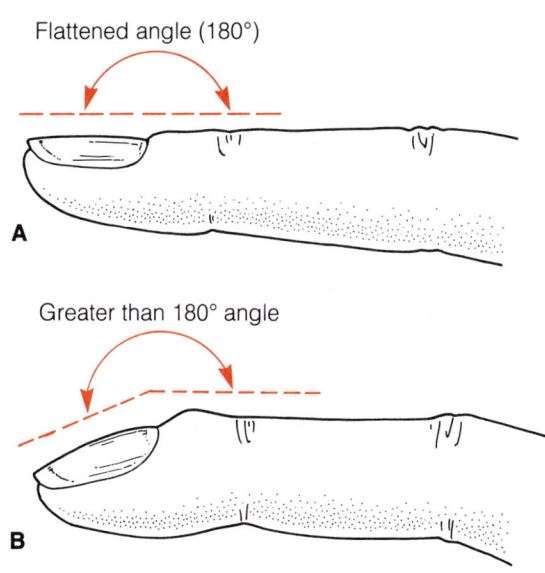

Flattened angle (180°)

A

Greater than 180° angle

B

Figure 19–16   A, early clubbing; B, late clubbing.

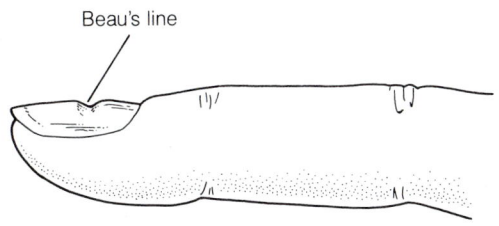

Beau's line

Figure 19–17   Beau's line on a nail.

tint to the nail bed may reflect cyanosis, and pallor may reflect poor arterial circulation.

The tissue surrounding the nails is normally intact epidermis. **Paronychia** is an inflammation of the tissues surrounding a nail. The tissues appear inflamed and swollen, and tenderness is usually present.

A **blanch test** can be carried out to test the capillary refill, i.e., peripheral circulation. Normal nail bed capillaries blanch when pressed but quickly turn pink (in Caucasians) or their usual color when pressure is released. In dark-skinned people, the rate of return of nail bed color may be more significant than the color. A slow rate of capillary refill may indicate circulatory problems. See the box above for a description of nail changes in elderly people.

HEAD

During an examination of the head, the nurse often uses inspection and palpation simultaneously, as well as auscultation. The nurse examines the skull, face, eyes, ears, nose, sinuses, mouth, and pharynx.

Skull

There is a large range of normal shapes of skulls. A normal head size is referred to as normocephalic. Names of areas of the head are derived from underlying bones: frontal, parietal, occipital, mastoid process, mandible, maxilla, and zygomatic. See Figure 19–18. Inspect the skull at all angles for size, shape, and symmetry. Note particularly areas of local trauma, lumps or bumps, and overall size. Abnormal findings include lack of symmetry and unusual size. If the skull appears to be of abnormal size, measure its circumference just above the eyebrows. Auscultate over the occipital, temporal, and orbital regions for **bruits** (audible pulsations). See Figure 19–19. To listen for an ocular bruit, apply the bell of the stethoscope around the orbit of the eye, forming a tight seal.

Face

Inspect the face for skin color, hair distribution, and symmetry of the structures. Ask the client to elevate the eyebrows, frown or lower the eyebrows, close the eyes tightly, puff the cheeks, and smile and show the teeth. These movements determine the function of the muscles of facial expression and the seventh cranial (facial) nerve. Sensation of the face, supplied by the fifth cranial (trigeminal) nerve, is tested as part of the neurologic examination, discussed later in this chapter.

Inspect the face for the presence of edema. Edema around the eyes (periorbital edema) and involuntary facial movements, i.e., tics or tremors, are abnormal findings. Abnormal facial contours, e.g., **moon face** (a rounded facial contour), can result from increased adrenal hormone production. Prolonged illness, starvation, and dehydration can result in sunken eyes, cheeks, and temples.

Eyes and Vision

Many people consider vision the most important sense, since

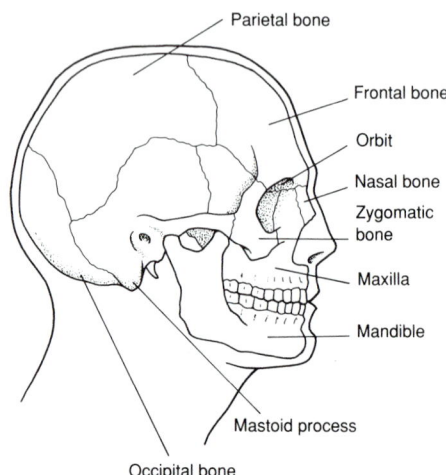

Figure 19–18   The bones of the head.

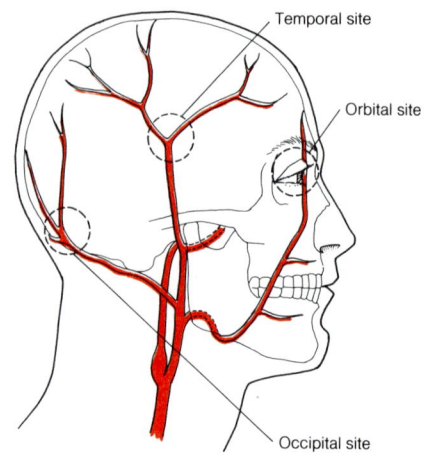

Figure 19–19   Auscultation sites for bruits.

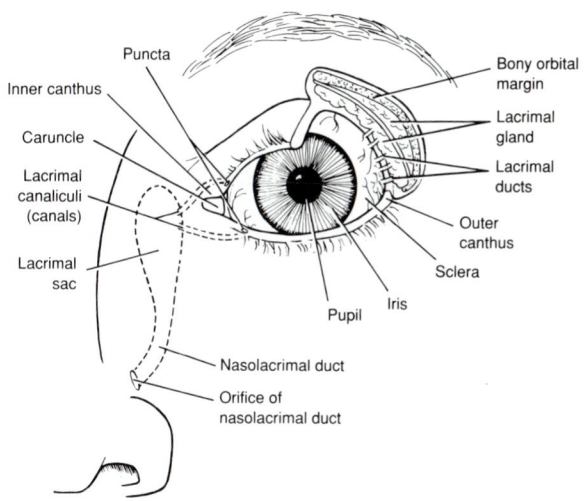

Figure 19–20 The left eye showing the external structures and the lacrimal apparatus.

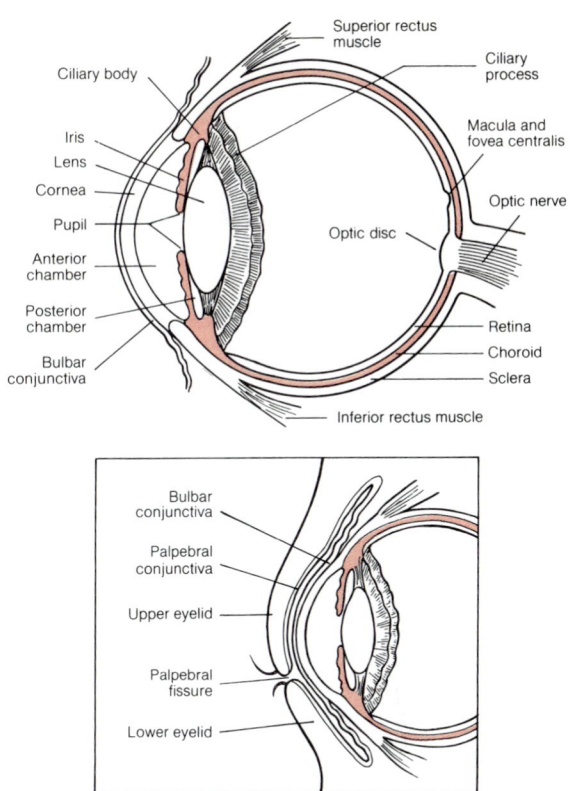

Figure 19–21 Anatomic structures of the right eye, lateral view.

it allows them to interact freely with their environment and enjoy the beauty of life around them. To maintain optimum vision, people need to have their eyes examined throughout life. It is recommended that people under age 40 have their eyes tested every 3 to 5 years, or more frequently if there is a family history of diabetes, hypertension, blood dyscrasia, or eye disease (e.g., glaucoma). After age 40, an eye examination is recommended every 2 years to rule out the possibility of glaucoma.

An eye assessment should be carried out as part of the client's initial physical examination; periodic reassessments need to be made for long-term care clients. Examination of the eyes includes assessment of visual acuity, ocular movement, visual fields, external structures, and the fundus. Most eye assessment procedures involve inspection. Consideration is also given to developmental changes and to individual hygienic practices, if the client wears contact lenses or an artificial eye. For the anatomic structures of the eye, see Figures 19–20 and 19–21.

Many people wear eyeglasses or contact lenses to correct common refractive errors of the lens of the eye. These errors include myopia (nearsightedness), **hyperopia** (farsightedness), and **presbyopia** (loss of elasticity of the lens and thus loss of ability to see close objects). Presbyopia begins at about 45 years of age. People notice that they have difficulty reading newsprint. Often two corrective lenses (bifocals) are required—one for near vision or reading, the other for far vision. **Astigmatism,** an uneven curvature of the cornea that prevents horizontal and vertical rays from focusing on the retina, is a common problem that may occur in conjunction with myopia and hyperopia.

Common inflammatory visual problems that nurses may encounter in clients include conjunctivitis, dacryocystitis, hordeolum, iritis, and contusions or hematomas of the eyelids and surrounding structures. **Conjunctivitis** (inflammation of the bulbar and palpebral conjunctiva) may result from foreign bodies, chemicals, allergenic agents, bacteria, or viruses. Redness, itching, tearing, and mucopurulent discharge occur. After sleep, the eyelids may be encrusted and matted together. **Dacryocystitis** (inflammation of the lacrimal sac) is manifested by tearing and a discharge from the nasolacrimal duct. **Hordeolum** (sty) is a redness, swelling, and tenderness of the hair follicle and glands that empty at the edge of the eyelids. **Iritis** (inflammation of the iris) may be caused by local or systemic infections and results in pain, tearing, and **photophobia** (sensitivity to light). **Contusions** or **hematomas** are "black eyes" resulting from injury.

Cataracts tend to occur in those over 65 years old. This opacity of the lens or its capsule, which blocks light rays, is frequently corrected by surgery. Cataracts may also occur in infants due to a malformation of the lens if the mother contracted rubella in the first trimester of pregnancy. **Glaucoma** (a disturbance in the circulation of aqueous fluid, which causes an increase in intraocular pressure) is the most frequent cause of blindness in people over 40. It can be controlled if diagnosed early. Danger signs of glaucoma include blurred or foggy vision, loss of peripheral vision, difficulty focusing on close objects, difficulty adjusting to dark rooms, and seeing rainbow-colored rings around lights.

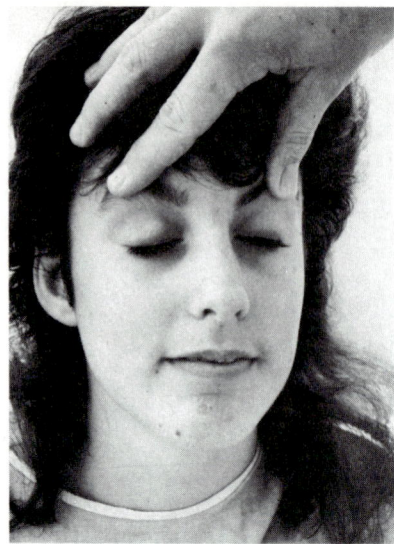

Figure 19–22 Inspecting the upper eyelids.

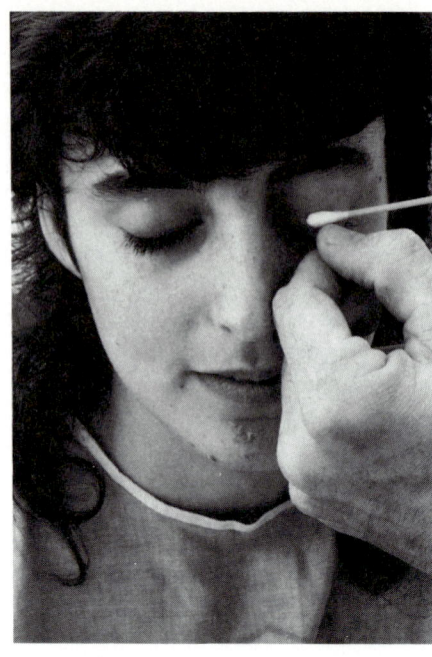

Figure 19–23 Everting the upper eyelid.

External Eye Structures   Assess the external eye structures as the client sits at eye level directly in front of you. Inspect the *eyebrows* for hair distribution and alignment, skin quality, and movement. Ask the client to raise and lower the eyebrows. Note loss of hair, and scaling or flakiness of the skin. Inspect the *eyelashes* for evenness of distribution and direction of curl. Normally, eyelashes are equally distributed and curled slightly outward. Inward turning of the eyelashes occurs with inversion of the eyelid.

Inspect the *eyelids* for surface characteristics (e.g., skin quality and texture), position, ability to blink, and frequency of blinking. Eyelids that lie at or below the pupil margin are referred to as **ptosis** and are usually associated with aging, edema from drug allergy or systemic disease (e.g., kidney disease), congenital lid muscle dysfunction, neuromuscular disease (e.g., myasthenia gravis), and third cranial nerve impairment. Eversion, an outturning of the eyelid, is called **ectropion;** inversion, an inturning of the lid, is called **entropion.** These abnormalities are often associated with scarring injuries or the aging process.

To inspect the *upper lids,* ask the client to close the eyes. Elevate the eyebrows with the thumb and index finger. Elevation stretches the skin folds for proper visual examination. See Figure 19–22. Note skin color, skin texture, and eyelid closure. The skin should be intact, there should be no discharge or discoloration, and the eyelids should close symmetrically. Document any redness, swelling, flaking, crusting, plaques, discharge, nodules, or lesions.

To inspect the *lower lids,* ask the client to open the eyes. Note the characteristics listed for the upper lids, ability to blink, frequency of blinking, and the position of the eyelids in relation to the cornea. Normally, there are approximately 15 to 20 involuntary blinks per minute, blinking is bilateral, and there is no visible sclera above corneas when the lids

open. The upper and lower borders of the cornea are slightly covered. A visible rim of sclera between the lid and the iris is often associated with hyperthyroidism. Asymmetric lid closure; incomplete or painful closure; and blinking that is rapid, monocular, absent, or infrequent must be reported.

The conjunctiva is a continuous transparent structure with two parts: the bulbar and the palpebral. The bulbar portion lies over the sclera and appears clear; however, some blood vessels are normally visible. The palpebral portion lines the eyelids and appears shiny, smooth, and pink or red.

To assess the *bulbar conjunctiva,* retract the client's eyelids with the thumb and index finger, exerting pressure over the upper and lower bony orbits. Ask the clients to look up, down, and from side to side. Inspect the conjunctiva for color, texture, and the presence of lesions.

To examine the *palpebral conjunctiva,* evert both lower lids and ask the client to look up. Then gently retract the lower lids with the index fingers. Inspect the conjunctiva for color, texture, and the presence of lesions.

Evert the *upper* lids *only if a problem is suspected.*

- Ask the client to look down and to keep the eyes slightly open. Closing the eyelids contracts the orbicular muscle, which prevents lid eversion.

- Gently grasp the client's eyelashes with the thumb and index finger. Pull the lashes gently downward. Upward or outward pulling on the eyelashes causes muscle contraction.

- Place a cotton-tipped applicator stick about 1 cm above the lid margin, and push it gently downward while still holding the eyelashes. See Figure 19–23. These actions

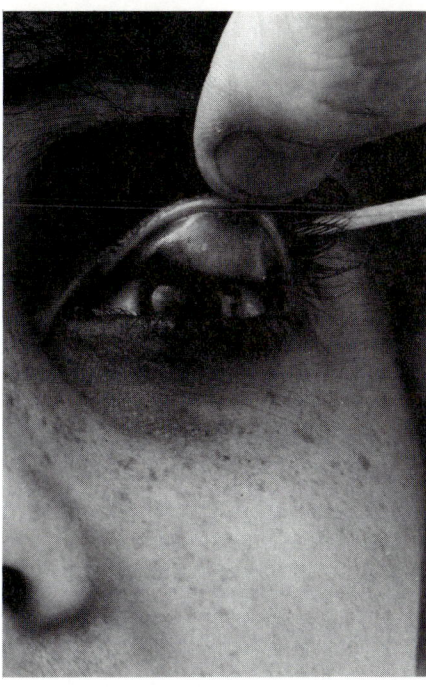

Figure 19–24 Holding the margin of the everted upper eyelid.

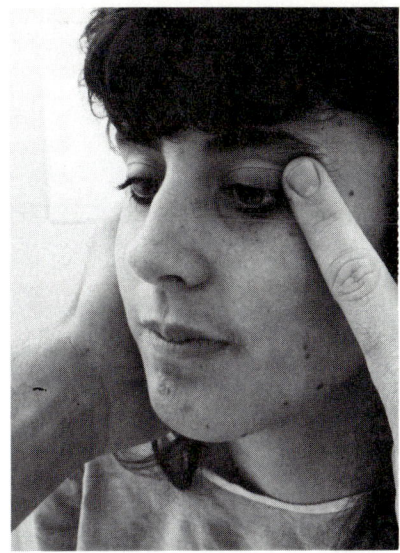

Figure 19–25 Palpating the lacrimal gland.

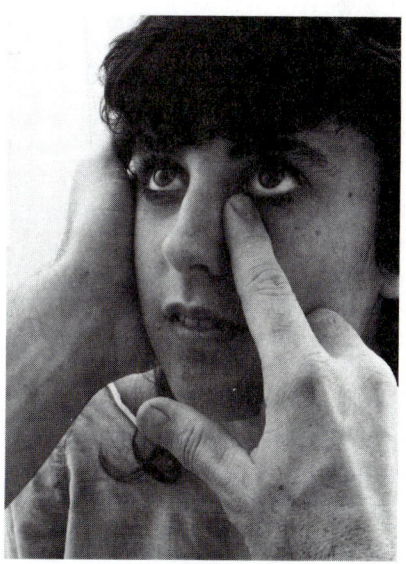

Figure 19–26 Palpating the lacrimal sac and nasolacrimal duct.

evert the lid, i.e., flip the lower part of the lid over on top of itself.

■ Hold the margin of the everted lid or the eyelashes against the ridge of the upper bony orbit with the applicator stick or the thumb. See Figure 19–24.

■ Inspect the conjunctiva for color, texture, lesions, and foreign bodies.

■ To return the lid to its normal position, gently pull the lashes forward, and ask the client to look up and to blink.

The *lacrimal apparatus* is shown in Figure 19–20 on page 375. Inspect and palpate the lacrimal gland. See Figure 19–25. Note any edema or tenderness. Inspect and palpate the lacrimal sac and nasolacrimal duct. See Figure 19–26. Observe for edema between the lower lid and the nose and for evidence of increased tearing. Using the tip of your index finger, palpate inside the lower orbital rim near the inner canthus, not on the side of the nose. Regurgitation of fluid on palpation of the lacrimal sac is abnormal.

To assess the *cornea,* ask the client to look straight ahead. Then hold a penlight at an oblique angle to the eye, and move the light slowly across the corneal surface. Inspect the cornea for clarity and texture. Normally, the cornea is transparent, shiny, and smooth. Details of the iris are visible. In older people, a thin, grayish white ring around the margin, called *arcus senilis,* may be evident. Arcus senilis in clients under age 40 is abnormal. An opaque or uneven surface of the cornea may be the result of trauma or an abrasion.

The *corneal sensitivity (reflex) test* determines the function of the fifth (trigeminal) cranial nerve. Ask the client to keep both eyes open and look straight ahead. With a wisp of cotton, approach from behind and beside the client and lightly touch the cornea with the cotton wisp. The blink response normally occurs when the cornea is touched, indicating that the trigeminal nerve is intact.

To inspect the *anterior chamber,* use the same oblique lighting technique used to test the cornea. Inspect the anterior chamber for transparency and depth. Normally, the anterior chamber is transparent and not cloudy. No shadows of light should appear on the iris. A crescent-shaped shadow on the far side of the iris indicates a bulging iris, a shallow anterior chamber, and a predisposition to glaucoma. The anterior chamber normally has a depth of about 3 mm. Deep chambers are indicative of glaucoma.

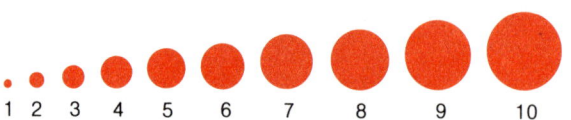

Figure 19–27 Variations in pupil diameters in millimeters.

Pupils are normally black, are equal in size (about 3 to 7 mm in diameter), and have round, smooth borders. Cloudy pupils are often indicative of cataracts. Enlarged pupils (**mydriasis**) may indicate injury, glaucoma, or be the result of certain drugs (e.g., atropine). Constricted pupils (**miosis**) may indicate an inflammation of the iris or be the result of such drugs as morphine or pilocarpine. Unequal pupils (**anisocoria**) may result from a central nervous system disorder; however, slight variations may be normal. Steps in assessing the pupil are shown in the accompanying box. The iris is normally flat and round. A bulging toward the cornea can indicate increased intraocular pressure.

Visual Acuity   The child acquires normal 20/20 vision by 6 years of age. Persons with denominators of 40 or more on the Snellen chart with or without corrective lenses need to be referred to an ophthalmologist. To assess visual acuity, the nurse requires the following equipment:

- Newsprint for testing near vision.
- A Snellen eye chart; for a person unable to read, a Snellen E chart; for a child of 3 years, a chart with identifiable pictures. See Figure 19–28.
- An eye cover or opaque index card.
- A penlight.

To test *near vision,* provide adequate lighting and ask the client to read from a magazine or newspaper held at a distance of 36 cm (14 in). If the client normally wears corrective lenses, the glasses or lenses should be worn during the test.

To test *distance vision,* ask the client to wear any corrective lenses, unless they are used for reading only, i.e., for

---

Assessing the Pupils

- Ask the client to look straight ahead.

- Inspect the pupils for color, shape, and symmetry of size. Pupil charts are available in some agencies. See Figure 19–27 for variations in pupil diameters in millimeters.

- Assess each pupil's direct and consensual reaction to light to determine the function of the third (oculomotor) and fourth (trochlear) cranial nerves.
  a. Partially darken the room.
  b. Ask the client to look straight ahead.
  c. Using a penlight or flashlight and approaching from the side, shine a light on the pupil.
  d. Observe the response of the illuminated pupil. It should constrict (direct response).
  e. Again shine the light on the pupil, and observe the response of the other pupil. It should also constrict (consensual response).

- Assess each pupil's reaction to accommodation.
  a. Hold an object (a penlight or pencil) about 10 cm (4 in) from the bridge of the client's nose.
  b. Ask the client to look first at the top of the object and then at a distant object (e.g., the far wall) behind the penlight. Alternate the gaze from the near to the far object.
  c. Observe the pupil response. The pupils should constrict when looking at the near object and dilate when looking at the far object.
  d. Next, move the penlight or pencil toward the client's nose. The pupils should converge.

- To record normal assessment of the pupils, use the abbreviation PERRLA (pupils equally round and react to light and accommodation).

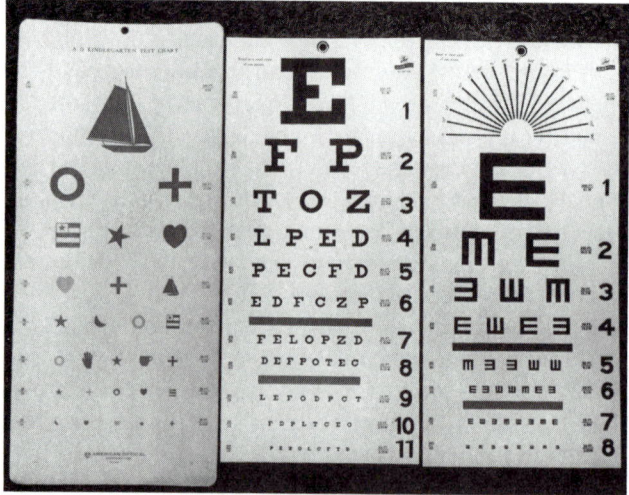

Figure 19–28   Three types of eye charts: the preschool children's chart (left), Snellen standard chart (center), and the Snellen E chart for clients unable to read (right).

distances of only 30 to 36 cm (12 to 14 in). Ask the client to stand or sit 6 m (20 ft) from a Snellen chart, cover the eye not being tested, and identify the letters on the Snellen chart. Take three readings.

If the client is unable to see the top line (20/200) of the Snellen chart, functional vision tests can be done. For the *light perception test,* shine a penlight into the client's eye from a lateral position, and then turn the light off. If the client knows when the light is on and off, light perception is present; the vision is recorded as LP. To test hand movements (H/M), hold a hand 30 cm (1 ft) from the client's face, and move it slowly back and forth, stopping periodically. If the client knows when the hand stops moving, record the vision as "H/M 1 ft."

A third functional vision test is counting fingers (C/F). Hold several fingers 30 cm (1 ft) from the client's face, and ask the client to count them. If the client can do so, record "C/F 1 ft." Clients who can pass these three functional tests are usually able to manage independently. A person unable to perform these tests with either eye is considered blind. Legal blindness is a visual acuity of 20/200 or less in both eyes with corrective lenses.

Visual Fields

Peripheral visual fields refer to sight on the periphery of a person's vision. Normally, when people look straight ahead, they can also see objects in the periphery. The peripheral visual field is assessed as the client sits 60 to 90 cm (2 to 3 feet) directly in front of the nurse. The client covers the left eye with a card, and the nurse covers the eye opposite (in this case, the nurse's right eye) with a card or the hand. The client then stares at the nurse's open eye. The nurse carrying out the assessment acts as a control and is presumed to have normal visual fields.

The nurse holds a small object, such as a pencil, in one hand and moves it into the visual field from various points in the periphery. The object should be an equal distance from the client and the nurse so that both can see it at the same time. The client tells the nurse when the client first sees the moving object.

- To test the *temporal field* of the right eye, the nurse extends and moves the left arm in from the client's right periphery. Temporally, peripheral objects can normally be seen at right angles (90°) to the central point of vision.

- To test the *upward field* of the right eye, the nurse extends and moves the left arm down from the upward periphery. The upward field of vision is normally only 50°, since the orbital ridge is in the way.

- To test the *downward field* of the right eye, the nurse extends and moves the left arm up from the lower periphery. The downward field of vision is normally 70°, since the cheekbone is in the way.

- To test the *nasal field* of the right eye, the nurse extends and moves the right arm in from the periphery. The nasal field of vision is normally 50° away from the central point of vision, since the nose is in the way.

The above steps are repeated for the left eye; the process is reversed.

Extraocular Muscle Tests

Normally, both eyes are coordinated, move in unison, and have parallel alignment. There may also be end-point nystagmus. **Nystagmus** is involuntary rapid movement of the eyeball. Three tests can be performed on clients over 6 months of age: the six ocular movements, the cover-uncover patch test, and the corneal light reflex test.

The *six ocular movements* test relates to the six muscles that guide each eye (see Figure 19–29). It tests eye coordination and alignment. To perform this test, stand directly in front of the client, and hold a penlight at a comfortable distance, e.g., 30 cm (1 ft) in front of the client's eyes. Ask the client to hold the head in a fixed position facing you and to follow the movements of the penlight with the *eyes only.* Move the penlight in a slow, orderly manner through the six ocular movements: from the center of the eye along the lines of the arrows in Figure 19–29 and back to the center. Stop the movement of the penlight periodically so that **nystagmus** can be detected. Slight nystagmus on the extreme lateral gaze (end-point nystagmus) occurs normally in many people. Other nystagmus is abnormal. Eye movements that are not coordinated or parallel and failure of one or both eyes to follow the penlight in specific directions are other abnormal findings.

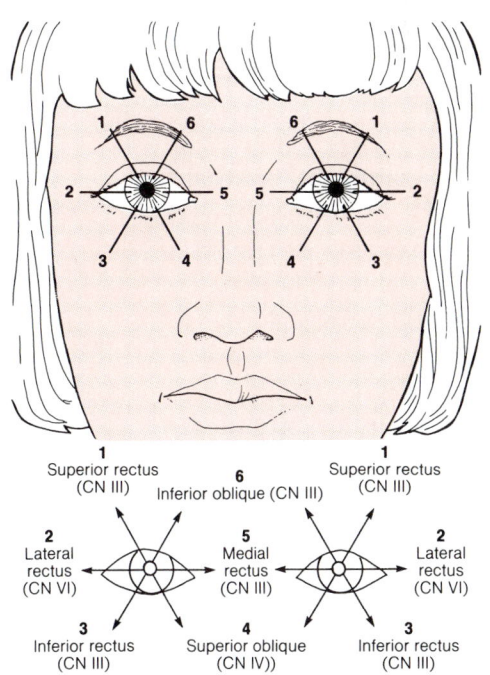

Figure 19–29   The six muscles that govern eye movement.

The *cover-uncover patch test* determines eye alignment. Ask the client to stare straight ahead at a fixed point, e.g., at a penlight held 15 cm (6 in) in front of the eyes. Cover one of the client's eyes with an eye cover or index card while observing the uncovered eye. If well aligned, the uncovered eye should not move from the fixed point when the other eye is covered. If it does move, to focus on the fixed point, it was *not* well aligned before the other eye was covered; it is shifting from a medial or lateral to central gaze.

Remove the eye cover, and observe the newly uncovered eye for movement. The newly uncovered eye, if well aligned, should not move. If it does move to focus on the fixed point when uncovered, it was *not* well aligned when covered. Muscle weakness is apparent when the eye turns inward or outward while covered. As the eye is uncovered, a quick inward or outward movement occurs to bring it back to alignment.

Repeat these steps for the other eye. It is important to test each eye several times to confirm the findings.

A nurse can also use the *corneal light reflex test* to determine eye alignment. To perform this test, darken the room and ask the client to stare straight ahead. Shine a penlight on the bridge of the nose, and observe the light reflection in both corneas. Light reflection is normally situated in the same spot on both eyes.

Internal Eye Structures   The internal part of the eye posterior to the lens, visible through the pupil by an ophthalmoscope, is called the *fundus* of the eye. Structures of the fundus include the retina, choroid, fovea, macula, disc, and retinal vessels.

Ophthalmic or funduscopic examination of the eye requires practice and skill. See Procedure 19–1. Refer also to Table 19–8 on page 382 for a review of normal and abnormal findings. In some practice settings, the nurse does not perform ophthalmic examination of the eye. See the box on page 383 for a description of changes in the eyes and vision in elderly people.

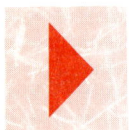

PROCEDURE 19–1

INSPECTING THE INTERNAL EYE STRUCTURES

Equipment ✓

Ophthalmoscope (see Figure 19–30)

Intervention

1. **First, assemble the ophthalmoscope.**

- Align the base of the head with the lugs on the top of the handle.

- Push the head down, and rotate it until you hear it click into place.

- Adjust the aperture selection dial on the back of the ophthalmoscope head to regulate the amount of light. Use the largest round light at first.

- Select the appropriate lens by adjusting the lens selection wheel on the side of the ophthalmoscope head. To begin, you may set the lens wheel at the 0 setting.

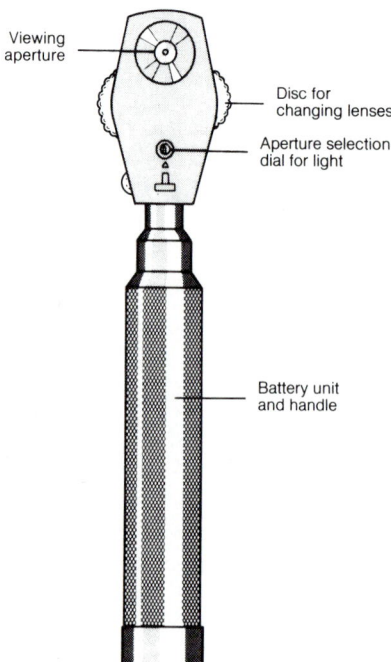

Viewing aperture

Disc for changing lenses

Aperture selection dial for light

Battery unit and handle

Figure 19–30   An ophthalmoscope, used to examine the interior of the eye.

2. **Prepare the client.**

- Darken the room to dilate the pupils.

- Have the client remove eyeglasses. Contact lenses may be left in, but their presence can increase light reflection.

- Ask the client to sit or stand in front of you.

3. **Inspect the red reflex through the pupil.**

- To examine the right eye, hold the ophthalmoscope against your right eye with your right hand. Reverse the position to examine the left eye.

- Hold the ophthalmoscope at least 30 cm (1 ft) from the client's pupil and at an angle of about 25° lateral to the client's line of central vision.

- Ask the client to keep both eyes open and to focus on a distant object.
- Shine the light on the client's pupil.
- Observe the bright round orange glow through the pupil (the red reflex). In dark-skinned persons, the fundus may appear brown or purplish. Grayish white opacities of the lens (cataracts) may impair visualization of the retina.

4. Inspect the optic disc and cup.

- Keeping the red reflex in sight, slowly move the ophthalmoscope close to the client's pupil. *Slow movement promotes dilation of the pupil and prevents eye movement.*
- Locate some retinal structure, such as a blood vessel, and focus the image. Adjust the lens until the margins of the structure appear sharp.
- Locate the optic disc by following the blood vessels toward the midline. See Figure 19–31.

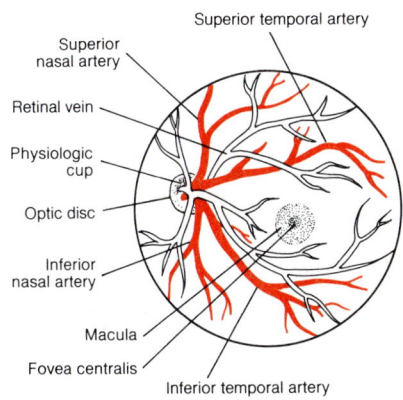

Superior temporal artery

Superior nasal artery

Retinal vein

Physiologic cup

Optic disc

Inferior nasal artery

Macula

Fovea centralis

Inferior temporal artery

Figure 19–31 The fundus of the left eye.

- Note the color, size, and shape of the disc, the distinctness of its margins, and its physiologic cup (the depressed central area of the disc).

5. Inspect the retinal blood vessels.

- Follow the blood vessels peripherally in each of four quadrants: superior temporal, inferior temporal, superior nasal, and inferior nasal. *The central retinal artery arises from the depth of the optic disc and divides into four main branches, which supply each retinal quadrant. The central retinal vein leaves the disc in company with the central artery and has similar branches in each quadrant. The four quadrants are scanned, since blood vessel abnormalities are not evenly distributed.*
- Inspect the vessels for size, color, pattern, and arteriovenous crossings. The color of the vessels is an indication of the oxygenated or deoxygenated blood they carry.

6. Examine the retinal background (periphery).

- Ask the client to look up, down, and from side to side.
- Inspect the retinal background of the four quadrants.
- Note color and surface characteristics.

7. Inspect the macula and fovea centralis retinae.

- Avoid directing light on the macula for long periods. *The macula is the center of most acute vision and is sensitive. Prolonging the time the light is on the macula can cause the client discomfort.*
- Locate the macula by first locating the optic disc and then looking two disc diameters (DD) away toward the client's temple. It is a small circular structure 1 DD in size.
  or
- Ask the client to look directly at the light.
- Inspect the macula for color and surface characteristics. Note the tiny glistening spot of reflected light in the center of the macula. This spot is the fovea centralis retinae.

8. Document your findings on the appropriate records.

- Identify the right eye as OD (oculus dexter), the left as OS (oculus sinister), and both eyes as OU (oculus uterque).

Sample Recording

Date: May/7/91	Time: 0900

Ophthalmic exam: Discs round and creamy pink; cups equal in size and color. Retinal vessels even caliber and intact. Retinal background has uniform orange-pink color. Maculae 2 DD from discs; no lesions apparent.—Simone L. White, RN

TABLE 19-8 *Summary Assessment Data: Internal Eye*

Structure Test	Normal Findings	Abnormal Findings
Red reflex	Bright, round, red-orange glow through pupil	Decreased redness or roundness
		Opacities
Optic disc and cup	Yellowish or creamy pink, almost round disc; lighter than retina	Pale disc
	Distinct regular outline (nasal edge less distinct than temporal edge)	Blurred disc margins and reddened disc
	About 1.5 mm in diameter but appears larger with magnification × 15	Discs unequal in size and shape
	Physiologic cup occupies one-third to one-half of disc area	Cup extends to disc border, is asymmetrical
	Cups equal in size	Cups unequal in size
	Cup paler than disc (yellow-white)	
Retinal vessels	Arteries	
	Light red color	Copper or silver color
		Pale or white vessel
	Narrow band of light in center (arteriolar light reflex) about one-fourth diameter of blood column	Narrowed light reflex
	Arteries two-thirds to four-fifths diameter of veins	
	Regular caliber, decreasing in size toward periphery	Irregularities in caliber (dilations or constrictions)
	Veins	
	Larger than arteries	Dilated and tortuous veins
	Darker color than arteries	
	No prominent light reflex	
	Arteriovenous crossings	
	Caliber of underlying vessel; not indented, pinched, or displaced	
Retinal background (periphery)	Uniform orange-pink color; lighter in fair people, darker in black people	Pallor
		Linear, or large or small dark or red patches
		Discrete tiny red dots
		Fuzzy white patches
Macula and fovea	Slightly darker than retina	Same as for retinal background, above
	Tiny capillaries may be evident on surface	
	Fovea seen as tiny bright light in center	

Ears and Hearing

Assessment of the ear includes direct inspection and palpation of the external ear, inspection of the remaining parts of the ear by an otoscope, and determination of auditory acuity. The ear is usually assessed during an initial physical examination; periodic reassessments may be necessary for long-term clients or those with hearing problems.

The ear is divided into three parts: external ear, middle ear, and inner ear. The external ear includes the **auricle** or **pinna,** the external auditory canal, and the tympanic membrane (eardrum). See Figure 19-32. Landmarks of the auricle include the lobule (earlobe), helix, anthelix, tragus, triangular fossa, and external auditory meatus. Although not part of the ear, the mastoid, a bony prominence behind the ear, is another important landmark. See Figure 19-33. The external ear canal is curved, is about 2.5 cm (1 in) long in the adult, and ends at the tympanic membrane. It is covered with skin that has many fine hairs, glands, and nerve endings. The glands secrete cerumen (earwax), which lubricates and protects the canal.

The Elderly: Physical Changes of the Eyes and Vision

Visual acuity

- Visual acuity is decreased as the lens of the eye ages and becomes more opaque and loses elasticity.
- The ability of the iris to accommodate to darkness and dim light diminishes.
- Peripheral vision is diminished.
- There is a decrease in adaptation to light (glare) and dark.
- Accommodation to far objects often improves, but accommodation to near objects decreases.
- Color vision is reduced; older people are less able to perceive purple colors and to discriminate pastel colors.
- Many older people wear corrective lenses; they are most likely to have hyperopia. Visual changes are due to loss of elasticity and transparency of the lens.
- The number of vitreous floaters increases with age.

External eye structures

- The skin around the orbit of the eye may be darkened.
- There may be a sunken appearance of the eyeball due to the decrease in orbital fat.
- Skin folds of the upper lids may seem more prominent, and the lower lids may sag.
- The eyes may appear dry and lusterless due to the decrease in tear production from the lacrimal glands.
- A thin, grayish white arc or ring (*arcus senilis*) is commonly seen around part or all of the cornea. It results from an accumulation of a lipid substance on the cornea. The cornea tends to cloud with age.
- The iris may appear pale with pale brown discolorations as a result of pigment degeneration.
- The conjunctiva of the eye may appear paler than in younger adults and may take on a slightly yellow appearance because of the deposition of fat.
- Pupil reaction to light and accommodation is normally symmetrically equal but may be less brisk.
- The pupils can appear smaller in size, unequal, and irregular in shape because of sclerotic changes in the iris.

Internal eye structures

- The fundus may be yellower in appearance and lack luster.
- The blood vessels are slightly narrowed.
- The macula and fovea are less bright.

The middle ear is an air-filled cavity that starts at the tympanic membrane and contains three ossicles (bones of sound transmission): the malleus (the most easily seen), the incus, and the stapes. See Figure 19–32. The eustachian tube, another part of the middle ear, connects the middle ear to the nasopharynx. The tube stabilizes the air pressure between the external atmosphere and the middle ear, thus preventing rupture of the tympanic membrane and discomfort produced by marked pressure differences.

The inner ear contains the cochlea, a seashell-shaped structure essential for sound transmission and hearing, and the vestibule and semicircular canals, which contain the organs of equilibrium. See Figure 19–32.

Sound transmission and hearing are complex processes. In brief, sound can be transmitted by air conduction or bone conduction. Air-conducted transmission occurs when

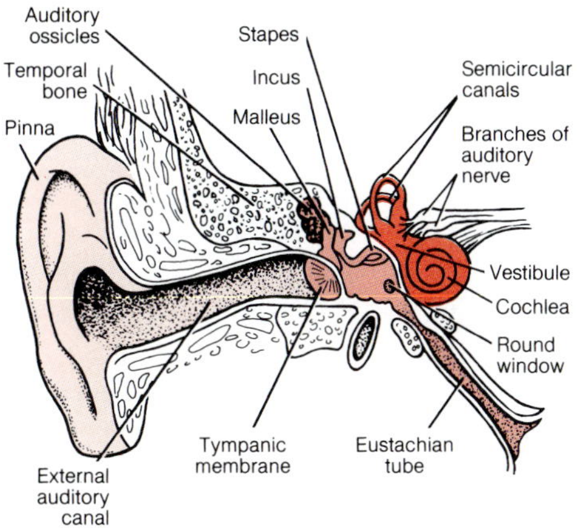

Figure 19–32 Anatomic structures of the external, middle, and inner ear.

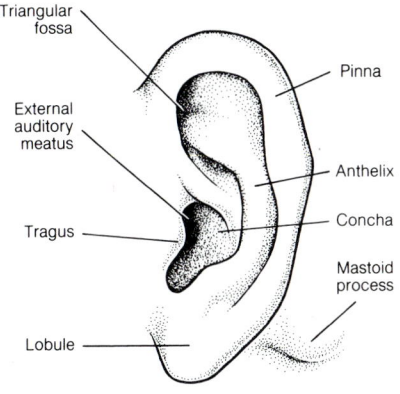

Figure 19–33 Landmarks of the external ear.

1. A sound stimulus enters the external canal and reaches the tympanic membrane.

2. The sound waves cross the tympanic membrane and reach the ossicles.

3. The sound waves travel from the ossicles to the opening in the inner ear (oval window).

4. The cochlea receives the sound vibrations.

5. The stimulus travels to the auditory nerve (the eighth cranial nerve) in the cerebral cortex.

Bone-conducted sound transmission occurs when skull bones transport the sound directly to the auditory nerve.

The curvature of the external ear canal differs with age. In the infant and toddler, the canal has an upward curvature. By age 3, the ear canal assumes the more downward curvature of adulthood.

Audiometric evaluations, which measure hearing at various decibels, are recommended for the elderly. A common hearing deficit with age is loss of ability to hear high-frequency sounds, such as *f, s, sh,* and *ph.* This neurosensory hearing deficit does not respond well to use of a hearing aid.

Auricles   To assess the *auricles,* assist the client to a comfortable sitting position. Inspect the auricles for color and texture. Normally, the auricles are the same color as the facial skin. Excessive redness may be associated with fever; bluish earlobes, with cyanosis; and extreme pallor, with frostbite. Normal texture is smooth. Note flaky, scaly skin, cysts, or other lesions.

Inspect the auricles for symmetry of size, position, and angle. To inspect position, note the level at which the superior aspect of the auricle attaches to the head. Relate this

point to the position of the eye. One should be able to visualize an imaginary horizontal line from the lateral angle of the eye to the point where the superior aspect of the auricle joins the head. Low-set ears are indicative of a congenital abnormality, e.g., mongolism. An imaginary line drawn from the top to the bottom of the ear should not vary more than 10° from the vertical. See Figure 19–34.

Palpate the auricle for texture, elasticity, and areas of tenderness: (a) pull the auricle upward, downward, and backward; (b) fold the pinna forward (it should recoil); (c) push in on the tragus; and (d) apply pressure to the mastoid process. Normally the auricle is mobile, firm, and not tender. Tenderness with motion or pressure can indicate an inflammation or infection of the external ear.

External Ear Canal and Tympanic Membrane   The nurse uses an otoscope to inspect the external ear canal and tympanic membrane for skin lesions, pus, and blood. An **otoscope** is a lighted instrument with a funnel-shaped part that is inserted into the external auditory canal. When performing an otoscopic examination, the nurse must be able to identify the four quadrants in the tympanic membrane: the anterior superior, anterior inferior, posterior superior, and posterior inferior. The anterior-posterior division is an imaginary straight line running through the handle of the malleus. See Figure 19–35. The nurse must also be able to identify the specific landmarks in the tympanic membrane:

- The *annulus* (tympanic ring) is the thickened cartilaginous ring surrounding the membrane.

- The *pars flaccida* is a triangular, lax, thin part of the tympanic membrane located at the top between two folds (anterior and posterior malleolar folds).

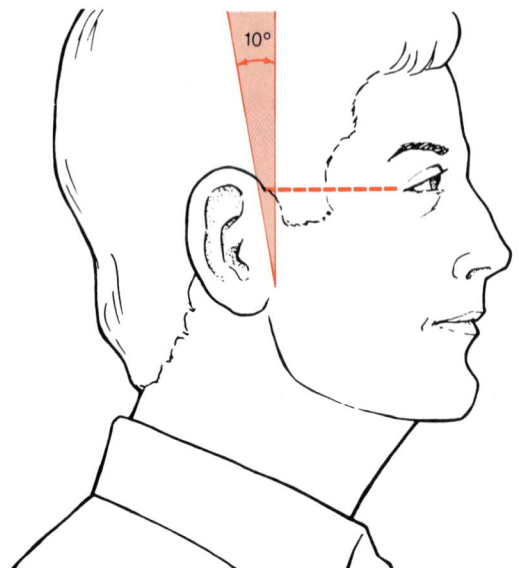

Figure 19–34   Normal ear alignment and ear angle.

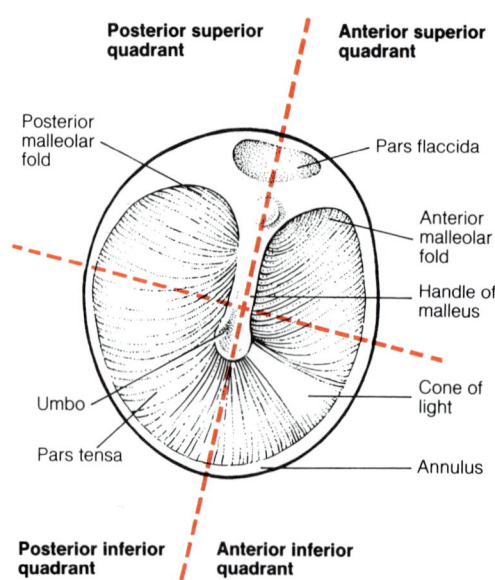

Figure 19–35   Landmarks of the tympanic membrane.

- The *pars tensa,* which is large and taut, is the remaining part of the membrane.

- The *malleus* (hammer) originates in the anterior superior quadrant of the membrane and extends approximately to its center. The handle of the malleus is firmly attached to the inner surface of the tympanic membrane as far as its center, which projects inward toward the tympanic cavity, making the inner surface of the membrane convex.

- The *umbo* is the point of greatest convexity of the malleus in the center of the membrane.

- The *light reflex* (a cone of light) is seen in the anterior inferior quadrant. Its point is directed toward the umbo, and its broad base is at the periphery of the tympanic annulus.

See Procedure 19–2 for the steps in an otoscopic examination. For normal and abnormal findings, see Table 19–9 on page 387. In some practice settings, the nurse does not perform otoscopic examinations. In others, the nurse's examination is limited to inspection of the external ear canal and the color of the tympanic membrane.

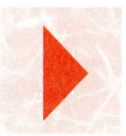

PROCEDURE 19–2

ASSESSING THE EXTERNAL EAR CANAL AND TYMPANIC MEMBRANE

Equipment ☑

Otoscope with several sizes of ear specula and an air insufflator to test tympanic membrane movement (optional) (see Figure 19–36)

Intervention

1. **Assemble the otoscope.**

- Attach a speculum to the otoscope.

- Use the largest diameter that will fit the ear canal without causing discomfort. *This achieves maximum vision of the entire ear canal and tympanic membrane.*

2. **Inspect the external ear canal.**

- Hold the otoscope either (a) right side up, with your fingers between the otoscope handle and the client's head or (b) upside down, with your fingers and the ulnar surface of your hand against the client's head. See Figure 19–37. *Holding the fingers and/or ulnar surface of the hand between the otoscope and the client's*

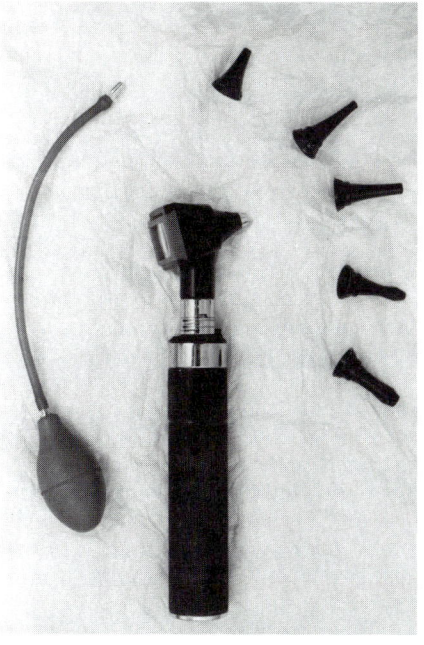

Figure 19–36 An otoscope with ear specula and an air insufflator.

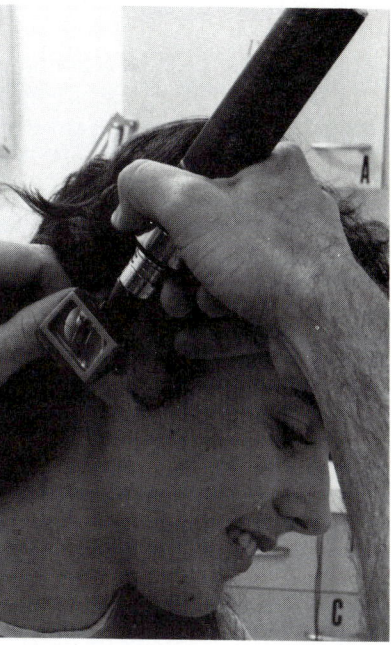

Figure 19–37 Inserting an otoscope.

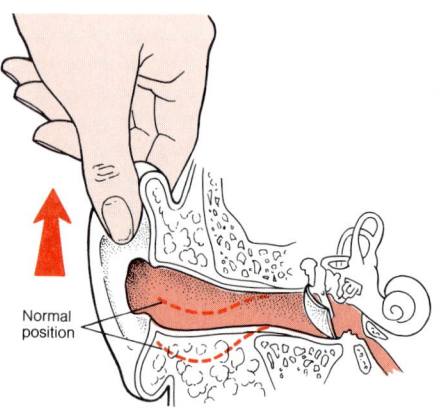

Figure 19–38 To straighten the ear canal of an adult, pull the pinna up and back.

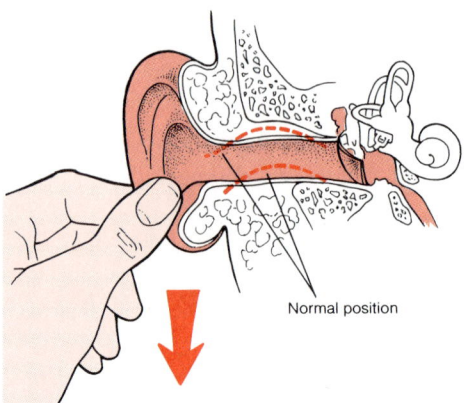

Figure 19–39 To straighten the ear canal of a child, pull the pinna down and back.

head stabilizes the head and protects the eardrum and canal from injury if a quick head movement occurs.

■ Tip the client's head away from you and straighten the ear canal. For an adult, straighten the ear canal by pulling the pinna up and back. See Figure 19–38. For a child under 3 years of age, pull the pinna down and then back. See Figure 19–39. *Straightening the ear canal facilitates vision of the ear canal and the tympanic membrane.*

Ⓢ ■ Gently insert the tip of the otoscope into the ear canal, avoiding pressure by the speculum against either side of the ear canal. *The inner two-thirds of the ear canal is bony; if the speculum is pressed against either side, the client will experience discomfort.*

■ Inspect the ear canal for cerumen, inflammation, scaling, foreign bodies, or other lesions.

3. If there is excessive cerumen, remove it.

■ Remove dry cerumen by irrigating the ear canal. *Removal of the cerumen is essential for proper visualization of the canal and tympanic membrane.*

■ Remove wet and waxy cerumen using a curette (cerumen spoon) or a cotton-tipped applicator. Use of a curette requires special skill.

4. Locate the tympanic membrane.

■ If you have difficulty seeing the tympanic membrane, try repositioning the client's head and pulling the pinna in a slightly different direction. The tympanic membrane is nearly oval, measuring about 9 to 10 mm in its downward and forward diameter, and 8 to 9 mm in its shorter diameter.

5. Inspect the tympanic membrane.

■ Inspect the membrane systematically in the four quadrants.

■ Inspect the membrane for color and gloss. Normally it is pearly gray and semitransparent.

■ Assess the appearance of the specific landmarks: the annulus, pars flaccida, pars tensa, malleus, umbo, and light reflex. This requires skill and experience.

6. Test the mobility of the tympanic membrane (pneumatic otoscopy) (optional).

■ Attach the rubber bulb and connecting tube to the otoscope.

■ Alternately squeeze and release the bulb a few times while observing the tympanic membrane. *Squeezing the bulb pushes air into the canal, causing the membrane to move inward. Releasing the bulb removes air, causing the membrane to move outward.* No movement or jerky movement of the tympanic membrane suggests a middle ear disorder or an obstructed eustachian tube.

A child must be carefully restrained during otoscopic assessment. An infant under 1 year of age can lie on the back on the examining table with the head turned to one side and the arms over the head. An adult holds the infant's arms securely at the elbows. The nurse then leans over the infant's chest and uses both hands when examining the ear. A young child sits on an adult's lap. The adult restrains the child's legs between the adult's knees and restrains the child's arms against the child's chest. The adult uses the free hand to hold the child's head against the adult's chest. Older children generally cooperate when standing or sitting.

TABLE 19–9 *Summary Assessment Data: External Ear Canal and Tympanic Membrane*

Structure	Normal Findings	Abnormal Findings
External ear canal	Distal third contains hair follicles and glands	Redness and discharge
		Scaling
	Dry cerumen, grayish tan in color; or wet cerumen, sticky and various shades of brown	Excessive cerumen obstructing canal
Tympanic membrane	Pearly gray color, semitransparent	Pink to red, some opacity
		Yellow-amber
		White
		Blue or deep red
		Dull surface
	Superior aspect is more anterior than lower rim; dimension is slightly conical	Loss of conical dimension and convex bulging
	Fluctuates (vibrates) slightly when client swallows	Membrane fixed, does not fluctuate
	Light reflex (cone of light) bright to dim	Light reflex dimmed or absent
	Malleus is dense whitish streak	Malleus poorly defined or not visible
	Umbo appears regressed	Umbo not visible
	Annulus is defined and whitish gray	Annulus poorly defined or not visible

Hearing Acuity

Gross hearing acuity tests *Gross hearing acuity* can be assessed by the client's response to voice tones and the ticking of a watch. First observe generally how well the client hears the voice. If the client has difficulty, assess the client's response to the whispered voice. Requesting that the nurse repeat words or statements, leaning toward the speaker, turning the head, cupping the ears, and speaking in a loud or unvaried tone of voice all suggest hearing problems.

To test the client's response to the whispered voice, stand 30 to 60 cm (1 to 2 ft) from the client in a position where the client cannot read your lips. Ask the client to occlude one ear by putting the finger in it. Whisper some nonconsecutive numbers and have the client repeat what was heard. The numbers are nonconsecutive so that the client cannot anticipate the sequence of numbers. Increase the loudness of the whisper until the client can identify at least 50% of the numbers. Repeat the process with the other ear. This is used only for screening, since it is difficult to maintain consistency in the whispered voice.

Another screening test is the watch tick test. The ticking of a watch has a higher pitch than the human voice. For this test, ask the client to occlude one ear. Out of the client's sight, place a ticking watch 2 to 5 cm (1 to 2 in) from the unoccluded ear. Ask whether the client can hear it. Repeat with the other ear.

Tuning fork tests Tuning fork tests are used by advanced practitioners to assess whether the client's hearing loss is a conduction, sensorineural, or mixed problem. **Conduction hearing loss** is the result of interrupted transmission of sound waves through the outer and middle ear structures. Possible causes are a tear in the tympanic membrane or an obstruction, due to swelling or other causes, in the auditory canal. **Sensorineural hearing loss** is the result of damage to the inner ear, the auditory nerve, or the hearing center in the brain. **Mixed hearing loss** is a combination of conduction and sensorineural loss.

Weber's test assesses bone conduction by testing the lateralization (sideward transmission) of sounds. Hold the tuning fork at its base, and activate it by tapping the fork gently against the back of the hand near the knuckles or by stroking the fork between the thumb and index fingers so that it rings softly. Then place the base of the vibrating fork on top of the client's head (see Figure 19–40 on the following page), and ask where the client hears the noise. Normally the sound is heard in both ears or localized at the center of the head (Weber negative). Clients with a unilateral conductive hearing loss hear the sound better in the poor or damaged ear. Clients with a sensorineural loss hear the sound better in the ear without a problem. Record positive findings as Weber right or Weber left.

The **Rinne test** compares air conduction to bone conduction. Ask the client to block the hearing in one ear inter-

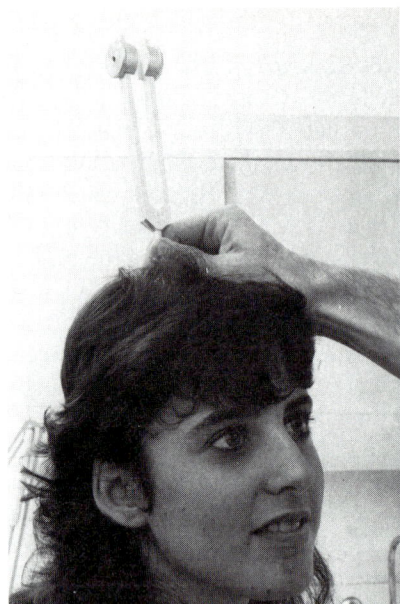

Figure 19–40 Placing the base of the tuning fork on the client's skull.

mittently by moving a fingertip in and out of the ear canal. Hold the *handle* of the activated tuning fork on the mastoid process of one ear until the client states that the vibrations can no longer be heard. Then immediately hold the still vibrating fork *prongs* in front of the client's ear canal. Push aside the client's hair if necessary. Ask whether the client

---

The Elderly: Physical Changes of the Ears and Hearing

- The skin of the ear may appear dry and be less resilient because of the loss of connective tissue.
- Increased coarse and wirelike hair growth may be seen along the helix, anthelix, and tragus.
- The pinna increases in both width and length, and the earlobe elongates.
- Earwax is drier.
- The tympanic membrane is more translucent and less flexible. The intensity of the light reflex may be slightly diminished.
- Sensorineural hearing loss occurs.
- Generalized hearing loss occurs in all frequencies, although the first symptom is the loss of high-frequency sounds: the *f, s, sh,* and *ph* sounds. To such persons, conversation can be distorted and result in what appears to be inappropriate or confused behavior.

---

now hears the sound. Sound conducted by air is heard more readily than sound conducted by bone. The tuning fork vibrations conducted by air are normally heard longer.

Repeat the procedure with the other ear. When air-conducted hearing is greater than bone-conducted hearing, the Rinne test is normal and is said to be positive, i.e., AC > BC. When there is a conductive loss, the bone conduction time is equal to or longer than the air conduction time, i.e., negative Rinne test, BC = AC or BC > AC.

The **Schwabach test** compares the client's bone conduction to the nurse's. The nurse, who is presumed to have normal hearing, places the handle of a vibrating tuning fork alternately on the client's and nurse's mastoid process and asks the client to indicate when the vibrations are no longer heard.

The client's other ear is then tested. Normally, the client and nurse hear the vibrations for the same length of time. The client with conductive hearing loss hears the tones longer than the nurse; the client with sensorineural hearing loss does not hear the tones as long.

See the accompanying box for a description of changes in the ears and hearing in elderly people.

Nose and Sinuses

The upper third of the nose is bone; the remainder is cartilage. Inspect the *external nose* for any deviations in shape, size, or color and flaring or discharge from the nares. Normally the nose is symmetrical and straight and there is no discharge or flaring. Lightly palpate the nose to determine areas of tenderness, masses, and displacement of bone and cartilage.

Air should move freely as the client breathes through the nares. To determine *patency* of the nasal cavities, ask the client to (a) close the mouth, (b) exert pressure on one naris, and (c) breathe through the opposite naris. Repeat the procedure to assess patency of the opposite naris. Adequacy of function of the olfactory nerve may also be assessed (see the neurologic assessment later in this chapter).

The nasal cavities can be inspected very simply with a flashlight while using the thumb of the nondominant hand to push the tip of the nose upward. However, for a more thorough assessment, the advanced practitioner uses a **nasal speculum,** a lighted instrument that facilitates examination of the nasal chambers.

The nasal cavities are assessed as follows:

1. Tip the client's head back.

2. If using a speculum, hold it in the nondominant hand and place the index finger on the side of the nose to stabilize its position. Use your dominant hand to position the head and hold the light.

3. Inspect the lining of the nares (mucosa) and the coarse hairs that filter the air. Observe the presence of redness, swelling, growths, and discharge. The mucosa is usually pink with clear watery discharge.

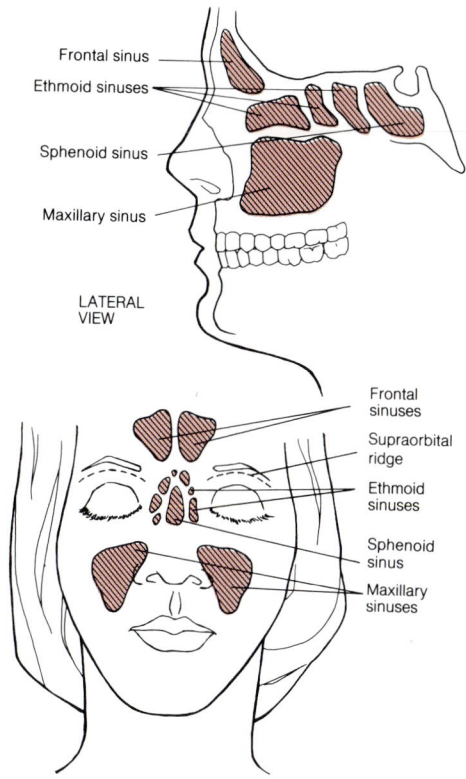

Figure 19–41   The facial sinuses.

The Elderly: Physical Changes of the Nose and Sense of Smell

- The sense of smell is markedly diminished because of a decrease in the number of olfactory nerve fibers and atrophy of the remaining fibers. Older persons are less able to identify and discriminate odors.

- Nosebleeds may result from hypertensive disease or other arterial vessel changes.

---

4. Inspect the position of the nasal septum between the nasal chambers, in particular any deviation to right or left. The nasal septum is normally intact and in the midline.

5. Inspect the inferior and middle turbinates when visible. The superior turbinate is difficult to inspect because of its position. These bones increase the surface of the mucous membrane in the nares. The mucous membranes warm and moisten the inspired air. The clefts between the turbinates are called meati. Each meatus is named for the adjacent turbinate, e.g., the inferior meatus is near the inferior turbinate.

6. Inspect the mucous membranes for purulent drainage and nasal polyps. These are an abnormal finding.

Palpate the maxillary and frontal *sinuses*. See Figure 19–41. Palpation can reveal tenderness. Normally, the sinuses are not tender.

Transillumination may be performed by advanced practitioners. Transilluminate the frontal sinuses by placing a penlight against the inner aspect of the supraorbital ridge of the frontal bone. This is best done in a darkened room. Normally, the light shines through the bone and outlines the sinus. Transillumination can reveal the presence of air or fluid in the sinuses. Normally, the sinuses contain air; they appear darker when fluid is present. Transilluminate the maxillary sinuses by placing a penlight in the client's mouth and shining it to the left and to the right. The sinuses should light up equally.

See the box above for a description of changes in the nose and sense of smell in the elderly.

Mouth and Oropharynx

The mouth and pharynx are composed of a number of structures: lips, inner and buccal mucosa, the tongue and floor of the mouth, teeth and gums, hard and soft palate, uvula, salivary glands, tonsillar pillars, and tonsils. Risk factors to be considered during the examination include poor oral hygiene, smoking, lack of regular dental care, and the use of dentures. The CDC recommends that the nurse wear gloves when in contact with the buccal mucosa. Physical examination of the mouth includes inspection and palpation techniques. See Table 19–10 for normal and abnormal findings.

Equipment needed for assessment of the mouth and pharynx includes tongue blade, gauze squares (2 × 2), a penlight or flashlight, and disposable gloves.

Lips   The lips are inspected for symmetry of contour, color, and texture. Ask the client to purse the lips as if to whistle. Normally people can purse their lips. The lips are usually soft, moist, and smooth in texture, with symmetric contour and uniform pink color, although the color may be darker in Mediterranean groups and blacks.

Inner and Buccal Mucosa   The inner mucosa and buccal mucosa are inspected and palpated. The *inner mucosa* is situated inside the upper and lower lips. Ask the client to relax the mouth, and pull the lower lip away from the lower teeth. See Figure 19–42 on page 391. The process is repeated for the upper lip. The mucosa is inspected for color, moisture, texture, and the presence of lesions such as ulcers or abrasions. Any lesions present are gently palpated for size, tenderness, and consistency.

To assess the *buccal mucosa,* which lines the cheeks, ask the client to open the mouth; then, using a tongue blade, retract the cheek (see Figure 19–43 on page 391). The sur-

TABLE 19–10 *Summary Assessment Data: Mouth and Oropharynx*

Structure	Normal Findings	Abnormal Findings
Lips	Uniform pink color (darker in Mediterranean groups and blacks, e.g., bluish hue)	Pallor
		Bluish discoloration
	Soft, moist, smooth texture	Blisters
	Symmetry of contour	Generalized swelling
	Ability to purse lips	Localized swelling
		Fissures, crusts, scales
		Inability to purse lips
Inner lips and buccal mucosa	Uniform pink color (brown freckled pigmentation in blacks)	Pallor
		White patches (leukoplakia)
	Moist, smooth, soft and elastic texture (drier oral mucosa in elderly due to decreased salivation)	Excessive dryness
		Mucosal cysts
		Irritations
		Abrasions
		Ulcerations, nodules
Teeth	32 adult teeth	Missing teeth, bridges, full or partial dentures
		Dental caries
	Smooth, white tooth enamel	Discoloration of enamel
Gums	Pink color (bluish or dark patches in blacks)	Excessive redness
	Moist, firm texture	Spongy texture, bleeding, tenderness
	No retraction (pulling away from the teeth)	Receding atrophied gums
		Swelling that partially covers the teeth
Tongue	Central position	Deviated from center
	Pink color (some brown pigmentation on tongue borders in blacks), moist, slightly rough, thin whitish coating	Dry, furry
		Smooth and red
	Moves freely	Nodes, ulcerations, discolorations, restricted mobility
	Smooth tongue base with prominent veins	Varicosities (tiny bluish black or purple swollen areas)
Palates	Light pink, smooth, soft palate	Discolorations
	Lighter pink hard palate, more irregular texture	Palates the same color
		Irritations
Uvula	Positioned in midline of soft palate	Deviation to one side
		Immobility
Oropharynx and tonsils	Pink and smooth posterior wall	Reddened, lesions, plaques
	Tonsils pink and normal size	Tonsillar crypts inflamed, filled with exudate, swollen

face buccal mucosa should be viewed completely from top to bottom and back to front. A flashlight or penlight will help illuminate the surface. Repeat the procedure for the other side. Normal buccal mucosa is a uniform pink color; brown freckled pigmentation (hyperpigmentation), however, is seen in some people. Hyperpigmentation appears after the age of 50 years in up to 90% of blacks and 10% of whites. The buccal mucosa is normally moist, smooth, soft, glistening, and elastic in texture. The elderly may experience reduced salivation; this factor, in addition to the use of prescribed medications, e.g., diuretics, may cause the mucosa to appear drier.

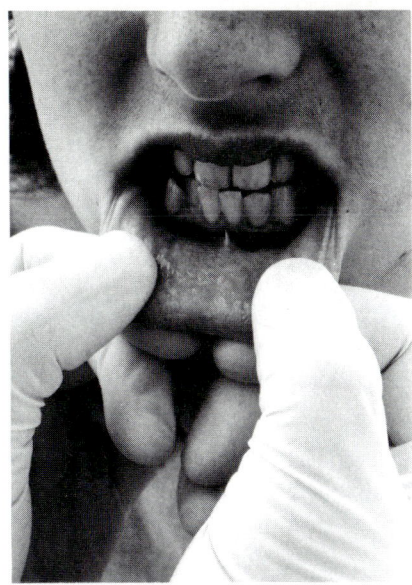

Figure 19–42 Inspecting the lower inner lip mucosa.

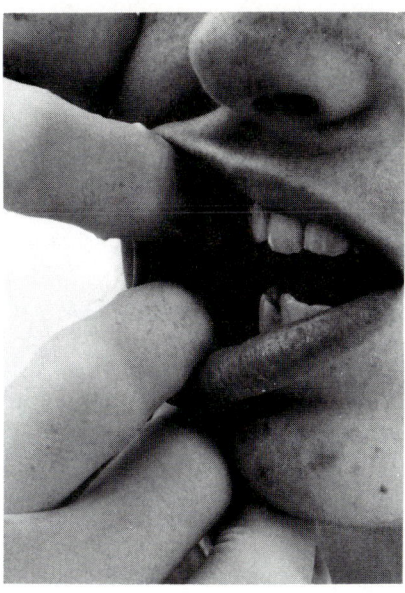

Figure 19–43 Inspecting the buccal mucosa.

 Teeth and Gums   As the cheeks are retracted, the gums and teeth should be inspected. The gums should be inspected for bleeding, color, retraction (pulling away from the teeth), edema, and lesions. The gums around the molars at the back of the mouth should be viewed carefully; they are prone to problems because of difficulty cleaning in that area. Normally, gums are pink, moist, and firm. No retraction should be apparent. Some black clients may have bluish or dark patches, and elderly people may have pale gums.

The nurse also palpates the gums using a tongue blade to determine texture. Sponginess may indicate the presence of periodontal disease. Spongy gums often bleed readily.

The teeth should be examined for color, the presence of fillings, dental caries, partial or complete dentures, and tartar along the base of the teeth. Normally, teeth are smooth, white, and shiny. Brown or black discoloration of the enamel can indicate staining or the presence of caries. Adults normally have 32 teeth; any missing teeth should be noted. Elderly people often have fewer teeth; 60% of people over the age of 75 years have no teeth.

Any lesion under dentures can cause discomfort and difficulty in chewing. Ask the client to remove the dentures, and inspect them for broken and worn areas. Also inspect the areas under the dentures for irritated and excoriated areas.

 Tongue and Floor of the Mouth   To inspect the surface of the tongue, ask the client to protrude it partially. Protruding the tongue excessively can elicit the gag reflex. Using a penlight for illumination, inspect the tongue for color, size, texture, position, mobility, and any coating. The tongue is normally positioned centrally; it is pink in color,

moist, and slightly rough on the top surface and has a thin whitish coating. The lateral margins are usually smooth. The prominent veins on the undersurface of the tongue are apparent when the client raises the tongue to the roof of the mouth. The undersurface should be smooth and free of lesions.

To palpate the tongue, grasp its tip using a piece of gauze, and with the index finger palpate the full length of the tongue and from side to side, including the base. See Figure 19–44. Look for white or red areas, tenderness, and any

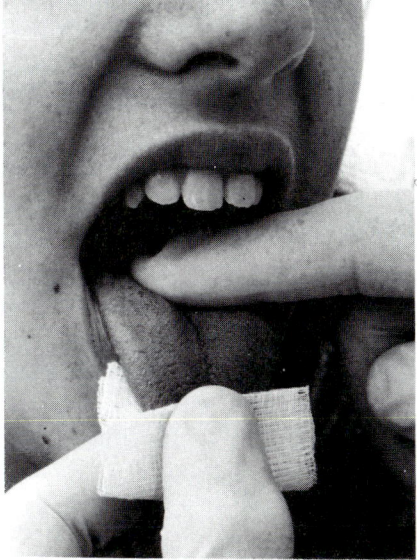

Figure 19–44 Palpating the tongue.

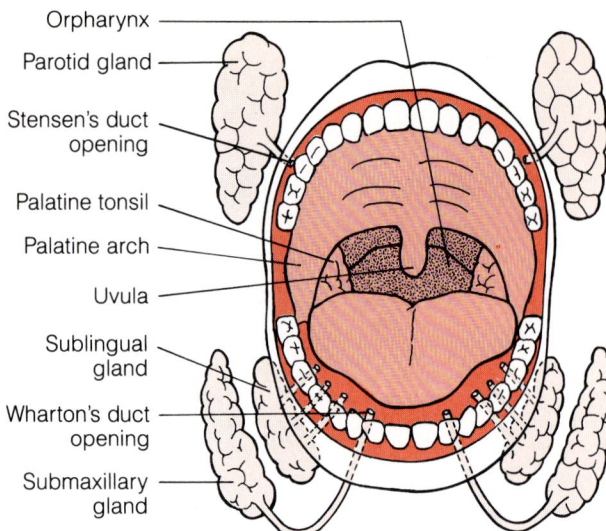

Figure 19–45 Anatomic structures of the mouth.

Labels for figure:
Orpharynx
Parotid gland
Stensen's duct opening
Palatine tonsil
Palatine arch
Uvula
Sublingual gland
Wharton's duct opening
Submaxillary gland

lesions such as cysts, growths, or nodules. At this time, palpate the floor of the mouth for any nodules, lumps, or excoriated areas. Sometimes varicosities appear on the floor of the mouth of the elderly but are rarely a problem.

To assess the function of the glossopharyngeal and hypoglossal nerves, see Table 19–25 later in this chapter.

Palates and Uvula   The client should extend the neck backward so that the hard and soft palates can be observed. The hard palate, or roof of the mouth, extends anteriorly, and the soft palate extends posteriorly toward the pharynx. It may be necessary to depress the tongue with a tongue blade and use a penlight to visualize the palates. Both palates are examined for color, shape, texture, and the presence of bony prominences. Normally the palates are pink; the hard palate is lighter in color and more irregular in texture. Some people have bony growths called *exostoses* growing from the hard palate. These are generally benign.

The uvula is normally centrally located and freely mobile. When the client says "ah," the soft palate rises, and the uvula should come into view (see Figure 19–45).

 Salivary Glands   Normally, three pairs of salivary glands empty into the oral cavity: the parotid, submandibular, and sublingual glands (see Figure 19–45). The parotid gland is the largest and empties through Stensen's duct opposite the second molar. The submandibular gland empties through Wharton's duct, which is situated at the side of the frenulum on the floor of the mouth. The sublingual salivary gland lies in the floor of the mouth and has numerous openings. The salivary gland opening should be inspected for any swelling or redness, which could indicate inflammation of the related gland.

 Oropharynx   Assessment of the oropharynx includes assessment of the tonsils. Equipment required includes a penlight or flashlight, tongue blade, and gloves. The client extends the head backward and opens the mouth. Press the tongue blade against the one side of the tongue about halfway back to expose one side of the oropharynx. Inspect the palatine arches. They are normally pink and smooth; any redness, lesions, or plaques should be noted. The tonsils, oval-shaped lymphoid tissue, are situated on either side between the posterior and anterior tonsillar pillars. The pillars are the soft tissues supporting the soft palate. Inspect the tonsils for color (normally pink and smooth), discharge, and size. A grading system can be used to describe the size of the tonsils:

Grade 1 (normal): The tonsils are behind the tonsillar pillars, i.e., the soft structures supporting the soft palate.

Grade 2: The tonsils are between the pillars and the uvula.

Grade 3: The tonsils are touching the uvula.

Grade 4: One or both tonsils are extending to the midline of the oropharynx.

When inspecting the tonsils, note any discharge around the tonsils and tonsillar pillars.

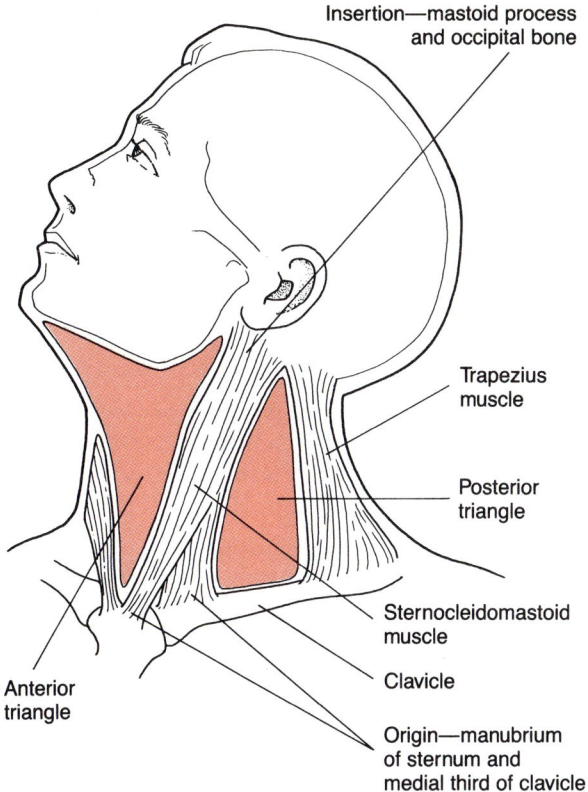

Figure 19–46   Major muscles of the neck.

Labels on Figure 19–46:
Insertion—mastoid process and occipital bone
Trapezius muscle
Posterior triangle
Sternocleidomastoid muscle
Clavicle
Origin—manubrium of sternum and medial third of clavicle
Anterior triangle

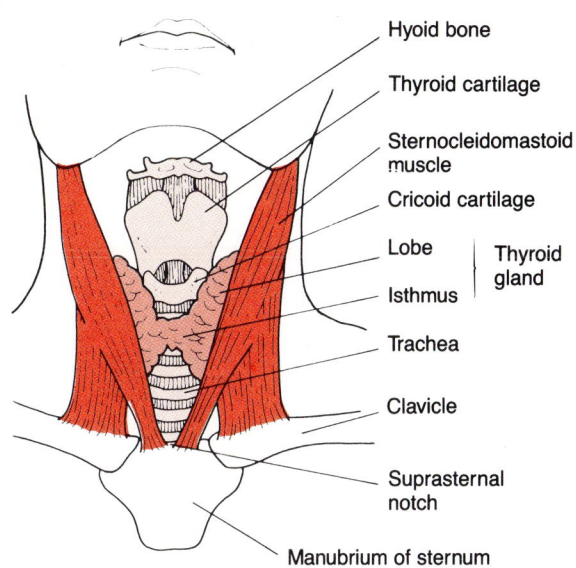

Figure 19–47   Structures of the neck.

Labels on Figure 19–47:
Hyoid bone
Thyroid cartilage
Sternocleidomastoid muscle
Cricoid cartilage
Lobe
Isthmus
Thyroid gland
Trachea
Clavicle
Suprasternal notch
Manubrium of sternum

The oropharynx is behind the tonsils. It is normally pink and smooth. Note the presence of any edema, inflammation, lesions, or exudate. Clients who have sinus problems may have an exudate that drains along the posterior wall of the pharynx. Part of the examination of the pharynx is to elicit the gag reflex by pressing the posterior tongue with a tongue blade. Lack of a gag reflex can indicate problems with glossopharyngeal or vagus nerves.

Physical changes of the mouth and sense of taste in elderly people are shown in the box on the previous page.

NECK

Examination of the neck includes the muscles, lymph nodes, trachea, thyroid gland, carotid arteries, and jugular veins. Areas of the neck are defined by the sternocleidomastoid muscles, which divide each side of the neck into two triangles: the anterior and posterior. See Figure 19–46. The trachea, thyroid gland, anterior cervical nodes, and carotid artery lie within the anterior triangle (the carotid artery runs parallel and anterior to the sternocleidomastoid muscle). See Figure 19–47. The posterior lymph nodes lie within the posterior triangle. See Figure 19–48.

Muscles   Ask the client to hold the head erect, and inspect the neck muscles (sternocleidomastoid and trapezius) for abnormal swellings or masses. Each sternocleidomastoid

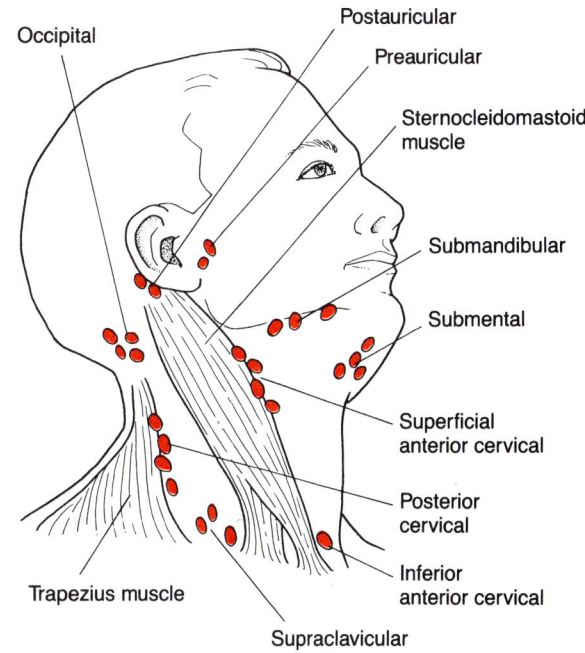

Figure 19–48   Lymph nodes of the neck.

Labels on Figure 19–48:
Occipital
Postauricular
Preauricular
Sternocleidomastoid muscle
Submandibular
Submental
Superficial anterior cervical
Posterior cervical
Inferior anterior cervical
Supraclavicular
Trapezius muscle

muscle extends from the upper sternum and the medial third of the clavicle to the mastoid process of the temporal bone behind the ear. See Figure 19–46. These muscles turn and laterally flex the head. Each trapezius muscle extends from the occipital bone of the skull to the lateral third of the clavicle. These muscles draw the head to the side and back, elevate the chin, and elevate the shoulders to shrug them.

Ask the client to

1. Move the chin to the chest (head flexion). This determines function of the sternocleidomastoid muscle.

2. Move the head back so that the chin points upward (head hyperextension). This determines function of the trapezius muscle.

3. Move the head so that the ear is moved toward the shoulder (lateral flexion) on each side. This determines function of the sternocleidomastoid muscle.

4. Turn the head to the right and to the left (lateral rotation). This determines function of the sternocleidomastoid muscle.

Ask the client to turn the head to one side against the resistance of your hand. Repeat with the other side. This determines the strength of the sternocleidomastoid muscle. Ask the client to shrug the shoulders against the resistance of your hands. This determines the strength of the trapezius muscles.

Lymph Nodes   Lymph nodes in the neck that collect lymph from the head and neck structures are grouped serially and referred to as chains. See Figure 19–48 and Table 19–11. The deep cervical chain is not shown in Figure 19–48, since it lies beneath the sternocleidomastoid muscle.

Palpate the entire neck for enlarged lymph nodes, using the following guidelines:

- Face the client, and bend the client's head forward slightly or toward the side being examined to relax the soft tissue and muscles.

- Palpate the nodes using the pads of the fingers. Move the fingertips in a gentle rotating motion.

- When examining the submental and submandibular nodes, place the fingertips under the mandible on the side nearest the palpating hand, and pull the skin and subcutaneous tissue laterally over the mandibular surface so that the tissue rolls over the nodes.

- When palpating the supraclavicular nodes, have the client bend the head forward to relax the tissues of the anterior neck and to relax the shoulders so that the clavicles are dropped. Use your hand nearest the side to be examined when facing the client, i.e., your left hand for the client's right nodes. Use your free hand to flex the client's head forward if necessary. Hook your index and third fingers over the clavicle lateral to the sternocleidomastoid muscle. See Figure 19–49.

TABLE 19–11   *Lymph Nodes of the Head and Neck*

Node Center	Location	Area Drained
Head		
Occipital	At the posterior base of the skull	The occipital region of the scalp and the deep structures of the back of the neck
Postauricular (mastoid)	Behind the auricle of the ear over or in front of the mastoid process	The parietal region of the head and part of the ear
Preauricular	In front of the tragus of the ear	The forehead and upper face
Floor of Mouth		
Submandibular (submaxillary)	Along the medial border of the lower jaw, halfway between the angle of the jaw and the chin	The chin, upper lip, cheek, nose, teeth, eyelids, part of the tongue and of the floor of the mouth
Submental	Behind the tip of the mandible, in the midline, under the chin	The anterior third of the tongue, gums, and floor of the mouth
Neck		
Superficial (anterior) cervical chain	Along and anterior to the sternocleidomastoid muscle	The skin and neck
Posterior cervical chain	Along the anterior aspect of the trapezius muscle	The posterior and lateral regions of the neck, occiput, and mastoid
Deep cervical chain	Under the sternocleidomastoid muscle	The larynx, thyroid gland, trachea, and upper part of the esophagus
Supraclavicular	Above the clavicle, in the angle between the clavicle and the sternocleidomastoid muscle	The lateral regions of the neck and lungs

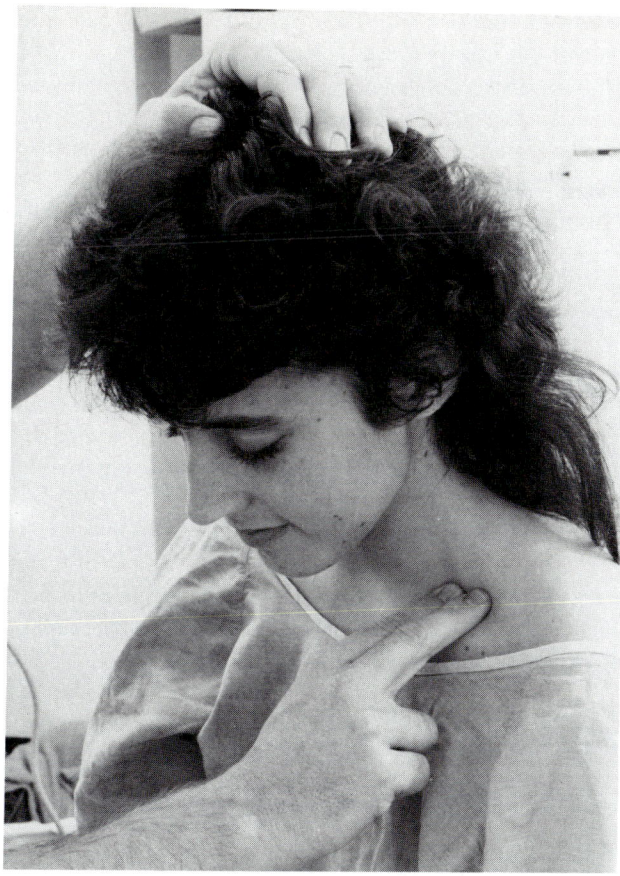

Figure 19–49 Palpating the supraclavicular lymph nodes.

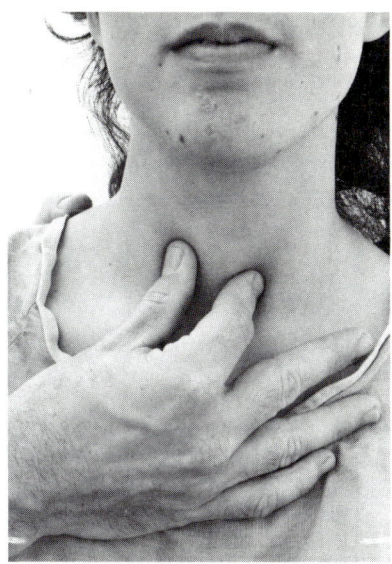

Figure 19–50 Palpating the trachea for lateral deviation.

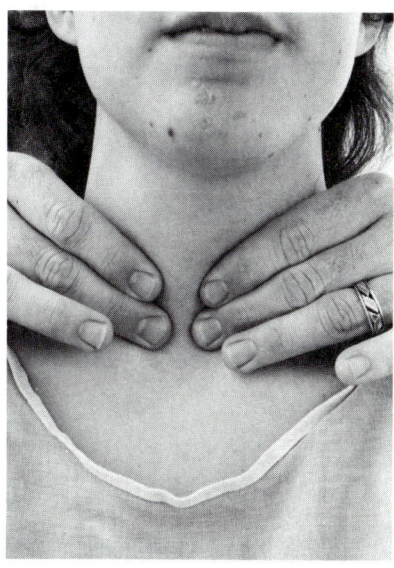

Figure 19–51 Palpating the thyroid: posterior approach.

■ When palpating the anterior cervical nodes and posterior cervical nodes, move your fingertips slowly in a forward circular motion against the sternocleidomastoid and trapezius muscles, respectively.

■ To palpate the deep cervical nodes, bend or hook your fingers around the sternocleidomastoid muscle.

Trachea　The trachea is normally located in the midline of the neck. It can be palpated for lateral deviation by placing a fingertip or a fingertip and thumb on the trachea in the suprasternal notch (see Figure 19–50) and then moving the finger(s) laterally to the left and the right in the spaces bordered by the clavicle, the anterior aspect of the sternocleidomastoid muscle, and the trachea. These spaces are normally equal on both sides, and the trachea is centrally placed. A deviation to one side could indicate a tumor or atelectasis.

Thyroid Gland　To inspect the thyroid gland, stand in front of the client, and observe the lower half of the neck overlying the thyroid gland for symmetry and visible masses. Ask the client to hyperextend the head and swallow. If necessary, offer a glass of water to make it easier for the client to swallow. This action determines how the thyroid and

cricoid cartilages move and whether swallowing causes a bulging of the gland. Normally the thyroid gland ascends during swallowing but is not visible.

To palpate the thyroid gland, stand either in front of or behind the client, and ask the client to lower the chin slightly. Lowering the chin relaxes the neck muscles, facilitating palpation.

For the posterior approach:

1. Place your hands around the client's neck, with your fingertips on the lower half of the neck over the trachea. See Figure 19–51.

2. Ask the client to swallow (taking a sip of water, if necessary), and feel for any enlargement of the thyroid isthmus, as it rises. The isthmus lies across the trachea below the cricoid cartilage. See Figure 19–47, earlier.

3. To examine the right thyroid lobe, have the client lower the chin slightly and turn the head slightly to the right (the side being examined). With your left fingers, displace the trachea slightly to the right. With your right fingers, palpate the right thyroid lobe for any enlargement, masses, or nodules. Have the client swallow while you are palpating.

4. Repeat step 3 in reverse to examine the left thyroid lobe.

For the anterior approach, place the tips of your index and middle fingers over the trachea, and palpate the thyroid isthmus as the client swallows. To examine the right thyroid lobe, ask the client to lower the chin slightly and turn the head slightly to the right. With your right fingers, displace the trachea slightly to the client's right (your left). With your left fingers, palpate the right thyroid lobe. To examine the left thyroid lobe, repeat the process in reverse. During palpation, check the surface of the thyroid gland for smoothness. Note any areas of roughness or nodules.

If enlargement of the gland is suspected, auscultate over the thyroid area for a bruit. Use the bell-shaped diaphragm of the stethoscope. In an enlarged hyperactive thyroid gland, blood flow through the thyroid arteries is increased and produces vibrations that may be heard as a soft rushing sound (bruit).

Carotid Arteries and Jugular Veins   See the discussion of the peripheral vascular system, later in this chapter.

Physical changes of the neck and associated structures in elderly people are shown in the accompanying box.

THORAX AND LUNGS

Assessing the thorax and lungs is frequently critical to assessing the client's aeration status. Changes in the respiratory system can come about slowly or quickly. In clients with chronic obstructive pulmonary disease (COPD), such as chronic bronchitis, emphysema, and asthma, changes are frequently gradual; however, in clients who are acutely ill, e.g., those who have a pneumothorax (accumulation of gas

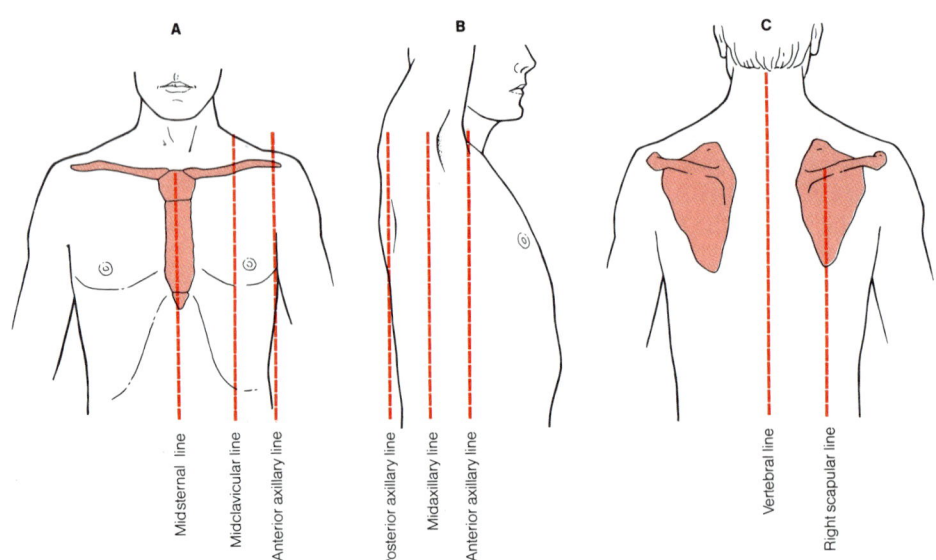

Figure 19–52   Chest wall landmarks: *A,* anterior chest; *B,* lateral chest; *C,* posterior chest.

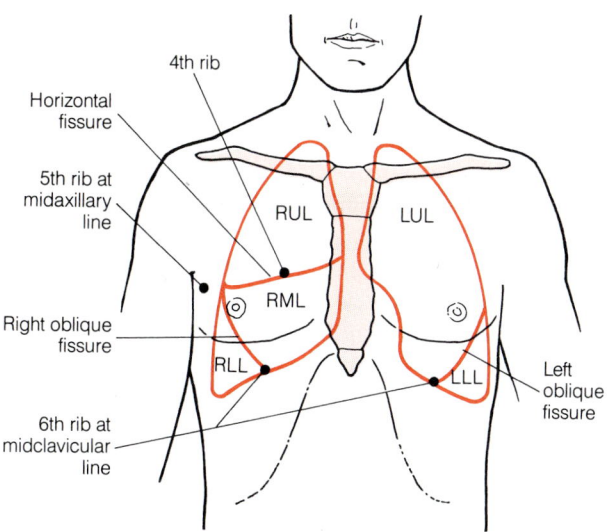

Figure 19–53 Anterior chest landmarks and underlying lungs.

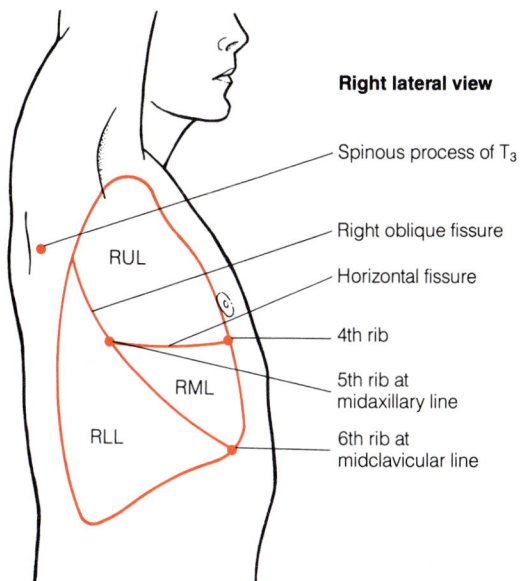

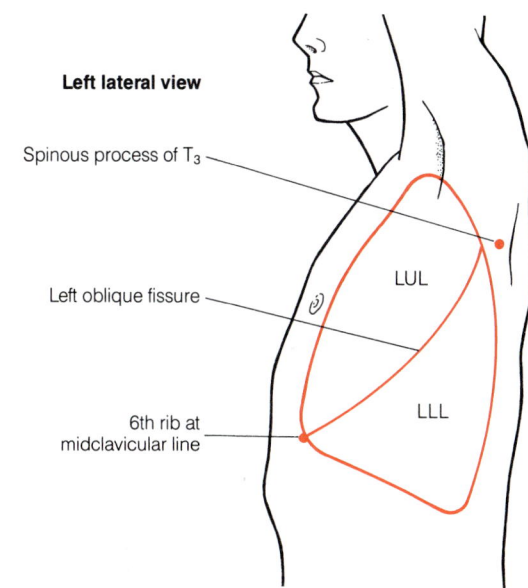

Figure 19–54 Lateral chest landmarks and underlying lungs.

or fluid in the pleural cavity), changes occur quickly, and death can result if immediate action is not taken. For information about the mechanics of breathing see Chapter 41.

The client's posture is important to note. Some people with chronic respiratory problems tend to bend forward or even prop their arms on a support to elevate their clavicles. This posture is an attempt to expand the chest fully and thus breathe with less effort.

Chest Wall Landmarks

Before beginning the assessment, the nurse must be familiar with a series of imaginary lines on the chest wall and be able to locate the position of each rib and some spinous processes. These landmarks help the nurse to identify the position of underlying organs, e.g., lobes of the lung, and to record abnormal assessment findings. Figure 19–52 shows the anterior, lateral, and posterior series of lines. The *midsternal line* is a vertical line running through the center of the sternum. The *midclavicular lines* (right and left) are vertical lines from the midpoints of the clavicles. The *anterior axillary lines* (right and left) are vertical lines from the anterior axillary folds. See Figure 19–52, *A*. Figure 19–52, *B* shows the three imaginary lines of the lateral chest. The *posterior axillary line* is a vertical line from the posterior axillary fold. The *midaxillary line* is a vertical line from the apex of the axilla. The anterior axillary line is described above. Figure 19–52, *C* shows the posterior chest landmarks. The *vertebral line* is a vertical line along the spinous processes. The *scapular lines* (right and left) are vertical lines from the inferior angles of the scapulae.

Locating the position of each rib and certain spinous processes is essential for visualizing underlying lobes of the lung. Figures 19–53, 19–54, and 19–55 show an anterior view, right and left lateral views, and a posterior view of the chest and underlying lungs. Each lung is first divided into the upper and lower lobes by an oblique fissure that runs from the level of the spinous process of the third thoracic vertebra (T-3) to the level of the sixth rib at the midclavicular line. See Figure 19–52. The right upper lobe is abbreviated RUL; the right lower lobe, RLL. Similarly, the left upper lobe is abbreviated LUL; the left lower lobe, LLL.

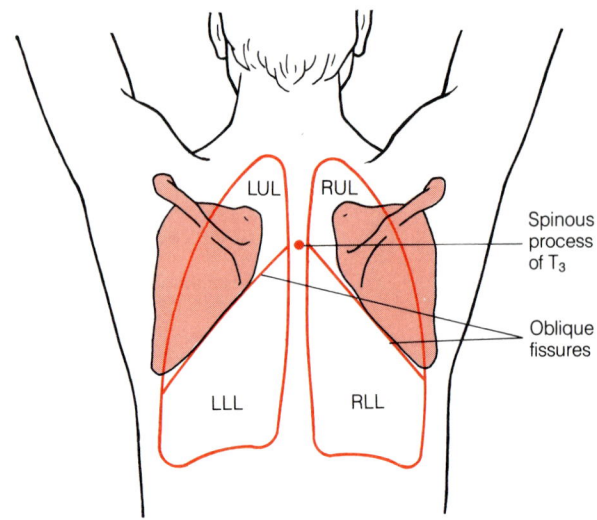

Figure 19–55 Posterior chest landmarks and underlying lungs.

The right lung is further divided by a minor fissure into the right upper lobe and right middle lobe (RML). This fissure runs anteriorly from the right midaxillary line at the level of the fifth rib to the level of the fourth rib.

These specific landmarks, i.e., T-3 and the 4th, 5th, and 6th ribs, are located as follows. The starting point for locating the ribs anteriorly is the *angle of Louis,* the junction between the manubrium and body of the sternum. The superior border of the second rib attaches to the sternum

at this manubriosternal junction. See Figure 19–56. Identification of the manubrium may be facilitated by first palpating the clavicle and following its course to its attachment at the manubrium. The nurse then palpates and counts distal ribs and intercostal spaces (ICS) from the second rib. It is important to note that an ICS is numbered according to the number of the rib immediately above the space. When palpating for rib identification, the nurse should palpate along the midclavicular line rather than the sternal border, since the rib cartilages are very close at the sternum. Only the first seven ribs attach directly to the sternum.

The counting of the ribs is more difficult on the posterior than on the anterior thorax. For identifying underlying lung lobes, the pertinent landmark is T-3. The starting point for locating T-3 is the spinous process of the seventh cervical vertebra (C-7), also referred to as the *vertebra prominens.* See Figure 19–57. When the client flexes the neck anteriorly, a prominent process can be observed and palpated. This is the spinous process of the seventh cervical vertebra. If two spinous processes are observed, the superior one is C-7, and the inferior one is the spinous process of the first thoracic vertebra (T-1). The nurse then palpates and counts the spinous processes from C-7 to T-3. Each spinous process up to T-4 is adjacent to the corresponding rib number; e.g., T-3 is adjacent to the third rib. After T-4, however, the spinous processes project obliquely, causing the spinous process of the vertebra to lie, not over its correspondingly numbered rib, but over the rib below. Thus, the spinous process of T-5 lies over the body of T-6 and is adjacent to the sixth rib.

Assessment of the lungs and thorax includes all methods of examination: inspection, palpation, percussion, and auscultation. The following are needed for the examination:

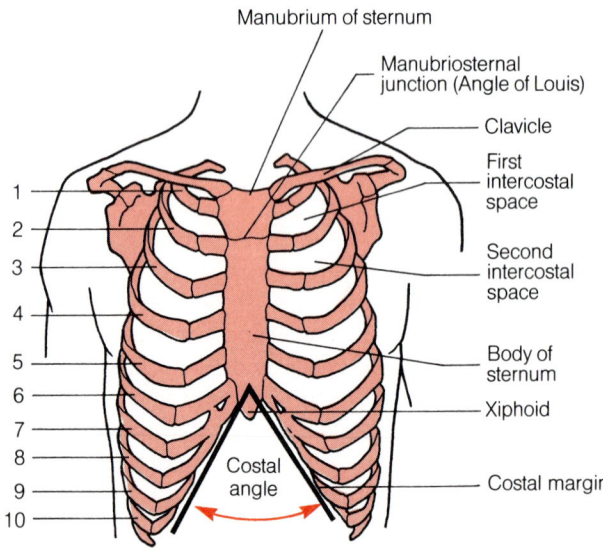

Figure 19–56 Location of the anterior ribs in relation to the angle of Louis and the sternum.

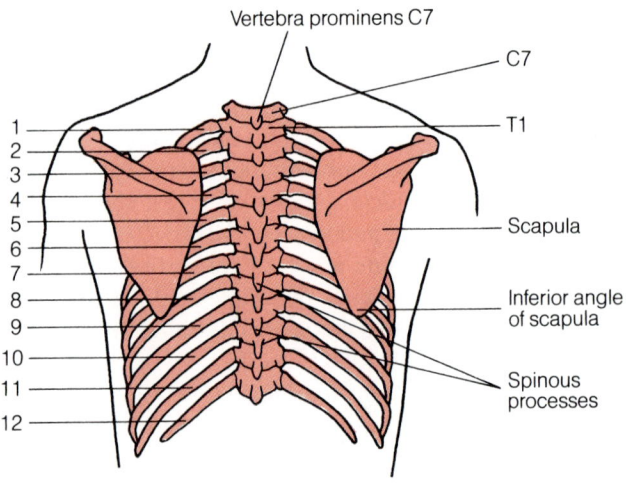

Figure 19–57 Location of the posterior ribs in relation to the spinous processes of the vertebrae.

TABLE 19–12 *Summary Assessment Data: Lungs*

Normal Findings	Abnormal Findings
Respiratory rate 16–20/min and regular (adult)	Increased or decreased rate
	Irregular pattern
	Retraction or bulging of intercostal muscles
Respiratory excursion is full and symmetrical	Impairment in movement
Vocal fremitus is symmetrical bilaterally	Decreased or increased fremitus
Percussion notes resonant except over liver, heart, sternum, scapula, and stomach	Asymmetry in percussion
	Areas of dullness
	Areas of hyperresonance
Auscultated vesicular breath sounds (see Table 19–14)	Auscultated adventitious breath sounds (see Table 19–15):
	Crackles
	Rhonchi
	Wheeze
	Friction rub

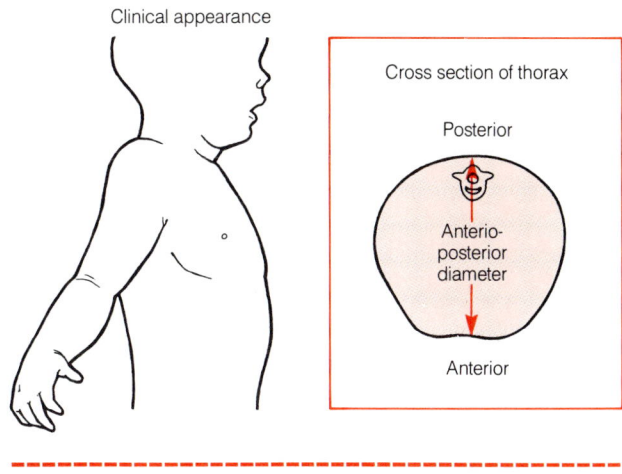

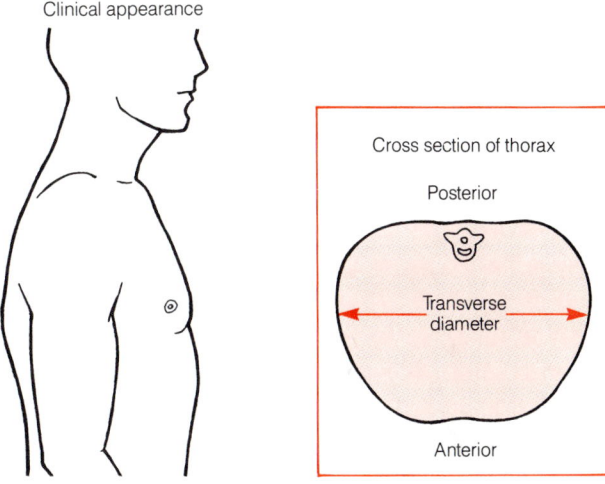

Figure 19–58 Configurations of the thorax showing anteroposterior diameter and transverse diameter: *A*, infant; *B*, adult.

(a) a stethoscope, (b) a marking pencil, and (c) a centimeter ruler. For efficiency, the posterior chest is usually examined first, then the anterior chest. For posterior and lateral chest examinations, the client is uncovered to the waist and in a sitting position. A sitting or lying position may be used for anterior chest examination. Good lighting is essential, especially for chest inspection. See Table 19–12 for normal and abnormal findings.

Posterior Thorax

Inspection   Inspection is performed to assess (a) the pattern of respirations, (b) the skin, and (c) the shape and symmetry of the thorax. Assessment of respirations is discussed in Chapter 18. Assessment of the skin is discussed earlier in this chapter. The nurse first observes the general *shape* of the thorax and its *symmetry*.

In the infant, the thorax is rounded; that is, the diameter from the front to the back (anteroposterior) is equal to the transverse diameter. It is also cylindrical, having a nearly equal diameter at the top and the base. When a child reaches 6 years, the anteroposterior diameter has decreased in proportion to the transverse one. In adults, the thorax is oval. Its anteroposterior diameter is two times smaller than its transverse diameter. See Figure 19–58. The overall shape of the thorax is elliptical; i.e., its diameter is smaller at the top than at the base. In the elderly, kyphosis and osteoporosis alter the size of the chest cavity as the ribs move downward and forward.

The shape of the chest is assessed from the front, sides, and back. There are several deformities of the chest. See Figure 19–59. **Pigeon chest** (pectus carinatum), a permanent deformity, may be caused by rickets. Pigeon chest is characterized by a narrow transverse diameter, an increased anteroposterior diameter, and a protruding sternum. A **funnel chest** (pectus excavatum), a congenital defect, is the opposite of pigeon chest in that the sternum is depressed, narrowing the anteroposterior diameter. Because the sternum points posteriorly in clients with a funnel chest, abnor-

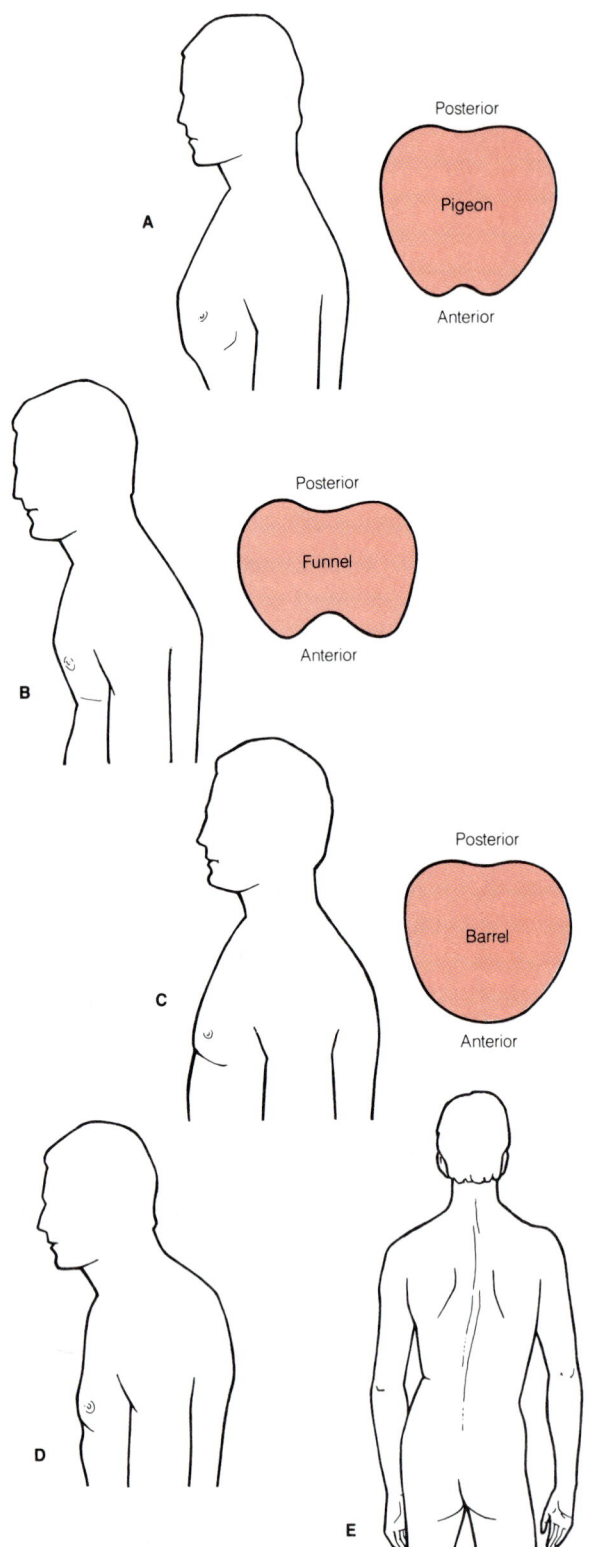

Figure 19–59 Chest deformities: *A,* pigeon chest; *B,* funnel chest; *C,* barrel chest; *D,* kyphosis; *E,* scoliosis.

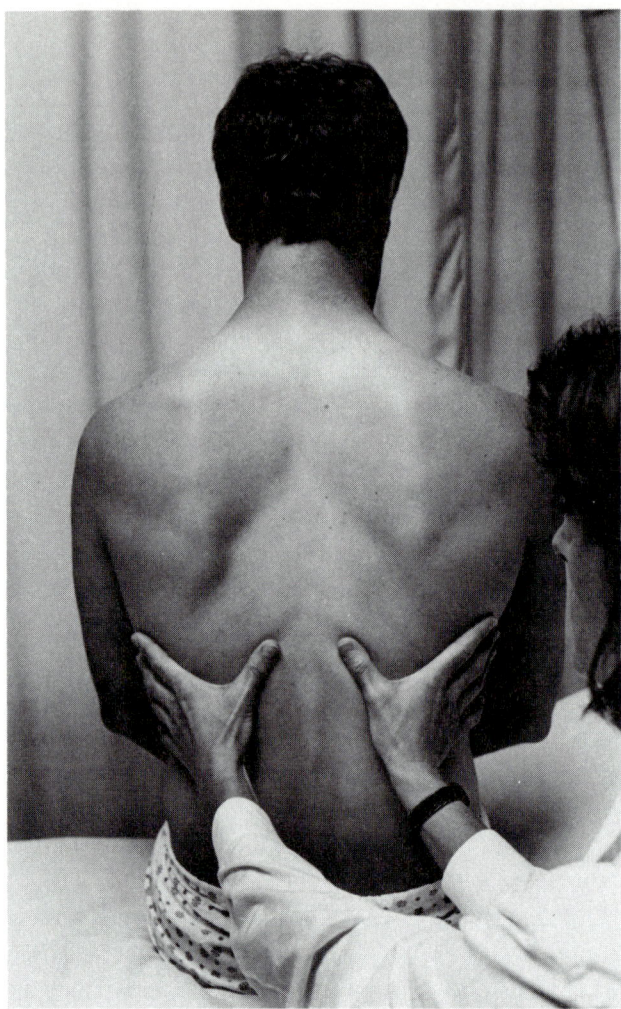

Figure 19–60 Position of the nurse's hands when assessing respiratory excursion on the posterior thorax.

mal pressure on the heart may result in altered function. A **barrel chest,** in which the ratio of the anteroposterior to lateral diameter is 1 to 1, is seen in clients with thoracic **kyphosis** (excessive convex curvature of the thoracic spine) and **emphysema** (chronic pulmonary condition in which the air sacs, or alveoli, are dilated and distended.)

The nurse notes spinal deformities, such as kyphosis or **scoliosis** (lateral deviation of the spine), during examination of the thorax. In addition, the nurse looks for changes in the exterior chest wall, such as intercostal bulges caused by cardiac enlargement, neoplasms, or obstruction to airflow. Depressions in the chest may be the result of the surgical removal of some ribs.

Palpation Palpation involves (a) general palpation, (b) assessment of respiratory excursion, and (c) assessment for vocal (tactile) fremitus. In *general palpation,* the nurse rapidly assesses the temperature, turgor, and integrity of all chest skin for clients who have no respiratory complaints. For clients who do have complaints, all chest areas should be palpated for bulges, tenderness, or abnormal movements. Any lumps or swollen areas noted by inspection should be lightly palpated for size, shape, and tenderness. Deep palpation should be avoided for painful areas, especially if a fractured rib is suspected; in such a case, deep palpation could lead to displacement of the bone fragment against the lungs.

To palpate the posterior chest for **respiratory excursion** (thoracic expansion), the nurse places the palms of both hands over the lower thorax, with the thumbs adjacent to the spine and the fingers stretched laterally. See Figure 19–60. The client is asked to take a deep breath while the nurse observes the movement of the hands and any lag in movement. When the client takes a deep breath, the nurse's thumbs should move apart an equal distance and at the same time, reflecting symmetric chest expansion. Normally, the thumbs are separated 3 to 5 cm (1½ to 2 in) during deep inspiration.

Vocal (tactile) **fremitus** is a faintly perceptible vibration on palpation produced by phonation (e.g., when the client speaks). Vibrations from speaking are normally felt most clearly at the apex of the lungs. Low-pitched voices of males are more readily palpated than the higher pitched voices of females. To assess vocal fremitus, the nurse places the palmar surface of the fingertips or the ulnar aspect of the hand or the ulnar aspect of the closed fist on the posterior chest, starting near the apex of the lungs. See Figure 19–61, *A*. To elicit vocal fremitus, the nurse asks the client to repeat words such as "blue moon," "ninety-nine," or "one-two-three." If fremitus is faint, the client may need to speak in a louder or lower tone of voice.

The nurse assesses and compares both sides of the thorax, moving sequentially to the base of the lungs. See Figure 19–61, *B* through *E*. The nurse compares the fremitus detected on one lung with that detected on the other, and the fremitus detected at the apex of each lung with that detected at the base. Increased fremitus occurs with consolidated lung tissue, as in pneumonia, since vibrations are transmitted more readily through solid matter than through air. Decreased or absent fremitus occurs in pneumothorax. Either one hand or two hands may be used for this exami-

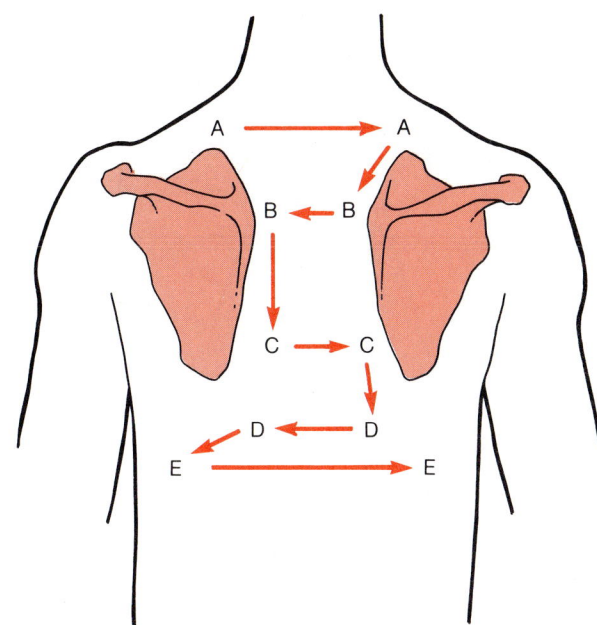

Figure 19–61 Areas and sequence for palpating tactile fremitus on the posterior chest.

nation (Malasanos, Barkauskas, and Stoltenberg-Allen 1990, p. 307). When one hand is used, it should be moved from one side of the chest to the corresponding area on the other side. Some nurses prefer this one-hand method, believing it ensures accuracy. When two hands are used, they should be placed simultaneously on the corresponding areas of each side of the chest.

Percussion   Percussion of the thorax determines (a) whether underlying lung tissue is filled with air, liquid, or solid material and (b) the positions and boundaries of certain organs. Because percussion penetrates to a depth of 5 to 7 cm (2 to 3 in), it detects relatively superficial rather than deep lesions. Chest percussion includes the indirect percussion method described earlier in this chapter and a measurement of diaphragmatic excursion. Percussion sounds and tones are described in Table 19–13.

TABLE 19–13   *Percussion Sounds and Tones*

Sound	Intensity	Pitch	Duration	Quality	Example of Location
Flatness	Soft	High	Short	Extremely dull	Muscle, bone
Dullness	Medium	Medium	Moderate	Thudlike	Liver, heart
Resonance	Loud	Low	Long	Hollow	Lung
Hyperresonance	Very loud	Very low	Very long	Booming	Emphysematous lung
Tympany	Loud	High (distinguished mainly by musical timbre)	Moderate	Musical	Stomach filled with gas (air)

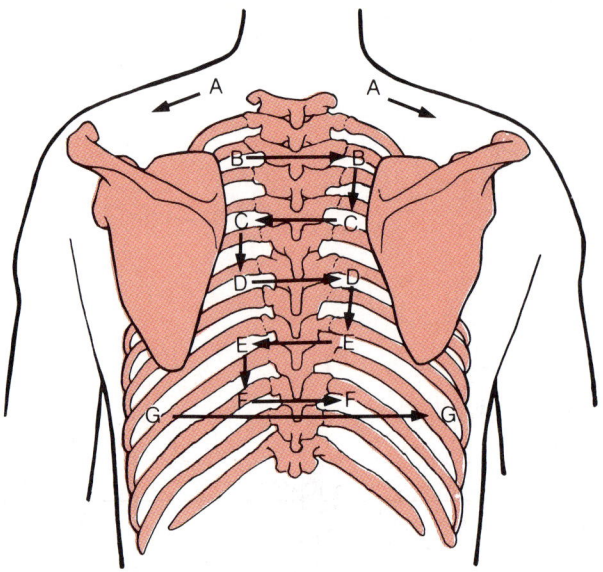

Figure 19–62 Sequence for posterior chest percussion.

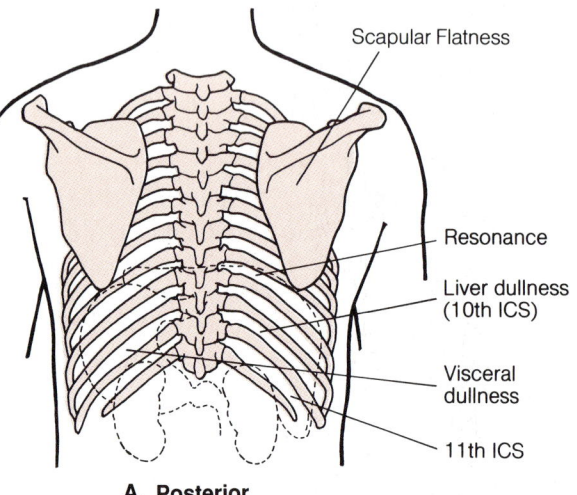

Scapular Flatness

Resonance

Liver dullness
(10th ICS)

Visceral
dullness

11th ICS

A. Posterior

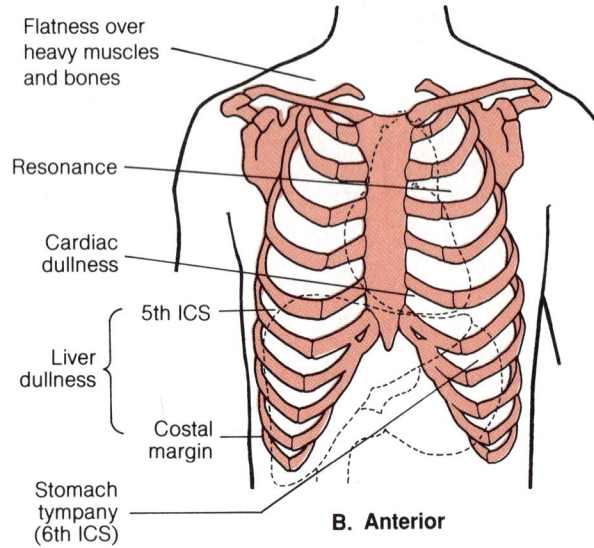

Flatness over
heavy muscles
and bones

Resonance

Cardiac
dullness

5th ICS

Liver
dullness

Costal
margin

Stomach
tympany
(6th ICS)

B. Anterior

Figure 19–63 Normal percussion sounds: *A*, posterior;
B, anterior.

To percuss the posterior thorax, the nurse asks the client to bend the head and fold the arms forward across the chest. This position separates the scapulae and exposes more lung tissue to percussion. The nurse percusses in the intercostal spaces at about 5-cm (2-in) intervals in a systematic sequence, starting at the apex of each lung and proceeding downward to the diaphragm. See Figure 19–62. One side of the lung is compared with the other. Normal percussion sounds are shown in Figure 19–63. The major percussion sound heard over the posterior thorax is resonance. The lowest point where resonance can be detected is at the diaphragm, i.e., at the level of the eighth to tenth rib posteriorly. Over bony areas or any solid area, the sound is flat; over organs the sound is normally dull. Areas of flatness or dullness over lung tissue indicate consolidation of lung tissue or a mass.

The *lateral* thorax is also percussed every few inches, starting at the axilla and working down to the eighth rib. Findings on each side are compared.

Diaphragmatic excursion (movement of the diaphragm during a maximal inspiration and expiration) is measured only on the posterior thorax. To determine diaphragmatic excursion, the nurse asks the client to take a deep breath and to hold it while the nurse percusses downward along the scapular line until dullness is produced. The percussion sounds change from resonance to dullness; dullness indicates the level of the diaphragm. With a marking pencil, the nurse places a mark on the skin on the scapular line at this level of dullness. The procedure is repeated on the other side of the chest. The client takes a few normal respirations, then expels the breath completely and holds it while the nurse percusses upward from the marked point to assess and mark the diaphragmatic excursion during deep expiration on each side. The distance between these two marks is then measured. Normal excursion is 3 to 5 cm (1 to 2 in) bilaterally in females and 5 to 6 cm (2 to 2.3 in) in males. The diaphragm is usually slightly higher on the right side.

Auscultation   The process of auscultation includes assessment of (a) breath sounds that occur as a result of the movement of air through the trachea, bronchi, and alveoli and (b) the sounds produced by the spoken voice. To auscultate the lungs, use the flat-disc diaphragm of the stethoscope, which best transmits high-pitched breath sounds in the adult. The bell-shaped disc, however, is often preferred for children because of their smaller chests. The systematic zigzag procedure used in percussion is also used for auscultating the posterior chest (see Figure 19–62). The client takes slow, deep breaths through the mouth while the nurse listens at each point to the breath sounds during a complete inspiration and expiration. Findings at each point are compared with the corresponding point on the opposite side of the chest. Sounds normally heard over the posterior thorax include vesicular and bronchovesicular sounds. Table 19–14.

Selected Skin Lesions

Nurses are responsible for describing skin lesions accurately, as shown below. Medical diagnoses are given in parentheses. See also Table 19–7 on page 371.

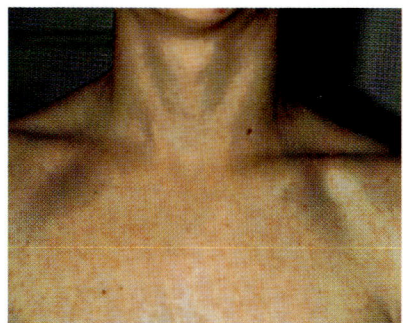

Diffuse discreet erythematous macules (rubella)

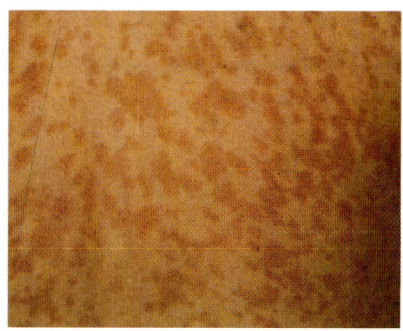

Diffuse varying-sized, confluent maculo-papular lesions (rubeola)

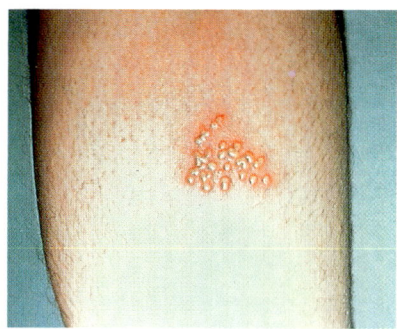

Clustered vesicles on an erythematous base (herpes simplex)

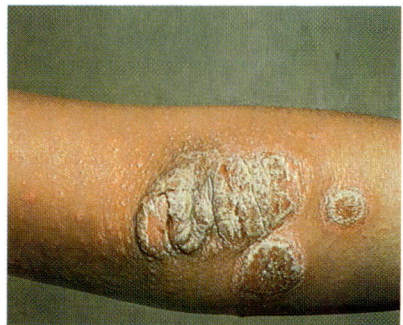

Grouped thick, silvery, scaly plaques (psoriasis)

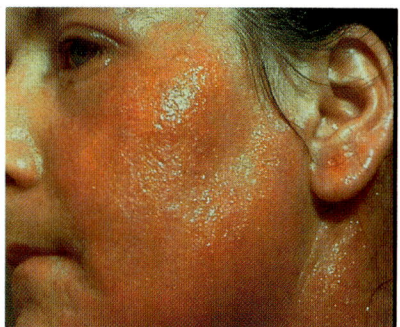

Diffuse edematous, bright erythema (contact dermatitis)

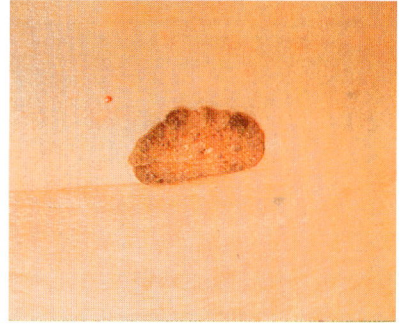

Circumscribed, oval, mottled, brown, slightly elevated lesion (sebborheic keratosis)

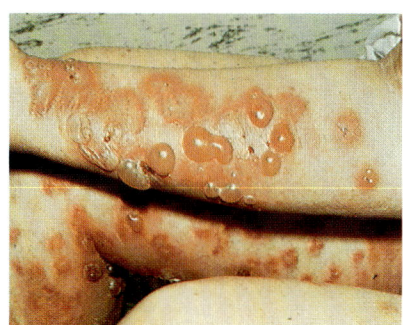

Grouped giant blisters on non-erythematous base (bullous pemphigoid)

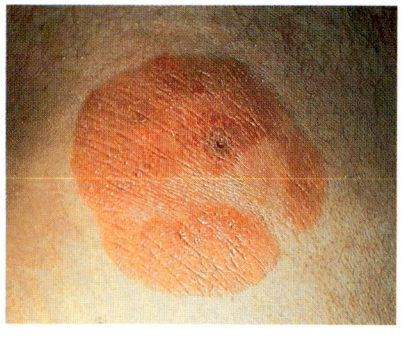

Coin-like, circumscribed, slightly elevated erythematous lesion (mycosis fungoides)

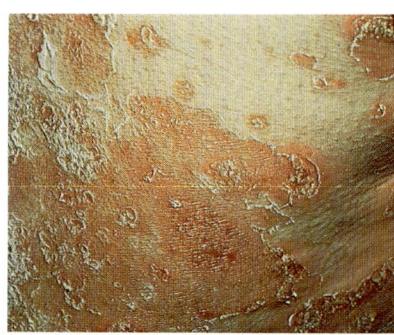

Irregular, varying-sized, pale erythematous patches with superficial fine scaling (pemphigus foliaceus)

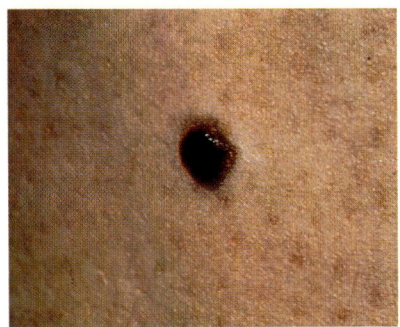

Solitary, deep brown, one-half inch nodule exhibiting a pale halo (malignant melanoma)

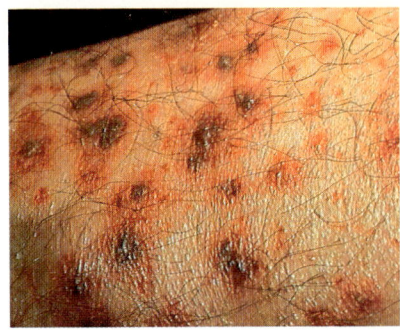

Purple discoloration with petechiae and ecchymoses (Henoch-Schönlein purpura)

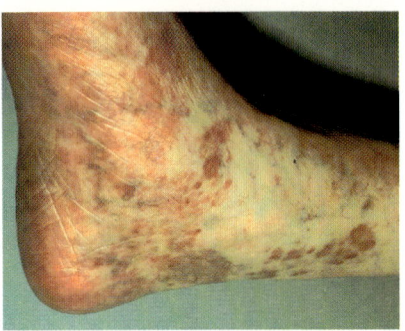

Extensive erythematous patches with small hemorrhagic nodules (Kaposi's sarcoma)

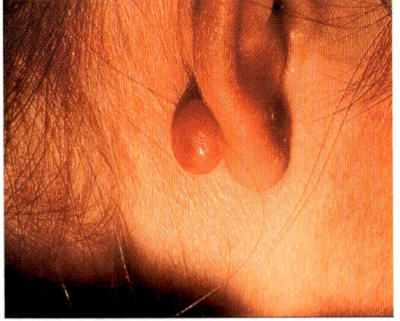

Solitary circumscribed, smooth, lentil-like papilloma (keloid)

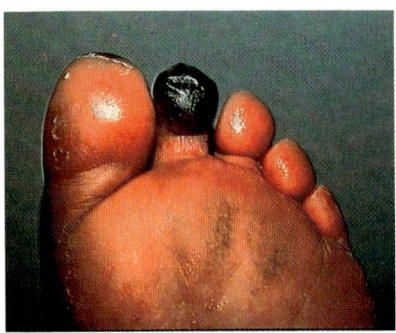

Distal half of toe exhibiting gangrene

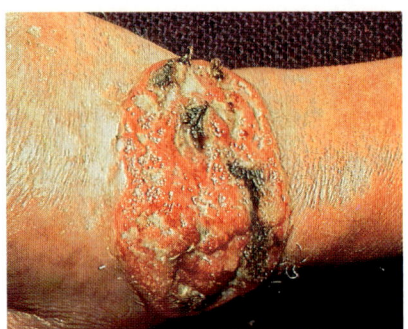

Fungating, ulcerating tumor exhibiting suppuration and necrosis (squamous cell carcinoma)

Decubitus Ulcers

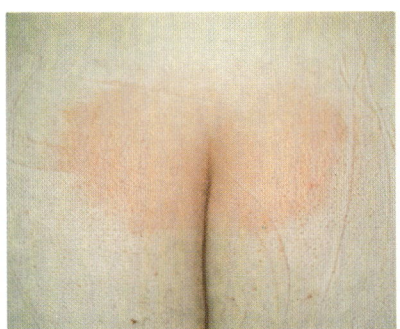

Stage I   Non-blanchable erythema signalling potential ulceration

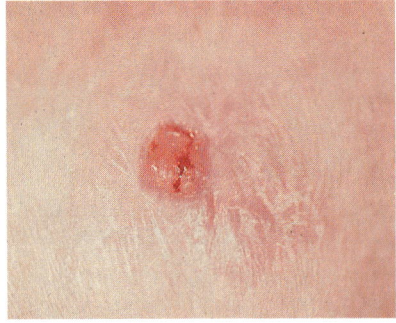

Stage II   Abrasion, blister, or shallow crater involving the epidermis and possibly the dermis

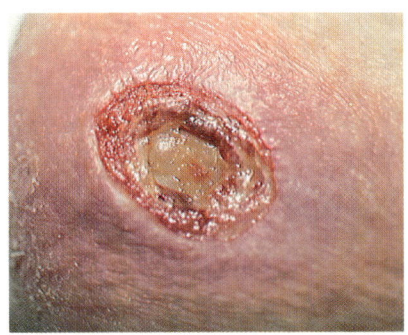

Stage III   Deep ulcer exhibiting necrotic tissue and extending through the subcutaneous layer

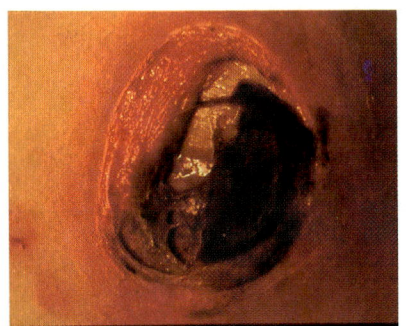

Stage IV   Tissue necrosis and damage involving muscle, bone, or supporting structures

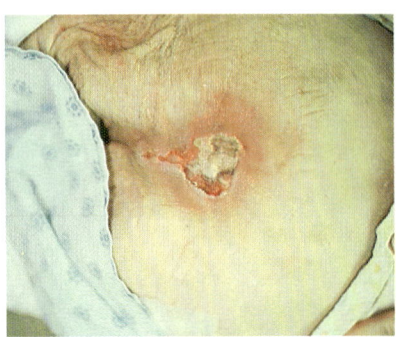

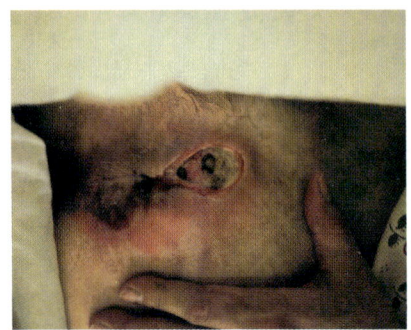

Kennedy terminal ulcer   A large, pear-shaped coccygeal or sacral ulcer of sudden onset. Exhibits red, yellow, and black colors and indicates imminent death (Kennedy 1989, First National Pressure Ulcer Advisory Panel, Washington, D.C.)

TABLE 19–14 *Normal Breath Sounds*

Type	Description	Location	Characteristics
Vesicular	Soft-intensity, low-pitched, "gentle sighing" sounds created by air moving through smaller airways (bronchioles and alveoli)	Over peripheral lung; best heard at base of lungs	Best heard on inspiration, which is about 2.5 times longer than the expiratory phase (5:2 ratio)
Bronchovesicular	Moderate-intensity and moderate-pitched "blowing" sounds created by air moving through larger airways (bronchi)	Between the scapulae and lateral to the sternum at the first and second intercostal spaces	Equal inspiratory and expiratory phases (1:1 ratio)
Bronchial (tubular)	High-pitched, loud, "harsh" sounds created by air moving through the trachea	Anteriorly over the trachea; not normally heard over lung tissue	Louder than vesicular sounds; have a short inspiratory phase and long expiratory phase (1:2 ratio)

Abnormal or adventitious breath sounds occur when air passes through narrowed airways or airways filled with fluid or mucus, or when pleural linings are inflamed. They are often superimposed over normal sounds. The four types of adventitious sounds—crackles (previously referred to as rales or **crepitations**), rhonchi, wheeze, and pleural friction rub—are described in Table 19–15. Absence of breath sounds over some lung areas is also a significant finding that is associated with collapsed and surgically removed lung lobes.

When abnormalities are found in inspection, palpation, percussion, or auscultation, the nurse may perform other auscultatory techniques for voice sounds or **vocal resonance** (transmitted voice sounds heard by stethoscope on the chest wall). In normal vocal resonance, voice sounds are nondistinct and muffled. An increase in the loudness

TABLE 19–15 *Adventitious Breath Sounds*

Name	Description	Cause	Location
Crackles (rales)	Fine, short, interrupted crackling sounds; alveolar rales are high-pitched; bronchial rales are lower-pitched. Sound can be simulated by rolling a lock of hair near the ear. Best heard on inspiration but can be heard on both inspiration and expiration. May not be cleared by coughing.	Air passing through fluid or mucus in any air passage.	Most commonly heard in the bases of the lower lung lobes.
Rhonchi	Continuous, low-pitched, coarse, gurgling, harsh, louder sounds with a moaning or snoring quality. Best heard on expiration but can be heard on both inspiration and expiration. May be altered by coughing.	Air passing through narrowed air passages as a result of secretions, swelling, tumors.	Loud sounds can be heard over most lung areas but predominate over the trachea and bronchi.
Wheeze	Continuous, high-pitched, squeaky musical sounds. Best heard on expiration. Not usually altered by coughing.	Air passing through constricted bronchi as a result of secretions, swelling, tumors.	Heard over all lung fields.
Friction rub	Superficial grating or creaking sounds heard during inspiration and expiration. Not relieved by coughing.	Rubbing together of inflamed pleural surfaces.	Heard most often in areas of greatest thoracic expansion (e.g., lower anterior and lateral chest).

and clarity of vocal resonance is called **bronchophony.** It may be present in any condition that causes consolidation of lung tissue. Two techniques performed when resonance is increased are whispered pectoriloquy and egophony. To detect *whispered pectoriloquy,* the nurse asks the client to whisper a series of words such as "one, two, three" while the nurse listens to the chest using the sequence described for assessing vocal fremitus. See Figure 19–61, earlier. To detect *egophony,* the nurse listens to the client's chest while the client repeats the sound of a long *e,* as in "she" or "e-e-e." Fluid in the lungs alters the sound from "ee" to an "ay," as in "say," when heard through the stethoscope. Change is often very subtle and may be detected only by the experienced nurse.

Anterior Thorax

The anterior thorax is examined in the same manner as the posterior thorax; however, the client may be positioned in either a supine or sitting position. The sitting position is preferred because it maximizes chest expansion.

Inspection   Breathing patterns such as respiratory rate and rhythm are usually assessed on the anterior chest. Abnormal breathing patterns, audible breath sounds, and abnormal chest movements indicating use of accessory muscles to breathe are detailed in Chapter 41, page 1098. In clients with obstructive lung disease, the **costal angle** (angle formed by the intersection of the costal margins) and the angle at which the ribs enter the spine are widened. Normally, the costal angle is less than 90°, and the ribs are inserted into the spine at approximately a 45° angle. See Figure 19–56, earlier.

Palpation   Palpation of the anterior chest also includes general palpation, measurement of diaphragmatic excursion, and assessment for tactile (vocal) fremitus. To palpate the anterior chest for *respiratory excursion,* the nurse places the palms of both hands on the lower thorax, with the fingers laterally along the lower rib cage and the thumbs along the costal margins. See Figure 19–64. When the client inhales, the thumbs normally separate 3 to 5 cm (1½ to 2 in), as in the posterior assessment.

Assessment of *tactile fremitus* is done in the same manner as for the posterior chest. The nurse assesses both sides of

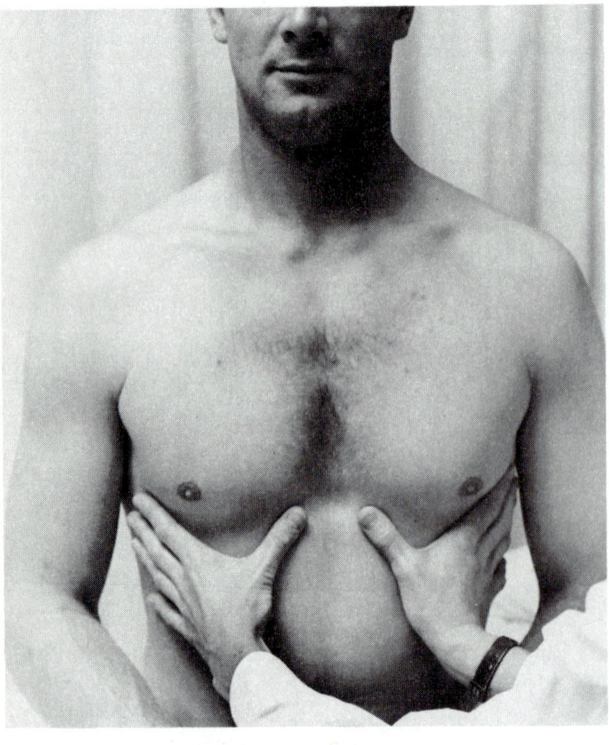

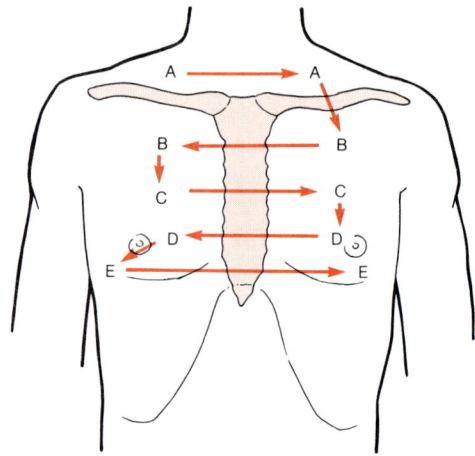

Figure 19–65   Areas and sequence for palpating tactile fremitus on the anterior chest.

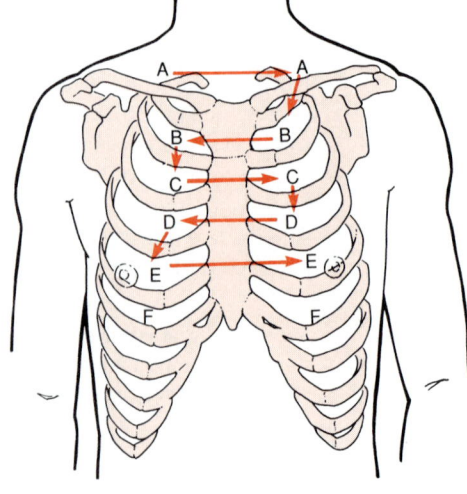

Figure 19–66   Sequence for anterior chest percussion.

Figure 19–64   Position of nurse's hands when assessing respiratory excursion on the anterior thorax.

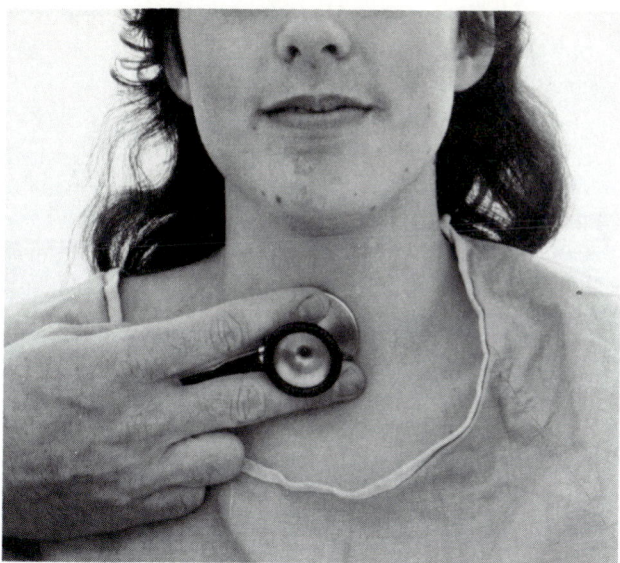

Figure 19–67 Auscultating the trachea.

the chest, moving sequentially to the base of the lungs, through positions *A* to *E* in Figure 19–65. Fremitus is normally decreased over the heart and breast tissue. If the breasts are large and cannot be retracted adequately for palpation, this part of the examination is usually omitted.

Percussion Systematic percussion of the anterior chest begins above the clavicles in the supraclavicular space and proceeds downward to the diaphragm. See Figure 19–66. Again, one side of the lung is compared with the other. The client may be positioned in either a supine or sitting position, but percussion is easier for the nurse if the client is supine. Female breasts may need to be displaced for proper examination. As in the posterior chest, the major percussion sound is normally resonance, down to the sixth rib anteriorly at the level of the diaphragm. However, flatness can be expected on areas over heavy muscle and bone, dullness on areas over the heart and liver, and tympany over the underlying stomach. See Figure 19–63, *B* earlier. See also Table 19–13 on page 401 for a description of percussion sounds and tones.

Auscultation Auscultation of the anterior chest starts over the trachea (see Figure 19–67), where bronchial or tubular breath sounds (described in Table 19–14) are heard. These sounds heard elsewhere are abnormal. Auscultation then proceeds in the sequence used for anterior chest percussion (see Figure 19–66), beginning over the bronchi between the sternum and the clavicles. In these areas, the normal bronchovesicular and vesicular sounds are heard. Any adventitious sounds (described in Table 19–15) must be identified.

Changes in the thorax and breathing patterns of elderly people are shown in the accompanying box.

The Elderly: Physical Changes of the Thorax and Breathing Patterns

- The thoracic curvature may be accentuated (kyphosis) because of osteoporosis and changes in cartilage, resulting in collapse of the verbebrae.

- The anteroposterior diameter of the chest widens, giving the person a barrel-chested appearance. This is due to loss of skeletal muscle strength in the thorax and diaphragm and constant lung inflation from excessive expiratory pressure on the alveoli.

- Breathing rate and rhythm are unchanged at rest; the rate normally increases with exercise but may take longer to return to the preexercise rate.

- Inspiratory muscles become less powerful, and the inspiration reserve volume is decreased. A decrease in depth of respiration is therefore apparent.

- Expiration may require the use of accessory muscles, and the expiratory reserve volume is significantly increased because of the increased amount of air remaining in the lungs at the end of a normal breath.

- Deflation of the lung is incomplete.

- Small airways lose their cartilaginous support and elastic recoil; as a result, they tend to close, particularly in basal or dependent portions of the lung.

- Elastic tissue of the alveoli loses its stretchability and changes to fibrous tissue. This thicker alveolar membrane decreases the pulmonary diffusion capacity. As a result, arterial oxyhemoglobin saturation and PaO_2 are slightly lower than those of young adults. Exertional capacity is also decreased.

- Cilia in the airways decrease in number and are less effective in removing mucus; elderly clients are therefore at greater risk for pulmonary infections.

CARDIOVASCULAR SYSTEM

Heart

Heart function can be assessed to a large degree by findings in the history, by symptoms such as shortness of breath, by the client's general appearance (e.g., cyanosis and edema of the legs suggest impaired function), and by pulse rate, rhythm, and quality. Direct examination of the heart, however, offers more specific information, including the heart sounds, the heart size, and findings such as lifts, heaves, or **murmurs** (more prolonged sounds during systole and diastole). Nurses assess heart functions through observations (inspection), palpation, and auscultation, in that

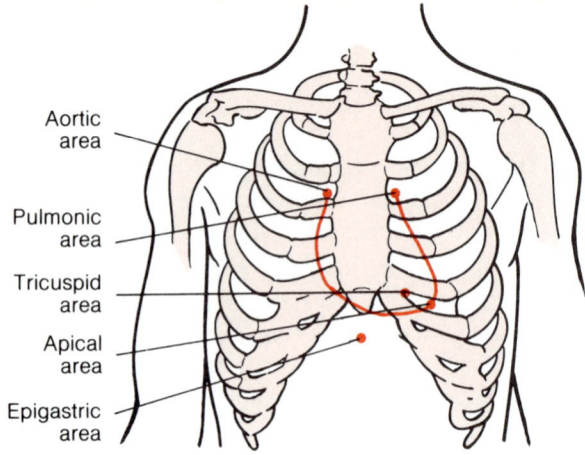

Aortic
area

Pulmonic
area

Tricuspid
area

Apical
area

Epigastric
area

Figure 19–68 Anatomic sites of the precordium.

sequence. Auscultation is more meaningful when other data are obtained first. The heart is usually assessed during an initial physical assessment; periodic reassessments may be necessary for long-term or at-risk clients or those with cardiac problems. Heart examinations are usually performed while the client is in a semi-reclined position. The practitioner stands at the client's right side.

To assess the client's heart, the nurse must first determine its exact location. In the average adult, most of the heart lies behind and to the left of the sternum. A small portion (the right atrium) extends to the right of the sternum. The upper portion of the heart (both atria), referred to as its **base,** lies toward the back. The lower portion (the ventricles), referred to as its **apex,** points forward. The apex of the left ventricle actually touches the anterior chest wall at or medial to the left midclavicular line (MCL) and at or near the fifth left intercostal space (LICS), which is slightly below the left nipple. See Figure 18–12 on page 336. This point where the apex touches the anterior chest wall is known as the **point of maximal impulse (PMI).**

Inspection and Palpation   The **precordium,** the area of the chest overlying the heart, is inspected and palpated simultaneously for the presence of abnormal pulsations or lifts or heaves. The terms *lift* and *heave,* often used interchangeably, refer to a rising along the sternal border with each heartbeat. A lift occurs when cardiac action is very forceful (overactive). It should be confirmed by palpation with the palm of the hand. Enlargement or overactivity of the left ventricle produces a heave lateral to the apex, while enlargement of the right ventricle produces a heave at or near the sternum. The precordium is inspected in a systematic manner at the following anatomic sites: *aortic* area, *pulmonic* area, *tricuspid* (or right ventricular) area, *apical* (or mitral) area, and *epigastric* area. See Figure 19–68. All pulsations are described by their location in an intercostal space and their distance from the midsternal, midclavicular, or axillary line. See the accompanying box for cardiac inspection and palpation.

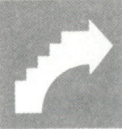

CLINICAL GUIDELINES
Cardiac Inspection and Palpation

■ Assist the client to a supine position with head elevated 30° to 45°, and stand at the client's right side. This position facilitates palpation of the cardiac area and allows for optimal inspection.

■ Locate the angle of Louis, the palpable ridge between the manubrium and the body of the sternum. It is felt as a prominence on the sternum.

■ Move your fingertips down each side of the angle until you can feel the second intercostal spaces. The client's *right* second intercostal space is the aortic area, and the *left* second intercostal space is the pulmonic area.

■ Inspect and palpate the aortic and pulmonic areas, observing them at an angle and to the side, to note the presence or absence of pulsations. Observing these areas at an angle increases the likelihood of seeing pulsations. Normally, these areas do not have pulsations, although some individuals may have aortic pulsations.

■ From the pulmonic area, move your fingertips down three left intercostal spaces along the side of the sternum. The left fifth intercostal space close to the sternum is the tricuspid or right ventricular area. Inspect and palpate the tricuspid area for pulsations and heaves or lifts. Normally pulsations, lifts, and heaves are absent.

■ From the tricuspid area, move your fingertips laterally 5 to 7 cm (2 to 3 in) to the left midclavicular line (LMCL). This is the apical or mitral area, or PMI.

■ Inspect and palpate the apical area for pulsation, noting its specific location (it may be displaced laterally or lower) and diameter.

■ Inspect and palpate the epigastric area at the base of the sternum for abdominal aortic pulsations. Pulsations are normally felt in this area; however, bounding pulsations are abnormal.

An apical impulse can be seen in about 50% of the adult population and is palpable in most people. The apical impulse is a good index of cardiac size. If the heart is enlarged, this impulse is lateral to the MCL and may be lower. Record the distance between the apex and the MCL in centimeters. If the apical beat cannot be observed, the apex may be located by palpation, but not always. If the nurse has difficulty locating the PMI, the client rolls onto the left side, thus moving the apex closer to the chest wall. Normally, no lifts or heaves are visible or palpable in this area. Diffuse lifts or heaves lateral to the apex indicate enlargement or overactivity of the left ventricle. Abdominal aortic pulsations are normally felt in the epigastric area; however, bounding pulsations are abnormal.

Auscultation   Several heart sounds can be heard by *auscultation*. Only the first and second heart sounds (S₁ and S₂) will be emphasized in this book. The normal first two heart sounds are produced by closure of the valves of the heart. The *first heart sound (S_1)* occurs when the atrioventricular (A-V) valves close. These valves close when the ventricles have been sufficiently filled. Although the right and left A-V valves do not close simultaneously, the closures occur closely enough to be heard as one sound (S₁), a dull, low-pitched sound described as "lub." After the ventricles empty their blood into the aorta and pulmonary arteries, the semilunar valves close, producing the *second heart sound (S_2),* described as "dub." S₂ has a higher pitch than S₁ and is also shorter. These two sounds, S₁ and S₂ ("lub-dub"), occur within 1 second or less, depending on the heart rate.

Auscultation is performed systematically, starting at the aortic area, then moving to the pulmonic, the tricuspid, and the apical. See Figure 19–68, earlier. Auscultation need not be limited to these areas, however. First locate these areas, and then move the stethoscope to find the most audible sounds for each particular client. The two heart sounds are audible anywhere on the precordial area, but they are best heard over these areas. Each area is associated with the closure of heart valves: the aortic area with the aortic valve (inside the aorta as it arises from the left ventricle); the pulmonic area with the pulmonic valve (inside the pulmonary artery as it arises from the right ventricle); the tricuspid area with the tricuspid valve (between the right atrium and ventricle); and the apical (mitral) area with the mitral valve (between the left atrium and ventricle).

Associated with these sounds are systole and diastole. **Systole** is the period in which the ventricles are contracted. It begins with the first heart sound and ends at the second heart sound. Systole is normally shorter than diastole. **Diastole** is the period in which the ventricles are relaxed.

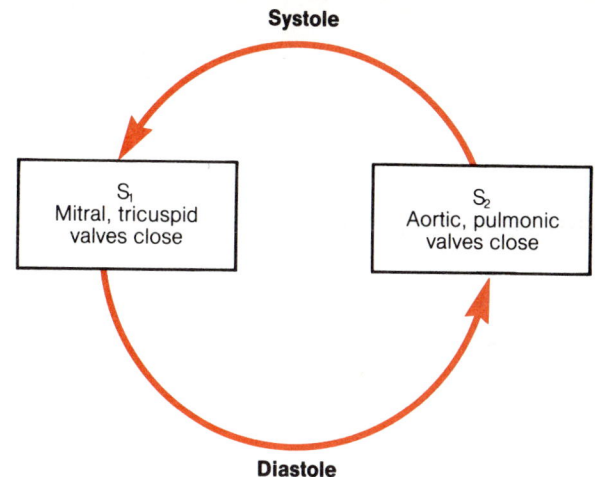

Figure 19–69   Relationship of heart sounds to systole and diastole.

It starts with the second sound and ends at the subsequent first sound. Normally no sounds are audible during these periods. See Figure 19–69. The experienced nurse, however, may perceive extra heart sounds (S₃ and S₄) during diastole. Both sounds are low in pitch and heard best at the apical site, with the bell of the stethoscope, and with the client lying on the left side. S₃ occurs early in diastole right after S₂ and sounds like "lub-dub-*ee*" (S₁, S₂, S₃) or "Ken-tuc-*ky*." It often disappears when the client sits up. S₃ is normal in children and young adults. In older adults it may indicate heart failure. S₄ is rarely heard in normal clients. It occurs near the very end of diastole just before S₁ and creates the sound of "*dee*-lub-dub" (S₄, S₁, S₂) or "*Ten*-nes-see." S₄ may be heard in many elderly clients and can be a sign of hypertension.

Normal heart sounds are summarized in Table 19–16. See Procedure 19–3 for the steps of heart auscultation and Table

---

TABLE 19–16   *Normal Heart Sounds*

Sound or Phase	Description	Area			
		Aortic	Pulmonic	Tricuspid	Apical
S₁	Dull, low-pitched, and longer than S₂; sounds like "lub"	Less intensity than S₂	Less intensity than S₂	Louder than or equal to S₂	Louder than or equal to S₂
S₂	High-pitched, snappy, and shorter than S₁; creates sound of "dub"	Louder than S₁	Louder than S₁; abnormal if louder than the aortic S₂ in adults over 40	Less intensity than or equal to S₁	Less intensity than or equal to S₁
Systole	Normally silent interval between S₁ and S₂				
Diastole	Normally silent interval between S₂ and next S₁				

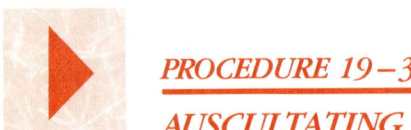

PROCEDURE 19–3

AUSCULTATING THE HEART

Equipment ☑

Stethoscope equipped with a bell diaphragm (for hearing low-pitched sounds) and a flat-disc diaphragm (for hearing high-pitched sounds)

Intervention

1. Prepare the environment and the client.

■ Eliminate all sources of room noise. *Heart sounds are of low intensity,*

and other noise hinders the nurse's ability to hear them.

■ Assist the client to a supine position with head elevated 30° to 45°, and stand at the client's right side. Later, reexamine the heart while the client is in the upright sitting position. *Certain sounds are more audible in certain positions.*

2. Auscultate the heart in all four anatomic sites: aortic, pulmonic, tricuspid, and apical (mitral).

■ Use both the flat-disc diaphragm and the bell to listen to all areas.

■ In every area of auscultation, distinguish both S_1 and S_2 sounds.

■ When auscultating, concentrate on one particular sound at a time in each area: the first heart sound, followed by systole, then the second heart sound, then diastole. Systole and diastole are normally silent intervals.

19–17 for a review of normal and abnormal findings. Physical changes in the heart of the elderly person are shown in the box on the next page.

Peripheral Vascular System

Assessment of the peripheral vascular system includes measurement of the blood pressure; palpation of peripheral pulses; inspection, palpation, and auscultation of the

carotid pulse; inspection of the jugular and peripheral veins; and inspection of the skin and tissues to determine perfusion to the extremities. Certain aspects of peripheral vascular assessment are often incorporated into other parts of the assessment procedure. For example, blood pressure is usually measured at the beginning of the physical examination (see the section on assessing blood pressure in Chapter 18).

Pulse sites and pulse assessments are described in Chap-

TABLE 19–17 *Summary Assessment Data: Heart Auscultation*

Auscultation sound	Normal Findings	Abnormal Findings	Possible Health Problem
S_1	Usually heard at all sites	Increased or decreased intensity	
	Usually louder at apical area	Varying intensity with different beats	Complete heart block
S_2	Usually heard at all sites	Increased intensity at aortic area	Arterial hypertension
	Usually louder at base of heart	Increased intensity at pulmonic area	Pulmonary hypertension
Systole	Silent interval	Sharp-sounding ejection clicks	Valvular deformities
	Slightly shorter duration than diastole at normal heart rate (60 to 90 beats/min)		
Diastole	Silent interval	S_3 in older adults	Heart failure
	Slightly longer duration than systole at normal heart rates		
	S_3 in children and young adults		
	S_4 in older adults		

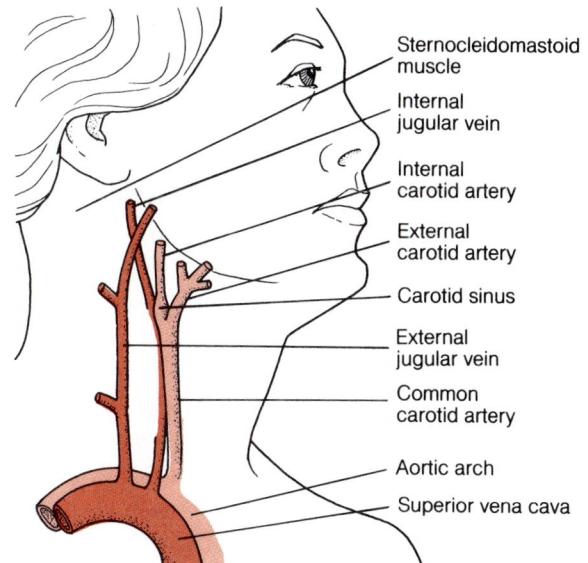

Figure 19–70 Arteries and veins of the right side of the neck.

ter 18. Figures 18–11 and 18–14 illustrate the sites for palpating the peripheral pulses. To assess the client's peripheral pulses:

1. Palpate the peripheral pulses (except the carotid pulse) on both sides of the client's body simultaneously and systematically to determine the symmetry of pulse volume; inequality may indicate arterial disease.
2. If you have difficulty palpating some peripheral pulses, use a Doppler ultrasound probe.

Note whether each pulse volume is absent; weak, thready, or decreased; normal; or increased and bounding. Normal findings are symmetric pulse volumes and easily palpable full pulsations. A scale for measuring pulse volumes is shown in Chapter 18, page 337. Asymmetric volumes indicate impaired circulation; absent pulsations indicate arterial spasm or occlusion. Decreased, weak, thready pulsations indicate impaired cardiac output, and increased pulse volumes may indicate hypertension, high cardiac output, or circulatory overload.

Carotid Arteries   The *carotid arteries* supply oxygenated blood to the head and neck. See Figure 19–70. Since they are the only source of blood to the brain, prolonged occlusion of one of these arteries can result in serious brain damage. The carotid pulses correlate with central aortic pressure, thus reflecting cardiac function better than the peripheral pulses. When cardiac output is diminished, the peripheral pulses may be difficult or impossible to feel, but the carotid pulse should be felt easily.

With the client in a sitting position, inspect the carotid arteries for obvious pulsations; sometimes a wave can be seen. *Extreme caution is required when palpating the carotid artery.* Only one carotid artery is palpated at a time to ensure adequate cerebral blood flow through the other and thus prevent possible cerebral ischemia. The nurse avoids exerting too much pressure and massaging the area, since pressure can occlude the artery and carotid sinus massage can

precipitate bradycardia. The *carotid sinus* is a small dilation at the beginning of the internal carotid artery just above the bifurcation of the common carotid artery, in the upper third of the neck.

Normally, carotid pulse volumes are symmetric, full, and thrusting. The thrusting quality remains the same when the client inhales or exhales, turns the head, and changes from a sitting to a supine position. The arterial wall normally feels elastic. Asymmetric volumes or decreased pulsations may indicate carotid artery stenosis or thrombosis, or inadequate left cardiac output. Thickened, hard, rigid, beaded, inelastic walls are indicative of arteriosclerosis. Normally the arterial wall is smooth and elastic.

To auscultate the carotid artery, turn the client's head slightly away from the side being examined to facilitate placement of the stethoscope. Auscultate the carotid artery on one side and then the other. Listen for the presence of a bruit (a blowing or swishing sound) created by turbulence of blood flow due either to a narrowed arterial lumen (a common development in older people) or to a condition, such as anemia or hyperthyroidism, that elevates cardiac output. Normally no sound is heard by auscultation. If a bruit is heard, gentle palpation of the artery is indicated to determine the presence of a thrill, which frequently accompanies a bruit. A **thrill** is a vibrating sensation like the purring of a cat or water running through a hose. It, too, indicates turbulent blood flow due to arterial obstruction.

Jugular Veins   The *jugular veins* drain blood from the head and neck directly into the superior vena cava and right side of the heart. See Figure 19–70. The external jugular veins are superficial and may be visible above the clavicle. The internal jugular veins lie deeper along the carotid artery and may transmit pulsations onto the skin of the neck. Normally, external neck veins are distended and visible when a person lies down; they are flat and not as visible when a person stands up, since gravity encourages venous drainage. By inspecting the jugular veins for pulsations and distention, the nurse can assess the adequacy of function of the right side of the heart and venous pressure. Bilateral jugular vein distention (JVD) may indicate right-sided heart failure. Unilateral distention may be caused by local obstruction.

To assess the jugular veins:

1. Remove clothing around the client's neck and thorax, and assist the client to semi-Fowler's position with the head supported on a small pillow. Clothing is removed to prevent constriction. Semi-Fowler's position is used, since at a 30° to 45° angle, neck veins should not be prominent if the right side of the client's heart is functioning normally. Veins may be visibly distended in clients with advanced cardiopulmonary disease. A small pillow aligns the head sufficiently to prevent neck hyperextension; a large pillow would create neck flexion.

2. If jugular distention is present, assess the jugular venous pressure (JVP) as follows:
   a. Locate the highest visible point of distention of the internal jugular vein. Although either the internal or the external jugular vein can be used, the internal jugular vein is more reliable. The external jugular vein is more easily affected by obstruction or kinking at the base of the neck.
   b. Measure the vertical height of this point in centimeters from the sternal angle (the point at which the clavicles meet). See Figure 19–71.
   c. Repeat steps a–b on the other side. Bilateral measurements above 3 cm are considered elevated and may indicate right-sided heart failure. Unilateral distention may be caused by local obstruction.

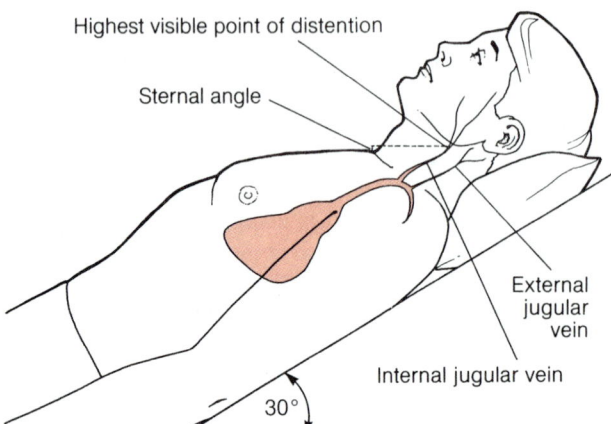

Figure 19–71 Assessing the highest point of distention of the internal jugular vein.

d. Note whether other veins in the neck, shoulder, and upper chest are distended.

Peripheral veins in the arms and legs are inspected for the presence and/or appearance of superficial veins when limbs are dependent and when limbs are elevated. When the limb is dependent, distention and nodular bulges in the calf veins are common, especially in older people. Distended veins in the anteromedial part of the thigh and/or lower leg or in the posterolateral part of the calf from the knee to the ankle are abnormal. When the legs are elevated, the veins normally collapse.

The nurse also assesses the peripheral leg veins for signs of phlebitis by inspecting the calves for redness and swelling over vein sites and palpating the calves for firmness or tension of the muscles, the presence of edema over the dorsum of the foot, and areas of localized warmth. Palpation augments inspection findings, particularly when the client is highly pigmented and redness may not be visible. Next, gently push the client's calves from side to side to test for tenderness and firmly dorsiflex the client's foot while supporting the entire leg in extension or have the person stand or walk. If forceful dorsiflexion of the foot produces pain in the calf muscles (positive **Homans's sign**), a deep phlebitis of the leg may be present.

Peripheral Perfusion   Peripheral or **tissue perfusion** is blood flow to the tissues in the extremities. To assess peripheral perfusion:

1. Inspect the skin of the hands and feet for color, temperature, edema, and skin changes.

2. Assess the adequacy of arterial flow if arterial insufficiency is suspected.
   a. Assist the client to a supine position. Ask the client to raise one leg or one arm about 30 cm (1 ft) above heart level, move the foot or hand briskly up and down for about 1 minute, and then sit up and dangle the leg or arm. This procedure is called **Buerger's test,** or the arterial adequacy test.
   b. Observe the time elapsed until return of original color and vein filling. Original color normally returns in 10 seconds, and the veins fill in about 15 seconds. Delayed color return indicates arterial insufficiency.

3. Test capillary refill:
   a. Squeeze a fingernail and a toenail between your fingers sufficiently to cause blanching.
   b. Release the pressure and observe how quickly normal color returns. Color normally returns immediately.

4. Inspect the fingernails for changes indicative of circulatory impairment. See the section on assessment of nails, earlier in this chapter. See Table 19–18 for clinical signs of adequate and altered tissue perfusion.

See the accompanying box for physical changes in the peripheral vascular system of older adults.

TABLE 19–18 *Clinical Signs of Adequate and Altered Tissue Perfusion*

Assessment Criterion	Normal Findings	Abnormal Findings	Possible Health Problem
Skin color	Pink	Cyanotic	Venous insufficiency
		Pallor that increases with limb elevation	Arterial insufficiency
		Dusky red color when limb lowered	Arterial insufficiency
		Brown pigmentation around ankles	Arterial insufficiency, chronic venous insufficiency
Skin temperature	Skin not excessively warm or cold	Skin cool	Arterial insufficiency
Edema	Absent	Marked edema	Venous insufficiency
		Mild or absent	Arterial insufficiency
Skin texture	Skin resilient, moist	Skin thin and shiny or thick, waxy, shiny, and fragile, with reduced hair and ulceration	Venous or arterial insufficiency
Arterial adequacy test	Original color returns in 10 seconds; veins in feet or hands fill in about 15 seconds	Delayed color return or mottled appearance; delayed venous filling; marked redness of arms or legs	Arterial insufficiency
Capillary refill test	Immediate return of color	Delayed return of color	Arterial Insufficiency
Peripheral pulse	Easily palpable	No pulse, decreased or absent	Arterial insufficiency

---

The Elderly: Physical Changes in the Peripheral Vascular System

- The overall effectiveness of blood vessels decreases as smooth muscle cells are replaced by connective tissue. The lower extremities are more likely to show signs of arterial and venous impairment because of the more distal and dependent position.

- Proximal arteries become thinner and dilate.

- Peripheral arteries become thicker and dilate less effectively because of arteriosclerotic changes in the vessel walls.

- Blood vessels lengthen and become more tortuous and prominent. Varicosities are seen more frequently.

- In some instances, arteries may be palpated more easily because of the loss of supportive surrounding tissues. Often, however, the most distal pulses of the lower extremities are more difficult to palpate because of decreased arterial perfusion.

- Systolic and diastolic blood pressures increase, but the increase in the systolic pressure is greater. As a result, the pulse pressure widens. Any client with a blood pressure reading above 140/90 should be referred for follow-up assessments.

- Peripheral edema is frequently observed and is most commonly the result of chronic venous insufficiency or low protein levels in the blood (hypoproteinemia).

- Carotid artery assessment is an essential aspect of peripheral vascular examination in the older adult.

BREASTS AND AXILLAE

The breasts of men and women need to be inspected and palpated. Men have some glandular tissue beneath each nipple, a potential site for malignancy, whereas mature women have glandular tissue throughout the breast. During adolescence, asymmetric development is not unusual, since one breast may develop more rapidly than the other. Boys may have some breast development in early adolescence. In females, the largest portion of glandular breast tissue is located in the upper outer quadrant of each breast. From this quadrant there is a projection of breast tissue into the axilla, called the **axillary tail of Spence.** See Figure 19–72. The majority of breast tumors are located in this upper outer breast quadrant and in the tail of Spence. During assessment, the nurse can localize specific findings by using this division of the breast into quadrants and the axillary tail.

Client teaching about breast self-examination (BSE) is exceedingly important for the early detection of breast cancer. Specific instructions for the client are shown in Chapter 26, page 650.

Inspection   For inspection of the breasts, the client needs to be in a sitting position. The nurse inspects the breasts for size, symmetry, and contour or shape; skin integrity; areolar characteristics; and integrity of the nipples.

Each breast is observed for *size, symmetry, and shape,* and the two breasts are then compared according to these criteria. Size varies according to age, heredity, endocrine functions, and amount of adipose tissue. Breast changes

during puberty are shown in the box below. In young adults, shape is generally symmetric, but the breasts may be slightly unequal in size. During pregnancy, both breasts enlarge, usually to two to three times the original size. In the second month, the areolae normally become raised and darken in color. The nipples too enlarge and may become erect. It is not unusual for some **colostrum** (a yellowish fluid) to be expressed from the breasts during the third month. During menopause, breasts shrink in size, and breast tissue becomes less firm and softer. In older females, the breasts sag, and the nipples decrease in size.

The male breast contains a nipple, an areola, and a small amount of breast tissue below the nipple. Normally male breasts are even with the chest wall; the breasts of obese men, however, may appear larger and similar in shape to female breasts.

The *skin of the breast* is the same in appearance as the skin of the abdomen or back. Some individuals may have a number of scattered hair follicles around the areola. In people with a light complexion, a diffuse horizontal or vertical vascular pattern may be noted. This pattern is normally symmetric. **Striae** or stretch marks (a result of rapid stretching of the skin) may also be present. These first appear reddish but become whitish with age. The skin should be inspected for the following:

- *Localized discolorations or hyperpigmentation.* Normally, breast tissue is uniform in color; only the areola and nipple are hyperpigmented. Localized hyperpigmentation is abnormal, although moles and nevi are common. The nurse should question the client about recent changes or problems with any skin lesion noted.

- *Retraction or dimpling.* This appears as a depression or puckering of the skin. See Figure 19–73. It can be the result of scar tissue formation or can be caused by an invasive growth process. Retraction can be accentuated by having the client raise the arms about the head and pushing the hands together with elbows flexed (see Figure 19–74) or pressing the hands down on the hips (see Figure 19–75).

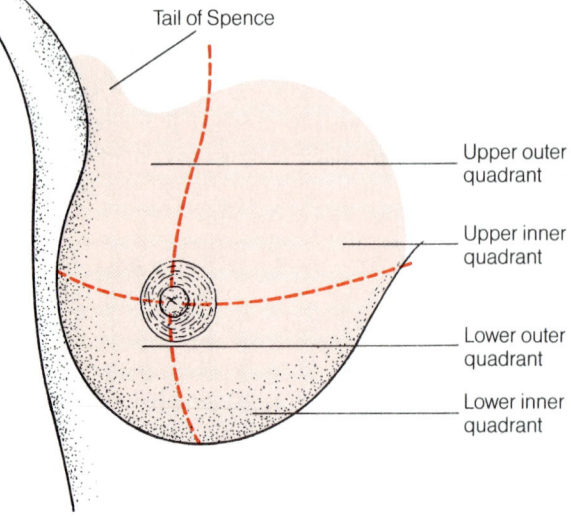

Figure 19–72   Four breast quadrants and the axillary tail of Spence.

Five Stages of Breast Development*
- Stage 1   Elevation of the nipple
- Stage 2   Enlargement of the areola
- Stage 3   Enlargement of the breast
- Stage 4   Projection of the areola and nipple
- Stage 5   Recession of the areola by about age 14 or 15, leaving only the nipple projecting

*The 2-year transient breast growth that occurs in males reaches only the second stage.

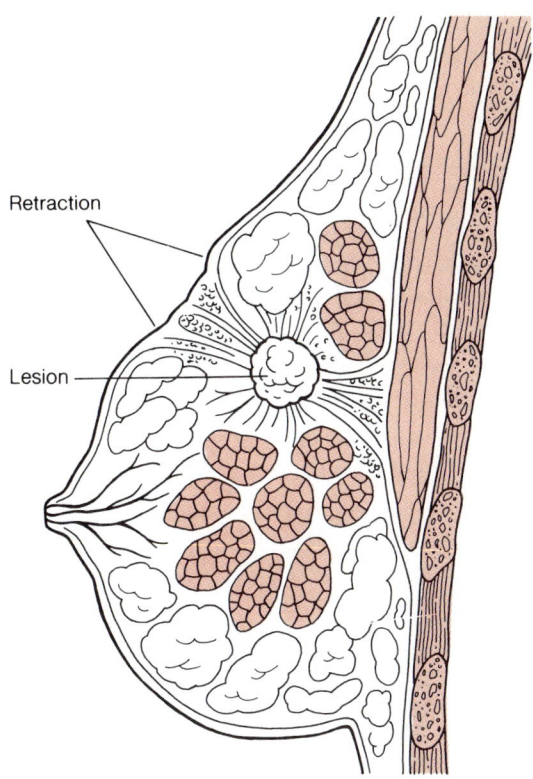

Figure 19-73 A lesion causing retraction of the skin.

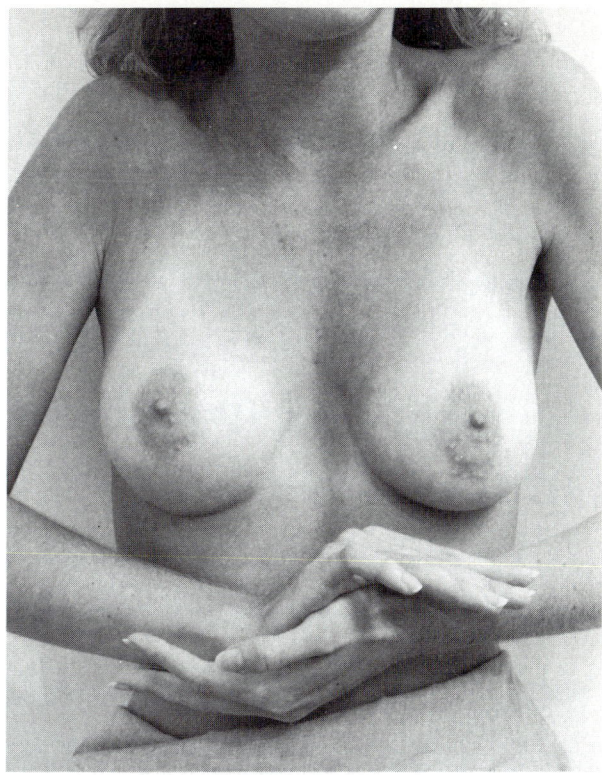

Figure 19-74 Pushing the hands together to accentuate retraction of breast tissues.

■ *Localized hypervascular areas.* Although hypervascular areas may be noted in pregnant or fair-skinned persons, unilateral localized areas are abnormal. These may be a result of dilated veins and increased blood flow associated with a malignancy.

■ *Swelling or edema.* Edema of the breast often produces a pitted appearance of the skin, since it causes an exaggeration of the pores. It appears like pigskin or an orange peel. The axilla and clavicle areas should also be inspected for any swelling or redness.

The *areolar area* is inspected for size, shape, symmetry, color, surface characteristics, and any masses or lesions. The areolar area should be round or oval and bilaterally the same. Areolar color normally varies widely from light pink to dark brown and is darker in brunettes and pregnant women than in fair-haired people. Any asymmetry, mass, or lesion is considered abnormal. **Montgomery's tubercles** (sebaceous glands on the surface of the areola) commonly assume an irregular placement, which is normal.

The *nipples* are assessed for size, shape, position, color, discharge, and lesions. The nipples should be round and equal in size, similar in color, and appear soft and smooth. Both nipples normally point in the same direction. *Inversion* of one or both nipples that is present from puberty is considered normal for that individual. However, recent inversion is likely to be associated with retraction and an underlying growth. There should be no discharge, crusts,

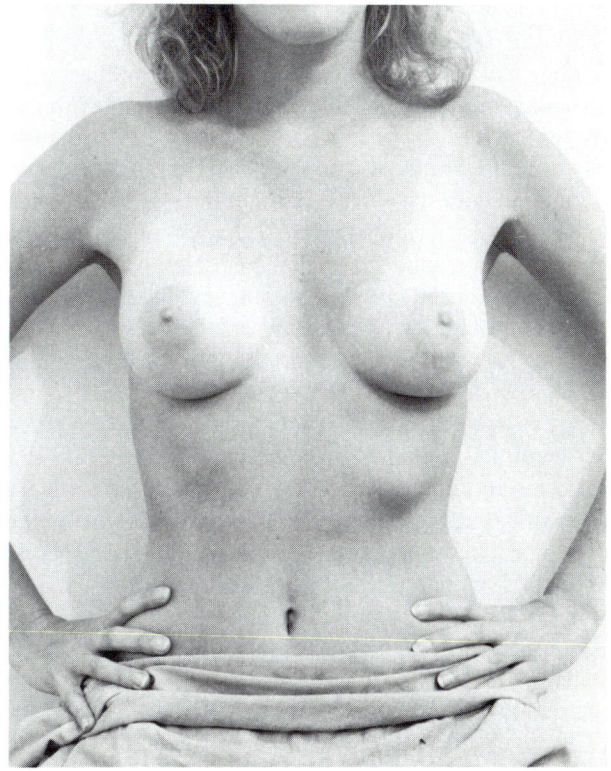

Figure 19-75 Pressing the hands down on the hips to accentuate retraction of breast tissue.

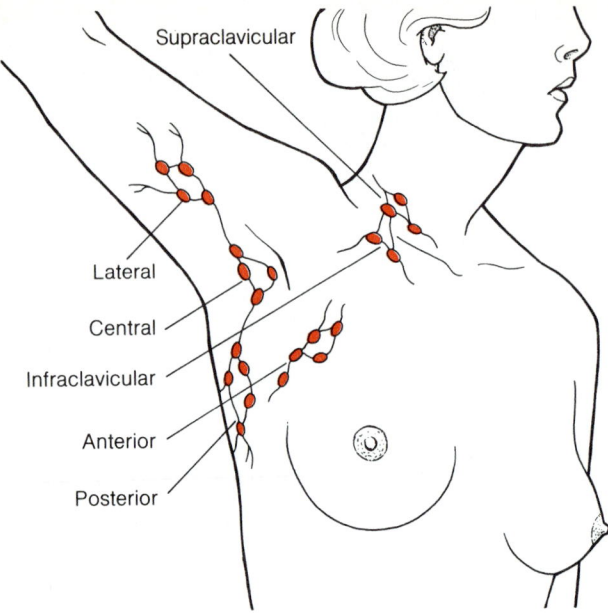

Figure 19–76 Lymph nodes that drain the breast tissues.

or cracks, although some colostrum (mentioned previously) may be expressed in pregnant females.

Palpation The primary purpose of breast palpation is to discover masses. It includes palpation of the axillary, subclavicular (infraclavicular), and supraclavicular lymph nodes, and palpation of the breast itself. The palpation procedure usually begins with palpation of the axillary and clavicular lymph nodes while the client is sitting with the arms at the side. These nodes, which drain the breast tissues, are often involved if cancerous breast lesions metastasize. See Figure 19–76. Palpation of the clavicular nodes is discussed earlier on page 394. Palpation of the axillary lymph nodes is facilitated when the muscles in the area are relaxed. Contracted muscles can obscure slightly enlarged nodes. The nurse helps the client achieve this relaxation by facing the client, abducting the client's arm and supporting it on the nurse's forearm. To palpate the axilla, the nurse uses the palmar surfaces of all fingertips and palpates four areas: (a) the edge of the greater pectoralis muscle (musculus pectoralis major) along the anterior axillary line, (b) the thoracic wall in the midaxillary area, (c) the upper part of the humerus, and (d) the anterior edge of the latissimus dorsi muscle along the posterior axillary line. The number of palpable nodes, consistency, movability, and size are assessed. Normally, nodes are not palpable. Nodes that are hard, tender, and immobile are suspect.

Palpation of the breast may be performed while the client is supine or sitting. For clients who have a past history of breast masses, who are at high risk for breast cancer, or who have pendulous breasts, examination in both positions is recommended (Malasanos, Barkauskas, and Stoltenberg-

Allen 1990, p. 289). When the client is in the *sitting position,* a bimanual technique is often preferred, particularly if the breasts are large. The nondominant hand is placed under the breast, and the dominant hand palpates the breast. This bimanual technique can be most effective in detecting small deep masses. It is performed as follows:

1. If the client reports a breast lump, start with the "normal" breast to obtain baseline data that will serve as a comparison to the reportedly involved breast.
2. Press the palmar surface of the middle three fingertips (held together) on the skin surface, starting at the periphery of the breast. See Figure 19–77.
3. Use a smooth rotary motion or back-and-forth technique to press the breast tissue against the other hand.
4. Palpate from the periphery to the areola.
5. Move from the peripheral starting point around the breast systematically until all breast surfaces are thoroughly surveyed.
6. Pay particular attention to the upper outer quadrant area and the tail of Spence, where about 50% of breast cancers develop.

In the *supine position,* the breasts flatten evenly against the chest wall, facilitating palpation. To enhance this flattening, the client abducts the arm and places her hand behind her head. In addition, the nurse can place a small pillow or rolled towel under the client's shoulder. Both of these maneuvers shift the breast tissue medially. To perform palpation in this position, the nurse uses fingertips of one hand and visualizes the breast as a clock (see Figure 19–78). The nurse palpates along the hands of the clock, moving from the periphery toward the areola. The starting point for palpation is arbitrary, but the nurse must start and end at a fixed point to ensure that all breast surfaces are assessed. If a mass is detected, the following data are recorded.

- *Location:* the exact location relative to the clock (as in Figure 19–78) and the distance from the nipple in centimeters.
- *Client's position:* whether the arms were raised or lowered and whether the client was sitting or supine. The position can change the perceived location of the mass.
- *Size:* the length, width, and thickness of the mass in centimeters. If you are unable to determine the discrete edges, record this fact.
- *Mobility:* whether the mass is movable or fixed. If it is fixed, determine whether it is firmly or moderately fixed, if possible.
- *Consistency:* whether the mass is hard or soft.
- *Surface:* whether the surface is smooth or irregular.
- *Tenderness:* whether palpation is painful to the client.
- *Shape:* whether the mass is round, discoid, regular, or irregular.

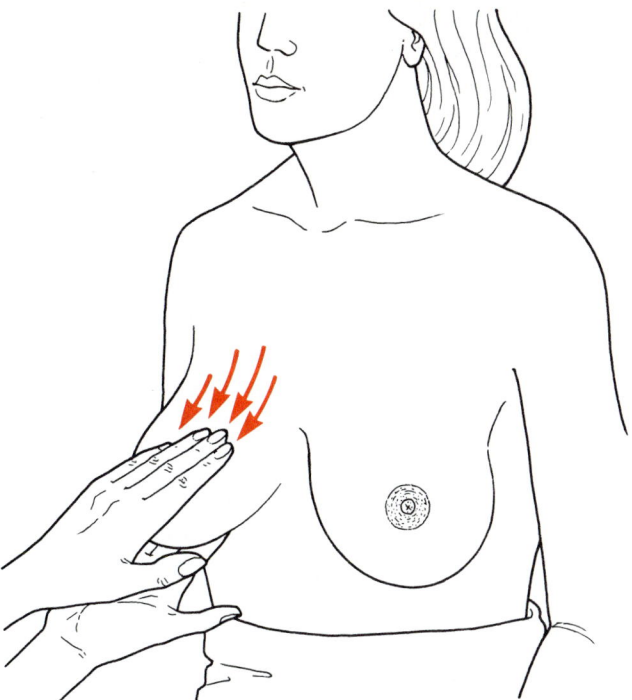

Figure 19–77 Bimanual breast palpation with the client in a sitting position.

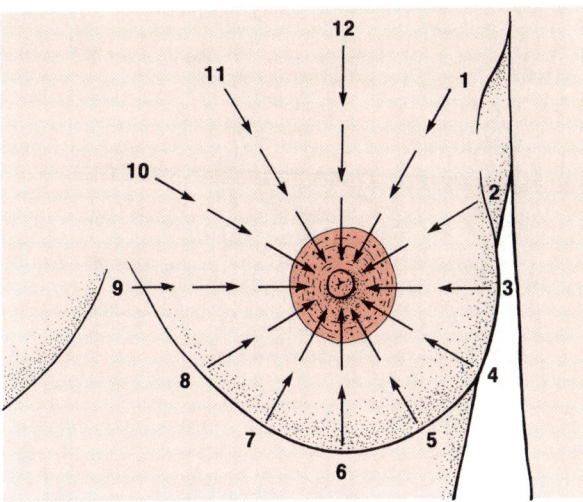

Figure 19–78 Pattern for palpating a breast and using the clock to describe the location of any masses.

The areolar areas and the nipples are also palpated for masses. Each nipple is gently compressed to determine the presence of any discharge. If discharge is present, the breast is milked along its radii to identify the discharge-producing lobe. Any discharge is assessed for amount, color, consistency, and odor. Any tenderness on palpation is also noted.

The male breast can be palpated when the client is supine. The axillary nodes should also be palpated. Male breast cancer, although rare, occurs most frequently in the areolar area. *Gynecomastia,* enlargement of the male breast, may occur as a result of pubertal changes, hormonal administration, cirrhosis of the liver, leukemia, thyrotoxicosis, or certain drugs.

Physical changes of the breasts in the elderly are shown in the accompanying box.

ABDOMEN

Description of abdominal findings is facilitated by two commonly used methods of subdivision: quadrants and nine regions. To divide the abdomen into quadrants, the nurse imagines two lines: a vertical line from the xiphoid process to the pubic symphysis, and a horizontal line across the umbilicus. See Figure 19–79. These quadrants are labeled upper right quadrant (*1*), upper left quadrant (*2*), lower right quadrant (*3*), and lower left quadrant (*4*). Using the

The Elderly: Physical Changes of the Breasts

■ In the postmenopausal female, breasts change in shape and often appear pendulous or flaccid; they lack the firmness they had in younger years.

■ The presence of breast lesions may be detected more readily because of the decrease in connective tissue.

■ General breast size remains the same. Although glandular tissue atrophies, the amount of fat in breasts (predominantly in the lower quadrants) increases in most women.

second method, division into nine regions, the nurse imagines two vertical lines, which extend superiorly from the midpoints of the inguinal ligaments, and two horizontal lines, one at the level of the edge of the lower ribs and the other at the level of the iliac crests. See Figure 19–80. Specific organs or parts of organs lie in each abdominal region. See Tables 19–19 and 19–20.

In addition, certain landmarks are often used to facilitate the location of abdominal signs and symptoms. These are the xiphoid process of the sternum, the costal margins, the midline (a line drawn from the tip of the sternum through the umbilicus to the pubic symphysis), the anterosuperior iliac spine, the inguinal ligaments (Poupart's ligaments), and the superior margin of the pubic symphysis. See Figure 19–81 on page 417.

Assessment of the abdomen involves all four methods of examination (inspection, auscultation, palpation, and per-

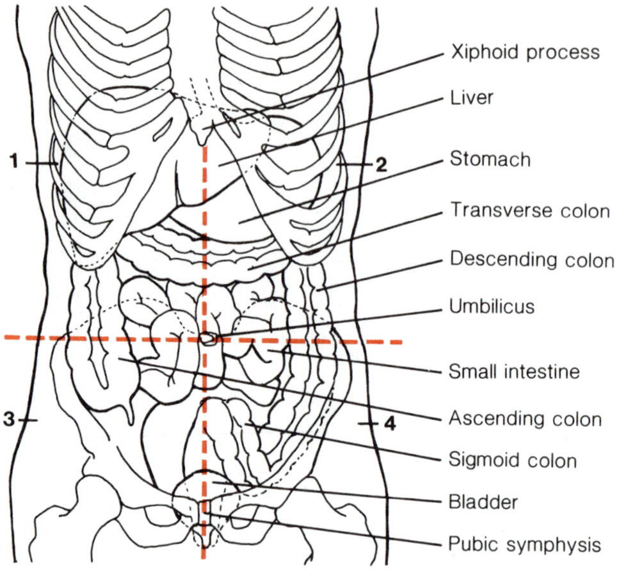

Xiphoid process
Liver
Stomach
Transverse colon
Descending colon
Umbilicus
Small intestine
Ascending colon
Sigmoid colon
Bladder
Pubic symphysis
1
2
3
4

Figure 19–79 The four abdominal regions and the underlying organs: *1,* right upper quadrant; *2,* left upper quadrant; *3,* right lower quadrant; *4,* left lower quadrant.

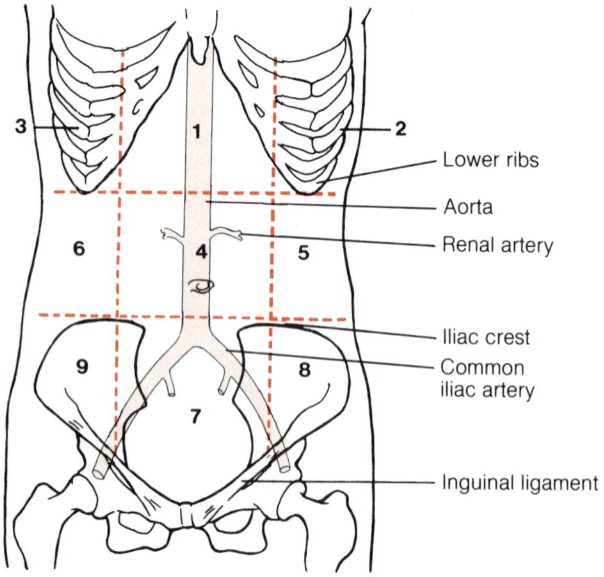

Lower ribs
Aorta
Renal artery
Iliac crest
Common iliac artery
Inguinal ligament
1
2
3
4
5
6
7
8
9

Figure 19–80 The nine abdominal regions: *1,* epigastric; *2, 3,* left and right hypochondriac; *4,* umbilical; *5, 6,* left and right lumbar; *7,* suprapubic and hypogastric; *8, 9* left and right inguinal or iliac.

TABLE 19–19 ***Organs in the Four Abdominal Quadrants***

Right Upper Quadrant	*Left Upper Quadrant*
Liver	Left lobe of liver
Gallbladder	Stomach
Duodenum	Spleen
Head of pancreas	Upper lobe of left kidney
Right adrenal gland	Pancreas
Upper lobe of right kidney	Left adrenal gland
Hepatic flexure of colon	Splenic flexure of colon
Section of ascending colon	Section of transverse colon
Section of transverse colon	Section of descending colon
Right Lower Quadrant	*Left Lower Quadrant*
Lower lobe of right kidney	Lower lobe of left kidney
Cecum	Sigmoid colon
Appendix	Section of descending colon
Section of ascending colon	Left ovary
Right ovary	Left fallopian tube
Right fallopian tube	Left ureter
Right ureter	Left spermatic cord
Right spermatic cord	Part of uterus (if enlarged)
Part of uterus (if enlarged)	

cussion). Of these, beginning practitioners usually perform only inspection and auscultation. If abnormalities are detected, the beginner consults a more experienced practitioner, who may perform palpation and percussion. Several body organs are assessed during the abdominal examination: the stomach, intestines, liver, spleen, kidneys, and, if it is distended or enlarged, the bladder.

When assessing the abdomen, inspection is done first, followed by auscultation, palpation, and/or percussion. **Auscultation is done before palpation and percussion,** since movement or stimulation of the bowel caused by palpation and percussion can increase bowel motility and thus heighten bowel sounds, creating false results.

To facilitate validity of observations and enhance client comfort, ask the client to urinate before beginning the assessment. Assist the client to a supine position with the arms placed comfortably at the sides. Place small pillows beneath the knees and the head. This position and an empty bladder prevent tension in the abdominal muscles. By contrast, the abdominal muscles tense when the client is sitting or supine with knees and arms extended and with hands clasped behind the head.

Ensure that the room is warm, and expose only the client's abdomen from chest line to the pubic area to avoid chilling

TABLE 19–20 *Organs in the Nine Abdominal Regions*

Right Hypochondriac	Epigastric	Left Hypochondriac
Right lobe of liver	Aorta	Stomach
Gallbladder	Pyloric end of stomach	Spleen
Part of duodenum	Part of duodenum	Tail of pancreas
Hepatic flexure of colon	Pancreas	Splenic flexure of colon
Upper half of right kidney	Part of liver	Upper half of left kidney
Suprarenal gland		Suprarenal gland
Right Lumbar	**Umbilical**	**Left Lumbar**
Ascending colon	Omentum	Descending colon
Lower half of right kidney	Mesentery	Lower half of left kidney
Part of duodenum and jejunum	Lower part of duodenum	Part of jejunum and ileum
	Part of jejunum and ileum	
Right Inguinal	**Hypogastric (Pubic)**	**Left Inguinal**
Cecum	Ileum	Sigmoid colon
Appendix	Bladder (if enlarged)	Left ureter
Lower end of ileum	Uterus (if enlarged)	Left spermatic cord
Right ureter		Left ovary
Right spermatic cord		
Right ovary		

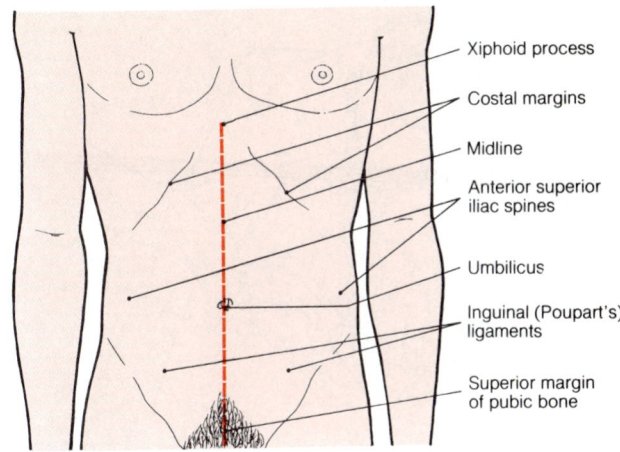

Figure 19–81 Landmarks commonly used to identify abdominal areas.

(labels: Xiphoid process; Costal margins; Midline; Anterior superior iliac spines; Umbilicus; Inguinal (Poupart's) ligaments; Superior margin of pubic bone)

and shivering, which can tense the abdominal muscles. An examining light, a tape measure (metal or unstretchable cloth), a water-soluble skin-marking pencil, and a stethoscope are necessary for the examination.

Inspection   The abdomen is inspected for skin integrity (refer to the discussion about skin assessment, earlier in this chapter); contour and symmetry; and any movements associated with respiration, peristalsis, or aortic pulsations. Before inspection, the nurse directs the examining light over the abdomen and inspects the abdominal surface, with the head only slightly higher than the client's abdomen.

Contour and symmetry   **Abdominal contour** (described as flat, rounded, or scaphoid) is the profile line

from the rib margin to the pubic bone viewed by the nurse at a right angle to the umbilicus when the client is supine. A *flat* contour lies in an approximately horizontal plane from the rib cage to the pubic area and is seen in well-muscled and well-nourished people. The *rounded* contour is convex to the horizontal plane and is generally the result of excessive subcutaneous fat deposits. The *scaphoid* contour is concave to the horizontal plane and indicates a relaxed or flaccid abdominal musculature and minimal fat deposits. After instructing the client to take a deep breath and to hold it, the nurse inspects the abdominal contour again. A deep breath forces the diaphragm downward, thus decreasing the size of the abdominal cavity and making masses such as an enlarged liver or spleen more obvious.

Symmetry of abdominal contour is more readily assessed from the foot of the bed. Asymmetric contours or *asymmetric distention* may result from a hernia, tumor, cysts, or bowel obstruction. When an umbilical or incisional hernia is suspected, the client raises the head and shoulders from the pillow without using the arms for support. This maneuver increases the intra-abdominal pressure, which may cause upward protrusion of the hernia.

Generalized or *symmetric abdominal distention* other than that caused by pregnancy is usually the result of obesity or the presence of fluid or gas within the bowel or abdominal cavity. The abdomen often appears taut and feels "tight" to the client in these situations. To differentiate fluid from gas as the cause of the distention, the nurse observes the flanks (they will bulge if fluid is the cause) and asks the client to roll onto one side. Fluid, if present, will flow to the dependent side and cause a protuberance. To obtain baseline data about the degree of distention, the nurse measures the abdominal girth by placing a tape measure

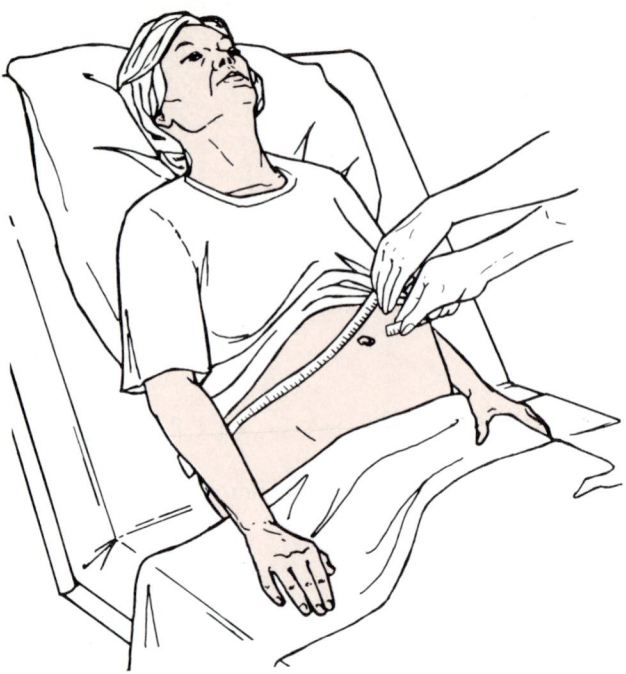

Figure 19–82 Measuring the abdominal girth at the level of the umbilicus.

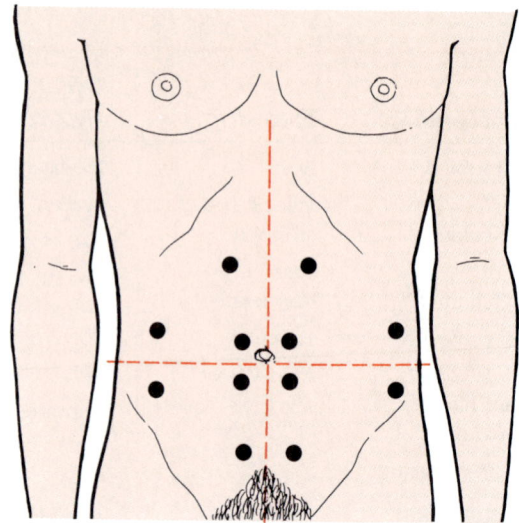

Figure 19–83 Auscultation sites of the abdomen.

around the abdomen at the level of the umbilicus. See Figure 19–82.

Abdominal movement Respiration causes abdominal movement, particularly in males, who breathe abdominally; females, by contrast, tend to breathe more costally. The presence of disease or pain, however, may limit this movement in the male client. *Visible peristalsis* can occur in the absence of disease in very lean people, but in other individuals it is abnormal. It is usually the result of a bowel obstruction, which causes strong contractions. To detect peristaltic waves, the nurse looks across the abdomen from the side for several minutes. *Aortic pulsations* may be normally visible in thin persons at the epigastric area.

Auscultation The nurse auscultates the abdomen for bowel sounds, vascular sounds, and friction rubs. In the pregnant woman, fetal sounds are also assessed. Before auscultating the abdomen, the nurse warms the hands and the stethoscope diaphragms. Cold hands and a cold stethoscope may cause the client to contract the abdominal muscles, and these contractions may be heard during auscultation.

When auscultating for *bowel sounds,* the nurse uses the flat-disc diaphragm, since intestinal sounds are relatively high-pitched and best accentuated by the flat diaphragm. Only light pressure with the stethoscope is adequate to detect sounds. The nurse asks when the client last ate, since the frequency of sounds relates to the state of digestion or the presence of food in the gastrointestinal tract. Shortly after or long after eating, bowel sounds may be normally increased. They are loudest when a meal is long overdue. Four to 7 hours after a meal, bowel sounds may be heard continuously over the ileocecal valve area while the digestive contents from the small intestine empty through the valve into the large intestine.

To auscultate, place the flat diaphragm of the stethoscope in each of the four quadrants of the abdomen over all the auscultatory sites shown in Figure 19–83. Many nurses begin in the lower right quadrant in the area of the cecum. Listen for active bowel sounds—irregular gurgling noises occurring about every 5 to 20 seconds. The duration of a single sound may range from less than a second to more than several seconds. Normal bowel sounds are described as *audible.* Alterations in sounds are described as *absent* or *hypoactive*, i.e., extremely soft and infrequent (e.g., one per minute), and *hyperactive* or increased (**borborygmi**), i.e., high-pitched, loud, rushing sounds that occur frequently (e.g., every 3 seconds). Absence of sounds indicates a cessation of intestinal motility. Hypoactive sounds indicate decreased motility and are usually associated with manipulation of the bowel during surgery, inflammation, paralytic ileus, or late bowel obstruction. Hyperactive sounds indicate increased intestinal motility and are usually associated with diarrhea, an early bowel obstruction, or use of laxatives.

If bowel sounds appear to be absent, listen for 3 to 5 minutes before concluding that they are absent. Because bowel sounds are so irregular, a longer time and more sites are used to confirm absence of sounds.

When auscultating for *vascular sounds* such as arterial bruits, use the bell of the stethoscope over the aorta, renal arteries, and iliac arteries as follows:

1. Auscultate the aorta superior to the umbilicus.

2. Auscultate the renal arteries at or to the left and right of the upper abdominal midline or farther toward the flank.

3. Auscultate the iliac arteries to the left and right of the abdominal midline below the umbilicus. See Figure 19–80 to locate these areas.

Bruits, normally absent, occur when an artery is partially obstructed, causing turbulent flow. A loud bruit over the aorta may also indicate an **aneurysm** (a sac formed by the dilation of the wall of the artery).

At the various auscultating sites, especially above the liver and spleen, listen for *peritoneal friction rubs,* which sound like two pieces of leather rubbing together. The liver and spleen have large surface areas in contact with the peritoneum; thus they are most frequently the beginning sites for friction rubs. To auscultate the *splenic site,* place the stethoscope over the left lower rib cage in the anterior axillary line, and ask the client to take a deep breath. A deep breath may accentuate the sound of a friction rub area. To auscultate the *liver site,* place the stethoscope over the lower right rib cage. Friction rubs may be caused by infectious or abnormal growth processes including metastases.

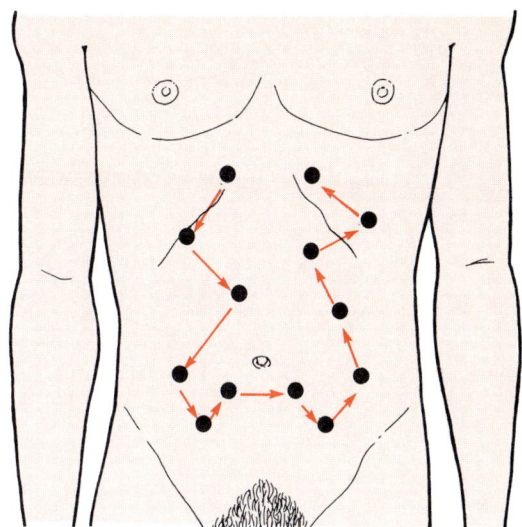

Figure 19–84 A systematic sequence for percussing the abdomen.

Percussion Percussion is used to detect gas, fluid, and/ or masses within the abdomen as well as the position and size of the liver and spleen. In some practice settings, the nurse does not perform abdominal percussion, with the exception of bladder percussion. In the absence of client complaints or a disease process, the major purpose of abdominal percussion is to identify the position and size of the liver and spleen. However many practitioners rely on the palpation method (discussed later) to detect enlargement of the spleen or liver.

The percussion procedure begins with light percussion of the entire abdomen in a systematic manner (see Figure 19–84). The nurse percusses from the right upper quadrant in a direction clockwise from the client's perspective (counterclockwise from the nurse's perspective). If the client is experiencing pain or tenderness in a specific area, the nurse percusses that area last. Pain felt early in the percussion sequence might cause the client to tense the abdominal muscles, making evaluation of percussion sounds more difficult. Normal percussion sounds over the abdomen include *tympany* and *dullness.* Tympanic sounds predominate in the abdomen because of the presence of gas in the stomach and intestines. Dullness (a decrease, absence, or flatness or resonance) is heard over solid masses, such as an enlarged liver or spleen, a sigmoid colon filled with stool, a distended bladder, and ascites.

A percussion test for *shifting dullness* is performed to detect free-floating intra-abdominal fluid (ascites) in the peritoneal cavity. It differentiates ascites from cysts or edema fluid contained in the abdominal wall. This test is performed in two stages: when the client is supine and when the client is turned onto the side. While the client is supine, the nurse percusses the abdomen, progressing laterally from the umbilicus toward the flank and marking the point where dullness is first heard. From the umbilical area, tympanic sounds are elicited over gas-filled structures until the area of fluid is reached; at this point, dullness is heard. When the client is supine, free-floating fluid in the abdomen moves to the flank areas because of gravity. The level of the fluid-filled area is determined by percussing the height of dullness. The client turns onto the side facing the nurse, who again percusses the abdomen as above, marking the new line between the areas of tympany and dullness. When the client lies on one side, ascitic fluid that rested in the opposite flank area flows by gravity to the dependent flank and shifts the line of dullness closer to the umbilicus. If the area of dullness does not shift significantly, the fluid is not free-floating and may be confined within the bowel, cysts, or the abdominal wall. This technique also helps the nurse to make a rough estimate of fluid volume.

Liver and spleen size Percussion to determine liver size begins in the right midclavicular line at or below the level of the umbilicus and proceeds as follows:

1. Percuss upward over tympanic areas until a dull percussion sound indicates the lower liver border. Mark the site with a skin-marking pencil. See Figure 19–85.

2. Then percuss downward at the right midclavicular line, beginning from an area of lung resonance and progressing downward until a dull percussion sound indicates the upper liver border. Mark this site.

3. Measure the distance between the two marks (upper and lower liver border) in centimeters to establish the liver

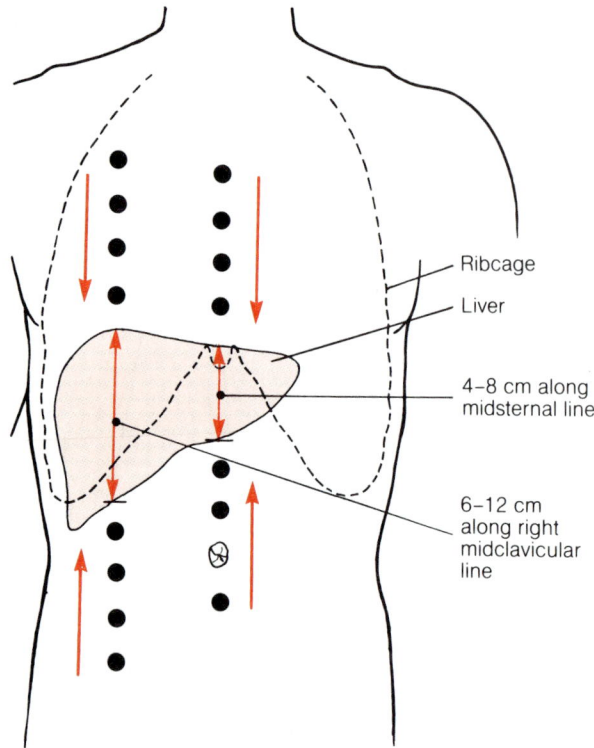

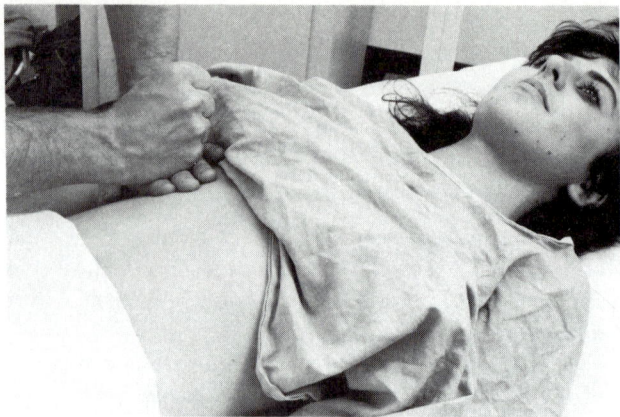

Figure 19–86 The indirect method of fist percussion is used to assess tenderness of the liver.

Figure 19–85 To locate the liver borders, the nurse percusses along the midclavicular line and the midsternal line.

span or size. Normally, the range of liver span in the midclavicular line is 6 to 12 cm (2½ to 3½ in), and the lower liver border is at or just below the rib cage.

4. Repeat the three above steps at the midsternal line. Normally, the range of liver span at the midsternal line is 4 to 8 cm (1½ to 3 in).

On inspiration, the diaphragm moves downward and shifts the span of liver dullness downward 2 to 3 cm (about 1 in). To assess this liver descent, ask the client to take a deep breath and hold it, again percuss upward in the midclavicular line, and estimate liver descent in centimeters.

The spleen is most easily percussed when it is enlarged. Percuss upward and downward along the left *midaxillary* line, and note where a dull tone is heard. Normally, a dullness is heard between the sixth and tenth ribs for a span of about 7 cm (2½ to 3 in).

Fist percussion   Fist percussion is used to detect areas of tenderness over regions of dullness of the liver and kidney. It vibrates tissues rather than producing sounds. Two methods are used to apply fist percussion: indirect and direct. In the *indirect method,* the palm of the nondominant hand is placed over the specific region and is then struck with a

light blow by the fisted dominant hand. In the *direct method,* the side of the fisted hand is applied directly to the specific region, e.g., the kidney. Fist percussion is not applied until the end of the examination, since it may produce discomfort and tenderness. The nurse assesses the tenderness by the client's reaction and always alerts the client before fist percussion. Otherwise, the nurse may interpret the client's reaction, even though it may only be surprise, as an indication of tenderness.

For the *liver,* only indirect fist percussion is applied. The nurse places the palm of the nondominant hand parallel to and below the right costal margin and strikes it with the back of the fist of the other hand (see Figure 19–86), noting any tenderness.

For the *kidney,* the nurse applies either direct or indirect fist percussion while the client is sitting upright or lying on the side. The nurse places the palm of the nondominant hand or the back of the clenched fist over the costovertebral angle between the spine and the twelfth rib. See Figure 19–87.

Bladder percussion   Percussion may be used to define the outline of a distended bladder. A distended bladder will emit a dull percussion sound above the pubic symphysis. The distance below the umbilicus is measured.

Palpation   Palpation is used to detect tenderness, the presence of masses or distention, and the outline and position of abdominal organs (e.g., the liver, spleen, and kidneys). Two types of palpation are used: light and deep. In some practice settings, palpation is limited to light abdominal palpation to assess tenderness and bladder palpation to assess for distention. Before palpation, (a) ensure that the client's position is appropriate for relaxation of the abdominal muscles, and (b) warm the hands. Cold hands can elicit muscle tension that impedes palpatory evaluation.

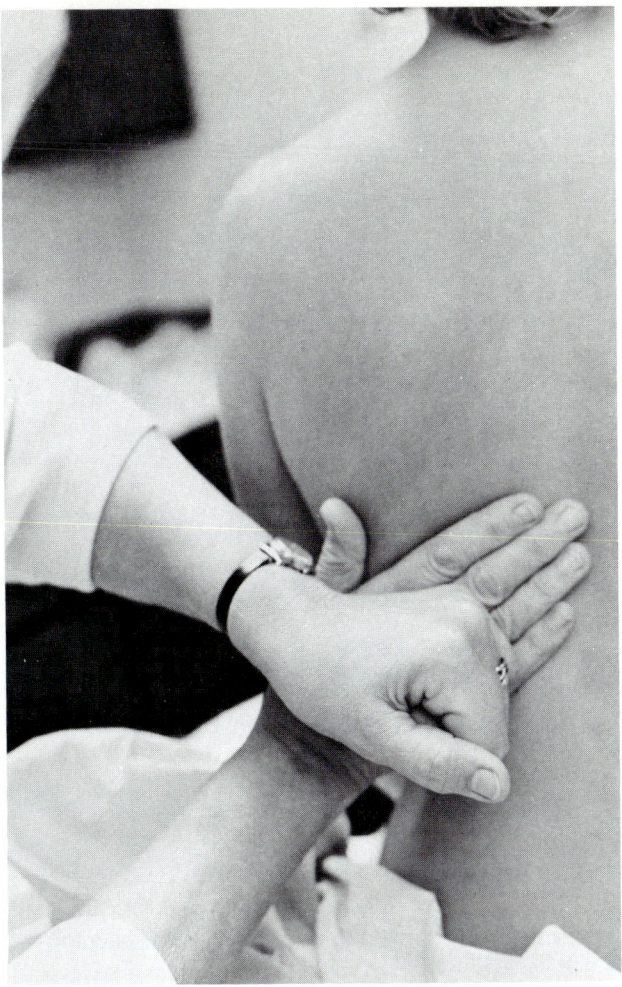

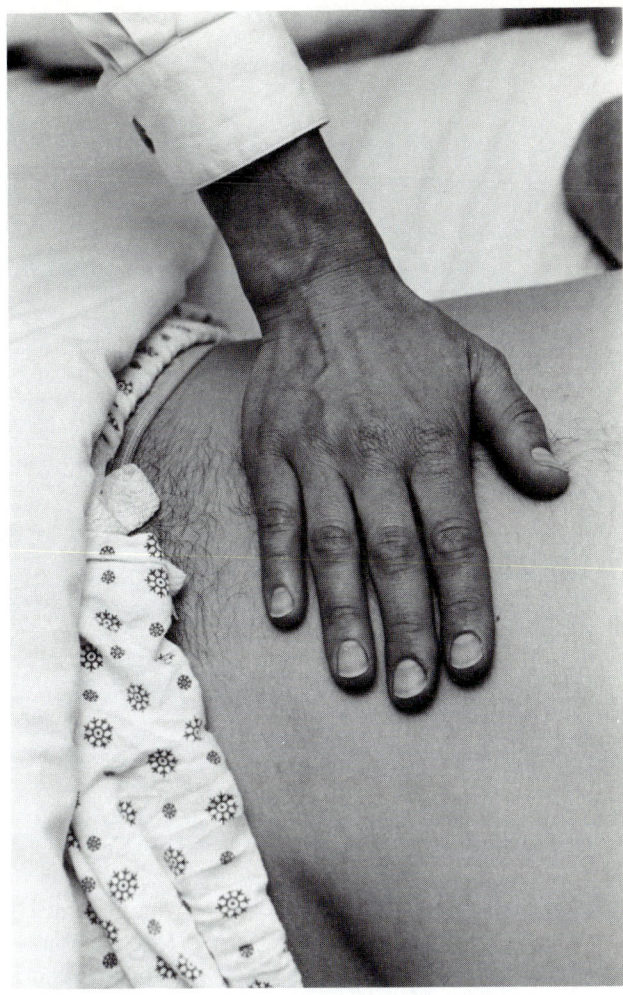

Figure 19–87   Applying indirect fist percussion at the costovertebral junction to assess kidney tenderness.

Figure 19–88   Light palpation of the abdomen.

Light palpation   *Light palpation* is performed before deep palpation to alert the nurse to areas of tenderness and/or muscle guarding (stiffening) before more vigorous palpation is performed. All four quadrants of the abdomen are systematically explored. Light palpation is performed as follows:

1. Hold the palm of your hand slightly above the client's abdomen with your fingers parallel to the abdomen.
2. Depress the abdominal wall lightly, about 1 cm or to the depth of the subcutaneous tissue, with the pads of the fingers. See Figure 19–88.
3. Move the finger pads in a slight circular motion.
4. If the client is extremely ticklish, place the client's hand under or over your own hand. This may decrease the degree of ticklishness and resulting muscle tenseness.
5. Note areas of slight tenderness or superficial pain, large masses, and muscle guarding. To determine areas of

tenderness, ask the client to tell you about them, watch for changes in the client's facial expressions, and note areas of muscle guarding. When the client complains of overall abdominal tenderness, use a cotton wisp for palpation to help the client identify specific pain areas.

Deep palpation   *Deep palpation* is also performed systematically over all four quadrants as follows:

1. Palpate sensitive areas last.
2. Press the distal half of the palmar surface of the fingers of one hand into the abdominal wall.

   or

   Use the bimanual method of palpation discussed earlier in this chapter, page 365.
3. Depress the abdominal wall about 4 to 5 cm (1.5 to 2.0 in) or an appropriate distance beyond subcutaneous tissue. See Figure 19–89.

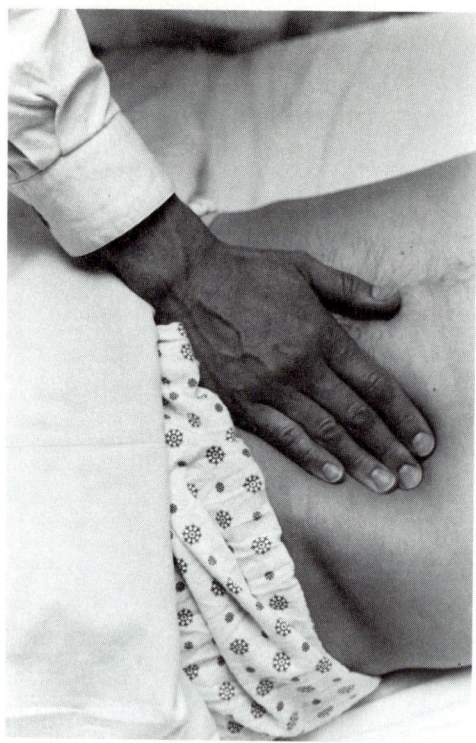

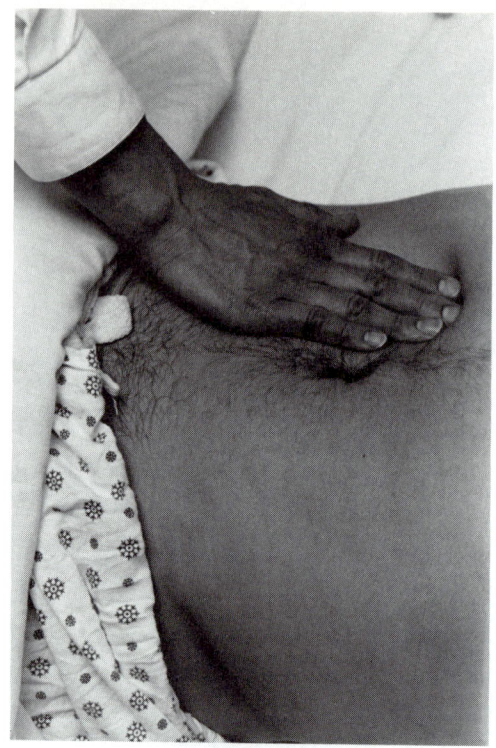

Figure 19−89   Deep palpation of the abdomen.

Figure 19−90   Palpating the liver.

4. Note masses and the structure of underlying contents. If a mass is present, determine its size, location, mobility, contour, consistency, and tenderness. Normal abdominal structures that may be mistaken for masses include: the lateral borders of the rectus abdominis muscles; the feces-filled ascending, descending, or sigmoid colon; the aorta; the uterus; the common iliac artery; and the sacral promontory.

Liver palpation   The liver is palpated to detect enlargement and tenderness. Two bimanual approaches are used. The first involves placement of one hand along the anterior rib cage and the other on the posterior rib cage. When using this method, the nurse stands on the client's right side and places the left hand on the posterior thorax at about the eleventh or twelfth rib. This hand is used to push upward and provide support of underlying structures for the subsequent anterior palpation. The right hand is then placed along the rib cage at about a 45° angle to the right of the rectus abdominis muscle or parallel to the rectus muscle with the fingers pointing toward the rib cage. See Figure 19−90. The nurse observes the client's respirations and, while the client exhales, exerts a gradual and gentle downward and forward pressure beneath the costal margin until a depth of 4 to 5 cm (1½ to 2 in) is reached. During expiration, the abdominal wall relaxes, facilitating deep palpation. Because inspiration makes the liver border descend and moves the liver into a palpable position, the liver is

also palpated after the client inhales deeply. Maintaining the hand position as above, the nurse asks the client to take a deep breath. While the client inhales, the nurse feels the liver border move against the hand. It should feel firm and have a regular contour. If the liver is not palpated initially, the client takes two or three more deep breaths, while the nurse maintains or applies slightly more palpation pressure.

Livers are difficult to palpate in obese, tense, or very physically fit people. If the liver is enlarged, i.e., palpable below the costal margin, the nurse measures the number of centimeters it extends below the costal region.

A second method is the bimanual palpation method discussed on page 365, in which one hand is superimposed on the other. The techniques and principles used above apply to that method as well.

Spleen palpation   Although the spleen is not palpable in the normal adult, the splenic area is palpated in the same manner as the liver. The nurse asks the client to turn onto the right side. This position brings the spleen forward and down by gravity and closer to the abdominal wall. The nurse palpates the spleen at the left costal margin.

Kidney palpation   The upper lobes of both kidneys touch the diaphragm, and the kidneys descend upon inhalation. Although both kidneys are difficult for the novice to palpate, the right kidney is normally more easily palpated than

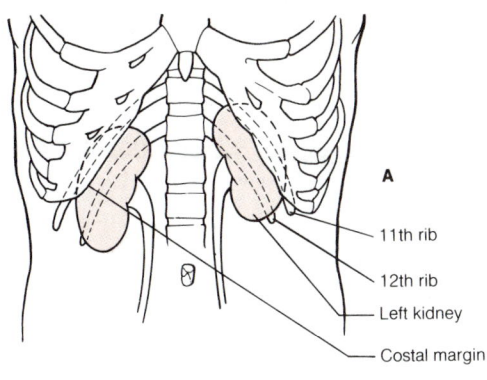

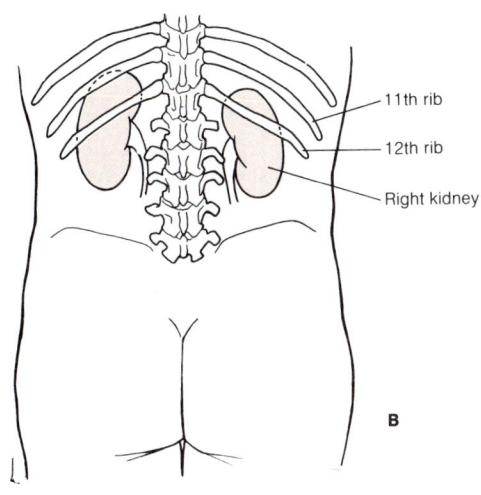

Figure 19–91 Normal position of the kidneys: *A,* anterior view; *B,* posterior view.

the left, because the right one lies a little lower than the left. The right kidney lies in line with the twelfth rib; the left kidney, with the eleventh rib. See Figure 19–91, *A* for the anterior view and Figure 19–91, *B* for the posterior view. The adult kidney is normally smooth, solid, firm, and shaped like a lima bean. It is generally about 11 cm (4.5 in) long, 5 to 7 cm (2 to 3 in) wide, and 2.5 cm (1 in) thick.

While the client lies supine, stand at the client's *right* side while assessing either kidney. To palpate the *right kidney,* place your left hand under the client's flank to elevate the kidney anteriorly. Place your right hand on the anterior abdominal wall at the midclavicular line and at the inferior edge of the costal margin. Press directly upward beneath the costal margin while the client takes a deep breath. Inhaling moves the diaphragm and the inferior aspect of the kidney downward, so that the kidney may be felt. Normally the kidneys of the adult are not palpable, but in very thin people the lower part of the right kidney may be felt. If the kidney is palpable, check it for contour (shape), size, tenderness, and lumps.

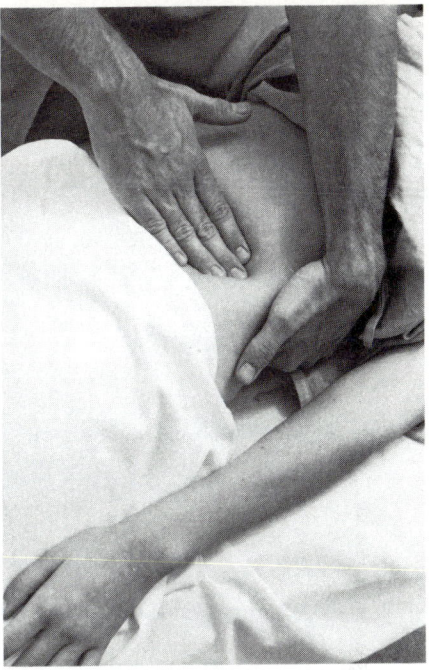

Figure 19–92 Palpating the left kidney.

To palpate the *left kidney,* reach across the client, and place your left hand under the client's flank (see Figure 19–92), and follow the above steps.

Bladder palpation If the client's history indicates possible urinary retention, palpate the bladder. With one or two hands, palpate the area above the pubic symphysis. See Figure 19–93. The bladder is palpable only when distended with urine. If it is distended, percuss the area for level of dullness.

Table 19–21 provides an overview of normal and abnormal abdominal assessment findings. Physical changes in the gastrointestinal tract of elderly people are shown in the box on page 425.

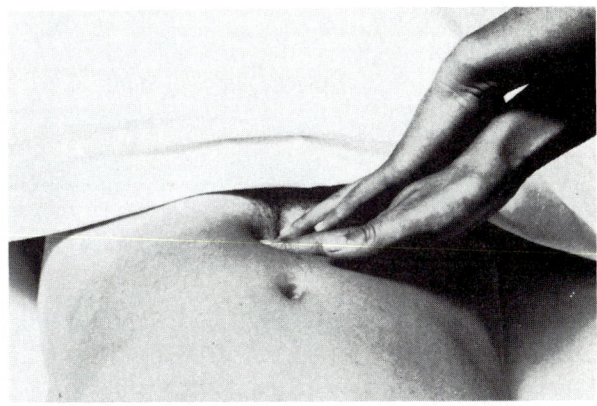

Figure 19–93 Palpating the bladder.

TABLE 19–21 *Summary Assessment Data: Abdomen*

Method and Structure	Normal Findings	Abnormal Findings
Inspection		
Abdomen	Smooth, soft; flat, rounded, or scaphoid contour	Tense, glistening skin
		Distention
		Visible peristalsis
		Visible midline pulsations
	Symmetric contour	Asymmetrical contour, e.g., localized protrusions around umbilicus, around inguinal ligaments, or near scars
	Silver-white striae or surgical scars	Purple striae
	Unblemished skin	Rash or other skin lesions
	After deep breath, smooth, even, symmetric movements	After deep breath, bulges or masses appear
		After deep breath, abdominal movement is restricted
	After raising head and shoulders, little or no midline bulge	After raising head and shoulders, marked ridge or bulge
Auscultation		
Abdomen	Audible bowel sounds	Absent or hypoactive bowel sounds
		Hyperactive bowel sounds
	Absence of arterial bruits	Loud bruit over aortic area
		Bruit over renal or iliac arteries
	Absence of venous hum	Medium-pitched hum in periumbilical region
		Friction rub
Percussion		
Abdomen	Predominantly tympanic percussion sound; suprapubic dullness over distended bladder	Dullness in localized area
Liver	Span of 6–12 cm at midclavicular line and 4–8 cm at midsternal line	Span exceeding 12 cm at midclavicular line and 8 cm at midsternal line
		Midsternal line span is equal to midclavicular line span
		Lower liver border displaced inferiorly
		Lower liver border displaced superiorly
Spleen	Span of about 7 cm at left midaxillary line between sixth and tenth ribs	Span exceeds 7 cm
Shifting dullness test		Change in first and second demarcation lines (between tympany and dullness)
Fist percussion	No tenderness of liver or kidney	Tenderness of liver
		Tenderness of kidney
Palpation		
Light abdominal	No tenderness; relaxed abdomen with smooth, consistent tension	Tenderness and hypersensitivity
		Superficial masses
		Localized areas of increased tension
Deep abdominal	Tenderness may be present near xiphoid process, over cecum, and over sigmoid colon	Generalized or localized areas of tenderness
		Mobile or fixed masses
Liver	May not be palpable	Enlarged but smooth and not tender
	Border feels smooth	Smooth but tender
		Nodular
		Hard

TABLE 19–21 *Summary Assessment Data: Abdomen (continued)*

Method and Structure	Normal Findings	Abnormal Findings
Palpation (continued)		
Spleen	Not palpable	Palpated
Kidney	Neither kidney palpable	Either or both kidneys palpable
	Pole of right kidney palpable, feels smooth and firm	Enlarged, hard, tender, or nodular
Bladder	Not palpable	Distended and palpable as smooth, round, tense mass

The Elderly: Physical Changes in the Gastrointestinal Tract

- The rounded abdomens of many older persons are due to greater amounts of adipose tissue and to decreased muscle tone.

- The abdominal wall is slacker and thinner making palpation easier and more accurate than in younger clients. Muscle wasting and loss of fibroconnective tissue occur.

- The side-effects of drugs are often manifested in the gastrointestinal tract, e.g., nausea, vomiting, and diarrhea.

- The pain threshold in the elderly is often increased; major abdominal problems such as appendicitis or other acute emergencies may therefore go undetected.

- Gastrointestinal pain needs to be differentiated from cardiac pain. Gastrointestinal pain may be located in the chest or abdomen, whereas cardiac pain is usually in the chest. Factors aggravating gastrointestinal pain are usually related to either ingestion or lack of food intake; gastrointestinal pain is usually relieved by antacids, food, or assuming an upright position. Common factors aggravating cardiac pain are activity or anxiety; cardiac pain is relieved by rest or nitroglycerine.

Esophagus

- Esophageal motility may be decreased and, if severe, can cause discomfort as food passes through the esophagus.

- Difficulty swallowing (dysphagia), a common complaint of older adults, must be differentiated from heartburn or regurgitation. Questions about food getting "stuck in the throat" or the ability to swallow liquid foods versus solid foods can clarify these symptoms.

- Many older individuals have increased esophageal spasms and less efficient action of the lower esophageal sphincter.

Stomach

- Gastric acid secretion is decreased, and emptying time of the stomach is delayed, resulting in indigestion and intolerance to certain foods. Decreases in the production of pancreatic enzymes also contribute to complaints of indigestion and anorexia.

Intestines

- Stool passes through the intestines at a slower rate in elderly clients, and the perception of stimuli that produce the urge to defecate is often diminished.

- Fecal incontinence may occur in confused or neurologically impaired older adults.

- Many older persons erroneously believe that the absence of a daily bowel movement signifies constipation. When assessing for constipation, the nurse must consider the client's diet, activity, medications, characteristics, and ease of passage of feces, as well as the frequency of bowel movements.

- The incidence of colon cancer is higher among older adults than younger adults. Symptoms include a change in bowel function, rectal bleeding, and weight loss. Changes in bowel function, however, are associated with many factors, such as diet, exercise, and medications.

- Decreased absorption of oral medications often occurs with aging.

Liver

- The liver changes minimally with age, as does the gall bladder. Liver function tests are unaltered.

- Impaired metabolism of some drugs may occur with aging.

Kidneys

- The kidneys become less effective in older clients, but signs of renal tenderness or impairment occur only when renal disease is present.

- Decreased renal excretion of medications often occurs.

MUSCULOSKELETAL SYSTEM

The musculoskeletal system encompasses the muscles, bones, and joints. The completeness of an assessment of this system depends largely on the needs and problems of the individual client. The nurse usually assesses the musculoskeletal system for muscle strength, tone, and size and symmetry of muscle development. Bones are assessed for normalcy of form. Joints are assessed for tenderness, swelling, thickening, crepitation, presence of nodules, and range of motion. Body posture is assessed for normalcy in standing and sitting positions. For information about body posture see Chapter 36.

Inspect the muscles for size. Compare the muscle on one side of the body, e.g., arm, thigh, calf, to the same muscle on the other side. Determine if there is any **atrophy** (a decrease in size or wasting away) or **hypertrophy** (an increase in size). If there appears to be a discrepancy between the sides, measure the muscles with a tape.

Observe muscles and tendons for contractures. These can be indicated by malposition of a body part, e.g., a foot fixed in dorsiflexion. Also, observe muscles for fasciculations and tremors. A **fasciculation** is an abnormal contraction (shortening) of a bundle of muscle fibers. A **tremor** is an involuntary trembling of a limb or body part. Tremors may involve large groups of muscle fibers or small bundles of muscle fibers. An *intention tremor* becomes more apparent when an individual attempts a voluntary movement, e.g., holding a cup of coffee. A *resting tremor* is more apparent when the client is at rest and diminishes with activity.

Inspect any tremors of the hands and arms by having the client hold the arms out in front of the body. Palpate muscles at rest to determine muscle tonicity. Muscle **tonicity** is the normal condition of tension (tone) of a muscle at rest. Muscles are normally firm. Palpate muscles while the client is active and passive for flaccidity, spasticity, and smoothness of movement. **Flaccidity** is weakness or laxness. **Spasticity** is a sudden involuntary muscle contraction.

Tests for muscle strength are shown in Table 19–22. Compare the right side with the left side. An individual normally has equal strength on each body side. Muscle strength is graded from zero (complete paralysis) to five (normal). See Table 19–23.

Inspect the skeleton for normal structure and deformities. Palpate the bones to locate any areas of edema or tenderness. The client's facial or verbal expressions are good indicators of discomfort. Tenderness can reflect such conditions as fractures, neoplasms, and osteoporosis.

Inspect each joint for swelling, which might indicate arthritis. Palpate each joint for tenderness, smoothness of movement, swelling, crepitation (a crackling, grating sound), and the presence of nodules. Normally, joints are not tender, move smoothly, and have no swelling, crepitation, or nodules.

Establish the range of motion of the body joints, as needed. The **range of motion** of a joint is the maximum movement that joint allows. Each person's range of motion is determined by genetic makeup, developmental patterns, the presence or absence of disease, and that person's degree of physical activity. Table 35–2, page 839, lists the types of joint movements.

When assessing joint movement, ask the client to move

TABLE 19–22 *Testing Muscle Strength*

Muscle	Client/Nurse Activity
Deltoid	Client holds arm up and resists while nurse tries to push it down.
Biceps	Client fully extends each arm and then tries to flex it while nurse attempts to hold arm in extension.
Triceps	Client flexes each arm and then tries to extend it against the nurse's attempt to keep arm in flexion.
Wrist and finger muscles	Client spreads the fingers and then resists as the nurse attempts to push the fingers together.
Grip strength	Client grasps the index and middle fingers of the examiner while the nurse tries to pull the fingers out.
Hip muscles	Client is supine, both legs extended; client raises one leg at a time while the nurse attempts to hold it down.
Hip abduction	Client is supine, both legs extended. Nurse's hands are on the lateral surface of each knee; client is asked to spread the legs apart against the nurse's resistance.
Hip adduction	Client is in same position as for hip abduction; the nurse's hands are now placed between the knees; client is asked to bring the legs together against the nurse's resistance.
Hamstrings	Client is supine with both knees bent. Client resists while the nurse attempts to straighten them.
Quadriceps	Client is supine with knee partially extended; client resists while the nurse attempts to flex the knee.
Muscles of the ankles and feet	Client resists while the nurse attempts to dorsiflex the foot and again resists while the nurse attempts to flex the foot.

TABLE 19–23 *Grading Muscle Strength*

Scale	Percentage of Normal Strength	Characteristics
0	0	Complete paralysis
1	10	No movement
		Contraction of muscle is palpable or visible
2	25	Full muscle movement against gravity, with support
3	50	Normal movement against gravity
4	75	Normal full movement against gravity and against minimal resistance
5	100	Normal strength
		Normal full movement against gravity and against full resistance

selected body parts as shown in Table 35–3, page 850. The amount of movement can be measured by a **goniometer,** a device that measures the angle of the joint in degrees. See Figure 19–94.

Physical changes in the musculoskeletal system of elderly people are shown in the box below.

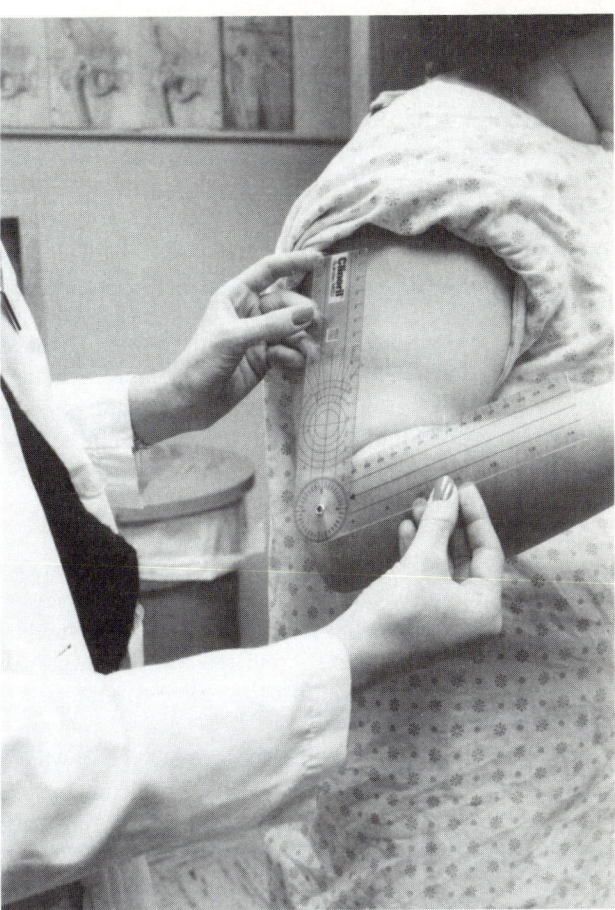

Figure 19–94   A goniometer used to measure joint range of motion.

The Elderly: Physical Changes in the Musculoskeletal System

- Muscle mass decreases progressively with age, but there are wide variations among different individuals.

- The decrease in speed, strength, resistance to fatigue, reaction time, and coordination in the older person is due to a decrease in nerve conduction and muscle tone.

- The bones become more fragile, and osteoporosis leads to a loss of total bone mass. As a result, elderly people are predisposed to fractures and compressed verbebrae.

- In most elderly people, osteoarthritic changes in the joints can be observed.

NEUROLOGIC SYSTEM

The nervous system integrates all other body systems, but it also depends on the appropriate functioning of peripheral organs from which it receives internal and external environmental stimuli. A thorough neurologic examination may take 1 to 3 hours; however, routine screening tests are usually done first. If the results of these tests are questionable, more extensive evaluations are made.

Examination of the neurologic system is not usually performed by the beginning student. It includes assessment of (a) mental status, (b) level of consciousness, (c) the cranial nerves, (d) deep tendon reflexes, (e) the motor system, and (f) the sensory system.

Mental Status

Assessment of mental status reveals the client's general cerebral function. These functions include intellectual (cognitive) as well as emotional (affective) functions. Affective behavior is discussed in the general survey at the beginning of this chapter.

A large part of the mental status assessment is performed during the taking of the history and when observing the client's general appearance. If problems are noted with use of language, memory, concentration, thought processes, or attention span and memory, a more extensive examination is required during neurologic assessment. Major areas of mental status assessment include language, orientation, memory, attention span and calculation, judgment, and abstract reasoning.

Language　　Any defects in or loss of the power to express oneself by speech, writing, or signs or to comprehend spoken or written language due to disease or injury of the cerebral cortex is called **aphasia.** Aphasias can be categorized as sensory or receptive aphasia and motor or expressive aphasia.

Sensory/receptive aphasia is the loss of the ability to comprehend written or spoken words. Two types of sensory aphasia are auditory or acoustic aphasia and visual aphasia. With *auditory aphasia* clients have lost the ability to understand the symbolic content associated with sounds. With *visual aphasia* clients have lost the ability to understand printed or written figures.

Motor/expressive aphasia involves loss of the power to express oneself by writing, making signs, or speaking. Clients may find that even though they can recall words, they have lost the ability to combine speech sounds into words.

To assess language deficits related to aphasia:

1. Point to common objects, and ask the client to name them.

2. Ask the client to read some words and to match the printed and written words with pictures.

3. Ask the client to respond to simple verbal and written commands, e.g., "point to your toes" or "raise your left arm."

It is also important to identify speech patterns. A pattern of repeating the same response as different questions are asked is called **perseveration. Paraphasia** is speech in which there are many incorrect words although it is appropriately expressive.

Orientation　　The client's orientation to *time, place,* and *person* is determined by tactful questioning. Orientation is easily assessed by asking the client the city and state or residence, time of day, date, day of the week, duration of illness, and names of family members. More direct questioning may be necessary for some people, e.g., "Where are you now? "What day is it today?" Most people readily accept these questions if initially the nurse asks, "Do you get confused at times?"

Memory　　Listen for lapses in memory. First, ask the client about difficulty with memory. If problems are apparent, three categories of memory are tested: immediate recall, recent memory, and remote memory.

To assess *immediate recall:*

1. Ask the client to repeat a series of three digits, e.g., 7-4-3, spoken slowly.

2. Gradually increase the number of digits, e.g., 7-4-3-5, 7-4-3-5-6, and 7-4-3-5-6-7-2, until the client fails to repeat the series correctly.

3. Start again with a series of three digits, but this time ask the client to repeat them backward. The average person can repeat a series of five to eight digits in sequence and four to six digits in reverse order.

To assess *recent memory:*

1. Ask the client to recall the recent events of the day, such as how the client got to the clinic. This information must be validated, however.

2. Ask the client to recall information given early in the interview, such as the name of a doctor.

3. Provide the client with three facts to recall, e.g., a color, an object, an address, or a three-digit number, and ask the client to repeat all three. Later in the interview, ask the client to recall all three items.

To assess *remote memory,* ask the client to describe a previous illness or surgery, e.g., 5 years ago, or a birthday or anniversary.

Attention Span and Calculation　　The ability to concentrate or attention span can be tested by asking the client to recite the alphabet or to count backward from 100. The ability to calculate can be tested by asking the client to subtract 7 or 3 progressively from 100; i.e., 100, 93, 86, 79, or 100, 97, 94, 91. This standard test is often referred to as the serial sevens or serial threes test. Normally, an adult can complete the serial sevens test in about 90 seconds with three or fewer errors. Because calculating ability is affected by educational level and by language or cultural differences, this test may be inappropriate for some people.

Judgment　　To test judgment, the nurse asks relatively simple questions and judges the response, always considering the person's sociocultural background.

1. Ask what the client would do in certain situations, e.g., "What would you do if a policeman pulled you over for not observing a stop sign? If you broke a shovel you had borrowed from your neighbor?"

2. Have the person pick from a series a word that does not relate to the others. For example, large, small, and red; or up, left, and down.

Abstract Reasoning　　To assess abstract reasoning:

1. Give the client a proverb to interpret, e.g., "A stitch in time saves nine" or "People who live in glass houses should not throw stones."

TABLE 19–24   *Levels of Consciousness: Glasgow Coma Scale*

Faculty Measured	Response	Score*
Eye opening	Spontaneous	4
	To verbal command	3
	To pain	2
	No response	1
Motor response	To verbal command	6
	To painful stimuli:	
	• Localizes pain	5
	• Flexes and withdraws	4
	• Assumes decorticate posture	3
	• Assumes decerebrate posture	2
	• No response	1
Verbal response (arouse client with painful stimuli, if necessary)	Oriented, converses	5
	Disoriented, converses	4
	Uses inappropriate words	3
	Makes incomprehensible sounds	2
	No response	1

*Coma is defined as a score of 7 or less. A score of 3 or 4 indicates an 85% chance of dying or remaining vegetative. A score of 11 or more suggests an 85% chance of moderate disability or good recovery.

Source: Adapted from G. Teasdale and B. Bennett, Assessment of coma and impaired consciousness: A practical scale, *Lancet* 1974; 2(7872):81.

2. Ask the client to explain how two words, e.g., "climate and season" or "orange and apple," differ or relate. Normally, an abstract or semiabstract response is expected. Concrete interpretations may indicate a problem or may indicate level of education.

Changes in mental function in elderly people are shown in the box above.

Level of Consciousness

Level of consciousness (LOC) can lie anywhere along a continuum from a state of alertness to coma. A fully alert client responds to questions spontaneously; a comatose client may not respond to verbal stimuli. The Glasgow Coma Scale was originally developed to predict recovery from a head injury; however, it is used today to assess LOC. It tests in three major areas: eye response, motor response, and verbal response. An assessment totaling 15 points indicates the client is alert and completely oriented. A comatose client scores 7 or less. See Table 19–24.

Cranial Nerves

For the specific functions and assessment methods of each cranial nerve, see Table 19–25. The nurse needs to be aware of these functions to detect abnormalities. (The names and order of the cranial nerves can be recalled by remembering this sentence: "On old Olympus's treeless top, a Finn and German viewed a hop." The first letter of each word in the phrase is the same as the first letter of the names of the cranial nerves.)

Reflexes

A **reflex** is an automatic response of the body to a stimulus. It is not voluntarily learned or conscious. The deep tendon reflex (DTR) is activated when a tendon is stimulated (tapped) and its associated muscle contracts. The quality of a reflex response varies among individuals and by age. As a person ages reflex responses may become less intense.

Reflexes are tested using a percussion hammer. The response is described on a scale of 0 to +4. See the box on page 431 for a scale describing reflex responses. Experience is necessary to determine appropriate scoring for an individual. It is important to compare one side of the body with the other when assessing reflexes to evaluate the symmetry of response.

Several reflexes are normally tested during a physical examination. These are (a) the biceps reflex, (b) the triceps reflex, (c) the bradioradialis reflex, (d) the patellar reflex, (e) the Achilles reflex, and (f) the plantar reflex.

TABLE 19–25 *Cranial Nerve Functions and Assessment Methods*

Cranial Nerve	Name	Type	Function	Assessment Methods
I	Olfactory	Sensory	Smell	Ask client to close eyes and identify different mild aromas, such as coffee, tobacco, vanilla, oil of cloves, peanut butter, orange, lemon, lime, chocolate.
II	Optic	Sensory	Vision and visual fields	Ask client to read Snellen chart; check visual fields by confrontation; and conduct an ophthalmoscopic examination.
III	Oculomotor	Motor	Extraocular eye movement (EOM); movement of sphincter of pupil; movement of ciliary muscles of lens	Assess six ocular movements and pupil reaction.
IV	Trochlear	Motor	EOM, specifically moves eyeball downward and laterally	Assess six ocular movements.
V	Trigeminal			
	Ophthalmic branch	Sensory	Sensation of cornea, skin of face, and nasal mucosa	While client looks upward, lightly touch lateral sclera of eye to elicit blink reflex; to test light sensation, have client close eyes, wipe a wisp of cotton over client's forehead and paranasal sinuses; to test deep sensation, use alternating blunt and sharp ends of a safety pin over same areas.
	Maxillary branch	Sensory	Sensation of skin of face and anterior oral cavity (tongue and teeth)	Assess skin sensation as for ophthalmic branch above.
	Mandibular branch	Motor and sensory	Muscles of mastication; sensation of skin of face	Ask client to clench teeth.
VI	Abducens	Motor	EOM; moves eyeball laterally	Assess directions of gaze.
VII	Facial	Motor and sensory	Facial expression; taste (anterior two thirds of tongue)	Ask client to smile, raise the eyebrows, frown, puff out cheeks, close eyes tightly; ask client to identify various tastes placed on tip and sides of tongue: sugar (sweet), salt, lemon juice (sour), and quinine (bitter); identify areas of taste.
VIII	Auditory			
	Vestibular branch	Sensory	Equilibrium	Assessment methods are discussed with cerebellar functions (in next section).
	Cochlear branch	Sensory	Hearing	Assess client's ability to hear spoken word and vibrations of tuning fork.
IX	Glossopharyngeal	Motor and sensory	Swallowing ability and gag reflex, tongue movement, taste (posterior tongue)	Use tongue blade on posterior tongue while client says "ah" to elicit gag reflex; apply tastes on posterior tongue for identification; ask client to move tongue from side to side and up and down.
X	Vagus	Motor and sensory	Sensation of pharynx and larynx; swallowing; vocal cord movement	Assessed with cranial nerve IX; assess client's speech for hoarseness.
XI	Accessory	Motor	Head movement; shrugging of shoulders	Ask client to shrug shoulders against resistance from your hands and turn head to side against resistance from your hand (repeat for other side).
XII	Hypoglossal	Motor	Protrusion of tongue	Ask client to protrude tongue at midline, then move it side to side.

Biceps Reflex
This reflex tests the spinal cord level C-5, C-6.

1. Partially flex the client's arm at the elbow, and rest the forearm over the thighs, placing the palm of the hand down.
2. Place the thumb of your nondominant hand horizontally over the biceps tendon.
3. With your other hand, hold the percussion hammer between thumb and index finger.
4. Deliver a blow (slight downward thrust) with the percussion hammer to your thumb.
5. Observe the normal slight flexion of the elbow and feel the bicep's contraction through your thumb. See Figure 19–95.

Triceps Reflex
This reflex tests the spinal cord level C-7, C-8.

1. Flex the client's arm at the elbow, and support it in the palm of your nondominant hand.
2. Palpate the triceps tendon about 2 to 5 cm (1 to 2 in) above the elbow.
3. Deliver a blow with the percussion hammer directly to the tendon. See Figure 19–96.
4. Observe the normal slight extension of the elbow.

Brachioradialis Reflex
This reflex tests the spinal cord level C-3, C-6.

1. Rest the client's arm in a relaxed position on your forearm or on the client's own leg.
2. Deliver a blow with the percussion hammer directly on the radius 2 to 5 cm (1 to 2 in) above the wrist or the styloid process (bony prominence on the thumb side of the wrist). See Figure 19–97.
3. Observe the normal flexion and supination of the forearm. The fingers of the hand may also extend slightly.

Patellar Reflex
This reflex tests the spinal cord level L-2, L-3, L-4.

1. Ask the client to sit on the edge of the examining table so that the legs hang freely.
2. Locate the patellar tendon directly below the patella (kneecap).
3. Deliver a blow with the percussion hammer directly to the tendon. See Figure 19–98.
4. Observe the normal extension or kicking out of the leg as the quadriceps muscle contracts.
5. If no response is obtained and you suspect the client is not relaxed, ask the client to interlock the fingers and pull. This action often enhances relaxation so that a more accurate response is obtained.

Scale for Grading Reflex Responses
- ▪ 0 No reflex response
- ▪ +1 Minimal activity (hypoactive)
- ▪ +2 Normal response
- ▪ +3 More active than normal
- ▪ +4 Maximum activity (hyperactive)

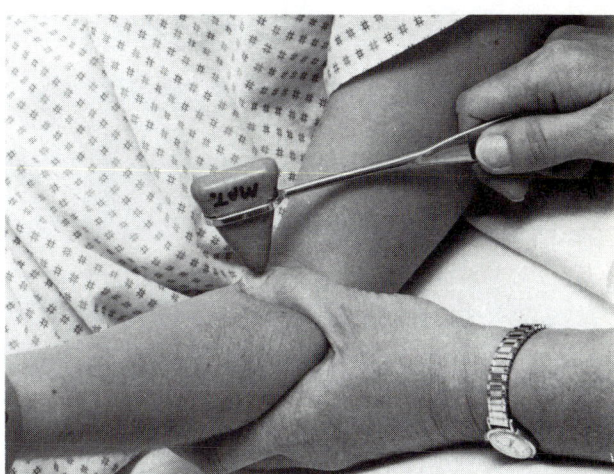

Figure 19–95 Assessing the biceps reflex.

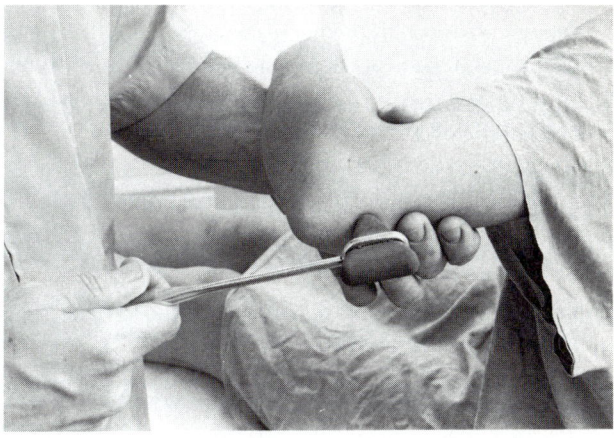

Figure 19–96 Assessing the triceps reflex.

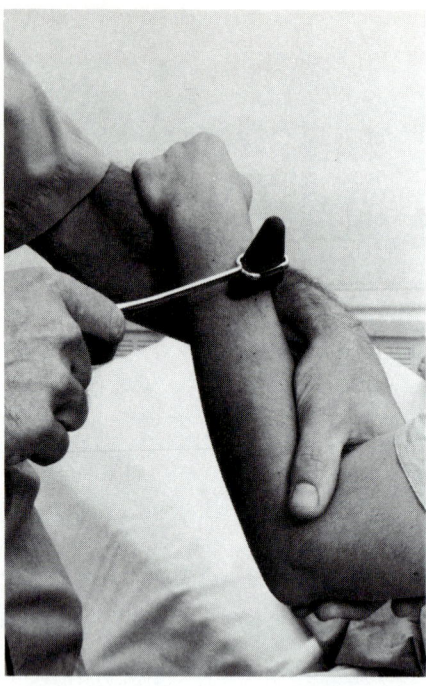

Figure 19-97 Assessing the brachioradialis reflex.

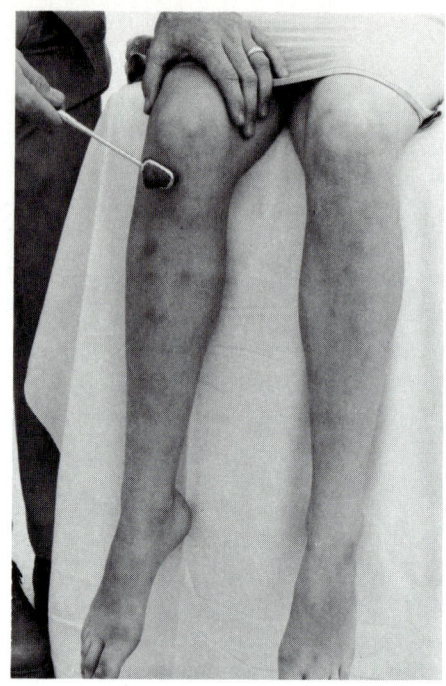

Figure 19-98 Assessing the patellar reflex.

Achilles Reflex   This reflex tests the spinal cord level S-1, S-2.

1. With the client in the same position as for the patellar reflex, slightly dorsiflex the client's ankle by grasping the toes in the palm of your hand.

2. Deliver a blow with the percussion hammer directly to the Achilles tendon just above the heel. See Figure 19-99.

3. Observe and feel the normal plantar flexion (downward jerk) of the foot.

Plantar (Babinski) Reflex   This reflex is superficial. It may be absent in adults without pathology or overridden by voluntary control.

1. Use a moderately sharp object, such as the handle of the percussion hammer, a key, or the dull end of a pin or applicator stick.

2. Stroke the lateral border of the sole of the client's foot, starting at the heel, continuing to the ball of the foot, and then proceeding across the ball of the foot toward the big toe. See Figure 19-100.

3. Observe the response. Normally, all five toes bend downward; this reaction is negative Babinski. In an abnormal Babinski response the toes spread outward and the big toe moves upward. Positive Babinski is abnormal after the child ambulates.

Motor Function

Neurologic assessment of the motor system evaluates proprioception and cerebellar function. Structures involved in proprioception are the proprioceptors, the posterior columns of the spinal cord, the cerebellum, and the vestibular apparatus (which is innervated by cranial nerve VIII) in the labyrinth of the internal ear.

Proprioceptors are sensory nerve terminals, occurring chiefly in the muscles, tendons, joints, and the internal ear, that give information about movements and position of the body. Stimuli from the proprioceptors travel through the posterior columns of the spinal cord. Deficits of function of the posterior columns of the spinal cord result in impairment of muscle and position sense. Clients with such an impairment often must watch their own arm and leg movements to ascertain the position of the limbs.

The cerebellum (a) helps to control posture; (b) acts with the cerebral cortex to make body movements smooth and coordinated; and (c) controls skeletal muscles to maintain equilibrium.

Cerebellar disorders cause certain characteristics and common symptoms: **ataxia,** impairment of position sense, lack of muscle coordination, tremors, disturbance of equilibrium, disturbance in the timing of movements, and disturbance of gait. Tremors are especially pronounced toward the end of movements. Clients with cerebellar disease also

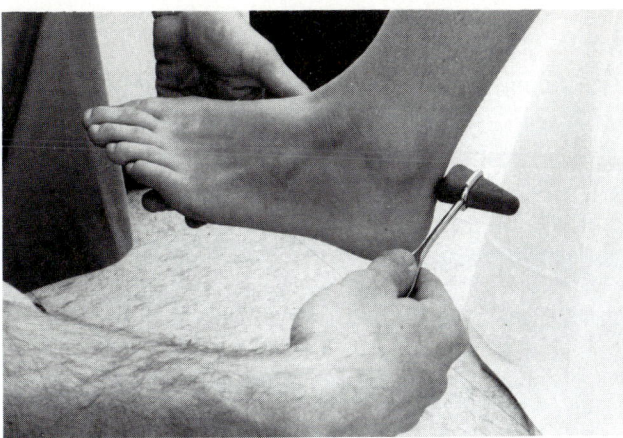

Figure 19–99 Assessing the Achilles reflex.

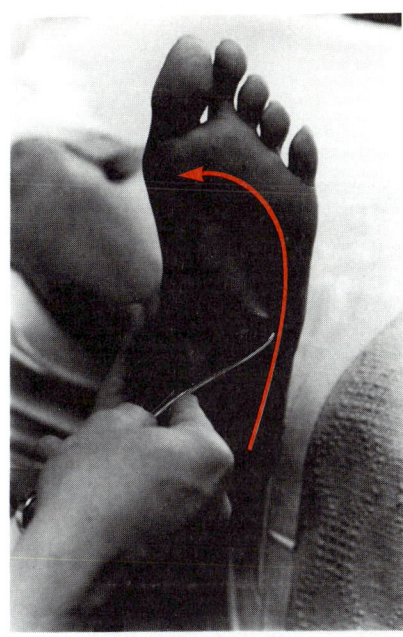

Figure 19–100 Assessing the plantar (Babinski) reflex.

have difficulty performing rapid skilled movements, alternating movements such as supinating and pronating the hands, and starting and stopping motions.

Gross Motor and Balance Tests

There are several gross motor function and balance tests (generally the Romberg test and one other is used):

1. Ask the client to walk across the room and back, and assess the client's gait.
2. Romberg test: Ask the client to stand with feet together and arms resting at the sides, first with eyes open, then closed. Stand close during this test to prevent the client from falling. A positive **Romberg's sign** is indicated by excessive swaying or an inability to maintain the stance without widening the foot base (with eyes open or shut). If the client has trouble maintaining balance with the eyes shut, the client has a loss of position sense referred to as sensory ataxia. If balance cannot be maintained whether the eyes are open or shut, the condition is referred to as cerebellar ataxia.
3. Ask the client to close the eyes and stand on one foot and then the other. Stand close to the client during this test.
4. Ask the client to walk a straight line, placing the heel of one foot directly in front of the toes of the other foot.
5. Ask the client to walk several steps on the toes and then on the heels.
6. Instruct the client to hop in place on one foot and then the other. A certain amount of muscle strength is required for this test and is not indicated for a frail or elderly client.
7. Ask the client to stretch the arms forward (in front of the body at shoulder level) and then do several knee

bends. This test also requires muscle strength and is not indicated for weak clients. See Table 19–26 for normal and abnormal findings.

Fine Motor Tests for the Upper Extremities

There are several tests of coordination of the upper extremities. In one test, the client is seated and asked to abduct and extend the arms at shoulder height and rapidly touch the nose alternately with one index finger and then the other. The client repeats the test with the eyes closed if the test is performed easily. An abnormal response is missing the nose and bringing the finger beyond the nose (past-pointing). See Figure 19–101 on page 435.

Another test is to pat both knees with the palms of both hands and then with the backs of the hands alternately at an ever-increasing rate, or to touch the nose and then the nurse's index finger, held at a distance at about 45 cm (18 in), at a rapid and increasing rate. Spreading the arms broadly at shoulder height and then bringing the fingers together at the midline, first with the eyes open and then closed, first slowly and then rapidly, also tests fine motor coordination.

In another test of fine motor coordination, the client is asked to touch each finger of one hand to the thumb of the same hand as rapidly as possible. See Figure 19–102 on page 435.

Fine Motor Tests for the Lower Extremities

Ask the client to lie supine and to carry out these actions:

TABLE 19–26 *Summary Assessment Data: Proprioception and Cerebellum*

Test	Normal Findings	Abnormal Findings
Gross Motor Function and Balance		
Walking gait	Has upright posture and steady gait with opposing arm swing; walks unaided maintaining balance	Has poor posture and unsteady, irregular, staggering gait with wide stance; bends legs only from hips; has rigid or no arm movements
Romberg test	May sway slightly but is able to maintain upright posture and foot stance	Cannot maintain foot stance; moves the feet apart to maintain stance
Standing on one foot with eyes closed	Maintains stance for at least 5 seconds	Cannot maintain stance for 5 seconds
Heel-toe walking	Maintains heel-toe walking along a straight line	Assumes a wider foot gait to stay upright
Toe or heel walking	Able to walk several steps on toes or heels	Cannot maintain balance on toes or heels
Hopping in place	Has adequate muscle strength to hop on one foot	Cannot hop or maintain single leg balance
Knee bends	Has adequate balance and muscle strength to perform knee bends	Does not have adequate balance or muscle strength to perform knee bends
Fine Motor Function: Upper Extremities		
Finger-to-nose test	Repeatedly and rhythmically touches the nose	Misses the nose or gives lazy response
Alternating supination and pronation of hands on knees	Can alternately supinate and pronate hands at rapid pace	Performs with slow, clumsy movements and irregular timing, has difficult alternating from supination to pronation
Finger to nose and to the nurse's finger	Performs with coordination and rapidity	Misses the finger and moves slowly
Fingers to fingers	As above	Moves slowly and is unable to touch fingers consistently
Fingers to thumb (same hand)	Rapidly touches each finger to thumb with each hand	Cannot coordinate this fine discrete movement with either one or both hands
Patting and polishing the nurse's hand	Performs these maneuvers smoothly and rapidly	Performs with clumsy movements and irregular timing
Fine Motor Function: Lower Extremes		
Heel down opposite shin	Demonstrates bilateral equal coordination	Has tremors, is awkward, heel moves off shin
Toe or ball of foot to the nurse's finger	Moves smoothly, with coordination	Misses the nurse's finger, is unable to coordinate movement
Figure-eight	Can perform this test	Unable to perform the test

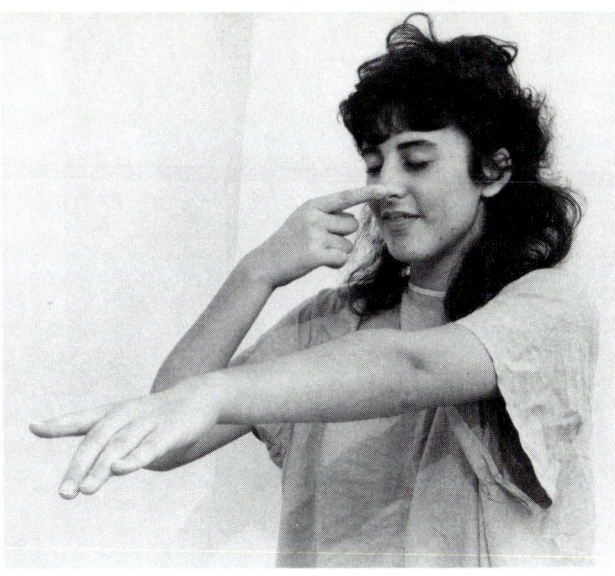

Figure 19–101   A test of fine motor coordination: touching the nose.

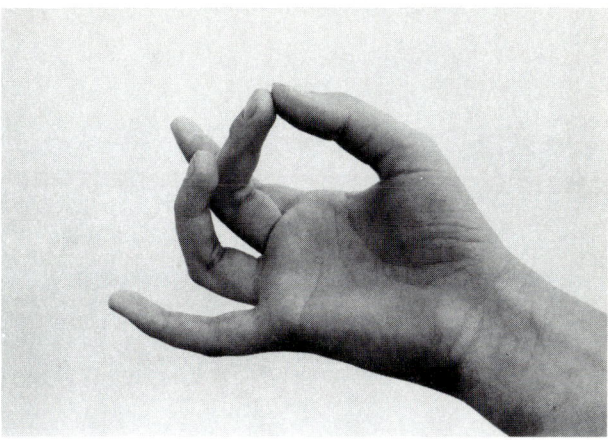

Figure 19–102   A test of fine motor coordination: touching the tip of each finger with the thumb.

1. Place the heel of one foot just below the opposite knee and run the heel down the shin to the foot. Repeat with the other foot. See Figure 19–103. (The client may also use a sitting position for this test.)
2. Touch the nurse's finger with the large toe of each foot. See Figure 19–104.

Sensory Function

Sensory functions include touch, pain, temperature, vibration, position, and tactile discrimination. The first three are routinely tested in a few locations. Vibration is tested at the wrists, elbows, knees, and ankles. Generally the face, arms, legs, hands, and feet are tested for touch and pain, although all parts of the body can be tested. If the client complains of numbness, peculiar sensations, or paralysis, sensation should be checked more carefully over flexor and extensor surfaces of limbs. Abnormality of touch or pain should then be mapped out clearly by examining responses in the area about every 2 cm (1 in). This is a lengthy procedure. A more detailed neurologic examination includes position sense, temperature sense, and tactile discrimination.

To assess sensory function, the nurse needs the following equipment:

- Wisps of cotton to assess light touch sensation
- Sterile safety pin or sterile hypodermic needle to assess pain sensation
- Large low-frequency tuning fork to assess vibratory sense
- Test tubes of hot and cold water for skin temperature assessment (optional)

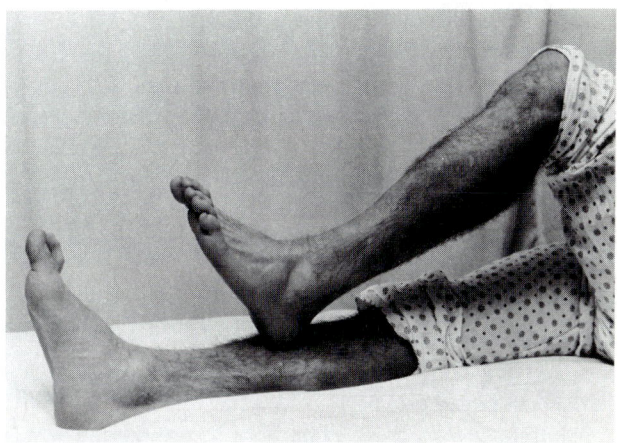

Figure 19–103   Running the heel down the shin to the foot.

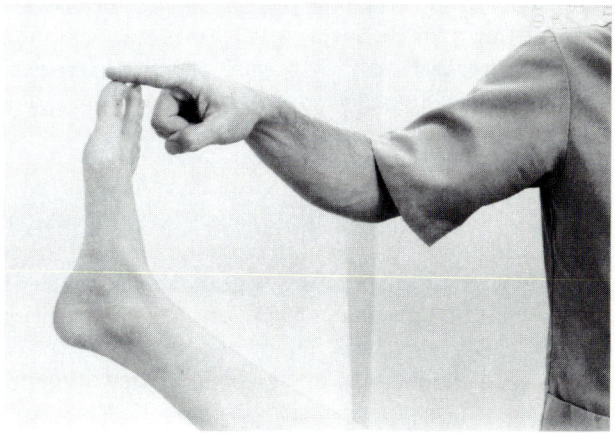

Figure 19–104   Touching the toes to the nurse's finger.

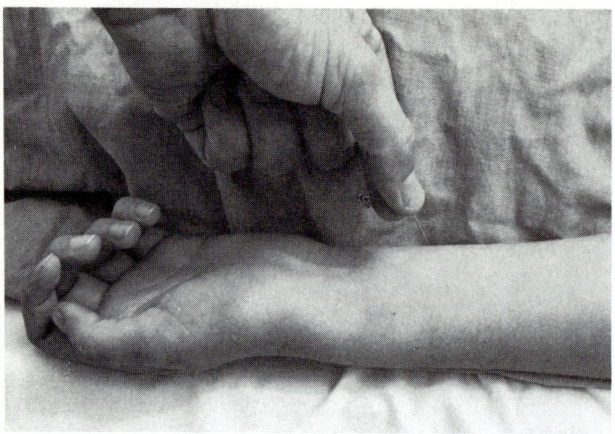

Figure 19–105 Assessing pain sensation with a pin.

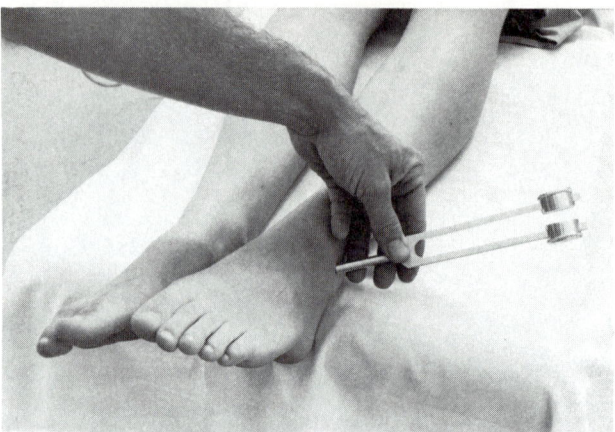

Figure 19–106 Assessing the vibratory sense.

Light Touch Sensation

To assess light touch sensation, ask the client to close the eyes and to respond by saying "yes" or "now" whenever the cotton wisp touching the skin is felt. With a wisp of cotton, lightly touch one specific spot and then the same spot on the other side of the body. Normally, a light tickling or touch sensation occurs. Sensitivity to touch varies at different skin areas, so it is important to compare the sensation of symmetric areas of the body. Test areas on the forehead, cheek, hand, lower arm, abdomen, foot, and lower leg. This ensures assessment of the major dermatome zones and peripheral nerves. A specific area of the limb is checked first (e.g., the hand before the arm and the foot before the leg), since the sensory nerve may be assumed to be intact if sensation is felt at its most peripheral part.

Ask the client to point to the spot where the touch was felt. This demonstrates whether the client is able to determine *tactile location* (point localization), i.e., can accurately perceive where the client was touched. If areas of sensory dysfunction are found, determine the boundaries of sensation by testing responses about every 2.5 cm (1 in) in the area. Make a sketch of the sensory loss area for recording purposes. Note if the response is loss of sensation to touch stimuli (**anesthesia**); more than normal sensation (**hyperesthesia**); less than normal sensation (**hypoesthesia**); or an abnormal sensation such as burning, pain, or the feel of an electric shock (**paresthesia**).

Pain Sensation

To assess the client's response to painful stimuli, ask the client to close the eyes and to say "sharp," "dull," or "don't know" when the sharp or dull end of the safety pin or needle is felt. Alternately use the sharp and dull end of the sterile pin or needle to lightly prick designated anatomic areas at random, e.g., hand, forearm, foot, lower leg, abdomen. See Figure 19–105. The face is not tested in this manner. Alternating the sharp and dull

ends of the instrument more accurately evaluates the client's response. A sterile safety pin or needle is used to avoid the risk of infection. Allow at least 2 seconds between each test to prevent summation effects of stimuli, i.e., several successive stimuli perceived as one stimulus. Note areas of reduced, heightened, or absent sensation, and map them out for recording purposes. If pain sensation is dulled or lost, assess temperature sensation in these areas. When sensations of pain are dulled, temperature sense is usually also impaired because distribution of these nerves over the body is similar.

Temperature Sensation

Temperature sensation is not routinely tested if pain sensation is found to be within normal limits. If pain sensation is not normal or is absent, testing sensitivity to temperature may prove more reliable. Touch skin areas with test tubes filled with hot or cold water. Have the client respond by saying "hot," "cold," or "don't know."

Vibratory Sense

The vibratory sense is tested with a vibrating tuning fork held firmly against a bone. Bones commonly used are in the ankle, the knee, the thumb side of the wrist, and the outside of the elbow. Routinely, the distal bones of an extremity are tested first. A person normally perceives the vibration as a buzzing or tingling sensation. In older persons (over 65 years of age), vibratory sensation may be diminished, particularly in the extremities. A large tuning fork is recommended because vibration cycles decline more slowly in a larger instrument.

1. Ask the client to close the eyes and to tell you (a) when vibrations are first felt by indicating "yes" or "now" and (b) when vibrations stop by indicating "not now" or "gone."

2. Apply the vibrating tuning fork to the designated area. See Figure 19–106.

3. Stop the vibrations between successive tests to facilitate more rapid assessment.

4. Compare the client's response to your own to confirm a normal response.

5. Compare the vibratory sensations felt on symmetric sides of the body.

6. If you believe the client is confusing the pressure of the fork against the skin with its vibrations, strike the tuning fork but place it on the client only after the vibrations stop; the client then should not report vibrations.

Position or Kinesthetic Sensation

Commonly, the middle fingers and the large toes are tested for the *kinesthetic sensation* (sense of position).

1. To test the fingers, support the client's arm with one hand, and hold the client's palm in the other; to test the toes, place the client's heels on the examining table.

2. Ask the client to close the eyes.

3. Grasp a middle finger or big toe firmly between your thumb and index finger, and exert the same pressure on both sides of the finger or toe while moving it.

4. Move the finger or toe until it is up, down, or straight out, and ask the client to identify the position.

5. Use a series of brisk up-and-down movements before coming to rest suddenly in one of the three positions. Normal persons can readily determine the position of their fingers and toes.

Tactile Discrimination

Three types of tactile discrimination are generally tested: **one- and two-point discrimination,** the ability to sense whether one or two areas of the skin are being stimulated by pressure; **stereognosis,** the act of recognizing objects by touching and manipulating them; and **extinction,** the failure to perceive touch on one side of the body when two symmetrical areas of the body are touched simultaneously. For all tests, the client's eyes need to be closed.

To assess *one- and two-point discrimination,* alternately stimulate the skin with two pins simultaneously and then with one pin. Ask whether the client feels one or two pinpricks. Wide perceptual variability occurs in adults over different parts of the body. Normally, a person can distinguish between a one- and two-point stimulus within the following minimum distances:

- Fingertips, 2.8 mm
- Palms of hands, 8 to 12 mm
- Chest, forearm, 40 mm
- Back, 50 to 70 mm
- Upper arm, thigh, 75 mm
- Toes, 3 to 8 mm

To assess *stereognosis,* place familiar objects, such as a key, paper clip, or coin, in the client's hand, and ask the client to identify them. If the client has a motor impairment of the hand and is unable to voluntarily manipulate an object, write a number or letter on the client's palm, using a blunt instrument, and ask the client to identify it. Recognition of a figure drawn on the hand is called **graphesthesia.**

To assess the *extinction phenomenon,* simultaneously stimulate two symmetrical areas of the body, such as the thighs, the cheeks, or the hands. Normally, both points of stimulus are felt. Extinction is frequently noted in clients with lesions of the sensory cortex.

Changes in the neurologic system of older adults are described in the box below.

The Elderly: Changes in the Neurologic System

- Since older clients tire more easily than younger clients, a total neurologic assessment is often done at a different time than the rest of the physical assessment.

- Although there is a progressive decrease in the number of functioning neurons in the central nervous system and sense organs, the older client usually functions well because of the abundant reserves in the number of brain cells.

- Impulse transmission and reaction to stimuli are slower in elderly clients.

- Many elderly clients generally have some impairment of hearing, vision, smell, temperature and pain sensation, memory, and mental endurance.

- Coordination changes in older clients include a reduced speed of fine finger movements. Standing balance remains intact, and Romberg's test remains negative.

- Reflex responses may be slightly increased or decreased in the older client. Many show loss of the Achilles reflex, and the plantar reflex may be difficult to elicit.

- When testing sensory function, the nurse needs to give the older client time to respond. Normally, older clients have unaltered perception of light touch and superficial pain, decreased perception of deep pain, decreased perception of temperature stimuli, and decreased vibratory sense at the ankle. Many also reveal a decrease or absence of position sense in the large toes.

FEMALE GENITALS AND REPRODUCTIVE TRACT

In adult females, the examination of the genitals and reproductive tract includes assessment of the inguinal lymph nodes, inspection and palpation of the external genitals, examination of the internal genitals by vaginal speculum, and collection of specimens.

Completeness of the assessment of the genitals and reproductive tract depends on the needs and problems of the individual client. In many practice settings, nurses perform *only* inspection of the external genitals.

Assessment of adolescent girls is limited to an inspection of the external genitals, unless the girl is sexually active. If so, an annual Papanicolaou test (Pap test) is advised for detecting cancer of the cervix and uterus. See the following section for information about taking a specimen for a Papanicolaou test. If the adolescent is sexually active and has an increased or abnormal vaginal discharge, specimens should be taken to check for sexually transmitted disease.

Examination of the genitals usually creates uncertainty and apprehension in females, and the lithotomy position required can cause embarrassment. The nurse must explain each part of the examination in advance and perform the examination in an objective and efficient manner. Appropriate draping is essential to prevent undue exposure of the client, and good lighting is essential for the nurse to ensure accuracy of inspection. The nurse wears disposable gloves for this genital examination to prevent the transfer of microorganisms from the client to the nurse and from the nurse to other clients.

Inguinal Lymph Nodes

There are two groups of superficial lymph nodes in the inguinal area: the superior (horizontal) group, and the inferior (vertical) group. See Figure 19–107. The superior group drains the skin of the abdominal wall, the external genitals, anal canal, and lower vagina. The inferior group receives lymph from the medial aspect of the leg and foot.

While the client is in a back-lying position, the nurse palpates the lymph nodes using the pads of the fingers in a rotary motion. Any enlargement or tenderness is noted.

External Genitals

Inspection of the external female genitals begins by observing the distribution, amount, and characteristics of pubic hair. Hair should be distributed in the shape of an inverse triangle. Generally, the pubic hair of menstruating adults is kinky; after menopause, it becomes sparser, straighter, more brittle, and gray in color. In the adolescent female, developmental maturity should be assessed. See the box below for the five stages of pubic hair development during puberty. Hair growth should not extend over the abdomen.

The skin of the pubic area is observed for parasites (e.g., lice), inflammation, swelling, and lesions (e.g., fissures excoriations, scars from episiotomies, varicosities, leukoplakia). To assess the pubic skin adequately, the nurse separates the labia majora. The skin of the vulvar area is slightly darker than the rest of the body. In adult females, the labia have a round, full appearance and should be relatively sym-

Figure 19–107 Lymph nodes of the groin area.

Superior or horizontal group

Inferior or vertical group

Five Stages of Pubic Hair Development in Females

- Stage 1 Preadolescence. No pubic hair except for fine body hair.

- Stage 2 Usually occurs at ages 11 and 12. Sparse, long, slightly pigmented curly hair develops along the labia.

- Stage 3 Usually occurs at ages 12 and 13. Hair becomes darker in color and curlier and develops over the pubic symphysis.

- Stage 4 Usually occurs between ages 13 and 14. Hair assumes the texture and curl of the adult but is not as thick and does not appear on the thighs.

- Stage 5 Sexual maturity. Hair assumes adult appearance and appears on the inner aspect of the upper thighs.

metric. In older females, the labia atrophy and appear flatter.

To inspect the clitoris, urethral orifice, and vaginal orifice, the nurse separates the labia minora. The *clitoris* is inspected for size and lesions. Normally, the clitoris does not exceed 1 cm in width and 2 cm in length. The clitoris is a common site for syphilitic chancres in younger females and for cancerous lesions in older females. The *urethral orifice* normally appears as a small slit just above the vaginal opening and is the same color as surrounding tissues. There should be no inflammation, swelling, or discharge. The tiny openings of *Skene's glands* (paraurethral glands) at either side of the urethral orifice are not normally visible or palpable. If inflammation or discharge is noted, these glands should be palpated (milked) to express any urethral discharge. This is done by (a) inserting a gloved index finger, palm uppermost, into the entrance of the vagina about 2.5 cm (1 in) and (b) while pressing gently upward, palpating for Skene's glands and then drawing the finger outward. This maneuver will milk the urethra of any discharge. See Figure 19–108. If discharge is present, the nurse should take a specimen and then change gloves before proceeding with further examination.

The nurse next palpates Bartholin's glands, which are normally located on the posterior aspect of the vaginal orifice and are not normally tender or palpable. See Figure 19–109. To palpate the area of Bartholin's glands, (a) insert a gloved finger into the entrance of the vagina, (b) move the finger to the side and posterior aspect of the vagina, and (c) palpate against the thumb at the posterior aspect of the labia majora. Repeat for the other side.

During this part of the examination, the integrity of the pelvic musculature is also assessed. The nurse places two gloved fingers (index and middle finger) into the vagina and proceeds as follows:

1. Ask the client to constrict her vaginal orifice. A nulliparous female (one who has never had a child) will probably have a high degree of muscle tone, whereas a multiparous female will have less tone.

2. Ask the client to bear down while the fingers spread the vaginal wall laterally. Observe the vaginal wall for bulges. A **cystocele** is a bulging of the anterior vaginal wall as a result of a prolapse of the anterior wall and the bladder. A **rectocele** is a bulging of the posterior vaginal wall as a result of a prolapse of the posterior wall and the rectum. An **enterocele** is a bulging from the posterior fornix as a result of prolapse of the pouch of Douglas into the vagina.

Internal Genitals

Examination of the internal genitals is achieved by vaginal speculum examination, which requires considerable skill and competence to prevent undue discomfort and trauma.

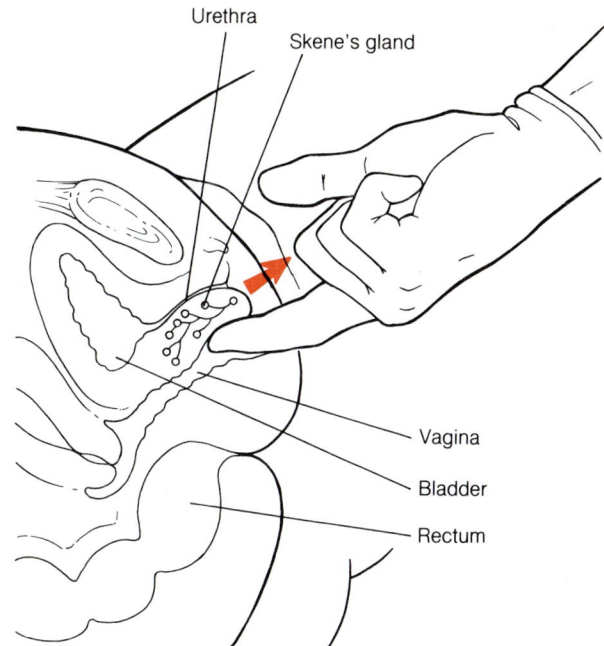

Figure 19–108   Palpating Skene's glands.

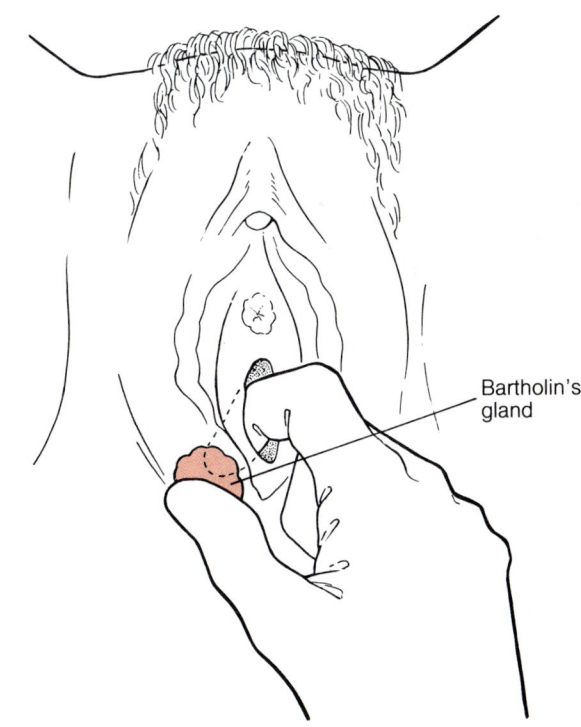

Figure 19–109   Palpating Bartholin's gland.

To perform this examination, see Procedure 19–4. Nurses do not perform vaginal examinations in some practice settings.

Changes in the genitourinary system of older females are described in the box on page 442.

PROCEDURE 19–4

PERFORMING A VAGINAL SPECULUM EXAMINATION

Equipment ☑

Good lighting (A flashlight may be necessary to view the cervix.)

Drapes to avoid undue exposure of the client

Disposable gloves

A vaginal speculum of the correct size (A virgin or a sexually inactive elderly woman will probably require a small speculum; otherwise, the size of the speculum required depends on the individual's sexual and obstetric history. See Figure 19–110.)

Warm water to lubricate the speculum

Lubricant

Supplies for cytology studies: cotton applicators, normal saline solution, an Ayre spatula (for a cervical scrape), slides, and fixative spray or solution for the specimen

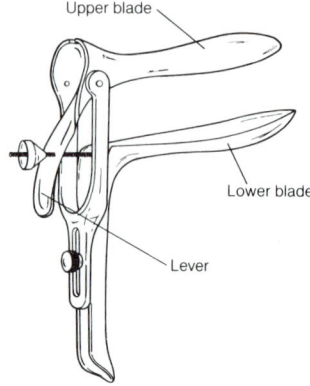

Figure 19–110 A vaginal speculum.

Intervention

1. **Prepare the client and the equipment.**

■ Assist the client to a lithotomy position as needed, and drape her appropriately.

■ Warm the speculum by running warm water over it.

■ Lubricate the vaginal speculum. Use warm water rather than lubricating jelly if a specimen is to be taken. *Lubricants can interfere with cytologic studies.*

 ■ Don gloves.

2. **Insert the vaginal speculum.**

■ Insert the index and middle fingers of the nondominant hand 2.5 cm (1 in) into the vaginal entrance.

■ Spread these fingers, and exert pressure down on the posterior wall.

■ Hold the speculum in the opposite hand, with the blades between curled index and middle fingers. See Figure 19–111.

■ Ask the client to bear down. *This helps to open the vaginal orifice more and to relax the perineal muscles.*

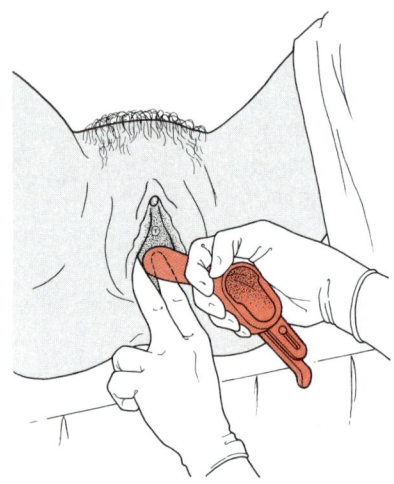

Figure 19–111 Inserting a speculum at an oblique angle into the vagina.

■ Insert the speculum obliquely and downward at a 45° angle toward the posterior wall. *This angle corresponds to the downward direction of the vagina and prevents trauma to the vaginal wall.*

■ Take care to avoid pulling pubic hair at the vaginal entrance during insertion of the speculum.

■ Once the speculum is inserted beyond the wide portions of the blade, turn it so that the handle is down, i.e., the blades are in a horizontal position. The fingers are removed simultaneously.

■ After full insertion, open the blades slowly, and observe the cervix between the blades. If the cervix is not in full view, the speculum may be either anterior or posterior to the cervix; withdraw the speculum about halfway, and reinsert it on a different plane to move it to the correct position.

■ Lock the blades in the open position.

3. **Inspect the cervix.**

■ Observe the following:

a. *Shape of the os.* The normal nulliparous cervical os is round or oval (see Figure 19–112, *A*); the normal parous os is slitlike (see Figure 19–112, *B*).

b. *Color.* Normally, the cervix glistens and is pink in color. It becomes pale after menopause. Hyperemia may indicate an inflammation.

c. *Size.* Normally, the cervix is 2 to 3 cm (about 1 in). A cervix longer than 4 cm (almost 2 in) may indicate an inflammatory condition or a tumor.

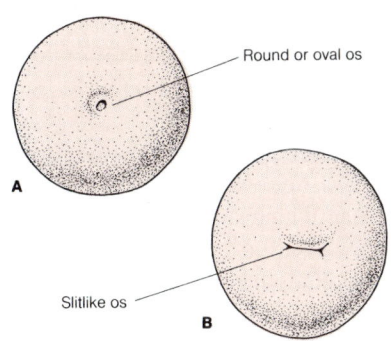

Figure 19–112 A, Appearance of the normal nulliparous cervical os. *B,* Appearance of the normal parous os.

d. *Position.* Normally, the cervix projects only slightly into the vaginal vault. One that projects further is indicative of uterine prolapse, and one that is malpositioned on a lateral wall can indicate a tumor or an adhesion.

e. *Surface characteristics.* Normally, the cervix is smooth and intact. Lacerations, erosions, nodules, masses, and discharge are abnormal.

f. *Discharge.* Characteristics of normal cervical mucus vary throughout the menstrual cycle from clear to white and from thin to thick, even stringy. Any colored or purulent discharge is abnormal.

4. Obtain a specimen for a Papanicolaou smear.

■ Collect smear samples from the three sites shown in Figure 19–113.

■ Place each smear on separate glass slides labeled 1, 2, and 3, and indicate its source.

■ Fix the specimen with a fixative spray or solution.

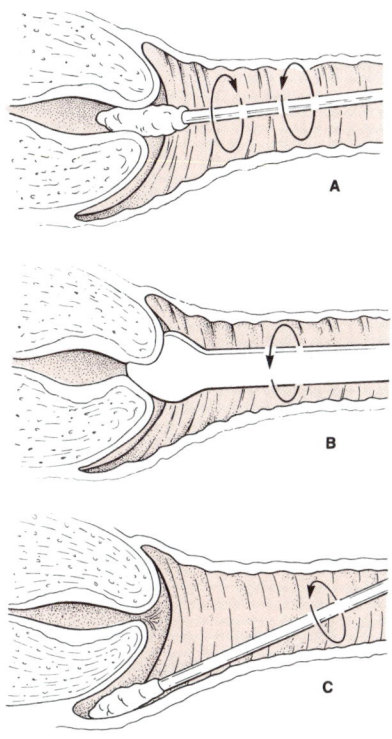

Figure 19–113 Methods for obtaining Pap smears: *A,* Endocervical. A cotton swab is inserted into the cervical os and rotated clockwise and counterclockwise in the os. *B,* Cervical scrape. An Ayre spatula with the longer end inserted into the cervical os is rotated to scrape cells from the outer surface. *C,* Vaginal smear or pool. A cotton-tipped applicator or elongated spatula is inserted along the vaginal floor.

5. Inspect the vagina while slowly withdrawing the speculum.

■ When the speculum is clear of the cervix, release the screws, and keep the blade open with the thumb.

■ During withdrawal, carefully rotate the speculum, and inspect the vaginal walls for color, texture, and vaginal secretions. Color is normally pink, texture is consistent, and vaginal secretions are thin or mucoid and odorless. Three common types of vaginal infections produce characteristic discharge. Monilial or yeast infections produce a thick, white, curdy, patchy discharge; trichomonal infections produce a profuse, watery, gray or green, frothy, odorous discharge; bacterial infections produce an odorous gray discharge.

■ Close the blades gradually as you remove the speculum, being careful not to pinch vaginal tissues or hairs in the blades. It should be closed completely when it is withdrawn from the vaginal opening.

6. Dispose of the equipment appropriately.

■ Discard a plastic speculum.

■ Rinse and soak a metal speculum in disinfectant solution.

■ Dispose of gloves unless bimanual vaginal examination is to follow.

7. Provide client comfort.

■ Clean and dry the client's perineum.

■ Assist the client as needed to a sitting position on the examining table.

MALE GENITALS

In adult males, complete examination should include assessment of the external genitals, the presence of any hernias, and the prostate gland. As with females, nurses in some practice settings performing routine assessment of clients may assess only the external genitals. The male reproductive and urinary systems (see Figure 19–114) share the urethra, which is the passageway for both urine and semen. Therefore, in physical assessment of the male, these two systems are frequently assessed together.

Examination of the male genital organs by a female practitioner (physician or nurse) is becoming increasingly common. Formerly, most examinations of men were done by men. Most male clients accept examination by a female, especially if she is emotionally comfortable herself about performing it and does so in a matter-of-fact and competent manner. If the female nurse does not feel comfortable about this part of the examination or if the client is reluctant to be examined by a female, the nurse should refer this part of the examination to a male practitioner.

The techniques of inspection and palpation are used to examine the male genitals. Equipment needed includes gloves and a penlight to transilluminate any mass. The client may be in a lying or sitting position.

Inspection of the male genitals begins with an assessment of the distribution, amount, and characteristics of pubic hair. Normal pubic hair distribution is triangular, often spreading up the abdomen. Very thin hair or absence of hair in adults should be reported. Development of secondary sex characteristics is also assessed in relationship to the client's age. See Table 19–27 for the five stages of the development of pubic hair, the penis, and the testes/scrotum during puberty.

Penis

The penile shaft, glans, and urethral meatus are inspected for lesions, nodules, swelling, inflammation, and discharge. The penile skin normally appears slightly wrinkled and varies in color as widely as other body skin. The *foreskin* (if present) should be easily retractable from the glans penis. To assess this retractability, the nurse retracts the foreskin or asks the client to do so. A small amount of thick white smegma is normally seen between the glans and the foreskin. The *urethral meatus* should appear pink and slitlike and should be positioned at the tip of the penis. Variations in its location are **hypospadias,** on the underside of the penile shaft, and **epispadias,** on the upper side of the penile shaft. Inspect the urethral meatus and the glans for ulcers, scars, nodules, inflammation, and discharge. Compress or ask the client to compress the glans slightly to open the urethral meatus to inspect it for discharge. If the client has reported a discharge, instruct the client to *strip the penis* from the base to the urethra. To strip the penis, the client grasps the base of the penis with thumb at the front and fingers behind and, while applying a moderate pressure, moves the thumb and fingers slowly down the shaft of the penis. If there is evidence of abnormal discharge, a specimen for culture is usually obtained. The shaft of the penis may be palpated (using the thumb and first two fingers) for tenderness, thickening, and nodules. The penis should feel smooth and semifirm and is slightly movable over the underlying structures.

Scrotum

Monthly testicular self-examination is an essential practice for detecting testicular cancer. Client instructions for this examination are provided in Chapter 26, page 650. To facilitate inspection of the scrotum during a physical examination, the nurse instructs the client to hold the penis out of the way. Observations of appearance, general size, and symmetry are made. Scrotal skin is darker in color than that of the rest of the body and is loose (any tightening may indicate edema or a mass). All skin surfaces are inspected by spreading the rugated surface skin and lifting the scrotum as needed to observe posterior surfaces. The size of the scrotum normally varies with temperature changes since the dartos muscles contract when the area is cold and relax when the area is warm. The scrotum normally appears asymmetric because the left testis is usually lower than the right testis.

The scrotum is palpated to assess the status of the underlying testes, epididymis, and spermatic cord. Both testes are often palpated simultaneously for comparative purposes. The nurse carries out the palpation procedure as follows:

1. Palpate the scrotum and testicles. Using your first two fingers and thumb, palpate each testis for size, consistency, shape, smoothness, and masses. The testicle normally feels rubbery and smooth and is free of nodules or masses. Each testis is normally about 2 × 4 cm (0.7 × 1.5 in). During assessment of male adolescents, it is most important to establish the descent of the testicles into the scrotum; undescended testes are noted.

2. Palpate the epididymis between your thumb and index finger. It is located at the top of the testis and extends behind it. The epididymis is resilient, normally tender, and softer than the spermatic cord.

3. Palpate the spermatic cord between thumb and index finger. It is usually found at the top lateral portion of the scrotum and feels firm.

If swelling, irregularities, or nodules are detected during the scrotal examination, the nurse attempts to transillumi-

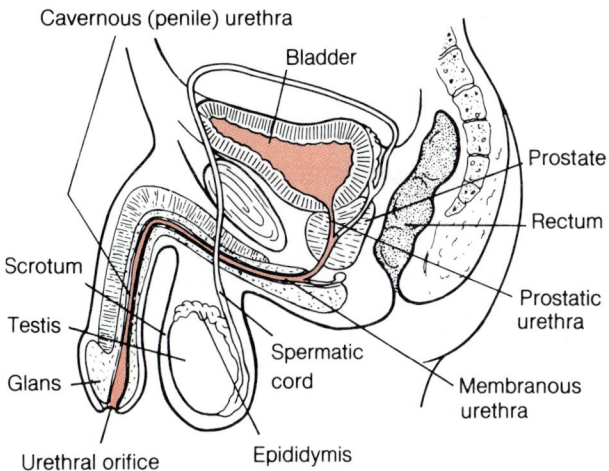

Figure 19–114 The male urogenital tract.

nate the lesion. This is done by darkening the room and shining a flashlight from behind the scrotum through the mass. Serous fluid causes the light to show with a red glow; tissue or blood does not transilluminate. The description of all scrotal masses should include their size, shape, placement, consistency, tenderness, and presence of transillumination.

Inguinal Area

All clients should be screened for the presence of inguinal or femoral hernias. A **hernia** is a protrusion of the intestine through the inguinal wall or canal. The loop of bowel may even extend down to the scrotum. Structures of the inguinal canal are shown in Figure 19–115. An *indirect inguinal*

TABLE 19–27 *Five Stages of Development of Pubic Hair, Penis, and Testes/Scrotum (12 to 16 Years)*

Stage	Pubic Hair	Penis	Testes/Scrotum
1 (pre-adolescent)	None, except for body hair like that on the abdomen	Size is relative to body size, as in childhood	Size is relative to body size, as in childhood
2	Scant, long, slightly pigmented at base of penis	Slight enlargement occurs	Becomes reddened in color and enlarged
3	Darker, begins to curl and becomes more coarse; extends over pubic symphysis	Elongation occurs	Continuing enlargement
4	Continues to darken and thicken; extends on the sides, above and below	Increase in both breadth and length; glans develops	Continuing enlargement; color darkens
5	Adult distribution that extends to inner thighs, umbilicus, and anus	Adult appearance	Adult appearance

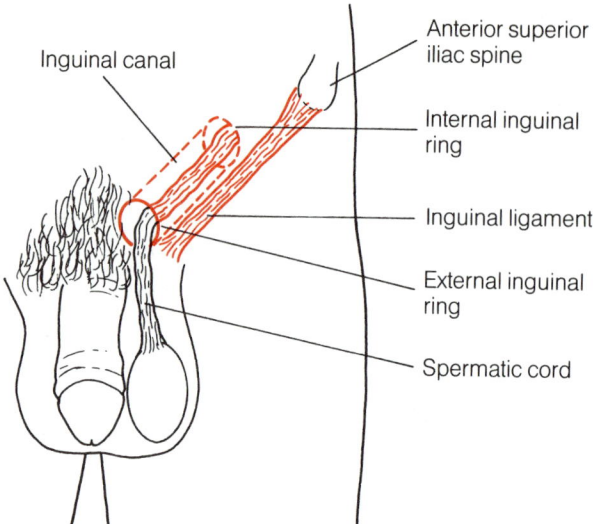

Figure 19–115   Structures of the inguinal area.

The Elderly: Changes in the Male Genitourinary System

Genitals

- The penis decreases in size with age; the size and firmness of the testes decrease.

- Testosterone is produced in smaller amounts.

- More time and direct physical stimulation are required for the older male to achieve an erection, but the elderly man can maintain the erection for longer periods before ejaculation than he could at a younger age.

- Seminal fluid is reduced in amount and viscosity.

Urinary Bladder

- In the elderly male client, urinary frequency, nocturia, dribbling, and problems with beginning and ending the stream are usually the result of prostatic enlargement.

hernia is a loop of bowel that enters the internal inguinal ring. It may stay in the canal, exit through the external ring, or pass into the scrotum. A *direct inguinal hernia* enters the inguinal canal directly through a weakness in the abdominal wall just behind the external inguinal ring. It does not pass through the inguinal canal. A *femoral hernia* is more common in women. It is lower and more lateral than an inguinal hernia and may look like an enlarged lymph node.

Assessment for hernias involves both inspection and palpation techniques. Whenever possible, these assessments are performed when the client is standing. Both inguinal

areas are observed for bulges (a) while the client is at rest and (b) while the client holds the breath and strains or bears down as though having a bowel movement. Bearing down may make the hernia more visible.

To palpate a *direct* inguinal hernia, the nurse advances the index finger into the loose scrotal skin and over the external inguinal ring. See Figure 19–116. The left finger is used to examine the client's left side; the right finger is used to examine the client's right side. The client is then instructed to bear down. If a hernia is present, a palpable bulge will appear in the area. To palpate an *indirect* inguinal hernia, the nurse attempts to move the index or little finger into the path of the inguinal canal while the client flexes the knee on the same side. When the examining finger has moved as far as possible the client is again asked to bear down. This indirect hernia, if present, will be felt as a mass of tissue touching the finger and withdrawing from it. To detect a *femoral* hernia, the nurse palpates the inguinal area directly, again both at rest and while bearing down.

Changes in the genitourinary system of elderly males are described in the box above.

RECTUM AND ANUS

Rectal examination, an essential part of every comprehensive physical examination, involves inspection and palpation (digital examination). The extent of the assessment of the rectum and anus depends on the rectal problems stated by the client in the nursing history. In many practice settings, the nurse performs only inspection of the anus. An

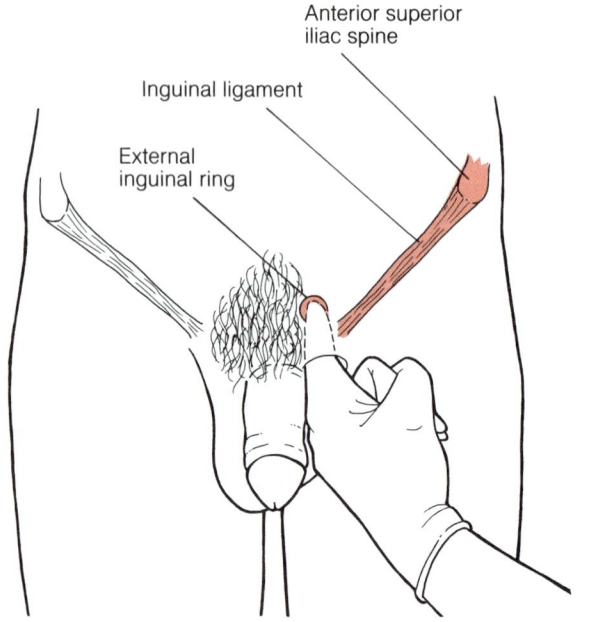

Figure 19–116   Palpating for the presence of an inguinal hernia.

interior view of the rectum and anal canal are shown in Figure 42–4 on page 1157.

A left lateral or Sims position with the upper leg acutely flexed is required for the examination. For females, a dorsal recumbent position with hips externally rotated and knees flexed or a lithotomy position may also be used. For males, a standing position while the client bends over the examining table may also be used. This position is commonly used to examine the prostate gland. For all rectal examinations the nurse should wear gloves (Malasanos, Barkauskas, and Stoltenberg-Allen 1990, p. 389).

Inspection

To inspect the anus and surrounding tissue, the nurse spreads the buttocks with both hands. Anal skin is normally more pigmented, coarser, and moister than the perianal skin. It is also usually hairless. The perianal skin should be intact and is usually slightly more pigmented than the skin of the buttocks. During inspection, the nurse assesses the perianal region for skin lesions such as fissures (cracks), ulcers, excoriations, inflammation, abscesses; protruding *hemorrhoids* (dilated veins seen as reddened protrusions of the skin); lumps or tumors; fistula openings; and *rectal prolapse* (varying degrees of protrusion of the rectal mucous membrane through the anus).

The nurse then instructs the client to bear down as though defecating. Bearing down creates slight pressure on the skin that may accentuate rectal fissures, rectal prolapse, polyps or internal hemorrhoids. The location of all abnormal findings are described in terms of a clock, with the 12 o'clock position toward the pubic symphysis.

Palpation (Digital Examination)

Because digital examination can cause apprehension and embarrassment in the client, it is important that the nurse (a) help the client relax by encouraging the client to take slow, deep breaths (tension can cause spasms of the anal sphincters, making the examination uncomfortable), (b) inform the client about potential sensations such as feelings of defecation or passing gas, (c) assure the client that an accident is very unlikely, (d) proceed with the examination in a competent and gentle way, and (e) drape the client appropriately to prevent undue exposure of body parts.

To perform rectal palpation, the nurse lubricates the index finger, instructs the client to bear downward as though having a bowel movement (this relaxes the anal sphincter), and slowly inserts the finger into the anus and into the rectum in the direction of the umbilicus. The anal canal (distance from the anal opening to the anorectal junction) is short—less than 3 cm (about 1 in). The posterior wall of the rectum follows the curve of the coccyx and sacrum. The nurse's finger is usually able to palpate a distance of 6 to 10 cm (over 2 to 4 in). The nurse should never force digital insertion. If lesions are painful or bleeding occurs, the examination should be discontinued.

In this palpation procedure, the nurse initially instructs the client to tighten the anal sphincter around the nurse's

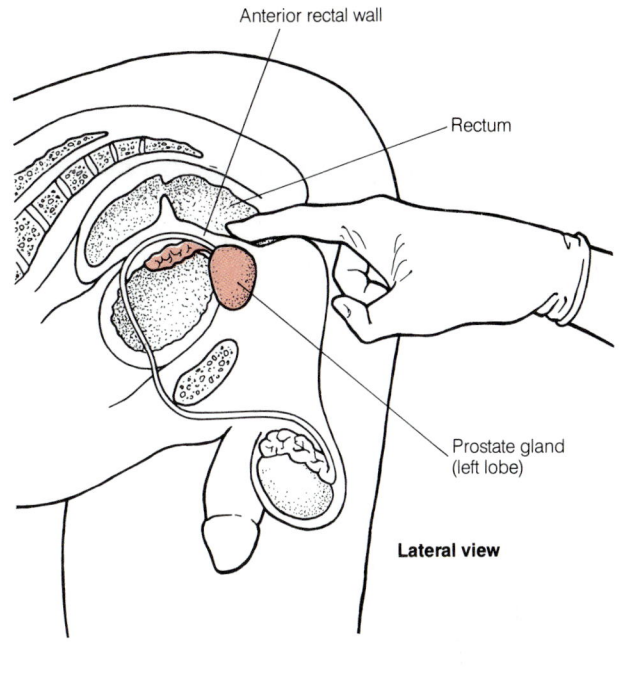

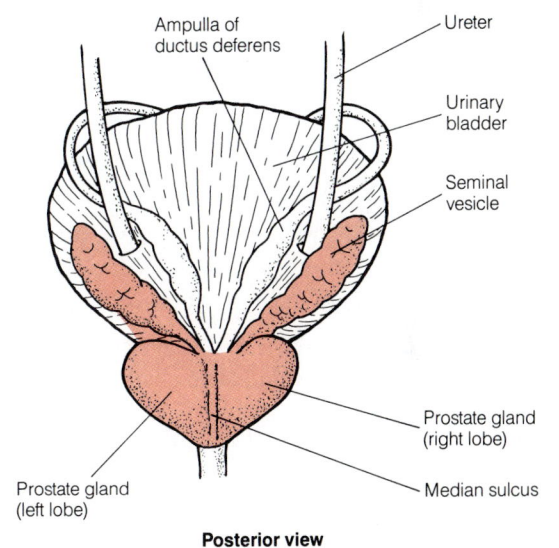

Figure 19–117 Palpating the prostate gland through the anterior wall of the rectum.

finger and notes the tone of the anal sphincter. Hypertonicity of the sphincter may occur in the presence of an anal fissure or other lesion that causes contraction; hypotonicity may occur after rectal surgery or result from a neurologic deficiency. The nurse then rotates the pad of the index finger along the anal and rectal walls, feeling for nodules, masses, and tenderness. Normally, the wall is smooth and not tender. Note the location of any abnormalities of the rectum (e.g., anterior wall, 2 cm proximal to the internal anal sphincter). The coccyx is also palpated to determine mobility and sensitivity.

In the male, the prostate gland can be palpated through the anterior wall of the rectum. See Figure 19–117. The

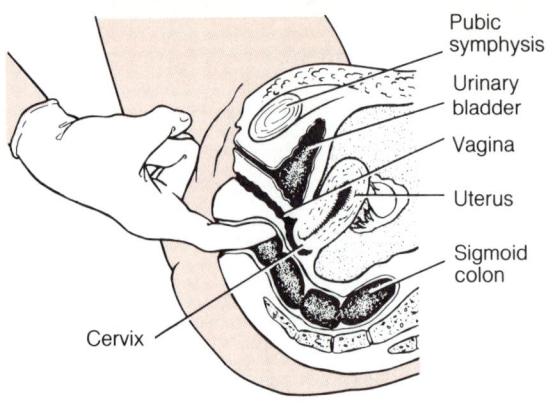

Figure 19–118 Palpating the cervix through the anterior rectal wall.

nurse should be able to feel the median sulcus, which divides the gland into two lobes. The prostate should be about 4 cm (1½ in) in diameter, firm and rubbery, smooth, and mobile. The edges are discrete. The client does not normally experience tenderness during the exam.

In the female, the cervix of the uterus can be palpated through the anterior rectal wall. See Figure 19–118. The cervix normally feels smooth, round, firm, and movable. It is not normally tender.

Upon withdrawing the finger from the rectum and anus, observe it for feces. Feces are normally brown. Observe the feces for the presence of any mucus, blood, or black tarry stool. A small quantity of feces can be tested for occult blood. See Chapter 42, page 1164.

CHAPTER HIGHLIGHTS

▶ The health examination is conducted to assess the function and integrity of the client's body parts.

▶ It may entail a complete head-to-toe assessment or individual assessment of a body system or body part.

▶ The health assessment is conducted in a systematic manner that requires the fewest position changes for the client.

▶ Aspects of physical assessment procedures should be incorporated in the assessment, intervention, and evaluation phases of the nursing process.

▶ Data obtained in the physical health examination supplement, confirm, or refute data obtained during the nursing history.

▶ Nursing history data help the nurse focus on specific aspects of the physical health examination.

▶ Data obtained in the physical health examination help the nurse establish nursing diagnoses, plan the client's care, and evaluate the outcomes of nursing care.

▶ Initial assessment findings provide baseline data about the client's functional abilities against which subsequent assessment findings are compared.

▶ Skills in inspection, palpation, percussion, and auscultation are required for the physical health examination; these skills are used in that order throughout the examination except during abdominal assessment, when auscultation follows inspection and precedes percussion and palpation.

▶ Knowledge of the normal structure and function of body parts and systems is an essential requisite to conducting physical assessment.

READINGS AND REFERENCES

SUGGESTED READINGS

Berliner, H. October 1986 and November 1986. Aging skin. (2 parts.) *American Journal of Nursing* 86:1138–41; 1259–61.

In the first article of this two-part series, Berliner focuses on "itchy" skin lesions. Included are asteatoic eczema, contact dermatitis, tinea pedis, onychomycosis, seborrheic dermatitis, seborrheic keratosis, bullous pemphigoid, herpes zoster, and psoriasis. Color photographs of most lesions are provided.

In the second article, Berliner discusses skin lesions of unusual consistency, color, or shape. Included are xanthelasma (fatty deposits on the eyelids), lentigo (freckles or liver spots), acrochordons (skin tags), actinic (solar) keratosis, corns, leukoplakia, stasis dermatitis, rhinophyma (cobblestone nose), various blood lesions such as spider angiomas and senile purpura, and basal and squamous cell carcinoma. Color photographs of most lesions are provided.

McConnell, E. A. August 1988. Getting the feel of lymph node assessment. *Nursing 88* 18:54–57.

An enlarged lymph node can be the first sign of a serious problem. McConnell reviews the proper technique for detecting this early warning sign. She discusses characteristics of lymph nodes, major lymph node groups and the areas they drain, and inspection and palpation techniques.

Smith, C. E. February 1988. Assessing bowel sounds: More than just listening. *Nursing 88* 18:42–43.

In this article, Smith discusses when to assess bowel sounds, how to inspect the abdomen, the sounds of peristalsis, hypoactive and hyperactive sounds, and percussion and palpation techniques.

Stevens, S. A., and Becker, K. L. September 1988 and October 1988. A simple, step-by-step approach to neurologic assessment. (2 parts.) *Nursing 88* 18:53–61; 51–58.

The first article of this two-part series discusses the first three of five areas in a neurologic screening examination: mental status, cranial nerves, and deep tendon reflexes. The second article provides a discussion of tests for assessing the client's motor and sensory systems.

SELECTED REFERENCES

Bates, B. 1987. *A guide to physical examination.* 4th ed. Philadelphia: J. B. Lippincott.

Becker, K. L. March 1988. Get in touch and in tune with cardiac assessment, Part 1. *Nursing 88* 18:51–55.

Becker, K. L., and Stevens, S. A. June 1988. Performing in-depth abdominal assessment. *Nursing 88* 18:59–63.

Block, G. J., and Nolan, J. W. 1986. *Health assessment for professional nursing: A developmental approach.* 2d ed. Norwalk, Conn.: Appleton-Century-Crofts.

Bowers, A. C., and Thompson, J. M. 1988. *Clinical manual of health assessment.* 3d ed. St. Louis. C. V. Mosby Co.

Burggraf, V., and Donlon, B. September 1985. Assessing the elderly, system by system. Part 1. *American Journal of Nursing* 85:974–84.

Dennison, R. April 1986. Cardiopulmonary assessment. *Nursing 86* 16:34–39.

Ebersole, P., and Hess, P. 1989. *Toward healthy aging.* 3d ed. St. Louis: C. V. Mosby Co.

Erickson, B. A. January 1986. Detecting abnormal heart sounds. *Nursing 86* 16:58–64.

Hays, A. M., and Borger, F. October 1985. Assessing the elderly: A test in time. Part 2. *American Journal of Nursing* 85:1107–11.

Henderson, M. L. October 1985. Assessing the elderly: Altered presentations. Part 2. *American Journal of Nursing* 85:1103–6.

Malasanos, L.; Barkauskas, V.; and Stoltenberg-Allen, K. 1990. *Health assessment.* 4th ed. St. Louis: C. V. Mosby Co.

Miracle, V. A. April 1988. Get in touch and in tune with cardiac assessment, Part 2. *Nursing 88* 18:41–47.

Nettles-Carlson, B. September/October 1989. Early detection of breast cancer . . . mammography, clinical breast examination (CBE) and breast self-examination. *Journal of Obstetric, Gynecologic, and Neonatal Nursing* 18:373–81.

Parrino, T. A. September 30, 1987. The art and science of percussion. *Hospital Practice* 22:25–28, 32, 34.

Rice, E. M. May/June 1989. Geriatric assessment. *Advances in Clinical Care* 4:8–15.

Robson, J. K.; Larkin, F.; Bursick, J. H.; and Perri, K. P. December 1975. Growth standards for infants and children: A cross-sectional study. *Pediatrics* 56:1017–18.

Santo-Novak, D. A. August 1988. Seven keys to assessing the elderly. *Nursing 88* 18:60–63.

Saul, L. December 1983. Heart sounds and common murmurs. *American Journal of Nursing* 83:1679–89.

Stark, J. L. July 1988. A quick guide to urinary tract assessment. *Nursing 88* 18:56–58.

Stevens, S. A., and Becker, K. L. January 1988. How to perform picture-perfect respiratory assessment. *Nursing 88* 18:57–63.

Taylor, D. L. January 1985. Clinical applications: Assessing heart sounds. *Nursing 85* 15:51–53.

———. March 1985. Clinical applications: Assessing breath sounds. *Nursing 85* 15:60–62.

PROTECTING HEALTH

CHAPTER

20

Preventing the Transfer of Microorganisms

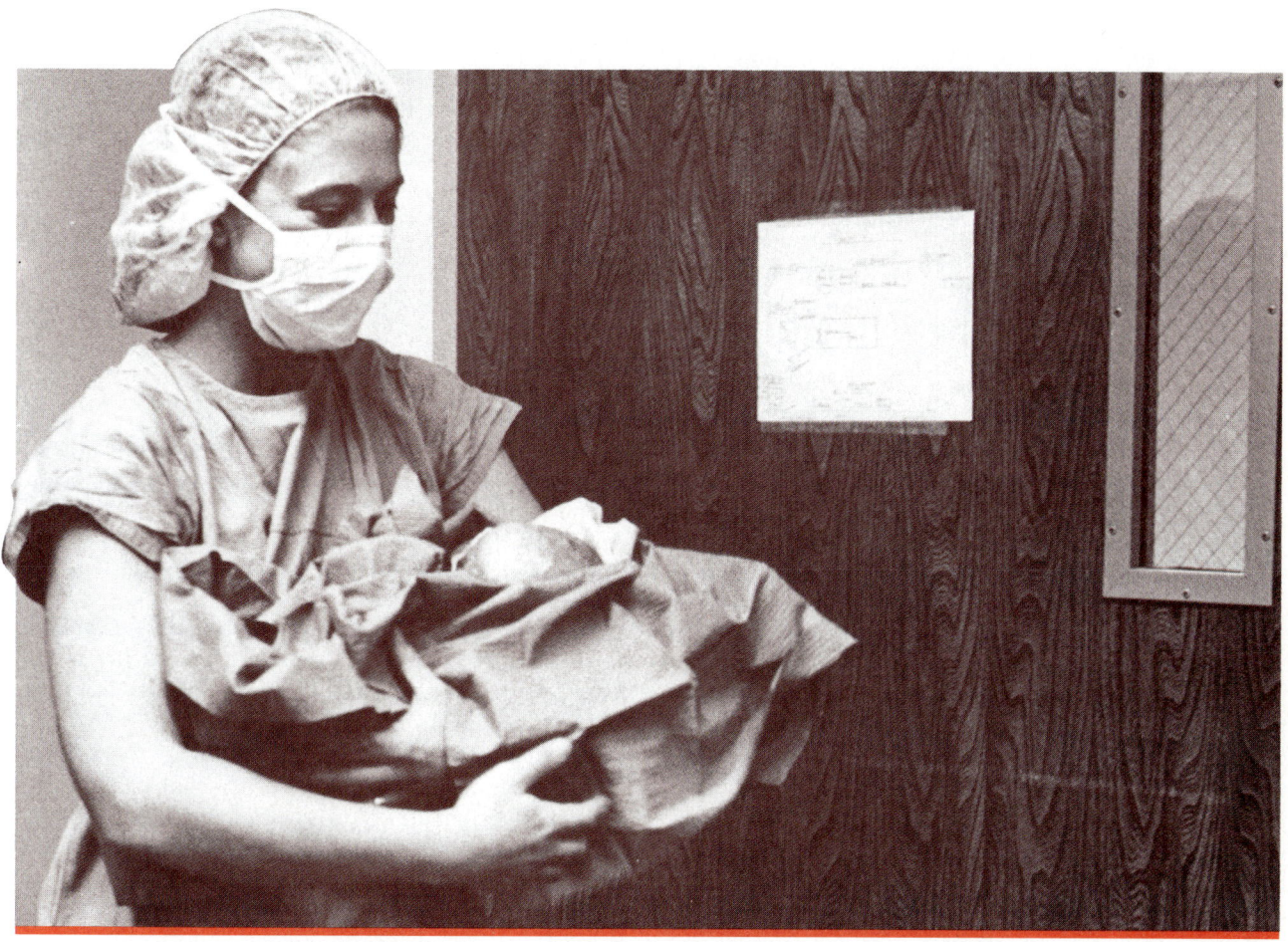

CONTENTS

CONTENTS (continued)

OBJECTIVES

▸ Describe the importance of biologic safety.

▸ Identify anatomic and physiologic barriers that defend the body against microorganisms.

▸ Describe the difference between nonspecific and specific defenses of the body.

▸ Differentiate active from passive immunity.

▸ Identify six links in the chain of infection.

▸ Identify measures that break each link in the chain of infection.

▸ Identify factors influencing a microorganism's capability to produce an infectious process.

▸ Identify people at risk of acquiring an infection.

▸ Describe four stages of an infectious process.

▸ Identify causal factors of nosocomial infections.

▸ Identify signs of localized and systemic infections.

▸ Identify relevant nursing diagnoses and contributing factors for clients at risk for infection and who have an infection.

▸ Develop outcome criteria to evaluate a client's response to nursing interventions and achievement of goals.

▸ Explain the concepts of medical and surgical asepsis.

▸ Identify interventions to prevent infections.

▸ Identify interventions to protect body defenses.

▸ Discuss methods for evaluating the effectiveness of protective measures.

IMPORTANCE OF BIOLOGIC SAFETY

Nurses are directly involved in providing a biologically safe environment and promoting health. Microorganisms exist everywhere in the environment: in water, soil, and on body surfaces such as the skin, intestinal tract, and other areas open to the outside (e.g., mouth, upper respiratory tract, vagina, and lower urinary tract). Most microorganisms are harmless, and some are even beneficial in that they perform essential functions in the body. Some microorganisms found in the intestines, i.e., enterobacteria, produce substances called **bacteriocins,** which are lethal to related strains of bacteria. Others produce antibiotic-like substances and toxic metabolites that repress the growth of other microorganisms. Some microorganisms are normal **flora** (the collective vegetation in a given area) in one part of the body and produce infection in another. For example, *Escherichia coli* is a normal inhabitant of the large intestine but a common cause of infection of the urinary tract.

An **infection** is an invasion of body tissue by microorganisms and their proliferation there. Such a microorganism is called an infectious agent. If the microorganism produces no clinical evidence of disease, the infection is called *asymptomatic* or *subclinical*. Some subclinical infections can cause significant damage to the host, e.g., cytomegalovirus (CMV) infection in a pregnant woman. A detectable alteration in normal tissue function, however, is

called **disease.** Microorganisms vary in their **virulence** (i.e., their ability to produce disease). In general, five groups of microorganisms normally can cause disease: bacteria, viruses, fungi, protozoa, and *Rickettsia.*

Microorganisms also vary in the severity of the diseases they produce and their degree of communicability. For example, the common cold virus is more readily transmitted than the bacillus that causes leprosy (*Mycobacterium leprae*). If the infectious agent can be transmitted to an individual by direct or indirect contact, through a vector or vehicle, or as an airborne infection, the resulting condition is called a **communicable disease.**

Trauma is injury to the body. Trauma can be physical, such as a cut by a piece of glass; trauma also describes injury caused by invading microorganisms. Thus, an infectious process can be described as trauma. Often, the trauma of infection follows physical trauma, as when a cut becomes infected.

Pathogenicity means the ability to produce disease; thus, a pathogen is a microorganism that causes disease. No microorganism produces disease 100% of the time. However, many microorganisms that are normally harmless can cause disease under certain circumstances. A "true" pathogen causes disease or infection in a healthy individual. An **opportunistic pathogen** causes disease only in a susceptible individual.

Etiology is the study of causes; the etiology of an infectious process is the identification of the invading microorganisms. The control of the spread of microorganisms and the protection of people from communicable diseases and infections are practiced on four levels: international, national, community, and individual. An example of infectious disease control at the international level is required immunization against certain diseases, such as cholera, before travel to certain countries. Similarly, international health regulations govern the immunizations required of American and Canadian citizens returning home. National regulations govern, for example, the interstate and interprovincial transportation of food. These regulations protect people from receiving contaminated food. Also, national regulations attempt to control pollution of water, the air, and the environment, subjects currently receiving much publicity.

Communities regulate the disposal of sewage and the purity of drinking water, for example. Such community regulations protect people from infectious disease. Protection from infection is also an individual responsibility. Individuals protect themselves not only by practicing good hygiene (see Chapter 22) but also by eating a balanced diet and exercising.

NORMAL BODY DEFENSES

The human normally has microbial flora that reside in and outside the body, e.g., on the skin, on mucous membranes, inside the respiratory passages, and inside the gastrointestinal tract. These microorganisms are called **resident flora** because they are always present, usually in numbers compatible with the individual's health. See Table 20–1 on page 454. In contrast to resident flora, **transient flora** are microorganisms that are present episodically.

Individuals normally have defenses that protect the body from infection. These defenses can be categorized as nonspecific and specific. **Nonspecific defenses** protect the person against all microorganisms, regardless of prior exposure. **Specific (immune) defenses,** by contrast, are directed against identifiable bacteria, viruses, fungi, or other infectious agents.

Nonspecific Defenses

Nonspecific body defenses include anatomic and physiologic barriers. *Intact skin and mucous membranes* are the body's first line of defense against microorganisms. Unless the skin and mucosa become cracked and broken, they are an effective barrier against bacteria. Fungi can live on the skin, but they cannot penetrate it. The dryness of the skin also is a deterrent to bacteria; they are most plentiful in moist areas, e.g., perineum and axillae. Another deterrent is sebum, which contains an unsaturated fatty acid that kills

some bacteria. Resident bacteria of the skin also prevent other bacteria from multiplying. They use up the available nourishment, and the end products of their metabolism inhibit other bacteria. Normal secretions make the skin slightly acidic; acidity also inhibits bacterial growth.

The *nasal passages* have a defensive function. As entering air follows the tortuous route of the passage, it comes in contact with moist mucous membranes and small hairlike projections called *cilia*. These trap microorganisms, dust, and foreign materials. The *lungs* have alveolar **macrophages** (large phagocytes). **Phagocytes** are cells, e.g., white blood cells, that ingest microorganisms, other cells, and foreign particles. Healthy lungs are free of microorganisms. The central nervous system is protected by the skull and spinal column, which prevent microbial entry.

Each body orifice also has protective mechanisms. The *oral cavity* regularly sheds mucosal epithelium to rid the mouth of colonizers. The flow of saliva and its partially buffering action help prevent infections. Saliva contains microbial inhibitors, e.g., lactoferrin, lysozyme, and secretory IgA. **Lactoferrin** is an iron-binding protein that inhibits the growth of invading microorganisms by making iron unavailable to them. The enzyme **lysozyme,** present in saliva and tears, functions as an antibacterial agent. Secretory IgA (SIGA) is an immunoglobulin that coats bacteria and thus prevents their attachment to the oral epithelium and to the teeth.

The *eye* is protected from infection by tears, which continually wash microorganisms away and contain inhibiting lysozyme. The *gastrointestinal tract* also has defenses against infection. The high acidity of the stomach normally prevents microbial growth. The role that the normal microorganisms of the small intestine play in the body's defense is unknown. However, the resident flora of the large intestine help prevent the establishment of disease-producing microorganisms. Many enterobacteria produce bacteriocins that are lethal to closely related bacterial strains. Some enterobacteria release an antibiotic-like substance that kills or inhibits the growth of some bacteria.

The *vagina* also has natural defenses against infection. When a girl reaches puberty, lactobacilli ferment sugars in the vaginal secretions, creating a vaginal pH of 3.5 to 4.5. This low pH inhibits the growth of many disease-producing microorganisms. A reasonably healthy female normally has a relatively constant number of these lactobacilli in the vagina. However, antibiotic therapy can upset the bacterial balance because the lactobacilli are highly susceptible to antibiotics. **Colonization** (the process by which strains of bacteria become resident flora) by *Candida albicans* (yeast) often results. The *entrance to the urethra* normally harbors many microorganisms, e.g., "negative staph" (*Staphylococcus epidermidis* coagulase from the skin) and *Escherichia coli* (from feces). It is believed that the urine has a flushing and bacteriostatic action that keeps the bacteria from ascending the urethra.

TABLE 20–1 *Common Resident Bacteria of the Body*

Body Area	Bacteria	Comment
Skin	*Staphylococcus epidermidis*	Normally nonpathogenic
	Propionibacterium acnes	Uses skin fat and oil for growth
	Staphylococcus aureus	Potential pathogen
	Corynebacterium xerosis	Most numerous in axilla
	Pityrosporum oxale (yeast)	Found on scalp and oily skin
Nasal passages	*Staphylococcus aureus*	Potential pathogen
	Staphylococcus epidermidis	
Oropharynx	*Streptococcus pneumoniae*	Potential pathogen
Bronchi, lungs	None	
Mouth	*Streptococcus*	Adhere to tooth enamel
		Component of plaque
	Lactobacillus	Involved in tooth decay
	Neisseria	
	Branhamella	
	Bacteroides	Increased with gum disease
	Actinomycetales	May cause deposition of calcium salts in plaque
Stomach	None	
Esophagus	None	
Small intestine	(See large intestine)	Fewer microorganisms than in large intestine
Large intestine	*Bacteroides*	Ferment food residues
	Fusobacterium	
	Eubacterium	
	Lactobacillus	Produce lactic acid
	Streptococcus	Low pathogenicity
	Enterobacteriaceae	Produce bacteriocins
	Vibrio	
	Escherichia coli	
Urethral orifice	*Staphylococcus epidermidis*	
Urethra	None	
Bladder	None	
Ureters	None	
Kidneys	None	
Vagina	*Lactobacillus*	Balance can be upset by antibiotics
	Bacteroides	
	Clostridium	
Nervous system	None	
Blood, lymph system	None	

Inflammation is a local and nonspecific defensive response of the tissues to injury or infection. It is an adaptive mechanism that destroys or dilutes the injurious agent, prevents further spread of the injury, and promotes the repair of damaged tissue. It is characterized by five signs: (a) pain, (b) swelling, (c) redness, (d) heat, and (e) impaired function of the part, if the injury is severe. Commonly, words with the suffix *-itis* describe an inflammatory process. For example, *appendicitis* means inflammation of the appendix; *gastritis* means inflammation of the stomach.

Injurious stressors (inflammatory agents) to body tissues can be categorized as physical agents, chemical agents, and microorganisms. *Physical agents* include mechanical objects causing trauma to tissues, excessive heat or cold (causing burns or frostbite), and radiation. *Chemical agents* include external irritants (e.g., strong acids, alkalis, poisons, and irritating gases) and internal irritants (substances manufactured within the body such as excessive hydrochloric acid in the stomach due to altered function). *Microorganisms* include the broad groups of bacteria, viruses, fungi, protozoa, and *Rickettsia.*

The inflammatory response involves a series of dynamic events commonly referred to as the three stages of the inflammatory response:

First stage: Vascular and cellular responses

Second stage: Exudate

Third stage: Reparative

At the start of the *first stage,* constriction of the blood vessels occurs at the site of injury, lasting only a few moments. This initial constriction is rapidly followed by dilation of small blood vessels (occurring as a result of histamine released by the injured tissues). Thus, more blood flows to the injured area. This marked increase in blood supply is referred to as **hyperemia** and is responsible for the characteristic signs of redness and heat.

Vascular permeability is increased at the injured site with the dilation of the vessels in response to tissue necrosis, the release of chemical mediators (e.g., bradykinin, serotonin, and prostaglandin), and the release of histamine. The result of this altered permeability is an outpouring of fluid, proteins, and leukocytes into the interstitial spaces, clinically manifested by the characteristic inflammatory signs of swelling (edema) and pain. The pain is caused by the pressure of accumulating fluid on local nerve endings and the chemical mediators, which are thought to irritate the nerve endings. Too much fluid pouring into areas such as the pleural or pericardial cavity can seriously affect organ function. In other areas, such as joints, mobility is impaired.

During the first stage of the inflammatory response, blood flow slows in the dilated vessels. This altered rate of flow facilitates the mobilization of the increased number of leukocytes to the injured tissues. Mobilization of leukocytes includes the two processes of margination and emigration. Normally, blood cells (erythrocytes, leukocytes, and platelets) flow along the center of a blood vessel, while a cellless stream of plasma flows around them against the walls of the blood vessel. When the blood flow slows, **leukocytes** (white blood cells) aggregate or line up along this inner surface of the blood vessels. This process is known as **margination.** Leukocytes then move through the blood vessel wall into the affected tissue spaces, a process called **emigration.**

The actual passage of blood corpuscles through the blood vessel wall is referred to as **diapedesis.** Leukocytes are attracted to injured cells by **chemotaxis.** The action of chemotaxis is not fully understood, but basically leukocytes are drawn toward the source of chemicals released in the injured cells (positive chemotaxis), or they are propelled away from released chemicals (negative chemotaxis).

In a compensatory response to the exit of leukocytes from the blood vessels, the bone marrow produces large numbers of leukocytes and releases them into the bloodstream (**leukocytosis**). The exact mechanism stimulating this increase is unknown, but it is another sign associated with inflammation. A normal leukocyte count of 4500 to 11,000 per cubic millimeter of blood can rise to 20,000 or more when inflammation occurs.

In the *second stage* of inflammation, fluid that escaped from the blood vessels, dead phagocytic cells, as well as dead tissue cells and products that they release, produce the inflammatory **exudate.** A plasma protein called **fibrinogen** (which is converted to fibrin when it is released to the tissues), thromboplastin (a product released by injured tissue cells), and platelets together form an interlacing network to form a barrier, wall off the area, and prevent its spread. During the second stage, the injurious agent is overcome, and the exudate is cleared away by lymphatic drainage.

The nature and amount of exudate vary in accordance with the tissue involved and the intensity and duration of the inflammation. The major types of exudate are serous, purulent, and hemorrhagic (sanguineous). A **serous exudate** is comprised chiefly of serum (the clear portion of the blood) derived from the blood and serous membranes of the body, such as the peritoneum, pleura, pericardium, and meninges. It is watery in appearance and has few cells. An example is the fluid in a blister from a burn.

A **purulent exudate** is thicker than serous exudate due to the presence of pus. It consists of leukocytes, liquefied dead tissue debris, and dead and living bacteria. The process of pus formation is referred to as **suppuration,** and the bacteria that produce pus are called **pyogenic bacteria.** Not all microorganisms are pyogenic. Purulent exudates vary in color, some acquiring tinges of blue, green, or yellow. The color may depend on the causative organism.

A **sanguineous (hemorrhagic) exudate** consists of large amounts of red blood cells, indicating damage to capillaries that is severe enough to allow the escape of red blood cells from plasma. This type of exudate is frequently seen in open wounds. Nurses often need to distinguish whether the sanguineous exudate is dark or bright. A bright sanguineous exudate indicates fresh bleeding, whereas dark sanguineous exudate denotes older bleeding. Mixed types of exudates are often observed. A serosanguineous (consisting of clear and blood-tinged drainage) exudate is commonly seen in surgical incisions.

The *third stage* of the inflammatory response, also referred to as the *reparative phase,* involves the repair of injured tissues by regeneration or replacement with fibrous tissue (scar) formation. **Regeneration** is the replacement of destroyed tissue cells by cells that are identical or similar in structure and function. It involves not only replacement of damaged cells one by one but also organization of these cells so that the architectural pattern of the tissue and function are restored.

The **stroma** is the tissue that forms the framework (connective tissue) or ground substance of an organ. The **parenchyma** is the essential functional elements of an organ. Functional cells must have proper relationships between stroma and parenchyma, and among their blood vessels, lymph vessels, nerves, and ducts. All must regenerate concurrently. If one component lags behind the others, a normal product will not be formed.

The ability to reproduce cells varies considerably from one type of tissue to another. For example, epithelial tissues of the skin and of the digestive and respiratory tracts have a good regenerative capacity, provided that their underlying support structures are intact. The same holds true for osseous, lymphoid, and bone marrow tissues. Tissues that have little regenerative capacity include nervous, muscular, and elastic tissues.

When regeneration is not possible, repair occurs by *fibrous tissue formation.* **Fibrous (scar) tissue** has the capacity to proliferate under the unusual conditions of ischemia and altered pH. The inflammatory exudate with its interlacing network of fibrin provides the framework for this tissue to develop. Damaged tissues are replaced with the connective tissue elements of collagen, blood capillaries, lymphatics, and other tissue ground substances. In the early stages of this process, the tissue is called **granulation tissue.** It is a fragile, gelatinous tissue, appearing pink or red because of the many newly formed capillaries. Later in the process, the tissue shrinks (the capillaries are constricted, even obliterated) and the collagen fibers contract, so that a firmer fibrous tissue remains. This is called a **cicatrix** or scar.

Although scar tissue has the positive attribute of repairing the injured area, it also can present problems. It can reduce the functional capacity of the tissue or organ. For example, scar tissue in cardiac muscle renders that area weaker. Mechanical obstructions can also arise, for example, in the healing of a duodenal ulcer. Sometimes the pyloric sphincter becomes stenosed as granulation tissue contracts into scar tissue.

Specific Defenses

Specific defenses of the body involve the immune system, which responds to foreign protein in the body (e.g., bacteria or transplanted tissues) or, in some cases, even the body's own proteins. Foreign proteins in the body are called **antigens** and are considered invaders. If the proteins originate in a person's own body, the antigen is called an **autoantigen. Immunity** is the specific resistance of the body to infection (pathogens or their toxins). There are two major types of immunity: active and passive. See Table 20–2. Through **active immunity,** the host produces its own antibodies in response to natural (e.g., infection) or artifi-

TABLE 20–2 *Types of Acquired Immunity*

Type	Antigen or Antibody Source	Duration
1. Active	Antibodies are produced by the body in response to infection	Long
a. Natural	Antibodies are formed in the presence of active infection in the body	Lifelong
b. Artificial	Antigens (vaccines or toxoids) are administered to the person to stimulate antibody production	Many years; the immunity must be reinforced by booster inoculations
2. Passive	Antibodies are produced by another source, animal or human	Short
a. Natural	Antibodies are transferred naturally from an immune mother to her baby through the placenta or in colostrum	6 months to 1 year
b. Artificial	Immune serum (antibody) from an animal or another human is injected	2 to 3 weeks

cial (e.g., vaccines) antigens. With **passive immunity,** the host receives natural (e.g., from a nursing mother) or artificial (e.g., from an injection of immune serum) antibodies produced by another source.

The immune response has two components: antibody-mediated defenses and cell-mediated defenses. These two systems provide distinct but overlapping protection. The *antibody-mediated defense* is also referred to as **humoral (circulating) immunity,** since it resides ultimately in the B-lymphocytes and is mediated by antibodies produced by B cells. **Antibodies,** also called **immunoglobulins,** are part of the body's plasma proteins. B cells are one type of lymphocyte; they comprise 30% of blood lymphocytes and are short-lived, having a life span of 15 days. The antibody-mediated response defends primarily against the extracellular phases of bacterial and viral infections.

B cells are activated when they recognize a foreign invader, an antigen. They then differentiate into plasma cells, which secrete antibodies, and serum proteins, which bind specifically to the foreign substance and initiate a variety of elimination responses. The B-cell response to an antigen may produce antibody molecules of five classes of immunoglobulins designated by the letters G, A, M, D, and E and

TABLE 20–3 *Antibodies and Their Functions*

Antibody	Description	Function
IgM	Principally an antibody of the blood; the first antibody produced in response to an antigen	Provides an early immune response
		Activates the complement system
		Stimulates ingestion by macrophages
		Serves as A, B, and O blood groups' isoantibodies and antibodies to serious infections, such as by Gram-negative microorganisms
		Responds to artificial immunization
IgG	The most prevalent antibody in the blood and a major antibody in tissue spaces; produced later in the immune response than IgM	Triggers complement fixation
		Activates macrophage ingestion
		The only antibody to cross the placental barrier
		Neutralizes microbial toxins and has antiviral and some antibacterial actions
IgA	Resides under the epithelial mucosal cells, especially of the gastrointestinal tract, but also found in tears, saliva, sweat, colostrum, and breast milk; also produced later in the immune response than IgM	Acts as a protective barrier against microorganisms at several points of entrance
		Easily crosses cell barriers
		Protects the mucous membranes of the gastrointestinal and the respiratory tracts
		Because it is a major antibody of milk and colostrum, may function to protect the gastrointestinal tracts of nursing infants
IgD	Normally present in only minute concentrations in the blood	Unknown
IgE	Normally present in only minute concentrations in the blood	Responds primarily to allergic reactions

usually written as follows: IgG, IgA, IgM, IgD, and IgE. See Table 20–3. The presence of IgM on laboratory analysis shows current infection. Before an antibody response, the phagocytic cells of the blood bind and ingest foreign substances. The rate of binding and phagocytosis increases if IgG antibodies (which indicate past infection and subsequent immunity) are present.

The first interaction between an antigen and antibody is known as the **primary immune response.** The principal characteristics of this response are a latent period before the appearance of an antibody, the production of only a small amount of antibody (chiefly IgM), and, most importantly, the creation of a large number of memory cells capable of responding to the same antigen in the future. The **secondary immune (booster) response** takes place on subsequent encounters with the same antigen. The principal characteristics of this response are: rapid proliferation of B cells, rapid differentiation of B cells into plasma cells that promptly produce large quantities of antibody (chiefly class IgG), and release of antibody into the blood and other body tissues, where it can react with the antigen.

The **cell-mediated defense** or **cellular immunity** occurs through the T-cell system. T cells (thymic-lymphoid cells) are present in the thymus gland at birth. These cells leave the thymus to circulate in the blood as long-lived lymphocytes with a life span of up to 5 years. Some settle in lymph nodes and the spleen. T cells comprise 70% of circulating blood lymphocytes. The cell-mediated response defends against viral infection, fungal infection, some bacterial infections, and malignant cells. Malignant cells are thought to arise from changes in normal body cells and therefore are regarded as foreign cells. The response is also responsible for graft rejection.

T cells serve as an immune regulator, primarily by activating the B cells. There are three types of T cells: T helper (Th) cells, which enhance the production of antibodies by the B cells (specifically IgG, IgA, and IgE); T suppressor (Ts) cells, which inhibit antibody production by the B cells; and T cytolytic (Tc) cells, cell-destroying cells, some of which are now called killer T cells. The cytolytic cells travel to the invading antigen, where they produce a variety of powerful chemicals or factors called **lymphokines.** The types and functions of some T-cell lymphokines are shown in Table 20–4. When cell-mediated immunity is lost, as occurs with

TABLE 20–4 *Types and Functions of Some T-Cell Lymphokines*

Lymphokine	Functions
Chemotactic factor (CF)	Attracts macrophages and monocytes to the antigen site
Migration inhibition factor (MIF)	Prevents departure of macrophages from the site
Macrophage activation or aggregation factor (MAF)	Increases phagocytosis of macrophages and agglutinates (clumps) them
Lymphotoxin factor (LT)	Acts as a cytotoxin and directly destroys microorganisms
Transfer factor	Causes nonsensitized lymphocytes at the site to act as a sensitized cell
Interferon (also produced by cells other than lymphocytes)	Blocks viral infection of tissue cells

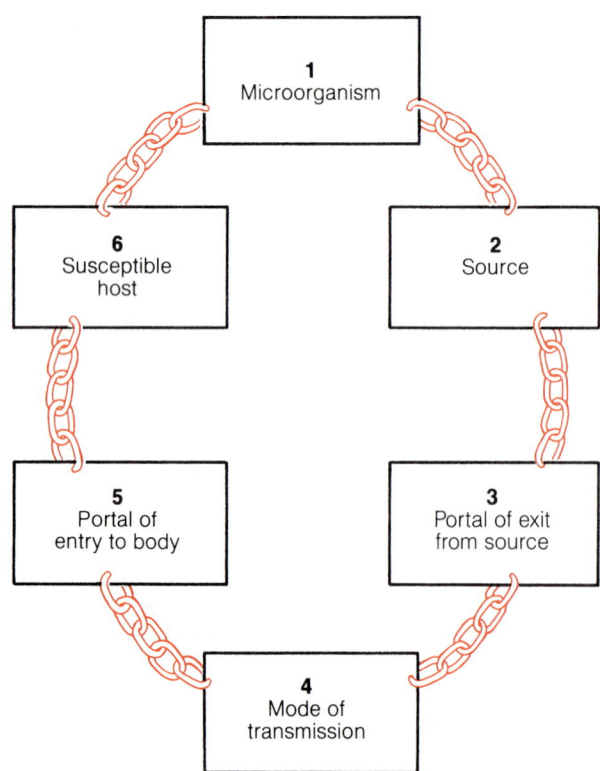

Figure 20–1 The chain of infection.

human immunodeficiency virus (HIV), the individual is "defenseless" against most viral, bacterial, and fungal infection.

CHAIN OF INFECTION

There are six links in the chain of infection: the etiologic agent, or microorganism; the place where the organism naturally resides (reservoir); a portal of exit from the reservoir; a method (mode) of transmission; a portal of entry into a host; and the susceptibility of the host. See Figure 20–1.

Etiologic Agent

A **parasite** is a microorganism that lives in or on another and obtains its nourishment from it. All viruses are parasites. The extent to which any microorganism or parasite is capable of producing an infectious process depends on the number of organisms present, the virulence and potency of the organisms (pathogenicity), the ability of the organisms to enter the body, the susceptibility of the host, and the ability of the organisms to live in the host's body.

Some microorganisms, such as the smallpox virus, have the ability to infect almost all susceptible people after exposure. By contrast, microorganisms such as the tuberculosis bacillus infect a relatively small number of the population who are susceptible and exposed, usually people who are poorly nourished and living in unsanitary conditions. Some animals and humans are **carriers,** i.e., they carry disease-producing organisms in their bodies although they are not ill themselves. Carriers can pass the microorganisms along to other people. For example, some persons harbor the typhoid bacillus in the gallbladder, excrete it in feces, but manifest no symptoms of the disease.

Reservoir

There are many **reservoirs,** or sources of microorganisms. Common sources are other humans, the client's own microorganisms, plants, animals, or the general environment. See Table 20–5. People are the most common source of infection for others and for themselves. The person with, for example, an influenza virus frequently spreads it to others. When resistance is lowered by fatigue and other factors, an infection emerges.

Insects, birds, and other animals are common reservoirs of infection. The *Anopheles* mosquito carries the malaria parasite. Food, water, milk, and feces also can be reservoirs. An example is contaminated chicken at a club luncheon. The reservoir must have certain characteristics for the organisms to live and grow. Among these characteristics are: food, water, oxygen (or, for some organisms, absence of oxygen), optimal temperature and pH, and minimal light.

TABLE 20–5 *Human Sources and Methods of Transmission of Common Microorganisms*

Body Area (Source)	Transport Vehicle	Common Infectious Organisms
Respiratory tract	Droplets expelled while sneezing and coughing	Parainfluenza virus *Klebsiella* species *Staphylococcus aureus*
Gastrointestinal tract	Emesis, feces, drainage (such as from the gallbladder), saliva	Viral hepatitis A *Shigella* species *Salmonella enteritidis*
Urinary tract	Urine	*Escherichia coli* enterococci *Pseudomonas aeruginosa*
Reproductive tract (including genitals)	Urine and semen	*Neisseria gonorrhoeae* *Treponema pallidum* Herpes simplex virus type 2 Viral hepatitis B
Blood	Blood sample, needle used for venipuncture	*Escherichia coli* *Staphylococcus aureus* *Klebsiella* species *Staphylococcus epidermidis*
Tissue	Drainage from a cut or wound	*Staphylococcus aureus* *Escherichia coli* enterococci *Proteus* species

Portal of Exit

Before an infection can establish itself in a host, the microorganisms must leave the reservoir. If the reservoir is within a human, the microorganisms have a number of exits, depending on the site of the reservoir. Common human reservoirs and their associated portals of exit are summarized in Table 20–6.

Method of Transmission

Microorganisms are transmitted by a number of routes, and the same microorganisms can be transmitted by more than one route. There are four main routes of transmission: contact, vehicle, airborne, and vectorborne. **Contact transmission** is the most important and frequent means of transmission of microorganism (Williams 1983, p. 341). There are three types of contact transmission: direct contact (physical transfer between an infected person and a susceptible host), indirect contact (contact with a contaminated object, e.g., the soiled hands of health care personnel), and droplet contact (close contact with contaminated secretions from an infected person). Most respiratory infections are transmitted by droplet contact.

Vehicle transmission is accomplished through a transporting agent of medium such as food, water, or blood. **Airborne transmission** occurs by dissemination of droplet nuclei or dust particles that contain microorganisms and

TABLE 20–6 *Human Reservoirs and Portals of Exit*

Reservoir	Portals of Exit
Respiratory tract	Nose/mouth through sneezing, coughing, breathing, or talking; endotracheal tubes or tracheostomies
Gastrointestinal tract	Mouth: through saliva, vomitus; anus/ostomies: feces; drainage tubes: e.g., nasogastric or T-tubes
Urinary tract	Urethral meatus and urinary diversion ostomies
Reproductive tract	Vagina: vaginal discharge; may be further transported by urine; urinary meatus: semen, urine
Blood	Open wound, needle puncture site, any disruption of intact skin or mucous membrane surfaces

remain in the air. The microorganisms are then inhaled by a susceptible host. Tuberculosis and varicella are two diseases transported by the airborne route. A **vector** is an animal that transfers microorganisms from a reservoir to a host. Insects and other animals can spread such organisms

TABLE 20−7 *Nursing Interventions That Break the Chain of Infection*

Link	Interventions	Rationale
Etiologic agent	Ensure articles are properly cleaned and disinfected or sterilized before use.	Proper cleaning, disinfecting, and sterilizing reduce or eliminate microorganisms.
	Educate clients and family members about appropriate methods to clean, disinfect, and sterilize articles.	Knowledge of ways to reduce or eliminate microorganisms reduces the numbers of microorganisms present and the likelihood of disease.
Source	Change dressings and bandages when they are soiled or wet.	Moist dressings are ideal environments for microorganisms to grow and multiply.
	Assist clients to carry out appropriate skin and oral hygiene.	Hygienic measures reduce the numbers of resident and transient microorganisms and the likelihood of infection.
	Dispose of damp, soiled linens appropriately.	Damp, soiled linens harbor more microorganisms than dry linens.
	Dispose of feces and urine in appropriate receptacles.	Urine and feces, in particular, contain many microorganisms. Feces may also be the source of certain virulent microorganisms, such as the hepatitis A virus in asymptomatic carriers.
	Ensure that all fluid containers, such as bedside water jugs and suction and drainage bottles, are covered or capped.	Prolonged exposure increases the risk of contamination and promotes microbial growth.
	Empty suction and drainage bottles at the end of each shift.	Drainage harbors microorganisms that, if left for prolonged periods, proliferate.
Portal of exit	Avoid talking, coughing, or sneezing over open wounds or sterile fields and cover the mouth and nose when coughing and sneezing.	These measures limit the number of microorganisms that escape from the respiratory tract.
Mode of transmission	Wash hands between client contacts, after touching infectious material, and before performing invasive procedures or touching open wounds. Instruct clients and family members to wash hands before handling food or eating, after eliminating, and after touching infectious material.	Hand washing is the most effective means of controlling and preventing the spread of microorganisms.
	Place discarded soiled materials in moisture-proof refuse bags.	Moisture-proof bags contain the spread of microorganisms to others.
	Hold used bedpans steadily to prevent spillage and dispose of urine and feces in appropriate receptacles.	Urine and feces, in particular, contain many microorganisms.
	Initiate and implement aseptic precautions for infected clients.	Controlling the mode of transmission of specific microorganisms prevents their spread.
	Wear masks when in close contact with clients who have infections transmitted by droplets from the respiratory tract.	Masks prevent the transmission of airborne microorganisms.
	Wear gloves when handling infectious secretions and excretions. Wear gowns if there is danger of soiling clothing with infectious material.	Gloves and gowns prevent soiling of the hands and clothing.
	Wear goggles when sprays of body fluid are possible, e.g., during irrigation procedures.	Goggles protect the eyes from infectious microorganisms in clients' body fluid.
Portal of entry	Use sterile technique for invasive procedures such as injections and catheterizations.	Invasive procedures penetrate the body's natural protective barriers to microorganisms.
	Use sterile technique when exposing open wounds or handling dressings.	Open wounds are vulnerable to microbial infection.

▶

TABLE 20-7 *(continued)*

Link	Interventions	Rationale
Portal of entry *(continued)*	Place used disposable needles and syringes in puncture-resistant containers for disposal.	Injuries from needles contaminated by blood or body fluids from an infected client or carrier are a primary cause of serum hepatitis and AIDS.
	Provide all clients with their own personal care items.	People have less resistance to another person's microorganisms than to their own.
Susceptible host	Maintain the integrity of the client's skin and mucous membranes.	Intact skin and mucous membranes protect against invasion by microorganisms.
	Ensure that the client receives a balanced diet.	A balanced diet supplies essential proteins and vitamins necessary to build or maintain body tissues.
	Educate the public about the importance of immunizations.	Immunizations protect people against virulent infectious diseases.

as certain *Salmonella* species, which are part of the normal flora of some domestic animals but cause gastroenteritis in humans.

Portal of Entry

Before a person can become infected, microorganisms must enter the body. The skin is a barrier to infectious agents; however, any break in the skin can readily serve as a portal of entry. Microorganisms can enter the body through the same routes they use to leave the body. Often, microorganisms enter the body by the same route they used to leave the source.

Susceptible Host

A **susceptible host** is any person who is at risk for infection. **Compromised hosts** are persons "at increased risk," individuals who for one or more reasons are more likely than others to acquire an infection. Impairment of the body's natural defenses and a number of other factors can affect susceptibility to infection. See "Factors Affecting Risk of Infection."

Breaking the Chain of Infection

Various practices break the chain of infection or interrupt the infectious disease process. For example, the first link in the chain, the etiologic agent, is interrupted by the use of **antiseptics** (agents that inhibit the growth of some microorganisms) and **disinfectants** (agents that destroy pathogens other than spores), and by sterilization. Nurses carry out practices that break other links in the chain. See Table 20-7. The aim of most hospital precautions is breaking the chain during the mode of transmission phase of the cycle.

FACTORS AFFECTING RISK OF INFECTION

Whether a microorganism causes an infection depends on a number of factors already mentioned. One of the most important factors is host susceptibility, which is affected by age, heredity, level of stress, nutritional status, immunization status, current medical therapy, and preexisting disease processes.

Age is a factor influencing the risk of infection. Newborns and elderly people have reduced defenses against infection. Infections are a major cause of death of newborns, who have immature immune systems and are protected only for the first 2 or 3 months by immunoglobulins passively received from the mother. Between 1 to 3 months of age, infants begin to synthesize their own immunoglobulins; about 40% of adult levels are reached by 1 year of age (Whaley and Wong 1989, pp. 270-71). Immunizations against diphtheria, tetanus, and pertussis are usually started at 2 months, when the infant's immune system can respond.

With advancing age, the immune responses again become weak. The immune response (cell-mediated immunity) is reduced. Lymphocytes become more diverse with age, and there is a progressive loss of cellular regulation in the body. Although there is still much to learn about aging, it is known that immunity to infection decreases with advancing age. Because of the prevalence of influenza and its potential for causing death, the CDC recommends immunization against influenza for the elderly and for persons with chronic cardiac, respiratory, metabolic, and renal disease. Pneumococcal vaccine is also recommended. Immunization is usually provided in early October or November; annual boosters are required to maintain immunity.

Heredity is a factor influencing the development of infection in that some people have a genetic susceptibility to certain infections. For example, some people may be deficient in serum immunoglobulins, which play a significant role in the internal defense mechanism of the body. The nature, number, and duration of physical and emotional *stressors* can influence susceptibility to infection. Stressors elevate blood cortisone. Prolonged elevation of blood cortisone decreases anti-inflammatory responses, depletes energy stores, leads to a state of exhaustion, and decreases resistance to infection. For example, a person recovering from a major operation or injury is more likely to develop an infection than a healthy person.

Resistance to infection depends on adequate *nutritional status*. Because antibodies are proteins, the ability of the body to synthesize antibodies may be impaired by inadequate nutrition, especially when protein reserves are depleted (e.g., as a result of injury, surgery, or debilitating diseases such as cancer). Some *medical therapies* predispose a person to infection. For example, radiation treatments for cancer destroy not only cancerous cells but also some normal cells, thereby rendering them more vulnerable to infection.

Certain *medications* also increase susceptibility to infection. Antineoplastic (anticancer) medications may depress bone marrow function, resulting in inadequate production of white blood cells and lymphocytes necessary to combat infections. Anti-inflammatory medications, such as adrenal corticosteroids, inhibit the inflammatory response, an essential defense against infection. Even some antibiotics used to treat infections can have adverse effects. Antibiotics may kill resident flora, allowing the proliferation of strains that would not grow and multiply in the body under normal conditions. Certain antibiotics can also induce resistance in some strain of organisms. Some *diagnostic procedures* may also predispose the client to an infection, especially when the skin is broken or sterile body cavities are penetrated during the procedure.

Any *disease* that lessens the body's defenses against infection places the client at risk. Examples are chronic pulmonary disease, which impairs ciliary action and weakens the mucous barrier; peripheral vascular disease, which inhibits blood flow; burns, which impair skin integrity; chronic or debilitating diseases, which deplete protein reserves; and such immune system diseases as leukemia and aplastic anemia, which alter the production rate of white blood cells. Diabetes mellitus is a major underlying disease predisposing clients to infection, since compromised peripheral vascular status and increased serum glucose levels increase susceptibility.

STAGES OF AN INFECTIOUS PROCESS

The course of an infection has four stages: the incubation period, the prodromal period, the illness period, and the convalescent period.

Incubation Period

The **incubation period** is the time between the entry of the microorganisms into the body and the onset of the symptoms. During this time, the organism adapts to the person and multiplies sufficiently to produce an infection. The length of incubation varies greatly, depending on the microorganism. For example, rubella (measles) develops in 10 to 14 days, whereas tetanus (lockjaw) takes from 4 to 21 days to develop. An average incubation period is 7 to 10 days. In many viral diseases (e.g., chickenpox and measles), persons can transmit infection during the incubation period. A person with hepatitis A is most infectious *before* the onset of any symptoms.

Prodromal Period

The **prodromal period** is the time from the onset of nonspecific symptoms, e.g., fatigue, malaise, elevated temperature, and irritability, until the specific symptoms of the infection appear. Infected persons are most infectious and most likely to spread the infecting organisms during this stage. Because the symptoms are general, precautions to prevent spread are often not taken at this time. A prodromal stage usually lasts a short time, hours or days at the most.

Illness Period

During the **illness period,** specific symptoms develop and become evident. The symptoms of most infectious processes are manifested both in the affected body organ or area (the local inflammatory response or **localized symptoms**) and in the entire body (**systemic symptoms**). During this period, the person often has fever and headache and feels fatigued. Sometimes a skin rash (**exanthema**) or a rash of the mucous membrane (**enanthema**) appears at this stage. The severity of the symptoms and the length of the illness vary with the susceptibility of the person to the etiologic agent.

Convalescent Period

The **convalescent period** extends from the time the symptoms start to abate until the person returns to a normal state of health. Depending on the severity of the illness and the person's general health, convalescence can last from a few days to months. Often it is longer than the person expects.

NOSOCOMIAL INFECTIONS

Nosocomial infections are infections that were not present or were incubating at the time of admission to a hospital or other medical facility. They include infections clients acquire during their stay in a facility or manifest after discharge. Nosocomial infections may also be acquired by health personnel working in the facility. These infections have received increasing attention in recent years. They are considered more difficult to prevent and treat, more unpredictable, and more resistant to cure than infections contracted in the community (Norton 1986, p. 774). U.S. surveys reveal that nosocomial infections occur in about 5% of all persons admitted to acute care hospitals and in about 8% of persons in long-term care facilities (Norton 1986, p. 774). Clients undergoing surgical procedures have a higher incidence of nosocomial infections than others. One survey indicated that about 70% of all nosocomial infections in a hospital developed in postoperative clients (Simmons 1983, p. 133).

The source of microorganisms that cause nosocomial infections can be the clients themselves (an **endogenous** source) or the hospital environment and hospital personnel (**exogenous** sources). Most infections appear to have endogenous sources (Simmons 1983, p. 134). The National Nosocomial Infections study, conducted between 1979 and 1983, found that *Escherichia coli* was the most common infecting organism, followed by *Staphylococcus aureus* and enterococci (Pickering and DuPont 1986, p. 28).

A number of factors contribute to nosocomial infections. **Iatrogenic** (meaning illness due to any aspect of medical therapy) infections are as a direct result of a diagnostic or therapeutic procedure. An example of an iatrogenic infection is bacteremia that results from an intravascular line. Not all nosocomial infections (e.g., the development of a respiratory infection in an immobilized elderly female) are iatrogenic.

Another factor contributing to the development of nosocomial infections is the presence of compromised hosts, i.e., clients whose normal defenses have been lowered by surgery or illness. *Insufficient hand washing* by personnel is perhaps the greatest factor contributing to the spread of nosocomial infections. Personnel can acquire microorganisms from infected clients and pass them on to other clients. The hands of personnel are a common vehicle for the spread of microorganisms. The cost of nosocomial infections to the client, the facility, and funding bodies (e.g., insurance companies and federal, state, or local governments) is very great. Nosocomial infections extend hospitalization time, increase clients' time away from work, cause disability and discomfort, and even result in loss of life.

ASSESSING

Nursing History

During the nursing history, the nurse assesses (a) the degree to which a client is at risk of acquiring an infection and (b) any client complaints suggesting the presence of an infection. To identify clients at risk, the nurse reviews the client's chart and structures the nursing interview to collect data regarding the factors influencing the development of infection, especially existing disease process, history of recurrent infections, current medications and therapeutic mea-

ASSESSMENT INTERVIEW
Clients at Risk for Infections

- When were you last immunized for diphtheria, tetanus, poliomyelitis, rubella, influenza, and pneumococcal pneumonia?

- What infections have you had in the past, and how were these treated?

- Have any of these been recurrent?

- Are you taking any of the following medications (antineoplastic, anti-inflammatory, antibiotic)?

- Have you had any recent diagnostic procedure or therapy that penetrated through your skin or a body cavity?

- How would you describe your nutritional status in terms of a well-balanced diet?

- On a scale of 1 to 10, how would you rate the stress you have experienced in the last 6 months?

sures, current emotional stressors, nutritional status, and history of immunizations. See the box above for a sample assessment interview.

To obtain subjective data that may indicate the presence of an infection, the nurse asks whether the client has experienced loss of energy, loss of appetite, nausea, headache, or other signs associated with specific body systems (e.g., difficulty in urinating, urinary frequency, or a sore throat).

Physical Health Data

Signs and symptoms of an infection may be either localized or systemic. The signs of *localized infection* vary according to the body area involved (see Table 20–8) and are caused by the inflammatory response. Commonly the skin and mucous membranes are involved, resulting in

- Localized swelling
- Localized redness
- Pain or tenderness with palpation or movement
- Palpable heat at the infected area
- Loss of function of the body part affected, depending on the site and extent of involvement

In addition, open wounds may exude drainage of various colors. For additional information regarding localized responses and description of exudate, see the discussion about inflammatory responses, earlier in this chapter.

Signs of *systemic infection* include

- Fever
- Increased pulse and respiratory rate, if the fever is high

TABLE 20–8 *Guide to Detect Infection of Various Body Parts*

Body Part	Common Signs and Symptoms
Respiratory Tract	
Nose and sinuses	Sneezing; watery or mucoid discharge from nose; swollen and inflamed nasal turbinates; nasal stuffiness; sensation of pressure over infected sinus; palpable tenderness over involved sinus (e.g., in the cheek for maxillary sinus, in the nasal bridge or around the eyes for ethmoid sinus)
Throat and pharynx	Inflamed throat and pharynx; dry, scratchy, or sore throat; reddened and enlarged tonsils with accumulation of leukocytes, dead cells, and bacteria in the crypts; possible swollen cervical lymph nodes; fever; chills
Larynx	Hoarseness or loss of voice; feeling of roughness or tickling in throat; dry cough; possible fever
Bronchi	Productive cough; burning substernal sensation that may be aggravated by a deep breath; auscultatory crackles, rhonchi, and wheeze; malaise
Lungs	Hacking cough initially, followed by productive cough with sputum; possible hemoptysis; chills; severe pleural pain; rapid, shallow respirations; fever; malaise; weakness
Gastrointestinal Tract	
Stomach	Epigastric discomfort; bloating; anorexia; nausea; vomiting; eructation; abdominal cramps; possible diarrhea
Intestines	Diarrhea; watery or purulent stools; abdominal cramps; nausea and vomiting
Urinary Tract	
Urethra and bladder	Reddened and inflamed urethra; discomfort with urination; urinary frequency; possible stress incontinence; suprapubic tenderness; cloudy or discolored urine; fever; fatigue
Kidneys	Severe pain or constant dull aching over the flank area; fever and chills; nausea and vomiting

- Lassitude, malaise, and loss of energy
- Anorexia and, in some situations, nausea and vomiting
- Enlargement and tenderness of lymph nodes that drain the area of infection

Laboratory Data

Laboratory data that indicate the presence of an infection include:

1. Elevated leukocyte (white blood) cell (WBC) count (4500 to 11,000/cu mm is normal).
2. Increases in specific types of leukocytes as revealed in the differential white blood cell count. Specific types of white blood cells are increased or decreased in certain infections. Normal values are cited for the adult.
   a. **Neutrophils** are increased in acute suppurative infections but may be decreased in acute bacterial infection, especially in older people. Normal range is 54 to 75%.
   b. **Lymphocytes** are increased in chronic bacterial and viral infections. Normal is 25 to 40%.
   c. **Monocytes** are increased in some protozoal and rickettsial infections and in tuberculosis. Normal is 2 to 8%.
   d. **Eosinophils** are generally unaltered in an infectious process. Normal is 1 to 4%.
   e. **Basophils** are generally unaltered in an infectious process. Normal is 0 to 1% (Byrne et al. 1986, p. 78).
3. Elevated **erythrocyte sedimentation rate (ESR),** commonly referred to as sedimentation rate. The ESR is a measure of the speed with which red blood cells in anticoagulated whole blood settle to the bottom of a calibrated tube. Sedimentation normally takes place slowly, but the rate increases in the presence of an inflammatory process.
4. Urine, blood, sputum, or other drainage **cultures** (cultivations of microorganisms in a special growth medium) that indicate the presence of pathogenic microorganisms.

DIAGNOSING

Potential for infection is the nursing diagnosis given to clients at risk for infection. According to NANDA, the presence of one or more of the following risk factors is a defining characteristic of this diagnosis:

- *Inadequate primary defenses,* such as broken skin, traumatized tissue, decrease of ciliary action, stasis of body fluids, change in pH of secretions, and/or altered peristalsis
- *Inadequate secondary defenses,* such as decreased hemoglobin, leukopenia, suppressed inflammatory response, immunosuppression or inadequate acquired immunity, tissue destruction and increased environmental exposure, chronic disease, invasive procedures, malnutrition, pharmaceutical agents, trauma, rupture of amniotic membranes, and/or insufficient knowledge to avoid exposure to pathogens

For clients who have an existing infection and require isolation or other protective measures, other nursing diagnoses may be relevant. These include potential **Social isolation,** a condition of aloneness experienced by the individual who desires contact with others but is unable to make that contact; potential **Diversional activity deficit,** the state in which an individual experiences a decrease in stimulation from interest or engagement in recreational or leisure activities; and **Self-esteem disturbance,** which is discussed in Chapter 29.

Some clients who have acquired immune deficiency syndrome (AIDS) may feel a sense of anxiety and frustration over the poor prognosis of this disease. In these situations, other diagnoses such as **Anxiety, Fear, Hopelessness,** and **Powerlessness** may apply. See Chapters 33 and 34 for details about these diagnoses.

Examples of contributing factors for selected nursing diagnoses are shown below. Examples of assessment data clusters and related nursing diagnoses are shown in Table 20–9.

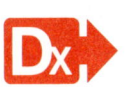

Nursing Diagnoses
Clients at Risk for Infection and
Clients with an Infection

Potential for infection related to:

- Lack of immunization
- Impaired skin integrity
- Chronic disease (e.g., cancer, diabetes, respiratory disorder)
- Suppressed inflammatory response secondary to cortisone therapy
- Immunosuppression secondary to chemotherapy
- Recent surgery
- Presence of invasive lines (e.g., intravenous line, Foley catheter, enteral feeding tube)
- Malnutrition

Potential social isolation related to misinformation about transmission of the infective organism (specify)

Potential diversional activity deficit related to:

- Confinement for communicable disease
- Monotonous hospital environment

PLANNING CARE FOR SUSCEPTIBLE CLIENTS

After deriving pertinent causative factors from the data base, nurses plan specific strategies to prevent or treat infection. Overall goals for clients at risk of acquiring an infection or for those with infections include the following:

TABLE 20–9   *Examples of Assessment Data Clusters and Related Nursing Diagnoses*

Data Cluster	Nursing Diagnosis
Kim Bradley, a 40-year-old shipyard worker, was admitted to emergency with a puncture wound on his foot. He reports stepping on a rusty nail that penetrated his shoe. Wound is 6 mm in diameter, unclean, and inflamed with slight serosanguineous discharge. Reports no immunization since childhood.	**Potential for infection** related to lack of immunization (tetanus) and **Impaired skin integrity**
Kuniko Tanaka, 12 years old, has had a diagnosis of chickenpox confirmed and must stay home from school until her lesions are dry. She anticipates "feelings of boredom," missing her friends and school, and, in particular, missing her art classes.	**Potential diversional activity deficit** related to confinement for communicable disease
Grant Madigan, a 28-year-old teacher who has AIDS, reports an increasing sense of aloneness. His health status does not allow him to work, and most of his former colleagues and friends no longer visit him.	**Social isolation** related to misinformation by others about the transmission of the AIDS virus

1. Maintain or restore body defenses
2. Prevent the spread of an infection
3. Reduce or alleviate problems associated with the infection

Supporting Body Defenses   Nursing plans to maintain or restore the client's body defenses include providing adequate fluids and nutrition, promoting rest, and administering and monitoring prescribed antimicrobial therapy. The immunologic system is the body's major defense against infections. The body gradually builds up natural defenses against pathogens with which it comes in contact; *immunizations* give additional protection. A balanced diet enhances the health of all body tissues. Adequate *nutrition* enables tissues to maintain and rebuild themselves and helps keep the reticuloendothelial system functioning well. Adequate *rest and sleep* are essential to health and to one's ability to perform usual activities. In addition, regular and thorough hygienic practices by or for the client remove transient microorganisms, thereby reducing the likelihood of infection. Hygiene is discussed in Chapter 22. Because *stress* predisposes a person to infection, a balance, for example, between work and recreation is important. See the section on psychologic homeostasis in Chapter 33.

Preventing Infection

Preventing Infection Planned nursing strategies to prevent the spread of an infection include use of meticulous medical and surgical asepsis. **Asepsis** is the freedom from infection or infectious material. Hands washed with soap and water or an antiseptic can be considered aseptic, i.e., free from infectious organisms. However, some microorganisms in all probability are still present on washed hands. There are two basic types of asepsis: medical and surgical. **Medical asepsis** includes all practices intended to confine a specific microorganism to a specific area, limiting the number, growth, and spread of microorganisms.

In medical asepsis, objects are often referred to as clean or dirty. **Clean** denotes the presence of some microorganisms but the absence of potentially infectious agents. **Dirty** (soiled) denotes the likely presence of disease-producing microorganisms. Aseptic measures are protective as they are designed to reduce the number of potentially infectious agents.

Surgical asepsis, or sterile technique, refers to those practices that keep an area or objects free of all microorganisms; it includes practices that destroy all microorganisms and spores. (A **spore** is a round or oval structure enclosed in a tough capsule. Some microorganisms assume this structure in response to adverse conditions; in this form, they are highly resistant to destruction.) Surgical asepsis is required for invasive procedures, such as injections, intravenous therapy, or urinary catheterization. Initiation of appropriate barrier precautions and client education about immunization, hygiene, sanitation, nutrition, and appropriate food handling practices are other examples of planned nursing strategies to prevent infection.

Alleviating Associated Problems Because malaise, fever, pain, and dehydration are often associated with an infection, plans need to incorporate interventions that promote comfort and reduce or prevent these problems.

Examples of outcome criteria to evaluate the achievement of client goals and the effectiveness of nursing interventions are shown below.

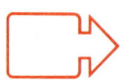

Outcome Criteria
Clients at Risk for Infection and Clients with an Infection

The client with **Potential for infection:**

- Verbalizes understanding of individual risk factors.
- Identifies measures to prevent or reduce the risk of infection.
- Practices appropriate precautions to prevent infection.
- Remains free of nosocomial infection during hospitalization.
- Obtains recommended immunization(s).
- Experiences no signs of infection in surgical wound.

- Has negative cultures of body secretions, excretions, and exudates.
- Has a WBC within normal limits.

The client with **Social isolation:**

- Verbalizes fears, limitations, and barriers to interaction with others.
- Identifies reasons for feelings of isolation.
- Identifies actions to correct isolation.

The client with **Diversional activity deficit:**

- Describes usual pattern of diversional activities.
- Identifies at least five activities that provide enjoyment within personal limitations.
- Chooses one usual activity to continue.
- Identifies new diversional activity.
- Expresses satisfaction with chosen activity.
- Relates available community services and agencies that can be used for hobbies or recreational activities.

IMPLEMENTING NURSING STRATEGIES

Nursing Actions to Prevent Infections

Among the interventions to prevent and/or promptly identify potential infections are the following:

- Wash hands before and after any direct client contact, before any invasive procedure (e.g., urinary catheterization), and after contact with any body substance (e.g., feces, urine, and wound drainage).
- Employ practices to reduce the number of organisms in the environment, e.g., change moist dressings frequently. (Drainage on dressings often has a heavy concentration of microorganisms.)
- Place soiled materials (e.g., tissues and dressings) in moisture-resistant containers for appropriate disposal.
- Handle needles and syringes carefully to avoid needle-prick injuries. *Do not recap* needles. Many facilities now provide disposal units in all clients rooms.
- Use surgical asepsis when inserting any intravenous needle or catheter; change intravenous tubing and solution containers according to hospital policy (e.g., every 24 to 72 hours); and check intravenous solutions for expiration date and clarity.
- Inspect skin surfaces every shift or more frequently to check for skin lesions, ulcers, pressure areas, presence

of peripheral edema and/or bulging leg veins, and changes in temperature or color of any extremity.

- Dry the skin thoroughly after bathing the client, and apply lotion to roughened or especially dry areas.

- Use pressure-relieving devices and turn clients with impaired physical mobility every 2 hours to maintain adequate circulation to all pressure points.

- Apply prescribed measures to decubitus ulcers (e.g., Maalox, heat lamp, Op Site) according to the physician's order and/or hospital procedure.

- Use surgical asepsis when changing dressings.

- Monitor for significant changes in vital signs that might indicate the presence of infection (e.g., systemic inflammatory signs: elevated temperature, pulse, and/or respirations; decreased blood pressure).

- Place clients at risk for infection in private rooms if possible; at least, move them away from clients with known infection.

- Ask the client to move, cough, and breathe deeply at least every 2 hours and use aseptic technique when suctioning clients.

- Report the amount and character of secretions expectorated or suctioned and monitor laboratory studies for sputum culture results.

- Provide a fluid intake of 2000 to 3000 ml/day, unless contraindicated; assist the client to obtain an optimal nutritional intake.

- Prevent urinary infections by using surgical asepsis when inserting the catheter; maintain a closed urinary drainage system with a downhill flow of urine; do not irrigate a catheter unless ordered to do so; provide regular catheter care, cleaning the perineal area with soap and water; and keep the drainage bag and spout off the floor.

- Measure urinary output and observe the characteristics of the urine; obtain specimens by aspiration and monitor lab results; and report to the physician any of the following: client complaints of itching or burning on urination, diminished urinary output or increased specific gravity, urinary frequency, or cloudy, foul-smelling urine.

Nursing Actions for Clients with Infections

 Nursing interventions for clients with infections include the following:

- Obtain blood specimens for differential white blood cell counts or serum immunoglobulins as ordered.

- Perform intradermal skin tests for diagnostic reactions as directed by the physician.

- Initiate and maintain barrier precautions specific to the infecting organism and its mode of transmission.

- Administer prescribed antimicrobial medications and monitor for effectiveness.

- Administer specific immune therapies ordered by the physician, e.g., vaccines, antitoxins or toxoids, and immune antiserums.

- Implement nursing strategies for clients with elevated temperature (see Chapter 18).

- Provide a humidifier to moisten and loosen respiratory secretions and soothe respiratory membranes for clients with coughs and administer expectorants or cough suppressants as prescribed.

- Limit the client's physical activity.

- Immobilize painful body parts, provide relaxation and comfort measures, and administer prescribed analgesics.

- Minimize fluid loss through excessive perspiration, diarrhea, or vomiting by offering fluids; and monitor the client's urinary output in comparison to intake.

- Measure and record the client's vital signs regularly.

- Assess breath sounds if the client has a respiratory infection.

- Obtain specimens for periodic sputum, wound drainage, blood, urine, or fecal cultures to determine the effectiveness of antimicrobial and other therapies.

- Teach the client and family members about the infectious organism, its mode of transmission, and ways to control and prevent its spread. Client education should stress the need for meticulous hand washing after contact with body substances, keeping hands away from drainage areas, and disposing of infectious materials properly. Some clients may need to learn how to take body temperature to monitor a fever; others, how to apply hot or cold compresses to localized infections.

Hand Washing   Hand washing is important in every setting where people are ill, including hospitals. It is considered one of the most effective infection control measures. The goal of hand washing is to remove transient microorganisms that might be transmitted to clients, visitors, or other health care personnel.

Any client may harbor microorganisms that are currently harmless to the client yet potentially harmful to another person or to the same client if they find a portal of entry. It is important that hands be washed at the following times to prevent the spread of these microorganisms: before eating, after using the bedpan or toilet, and after the hands have come in contact with any body substances, such as sputum or drainage from a wound. In addition, health care workers should wash their hands before and after any direct client contact.

For routine client care, the CDC recommends a vigorous hand washing under a stream of water for at least 10 seconds using bar soap, granule soap, soap-filled tissues, or antimicrobial liquid soap (Garner and Favero 1985, p. 7). Liquid soaps are frequently supplied in dispensers at the sink. Antimicrobial soaps are usually provided in high-risk areas, e.g., the newborn nursery. The CDC recommends

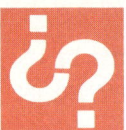

How Well Do Health Care Workers Meet Recommended Hand Decontamination Practices?

Graham observed the frequency and duration of hand washing in an 18-bed intensive care unit of a 663-bed acute care metropolitan teaching hospital in Perth, Australia. The 18-bed unit consisted of two wings of identical design. Each wing contained three single rooms with individual sinks for hand washing, and a bay with six beds that had a sink for hand washing at each end.

Stage one of the study consisted of six 3-hour observation periods during a 2-week period. Nursing, medical, physiotherapy, radiology, and orderly staff members were observed. Staff members were told that an audit of infection control procedures would be carried out but were not told that hand washing practices were being specifically observed. Stage two of the study included further observation during six additional 3-hour periods *after* an antiseptic handrub lotion was supplied for each bed in the unit. The lotion, which contained chlorhexidine gluconate 0.5% and isopropyl alcohol 60% and was packaged in a dispenser, did not require water for use because it was rubbed onto the hands until dry.

Client care activities before hand washing were classified as high or low according to the degree of contact with the clients and their equipment. For example, high-contact activities include invasive procedures, handling wounds or mucous membranes and body fluids, and prolonged client contact. Low-contact activities include taking observations, giving medications, and adjusting equipment. Hand washing frequency was measured by counting the number of hand washes with the use of soap and water or the handrub lotion by each observed staff member. Hand washing duration was measured by a concealed stopwatch.

A total of 884 client contacts and 341 hand decontamination episodes were observed: 440 contacts and 140 hand washes in stage one (32%), and 444 contacts and 201 hand washes in stage two (45%). There was an increase of 13% hand decontamination frequency after the introduction of the handrub lotion. Data indicate that the frequency of hand washing is below levels recommended by infection control authorities. Moreover, the recommended hand washing duration of 15 to 30 seconds was not met.

Implications: This study suggests that increasing the accessibility of hand decontamination facilities did result in a slight increase in hand washing compliance and that in-service education of health care workers regarding hand washing habits must be continually reinforced.

M. Graham. Frequency and duration of hand washing in an intensive care unit, *American Journal of Infection Control* April 1990, 18:77–81.

antimicrobial hand-washing agents with any chemical germicides listed with the Environmental Protection Agency:

1. When there are known multiple resistant bacteria
2. Before invasive procedures
3. In special care units, such as nurseries and ICUs

This book recommends that the hands be held down (below the elbows) when washing off infectious materials and during routine hand washing so that the microorganisms are washed directly into the sink. For surgical asepsis, the hands should be held above the elbows so that the water runs from the cleanest to least clean area. Nurses usually dry their hands with paper towels, discarding them in an appropriate container immediately after use. Procedure 20–1 provides instructions for hand washing.

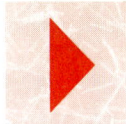

PROCEDURE 20–1

HAND WASHING

Equipment ☑

Soap
Warm running water
Towels

Intervention

1. **Prepare and assess your hands.**

- File the nails short. *Short nails are less likely to harbor microorganisms or scratch a client. Long nails are hard to clean.*

- Remove jewelry, except a plain wedding ring or band, from the hands and arms. Some nurses slide their watches up above their elbows. Others pin the watch to the uniform. *Microorganisms can lodge in the settings of jewelry. Removal facilitates proper cleaning of the hands and arms.*

- Check hands for breaks in the skin, such as hangnails or cuts. Report cuts to the instructor or nurse in charge before beginning work, or check agency policy about cuts. Use lotions to prevent hangnails and cracked, dry skin. A nurse who has open sores may have to change work assignments or wear gloves to avoid contact with infectious material.

2. **Turn on the water, and adjust the flow.**

- There are four common types of faucet controls:
  a. Hand-operated handles.
  b. Knee levers. Move these with the knee to regulate flow and temperature. See Figure 20–2.
  c. Foot pedals. Press these with the foot to regulate flow and temperature. See Figure 20–3.
  d. Elbow controls. Move these with the elbows instead of the hands.

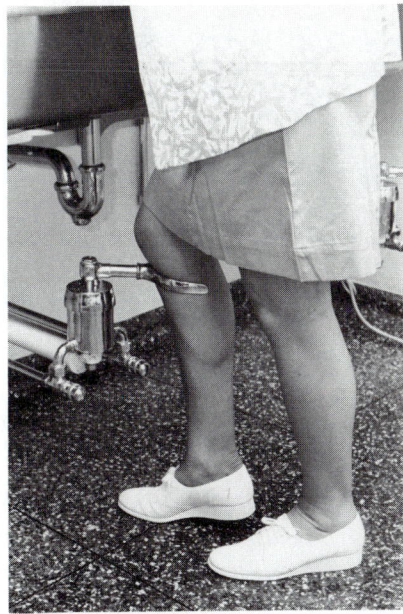

Figure 20–2 A knee-lever faucet control.

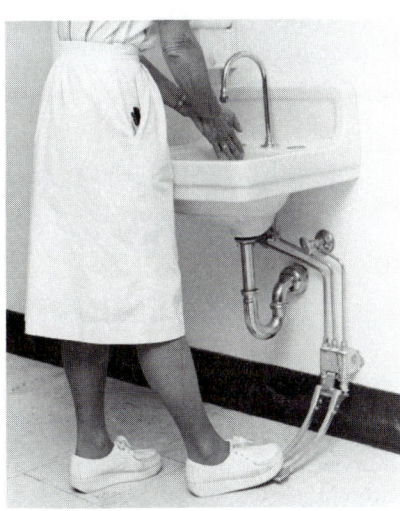

Figure 20–3 A foot pedal faucet control.

This type of handle is most frequently used for surgical asepsis.

- Adjust the flow so that the water is warm. *Warm water removes less of the protective oil of the skin than hot water.*

3. **Wet the hands thoroughly by holding them under the running water, and apply soap to the hands.**

- Hold the hands lower than the elbows so that the water flows from the arms to the fingertips. *The water should flow from the least contaminated to the most contaminated area; the hands are more contaminated than the lower arms.*

- If the soap is liquid, apply 2 to 4 ml (1 tsp). If it is bar soap, rub it firmly between the hands, and rinse the bar before returning it to the dish. *Rinsing the bar removes microorganisms.*

4. **Thoroughly wash and rinse the hands.**

- Use firm, rubbing, circular movements to wash the palm, back, and wrist of each hand. Interlace the fingers and thumbs, and move the hands back and forth. See Figure 20–4. Continue this motion for 10 to 15 seconds. *The circular action helps remove microorganisms mechanically. Interlacing the fingers and thumbs cleans the interdigital spaces.*

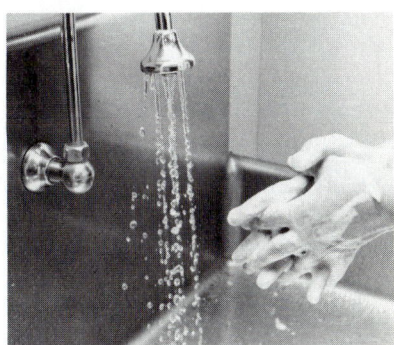

Figure 20–4 Interlacing the fingers during hand washing.

- Rinse the hands.

- Wash hands for a minimum of 15 seconds. For a more thorough hand washing, extend the time for wetting, washing, and rinsing.

5. Thoroughly dry the hands and arms.

- Dry the hands and arms thoroughly with the paper towel. *Moist skin becomes chapped readily; chapping produces lesions.*

- Discard the paper towel in the appropriate container.

6. Turn off the water.

- Use paper towels to grasp a hand-operated control. See Figure 20–5. *This prevents picking up microorganisms from the faucet handles.*

Variation: Hand washing before sterile techniques

- Hold the hands higher than the elbows during this hand wash. Wet the hands and forearms under the running water, letting it run from the fingertips to the elbows so that the hands become cleaner than the

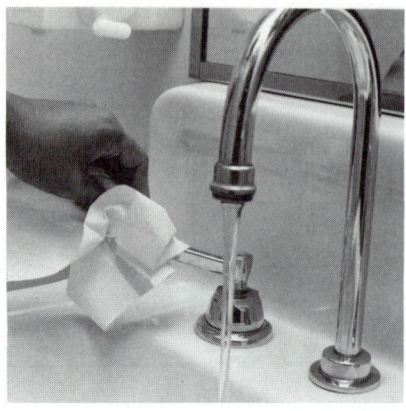

Figure 20–5 Using a paper towel to grasp the handle of a hand-operated faucet.

elbows. See Figure 20–6. *In this way, the water runs from the area with the fewest microorganisms to areas with a relatively greater number.*

- Apply the soap and wash as described earlier in Step 4, maintaining the hands uppermost.

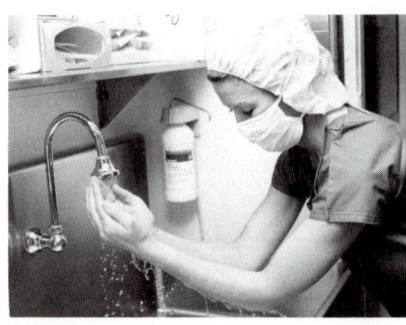

Figure 20–6 The hands are held higher than the elbows during a hand wash before sterile technique.

- After washing and rinsing, use a towel to dry one hand thoroughly in a rotating motion from the fingers to the elbow. Use a clean towel to dry the other hand and arm. *A clean towel prevents the transfer of microorganisms from one elbow (least clean area) to the other hand (cleanest area).*

TABLE 20–10 *Category-Specific Isolation Precautions*

Isolation Category	Purpose	Private Room	Gowns
Strict isolation, e.g., for diphtheria pneumonic plague, smallpox, varicella (chickenpox), zoster	To prevent airborne or contact transmission of highly contagious or virulent microorganisms	Necessary; door must be kept closed	Must be worn by all persons entering room; for smallpox, coverings for cap and shoes are also recommended
Contact isolation, e.g., for acute respiratory infections and influenza in children, pediculosis, wound infections, herpes simplex, impetigo, rubella, scabies	To prevent highly transmissible infections not requiring strict isolation but spread by close or direct contact	Necessary	Must be worn if soiling is likely
Respiratory isolation, e.g., for epiglottitis, measles, meningitis, mumps, pertussis, pneumonia in children	To prevent infections spread by contaminated articles (e.g., tissues) and respiratory droplets that are coughed, sneezed, or exhaled	Necessary	Not necessary

Isolation Precautions Isolation practices are indicated when a client has an infection that can be transmitted to others. In 1983, the CDC published recommendations regarding isolation practices in hospitals. Seven categories for isolation were described: strict isolation, contact isolation, respiratory isolation, tuberculosis isolation, enteric precautions, drainage/secretion precautions, and blood/body fluid precautions (see Table 20–10). In 1987, the CDC also presented recommendations for universal precautions on all clients to decrease the risk of transmitting unidentified pathogens. The CDC guidelines for universal precautions are shown on the inside front cover.

Associated psychologic problems Clients requiring isolation precautions can develop several problems as a result of the separation from others and of the special precautions taken in their care. Two of the most common are sensory deprivation and decreased self-esteem related to feelings of inferiority. *Sensory deprivation* occurs when the environment lacks normal stimuli for the client, e.g., frequent communications with others. The client is usually in a private room and thus has no contact with other clients. Because support persons may need to put on gowns before entering the room, they may not visit as often as usual. Visits by other clients are usually discouraged. Nurses should therefore be alert to common clinical signs of sensory deprivation: boredom, inactivity, slowness of thought, daydreaming, increased sleeping, thought disorganization, anxiety, panic, and hallucinations.

Chapter 29 provides information on the development of self-esteem and self-esteem disturbances. A client's *feeling of inferiority* can be due to the perception of the infection itself or to the required precautions. In North America, many people place a high value on cleanliness, and the idea of being "soiled," "contaminated," or "dirty" can give clients the feeling that they are at fault and substandard. While this is obviously not true, the infected persons may feel "not as good" as others and blame themselves.

Nurses need to provide care that prevents these two problems and/or deals with them positively. Nursing interventions include the following:

1. Assess the individual's need for stimulation.

2. Initiate measures to help meet the need, including regular communication with the client and diversionary activities, e.g., toys for a child and books, television, or radio for an adult; provide a variety of foods to stimulate the client's sense of taste; stimulate the client's visual sense by providing a view or an activity to watch.

3. Explain the infection and the associated procedures to help clients and their support persons understand and accept the situation.

4. Demonstrate warm, accepting behavior. Avoid conveying to the client any sense of annoyance about the precautions or any feelings of revulsion about the infection.

Donning and removing face masks Masks are worn to prevent the spread of organisms by the droplet contact

Masks	Gloves	Hand Washing	Disposal of Contaminated Articles
Must be worn by all persons entering room	Must be worn by all persons entering room	Necessary after touching client or potentially contaminated articles and before caring for another client	Discard in plastic-lined container or bag and label before sending for decontamination and reprocessing
Must be worn if person comes near the client	Worn if touching infected material	Same as for strict isolation	Same as for strict isolation
Must be worn by all persons in close contact	Not necessary	Same as for strict isolation	Same as for strict isolation

and airborne routes. The CDC recommends that masks be worn (Garner and Simmons 1983, p. 254):

1. Only by those close to the client if the infection (e.g., acute respiratory diseases in children, measles, or mumps) is transmitted by large-particle aerosols (droplets). Large-particle aerosols are transmitted by close contact and generally travel short distances (about 1 m, or 3 ft).

2. By all persons entering the room if the infection (e.g., diphtheria) is transmitted by small-particle aerosols (droplet nuclei). Small-particle aerosols remain suspended in the air and thus travel greater distances by air.

Masks are worn by all persons entering the rooms of clients who require strict isolation. They are also worn during certain techniques requiring surgical asepsis. During a procedure requiring sterile technique, masks are worn to prevent the airborne or droplet contact transmission of exhaled microorganisms to the sterile field or to a client's open wound. Nurses should wear masks when they are in close contact with clients who require contact isolation, respiratory isolation, and tuberculosis isolation when the client does not cover the mouth when coughing.

Masks must cover the nose and mouth (see Figure 20–7). To don a mask, first hold it by the top strings or loops, position the mask over the bridge of the nose, and tie the upper strings at the top back of the head so that the ties lie above the ears. If glasses are worn, fit the top edge of the mask under the glasses to minimize fogging of the glasses. Then make sure the lower part of the mask is well under the chin, and tie the lower ties at the nape of the neck. If the mask has a metal strip, adjust it firmly over the bridge of the nose. While wearing the mask, avoid talking as much as possible to keep respiratory airflow at a minimum. Masks become moist and ineffective after a few hours. For this reason, masks should be worn only once and disposed of appropriately. If a mask becomes moist during a lengthy procedure, e.g., an operation, it may be necessary to have another nurse who is not gowned and gloved put a clean, dry mask over the one being worn. Before removing a mask, remove gloves, if used, or wash the hands if they have been in contact with infectious material. After removing the mask, fold it in half with the moist inner surfaces together to contain the microorganisms. Dispose of the mask in the appropriate waste or laundry container.

Gowning for isolation precautions   Clean or disposable gowns or plastic aprons are worn for isolation precautions when the nurse's uniform is likely to become soiled. Gowns are also required when persons enter the room of a client who has an infection, for example, varicella (chickenpox), that could cause serious illness if spread to others, even though soiling of the clothing is not likely (Garner and Simmons 1983, p. 254). Sterile gowns may be indicated when the nurse is changing the dressings of a client with extensive wounds, e.g., burns. It is recommended that a

TABLE 20–10   *Category-Specific Isolation Precautions (continued)*

Isolation Category	Purpose	Private Room	Gowns
Tuberculosis isolation (AFB isolation) for pulmonary tuberculosis when clients have positive sputum smear or suggestive chest x-ray film	To prevent spread of acid-fast bacilli (AFB)	Necessary, with special ventilation	Necessary only if clothing may become contaminated
Enteric precautions, e.g., for hepatitis A, some gastroenteritis, typhoid fever, cholera, diarrhea with suspected infectious etiology, encephalitis, meningitis	To prevent infections spread through direct or indirect contact with feces	Necessary if client hygiene is poor, e.g., client is incontinent	Same as for tuberculosis isolation
Drainage/secretion precautions, e.g., for any draining lesion, abscess, infected burn, infected skin, decubitis ulcer, conjunctivitis	To prevent infections, spread through direct or indirect contact with material or drainage from body site	Not necessary unless client hygiene is poor	Same as for tuberculosis isolation
Blood/body fluid precautions, e.g., for hepatitis B, syphilis, AIDS, malaria	To prevent infections spread through direct or indirect contact with infected blood or body fluids	Necessary if client hygiene is poor	Same as for tuberculosis isolation

Source: Adapted from J. S. Garner and B. P. Simmons, CDC guidelines for isolation precautions in hospitals, *Infection Control,* July/August 1983. 4(4):258–60.

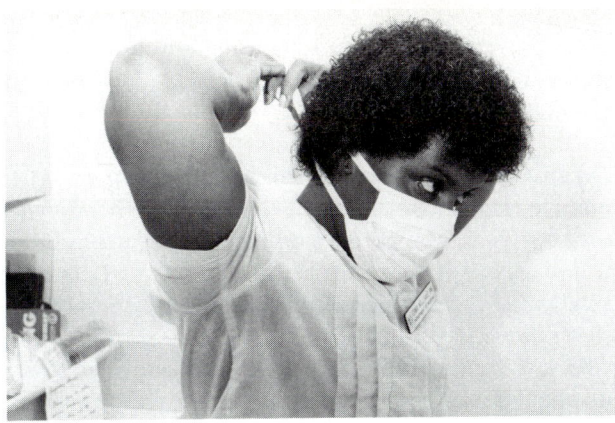

Figure 20−7 A face mask covering the nose and mouth.

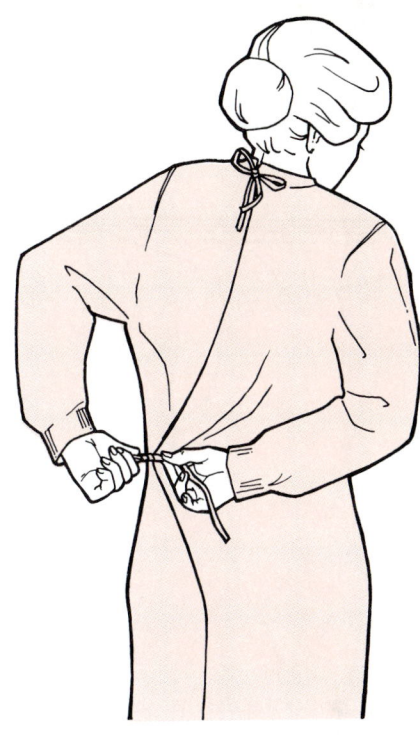

Figure 20−8 Overlapping the gown at the back to cover the nurse's uniform.

clean gown be used only once and then discarded in the receptacle designated for the purpose. Gowns may be disposable or reusable after laundering.

Before donning a gown, the nurse washes the hands thoroughly and dons a face mask, if required. When donning the gown the nurse fastens the ties at the neck, overlaps the gown at the back as much as possible, and fastens the waist ties. Overlapping securely covers the uniform at the back. See Figure 20−8. No special precautions are necessary when

Masks	Gloves	Hand Washing	Disposal of Contaminated Articles
Necessary if client is coughing and does not always cover mouth	Not necessary	Same as for strict isolation	Clean and disinfect, although these articles rarely transmit disease
Not necessary	Necessary if touching infected material	Same as for strict isolation	Same as for strict isolation
Not necessary	Same as for enteric precautions	Same as for strict isolation	Same as for strict isolation
Not necessary Goggles are used if spatter is considered likely	Necessary if touching infected blood or body fluid with visible blood	Necessary if hands can become contaminated and before caring for another client	Same as for strict isolation; used needles must be placed in puncture-proof container for disposal

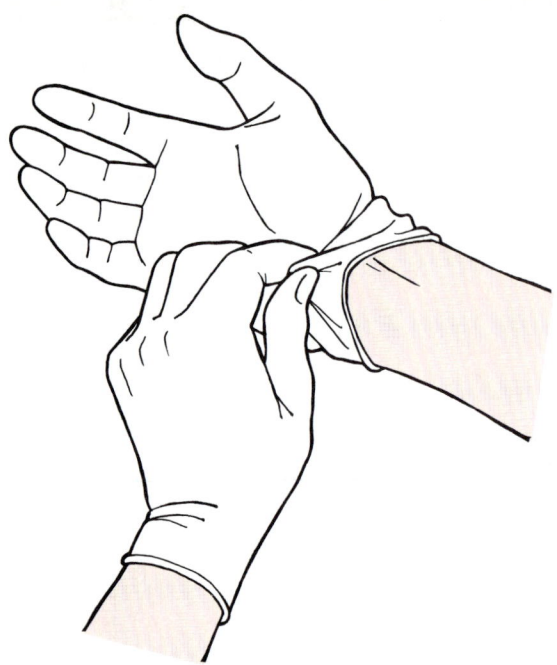

Figure 20–9 Removing the first soiled disposable glove.

removing a gown unless the gown is soiled with infectious materials. When a gown is soiled with infectious material, the nurse removes the gown so that it does not contaminate the uniform.

Donning and removing disposable gloves   Disposable clean gloves are worn to protect the hands when the nurse is likely to handle any body substances, e.g., blood, urine, feces, sputum, mucous membranes, and nonintact skin. Nurses who have open sores or cuts on the hands should wear gloves for protection. Sterile gloves are used when the hands will come in contact with an open wound or when the hands might introduce microorganisms into a body orifice (see Procedure 20–3, later).

Before donning gloves, don a mask (if required), wash and dry the hands, and don a gown. No special technique is required to don disposable gloves, since they are relatively shapeless and either glove fits either hand. They need to be donned carefully, however, so that they do not tear. If a gown is worn, pull up the gloves to cover the cuffs of the gown. If a gown is not worn, pull up the cuffs to cover the wrists.

No special technique is required to remove gloves, since hands should be washed afterward. However, if there is a reason to prevent soilage of the hands (e.g., the nurse has a cut), grasp the first glove to be removed on its palmar surface just below the cuff, taking care that only glove touches glove and not the skin of the wrist or hand, which is considered clean. See Figure 20–9. Pull the first glove completely off by inverting or rolling the glove inside out. Continue to hold the inverted removed glove with the fingers of the gloved hand. Then place the first two fingers of the bare hand inside the cuff of the second glove and pull the second glove off to the fingers by turning it inside out. This action pulls the first glove inside the second. See Figure 20–10. Using the bare hand, continue to remove the gloves, which are now inside out, and put them in the refuse container. See Figure 20–11. The bare hands, which are con-

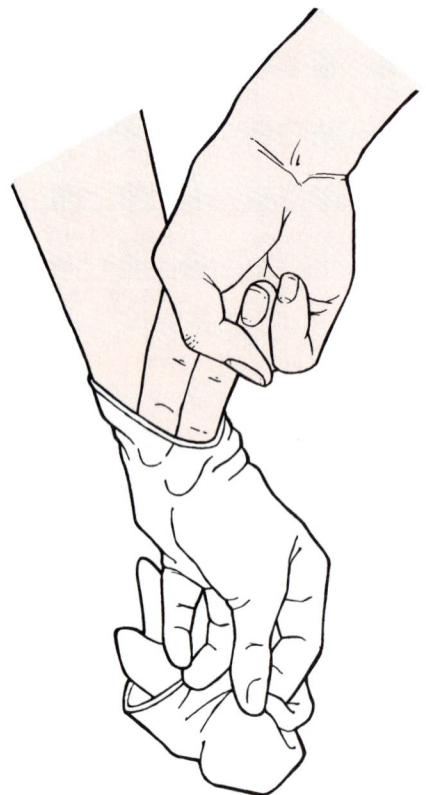

Figure 20–10 Removing the second soiled disposable glove.

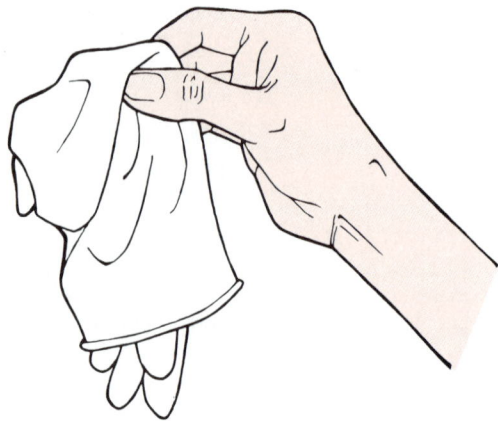

Figure 20–11 Holding soiled disposable gloves with the inside outermost.

sidered clean, touch only the insides of the gloves, which are also considered clean. Wash the hands well. Even though gloves were worn, it is considered essential practice to wash the hands following contact with body substances, mucous membranes, or open skin lesions.

Bagging articles   Articles contaminated with body substances must be bagged before they are removed from the client's unit. The 1983 CDC guidelines recommend the following methods:

1. A single bag, if it is sturdy and impervious to microorganisms, and if the contaminated articles can be placed in the bag without soiling or contaminating its outside

2. Double-bagging (placing items into bags inside the client's room and in turn placing those bags inside clean bags held outside the room by another person) if the above conditions are not met

The nurse who cares for the client is responsible for ensuring that all items are placed in the appropriate containers inside the client's room. General guidelines are shown in the accompanying box.

Recommendations for severely compromised clients   Compromised clients are often infected by their own microorganisms, by microorganisms on the inadequately washed hands of health personnel, and by nonsterile items (food, water, air, and client care equipment). See the accompanying box for the 1983 CDC guidelines for severely compromised clients (Garner and Simmons 1983, p. 254).

Maintaining Surgical Asepsis

An object is sterile only when it is free of all microorganisms. It is well known that surgical asepsis is practiced in operating rooms, labor and delivery rooms, and special diagnostic areas. Less known perhaps is that surgical asepsis is also employed for many procedures in general care areas (i.e., procedures such as administering injections, changing wound dressings, performing urinary catheterizations, and administering intravenous therapy). In these situations, all of the principles of surgical asepsis are applied as in the operating or delivery room; however, not all of the sterile techniques that follow are always required. For example, before an operating room procedure, the nurse generally puts on a mask and cap, performs a surgical hand scrub, and then dons a sterile gown and gloves. In a general care area, the nurse may only perform a hand wash and don sterile gloves. The nine basic principles of surgical asepsis, and practices that relate to each principle, appear in Table 20–11 on page 476.

Using Sterile Equipment and Supplies   Equipment is wrapped in a variety of materials to maintain its sterility. Commercially prepared items are frequently

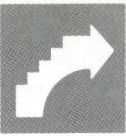

CLINICAL GUIDELINES
Handling Soiled Items

- Handle soiled linen as little as possible and with the least agitation possible, to prevent gross microbial contamination of the air and/or persons handling the linen.

- Place garbage and soiled *disposable* equipment in the plastic bag that lines the waste container. Some agencies separate dry and wet waste material and incinerate dry items, e.g., paper towels and disposable items. They place other waste materials in a central garbage chute or storage area.

- Place glass bottles or jars in separate plastic or paper containers.

- Place leftover food in the wet garbage container, or flush it down the toilet.

- Food trays and dishes do not require special precautions unless they are visibly soiled with infectious material. If the client's hygienic practices are unsafe, use disposable dishes (if available), and discard them in the appropriate waste receptacle in the client's unit. Bag and label contaminated nondisposable (reusable) dishes, utensils, and trays before sending them to the food service department.

- Place dressings in either the wet or the dry waste container, depending on how soiled they are.

- Place special *nondisposable* equipment in a separate bag to be sent to the central supply area. Place glass and metal equipment in separate bags from rubber and plastic items. Glass and metal can be sterilized in an autoclave, but rubber and plastic are damaged by this process and must be cleaned by other methods, e.g., gas sterilization.

- Disassemble special procedure trays into component parts. Some components can be discarded; others need to be sent to the laundry or central services for cleaning and decontaminating.

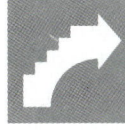

CLINICAL GUIDELINES
Severely Compromised Clients (CDC)

- Frequent and appropriate hand washing by all personnel before, during, and after client care

- Private rooms whenever possible

- Use of sterile gloves, sterile gowns, and masks by people caring for clients with major wounds or burns that cannot be enclosed by dressings.

TABLE 20–11 *Principles and Practices of Surgical Asepsis*

Principles	Practices
All objects used in a sterile field must be sterile.	All articles are sterilized appropriately by dry or moist heat, chemicals, or radiation before use.
	Sterile articles can be stored for only a prescribed time; after that, they are considered unsterile.
	Always check a package containing a sterile object for intactness, dryness, and expiration date. Any package that appears already open, torn, punctured, or wet is considered unsterile. Never assume an item is sterile.
	Storage areas should be clean, dry, off the floor, and away from sinks.
	Always check the sterilization dates and periods on the labels of wrapped items before using the items.
	Always check chemical indicators of sterilization before using a package. The indicator is often a tape used to fasten the package or contained inside the package. The indicator changes color during sterilization, indicating that the contents have undergone a sterilization procedure. If the color change is not evident, the package is considered unsterile. Commercially prepared sterile packages may not have indicators but are marked with the word *sterile*.
Sterile objects become unsterile when touched by unsterile objects.	Handle sterile objects that will touch open wounds or enter body cavities only with sterile forceps or sterile gloved hands.
	Discard or resterilize objects that come into contact with unsterile objects.
	Whenever the sterility of an object is questionable, assume the article is unsterile.
Sterile items that are out of vision or below the waist level of the nurse are considered unsterile.	Once left unattended, a sterile field is considered unsterile.
	Sterile objects are always kept in view. Nurses do not turn their backs on a sterile field.
	Only the front part of a sterile gown (from the waist to the shoulder) and two inches above the elbows to the cuff of the sleeves are considered sterile.
	Always keep sterile gloved hands in sight and above waist level; touch only objects that are sterile.
	Sterile draped tables in the operating room or elsewhere are considered sterile only at surface level.
	Once a sterile field becomes unsterile, it must be set up again before proceeding
Sterile objects can become unsterile by prolonged exposure to airborne microorganisms.	Doors are closed and traffic is kept to a minimum in areas where a sterile procedure is being performed because moving air can carry dust and microorganisms.
	Areas in which sterile procedures are carried out are kept as clean as possible by frequent damp cleaning with detergent germicides to minimize contaminants in the area.
	The nurse's hair is kept clean and short or enclosed in a net to prevent hair from falling on sterile objects. Microorganisms on the hair can make a sterile field unsterile.
	Surgical caps are worn in operating rooms, delivery rooms, and burn units.
	Sneezing or coughing over a sterile field can make it unsterile because droplets containing microorganisms from the respiratory tract can travel 3 feet. Some nurses recommend that masks covering the mouth and the nose should be worn by anyone working over a sterile field or an open wound.
	Nurses with mild upper respiratory tract infections refrain from carrying out sterile procedures or wear masks.
	Anyone working over a sterile field keeps talking to a minimum. The nurse averts the head from the field if talking is necessary.
	The nurse refrains from reaching over a sterile field unless sterile gloves are worn and from moving unsterile objects over a sterile field because microorganisms can fall onto it. Always reach around a sterile field or carefully turn it by reaching under the wrapper or by touching the wrapper edges.

TABLE 20–11 *(continued)*

Principles	Practices
Fluids flow in the direction of gravity.	Unless the nurse is wearing gloves, wet forceps are always held with the tips below the handles. When the tips are held higher than the handles, fluid can flow onto the handle and become contaminated by the hands. When the forceps are again pointed downward, the fluid flows back down and contaminates the tips.
	During a surgical hand wash, the hands are held higher than the elbows to prevent contaminants from the forearms from reaching the hands.
Moisture that passes through a sterile object draws microorganisms from unsterile surfaces above or below to the sterile surface by capillary action.	Sterile waterproof barriers are used beneath sterile objects. Liquids (sterile saline or antiseptics) are frequently poured into containers on a sterile field. If they are spilled onto the sterile field, the barrier keeps the liquid from seeping beneath it.
	The sterile covers on sterile equipment are kept dry. Damp surfaces can attract microorganisms in the air.
	When pouring sterile solutions into sterile containers, care is taken to avoid dampening the sterile field.
	One must replace sterile drapes that do not have a sterile barrier underneath when they become moist.
The edges of a sterile field are considered unsterile.	A 2.5 cm (1 in) margin at each edge of an opened drape is considered unsterile, since the edges are in contact with unsterile surfaces.
	All sterile objects are placed more than 2.5 cm (1 in) inside the edges of a sterile field.
	Any article that falls outside the edges of a sterile field is considered unsterile.
The skin cannot be sterilized and is unsterile.	Sterile gloves are worn and/or sterile forceps are used to handle sterile items.
	Prior to a surgical aseptic procedure, the hands are washed to reduce the number of microorganisms on them.
Conscientiousness, alertness, and honesty are essential qualities in maintaining surgical asepsis.	When a sterile object becomes unsterile, it does not necessarily change in appearance.
	The person who sees a sterile object become contaminated must correct or report the situation.
	A sterile field should not be set up ahead of time for future use.

wrapped in plastic, paper, or glass. Commercially prepared sterile liquids for both internal and external use are often supplied in plastic or glass containers. Plastics are often pliable, usually transparent, impervious to dust, and relatively resistant to tearing. Intravenous solutions are commonly packaged in plastic bags. Liquid medications are sterilized in glass containers. Liquids used in hospitals may be prepared commercially or in the hospital. In the past it was not unusual for sterile liquids, e.g., sterile water for irrigations, to be supplied in large glass containers and used many times. This practice is considered undesirable today because once a container has been opened, there can be no assurance that it is sterile. Liquids are preferably packaged in amounts adequate for one use only. Any leftover liquid is discarded. Hospital-packaged liquids are often sterilized in reusable containers; commercially packaged liquids are supplied in disposable containers. These containers normally have a seal over the cap, and often the word *sterile* is clearly marked on the top. If the cap has been tampered with or if the seal is broken, the liquid is considered unsterile. All containers should also be inspected for cracks.

Handling Sterile Forceps Many styles of forceps are used to handle sterile supplies. Forceps used commonly by nurses are (a) hemostat or artery forceps (see Figure 20–12); (b) tissue forceps (see Figure 20–13); and (c) sponge or transfer (lifting) forceps.

Hemostats and tissue forceps are commonly used for such techniques as changing a sterile dressing and shortening a

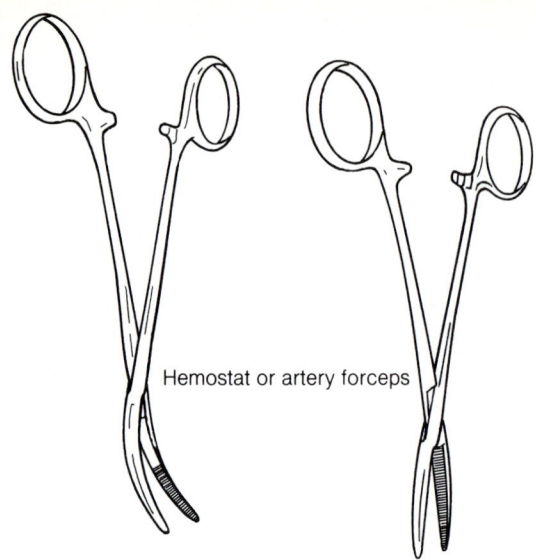

Figure 20–12   Hemostat forceps (curved and straight).

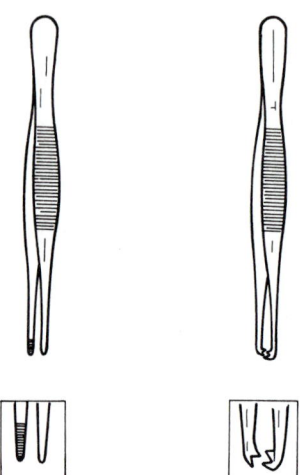

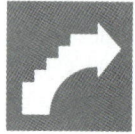

Figure 20–13   Tissue forceps (plain and toothed).

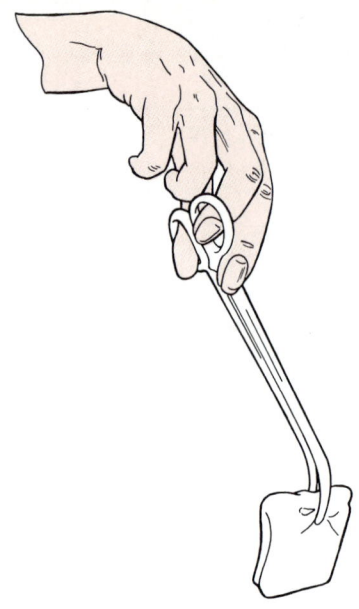

Figure 20–14   Holding forceps with tips lower than the hand.

drain. Transfer forceps are used to move a sterile article from one place to another, e.g., transferring sterile gauze from its package to a sterile dressing tray. Forceps are usually packaged and discarded or resterilized after use.

See the accompanying box for guidelines applying to the use of all types of forceps.

Establishing a Sterile Field   A **sterile field** is a microorganism-free area that can receive sterile supplies. It is often established by using the innermost side of a sterile wrapper or by using a sterile drape. When the field is established, sterile supplies and sterile solutions can be placed on it. Sterile forceps are used in many instances to handle and transfer the sterile supplies.

Procedure 20–2 provides guidelines for using sterile equipment and establishing a sterile field.

CLINICAL GUIDELINES
Using Forceps

■ Keep the tips of wet forceps lower than the wrist at all times, unless wearing sterile gloves. See Figure 20–14. Gravity prevents liquids on the tips from flowing to the handles and later back to the tips, thus making the forceps unsterile. The handles are unsterile once they are held by the bare hand.

■ Hold sterile forceps above waist level. There is less danger of contamination if the forceps are held nearer to eye level.

■ Hold sterile forceps within sight. While out of sight, forceps may inadvertently become unsterile. Any such forceps should be considered unsterile.

■ Remove transfer forceps from their package by lifting the forceps directly upward. Make sure that the forceps do not touch the edge or inside of the container or the outside of the wrapper. These areas are not sterile.

■ When using forceps to lift sterile supplies out of a commercially prepared package, be sure that the forceps do not touch the edges or outside of the wrapper which have been handled, and are thus unsterile.

■ When placing forceps whose handles were in contact with the bare hand on a sterile field, position the handles outside the sterile area.

■ Deposit a sterile item on a sterile field without permitting moist forceps to touch the sterile field.

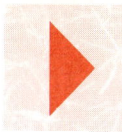

ESTABLISHING AND MAINTAINING A STERILE FIELD

Equipment ☑

Package containing a sterile drape

Sterile equipment as needed, e.g., wrapped sterile gauze, wrapped sterile bowl, antiseptic solution, sterile forceps

Intervention

1. Confirm the sterility of the package.

- Ensure that the package is clean and dry; if moist, it is considered contaminated and must be discarded.

- Check the sterilization expiration dates on the package, and look for any indications that it has been previously opened.

- Follow agency practice about the disposal of possibly contaminated packages.

2. Open the package.

To open a wrapped package on a surface:

- Place the package in the center of the work area so that the top flap of the wrapper opens away from you. *This position prevents subsequent reaching directly over the exposed sterile contents, which could contaminate them.*

- Reaching around the package (not over it), pinch the first flap on the outside of the wrapper between your thumb and index finger. See Figure 20–15. With some folded packages, it may be necessary to grasp the uppermost flap at each corner. *Touching only the outside of the wrapper maintains the sterility of the inside of the wrapper.* Pull the flap open, laying it flat on the far surface.

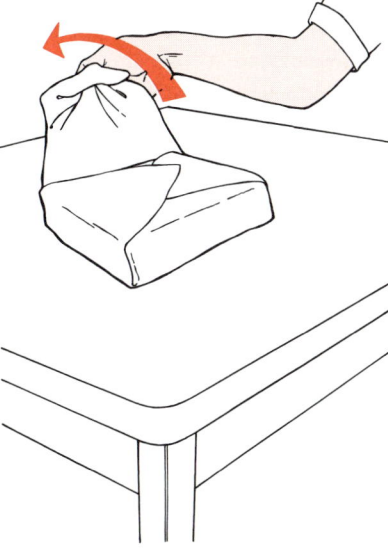

Figure 20–15 Opening the first flap of a sterile wrapped package.

- Repeat for the side flaps, opening the top one first. Use the right hand for the right flap, and the left hand for the left flap. See Figure 20–16. *By using both hands, you avoid reaching over the sterile contents.*

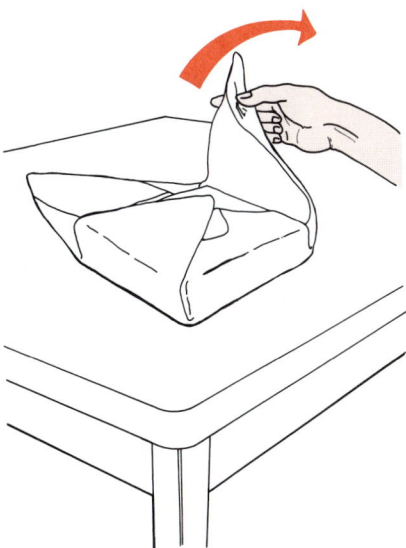

Figure 20–16 Opening the second flap to the side.

- Pull the fourth flap toward you by grasping the corner that is turned down. See Figure 20–17. Make sure that the flap does not touch your uniform. *If the inner surface touches any unsterile article, it is contaminated.*

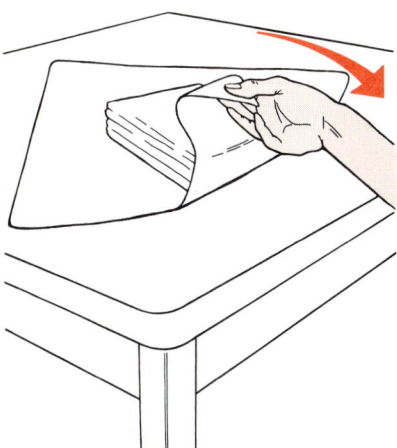

Figure 20–17 Pulling the last flap toward the nurse by grasping the corner.

To open a wrapped package while holding it:

- Hold the package in one hand with the top flap opening away from you.

- Using the other hand, open the package as described above, pulling the corners of the flaps well back. See Figure 20–18. *The hands are considered contaminated, and*

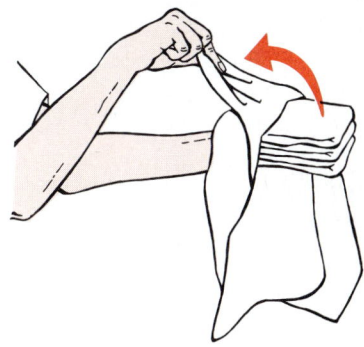

Figure 20–18 Opening a wrapped package while holding it.

at no time should they touch the contents of the package.

To open commercially prepared packages:

Commercially prepared sterile packages and containers usually have manufacturer's directions for opening.

- If the flap of the package has an unsealed corner, hold the container in one hand, and pull back on the flap with the other hand. See Figure 20−19.

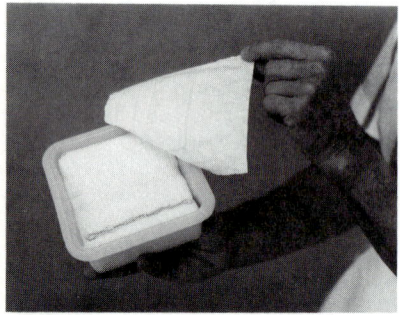

Figure 20−19 Opening a sterile package with an unsealed corner.

- If the package has a partially sealed edge, grasp both sides of the edge, one with each hand, and pull apart gently. See Figure 20−20.

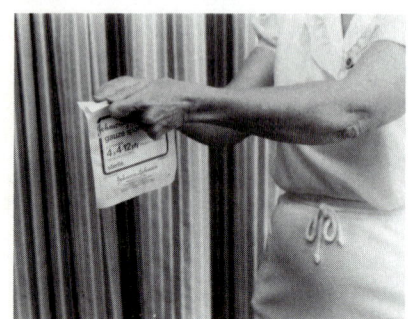

Figure 20−20 Opening a sterile package with a partially sealed edge.

3. **Rewrap the sterile package as required, e.g., for transport to the bedside.**

- Rewrap in the *reverse* order to unwrapping. Close the proximal flap first to prevent reaching across the sterile field, the side flaps next, and the distal flap last.

4. **Establish a sterile field by using a drape.**

- Open the package containing the drape as described above.
- With one hand, pluck the corner of the drape that is folded back on the top.
- Lift the drape out of the cover, and permit it to open freely without touching any articles. See Figure 20−21. *If the drape touches the outside of the package, the nurse's uniform, or any unsterile surface. It is considered contaminated.*

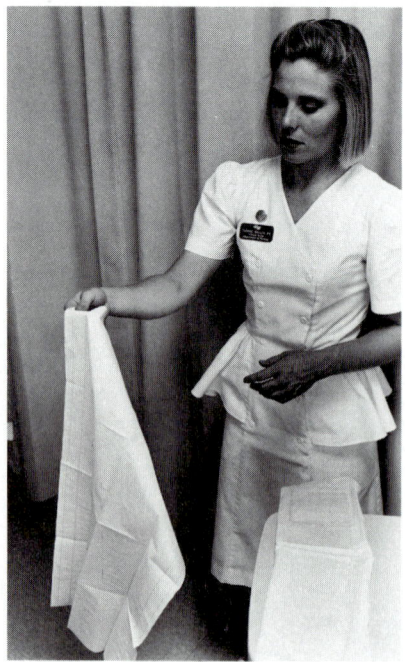

Figure 20−21 Permit a drape to open freely without touching any articles.

- Discard the cover.
- With the other hand, carefully pick up another corner of the drape, holding it well away from yourself.
- Lay the drape on a clean, dry surface, placing the bottom (i.e., the freely hanging side) farthest from you. See Figure 20−22. *By placing the lowermost side farthest away, the nurse avoids leaning over the sterile field and contaminating it.*

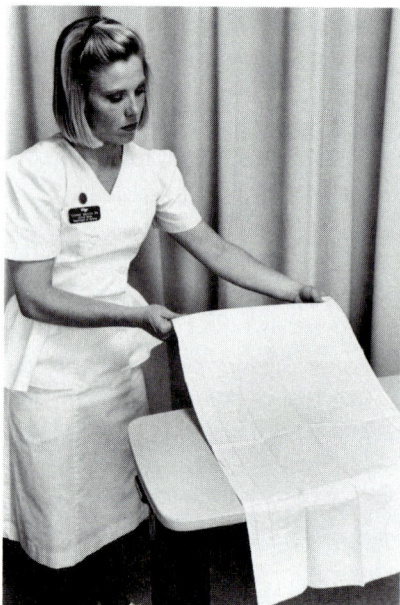

Figure 20−22 Placing a drape on a surface.

5. **Add necessary sterile supplies.**

To add wrapped supplies to a sterile field:

- Open each wrapped package as described in the preceding steps.
- With your free hand, grasp the corners of the wrapper and hold them against the wrist of the hand holding the package. See Figure 20−23. *The unsterile hand is now covered by the sterile wrapper.*

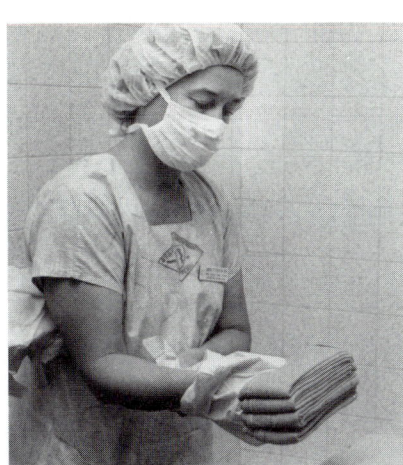

Figure 20–23 Adding wrapped sterile supplies to a sterile field.

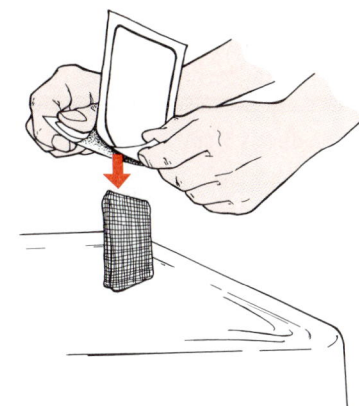

Figure 20–24 Adding a commercially packaged supply to a sterile field.

- Place the sterile bowl, drape, or other supply on the sterile field by approaching from an angle rather than holding your arm over the field.

- Discard the wrapper.

To add commercially packaged supplies to a sterile field:

- Open each package, e.g., gauze, as described above.

- Hold the package 15 cm (6 in) above the field, and permit the contents to drop on the field. See Figure 20–24. Keep in mind that 2.5 cm (1 in) around the edge of the field is considered contaminated. *At a height of 15 cm (6 in), the outside of the package is not likely to touch and contaminate the sterile field.*

To add sterile solution to a sterile bowl:

Sterile liquids (e.g., normal saline) frequently need to be poured into metal or nonabsorbent containers within a sterile field. Unwrapped bottles or flasks that contain sterile solution are considered sterile on the inside and contaminated on the outside, since the bottle may have been handled. Bottles used in an operating room may be sterilized on the outside as well as the inside, however, and these are handled with sterile gloves.

Before pouring any liquid, **read the label three times to make sure you have the correct solution.**

- Obtain the exact amount of solution, if possible. *Once a sterile container has been opened, its sterility cannot be assured for a future use unless it is used again immediately.*

- From the label, confirm the name of solution and its strength.

- Remove the lid or cap from the bottle and invert the lid before placing it on a surface that is not sterile. *Inverting the lid maintains the sterility of the inside surface because it is not allowed to touch an unsterile surface.*

- Hold the bottle so that the label is uppermost. *Any solution that flows down the outside of the bottle during pouring will not damage or obliterate the label.*

- Hold the bottle of fluid at a height of 10 to 15 cm (4 to 6 in) over the bowl and to the side of the sterile field so that as little of the bottle as possible is over the field. *At this height, there is less likelihood of contaminating the sterile field by touching the field or by reaching an arm over it.*

- Pour the solution gently so as not to splash the liquid. *If the sterile drape is on an unsterile surface, any moisture will contaminate the field by facilitating the movement of microorganisms through the sterile drape.*

- Replace the lid securely on the bottle if you plan to use it again, and provide date and time of opening. See agency protocol. *Replacing the lid immediately maintains the sterility of the inner aspect of the lid and the solution.* In many agencies a sterile container of solution that is opened is used only once and then discarded.

Donning Sterile Gloves (Open Method)   Sterile gloves may be donned by the open method or the closed method. The open method is most frequently used outside the operating room, since the closed method requires that the nurse wear a sterile gown. Gloves are worn during many sterile procedures to maintain the sterility of equipment and protect a client's open wound.

Sterile gloves are packaged with a cuff often about 5 cm (2 in) and with the palms facing upward when the package is opened. The package usually indicates the size of the glove (e.g., size 6 or 7½). Gloves may or may not be used with sterile forceps. For example, when inserting a catheter, the nurse generally wears gloves and uses sterile forceps; when changing a dressing, the nurse uses sterile forceps but may not wear gloves. Procedure 20–3 provides instructions for donning sterile gloves.

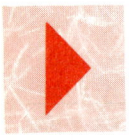

PROCEDURE 20–3

DONNING AND REMOVING STERILE GLOVES (OPEN METHOD)

Equipment

Package of sterile gloves

Intervention

1. Open the package of sterile gloves.

- Place the package of gloves on a clean dry surface. *Any moisture on the surface could contaminate the gloves.*

- Some gloves are packed in an inner as well as an outer package. Open the outer package without contaminating the gloves or the inner package. See Procedure 20–2.

- Remove the inner package from the outer package.

- Open the inner package as above or according to the manufacturer's directions. Some manufacturers provide a numbered sequence for opening the flaps and folded tabs to grasp for opening the flaps. If no tabs are provided, pluck the flap so that your fingers do not touch the inner surfaces. *The inner surfaces, which are next to the sterile gloves, will remain sterile.*

2. Put the first glove on your dominant hand.

- If the gloves are packaged so that they lie side by side, grasp the glove

for your dominant hand by its cuff (on the palmar side) with the thumb and first finger of the nondominant hand. Touch only the inside of the cuff. See Figure 20–25. *The hands are not sterile. By touching only the inside of the glove, the nurse avoids contaminating the outside.*

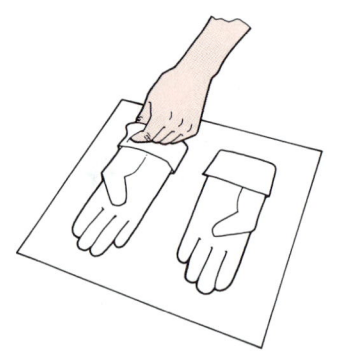

Figure 20–25   Picking up the first sterile glove.

or

If the gloves are packaged one on top of the other, grasp the cuff of the top glove as above, using the opposite hand.

- Insert the dominant hand into the glove and pull the glove on. Keep the thumb of the inserted hand against the palm of the hand during insertion. See Figure 20–26. *If the thumb is kept against the palm,*

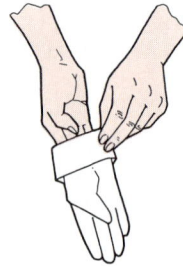

Figure 20–26   Putting on the first sterile glove.

it is less likely to contaminate the outside of the glove.

- Leave the cuff turned down.

3. Put the second glove on your nondominant hand.

- Pick up the other glove with the sterile gloved hand, inserting the gloved fingers under the cuff and holding the gloved thumb close to the gloved palm. See Figure 20–27. *This helps prevent accidental contamination of the glove by the bare hand.*

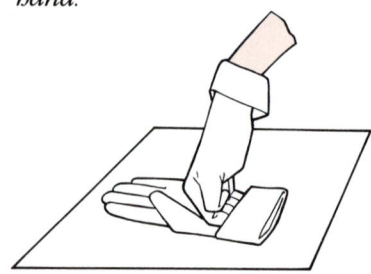

Figure 20–27   Picking up the second sterile glove.

▶

- Pull on the second glove carefully. Hold the thumb of the gloved first hand as far as possible from the palm. See Figure 20–28. *In this position, the thumb is less likely to touch the arm and become contaminated.*

- Adjust each glove so that it fits smoothly, and carefully pull the cuffs up by sliding the fingers under the cuffs.

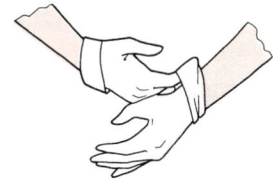

Figure 20–28 Putting on the second sterile glove.

4. **Remove and dispose of used gloves.**

- There is no special technique for removing sterile gloves. If they are soiled with secretions, remove 🔴 them by turning them inside out. See "Donning and Removing Disposable Gloves" earlier.

Donning a Sterile Gown and Sterile Gloves (Closed Method) Sterile gowning and closed gloving are chiefly carried out in operating or delivery rooms, where surgical asepsis is necessary. The closed method of gloving can be used only when a sterile gown is worn because the gloves are handled through the sleeves of the gown. In some agencies, gown and gloves are provided in a single sterile pack; in others, the gloves are provided in a separate package. Prior to these procedures, the nurse dons a hair cover and a mask, and performs a surgical hand wash. See Procedure 20–4.

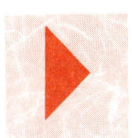

PROCEDURE 20–4

DONNING A STERILE GOWN AND STERILE GLOVES (CLOSED METHOD)

Equipment ☑

A sterile pack containing a sterile gown and sterile gloves.

Intervention

Donning a sterile gown:

1. **Open the sterile pack.**

- Remove the outer wrap from the sterile gloves, and drop the gloves in their inner sterile wrap on the sterile field established by the sterile outer wrapper. *By not touching the inner wrapper, it remains sterile.* See Procedure 20–3, Step 1.

2. **Carry out a surgical scrub for the length of time required by the agency.**

- See Procedure 20–1, page 469.

3. **Put on the sterile gown.**

- Grasp the sterile gown at the crease near the neck, hold it away from you, and permit it to unfold freely without touching anything, including your uniform. *The gown will be unsterile if its outer surface touches any unsterile articles.*

- Put your hands inside the shoulders of the gown, and work your arms partway into the sleeves without touching the outside of the gown. See Figure 20–29.

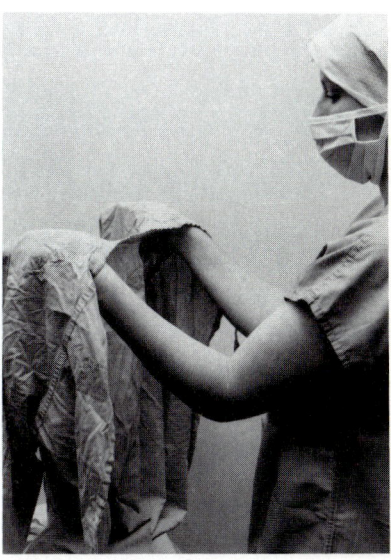

Figure 20–29 Putting on a sterile gown.

■ If donning sterile gloves by using the *closed* method (see below), work your hands down the sleeves only to the proximal edge of the cuffs.

or

If donning sterile gloves by using the *open* method, work your hands down the sleeves and through the cuffs.

■ Have a coworker wearing a hair cover and mask grasp the neck ties without touching the outside of the gown and pull the gown upward to cover the neckline of your uniform in front and back. The coworker ties the neck ties. Gowning continues at step 7.

Donning sterile gloves (closed method):

4. Open the sterile wrapper containing the sterile gloves.

■ Open the glove wrapper while the hands are still covered by the sleeves. See Figure 20–30.

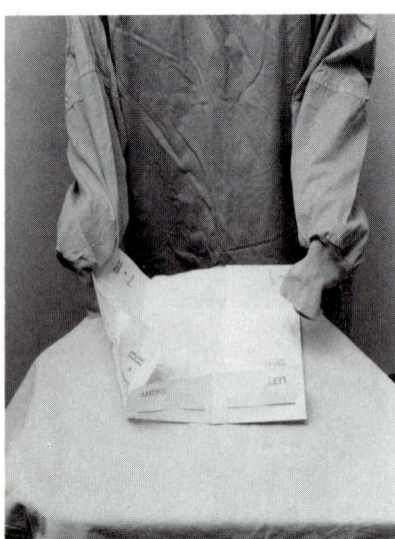

Figure 20–30 Opening the sterile glove wrapper.

5. Put the glove on your non-dominant hand.

■ With your *dominant* hand, pick up the *opposite* glove with your thumb and index finger, handling it through the sleeve.

■ Lay the glove on the opposite gown cuff, thumb side down, with the glove opening pointed toward the fingers. See Figure 20–31. Position your nondominant hand palm upward inside the sleeve.

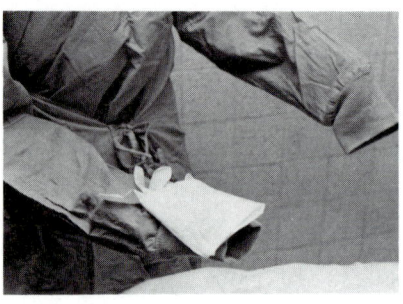

Figure 20–31 Positioning the first sterile glove for the nondominant hand.

■ With the nondominant hand, grasp the cuff of the glove through the gown cuff, and firmly anchor it.

■ With your dominant hand working through its sleeve, grasp the upper side of the glove's cuff, and stretch it over the cuff of the gown.

■ Pull the sleeve up to draw the cuff over the wrist as you extend the fingers of the nondominant hand into the glove's fingers. See Figure 20–32.

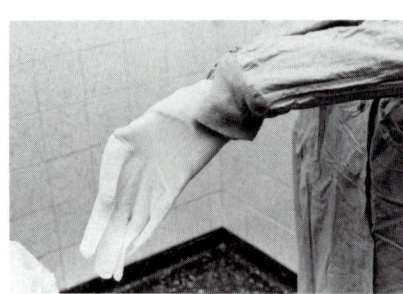

Figure 20–32 Pulling on the first sterile glove.

6. Put the glove on your dominant hand.

■ Place the fingers of the gloved hand under the cuff of the remaining glove.

■ Place the glove over the cuff of the second sleeve.

■ Extend he fingers into the glove as you pull the glove up over the cuff. See Figure 20–33.

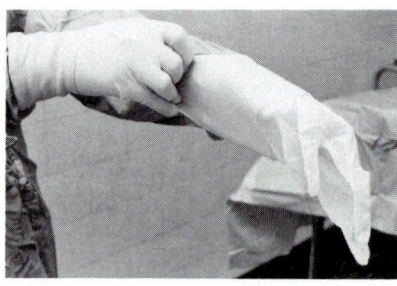

Figure 20–33 Extending the fingers into the second glove for the dominant hand.

Completion of gowning:

7. Complete gowning as follows.

■ Have a coworker who is masked and whose hair is covered hold the waist tie of your gown, using sterile gloves or a sterile wrapper or drape. *This approach keeps the ties sterile.*

■ Make a three-quarter turn, then take the tie, and secure it in front of the gown.

or

Have a coworker wearing sterile gloves take the two ties at each side of the gown and tie them at the back of the gown, making sure that your uniform is completely covered. *Both methods ensure that the back of the gown remains sterile.*

EVALUATING THE EFFECTIVENESS OF PROTECTIVE MEASURES

To evaluate the achievement of client goals, the nurse may need to perform the following evaluative activities:

- Question the client about causative or risk factors for infection, measures to reduce the risk of infection, practices implemented to prevent infection, immunizations received, and the presence of specific signs and symptoms of infection.
- Observe the client for signs of infection, e.g., the status of a surgical incision.
- Review recent laboratory data, e.g., cultures of body secretions, excretions, and exudates and white blood cell counts.

Examples of evaluative statements indicating goal achievement are "The client verbalized five measures to reduce the risk of infection," "The client stated she obtained diphtheria immunization September 20, 19xx," and "Surgical incision dry and free of inflammation (September 30, 19xx)."

Many health facilities have infection control committees whose responsibility is to investigate, control, and prevent infections in the facility. In 1958, the Joint Commission on Accreditation of Hospitals (JCAH) recommended that every hospital set up an infection control committee. The responsibilities of the infection control committee are

1. To establish a system for reporting infections
2. To keep records of infections
3. To review the hospital's bacteriologic services
4. To review and make recommendations about the hospital's aseptic practices
5. To undertake an educational program for hospital employees

An infection control nurse is a member of the committee. The responsibilities of this nurse, often referred to as a nurse epidemiologist, are to

1. Promote personnel behaviors that help control infection
2. Provide facts and statistical data regarding epidemiologic investigations
3. Supervise the hospital infection control program

How the infection control nurse performs these responsibilities varies from agency to agency. The following are common ways:

- Conveying, promoting, and supporting positive attitudes toward infection control
- Reporting relevant information to the hospital infection control committee, e.g., problems with implementing specific control measures
- Initiating and presenting proposals regarding infection control to the committee
- Carrying out an infection control education program for staff
- Collecting and analyzing data regarding nosocomial infections among clients and staff
- Teaching clients, support persons, and staff specific protective measures for clients
- Investigating unusual occurrences of infection
- Consulting with staff regarding infection control
- Coordinating the hospital program with the community
- Acting as the hospital liaison to public health agencies

CHAPTER HIGHLIGHTS

- Microorganisms are everywhere. Most are harmless and some are beneficial; however, many can cause infection in susceptible persons.
- Effective control of infectious disease is an international, national, community, and individual responsibility.
- Asepsis is the freedom from infection or infectious material.
- Medical aseptic practices limit the number, growth, and spread of microorganisms.
- Surgical aseptic practices keep an area or objects free of all microorganisms.

- An infection can develop if the six links in the chain of infection—infectious agent, reservoir, portal of exit, mode of transmission, portal of entry, and susceptible host—are not interrupted.
- Aseptic practices can be used to break any of the six links in the chain of infection.
- Humans have both nonspecific and specific defenses that combat infectious agents.
- Intact skin and mucous membranes are the body's first line of defense against microorganisms.
- Some normal body flora release bacteriocins and anti-

▶

CHAPTER HIGHLIGHTS (continued)

biotic-like substances that inhibit microbial growth and destroy foreign bacteria.

▸ Some body secretions (e.g., saliva and tears) contain enzymes that act as antibacterial agents.

▸ The inflammatory response limits physical, chemical, and microbial injury and promotes repair of injured tissue.

▸ The immune defense responds to specific antigens; it is mediated either by antibodies produced by lymphoid B cells circulating in blood serum or by lymphoid T cells residing in cells of the lymphoid system.

▸ Both B cells and T cells are cells that defend against invasions by the same antigen.

▸ Immunity is the specific resistance of the body to infectious agents.

▸ Acquired immunity is active or passive and in either case may be naturally or artifically induced.

▸ Especially at risk of acquiring an infection are the very young or old; those with poor nutritional status, a defi-ciency of serum immunoglobulins, multiple stressors, insufficient immunizations, or an existing disease process; and those receiving certain medical therapies.

▸ The incidence of nosocomial infections is significant. Major sites for these infections are the respiratory and urinary tracts, the bloodstream, and surgical or open wounds.

▸ Factors that contribute to nosocomial infections are invasive procedures, medical therapies, the existence of a large number of susceptible persons, inappropriate use of antibiotics, and insufficient hand washing after client contact and after contact with body substances.

▸ Preventing infections in healthy or ill persons and preventing the spread of microorganisms from infected clients to others are major nursing functions.

▸ The nurse must be knowledgeable about sources and modes of transmission of microorganisms.

▸ Microorganisms are invisible, and nurses have an ethical obligation to ensure that appropriate aseptic measures are taken to protect clients, support persons, and health personnel, including themselves.

READINGS AND REFERENCES

SUGGESTED READINGS

Brennan, L., and the Editors of *Nursing 88*. April 1988. The battle against AIDS: A report from the nursing front. *Nursing 88* 18:60–64.

The authors surveyed 18 hospitals to learn how nurses feel about caring for AIDS patients. The report includes ways nurses are protecting themselves and discusses their major concerns.

Crow, S. March 1990. Calling in sick: How to decide. *Nursing 90* 20:63–64.

The author describes some of the common illnesses of nurses and suggests not going to work when, for example, coughing up heavy mucus, running a fever, and experiencing a severe sore throat, jaundice, or draining lesion. The article offers nurses guidelines for action when experiencing certain symptoms.

Jackson, M. M.; Lynch, P.; McPherson, D. C.; Cummings, M. J.; and Greenawalt, N. C. September 1987. Why not treat all body substances as infectious? *American Journal of Nursing* 87:1137–39.

The authors present a case for treating all blood and body substances from all clients as infectious. In 1987, the American Hospital Association and the Association for Practitioners of Infection Control recommended the practice of universal blood and body fluid precautions. The authors contend that this system would reduce cross-infection from infected clients and cross-transmission from clients who are colonized but show no signs of infection.

Jones, I. April 1985. You can drive back infection . . . if you know where to make your stand. *Nursing 85* 15:50–52.

Jones discusses the process by which an infection takes hold. Colonization by the microorganism, the barriers to infection, two methods of transmission, and the targets of infection are explained. Included is a chart indicating the normal flora of each system, common signs and symptoms of an infection of each system, laboratory data, and special nursing considerations.

RELATED RESEARCH

Butz, A. M.; Laughon, B. E.; Gullette, D. L.; and Larson, E. L. April 1990. Alcohol-impregnated wipes as an alternative in hand hygiene. *American Journal of Infection Control* 18:70–76.

Graham, M. April 1990. Frequency and duration of handwashing in an intensive care unit. *American Journal of Infection Control* 18:77–81.

Jackson, M. M.; Dechairo, D. C.; and Gardner, D. F. February 1986. Perceptions and beliefs of nursing and medical personnel about needle-handling practices and needlestick injuries. *American Journal of Infection Control* 14:1–10.

LeClair, S. M.; Schicker, J. M.; Duthie, E. H.; Hoffman, R. G.; and Franson, T. R. August 1988. Survey of nursing personnel attitudes toward infections and their control in the elderly. *American Journal of Infection Control* 16:159–66.

Williamson, K. M.; Selleck, C. S.; Turner, J. G.; Brown, K. C.; Newman, K. D.; and Sirles, A. T. Spring 1988. State of the science: Occupational health hazards for nurses: Infection. *Image: Journal of Nursing Scholarship* 20:48–53.

SELECTED REFERENCES

Benenson, A. S., editor. 1985. *Control of communicable diseases in man.* 14th ed. An official report of the American Public Health Association. Washington, D.C.: The American Public Health Association.

Byrne, J. C.; Saxton, D. F.; Pelikan, P. K.; and Nugent, P. M. 1986. *Laboratory tests: Implications for nursing care.* Menlo Park, Calif.: Addison-Wesley Publishing Co.

Carpenito, L. J. 1989. *Nursing diagnosis: Application to clinical practice.* 3d ed. Philadelphia: J. B. Lippincott Co.

Carroll, M. March/April 1984. Infection control in long-term care. *Geriatric Nursing* 5:100–103.

Centers for for Disease Control. 1987. Recommendations for prevention of HIV transmission in health-care settings. *Morbidity and Mortality Weekly Report* (suppl) 36:3s–18s.

————. Recommendations for prevention of HIV transmission in health care settings. June 24, 1988. *Morbidity and Mortality Weekly Report* 37:1–7.

Doenges, M. E., and Moorhouse, M. F. 1988. *Nurse's pocket guide: Nursing diagnoses with interventions.* 2d ed. Philadelphia: F. A. Davis Co.

Garner, J. S., and Favero, M. S. 1985. *Guideline for handwashing and hospital environmental control 1985.* Washington, D.C.: U.S. Government Printing Office.

Garner, J. S., and Simmons, B. P. July/August 1983. CDC guidelines for isolation precautions in hospitals. *Infection Control* 4:245–325. Special Supplements.

Jackson, M. M.; Lynch, P.; McPherson, D. C.; Cummings, M. J.; and Greenawalt, N. C. September 1987. Why not treat all body substances as infectious? *American Journal of Nursing* 87:1137–39.

Jones, I. April 1985. You can drive back infection . . . if you know where to make your stand. *Nursing 85* 15:50–52.

Kim, M. J.; McFarland, G. K.; and McLane, A. M. 1989. *Pocket guide to nursing diagnoses.* 3d ed. St. Louis: C. V. Mosby Co.

Larson, E. January 1984. Current handwashing issues. *Infection Control* 5:15–17.

Maki, D. G.; Alvarado, C.; Hassemer, C. 1986. Double-bagging of items from isolation rooms is unnecessary as an infection control measure: A comparative study of surface contamination with single- and double-bagging. *Infection Control* 7:535–37.

NANDA approved nursing diagnostic categories for clinical use and testing. Summer 1988. *Nursing Diagnosis Newsletter* 15:1–3.

Norton, C. F. 1986. *Microbiology.* 2d ed. Reading, Mass.: Addison-Wesley Publishing Co.

Parent, B. December 1985. Moral, ethical, and legal aspects of infection control. *American Journal of Infection Control* 13:278–80.

Pickering, L. K., and DuPont, H. L. 1986. *Infectious diseases of children and adults: A step-by-step approach to diagnosis and treatment.* Menlo Park, Calif.: Addison-Wesley Publishing Co.

Setia, U.; Serventi, I.; and Lorenzo, P. April 1985. Nosocomial infection among patients in a long-term care facility: Spectrum, prevalence, and risk factors. *American Journal of Infection Control* 13:57–62.

Simmons, B. P. August 1983. CDC guidelines for the prevention and control of nosocomial infections. Guidelines for prevention of surgical wound infections. *American Journal of Infection Control* 11:133–41.

Stark, J. L., and Hunt, V. January 1985. Don't let nosocomial infections get your patients down. *Nursing 85* 15:10–11.

Turner, J. G., and Williamson, K. M. June and August 1986. AIDS: A challenge for contemporary nursing. (2 parts) *Focus* 13:53–61; 41–50.

Whaley, L. F., and Wong, D. L. 1989. *Essentials of pediatric nursing.* St. Louis: C. V. Mosby Co.

William, A. R. October 1985. Cost-effective application of the Centers for Disease Control guideline for handwashing and hospital environment control. *American Journal of Infection Control* 13:218–23.

Williams, P., and Bierer, B. March/April 1984. Wash your hands! *Geriatric Nursing* 5:103–4.

Williams, W. W. July/August 1983. CDC guideline for infection control in hospital personnel. *Infection Control* 4:326–49.

————. February 1984. CDC guidelines for the prevention and control of nosocomial infections: Guideline for infection control in hospital personnel. *American Journal of Infection Control* 12:34–57.

CHAPTER

21

Providing a Safe Environment

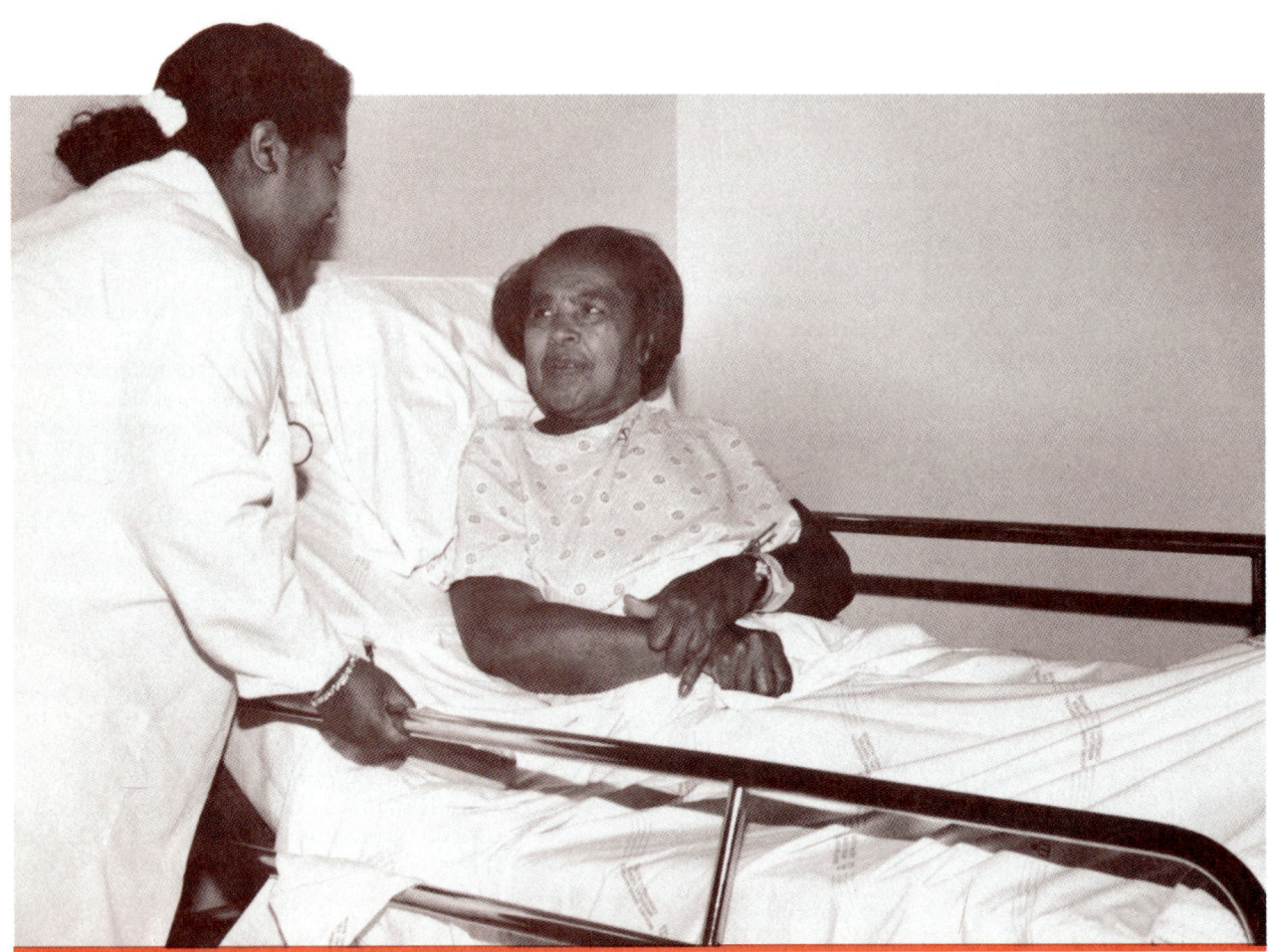

OBJECTIVES

▶ Identify clients at risk of physical injury.

▶ Identify common hazards in the home.

▶ Give examples of nursing diagnoses for clients at risk for accidental injury.

▶ List outcome criteria for evaluating

selected strategies for preventing injury.

▸ Describe nursing responsibilities regarding fires.

▸ Identify common causes of scalds and burns in home and hospital settings.

▸ Identify precautions to prevent falls of hospitalized clients.

▸ Describe legal implications of restraining clients.

▸ State guidelines for selecting and applying restraints.

▸ Identify essential precautions to prevent poisoning.

▸ Identify measures to reduce electrical hazards.

▸ Describe measures to minimize noise.

▸ List precautions to prevent exposure to radiation.

ASSESSING CLIENTS AT RISK FOR INJURY

The ability of people to protect themselves from injury is affected by a number of factors, such as age, life-style, sensory perception, awareness, mobility, emotional state, ability to communicate, history of previous accidents, safety knowledge, and the existence of safety hazards in the home. Nurses need to assess each of these factors when they plan care or teach clients to protect themselves.

Age
Through knowledge and accurate assessment of the environment, people learn to protect themselves from many injuries. Children walking to school learn to stop before crossing the street and wait for oncoming traffic. They also learn not to touch a hot stove. For the very young, learning about the environment is essential. Only through knowledge and experience do children learn what is potentially harmful.

Elderly people also can have special problems protecting themselves from injury. Often the balance of elderly people is impaired by their flexed posture, which places their center of gravity forward. Once balance is lost, it is not readily regained. An elderly person may need to learn to stand up slowly, thus avoiding the fall that can result from a quick, sudden movement. Slowness of movement and diminished sensual acuity also contribute to the likelihood of injury. Elderly persons may neither see nor hear an oncoming car. They may not see a footstool. They may also be unable to pull themselves out of a bathtub safely.

Life-Style
Life-style factors that place people at risk are unsafe work environments, where workers are in danger from machinery, industrial belts and pulleys, and chemicals; residence in neighborhoods with high crime rates; access to guns and ammunition; insufficient income to buy safety equipment or make necessary repairs; and access to illicit drugs, which may also be contaminated by harmful additives. Risk-taking behavior is a factor in accidents. For example, some people disregard safety recommendations by driving automobiles at high speeds and refusing to wear seat belts in automobiles, headgear on motorcycles, or flotation jackets in boats.

Sensory/Perceptual Alterations
Accurate sensory perception of environmental stimuli is vital to safety. These stimuli, which are received by sensory receptors of the body, travel through the nerves to the central nervous system. In a reflex action, such as jerking the hand away from a hot object, some of the impulses travel directly to motor neurons, which then convey the impulses to the muscles that cause the sudden, quick withdrawing of the hand. At the same time, other sensory impulses travel to the cerebral cortex; and the person, now aware of the stimulus, initiates further impulses that result in voluntary muscle movement. Impairment of any of these areas—the sensory receptors, sensory pathways, the internuncial neurons that transmit the impulses from the sensory pathways to the motor pathways, the motor pathways, or the cerebral cortex—can diminish ability to respond normally to environmental stimuli.

People with impaired touch perception, hearing, taste, smell, and vision are highly susceptible to injury. A person who does not see well may trip over a toy or not see a signal cord at a hospital bed unit. Deaf persons do not hear a siren in traffic, and persons with impaired olfactory sense may not smell burning food or escaping gas. Paralysis and other neurologic impairments diminish touch perceptions. A paralyzed person may not feel a burn from a burning hot-water bottle, and a person whose sense of taste is impaired may not detect contaminated food.

Some neurologic diseases cause changes in kinesthetic sense and tactile perceptions. Disease of the inner ear, for example, can cause loss of kinesthetic sense. Spinal cord injuries and cerebrovascular accidents cause paralysis and loss of tactile perception. Certain problems create sensations that do not arise from normal external or internal stimuli. For example, a client who has a disease of the auditory nerve may hear sounds that correspond to no external stimulus. Hallucinations (perceptions of external stimuli in the absence of such stimuli) can result, for example, from a disease process or hallucinogenic drugs. Illusions are misinterpretations of external stimuli. For example, a person may interpret a shadow cast by a lamp as a person.

Level of Awareness
Awareness is the ability to perceive environmental stimuli and body reactions and to

respond appropriately through thought and action. The normal, alert person assimilates many kinds of information at one time, perceives reality accurately, and acts on those perceptions. Part of this process is separating necessary stimuli from extraneous ones and reaching logical conclusions by correlating information. Most people do this with little or no awareness of the mental processes involved. Occasionally, people exhibit abnormalities of thought; they may become absent-minded or lose their sense of direction. Often these episodes are due to intense concentration on one subject to the exclusion of others.

Illness and age can affect **consciousness** (the awareness of environment, self, and others), as can hospitalization. Mildly confused hospitalized clients may momentarily forget they are not at home, wander from their rooms, misplace personal belongings, and so forth. Severely confused (disoriented) persons may not know family members or may think the nurse is a relative. Such persons may act atypically: Confused, usually docile people may become combative with nurses and others. Severely confused people do not know where they are or what time of day or day of the week it is. Clients with impaired awareness include persons lacking in sleep, unconscious or semiconscious persons, disoriented persons, (i.e., those who may not understand where they are or what to do to help themselves), persons who perceive stimuli that do not exist, and persons whose judgment is altered by medications, such as narcotics, tranquilizers, hypnotics, and sedatives.

Mobility Status

Persons who have impaired mobility due to paralysis, muscle weakness, and poor balance or coordination are obviously prone to injury. Clients with spinal cord injury and paralysis of both legs may be unable to move even when they perceive discomfort. Hemiplegic clients or clients with leg casts often have poor balance and fall easily. Clients weakened by illness or surgery are not always fully aware of their condition. It is not uncommon for clients to believe themselves able to walk and fall while trying.

Emotional State

Extreme emotional states can alter the ability to perceive environmental hazards. The acutely anxious or angry person has reduced perceptual awareness. Depressed persons may think and react to environmental stimuli more slowly than usual. People worried about their own or loved ones' illnesses are less aware than usual of potential dangers in the environment, such as a street curb or an oncoming automobile.

Ability to Communicate

People with diminished ability to receive and convey information are also at risk for injury. Aphasic clients, people with language barriers, and those unable to read are among them. For example, the person unable to interpret the sign "No smoking—oxygen in use" may cause a fire.

Previous Accidents

It is helpful to know if a client has a previous history of accidents. It has been recognized for some time that some people are accident prone. Predisposition to accidents is thought to have an emotional basis. One theory is that emotional tension impairs a person's perceptions and judgments, thus making that person more likely to have an accident. Some propose that accidents may fulfill masochistic and hostile needs or fulfill desires to be cared for by others.

Safety Knowledge

Information is crucial to safety. Clients in hospitals and other unfamiliar environments frequently need specific safety information. Lack of knowl-

---

Adult Home Hazard Appraisal

Assess:
- *Walkways and stairways (inside and outside)*. Note uneven sidewalks or paths, broken or loose steps, absence of hand rails or placement on only one side of stairways, insecure hand rails, congested hallways or other traffic areas, and adequacy of lighting at night.
- *Floors*. Note uneven and highly polished or slippery floors and any unanchored rugs or mats.
- *Furniture*. Note hazardous placement of furniture with sharp corners. Note chairs or stools that are too low to get into and out of or that provide inadequate support.
- *Bathroom(s)*. Note presence of grab bars around tubs and toilets, nonslip surfaces in tubs and shower stalls, adequacy of night lighting, adequacy of lighting for medicine cabinet, and need for raised toilet seat or bath chair in tub or shower.
- *Kitchen*. Note pilot lights (gas stove) in need of repair, inaccessible storage areas, and hazardous furniture.
- *Bedrooms*. Note adequacy of lighting, in particular the availability of night lights and accessibility of light switches. Assess floors and furniture as above.
- *Electrical*. Note unanchored and/or frayed electrical cords and overloaded outlets or those near water.
- *Fire protection*. Note presence or absence of fire extinguisher and fire escape plan, improper storage of combustibles, e.g., gasoline, or corrosives, e.g., rust remover (phosphoric acid), and accessibility of emergency telephone numbers (fire, police).
- *Toxic substances*. Note medications kept beyond date of expiration and improperly labeled cleaning solutions.

edge about unfamiliar equipment, such as oxygen tanks, intravenous tubing, and hot packs, is a potential hazard. Nurses need to teach clients what safety precautions to take when oxygen is in use and how to maintain intravenous infusions.

 Home Hazard Appraisal　　Hazards in the home are major causes of falls, fire, poisoning, **suffocation** (smothering), and other accidents, such as those caused by improper use of household equipment (e.g., tools and cooking utensils). The appraisal of such hazards is an essential nursing function. See the accompanying box for a home hazard appraisal for the adult. See Chapters 25 and 26 for potential hazards and preventive actions for children and adolescents.

DIAGNOSING

The nursing diagnostic category applicable to clients at risk for physical injury is **Potential for injury**. This is defined as "the state in which an individual is at risk for harm because of a perceptual or physiologic deficit, a lack of awareness of hazards or maturational age" (Carpenito 1989, p. 472).

Three subcomponents of the diagnostic label **Potential for injury** accepted by NANDA are **Potential for trauma**, "an accentuated risk of accidental tissue injury such as a wound, burns, or fracture"; **Potential for poisoning**, "the state in which an individual is at high risk of accidental exposure to or ingestion of drugs or dangerous substances"; and **Potential for suffocation**, "the state in which an individual is at risk for smothering and asphyxiation" (Carpenito 1989, p. 472).

Examples of these nursing diagnoses and contributing factors are shown below. Examples of assessment data clusters and related nursing diagnoses are shown in Table 21–1.

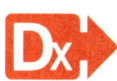 **Nursing Diagnoses**
Clients at Risk for Physical Injury

Potential for injury related to:
- Impaired physical mobility associated with musculoskeletal disability or prescribed therapy
- Altered thought processes (e.g., faulty judgment)
- Impaired sensory function
- Household hazards
- Automotive hazards
- Fire hazards
- Thermal hazards
- Chemical hazards
- Radiation hazards
- Substance abuse

- History of accidents
- Improper use of household, recreational, or occupational equipment
- Medications that affect cerebral functioning
- Unfamiliar setting (e.g., hospital, nursing home)
- Improper use of cane, walker, crutches, or wheelchair
- Knowledge deficit (safety education)
- Lack of safety precautions

Potential for trauma related to the above

Potential for poisoning related to:
- Lack of education
- Dangerous products accessible to children
- Chemical contamination of food or water
- Presence of poisonous vegetation
- Presence of atmospheric pollutants

Potential for suffocation related to:
- Lack of safety education (e.g., water safety)
- Lack of safety precautions
- External factors (e.g., playing with plastic bags, pillow in infant's crib, warming automobile in closed garage, nonvented fuel-burning heaters)

TABLE 21–1　*Examples of Assessment Data Clusters and Related Nursing Diagnoses*

Data Clusters	Nursing Diagnosis
Edith Dalton, an elderly widow, lives alone in her own home. She has a history of glaucoma, for which she takes eye drops twice daily. She reports difficulty in focusing, loss of side vision, and inability to adjust to darkness.	**Potential for injury** related to sensory deficit (impaired visual ability)
David Gagnon suffered a stroke one month ago and has been discharged to his apartment. Home assessment revealed lack of bathroom safety (no grab bars or nonskid shower floor), unanchored rugs, inadequate light at night, and several cluttered traffic areas	**Potential for injury** related to altered mobility and lack of home safety precautions

PLANNING CARE TO PREVENT CLIENT INJURY

The nurse planning health protective measures must consider the age, knowledge, and sensory deficits of the client. Potential hazards and preventive measures for people of all ages are discussed in Chapters 25, 26, and 27. The nursing care plan should include two aspects: (a) educating clients about preventive actions and (b) modifying the environment to make it safe. The latter can involve not only arranging the environment but also limiting the environment in some ways.

The overall client goal is to prevent injury by helping the client to identify hazards and to take related safety measures.

Education is a major factor in preventing accidents. It is directed toward helping people identify potential hazards and changing their health practices and habits accordingly. The environment contains many hazards, both seen and unseen. The automobile is an obvious hazard. Radiation is an unseen hazard.

The need for a safe environment is a national, community, and individual concern. Nurses are voicing their thoughts individually and collectively about such issues as air and water pollution and the safety of foods, cosmetics, and medications. The need for safety on the highways is underscored by newspaper reports of morbidity and mortality from automobile accidents. Increasingly, governments are being pressed to take action and legislate in these areas to make the environment safer. In addition, people are also becoming aware of safety hazards in their communities. Regulations to control the speed of boats on lakes used for swimming, local ordinances curbing the burning of refuse, and stricter local regulation of industrial pollution are all indications of increasing awareness of the need for safety in the environment.

Traditionally, nurses have thought of safety in relation to a client's immediate environment, and this awareness is no less important today in spite of the broader focus on human protection. A primary concern of nurses is awareness of what constitutes a safe environment for a particular person and how this environment can be achieved. The blind person may need railings; the crawling baby, a protective gate at the head of the stairs; and the person who has impaired sight, a secure footing and an uncluttered floor. Nurses thus focus attention on preventing accidents and injury as well as on assisting the injured.

To provide a safe environment, it may be necessary for the nurse and/or client to modify the environment. Older clients with sensory deficits are particularly susceptible to injury. As a result, they may require assistance from nurses in taking precautions to prevent accidents. A client with loss of vision may require assistance walking. A nurse should stand on the client's nondominant side about one step ahead of the client. A blind person should grasp the nurse's arm with the nondominant arm. In addition, nurses can make the environment safe by (a) arranging furniture and other objects so the client will not trip over them and explaining the location of furniture and (b) leaving bedside articles as the client arranges them and within easy reach.

The client whose level of consciousness is altered also requires special protection. Side rails to prevent falls, appropriate positioning in bed, appropriate lighting, and reduced noise level are all common measures nurses employ to ensure client safety. If the client is unconscious, necessary nursing interventions include bathing, giving skin care, feeding, and meeting elimination needs. If the client is disoriented but conscious, the nurse may need to give instructions on how to perform these activities. Unless the person is totally incapacitated, nurses should foster independence and feelings of self-worth by helping the individuals care for themselves.

Planning also involves the development of outcome criteria to evaluate the achievement of client goals and the effectiveness of nursing interventions. Examples of outcome criteria follow.

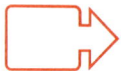

Outcome Criteria
Clients at Risk for Physical Injury

The client:

- Relates factors (e.g., physiologic) that increase the potential for injury.
- Identifies potentially hazardous factors in the environment.
- Identifies preventive measures for specific hazards (e.g., fire, falls, poisoning, burns).
- Reports an intent to carry out selected preventive measures.
- Demonstrates appropriate use of countermeasures to protect self from injury.
- Teaches children safety precautions and habits.
- Reports or demonstrates safety practices in the home.
- Alters physical environment to reduce risk of injury.
- Seeks instruction to (a) handle new equipment (e.g., household, occupational, or recreational) or (b) implement safe child-rearing practices.

IMPLEMENTING STRATEGIES IN RESPONSE TO SPECIFIC HAZARDS/CONDITIONS

Fire

Fire is a constant danger in homes and hospitals. Common causes of hospital fires are smoking in bed and faulty electrical equipment. Hospital fires are particularly hazardous to clients who are incapacitated and unable to leave the building without assistance. Many health care agencies have instituted no smoking policies both to decrease the chances of fire and to promote employee health.

A fire can burn only if three elements are present: sufficient heat to start the fire, a combustible material, and sufficient oxygen to support the fire. To prevent fires, the nurse controls the environment to ensure that the three essential elements are not simultaneously present.

Health care agencies usually follow established procedures in an emergency or during a fire. Nurses need to become familiar with the practices of their employing agency. When a fire occurs, the nurse has two major goals:

1. To protect clients from injury
2. To contain and put out the fire

 General protective practices to meet these goals include the following:

- Making sure the telephone numbers of emergency services are displayed on all telephones
- Knowing the location of fire exits
- Knowing the location and types of fire extinguishers and learning to operate them
- Learning the agency's fire drill or fire evacuation procedure
- Keeping access to firehoses clear at all times
- Keeping hallways free of unnecessary furniture and equipment
- Posting signs on elevator doors so that people will know to use the stairs in the event of fire
- Making sure the location of fire exits is clearly marked.

In the event of fire, nurses follow the guidelines in the accompanying box.

Carrying Clients from Fires

There are a number of methods of carrying persons from the scene of a fire. Generally, nurses use these carries when they cannot wheel out clients confined to their beds or transfer them out on stretchers. Nonnursing hospital personnel (e.g., maintenance, housekeeping, and dietary staff) may assist with evacuating clients and should receive inservice education on using these carries.

- *Swing carry.* The swing is a two-person carry used for heavy clients. The client, in a sitting position, places the arms around each nurse's shoulders. Each nurse holds the client's wrists, which are over each nurse's shoulders, to support the client. The nurses then reach behind the client and grasp each other's shoulder or upper arm. The nurses then release the client's wrists, reach under the client's thighs, and grasp each other's wrists. They lift and carry the client in this sitting position. See Figure 21–1. This carry is sometimes referred to as the two-handed seat, in which a hand-forearm interlock is used. A varia-

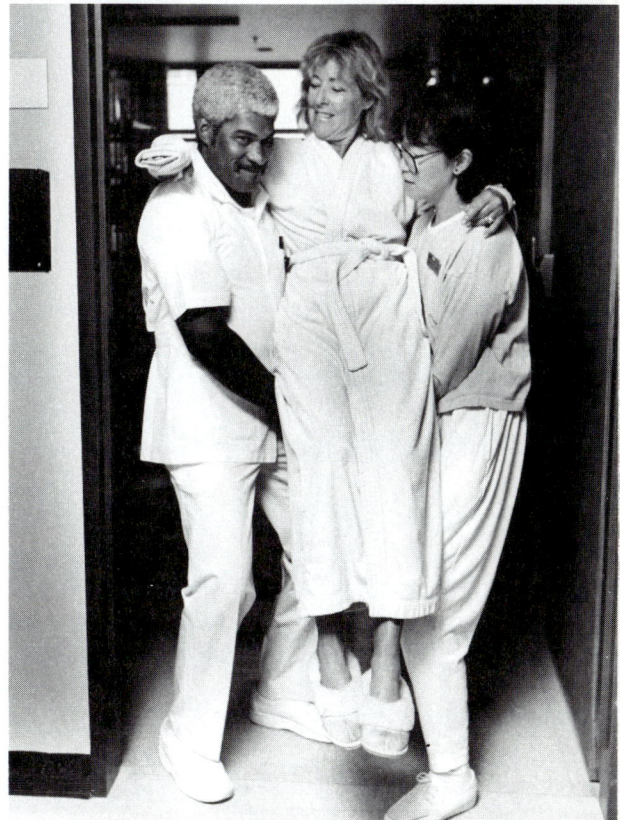

Figure 21–1 The swing carry.

Steps to Follow in the Event of Fire

- Evacuate clients who are in immediate danger. First, direct ambulatory clients to a safe area, or enlist their help in moving clients in wheelchairs. This clears the area for the evacuation of nonambulatory clients, who can be moved in a stretcher or bed, carried, or dragged on sheets and blankets.
- Activate the fire alarm if one is nearby.
- Notify the hospital switchboard of the location of the fire.
- If the fire is small, use the fire extinguisher on the fire.
- Close windows and doors in the area of the fire to reduce ventilation.
- Turn off oxygen and any electrical appliances in the vicinity of the fire.
- Clear fire exits, if necessary.
- Contain smoke as necessary by placing damp cloths or blankets around the outside edges of doors.
- Protect clients from smoke inhalation by giving them wet washcloths through which to breathe.

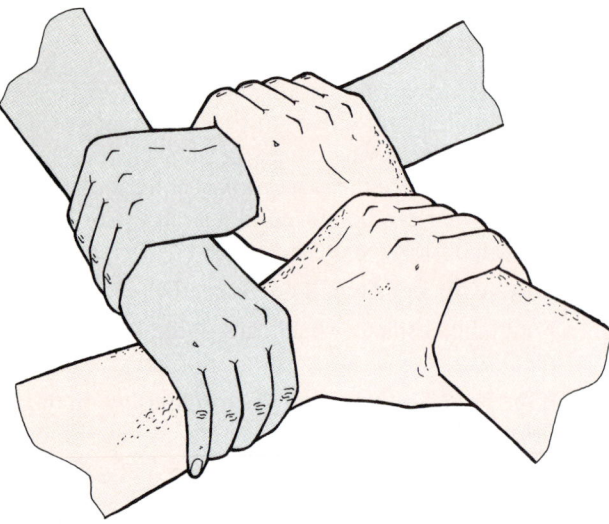

Figure 21–2 Position of hands for a four-handed seat.

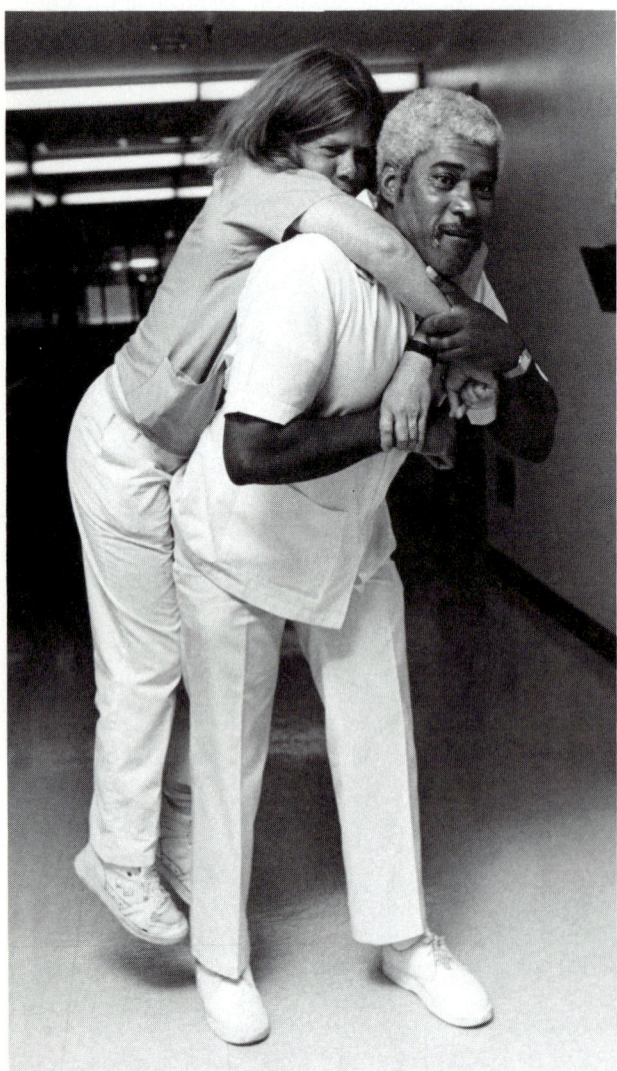

Figure 21–3 The pack strap carry.

tion is the four-handed seat, used for clients who are able to sit up with less support. See Figure 21–2.

- *Pack strap carry.* The packstrap is a one-person carry. The nurse faces the seated client and grasps the wrists. The nurse's right hand grasps the client's left wrist; the left hand grasps the client's right wrist. The nurse then pivots and slips under one of the client's arms so that the nurse's back is to the client and the client's arms are crossed in front of the nurse. The nurse assumes a broad stance, one leg in front of the other, and rolls the client onto the nurse's back. See Figure 21–3.

- *Piggy-back carry.* This carry is used for clients who are conscious and have some strength to help. The client sits at the edge of the bed. The nurse stands in front of the client with the back toward the client. The client reaches over the nurse's shoulders, and clasps the hands in front of the nurse while the nurse grasps the backs of the client's legs above the knees. With this carry, the nurse can support the client's weight more easily than with the pack strap carry.

- *Cradle carry.* The cradle carry is used for children or adults who are light in weight. The nurse lifts the client by placing one arm beneath the person's knees and the other around the back.

Containing the Fire   Fires are categorized into four classes according to the type of material burning. Several types of fire extinguishers are in use today. The right type of extinguisher must be used to fight a fire. See Table 21–2 for various types of extinguishers and indications for their use. Fire extinguishers are now commonly labeled with picture symbols showing on which fires they should and should not be used. Directions for use are also attached to the extinguisher.

Scalds and Burns

A **scald** is a burn from a hot liquid or vapor, such as steam. A **burn** results from excessive exposure to thermal, chemical, electrical, or radioactive agents.

Common home hazards causing scalds are

- Pot handles that protrude over the edge of a stove
- Electrical appliances used to heat liquids or oils, especially those that have dangling cords within reach of crawling infants and young children
- Excessively hot bath water
- Excessively hot coffee or other beverages that are accidentally spilled

Burns in the home setting are usually caused by

- Improper use of matches
- Cigarettes
- Improper use of gasoline or lighter fluid in barbecue grills

TABLE 21–2   Types of Fire Extinguishers: Indications and Procedures for Use

Type of Extinguisher	Class and Kind of Fire	Procedure	Comments
Water: a) Stored pressure type b) Gas cartridge type c) pump type d) Soda acid type	Class A: paper, wood, draperies, upholstery, and ordinary rubbish	Stored Pressure Type: Pull locking pin, then squeeze handle. Gas Cartridge Type: Pull locking pin, then squeeze handle (or) turn unit upside down. Pump Type: Release lock latch if present, then pump plunger rapidly. Soda Acid Type: Turn unit upside down to mix chemicals (do *not* invert extinguisher until *ready* to use.) -Direct water stream at the base of the fire, not at the smoke. -Use side-to-side sweeping motions to wet all surfaces.	-Water soaks and cools the burning material below its ignition temperature. -Do not use on electrical or flammable liquid fires (e.g., grease); water conducts electricity and causes grease to splatter, thus spreading the fire. -For home use this type of extinguisher could be placed in a living room, den, or office.
Carbon dioxide (CO_2)	Classes B and C: flammable liquids and gases and electrical fires	Self-Expellent type: Pull locking pin, then squeeze the operating handle. Avoid touching the discharge horn, since it gets very cold and may accumulate static electricity. -For *flammable liquid fires,* get close to the fire, point the nozzle at the near edge, and slowly sweep the nozzle side to side. -When the fire is out, continue the extinguisher discharge to prevent reflash of flames. -For *electrical fires,* first shut off power to remove possible fire source.	-Carbon dioxide smothers flames and cuts off the oxygen supply to the fire. -Because it has a limited range, the extinguisher must be used close to the flames. -For home use, this type of extinguisher should be placed in the kitchen.
Regular dry chemical: 1) Stored pressure type b) Gas cartridge type	Classes B and C: flammable liquids and gases and electrical fires	Stored Pressure Type: Pull locking pin, then squeeze handle. Gas Cartridge Type: Pull locking pin, and press cartridge puncture lever. Then squeeze operating handle. -Stand relatively far away, and direct the discharge of dry chemical across the entire fire front. -Move toward the fire, and use quick side-to-side motions. -When the fire is out, continue the extinguisher discharge to prevent reflash of flames. -For an *electrical fire,* shut off the power as soon as possible to remove potential fire source.	-Regular dry chemical extinguishers interrupt and smother the flames. -Starting far enough away avoids splashing and allows the discharge stream to flare out. -For home use, see comment about CO_2 extinguisher.
Multipurpose dry chemical: a) Stored pressure type b) Gas cartridge type	Classes A, B and C: paper, wood, cloth, flammable liquids, and electrical equipment	-As above for regular dry chemical. -Use the same as the regular dry chemical extinguishers on class B and class C fires. -On class A fires, coat all exposed surfaces, and wet thoroughly to prevent rekindling.	-Multiple-purpose dry chemicals interrupt and smother the flames, cutting off the oxygen supply. -These extinguishers are good anywhere in the home since they put out most types of fires.

Type of Extinguisher	Class and Kind of Fire	Procedure	Comments
Foam	Class B: flammable liquid fires only	-Operate like the soda-acid water extinguisher. Turn the unit upside down to operate. (Do *not* invert unit until *ready* to use.)	-Foam smothers and cools the fire. -For home use this type of extinguisher could be placed in a garage or basement.
		-To avoid splashing, curve the stream upward so foam falls lightly, *or* direct the foam at the floor to spread it. -For *fires in containers,* direct the stream at the back wall so that the foam flows forward.	
Special dry powder extinguishants	Class D: metal	Used for designated metals. May be applied by scoop, shovel, or extinguisher.	Special dry powder extinguishants absorb heat.
Loaded stream	Classes A and B	Follow instructions on device.	Uses a water-chemical mixture.
Liquified gas	Classes B and C	Follow instructions on device.	Chemical turns to gas when discharged.

- Uncontrolled fires in fireplaces
- Faulty electrical wiring
- Excessively hot heating pads

    In health care agencies, the risk of scalds and burns is greater for clients whose skin sensitivity to temperature is impaired. Scalds can occur from overly hot bath water or from overly hot moist dressings. Heat lamps can cause burns. (The therapeutic application of heat is discussed in Chapter 46.) It is important for the nurse to assess how well clients can protect themselves and what special precautions, if any, need to be taken.

Falls

 Falls are common among the ill or injured, who are weakened and frequently lose their balance. To prevent falls and self-inflicted injury of hospitalized clients, the nurse should consider the guidelines in the accompanying box.

Restraining Clients

Restraints are protective devices used to limit the physical activity of the client or a part of the body. They are applied only to enable the reception of treatment and to allow the treatment to proceed without client interference, e.g., to prevent movements that would disrupt therapy to a limb connected to tubes or appliances (Houston and Lach 1990, p. 231). Experience has shown that restraints do not prevent falls or injury (Innes and Turman 1983, p.35).

Preventing Falls in Hospitals

- Orient clients on admission to their surroundings, and explain the call system.
- Carefully assess the client's ability to ambulate and transfer; provide walking aids and assistance as required.
- Closely supervise the clients at risk for falls during the first few days, especially at night.
- Encourage the client to use call bell to request assistance; ensure that the bell is within easy reach.
- Place bedside tables and overbed tables near the bed or chair so that clients do not overreach and consequently lose their balance.
- Always keep hospital beds in the low position when not providing care so that clients can move in or out of bed easily.
- Encourage clients to use grab bars mounted in toilet and bathing areas and railings along corridors.
- Make sure nonskid bath mats are available in tubs and showers.
- Encourage the client to wear nonskid footwear.
- Keep the environment tidy, especially keep light cords from underfoot and furniture out of the way.
- Attach side rails to the beds of confused, sedated, restless, and unconscious clients, and keep the rails in place when the client is unattended.

RESEARCH NOTE

Which Clients Are Most Likely to Fall?

Falls account for 29% to 89% of all incidents reported in hospitalized patients. In 1984, this represented 8769 deaths as a result of falls. The authors reviewed the research regarding the prediction and prevention of falls. Their conclusions are (a) no high-risk profiles have yet been developed with adequate sensitivity and specificity to be useful as predictive instruments; (b) current fall interventions are rarely research-based; and (c) the four intervention studies conducted to date seem to reduce the incidence of falls through consciousness raising rather than specific changes in practice.

Implications: More research is needed to help nurses predict clients at risk for falling.

M. B. Whedon and P. Shedd, State of the science: Prediction and prevention of patient falls, *Image: Journal of Nursing Scholarship,* Summer 1989, 21:108–14.

Restraints can be classified as physical or chemical. *Physical restraints* are any manual method or physical or mechanical device, material, or equipment attached to the client's body; they cannot be removed easily and they restrict the client's movement. *Chemical restraints* are medications such as neuroleptics, anxiolytics, sedatives, and psychotropic agents used to control socially disruptive behavior.

Because restraints restrict an individual's ability to move freely, their use has legal implications. In some settings, the decision to use a restraint is made by the nurse; in others, it must be made by a physician. Often a nurse can apply a restraint as a temporary emergency measure. Nurses need to know their agency's policies and the state or provincial laws about restraining clients. Increasingly the need for safety measures is viewed as an independent nursing function.

Restrained clients often become restless and anxious as a result of the loss of self-control. Nurses may need to remain with the restrained client and speak quietly to give reassurance and allay distress. Understanding why the body part has to be kept relatively still helps the client to view the restraint as a protective measure.

The nurse must document the type of restraint used, the exact times the restraint was applied and removed, the client's behavior before and with the restraint, care given while the restraint was applied, and notification of the physician. Nurses must explain the need for the restraint, both to the client and to support persons, and document the substance of these explanations.

Selecting a Restraint

Before selecting a restraint, nurses need to understand its purpose clearly. A restraint should be measured against the following five criteria in the process of selection:

1. It restricts the client's movement as little as possible. If a client needs to have one arm restrained, do not restrain the entire body.

2. It is the least obvious to others. Both clients and visitors are often embarrassed by a restraint, even though they understand why it is being used. The less obvious the restraint, the more comfortable people feel.

3. It does not interfere with the client's treatment or health problem. If a client has poor blood circulation to the hands, apply a restraint that will not aggravate that circulatory problem.

4. It is readily changeable. Restraints need to be changed frequently, especially if they become soiled. Keeping other guidelines in mind, choose a restraint that can be changed with minimal disturbance to the client.

5. It is safe for the particular client. Choose a restraint with which the client cannot self-inflict injury. For example, a physically active child could incur injury trying to climb out of a crib if one wrist is tied to the side of the crib. A jacket restraint would restrain the child more safely.

Kinds of Restraints

There are a number of kinds of restraints. Among the most common in use in health care settings are the jacket restraint, the belt restraint, the mitt or hand restraint, limb restraints, elbow restraints, mummy restraints, and crib nets. Geri chairs, wheelchairs, and bedsheets used to confine client activity can also be considered restraints. While *jacket restraints* vary, they are all essentially sleeveless jackets (vests) with straps (tails) that can be tied to the bed frame under the mattress or to the legs of a chair. The jacket may be put on with the ties at the front or at the back, depending on the type. See Figure 21–4. Jackets intended to open at the front must be applied in this manner. These body restraints are used for confused or sedated clients.

Belt or safety strap body restraints are used to ensure the safety of all clients who are being moved on stretchers or in wheelchairs. They may also be used for certain clients confined to bed or to chairs. A *mitt or hand restraint* is used to prevent confused clients from using their hands or fingers to scratch and injure themselves. For example, a confused client may need to be prevented from pulling at intravenous tubing or a head bandage following brain surgery. Hand or mitt restraints allow the client to be ambulatory and/or to move the arm freely rather than be confined to a bed or a chair.

Mitt restraints are commercially available. See Figure 21–5. Hand restraints can also be made using large dressings and stockinette. The nurse asks the client to grasp a small pad, so that the hand assumes a natural position. The client's wrist is padded with large dressings to prevent skin abrasions, and all skin surfaces are carefully separated, also to prevent abrasions. The nurse then places two large dress-

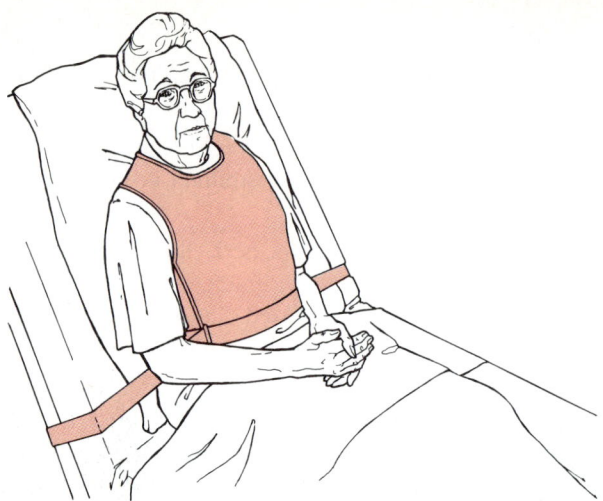

Figure 21–4 Poncho-type jacket restraint.

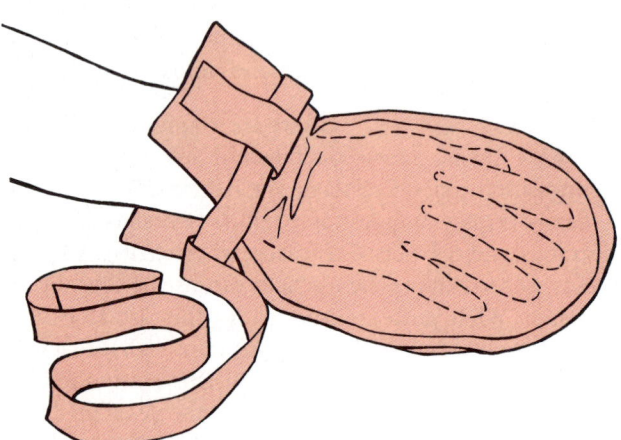

Figure 21–5 A commercially made mitt restraint.

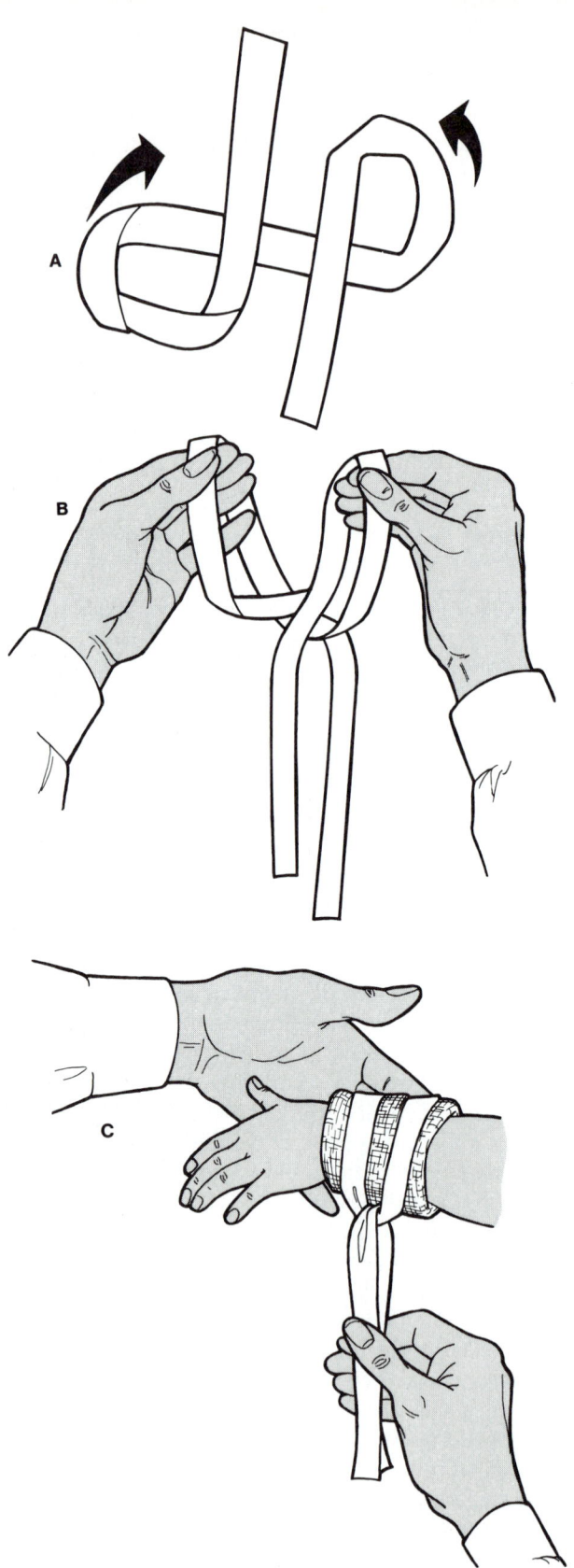

Figure 21–6 To make a clove hitch: *A,* Make a figure-eight; *B,* pick up the loops; *C,* put the limb through the loops, and secure it.

ings over the hand, one from side to side and the other from the ventral surface to the dorsal surface. The dressings are secured with gauze bandage and adhesive tape. Stockinette is then put over the hand and secured just above the wrist pad with adhesive tape. Mittens need to be removed at least every two hours to permit the client to wash and exercise the hands. The nurse also needs to take off the mitten to check the circulation to the hand regularly.

Limb restraints, generally made of cloth, may be used to immobilize a limb, primarily for therapeutic reasons (e.g., to maintain an intravenous infusion). Some commercially prepared restraints are available. A clove hitch limb restraint can also be improvised using padded dressings and gauze. See Figure 21–6.

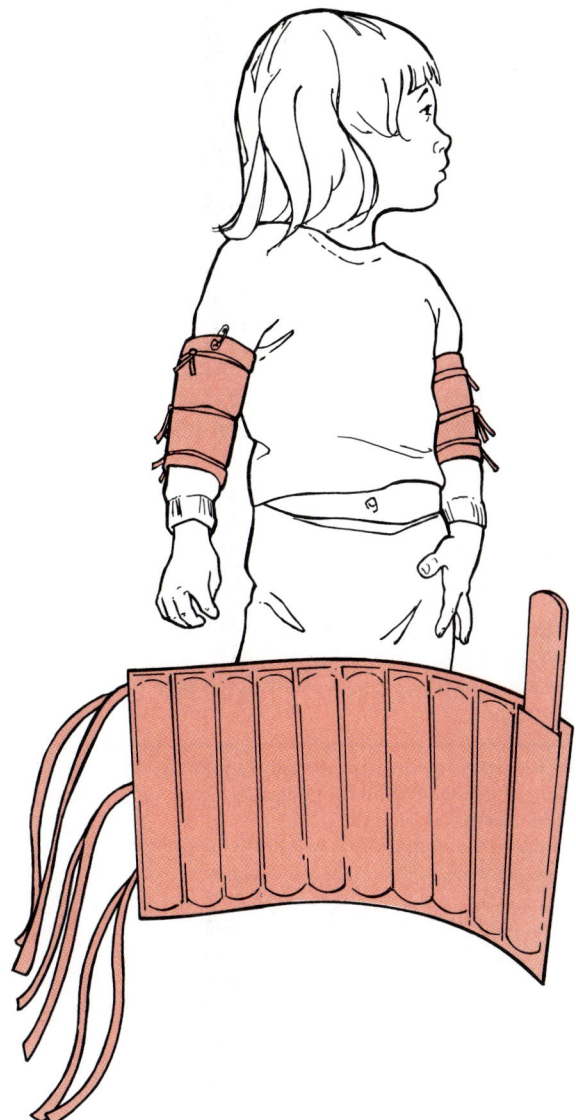

Figure 21–7 An elbow restraint for a young child.

Elbow restraints are used to prevent infants or small children from flexing their elbows to touch or scratch a surgical incision or skin lesion, e.g., eczema. See Figure 21–7. This restraint consists of a piece of material with pockets into which plastic or wooden tongue depressors are inserted to provide rigidity. After the restraint is applied, it is sometimes pinned to the child's shirt to prevent it from sliding down the arm.

The *mummy restraint* is a special folding of a blanket or sheet around the child to prevent movement during a procedure such as gastric washing, eye irrigation, or collection of a blood specimen. A *crib net* is simply a net placed over the top of a crib to prevent active young children from climbing out of the crib. At the same time, it allows them freedom to move about in the crib.

When using restraints, the nurse may find the guidelines in the accompanying box helpful.

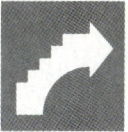

CLINICAL GUIDELINES
Applying Restraints

- Assure the client and the client's support persons that the restraint is temporary and protective. A restraint must never be applied as punishment for any behavior or merely for the nurse's convenience.

- Apply the restraint in such a way that the client can move as freely as possible without defeating the purpose of the restraint.

- Ensure that limb restraints are applied securely but not so tightly that they impede blood circulation to any body area or extremity.

- Pad bony prominences (e.g., wrists and ankles) before applying a restraint over them. The movement of a restraint without padding over such prominences can quickly abrade the skin.

- Always tie a limb restraint with a knot, e.g., a clove hitch that will not tighten when pulled.

- Tie the ends of a body restraint to the part of the bed that moves when the head is elevated. Never tie the ends to a side rail or to the fixed frame of the bed if the bed position is to be changed.

- Assess the restraint every 30 minutes. Some facilities have specific forms to be used to record ongoing assessment.

- Release all restraints at least every 2 hours, and provide range-of-motion (ROM) exercises (see Chapter 35) and skin care (see Chapter 22).

- Reassess the continued need for the restraint every 8 hours. Include an assessment of the underlying cause of the behavior necessitating use of the restraints.

- When a restraint is temporarily removed, do not leave the client unattended.

- Immediately report to the nurse in charge and record on the client's chart any persistent reddened or broken skin areas under the restraint.

- At the first indication of cyanosis or pallor, coldness of a skin area, or a client's complaint of a tingling sensation, pain, or numbness, loosen the restraint and exercise the limb.

- Apply a restraint so that it can be released quickly in case of an emergency and with the body part in a normal anatomic position.

- Provide emotional support verbally and through touch.

Poisonous*		Nonpoisonous†	
Avocado (leaves)	Morning glory	African violet	Honeysuckle
Azaleas	Mushrooms (some	Aster	Impatiens
Buttercups	varieties)	Baby's tears	Jade plant
Cherries (pits)	Narcissus	Bamboo	Lipstick plant
Crocus, autumn	Oleander	Begonia	Magnolia
Daffodil	Philodendron	California poppy	Marigold
English ivy	Poison hemlock	Camellia	Orchid
Foxglove	Poison ivy	Christmas cactus	Petunia
Holly berries	Poison oak	Chrysanthemum	Piggy-back plant
Horsetail reed	Poppy (California	(dermatitis)	Prayer plant
Hyacinth	poppy excepted)	Crabapples	Rose
Hydrangea	Potato (sprouts)	Dahlia	Rubber plant
Iris	Rhododendron	Daisies	(dermatitis)
Ivy (Boston, English,	Rhubarb (leaves)	Dandelion	Umbrella tree
and others)	Tobacco	Easter lily	Wandering Jew
Larkspur	Tomato (except fruit)	Eucalyptus (caution)	Weeping fig
Lily-of-the-valley	Tulip	Gardenia	Yucca
Lobelia	Wisteria	Gloxinia	Zebra plant
Mistletoe	Yew berries	Hibiscus	

*These plants are considered poisonous and possibly dangerous. They contain a wide variety of poisons, and symptoms of ingestion may very from a mild stomachache, skin rash, and swelling of the mouth and throat to involvement of the heart, kidneys, or other organs. Many plants are not toxic unless ingested in very large amounts.

†These plants are considered essentially safe, not poisonous. It is unlikely that an individual will develop symptoms from eating or handling these plants, but any plant may cause an unexpected reaction in certain individuals.

Poisoning

A **poison** is any substance that injures or kills through its chemical action when inhaled, injected, applied, or absorbed in relatively small amounts. For certain poisons, specific antidotes or treatments are available; for many, there is no specific therapy.

In response to the ever-increasing number of poison hazards, many countries have established poison centers. The American and Canadian Association of Poison Control Centers is a nationwide network of poison control centers and concerned individuals, who work together and with government and industry to make life safer from the hazards of poisons. Poison control centers provide accurate, up-to-date information about potential hazards and recommend treatment as needed. Selected poisonous plants are shown in the box above. Additional information is available from poison control centers.

The major reasons for poisoning in children are inadequate supervision and improper storage of many household toxic substances (over 500 in the average home). Adolescent and adult poisonings are usually caused by insect or snake bites and drugs used for recreation or in suicide attempts. Poisoning in elderly people usually is a result of accidental ingestion of a toxic substance due to failing eyesight or an overdose of a prescribed medication due to impaired memory.

Nurses can intervene by educating the public about what to do in the event of poisoning. Identify the specific poison by searching for an opened container, empty bottle, or other evidence. Contact the poison control center, indicate the exact quantity of poison the person ingested, and state the person's age and apparent symptoms. Keep the person as quiet as possible on one side or with head placed between the legs to prevent aspiration of vomitus.

The accompanying box provides additional guidelines in teaching clients to prevent poisoning.

Electric Shock

Nurses need to use electrical equipment that is properly **grounded** (that transmits an electric current from an object or surface to the ground). The electrical plug of grounded

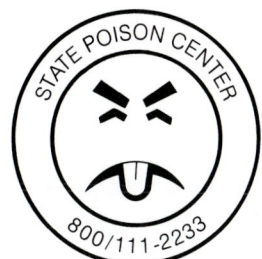

Figure 21–8 The "Mr. Yuk" poison label.

equipment has three prongs. The two short prongs transmit the power to the equipment. The third, longer prong is the grounding device, which carries short circuits or stray electric current to the ground. See Figure 21–9. Grounding prongs offer a path of least resistance to stray electric currents.

If the equipment is faulty, e.g., if a cord is frayed, there is a danger of electric shock. Also, faulty electrical equipment can start fires. For example, an electric spark near certain anesthetic gases or a high concentration of oxygen may cause a serious fire.

If an individual receives a macroshock, it is important not to touch that person until the electricity is shut off and the person is safely away from the electric current. A macroshock can cause both superficial and deep burns, muscle contractions, and cardiac and respiratory arrest. Using machines in good repair, wearing shoes with rubber soles, standing on a nonconductive floor, and using nonconductive gloves can prevent macroshock.

To prevent explosions caused by the buildup of static electricity in operating rooms, personnel do not use nylon,

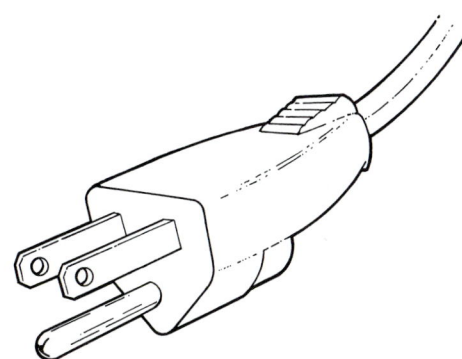

Figure 21–9 Three-pronged ground plug.

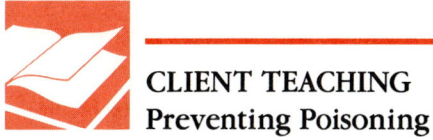

CLIENT TEACHING
Preventing Poisoning

- Place potentially toxic agents, including drugs and cleaning agents, out of reach of crawling infants.

- Lock cleaning agents in a cupboard, or attach special plastic hooks to the inside of cabinet doors to keep them securely closed. Unlatching these hooks requires firmer thumb pressure than small children can usually exert.

- Avoid storing toxic liquids or solids in food containers, such as soft drink bottles, peanut butter jars, or milk cartons.

- Do not remove container labels or reuse empty containers to store different substances. Laws mandate that the labels of all poisons specify antidotes.

- Keep poisonous house plants out of reach of young children. Be able to identify the poisonous plants in your neighborhood.

- Do not rely on cooking to destroy toxic chemicals in plants. Never use anything prepared from nature as a medicine or "tea."

- Teach children never to eat any part of an unknown plant or mushroom and not to put leaves, stems, bark, seeds, nuts, or berries from any plant into their mouths.

- Place poison warning stickers designed for children on containers of bleach, lye, kerosene, solvent, and other toxic substances. See Figure 21–8. Teach children that the Mr. Yuk label means danger.

- Do not take medications in front of children. They may imitate you.

- Never call medicine candy when giving medications to children.

- Read and follow label directions on all products before using them.

- Keep syrup of ipecac on hand at all times. Syrup of ipecac is a nonprescription emetic available in single-dose 15 ml vials in all drugstores. Use it only after advice from the local poison control center or the family physician.

- Display the phone number of the poison control center near or on all telephones in the home so that it is available to baby-sitters, family, and friends.

CLIENT TEACHING
Reducing Electrical Hazards

- Check cords for fraying or other signs of damage before using an appliance. Do not use if damage is apparent.

- Avoid overloading outlets and fuse boxes with too many appliances.

- Use only grounded outlets and plugs.

- Always pull a plug from the wall outlet by firmly grasping the plug and pulling it straight out. Pulling a plug by its cord can damage the cord and plug unit.

- Never use electrical appliances near sinks, bathtubs, showers, or other wet areas since water readily conducts electricity.

- Keep electrical cords and appliances out of the reach of young children.

- Place protective covers over wall outlets to protect young children (see Figure 21–10).

- Have all noninsulated wiring in the home altered to meet safety standards.

- Carefully read instructions before operating electrical equipment. Clients who do not understand how to operate the equipment should seek advice.

- Always disconnect appliances before cleaning or repairing them.

- Unplug any appliance that has given a tingling sensation or shock and have an electrician evaluate it for stray current.

- Keep electrical cords coiled or taped to the ground away from areas of traffic to prevent others from damaging the cord or tripping over it.

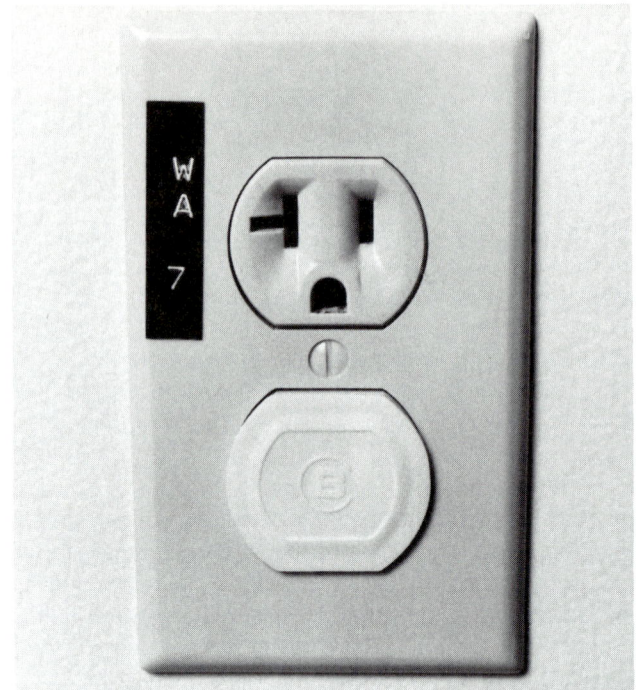

Figure 21–10 Safety cover for an electrical outlet.

dacron, and other materials that tend to build up static charges. Also, the air is humidified, and antistatic sprays are used in such areas. Actions to reduce electrical hazards are shown in the box above.

Excessive Noise

Excessive noise is a health hazard that can cause hearing loss, depending on (a) the overall level of noise, (b) the frequency range of the noise, and (c) the duration of exposure and individual susceptibility. Sound levels above 120 decibels (units of loudness) are painful and may cause hearing damage even if a person is exposed for only a short period. Exposure to 85 to 95 decibels for several hours a day can lead to progressive or permanent hearing loss. Noise levels below 85 decibels usually do not affect hearing.

Tolerance of noise is largely individual. The rural dweller may find the city noisy, whereas the city dweller may be oblivious to urban sounds. Adults often find teenager's music uncomfortably loud. Noise has psychosocial effects, such as feelings of annoyance, disrupted sleep and relaxation, and interruption of thought and conversation patterns. Noise can also interfere with job performance and safety.

The ill and injured are frequently sensitive to noises that normally would not disturb them. Loud voices, the clatter of dishes, and even a nearby television can disturb clients, some of whom react angrily. Physiologic effects of noise include (a) increased heart and respiratory rates, (b) increased muscular activity, (c), nausea, and (d) hearing loss, if the noise is sufficiently loud.

Noise can be minimized in several ways. Acoustic tile on ceilings, walls, and floors as well as drapes and carpeting absorb sound. Background music can mask noise and have a calming effect on some people. It is important for nurses to minimize noise in the hospital setting and to encourage clients to protect their hearing as much as possible.

Radiation

Radiation as a health hazard is a recent source of concern. Nurses are concerned specifically with those radioactive materials used in diagnostic and therapeutic practices. Radiation injury can occur from overexposure or from exposure to radiation that treats specific tissues and at the same time injures other tissues.

Radioactive materials are used in diagnostic procedures such as radiography, fluoroscopy, and nuclear medicine. In nuclear medicine, radioactive isotopes that have an affinity for specific tissues are given orally or intravenously. Some of the isotopes of the elements used are:

- Calcium, which has an affinity for bones
- Iodine, which is attracted to the thyroid gland
- Phosphorus, which is attracted to blood

Radioactive materials are provided in sealed sources and unsealed liquid sources. For example, cobalt implants are sealed; iodine 131 and phosphorus 32 are unsealed liquids. Principles governing the degree of exposure to radiation are as follows:

- The longer the time in the presence of radiation, the greater the exposure.
- The closer a person is to the radioactive source, the greater the exposure.
- The more extensive the use of lead and other radiation shields, the greater the protection against radiation.

Often nurses help care for clients treated or diagnosed with radioactive substances. The client diagnosed through radiography or fluoroscopy generally receives minimal exposure, and few precautions are necessary. The nurse restraining a small child during radiography needs to wear a lead apron. Clients with radioactive implants are a source of radiation to the immediate environment. The nurse who is in close contact with such clients also needs to wear a lead apron.

Nurses must deal safely with radioactive body discharges by wearing gloves and in some instances placing excreta in containers for special disposal. The nurse must wash gloved hands well before and after removing the gloves and place contaminated materials in a special container for disposal.

Hospitals in which radioactive materials are used usually have a radioisotope committee. This committee establishes policies and procedures to be used in the care of clients who receive radioactive materials. Nurses must be cognizant of these policies.

One important aspect of caring for clients receiving radiation treatment is making sure they understand the treatment and the precautions they need to take. Often such clients are restricted to bed or to a confined area to protect others. These clients need emotional support to deal with the precautions and will likely accept treatments and precautions better when they know what will happen, when, and why.

EVALUATING

To evaluate the achievement of client goals, the nurse collects data pertaining to the outcome criteria established by (a) questioning the client about factors that increase the potential for self-injury, especially those in the environment; (b) observing the client's use of safety measures (e.g., wearing a bicycle helmet) or alterations the client has made in the home environment to ensure safety; and (c) listening as the client verbalizes appropriate safety measures taken. Examples of evaluative statements indicating partial or complete goal achievement are "The client identified ten out of sixteen hazards in his home," "The client reported carrying out all preventive measures discussed June 5, 19xx," and "The client reported installing grab bars in bathroom and hand rails for inside and outside stairways June 15, 19xx."

CHAPTER HIGHLIGHTS

- The provision of a safe external environment is a constant concern of the nurse.

- Education is a major health protection strategy in preventing accidents.

- When planning to meet safety needs of clients, nurses need to consider physical factors in the environment and the psychologic and physiologic state of the individual.

- Accidents are a major cause of death among individuals of all ages in the United States and Canada. The seven major causes of accidental deaths in the United States are motor vehicle accidents, falls, fires, drowning, poisoning, suffocation, and firearms. Most accidents are due to negligence and are preventable.

- Nursing assessment of the clients at risk includes assessment of age, life-style, sensory-perceptual alterations, level of awareness, mobility, emotional state, language barriers, history of previous accidents, and knowledge and use of safety precautions.

- Nursing diagnoses for clients at risk of accidental injury can be categorized as **Potential for injury**, with three subcategories: **Potential for trauma**, **Potential for poisoning**, and **Potential for suffocation**.

- Nursing intervention must include education in accident prevention and modification of the environment to make it safe.

- Nurses must be familiar with the fire procedures in

CHAPTER HIGHLIGHTS (continued)

their employing agency. In the event of a fire, the nurse must protect clients from injury and contain and put out the fire.

▶ Falls are a common cause of injury among the very young, the elderly, and the ill or injured.

▶ To prevent falls, the nurse must provide constant surveillance for infants and young children and carefully assess older clients' safety needs.

▶ Side rails and hand rails protect hospitalized clients from falls; restraints keep clients from falling and from inflicting injuries on themselves and others.

▶ Because restraints restrict a client's basic freedom to move, careful assessment and accurate, complete documentation are important when restraints are used.

▶ Poisoning from numerous plants, household chemicals, and medications is a major threat to young, curious children.

▶ Major reasons for poisoning in children are inadequate supervision and improper storage of household toxic substances.

▶ Faulty electrical equipment and improper grounding pose health hazards in the hospital and the home.

▶ Electrical accidents can be prevented by using grounded outlets and plugs, putting protective covers over outlets, keeping appliances in good repair, and making sure that electrical wiring and circuits meet safety standards.

▶ Prolonged exposure to excessive noise can produce hearing loss.

▶ In hospitals, radioactive substances are used for both diagnostic and treatment purposes; agency policy should be followed to safeguard clients and staff from inadvertent exposure.

▶ Because of their diminished sensory acuity and balance, elderly people need to make the home safe. They also need education about ways to prevent automobile and pedestrian accidents.

READINGS AND REFERENCES

SUGGESTED READINGS

Hernandez, M., and Miller, J. March/April 1986. How to reduce falls. *Geriatric Nursing* 7:97–102.

Hernandez and Miller collected data on falls on a geropsychiatric unit to identify precipitants and predictors of falls, to develop and test levels of all precautions, and to decrease the incidence of falls. Findings are shown in a Falls Assessment Tool. Included are risk factors identified, a comparison of nonfallers and fallers, precautions to prevent falls, and recommendations for nurse administrators and staff.

Widder, B. September/October 1985. A new device to decrease falls. *Geriatric Nursing* 6:287–88.

A new device called the Ambularm, developed by the associate director of medicine at the Saint Vincent Hospital and Medical Center in Portland, Oregon, and a colleague, summons help when the client is in the act of arising. It has reduced falls by 45%.

Wyatt, D. M. February 1985. Are you prepared for a hospital fire? *Nursing 85* 15:51.

This article describes a situation in which a fire was discovered in a hospital. The author describes two mistakes made in this situation and a number of safety tips for nurses who encounter a hospital fire.

RELATED RESEARCH

Craven, R., and Bruno, P. August 1986. Teach the elderly to prevent falls. *Journal of Gerontological Nursing* 12:27–33.

Johnston, J. E. November 1988. The elderly and fall prevention. *Applied Nursing Research* 1:140.

Wolf-Klein, G. B.; Silverstone, F. A.; Basavaraju, N.; et al. September 1988. Prevention of falls in the elderly population. *Archives of Physical Medicine and Rehabilitation* 69:689–91.

SELECTED REFERENCES

Barbieri, E. B. March 1983. Patient falls are not patient accidents. *Journal of Gerontological Nursing* 9:164–73.

Berger, M. E., and Hubner, K. F. August 1983. Hospital hazards: Diagnostic radiation. *American Journal of Nursing.* 83:1155–59.

Campbell, E. B.; Williams, M. A.; and Mlynarczyk, S. M. February 1986. After the fall: Confusion. *American Journal of Nursing* 86:151–53.

Carpenito, L. J. 1989. *Nursing diagnosis: Application to Clinical practice.* 3d ed. Philadelphia: J. B. Lippincott Co.

Dallaire, L. B., and Burke, E. V. January 1989. A new program for reducing patient falls. *Nursing 89* 19:65.

Denomy, E. B. April 1990. Accidental killers. *Canadian Nurse* 86:22–4.

Easterling, M. L. January 1990. Which of your patients is headed for a fall? *RN* 53:56–59.

Fitzgibbon, M., and Roberts, F. M. 1988. Prevention of accidents to hospital patients. *Recent Advances in Nursing* (22): 33–48.

Friedman, F. B. January 1983. Restraints: When all else fails, there still are alternatives, *RN* 46:79–80, 82, 84.

Gray-Vickrey, M. May/June 1984. Education to prevent falls. *Geriatric Nursing* 5:179–83.

Hernandez, M., and Miller, J. March/April 1986. How to reduce falls. *Geriatric Nursing* 7:97–102.

Houston, K. A. and Lach, H. W. September/October 1990. Restraints: How do you score? *Geriatric Nursing* 11:231–232.

Innes, E. M. and Turman, W. G. February 1983. Evaluation of patient falls. *Quality Review Bulletin* 9:30–35.

Jackson, M. M.; Dechairo, D. C.; and Gardner, D. F. February 1986. Perceptions and beliefs of nursing and medical personnel about needle-handling practices and needle-stick injuries. *American Journal of Infection Control* 14:1–10.

Kim, M. J.; McFarland, G. K.; and McLane, A. M. 1989. *Pocket guide to nursing diagnoses*. 3d ed. St. Louis: C. V. Mosby Co.

Louis, M. March 1983. Falls and their causes. *Journal of Gerontological Nursing* 9:142–56.

McHutchion, E., and Morse, J. M. February 1989. Releasing restraints: A nursing dilemma. *Journal of Gerontological Nursing* 15:16–21.

Nursing guidelines for the use of restraints in nonpsychiatric settings. March 1983. *Journal of Gerontological Nursing* 9:180–81.

Tideiksaar, R. July 1989. Restraint use declines as fall prevention options rise. *Provider* 15:35–36.

———. November/December 1989. Home safe home: Practical tips for fall-proofing. *Geriatric Nursing* 10:280–84.

Wyatt, D. M. February 1985. Are you prepared for a hospital fire? *Nursing 85* 15:51.

Hygiene

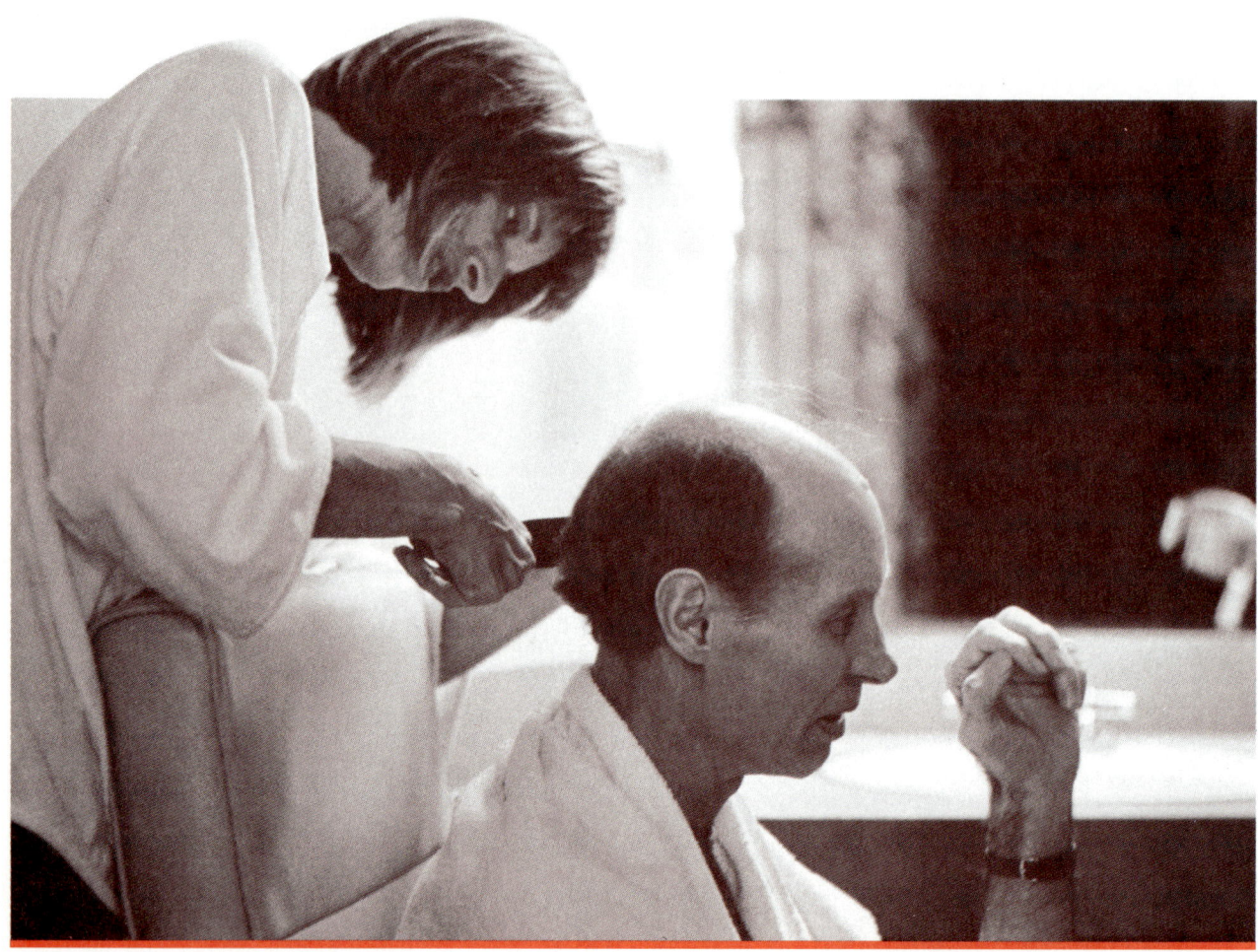

CONTENTS

OBJECTIVES

▸ Describe kinds of hygienic care
  nurses provide to clients.

▸ Identify factors influencing personal hygiene.

▶ Identify normal and abnormal findings obtained during inspection and palpation of the skin, feet, nails, mouth, hair, eyes, ears, and nose.

▶ Describe variations in the appearance of the skin, nails, and mucous membranes of light-skinned and dark-skinned clients.

▶ Identify common problems of the skin, feet, nails, mouth, hair, eyes, ears, and nose and formulate related nursing diagnoses.

▶ Describe guidelines for planning and implementing nursing interventions for the skin, feet, nails, mouth, hair, eyes, ears, and nose.

▶ List outcome criteria to evaluate goal achievement.

▶ Identify the purposes of bathing.

▶ Describe various types of baths.

▶ Describe steps in perineal and genital care.

▶ Explain five techniques used in back rubs.

▶ Explain specific ways in which nurses help hospitalized clients with oral hygiene.

▶ Identify steps in inserting and removing contact lenses and artificial eyes.

▶ Describe steps in inserting and removing hearing aids.

▶ Identify safety and comfort measures underlying bedmaking procedures.

HYGIENIC CARE

Hygiene is the science of health and its maintenance. Personal hygiene is the self-care by which people maintain health. Hygiene is a highly personal matter determined by individual values and practices. It is influenced by cultural, social, familial, and individual factors, as well as by the person's knowledge of health and hygiene and perceptions of personal comfort and needs. People may or may not be aware of their individual needs. A person with particularly malodorous feet is likely to be aware of this problem; however, people with underarm perspiration odors may need assistance, for example, from a nurse, to cope with the problem.

When people are ill, hygienic practices frequently become secondary to other functions, such as breathing, which in health are taken for granted. One sign that a formerly ill or depressed client is feeling better is an interest in shaving, hair care, or make-up. Hygiene involves care of the skin, hair, nails, teeth, oral and nasal cavities, eyes, ears, and perineal and genital areas. It serves a number of purposes:

■ Promotes cleanliness, e.g., removes transient microorganisms and body secretions and excretions.

■ Provides comfort and relaxation, refreshes the client, and relaxes tired, tense muscles.

■ Improves self-image by improving appearance and eliminating offensive odors.

■ Conditions the skin, e.g., a warm bath causes peripheral vasodilation and thus increases the blood circulation to the skin.

People who are very ill often are unable or lack the energy to bathe or brush their teeth, for example. They require assistance to carry out many hygienic activities. It is important for nurses to know exactly how much a client can safely do and how much assistance is required. Clients may require care after urinating or defecating, after vomiting, and whenever they become soiled, e.g., from wound drainage or from profuse perspiration. Nurses must keep the hygiene needs of clients in mind and assist them whenever indicated.

Nurses commonly use the following terms to describe kinds of hygienic care.

Early morning care is provided to clients as they awaken in the morning. In a hospital, nurses on the night shift may provide early morning care. This care helps clients ready themselves for breakfast or for early diagnostic tests. Usually, it consists of providing a urinal or bedpan to the client confined to bed, washing the face and hands, and giving oral care. *Morning care* is provided after clients have breakfast. It usually includes the provision of a urinal or bedpan (to clients who are not ambulatory), a bath or shower, perineal care, back massage, and oral, nail, and hair care. Making the client's bed is part of morning care. *Afternoon care* may be provided, for example, when clients return from physiotherapy or diagnostic tests. Providing a bedpan or urinal, washing the hands and face, and assisting with oral care refresh clients. *Hour of sleep (HS) care* is provided to clients before they retire for the night. It usually involves providing for elimination needs, washing face and hands, giving oral care, and giving a back massage.

SKIN

The skin is the largest organ of the body. It serves five major functions:

1. It protects underlying tissues from injury by preventing the passage of microorganisms. The skin and mucous membrane are considered the body's first line of defense.

2. It regulates the body temperature. Cooling the body occurs through the heat loss processes of evaporation of perspiration, and by radiation and conduction of heat from the body when the blood vessels of the skin are vasodilated. Body heat is conserved through lack of perspiration and vasoconstriction of the blood vessels. See Chapter 18 for a detailed discussion of body heat losses and gains.

3. It secretes **sebum**, an oily substance that (a) softens and lubricates the hair and skin, (b) prevents the hair from becoming brittle, (c) decreases water loss from the skin when the external humidity is low. Because fat is a poor conductor of heat, sebum (d) lessens the amount of heat lost from the skin. Sebum also (e) has a **bactericidal** (bacteria-killing) action.

4. It transmits sensations through nerve receptors, which are sensitive to pain, temperature, touch, and pressure.

5. It produces and absorbs vitamin D in conjunction with ultraviolet rays from the sun, which activate a vitamin D precursor present in the skin.

The *normal skin* of a healthy person has transient microorganisms that are not usually harmful. Adults usually have some resident micrococci, bacteria of the genera *Corynebacterium* and *Propionibacterium,* and a genus of fungi, *Pityrosporon.* Children also have gram-positive, spore-forming rods and *Neisseria* bacteria. Transient microorganisms vary considerably from one person to another. They do not maintain themselves on the skin because of (a) the chemical effects of the fatty acids in the sebum and (b) the normal skin pH of 5 to 6, which is too acidic for many microorganisms.

Sudoriferous (sweat) glands are on all body surfaces except the lips and parts of the genitals. The body has from two to five million, which are all present at birth. They are most numerous on the palms of the hands and the soles of the feet. Sweat glands are classified as apocrine and eccrine. The **apocrine glands**, located largely in the axillae and anogenital areas, begin to function at puberty under the influence of androgens. Although their secretion is produced almost constantly, apocrine glands are of little use in thermoregulation. The secretion of these glands is odorless, but when decomposed or acted upon by bacteria on the skin, it takes on a musky, unpleasant odor. The **eccrine glands** are important physiologically. They are more numerous than the apocrine glands and are found chiefly on the palms of the hands, the soles of the feet, and forehead. The sweat they produce cools the body through evaporation. Sweat is made up of water, sodium, potassium, chloride, glucose, urea, and lactate.

Developmental Changes

In early embryonic life, the skin is a single layer of cells. Other layers develop quickly. The fetus's skin is covered by a substance called **vernix caseosa**, a whitish, cheesy material seen on newborns. It usually disappears in the first day. The skin of an infant is thinner than an adult's, is usually mottled, and in whites varies from pink to red and becomes ruddy when the baby cries. Babies who are genetically dark-skinned are lightly pigmented at birth. Skin pigmentation gradually increases until about 6 or 8 weeks. Sweat glands of babies begin to function at about 1 month of age.

In adolescence, the **sebaceous glands** (oil-supplying glands) increase in activity as a result of increased levels of hormones (androgens). This is thought to be one factor responsible for the development of acne, a common skin problem of adolescents.

The older adult also experiences skin changes. The skin tends to be thinner, drier, somewhat inelastic, and thus subject to fine wrinkling. This process usually begins any time after age 40. The elderly person's skin typically shows wrinkles, sagging, pigmentations, and keratotic spots, usually on areas exposed to the sun. The skin is less resilient, i.e., when pinched, it returns to place more slowly than the skin of a younger person does.

Assessing

Assessment of the client's skin and hygienic practices includes (a) a nursing history to determine the client's skin care practices, self-care abilities, and past or current skin problems; (b) physical assessment of the skin; and (c) identification of clients at high risk for developing skin impairments.

Nursing History   Data about the client's *skin care practices* enable the nurse to incorporate the client's needs and preferences as much as possible in the plan of care and to determine necessary learning needs. Assessment of the client's *self-care abilities* determines the amount of nursing assistance and the kind of bath (bed, tub, or shower) the client requires. Important considerations include the client's balance (for tub and shower), ability to sit unsupported (in the tub or bed), activity tolerance, coordination, adequate muscle strength, appropriate joint range-of-motion, and vision. Cognition and motivation are also essential. Clients whose cognitive function is impaired or whose illness alters energy levels and motivation will also need assistance. Functional levels of self-care are shown in Table 22–1. The *presence of past or current skin problems* alerts the nurse to specific nursing interventions or referrals the client may require. The client may provide descriptions of these problems during the nursing history, or the nurse may observe some during the physical examination that follows. Common skin problems and implications for nursing interventions are shown in Table 22–2. Frequently encountered skin problems are also shown in the color section on skin lesions, following page 402. Questions to elicit data about the client's skin care practices, self-care abilities, and skin problems are shown in the box on page 510.

Physical Assessment   Physical assessment of the skin, which involves inspection and palpation, is described in

TABLE 22–1 *Classification of Functional Levels of Self-Care**

Level	Behavioral Indicator
0	Independent; able to initiate and complete activity for self
1	Requires minimum assistance; may use equipment but manages it alone; does at least 75% of work
2	Requires moderate assistance, supervision, or teaching; does approximately 50% of work
3	Requires extensive assistance from another person *and* equipment or devices; does less than 25% of work
4	Dependent on caregivers, total care; does not participate actively

*Use of this scale to indicate level of dependence/independence further defines functional deficit and guides nursing intervention. Self-care deficits exist for levels 1 through 4.

Source: Thompson, J. M., McFarland, G. K., Hirsch, J. E., Tucker, S. M. and Bowers, A. C. 1989. *Mosby's manual of clinical nursing, 2d ed.* St. Louis: The C. V. Mosby Co., p. 1692. Reprinted with permission.

TABLE 22–2 *Common Skin Problems*

Problem and Appearance	Nursing Implications
Abrasion Superficial layers of the skin are scraped or rubbed away. Area is reddened and may have localized bleeding or serous weeping.	1. Prone to infection; therefore, wound should be kept clean and dry. 2. Do not wear rings or jewelry when providing care to avoid causing abrasions to clients. 3. Lift, do not pull, a client across a bed. See Chapter 36.
Excessive Dryness Skin can appear flaky and rough.	1. Prone to infection if the skin cracks; therefore, provide lotions to moisturize the skin and prevent cracking. 2. Bathe client less frequently; use no soap, or limit use of nonirritating soap. Rinse skin thoroughly, because soap can be irritating and drying. 3. Encourage increased fluid intake if health permits to prevent dehydration.
Ammonia Dermatitis (Diaper Rash) Caused by skin bacteria reacting with urea in the urine. The skin becomes reddened and is sore.	1. Keep skin dry and clean by applying protective ointments containing zinc oxide to areas at risk, e.g., buttocks and perineum. 2. Treat by exposing area to the warmth of a 40-watt gooseneck lamp, placed 30 cm (12 inches) away for 30 minutes, three times a day. This warmth helps to dry the rash. 3. Boil an infant's diapers or wash them with an antibacterial detergent to prevent infection. Rinse diapers well, because detergent is irritating to an infant's skin.
Acne Inflammatory condition with papules and pustules.	1. Keep the skin clean to prevent secondary infection. 2. Treatment varies widely.
Erythema Redness associated with a variety of conditions: e.g., rashes, exposure to sun, elevated body temperature.	1. Wash area carefully to remove excess microorganisms. 2. Apply antiseptic spray or lotion to prevent itching, promote healing, and prevent skin breakdown.
Hirsutism Excessive hair on a person's body and face, particularly in women.	1. Remove unwanted hair by using depilatories, shaving, electrolysis, or tweezing. 2. Enhance client's self-concept. See Chapter 29.

Skin Care Practices

■ What are your usual showering or bathing times?

■ What hygienic products do you routinely use (e.g., bath oils, powder, facial cleansing creams, body lotions or creams, deodorants, antiperspirants)?

■ What facial cosmetic products do you use?

■ How and when do you clean make-up applicators and puffs? (Applicators should be kept clean, and products used around the eyes, in particular, should be discarded after 4 months to prevent bacterial and fungal infections.)

■ What hygienic or cosmetic products do you *not* use because of the skin problems they create (e.g., skin dryness or allergic reactions)?

Self-Care Abilities

■ Do you have any problems managing your hygienic practices (e.g., baths and facial care)? If so, what are these?

■ How can the nurses best help you?

Skin Problems

■ Do you have any tendency toward skin dryness, itchiness, rashes, bruising, excessive perspiration, or lack of perspiration? Have you had lesions in the past?

■ Do you have any allergic tendencies? If so, what?

Positive responses to any of these require further exploration in terms of duration (when did it start?) frequency (how often have you had this?); description of lesion or rash; any associated signs, such as fever or nausea; aggravating factors (e.g., season of the year, stress, occupation, medication, recent travel, housing, personal contact); alleviating factors (e.g., medications, lotions, home remedies); and any family history of the problem.

Chapter 19, pages 370 to 372. A systematic head-to-toe assessment facilitates collection of data about skin color, uniformity of color, texture, turgor, temperature, intactness, and lesions.

 Identifying Clients at Risk When bathing clients, the nurse should be especially observant in noting any reddened areas (which might indicate increased pressure over a bony prominence) or blanched areas (indicative of inadequate circulation to the skin tissues). A number of conditions place clients at risk of developing skin impairments, as follows.

■ *Alterations in nutritional status,* such as emaciation and insufficient protein intake. **Emaciation** is a wasted appearance due to extreme weight loss. In emaciated individuals, subcutaneous fat is insufficient to provide padding or support over bony prominences to withstand normal stress or pressure. Individuals with inadequate protein intake are also prone to skin breakdown, since protein is essential for the building, maintenance, and repair of all body tissues.

■ *Immobility.* Normally, people change position frequently, even during sleep. When position cannot be altered, e.g., if the person is paralyzed or unconscious, or when it is not altered for prolonged periods (1 or 2 hours), blood circulation, which carries essential nutrients to the skin, is reduced. Without essential nutrients, tissues of the skin are ultimately destroyed.

■ *Altered hydration.* In dehydrated individuals, the skin becomes excessively dry, and skin turgor is diminished. Both conditions make the skin less resistant to injury.

■ *Altered sensation.* Loss of sensation in a body area may be the result of paralysis or other neurologic disease. Loss of sensation reduces a person's ability to discern injurious heat and cold and to feel the tingling (pins and needles) that signals loss of circulation. This loss makes the person prone to skin damage.

■ *Presence of secretions or excretions on the skin.* An accumulation of secretions, such as perspiration and sebum, or excretions, such as urine or feces, is irritating to the skin, harbors microorganisms, and makes an individual prone to skin breakdown and infection.

■ *Mechanical devices.* The presence of restraints, casts, or braces that create pressure or a shearing force can alter skin integrity considerably.

■ *Altered venous circulation.* Stasis of venous blood in the lower extremities, which is associated with varicose veins, can cause **stasis dermatitis** (inflammation of the skin) on the feet and around the ankles. This dermatitis is characterized by redness, dryness, itching, and swelling. Ultimately, skin tissues become **ischemic** (deficient of blood) and **necrotic** (dying), and ulcerations form. See Chapter 35, as well as the photographs of decubitus ulcers in the color section on skin lesions that follows page 402.

Diagnosing

Several nursing diagnoses relate to skin and hygienic problems. **Self-care deficit** is the nursing diagnosis given to clients who have problems performing hygienic care. This diagnosis is further specified, as, for example,

Self-care deficit: Bathing/hygiene or **Self-care deficit: Dressing/grooming.** Other possible nursing diagnoses include **Impaired skin integrity** (**Actual** or **Potential**), **Impaired tissue integrity, Knowledge deficit,** and **Self-esteem disturbance.** The most common discomfort caused by skin lesions is *pruritus* (itching).

Pain is discussed in Chapter 38. Examples of these nursing diagnoses and possible contributing factors are shown below. Examples of assessment data clusters and related nursing diagnoses are shown in Table 22–3.

Dx ▶ *Nursing Diagnoses*
Clients with Skin Problems

Self-care deficit: Bathing/hygiene related to:

■ Cognitive deficit (associated with aging, trauma, cerebrovascular accident)

■ Lack of motivation (associated with physical or mental disease process)

■ Visual deficit

■ Impaired limb(s) (associated with painful arthritis, contracture, paralysis, cast, spasticity)

■ Inability to use hands (associated with neuromuscular impairment)

■ Activity intolerance related to decreased cardiac output

Impaired skin integrity related to:

■ Immobility

■ Impaired venous circulation

■ Impaired arterial circulation

■ Nutritional and/or fluid deficit or excess

■ Exposure to irritant (chemical, thermal, mechanical radiation)

Impaired tissue integrity related to:

■ Immobility

■ Altered circulation

■ Fluid volume excess

■ Exposure to irritant (chemical, thermal, radiation, or mechanical)

Potential impaired skin integrity related to:

■ Imposed immobility

■ Altered circulation

■ Altered nutrition: Less than body requirements

■ Exposure to irritant (radiation)

■ Urinary incontinence

■ Reduced sensation in lower extremities

Self-esteem disturbance related to:

■ Body odor

■ Skin problem (acne)

Knowledge deficit related to:

■ Therapeutic regimen to manage skin problem

■ Lack of experience providing hygienic care to dependent person

TABLE 22–3 *Examples of Assessment Data Clusters and Related Nursing Diagnoses for Clients with Skin Problems*

Data Cluster	Nursing Diagnosis
Stan Bailey, 75 years old, suffered a "stroke" 2 weeks ago resulting in paralysis of his left side. States, "I don't want a bath. I can wash myself. I just want to be left alone." Is withdrawn and uncommunicative.	**Self care deficit: Bathing/hygiene** related to paralyzed left upper and lower limbs and lack of motivation
Juanita Perez, an 85-year-old, is newly admitted to the hospital. Appears pale, emaciated, and listless. Weight 90 lbs. Is incontinent of urine, has no bowel control, and is bedridden.	**Potential impaired skin integrity** related to incontinence and immobility
Mark Drake, a 15-year-old, has facial pustules and papules. Facial skin is inflamed. States, "I hate going to school or anywhere looking like this. I don't think any girl wants to go out with me. Can you do something to get rid of this?"	**Self-esteem disturbance** related to acne

Planning

Nursing interventions are identified that will assist the client to achieve the overall client goals of maintaining or improving skin cleanliness, maintaining or restoring skin integrity, maintaining circulation to the skin, and improving or maintaining a sense of well-being. Nursing interventions may include assisting dependent clients with bathing, skin care, and perineal care, providing back massages to promote circulation, and instructing clients about appropriate hygienic practices and therapies to prevent skin lesions. Although the focus of nursing interventions in this chapter is hygienic measures, the etiology of the nursing diagnoses established may point to other interventions that promote circulation, promote self-esteem, restore nutritional status, correct fluid deficits or excesses, or prevent problems associated with immobility. Nursing strategies to deal with these etiologies are provided in other chapters.

Planning to assist a client with personal hygiene includes consideration of the client's personal preferences, health, and limitations; the best time to give the care; and the equipment, facilities, and personnel available. Clients' personal preferences—about when and how they bathe, for example—should be followed as long as they are compatible with the clients' health and the equipment available. Nurses need to provide whatever assistance the client requires, either directly or by delegating this task to other nursing personnel. Examples of outcome criteria to evaluate the achievement of client goals and the effectiveness of nursing interventions are shown below.

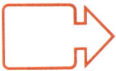

Outcome Criteria
Clients with Skin Problems

The client:

- Has intact, pink, smooth, soft, and hydrated skin.
- Has good tissue turgor.
- Has warm skin.
- Experiences less discomfort.
- Describes factors, when known, that contribute to skin alterations.
- Demonstrates hygienic and other interventions to maintain skin integrity.
- Describes interventions to prevent specific skin problems.
- Expresses positive statements about sense of well-being.
- Completes bathing/hygiene and dressing/grooming self-care activities independently.

Implementing
General Guidelines for Skin Care

1. *An intact, healthy skin is the body's first line of defense.* Nurses need to ensure that all skin care measures prevent injury and irritation. Scratching the skin with jewelry or long, sharp fingernails is avoided. Harsh rubbing or use of rough towels and washcloths can cause tissue damage, particularly when the skin is irritated or when circulation or sensation is diminished. Bottom bedsheets are kept taut and free from wrinkles to reduce friction and abrasion to the skin. Top bed linens are arranged to prevent undue pressure on the toes. When necessary, bed cradles or footboards are used to keep bedclothes off the feet.

2. *The degree to which the skin protects the underlying tissues from injury depends on the general health of the cells, the amount of subcutaneous tissue, and the dryness of the skin.* Skin that is poorly nourished and dry has less ability to protect and is more vulnerable to injury. When the skin is dry, lotions or creams with lanolin are applied, and bathing is limited to once or twice a week. For back rubs, lotion is used rather than alcohol. The greater the amount of subcutaneous tissue, the more padding there is, particularly over bony prominences.

Nurses also assess the client's nutritional and fluid intake. When either one is deficient, measures are taken to improve it.

3. *Moisture in contact with the skin for a period of time can result in increased bacterial growth and irritation.* After a bath, the client's skin is dried carefully. Particular attention is paid to areas such as the axillae, the groin, beneath the breasts, and between the toes, where the potential for irritation is greatest. A nonirritating dusting powder, such as cornstarch, tends to reduce moisture and can be applied to these areas after they are dried. If clients are incontinent of urine or feces or if they perspire excessively, immediate cleaning is provided to prevent skin irritation.

4. *Body odors are caused by resident skin bacteria acting on body secretions.* Cleanliness is the best deodorant. Commercial deodorants and antiperspirants can be applied only after the skin is cleaned. Deodorants diminish odors, whereas antiperspirants reduce the amount of perspiration. Neither is applied immediately after shaving, because of the possibility of skin irritation. Nor are they used on skin that is already irritated.

5. *Skin sensitivity to irritation and injury varies among individuals and in accordance with their health.* Generally speaking, skin sensitivity is greater in infants, very young children, and the elderly. A person's nutritional status also affects sensitivity. Emaciated or obese persons tend to experience more skin irritation and injury. The same tendency is seen in individuals with poor dietary habits and insufficient fluid intake. Even in healthy persons, skin sensitivity is highly variable. Some people's skin is sensitive to chemicals in skin care agents and cosmetics. Hypoallergenic cosmetics and soaps or soap substitutes are now available for these people. The nurse needs to ascertain whether the client has any sensitivities and what agents are appropriate to use.

6. *Agents used for skin care have selective actions and purposes.* Commonly used agents are described in Table 22–4.

Bathing and Skin Care Bathing has a number of functions. The skin continuously secretes sebum and perspiration, which have protective functions: Sebum prevents dryness, and perspiration makes the skin slightly acid, discouraging bacterial growth. Excessive accumulation of sebum, perspiration, and dead skin cells, however, can be injurious or disadvantageous. Excessive perspiration interacts with bacteria on the skin, causing body odor, considered offensive in some cultures. Overaccumulation of sebum on the skin can be irritating in itself, since it promotes the growth of bacteria. Large numbers of bacteria on the skin can cause problems, particularly when the skin integrity is interrupted, for example, by a cut. Dead skin cells also harbor bacteria. Bathing, then, removes accumulated oil, perspiration, dead skin cells, and some bacteria. The quantity of oil and dead skin cells produced can be appreciated when nurses observe the skin of a person after the removal of a cast that has been on for 6 weeks. The skin is crusty, flaky, and dry underneath the cast. Applications of oil over several days are usually necessary to remove the debris.

Excessive bathing, however, can interfere with the intended lubricating effect of the sebum, causing dryness of the skin. This is an important consideration of people, e.g., the elderly, who produce limited sebum.

In addition to cleaning the skin, bathing also stimulates circulation. A warm or hot bath dilates superficial arterioles, bringing more blood and nourishment to the skin. Vigorous rubbing has the same effect. Rubbing with long smooth strokes from the distal to proximal parts of extremities (from the point farthest from the body to the point closest) is particularly effective in facilitating venous blood flow.

Bathing also produces a sense of well-being. It is refreshing and relaxing and frequently improves morale, appearance, and self-respect. Some people take a morning shower for its refreshing, stimulating effect. Others prefer an evening bath because it is relaxing. These effects are more evident when a person is ill. For example, it is not uncommon for clients who have had a restless or sleepless night to feel relaxed, comfortable, and sleepy after a morning bath.

Bathing offers an excellent opportunity for the nurse to assess ill clients. The nurse can observe the condition of the client's skin and physical conditions such as sacral edema or rashes. While assisting a client with a bath, the nurse can also assess the client's psychosocial needs, e.g., orientation to time and ability to cope with the illness. Learning needs, such as a diabetic client's need to learn foot care, can also be assessed.

There are generally two categories of baths given to clients: cleaning and therapeutic. *Cleaning baths* are given chiefly for hygienic purposes and include these types:

■ *Complete bed bath.* The nurse washes the entire body of a dependent client in bed.

■ *Self-help bed bath.* Clients confined to bed are able to bathe themselves with help from the nurse for washing the back and perhaps the feet.

■ *Partial bath (abbreviated bath).* Only the parts of the client's body that might cause discomfort or odor, if neglected, are washed: the face, hands, axillae, perineal area, and back. Omitted are the arms, chest, abdomen, legs, and feet. The nurse provides this care for dependent clients and assists self-sufficient clients confined to bed by washing their backs. Some ambulatory clients prefer to take a partial bath at the sink. The nurse can assist them by washing their backs.

■ *Tub bath.* Tub baths are preferred to bed baths, since washing and rinsing are easier in a tub. Tubs are also used for therapeutic baths. The amount of assistance offered by the nurse depends on the abilities of the client. Many agencies have specially designed tubs for dependent

TABLE 22–4 *Agents Commonly Used on the Skin*

Type	Description
Soap	Lowers surface tension and thus helps in cleaning. Some soaps contain antibacterial agents, which can change the natural flora of the skin.
Detergent	Used instead of soap for cleaning. Some people who are allergic to soaps may not be allergic to detergents, and vice versa.
Bath oil	Used in bath water; provides an oily film on the skin that softens and prevents chapping.
Skin cream, lotion	Provides a film on the skin that prevents evaporation and therefore chapping.
Powder	Can be used to absorb water and prevent friction. For example, powder under the breasts can prevent skin irritation. Some powders are antibacterial.
Deodorant	Masks or diminishes body odors.
Antiperspirant	Reduces the amount of perspiration.

clients. These tubs greatly reduce the work of the nurse in lifting clients in and out of the tub and have greater benefits than a sponge bath in bed.

■ *Shower.* Many ambulatory clients are able to use shower facilities and require only minimal assistance from the nurse.

The water should feel comfortably warm to the client. People vary in their sensitivity to heat; generally, the temperature should be 43 to 46 C (110 to 115 F). Most clients will verify a suitable temperature. The water for a bed bath should be changed at least once.

Therapeutic baths, which are usually ordered by a physician, are given for physical effects, such as to soothe irritated skin or to treat an area (e.g., the perineum). Medications may be placed in the water. A therapeutic bath is generally taken in a tub one-third or one-half full, about 114 liters (30 gal). The client remains in the bath for a designated time, often 20 to 30 minutes. If the client's back, chest, and arms are to be treated, these areas need to be immersed in the solution. The bath temperature is generally included in the order; 37.7 to 46 C (100 to 115 F) may be ordered for adults and 40.5 C (105 F) is usually ordered for infants. See Table 22–5 for types of therapeutic baths.

Because of the increasing acuity of hospitalized clients, many clients receive intravenous therapy. The nurse needs to pay special attention when changing the client's gown after the bath (or whenever the gown becomes soiled). General guidelines (see the box on page 514) for changing the gown may be modified to suit the equipment in use.

Procedure 22–1 provides guidelines for bathing clients.

TABLE 22–5 *Types of Therapeutic Baths*

Bath Solution	Directions	Uses
Saline	4 ml (1 tsp) sodium chloride (NaCl) to 500 ml (1 pt) water.	Has a cooling effect. Cleans. Decreases skin irritation.
Oatmeal or Aveeno	720 ml (3 cups) cooked oatmeal in a cheesecloth bag. Tie the bag securely and twirl it in the tub until the water is opalescent.	Soothes skin irritations. Softens and lubricates dry, scaly skin.
Cornstarch	0.45 kg (1 lb) cornstarch in sufficient cold water to dissolve it; then add boiling water until the mixture is thick. Add to the tub water.	Soothes skin irritation.
Sodium bicarbonate	4 ml (1 tsp) sodium bicarbonate to 500 ml (1 pt) water, or 120–360 ml (4–12 oz) to 120 liters (30 gal).	Has a cooling effect. Relieves skin irritation.
Potassium permanganate ($KMnO_4$)	Available in tablets, which are crushed, dissolved in a little water, and added to the bath.	Cleans and disinfects. Treats infected skin areas.

Changing a Hospital Gown for a Client with an Intravenous Infusion

- Slip the gown completely off the arm without the infusion and onto the tubing connected to the arm with the infusion.

- Holding the container above the client's arm, slide the sleeve up over the container to remove the used gown.

- Place the clean gown sleeve for the arm with the infusion over the container as if it were an extension of the client's arm, from the inside of the gown to the sleeve cuff.

- Rehang the container. Slide the gown carefully over the tubing toward the client's hand.

- Guide the client's arm and tubing into the sleeve, taking care not to pull on the tubing.

- Assist the client to put the other arm into the second sleeve of the gown, and fasten as usual.

- Count the rate of flow of the infusion to make sure it is correct before leaving the bedside.

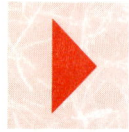

PROCEDURE 22–1

BATHING AN ADULT

Equipment ☑

Two bath towels
Washcloth
Soap
Basin

Hygienic supplies such as lotion, powder, and deodorant
Bath blanket
Water between 43 and 46 C (110 and 115 F) for adults

Clean gown or pajamas as needed
Additional bed linen and towels, if required
Bedpan or urinal
Gloves (optional)

Intervention

1. Prepare the client and the environment.

- Before beginning the bath, determine (a) other care the client is receiving, such as roentgenography or physiotherapy, so that the bath can be coordinated with those activities to prevent undue fatigue to the client; and (b) aspects of the client's health that affect the bathing process. For example, some clients may have limited range of motion of the joints, muscle pain, or a cast or intravenous therapy that interferes with abilities to provide self-care.

■ Close the windows and doors to make sure that the room is free from drafts. *Air currents increase loss of heat from the body by convection.*

■ Provide privacy by drawing the curtains or closing the door. *Hygiene is a personal matter.* Some agencies provide signs indicating the need for privacy.

■ Offer the client a bedpan or urinal or ask whether the client wishes to use the toilet or commode. *The client will be more comfortable after voiding, and voiding before cleaning the perineum is advisable.*

■ During the bath, assess each area of the skin carefully.

For a bed bath:

2. Prepare the bed, and position the client appropriately.

■ Place the bed in the high position. *This avoids undue strain on the nurse's back.*

■ Remove the top bed linen, and replace it with the bath blanket. If the bed linen is to be reused, place it over the bedside chair. If it is to be changed, place it in the linen hamper.

■ Assist the client to move near you. This facilitates access without undue reaching and straining.

■ Remove the gown.

3. Make a bath mitt with the washcloth (see Figure 22–1). *A bath mitt retains water and heat better than a cloth loosely held.*

■ Triangular method: (1) Lay your hand on the washcloth; (2) fold the top corner over your hand; (3,4) fold the side corners over your hand; (5) tuck the second corner under the cloth on the palmar side to secure the mitt.

■ Rectangular method: (1) Lay your hand on the washcloth, and fold one side over your hand; (2) fold

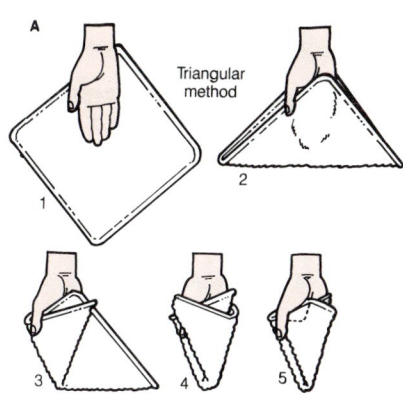

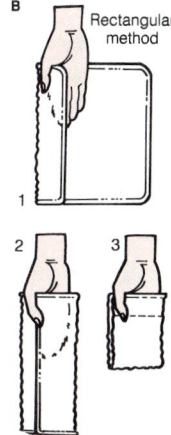

Figure 22–1   Making a bath mitt: *A,* triangular method; *B,* rectangular method.

the second side over your hand; (3) fold the top of the cloth down, and tuck it under the folded side against your palm to secure the mitt.

4. Wash the face.

■ Place one towel across the client's chest.

■ Wash the client's eyes with water only, and dry them well. Use a separate corner of the washcloth for each eye. *Using separate corners prevents transmitting microorganisms from one eye to the other.* Wipe from the inner to the outer canthus. *Cleaning from the inner to*

the outer canthus prevents secretions from entering the nasolacrimal ducts.

■ Ask whether the client wants soap used on the face. *Soap has a drying effect, and the face, which is exposed to the air more than other body parts, tends to be drier.*

■ Wash, rinse, and dry the client's face, neck, and ears.

5. Wash the arms and hands.

■ Place the bath towel lengthwise under the arm. *It protects the bed from becoming wet.*

■ Wash, rinse, and dry the arm, using long, firm strokes from distal to proximal areas (from the point farthest from the body to the point closest). *Firm strokes from distal to proximal areas increase venous blood return.*

■ Wash the axilla well. Repeat for the other arm. (Omit the arms for a partial bath.) Exercise caution if an intravenous infusion is present, and check its flow after moving the arm.

■ Place a towel directly on the bed, and put the basin on it. Place the client's hands in the basin. *Many clients enjoy immersing their hands in the basin and washing themselves.* Assist the client as needed to wash, rinse, and dry the hands, paying particular attention to the spaces between the fingers.

6. Wash the chest and abdomen.

■ Fold the bath blanket down to the client's pubic area, and place the towel alongside the chest and abdomen.

■ Wash, rinse, and dry the chest and abdomen, giving special attention to the skinfold under the breasts. Keep the chest and abdomen covered with the towel between the wash and the rinse.

■ Replace the bath blanket when the areas have been dried. (Omit the chest and abdomen for a partial bath. However, the creases under a woman's breasts may require bathing if they are irritated.) Avoid undue exposure when washing the chest and abdomen. For some clients, it may be preferable to wash the chest and the abdomen separately. In that case, place the bath towel horizontally across the abdomen first and then across the chest.

7. Wash the legs and feet.

■ Wrap one of the client's legs and feet with the bath blanket, ensuring that the pubic area is well covered. See Figure 22–2.

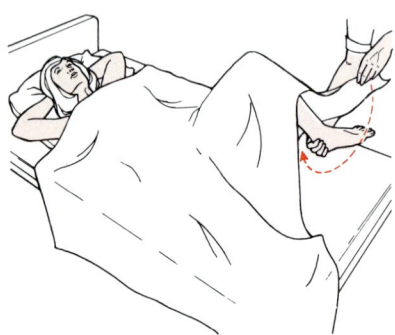

Figure 22–2 Draping one leg of the client.

■ Place the bath towel lengthwise under the other leg, and wash that leg. Use long, smooth, firm strokes, washing from the ankle to the knee to the thigh. *Washing from distal to proximal areas stimulates venous blood flow.*

■ Rinse and dry that leg, reverse the coverings, and repeat for the other leg. (Omit legs and feet for a partial bath.)

■ Wash the feet by placing them in the basin of water.

■ Dry each foot. Pay particular attention to the spaces between the toes.

If you prefer, wash one foot after that leg, before washing the other leg.

■ Obtain fresh, warm bath water now or when necessary. *The temperature of the water in the basin cools relatively rapidly, and the water becomes soapy.*

8. Wash the back and perineum.

■ Assist the client to turn to a prone position or side-lying position facing away from you, and place the bath towel lengthwise alongside the back and buttocks.

■ Wash and dry the back, buttocks, and upper thighs, paying particular attention to the gluteal folds. Give a back rub (see Procedure 22–3). Avoid undue exposure of the client, as for the abdomen and chest. See above.

■ Assist the client to the supine position, and determine whether the client can wash the genital-perineal area independently. If the client cannot do so, drape the client as shown in Figure 22–3, and wash the area. See Procedure 22–2.

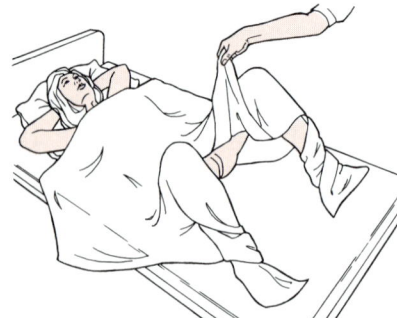

Figure 22–3 Draping the client for perineal-genital care.

9. Assist the client with grooming aids such as powder, lotion, or deodorant.

■ Use powder sparingly, because it tends to accumulate.

■ Help the client to put on a clean gown or pajamas.

■ Assist the client with hair, mouth, and nail care. Some people prefer or need mouth care prior to the bath.

10. Document pertinent data.

■ Record assessments, such as excoriation in the folds beneath the breasts or reddened areas over bony prominences and progress in relief of previous problems.

■ Record the type of bath given (i.e., complete, partial, or self-help). This is usually recorded on a flow sheet.

For a tub bath or shower:

11. Prepare the client and the tub.

■ Fill the tub about one-third to one-half full of water at 43 to 46 C (110 to 115 F). *Sufficient water is needed to cover the perineal area.*

■ Assist the client to the tub or shower.

■ Provide any needed assistance. Many people can manage a tub bath or shower independently; others require assistance only to wash their backs. The person taking a standing shower may need help initially to adjust the temperature and flow of the water.

■ Explain how the client can signal for help, and then leave the client for 2 to 5 minutes.

12. Implement safety precautions.

■ If the client requires considerable assistance, a second nurse may be needed to help the client into and out of the tub and/or to hold the client in a sitting position throughout the bath. When assisting people into and out of tubs, take safety measures to prevent falling or slipping. For example, if the client can step into the tub, the client should hold the handbar while you support the upper trunk under the axillae. To provide support as the client sits down in the tub, fold a towel lengthwise, and place it around the chest, under both axillae; then hold the ends securely at the back as the client sits.

■ Other people may need to sit on the edge of the tub or on a chair beside the tub before transferring into the tub. Some tubs have a nonskid surface to prevent the feet

from slipping. A rubber mat or a towel placed in the bottom of the tub can provide a secure base for the feet.

13. **Wash the client.**

■ Wash the client's back, if necessary, and assist the client out of the tub. If the client is unsteady, drain the tub of water before the client attempts to get out of it, and place a bath towel over the client's shoulders. *Draining the water first lessens the likelihood of a fall. The bath blanket prevents chilling.*

14. **Assist with follow-up care.**

■ Assist the client as necessary to dry and to put on a clean gown or pajamas.

■ Assist the client back to the room, and provide a back rub if the client is spending long periods in bed. See Procedure 22–3.

■ Follow steps 9 and 10.

■ Clean the tub or shower in accordance with agency practice, discard used linen in the laundry hamper, and place the "unoccupied" sign on the door.

Perineal-Genital Care Perineal-genital care is also referred to as *perineal care* or *peri-care*. Perineal care is a part of the bed bath that may be an embarrassing procedure for many clients. Nurses also may find it embarrassing initially, particularly when the client is of the opposite sex. Most clients who require a bed bath from the nurse are able to clean their own genital areas with minimal assistance. The nurse may need to hand a moistened washcloth and soap to the client, rinse the washcloth, and provide a towel.

Because some clients are unfamiliar with terminology for the genitals and perineum, it may be difficult for nurses to

explain what is expected. Most clients, however, understand what is meant if the nurse simply says, "I'll give you a washcloth to finish your bath." Older clients may be familiar with the term *private parts*. Whatever expression the nurse uses, it needs to be one that the client understands and one that is comfortable for the nurse to use.

The nurse needs to provide perineal care efficiently and matter-of-factly. Some nurses wear gloves while providing this care for the comfort of the client and to protect themselves from infection. Procedure 22–2 explains how to provide perineal-genital care.

PROCEDURE 22–2

PROVIDING PERINEAL-GENITAL CARE

Equipment ☑

When perineal-genital care is provided in conjunction with the bed bath, the following bed bath equipment is used:

Bath basin two-thirds filled with water at 43 to 46 C (110 to 115 F)

Soap

Washcloth

Bath towel

Bath blanket

Disposable gloves

Protective ointment as required

When special perineal-genital care is provided, the equipment listed below may be needed.

Bath towel

Bath blanket

Disposable gloves

Cotton balls or swabs

Solution bottle, pitcher, or container filled with warm water or a prescribed solution

Bedpan to receive the rinse water

Moisture-resistant bag or receptacle for used cotton swabs

Perineal pad

Intervention

1. Prepare the client.

- Offer an appropriate explanation, being particularly sensitive to any embarrassment felt by the client.

- Determine whether the client is experiencing any discomfort in the genital-perineal area.

- Fold the top bed linen to the foot of the bed, and fold the gown up to expose the genital area.

- Place a bath towel under the client's hips so that the lower end can be used to dry the anterior perineum, while the upper end can dry the rectal area. *The bath towel also prevents the bed from becoming soiled.*

2. Position and drape the client, and clean the upper inner thighs.

For females:

- Position the female in a back-lying position, with the knees flexed and spread well apart (abducted).

- Cover her body and legs with the bath blanket. Drape the legs by tucking the bottom corners of the bath blanket under the inner sides of the legs. *Minimum exposure lessens embarrassment and provides warmth.* See Figure 22–3. Bring the middle portion of the base of the blanket up over the pubic area.

- 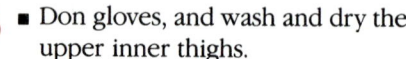 Don gloves, and wash and dry the upper inner thighs.

For males:

- Position the male client in a supine position with knees slightly flexed and hips slightly externally rotated.

- Don gloves and wash and dry the upper inner thighs.

3. Inspect the perineal area.

- Note particular areas of inflammation, excoriation, or swelling, especially between the labia in females and the scrotal folds in males.

- Also note excessive discharge or secretions from the perineal-genital orifices and the presence of odors.

4. Wash and dry the perineal-genital area.

For females:

- Clean the labia majora. Then spread the labia to wash the folds between the labia majora and the labia minora. See Figure 22–4. *Secretions that tend to collect around the labia minora facilitate bacterial growth.*

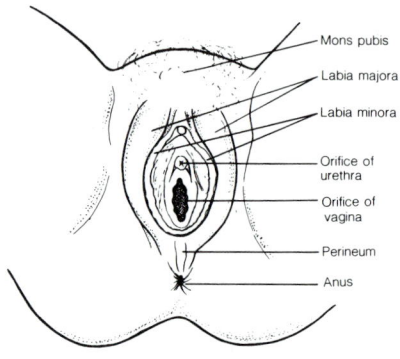

Figure 22–4 Female genitals.

- Use separate quarters of the wash-cloth for each stroke, and wipe from the pubis to the rectum. For menstruating women and clients with indwelling catheters, use cotton balls or gauze. Take a clean ball for each stroke. *Using separate quarters of the washcloth or new cotton balls or gauzes prevents the transmission of microorganisms from one area to the other. Wiping is done from the area of least contamination (the pubis) to the area of greatest contamination (the rectum).*

- Rinse the area well. You may place the client on a bedpan and pour a pitcher of warm water over the area. Dry the perineum thoroughly, paying particular attention to the folds between the labia. *Moisture supports the growth of many microorganisms.*

For males:

- Wash and dry the penis, using firm strokes. *By handling the penis firmly, the nurse may prevent an erection.*

- If the client is uncircumcised, retract the prepuce (foreskin) to expose the glans penis (the tip of the penis) for cleaning. Replace the foreskin after cleaning the glans penis. See Figure 22–5. *Retracting the foreskin is necessary to remove the smegma that collects under the foreskin and facilitates bacterial growth.*

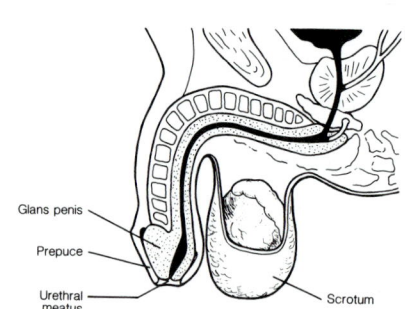

Figure 22–5 Male genitals.

- Wash and dry the scrotum. The posterior folds of the scrotum may need to be cleaned with the buttocks. *The scrotum tends to be more soiled than the penis because of its proximity to the rectum; thus it is usually cleaned after the penis.*

5. Inspect perineal orifices for intactness.

- Inspect particularly around the urethra in clients with indwelling catheters. *A catheter may cause excoriation around the urethra.*

- Apply protective ointment, if necessary.

6. Clean between the buttocks.

- Assist the client to turn on the side facing away from you.

- Pay particular attention to the anal area and posterior folds of the scrotum in males. Clean the anus

with toilet tissue before washing it, if necessary.

- Dry the area well.

- Apply protective ointments, such as petroleum jelly, if necessary.

- For postdelivery females, apply a perineal pad as needed from front to back. *This prevents contamination of the vagina and urethra from the anal area.*

7. Document any significant assessments, such as redness, swelling, or discharge.

Sample Recording

Date 7/10/91	Time: 0900

Perineal care given. Circular reddened area about 2.5 cm diameter to left of urethral orifice. No discharge apparent. ⎯⎯
⎯⎯⎯⎯⎯⎯⎯⎯ Patricia L. Snow, SN

Back Rubs   Back rubs, or massage of the back, have two chief objectives: to relax and relieve tension (sedative effect), and to stimulate blood circulation to the tissues and the muscles. Friction from the rubbing produces heat at the skin surface. Heat dilates the peripheral blood vessels in the area, thus increasing the blood supply to the area. Because tissues are under pressure when a client is in bed and muscles are usually relaxed, stimulation of the circulation is essential so that the tissues obtain nutrients and oxygen.

Five massage methods can be used to rub the back and the bony prominences of the body:

1. In the **tapotement**, the little-finger side of each hand is used in a sharp, hacking movement on the back. Care must be taken not to bruise the client. This method is *not* advised for elderly, debilitated clients, or clients who have disease conditions of the back.

2. The **petrissage** is a kneading or large, quick pinch of the skin, subcutaneous tissue, and muscle. Pinches are taken first up the vertebral column and then over the entire back. The tapotement and the petrissage are primarily stimulating, especially if done quickly and with firm pressure.

3. The **friction stroke** is a circular stroke accomplished with both thumbs. The nurse massages the back from the buttocks to the shoulders, using smooth, tiny circles.

4. The **effleurage** is a smooth, long stroke: a moving of the hands up and down the back. The hands move lightly down the sides of the back, maintaining contact with the skin, but move firmly up the back. This rub has a relaxing, sedative effect if slow movement and light pressure are used.

5. The **three-handed effleurage** is a smooth, stroking motion that gives the client an impression of being rubbed

by three hands. The nurse starts with one hand at the base of the client's neck and moves the hand to the lateral aspect of the shoulder. The nurse then makes the same movement with the other hand, moving it to the other shoulder before removing the first hand from the shoulder and returning it to the base of the neck. This rub is particularly effective in relieving tension of the neck muscles.

During the back rub, the nurse observes any reddened areas that do not disappear after a few minutes of massage, any breaks in the skin, and any bruises. They should be reported and recorded. Often, these conditions predispose to decubitus ulcers.

Emollient creams and lotions are frequently used to lubricate the skin during back rubs. Unless another agent is specifically ordered by the physician, lotion is preferred because of its lubricating action on the skin. Powder is sometimes used. Alcohol preparations are cooling, but they are used infrequently today. They are refreshing, and they toughen skin by hardening the skin protein, but they tend to dry the skin, and very dry skin is likely to crack. Alcohol preparations are particularly undesirable for use on elderly clients, whose skin is usually dry. Dehydrated and poorly nourished clients may also not benefit from an alcohol back rub.

The position of choice for a back rub is the prone position (lying on the stomach). The second preferred position is the side-lying position; its disadvantage is the difficulty of massaging the lateral aspect of the hip on which the client is lying, and the client must be turned to the other side.

Other pressure points on the body that generally benefit from massage and the application of lotions are the elbows, knees, and heels. Sometimes massage of the anterior aspects of both iliac crests of very thin clients is also indicated.

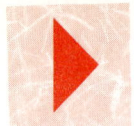

GIVING A BACK RUB

Equipment

Lotion, alcohol, or powder
Towel

Intervention

1. Prepare the client.

- Assist the client to move to the near side of the bed within your reach.
- Establish which position the client prefers. The prone position is recommended for a back rub. A client who cannot assume this position assumes a side-lying position but will need to turn to the other side for you to complete the massage.
- Expose the back from the shoulders to the inferior sacral area.

2. Massage the back.

- Pour a small amount of lotion onto the palms of your hands, and hold it for a minute, or place the container in a bath basin filled with warm water. *Back rub preparations tend to feel uncomfortably cold to people. Holding warms the*

solution, so that it will be more comfortable.

- Rub in a circular motion over the sacral area.
- Move your hands up the center of the back and then over both scapulae.
- Massage in a circular motion over the scapulae.
- Move your hands down the sides of the back.
- Massage the areas over the right and left iliac crests. See Figure 22–6.
- Repeat above for 3 to 5 minutes, obtaining more lotion as necessary.
- While massaging the client's skin, inspect for (a) whitish or reddened skin areas that do not disappear after rubbing and (b) broken or raw skin areas, especially on the elbows or heels.
- Massage directly over pressure areas gently and only if there is no evidence of underlying tissue damage. If there is evidence of pressure, massage around the area, not directly on it. *Vigorous massage over bony prominences can*

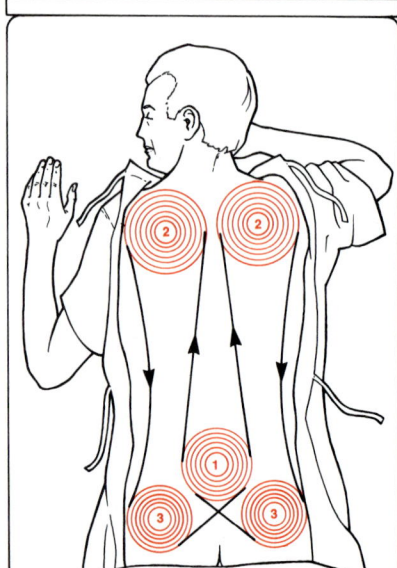

Figure 22–6 One suggested pattern for a back massage.

increase damage in nutrient-deprived tissues.

- Pat dry any excess solution with a towel.

3. Document assessments such as redness, broken skin areas, and bruises.

 Nurses are advised not to rub tender, reddened areas on the lower legs of clients, particularly the calves. Redness, tenderness, and heat, particularly along the course of a vein, may indicate a thrombus (blood clot) in the area. Massage might dislodge the clot, which could travel to the heart or the lung, causing a myocardial or pulmonary embolus. This can present a very serious problem. Procedure 22–3 provides guidelines for giving a back rub.

Client Teaching   Clients often need information about dry skin, skin rashes, diaper rash, and acne (a condition described in Chapter 26, page 638). The accompanying box provides some guidelines for these problems.

Evaluating

To evaluate the achievement of client goals, the nurse inspects the client's skin, palpates specific areas to assess circulatory

status, listens to the client's statements about sense of well-being, observes the client's hygienic self-care, and asks the client to discuss specific information or demonstrate specific skills. Goal achievement is then documented. Examples of evaluative statements are "The client's skin is intact, warm, smooth and soft," "The client described three factors that contributed to his skin problem," and "The client completed 75% of bathing/hygiene self-care independently." See also the nursing care plan at the end of this chapter and the section on decubitus ulcers in Chapter 35.

FEET

Healthy feet are essential for ambulation and for comfort when standing and performing daily activities. Foot care that involves regular nail trimming, cleanliness, the wear-

CLIENT TEACHING
Skin Problems and Care

Dry Skin

- Use cleansing creams to clean the skin rather than soap or detergent, which cause drying and, in some cases, allergic reactions.
- Use bath oils, but take precautions to prevent falls caused by slippery tub surfaces.
- Thoroughly rinse soap or detergent, if used, from the skin.
- Bathe less frequently when environmental temperature and humidity are low.
- Increase fluid intake.
- Humidify the air with a humidifier or by keeping a tub or sink full of water.
- Use moisturizing or emollient creams that contain lanolin, petroleum jelly, or cocoa butter to retain skin moisture.

Skin Rashes

- Keep the area clean by washing it with a mild soap. Rinse the skin well, and pat it dry.
- To relieve itching, try a tepid bath or soak. Some over-the-counter preparations, such as Caladryl lotion, may

help but should be used with full knowledge of the product.
- Avoid scratching the rash to prevent inflammation, infection, and further skin lesions.
- Choose clothing carefully. Too much can cause perspiration and aggravate a rash.
- Consult a physician if symptoms persist.

Acne

- Wash the face frequently with soap or detergent and hot water to remove oil and dirt.
- Avoid using oily creams, which aggravate the condition.
- Avoid using cosmetics that block the ducts of the sebaceous glands and the hair follicles.
- Never squeeze or pick at the lesions. This increases the potential for infection and scarring.
- Avoid foods such as chocolate, nuts, and colas, *if* they exaggerate the problem after they are ingested.
- Obtain adequate rest and moderate exercise.
- Consult a physician if the problem is severe.

---

ing of properly fitted shoes, and protection from injurious agents can prevent common foot problems such as odor, infection, and injury. For normal development, the arches must be supported and the bony structures of the feet allowed to grow with no external restraints. Discomfort or pain is often the first warning of foot problems. Because foot discomfort usually alters the way a person walks, various muscle groups of the body can become strained and emotional well-being adversely affected.

Developmental Variations

At birth, a baby's foot is relatively unformed. The arches are supported by fatty pads and do not take their full shape until 5 or 6 years of age. Feet are not fully grown until about age 20. Healthy feet remain relatively unchanged during life. However, the feet of elderly people often require special attention. Reduced blood supply and accompanying arteriosclerosis, for example, can predispose the foot to infection following trauma.

Assessing

Nursing History   The nurse determines the client's history of (a) normal nail and foot care practices; (b) type of footwear worn; (c) self-care abilities; (d) presence of

factors that place the client at risk of foot problems; (e) any foot discomfort; and (f) any perceived problems with foot mobility. To elicit such data, the nurse asks the client the questions in the box on page 522.

Physical Assessment   Each foot and toe is inspected for shape, size, and presence of lesions and is palpated to assess areas of tenderness, edema, and circulatory status. Normally, the toes are straight and flat. The plantar surface of each foot should have the following landmarks: the medial longitudinal arch, an apparent heel, and an apparent ball of the foot (metatarsophalangeal joints). See Table 22–6 on page 523 for physical assessment methods and normal and abnormal findings. Common foot problems include calluses, corns, unpleasant odors, plantar warts, fissure between the toes, fungal infections such as athlete's foot, and deviations in toe contour.

A **callus** is a thickened portion of epidermis, a mass of keratotic material. Calluses are usually painless and flat and found on the bottom or side of the foot over a bony prominence. Calluses are usually caused by pressure from shoes. They can be softened by soaking the foot in warm water with Epsom salts, and they can be abraded by pumice stones or similar abrasives. Creams with lanolin help to keep the skin soft and prevent the formation of calluses.

A **corn** is a keratosis caused by friction and pressure from a shoe. It commonly occurs on a toe, usually the fourth or fifth toe, and usually on a bony prominence such as a joint. Corns are usually conical (circular and raised). The base is the surface of the corn and the apex is in deeper tissues, sometimes even attached to bone. Corns are generally removed surgically. They are prevented from reforming by relieving the pressure on the area (i.e., wearing comfortable shoes), and massaging the tissue to promote circulation. The use of oval corn pads should be avoided, since they increase pressure and decrease circulation.

Unpleasant odors occur as a result of perspiration and its interaction with microorganisms. Regular and frequent washing of the feet and wearing clean hosiery help to minimize odor. Foot powders and deodorants also help to prevent this problem.

Plantar warts appear on the sole of the foot. These warts are caused by the virus papovavirus hominis. They are moderately contagious. The warts are frequently painful and often make walking difficult. The treatment ordered by a physician may be curettage, freezing with solid carbon dioxide several times, or repeated applications of salicylic acid.

Fissures between the toes occur frequently as a result of dryness and cracking of the skin. A **fissure** is a deep groove. The treatment of choice is good foot hygiene and application of an antiseptic to prevent infection. Often a small piece of gauze is inserted between the toes in applying the antiseptic and left in place to assist healing by allowing air to reach the area.

Athlete's foot or **tinea pedis** (ringworm of the foot) is caused by a fungus. The symptoms are scaling and cracking of the skin, particularly between the toes. Sometimes small blisters form, containing a thin fluid. In severe cases the lesions may also appear on other parts of the body, particularly the hands. Treatments vary from potassium permanganate soaks, using a 1:8000 solution, to application of commercial antifungal ointments or powders. Prevention is important. Common preventive measures are keeping the feet well ventilated, drying the feet well after bathing, wearing clean socks or stockings, and not going barefoot in public showers.

An **ingrown toenail**, the growing inward of the nail into the soft tissues around the nails, most often results from improper nail trimming. Pressure applied to the area causes localized pain. Treatment involves frequent, hot antiseptic soaks and surgical removal of the portion of nail embedded in the skin. Prevention of recurrence involves appropriate instruction and adherence to proper nail-trimming techniques.

Common deviations in toe contour include hallux valgus and hammer toe. **Hallux valgus** (bunion) is a lateral deviation of the big toe at its metatarsophalangeal joint, with enlargement and development of a bursa or callus over the area, which constitutes the bunion. See Figure 22–7, *A* on page 524. If the deviation is severe, the great toe may overlap the second toe. Displacement may cause the second toe to develop hammer toe. A familial tendency toward hallux valgus is apparent, and it is more common in females than in males. Contributing causes include poorly fitted shoes, flat feet, and degenerative arthritic changes. Conservative treatment consists of well-fitted shoes with ample room for the forefoot and use of bunion pads to relieve shoe pressure. A severe, painful bursitis may require incising and applying hot, moist compresses. Surgical correction is sometimes necessary. Intra-articular injections of corticosteroids may be given if there is osteoarthritic joint involvement.

Hammer toe is characterized by hyperextension of the metatarsophalangeal joint, flexion of the proximal interphalangeal joint, and hyperextension of the distal interphalangeal joint. See Figure 22–7, *B*. The second toe is most

TABLE 22–6 *Assessment Data: Feet*

Physical Assessment	Data	Method	Normal Findings	Abnormal Findings
Inspection	1. Skin surfaces, for cleanliness, odor, dryness, inflammation, swelling, abrasions, or other lesions	Carefully check all skin surfaces, paying particular attention to areas between toes.	Intact skin Absence of swelling or inflammation	Excessive dryness Areas of inflammation or swelling, e.g., corns, calluses Fissures Scaling and cracking of skin, e.g., athlete's foot Plantar warts
	2. Status of toenails	See discussion of nails.		
	3. Toe contour	Observe toe profile.	Toes extended (straight and flat)	Bunion (hallux valgus) Hammer toe Claw toe
	4. Longitudinal foot arch	Observe medial foot profile when client is standing.	Presence of medial longitudinal arch, i.e., medial concavity, with prominent heel and ball of foot	Flat foot (pes planus) High arch (pes cavus)
	5. Foot alignment	Observe alignment of foot to ankle and tibia, and metatarsal alignment (alignment of forefoot to heel).	Foot in straight alignment	Toeing-in (pes vargus) Toeing-out (pes valgus) Abduction of forefoot (metatarsus varus) Adduction of forefoot (metatarsus valgus) Clubfoot
	6. Ability to stand, walk, and perform range-of-motion exercises with each ankle and set of toes	See Chapters 35 and 36.	Full range of motion	Deformity (e.g., foot drop) Impaired range of motion in ankle or toes
Palpation	7. Areas of tenderness on body or muscular structures or on plantar surface.	Palpate bony and muscular structures of foot and plantar surface to locate points of tenderness.	Absence of tenderness and nodules Smooth, firm, fleshy plantar surface	Tenderness in certain areas, related to arthritic changes, muscle strain, or lesions, e.g., plantar warts or bunions
	8. Ankle edema	Palpate anterior and posterior surfaces of ankle.	No swelling	Swelling or pitting edema
	9. Circulatory status	Palpate dorsalis pedis pulse on dorsal surface of foot just above longitudinal arch. Compare skin temperatures of two feet.	Strong, regular pulses in both feet Warm skin temperature	Weak or absent pulses Cool skin temperature in one or both feet.

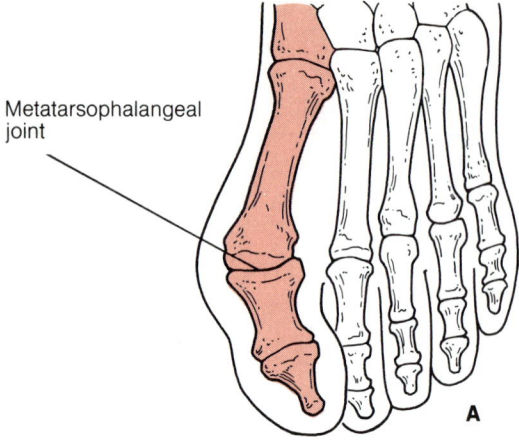

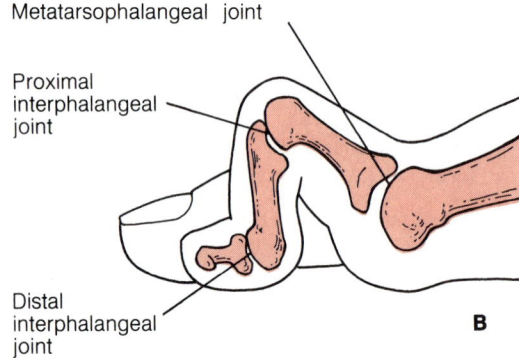

Figure 22–7 Toe deviations: *A,* hallux valgus; *B,* hammer toe.

frequently involved, often bilaterally, and it may be associated with hallux valgus. Painful calluses often develop over the proximal interphalangeal joint. Hammer toes may be congenital, linked to a familial tendency, or acquired. If acquired, they are caused most frequently by poorly fitted shoes that force the involved toe into a flexion deformity. Conservative treatment for hammer toe includes passive stretching exercises and well-fitted shoes, perhaps with padding and inserts to decrease pressure over the proximal interphalangeal joint. Surgery to correct the flexion of the joint and splinting are sometimes necessary.

Diagnosing

A number of nursing diagnoses may be developed for clients with foot or foot care problems. **Self-care deficit: Bathing/hygiene** may be the diagnosis given. Other possible diagnoses include **Impaired skin integrity, (Actual** or **Potential), Potential for infection, Pain, Knowledge deficit,** and **Impaired physical mobility**. Examples of these nursing diagnoses and possible contributing factors are shown below. Examples of assessment data clusters and related nursing diagnoses are shown in Table 22–7.

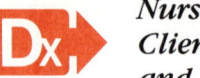 **Nursing Diagnoses**
Clients with Foot Hygiene and Foot Problems

Self-care deficit related to:

■ Visual impairment

■ Impaired hand coordination

■ Other factors contributing to skin problems (see page 511)

Potential impaired skin integrity related to:

■ Altered tissue perfusion: Peripheral (associated with edema, inadequate arterial circulation)

■ Improper foot care practices

Impaired skin integrity related to:

■ Ineffective hygienic practices

■ Altered tissue perfusion: Peripheral

Potential for infection related to:

■ Impaired skin integrity (ingrown toenail, corn, trauma)

■ Deficient nail or foot care.

Pain related to: Impaired skin integrity (corn, ingrown toenail)

Knowledge deficit (diabetic foot care) related to:

■ Lack of exposure to information

■ Misinterpretation of information

■ Ineffective individual coping

Impaired physical mobility related to:

■ Painful foot lesion (corn, ingrown toenail, plantar wart)

■ Altered foot alignment (contracture)

Planning

Planning involves (a) identification of nursing interventions that will achieve the overall client goals of maintaining or restoring healthy foot care practices and (b) establishing specific outcome criteria for each client. Interventions may include teaching the client about correct nail and foot care, proper foot wear, and ways to prevent potential foot problems (e.g., infection, injury, and decreased circulation). For clients with self-care difficulties, the nurse plans a schedule for soaking the client's feet and assisting with regular cleaning and trimming of nails (if not contraindicated). Foot and nail care is often provided during the client's bath but may be provided at any time in the day to accommodate the client's preference. The frequency of foot care is deter-

TABLE 22–7 *Examples of Assessment Data Clusters and Related Nursing Diagnoses for Clients with Foot Problems*

Data Cluster	Nursing Diagnosis
Sally Brown, an 83-year-old widow, lives alone. Has homemaker services 2 times per week and Meals-On-Wheels service daily. Manages a shower once per week with daughter's help. Has pronounced hand tremors and obvious cataracts. States, "I can't see well enough to cut my nails, and even if I could see, my hands shake so badly."	**Self-care deficit: Foot hygiene** related to impaired hand coordination and visual impairment
Kyle Stevens, 14-year-old, lives with his mother and 8 sisters and brothers in a 3-room walk-up. Bathroom down the hall is shared with other tenants in the building. Shoes are ragged and poorly fitted. States, "I can't get new ones."	**Potential impaired skin integrity** related to improper foot care practices
Jim Wakefield, 64 years old, was recently diagnosed with diabetes mellitus. States has heard of "diabetes" and is worried, since a friend of his father's had diabetes and, after cutting his foot, had his leg amputated.	**Knowledge deficit** (diabetic foot care) related to misinterpretation of information

mined by the nurse and client and is based on objective assessment data and the client's specific problems. For some clients, the feet need to be bathed daily; for those whose feet perspire excessively, bathing more than once a day may be necessary. Examples of outcome criteria to evaluate the achievement of goals and effectiveness of nursing interventions are shown below.

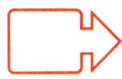

Outcome Criteria
Clients with Foot Hygiene and Foot Problems

The client:

- Has intact, pink, smooth, soft, and hydrated skin.
- Has warm skin.
- Experiences less pain or discomfort.
- Has intact cuticles and skin surrounding nails.
- Has quick return of nail bed color after blanch test.
- Wears appropriate shoes and walks without discomfort.
- Describes hygienic and other interventions to maintain skin integrity and peripheral tissue perfusion.
- Describes interventions to prevent specific foot problems.
- Demonstrates correct foot and nail care practices.
- Performs self-care (foot hygiene) practices independently.

Implementing

Foot care is described in Procedure 22–4. See also the discussion of nails. During these procedures, the nurse has the opportunity to teach the client appropriate methods for

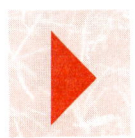

PROCEDURE 22–4

PROVIDING FOOT CARE

Equipment ☑

Washbasin

Soap

Washcloth

Towels

Moisture-resistant disposable pad

Lotion or foot powder

Toenail cleaning and trimming equipment

Intervention

1. Prepare the equipment and the client.

- Fill the washbasin with warm water at about 40 to 43 C (105 to 110 F). *Warm water promotes circulation, comforts, and refreshes.*

- Assist the ambulatory client to a sitting position in a chair, or the bed client to a supine or semi-Fowler's position.

- Place a pillow under the bed client's knees. *This provides support and prevents muscle fatigue.*

- Place the washbasin on the moisture-resistant pad at the foot of the bed for a bed client or on the floor in front of the chair for an ambulatory client.

- For a bed client, pad the rim of the washbasin with a towel. *This towel prevents undue pressure on the skin.*

2. Wash the foot, and soak it as required.

- Place one of the client's feet in the basin, and wash it with soap, paying particular attention to the interdigital areas.

- Rinse the foot well to remove soap.

Soap irritates the skin if not properly removed.

- Rub callused areas of the foot with the washcloth. *This helps remove dead skin layers.*

- If the nails are brittle or thick and require trimming, replace the water and allow the foot to soak for 10 to 20 minutes. *Soaking softens the nails and loosens debris under them.*

- Clean the nails as required with an orange stick or the blunt end of a toothpick. *This removes excess debris that harbors microorganisms.*

- Remove the foot from the basin, and place it on the towel.

3. Dry the foot thoroughly, and apply lotion or foot powder.

- Blot the foot gently with the towel to dry it thoroughly, particularly between the toes. *Harsh rubbing can damage the skin. Thorough drying reduces the risk of infection.*

- Apply lotion or lanolin cream. *This lubricates dry skin.*
  or

- Apply a foot powder containing a

nonirritating deodorant if the feet tend to perspire excessively. *Foot powders have greater absorbent properties than regular bath powders; some also contain menthol, which makes the feet feel cool.*

4. If agency policy permits, trim the nails of the first foot while the second foot is soaking.

- See the discussion on nails for the appropriate method to trim nails. Note that in many agencies toenail trimming is contraindicated for clients with diabetes mellitus, toe infections, and peripheral vascular disease, unless performed by a podiatrist or general practice physician.

5. Document any foot problems observed.

- Foot care is not generally recorded unless problems are noted.

- Record any signs of inflammation, infection, breaks in the skin, corns, troublesome calluses, bunions, and pressure areas. This is of particular importance for clients with peripheral vascular disease and diabetes.

---

foot care, i.e., those designed to prevent tissue injury and infection. Because of reduced peripheral circulation to the feet, clients with diabetes or peripheral vascular disease are particularly prone to infection if skin breakage occurs. Many foot problems can be prevented when the client follows simple foot care guidelines. See the accompanying Client Teaching box.

Evaluating

At designated intervals, the nurse evaluates whether the client has achieved the outcome criteria established during the planning phase. Examples of evaluative statements are "The client described interventions to prevent corns and infection," or "The client demonstrated foot and nail care practices as taught." These observations need to be dated and documented appropriately.

NAILS

Nails are normally present at birth. They continue to grow throughout life and change very little until people are old. At that time, the nails tend to be tougher, more brittle, and in some cases thicker. The nails of an elderly person normally grow less quickly than those of a younger person and may be ridged and grooved.

Assessing

During the nursing history, the nurse explores the client's usual nail care practices, self-care abilities, and any problems associated with them. See the accompanying assessment box. Physical assessment involves inspection of the nails (see also Chapter 19, page 373).

CLIENT TEACHING
Foot Care

- Wash the feet daily, and dry them well, especially between the toes.

- When washing, check the skin of the feet for breaks or red or swollen areas.

- To prevent burns, check the water temperature before immersing the feet.

- Use creams or lotions to moisten the skin, or soak the feet in warm water with Epsom salts to avoid excessive drying of the skin of the feet. Lotion will also soften calluses. A lotion that reduces dryness effectively is a mixture of lanolin and mineral oil.

- To prevent or control an unpleasant odor due to excessive foot perspiration, wash the feet frequently, and change socks and shoes at least daily. Special deodorant sprays or absorbent foot powders are also helpful.

- File the toenails rather than cutting them to avoid skin injury. File the nails straight across the ends of the toes. If the nails are too thick or misshapen to file, consult a podiatrist.

- Wear clean stockings or socks daily. Avoid socks with holes or darns that can cause pressure areas.

- Wear correctly fitting shoes that neither restrict the foot nor rub on any area; rubbing can cause corns and calluses. Check worn shoes for rough spots in the lining. Break in new shoes gradually by increasing the wearing time 30 to 60 minutes each day.

- Avoid walking barefoot, since injury and infection may result. Wear slippers in public showers and change areas to avoid contracting athlete's foot or other infections.

- Several times each day, exercise the feet to promote circulation. Point the feet upward, point them downward, and move them in circles.

- Avoid wearing constricting garments such as kneehigh elastic stockings or sitting with the legs crossed at the knees, which may decrease circulation.

- When the feet are cold, use extra blankets and wear warm socks rather than using heating pads or hot water bottles, which may cause burns.

- Wash any cut on the foot thoroughly, apply a mild antiseptic, and notify the physician.

- Avoid self-treatment for corns or calluses. Pumice stones and some callus and corn applications are injurious to the skin. Consult a podiatrist.

ASSESSMENT INTERVIEW
Nail Hygiene

- What are your usual nail care practices?

- Do you have any problems managing your nail care? If so, what are these?

- Have you had any problems associated with your nails (e.g., inflammation of the tissue surrounding the nail, injury, prolonged exposure to water or chemicals, circulatory problems)?

Diagnosing

Nursing diagnoses related to nail care and nail problems include **Self-care deficit, Potential for infection,** and **Pain.** Examples of these nursing diagnoses and contributing factors are shown below.

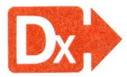

Nursing Diagnoses
Clients with Nail Hygiene and Nail Problems

Self-care deficit: Grooming related to:
- Impaired vision
- Impaired hand coordination

Potential for infection around the nail bed related to:
- Impaired skin integrity of cuticles
- Altered peripheral circulation

Pain related to inflamed cuticle and/or skin surrounding the nails.

Planning

The nurse identifies measures that will assist the client to achieve the overall client goals of developing or maintaining healthy nail care practices. A schedule of nail care needs to be established. Examples of outcome criteria to evaluate the achievement of client goals and the effectiveness of nursing interventions are shown on the following page.

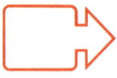

Outcome Criteria
Clients with Nail Hygiene and Nail Problems

The client:

- Has smooth, convex, clean nails.
- Has pink nail beds.
- Has intact cuticles and hydrated surrounding skin.
- Has quick return of nail bed color after the blanch test.
- Experiences less or no pain and inflammation.
- Has short nails with smooth edges.
- Describes factors contributing to the nail problem.
- Describes preventive interventions for the specific nail problem.
- Demonstrates nail care as instructed.

Implementing

To provide nail care, the nurse needs a nail cutter or sharp scissors, a nail file, an orange stick to push back the cuticle, hand lotion or mineral oil to lubricate any dry tissue around the nails, and a basin of water to soak the nails if they are particularly thick or hard.

One hand or foot is soaked, if needed, and dried; then the nail is cut or filed straight across beyond the end of the finger or toe. See Figure 22–8. Avoid trimming or digging into nails at the lateral corners. This predisposes the client to ingrown toenails. Clients who have diabetes or circulatory problems should have their nails filed, rather than cut. Inadvertent injury to tissues can occur if scissors are used. After the initial cut or filing, the nail is filed to round the corners, and the nurse cleans under the nail. The nurse then gently pushes back the cuticle, taking care not to injure it. The next finger or toe is cared for in the same manner. Any abnormalities, such as an infected cuticle or inflammation of the tissue around the nail, are recorded and reported.

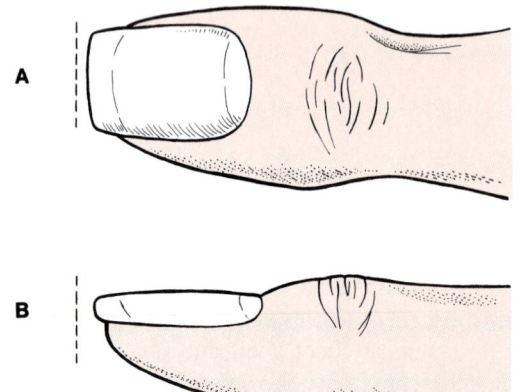

Figure 22–8 Fingernails are trimmed straight across.

Evaluating

Using the preestablished outcome criteria at a designated time, the nurse determines whether the client has achieved the goals. To evaluate, the nurse inspects the client's nails, asks the client about any discomfort, questions the client about specific information taught, asks for a demonstration of nail care, and perhaps performs the blanch test. Goal achievement is then documented, for example, "The client's cuticles were not inflamed and were intact," or "The client reported, 'My nail is not painful today.' "

MOUTH

Developmental Variations

Teeth usually appear 5 to 8 months after birth. Each tooth has a number of parts: the crown, the root, and the pulp cavity. The **crown** is the exposed part of the tooth, which is outside the gum. It is covered with a hard substance called **enamel**. The ivory-colored internal part of the crown below the enamel is the **dentin**. See Figure 22–9. The root of a tooth is embedded in the jaw and covered by a bony tissue called **cementum**. The **pulp cavity** in the center of the tooth contains the blood vessels and nerves.

By the time children are 2 years old, they usually have all 20 of their temporary teeth. See Figure 22–10. At about age 6 or 7, children start losing their deciduous teeth, and these are gradually replaced by the 32 permanent teeth. See Figure 22–11. By age 25, most people have all their permanent teeth.

The incidence of periodontal disease increases during pregnancy, since an increase in female hormones affects gingival tissue and increases its reaction to bacterial plaque. Many pregnant women manifest increased bleeding from the gingival sulcus during brushing and increased redness and swelling of the **gingiva** (the gum). These gingival changes heighten the pregnant woman's chances of acquiring periodontal disease (Martin and Reeb 1982, p. 391).

Elderly people may have few permanent teeth left, and many have **dentures**. Most people have lost all their own teeth by age 70, mainly because of periodontal disease rather than dental caries; however, caries are also common in the middle-aged adult. Preventive dental care is important.

Some receding of the gums and a brownish pigmentation of the gums occur with age. Because saliva production decreases with age, dryness of the oral mucosa is a common finding in older people.

Assessing

Assessment of the client's mouth and hygienic practices includes (a) a nursing history, (b) physical assessment of the mouth, and (c) identification of clients at risk for developing oral problems.

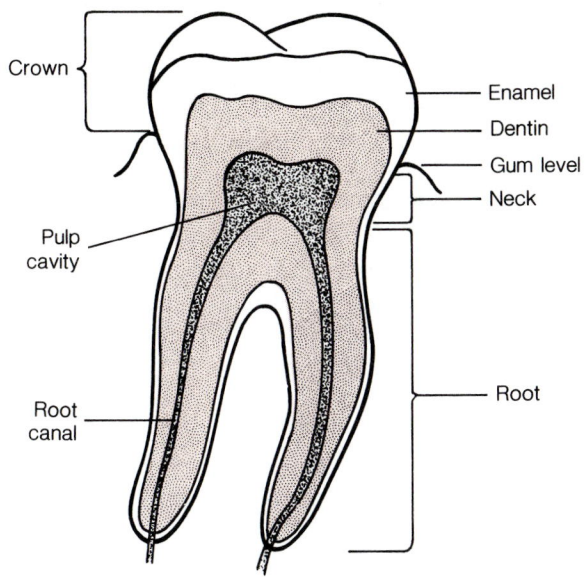

Figure 22–9 The anatomic parts of a tooth.

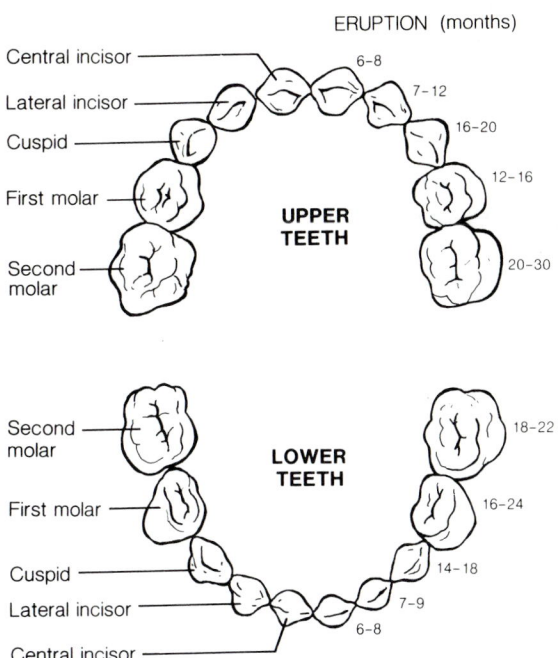

Figure 22–10 Temporary teeth and their times of eruption (stated in months).

Nursing History During the nursing history, the nurse obtains data about the client's oral hygiene practices, including dental visits, self-care abilities, and past or current mouth problems. Data about the client's oral hygiene helps the nurse determine necessary learning needs and to incorporate the client's needs and preferences in the plan of care. Assessment of the client's *self-care abilities* determines the amount and type of nursing assistance to provide. Clients whose hand coordination is impaired, whose cognitive function is impaired, whose illness alters energy levels and motivation, or whose therapy imposes restrictions on activities will need assistance from the nurse. Data about *past or current problems* alerts the nurse to specific interventions required or referrals that may be necessary. Questions to elicit the above data are shown in the box on page 530.

Physical Assessment For information about mouth assessment, see Chapter 19, pages 389 to 392. Dental **caries** (cavities) and **periodontal disease** (pyorrhea) are two problems that most frequently affect the teeth. Both problems are commonly associated with plaque and tartar deposits. **Plaque** is an *invisible* soft film that adheres to the enamel surface of teeth; it consists of bacteria, molecules of saliva, and remnants of epithelial cells and leukocytes. When plaque is unchecked, tartar (dental calculus) is formed. **Tartar** is a visible, hard deposit of plaque and dead bacteria that forms at the gum lines. Tartar buildup can alter the fibers that attach the teeth to the gum and eventually disrupt bone tissue. Periodontal disease is characterized by **gingivitis** (red, swollen gingiva), bleeding, receding gum lines, and the formation of pockets between the teeth and

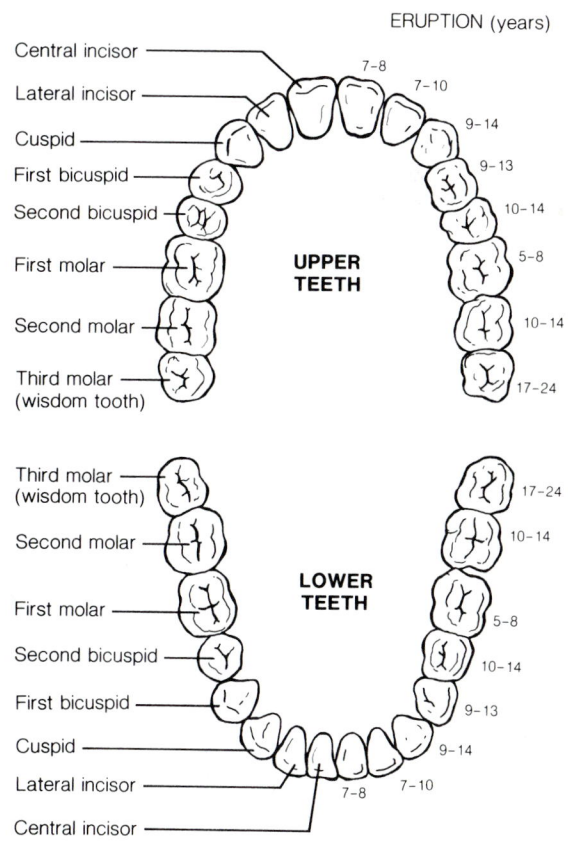

Figure 22–11 Permanent teeth and their times of eruption (stated in years).

ASSESSMENT INTERVIEW
Oral Hygiene

Oral Hygiene Practices

■ What are your usual mouth care and/or denture care practices?

■ What oral hygiene products do you routinely use (e.g., mouthwash, type of toothpaste, dental floss, denture cleaner)?

■ When was your last dental examination, and how often do you see your dentist?

Self-Care Abilities

■ Do you have any problems managing your mouth care?

Past or Current Mouth Problems

■ Have you had or do you have any problems such as bleeding, swollen or reddened gums, ulcerations, lumps, or tooth pain?

or the inability to maintain oral hygiene. Among these are seriously ill, confused, comatosed, depressed, and dehydrated clients. In addition, persons with nasogastric tubes or receiving oxygen are likely to develop dry oral mucous membranes, especially if they breathe through their mouths. Clients who have had oral or jaw surgery must have meticulous oral hygiene care to prevent the development of infections.

Healthy-appearing individuals, too, may be at risk. High-risk variables such as inadequate nutrition, excessive intake of refined sugars, and family history of periodontal disease also need to be identified. Some elderly people may also be at risk, e.g., those who choose salty and enamel-eroding sugary foods because of a decline in their number of taste buds. The decreased saliva production in the aged, which produces a dry mouth and thinning of the oral mucosa, is another factor (Pettigrew 1989, p. 22).

A dry mouth can be aggravated by poor fluid intake, heavy smoking, alcohol use, high salt intake, anxiety, and many medications. Medications that can cause a dryness of the mouth include diuretics; laxatives, if used excessively; all major tranquilizers, e.g., chlorpromazine (Thorazine); some minor tranquilizers, e.g., diazepam (Valium), chlordiazepoxide (Librium); some antidepressants, e.g., amitriptyline (Elavil), imipramine (Tofranil); some antihypertensives, e.g., trimethaphan (Arfonad); some antispasmodics, e.g., propanthaline (Pro-Banthine); and antihistamines used in cold and cough remedies and in analgesics (Todd 1982, p. 122). Some chemotherapeutic agents used to treat cancer also cause dryness and oral lesions.

gums. In advanced periodontal disease, the teeth are loose, and pus is evident when the gums are pressed.

Other problems nurses may see are **glossitis** (inflammation of the tongue), **stomatitis** (inflammation of the oral mucosa), and **parotitis** (inflammation of the parotid salivary gland). The accumulation of foul matter (food, microorganisms, and epithelial elements) on the teeth and gums is referred to as **sordes**. See also Table 22–8 for common problems of the mouth.

Identifying Clients at Risk   Certain clients are prone to oral problems often because of lack of knowledge

Diagnosing

Nursing diagnoses related to problems with oral hygiene and the oral cavity may include **Self-care deficit, Impaired tissue integrity, Potential for infection, Altered**

TABLE 22–8   *Common Problems of the Mouth*

Problem	Description	Nursing Implications
Halitosis	Bad breath	Teach or provide regular oral hygiene.
Glossitis	Inflammation of the tongue	As above
Gingivitis	Inflammation of the gums	As above
Periodontal disease	Gums appear spongy and bleeding	As above
Reddened or excoriated mucosa		Check for ill-fitting dentures.
Excessive dryness of the buccal mucosa		Increase fluid intake as health permits.
Chilosis	Cracking of lips	Lubricate lips, use antimicrobial ointment to prevent infection.
Dental caries	Teeth have darkened areas, may be painful	Advise client to see a physician and/or dentist.

nutrition: Less than body requirements and **Knowledge deficit**. Examples of these diagnoses and possible contributing factors are shown below. Examples of assessment data clusters and related nursing diagnoses are shown in Table 22–9.

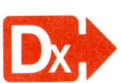

Nursing Diagnoses
Clients with Oral Hygiene and Mouth Problems

Self-care deficit (oral hygiene) related to:

- Lack of upper limb dexterity associated with neuromuscular impairment
- Cognitive inability associated with trauma
- Low value placed on regular oral care and dental visits

Altered oral mucous membrane related to:

- Ineffective oral hygiene
- Dehydration

Impaired tissue integrity related to:

- Radiation therapy involving oral cavity
- Medication
- Ill-fitting dentures

Potential for infection related to:

- Ineffective oral hygiene practices
- Impaired oral mucosa

Altered nutrition: Less than body requirements related to:

- Painful oral lesions
- Ill-fitting dentures

Knowledge deficit (correct oral hygiene practices) related to lack of exposure to information on correct oral hygiene

Planning

The nurse and the client establish relevant goals and outcome criteria and identify interventions that will assist the client to achieve the goals. Nursing interventions may include assisting dependent clients to clean their teeth and oral cavity, teaching the client about good oral hygienic practices and other measures to prevent tooth decay (e.g., use of fluoride, adequate nutrition, and regular visits to a dentist). Examples of outcome criteria to evaluate the degree of goal achievement are outlined below.

TABLE 22–9 *Examples of Assessment Data Clusters and Related Nursing Diagnoses for Clients with Oral Cavity Problems*

Data Cluster	Nursing Diagnosis
Mary Brown, 77 years old, suffered a cerebrovascular accident. Is unconscious and breathing through the mouth via O_2 face mask. 2500 ml intravenous fluid ordered daily.	**Self care deficit: Oral hygiene** related to cognitive inability (unconsciousness)
Joe Kwan, 46 years old, was admitted with a fractured femur. Teeth stained from heavy smoking. One large cavity evident in 2nd lower left molar, tartar buildup along gum margins, and pronounced halitosis. Gums are reddened in some areas and bleed when flossed. States, "I can't remember when I last saw a dentist."	**Impaired tissue integrity** related to ineffective oral hygiene

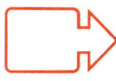

Outcome Criteria
Clients with Oral Hygiene and Mouth Problems

The client:

- Has an intact, smooth, well-hydrated oral mucosa of uniform color.
- Has no inflammation of the oral mucosa.
- Has firm, well-hydrated, nonbleeding gums of uniform color.
- Has a well-hydrated tongue without inflammation.
- Has smooth and well-hydrated lips.
- Experiences no oral discomfort.
- Has teeth free of food particles and plaque.
- Demonstrates appropriate brushing and flossing techniques.
- Describes interventions that prevent tooth decay and dental plaque.
- Expresses positive feelings about sense of well-being and appearance.

CLIENT TEACHING
Measures to Prevent Tooth Decay

- Brush the teeth thoroughly after meals and at bedtime. Assist children or inspect their mouths to be sure the teeth are clean. If the teeth cannot be brushed after eating, vigorous rinsing of the mouth with water is recommended.

- Floss the teeth daily.

- Ensure an adequate intake of nutrients, particularly calcium, phosphorus, vitamins A, C, and D, and fluoride.

- Avoid sweet foods and drinks between meals. Take them in moderation at meals.

- Eat coarse, fibrous foods (cleansing foods), such as fresh fruits and raw vegetables.

- Take a fluoride supplement daily until age 14 or 16, unless the drinking water is fluoridated.

- Have topical fluoride applications as prescribed by the dentist.

- Have a checkup by a dentist every 6 months.

- A child's first visit to the dentist should occur at about age 2½ or 3, so that the child learns not to fear such visits.

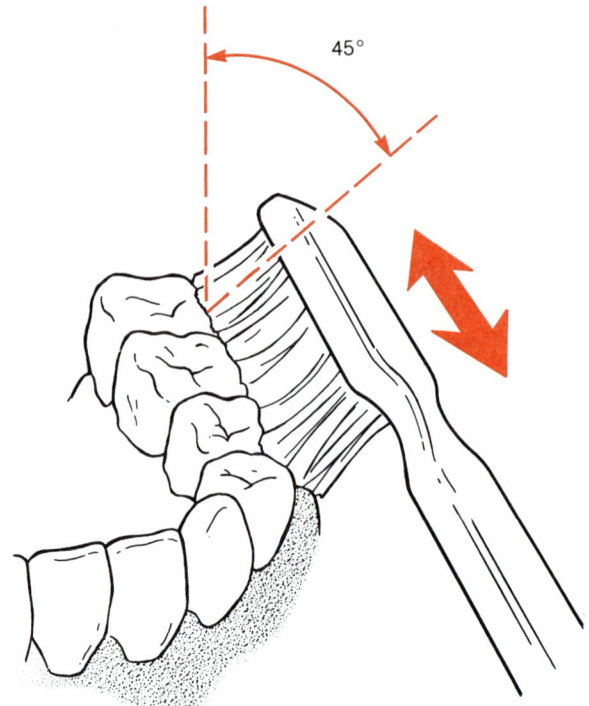

Figure 22–12 In using the sulcular technique, place the bristles at a 45° angle against the teeth.

Implementing

Good oral hygiene includes daily stimulation of the gums, mechanical scrubbing of the teeth, flushing of the mouth, and regular checkups by a dentist. The nurse is often in a position to help people to maintain oral hygiene by helping or teaching them to clean the teeth and oral cavity, by inspecting whether clients (especially children) have done so, or by actually providing mouth care to clients who are ill or incapacitated. The nurse can also be instrumental in identifying and referring problems that require the intervention of a dentist or oral surgeon. Specific measures to prevent tooth decay and periodontal disease are shown in the box above.

Brushing and Flossing the Teeth Thorough brushing of the teeth is important in preventing tooth decay. The mechanical action of brushing removes food particles that can harbor and incubate bacteria. It also stimulates circulation in the gums, thus maintaining their healthy firmness. The brushing of teeth needs to be demonstrated to children by age 2, when their teeth appear. Until the child can manipulate the toothbrush effectively, however, parents need to help the child to do this. The technique most recently recommended for brushing teeth is called the **sulcular technique**, which removes plaque and cleans under

the gingival margins. Many toothpastes are marketed, any of which can be used. However, an effective dentifrice can be made by combining two parts of table salt to one part of baking soda.

When providing mouth care for the client, the nurse should wear gloves to guard against infectious diseases such as AIDS. Other required equipment includes a curved basin that fits snugly under the client's chin (e.g., a kidney basin) to receive the rinse water and a towel to protect the client and the bedclothes.

The *sulcular technique* is taught to or performed for the client as follows:

1. Moisten the bristles of a *soft* toothbrush with tepid water, and apply the dentifrice.

2. Hold the brush against the teeth with the bristles at a 45° angle. See Figure 22–12. The tips of the outer bristles should rest against and penetrate under the gingival sulcus. See Figure 22–13. The brush will clean under the sulcus of two or three teeth at one time.

3. Move the bristles back and forth using a vibrating or jiggling motion, from the sulcus to the crowns of the teeth.

4. Repeat until all outer and inner surfaces of the teeth and sulci of the gums are cleaned.

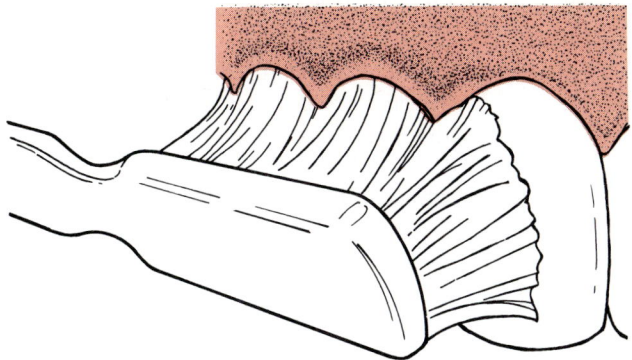

Figure 22–13 Direct the tips of the outer bristles under the gingival margins.

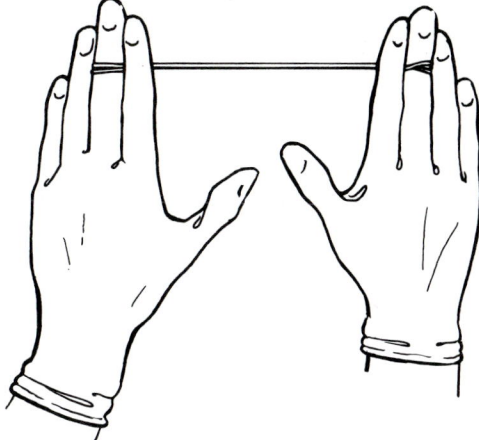

Figure 22–14 Securing dental floss around the third fingers.

5. Clean the biting surfaces by moving the brush back and forth over them in short strokes.

6. After the teeth are brushed, rinse the mouth with water to remove dislodged food particles and excess dentifrice. Many antiseptic mouthwashes are marketed, and some people prefer these for rinsing.

Flossing of the teeth is especially beneficial in preventing the formation of plaque and removing it from the teeth, particularly at the gum line. A method for flossing follows:

1. Wrap one end of floss around the third finger of each hand. See Figure 22–14.

2. To floss the upper teeth, use your thumb and index finger to stretch the floss. See Figure 22–15. Move the floss up and down between the teeth from the tops of the crowns to the gum and along the gum lines as far as possible. Make a figure "C" with the floss around the tooth edge being flossed. Start at the back on the right side and work around to the back of the left side, or work from the center teeth to the back of the jaw on either side.

3. To floss the lower teeth, use your index fingers to stretch the floss. See Figure 22–16.

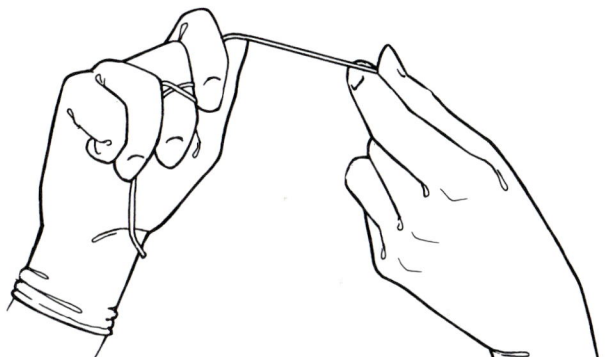

Figure 22–15 To floss the upper teeth, use the thumbs and index fingers to stretch the floss.

Care of Dentures   Most clients in a hospital can clean their own dentures. However, if the client is incapacitated, elderly, confused, or confined to bed, care of dentures becomes the nurse's responsibility.

To remove upper dentures, the nurse dons gloves, then grasps the dentures at the front with the thumb and index finger, using a piece of tissue or gauze to prevent slippage. They may need to be moved slightly up and down to overcome the suction on the roof of the mouth. Lower dentures are readily removed by retracting the cheek, turning them slightly, and pulling them out between the lips on one side and then the other. Partial plates and removable bridges may also need to be taken out by the nurse. These are

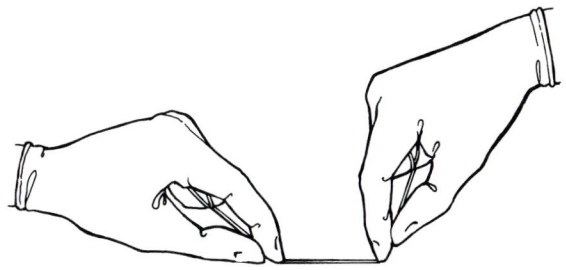

Figure 22–16 To floss the lower teeth, use the index fingers to stretch the floss.

removed by exerting equal pressure on the border of each side of the denture, not on the clasps, which can bend or break.

Dentures must be handled carefully, since they can break if dropped or knocked against metal water taps. When handling dentures, the nurse always transports them in the client's denture container and before cleaning them places a washcloth in the bowl of the sink. A washcloth prevents damage to the dentures if the nurse drops them.

Dentures are cleaned with a toothbrush or special stiff-bristled brush, a dentifrice, and tepid water. Hot water is not used because heat can change the shape of some dentures. The dentures are rinsed well and replaced in the client's mouth.

If the dentures are stained, the nurse soaks them in a commercial cleaner, following the manufacturer's directions. To prevent corrosion, dentures with metal parts should not be soaked overnight. Home substitutes for commercial cleaner are the following mixtures:

1. 5 to 10 ml (1 to 2 tsp) white vinegar and 240 ml (1 cup) warm water *or*

2. 5 ml (1 tsp) chlorine bleach, 10 ml (2 tsp) water softener, and 240 ml (1 cup) warm water. It is essential to mix water softener with the bleach to prevent denture corrosion and to rinse well before replacing in the mouth.

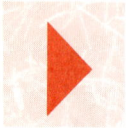
Before reinserting the dentures, the nurse observes the dentures for any rough, sharp, or worn areas that could irritate the tongue or mucous membranes of the mouth, lips, and gums and inspects the client's mouth for any redness, irritated areas, or indications of infection. The nurse offers some mouthwash and a curved basin to rinse the mouth. If the client cannot insert the dentures independently, the nurse inserts the plates one at a time. Hold each plate at a slight angle while inserting it, to avoid injuring the lips.

Dentures that are not reinserted because the client either does not want to or cannot wear them are stored in a denture container with water. The container should be labeled with the client's name and identification number.

Special Mouth Care   It may be necessary to clean a client's oral mucosa and tongue, in addition to cleaning the teeth, if the person is unconscious or has excessive dryness, sores, or irritations of the mouth. Agency practices differ in regard to special mouth care and the frequency with which it is provided. Depending on the health of the client's mouth, special care may be needed every two to eight hours.

Mouth care for unconscious people is very important, since their mouths tend to become dry and consequently predisposed to infections. Dryness occurs because the client cannot take fluids by mouth, is often breathing through the mouth, or may be receiving oxygen, which tends to dry the mucous membranes.

The nurse can use commercially prepared applicators of lemon juice and oil to clean the mucous membranes. If these are unavailable, a gauze square rolled around the index finger and dipped into lemon juice and oil or into mouthwash solution usually suffices. Applicator swabs or tongue blades covered with gauze may also be used. Mineral oil is generally contraindicated, because aspiration of it can initiate an infection (lipid pneumonia). Hydrogen peroxide can be used prior to the lemon juice and oil, if necessary. This agent, which should be diluted 1:1 with water, is effective in removing encrustations that coat the tongue.

Procedure 22–5 focuses on oral care for the unconscious person but may be adapted for conscious persons who are seriously ill or have mouth problems.

PROCEDURE 22–5

PROVIDING SPECIAL ORAL CARE

Equipment ☑

Dentifrice or denture cleaner

Toothbrush

Cup of tepid water

Curved basin

Towel

Mouthwash

Denture container as needed

Tissue or piece of gauze to remove dentures (optional)

Applicators and cleaning solution for cleaning the mucous membranes

Rubber-tipped bulb syringe

Petroleum jelly (Vaseline) or cold cream

Cleaning agent such as hydrogen peroxide for use prior to the lemon juice and oil, if necessary.

Bite-block to hold the mouth open and teeth apart (optional).

Gloves to protect the nurse

Intervention

1. Prepare the client.

- Position the unconscious client on the side with the head of the bed lowered, so that the saliva automatically runs out by gravity rather than being aspirated into the lungs. This position is the one of choice for the unconscious client receiving mouth care. If the client's head cannot be lowered, turn it to one side so that fluid will readily run out of the mouth or pool in the side of the mouth where it can be suctioned.
- Place the towel under the client's chin.
- Place the curved basin against the client's chin and lower cheek to receive the fluid from the mouth. See Figure 22−17.
- 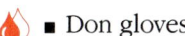 Don gloves.

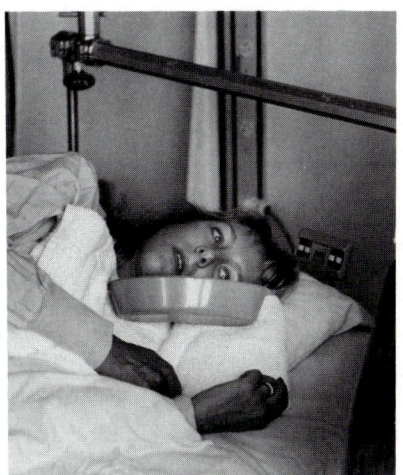

Figure 22−17 Position of client and placement of kidney basin when providing special mouth care.

2. Clean the teeth, and rinse the mouth.

- If the person has natural teeth, brush the teeth as described earlier. Brush gently and carefully to avoid injuring the gums. If the client has artificial teeth, clean them as described earlier.
- Rinse the client's mouth by drawing about 10 ml (3 oz) of water or mouthwash into the syringe and injecting it gently into each side of the mouth. *If the solution is injected with force, some of it may flow down the client's throat and be aspirated into the lungs.*
- Watch carefully to make sure that all the rinsing solution has run out of the mouth into the basin. If not, suction the fluid from the mouth. See the section on oropharyngeal suctioning in Chapter 41. *Fluid remaining in the mouth may be aspirated into the lungs.*
- Repeat the rinsing until the mouth is free of dentifrice, if used.

3. Inspect and clean the oral tissues.

- If the tissues appear dry or unclean, clean them with the applicators or gauze and cleaning solution. If hydrogen peroxide is used, rinse the mouth thoroughly before applying oil and lemon juice. *Oil and lemon juice are recommended for short term use. The gums and mucosa can become spongy from prolonged action of hydrogen peroxide.*
- Picking up one oil applicator, wipe the mucous membrane of one cheek. In the absence of commercially prepared applicators, wrap a small gauze square around your gloved finger, and moisten it with oil and lemon solution. Discard the applicator or gauze in a waste container, and with a fresh one clean the next area. *Using separate applicators for each area of the mouth prevents the transfer of microorganisms from one area to another.*
- Clean all the mouth tissues in an orderly progression using separate applicators: the cheeks, roof of the mouth, base of the mouth, and tongue.
- Observe the tissues closely for inflammation and dryness.
- Rinse the client's mouth as above.
- Remove gloves, and discard.

4. Ensure client comfort.

- Remove the basin, and dry around the client's mouth with the towel. Replace artificial dentures if indicated.
- Lubricate the client's lips with petroleum jelly or cold cream. *Lubrication prevents cracking and subsequent infection.*

5. Document pertinent data.

- Record special oral hygiene and pertinent observations
- Report problems to the nurse in charge.

Sample Recording

Date 4/7/91	Time: 1500

Special mouth care using oil and lemon q1h. Outer aspect of lower right gum remains reddened and swollen. _____
_____ Sally R. Nolan, SN

Evaluating

To evaluate the achievement of client goals, the nurse inspects the client's teeth and oral cavity, asks about any discomfort, listens to the client's expressions of feelings, and asks the client to describe specific information as instructed and/or to demonstrate specific skills. Examples of evaluative statements indicating goal achievement are "The client's oral mucous membrane was intact, smooth, and uniform in color," or "The client described five ways to prevent tooth decay."

HAIR

The appearance of the hair often reflects a person's feelings of well-being. A person who feels ill may not groom hair as before. The hair may also reflect state of health, e.g., endocrine changes can affect the pattern of hair growth, and color changes may reflect aging. In addition, hair texture can also reflect health status, e.g., excessive coarseness and dryness may be associated with endocrine disorders such as hypothyroidism.

In elderly people, the hair is generally thinner, grows more slowly, and loses its color as a result of aging tissues and diminishing circulation. Men often lose their scalp hair and may become completely bald. Even relatively young men may be bald. The older person's hair also tends to be drier than normal. With age, axillary and pubic hair becomes finer and scanter, in contrast to the eyebrows, which become bristly and coarse. Most women develop hair on their faces, which some view as a problem.

Each person has particular ways of caring for hair, influenced by a number of factors. Some shampoo it daily; others shampoo once a week or even less often. Black-skinned people often need to oil their hair daily because it tends to be dry. Oil prevents the hair from breaking and the scalp from drying. A wide-toothed comb is usually used, because finer combs pull and break the hair. Some people brush their hair vigorously before retiring, others comb their hair frequently.

Assessing

Nursing History   During the nursing history, the nurse elicits data about usual hair care, self-care abilities, history of hair or scalp problems, and conditions known to affect the hair. Chemotherapeutic agents and radiation of the head may cause **alopecia** (hair loss). Hypothyroidism may cause the hair to be thin, dry, and/or brittle. Use of some hair dyes and curling or straightening preparations can cause the hair to become dry and brittle. Questions to elicit these data are shown in the accompanying box.

Physical Assessment   Physical assessment of the hair is discussed in Chapter 19, page 372. Problems include dandruff, hair loss, ticks, pediculosis, and hirsutism.

Dandruff   Dandruff appears as a diffuse scaling of the scalp often accompanied by itching. In severe cases it involves the auditory canals and the eyebrows. Mild cases of dandruff can usually be treated effectively with a commercial shampoo specifically recommended for dandruff. In severe or persistent cases, the client may need the advice of a physician.

Hair loss   Hair loss and growth are continual processes. Some permanent thinning of hair normally occurs with aging. Baldness, common in men, is thought to be a hereditary problem for which there is no known remedy other than the wearing of a hairpiece or a costly surgical hair transplant, in which hair is taken from the back or the sides of the scalp and surgically moved to the hairless area. Although some external medications are being developed, their long-term outcomes are unknown.

Ticks   Ticks are small parasites that bite into tissue and suck blood. They take many forms and can adapt themselves to various conditions. The genera *Ornithodoros* and *Dermacentor* are found in North America. They can attach to human beings and are found frequently in the hair. They can be as large as 1.3 cm (0.5 in) and appear gray-brown. They attach to a person with the apparatus by which they suck blood and should not be torn off, because the sucking apparatus may be left in the skin and become infected. Pouring oil on the tick causes it to lose its hold, because it is deprived of oxygen, and it withdraws its sucker.

Ticks transmit several diseases to people, in particular, Rocky Mountain spotted fever and tularemia.

Pediculosis (lice)   Lice are parasitic insects that infest mammals. Infestation with lice is called **pediculosis**. Hundreds of varieties of lice infest humans. Three common kinds are *Pediculus capitis* (the head louse), *Pediculus corporis* (the body louse), and *Pediculus pubis* (the crab louse).

Pediculus capitis is found on the scalp and tends to stay hidden in the hairs; similarly, *Pediculus pubis* stays in pubic hair. *Pediculus corporis* tends to cling to clothing, so that, when a client undresses, the lice may not be in evidence on the body; these lice suck blood from the person and lay their eggs on the clothing. The nurse can suspect their presence in the clothing if (a) the person habitually scratches, (b) there are scratches on the skin, and (c) there are hemorrhagic spots on the skin where the lice have sucked blood.

Head and pubic lice lay their eggs on the hairs; the eggs look like oval particles, similar to dandruff, clinging to the hair. Bites and pustular eruptions may also be noticed at the hair lines and behind the ears.

Lice are very small, grayish white, and difficult to see.

The crab louse in the pubic area has red legs. Lice may be contracted from infested clothes and direct contact with an infested person.

The treatment now used in most areas is gamma benzene hexachloride (Kwell), available as a cream, a lotion, and a shampoo. If the client has head lice, the hair is washed with the shampoo and the bed linens are changed. This treatment is repeated 12 to 24 hours later if needed. A client with pubic or body lice takes a bath or shower, dries, and applies the lotion or cream—to the entire body surface for body lice, and to the pubic area and adjacent areas for pubic lice. After 12 to 24 hours, the lotion is washed off, and clean clothing and linens are supplied.

Hirsutism **Hirsutism** is the growth of excessive body hair. The acceptance of body hair in the axillae and on the legs is largely dictated by culture. In North America, the well-groomed woman, as depicted in magazines, has no hair on her legs or under her axillae (although this idea is changing). In many European cultures, it is not customary for well-groomed women to remove this hair.

Excessive facial hair on a woman is thought unattractive in most Western and Oriental cultures. For example, some Japanese brides follow the custom of shaving their faces the day before the wedding.

The cause of excessive body hair is not always known. Elderly women may have some on their faces, and women during menopause may also experience the growth of facial hair. These conditions may be due to the action of the endocrine system. It is also thought heredity influences both the pattern of hair distribution and the production of androgens by the adrenal glands.

There are a number of ways of removing hair: waxing, pulling with tweezers, shaving with a razor, applying depilatory lotions, and electrolysis. In the waxing process, warm wax is poured on the area and allowed to harden. The hairs become embedded in the wax and come away from the skin when the wax is removed. Tweezers are commonly used to remove excess hair from the eyebrows and the face. This can be a time-consuming project if there is a great deal of hair, and it needs to be repeated when the hair grows back, often in 2 to 3 weeks. Shaving with a razor is done frequently for leg and axilla hair. It is an inexpensive and effective method, but it must be repeated frequently. Depilatory creams and lotions destroy the hair shaft through a chemical action, so that the hair wipes away easily. This method of hair removal is expensive compared to shaving. In the initial use of a product, it is important to assess the amount of skin irritation it causes. It is advisable to put lotion on a small area initially and observe for signs of irritation. Electrolysis is the only permanent way of removing hair. The hair follicle is destroyed by means of an electric current. Usually, repeated treatments are needed before a follicle is completely destroyed. This method of treatment is relatively expensive.

ASSESSMENT INTERVIEW
Hair Care

Hair Care Practices

■ What are your usual hair care practices?

■ What hair care products do you routinely use (e.g., hair spray, lubricant, shampoo, conditioners, hair dye, curling or straightening preparations)?

Self-Care Abilities

■ Do you have any problems managing your hair?

Past or Current Hair Problems

■ Have you had any of the following conditions or therapies: recent chemotherapy, hypothyroidism, radiation of the head, unexplained loss of hair, growth of excessive body hair?

Diagnosing

Nursing diagnoses related to hair hygiene and hair and scalp problems include **Self-care deficit** (grooming), **Impaired skin integrity, Potential for infection,** and **Body image disturbance**. Examples of these nursing diagnoses with contributing factors are shown below.

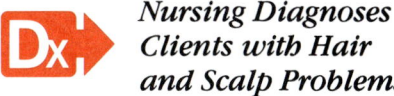

Nursing Diagnoses
Clients with Hair
and Scalp Problems

Self-care deficit (grooming) related to:

■ Activity intolerance

■ Imposed immobility (bed rest)

■ Pain in upper extremities

■ Altered level of consciousness

■ Lack of motivation associated with depression

Impaired skin integrity related to:

■ Scalp laceration

■ Insect bite

Potential for infection related to:

■ Scalp laceration

■ Insect bites

Body image disturbance related to alopecia

Planning

Nursing interventions are identified that will assist the client to achieve the overall goals of maintaining or improving hair texture, growth, and cleanliness; maintaining or improving a sense of well-being; and preventing specific hair and scalp problems. Plans for assisting the client include consideration of personal preferences, health, and energy resources and the time, equipment, and personnel available. Often, clients like to receive hair care after a bath, before receiving visitors, and/or before retiring. At some agencies, shampoos can be given to clients only after a physician's order. Examples of outcome criteria to evaluate the achievement of goals and the effectiveness of nursing interventions are shown below.

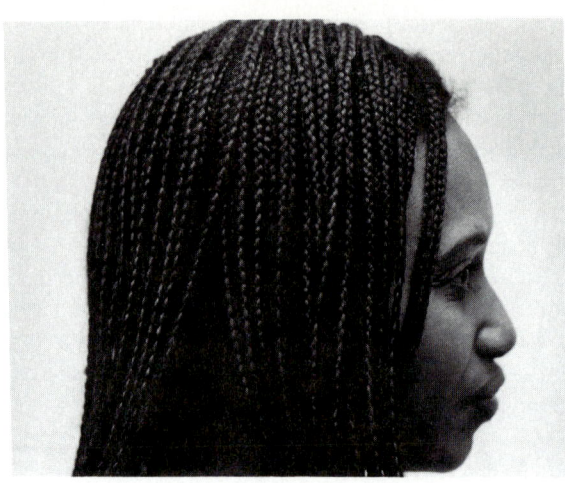

Figure 22–18   A black person's hair styled with cornrow braids.

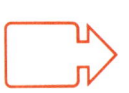

Outcome Criteria
Clients with Hair
and Scalp Problems

The client:

■ Has resilient hair with a healthy sheen.

■ Has reduced or absent scalp lesions or infestations.

■ Describes contributing factors and interventions for dandruff (or other hair problem).

■ Expresses positive statements about sense of well-being.

Implementing

Brushing and Combing Hair   To be healthy, hair needs to be brushed daily. Brushing has three major functions: It stimulates the circulation of blood in the scalp, it distributes the oil along the hair shaft, and it helps to arrange the hair, although many people use a comb for that purpose.

Long hair may present a problem for hospitalized clients. To prevent hair from matting, the client or nurse needs to comb it at least daily. Some clients are pleased to have it tied neatly in the back or braided until other assistance is available or until they feel better and can look after it. Others may consider such styles unattractive or juvenile. The nurse should work with the client to find an acceptable style.

Dark-skinned people often have thicker, drier, curlier hair than light-skinned people. Spiraled or very curly hair may stand out from the scalp. Although the shafts of spiraled hair look strong and wiry, they have less strength than straight hair shafts and are easily broken.

Some black clients have their spiraled hair straightened. Even if straightened, the hair tends to tangle and mat easily, especially at the back and the sides if the client is confined to bed. Other blacks style their hair in cornrows. See Figure

22–18. These cornrows do not have to be unbraided before shampooing and washing. The nurse should obtain the client's permission before any such unbraiding.

To comb black hairstyles, apply a lubricant as the client indicates or as needed. Then, using a large opentoothed comb, start at the neckline and lift and fluff the hair outward, moving upward toward the forehead. Continue to fluff the hair outward and upward until all of the hair is combed on one half of the head. Then repeat for the other half of the head. To remove tangles:

1. After the hair is lubricated, weave and lift your open fingers through the hair to ease the tangles free.

   or

2. Support the hair securely at the base of the scalp, if possible, to prevent pulling and discomfort. Insert a long-toothed comb into the ends of the hair and carefully comb out the ends of the tangles. See Figure 22–19. Repeat this step, each time working the comb farther up the hair shaft toward the scalp, until the hair is untangled.

Shampooing Hair   When a client is hospitalized for extended periods or the hair becomes soiled, the nurse needs to help shampoo the client's hair. There are several ways to shampoo clients' hair, depending on their health, strength, and age. The client who is well enough to take a shower can shampoo while in the shower. The client who is unable to shower may be given a shampoo while sitting on a chair in front of a sink. The back-lying client who can move to a stretcher can be given a shampoo on a stretcher wheeled to a sink. The client who must remain in bed can be given a shampoo with water brought to the bedside. This method is the least convenient, but it allows the person who is confined to bed to receive a shampoo. Some hospitals

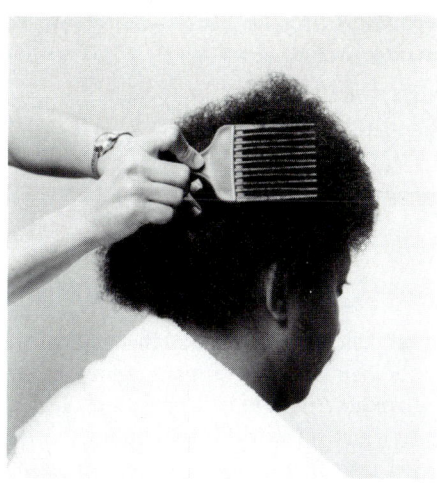

Figure 22–19 Removing tangles with a long-toothed comb.

have volunteer beauticians with portable shampoo chairs who assist with hair care.

How often a person needs a shampoo is highly individual, depending to a large degree on the person's activities and the amount of sebum secreted by the scalp. Oily hair tends to look stringy and dirty, and it feels unclean to the person.

A nurse who assists a client with a shampoo should wet the hair with warm water, apply the shampoo, and make a good lather while massaging the scalp with the pads of the fingertips. Massaging stimulates the blood circulation in the scalp. The pads of the fingers are used so as not to scratch the scalp with the fingernails. The nurse then rinses the hair thoroughly, making sure no shampoo remains in the hair to dry and irritate the scalp. The hair is then combed to prevent tangles and dried thoroughly, often with a hair drier.

Beard and Mustache Care   Beards and mustaches also require daily care. The most important aspect of the care is to keep them clean. Food particles tend to collect in beards and mustaches, and they need washing and combing periodically. Clients may also wish a beard or mustache trim to maintain a well-groomed appearance. A beard or mustache should not be shaved off without the client's consent.

Male clients often shave or are shaved after a bath. Frequently clients supply their own electric or safety razors. When using a safety razor to shave a client's beard, apply shaving cream or shaving soap and water first to soften the bristles and make the skin more pliable. Hold the razor so that the blade is at a 45° angle to the skin and shave in short, firm strokes in the direction of hair growth. Hold the skin taut, particularly around creases, to prevent cutting the skin. After shaving the entire area, wipe the client's face with a wet washcloth to remove any remaining shaving cream and

hair. Dry the face well, then apply after-shave lotion or powder as the client prefers. To prevent irritating the skin, pat on the lotion with the fingers and avoid rubbing the face.

Evaluating

To evaluate the achievement of client goals, the nurse inspects the client's hair and scalp, listens to expressions of feelings, and asks the client to state specific interventions as taught. Examples of evaluative statements indicating goal achievement are "The client's scalp is free of lesions," or "The client stated, 'I feel so much better after that shampoo.'"

EYES

Normally, eyes require no special hygiene, since lacrimal fluid continually washes the eyes, and the eyelids and lashes prevent the entrance of foreign particles. Special interventions are needed, however, for unconscious clients and for clients recovering from eye surgery or having eye injuries, irritations, or infections. In unconscious clients, the blink reflex may be absent, and excessive drainage may accumulate along eyelid margins. In clients with eye trauma or eye infections, excessive discharge or drainage is common. Excessive secretions on the lashes need to be removed before they dry on the lashes as crusts. Clients who wear eyeglasses, contact lenses, or an artificial eye also may require instruction from and care by the nurse.

Assessing

Nursing History   During the nursing history, the nurse obtains data about the client's eyeglasses or contact lenses, recent examination by an ophthalmologist, and any history of eye problems and related treatments. Questions to elicit these data are shown in the box on page 540.

Physical Assessment   In physical assessment, all external eye structures are inspected for signs of inflammation, excessive drainage, encrustations, or other obvious abnormalities. Inspection of the external eye structures is discussed in Chapter 19.

Diagnosing

Nursing diagnoses related to eye problems may include **Potential for infection, Self-care deficit,** and **Potential for injury**. Examples of these diagnoses and possible contributing factors are shown below.

For Clients Who Wear Eyeglasses

■ When were the glasses/lenses prescribed?

■ What is your vision like with and without the corrective device?

For Clients Who Wear Contact Lenses

■ How often do you wear lenses? Daily? On special occasions?

■ How long do you wear your lenses in a given day, including sleep time?

■ Do you have any problems with the lenses, e.g., cleaning, insertion, removal, damage?

■ Do you carry an emergency identification label to alert others to remove the lenses and ensure appropriate care in an emergency? (If not, advise the client to acquire one.)

■ What are your insertion and removal procedures?

■ What are your cleaning and storage procedures?

■ Have you had any problems with either or both eyes or eyelids, such as excessive tearing, burning, redness, sensitivity to light, swelling, or feelings of dryness? Describe them.

■ Are you using any eyedrops or ointments? (These medications can combine chemically with *soft* lenses and cause lens damage and eye irritation.)

For All Clients

■ When did you last visit an ophthalmologist?

■ Are you currently taking any eye medication? If so, provide name, dosage, and frequency.

■ Do you have any of the following eye problems: difficulty reading or seeing objects, blurring of vision, tearing, spots or floaters, photophobia (sensitivity to light), burning, itching, pain, double vision, flashing lights, or halos around lights?

Dx ▶ *Nursing Diagnoses*
Clients with Eye Problems

Potential for infection related to:

■ Improper contact lens hygiene

■ Accumulation of secretions on eyelids

Potential for injury related to:

■ Prolonged wearing of contact lenses

■ Absence of blink reflex associated with unconsciousness

Self-care deficit (contact lens insertion, removal, and cleaning) related to:

■ Knowledge deficit

■ Impaired vision associated with cataracts

Planning

Nursing interventions are identified that will assist the client to achieve the overall goals of maintaining the integrity of the cornea, conjunctiva and/or a prosthesis and of preventing eye injury and infection from contact lenses. Nursing interventions may include teaching clients about proper insertion, cleaning, and removal of contact lenses or a prosthesis and ways to protect the eyes from injury and strain. Examples of outcome criteria to evaluate the achievement of client goals and the effectiveness of nursing interventions are shown below.

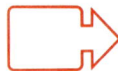

Outcome Criteria
Clients with Eye Problems

The client:

■ Has clear conjunctiva and white sclera without inflammation.

■ Has reduced secretions on eyelids.

■ Experiences no tearing.

■ Experiences no eye discomfort.

■ Demonstrates appropriate methods of caring for contact lenses.

■ Describes interventions to prevent eye injury and infection.

Implementing

Eye Care   *Dried secretions* that have accumulated on the lashes, need to be softened and wiped away. Hospital nurses soften dried secretions by placing a sterile cotton ball moistened with sterile water or normal saline over the lid margins. The nurse then wipes the loosened secretions from the inner canthus of the eye to the outer canthus to prevent the particles and fluid from draining into the lacrimal sac and nasolacrimal duct.

If the client is *unconscious* and lacks a blink reflex or cannot close the eyelids completely, drying and irritation of the cornea must be prevented. Lubricating eye drops may be administered if ordered by the physician. An eye patch may also be placed over the affected eye or eyes.

Eyeglass Care

Caution is essential when cleaning eyeglasses to prevent breaking or scratching the lenses. Glass lenses can be cleaned with warm water and dried with a soft tissue that will not scratch the lenses. Plastic lenses are easily scratched and require special cleaning solutions and drying tissues. When not being worn, all glasses should be placed in a case labeled appropriately, and stored in the client's bedside table drawer.

Contact Lens Care

Contact lenses, thin curved discs of hard or soft plastic, fit on the cornea of the eye directly over the pupil. They float on the tear layer of the eye. For some people, there are several advantages of contact lenses over eyeglasses: (a) they cannot be seen and thus have cosmetic value; (b) they are highly effective in correcting some astigmatisms; (c) they are safer than glasses for some physical activities; (d) they do not fog, as eyeglasses do; and (e) they provide better vision in many cases.

Contact lenses may be either hard or soft or a compromise between the two—gas-permeable lenses. *Hard contact lenses,* introduced in the 1940s, cover part of the cornea and can endure up to 20 years of use. They are made of a rigid, unwettable, airtight plastic that does not absorb water or saline solutions. The portion of the eye beneath the hard lens is lubricated and oxygenated by tears. Disadvantages are that they restrict oxygen supply to the cornea, usually cannot be worn for more than 12 to 14 hours, and are rarely recommended for first-time wearers.

Soft contact lenses, introduced in the early 1970s, cover the entire cornea. Being more pliable and soft, they mold to the eye for a firmer fit. They are composed of polymers that absorb water, allow through-the-lens oxygen transmission, and are easier on the eyes. There are many varieties: bifocal, toric (for high astigmatism), tinted (to enhance eye color), and extended-wear. The duration of extended-wear varies by brand from 1 to 30 days or more. Eye specialists recommend that long-wear brands be removed and cleaned at least once a week. Extended-wear soft lenses that are ultrathin are comfortable but very flimsy and difficult to keep clean. Disadvantages of soft lenses are that they do not provide vision as crisp as the hard lenses, are more prone to bacterial buildup, are easily ripped, and need to be replaced every year or so. They require scrupulous care and handling.

Gas-permeable lenses, introduced in the late 1970s, are rigid enough to provide clear vision but are more flexible than the traditional hard lens. They permit oxygen to reach the cornea, thus providing greater comfort, and will not cause serious damage to the eye if left in place for several days.

Most clients normally care for their own contact lenses. There are a number of ways to place contact lenses on the eyes and to remove them. Clients learn the method that best suits them from their eye specialists. In certain cases or emergencies, the nurse may need to remove a client's lenses. A hard contact lens wearer who is unconscious and unable to blink can develop corneal abrasions from lack of tears for lubrication. Clients with impaired judgment, e.g., due to substance abuse, are prone to eye damage from prolonged lens wearing. Proper handling of the lenses by the nurse is essential.

Contact lenses are cleaned relatively easily with chemical lens-cleaning solutions. Soft lenses can also be cleaned by electric heat disinfecting units. Each manufacturer provides detailed cleaning instructions. In general, lens cleaner is spread on both sides of the lens with the thumb and index finger or an absorbent applicator, or the lens is placed in the palm of the hand and the solution spread with the index finger. Cleaners remove surface deposits, such as dirt and cosmetics, which reduce the comfort and clarity of the lens. The lens is then rinsed, since cleaners are irritating to the eyes. Depending on the type of lens and cleaning method used, warm tap water, normal saline, or special rinsing or soaking solutions may be used.

When cleaned, the lenses are placed in their storage container. Disinfecting solutions, conditioning solutions, or no solution is added, according to the type of lens and the cleaning method used. Hard lenses and gas-permeable lenses can be stored dry. Soft lenses must be stored in a sterile normal saline solution to keep them hydrated. Unsterile solutions promote bacterial growth, and the minerals in tap water can damage a soft lens.

Soft daily wear contact lenses also require weekly removal of protein deposits that accumulate from tears. If left unchecked, these deposits reduce the clarity of the lens and may cause damage that reduces the life of the lens. Enzyme protein remover tablets are used.

Guidelines for teaching contact lens users cleaning and storage practices are shown in the box on pgae 542.

It is important for nurses to check the cleaning practices of clients who wear contact lenses, since many clients have difficulty in complying with recommended cleaning practices or are unable to perform the cleaning procedure themselves. Many elderly clients, for example, with impaired vision and/or manual dexterity wear extended-wear lenses. These clients usually schedule appointments with their eye care practitioners on a monthly basis, at which time their lenses are removed, cleaned, and reinserted for them. When these clients are hospitalized, the nurse needs to assume this responsibility. Hospital nursing units should provide cleaning and storage kits for this purpose. Check agency procedures.

Inserting Contact Lenses

Seriously ill clients whose contact lenses have been removed will not need them reinserted until they become more active in their care and require the lenses to see properly. Contact lenses need to be lubricated in a sterile, nonirritating wetting solution (usually a saline solution) before they are inserted. The wetting solution helps the lens to glide over the cornea, thus reducing the risk of injury. A few drops of wetting solution is placed on the lens and spread over both surfaces in the same man-

CLIENT TEACHING
Cleaning Contact Lenses

- Before handling your lenses, always wash and rinse your hands.

- Work over a flat surface covered with a soft towel.

- Avoid contaminating the exposed tips of solution containers. Keep solution bottles tightly closed when not in use.

- Use solutions only *before* the expiration date marked on the container.

- Clean lenses one at a time to make sure they are not put in the wrong storage slot or the wrong eye. Always start with the right lens. Getting into the habit of always starting with the right eye reduces the risk of inserting the wrong lens.

- Be sure the sink drain is closed when rinsing the lens over a sink.

- Clean hard and daily wear (dw) soft lenses *daily;* clean extended-wear (ew) lenses *weekly,* using the method demonstrated by your eye care professional.

- Remember that lens care products are *not* interchangeable. Do not switch products without first consulting your eye care practitioner. Never reuse solutions.

- Proper storage of the lens in the lens storage case is essential. Each case has two labeled slots indicating which lens should be stored there. It is essential to store each lens in the appropriate slot, since each lens is ground for a specific eye. *Soft* contact lenses must be kept hydrated and stored in solution (normal saline). They can become dry, brittle, and permanently damaged if left exposed to the air for an hour or less. *Hard* contact lenses and gas-permeable lenses can be stored dry.

- Be sure each lens is centered well in its storage case before tightening or closing the cover to avoid cracks or tears.

- Avoid exposing the lens (soft lenses in particular) and the case to direct sunlight or extreme heat, which can dry or warp them.

- After inserting *soft* lenses, always empty your lens storage case, rinse it, and allow it to air dry.

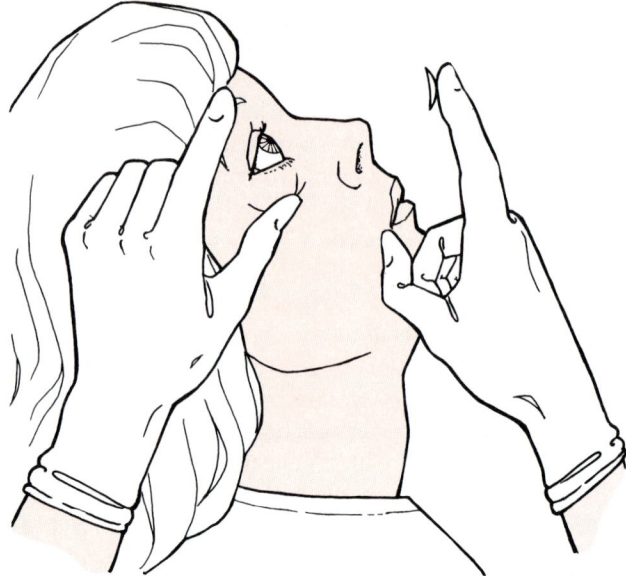

Figure 22–20 Inserting a hard contact lens.

eyelids of the client's eye with the thumb and index finger of your nondominant hand. See Figure 22–20. When separating the eyelids, exert gentle pressure with your fingers over the supraorbital and infraorbital bony prominences. This prevents direct pressure, discomfort, and injury to the eyeball. Place the lens as gently as possible on the cornea directly over the iris and pupil. If the lens is off center, center the lens as follows:

1. Separate the eyelids, using the index or middle finger of the left hand to lift the upper lid and the index or middle finger of the right hand to depress the lower lid.

2. Locate the lens, and ask the client to gaze in the opposite direction.

3. Gently push the lens in the direction of the cornea, using a finger or the eyelid margins.

4. Ask the client to look slowly toward the lens. The lens will slide easily onto the cornea as the client looks toward it.

To insert *soft* lenses, a few variations are necessary. First, the dominant finger must be kept dry for inserting the lens. Because "water-loving" soft contact lenses have a natural attraction to wet surfaces, the lens will adhere more readily to the moist eye if the finger is dry. Second, the lens must be positioned correctly for insertion. To check that the position is correct, hold the lens at the edge between your thumb and index finger, and flex it slightly. The lens is in the correct position if the edges point inward. It is in the wrong position (i.e., inside out) and must be reversed if the edges point outward. See Figure 22–21. A lens placed on the eye inside out is less comfortable, tends to fold on the eye, can drop to a lower position on the eye, and may

ner as the cleaning agent. Some clients use their saliva to wet their lenses. This practice is to be discouraged, since contaminants in saliva can cause bacterial buildup on the lens and infection.

To insert *hard* lenses, ask the client to tilt the head backward, place the lens convex side down on the tip of your dominant index finger, and separate the upper and lower

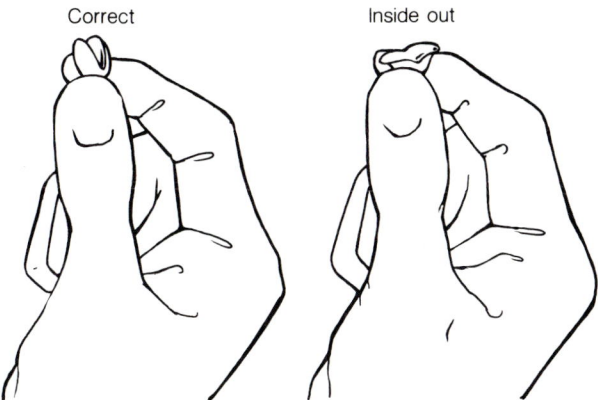

Figure 22–21 Checking the position of a soft contact lens before insertion.

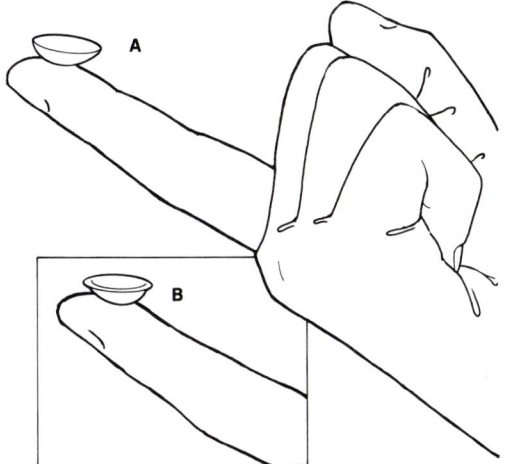

Figure 22–22 Checking the position of an ultrathin contact lens before insertion: *A,* correct position with edges turned upward; *B,* lens is inside out and must be reversed.

move excessively on blinking. If the lens is *ultrathin,* do not flex it; doing so may cause the lens to fold and stick together. Instead, put the lens on your placement finger, and allow it to dry slightly for a few seconds. Closely inspect the lens to see whether the edges turn upward. See Figure 22–22, *A.* If they turn downward, the lens is inside out and must be reversed. See Figure 22–22, *B.* Then lubricate the lens with wetting solution, and insert it in the same manner as a hard contact lens.

Removing Contact Lenses   *Hard* contact lenses must be positioned directly over the cornea for proper removal. If the lens is displaced, ask the client to look straight ahead, and gently exert pressure on the upper and lower lids to move the lens back onto the cornea. Figure 22–23 shows the steps needed to remove a hard lens. To avoid lens mix-ups, place the first lens in its designated cup in the storage case before removing the second lens.

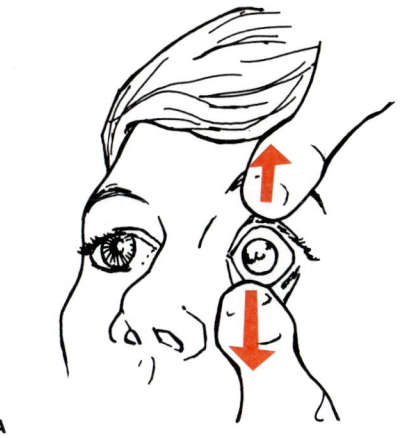

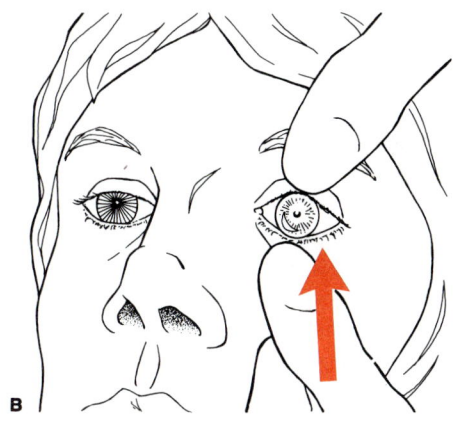

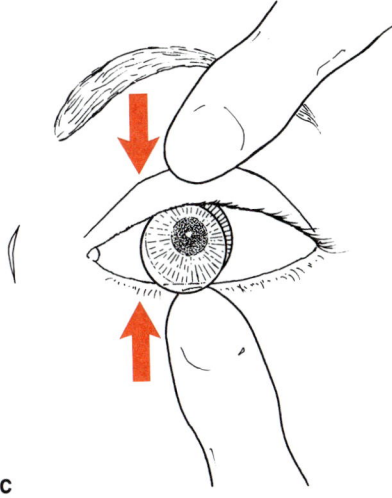

Figure 22–23 Removing hard contact lenses: *A,* separate the eyelids until they are beyond the edges of the lens; *B,* hold the top eyelid stationary at the edge of the lens, and lift the bottom edge of the contact lens by pressing the lower lid at its margin; *C,* After the lens is slightly tipped, slide the lens out of the eye by moving both eyelids toward each other.

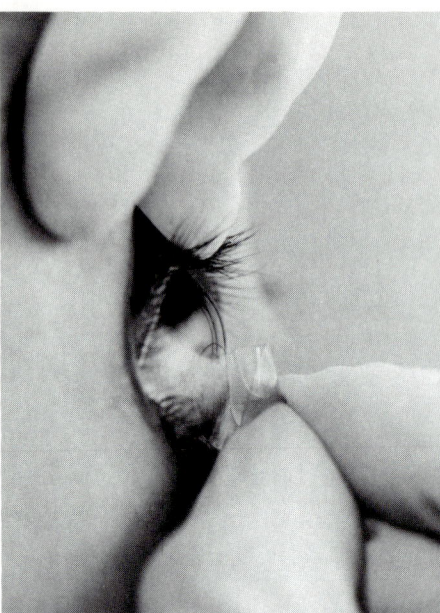

Figure 22–24 After moving the lens down onto the sclera, pinch a soft contact lens to remove it.

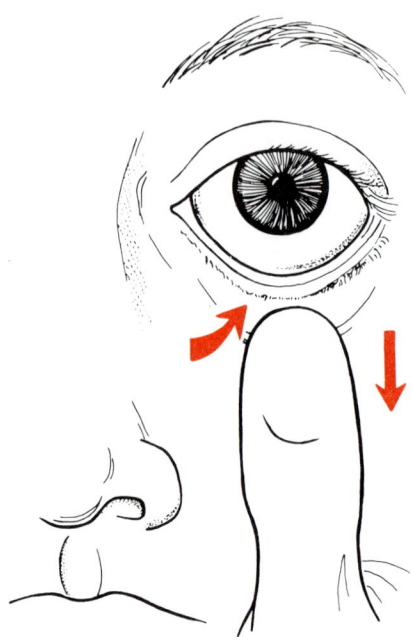

Figure 22–25 When removing an artificial eye, retract the lower eyelid and exert slight pressure below the eyelid.

Removal of *soft* lenses varies in two ways. First, after separating the eyelids with the nondominant hand, move the lens down to the inferior part of the sclera using the pad of the dominant index finger. This reduces the risk of damage to the cornea. Second, remove the lens by gently pinching the lens between the pads of the thumb and index finger of your dominant hand. See Figure 22–24. Pinching causes the lens to double up, so that air enters underneath the lens, overcoming the suction and allowing removal. Use the pads of the fingers to prevent scratching the eye or the lens with the fingernails.

Artificial Eyes Artificial eyes are usually made of glass or plastic. Some are permanently implanted; others are removed regularly for cleaning. Most clients who wear a removable artificial eye follow their own care regimen. Even for an unconscious client, daily removal and cleaning are not necessary. If the nurse notices problems, e.g., redness of the surrounding tissues, drainage from the eye socket, or crusting on the eyelashes, or if the client is scheduled for surgery, the nurse must remove the eye from the socket; clean the eye, the socket, and the surrounding tissues; and then reinsert the eye. Clients whose mobility is impaired by injury or paralysis may also require assistance. In addition, the nurse must determine the client's routine eye care practices so that these can be followed. Some clients may remove and clean the eye and socket daily.

To remove an artificial eye, the nurse dons clean gloves and uses the dominant thumb to pull the client's lower eyelid down over the infraorbital bone, exerting slight pressure below the eyelid to overcome the suction. See Figure 22–25. An alternate method is to compress a small rubber

bulb and apply the tip directly to the eye. As the nurse gradually releases the finger pressure on the bulb, the suction of the bulb counteracts the suction holding the eye in the socket and draws the eye out of the socket.

The eye is cleaned with warm normal saline. If the eye is not to be reinserted, the nurse places it in a container filled with water or saline solution, closes the lid, labels the container with the client's name and room number, and places it in the drawer of the bedside table. The nurse should also clean the socket and tissues around the eye with soft gauze or cotton wipes and normal saline or warm tap water. After inspecting these tissues, the nurse must report and record any abnormal findings. To reinsert the eye, the nurse uses the thumb and index finger of one hand to retract the eyelids, exerting pressure on the supraorbital and infraorbital bones. Holding the eye between the thumb and index finger of the other hand, the nurse slips the eye gently into the socket. See Figure 22–26.

General Eye Care Many clients may need to learn specific information about care of the eyes. Some examples are given below.

- Avoid home remedies for eye problems. Eye irritations or injuries at any age should be treated medically and immediately.

- If dirt or dust gets into the eyes, clean them copiously with clean, tepid water as an emergency treatment.

- Take measures to guard against eyestrain and to protect

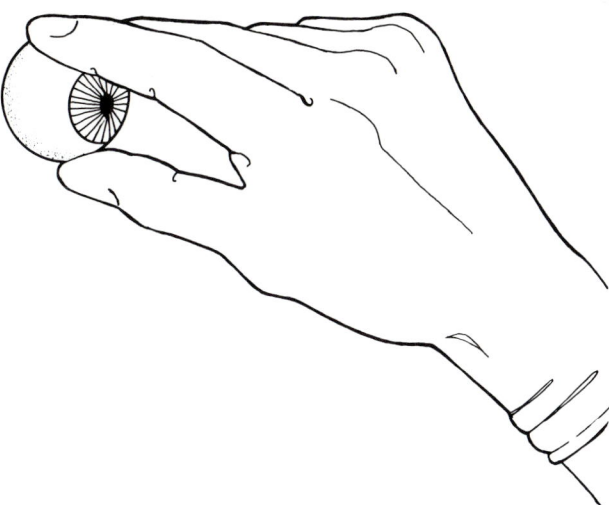

Figure 22–26 Hold an artificial eye between the thumb and index finger for insertion.

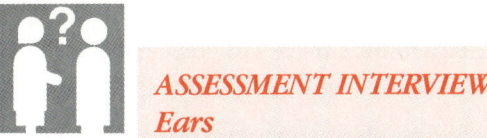

For Clients Who Wear Hearing Aids

- When and where was the hearing aid obtained, and from whom?
- How do you maintain and clean the hearing aid?
- Do you experience any problems with the hearing aid?
- Does wearing the hearing aid bother you? Describe.

For All Clients

- Do you have any ear problems, such as difficulty hearing, pain, itching, discharge, tinnitus (ringing in the ears)? If so, when did this start, and what do you think caused it?
- What medications are you taking for ringing in the ears?
- Are noise levels high in your work environment? If so, how do you protect your ears?

vision, such as maintaining adequate lighting for reading and obtaining shatterproof lenses for glasses.

- Schedule regular eye examinations, particularly over age 40, to detect problems such as cataracts and glaucoma.

Evaluating

To evaluate the achievement of client goals, the nurse inspects the client's eyes, asks the client about any eye discomfort, questions the client about ways to prevent eye injury and strain, and asks the client to demonstrate specific skills such as care of a prosthesis. Examples of evaluative statements indicating goal achievement are "The client states his eye is not painful anymore and is not tearing," or "The client demonstrated appropriate care of his eye prosthesis as taught."

EARS

Normal ears require minimal hygiene. Clients who have excessive **cerumen** (earwax) and dependent clients who have hearing aids may require assistance from the nurse.

Assessing

Nursing History During the nursing history, the nurse obtains data about any ear problems or hearing difficulty, presence of high noise levels in the work environment, and specifics about a hearing aid, if worn. Questions to elicit these data are shown in the accompanying box.

Physical Assessment Physical assessment involves inspection of the external ear structures for signs of inflammation, excessive drainage, discomfort, or other obvious abnormalities. Inspection of the external ear structures is discussed in Chapter 19, page 382.

Diagnosing

Nursing diagnoses related to ear problems may include **Potential for injury, Potential for infection, Self-care deficit** (hearing aid care and insertion), **Body image disturbance**, and **Sensory/perceptual alteration: Auditory.** Examples of these nursing diagnoses and possible contributing factors are listed below.

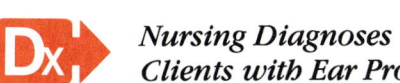

Nursing Diagnoses
Clients with Ear Problems

Potential for injury related to improper methods used to remove cerumen

Potential for infection related to ineffective practices for cleaning hearing aid

Self-care deficit (hearing aid removal, cleaning, and inserting) related to:
- Impaired manual dexterity
- Visual impairment
- Knowledge deficit

Self esteem disturbance related to need to wear hearing aid

Sensory/perceptual alteration: Auditory related to obstructed ear canal associated with impacted cerumen

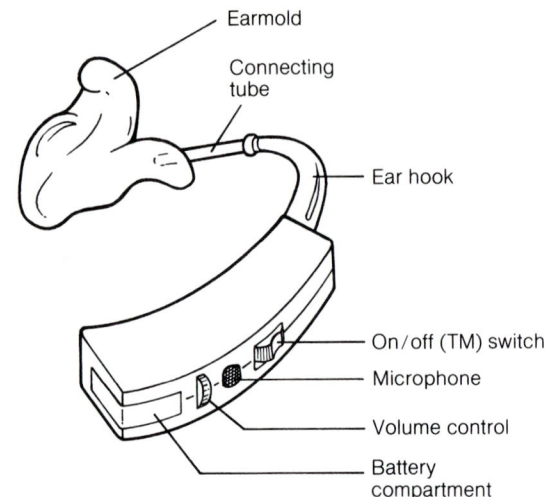

Figure 22–27   A behind-the-ear hearing aid.

Planning

Overall client goals include preventing ear injury and infection and maintaining hearing. Nursing interventions to achieve these goals often involve teaching the client about appropriate methods to remove cerumen and assisting dependent clients with hearing aid removal, cleaning, and insertion. Because some clients feel conspicuous or embarrassed about wearing hearing aids, the nurse may also need to assist the client in developing a more positive self-image (see Chapter 29). Examples of specific outcome criteria are shown below.

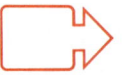

Outcome Criteria
Clients with Ear Problems

The client:

■ Describes measures to prevent ear injury and infection.

■ Demonstrates appropriate methods of caring for a hearing aid.

■ Experiences no ear discomfort.

■ Wears a hearing aid throughout the day.

■ Expresses positive feelings about wearing a hearing aid.

Implementing

Cleaning the Ears   The auricles of the ear are cleaned during the bed bath. The nurse or client must remove excessive cerumen that is visible or that causes discomfort or hearing difficulty. Visible cerumen may be loosened and removed by retracting the auricle downward. If this measure is ineffective, irrigation is necessary (see the section on otic irrigation in Chapter 45). Clients need to be advised never to use bobby pins, toothpicks, or cotton-tipped applicators to remove cerumen. Bobby pins and toothpicks can injure the ear canal and rupture the tympanic membrane; cotton-tipped applicators can cause wax to become impacted within the canal.

Care of Hearing Aids   A hearing aid is a battery-powered, sound-amplifying device used by hearing-impaired persons. It consists of a microphone that picks up sound and converts it to electric energy, an amplifier that magni-

fies the electric energy electronically, a receiver that converts the amplified energy back to sound energy, and an earmold that directs the sound into the ear. There are several types of hearing aids:

■ *Behind-the-ear aid.* This is the most widely used type, since it fits snugly over the ear. The hearing aid case, which holds the microphone, amplifier, and receiver, is attached to the earmold by a plastic tube. See Figure 22–27.

■ *In-the-ear aid.* This one-piece aid is the most compact hearing aid. All its components are housed in the earmold. See Figure 22–28.

■ *Eyeglasses aid.* This is similar to the behind-the-ear aid, but the components are housed in the temple of the eyeglasses. A hearing aid can be in one or both temples of the glasses. See Figure 22–29.

■ *Body hearing aid.* This pocket-sized aid, used for more severe hearing losses, clips onto an undergarment, shirt pocket, or harness carrier supplied by the manufacturer. See Figure 22–30. The case, containing the microphone and amplifier, is connected by a cord to the receiver, which snaps into the earpiece.

To ensure proper functioning, the wearer must handle the hearing aid appropriately during insertion and removal, clean the earmold regularly, and replace dead batteries. Although most clients can look after their hearing aids themselves, some debilitated clients may require assistance. Hearing aids must be removed before surgery. Guidelines for talking to the hearing-impaired person are outlined in Chapter 44. Procedure 22–6 outlines the steps involved in removing, cleaning, and inserting a hearing aid.

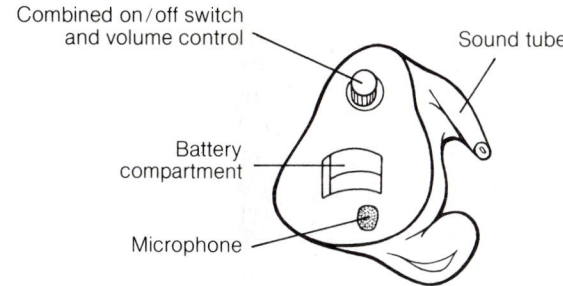

Figure 22–28 An in-the-ear hearing aid.

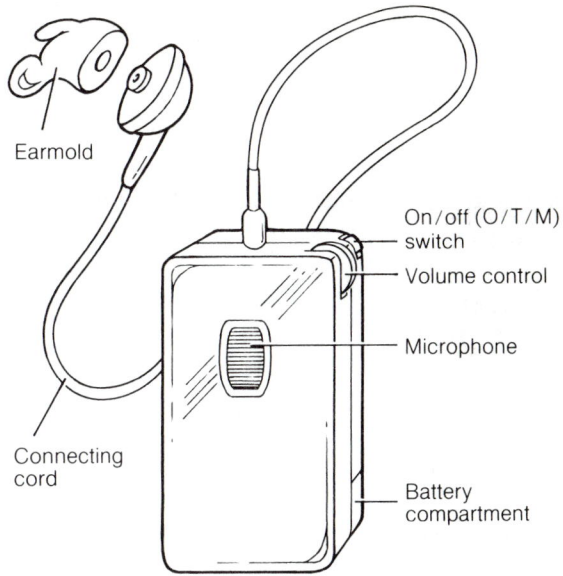

Figure 22–30 A body hearing aid.

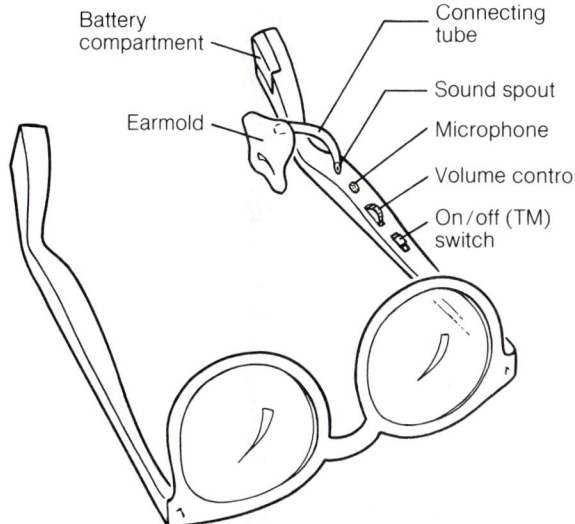

Figure 22–29 An eyeglasses hearing aid.

Evaluating

To evaluate the achievement of client goals, the nurse inspects the ear and asks the client about any ear discomfort. For a client who wears a hearing aid, the nurse questions the client about correct methods of caring for it or asks the client to demonstrate this skill; observes whether the client uses the aid; and listens to the client's comments about the aid. Examples of evaluative statements indicating goal achievement are "The client demonstrated the appropriate method of cleaning his hearing aid," or "The client wore his hearing aid from 0900 to 2200 for the past week."

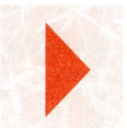

PROCEDURE 22–6

REMOVING, CLEANING, AND INSERTING A HEARING AID

Equipment ☑

Client's hearing aid

New battery (if needed)

Pipe cleaner or toothpick (optional)

Soap, water, and towels or a damp cloth

Intervention

1. **Remove the hearing aid.**

■ Turn the hearing aid off, and lower the volume. The on/off switch may be labeled "O" (off), "M" microphone, "T" (telephone), or "TM"
(telephone/microphone). *The batteries continue to be used if the aid is not turned off.*

■ Remove the earmold by rotating it slightly forward and pulling it outward.

■ If the aid is not to be used for several days, remove the battery. *Removal prevents corrosion of the aid from battery leakage.*

■ Store the hearing aid in a safe place. Avoid exposure to heat and moisture. *Proper storage prevents loss or damage.*

2. Clean the earmold.

■ Detach the earmold *if possible.* Disconnect the earmold from the receiver of a body hearing aid or from the hearing aid case of behind-the-ear and eyeglasses aids where the tubing meets the hook of the case. Do not remove the earmold if it is glued or secured by a small metal ring. *Removal facilitates cleaning and prevents inadvertent damage to the other parts.*

■ If the earmold is *detachable,* soak it in a mild soapy solution. Rinse and dry it well.

■ If the earmold is *not detachable* or is for an in-the-ear aid, wipe the earmold with a damp cloth.

■ Check that the earmold opening is patent. Blow any excess moisture through the opening or remove debris (e.g., earwax) with a pipe cleaner or toothpick.

■ Reattach the earmold if it was detached from the rest of the hearing aid.

3. Insert the hearing aid.

■ Determine from the client whether the earmold is for the left or the right ear.

■ Check that the battery is inserted in the hearing aid. Turn off the hearing aid, and make sure the volume is turned all the way down. *A volume that is too loud is distressing.*

■ Inspect the earmold to identify the ear canal portion. Some earmolds are fitted for only the ear canal and concha; others are fitted for all the contours of the ear. The canal portion, common to all, can be used as a guide for correct insertion.

■ Line up the parts of the earmold with the corresponding parts of the client's ear.

■ Rotate the earmold slightly forward, and insert the ear canal portion.

■ Gently press the earmold into the ear while rotating it backward.

■ Check that the earmold fits snugly by asking the client if it feels secure and comfortable.

■ Adjust the other components of a behind-the-ear or body hearing aid.

■ Turn the hearing aid on and adjust the volume according to the client's needs.

4. Correct problems associated with improper function.

■ If the sound is weak or there is no sound:
   a. Ensure that the volume is turned high enough.
   b. Ensure that the earmold opening is not clogged.
   c. Check the battery, by turning the aid on, turning up the volume, cupping your hand over the earmold, and listening. A constant whistling sound indicates the battery is functioning. If necessary, replace the battery. Be sure that the negative (−) and positive (+) signs on the battery match those on the aid.
   d. Ensure that the ear canal is not blocked with wax, which can obstruct sound waves.

■ If the client reports a whistling sound or squeal after insertion:
   a. Turn the volume down.
   b. Ensure that the earmold is properly attached to the receiver.
   c. Reinsert the earmold.

5. Document pertinent data.

■ Removal and insertion of a hearing aid are not normally recorded.

■ Report and record any problems the client has with the hearing aid.

NOSE

Nurses usually need not provide special care for the nose because clients can ordinarily clear nasal secretions by blowing into a soft tissue. However, clients with tubes that exit from the nares or those whose excessive secretions impair breathing may require special assistance.

Assessing

Nursing History   During the nursing history, the nurse obtains data about any problems associated with the nasal passages (e.g., difficulty breathing through the nose, sinus infections, injuries to the nose, and nosebleeds); medications; and any changes in the sense of smell.

Physical Assessment   Physical assessment of the nares is discussed in Chapter 19. If a client has a nasogastric tube or any tube exiting from the nares, the nurse inspects the nares, particularly the surfaces in contact with the tube, for signs of inflammation, tenderness, bleeding, and sloughing. Pressure and movement of these tubes can cause tissue irritation and damage.

Diagnosing

Nursing diagnoses related to nose problems may include potential or actual **Impaired tissue integrity, Potential for infection**, and **Ineffective breathing pattern**. Examples of these nursing diagnoses and possible contributing factors are listed below.

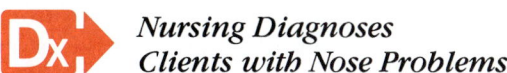

Nursing Diagnoses
Clients with Nose Problems

Impaired tissue integrity related to nasogastric tube

Potential for infection related to impaired integrity of nasal mucous membrane secondary to nasogastric tube

Ineffective breathing pattern related to excessive secretions in nasopharynx

Planning

The overall client goal related to nose care is the maintenance of nasal tissue integrity. Nursing interventions to achieve this goal include regular assessment and cleaning of the nares of clients with nasal tubes or excessive secretions (e.g., q4h or bid). Specific outcome criteria for clients with problems related to the nose are shown below.

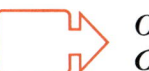

Outcome Criteria
Clients with Nose Problems

The client:
- Has intact nasal mucous membranes.
- Has pink nasal mucosa with clear, watery discharge.
- Experiences no tenderness.
- Has patent nares.

Implementing

Excessive nasal secretions can be removed by inserting a cotton-tipped applicator moistened with water or normal saline or by applying suction. A cotton-tipped applicator should be not inserted beyond the length of the cotton tip. Suctioning of the nares is discussed in Chapter 41.

The nares of clients with nasal tubes should be cleaned with a moistened, cotton-tipped applicator to prevent the accumulation of secretions around the tubing. The tape that anchors the tube should be changed when it becomes moist to prevent maceration of the skin and mucous membrane. Methods of taping tubes to minimize their movement are discussed in Chapter 39.

Evaluating

To evaluate the achievement of client goals, the nurse inspects the client's nares and asks the client about nasal comfort. Goal achievement is then documented. Examples of evaluative statements are "The client's nasal mucous membranes are intact," or "The client states he has no nasal tenderness."

SUPPORTING A HYGIENIC ENVIRONMENT

Because ill persons are confined to bed, sometimes for weeks or months, the bed unit becomes an important element in the client's life. A unit that is clean, safe, and comfortable contributes to the client's ability to rest and sleep and to a sense of well-being. Basic furniture in a hospital bed unit includes the bed, bedside table, overbed table, one or more chairs, and a storage space for clothing. Hospitals vary in the equipment provided as part of the bed unit. Basic to all are a call light, light fixtures, electrical outlets, and hygienic equipment in the bedside table. Long-term care facilities may have very little additional equipment, whereas an acute facility may have several commonly used devices built into each unit. Three types of equipment are often installed on the wall at the head of the bed: a *suction outlet* for several kinds of suction, an *oxygen outlet* for most oxygen equipment, and a *sphygmomanometer* to measure the client's blood pressure.

Some long-term care agencies also permit clients to have *personal equipment,* such as a television, a chair, and lamps, at the bedside. A major nursing responsibility is ensuring that the unit's equipment is functioning properly and is safe and comfortable.

Hospital Beds

A hospital bed has characteristics particularly suited to people who are in bed continuously or for a long time. Most hospitals use Gatch beds. When the gatches, or joints, are flexed, the client is raised to a sitting position with the knees elevated. The cranks that operate the gatches are usually at the bottom or side of the bed. When not in use, manual cranks are left in the retracted position under the bed. Otherwise, people walking by the bed might easily injure their legs against the cranks. Increasingly, hospitals are purchasing beds with electric motors to operate the gatches. The motor is activated by pressing a button or moving a small lever, located either at the side of the bed or on a small panel separate from the bed but attached to it by a cable.

Hospital beds are usually 66 cm (26 in) high and 0.9 m (3 ft) wide, narrower than the usual bed, so that the nurse can reach the client from either side of the bed without undue stretching. The length is usually 1.9 m (6.5 ft). Some beds can be extended in length, if required. Long-term care facilities for ambulatory clients usually have low beds to facilitate movement in and out of bed. Most hospital beds have "high" and "low" positions that can be adjusted either mechanically by a crank at the center of the foot of the bed or electrically by a button or lever on the same panel as the gatch controls. The high position permits the nurse to reach the client without undue stretching or stooping. The low position allows the client to step easily to the floor.

Mattresses

Most mattresses used in hospitals have innersprings, which give even support to the body. When changing a bed, nurses need to note any unevenness of the mattress surface, which might indicate a broken spring. Mattresses are usually covered with a water-repellent material that resists soiling and can be cleaned easily. Most mattresses have handles on the sides called lugs by which the mattress can be removed.

Foam rubber *egg crate mattresses* are also used in hospitals. See Figure 22–31. They provide support and have the advantage of relieving pressure on the body's bony prominences, such as the heels. Foam mattresses are particularly helpful for clients confined to bed for a long time. Another option is the air mattress (also called an *alternating pressure mattress*), which is attached to a motor that lowers or raises the air pressure inside the mattress. The

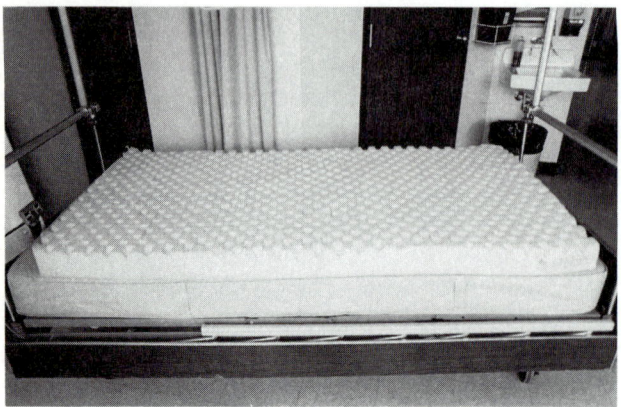

Figure 22–31 An egg crate mattress provides comfort and helps to distribute the body weight evenly, thus helping to reduce pressure on bony prominences.

water mattress is a plastic bag filled with water. This mattress employs the principle of weight displacement. If the body displaces 9 kg (20 lb) of water, there is 9 kg less pressure on the weight-bearing areas.

The surfaces of air and water mattresses must be intact so that the air or water will not escape. It is therefore inadvisable to use pins on the sheets covering these mattresses. Special mattresses are placed atop the standard bed mattress, although the water mattress may be placed on the base springs.

Side Rails

Side rails, or safety sides, are used on both hospital beds and stretchers. They are of various shapes and sizes and are usually made of metal. Devices to raise and lower them differ. Often one or two knobs are pulled to release the side and permit it to be moved. When side rails are being used, it is important that the nurse *never* leave the bedside while the rail is lowered. Some side rails have two positions: up and down. Others have three: high, intermediate, and low. The down and low positions are employed when a side rail is not needed. With some models, the bed foundation must be raised before the side rail can be put in the low position; otherwise, the side rail might hit the floor and be damaged. The intermediate position is used when the bed is in the low position and the nurse is present. The up or high side rail position is used when a client is in bed and requires protection from falling.

Footboards

A *footboard* is a flat panel, often made of wood or plastic, placed at the foot of a bed. It serves three purposes:

1. To provide support for the client's feet and maintain a natural foot position while the client is in bed. See Figure 22–32.

2. To keep the top bed covers off the client's feet, relieving the pressure of the weight of the covers.

3. To make the foot comfortable (for example, when a client has a painful foot).

Without the support of a footboard, a client's feet drop from their normal right angle to the legs and assume a plantar flexion position with the toes pointing toward the foot of the bed. See Figure 22–33. Prolonged assumption of this position results in permanent shortening of the muscles and tendons at the back of the legs. When that happens, the client is unable to stand flat-footed on the floor, and walking is seriously impaired.

Footboards are often made in an L shape so that the base of the L fits under the foot of the mattress. Some footboards can be moved along the mattress to adjust to the client's height. If a board cannot be adjusted, sandbags and rolled pillows or blankets can be used to fill the space between the client's feet and the board.

Bed Cradles

A *bed cradle,* sometimes called an Anderson frame, is a device designed to keep the top bed-

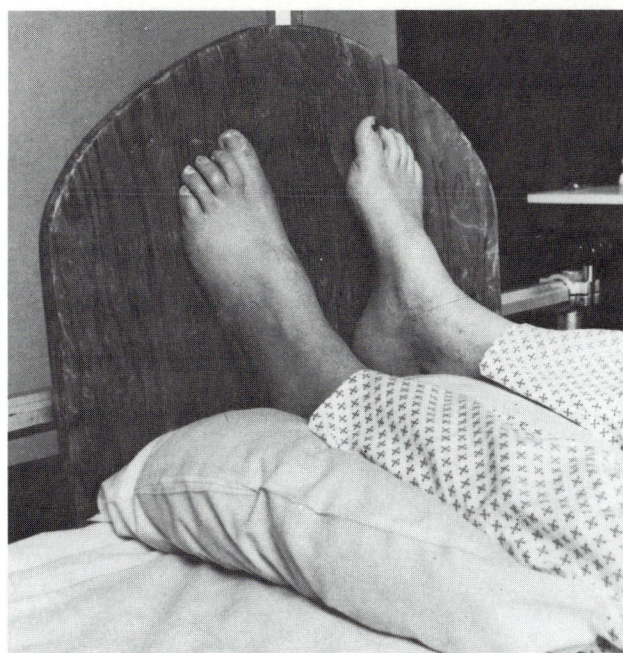

Figure 22–32 A footboard maintains dorsiflexion of the feet.

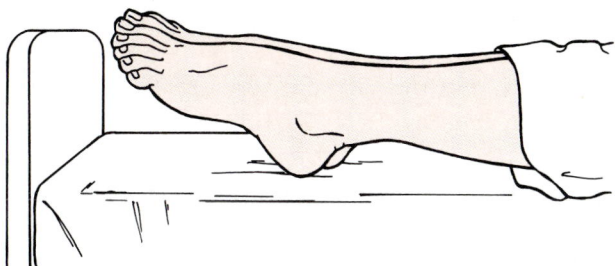

Figure 22–33 The feet in plantar flexion.

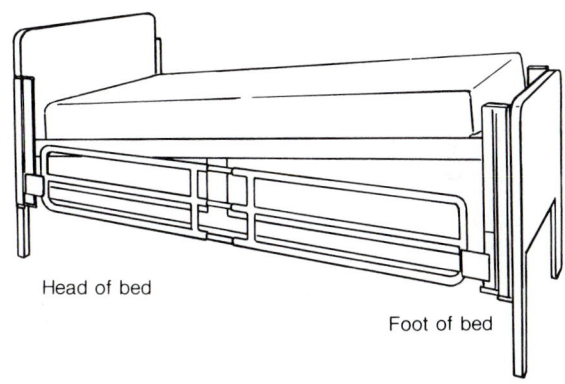

Head of bed

Foot of bed

Figure 22–34 A bed in Trendelenburg's position.

clothes off the feet, legs, and even abdomen of a client. The bedclothes are arranged over the device and may be pinned in place. There are several types of bed cradles. One of the most common is a curved metal rod that fits over the bed. Part of the cradle fits under the mattress, and small metal brackets press down on each side of the mattress to keep the cradle in place. The frame of some cradles extends over only half of the bed, above only one leg.

Intravenous Rods   Intravenous rods (poles, stands, standards), usually made of metal, support intravenous (IV) infusion containers while fluid is being administered to a client. These rods were traditionally freestanding on the floor beside the bed. Now, intravenous rods are often attached to the hospital beds. Some hospital units have overhead hanging rods on a track for IVs.

Bed Positions

When the bed is in the *flat position,* the mattress is completely horizontal. Pillows may or may not be used. *Fowler's position* is a semisitting bed position (the head of the bed is raised to at least 45°) frequently used in hospitals. It gives clients relief from the lying positions and is convenient for eating and reading. In *Trendelenburg's position,* the head of the bed is lowered and the foot of the bed is elevated in a straight incline. See Figure 22–34. If the foundation cannot be raised mechanically, this position may be obtained by placing blocks or special pins under the foot of the bed.

The blocks are often referred to as shock blocks, because this position was used some years ago for clients in shock. It is now contraindicated for clients suffering from head injuries, respiratory distress, chest injuries, or shock. Currently it is used for some postural drainage. *Reverse Trendelenburg's position* is a straight tilt in the opposite direction: The head of the bed is elevated, and the foot of the bed is lowered. Sometimes the legs at the head of the bed are raised by blocks or by pins if the foundation cannot be raised mechanically. This position may be used for clients experiencing problems with arterial circulation to the legs. In the *contour position,* both the head and foot of the bed are elevated about 15°. See Figure 22–35. It is necessary to raise both the knee and the foot sections of some hospital beds to obtain this position. For the *hyperextension position,* both the head and the foot sections are lowered 15°. See Figure 22–36. This position is sometimes used for clients with spinal fractures. It should be used only with specific orders, and continuous nursing assessment of the client is important. Not all hospital beds can be adjusted to this position.

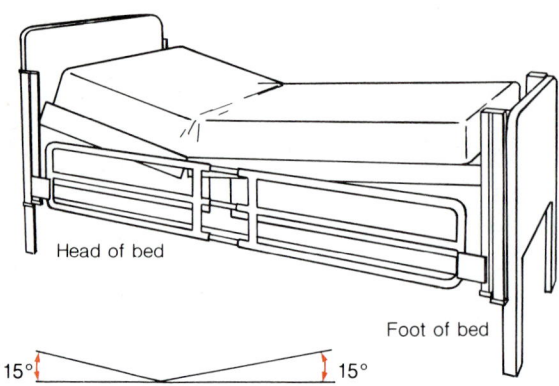

Figure 22–35 A bed in contour position.

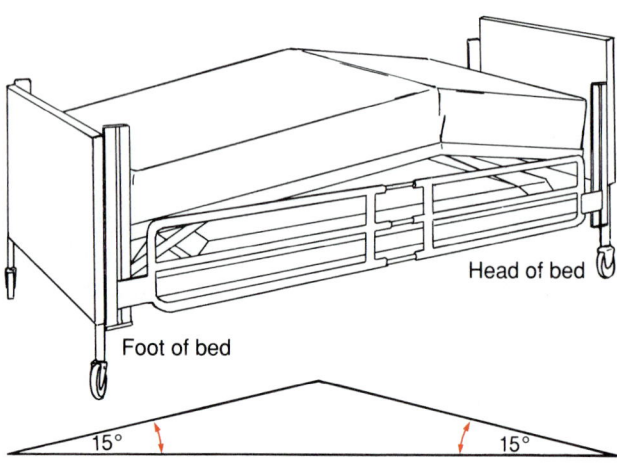

Figure 22–36 A bed in hyperextension position.

Specialized Beds   Whenever a client's body alignment must be strictly maintained, a specially designed bed that rotates on an axis is used to turn the client from the supine to the prone position and vice versa. Two such beds are the Stryker wedge frame and the CircOlectric bed. The Stryker wedge frame, which is manually operated by the nurse, turns the client laterally through the side-lying position. The CircOlectric bed, which is operated electrically by the nurse using a push button, rotates the client vertically through the standing position. These turning frames are used for clients with certain types of spinal injuries, e.g., extensive burns, arthritis, and pressure sores, who require position changes that cannot be effectively managed in the standard bed.

Making Beds

Nurses need to be able to prepare hospital beds in different ways for specific purposes. In most instances, beds are made after the client receives certain care and when beds are

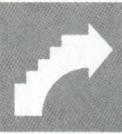

unoccupied. At times, however, nurses need to make an occupied bed or prepare a bed for a client who is having surgery (an anesthetic, postoperative, or surgical bed). Regardless of what type of bed equipment is available, whether the bed is occupied or unoccupied, or the purpose for which the bed is being prepared, certain guidelines pertain to all bed making. These are summarized in the box above.

An *unoccupied bed* can be either closed or open. Generally the top covers of an open bed are folded back (*open bed*) to make it easier for a client to get in. Open and closed beds are made the same way, except that the top sheet, blanket, and bedspread of a *closed* bed are drawn up to the top of the bed and under the pillows.

Hospital beds are often changed after bed baths. The linen can be collected before the bath. Nurses in some hospitals do not change all the linen unless it is soiled. Check the policy at each clinical agency. Unfitted sheets, blankets, and bedspread are mitered at the corners of the bed. The purpose of mitering is to secure the bedclothes while the bed is occupied. Figure 22–37 shows how to miter the corner of a bed.

Procedure 22–7 explains how to change an *unoccupied* bed.

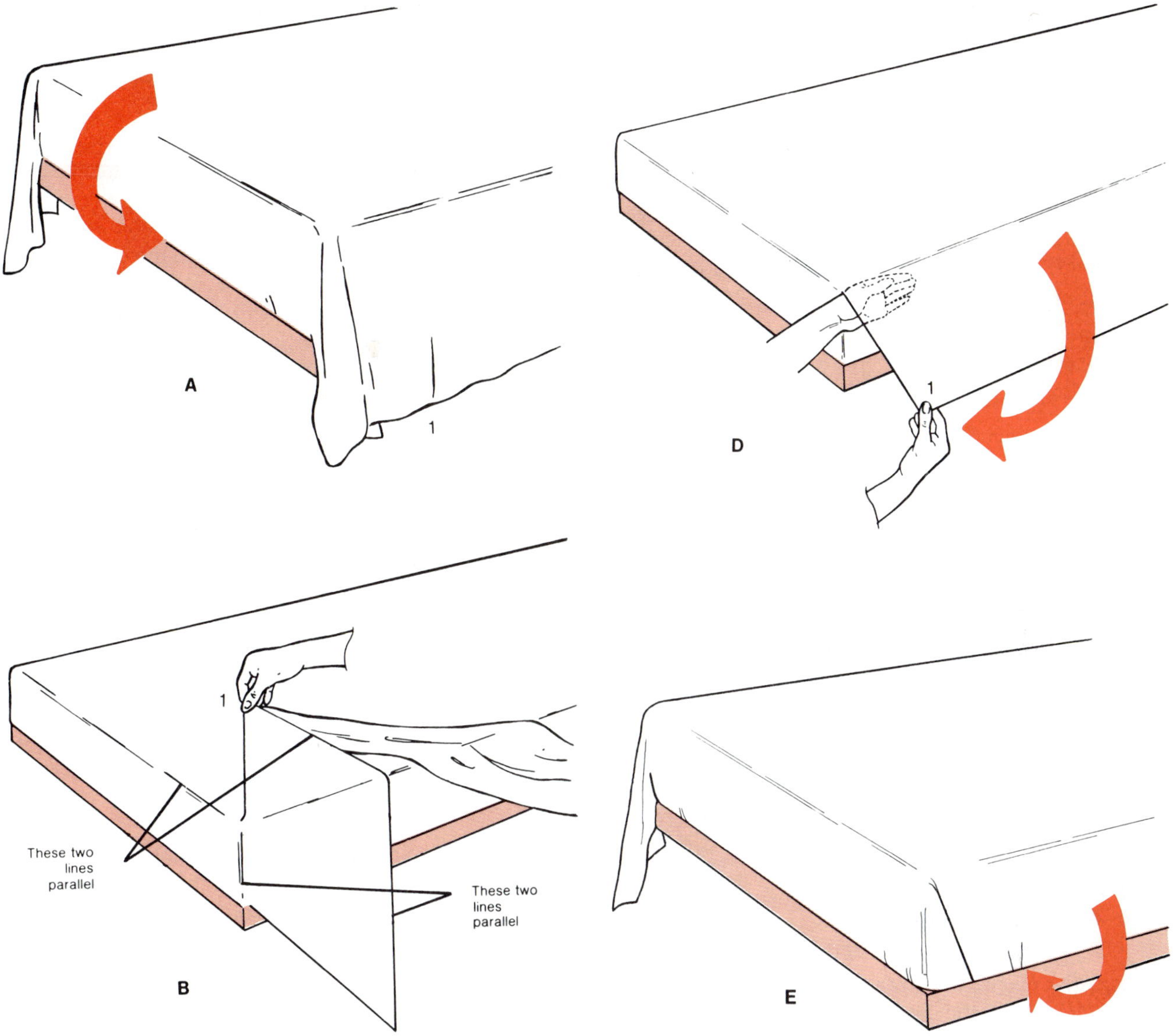

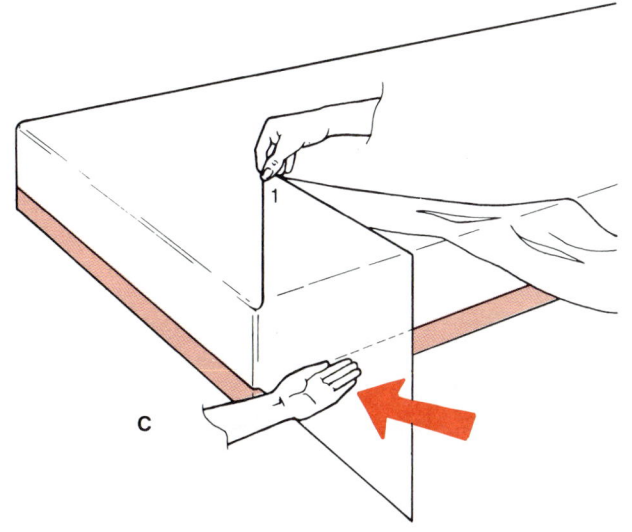

A

B

These two
lines
parallel

These two
lines
parallel

C

D

1

E

Figure 22–37 Mitering the corner of a bed: *A,* tuck the bedcover (sheet, blanket, and/or spread) in firmly under the mattress at the bottom or top of the bed; *B,* lift the bedcover at point 1 so that it forms a triangle with the side edge of the bed, and the edge of the bedcover is parallel to the end of the bed; *C,* tuck the part of the cover that hangs below the mattress under the mattress while holding the cover at point 1 against the mattress; *D,* bring point 1 down toward the floor while the other hand holds the fold of the cover against the side of the mattress; *E,* remove the hand, and tuck the remainder of the cover under the mattress, if appropriate. The sides of the top sheet, blanket, and bedspread may be left hanging freely rather than tucked in. The bedspread is mitered separately and left hanging freely if the top sheet and blanket are tucked in.

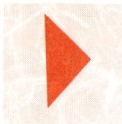

CHANGING AN UNOCCUPIED BED

Equipment

Two large sheets

Cloth drawsheet (optional)

One blanket

One bedspread

Waterproof drawsheet or waterproof pads (optional)

Pillowcase(s) for the head pillow(s)

Portable linen hamper, if available

Intervention

1. **Place the fresh linen on the client's chair or overbed table; do not use another client's bed.** *This prevents cross-contamination (the movement of microorganisms from one client to another) via soiled linen.*

2. **Assess and assist the client out of bed.**

■ Make sure that this is an appropriate and convenient time for the client to be out of bed.

■ Assess the client's health status to determine that the person can safely get out of bed. In some hospitals it is necessary to have a written order if the client has been in bed continuously.

■ Assess the client's pulse and respirations.

■ Assist the client to a comfortable chair.

3. **Strip the bed.**

■ Check bed linens for any of the client's misplaced personal items, and detach the call bell or any drainage tubes from the bed linen.

■ Loosen all bedding, starting at the head of the bed, moving down the bed, working around the foot, and moving up to the other side of the head. *Moving around the bed sys-*

tematically prevents stretching and reaching and possible muscle strain.

■ Remove the pillowcases, if soiled, and place the pillows on the bedside chair near the foot of the bed.

■ Fold reusable linens, such as the bedspread and top sheet on the bed, into fourths. First, fold the linen in half by bringing the top edge even with the bottom edge, and then grasp it at the center of the middle fold and bottom edges. See Figure 22−38. *Folding linens on the bed prevents strain on the nurse's arms and saves time and energy when reapplying the linens on the bed.*

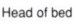

Head of bed

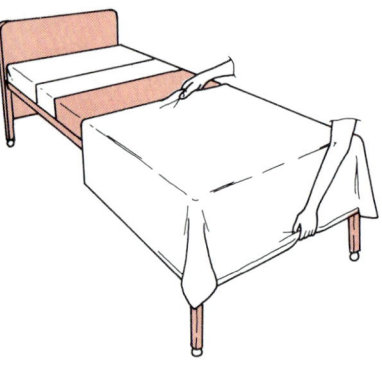

Figure 22−38 Reusable linens are folded into fourths when removing them from the bed.

■ Remove the waterproof pad, and discard it if soiled.

■ Roll all soiled linen inside the bottom sheet, hold it away from your uniform, and place it directly in the linen hamper. *These actions are essential to prevent the transmission of microorganisms to yourself and others.*

■ Grasp the mattress securely, using the lugs if present, and move the mattress up to the head of the bed.

4. **Apply the bottom sheet and drawsheet.**

■ Place the folded bottom sheet with its center fold on the center of the bed. Make sure the sheet is hemside down for a smooth foundation. Spread the sheet out over the mattress, and allow a sufficient amount of sheet at the top to tuck under the mattress. *The top of the sheet needs to be well tucked under to remain securely in place, especially when the head of the bed is elevated.* Place the sheet along the edge of the mattress at the foot of the bed, and do not tuck it in (unless it is a contour sheet).

■ Miter the sheet at the top corner on the near side (see Figure 22−37, earlier), and tuck the sheet under the mattress, working from the head of the bed to the foot.

■ If a waterproof drawsheet is used, place it over the bottom sheet so that the center fold is at the center line of the bed and the top and bottom edges will extend from the middle of the client's back to the area of the midthigh or knee. Fanfold the uppermost half of the folded drawsheet at the center or far edge of the bed, and tuck in the near edge.

■ Lay the cloth drawsheet over the waterproof sheet in the same manner described above.

■ *Optional:* Before moving to the other side of the bed, place the top linens on the bed, hem-side up, unfold them, tuck them in, and miter the bottom corners. *Completing the entire side of the bed saves time and energy.*

5. **Move to the other side of the bed, and secure the bottom linens.**

- Tuck in the bottom sheet under the head of the mattress, pull the sheet firmly, and miter the corner.
- Pull the remainder of the sheet firmly so that there are no wrinkles. *Wrinkles can cause discomfort for the client.* Tuck the sheet in at the side.
- Do the same for the drawsheet(s).

6. Apply or complete the top bedding.

- Place the top sheet, hem-side up, on the bed so that its center fold is at the center of the bed and the top edge is even with the top edge of the mattress.
- Unfold the sheet over the bed.
- *Optional:* Make a vertical or a horizontal toe pleat in the sheet to provide additional room for the client's feet.
  - a. *Vertical toe pleat:* Make a fold in the sheet 5 to 10 cm (2 to 4 in) perpendicular to the foot of the bed. See Figure 22–39.

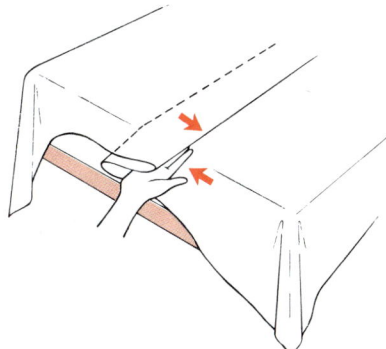

Figure 22–39 A vertical toe pleat.

  - b. *Horizontal toe pleat:* Make a fold in the sheet 5 to 10 cm (2 to 4 in) across the bed near the foot. See Figure 22–40.

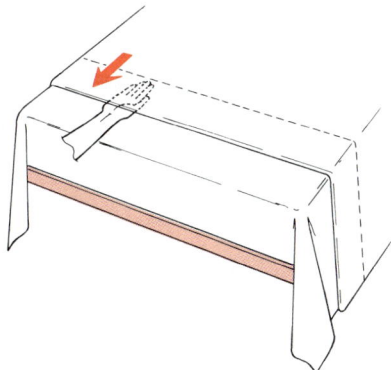

Figure 22–40 A horizontal toe pleat.

Loosening the top covers around the feet after the client is in bed is another way to provide additional space.

- Follow the same procedure for the blanket and the spread, but place the top edges about 15 cm (6 in) from the head of the bed to allow a cuff of sheet to be folded over them.
- Tuck in the sheet, blanket, and spread at the foot of the bed, and miter the corner, using all three layers of linen. Leave the sides of the top sheet, blanket, and spread hanging freely unless toe pleats were provided.
- Fold the top of the top sheet down over the spread, providing a cuff of about 15 cm (6 in). *The cuff of sheet makes it easier for the client to pull the covers up.*
- Move to the other side of the bed, and secure the top bedding in the same manner.

7. Put clean pillow cases on the pillows as required.

- Grasp the closed end of the pillowcase at the center with one hand.
- Gather up the sides of the pillowcase, and place them over the hand

grasping the case. Then grasp the center of one short side of the pillow through the pillowcase. See Figure 22–41.

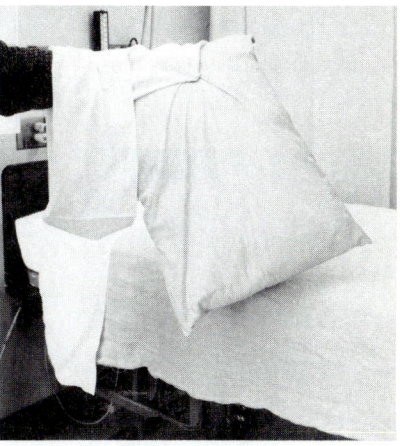

Figure 22–41 Method for putting a clean pillowcase on a pillow.

- With the free hand, pull the pillowcase over the pillow.
- Adjust the pillowcase so that the pillow fits into the corners of the case and the seams are straight. *A smoothly fitting pillowcase is more comfortable than a wrinkled one.*
- Align and place the pillows at the head of the bed in the center, with the open ends of the pillowcase facing away from the door of the room. *This provides a neat appearance.*

8. Provide for client comfort and safety.

- Attach the signal cord so that the client can conveniently use it. Some cords have clamps that attach to the sheet or pillowcase. Others are attached by a safety pin.
- If the bed is currently being used by a client, either fold back the top covers at one side or fanfold them down to the center of the bed. *This makes it easier for the client to get into the bed.*

■ Put the bedside table and the overbed table in order so that they are available to the client.

■ Leave the bed in the high position if the client is returning by stretcher, or place in the low position if client is returning to bed after being up.

9. **Document and report pertinent data.**

■ Bed-making is not normally recorded.

■ Record nursing assessments such as the client's physical status and pulse and respiratory rates before and after being out of bed.

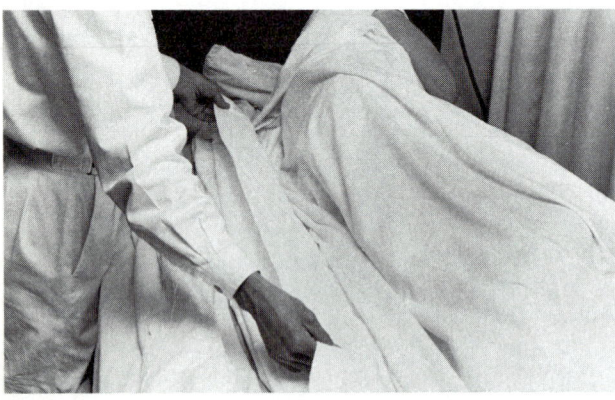

Figure 22–42   Fanfolding soiled linen as close to the client as possible.

Changing an Occupied Bed   When changing an occupied bed, the nurse must work quickly and disturb the client as little as possible. Guidelines for changing an occupied bed are listed in the box below.

Making a Surgical Bed   A surgical bed is made for clients who are having surgical or diagnostics procedures that require use of an anesthetic agent. See Chapter 47 for information about how to prepare a surgical bed.

CLINICAL GUIDELINES
Changing an Occupied Bed

■ Maintain the client in good body alignment. Never move or position a client in a manner that is contraindicated by the client's health. Obtain help if necessary to ensure safety.

■ Move the client gently and smoothly. Rough handling can cause the client discomfort and abrade the skin.

■ Throughout the procedure, explain what you plan to do before you do it. Use terms that the client can understand.

■ Use the bed-making time, like the bed bath time, to assess and meet the client's needs.

■ Loosen all the top linen at the foot of the bed, and remove the spread and blanket.

■ Leave the top sheet over the client (the top sheet can remain over the client if it is being changed and if it will provide sufficient warmth) *or* replace it with a bath blanket as follows:
   a. Spread the bath blanket over the top sheet.
   b. Ask the client to hold the top edge of the blanket.

   c. Reaching under the blanket from the side, grasp the top edge of the sheet and draw it down to the foot of the bed, leaving the blanket in place.
   d. Remove the sheet from the bed and place it in the soiled linen hamper.

■ Place the bed in the flat position if the client's health permits.

■ Grasp the mattress lugs and, using good body mechanics, move the mattress up to the head of the bed. Ask the client to assist, if permitted, by grasping the head of the bed and pulling as you push. If the client is heavy, you may need help from another nurse.

■ Assist the client to turn on the side facing away from the side where the clean linen is. Raise the side rail nearest the client.

■ Loosen the foundation linen on the side of the bed near the linen supply. Fanfold the drawsheet and the bottom sheet at the center of the bed, as close to the client as possible. Doing this leaves the near half of the bed free to be changed. See Figure 22–42.

(continued)

- Place the new bottom sheet on the bed, and vertically fanfold the half to be used on the far side of the bed as close to the client as possible. Tuck the sheet under the near half of the bed, and miter the corner if a contour sheet is not being used.

- Place the clean drawsheet on the bed with the center fold at the center of the bed. Fanfold the uppermost half vertically at the center of the bed, and tuck the near side edge under the side of the mattress.

- Assist the client to roll over toward you onto the clean side of the bed. The client rolls over the fanfolded linen at the center of the bed.

- Move the pillows to the clean side for the client's use. Raise the side rail before leaving the side of the bed.

- Move to the other side of the bed, and lower the side rail.

- Remove the used linen, and place it in the portable hamper.

- Smooth out the mattress cover to remove any wrinkles. Unfold the fanfolded bottom sheet from the center of the bed.

- Facing the side of the bed, use both hands to pull the bottom sheet so that it is smooth, and tuck the excess under the side of the mattress.

- Unfold the drawsheet fanfolded at the center of the bed, and pull it tightly with both hands. Pull the sheet in three sections: (a) face the side of the bed to pull the middle section; (b) face the far top corner to pull the bottom section; and (c) face the far bottom corner to pull the top section.

- Tuck the excess drawsheet under the side of the mattress.

- Reposition the pillows at the center of the bed.

- Assist the client to the center of the bed. Determine what position the client requires or prefers, and assist the client to that position.

- Spread the top sheet over the client, and ask the client to hold the top edge of the sheet or tuck it under the shoulders. The sheet should remain over the client when the bath blanket or used sheet is removed.

- Complete the top of the bed.

- Raise the side rails, and place the bed in the low position before leaving the bedside.

NURSING CARE PLAN FOR ANN RODGERS

ASSESSMENT DATA

Nursing Assessment

Mrs. Ann Rodgers is a 55-year-old sales clerk who has been admitted to Fairfax County Hospital for treatment of a leg ulcer. She is married and has six children. Her full-time position entails standing for long periods of time. She is always well groomed and meticulous about her appearance. She has a history of varicose veins and venous problems, and last week, while at work, she accidentally struck her leg against the sales counter. A leg ulcer began to develop at the site of the injury, and yesterday she saw her physician, who suggested hospitalization for the treatment of the ulcer. Now that she is in the hospital, her physician has written orders for bed rest and Betadine solution to be applied daily.

Physical Examination
Height: 167.6 cm (5'6")
Weight: 61.2 kg (135 lb)
Temperature: 37.5 C (97.5)
Pulse rate: 90 BPM
Respirations: 20 per minute at rest
Blood pressure: 132/82 mm Hg
Left ankle edematous with a 5.5 cm ulcer present above the medial malleolus
Veins of both legs dilated and visible
Skin from ankles to mid calf area, scaly, dry, pigmented

Diagnostic Data
Chest x-ray film: Negative
WBC: 11,500 cu mm
Urine: Negative

CARE PLAN

Nursing Diagnosis	Client Goals and Outcome Criteria	Nursing Interventions and Rationales	Evaluation
Impaired skin integrity related to altered venous circulation resulting in destruction of skin layers by ulceration, edema, redness.	Client Goals: Improved venous circulation. Healed ulcer. Outcome Criteria: Reduced size of impairment is noted by day 7. Skin temperature of both feet is warm to touch. Skin is intact, pink and moist by day 21. Temperature is 37 C by day 3.	Apply wet to dry dressings to debride ulcer. *Rationale:* Wet to dry dressings entrap infected and necrotic material. Cleanse ulcer daily at 1000 hrs with Betadine solution. *Rationale:* Betadine is an antiseptic that is effective for cleaning ulcers and removing dead tissue. Assess nutritional status and encourage intake of foods high in protein and vitamin C. *Rationale:* Good nutrition is essential to promote healing. Change dressings 4 times daily employing sterile technique. *Rationale:* Sterile technique prevents infection. Keep affected leg above heart level whenever possible. *Rationale:* Facilitates venous circulation and decreases edema formation. Instruct client on care of ulcer. *Rationale:* Instruction will prevent complications of skin disruption.	Skin temperature of both feet was warm to touch by day 3. The circumference of both ankles was equal—20 cm by week's end. Body temperature was 36.5 C by day 4. The size of the ulcer was reduced by 3 cm.
Self-care deficit related to impaired mobility status, resulting in inability to get to bathroom, to bathe and dress independently.	Client Goal: Client cares for self as much as possible. Outcome Criteria: States feeling of comfort and satisfaction with body cleanliness. Demonstrates coping ability with inability to toilet self. Uses bedpan as scheduled. Assists with daily grooming.	Involve client in plan of care. *Rationale:* Enhances sense of control. Encourage self-care in bathing. *Rationale:* Enhances feeling of self-worth. Change client's position every 2 hours. *Rationale:* Body surfaces will bear weight alternately. Keep client's skin clean and dry *Rationale:* Prevents skin breakdown. Offer toileting devices as necessary. *Rationale:* Prevents constipation and urinary retention. Provide privacy. *Rationale:* Important to self-esteem.	Client participates in partial bed bath daily. States she feels comfortable and refreshed after bathing. Has adjusted to use of bedpan and voids several times each day. Has a daily bowel movement.

CHAPTER HIGHLIGHTS

▶ Clients' hygiene is influenced to a large degree by their sociocultural background.

▶ When people become ill, hygiene is often of secondary importance to vital body needs, such as breathing and rest.

▶ When clients cannot meet their hygiene needs, the nurse usually assumes them.

▶ The major functions of the skin are to help regulate body temperature, to protect underlying tissues, to secrete sebum, to contain nerve receptors that act in sensory perception.

▶ While assisting a client with hygiene measures, the nurse has an opportunity to assess the client's health.

▶ While planning hygiene care, the nurse must take the client's preferences into consideration.

▶ The back rub is an essential part of hygiene care for clients confined to bed.

▶ Nurses provide perineal-genital care for clients who are unable to do so for themselves.

▶ Nurses can often teach clients how to prevent foot problems.

▶ Oral hygiene should include daily dental flossing and mechanical brushing of the teeth.

▶ Regular dental checkups and fluoride supplements are recommended to maintain healthy teeth.

▶ Nurses provide special oral care to clients who are helpless, e.g., unconscious, and who have oral problems.

▶ Hair care includes daily combing and brushing and regular shampooing.

▶ A black person's hair may require special care.

▶ Nurses may need to assist helpless clients with their artificial eyes, eyeglasses, and contact lenses.

▶ The deaf client may require nursing assistance with his or her hearing aid.

▶ Changing beds is a part of maintaining hygiene.

▶ It is important to keep beds clean and comfortable for clients.

READINGS AND REFERENCES

SUGGESTED READINGS

Blaney, G. M. September/October 1986. Mouth care—basic and essential. *Geriatric Nursing* 7:242–43.
    Blaney reviews some of the conditions that predispose clients to oral problems and some of the products in current use. Normal saline is thought to be universally available and the oral cleanser least likely to cause irritation. The author stresses the importance of regular mouth care.

Davis, M. April 1977. Getting to the root of the problem. *Nursing 77* 7:60–65.
    Davis describes hair care for a black client. It is important to select the right comb and learn some basic grooming techniques. Removing tangles and preventing matting are discussed.

Gannon, E. P., and Kadezabek, E. March 1980. Giving your patients meticulous mouth care. *Nursing 80* 10:14–19.
    The authors describe examining the mouth and throat, helping with mouth care, providing mouth care to unconscious clients, removing and cleaning dentures, and using special aids. Photographs clarify the content.

Michelsen, D. July 1978. Giving a great back rub. *American Journal of Nursing* 78:1197–99.
    The author describes a 15-step technique, referred to as a *back massage,* that stimulates circulation and relieves muscle tension. Photographs illustrate the steps of the technique.

Schaeffer, A. M. May/June 1982. Nursing measures to maintain foot health. *Geriatric Nursing* 3:182–83.
    Schaeffer discusses early clues to decreased foot circulation and what to do about them.

Smiler, I. May/June 1982. Foot problems of elderly diabetics. *Geriatric Nursing* 3:177–81.
    Conserving the feet of the person who has diabetes mellitus is an important goal of the nurse. Smiler discusses ulcers of the foot, vascular impairment, foot health rules, orthotics, and various types of shoes that decrease pressure on the foot.

Wells, R., and Trostle, K. January 1984. Creative hairwashing techniques for immobilized patients. *Nursing 84* 14:47–51.
    These authors include photographs that illustrate inventive ways to wash the hair of clients, including those confined to bed, those wearing cervical collars, braces, or halo vests; and those on Stryker frames.

RELATED RESEARCH

DeWalt, E. M., and Haines, Sr. A. K. January/February 1969. The effects of specified stressors on healthy oral mucosa. *Nursing Research* 18:22–27.

Poland, J. M. April 1987. Comparing moi-stir to lemon glycerin swabs. *American Journal of Nursing* 87:422,424.

SELECTED REFERENCES

Bates, B. 1987. *A guide to physical examination.* 4th ed. Philadelphia: J. B. Lippincott Co.

Blaney, G. M. September/October 1986. Mouth care—basic and essential, *Geriatric Nursing* 7:242–43.

Carden, R. G. February 1985. The ins and outs of contact lenses. *RN* 48:48–50.

Edelstein, J. E. December 1988. Foot care for the aging. *Physical Therapy* 68:1882–86.

Eliopoulos, C., editor, 1984. *Health assessment of the older adult.* Menlo Park, Calif.: Addison-Wesley Publishing Co.

Freinkel, R. K. July 1988. Caring for your skin. *Diabetes Forecast* 41:76–78, 81.

Gannon, E. D., and Kadezabek, E. March 1980. Giving your patients meticulous mouth care. *Nursing 80* 10:14–19.

Giles, S. F. 1972. Hair, the nursing process and the black patient *Nursing Forum* 11(1):78–88.

Hauk, L. September/October 1986. Enabling clients to manage dentures. *Geriatric Nursing* 7:254–55.

Holder, L., April 1982. Hearing aids: Handle with care. *Nursing 82* 12:64–67.

Joachim, G. April 1983. Step-by-step massage techniques. *Canadian Nurse* 79:32–33.

Kamenir, S., and Fothergill, R. December 1982. Hands-on skills for dealing with hearing aids. *Canadian Nurse* 78:44–45.

King, P. A. September/October 1980. Foot problems and assessment. *Geriatric Nursing* 1:182–86.

Longman, A. L. and Dewalt, E. M. September/October 1986. A guide for oral assessment: Nursing assistants working in long-term care facilities. *Geriatric Nursing* 7:252–53.

MacMillan, K. March 1981. New goals for oral hygiene. *Canadian Nurse* 77:40–43.

Marieb, E. N. 1989. *Human anatomy and physiology.* Redwood City, Calif.; Benjamin/Cummings.

Martin, B. J., and Reeb, R. M. November/December 1982. Oral health during pregnancy: A neglected nursing area. *American Journal of Maternal and Child Nursing* 7:391–92.

Meissner, J. E. April 1980. A simple guide for assessing oral health. *Nursing 80* 10:70–75 (Canadian ed., pp. 24–25).

Ofstehage, J. C., and Magilvy, K. September/October 1986. Oral health and aging. *Geriatric Nursing* 7:238–41.

Ophthalmic issues. April 1988. Facts and myths: Misconceptions about eye care. *American Association of Occupational Health Nurses Journal* 36:174–77.

Osguthorpe, N. C. October 1984. If your patient has contact lenses. *American Journal of Nursing* 84:1255–56.

Parrott, T. E. September/October 1987. Care of long hair. *Associate Degree Nurse* 2:8–10.

Pettigrew, D. January/February 1989. Investigating in mouth care. *Geriatric Nursing* 10:22–24.

Todd, B. March/April 1982. Drugs and the elderly: Dry mouth—causes and cures. *Geriatric Nursing* 3:122–23.

Wagnild, G., and Manning, R. W. December 1985. Convey respect during bathing procedures. *Journal of Gerontological Nursing* 11:6–10.

Wells, R., and Trostle, K. January 1984. Creative hairwashing techniques for immobilized patients. *Nursing 84* 14:47–51.

PROMOTING HEALTH THROUGH THE LIFESPAN

Health Promotion

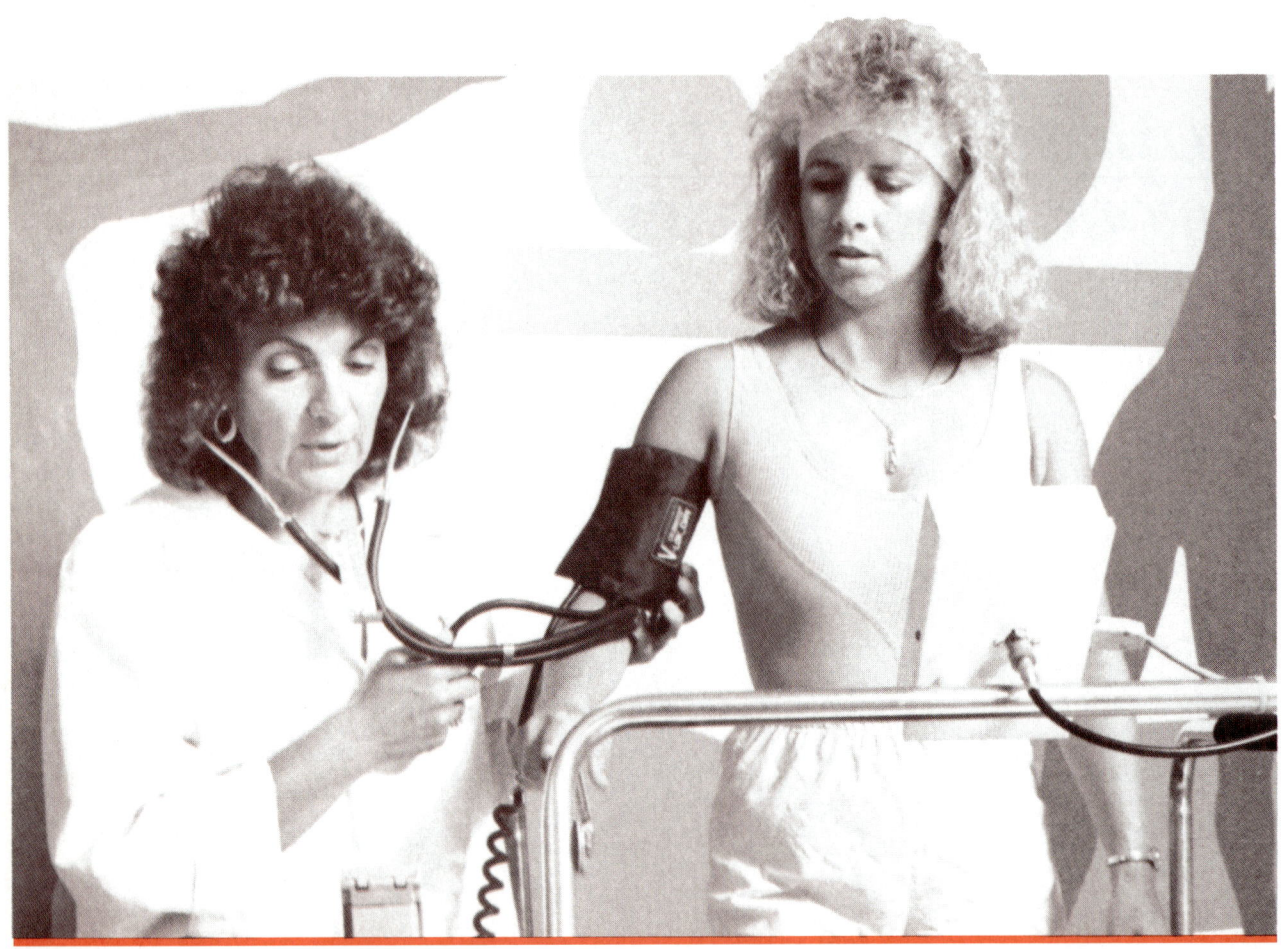

OBJECTIVES

▶ Explain the essential facts about health promotion.

▶ Compare Pender's concept of health promotion with that of Leavell and Clark.

▶ List the various types of health promotion programs.

▶ Describe the common sites for health promotion activities.

▶ Discuss the nurse's role in health promotion.

CONCEPT AND SCOPE OF HEALTH PROMOTION

Considerable differences appear in the literature regarding the use of the terms *health; wellness; health promotion; primary, secondary, and tertiary prevention; health protection;* and *illness prevention.* These differences are confusing to both health professionals and the consumers of health care services. Authors in nursing and the health care fields present different definitions of health promotion and primary prevention and offer different ideas about their application. See Table 23–1.

Leavell and Clark (1965, p. 21) define three levels of prevention: primary, secondary, and tertiary. There are five steps that describe these levels: (1) health promotion and (2) specific protection are *primary preventions;* (3) early diagnosis and (4) prompt treatment to limit disability are *secondary preventions;* and (5) restoration and rehabilitation are *tertiary preventions.*

In the model used by Leavell and Clark, primary prevention precedes any disease symptoms. The purpose of **primary prevention** is to encourage optimal health and to increase the person's resistance to illness (Edelman and Mandle 1986, p. 9). Examples of primary prevention include health education concerning the hazards of smoking and specific protection against a particular disease, such as the vaccine against poliomyelitis.

The second level, **secondary prevention,** presumes the presence of a disease or illness. Screening procedures, such as a blood sugar test for a client with diabetes mellitus, and the Denver Developmental Screening Tests to assess developmental delays, are facets of secondary prevention. Screening procedures facilitate early discovery and allow treatment to begin before the illness progresses. Disability limitation, another step in secondary prevention, is also more effective in the early stages of a disease.

Tertiary prevention relates to situations where a disability is already present. The goal of tertiary prevention is to restore individuals to their optimal level of functioning within the limitations imposed by their condition.

Pender (1987, p. 4) considers health promotion separate from primary prevention. She defines **health promotion** as "activities directed toward increasing the level of well being," and primary prevention as "activities directed toward decreasing the probability of specific illnesses." In this

TABLE 23–1 *Definitions of Health Promotion*

Author	Definition
Pender (1987)	Activities directed toward increasing the level of well being and actualizing the potential of individuals, families, and groups; a category separate from primary prevention
Leavell and Clark (1965)	Maintaining or improving the general level of health of individuals, families, and groups; part of primary prevention
Julius Richmond, U.S. Surgeon General (1979)	Individual and community activities to promote healthful lifestyles
Amelia Mangay Maglacas, Chief Nurse WHO (1988)	*Positive* health promotion is the process of enabling people to increase control over and improve their own health; aimed primarily at improving health potential and maintaining health balance

Sources: N. J. Pender, *Health promotion in nursing practice,* 2d ed. (Norwalk, Conn.: Appleton & Lange, 1987), p. 4; H. R. Leavell and E. G. Clark, *Preventive medicine for the doctor in the community,* 3d ed. (New York: McGraw-Hill, 1965), p. 21; *Healthy people: The Surgeon General's report on health promotion and disease prevention* (Washington, D. C.: U.S. Department of Health, Education, and Welfare, 1979), p. 119; A. M. Maglacas, Health for all: Nursing's role, *Nursing Outlook,* November 1988, 88:67.

instance, health promotion is considered to be an approach behavior, whereas primary prevention is considered avoidance behavior. Health promotion is not disease oriented; that is, no specific problem is being avoided. By contrast, primary prevention activities are geared toward avoiding specific problems (Pender 1987, p. 5). Having analyzed the terms used in the health promotion literature, Brubaker (1983, p. 4) agrees with Pender's definition and further argues that even dictionary definitions support differences between the terms health promotion and primary or illness prevention. Brubaker notes that promotion is geared to "helping and encouraging to flourish," whereas to prevent is defined as "to keep from occurring." For example, a 40-year-old male may begin a program of walking 3 miles each day. If the goal of his program is to "decrease the risk of heart disease," then the activity would be considered prevention. By contrast, if his walking regime is instituted to "increase his overall health and feeling of well being," then the activity would be considered health promotion behavior. Most authors do not take health promotion to mean simply the avoidance of risk factors or the maintenance of stability. Rather, health promotion is seen as being directed toward self-development, growth, and a high level of wellness (Brubaker 1983, pp. 4–5).

In a 1979 document called *Healthy People,* the Surgeon General of the United States differentiates health promotion, health protection, and preventive health services. He outlines specific activities for each category:

- *Health promotion*—individual and community activities to promote healthful life-styles. Examples of health promotion activities include improving nutrition, preventing alcohol and drug misuse, maintaining fitness, and exercising.

- *Health protection*—actions by government and industry to minimize environmental health threats. Health protection relates to activities such as maintaining occupational safety, controlling radiation and toxic agents, and preventing infectious diseases and accidents.

- *Preventive health services*—actions of health care providers to prevent health problems. These services include control of high blood pressure, control of sexually transmitted diseases, immunization, family planning, and health care during pregnancy and infancy.

The chief scientist for nursing from the World Health Organization (WHO), Amelia Mangay Maglacas, uses the terms *positive health* and *positive health promotion* and presents them in a broader context. According to Maglacas, *positive* health for all does not mean the eradication of every disease or the healing of every body part. Rather, health should be considered in the context of its contribution to social and economic development, so that all people have the necessary social and economic support to lead satisfying lives (1988, p. 67). *Positive* health promotion is the process of enabling people to improve and to increase their control over their own health. The aim of positive health promotion is the improvement of health potential and the maintenance of health balance. This goal of positive health is attained by caring for ourselves and for others, by controlling life's circumstances with careful and conscientious decision making, and by ensuring that conditions in society allow people to attain health.

Health promotion organizations, wellness centers, and traditional health care centers all offer a different approach to client care. Table 23–2 demonstrates these differences. Health promotion activities take place before any disease occurs and can be considered a part of primary prevention. Health promotion strategies are geared toward raising the level of the health and well-being of the individual, family, or community. These activities can be carried out on a governmental level (e.g., a national program to improve knowledge of nutrition) or on a personal level (e.g., an individual exercise program).

Health promotion programs on an individual level can be active or passive. With *passive* strategies, the client is a recipient of the health promotion effort. Many health professionals participate in national programs to define and institute these passive strategies. Examples of passive government strategies are maintaining the cleanliness of water

TABLE 23–2 *Focus of Traditional Health Care Contrasted with Health Promotion and Wellness*

	Traditional	Health Promotion	Wellness
Primary goal	Identify and correct problem	Disease prevention and risk reduction	Increased health
Dominant message	"Health care professionals will take care of you."	"You will live longer if you avoid illness."	"You are responsible, and your efforts to be well will be supported."
Change agent	Treatment	Information and behavior change	Positive experience and cultural influences
Target	The problem	Individuals, families, and communities	Clients within cultures
Duration of intervention	Ends when the problems clear up	Length of class or program	Ongoing

Source: Adapted from J. P. Opatz, *A primer of health promotion: Creating healthy organizational cultures* (Washington, D.C.: Oryn Publications, 1985), p. 101.

and promoting a healthy environment by enforcing sewage regulations to decrease the spread of disease. *Active* strategies depend on individuals' commitment to and involvement in adopting a program directed toward their health promotion. Active strategies are more important in that they encourage individuals to take control of their lives and assume the responsibility for their health. Examples of active strategies that involve changes in life-style are (1) a diet management program to improve nutrition, (2) a self-help program to reduce stress related to parenting, (3) an exercise program to improve muscle strength and endurance, or (4) a combination diet and exercise regime for weight reduction or control. For optimal health and well-being, a combination of both active and passive strategies is suggested (Edelman and Mandle 1986, p. 10).

Types of Health Promotion Programs

A variety of programs can be used for the promotion of health, including (1) information dissemination, (2) health appraisal and wellness assessment, (3) life-style and behavior change, (4) worksite wellness programs, and (5) environmental control programs.

Information dissemination is the most basic type of health promotion program. This method makes use of a variety of media to offer information to the public about the risk of particular life-style choices and personal behavior, as well as the benefits of changing that behavior and improving the quality of life. Billboards, posters, brochures, newspaper features, books, and health fairs all offer opportunities for the dissemination of health promotion information. Alcohol and drug abuse, driving under the influence of alcohol, good nutrition, and hypertension are some of the topics frequently discussed. Recently, information about AIDS, including how it is transmitted, techniques for prevention, and the issue of sexual responsibility, has been distributed. The intent is to reduce unjustified fear, correct misinformation, and educate the public about this disease. Information dissemination is a useful strategy for raising the level of knowledge and awareness of individuals and groups about health habits.

Health appraisal/wellness assessment programs are used to apprise individuals of the risk factors that are inherent in their lives in order to motivate them to reduce specific risks and develop positive health habits. Wellness assessment programs are focused on more positive methods of enhancement, in contrast to the risk factor approach used in the health appraisal. A variety of tools are available to facilitate these assessments. Some of these tools are computer based and can therefore be offered to educational institutions and industries at a reasonable cost.

Life-style and behavior change programs require the participation of the individual and are geared toward enhancing the quality of life and extending the life span. Individuals generally consider life-style changes after they have been informed of the need to change their health behavior and become aware of the potential benefits of the process. Many programs are available to the public, both on a group and individual basis, some of which address stress management, nutrition awareness, weight control, smoking cessation, and exercise.

Worksite wellness programs are found in a variety of settings and are generally developed to serve the needs of individuals spending a great deal of time in the work environment. These include programs that address air quality standards for the office, classroom, or plant; programs aimed at specific populations, such as accident prevention for the machine worker or back-saver programs for the individual involved in heavy lifting; programs to screen for high blood pressure; or health enhancement programs, such as fitness information and relaxation techniques.

Environmental control programs have been developed in response to the recent growth in the number of contaminants of human origin that have been introduced into our environment (Logan and Dawkins 1986, p. 313). The amount of contaminants that are already present in the air, food, and water will affect the health of our descendants for several generations. The most common concerns of community groups are toxic and nuclear wastes, nuclear power plants, air and water pollution, and herbicide and pesticide spraying.

Sites for Health Promotion Programs

Health promotion programs are found in many settings. Programs and activities may be offered to individuals and families in the home or in the community setting, at schools, hospitals, or worksites. Some individuals may feel more comfortable having the nurse, diet counselor, or fitness expert come to their home for teaching and following up individual needs. This type of program, however, is not cost-effective for most individuals. Many people prefer the group approach, find it more motivating, and enjoy the socializing and group support. Most programs offered in the community are group oriented.

Community programs are frequently offered by cities and towns. The type of program depends on the current concerns and the expertise of the sponsoring department or group. Program offerings may include health promotion, specific protection, and screening for early detection of disease. The local health department may offer a townwide immunization program or blood pressure screening. The fire department may disseminate fire prevention information; the police may offer a bicycle safety program for children or a safe-driving campaign for young adults.

Hospitals began the emphasis on health promotion and prevention by focusing on the health of their employees. Because of the stress involved in caring for the sick and the various shifts that nurses and other health care workers must work, the life-styles and health habits of health care employees was seen as a priority.

Programs offered by health care organizations initially began with the specific focus of prevention, i.e., infection control, fire prevention and fire drills, limiting exposure to x rays, and the prevention of back injuries. Gradually, issues related to the health and life-style of the employee were addressed with programs such as smoking cessation, exercise and fitness, stress reduction, and time management. Increasingly, hospitals have offered a variety of these programs and others (e.g., women's health) to the community as well as to their employees. This community activity of the health care institution enhances the public image of the hospital, increases the health of the surrounding population, and generates some additional income.

School health promotion programs may serve as a foundation for children of all ages to learn basic knowledge about personal hygiene and issues in the health sciences. Because school is the focus of a child's life for so many years, the school provides a cost-effective and convenient setting for health-focused programs. The school nurse may teach programs about basic nutrition, dental care, activity and play, drug and alcohol abuse, domestic violence, child abuse, and issues related to sexuality and pregnancy. Classroom teachers may include health-related topics in their lesson plans, e.g., the way the normal heart functions or the need for clean air and water in the environment.

Worksite programs for health promotion have developed out of the need for businesses to control the rising cost of health care and employee absenteeism (Greiner 1987, p. 53). Many industries feel that both employers and employees can benefit from healthy life-style behavior. The convenience of the worksite setting makes these programs particularly attractive to many adults who would otherwise not be aware of them or motivated to attend them. Health promotion programs may be held in the company cafeteria so that employees can watch a film or have a discussion group during their lunch break. Program offerings include diet, relaxation techniques, or physical fitness. Benefits to the worker may include an increased feeling of well-being, fitness, weight control, and decreased stress. Benefits to the employer may include an increase in employee motivation and productivity, an increase in employee morale, a decrease in absenteeism, and a lower rate of employee turnover, all of which may decrease business and health care costs.

The Nurse's Role in Health Promotion

Changes in the health care system, the demands of society, environmental and social issues, and the increased use of modern technology have all affected the role of the nurse. Clients are spending less time in acute care facilities. The focus is shifting to community and preventive nursing services. Nurses, as the largest group of health care workers, must prepare for the shift in emphasis and anticipate the nursing services that consumers will require. The nurse

---

The Nurse's Role in Health Promotion

- Model healthy life-style behaviors and attitudes.
- Facilitate client involvement in the assessment, implementation, and evaluation of health goals.
- Teach clients self-care strategies to enhance fitness, improve nutrition, manage stress, and enhance relationships.
- Assist individuals, families, and communities to increase their levels of health.
- Teach clients to be effective health care consumers.
- Assist clients, families, and communities to develop and choose health-promoting options.
- Guide clients' development in effective problem solving and decision making.
- Reinforce clients' personal and family health-promoting behaviors.
- Advocate in the community for changes that promote a healthy environment.

---

may act as advocate, consultant, teacher, or coordinator of services. For examples of the nurse's role in health promotion, see the accompanying box. In this role, the nurse may work with all age groups or be limited to a specific population, e.g., new parents, school-age children, or senior citizens. In any case, the nursing process is a basic tool for the nurse in a health promotion role. Although the process is the same, the emphasis is on teaching the client self-care responsibility. The clients decide the goals, determine the health promotion plans, and take the responsibility for the success of the plans. The steps of the nursing process in health promotion are health assessment, formulation of a nursing diagnosis, development of a health promotion/protection plan, implementation of the plan, and evaluation.

ASSESSING

A thorough assessment of the client's health status is basic to health promotion. Components of this assessment are the health history and physical examination, physical-fitness assessment, nutrition assessment, health risk appraisal, life-style assessment, health beliefs review, and life-stress review (Pender 1987, p. 103). As nurses move toward greater autonomy in providing client care, expanded assessment skills are essential to provide the meaningful data needed for health planning.

Health History and Physical Examination

The health history and physical examination provide a means for detecting any existing problems. See Chapter 19 for detailed information about the health history and physical examination.

Physical-Fitness Assessment

During an evaluation of physical fitness, the nurse takes girth and skinfold measurements, administers the step test, and assesses strength and endurance of muscles and flexibility of joints.

Girth Measurements   The nurse measures the girth of the chest, waist, hips, upper arm (biceps), thigh, calf, and ankle. Guidelines for appropriate body proportions are shown in Table 23–3.

Skinfold Measurements   Skinfold measurements indicate the amount of body fat. To take skinfold measurements, the nurse grasps the skinfold (skin layers and subcutaneous fat) between the thumb and forefinger and measures the skinfold with special calipers. Skinfold sites are the triceps, subscapula, suprailiac, and thigh. See Chapter 39 for further information about skinfold procedures and norms.

The Step Test   For this test, the client steps up and down a 17-inch step for 3 minutes. The following movements constitute one step: left foot up, right foot up, left foot down, right foot down. The rate should be 24 steps per minute for women and 30 steps for men (Getchell 1979, pp. 72–73). After the test, the client sits in a chair while the nurse assesses the pulse rate for 30 seconds at prescribed intervals:

1. 1 to 1½ minutes after the test
2. 2 to 2½ minutes after the test
3. 3 to 3½ minutes after the test

The sum of these three 30-second pulse rates is referred to as the **recovery index.** Normal values for women are 154–170; for men, 149–165 (Getchell 1979, pp. 72–73).

Muscle Strength and Endurance   There are several tests of muscle strength and endurance. One is performing sit-ups with knees bent (bent-knee sit-ups). Women are asked to do these for 1 minute; men, for 2 minutes. The average rate for women is about 20 to 25 sit-ups per minute; for men, 50 to 60 per 2 minutes (Getchell 1979, p. 56).

Joint Flexibility   Range of motion in joints can be assessed quickly by asking the person to touch the toes several times. The average touch point is 1 to 3 inches in front of the toes. See Chapter 35 for detailed discussion of joint range of motion.

Nutritional Assessment

To assess nutritional status, the nurse compares the client's weight to body build and height (see Chapter 19), measures mid-upper arm circumference to determine muscle mass, observes for signs of malnutrition, and takes a dietary history. The latter three are discussed in Chapter 39.

Health Risk Appraisal

A **health risk appraisal** (HRA) or health hazard appraisal (HHA) is an assessment and educational tool that indicates a client's risk of disease or injury over the next 10 years by comparing the client's risk with the mortality risk of the corresponding age, sex, and racial group. The client's health behavior and demographic data are compared to behaviors of and data about a large national sample. The principle behind risk appraisal is that each person, as a member of a specific group, faces certain quantifiable health hazards and that average risks are applicable to a client if the health professional knows the client's characteristics and the mortality of a large group of cohorts with similar characteristics (Pender 1987, p. 119).

Many HRA instruments are available today. In 1970, Drs. Lewis Robbins and Jack Hall used the medical health model to develop an HRA called Health Hazard Appraisal. Since that time, other health care groups have adapted this tool and marketed it under several names. More recently HRAs have begun to reflect a broader approach to health. The

TABLE 23–3   *Guidelines for Appropriate Girth Measurements*

	Males	Females
Chest or bust	Same size as hips	Same size as hips
Waist	About 13 to 18 cm less than chest	About 25 cm less than bust
Upper arm	Twice the wrist size	Twice the wrist size
Thigh	20 to 25 cm less than abdomen	15 cm less than abdomen
Calf	18 to 20 cm less than thigh	15 to 18 cm less than thigh
Ankle	15 to 18 cm less than calf	13 to 15 cm less than calf

Source: N. J. Pender, *Health promotion in nursing practice,* 2d ed. (Norwalk, Conn.: Appleton & Lange, 1987), p. 112. Used by permission.

new focus is on the assessment of life-style factors and health behaviors. The objectives of most HRAs are twofold:

1. To assess risk factors that may lead to health problems. A **risk factor** is a phenomenon (e.g., age or life-style behavior) that increases a person's chance of acquiring a specific disease. The concept of at-risk aggregate is increasingly being used in community nursing practice. An **at-risk aggregate** is a subgroup within the community or population that is at greater risk of illness or poor recovery (Logan and Dawkins 1986, p. 18).

2. To change health behaviors that place the client at risk of developing an illness.

An HRA may have from 25 to 300 or more questions. Clients either score their responses themselves or send them to an organization for computer printouts. Scores are often tabulated according to an overall life-style profile, levels of health risk, and life expectancy.

Risk factors may be categorized according to (a) age, (b) genetic factors, (c) biologic characteristics, (d) personal health habits, (e) life-style, and (f) environment. Clients cannot control some of the risk factors appraised, such as age, sex, and family history; others, such as blood pressure, stress, and cigarette smoking, can be partially or totally controlled.

Pender (1987, pp. 123–130) developed a comprehensive risk factor assessment tool. She classifies risk factors into five categories: (a) risk of cardiovascular disease, (b) risk of malignant disease, (c) risk of automobile accidents, (d) risk of suicide, and (e) risk of diabetes. Contributing factors, such as family and personal medical history, habits, sex, age, environment, and life-style patterns, are included. See Figure 23–1 for part of Pender's risk appraisal form, i.e., the section related to risk of cardiovascular disease.

A client is usually appraised as being at high risk of developing a specific disease when two or three of the risk factors are at the highest level or four of the risk factors are at the two highest levels.

Life-Style Assessment

Life-style assessment focuses on the personal life-style and habits of the client as they affect health. Categories of life-style generally assessed are physical activity, nutritional practices, stress management, and such habits as smoking, alcohol consumption, and drug use. Other categories may be included.

Several tools are available to assess life-style. Pender (1987, pp. 138–143) outlines a comprehensive 10-category, 100-item tool that includes the following:

1. Competence in self-care, including dental hygiene, breast self-examination, knowledge about the danger signs of cancer, blood pressure, and other health care practices

2. Nutritional practices

3. Physical or recreational activity

4. Sleep patterns

5. Stress management

6. Self-actualization, including outlook on life and feelings about self, work, and accomplishments

7. Sense of purpose in life and knowledge of what is important in one's life

8. Relationships with others

9. Environmental control to make living areas free of hazards

10. Use of the health care system

The number of statements in each category range from 4 to 16. The reader is referred to Pender 1987 (see Selected References) for detailed information.

Walker, Sechrist, and Pender (1987) have developed the Health-Promoting Lifestyle Profile (HPLP), a 48-item tool that measures six dimensions of a healthy life-style: nutrition, exercise, health responsibility, stress management, interpersonal support, and self actualization. This tool allows researchers to investigate patterns of a healthy life-style and measure the effects of health promoting interventions.

Ryan and Travis (1981) have developed a shorter, 16-item life-style assessment form entitled the Wellness Index. This tool may be used for initial assessments when client time is limited. See Figure 23–2 on page 571.

The goals of life-style assessment tools are

1. To provide an opportunity for clients to assess the impact of their present life-style on their health

2. To provide a basis for decisions related to desired behavior and life-style change.

Health Care Beliefs

Clients' health care beliefs need to be clarified, particularly those beliefs that determine how they perceive control of their own health care status.

Locus of control is a concept from social learning theory. It is also relevant when determining who is most likely to take action regarding health, i.e., whether clients believe that their health status is under their own or others' control. People who believe that they have a major influence on their own health status, i.e., who believe health is largely self-determined, are called *internals*. Persons who are internally controlled are more likely than others to take the initiative in their own health care, be more knowledgeable about their health, and adhere to prescribed health care regimens. By contrast, people who believe their health is largely controlled by outside forces (e.g., chance, luck, or powerful others) and is beyond their control are referred to as *externals*. Edelman and Mandle (1986, p. 53) suggest that externally controlled people may need assistance to become more internally controlled if behavior changes are to be successful.

In each row, place a check in the box that best describes your current life situation or behavior.

Risk for Cardiovascular Disease

Risk factor:		Increasing risk ⟶					
Sex and age:		Female under 40	Female 40–50	Male 25–40	Female after menopause	Male 40–60	Male 61 or over
Family history (mother, father, brothers, sisters)	High blood pressure	No relatives with condition		One relative		Two relatives	Three relatives
	Heart attack	No relatives with condition	One relative with condition after 60	Two relatives with condition after 60	One relative with condition before 60	Two relatives with condition before 60	
	Diabetes	No relatives with condition		One or more relatives with maturity onset diabetes		One or more relatives with preadolescent or adolescent onset	
Blood pressure*	Systolic	120 or below	121–140	141–160	161–180	181–200	above 200
	Diastolic	70 or below	71–80	81–90	91–100	101–110	above 110

Risk factor:		Increasing risk ⟶				
Diabetes*		No diagnosis	Maturity onset, controlled	Maturity onset, uncontrolled	Adolescent onset, controlled	Adolescent onset, uncontrolled
Weight*		At or slightly below recommended weight	10% overweight	20% overweight	30% overweight	40% overweight	50% overweight
Cholesterol*† level (mg/100 ml)		Below 180	181–200	201–220	221–240	241–260	261–280	Above 280
Serum triglycerides* (mg/100 ml) fasting		150 or below		151–400		401–1000	Above 1000
Percent of fat in diet*		20–30%		31–40%		41–50%	Above 50%
Frequency of exercise*	Recreational	Intensive recreational exertion (35–45 min at least 4 times/wk)		Moderate recreational exertion		Minimal recreational exertion	No recreational exertion
	Occupational	Intensive occupational exertion		Moderate occupational exertion		Minimal occupational exertion	Sedentary occupation

Figure 23–1 Risk assessment tool for cardiovascular disease. *Source:* N. J. Pender, *Health promotion in nursing practice,* 2d ed. (Norwalk, Conn.: Appleton & Lange, 1987), pp. 123–125. Used by permission.

In each row, place a check in the box that best describes your current life situation or behavior.						
Risk for Cardiovascular Disease						
Sleep patterns*		7 or 8 hr sleep/night		More than 8 hr sleep/night		4–6 hr sleep/night
Cigarette smoking*	No./day	Nonsmoker	1–10/day	11–20/day	21–30/day	31–40/day Over 40/day
	No. of yr smoked	Nonsmoker	Less than 10 yr	11–15 yr	16–20 yr	21–30 yr 31 yr or more
Stress*	Domestic	Minimal	Moderate		High	Very high
	Occupational	Minimal	Moderate		High	Very high
Behavior pattern* (particularly males)		**Type B** Relaxed, appropriately assertive, not time dependent, moderate to slow speech		**Type A** Excessively competitive, aggressive, striving, hyperalert, time dependent, loud, explosive speech		
Air pollution*		Low		Moderate		High
Use of oral contraceptives* (females)		Do not use oral contraceptives		Under 40 and use oral contraceptives		Over 40 and use oral contraceptives
*Indicates risk factors that can be fully or partially controlled. †Serum lipid analysis is also recommended to determine low-density (beta) and high-density (alpha) lipoprotein levels. Evidence suggests that high-density lipoprotein (HDL) carries cholesterol from tissues for metabolism and excretion. An inverse correlation appears to exist between HDL and coronary artery disease.						

Figure 23–1   Risk assessment tool for cardiovascular disease *(continued)*

Locus of control is a measurable concept that can be used to predict which people are most likely to change their behavior. Wallston, Wallston, and DeVellis (1978) have developed two Multidimensional Health Locus of Control (MHLC) instruments to assess perceptions of health control. See Figure 23–3 on page 572 for one such instrument. Assessment of clients' health care beliefs provides the nurse with an indication of how much the clients believe they can influence or control health through personal behaviors.

The results of a study by Lewis suggest that greater personal control over one's life is associated with higher levels of self-esteem, greater purpose in life, and decreased self-report of anxiety (Lewis 1982, p. 113). Nurses can use this information about a client's locus of control to plan internal reinforcement training if necessary in order to improve client compliance. However, according to Shillinger (1983, p. 63):

> Greater emphasis should be placed on assisting the client to make his own informed decisions, helping to identify and find solutions to problems that may interfere with compliance, and giving support and guidance as needed. In essence, this means building a partnership, an alliance, with the client rather than having compliance as the major goal.

The Health Belief Model (HBM) discussed in Chapter 5 on page 92 suggests that the motivation to engage in a behavior is based on the person's belief that (a) one is vulnerable to the health problem, (b) the illness or problem is a threat, (c) the recommended health action will reduce the threat without substantial inconvenience, and (d) people should be generally concerned about health matters and be willing to accept medical advice (Becker et al. 1972, p. 852). The HBM is focused on susceptibility to disease and is therefore considered appropriate to explain health-protecting or preventive behaviors. It is not considered an appropriate model for health promoting behaviors.

Researchers have not been able to validate a significant association between a person's health beliefs and behaviors (Muhlencamp et al. 1985, p. 327). Cox (1985, p. 178) therefore has developed a new measure of motivation called the Health Self-Determination Index (HSDI). She believes that motivation is multidimensional, i.e., based on many factors. The process of choosing between behaviors is a primary factor.

Cox's HSDI includes a 20-item scale that has four interrelated subscales or factors:

1. *Self-determined health judgments.* Self-determinism in health judgments is assessed by the client's responses to statements such as:

   "Whatever the doctor suggests is OK with me."

Circle the category that most closely answers the question.

1. I am conscious of the ingredients of the food I eat and their effect on me.   Rarely, Sometimes, Very Often (R, S, VO)
2. I avoid overeating and abusing alcohol, caffeine, nicotine, and other drugs.   R, S, VO
3. I minimize my intake of refined carbohydrates and fats.   R, S, VO
4. My diet contains adequate amounts of vitamins, minerals, and fiber.   R, S, VO
5. I am free from physical symptoms.   R, S, VO
6. I get aerobic cardiovascular exercise.   R, S, VO   (Very Often is at least 12–20 minutes 5 times per week vigorously running, swimming, or bike riding)
7. I practice yoga or some other form of limbering/stretching exercise.   R, S, VO
8. I nurture myself.   R, S, VO   (Nurturing means pleasuring and taking care of oneself, for example, massages, long walks, buying presents for self, "doing nothing," sleeping late without feeling guilty, etc.)
9. I pay attention to changes occurring in my life and am aware of them as stress factors.   R, S, VO   (See Life-Change Index—a score of over 300 is considered very stressful)
10. I practice regular relaxation.   R, S, VO   (Suggested: 20 minutes a day "centering" or "letting go" of thoughts, worries, etc.)
11. I am without excess muscle tension.   R, S, VO
12. My hands are warm and dry.   R, S, VO
13. I am both productive and happy.   R, S, VO
14. I constructively express my emotions and creativity.   R, S, VO
15. I feel a sense of purpose in life and my life has meaning and direction.   R, S, VO
16. I believe I am fully responsible for my wellness or illness.   R, S, VO

Using your answers at the left to guide you, you can synthesize a graphic picture of your wellness. Each numbered pie-shaped segment of the circle below corresponds to the same numbered question on the preceding page. (They are divided into quarters representing four major dimensions of wellness.) Color in an amount of each segment corresponding to your answer to the question with the same number. The inner broken circle corresponds to "rarely," the next one to "sometimes," and third to "very often." You don't need to restrict yourself to these categories, however, and can fill in any amount in between. You may use different colors for each section if you like.

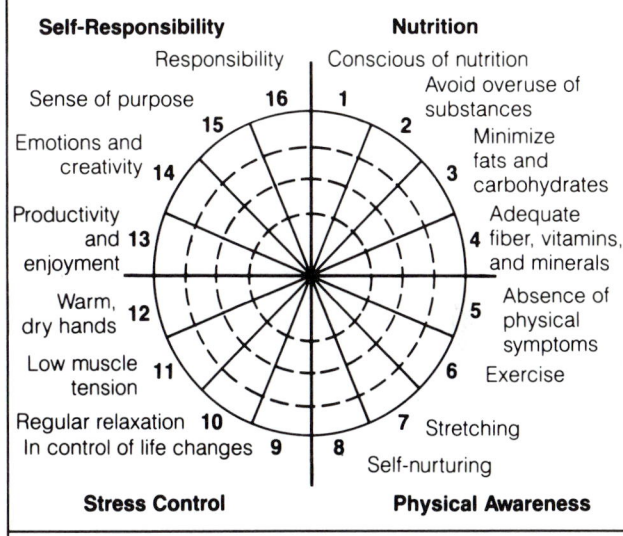

Now look at the shape of your index. Is it lopsided or balanced? This should provide beginning suggestions for improving your lifestyle and health habits.

Figure 23–2   Wellness index.   *Source:*   R. S. Ryan and J. W. Travis, *Wellness workbook for health professionals* (Berkeley, Calif.: Ten Speed Press, 1981). Used by permission.

"Only the doctor knows if I am in good health."

"What the doctor thinks is more important than what I think."

"I do things to help my health without a doctor's or nurse's input."

2. *Self-determined health behavior.* Self-determinism in health behavior is assessed by the client's responses to statements such as:

"I know without a doctor's telling me so that I'm doing the right things for my health."

"I know without someone telling me so when I am in good health."

"My own ideas are better than the doctor's."

"I know what I am doing when it comes to taking care of my health."

3. *Perceived competency in health matters.* Perceived com-

petency is determined by the client's responses to statements such as:

"I feel good about how I take care of my health."

"I do things to help my health without a doctor's or nurse's input."

"I don't do as well at taking care of my health as others."

4. *Responsiveness to internal and external cues.* Responsiveness is measured by response to statements such as:

"Some people think the doctor should decide about their health, but I think I should."

"I worry about my health."

"I'm never sure I'm doing the right things for my health unless I check with a doctor."

Although this tool has not been tested sufficiently to be used as a diagnostic aid, the data obtained in Cox's study

This questionnaire is designed to determine the way in which different people view certain important health-related issues. Each item is a belief statement with which you may agree or disagree. Beside each statement is a scale that ranges from strongly disagree (1) to strongly agree (6). For each item we would like you to circle the number that represents the extent to which you disagree or agree with the statement. The more strongly you agree with a statement, the higher will be the number you circle. The more strongly you disagree with a statement, the lower will be the number you circle. Please make sure that you answer every item and that you circle *only one* number per item. This is a measure of your personal beliefs; obviously, there are no right or wrong answers.

Please answer these items carefully, but do not spend too much time on any one item. As much as you can, try to respond to each item independently. When making your choice, do not be influenced by your previous choices. It is important that you respond according to your actual beliefs and not according to how you feel you should believe or how you think we want you to believe.

**1 = Strongly Disagree; 2 = Moderately Disagree;
3 = Slightly Disagree; 4 = Slightly Agree;
5 = Moderately Agree; 6 = Strongly Agree.**

1. If I become sick, I have the power to make myself well again.   1 2 3 4 5 6
2. Often I feel that no matter what I do, if I am going to get sick, I will get sick.   1 2 3 4 5 6
3. If I see an excellent doctor regularly, I am less likely to have health problems.   1 2 3 4 5 6
4. It seems that my health is greatly influenced by accidental happenings.   1 2 3 4 5 6
5. I can only maintain my health by consulting health professionals.   1 2 3 4 5 6
6. I am directly responsible for my health.   1 2 3 4 5 6
7. Other people play a big part in whether I stay healthy or become sick   1 2 3 4 5 6
8. Whatever goes wrong with my health is my own fault.   1 2 3 4 5 6
9. When I am sick, I just have to let nature run its course.   1 2 3 4 5 6
10. Health professionals keep me healthy.   1 2 3 4 5 6
11. When I stay healthy, I'm just plain lucky.   1 2 3 4 5 6
12. My physical well-being depends on how well I take care of myself.   1 2 3 4 5 6
13. When I feel ill, I know it is because I have not been taking care of myself properly.   1 2 3 4 5 6
14. The type of care I receive from other people is what is responsible for how well I recover from an illness.   1 2 3 4 5 6
15. Even when I take care of myself, it's easy to get sick.   1 2 3 4 5 6
16. When I become ill, it's a matter of fate.   1 2 3 4 5 6
17. I can pretty much stay healthy by taking good care of myself.   1 2 3 4 5 6
18. Following doctor's orders to the letter is the best way for me to stay healthy.   1 2 3 4 5 6

Figure 23–3   Multidimensional health locus of control scale (Form B).   *Source:* K. A. Wallston, B. S. Wallston, and R. DeVellis, Development of multidimensional health locus of control (MHLC) scales, *Health Education Monographs,* Spring 1978, 6:164–65.

strongly support the multidimensionality of motivation and the contributing roles of judgment, behavior, sense of competency, and responsiveness to internal or external cues. With further refinement and research, the HSDI will enable nurses to (Cox 1985, p. 182)

- Identify people at risk for decreased health and well-being owing to specific motivational responses
- Examine the motivational responses of clients throughout the life span for trends and changes
- Evaluate the differential effects of chronic versus acute illness on a person's motivational response
- Examine the effectiveness of interventions on specific health outcomes

Life-Stress Review

There is abundant literature about the impact of stress on mental and physical well-being. Assessment of stressors, signs of anxiety, and stress is discussed in Chapter 33.

Validation of Assessment Data

Following the collection of assessment data, the nurse and client need to review, validate, and summarize the information. This step is carried out jointly by the nurse and the client. During this process, the nurse verbally reviews the current practices and attitudes of the client. This allows validation of the information by the client and may increase awareness of the need to change behavior. The following information should be considered (Pender 1987, p. 214):

- Any existing health problems
- The client's perceived degree of control over health status
- Level of physical fitness and nutritional status
- Illnesses for which the client is at risk
- Current positive health practices
- Ability to handle stress
- Information needed to enhance health care practices

DIAGNOSING

Following assessment, validation, and summarizing of data, nursing diagnoses are identified. The nurse and client may agree on potential nursing diagnoses that will assist the client in decreasing the risk of developing specific diseases. Diagnoses such as **Altered nutrition: potential for more**

than body requirements are meaningful to a client who is interested in decreasing the risk factors related to cardiac disease.

Nursing diagnoses accepted by NANDA (North American Nursing Diagnosis Association) have generally focused on altered health patterns. Nurses caring for basically healthy individuals would find it necessary to use statements such as **Potential altered nutrition** to describe a healthy client on a moderate weight-loss program, or **Potential altered parenting** to describe new parents wanting information about child care. Houldin, Saltstein, and Ganley find the use of problem-oriented diagnoses somewhat inappropriate for a healthy population and suggest using a wellness-oriented classification system. Nursing diagnoses statements that describe motivational and wellness behaviors will identify client strengths, recognize self-care potential, reinforce healthy life-styles, assist the nurse in providing comprehensive, meaningful nursing care, and achieve the goals of health promotion and the prevention of illness (1987, pp. 16–17).

Wellness- or strength-oriented diagnoses can be applied at all levels of prevention but are particularly useful in primary care settings such as schools, industries, clinics, and community health facilities. When the nurse and client conclude that the client has positive function in a certain pattern area, such as adequate nutrition or effective coping, the nurse can use this information to help the client reach a higher level of functioning. Some examples of wellness nursing diagnoses adapted from Houdin, Saltstein, and Ganley (1987) are listed in the box in the left column. NANDA nursing diagnoses written as *potential* diagnostic statements can also direct activities related to health promotion. See the examples of NANDA diagnoses in the box below.

Wellness Nursing Diagnoses

- Appropriate health maintenance related to balanced pattern of activity and rest
- Potential for adequate health maintenance related to good parenting skills
- Potential for adequate safety precautions related to knowledge of unsafe and unhealthy practices
- Adequate nutrition for body requirements related to support of spouse and awareness of balance between nutrition and exercise
- Satisfactory bowel elimination related to effective intestinal function and adequate fluids
- Optimal physical fitness related to regular exercise routine and motivation
- Potential for adequate physical fitness related to motivation
- Effective sleep pattern related to ability to fall asleep and adjust to interruptions in sleep
- Potential for successful coping of diminished sensory abilities related to willingness to change and ability to develop new coping skills
- Productive family processes related to adequate physical health of family members and ability to accept family responsibilities
- Positive social functioning related to personal maturity and respect for others
- Satisfactory sexual functioning related to healthy relationship with spouse
- Adequate personal coping related to appropriate emotional control and balance of work and recreational activities

---

NANDA Nursing Diagnoses Related to Health Promotion

- Health-seeking behaviors related to new role as parent
- Health-seeking behaviors related to optimal nutrition for age and body size
- Altered nutrition: More than body requirements related to young-adult eating habits and adjustment to college life
- Altered nutrition: Less than body requirements related to lack of scheduled meals
- Potential altered health maintenance related to tobacco use
- Potential altered health maintenance related to insufficient finances
- Potential altered growth and development related to school-related stressors
- Potential diversional activity deficit related to post-retirement status
- Potential ineffective individual coping related to new parenting role
- Potential decisional conflict related to college and career choices
- Potential altered sexuality patterns related to job stress
- Potential for injury related to knowledge deficit of environmental hazards
- Potential impaired adjustment related to divorce and inadequate support from family members
- Potential activity intolerance related to lack of motivation

PLANNING

During the diagnosis phase of the health promotion process, the client has determined areas of potential problems and risks as well as areas of strength or positive health. The client then determines a health promotion plan. Health promotion plans need to be developed according to the needs, desires, and priorities of the client. The client decides on health promotion goals, the activities or interventions to achieve those goals, the frequency and duration of the activities, and the method of evaluation. During the planning process the nurse acts as a resource person rather than as an adviser or counselor. The nurse provides information when asked, emphasizes the importance of small steps to behavioral change, and reviews the client's goals and plans to make sure they are realistic, measurable, and acceptable to the client.

Steps in Planning

Pender (1987, p. 214) outlines several steps in the process of health promotion planning, which are carried out jointly by the nurse and the client:

1. *Identify health care goals.* The client selects two or three top priority goals or areas for improvement. Common goals are:
   a. To reduce the risk of cardiovascular disease
   b. To achieve or maintain a desired weight
   c. To improve or increase physical fitness
   d. To initiate and maintain relationships with a peer group
   e. To adjust to life-style changes effectively
   f. To decrease the amount of tobacco use
   g. To maintain an optimal balance between activity and rest
   h. To increase knowledge of safety practices in the home
   i. To improve relationships with family members

2. *Identify possible behavior changes.* For each of the selected goals or areas in step 1, determine what specific behavioral changes are needed to bring about the desired outcome. For example, to reduce the risk of cardiovascular disease, the client may need to change these specific behaviors:
   a. Stop smoking
   b. Lose weight
   c. Increase activity level
   d. Learn to relax
   e. Decrease animal fat in diet
   f. Discontinue use of oral contraceptives
   g. Sleep 7 to 8 hours per night

3. *Assign priorities to behavior changes.* Behavior must be acceptable to the client if it is to be adopted and integrated. From the list of behavior options in step 2, the clients select and assign priorities to those changes they are most willing to try. For example, the client may select

increasing activity level, losing weight, and stopping smoking, in that order. It is helpful if the client first selects a behavior change area in which change is most readily perceived as positive. A successful beginning experience is important.

4. *Make a commitment to change behavior.* In the past, commitments to change behavior have usually been verbal. Increasingly, a formal, written **behavioral contract** is being used to motivate the client to follow through with selected actions. Motivation to follow through is provided by a positive reinforcement or reward stated in the contract. Contracting is based on the belief that all persons have the potential for growth and the right of self-determination, even though their choices may be different from the norm. Contracts are of two types: nurse-client contracts or self-contracts. Here is a sample of a self-contract:

   I, Amy Martin will exercise strenuously for 20 minutes three times per week for a period of 2 weeks and will then buy myself six yellow roses.

   > Amy Martin
   > July 30, 1991

   To ensure that a contract is explicit and meaningful, Kort (1984, p. 25) recommends that the client review it against the SMART checklist:

   Specific: Do I know how, when, where, with whom, and how long I will do this?

   Measurable: Will I know when it's done?

   Acceptable: Will I feel good about doing this?

   Realistic: Am I able to do this?

   Truthful: Do I really want to?

   Before a contract can be made, the client needs to identify actions that will bring about the desired behavior change. If, for example, the behavior change is to increase activity level, the client needs to consider and adopt specific actions. The client may consider swimming for 30 minutes three times a week, walking briskly for 1 hour daily, or some similar activity.

5. *Identify effective reinforcements and rewards.* Rewards tend to provide an incentive for behavior change, more so than individual willpower, provided the reward is meaningful to and selected by the client. Rewards can be objects, experiences, family activities, or praise. Examples of objects used as rewards are books, educational pamphlets, and personal care items. Examples of experiences used as rewards are having a 15-minute talk with a consultant, renting a cassette about a specific health matter, or going to a concert or health spa. Family trips, sports, or picnics are strong reinforcement for some people.

6. *Determine barriers to change.* Some specific barriers to change are
   a. Lack of support from family members

b. Lack of space to carry out a certain activity
c. Inappropriate weather
d. Lack of motivation
e. Fatigue or boredom
f. Strong anxiety
g. Cost of change
h. Inconvenience
i. Lack of time
j. Culture or peer pressure

7. *Develop a schedule for implementing the behavior change.* Clients need to set up a time frame to make the behavior changes required to meet each goal. Time frames may be several weeks or months. Scheduling short-term goals and rewards can offer encouragement to achieve long-term objectives. Clients may need help to be realistic and to deal with one behavior at a time.

Exploring Available Resources

Another essential aspect of planning is identifying support resources available to the client. These may be community resources, such as a fitness program at a local gymnasium, or educational programs, such as stress management, breast self-examination, nutrition, smoking cessation, and health lectures. The nurse, too, may meet some of the client's educational needs. A major nursing role is to support the client. The nurse can contact the client or be available at specified intervals to review the contract and to assist with problem solving.

IMPLEMENTING

Implementing is the "doing" part of behavior change. Self-responsibility is emphasized for implementing the plan. The client, therefore, is the primary decision maker, seeking out the expertise of the nurse where it will assist in goal achievement. The strategies to be used, their frequency, and the priorities have all been determined in the plan. To increase the likelihood of a successful implementation, the nurse ascertains that the assessment has been accurate and complete and that the goals are individualized and attainable. Depending on the clients' needs, the nursing strategies may include supporting, teaching, consulting, coordinating, facilitating, counseling, and enhancing the behavior change.

Providing and Facilitating Support

A vital component of life-style change is ongoing support that focuses on the desired behavior change and is provided in a nonjudgmental manner. Support can be offered by the nurse on an individual basis or in a group setting. The nurse can also facilitate the development of support networks for the client, such as family members and friends.

Individual counseling sessions Counseling sessions may be routinely scheduled as part of the plan or may be provided if the client encounters difficulty in carrying out interventions or meets insurmountable barriers to change. In a counseling relationship, the nurse and client share ideas. In this sharing relationship, the nurse acts as a facilitator, promoting the client's decision making regarding the health promotion plan.

Telephone counseling Regular telephone sessions may be provided to the client to help in answering questions, reviewing goals and strategies, and reinforcing progress. The client may find that scheduling a weekly telephone session is helpful or may wish to initiate a call if a problem occurs. The client is asked, "Is your plan working?" If the plan is not working, the nurse asks, "What would you like to do?" The client may wish to continue or may wish to change the plan to a more realistic one. Telephone support is efficient for the busy client who may not have the time for regular, in-person sessions.

Group support Group sessions provide an opportunity for participants to learn the experiences of others in changing behavior. Group contact gives individuals a renewed commitment to their goals. Groups can be scheduled at monthly or less frequent intervals for over a year.

Facilitating social support Social networks, such as families and friends, can facilitate or impede the efforts directed toward health promotion and prevention. The nurse's role is to assist the client to assess, modify, and develop the social support necessary to achieve the desired change (Pender 1987, p. 393). In order to provide the necessary support, families must communicate effectively, be aware of and support each other's needs and goals, and provide help and assistance to one another to achieve those goals. The client may wish the nurse to meet with the family or significant others and help in enlisting their understanding and support.

Providing Health Education

Health education programs on a variety of topics can be provided to groups, individuals, or communities. Group programs need to be planned carefully before they are implemented. The decision to establish a health promotion program must be based on the assessed health needs of the people; also, specific health promotion goals must be set. After the program is implemented, program outcomes must be evaluated.

In the evaluation of health promotion programs, the client's understanding must be ascertained. Simply asking clients if they understand may be inappropriate (Byham and Vickery 1988, p. 10). In some cases, the client may understand the information but may not be able to apply it or may have anxiety about doing a particular task. For instance, a new parent may understand all the principles of giving an infant

What Are the Health Promotion Practices of Nursing Students?

Nursing students have the power to act as role models for classmates, family, friends, and clients. How well do they play this role? The purpose of this study was to identify the health practices of nursing students and to find out their overall opinion toward primary preventive practices. The sample for this study consisted of 1081 female nursing students from ten schools in the Buffalo, New York area. The ten schools included diploma, associate degree, and baccalaureate programs. The ages of the students ranged from 17 to 55 years, with a mean age of 24.

The results showed considerable variation in the extent to which students practiced health promotion and prevention. On the positive side, the majority of students obtained 6–8 hours of sleep per night, did not or had never smoked, brushed their teeth regularly, exercised regularly, had routine dental care, and had a yearly physical examination. However, less than half of the students ate breakfast daily, three-fourths of those surveyed ate between meals, and less than half limited fats, salt, and sugar in their diets. Breast self-examination was done by only one-third of the group; most did not wear seat belts; and 90% consumed alcoholic beverages.

The preventive health orientation (PHO) of the sample was measured by a 14-item index. The scores ranged from 1 to 13, with a mean of 7.1. Thus, the typical nursing student practiced about half the desired behaviors. Both age and type of educational program were significant factors with respect to preventive health practices. Scores on the PHO index were significantly higher for older students versus younger ones, and for associate degree and baccalaureate students versus diploma students.

These findings indicate that although nursing students, as future health care professionals, are expected to act as role models, their own health practices need improvement.

Implications: The authors suggest that faculty take a more active role in promoting positive health promotion behaviors by (a) increasing students' awareness regarding the information and resources that are available for facilitating behavior change, (b) increasing content related to health promotion and prevention within the core curriculum and in courses relating to health and life-styles, and (c) instituting no-smoking policies in classrooms and school buildings. In addition, nursing faculty members should be aware of their role in setting the appropriate example by practicing health promotion and prevention.

S. Dittmar, B. Hoyghey, R. O'Shea, and J. Brasure. Health practices of nursing students. *Health Values,* March/April 1989, 13:24–31.

a bed bath but have considerable anxiety about safely managing the procedure. Giving clients ample opportunity to demonstrate or practice routines and procedures, asking them to repeat important steps or information, and clarifying any unclear statements allows the nurse to evaluate the clients' knowledge and competence more fully.

Nurses may offer an abundance of information less formally. To do so, however, nurses need up-to-date knowledge, the ability to assess learning needs, and effective teaching skills. See Chapter 16 for detailed information. For example, nurses often disseminate information about parenting, breast and testicular self-examination, prevention of sexually transmitted disease, nutritional needs, and monitoring blood pressure and pulse rates.

Health fairs are a recent method being used to disseminate information to the public about health promotion and disease prevention and early detection. Nurses are often the initiators of health fairs and may provide participants of all age groups with information, teaching, counseling, or screening. Health fairs are usually offered in convenient locations such as shopping malls, schools, hospitals, and business settings in order to encourage maximum participation.

Enhancing Behavior Change

Whether people will make and maintain changes to improve health or prevent disease depends on many interrelated factors. See the section on assessing health care beliefs, earlier in this chapter. Murphy (1982, p. 427) says that the distances between wanting to change, attempting to change, and being able to change can be enormous. She emphasizes this statement by pointing out the difficulty many people have in acquiring regular dental flossing habits. When a client succeeds in making healthy behavior changes because of information the nurse has provided, the nurse feels satisfied and pleased. When, however, the client does not succeed in planned behavioral changes, the nurse tends to feel frustrated and often describes the person as "resistant," "uninterested," "unmotivated," or "noncompliant."

Murphy (1982) says the nurses are erroneously inclined to believe (a) that change will occur simply by bringing unhealthy behavior to the client's attention and (b) that when the client does not change, the desire to change is absent.

To help clients succeed in implementing behavior changes, the nurse needs to understand the process of change and the nature of the client's motivation or the client's current situation. An application of Lewin's stages of change (Lewin 1951) can help the nurse recognize the client's needs (Murphy 1982, p. 428). See Chapter 16 for additional information on Lewin's stages.

In *Stage 1 (unfreezing),* the client's motivation to change emerges. The client recognizes the need to change and becomes uneasy about the present way of doing things. At this stage, the nurse must help the client feel safe enough to explore and consider alternatives. Murphy says, "'Unfreezing' or 'unlearning' old habits is probably the most important stage of change but it is also the most difficult and challenging for the health promoter" (1982, p. 428). The nurse can best help the client by emphasizing what that person values. Loss of an unhealthy behavior may then become tolerable. For example, a client may start to "unfreeze" a habit of eating excessive carbohydrates if emphasis is placed on maximizing energy potential through a balanced food intake rather than just on the components of a healthy diet. In *Stage 2 (moving)*, the client is ready to change and develop new responses. Many health promoters tend to focus their efforts on this stage of eliciting new desired responses (Murphy 1982). In *Stage 3 (refreezing)*, the client internalizes behavior changes and stabilizes a new level of functioning.

The response of the nurse to lack of change in the client is generally to provide more information or to withdraw from the interaction after concluding that there is no point wasting time on people who do not want to change. Both responses deny such clients the opportunity to improve their health. By providing more information to the client, the nurse assumes that the client lacks knowledge. If, however, the client has understood the information, repeating or amplifying the information more than likely will annoy the client. The nurse has failed to identify the problem clearly. Withdrawal from clients who have difficulty changing implies that the nurse's health promotion efforts will be directed toward persons who readily and willingly comply. Such people, however, are probably the ones who least need the nurse's help. Additional guidelines for assisting the client toward behavior change are offered in the accompanying box.

Modeling

Modeling consists of observing the behavior of other people who have successfully achieved the goal that clients have set for themselves (Pender 1987, p. 265). Modeling is not imitating. Through observing a model, the client acquires ideas for behavior and coping strategies for specific problems. The client is not expected to mimic the sequence of actions or behavior patterns of the model.

The nurse and client should mutually select models with whom the client can identify, since the cultural and ethnic backgrounds of the nurse and client often differ. Models should be frequently available during the early learning and change stages of unfreezing and moving. Models should also be people the client respects.

Nurses should serve as models of wellness. In order to model effectively, nurses need to have a philosophy and life-style that demonstrate good health habits. Pender (1987, p. 463) believes that undergraduate nursing students should work with faculty and college health services to develop a wellness program. Through such a plan, students can assess their own life-styles, develop a health promotion plan, and

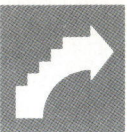

CLINICAL GUIDELINES
Enhancing Behavior Change

(Murphy 1982, p. 429):

- Recognize that motivation is the basis of all behavior whether it is healthy or unhealthy, good or bad.

- Recognize that people are motivated by their needs.

- Avoid labeling people as unmotivated. The label simply means that the person does not comply with the wishes of the nurse who applies the label.

- Focus on the sources or factors that motivate the person's behavior rather than on the presence or absence of motivation.

- Remember that resistance is a normal part of change and a healthy response to a threat.

- Understand that a client may choose to keep unhealthy habits for many reasons.
  a. The habit may be a culturally learned response such as cigarette smoking and alcohol consumption. In North America, these habits were once associated with a glamorous or sophisticated life-style and a certain kind of satisfaction.
  b. The client may be directing all available energies to meet other needs. A person who is grieving the loss of a loved one, or a recently divorced person, for example, may not have the energy to follow a weight-loss diet.
  c. The conditions required to change may be absent. For example, clients need help first to "unlearn" or "unfreeze" old habits and recognize the benefits of new habits before they can consider or undertake action.

- Cast aside the idea that the client *must* change. This attitude is not conducive to a helping relationship with the client and does not convey respect for the client. The client who does not change is entitled to the nurse's interest and nonjudgmental response.

- Measure your competence in terms of how well you understand clients' needs and implement clients' care rather than by the extent to which clients change their behavior.

actually carry out the implementation strategies. The college years offer access to facilities and health services that may not be available when students begin their working life. Once students have had a firsthand experience with creating a health promotion plan and with the difficulties involved with behavior change, they will be able to work more effectively with peers and clients. Clients are more likely to respect and trust the nurse who can tell them what worked in the nurse's personal situation.

EVALUATING

Evaluation takes place on an ongoing basis, both during the attainment of short-term goals and after the completion of long-term goals. During evaluation, the client may decide to continue with the plan, reorder priorities, change strategies, or revise the health promotion contract. Evaluation of the plan is a collaborative effort between the nurse and the client. Goals are written during the planning phase and a date determined for attaining the specific results or behaviors that are desired to promote health or prevent illness. The following is an example of a nursing diagnosis, goal statements, planned interventions, and evaluative statements.

■ *Nursing Diagnosis*
  Health-seeking behaviors related to desire for information on breast self-examination

■ *Long-Term Goal*
  The client performs breast self-examination regularly by 10/15/19xx.

■ *Short-Term Goals*
  #1. The client passes a test on the basic facts about breast cancer by 2/2/19xx.
  #2. The client performs breast self-examination accurately by 3/4/19xx.

■ *Interventions*
  The client attends two educational sessions to learn basic information on breast cancer.
  The client practices and demonstrates procedures on models.
  The client demonstrates procedure on self.

■ *Evaluation*
  Goal #1 attained. By the date specified, the client was able to pass a test on basic knowledge of the subject. Because this is an objective measure of cognitive knowledge, the nurse can clearly evaluate whether the client has learned the material and met this short-term goal.

  Goal #2 attained. By the date specified, the client was able to perform the breast self-examination accurately. This is a psychomotor objective that the nurse can evaluate by having the client demonstrate breast self-examination using the appropriate techniques.

■ *Evaluation of the Long-Term Goal*
  In this example, the long-term goal may be evaluated during a meeting or planned telephone conversation with the client. Achievement of the long-term goal is ascertained by asking the client if she performed accurate breast self-examination each month. The client states, "Yes, I have done the procedure every month for the past five months." In this example, goal achievement is measured solely on the basis of information the client gives the nurse. There is no objective measure to ascertain that this was done. It is up to the client to be honest in her self-assessment and commitment to the health promotion goal.

Using the nursing process for promotion of health and prevention of illness assumes that the client is a motivated, self-directed, responsible consumer. The nurse's role is to assist clients in achieving their goals. The nurse is available to lend expertise in the assessment of health, the implementation of a health promotion plan, and the evaluation of the goals. The nurse also enhances the potential for client success in goal achievement by using strategies such as teaching, counseling, support, and the modeling of good health behaviors.

CHAPTER HIGHLIGHTS

▶ Health promotion activities are directed toward developing client resources that maintain or enhance well-being.

▶ The goal of health promotion is to raise the client's level of health.

▶ Health protection activities are geared toward the prevention of specific diseases, such as obtaining immunizations to prevent poliomyelitis.

▶ Health promotion programs can be categorized as information dissemination, health appraisal and wellness assessment, life-style and behavior change, worksite wellness, and environmental control programs.

▶ Wellness-oriented nursing diagnoses identify client strengths, recognize self-care abilities, and enhance health promotion goals.

▶ A thorough assessment of the client's health status is basic to health promotion.

▶ Health risk or hazard appraisals provide the data that often spur the client to adopt a healthier life-style.

▶ Life-style assessment tools give clients the opportunity to assess the impact of their present life-styles on their health and to make decisions about life-style changes.

▶ Clients' health care beliefs provide the nurse with an indication of how much clients believe they can influence or control health through personal behaviors.

▸ To help clients change their life-styles or health behaviors, the nurse provides ongoing support, supplies additional information and education, and explores the motivating sources of the client's behavior.

▸ During planning the client may wish to make a behavioral contract. A contract usually includes the client goal, activities to achieve the goals, and the methods of evaluation to measure goal achievement.

▸ Nurses, in order to be role models for their clients, should develop attitudes and behaviors that reflect healthy lifestyles.

▸ During the evaluation phase of the health promotion process, the nurse assists clients in determining whether they will continue with the plan, reorder priorities, or revise the plan.

READINGS AND REFERENCES

SUGGESTED READINGS

Ireland, D. November 1988. Reading, writing and reasons for health. *American Journal of Nursing* 88:1506.

Ireland describes the development, philosophy, staffing, and types of services offered at an adolescent health center located on the grounds of a high school. Each visit to the clinic is seen as an opportunity for health teaching. The staff also reaches out to the classroom and community centers with career days, tutoring, film festivals, walking programs, and other such "sideline sessions."

McMahon, A., and Maibush, R. M. November 1988. How to send quit-smoking signals: Timing is everything when encouraging a patient to decide to quit smoking. *American Journal of Nursing* 88:1498–99.

McMahon and Maibush outline a three-step process nurses can use to assist clients to quit smoking. The authors suggest using quit-smoking messages that are brief, direct, and informative. A chart with examples of "the do's and don'ts of quit-smoking messages" is provided.

Maglacas, A. M. March/April 1988. Health for all: Nursing's role. *Nursing Outlook* 36:66–71.

This author shares her vision of health for all in the 21st century and describes the role and responsibility of the nurse if the vision is to become reality. The future role of the nurse will emphasize not interventions related to disease but support of the total person to meet all the individual's needs. To prepare for this new role, the nurse must develop new skills that enable people to accept responsibility for self-care, self-help, environmental improvement, and positive health promotion.

RELATED RESEARCH

Boyd, A. September/October 1988. Level of wellness of nursing students. *Health Values* 12:14–20.

Byham, L. D., and Vickery, C. E. July/August 1988. Compliance and health promotion. *Health Values* 12:5–13.

Campion, V. Summer 1989. Effect of knowledge, teaching method, confidence and social influence on breast self-examination. *Image: Journal of Nursing Scholarship* 21:76–80.

SELECTED REFERENCES

Becker, M.; Drachman, R; and Kirscht, J. 1972. Motivation as predictors of health behavior. *Health Services Reports* 87:852–62.

Brubaker, B. H. April 1983. Health promotion: A linguistic analysis. *Advances in Nursing Science* 5:1–14.

Byham, L. D., and Vickery, C. E. July/August 1988. Compliance and health promotion. *Health Values* 12:5–12.

Clark, C. C. 1986. *Wellness Nursing.* New York: Springer Publishing Co.

Cox, C. L. May/June 1985. The health self-determinism index. *Nursing Research* 34:177–83.

Donoghue, J., Duffield, C., Pelletier, D. et al. 1990. Health promotion as a nursing function: Perceptions held by university students of nursing. *International Journal of Nursing Studies* 27:51–60.

Edelman, C., and Mandle, C. L. 1986. *Health promotion throughout the life span.* St. Louis: C. V. Mosby Co.

Getchell, B. 1979. *Physical fitness: A way of life.* 2d ed. New York: John Wiley and Sons.

Greiner, P. A. November 1987. Nursing and worksite wellness. *Holistic Nursing Practice* 2:53–60.

Hales, D. 1989. *An invitation to health.* 4th ed. Redwood City, Calif.: Benjamin/Cummings Publishing Co.

Healthy People: The Surgeon General's Report on Health Promotion and Disease Prevention. 1979. Washington, D.C.: U.S. Department of Health, Education and Welfare.

Houldin, A.; Saltstein, S.; and Ganley, K. 1987. *Nursing Diagnosis for Wellness.* Philadelphia: J. B. Lippincott Co.

Ireland, D. F. November 1988. Reading, writing and reasons for health. *American Journal of Nursing* 88:1506.

Kort, M. April 1984. Support: An important component of health promotion. *Canadian Nurse* 80:24–26.

Leavell, H. R., and Clark, E. G. 1965. *Preventive medicine for the doctor in the community.* 3d ed. New York: McGraw-Hill.

Lewin, K. 1951. *Field theory in social science.* New York: Harper and Row.

Lewis, F. M. March/April 1982. Experienced personal control and quality of life in late-stage cancer patients. *Nursing Research.* 31:113–18.

Logan, B. B., and Dawkins, C. E. 1986. *Family-centered nursing in the community.* Menlo Park, Calif.: Addison-Wesley.

Maglacas, A. M. March/April 1988. Health for all: Nursing's role. *Nursing Outlook* 36:266–71.

Montoye, H. J.; Christian, J. L.; Nagle, F. J.; and Levin, S. M. 1988. *Living Fit.* Menlo Park, Calif.: Benjamin/Cummings Publishing Co.

Muhlenkamp, A. F.; Brown, N. J.; and Sands, D. November/December 1985. Determinants of health promotion activities in nursing clinic clients. *Nursing Research* 34:327–32.

Murphy, M. M. November/December 1982. Why won't they shape up? Resistance to the promotion of health. *Canadian Journal of Public Health* 73:427–30.

Murray, R. B., and Zentner, J. P. 1989. *Nursing assessment and health promotion strategies through the life span.* 4th ed. Norwalk, Conn.: Appleton & Lange.

Noack, H. 1987. Concepts of health and health promotion. In Abelin, T., editor. pp. 5–28. *Measurement in health promotion and disease protection.* Copenhagen: World Health Organization, Regional Publication, Ser. No. 22.

Pender, N. J. 1987. *Health promotion in nursing practice.* 2d ed. Norwalk, Conn.: Appleton & Lange.

Ryan, R. S., and Travis, J. W. 1981. *Wellness workbook for health professionals.* Berkeley, Calif.: Ten Speed Press.

Shillinger, F. L. Spring 1983. Locus of control: Implications for clinical nursing practice. *Image: Journal of Nursing Scholarship* 25:58–63.

Walker, S. N.; Sechrist, K. R.; and Pender, N. J. March/April 1987. The health-promoting lifestyle profile: Development and psychometric characteristics. *Nursing Research* 36:76–81.

Wallston, K. A.; Wallston, B. S.; and DeVellis, R. Spring 1978. Development of the multidimensional health locus of control (MHLC) scales. *Health Education Monographs* 6:164–65.

Concepts of Growth and Development

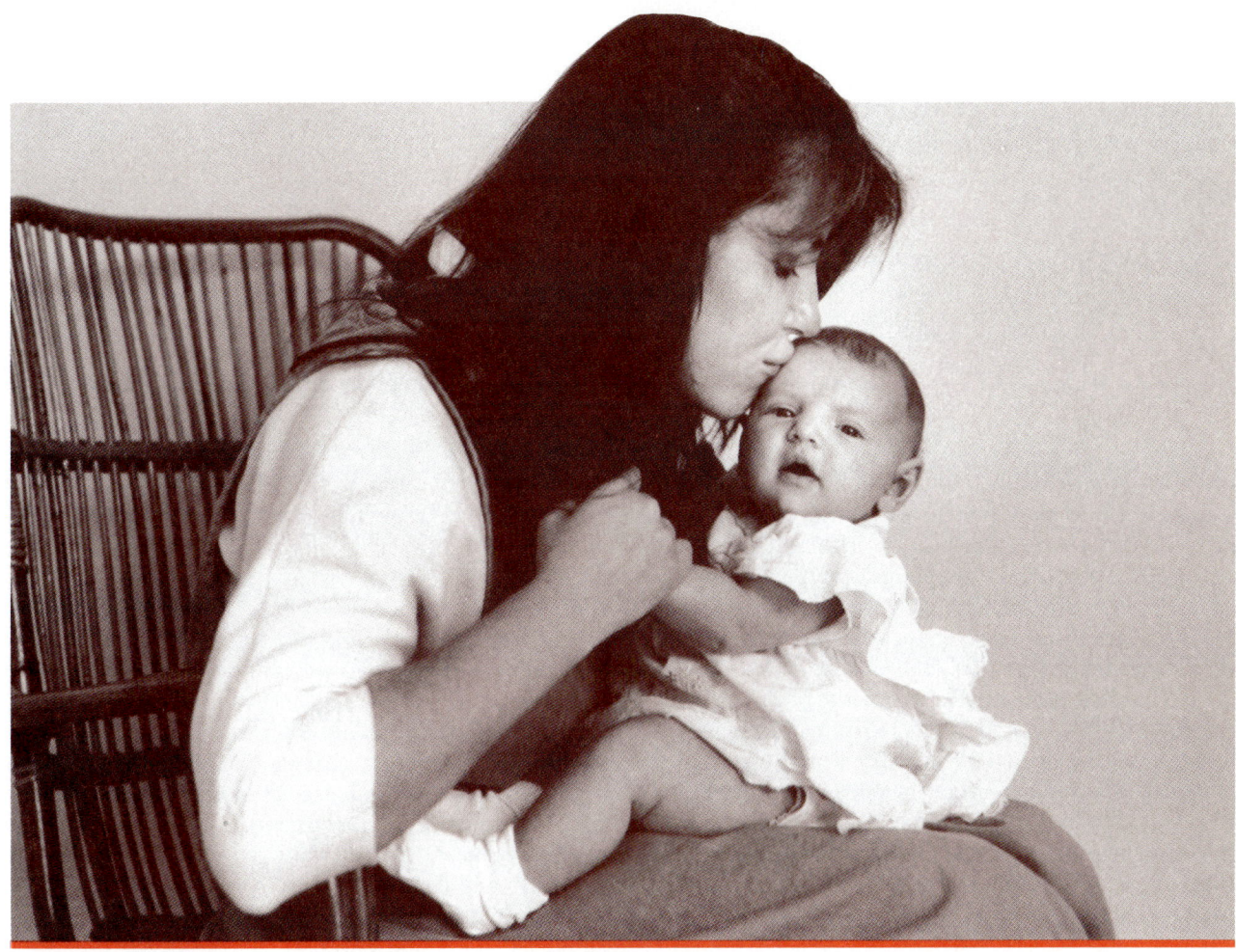

CONTENTS

GROWTH, DEVELOPMENT, AND MATURATION

The terms *growth* and *development* both refer to dynamic processes. Often used interchangeably, these terms have different denotations. **Growth** is physical change and increase in size. Growth can be measured quantitatively. Indicators of growth include height, weight, bone size, and dentition. **Development** is an increase in the complexity of function and skill progression (James and Mott 1988, p. 58). It is the capacity and skill of a person to function. Development is the behavioral aspect of growth; for example, a person develops the ability to walk, to talk, and to run. Growth and development are independent, interrelated processes. For example, an infant's muscles, bones, and nervous system must grow to a certain point before the infant can sit up or walk. Growth generally takes place during the first 20 years of life; development continues after that.

Maturation refers to the development of inherited characteristics, such as stature. **Maturation** is the sequence of physical changes that are related to genetic influences (James and Mott 1988, p. 58). Maturation is independent of the environment, but its timing can be influenced by environmental factors. For example, inadequate nutrition can delay walking and growth.

Stages of Growth and Development

The rate of a person's growth and development is highly individual; however, the sequence of growth and development is predictable. Stages of growth usually correspond to certain developmental changes. See Table 24–1. It is generally accepted that those aspects of growth and development that are not determined genetically are influenced by the environment.

Growth and development are commonly thought of as having five major components: physiologic, cognitive, psychosocial, moral, and spiritual.

TABLE 24–1   *Stages of Growth and Development*

Stage	Age	Significant Characteristics	Nursing Implications
Neonatal	Birth to 28 days	Behavior is largely reflexive and develops to more purposeful behavior.	Assist parents to identify and meet unmet needs.
Infancy	1 month to 1 year	Physical growth is rapid.	Control the infant's environment so that physical and psychological needs are met.
Toddlerhood	1 to 3 years	Motor development permits increased physical autonomy. Psychosocial skills increase.	Safety and risk-taking strategies must be balanced to permit growth.

TABLE 24–1 *(continued)*

Stage	Age	Significant Characteristics	Nursing Implications
Preschool	3 to 6 years	The preschooler's world is expanding. New experiences and the preschooler's social role are tried during play. Physical growth is slower.	Provide opportunities for play and social activity.
School age	6 to 12	Stage includes the preadolescent period (10 to 12 years). Peer group increasingly influences behavior. Physical, cognitive, and social development increases, and the child has increased competence in communication.	Allow time and energy for the school-age child to pursue hobbies and school activities. Recognize and support child's achievement.
Adolescence	12 to 20 years	Self-concept changes with biologic development. Values are tested. Physical growth accelerates. Stress increases, especially in face of conflicts.	Assist adolescents to develop coping behaviors. Help adolescents develop strategies for resolving conflicts.
Young adulthood	20 to 40 years	A personal life-style develops. Person establishes a relationship with a significant other, a commitment to something, and competence.	Accept adult's chosen life-style and assist with necessary adjustments relating to health. Recognize the person's commitment and the function of competence in life. Support change as necessary for health.
Middle adulthood	40 to 65 years	Life-style changes because of other changes, e.g., children leave home, occupational goals change.	Assist clients to plan for anticipated changes in life, to recognize the risk factors related to health, and to focus on strengths rather than weaknesses.
Older adulthood Young old	65 to 74 years	Adaptation to retirement and changing physical abilities is often necessary. Chronic illness may develop.	Assist clients to keep physically and socially active and to maintain peer group interactions.
Middle old	75 to 84 years	Adaptation to decline in speed of movement, reaction time, and sensory abilities and increasing dependence on others may be necessary.	Assist clients to cope with loss, e.g., hearing, eyesight, death of loved one. Provide necessary safety measures.
Old old	85 and over	Increasing physical problems may develop.	Assist clients with self-care as required, and with maintaining as much independence as possible.

Factors Influencing Growth and Development

The factors that influence growth and development are both genetic and environmental. Theorists assign different importance to the respective roles of heredity and environment. Theorists usually hold one of the following three beliefs:

1. Heredity determines most if not all growth.
2. The environment is the primary determinant of development.
3. Heredity and environment contribute to development, each affecting the individual to a greater or lesser extent during differing aspects of development.

The genetic inheritance of an individual is established at conception. This genetic inheritance remains unchanged throughout life. Genetic inheritance determines such characteristics as sex, physical stature, and race.

Many environmental factors affect an individual's growth and development. Some of these are family, religion, climate, culture, school, community, and nutrition. For example, poorly nourished children are more likely to have infections than are well-fed children and may not attain their full height potential.

Whether one favors heredity, environment, or an interactive approach (i.e., an interrelationship between heredity and environment) to understand growth and development, some basic principles are commonly accepted. These are summarized in the box on the following page.

PHYSIOLOGIC GROWTH AND DEVELOPMENT

Physiologic growth refers to an individual's size and body functioning. The pattern of physiologic growth is similar for all people. However, growth rates vary during different stages of growth and development. See Table 24–1. For example, the growth rate is very rapid during the prenatal, neonatal, infancy, and adolescent stages. The growth rate slows during childhood, and physical growth is minimal during adulthood. Specific growth trends throughout life are discussed in detail in Chapters 25, 26, and 27.

MATURATION THEORIES

Gesell

Arnold Gesell extensively observed, described, and recorded the changes in the growth and behavior of children from birth to adolescence. He believes that changes in a child are the result of heredity. In other words, genes determine the build of a child's body and the schedule for the appearance of individual characteristics (Gesell and Ilg, 1949). According to Gesell, the environment has very little effect on the individual's development.

Gesell describes cycles of behavior that he found to be essentially the same for all children; these cycles tend to coincide with a child's chronologic age. He categorizes periods of six months to one year as *better* or *worse* stages. During a *better stage,* the child appears to be in balance with the outside world and the people in it. In a *worse stage,* the child seems unhappy and frustrated with both the physical aspects of the environment and the people in it. Gesell considers these stages a necessary part of the normal maturation process. Thus, parents are urged to be tolerant of difficult behavior and to view these stages as part of a child's normal development.

Gesell utilizes Sheldon's (1942) theory of somatotypes to explain individual differences in the development of personality. **Somatotypes** describe body type and personal tendencies among people. The three body types are endomorph, mesomorph, and ectomorph. The **endomorph** is described as soft, round, fat, with a love of comfort, food, and the approval of others. The **mesomorph** has big bones and heavy muscles, loves activity, and prefers to dominate in social situations. The **ectomorph** is thin, fragile, and sensitive and withdraws in social situations.

Gesell describes what the typical child is like at different ages. His work provides an informative resource that nurses, parents, and teachers can use to assess the status of the child in relation to what is considered average or normal. In addition, such information can be very helpful in anticipating the changes in a child's behavior over the years.

Havighurst

Robert Havighurst believes that learning is basic to life and that people continue to learn throughout life. He describes growth and development as occurring during six stages, each associated with from six to ten tasks to be learned. See Table 24–2. Havighurst believes that once a person learns to talk, it is mastered for life.

Havighurst promoted the concept of developmental tasks in the 1950s. A **developmental task** is "a task which arises at or about a certain period in the life of an individual, successful achievement of which leads to his happiness and to success with later tasks, while failure leads to unhappiness in the individual, disapproval by society, and difficulty with later tasks" (Havighurst 1972, p. 2).

TABLE 24–2 *Havighurst's Age Periods and Developmental Tasks*

Infancy and Early Childhood

1. Learning to walk
2. Learning to take solid foods
3. Learning to talk
4. Learning to control the elimination of body wastes
5. Learning sex differences and sexual modesty
6. Achieving psychologic stability
7. Forming simple concepts of social and physical reality
8. Learning to relate emotionally to parents, siblings, and other people
9. Learning to distinguish right from wrong and developing a conscience

Middle Childhood

1. Learning physical skills necessary for ordinary games
2. Building wholesome attitudes toward oneself as a growing organism
3. Learning to get along with age-mates
4. Learning an appropriate masculine or feminine social role
5. Developing fundamental skills in reading, writing, and calculating
6. Developing concepts necessary for everyday living
7. Developing conscience, morality, and a scale of values
8. Achieving personal independence
9. Developing attitudes toward social groups and institutions

Adolescence

1. Achieving new and more mature relations with age-mates of both sexes
2. Achieving a masculine or feminine social role
3. Accepting one's physique and using the body effectively
4. Achieving emotional independence from parents and other adults
5. Achieving assurance of economic independence
6. Selecting and preparing for an occupation

7. Preparing for marriage and family life
8. Developing intellectual skills and concepts necessary for civic competence
9. Desiring and achieving socially responsible behavior
10. Acquiring a set of values and an ethical system as a guide to behavior

Early Adulthood

1. Selecting a mate
2. Learning to live with a partner
3. Starting a family
4. Rearing children
5. Managing a home
6. Getting started in an occupation
7. Taking on civic responsibility
8. Finding a congenial social group

Middle Age

1. Achieving adult civic and social responsibility
2. Establishing and maintaining an economic standard of living
3. Assisting teenage children to become responsible and happy adults
4. Developing adult leisure-time activities.
5. Relating oneself to one's spouse as a person
6. Accepting and adjusting to the physiologic changes of middle age
7. Adjusting to aging parents

Later Maturity

1. Adjusting to decreasing physical strength and health
2. Adjusting to retirement and reduced income
3. Adjusting to death of a spouse
4. Establishing an explicit affiliation with one's age group
5. Meeting social and civil obligations
6. Establishing satisfactory physical living arrangements

Source: Developmental tasks and education, 3d ed., by Robert J. Havighurst. Copyright © 1972 by Longman Inc. Reprinted by permission of Longman, Inc., New York.

Havighurst's developmental tasks provide a framework that the nurse can use to evaluate a person's general accomplishments. However, some nurses find that the broad categories limit its usefulness as a tool in assessing specific accomplishments, particularly those of infancy and childhood.

PSYCHOSOCIAL THEORIES

Psychosocial development refers to the development of personality. **Personality** is a complex concept that is difficult to define. It can be considered as the outward (interpersonal) expression of the inner (intrapersonal) self. It encompasses a person's temperament, feelings, character traits, independence, self-esteem, self-concept, behavior, ability to interact with others, and ability to adapt to life changes.

Many theorists attempt to account for psychosocial development in humans. Many of these theories explain the development of a person's personality and the causes of behavior. The theorists discussed in this book are Freud, Sullivan, Erikson, Skinner, Bandura, Peck, and Gould.

Freud

Sigmund Freud, whose writings and research were very popular in the 1930s, introduced a number of concepts about development that are still used today. The concepts of the unconscious mind, defense mechanisms, and the id, ego, and superego are Freud's. The **unconscious mind** is the mental life of a person of which the person is unaware. This concept of the unconscious is one of Freud's major contributions to the field of psychiatry. **Defense mechanisms,** or **adaptive mechanisms** as they are more commonly called today, are the result of conflicts between inner impulses and the anxiety that attends these conflicts. The **id** is the source of instinctive and unconscious urges, which Freud considers chiefly sexual in nature. The id is also the source of all pleasure and gratification. The **ego** is formed by the person to make effective contact with social and physical needs. Through the ego, the id impulses are satisfied. The third aspect of the personality, according to Freud, is the **superego.** This is the conscience of the personality, a control on the id. The superego is the source of feelings of guilt, shame, and inhibition. See Chapter 33 for additional information on adaptive processes and ego defense mechanisms. Freud proposes that the underlying motivation to human development is an energy form or life instinct, which he calls **libido.**

According to Freud's theory of psychosexual development, the personality develops in five overlapping stages from birth to adulthood. The libido changes its location of emphasis within the body from one stage to another. Therefore, a particular body area has special significance to a client at a particular stage. See Table 24–3. If the individual does not achieve a satisfactory resolution at each stage, the personality becomes fixated at that stage. **Fixation** is immobilization or the inability of the personality to proceed to the next stage because of anxiety.

The first three stages (oral, anal, and phallic) are called the pregenital stages. During the first, or *oral stage,* the mouth is the principal source of pleasure, primarily as a result of eating. Feelings of dependence arise in the oral stage, and they tend, according to Freud, to persist through-

TABLE 24–3 *Freud's Five Stages of Development*

Stage	Age	Characteristics	Implications
Oral	0 to 1 year	Mouth is the center of pleasure.	Feeding produces pleasure and sense of comfort and safety. Feeding should be pleasurable and provided when required.
Anal	2 and 3 years	Anus and rectum are the centers of pleasure.	Controlling and expelling feces provide pleasure and sense of control. Toilet training should be a pleasurable experience, and appropriate praise can result in a personality that is creative and productive.
Phallic	4 and 5 years	The child's genitals are the center of pleasure.	The child identifies with the parent of the opposite sex and later takes on a love relationship outside the family. Encourage identification.
Latency	6 to 12 years	Energy is directed to physical and intellectual activities.	Encourage child with physical and intellectual pursuits.
Genital	13 years and after	Energy is directed toward attaining a mature heterosexual relationship.	Encourage separation from parents, achievement of independence, and making decisions.

Source: Adapted from Patricia H. Miller, *Theories of developmental psychology.* Copyright © 1983 W. H. Freeman and Company. Used by permission.

out life. A person who is fixated at the oral stage may have difficulty trusting others and may demonstrate such behaviors as nail biting, drug abuse, smoking, overeating, alcoholism, argumentativeness, and overdependency. The *anal stage* occurs when the child is learning toilet training. Fixation at this stage can result in obsessive-compulsive personality traits such as obstinance, stinginess, cruelty, and temper tantrums. During the *phallic stage,* sexual and aggressive feelings associated with the genitals come into focus. Masturbation offers pleasure at this time, and the child experiences the Oedipus or Electra complex. The **Oedipus complex** refers to the male child's attraction for his mother and his hostile attitudes toward his father. The **Electra complex** is the female child's attraction for her father and her hostility toward her mother. Fixation at the phallic phase can result in such traits as problems with sexual identity and problems with authority.

During the *latency stage,* the sexual impulses tend to be repressed. Unresolved conflict at this stage may be reflected in obsessiveness and lack of self-motivation. Following latency come adolescence and the reactivation of the pregenital impulses. The person usually displaces these impulses and subsequently passes into the final stage of adult maturity, the *genital stage.* The inability to resolve conflicts during this stage can result in sexual problems, such as frigidity, impotence, and the inability to be satisfied in a heterosexual relationship.

Nurses can assist an infant's development by, for example, making feeding a pleasurable experience and by making toilet training a positive experience, thereby enhancing the child's feeling of self-control. See implications of the five stages in Table 24–3.

Freud also emphasizes the importance of infant-parent interaction. Therefore, the nurse, as a caregiver, should provide a warm, caring atmosphere for an infant and assist parents to do so also when the infant returns to their care.

Sullivan

Harry Stack Sullivan delineates six stages of interpersonal development that span the period from infancy to adulthood. He sees the growth of the personality from a sociopsychologic viewpoint. Although he does not reject the role of heredity (biology) in development, he believes that sociologic factors have greater influence. Sullivan defines interpersonal behavior as "all that can be observed as personality" (Hall and Lindzey 1970, p. 137). He views interpersonal development as a series of stages. In the second stage, for example, he believes that a child develops **malevolent transformation,** which is the feeling that one lives among enemies. Sullivan considers his six stages as applicable to people in Western European cultures; stages in other cultures may differ. See Table 24–4.

Erikson

Erik H. Erikson adapts and expands Freud's theory of development to include the entire life span, believing that people continue to develop throughout life. He describes eight stages of development. In contrast to Freud, Erikson believes the ego to be the conscious core of the personality. See Table 24–5 on page 588.

Erikson envisions life as a sequence of levels of achievement. Each stage signals a task that must be achieved. The resolution of the task can be complete, partial, or unsuccessful. Erikson believes that the greater the task achievement, the healthier the personality of the person; failure to achieve a task influences the person's ability to achieve the

TABLE 24–4 *Sullivan's Stages of Interpersonal Development*

Stage	Age	Selected Characteristics
Infancy	Birth to the appearance of articulate speech	Activity is primarily mouth-centered. Nursing is the infant's first interpersonal experience.
Childhood	Articulate speech to the need for playmates	The child integrates self-esteem and develops malevolent transformation (the feeling that one lives among enemies).
Juvenile	First 5 to 6 years	The child becomes social, competitive, and cooperative and learns to supervise own behavior by external controls.
Preadolescence	7 years to adolescence	Child begins to form genuine human relationships. The child forms peer relationships.
Early adolescence	12 to 14 years	The child develops a pattern of heterosexual activity. The erotic need is focused on a member of the opposite sex. The need for intimacy is focused on a member of the same sex.
Late adolescence	15 to 18 years	The person is initiated into the privileges, duties, satisfactions, and responsibilities of social living.

Source: Adapted from C. S. Hall and G. Lindzey, *Theories of personality,* 2d ed. (New York: John Wiley and Sons, 1970). Copyright © 1970 John Wiley & Sons, Inc. Reprinted by permission.

TABLE 24-5   Erikson's Eight Stages of Development

Stage	Age	Central Task	Indicators of Positive Resolution	Indicators of Negative Resolution
Infancy	Birth to 18 months	Trust versus mistrust	Learning to trust others	Mistrust, withdrawal, estrangement
Early childhood	18 months to 3 years	Autonomy versus shame and doubt	Self-control without loss of self-esteem Ability to cooperate and to express oneself	Compulsive self-restraint or compliance Willfulness and defiance
Late childhood	3 to 5 years	Initiative versus guilt	Learning the degree to which assertiveness and purpose influence the environment Beginning ability to evaluate one's own behavior	Lack of self-confidence Pessimism, fear of wrongdoing Overcontrol and overrestriction of own activity
School age	6 to 12 years	Industry versus inferiority	Beginning to create, develop, and manipulate Developing sense of competence and perseverence	Loss of hope, sense of being mediocre Withdrawal from school and peers
Adolescence	12 to 20 years	Identity versus role confusion	Coherent sense of self Plans to actualize one's abilities	Confusion, indecisiveness, and inability to find occupational identity
Young adulthood	18 to 25 years	Intimacy versus isolation	Intimate relationship with another person Commitment to work and relationships	Impersonal relationships Avoidance of relationship, career, or life-style commitments
Adulthood	25 to 65 years	Generativity versus stagnation	Creativity, productivity, concern for others	Self-indulgence, self-concern, lack of interests and commitments
Maturity	65 years to death	Integrity versus despair	Acceptance of worth and uniqueness of one's own life Acceptance of death	Sense of loss, contempt for others

Sources: Adapted from E. H. Erikson, *Childhood and society,* 2d ed. (New York: W. W. Norton and Co., 1963); and H. S. Wilson and C. R. Kneisl *Psychiatric nursing,* 3d ed. (Menlo Park, Calif.: Addison-Wesley Publishing Co., 1988). Used by permission.

next task. These developmental tasks can be viewed as a series of crises, and successful resolution of these crises is supportive to the person's ego. Failure to resolve the crises is damaging to the ego. After attaining one stage, the person may fall back and need to approach it again.

Erikson's eight stages reflect both positive and negative aspects of the critical life periods. The resolution of the conflicts at each stage enables the person to function effectively in society. Each phase has its developmental task, and the individual must find a balance between, for example, trust versus mistrust (stage 1) or generativity versus stagnation (stage 7).

When using Erikson's developmental framework, nurses should be aware of indicators of positive and negative resolution of each stage. It is also important to be aware that, according to Erikson, the environment is highly influential

in development. Nurses can enhance people's development by being aware of their developmental stage, by providing opportunities for the individual to resolve his or her developmental task, and by helping the person develop coping skills relative to stressors experienced at that level. Nurses can enhance a client's positive resolution of a developmental task by providing the individual with appropriate opportunities and encouragement. For example, a 10-year-old child can be encouraged to be creative, to finish schoolwork, and to learn how to accomplish these tasks within the limitations imposed by health.

Erikson emphasizes that people must change and adapt their behavior to maintain control over their lives. In his view, no stage in personality development can be bypassed, but people can become fixated at one stage or regress to a previous stage. For example, a middle-aged woman who has never satisfactorily accomplished the task of resolving identity versus role confusion might regress to an earlier stage when stressed by an illness with which she cannot cope.

Skinner

B. F. Skinner is of the behaviorist school of thought. He considers thoughts and feelings inappropriate for scientific study and therefore examines only observable behavior in a laboratory where variables can be controlled. Behaviorists believe that human behavior is the result of learned responses to environmental stimuli. Behaviorists concentrate on research that identifies general laws of human behavior applicable to everyone rather than on individual personality development and on the present rather than the past as the root of all behavior. How environment influences behavior and how a person controls it are the essential factors that determine human action. An act is often called a *response* when it can be traced to the effects of a stimulus.

Skinner postulates two types of **conditioning** (behavioral responses to a stimulus) that cause the response or behavior. The first type of conditioning, termed classical conditioning, is illustrated by Pavlov's well-known experiments with dogs. Pavlov (1849–1936) conditioned dogs to salivate in response to the sound of a tuning fork, a sound they heard when they received food. *Classical conditioning* is a procedure in which conditioned responses are established by the association of a new stimulus that is known to cause an unconditioned response. The resulting response is the conditioned response to the *new* (unrelated) stimulus.

An early experience in the life of a newborn infant can be used to illustrate this process. A newborn who has not been fed for several hours becomes increasingly restless and cries. The infant continues to cry until the nipple is placed in the mouth, then quiets down and begins to suck. In the same situation a few weeks later, the infant again becomes restless and cries but now, upon hearing the mother's footstep, quiets down and stops crying.

The second type of conditioning is what Skinner refers to as *operant conditioning,* a process by which the frequency of a response can be increased or decreased depending on when, how, and to what extent it is reinforced. Skinner believes that humans, like animals, will always repeat actions that bring pleasure. He considers the consequences of an action, what he terms **reinforcement,** to be all-important. Positive consequences foster repetition of the action; the absence of consequences causes the action to cease.

A learning experience of a young child can be used to illustrate operant conditioning. A nine-month-old boy babbles meaningless sounds. One day, in the midst of many other sounds, the child utters the syllables "ma-ma". Suddenly the mother stops what she is doing, picks up the child, and cuddles and kisses him. Perhaps the child repeats the syllables, to the mother's delight. That evening, the mother reports to the father that the child said his first words.

Extinction is the process in which a conditioned behavior is "unlearned" because the reinforcement has been removed. Greater effort, however, is required to extinguish a behavior than to condition it. The procedure involves removing the *unconditional stimulus* or the reward from the training situation. When the conditioning procedure is again instigated following complete extinction, it does not take the subject as long to show the conditioned response as it did in the original conditioning.

Skinner and his associates subsequently discovered that learning is more permanent if reinforcers are provided intermittently rather than continuously. For example, if a child asks for candy or a toy during every trip to the grocery store but receives it only part of the time, this behavior is more apt to continue. In addition, teaching complicated behaviors requires time, patience, and the grading of steps from simple to complex.

This technique of breaking down complex concepts into simpler parts is applied in educational programs today. For example, in programmed instruction and the use of teaching machines or computers, the learners read a short passage, answer a question, then turn a knob or push a button to see whether they are correct.

Studies of conditioning produced a number of laws of learning that were thought to be universal; i.e., they were thought to apply to all ages, all cultures, and all types of behavior—motor, cognitive, emotional, and social. Examples include the following (Miller 1989, p. 218):

- The more quickly reinforcement occurs after response, the more effective the reinforcement.
- A response made in the presence of one stimulus generalizes to similar stimuli.
- Behavior that is reinforced only part of the time takes longer to extinguish than behavior that is reinforced continuously.

Nurses can apply these principles of behavior to change certain actions of some children. This approach is referred to as *behavior modification*. Positive, desirable actions are praised and rewarded. Disobedience or undesirable actions are ignored and thereby weakened; they are *not* punished. To use behavior modification effectively, the nurse must accurately identify what behavior is being reinforced and what will be the positive reinforcer.

Bandura

Social learning theorists such as Bandura agree with Skinner that the environment exerts a great deal of control over overt behavior; however, they believe that the entire learning process involves three highly interdependent factors:

1. Characteristics of the person

2. The person's behavior

3. The environment

These factors influence and control each other through a process that Bandura calls *reciprocal determinism*. The major contribution of Bandura's reciprocal determinism is the concept that the child's behavior affects or "creates" that child's environment. This differs from Skinner's belief that the environment, viewed as a set of stimuli, controls behavior.

Bandura considers Skinner's classification of learning into two types (classical and operant conditioning) to be too simplistic. He does not discount Skinner's types of learning but claims that most learning comes from observational learning and instruction rather than from overt trial-by-error behavior. **Observational learning** is the acquisition of new skills or the alteration of old behaviors simply by watching other children and adults. It is especially important for acquiring behavior in situations where mistakes are life-threatening or costly, e.g., driving a car or performing brain surgery. Although operant conditioning (trial-by-error) learning can produce relatively new behaviors, it is inappropriate for learning complex behaviors such as these.

Bandura's research focuses on **imitation,** the process by which individuals copy or reproduce what they have observed, and **modeling,** the process by which a person learns by observing the behavior of others.

Imitation was first introduced by Miller and Dollard (1941), who set out to demonstrate that imitation is one of the most powerful socialization forces. It is natural to human beings from childhood. They propose that a tendency to imitate is learned because various imitative behaviors are reinforced by a process of operant conditioning. For example, a boy may be praised for being "just like his father". The child may even self-reinforce the imitations by repeating an adult's words of praise.

Bandura and Walters (1963) carry the concept of imitation one step further by demonstrating that children can acquire relatively new behaviors by simply watching a model. The child or observer does not need to make an overt response or be reinforced, since punishment or reinforcement of the model's behavior has the same effect on the observer as it does on the model. For example, a child who sees a hard-working classmate praised by the teacher learns to reproduce that behavior. Bandura and Walters call this process **vicarious reinforcement.** Observing that others are reinforced for a particular behavior may convey to the child the perception that the behavior is desirable in that situation and may encourage imitation of it. Seeing others punished has the opposite effect. However, Bandura has found that reinforcement or punishment to the model or child is not necessary for observational learning to occur.

Much of a child's learning comes from observing models such as older children, parents, coaches, and professional athletes or movie stars in action. Perceived characteristics that encourage modeling are high status, competence, and power (Bandura 1986). After children acquire new behaviors by observing various models, they can combine these behaviors to form complex behaviors. According to Bandura, models influence others mainly by providing information rather than by eliciting matching behavior, so that learning can occur without even once performing the model's behavior.

In recent years, Bandura's theory has become more cognitive, and he now calls his theory a "social cognitive theory." Learning is defined as "knowledge acquisition through cognitive processing information" (1986, p. xii). For example, television's effects on children depend on both cognitive and imitative processes. Whether the child can comprehend the story affects the child's perceptions of the model and the tendency to imitate the model. See also the cognitive and moral theories of Piaget and Kohlberg in this chapter.

Peck

Theories and models about adult development are relatively recent compared with theories of infant and child development. Research into adult development has been stimulated by a number of factors, including increased longevity and healthier old age. In the past, development was viewed as complete by the time of physical maturity, and aging was considered a decline following maturity. The emphasis was on the decremental aspects rather than the incremental aspects of aging. However, Peck believes that although physical capabilities and functions decrease with old age, mental and social capacities tend to increase in the latter part of life (Peck 1968).

Peck proposes three developmental tasks during old age, in contrast to Erikson's one (integrity versus despair). Peck believes that the older person must accomplish these three tasks:

1. *Ego differentiation versus work-role preoccupation.* An adult's identity and feelings of worth are highly dependent on that person's work role. Upon retirement, some people experience feelings of worthlessness, unless they derive their sense of identity from a number of roles so that one such role can replace the work role or occupation as a source of self-esteem. For example, a man who likes to garden or golf can obtain ego rewards from those activities, replacing rewards formerly obtained from his occupation.

2. *Body transcendence versus body preoccupation.* This task calls for the individual to adjust to decreasing physical capacities and at the same time maintain feelings of well-being. Preoccupation with declining body function reduces happiness and satisfaction with life.

3. *Ego transcendence versus ego preoccupation.* Ego transcendence is the acceptance without fear of one's death as inevitable. This acceptance includes being actively involved in one's own future beyond death. Ego preoc-

cupation, by contrast, results in holding on to life and a preoccupation with self-gratification.

Gould

Gould also studied adult development. He believes that transformation is a central theme during adulthood: "Adults continue to change over the period of time considered to be adulthood and ... developmental phases may be found during the adult span of life" (Gould 1972, p. 33). According to Gould, the twenties is the time when a person assumes new roles; in the thirties, role confusion often occurs; and in the forties, time limitations are realized in relation to accomplishing life's goals. In the fifties, according to Gould, the acceptance of each stage as a natural progression of life marks the path to adult maturity. Gould's study of 524 men and women led him to describe the seven stages of adult development:

- *Stage 1 (age 16–18):* Individuals consider themselves part of the family rather than individuals, and want to separate from their parents.

- *Stage 2 (ages 18–22):* Although the individuals have established autonomy, they feel it is in jeopardy; they feel they could be pulled back into their families.

- *Stage 3 (ages 22–28):* Individuals feel established as adults and autonomous from their families. They see themselves as well-defined but still feel the need to prove themselves to their parents. They see this as the time for growing and building for the future.

- *Stage 4 (ages 29–34):* Marriage and careers are well established. Individuals question what life is all about and wish to be accepted as they are, no longer finding it necessary to prove themselves.

- *Stage 5 (ages 35–43):* This is a period of self-reflection. Individuals question values and life itself. They see time as finite, with little time left to shape the lives of adolescent children.

- *Stage 6 (ages 43–50):* Personalities are seen as set. Time is accepted as finite. Individuals are interested in social activities with friends and spouse and desire both sympathy and affection from spouse.

- *Stage 7 (ages 50–60):* This is a period of transformation, with a realization of mortality and a concern for health. There is an increase in warmth and a decrease in negativism. The spouse is seen as a valuable companion (Gould 1972, pp. 525–527).

COGNITIVE THEORY

Cognitive development refers to the manner in which people learn to think, reason, and use language. It involves a person's intelligence, perceptional ability, and ability to process information. Cognitive development represents a progression of mental abilities from illogical to logical thinking, from simple to complex problem solving, and from understanding concrete ideas to understanding abstract concepts.

Piaget

The most widely known cognitive theorist is Jean Piaget (1896–1980). His theory of cognitive development has contributed to other theories, such as Kohlberg's theory of moral development and Fowler's theory of the development of faith, both discussed in this chapter.

According to Piaget, cognitive development is an orderly, sequential process in which a variety of new experiences (stimuli) must exist before intellectual abilities can develop. Piaget's cognitive developmental process is divided into five major phases: the sensorimotor phase, the preconceptual phase, the intuitive phase, the concrete operations phase, and the formal operations phase. A person develops through each of these phases; each phase has its own unique characteristics. See Table 24–6.

TABLE 24–6 *Piaget's Phases of Cognitive Development*

Phases and Stages	Age	Significant Behavior
Sensorimotor	Birth to 2 years	
Stage 1 Use of reflexes	Birth to 1 month	Most action is reflexive.
Stage 2 Primary circular reaction	1 to 4 months	Perception of events is centered on the body.
		Objects are extension of self.
Stage 3 Secondary circular reaction	4 to 8 months	Acknowledges the external environment.
		Actively makes changes in the environment.
Stage 4 Coordination of secondary schemata	8 to 12 months	Can distinguish a goal from a means of attaining it.

Source: Adapted from Jean Piaget, *The Origin of intelligence in children.* International Universities Press, Inc. Copyright © 1966. Used by permission.

TABLE 24–6 *Piaget's Phases of Cognitive Development* (continued)

Phases and Stages	Age	Significant Behavior
Stage 5 Tertiary circular reaction	12 to 18 months	Tries and discovers new goals and ways to attain goals.
		Rituals are important.
Stage 6 Inventions of new means	18 to 24 months	Interprets the environment by mental image.
		Uses make-believe and pretend play.
Preconceptual	2 to 4 years	Uses an egocentric approach to accommodate the demands of an environment.
		Everything is significant and relates to "me."
		Explores the environment.
		Language development is rapid.
		Associates words with objects.
Intuitive thought	4 to 7 years	Egocentric thinking diminishes.
		Thinks of one idea at a time.
		Includes others in the environment.
		Words express thoughts.
Concrete operations	7 to 11 years	Solves concrete problems.
		Begins to understand relationships such as size.
		Understands right and left.
		Cognizant of viewpoints.
Formal operations	11 to 15 years	Uses rational thinking.
		Reasoning is deductive and futuristic.

In each phase, the person uses three primary abilities: assimilation, accommodation, and adaptation. **Assimilation** is the process through which humans encounter and react to new situations by using the mechanisms they already possess. In this way, people acquire new knowledge and skills as well as insights into the world around them. **Accommodation** is a process of change whereby cognitive processes mature sufficiently to allow the person to solve problems that were unsolvable before. This adjustment is possible chiefly because new knowledge has been assimilated. **Adaptation** or coping behavior, is the ability to handle the demands made by the environment.

Nurses can employ Piaget's theory of cognitive development when developing teaching strategies. For example, a nurse can expect a toddler to be egocentric and literal; therefore, explanations to the toddler should focus on the needs of the toddler rather than on the needs of others. Further, a 13-year-old can be expected to use rational thinking and to reason; therefore, when explaining the need for a medication, a nurse can outline the consequences of taking and not taking the medication, enabling the adolescent to make a rational decision. Nurses must remember, however, that the range of normal cognitive development is very broad, despite the ages arbitrarily associated with each level. When teaching adults, nurses may become aware that some adults are more comfortable with concrete thought and slower to acquire and apply new information than are other adults.

MORAL THEORIES

Moral development, a complex process not fully understood, involves learning what ought to be and what ought not to be done. It is more than imprinting parents' rules and virtues or values upon children. The term **moral** means relating to right and wrong. Distinctions need to be made between the terms *morality, moral behavior,* and *moral development.* **Morality** refers to the requirements necessary for people to live together in society; **moral behavior** is the way a person perceives those requirements and responds to them; **moral development** is the pattern of change in moral behavior with age (White 1975).

Freud

Freud (1961) believes that the mechanism for right and wrong within the individual is the superego, or conscience. He hypothesizes that a child internalizes and adopts the moral standards and character or character traits of the model parent through the process of identification during resolution of the Oedipus complex. To Freud, children acquire morals unconsciously from parental standards, specifically from the model parent with whom the child identifies. Freud believes moral behavior results from the strength of the superego, which strives to be "supermoral," in conflict with the ego, which strives to be "moral," and the id, which is totally "nonmoral." The strength of the superego depends on the intensity of the child's feelings of aggression and attachment toward the model parent rather than on the actual standards of the parent.

As a psychoanalyst, Freud focuses on human failings, including moral failure and failure to mature. He notes that some people fixate a certain level and develop a fixated character. His theory implies that moral development is completed in childhood and focuses on an emotional component. Because, in Freud's view, morals develop unconsciously, there is no rational conscious component in moral development. Through feelings of love or affection for the mother or father and identification with that parent's character traits, the child develops feelings of guilt, self-respect, praise, or blame.

Erikson

Erikson's theory of the development of virtues or unifying strengths of the "good man" suggests that moral development continues throughout life. Erikson (1964) believes that if the conflicts of each psychosocial developmental stage are favorably resolved, then an "ego-strength" or virtue emerges. See Table 24–7. This theory of virtues or moral development focuses on goals that can be achieved at various stages of life. It implies that fidelity, love, care, and wisdom are adult phenomena only.

Kohlberg

Kohlberg suggests three levels of moral development that encompass six stages (Berkowitz and Oser 1985, p. 28). He focuses on the reasons for the making of a decision, not on the morality of the decision itself. At Kohlberg's first level, called the *premoral* or *preconventional level,* children are responsive to cultural rules and labels of good and bad, right and wrong. However, children interpret these in terms of the physical consequences of their actions, i.e., punishment or reward. At the second level, the *conventional level,* the individual is concerned about maintaining the expectations of the family, group, or nation and sees this as right. The emphasis at this level is conformity and loyalty to one's own expectations as well as society's. Level three is called the *postconventional, autonomous,* or *principled level.* At this level, people make an effort to define valid values and principles without regard to outside authority or to the expectations of others. For additional information about Kohlberg's levels, see Table 24–8 on page 594.

With reference to Kohlberg's six stages, Munhall writes that stage four, the "law and order" orientation, is the dominant stage of most adults (Munhall 1982, p. 14). It is recognized that there is a difference in action between nurses who act at the conventional level (level II) and those who act at the postconventional or principled level (level III). Nurses who are conventional thinkers base perceptions of moral obligations and rights on the maintenance of the social system and loyalty to established institutions and social groups. However, the postconventional nurse understands that societies and social relationships can be arranged in many ways, and that these different ways can maximize or minimize values (Munhall 1982, p. 13). Therefore, the nurse at level III questions authority and follows social norms as long as they support human values.

Peters

Peters combines aspects of existing theories to arrive at a concept of morality and moral behavior. He proposes a concept of rational morality based on principles. Moral development is usually considered to involve three separate components: *moral emotion* (what one feels), *moral judgment* (how one reasons), and *moral behavior* (how one acts). Various theorists of moral development emphasize

TABLE 24–7 *Erikson's Virtues or Ego-Strengths*

Stage of Development	Virtue
Trust versus mistrust	*Hope* or *confidence.* Belief that fervent wishes will be attained
Autonomy versus doubt	*Will.* Determination to exercise free choice as well as self-restraint
Initiative versus guilt	*Purpose.* Courage to envisage and pursue valued goals
Industry versus inferiority	*Competence.* Free exercise of dexterity and intelligence in the completion of tasks
Identity versus identity diffusion	*Fidelity.* Ability to sustain loyalties freely pledged in spite of the inevitable contradictions of value systems
Intimacy versus isolation	*Love.* Mutuality of devotion
Generativity versus stagnation or self-absorption	*Care.* Widened concern for what has been generated by love extending to whatever a person generates, creates, produces, or helps to produce
Integrity versus despair	*Wisdom.* Detached concern with life in the face of death

Source: E. H. Erikson, *Insight and responsibility: Lectures on the ethical implications of psychoanalytic insight* (New York: W. W. Norton and Co., 1964).

TABLE 24-8 *Kohlberg's Stages of Moral Development*

Level and Stage	Definition	Example
Level I *Preconventional*		
Stage 1: Punishment and obedience orientation	The activity is wrong if one is punished, and the activity is right if one is not punished.	A nurse follows a physician's order so as not to be fired.
Stage 2: Instrumental-relativist orientation	Action is taken to satisfy one's needs.	A client in hospital agrees to stay in bed if the nurse will buy the client a newspaper.
Level II *Conventional*		
Stage 3: Interpersonal concordance (good boy, nice girl)	Action is taken to please another and gain approval.	A nurse gives elderly clients in hospital sedatives at bedtime because the night nurse wants all clients to sleep at night.
Stage 4: Law and order orientation	Right behavior is obeying the law and following the rules.	A nurse does not permit a worried client to phone home because hospital rules stipulate no phone calls after 9:00 P.M.
Level III *Postconventional*		
Stage 5: Social contract, legalistic orientation	Standard of behavior is based on adhering to laws that protect the welfare and rights of others. Personal values and opinions are recognized, and violating the rights of others is avoided.	A nurse arranges for an East Indian client to have privacy for prayer each evening.
Stage 6: Universal-ethical principles	Universal moral principles are internalized. Person respects other humans and believes that relationships are based on mutual trust.	A nurse becomes an advocate for a hospitalized client by reporting to the nursing supervisor a conversation in which a physician threatened to withhold assistance unless the client agreed to surgery.

Source: Adapted from *Moral development: A guide to Piaget and Kohlberg* by Ronald Duska and Mariaellen Whelan. Copyright © 1975 by The Missionary Society of St. Paul the Apostle in the State of New York. Used by permission of Paulist Press.

one component above the other two. For example, Freud emphasizes the moral emotional component by focusing on the role of one's conscience or ego-strength and feelings such as guilt or self-respect. Piaget and Kohlberg emphasize the moral judgment or reasoning component. They see moral behavior as resulting from either the feelings or reasoning components, or both. Peters (1981, p. 83) states that much of moral philosophy in the past has not addressed *what* is morally important.

Facets of Moral Life   Peters (1981, p. 69) holds that morality and moral development are complex phenomena and that at least five facets of moral life must be distinguished:

1. Under the concepts of *good, worthwhile,* and *desirable* fall those activities that are thought to be so important that time must be spent on initiating children into them. Examples are poetry, science, engineering, and a variety of games and pastimes. Most of these activities are intimately connected with possible vocations and ideals of life.

2. Under the concepts of *obligation* and *duty* fall ways of behaving connected with social roles. For example, much of a person's moral life is taken up with one's station and its duties, for instance, with what is required of that person as a parent, spouse, and citizen.

3. There are those duties, more prominent in an open society, that are not specifically connected with social roles but that relate to following the general *rules governing conduct* between members of society, e.g., unselfishness, honesty, and fairness. These are personalized as character traits.

4. There are equally wide-ranging goals of life that are personalized in the form of *motives* or *traits of character* thought of as *virtues,* such as honesty, fairness, gratitude, and benevolence, and *vices,* such as meanness, selfishness, greed, and lust. These motives or purposes are not confined to a particular activity or role.

5. Finally, there are those very general traits of character that relate to the *manner in which a person follows rules or pursues purposes,* e.g., integrity, persistence, deter-

mination, conscientiousness, and consistency. These are all connected with what people call "the will."

Peters says the reason for spelling out this complexity of moral life is to rid persons of simple-minded views of morality, e.g., morality is just good interpersonal relationships or simply observing rules about stealing, sex, and the like. He believes that getting someone committed to a worthwhile activity is no less a part of morality than is the curbing of selfishness (Peters 1981, p. 70).

Hierarchy of Virtues   Peters's formulations contrast with Kohlberg's, who maintains that character traits such as honesty are comparatively unimportant in morals and that processes of habit formation by which traits are assumed to be established are of secondary importance. Peters, however, believes that the development of character traits or virtues is an essential aspect of moral development. He believes that virtues or character traits can be learned from others and encouraged by the example of others. For example, Peters states that a child develops concern for others much earlier than a sense of justice or honesty; further, concern for others does not require the same level of conceptual development as justice and honesty do. In the early stages of their lives, children cannot grasp the principle of justice.

In addition, Peters believes that some virtues can be described as habits because they are in some sense automatic and therefore are performed habitually. Examples are punctuality, politeness, chastity, tidiness, thrift, and honesty (Peters 1981, p. 93). Peters believes that habits need to be established in moral life. A **habit** is a behavior that a person can perform without deliberation or concentration: "Life would be exhausting if, in moral situations, people always had to reflect, deliberate, and make decisions. It would be difficult for people to conduct their social lives if they could not rely on a fair stock of habits such as politeness and punctuality, for example (Peters 1981, p. 98). Kohlberg, by contrast, stresses that the most important features of moral education are cognitive.

Virtues that cannot be classed as habits include compassion, concern for others, caring, justice, tolerance, courage, integrity, perseverance, and consistency. The mind is actively involved in exercising these virtues.

Schulman and Mekler

Schulman and Mekler believe that morality is a measure of how people treat fellow humans and that a moral child is one who strives to be kind and just. Both terms refer to how a person's behavior affects other people. They believe that morality has two components (Schulman and Mekler 1985, p. 6):

1. The intention of the person acting must be good in the sense that the goal of the act is the well-being of one or more people.

2. The person acting must be fair or just in the sense that the person considers the rights of others without prejudice or favoritism. A person's acts may be moral, immoral, or amoral. An act is considered *immoral* if through it a person seeks to harm others or gain an unfair advantage over them. An *amoral* act is not performed specifically to benefit or harm others. Intention is crucial when judging the morality of an act. An act is judged to be *well-intentioned* when the person performs the act without being threatened or coerced and when the primary reward is the well-being of another.

Schulman and Mekler's (1985, pp. 5–9) theory of moral development is based on three foundations, which they believe can be taught:

1. *Internalizing parental standards of right and wrong.* Children internalize parental standards, such as "Share your toys," "Don't hit," and "Consider other people's feelings." Internalization is more than obeying rules to avoid punishment. It is the learning of standards rather than just rules (Schulman and Mekler 1985, p. 21). The child must "define certain actions as *right* or *wrong* based on the parent's rules and learn to apply to him or herself the same words he or she has heard from the parents on how to behave properly" (Schulman and Mekler 1985, p. 8). Internalization is the first stage of self-control over selfish and aggressive impulses and the first step toward an adult conscience. It is accomplished when the child hears the "inner voice" speaking *before* the child acts. It is based primarily on love for parents and the desire to please them.

2. *Developing empathic reactions.* Children need to learn to react with empathy to someone else's feelings, e.g., feeling good about another person's joy and feeling bad about another person's unhappiness. Schulman and Mekler say that empathy appears to be an inborn capacity and is surprisingly common in children. However, the capacity for empathy varies from person to person. Through empathy, children learn that harming others is bad and comforting them is good.

3. *Acquiring personal standards.* The third foundation of morality is the development of personal standards that guide how a person *should* treat fellow human beings and what kind of person the individual wants to be. When individuals develop personal standards, they begin to evaluate parental rules and those of other authorities in relation to the new standards.

    Personal standards are not based on the approval of others. Reliance on them depends on the person's confidence in the ability to reason about the long-term consequences of actions. The consequences that keep a person striving to treat others kindly and justly are based on one's personal judgments about whether actions will bring a better world into being. In developing personal moral standards, the child first discerns whether the moral standards acquired from other people, starting with parents, work or not. This process occurs as the child expands relationships and experiences with others. If the moral standards learned earlier seem to bring about a better way of life, the child adopts personal standards learned from others. If the standards do not work, the child formulates new principles and standards.

Gilligan

Carol Gilligan (1982), after more than 10 years of research with women subjects, found that women often considered the dilemmas that Kohlberg used in his research to be irrelevant. Women scored consistently lower on his scale of moral development, in spite of the fact that they approached moral dilemmas with considerable sophistication. Gilligan believed that most frameworks do not include the concepts of caring and responsibility. Yet it is from these frameworks that most research in moral development is done. The result is that male emphasis upon individualism and autonomy is central to most moral development theories.

Gilligan describes three stages in the process of developing an "ethic of care" (Gilligan 1982, p. 74). Each stage ends with a transitional period. A **transitional period** is a time when the individual recognizes a conflict or discomfort with some present behavior and considers new approaches.

Stage 1. Caring for oneself. In this first stage of development, the person is concerned with caring only for the self. The individual feels isolated, alone, and unconnected to others. There is no concern or conflict with the needs of others because the self is the most important. The focus of this stage is survival. The end of this stage occurs when the individual begins to view this approach as selfish. At this time, the person also begins to see a need for relationships and connections with other people.

Stage 2. Caring for others. During this stage, the individual recognizes the selfishness of earlier behavior and begins to understand the need for caring relationships with others. Caring relationships bring with them responsibility. The definition of *responsibility* includes self-sacrifice, where "good" is considered to be "caring for others." The individual now approaches relationships with a focus of not hurting others. This approach causes the individual to be more responsive and submissive to others' needs, excluding any thoughts of meeting one's own. A transition occurs when the individual recognizes that this approach can cause difficulties with relationships because of the lack of balance between caring for oneself and caring for others.

Stage 3. Caring for self and others. During this last stage, a person sees that there is a need for a balance between caring for others and caring for the self. One's concept of responsibility is now defined as including both responsibility for the self and for other people. In this final stage, care still remains the focus on which decisions are made. However, the person now recognizes the interconnections between the self and others and thus realizes that it is important to take care of one's own needs, because if those needs are not met, other people may also suffer.

Gilligan believes women see morality in the integrity of relationships and caring, so that the moral problems they encounter are different from those of men. Men consider what is right to be what is just, whereas for women what is right is taking responsibility for others as a self-chosen decision (Gilligan 1982, p. 140).

Gilligan feels that a blend of perspectives is necessary for a person to reach maturity. The ethic of justice, or fairness, is based on the idea of equality: that everyone should receive the same treatment. This is the development path usually followed by men. It is widely accepted by the theorists in the field. By contrast, the ethic of care is based on a premise of nonviolence: that no one should be harmed. This is the path typically followed by women. It is an approach that has been given very little attention in the literature.

In the development of maturity, according to Gilligan, both viewpoints blend "in the realization that just as inequality adversely affects both perspectives in an unequal relationship, so too violence is destructive for everyone involved" (Gilligan 1982, p. 174). The blending of these two perspectives could give rise to a new view of human development and a better understanding of human relations.

Gilligan and Murphy, in their studies of postcollege adults, found that these adults began to doubt whether it is possible to construct generalized rules about right and wrong. They found these people evolving a rather new way of thinking in which change and process are primary features of reality. They see contradictions as acceptable and not needing resolution at all costs (Kegan 1982, p. 229).

SPIRITUAL THEORY

Fowler

The spiritual component of growth and development refers to individuals' understanding of their relationship with the universe and their perceptions about the direction and meaning of life. James Fowler describes the development of faith. Fowler believes that faith, or the spiritual dimension, is a force that gives meaning to a person's life. Fowler uses the term *faith* as a form of knowing, a way of being in relation to "an ultimate environment" (Fowler and Keen 1978). To Fowler, **faith** is a relational phenomenon; it is "an active 'made-of-being-in-relation' to another or others in which we invest commitment, belief, love, risk and hope" (Fowler and Keen 1978). Fowler's stages in the development of faith are given in Table 24–9.

Fowler's theory and developmental stages were influenced by the work of Piaget, Kohlberg, and Erikson. Fowler believes that the development of faith is an interactive process between the person and the environment. In each of Fow-

TABLE 24-9   Fowler's Stages of Spiritual Development

Stage	Age	Description
0. Undifferentiated	0 to 3 years	Infant unable to formulate concepts about self or the environment
1. Intuitive-projective	4 to 6 years	A combination of images and beliefs given by trusted others, mixed with the child's own experience and imagination
2. Mythic-literal	7 to 12 years	Private world of fantasy and wonder; symbols refer to something specific; dramatic stories and myths used to communicate spiritual meanings
3. Synthetic-conventional	Adolescent or adult	World and ultimate environment structured by the expectations and judgments of others; interpersonal focus
4. Individuating-reflexive	After 18 years	Constructing one's own explicit system; high degree of self-consciousness
5. Paradoxical-consolidative	After 30 years	Awareness of truth from a variety of viewpoints.
6. Universalizing	Maybe never	Becoming an incarnation of the principles of love and justice

Source: Adapted from J. Fowler and S. Keen, *Life maps: Conversations in the journey of faith* (Waco, Texas: Word Books, 1978); and A. Hollander, *How to help your child have a spiritual life: A parents' guide to inner development* (New York: A and W Publishers, 1980). Used by permission.

ler's stages, new patterns of thought, values, and beliefs are added to those already held by the individual; therefore the stages must follow in sequence. Faith stages, according to Fowler, are separate from cognitive stages of Piaget. Faith stages evolve from a combination of knowledge and values.

TABLE 24-10   Westerhoff's Four Stages of Faith

Stage	Age	Behavior
Experience faith	Infancy/early adolescence	Experiences faith through interaction with others who are living a particular faith tradition
Affiliative faith	Late adolescence	Actively participates in activities that characterize a particular faith tradition; experiences awe and wonderment; feels a sense of belonging
Searching faith	Young adulthood	Through a process of questioning and doubting own faith, acquires a cognitive as well as an affective faith
Owned faith	Middle adulthood/ old age	Puts faith into personal and social action and is willing to stand up for what the individual believes even against the nurturing community

Source: Adapted from J. Westerhoff, *Will our children have faith?* (New York: Seabury Press, 1976), pp. 79–103.

Westerhoff

John Westerhoff has developed a four-stage theory of faith development (see Table 24–10) based largely on his own life experiences and the interpretation of those experiences. Westerhoff proposes that faith is a way of behaving.

APPLYING GROWTH AND DEVELOPMENT CONCEPTS TO NURSING PRACTICE

A variety of different theories explain one or more aspects of an individual's growth and development. Typically, theorists examine only one aspect of an individual's development, such as the cognitive, moral, or physical aspects. The area chosen for examination usually reflects the researcher's academic discipline and personal interest. The theorists may also limit the population that is studied to a particular part of the life span, such as infancy, childhood, or adulthood.

Although such theories can be useful, they also have limitations. First, the theory chosen may explain only one aspect of the growth and development process. Yet, a person does not develop in fragmented sections, but rather as a whole human being. Thus, the nurse may find it necessary to apply several theories for an adequate understanding of the growth and development of a client.

Another limitation of some theories is the suggestion that certain tasks are performed at a specific age. In most cases, the child or adult does accomplish the task at the time specified by the guidelines. In other cases, however, the nurse may find that an individual does not accomplish the task or meet the milestone at the exact time suggested by the theory. Such individual differences are not easily defined or categorized by a single theory. Human development is a complex synthesis of physiologic, cognitive, psychologic, moral, and spiritual development. Nurses should expect individual variations and take these into consideration when applying these theories about growth and development. In so doing, they will be better able to understand a client's development and plan effective nursing interventions.

In nursing, developmental theories can be useful in guiding assessment, explaining behavior, and providing a direction for nursing interventions. An understanding of a child's intellectual ability helps a nurse to anticipate and explain certain reactions, responses, and needs. Nurses can then encourage client behavior that is appropriate for that particular developmental stage.

Theories are also useful in planning a nursing intervention. For instance, choosing the appropriate toy for a 3-year-old boy requires some knowledge of the physical and cognitive development of the child, as well as a sensitivity for individual preferences.

In adult care, knowledge about the physical, cognitive, and psychologic aspects of the aging process is a fundamental aspect of administering sensitive nursing care. For example, nurses can use their familiarity with the theories of development to help clients understand and anticipate the psychosocial changes that take place after retirement or the physical limitations that come with old age.

CHAPTER HIGHLIGHTS

▶ Growth and development are independent, interrelated processes.

▶ Growth is physical change and increase in size. The pattern of physiologic growth is similar for all people.

▶ Development is an increase in the complexity of function and skill progression.

▶ Maturation refers to the sequence of physical changes that is primarily related to genetic influences.

▶ The rate of a person's growth and development is highly individual, but the sequence of growth and development is predictable.

▶ Heredity and environment are the primary factors influencing growth and development.

▶ Components of growth and development are generally categorized as physiologic, psychosocial, cognitive, moral, and spiritual.

▶ There are several theories about the various stages and aspects of growth and development, particularly in regard to infant and child development. Theories and models about adult development are more recent.

▶ Each developmental stage has its own characteristics and unique problems.

▶ A progression of sequential steps or tasks is proposed in most theories, so that successful achievement of tasks is required in early stages before success can be achieved with later tasks.

▶ The nurse's major role in relation to growth and development is to assess the client's growth and development using the standards proposed in these theories, to identify and report any problem areas, and to plan and implement nursing strategies that will maintain or promote the client's development.

READINGS AND REFERENCES

SUGGESTED READINGS

Erikson, E. H. 1985. *The life cycle completed: A review.* New York: W. W. Norton and Co.
    This small book by Erikson describes the relationship of psychoanalytic (Freudian) theory to psychosocial (Eriksonian) theory. Erikson's premise in this book is that all stages are interwoven. In Chapter 3, Erikson discusses the major stages of psychosocial development. The human attributes of hope, will, purpose, competence, fidelity, love, care, and wisdom that emerge from the life stages are explained.

McWeeny, M. March/April 1988. Life span growth and development: A review and application to nursing diagnosis. *Journal of Enterostomal Therapy* 15:81–86.
    This author reviews the developmental theories of Piaget, Erikson, and Duvall and outlines the physical, cognitive, emotional, and social competences associated with each phase of the life

cycle. McWeeny emphasizes the importance of assessing the psychosocial development of the client with an ostomy and suggests appropriate nursing diagnoses.

Schulman, M., and Mekler, E. 1985. *Bringing up a moral child: A new approach for teaching your child to be kind, just, and responsible.* Reading, Mass.: Addison-Wesley Publishing Co.

This book written for parents provides practical suggestions for teaching morality to children. It includes what to teach, how to teach, and when to teach. The book is divided into three parts. The first part explains how children actually develop a conscience and how to teach them moral values. The second part includes forces, such as jealousy, anger, and greed, that work against leading a moral life. The third part includes common moral issues and dilemmas that children face at different ages.

Trocchio, J. March/April 1989. Life as a bell-shaped curve. *Geriatric Nursing* 10:71.

This brief article outlines some parallels between aging and child development. The author suggests that application of some of the principles of child care to care of the elderly may create positive results.

SELECTED REFERENCES

Bandura, A. 1986. *Social foundations of thought and action.* Englewood Cliffs, NJ: Prentice-Hall.

Bandura, A., and Walters, R. H. 1963. *Social learning and personality development.* New York: Holt, Rinehart and Winston.

Berkowitz, M. W., and Oser, F., editors. 1985. *Moral education: Theory and application.* Hillsdale, NJ: Lawrence Erlbaum.

Bloom, M. 1985. *Life span development: Basis for preventive and interventive helping.* 2d ed. New York: Macmillan Co.

Duska, R., and Whelan, M. 1975. *Moral development: A guide to Piaget and Kohlberg.* New York: Paulist Press.

Ebersole, P., and Hess, P. 1985. *Toward healthy aging: Human needs and nursing response.* 2d ed. St. Louis: C. V. Mosby Co.

Erikson, E. H. 1963. *Childhood and society.* 2d ed. New York: W. W. Norton and Co.

———. 1964. *Insight and responsibility: Lectures on the ethical implications of psychoanalytic insight.* New York: W. W. Norton and Co.

———. 1985. *The life cycle completed: A review.* New York: W. W. Norton and Co.

Fowler, J. W. 1981. *Stages of faith: The psychology of human development and the quest for meaning.* New York: Harper and Row.

Fowler, J., and Keen, S. 1978. *Life maps: Conversations in the journey of faith.* Waco, Texas: Word Books.

Freud, S. 1961. *The ego and the id and other works* (Vol. 19, James Strachey, translator). London: Hogarth Press and the Institute of Psychoanalysis.

Gesell, A., and Ilg, F. L. 1949. *Child development: An introduction to the study of human growth.* New York: Harper and Row.

Gilligan, C. 1982. *In a different voice: Psychological theory and women's development.* Cambridge, Mass.: Harvard University Press.

Gould, R. L. November 1972. The phases of adult life: A study in developmental psychology. *American Journal of Psychiatry* 129:33–43.

Hall, C. S., and Lindzey, G. 1970. *Theories of personality.* 2d ed. New York: John Wiley and Sons.

Havighurst, R. J. 1972. *Developmental tasks and education.* 3d ed. New York: David McKay Co.

Hollander, A. 1980. *How to help your child have a spiritual life: A parents' guide to inner development.* New York: A. and W. Publishers.

James, S., and Mott, S. 1988. *Child health nursing: Essential care of children and families.* Menlo Park, Calif.: Addison-Wesley Publishing Co.

Kegan, R. 1982. *The evolving self: Problem and process in human development.* Cambridge, Mass.: Harvard University Press.

Miller, N. E., and Dollard, J. 1941. *Social learning and imitation.* New Haven, Conn.: Yale University Press.

Miller, P. H. 1989. *Theories of developmental psychology.* 2d ed. San Francisco: W. H. Freeman and Co.

Munhall, P. L. June 1982. Moral development: A prerequisite. *Journal of Nursing Education* 21:11–15.

Peck, R. 1968. Psychological developments in the second half of life. In Neugarten, B. L. *Middle age and aging.* Chicago: University of Chicago Press.

Peters, R. S. 1981. *Moral development and moral behavior.* London: George Allen and Unwin, Publishers.

Piaget, J. 1966. *Origins of intelligence in children.* New York: W. W. Norton and Co.

Schulman, M., and Mekler, E. 1985. *Bringing up a moral child: A new approach for teaching your child to be kind, just, and responsible.* Reading, Mass.: Addison-Wesley Publishing Co.

Sheldon, W. H. 1942. *Varieties of temperament.* New York: Harper and Row.

Schuster, C. S., and Ashburn, S. S. 1986. *The process of human development: A holistic approach.* 2d ed. Boston: Little, Brown and Co.

Skinner, B. F. 1948. *Walden Two.* New York: Macmillan Co.

———. 1971. *Beyond freedom and dignity.* New York: Alfred A. Knopf.

———. 1980. The experimental analysis of operant behavior: A history. In Rieber, R. W., and Salzinger, K., editors. *Psychology: Theoretical-historical perspectives.* New York: Academic Press.

Sugarman, L. 1986. *Life-span development: Concepts, theories and interventions.* New York: Methuen and Co.

Westerhoff, J. 1976. *Will our children have faith?* New York: Seabury Press.

White, R. 1975. *Lives in progress: A study of the natural growth of personality.* 3d ed. New York: Holt, Rinehart and Winston.

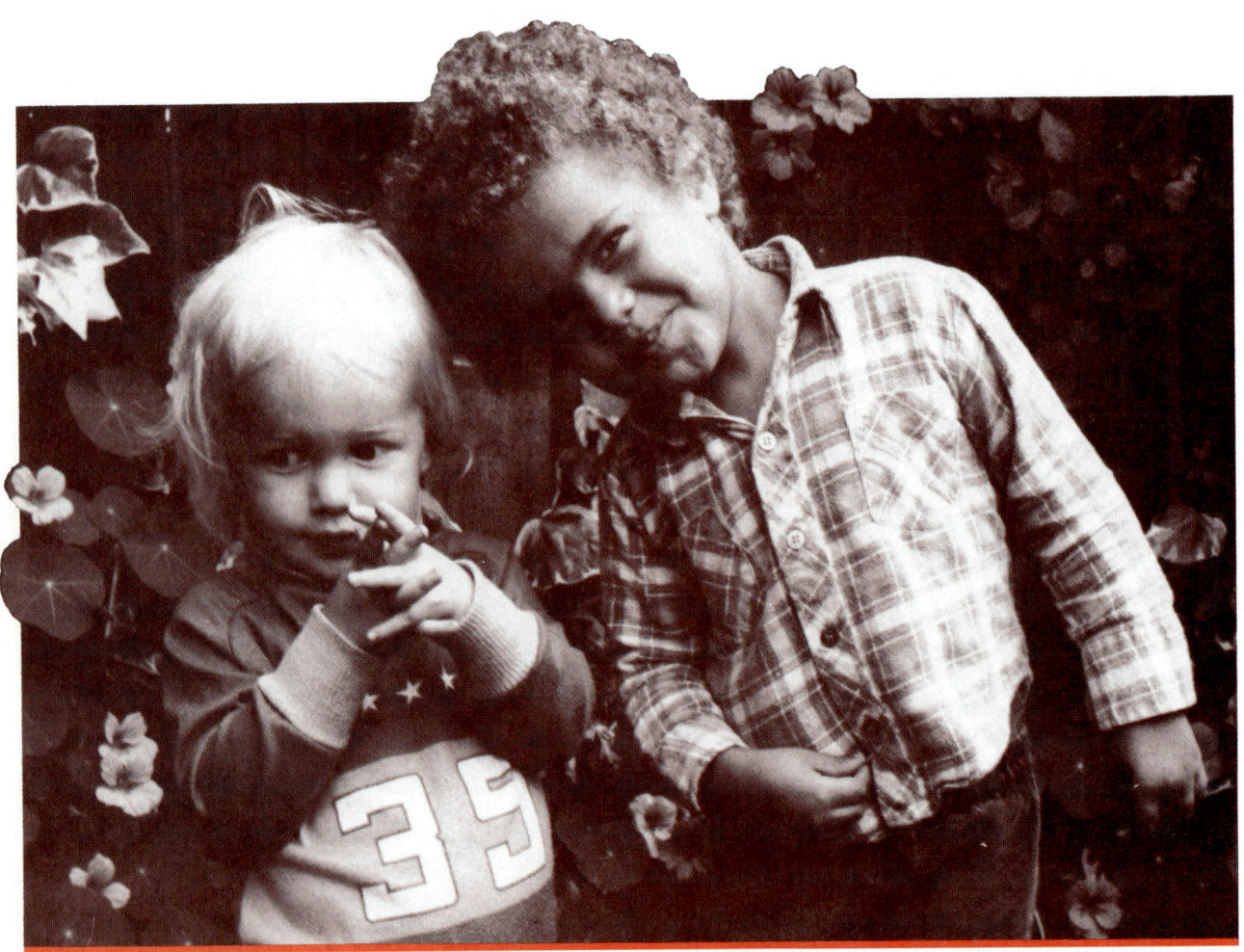

CONTENTS

OBJECTIVES

▶ Identify characteristic tasks at different stages of development during infancy and childhood.

▶ Describe usual physical development throughout infancy and childhood

▶ Trace psychosocial development according to Erikson through infancy and childhood. ▶

▶ Explain changes in cognitive development according to Piaget throughout infancy and childhood.

▶ Describe moral development according to Kohlberg throughout childhood.

▶ Describe spiritual development according to Fowler throughout childhood.

▶ Identify assessment activities and expected characteristics from birth through late childhood.

▶ Identify nursing diagnoses for health promotion from birth through late childhood.

▶ List examples of health promotion goals from birth through late childhood.

▶ Identify essential health promotion and protection activities to meet the needs of infants, toddlers, preschoolers, and school-age children.

INFANTS (BIRTH TO 1 YEAR)

Physiologic Growth and Development

An infant's basic task is survival, which requires breathing, sleeping, sucking, eating, swallowing, digesting, and eliminating. Because many of the infant's activities and pleasures are mouth-centered, this stage in development is often referred to as Freud's oral stage (see Chapter 24). Infants undergo significant physiologic change in these areas: weight, length, head growth, vision, and motor development

A number of factors can affect the *weight* at birth of a child. These include the mother's life-style (e.g., nutrition, substance abuse), age, heredity, and the weeks of gestation. At birth, most babies weigh from 2.7 to 3.8 kg (6.0 to 8.5 lb); white infants tend to weigh more than infants of other races. Just after birth, most infants lose 5% to 10% of their birth weight because of fluid loss. This weight loss is normal, and infants usually regain that weight in about 1 week. After several days, babies usually gain weight at the rate of 5 to 7 ounces weekly for 6 months. By 5 months of age infants usually reach twice their birth weight and three times their birth weight by age 12 months.

The average *length* of a white newborn in the United States is about 50 cm (20 in). At birth, black infants tend to be shorter than white infants. This range is from 47.5 to 52.5 cm (19 to 21 in). Female babies are on the average smaller than male babies.

Two recumbent lengths are the crown-to-rump length (the sitting length) and the head-to-heel length (from the top of the head to the base of the heels). See Figure 25–1. Normally the crown-to-rump length is approximately the same as the head circumference. By 6 months, infants gain another 13.75 cm (5.5 in) of height. By 12 months, they add another 7.5 cm (3 in). Rate of increase in height is largely influenced by the baby's size at birth and by nutrition.

Assessment of head *circumference* is of particular importance in infants and children to determine the growth rate of the skull and the brain. An infant's head should be measured at every visit to the physician or nurse until the child is 2 years. Head measurement of children 3 years or older usually does not need to be done routinely; however, this

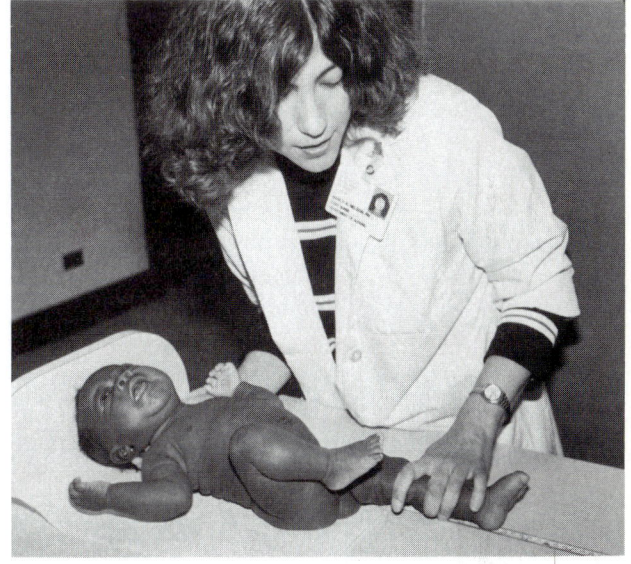

Figure 25–1 Measuring an infant, crown to rump.

measurement should be taken during initial examinations of young children. See Figure 25–2 on page 602.

Normal head circumferences (**normocephaly**) are often related to chest circumferences. At birth, the average infant's head circumference is 35 cm (14 in) and generally varies only 1 or 2 cm (0.5 in). The *chest circumference* of the newborn is usually less than the head circumference by about 2.5 cm (1 in). As the infant grows the chest circumference becomes larger than the head circumference. At about 9 or 10 months, the head and chest circumferences are about the same, and after 1 year of age the chest circumference is larger.

Abnormalities in head circumferences are referred to as **macrocephaly** (a large head) or **microcephaly** (a small head). The former is often the result of excessive cerebrospinal fluid within the skull (**hydrocephalus**).

The heads of most newborn babies are misshapen because of the molding of the head that occurs during vaginal deliveries. Molding of the head is made possible by **fontanelles** (unossified membranous gaps) in the bone structure of the

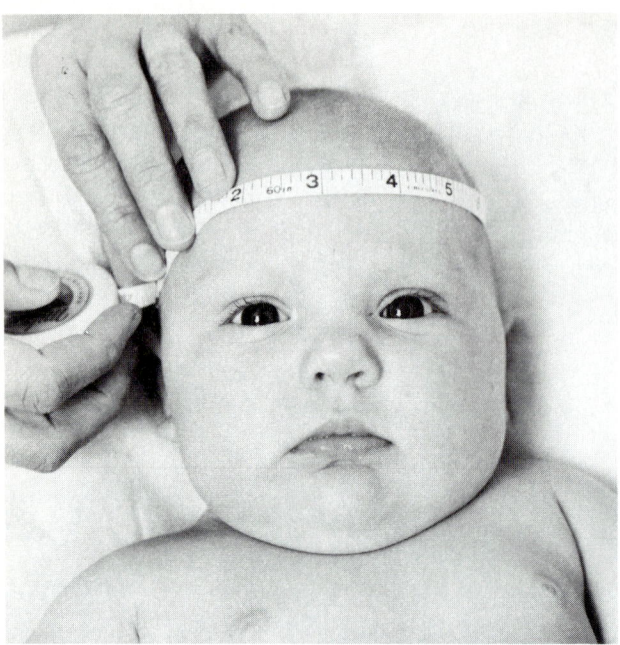

Figure 25–2 An infant's head circumference is measured around the skull, above the eyebrows.

skull and by overriding of the **sutures** (junction lines of the skull bones). Within a week, a newborn's head usually regains its symmetry, a fact that reassures parents.

The eight bones of the cranium are separated by sutures, which gradually ossify during childhood. These bones are the frontal bone, the occipital bone, two parietal and two temporal bones, and the sphenoid and ethmoid bones. See Figure 25–3. Six fontanelles are present at birth, but the two most prominent ones are the frontal (anterior) and the occipital (posterior) ones. The latter is the smaller of the two (1 to 2 cm in diameter) and is generally closed by 4 months. The posterior fontanelle may not be palpated for a few hours after birth because of the overriding of the sutures during delivery. The larger anterior fontanelle (4 to 6 cm in diameter and diamond-shaped) can increase in size for several months after birth. After 6 months, the size gradually decreases until closure occurs between 9 and 18 months (Behrman and Vaughan 1983, p. 16). The posterior fontanelle between the parietal bones and the occipital bone closes from 4 to 8 weeks after birth.

Examination of the head of infants for symmetry of shape and for palpation of the fontanelles is best achieved while the infant is sitting comfortably in the mother's lap. Normally, in a crying, coughing, or vomiting infant, the anterior fontanelle has a certain tenseness, fullness, and bulging, indicating increased intracranial pressure. Continual bulging is abnormal and associated with tumors or infections of the brain or hydrocephalus due to obstruction of the cerebrospinal fluid circulation in the ventricles. Depression of the anterior fontanelle generally indicates dehydration.

Visual abilities are present at birth; the newborn can follow large moving objects and can react to changes in the intensity of light. The baby blinks in response to bright light and to sound. The pupils of the newborn respond slowly, and the eyes cannot focus on close objects. During the first year, vision develops, so that the infant's eyes are coordi-

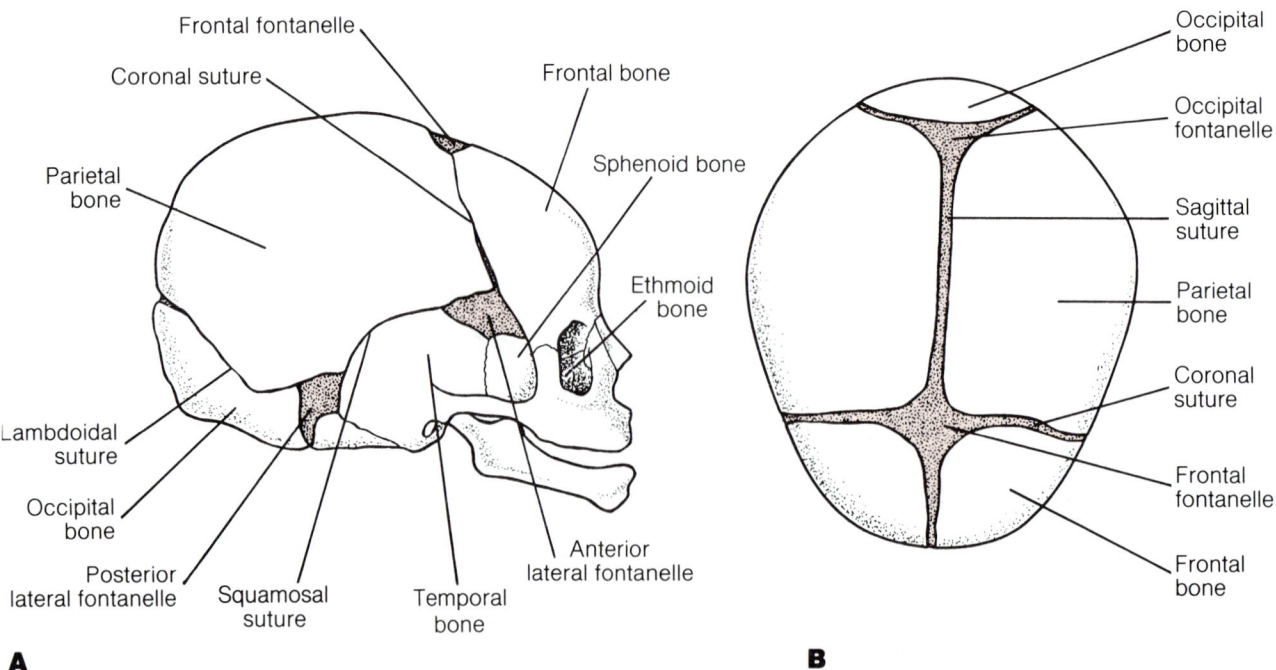

A **B**

Figure 25–3 The bones of the skull showing the fontanelles and the suture lines. *A,* lateral view; *B,* superior view.

nated both vertically and horizontally. At 4 months, the infant can recognize familiar objects and follow moving ones. By 6 months, the infant can perceive colors. After 9 months, most can recognize facial characteristics and often smile in response to a familiar face. By 12 months, depth perception has developed, and the infant will be able to recognize where a change in level occurs, such as at the edge of the bed.

The infant's *hearing* is indistinct at birth because of the retention of fluid in the middle ear. After the baby's first cry, this fluid is cleared out. Newborns with intact hearing will react with a startle to a loud noise, referred to as the Moro reflex (see the discussion of reflexes later in this chapter). Within a few days, they are able to distinguish different sounds. For example, they can tell the difference between their mother's voice and that of another woman (James and Mott 1988, p. 90). In addition, they have the ability to ignore many of the sounds in the environment. Their preference is for soft, high-pitched noises, such as that of the female voice. At about 5 months of age, the infant will pause while sucking in order to listen to the mother's voice. A 9-month-old infant is able to locate the source of sounds and recognizes familiar ones. By 1 year, the infant listens to sounds, begins to distinguish words, and responds to simple commands.

The senses of *smell* and *taste* are functional shortly after birth. Newborns prefer sweet tastes and tend to decrease their sucking in response to liquids with a salty content. They are able to recognize the smell of their mother's milk and respond to this smell by turning toward the mother.

The sense of *touch* is well developed at birth. Skin-to-skin touching is important for an infant's development. They respond positively i.e., perceive warmth, love, and security, when touched, held, and cuddled. The newborn is also sensitive to temperature extremes and pain; however, babies react diffusely and cannot isolate the discomfort. The pain of an open safety pin in the buttock, for example, is not isolated in the buttock.

The *reflexes* of the newborn are unconscious, involuntary responses. They are neither learned nor consciously carried out. They are nervous system reflexes in response to a number of stimuli. The degree of stimulation that is required to produce a reflex, for example the sucking reflex, varies considerably among newborns. Some newborns respond with vigor to the slightest stimulus, while others respond more slowly.

Ten main reflexes are normally present at birth. They are rooting, sucking, swallowing, Moro, palmar grasp, plantar, tonic neck, placing, stepping, and Babinski. These are described in the accompanying box. In addition, the abilities to yawn, stretch, sneeze, burp, and hiccup are all present at birth. Infant reflexes disappear during the first year of life.

Motor development is the development of the baby's ability to move and to control the body. Initially, body movement is uncoordinated. At 1 month of age, the infant

Infant Reflexes

- *Rooting* and *sucking reflexes*. Both used in feeding. The former is elicited by touching the baby's cheek, causing the baby's head to turn to the side that was touched. The sucking reflex occurs when the baby's lips are touched.

- *Swallowing reflex*. Can be observed when the infant swallows any liquid obtained from sucking.

- *Moro reflex* (startle reflex). Often assessed to estimate the maturity of the central nervous system. A loud noise, a sudden change in position, or an abrupt jarring of the crib elicits this reflex. The infant reacts by extending both arms and legs outward with the fingers spread, then suddenly retracting the limbs. Often the infant cries at the same time.

- *Palmar grasp reflex*. Occurs when a small object is placed against the palm of the hand, causing the fingers to curl around it.

- *Plantar reflex*. Similar to the palmar grasp reflex in that an object placed just beneath the toes causes them to curl around it.

- *Tonic neck reflex* (TNR) or fencing reflex. A postural reflex. When a baby who is lying on its back turns the head to the right side, for example, the left side of the body shows a flexing of the left arm and the left leg. This reflex is observed during the first week after birth.

- *Placing reflex*. Seen when a baby is held vertically with legs separated. When one foot is moved to touch the edge of a table, the baby automatically flexes the knee and hip of the same leg and tries to place the foot on the surface of the table.

- *Stepping reflex* (walking or dancing reflex). Can be elicited by holding the baby upright so that the feet touch a flat surface. The legs then move up and down as if the baby were walking. This reflex usually disappears at about 2 months.

- *Babinski reflex*. A newborn baby has a positive Babinski. When the sole of the foot is stroked, the big toe rises and the other toes fan out. After age 1, the infant exhibits a negative Babinksi, that is, the toes curl downward; positive Babinski after age 1 indicates brain damage.

lifts the head momentarily when prone, turns the head when prone, and has a head lag when pulled to a siting position. By 2 months, infants can raise their heads from a prone position. After 6 months, they can sit without support. See Figure 25–4. At 9 months, they can reach, grasp a rattle, and transfer it from hand to hand. At 12 months, they can turn the pages of a book, put objects into a container, walk with some assistance, and help to dress themselves. See Table 25–1 for details about motor development.

Psychosocial Development

According to Erickson, the central crisis at this stage is *trust versus mistrust*. Resolution of this stage determines how the person approaches subsequent developmental stages. An infant first learns trust from the parent or caregiver and then from others in the environment. Parents and caregivers can enhance a sense of trust by consistently responding promptly to an infant's needs and by providing a predictable environment in which routines are established.

Infants have no understanding of waiting and no time frame by which to measure waiting. The initial reaction of an infant to stress is crying, and crying is the infant's way of communicating distress. Infants learn gradually to tolerate stress. Tension is reduced by sucking and mouthing objects. Nurses and parents can reduce the stress of an infant by maintaining the infant's routine as much as possible and limiting the number of strangers interacting with the infant.

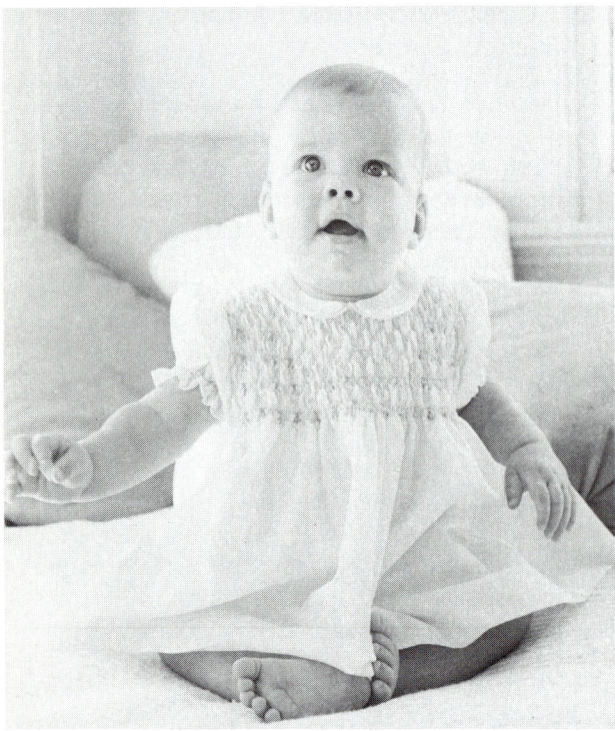

Figure 25–4 An infant sits without support at 6 months of age.

By 8 months, most infants seem to be attached to their parents and may show displeasure when left with strangers.

The newborn reacts socially by paying attention to the adult face or voice and by cuddling when held. They are able to interact with the environment by responding to various stimuli such as touch and sound. See Table 25–1 for details about social development.

Cognitive Development

Cognitive development involves remembering, thinking, perceiving, abstracting, and generalizing. It results in the development of a logical method of looking at the world and utilizing perceptual and conceptual abilities. *Intelligence,* by contrast, is the ability to learn.

According to Piaget, cognitive development is a result of interaction between an individual and the environment. Piaget refers to the initial period of cognitive development as the sensorimotor phase. See Table 24–6 on page 591. This phase has six stages, three of which take place during the first year. From 4 to 8 months, infants begin to have perceptual recognition. By 6 months, they respond to new stimuli, and they remember certain objects and look for them for a short time. By 12 months, infants have a concept of both space and time. They experiment to reach a goal, such as a toy on a chair.

An infant's cognitive development also proceeds from reflexive ability of the newborn to using one or two actions to attain a goal by the age of 1 year.

Moral Development

Infants associate right and wrong with pleasure and pain. What gives them pleasure is right, since they are too young to reason otherwise. When infants receive abundant positive responses from the parent such as smiles, caresses, and voice tones of approval in these early months, they learn that certain behaviors are wrong or good and that pain or pleasure is the consequence. In later months and years, children can tell easily and quickly by changes in parental facial expressions and voice tones that their behavior is either approved or disapproved. The less pleasure and more frustration the infant experiences in interactions with parents, the more important other sources of pleasure become. Children are then liable to risk parental anger and do things they like and desire even though others disapprove.

Health Promotion and Protection

Apgar Scoring Newborn babies can be assessed immediately by the **Apgar scoring system.** This provides a numeric indicator of the baby's physiologic capacities to adapt to extrauterine life. Each of five signs is assigned a maximum score of 2, so that the total score achievable is 10. A score under 7 suggests that the baby is having difficulty, and a score under 4 indicates that the baby's condition

TABLE 25-1 *Motor and Social Development in Infancy*

Age	Motor Development	Social Development
Newborn	Moves legs and arms randomly	Responds with eye contact
	Grasps objects in hands	Attends to adult face and voice
	Has substantial eye and mouth control but is unable to hold head up	Displays satisfaction
2 months	Lifts head off table when prone	Recognizes familiar face
	Turns from side to back	Attends to speaking voice
	Follows moving objects with eyes	Social smile appears
3 months	Actively holds rattle	Laughs aloud
	Holds head erect	Shows pleasure in vocalization
	Willfully places objects in mouth	Smiles in response to mother's face
		Makes prelanguage vocalizations: coos and babbles
4 months	Holds head steady in sitting position	Reaches out to people
	Rolls from back to side and abdomen to back	Squeals
	Grasps objects in two hands	
5 months	Grasps objects with whole hand	Discriminates between strangers and family
	Plays with toes	Vocalizes displeasure when a desired object is removed
	Rolls from stomach to back or vice versa	Smiles at image in mirror
6 months	Lifts cup by handle	Starts to imitate sounds
	Sits alone without support	Vocalizes one syllable sounds: *ma ma, da da*
		Plays peek-a-boo
7 months	Able to bear weight when held in standing position	Shows fear of strangers
	Bangs objects together	Imitates simple acts
	Grasps toys with one hand	
8 months	Feeds self with fingers	Is bashful and nervous with strangers
	Pulls toys	Opens arms to be picked up
		Responds to *no*
9 months	Creeps and crawls	Cries when scolded
	Sucks, chews, and bites objects	Complies to simple verbal requests
	Handles cup or glass with help	Displays fear of being alone, e.g., going to bed
	Pulls self to standing position	Waves bye-bye
	Uses pincer grasp with thumb and forefinger	
10 months	Sits by falling	Aware of own name
	Picks up objects	Presents toy to another person but will not release it
	Pulls self to standing position	
	Stands if holding onto support	
11 months	Pushes toys	Imitates speech sounds
	Puts objects into container	Reacts with frustration when restricted
	Tries to walk unsupported	
	Tries to hold spoon	
12 months	Hand dominance manifested	Knows own name
	Walks with help	Shakes head for *no*
	Uses spoon to feed self	Does things to attract attention

Source: Adapted from C. Edelman and C. L. Mandle, *Health promotion throughout the life span* (St. Louis: C. V. Mosby Co., 1986), pp. 318–19. Reproduced by permission of the C. V. Mosby Co.

is critical. Apgar scoring is usually carried out 60 seconds after birth and is repeated in 5 minutes. Those with very low scores require special resuscitative measures and care. See Table 25–2.

Developmental Screening Tests

Development can be assessed by observing the infant's behavior and by using standardized tests such as the **Denver Developmental Screening Test (DDST).** See Figure 25–5. The DDST is used to screen children from birth to 6 years of age. The test is intended to estimate the abilities of a child compared to those of an average group of children of the same age. The DDST does not provide diagnostic information about a child's problem, does not predict how a child will develop, and should not be used to assign a child to a developmental age group. Four main areas of development are screened: *personal-social, fine motor adaptive, language,* and *gross motor.* For each behavior, an age range is given that indicates whether 25%, 50%, 75%, or 90% of the children perform the task.

DDST manuals, kits, and scoring forms include directions for administering the test. The test is intended to be administered by professionals, such as nurses or psychologists. Usually, the child is asked to perform tasks of increasing difficulty. The child's performance is then scored according to the instructions.

Another screening tool, the **Denver Prescreening Developmental Questionnaire (PDQ)**, is completed by parents when the DDST cannot be administered. It consists of 97 questions grouped according to the child's age. The parents need to answer only 10 questions. In many situations, the PDQ is preferred as the initial screening tool because of its brevity. Depending on the results, the DDST can then be administered.

There are many other screening tests, for example, the Brazelton Neonatal Behavioral Assessment Scale, which focuses on neonatal behavior, and the Washington Guide to Promoting Development in Young Children.

Ongoing Nursing Assessments

During ongoing assessments, the nurse examines and observes the infant, actively listens to the parent for possible problems or areas of concern, and reviews with the parent the expected behavior or characteristics for the particular age group. This is an opportunity to allow the parent to discuss observations of the infant with the nurse. It is important for the parent to know that certain behaviors, responses, and activities of the infant are normal and expected. It is also important to discuss the many individual differences that can, quite normally, occur. The new parent needs to be given valid and accurate information to avoid undue concern with advice and comparisons from well-meaning friends.

The assessment interview is also a time to be supportive of the parent's role, to assess the attachment of the mother to the infant, and to observe the interactions between the infant and parent. Assessment activities may include the following:

- Observation of the skin for rashes or chafing.
- Measurement of weight, length, and head and chest circumferences.
- Palpation of the fontanelles for size, pulsations, and tenseness.
- Assessment of vital signs (see Chapter 18 for normal values): Remember that the pulse of the baby at birth is affected by the child's activity, rising up to 170 when the infant is crying and falling to as low as 70 during sleep. Blood pressure is difficult to measure in the newborn and may vary according to the instrument used and the skill of the practitioner taking the measurement.
- Assessment of vision and hearing. Inspect vision by observing the infant's ability to follow a moving object. Inspect hearing by observing response to clapping hands and talking.
- Assessment of reflexes and motor abilities.
- Observation of the infant's interaction with the parent and vocalizations.
- Discussion of the infant's nutrition, elimination, and rest/sleep patterns.

Examples of wellness diagnoses (see Chapter 23) and NANDA nursing diagnoses and goals for the infant are shown in Table 25–3. Outcome criteria also need to be developed.

TABLE 25–2 *Apgar Scoring System to Assess the Newborn*

	Score		
Sign	**0**	**1**	**2**
1. Heart rate	Absent	Slow (below 100 per minute)	Above 100 per minute
2. Respirations	Absent	Slow, irregular	Regular rate, crying
3. Muscle tone	Flaccid	Some flexion of extremities	Active movements
4. Reflex irritability	None	Grimace	Cries
5. Color	Body pale or cyanotic	Body pink (for black babies, pink mucous membranes), extremities blue	Body completely pink in whites, pink mucous membranes in blacks

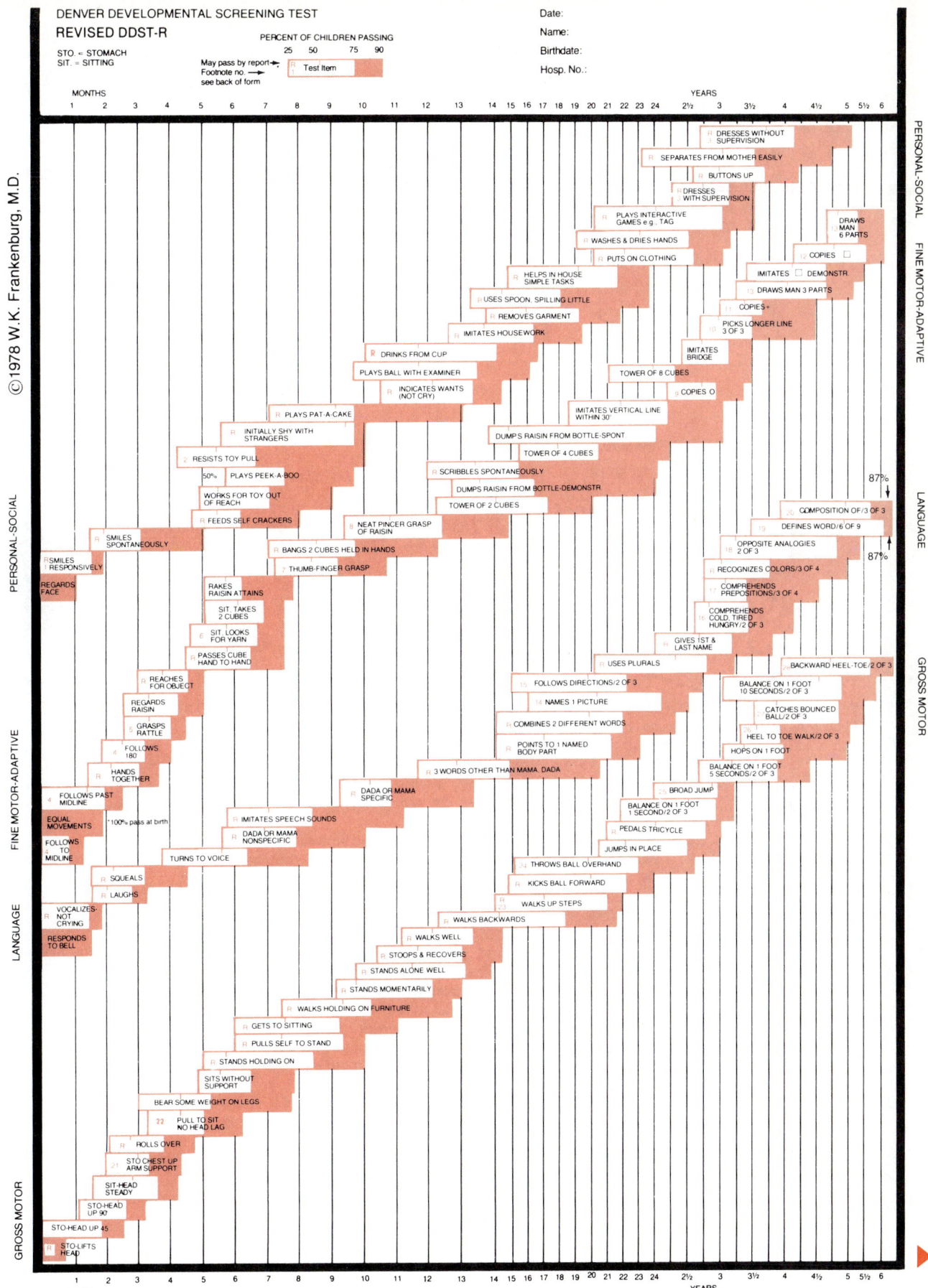

Figure 25-5 The Revised Denver Developmental Screening Test: Screening form.
Source: Reprinted with permission of W. K. Frankenburg, University of Colorado Medical Center.

607

1. Try to get child to smile by smiling, talking or waving to him. Do not touch him.
2. When child is playing with toy, pull it away from him. Pass if he resists.
3. Child does not have to be able to tie shoes or button in the back.
4. Move yarn slowly in an arc from one side to the other, about 6" above child's face. Pass if eyes follow 90° to midline. (Past midline; 180°)
5. Pass if child grasps rattle when it is touched to the backs or tips of fingers.
6. Pass if child continues to look where yarn disappeared or tries to see where it went. Yarn should be dropped quickly from sight from tester's hand without arm movement.
7. Pass if child picks up raisin with any part of thumb and a finger.
8. Pass if child picks up raisin with the ends of thumb and index finger using an over hand approach.

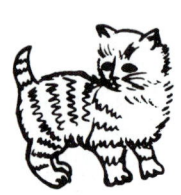 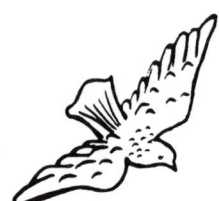 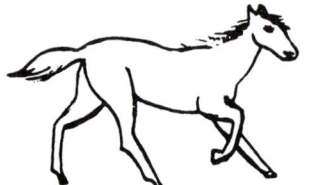 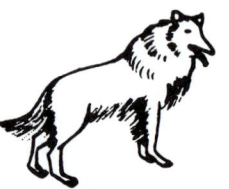

9. Pass any enclosed form. Fail continuous round motions.
10. Which line is longer? (Not bigger.) Turn paper upside down and repeat. (3/3 or 5/6)
11. Pass any crossing lines.
12. Have child copy first. If failed, demonstrate

When giving items 9, 11 and 12, do not name the forms. Do not demonstrate 9 and 11.

13. When scoring, each pair (2 arms, 2 legs, etc.) counts as one part.
14. Point to picture and have child name it. (No credit is given for sounds only.)

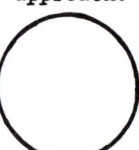 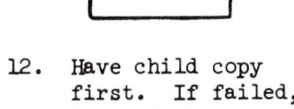 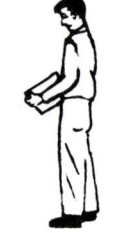

15. Tell child to: Give block to Mommie; put block on table; put block on floor. Pass 2 of 3. (Do not help child by pointing, moving head or eyes.)
16. Ask child: What do you do when you are cold? ..hungry? ..tired? Pass 2 of 3.
17. Tell child to: Put block on table; under table; in front of chair, behind chair. Pass 3 of 4. (Do not help child by pointing, moving head or eyes.)
18. Ask child: If fire is hot, ice is ?; Mother is a woman, Dad is a ?; a horse is big, a mouse is ?. Pass 2 of 3.
19. Ask child: What is a ball? ..lake? ..desk? ..house? ..banana? ..curtain? ..ceiling? ..hedge? ..pavement? Pass if defined in terms of use, shape, what it is made of or general category (such as banana is fruit, not just yellow). Pass 6 of 9.
20. Ask child: What is a spoon made of? ..a shoe made of? ..a door made of? (No other objects may be substituted.) Pass 3 of 3.
21. When placed on stomach, child lifts chest off table with support of forearms and/or hands.
22. When child is on back, grasp his hands and pull him to sitting. Pass if head does not hang back.
23. Child may use wall or rail only, not person. May not crawl.
24. Child must throw ball overhand 3 feet to within arm's reach of tester.
25. Child must perform standing broad jump over width of test sheet. (8-1/2 inches)
26. Tell child to walk forward, ⚬━⚬━⚬━➔ heel within 1 inch of toe. Tester may demonstrate. Child must walk 4 consecutive steps, 2 out of 3 trials.
27. Bounce ball to child who should stand 3 feet away from tester. Child must catch ball with hands, not arms, 2 out of 3 trials.
28. Tell child to walk backward, ◀━⚬━⚬━⚬ toe within 1 inch of heel. Tester may demonstrate. Child must walk 4 consecutive steps, 2 out of 3 trials.

DATE AND BEHAVIORAL OBSERVATIONS (how child feels at time of test, relation to tester, attention span, verbal behavior, self-confidence, etc,):

Figure 25−5 (continued) The Revised Denver Developmental Screening Test: Test instructions.

TABLE 25–3 Examples of Nursing Diagnoses and Goals for the Infant

	Diagnoses	Goal
Wellness diagnoses	**Appropriate health maintenance** related to good parenting skills	Over the next 2 months, parents continue to provide effective health maintenance for the infant.
	Optimal nutritional status related to knowledge of age-related nutritional needs	Over next 2 months, the infant continues to maintain optimal nutritional status.
NANDA diagnoses	**Health-seeking behaviors** related to knowledge of normal infant physical and social development	Parents learn normal growth and development patterns for first year of life.
	Altered nutrition: potential for more than body requirements related to lack of knowledge of infant cues of satiety	In 2 months, infant's weight gain is within normal limits.

The following are examples of criteria for the NANDA diagnosis **Health-seeking behaviors** in Table 25–3:

- Parents read instructional materials as assigned.
- Parents attend classes for new parents for one month.
- Parents obtain a passing grade on a comprehensive test related to infant care.

To give adequate *care to the infant,* the parent or caregiver needs teaching, support, and guidance from the nurse. The nurse may wish to discuss the following topics with the parents and also provide appropriate reading materials and references.

Immediate Protective Measures

Newborns have very little resistance to infection. For this reason, parents and caregivers should be instructed to wash their hands before handling the newborn and to avoid contact with the infant if they have a cold or skin infection. In some cases, it is possible for gonorrhea organisms to be transmitted to an infant during its passage through an infected vaginal canal. Two protective measures usually carried out immediately after birth are the use of antibiotics or the placement of 2 drops of 1% silver nitrate solution into each eye to protect against the gonorrhea organisms, and the administration of Vitamin K to protect the infant against trauma. Vitamin K, which is necessary for clotting, is not produced by intestinal bacteria for several days. In the female infant, the vaginal area is protected by a thin, bluish-white mucous coating known as **smegma.** This mucous substance protects the vaginal area from fungal and bacterial infections.

Health Maintenance Visits

Infants should have preventive health care visits 2 weeks after birth and at 2, 4, 6, 9, and 12 months of age. These health maintenance visits are necessary for health promotion activities such as maintaining proper diet, health protection activities such as obtaining immunizations, and for early detection of problems such as screening for tuberculosis. See the health maintenance schedule in Table 25–4.

TABLE 25–4 Health Maintenance Schedule

Nursing Activities	Ages
Assessments	2 weeks; 2, 4, 6, 9, 12, and 18 months; 2, 3, 5, 8, 11, 13, 15, and 17 years
Complete history and physical examination	First visit, interval history thereafter
Immunization (DTP, OPV, MMR, Td)	According to schedule
Rubella serology	Prepuberty (unvaccinated girls)
Haemophilus influenzae type B	24 months
Tuberculin (tine) test	1, 3, 5, 11, and 15 years
Hemoglobin/hematocrit	1, 4, 9, 12, 14, and 16 years
Lead screening	2 years
Urinalysis	6 months; 2, 3, 4, 5, 6, 9–10, 11–12, 13–15, and 15–18 years
Urine culture	3 and 8 years
Blood pressure	4 years and at each subsequent visit
Vision/hearing	1, 4, and 6 months; 1, 3, and 6 years and at each subsequent visit
Language	2, 3, and 5 years
Dental	6, 7–8, 13–15, and 15–18 years
Scoliosis	9–10, 11–12, and 13–15 years
Counseling (nutrition, physical care, psychosocial concerns, sex education, safety, family interaction)	Each visit

Source: S. R. James and S. R. Mott, *Child Health Nursing: Essential Care of Children and Families.* (Menlo Park, Calif.: Addison-Wesley Publishing Co., 1988), p. 314. Used with permission.

Immunization   Immunization against communicable diseases is a preventive health measure advocated by government agencies in the United States and Canada.

Newborn infants have limited ability to produce antibodies until they are about 3 months of age. However, during the last months of pregnancy, certain maternal antibodies pass through the placenta, thus providing the baby with some passive immunity. This immunity is temporary; so it is vital to practice good hygiene around infants, sterilize their formulas, and not expose them to infected people.

At 2 or 3 months of age, children should receive their first immunizations. Antigens in the form of **vaccines** (living or dead microorganisms) or **toxoids** (detoxified toxins) are administered to induce active immunity. Tables 25–5 and 25–6 show the immunizations advised in the United States and Canada. Immunizations are needed to protect infants from the microorganisms causing diphtheria, pertussis, and tetanus. Immunization is provided in a combined diphtheria, tetanus toxoids, and pertussis (DTP) vaccine. Infants also require the orally administered poliomyelitis vaccine. In the United States and Canada, infants usually receive DTP vaccines at approximately 2, 4, and 6 months and poliomyelitis vaccine at 2 and 4 months. Measles-rubella vaccine or a combined measles-mumps-rubella vaccine is recommended at age 1 year, as well as a tuber-culin test to determine exposure to the tuberculosis bacillus. In some areas, smallpox vaccine is also given between the third and twelfth months.

Haemophilus influenzae type B (Hib) is a bacterial infection that most commonly occurs in children under the age of 5 years. It is the major cause of bacterial meningitis (an infection of the covering of the brain) in this age group. Bacterial meningitis is fatal in about 5% of cases, and many of the children who survive have some permanent brain damage, which can cause mental retardation, deafness, paralysis, or other serious problems. Other forms of Hib infection include pneumonia and epiglottiditis (an inflammation of the entrance of the voice box in the throat), which when severe can require emergency surgery to prevent suffocation. Hib infection is spread by coughing, sneezing, or close face-to-face contact.

Immunizations are normally not given to persons with elevated temperatures; however, mild infections, such as a cold without a fever, do not contraindicate immunizations. The most frequent reaction to an immunization is slightly elevated temperature; occasionally a reaction can be more severe—high temperature, sleepiness, or even convulsion. Physicians needs to be consulted if the immunized person has a severe reaction or continues to feel ill 48 hours after the immunization.

TABLE 25–5   *Recommended Schedule for Active Immunization of Normal Infants and Children*

Recommended Age*	Vaccine(s)†	Comments
2 months	DTP-1‡, OPV-1§	Can be given earlier in areas of high endemicity
4 months	DTP-2, OPV-2	6-week to 2-month interval desired between OPV doses to avoid interference
6 months	DTP-3	Additional dose of OPV at this time optional for use in areas with a high risk of polio exposure
15 months¶	MMR**, DTP-4, OPV-3	Completion of primary series of DTV and OPV
24 months	*Haemophilus influenzae* type B	Can be given at 18–23 months for children at increased risk
4–6 years††	DTP-5, OPV-4	Preferably at or before school entry
11–13 years	MMR***	2nd dose of a 2-dose schedule
14–16 years	Td‡‡	Repeat every 10 years throughout life

* These recommended ages should not be construed as absolute; that is, 2 months can be 6–10 weeks, for example.

† For all products used, consult manufacturer's package enclosure for instructions for storage, handling, and administration. Immunobiologics prepared by different manufacturers might vary, and those of the same manufacturer might change from time to time. The package insert should be followed for a specific product.

‡ DTP—Diphtheria and tetanus toxoids and pertussis vaccine.

§ OPV—Oral, attenuated poliovirus vaccine contains poliovirus types 1, 2, and 3.

¶ Simultaneous administration of MMR, DTP, and OPV is appropriate for clients whose compliance with medical care recommendations cannot be assured.

**MMR—Live measles, mumps, and rubella viruses in a combined vaccine. For children living in high risk areas, vaccination is recommended at 12 months, 15 months, and between 11–13 years.

†† Up to the seventh birthday

‡‡ Td—Adult tetanus toxoid and diphtheria toxoid in combination, which contains the same dose of tetanus toxoid as DTP or DT and a reduced dose of diphtheria toxoid

Source: New immunization guidelines issued by the CDC, *Hospital Practice,* March 1983, 18:1000. Reprinted with permission. ***American Academy of Pediatrics revises measles vaccination policy. AAP News Release (July 1989).

TABLE 25-6 *Routine Immunization Schedule for Infants and Children—Canada*

Age	Immunization Agent
2 months	Diphtheria-pertussis-tetanus, poliomyelitis
4 months	Diphtheria-pertussis-tetanus, poliomyelitis
6 months	Diphtheria-pertussis-tetanus, poliomyelitis
12 months	Measles-mumps-rubella†
18 months	Diphtheria-pertussis-tetanus, poliomyelitis, *Haemophilus influenzae*, type B‡
4–6 years	Diphtheria-pertussis-tetanus, poliomyelitis
14–16 years	Diphtheria§

* This dose may be omitted if live (oral) polio vaccine is being used exclusively.

† Rubella vaccine is also indicated for all girls and women of childbearing age who lack proof of immunity. At all medical visits, the opportuntiy should be taken to check whether girls and women need rubella vaccine.

‡ A single dose of *Haemophilus influenzae* type B (Hib) conjugate vaccine should be administered to all children 18 to 24 months. Children 25 to 60 months should also be considered for vaccination, particularly those in daycare centers and at increased risk of invasive Hib disease. Conjugate vaccine should be given at the first visit for children over 18 months who are unlikely to return for further immunization. Conjugate vaccine and diphtheria-pertussis-tetanus (DPT) vaccines may be given simultaneously at different sites.

§ Tetanus and diphtheria toxoid (Td), a combined absorbed "adult type" preparation for use in persons 7 years of age or more, contains less diphtheria toxoid than preparations given to younger children and is less likely to cause reactions in older persons.

Source: National Advisory Committee on Immunization, Canada, *Canadian Immunization Guide* 3d ed., Catalog No. H49–8/1989 E (Ottawa: Minister of National Health and Welfare, Canada Health Protection Branch, Laboratory Centre for Disease Control 1989), pp. 26–27.

The risks of immunization include potential side-effects and complications, contamination of the serum with microorganisms other than the desired antigens, worsening of a natural disease, and failure to protect against the disease. Vaccinating a person whose resistance to infection is decreased or who is allergic to the vaccine could result in death. Nurses who administer immunizations must be knowledgeable about the indications, storage, dosage, preparation, and contraindications for each of the vaccines to be administered. Specific immunization guidelines and precautions are available from national public health service departments.

Safety   Accident prevention planning is essential. Although infants are completely dependent on others for care, they soon learn to roll from side to side, put objects in their mouths, and crawl. They are oblivious to such dangers as falling or ingesting harmful substances. Accidents are the sixth leading cause of death during infancy and one of the major causes of death after the first year of life. Parents should be advised that infants need to be watched con-stantly. To prevent falls, caregivers should never leave an infant unattended on a dressing table or on any raised surface without sides. To prevent burns, parents and caregivers need to check the temperature of bath water prior to bathing the infant, avoid handling hot liquids near the infant, and keep the infant protected from the sun. In addition, prior to taking the infant home from the hospital, parents need to acquire a federally approved infant car seat, which should then be used consistently.

In the United States, crib safety regulations were enacted in February 1974. All cribs manufactured after that date must comply with special standards. Regulations govern the space between slats (no more than 2⅜ in), the size of the crib and mattress, the height of the crib sides, and the use of lead-free paint. Parents should be warned that second-hand or borrowed furniture manufactured prior to 1974 may not comply with these standards.

Recently, the traditional playpen has been replaced by expandable wooden corrals, which provide for a larger and more portable play area. These play spaces have resulted in injury, because children can use the openings as footholds for climbing. Children have also sustained injuries by putting their heads through these openings and having the sides collapse on them. Playpens with sides made of netting decrease this type of injury, but even they are not without danger. The size of the netting must be small enough so that the infant cannot get buttons caught in it. The sides of the playpen should remain up whenever the child is left in it. Leaving one side down increases the risk of suffocation if the child gets caught between the mattress and the netting.

During the first year of life, infants learn to crawl and stand. This activity allows them access to a wide variety of potential hazards. Parents may need help in identifying potential hazards in and around the home and should be encouraged to remove many of the dangers in anticipation of the infant's development. The nurse should encourage parents to enroll in a first aid course that includes cardiopulmonary resuscitation, interventions for airway obstruction, and the identification of common household hazards. As a result of this, they will be more knowledgeable and better prepared to protect their children from accidents and injuries. Common accidents during infancy include burns, suffocation, automobile accidents, falls, poisoning, and choking. See Table 25–7 on page 612 for a list of potential hazards to infants and preventive measures.

Skin Care   The infant depends upon the parent or caregiver for care of the skin. Sponge baths are suggested for the newborn, since daily tub baths are not considered necessary. The frequency of bathing depends on the type of the infant's skin (dry, normal, or oily). For example, children with dry skin should be bathed less frequently. Other factors to be considered include the infant's schedule and the environmental temperature. After the bath, the infant should be immediately dried and wrapped. Parents need to be advised that the infant's ability to regulate body temperature has not yet fully developed. Infants perspire mini-

TABLE 25–7 *Potential Hazards and Preventive Measures for Newborns and Infants (Birth to 1 Year)*

Potential Hazard	Preventive Actions
Suffocation in crib	Do not put pillows, excess blankets, plastic, or anything that might suffocate a baby in the crib.
Strangulation by objects hung around the neck	Do not suspend a pacifier or anything that might cause strangulation around the infant's neck
Choking from aspirated milk or ingested objects	Hold the infant at feeding time. Do not leave the infant alone with a propped bottle.
	Provide only soft, large toys that do not have parts the infant can remove, swallow, and aspirate
	Cut solid foods into small pieces, and do not feed the child peanuts or popcorn.
	Do not leave infants unattended while they are eating
	Hold infants relatively upright while they are nursing or feeding from a bottle and have older infants eat only when sitting.
	Keep pins, needles, buttons, and nails out of reach of the baby. It is natural for infants to put such objects in their mouths.
Falling	Do not leave a baby alone in the bath, at the bed or table, or anywhere the infant may roll off or fall. Always keep a hand on the infant.
	Always keep the sides of the crib up when not handling the baby.
	On stairs, hold the baby with two hands.
	When the infant begins to crawl, place guard rails at the top and bottom of stairs and put screens on windows.
	Supervise children constantly when they are in a walker, jumper, swing, or high chair.
Automobile accidents	Use approved infant car seats to restrain infants in automobile.
	Place the infant in the back seat.
Burns	Always test bath water before immersing the infant.
	Remove potential hazards such as hot coffee while the baby is sitting in your lap.
	Turn pot handles toward the back of the stove and use back burners.
	Remove stove burner dials if they are within the infant's reach.
	Fence off wood-burning stoves and portable heaters.
	Protect the baby from sunburn.
	Avoid smoking around the infant.
Cuts, puncture wounds, bruises, and other injury	Place bumpers in the crib to prevent the infant from putting his or her head between the crib slats; slats should be no more than 2⅜ inches apart.
	Stuff towels between loose-fitting mattress and the sides of the crib to prevent infants from catching their arms or fingers between them.
	Keep the sharp points of diaper pins away from the baby's skin.
	Cut the baby's fingernails while the baby sleeps; sharp fingernails can scratch the infant.
	Use only plastic bottles and feeding cups; broken glass is a hazard.
	Make sure that toys have no sharp edges.
	Keep hazardous equipment such as fans and humidifiers off the floor and out of the infant's reach, and remove dangerous objects from counters and tables.
	Raise the sides of playpens and use corrals with net siding.
Electrical shock	Cover electrical outlets. Coil the cords of appliances to keep them out of reach.
Poisoning	Place plants, household cleaners, and wastebaskets out of the infant's reach.
	Lock cabinets that contain such potential poisons as medicines, paint, and gasoline.
	Store formula in a cool, dry place to prevent it from spoiling.

mally, and shivering starts at a lower temperature than it does in adults; therefore, they lose more heat before shivering begins. In addition, because the infant's body surface area is very large in relation to body mass, the body loses heat readily (Guyton 1986, p. 1003). Therefore, the infant should be dressed appropriately and covered with a blanket. A draft-free room with temperatures between 20.0 C and 24.4 C (60–76 F) is recommended.

Parents and caregivers must also be aware that infants can be dressed too warmly. **Miliaria rubra** (prickly heat) is a common skin problem that occurs on hot, humid days and is caused by blocked sweat glands. Newborns are particularly susceptible because they do not perspire until after 1 month of age. The rash can occur on any part of the body that is overheated. Prickly heat can be prevented by keeping the infant cool and dry. To reverse the rash, the caregiver can remove excess clothing, give a tepid sponge bath, or move the infant to a cooler environment.

Nutrition

Meeting an infant's nutritional needs is one of the prime concerns of parents and caregivers. Good nutritional habits begin in infancy and are one of the best preventive practices available (James and Mott 1988, p. 116). Nurses need to know the beliefs of the parents with respect to nutritional practices. These beliefs may include cultural and ethnic preferences as well as individual variations. The nurse also should discuss some of the common myths that parents may believe. One of these is that "a fat baby is a healthy one." Obesity is a common problem among infants, and some parents may still falsely believe that an overweight infant represents successful parenting and good health. Parents need to be educated regarding the dangers of overfeeding infants, since obesity can hinder normal development and place the infant at risk for future health problems.

The *neonate's* fluid and nutritional needs are met by breast milk or formula. Newborns may be hungry shortly after birth, or they may not develop an appetite for 1 to 2 days. Their stomach capacity is about 90 ml, and feedings are required every 2½ to 4 hours. Restlessness, crying, and head movement are behaviors that may indicate that the infant is hungry. The total daily nutritional requirement of the newborn is about 80 to 100 ml of breast milk, or formula, per kilogram of body weight. Neonates who perspire excessively in very warm environments may require additional fluids. In these cases, water may be prescribed. Practices vary with regard to the initial feeding of the newborn. Some newborns are fed immediately after birth; others are not given their first feeding for 12 hours. If feedings are withheld, sterile water or a solution of glucose in water should be substituted for them. Recently, it has been noted that babies fed early lose less weight and tend to coordinate their sucking and swallowing more effectively (Schuster and Ashburn 1986, p. 113).

The newborn infant is usually fed "on demand." A **demand-feeding** schedule usually means that the child is fed when hungry. This method tends to decrease the problem of overfeeding or underfeeding the infant.

The newborn infant typically requires up to eight feedings per day, at irregular time periods. The parent or caregiver needs to be able to recognize the infant's cues to hunger, the normal behavior during feeding, and signs of satisfaction or satiety. The newborn who is ready to eat usually cries, holds the fists tense, and exhibits tension in the entire body. During feeding, the infant sucks readily and needs burping after each ounce of formula or after 5 minutes of breast feeding. Burping is done by holding the infant in an upright position while gently patting the back. *Parents should be warned that infant bottles should never* *be propped up for feeding.* There is a real danger that aspiration or choking could result.

Infants demonstrate satisfaction by slowing their sucking activity, withdrawing their mouth from the nipple, or by falling asleep. Once satisfaction has been demonstrated, infants should not be coaxed into finishing the feeding. This could lead to discomfort or overfeeding. When feeding is completed, infants can be positioned prone or laterally; if positioned supine infants may aspirate some of the feeding.

Regurgitation, or spitting up, of predigested milk during or after a feeding is a common occurrence during the first year. Although this may be of concern to parents, it does not usually result in nutritional deficiency. Demonstration of adequate weight gain should reassure parents that the infant is receiving adequate nutrition.

Parents can help reduce the incidence of regurgitation by (a) placing the infant in an infant seat after the feeding to keep the head higher than the stomach, (b) holding the bottle tipped, so that the nipple is filled with formula, to prevent air swallowing, and (c) burping the infant frequently to prevent air bubbles. Regurgitation usually stops at about 3 months of age, when the sphincter muscle tone of the lower esophagus tightens (Schuster and Ashburn 1986, p. 144).

The *fluid needs* of infants are proportionately greater than those of adults because of a higher metabolic rate, immature kidneys, and greater water losses through the skin and the lungs. The last is largely due to rapid respirations. Therefore, fluid balance is a critical factor. Under normal environmental conditions, infants do not need additional water; adequate water intake should be provided in the infant formula. However, when limited volumes of milk are ingested during illness and when losses from vomiting and diarrhea occur, difficulties arise.

The addition of solid food to the diet usually takes place after 4 months of age. Some authorities suggest waiting until the child is 6 months old, when the first teeth appear. Six-month-old infants can consume solid food more readily because they can sit up, can hold a spoon, and have matured from the up-and-down tongue movements required for sucking to the lateral (side-to-side) tongue movements required for spoon feeding. Parents need to be given some instruction in basic nutrition and in the types of foods to give the infant. Solid foods (strained or pureed) are generally introduced in the following order: cereals (rice), fruits, vegetables (yellow before green), and strained meats. Foods are introduced one at a time, usually with only one new food introduced every 5 days. With the eruption of teeth at about 7 to 9 months, the infant is ready to chew and can begin to experience different textures of food. At this time, the infant enjoys finger foods, such as pieces of skinless fruit, dry cereal, or toast.

At about 6 months of age, infants require iron supplementation to prevent iron deficiency anemia. **Iron deficiency anemia** is a form of anemia caused by inadequate supply of iron for synthesis of hemoglobin. This anemia is manifested by a hematocrit of less than 30% at approximately 9 months of age. The low hematocrit may be accompanied by symptoms of pallor, anorexia, irritability, and lethargy. Iron-fortified cereals are usually recommended by 6 months of age and are continued until the child reaches 18 months.

Weaning from the breast or bottle to the cup takes place gradually and is usually achieved by age 1. Some infants enjoy drinking from a cup, while others have difficulty in giving up the bottle, particularly at nap time or bedtime. Parents should be warned that having the bottle in bed can lead to **bottle mouth syndrome.** The term describes the decay of the teeth caused by constant contact with the sweet liquid from the bottle. Some dentists advocate brushing or cleaning the infant's teeth to prevent bottle mouth syndrome, especially for the infant who requires a bottle only at nap or bedtime. Weaning from the bottle can be facilitated by increasingly diluting the formula with water until the infant is drinking plain water. Most infants do not like to drink plain water. By the age of 1, most infants can be completely fed on table food, and milk intake is about 20 ounces per day. See Chapter 39 for additional information on nutrition.

Elimination

Meconium is the first fecal material passed by the newborn, normally up to 24 hours after birth. It is black, tarry, odorless, and sticky. Transitional stools, which follow for about a week, are generally greenish yellow; they contain mucus and are loose.

Infants pass stool frequently, often after each feeding. Because the intestine is immature, water is not well absorbed, and the stool is soft, liquid, and frequent. When the intestine matures, bacterial flora increase. After solid foods are introduced, the stool becomes less frequent and firmer. Control is not established until the infant's neuromuscular systems are sufficiently developed.

Urine output varies according to fluid intake but usually is about 15 to 60 ml per day after birth, increasing to 250 to 500 ml per day during the first year. An infant may urinate as often as 20 times a day. The urine of the neonate is colorless and odorless and has a specific gravity of 1.008. Because newborns and infants have immature kidneys, they are unable to concentrate urine effectively.

Parents need to be informed that diarrhea (very watery stools occurring more than 5 times a day) may lead to dehydration. For infants, particularly those under 6 months old, medical treatment must be sought. The causes of diarrhea for the bottle-fed infant may include contamination of the formula or of the water supply or contamination during preparation. Diarrhea may also be caused by an infection in the infant. For the infant on solid foods, diarrhea may be the result of an intake of too much fruit or the introduction of a new food. For mild diarrhea of 1 or 2 days' duration, parents should be instructed to omit solid foods and to dilute the formula with water by up to one-half.

Rest/Sleep

An area of infant care of great concern to parents is rest and sleep. Some infants sleep as long as 22 hours a day, others as little as 10–12 hours a day. At first, they usually awaken every 3 or 4 hours, eat, and then go back to sleep. Periods of wakefulness gradually increase by the end of the first months. At about age 4 weeks, they may take three or four naps during the day and sleep for longer periods at night. By 4 months, most infants sleep through the night and establish a pattern of daytime naps that varies among individuals. They generally awaken early in the morning, however. At the end of the first year, an infant usually takes one or two naps per day and sleeps about 14 of every 24 hours.

About half of the infant's sleep time is spent in light sleep. During light sleep, the infant has a great deal of activity, e.g., movement, gurgles, and coughing. Parents need to ascertain that infants are truly awake before picking them up for feeding and changing. Most parents eagerly await the time when their infant begins to sleep through the night. Many infants, however, begin waking up again in the middle of the night between 5 and 9 months of age. Some parents are not bothered by these awakenings; others find this interruption in their own sleep difficult to tolerate. For parents who find this behavior a problem, the nurse needs to assess the infant's total sleep pattern and compare it with the parents' sleep schedule. Parents need reassurance that there is no correct way to handle this situation. The best solution is one that provides a continuous healthy environment for both the infant and the parents.

Crying

Crying is of great concern to parents. When an infant's crying cannot be alleviated, parents often feel a sense of failure and frustration. A crying and fussy period lasting from 1 to 2 hours a day is usually considered normal for most infants. Parents need to be given assurance that this crying period is considered a source of energy release for the infant and will stop as the infant replaces this activity with more interesting interactions.

Colic

A colicky infant is described as one having extended periods of crying, sometimes lasting up to 8 or 10 hours a day. Often the legs are extended, the body rigid, and the fists clenched. Colic is often associated with abdominal distention or passage of flatus. The crying results in the intake of more air, and the cycle of distention and pain continues. The cause of true colic is not known. Possible explanations include milk allergy, hyperactivity, parental anxiety, and feeding problems. The infant should be assessed for any underlying disease. If none is present, parents can be informed that their infant will outgrow colic after a few months. Parents with a colicky infant are often tired and stressed. The nurse should assure them that the behavior of the infant is not a result of any inadequacy on their part.

To help relieve the colic, the nurse can assess the infant during feeding and suggest possible changes. Suggestions may include decreasing environmental stimuli during and after feeding, changing the formula or nipple, and increasing the burping frequency. Other suggestions include increasing the water intake, cuddling the infant, and finding the position that provides the infant with the most comfort.

Sudden Infant Death Syndrome (SIDS)

Sudden infant death syndrome, also called "crib death," is the sudden and unexplained death of an infant who had previously been healthy. The cause of death remains unexplained even after a thorough postmortem examination. SIDS is currently the leading cause of postneonatal death in the United States, claiming over 10,000 lives annually. The etiology is unknown, but current research and debate is focused on the relationship between SIDS and infant apnea. SIDS primarily affects boys between 2 and 4 months of age. The risk is increased for infants of low birth weight and those whose mothers are younger than 20 years of age. Infants considered to be a high risk for SIDS include (a) siblings of SIDS victims, (b) premature infants with recurring episodes of apnea during sleep, and (c) survivors of SIDS (Edelman and Mandle 1986, p. 331).

With respect to prevention, monitors to detect apnea have been used in certain situations. Infants in high-risk categories with abnormal results from sleep studies are considered candidates for home apneic monitoring. The use of these monitoring systems is the subject of much debate and controversy. Parents often feel a great deal of anxiety as a result of being responsible for their infant's life. The nurse should support and counsel the family during this period.

Stimulation Through Play

The newborn can be stimulated by holding, touching, and looking at the infant, providing large, colorful hanging objects over the crib, and talking to the infant in a soothing voice. Infants also like to be rocked and stroked. All of these activities are enjoyable to the infant and promote healthy language, sensory, and cognitive development. Colorful hanging toys, toys that move, and musical toys enhance eye coordination and hearing and motivate the infant to reach and grasp. Play also provides the infant with activity and exercise. Playing, for the newborn, is moving the arms and legs, kicking, turning the head, and exploring the environment. Activity and exercise are enhanced by interaction from parents and others, including talking, rocking, and singing. Such toys and activities are

important stimulation opportunities until about 3 months of age. Later, infants explore objects by handling them and putting them in the mouth. They should have toys that they can grasp but not swallow, such as plastic blocks and rings, stuffed animals, rubber or plastic cars, or boats. By age 1, they like toys that pull apart, such as large plastic beads; those with wheels that they can push back and forth, such as a cart or wagon; and those that provide them with a variety of noises, such as musical instruments, bells, and whistles. Parent education should focus on the infant's developmental landmarks and the activities that can promote this development. For example, infants at 4 months need the opportunity to sit on the parent's lap so that they can learn to support their heads when upright. At 5 months, infants begin to roll from back to stomach. Parents can place toys out of reach to encourage this activity. As the infant begins to stand, parents can place an object of appropriate height within the infant's reach.

Infants need constant supervision during play and respond well to interaction and encouragement. For the young infant, a playpen provides a safe environment in which to crawl and move around. As the infant grows, a larger area is needed to promote and enhance development.

Trust

During the first year of life, infants show dissatisfaction by crying, and satisfaction by sleeping and playing. They depend on the parents for all their physiologic and psychologic needs. Fulfillment of these needs is required for the infant to develop a basic sense of trust. Parents can enhance this sense of trust by (1) responding consistently to an infant's needs, (2) providing a predictable environment in which routines are established, and (3) being sensitive to the infant's needs and meeting these needs skillfully and promptly. Mothering behavior such as loving care, handling, stroking, and cuddling are essential for healthy psychosocial development. Infants deprived of mothering, especially from months 3 to 15, will not learn to form significant relationships or to trust others.

Infants who fail to establish a loving, responsive relationship with an adult often fail to develop normally. The disturbed parent-child relationship can result in the **failure-to-thrive syndrome.** The infants show delayed development without any physical cause. They are often malnourished and fail to gain weight and grow normally. Another problem that can result from a disturbed parent-infant relationship is infant or child abuse. Abusing parents were often abused themselves as children.

Abuse

The problem of infant and child abuse is widespread in society. Some authorities place the figure at over 2 million cases of child abuse annually (James and Mott 1988, p. 393). About 6,000 children die each year from abuse, more than from any disease. Abuse is considered to be a symptom of severe family dysfunction. In such cases, each member of the family will require help and support from the nurse if the family is to move toward positive functioning.

Abuse can be physical, emotional, or sexual and includes neglect. The abused infant may appear dirty, have poor skin condition, or be inadequately dressed for the weather. The infant may be malnourished or listless and exhibit delays in meeting developmental milestones. Many parents who abuse their children have been abused themselves. Often, the parents feel inadequate in their role as parents and are overwhelmed by life itself.

Early recognition and reporting of child abuse, or suspected child abuse, is the key to promoting the health and well-being of children. All children in a potentially abusive situation should be protected until an investigation takes place. The following nursing interventions are suggested to prevent the abuse of infants:

■ During their high school years, teach adolescents about basic infant care, including the realities and pressures of 24-hour-a-day responsibilities.

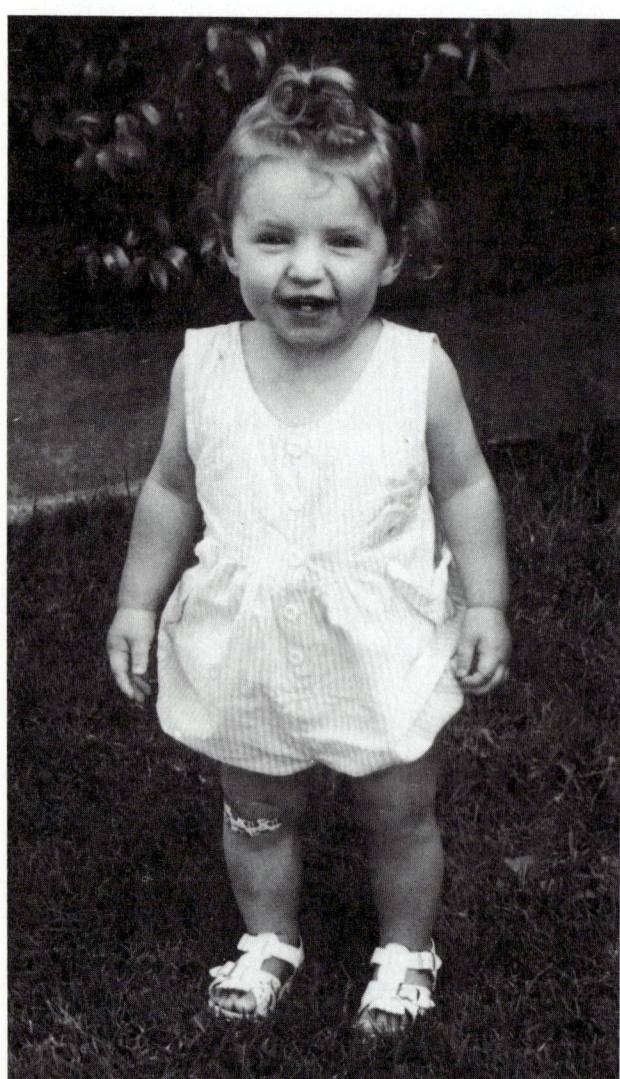

Figure 25–6 The toddler appears chubby with relatively short legs and a large head.

■ Offer prenatal classes to assist new parents in enhancing their child care knowledge and skills.

■ Assess and promote parent-infant bonding.

■ Schedule home visits for supervision and telephone contact hours for support.

TODDLERS (1 TO 3 YEARS)

Toddlers develop from having no voluntary control to being able both to walk and speak. They also learn to control their bladder and bowels, and they acquire all kinds of information about their environment.

Physical Development

Two-year-old children lose the baby look. Toddlers are usually chubby with relatively short legs and a large head. See Figure 25–6. The face appears small in comparison to the skull; but as the toddler grows, the face seems to grow from under the skull and appears better proportioned. Toddlers have a pronounced lumbar lordosis and a protruding abdomen. The abdominal muscles develop gradually as the toddler grows, and the abdomen flattens.

Two-year-olds can be expected to weigh approximately four times their birth weight. The *weight gain* is about 2 kg (5 lb) between 1 year and 2 years and about 1 to 2 kg (2 to 5 lb) between 2 and 3 years. The 3-year-old weighs about 13.6 kg (30 lb).

A toddler's *height* can be measured as height or length. Height is measured while the toddler stands, and length is measured while the toddler is in a recumbent position. Although the measurements differ slightly, nurses must specify which measurement is used to avoid confusion. Between ages 1 and 2 years the average growth in height is 10 to 12 cm (4 to 5 in), and between ages 2 and 3 years it slows to 6 to 8 cm (2½ to 3½ in).

The *head circumference* of the toddler increases on an average about 2.5 cm (1 in), and by 24 months the head is four-fifths of the average adult size. The brain is 70% of its adult size by the time the infant is 2 years old.

Visual acuity is fairly well established at 1 year; average estimates of acuity for the toddler are 20/70 at 18 months and 20/40 at 2 years of age. Accommodation to near and far objects is fairly well developed by 18 months and continues to mature with age. At 3 years of age, the toddler can look away from a toy prior to reaching out and picking it up. This ability requires the integration of visual and neuromuscular mechanisms.

The senses of *hearing, taste, smell,* and *touch* become increasingly developed and associated with each other. Hearing for the 3-year-old is at adult levels. The taste buds of the toddler are sensitive to the natural flavors of food, and the 3-year-old prefers familiar odors and tastes. Touch is a very important sense, and a distressed toddler is often soothed by tactile sensations.

Fine muscle coordination and *gross motor skills* improve during toddlerhood. At the age of 18 months, babies can pick up small beads and place them in a receptacle. They can also hold a spoon and a cup and walk upstairs with assistance. They will probably crawl down the stairs.

At 2 years, toddlers can hold a spoon and put it into the mouth correctly. They are able to run; their gait is steady; and they can balance on one foot and ride a tricycle. By 3 years, most children are toilet trained, although they still may have the occasional accident when playing or during the night.

Psychosocial Development

According to Freud, the ages of 2 and 3 years represent the *anal phase* of development, when the rectum and anus are the specially significant areas of the body. Erikson sees the period from 18 months to 3 years as the time when the central developmental task is autonomy versus shame and doubt (see Table 24–5 on page 588).

Toddlers begin to develop their **sense of autonomy** by asserting themselves with the frequent use of the word *no*. They are often frustrated by restraints to their behavior and between ages 1 and 3 may have temper tantrums. However, they slowly gain control over their emotions, usually with the guidance of their parents.

The period of the development of a sense of autonomy (1 to 3 years) is a time of expanding social contacts. Toddlers are curious and ask many questions. Children at this age are often creative, although the products of this activity may not be perfect.

Common responses of toddlers to stress are **separation anxiety** and **regression.** For example, toddlers may become highly anxious when separated from their parents and admitted to hospital. Regression or reverting to an earlier developmental stage may be indicated by bed-wetting or using baby talk. Nurses can assist parents by helping them understand that this behavior is normal and indicates that these toddlers are trying to establish their positions in the family. Toddlers assert their independence by saying no or by dawdling. During the toddler stage, receptive and expressive language skills are developing quickly. **Receptive language skill** is the ability to understand words. **Expressive language skill** refers to the ability to use or speak the words. At all ages, the ability to understand words is more advanced than the ability to express words and ideas. Children can understand words and follow directions long before they can actually form them into sentences (Castiligia 1987a, p. 165). By 1 year of age, toddlers can recognize their own names.

Cognitive Development

According to Piaget, the toddler completes the 5th and 6th stages of the *sensorimotor phase* and starts the *preconcep-*tual phase* at about 2 years of age. See Table 24–6 on page 591. In the fifth stage, the toddler solves problems by a trial-and-error process. By stage 6, toddlers can solve problems mentally. For example, when given a new toy, the toddler will not immediately handle the toy to see how it works but will look at it carefully to think about how it works.

During Piaget's preconceptual phase, toddlers develop considerable cognitive and intellectual skills. They learn about the sequence of time. They have some symbolic thought; for example, a chair may represent a place of safety, while a blanket may symbolize comfort. Concepts start to form in late toddlerhood. A concept develops when the child learns words to represent classes of objects or thoughts. An example of a concrete concept is *table,* representing a number of articles of furniture, which are all different but all tables.

Moral Development

According to Kohlberg, the first level of moral development is the preconventional when children respond to labels of "good" or "bad" (see Table 24–8, page 594). During the second year of life, children begin to know that some activities elicit affection and approval. They also recognize that certain rituals, such as repeating phrases from prayers, also elicit approval. This provides children with feelings of security. By 2 years of age, toddlers are learning what attitudes their parents hold about moral matters.

Spiritual Development

According to Fowler, the toddler's stage of spiritual development is undifferentiated (see Table 24–9 page 597). Toddlers may be aware of some religious practices, but they are primarily involved in learning knowledge and emotional reactions rather than establishing spiritual beliefs. A toddler may repeat short prayers at bedtime, conforming to a ritual, because praise and affection result. This parental response enhances the toddler's sense of security.

Health Promotion and Protection

Assessment activities for the toddler are similar to those for the infant in terms of measuring weight, length (height), and vital signs (see Chapter 18). The Snellen E chart (see page 378) can be used to assess the 2-year-old's vision. In addition, the nurse should obtain the following information from the parent:

- Motor skills, e.g., walking up stairs with assistance, putting beads into a container, balancing on foot, pedaling a tricycle, building a bridge from blocks, feeding skills
- Behavior when separated from parents
- Behavior when playing with other children
- Language abilities
- Nutrition, elimination, and rest/sleep patterns

Assessment guidelines for growth and development of the toddler are shown in the accompanying box.

Examples of wellness diagnoses (see Chapter 23) and NANDA nursing diagnoses and goals for the toddler are shown in Table 25–8. *Outcome criteria* also need to be developed. The following are examples of criteria for the NANDA diagnosis **Potential for injury** in Table 25–8:

- Within 1 week, parents remove all breakables and medicines from the toddler's reach.

- Within 1 week, all cleaning agents are moved to higher shelves.

- Within 1 week, all sharp-edged furniture is stored or removed from the toddler's play areas.

To facilitate the growth and development of the toddler and appropriate health maintenance, the nurse may choose to discuss the following topics with the parents.

Health Maintenance Visits and Immunizations

During the toddler period, health maintenance visits should be scheduled at 18 months and at 2 and 3 years of age (see Table 25–4). Immunizations continue to be an important aspect of health maintenance (see Tables 25–5 and 25–6).

Safety

Accidents are the leading cause of mortality of toddlers. They are curious and like to feel and taste everything. Because they are also fascinated by such potential dangers as garden pools and busy streets, they need constant supervision and protection. The most common causes of fatal injuries are automobile accidents, drowning, burns, poisoning, and falls. Parents need to provide the appropriate preventive measures to guard against these health threats. For example, in the United States, many states now require the use of federally approved car restraints for young children. For children under 40 pounds or 40 inches, a safety-tested car seat is recommended; children over 40 pounds can safely use a regular seat belt with a cushion to hold the belt in position and protect the abdomen from pressure. Children should be told that the car does not move until they are properly buckled up. Parents may also wish to reas-

ASSESSMENT GUIDELINES
The Toddler

Does the toddler:

- Indicate physical development within normal range?
- Eat and drink appropriately?
- Feed self?
- Start to develop bowel and bladder control?
- Exhibit physical skills appropriate for the age?

By 3 years of age, is the toddler able to:

- Pedal a tricycle?
- Balance on one foot, jump, and walk on tip toes?
- Copy a figure such as a circle?
- Build a bridge from blocks?
- Dress self?
- Express likes and dislikes or exhibit any other autonomous behavior?
- Understand words such as "up," "down," "cold," and "hungry"?
- Speak in sentences of three to four words?
- Stay dry both day and night?
- Accept separation from mother for short periods of time?
- Begin to play and communicate with children and others outside the immediate family?
- Display curiosity and ask many questions?
- Imitate religious rituals of the family?

sess their own behavior with respect to automobile safety and the use of seat belts.

Poisoning with lead, known as **plumbism**, remains a risk for the child under 6 years of age. Common sources of lead include paint chips from lead paint, fumes from leaded gasoline, and paper products and earthenware that have been

TABLE 25–8 *Examples of Nursing Diagnoses and Goals for the Toddler*

	Diagnosis	Goal
Wellness diagnoses	**Effective immune response** related to age-appropriate immunizations	During the next 6 months, toddler maintains effective immune response.
	Effective sleep and rest periods related to support of parents and caregivers	During the next 3 months, toddler maintains adequate sleep and rest periods.
NANDA diagnoses	**Health-seeking behaviors** related to knowledge of the effective methods of toilet training	Within 2 weeks, parent learns basic principles related to toilet training.
	Potential for injury related to age and motor development	Within 1 week, parents remove or secure major safety hazards from the toddler's reach.

decorated with lead paint. Parents should be aware that the ingestion of lead paint chips from windowsills and window frames painted with lead-based paint is the most common cause of lead poisoning in children. The nurse should provide the parents with the following guidelines:

- Children under 6 with a history of pica are at risk for lead poisoning.
- Homes built prior to 1957 should be tested for lead paint.
- Lead paint on walls must be removed professionally to the bare wood to a height of 4 feet from the floor.
- If paint cannot be removed, it must be covered with masonite or wood panels.
- Baseboards and moldings covered with peeling lead paint must be replaced.

Parents can prevent many accidents by "toddler proofing" the home or other setting where the child will be. This concept includes removing or securing all items that can pose a safety hazard to the child. All valuable or "precious" items should also be removed from the child's reach. Parents must keep in mind that the child's cognitive and motor skills increase quite quickly, and safety measures should keep up with these new skills. Training in safety should begin at this age. For example, toddlers should be taught not to run out on the street and taught the meaning of the Mr. Yuk sticker (available from the Poison Control Center) on cleaning solutions, insecticides, and other poisonous substances. A list of potential hazards along with their preventive measures is provided in Table 25–9.

Vision   Parents should be made aware that behaviors such as rubbing the eyes, squinting, blinking, or an inability to see things clearly may be indicative of a vision problem such as myopia or hyperopia. Myopia and hyperopia are refractive errors caused by alterations in the path of light

TABLE 25–9   *Potential Hazards and Preventive Measures for Toddlers (1 to 3 Years)*

Potential Hazard	Preventive Actions	Potential Hazard	Preventive Actions
Physical trauma from falling, banging into objects, or getting cut by sharp objects	Because accidents occur most frequently when parents are preoccupied, such as at mealtimes, parents need to share responsibility for preparing meals and supervising children.	Burns (*continued*)	Keep matches safely out of reach.
	If the child still sleeps in a crib, lower the sides while the child sleeps. Obtain a bed.		Place hot pots on the back burners, away from the toddler's reach.
	Keep the house free of clutter.		Test bath water before allowing the child to get in the tub.
	Keep furniture with sharp edges (e.g., glass-topped tables) out of the child's way.		Teach the dangers of charcoal fires.
	Place knives and other sharp tools out of reach.	Poisoning	Keep cleaning solutions, insecticides, and medicines in locked cupboards.
	Make sure that windows and balconies are made safe, for instance, sturdily screened.		Have house checked for lead paint.
	Make sure that pull-toy strings are no longer than 12 inches. Toys with longer strings can be lost from sight and pulled over hazardous objects.		Teach children not to put objects in their mouths. Especially warn against vegetation (e.g., leaves and berries), peeling paint, plaster, or objects picked up from the floor or street.
Motor vehicles	Make children wear seat belts and sit in the back seat while they are in the car.		Teach the child never to take pills unless they are given by a parent, nurse, or trusted adult.
	Teach the child not to ride a tricycle in the streets or behind cars.	Drowning	Do not leave toddlers unattended in bathtubs or pools.
Burns	Teach the words *no* and *don't.* Make the child understand that these words often signify danger and must be obeyed.		Do not overfill the bathtub.
			Do not let toddlers play near deep ditches and wells
			Teach the child to swim but never leave the child unsupervised at a pool or beach.
			Fence in pools.
		Electrical shock	Ensure that the toddler is protected from electrical outlets and equipment.

rays through the structure of the eye. **Myopia,** nearsightedness, is the inability to focus on objects that are far away. **Hyperopia,** or farsightedness, is the inability to focus on near objects. In severe cases of hyperopia and myopia, glasses may be prescribed.

During this period, the toddler should be screened for amblyopia and strabismus. **Amblyopia** (reduced visual acuity in one eye) may occur when there are unequal refractive errors in each eye, but it is usually the result of strabismus. The child with amblyopia has straight eyes, whereas the child with **strabismus** (cross-eye) has a deviant eye.

To detect amblyopia, visual testing is done with one eye occluded. The optimal time for correction of amblyopia is during early childhood. Treatment consists of patching the stronger eye so that the child is forced to use the weaker eye. This treatment is more difficult to encourage in school-age children because the poor visual acuity of the uncovered eye interferes with schoolwork and the patch may set them apart from their peers.

Strabismus is a deviation of the line of vision from the midline due to an imbalance or weakness in the extraocular muscles. Parents should be advised that strabismus must be treated as early as possible to prevent irreversible visual deficits. Methods of treatment include corrective surgery or the use of an eye patch over the nonaffected eye to require the deviated eye to fixate. Correction of these problems is important for future learning as well as for the optimum development of the toddler's concept of self.

Dental Health
Dental caries occur frequently during the toddler period, often as a result of the excessive intake of sweets or a prolonged use of the bottle during naps and at bedtime. The nurse should give parents the following instructions for promoting and maintaining dental health:

- Cleanse the child's teeth gently with a cotton ball moistened with hydrogen peroxide. This should begin when the first tooth erupts.

- Beginning at about 18 months of age, brush the child's teeth with a soft toothbrush.

- Schedule an initial dental visit for the child at about 2 years of age, and prepare the child for this experience.

- Seek professional dental attention for any problems such as discoloring of the teeth, chipping, or signs of infection such as redness and swelling.

Nutrition
Because of a maturing gastrointestinal tract, toddlers can eat most foods and adjust to three meals each day. In addition, by age 3, when most of the deciduous teeth have emerged, the toddler is able to bite and chew adult table food. Toddler's manipulative skills are sufficiently well developed for them to learn how to feed themselves. Before the age of 20 months, most toddlers require help with glasses and cups because their wrist control is limited.

Developing independence may be exhibited through the toddler's refusal of certain foods. Meals should be short because of the toddler's brief attention span and environmental distractions. Often toddlers display their liking of rituals by eating foods in a certain order, cutting foods a specific way, or accompanying certain foods with a particular drink.

The toddler is less likely to have fluid imbalances than the infant. Toddler's gastrointestinal function is more mature, and the percent of fluid body weight is lower. A healthy toddler weighing 15 kg (33 lb) needs about 1250 ml of fluid per 24 hours (James and Mott 1988, p. 638).

During the toddler stage, the caloric requirement is decreased (e.g., 1000 to 1500 kcal) because of a decrease in the rate of growth. From 1 to 2 years of age, the toddler may be eating a combination of prepared toddler foods and some table foods. Parents should be instructed to read labels carefully and be aware that the table foods offer more variety and are less expensive and more nutritious than prepared toddler foods. The basic four food groups should be used as a guide in discussing the toddler's diet with parents. The need for adequate iron, calcium, vitamins C and A, which are common toddler deficiencies, should also be discussed.

Three-year-olds often use mealtime to control the family conversation and gain attention by their constant chatter and disruption. Parents may need to anticipate the child's needs, make adjustments in their food preparation, and determine the acceptable level of table manners for the child's developmental level. The following suggestions may help parents to meet the child's nutritional needs and promote effective parent-child interactions: (a) make mealtime a pleasant time; avoid tensions at the table and discussions of bad behavior, (b) offer a variety of simple, attractive foods in small portions, and avoid meals that combine foods into one dish, such as a stew, (c) Do not use food as a reward or punish a child who does not eat, (d) schedule meals, sleep, and snack times that will allow for optimum appetite and behavior, and (e) avoid the routine use of sweet desserts.

Elimination
Control of the bladder and bowel is an important milestone of childhood. The average age for the completion of daytime toilet training is about 29 months; the average age for completion of day and night training is about 33 months. Parents need instruction early in the toddler period to avoid the pitfalls that can occur when toilet training is attempted too early. One-year-olds whose mothers put them on the potty every day at the right time are not trained; their mothers are trained. Toilet trained children independently go to the bathroom, undress, eliminate, and put their clothes back on. Children must be both interested and cooperative to complete this complex series of tasks. Parents need both instruction and support if they are to avoid the many frustrations that can occur in managing this first step toward the child's self-care. Children who are ready for toilet training are able to walk and balance well, climb onto the potty, and undress and dress themselves. The child also shows awareness of the need to defecate or urinate by either words or behavior. The read-

iness of the parent is also important. Toilet training requires time, patience, and a consistent approach. If a new sibling has entered the family or if the mother is returning to full-time work, the readiness of the child may be affected. After readiness has been determined, parents can promote and enhance development by using the following steps:

1. Introduce children to the potty chair, explain its use with words they can understand, and have them sit in it if they wish.

2. After a week or so, have the child sit in the potty chair with clothes off for 3 to 5 minutes, and explain what should be done, using the same words consistently.

3. If the child is interested, encourage potty use several times a day, praise the child's behavior, even for attempts, and do not scold or punish the child for undesired behavior.

4. When toddlers demonstrate their ability to achieve success, dress them in training pants that they can easily remove, and provide easy access to the potty chair.

Rest/Sleep   The sleep requirements of toddlers decrease to 10 to 14 hours per day. Most still need an afternoon nap, but the need for midmorning naps gradually decreases. The toddler may exhibit a great deal of resistance to going to bed. Parents need assurance that if the child has had adequate attention from them during the day, maintaining a consistent approach with respect to bedtime will promote good sleep habits for the entire family.

The child who awakens at night may be afraid of the dark or have experienced night terrors or nightmares. These fears should be respected and the child can be given a night light. When children awaken, the parents should talk with them and reassure them that they are all right and that the parents are close by. Bringing the children to the bed of the parents or lying down with them to help them get to sleep can cause difficulties, because children will expect those routines to continue. There are other points the nurse should emphasize to parents:

- Allow the child to bring a soft toy or blanket to bed.
- Activities prior to bedtime should be physically quieting and emotionally soothing.
- Sleep disturbances are a normal result of the developmental level as the child begins to deal with the idea of separation.

Autonomy/Sense of Self   The toddler period is the time when autonomy is developed. Parents need to have a great deal of patience coupled with an understanding of the importance of this developmental milestone. To be effective, parents need to give the child some measure of control and at the same time be consistent in setting limits so that the child learns the results of misbehavior. The nurse can also assist the parents and caregivers in promoting the tod-

---

Fostering the Toddler's Development

- Provide toys suitable for the toddler, including some toys challenging enough to motivate but not so difficult that the toddler will fail, as this will intensify feelings of self-doubt and shame.
- Make positive suggestions rather than commands. Avoid an emotional climate of negativism, blame, and punishment.
- Give the toddler choices, all of which are safe; however, limit number to two or three.
- When toddler has a temper tantrum, make sure the child is safe, and then leave.
- Help the toddler to develop inner control by setting and enforcing consistent, reasonable limits.
- Praise the toddler's accomplishments.

---

dler's development by suggesting the activities summarized in the box above.

Children learn to develop a sense of self through their immediate social environment, in which their parents play a significant role. If the children's social interactions with their parents are negative (e.g., constant disapproval regarding eating, toilet training, or other behavior), the children may begin to see themselves as bad. This perception is the basis of a negative self-concept. Parents need to give toddlers positive input so that they can develop a positive and healthy self-concept. With a healthy sense of self-esteem and security, the toddler is able to deal with periodic failures later in life without damage to self-esteem.

Although toddlers like to explore the environment, they always need to have a significant person nearby. Parents need to know that young children experience acute **separation anxiety,** the fear and frustration that comes with parental absences. Abandonment is their greatest fear. At this age, the child may have difficulty accepting a baby-sitter or strongly resist being left by the parents at a day-care center. Experience with separation helps the child cope with parental absences. Children need room for exploration and interaction with other children and adults. At the same time, they need to know that the parental bond of a loving and close relationship remains secure.

Stimulation Through Play   The child between 1 and 3 years of age seems to be engaged in endless activity. This activity is important for muscle development and the improvement of both motor skills and social skills. It is important for parents to help children pace their activity by providing outdoor games or swings and trips to the park, along with more quiet times, such as reading a book or having a nap. The main ingredient that the child needs to facilitate and enhance successful activity and play is freedom. Freedom implies that the child has adequate space to play and be active, without excess restraints on activity. During playtime, the child should also be free to act silly or to make mistakes without the restraint of parental evaluation (James and Mott 1988, p. 147).

The types of play toddlers engage in can be described as **onlooker play** (e.g., watching TV), **solitary play** (involvement in independent activities), **parallel play** (the child sits with other children but does not cooperate or interact with them), and **associative play** (e.g., building a tower of blocks with another child).

Most of the toddler's playing time is spent in solitary play. Young children like to move constantly and to move things constantly. They may empty bookcases and drawers, rearrange kitchen cupboards, change their clothes, imitate parental behavior such as sweeping or doing dishes, or run back and forth through the house. Parents should show enthusiasm for the toddler's activities, giving them praise for the "help," and smiling and clapping at the child's accomplishments. The amount of time a child spends watching TV should be monitored by parents. Parents may want to anticipate this problem and set limits early concerning the amount of time and the quality of programs they want their children to view.

Cognitive Stimulation   Parents need to be aware that the cognitive development of their child is a result of inherited ability, social interactions, and life experiences. Thus, cognitive development is enhanced by providing a variety of stimulating activities, interactions, and opportunities and by understanding the toddler's developmental skills. Parents can assist in the development of logic and reasoning by (a) playing simple games and solving puzzles (b) hiding objects and having the child find them, and (c) putting small objects in a container for the child to retrieve. Parents also need to be aware, and accepting, of any imaginary friends the child has created. The child often uses this make-believe behavior to do and say things that may sometimes be forbidden in the real world. Parents may experience some frustration when toddlers do not understand that they cannot have their own way or when it is difficult to understand what the child wants. Toddlers are very egocentric and do not realize that others may have thoughts that are different from their own.

PRESCHOOLERS (4 AND 5 YEARS)

During this period, physical growth slows, but control of the body and coordination increase greatly. The preschoolers' world gets larger as they meet relatives, friends, and neighbors.

Physical Development

By the time children are 4 or 5 years old, they appear taller and thinner than toddlers, because children tend to grow more in height than in weight. The preschooler's brain reaches its adult size by 5 years. The extremities of the body grow more quickly than the body trunk, making the child's body appear somewhat out of proportion. The posture of preschoolers gradually changes as the pelvis is straightened and the abdominal muscles become stronger. Thus the preschooler appears slender with erect posture.

Weight gain in preschool children is generally slow. By 5 years, they have added only another 3 to 5 kg (7 to 12 lb) to their 3-year-old weight, increasing it to somewhere between 18 and 20 kg (40 and 45 lb).

Preschool children grow about 5 to 6.25 cm (2.0 to 2.5 in) each year. Thus by 5 years of age, they double the birth length and measure 100 cm (40 in).

Preschool children are generally **hyperopic** (farsighted). As the eye grows in length, it becomes **emmetropic** (it refracts light normally). If the eyes become too long, the child becomes **myopic** (nearsighted). By the end of the preschool years, visual ability has improved; normal vision for the 5-year-old is approximately 20/30.

The hearing of the preschool child has reached optimal levels, and the ability to listen (attending to and comprehending what is said) has matured since the toddler age. In relation to the sense of taste, preschoolers show their preferences by asking for something "yummy," and may refuse something they consider "yucky."

By 5 years of age, children are able to wash their hands and face and brush their teeth. They are self-conscious about exposing their bodies and go to the bathroom without telling others. Typically, preschool children run with increasing skill each year. By 5 years of age, they run skillfully and can jump three steps. Preschoolers can balance on their toes and dress themselves without assistance.

Psychosocial Development

Erikson writes that the major developmental crisis of the preschooler is *initiative versus guilt*. See Table 24–5 on page 588. Preschoolers must solve problems in accordance with their consciences. Their personalities develop. Erikson views the crises at this time as important for the development of the individual's *self-concept*. Parents and caregivers can enhance the development of the preschoolers by praising effort at new activities and providing opportunities to repeat new activities until they are mastered. According to Erikson, preschoolers must learn what they can do. As a result, preschoolers imitate behavior, and their imagination and creativity become lively.

Preschoolers also become increasingly aware of themselves. They play with their bodies largely out of curiosity. They know where the body begins and ends as well as the correct names for the different parts. By 5 years of age, they are able to draw a person including all the features. Pre-schoolers also learn about their feelings; they know the words *cry, sad, laugh,* and the feelings related to them. They also begin to learn how to control their feelings and behavior.

Freud theorizes that the preschooler is in the *phallic stage* of development. The biologic focus of the child during this stage is the genital area.

The preschooler uses the same types of *coping mechanisms* in response to stress as the toddler does, although protest behavior (kicking, screaming) is less likely to occur in the older preschooler. Preschoolers usually have greater ability to verbalize stress.

By 4 years of age, children tend to believe that what they know is right. They tend to be dogmatic in their *speech.* Four-year-olds love nonsense words such as *jump-jump* and can string them together much to an adult's exasperation. At 4, children are aggressive in their speech and capable of long conversations, often mixing fact and fiction. By 5 years of age, speaking skills are well developed. Children use words purposefully and ask questions to acquire information. They do not merely practice speaking as 3- and 4-year-olds do, but speak as a means of social interaction. Exaggeration is common among 4- and 5-year-olds.

Preschool children gradually emerge as social beings. At the age of 3 or 4, they learn to play with a small number of their peers. They gradually learn to play with more people as they grow older. Preschoolers participate more in the family than they did previously. In associations with neighbors, family guests, and baby-sitters, too, they learn about social relationships.

The phase of close emotional relationship with both parents changes to the phase Freud referred to as the Electra or Oedipus complex (Engel 1962, pp. 90–104). At this time, the child focuses feelings of love chiefly on the parent of the opposite sex, and the parent of the same sex may receive some hostile feelings. At this time, the child begins to develop sexual interests. The child become interested in clothes and hair styles.

During the preschool years, four *adaptive mechanisms* are learned: identification, introjection, imagination, and repression. **Identification** occurs when the child perceives the self as similar to another person and behaves like that person. For example, a boy may internalize the attitudes and gender behavior of his father. **Introjection** is similar to identification. It is the assimilation of the attributes of others. When preschoolers observe their parents, they assimilate many of their values and attitudes. **Imagination** is an important part of preschoolers' life. The preschooler has an active imagination and fantasizes in play; for example, a chair becomes a beautiful throne to a girl, and she is the ruler. **Repression** is removing experiences, thoughts, and impulses from awareness. The preschooler generally represses thoughts related to the Oedipus or Electra complex.

Cognitive Development

The preschooler's cognitive development, according to Piaget, is the phase of *intuitive thought.* Children are still egocentric, but egocentrism gradually subsides as they encounter wider experiences. Preschoolers learn through trial and error, and they think of only one idea at a time. They do not understand relationships such as those between mother and father or sister and brother. Children start to form concepts in late toddlerhood or the early preschool years. Preschoolers become concerned about death as something inevitable, but they do not explain it. They also associate death with others rather than themselves.

Most children at the age of 5 years can count pennies; however, the opportunity to spend money usually does not occur until they attend school. Reading skills also start to develop at this age. Young children like fairy tales and books about animals and other children.

Moral Development

Preschoolers are capable of prosocial behavior, i.e., any action that a person takes to benefit someone else. See Figure 25–7 on page 624. The term *prosocial* is synonymous with *kind* and connotes sharing, helping, protecting, giving aid, befriending, showing affection, and giving encouragement (Schulman and Mekler 1985, p. 232).

At this stage of development, preschoolers do not have fully formed consciences; however, they do develop some internal controls. Moral behavior is largely learned by *modeling*, initially after parents and later after significant others. The preschooler usually behaves well in social settings.

Children who perceive their parents as strict may become resentful or overly obedient. Preschoolers usually control their behavior because they want love and approval from their parents. Moral behavior to a preschooler may mean taking turns at play or sharing. Nurses can assist parents by discussing moral development and encouraging parents to give preschoolers recognition for actions such as sharing. It is also important for parents to answer preschoolers' "why" questions and discuss values with them.

Spiritual Development

Many preschoolers enroll in Sunday school or faith-oriented classes. The preschooler usually enjoys the social interaction of these classes. According to Fowler, children from the ages of 4 to 6 years are at the intuitive-projective stage of spiritual development. See Table 24–9 on page 597.

Faith at this stage is primarily a result of the teaching of significant others, e.g., parents and teachers. Children learn to imitate religious behavior, e.g., bowing the head in prayer, although they don't understand the meaning of the behavior. Preschoolers require simple explanations, like those in picture books, of spiritual matters. Children at this age use

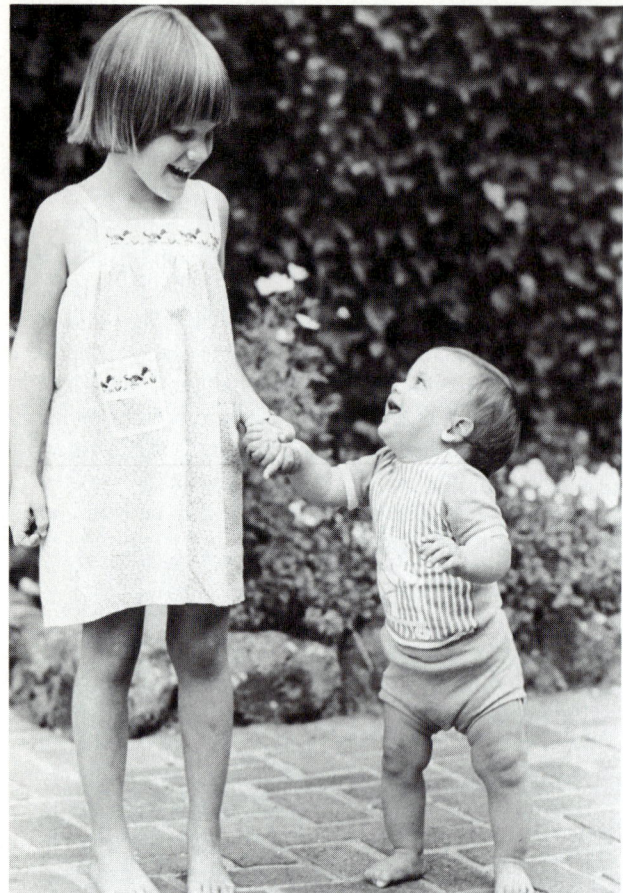

Figure 25–7 Preschoolers are capable of deriving pleasure from helping and encouraging others.

their imaginations to envision such ideas as angels or the devil.

Health Promotion and Protection

During assessment, the preschooler can participate in answering questions with some assistance from parents when appropriate. For instance, children who attend preschool can describe the typical lunch and how much of it they usually eat. Preschoolers can also describe the types of activities that they enjoy. Assessment activities may include

- Measurements of weight, height, and vital signs (see Chapter 18)
- Vision testing with Snellen E test (if the child is unable to read) or the alphabet test (if the child is able to identify letters)
- Listening to speaking skills (by 5 years the child uses complete sentences)
- Discussion with parents about the child's interaction with peers, parents, siblings; and patterns of nutrition, elimination, activity/exercise, and sleep/rest

Assessment guidelines for growth and development of the preschooler are shown in the box below.

Examples of wellness diagnoses (see Chapter 23) and NANDA nursing diagnoses and goals for the preschooler are shown in Table 25–10. *Outcome criteria* also need to be developed. The following are examples of criteria for the NANDA diagnosis **Potential for infection** in Table 25–10:

- Child learns preventive measures, such as not sharing food or drinks.
- Child maintains good health practices, such as proper diet, exercise, and rest.

The nurse may wish to discuss the following topics with the parents in order to help them facilitate the optimum development of their preschool child.

ASSESSMENT GUIDELINES
The Preschooler

Does the preschooler:

- Indicate physical development within a normal range?
- Possess physical skills appropriate for the age?

By 5 years of age, is the child able to:

- Jump rope and skip?
- Climb playground equipment?
- Ride a bicycle with training wheels?
- Demonstrate that the child is toilet trained?
- Perform simple hygiene measures and dress and undress self?
- Enjoy playing with peers in cooperative activities?
- Use complete sentences with all parts of speech?
- Identify four colors?
- Print letters and numbers?
- Separate easily from parents?
- Display imagination and creativity?
- Exhibit appropriate emotional expressions in different situations?
- Understand right and wrong, and respond to others' expectations about behavior?
- Ask questions and exhibit increasing vocabulary?
- Appear eager to do things, e.g., completing a household chore such as putting away toys, and to please others?
- Identify with people of own sex?

TABLE 25–10 *Examples of Nursing Diagnoses and Goals for the Preschooler*

	Diagnosis	Goal
Wellness diagnosis	**Nutrition intake appropriate for adequate growth** related to the parents' knowledge of the needs of the age group	Child maintains an appropriate nutritional intake over the next year.
NANDA diagnoses	**Potential for infection** related to exposures at nursery school.	Child maintains health during the school year.
	Potential altered growth and development related to the ages of the children and changes in the family situation	Child continues normal growth and development during family transition.

Health Maintenance Visits and Immunizations

Parents should schedule preventive health care visits and regular dental examinations during the preschool years. A suggested schedule for health maintenance is outlined in Table 25–4. Immunizations that are recommended between 4 and 6 years of age include diphtheria, tetanus toxoid, and pertussis (DTP) vaccine, and oral attenuated poliomyelitis (OPV) vaccine. See Tables 25–5 and 25–6, earlier in this chapter.

Safety

Accidents continue to be the major cause of mortality among preschool children. These children are active and often clumsy and are therefore susceptible to injury. Accidents can be prevented in two ways: control of the environment and education of the child. Parents may need to learn to control the environment, for instance, by keeping matches, household medicines, and other potential poisons out of the child's reach, by teaching the child to put toys away when they are not being used and by safeguarding swimming pools and other potentially dangerous areas. The education of the preschooler may involve learning how to cross streets, what traffic signals mean, and how to ride a bicycle safely. Preschoolers like to imitate their parents, so adults can teach safety through example. For a list of potential hazards and their preventive measures for preschoolers, see Table 25–11 on page 626.

Dental Health

Estimates are that 80% of children in this age group have some tooth decay. Deciduous teeth guide the entrance of permanent teeth. Therefore, abnormally placed or lost deciduous teeth can cause the misalignment of permanent teeth. Fluoridation of water in the community and in school water systems can significantly reduce the number of cavities in children. If the local water supply is not fluoridated, parents can provide rinses, toothpastes, or supplements to protect their children against cavities and gum disease. Children also need instruction in the care of their teeth, such as proper brushing and the avoidance of sugary snacks. Parental supervision is needed to assure the completion of these self-care activities. See Chapter 22 for additional information.

Nutrition

The preschooler eats adult foods and should have the required amounts from the four food groups. See Chapter 39 for specific information about these amounts. Parents should become informed about the diet of their child in day-care or preschool settings so that they can be sure of meeting the child's total nutritional needs. Children at this age are very active and may rush through the meal to return to playing. The 4-year-old still requires parent's help in cutting meat and may spill milk when pouring from a large container. Parents also need to teach the preschooler how to use utensils and should provide them with the opportunity to practice (e.g. buttering bread). However, 4- and 5-year-olds often use their fingers to pick food up. Table manners are marginal at best. Active children often require snacks between meals. Cheese, fruits, yogurt, raw vegetables, and milk are good choices. Children at this age may enjoy helping in the kitchen, and both girls and boys should be encouraged to do so.

The preschooler is even less susceptible than the toddler to fluid imbalances. The average 5-year-old weighing 20 kg (44 lb) requires at least 75 ml of liquid per kilogram of body weight per day, or 1500 ml every 24 hours (James and Mott 1988, p. 638).

Elimination

The preschooler is able to take responsibility for independent toileting. Parents need to realize that accidents do occur and the child should never be punished or chastised for this. Children often forget to wash their hands or flush the toilet and need instruction in wiping themselves. The female child should be taught to wipe from front to back to prevent contamination of the urinary tract by feces.

Rest/Sleep

The preschool child requires 12 hours of sleep per night, particularly during the school year. Many children of this age dislike bedtime and resist by requesting another story, game, or television program. The 4- to 5-year-old may become restless and irritable if sleep requirements are not met. A nap or quiet time during the day may be needed to restore energy levels.

TABLE 25–11 *Potential Hazards and Preventive Measures for Preschoolers (4 to 5 Years)*

Potential Hazards	Preventive Measures
Choking, suffocation, and obstruction of the airway and ear canal by foreign objects	Do not allow children to run while they have candy or other objects in mouth.
	Teach children not to put small objects in the mouth, nose, and ears.
	Remove doors from unused equipment such as refrigerators, which can entrap and asphyxiate the child who hides in them.
Injury from traffic, playground equipment, and other objects	Teach preschoolers to cross streets safely and to obey traffic signals.
	Teach them to play on sidewalks or grass rather than in driveways, in the street, or on railroad tracks.
	Teach them not to walk in front of swings and not to push others off playground equipment.
	Encourage them to put their toys away so that people will not trip over them.
Poisoning	Check Halloween treats before allowing the child to eat them; discard any loose or open candy.
	Reinforce that they should not eat any vegetation or objects from the street.
	Reinforce that they should not take pills without the parent's consent.
Drowning	Same as for the toddler, Table 25–9.
Fire and burns	Teach the preschooler the dangers of playing with matches and near charcoal or other controlled fires and heating appliances.
Harm from other people or animals	Teach children to avoid strangers and to keep parents informed of their whereabouts.
	Teach children to walk quietly near animals and to avoid approaching them if a trusted adult is not present.

Children in this age group still require bedtime rituals. Parents can help children who resist bedtime by warning them that bedtime is approaching and by continuing to use the same firm and consistent approach as suggested for the toddler. Preschool children wake up frequently at night. Knowing how commonly this behavior occurs and that it usually decreases by age 6 may be reassuring for many parents. The cause of this nighttime wakening may be night terrors or nightmares. During a *night terror* the child screams, is in obvious distress, and is difficult to console. The child never fully wakes up but goes back to sleep in about 10 minutes with no recollection of the frightening episode. During *nightmares,* which are far more common, children wake up and can describe the details of their dreams vividly. Children who wake up at night should be consoled by their parents, reminded that the dream was not real, and encouraged to return to sleep.

Sense of Self   Preschoolers emerge from the toddler years with a sense of self that they will continue to develop and refine. Parents can enhance the self-concept of the preschooler by providing opportunities for new achievements where the child can learn, repeat, and master. For example, a child obtains a two-wheel bike with safety wheels and quickly learns coordination, balance, use of the brakes, and bicycle safety. Mastery of these tasks provides the child with a sense of accomplishment. The child is soon ready for the new challenge of mastering the two-wheeler.

The self-concept of the preschooler is also based on gender identification. The preschooler is aware of the two sexes and identifies with the correct one. They often imitate sexual stereotypes and usually begin by identifying with the parent of the same sex. They may mimic the parent's behavior, attitudes, and appearance. Parents need to be aware that preschoolers are very curious about their own bodies and sexual functions, as well as those of others, and will often ask questions. Parents should not imply that a question is inappropriate or that a particular subject is bad.

Preschoolers need to feel that they are loved and that they are an important part of the family. The child who has to compete with siblings for parental attention will often display jealousy. Parents should be aware that preschoolers need time to adjust to a new baby and may need additional attention or special activities to help them through this adjustment period. Preschoolers with older siblings may also experience sibling rivalry. Siblings may fight and argue and become very aggressive because of their daily close proximity or competition for parental attention. Parents who can plan some special time or activity for each child will help that child to feel loved and may decrease the sibling rivalry.

Guidance and discipline are important parts of the parental role during the preschool years. As children seek independence from adults, they often test limits by refusing to cooperate and by repeatedly ignoring parental requests. Parents find themselves both frustrated and irritated. These power struggles can sometimes be avoided by encouraging children to be responsible for their own behavior as much as possible and by setting reasonable expectations and consistent limits. When conflict does occur, parents can employ the "no-lose" method of conflict resolution, which involves mutual discussion and compromise (James and Mott 1988, p. 175).

Stimulation through Play The preschooler's main activity continues to be play. Children of 4 to 5 years can separate easily from their parents and enjoy more interactive activities. Parents can facilitate their development by introducing new games to children, such as hide-and-seek, that have simple rules and require cooperation. Children also enjoy planning group activities, such as a picnic or visit to the zoo, and benefit from toys that encourage role playing, such as construction trucks, dress-up dolls, and make-believe games. Preschoolers are able to regulate their activity and usually do well in a group setting for several sessions per week.

Social Interaction Preschoolers enjoy playing with their peers and can even take part in some activities with older children. Social interaction is important for this age group. It provides them with opportunities to learn the rules of play and cooperation, such as taking turns and following directions. Parents should be encouraged to provide these situations for the preschooler in order to enhance social development and foster school readiness.

Language The preschooler uses language to express ideas. Parents can facilitate improved language skills by

- Encouraging the child to tell stories
- Never criticizing the child's speech, and remaining patient if the child stumbles over words
- Playing word games to teach the child new objects or names
- Reading and discussing stories with the child

Cognitive Stimulation Preschool children remain egocentric and cannot understand that other people have thoughts that are different from theirs. Parents who are aware of this will be prepared for the difficulty and the frustration that children experience when they cannot have their own way and are unable to understand that another way exists.

Preschoolers understand the concept of time, and memory and creativity are developing. When parents discuss the activities of last week or last winter, children can usually remember the sequence of events that took place. Cognitive development can be promoted by providing opportunities for memory games and by encouraging a variety of creative play activities.

The development of moral values is closely related to the cognitive development of the child. At the preschool age, children do not have a true conscience and basically do things in their own best interest. Parents can assist in their moral development by encouraging and praising actions such as sharing and by discussing values with them.

SCHOOL-AGE CHILDREN (6 TO 12 YEARS)

The school-age period starts when children are about 6 years of age, when the deciduous teeth are shed. This period includes the preadolescent (prepuberty) period. It ends at about 12 years, with the onset of puberty. Puberty is the age when the reproductive organs become functional and secondary sex characteristics develop. Because the average age of onset of puberty is 10 for girls and 12 for boys, some people define the school-age years as 6 to 10 for girls and 6 to 12 for boys. Skills learned during this stage are particularly important in relation to work later in life and willingness to try new tasks.

Starting school is significant for a number of reasons; for one, children are able to compare their skills to those of their peers. They also receive impressions of how their skills are perceived by others: the teacher, the school nurse, and their peers. These perceptions can bolster a child's self-image or can weaken feelings of self-worth. In general, the period from 6 to 12 years is one of rapid and dramatic change.

Physical Development

The school-age child gains weight rapidly and thus appears less thin than previously. Individual differences due to both genetic and environmental factors are obvious at this time. At 6 years, boys tend to weigh about 21 kg (46 lb), about 1 kg (2 lb) more than girls. The *weight gain* of school children from 6 to 12 years of age averages about 3.2 kg (7 lb) per year, but the major weight gains occur from age 10 to 12 for boys and from 9 to 12 for girls. By 12 years of age, boys and girls weigh on the average 40 to 42 kg (88 to 95 lb); girls are usually heavier.

At 6 years, both boys and girls are about the same *height*, 115 cm (46 in). They are about 150 cm (60 in) by 12 years. Before puberty, children of both sexes have a growth spurt, girls between 10 and 12 years and boys between 12 and 14 years. Thus, girls may well be taller than boys at 12 years, although the boys are usually stronger.

The extremities tend to grow more quickly than the trunk, thus school-age children's bodies appear somewhat ill-proportioned. By 6 years of age, the thoracic curvature starts to develop, and the lordosis disappears. Full adult *posture* is not assumed, however, until after the complete development of the skeletal musculature during the adolescent period.

The *depth and distance perception* of children 6 to 8 years of age is accurate. By age 6, children have full binocular vision: The eye muscles are well developed and coordinated, and both eyes can focus on one object at the same time. Because the shape of the eye changes during growth, the farsightedness of the preschool years gradually changes to 20/20 vision during the school-age years; 20/20 vision is usually well established between 9 and 11 years of age. In later childhood, myopia is not uncommon; that is, the child is able to see clearly only objects that are close. This problem is generally corrected by eyeglasses.

Auditory perception is fully developed in school-age children, who are able to identify very fine differences in voices, both in sound and in pitch. At this stage, children also have a well-developed sense of touch and are able to locate points of heat and cold on all body surfaces. They are also able to identify an unseen object, such as a pencil or a book, simply by touch. This ability is called **stereognosis** (Shuster and Ashburn 1986, p. 449).

Very little change takes place in the reproductive and endocrine systems until the prepuberty period. During *prepuberty,* at about ages 9 to 13, endocrine functions slowly increase. This change in endocrine function can result in increased perspiration and more active sebaceous glands. As a result, acne may develop, particularly on the face, neck, and back.

Certain physical changes occur in both boys and girls during prepuberty. Some of the changes in approximate sequence are as follows:

For the boy:

- The testes and scrotum increase in size.
- The skin over the scrotum changes color; it becomes reddened and stippled.
- The breasts may enlarge slightly, but this growth disappears in a few months.
- Sparse, downy pubic hair grows at the base of the penis.
- The penis gradually becomes wider and longer. Development of the genitals to adult size take about 5 to 6 years.
- The boy grows taller and his shoulders widen.
- Axillary sweating begins.

For the girl:

- The pelvis and hips broaden.
- The breast tissues develop and may be tender. At first the nipple is slightly elevated, at 7½ to 8 years of age. The areolae become somewhat protuberant and enlarged between the ages of 9 and 11 years.
- Axillary sweating begins.
- The initial growth of pubic hair occurs at 8 to 14 years.
- Vaginal secretions become milky and change from an alkaline to an acid pH, and vaginal flora change from mixed to Döderlein's lactic acid–producing bacilli (Murray and Zentner 1989, p. 296).

During the middle years (6 to 10), children perfect their *muscular skills* and coordination. By 9 years, most children are becoming skilled in games of interest, such as football or baseball. These skills are often associated with school, and many of them are learned there. By 9 years most children have sufficient fine motor control for such activities as building models or sewing.

Psychosocial Development

According to Erikson, the central task of school-age children is *industry versus inferiority.* At this time children begin to create and develop a sense of competence and perseverance. School-age children are motivated by activities that provide a sense of worth. They concentrate on mastering skills that will help them function in the adult world. Although children of this age work hard to succeed, they are always faced with the possibility of failure, which can lead to a sense of inferiority. If children have been successful in previous stages, they are motivated to be industrious and to cooperate with others toward a common goal (Erikson 1963).

Sullivan refers to this period (7 years to adolescence) as the preadolescent stage, during which genuine human relationships develop. Sullivan believes that peer relationships are highly significant at this time (Hall and Lindzey 1970, p. 148).

Freud describes the period from 6 through 12 years of age as the latency stage. During this time, the focus is directed toward physical and intellectual activities, while sexual tendencies seem to be repressed.

In school, children have the restraints of the school system imposed on their behavior, and they learn to develop controls. Children compare their skills with those of their peers in a number of areas, including motor development, social development, and language. This comparison assists in the development of self-concept. School children can sometimes be cruel in their honesty, and teachers often need to intercede to assist children who have limitations. The schoolchild develops a number of adaptive mechanisms. Four of these are regression, malingering, rationalization, and ritualistic behavior. **Regression** is returning to a form of behavior that was suitable at an earlier age. For example, the child who is anxious about starting school may start bed-wetting at night or perhaps revert to baby talk. **Malingering** is a familiar mechanism to schoolchildren. It is pretending to be ill rather than facing something unpleasant; the child who feels sick the morning before a test may be malingering. **Rationalization** is an attempt to justify behavior by logical reason and explanation. A girl who does not make the swimming team may rationalize to her parents by saying she really did not try because she doesn't want swimming to interfere with her piano lessons. **Ritualistic behavior** is demonstrated by schoolchildren in many settings. For example, a child may walk down the sidewalk without stepping on a crack. Clubs and gangs often have rituals of membership. These rituals become very important to schoolchildren even though they usually do not persist for a long time. For example, the boy who must have a shower every morning may forget this ritual after a few weeks.

As they grow older, schoolchildren learn to play with more children at one time. Usually the 6- or 7-year-old is a member of a peer group. This group can be a greater influence than the family in teaching attitudes. During late childhood, children join a gang, a small group of peers, which is formed by the children themselves. It is usually informal and transitory, and the leadership changes from time to time. During this period of socialization with others, children gradually become less self-centered and selfish and more cooperative and conscious of the group.

Cognitive Development

According to Piaget, the ages 7 to 11 years mark the phase of *concrete operations*. See Table 24–6 on page 591. During this stage, the child changes from egocentric interactions to cooperative interactions. See Figure 25–8. School-age children also develop an increased understanding of concepts that are associated with specific objects, for example, environmental conservation or wildlife preservation. Children at this time develop logical reasoning from intuitive reasoning. For example, they learn to add and subtract to obtain an answer to a problem. Children also learn about cause-and-effect relationships at this age, e.g., they know that a stone will not float because it is heavier than water.

Money is a concept that gains meaning for children when they start school. By time time they are 7 or 8 years old, children usually know the value of most coins. The concept of time is also learned at this age. By 6 years of age, children enter school; the schedule in school helps them learn time periods. However, it is not until 9 or 10 years of age that children are able to understand the long periods of time in the past. Knowing the time of day and the day of the week are relatively easy for children because they relate time to routine activities. For example, a girl may go to school Monday through Friday, play on Saturday, go to Sunday school on Sunday morning, and go out with her father Sunday afternoon. Children are beginning to read a clock by the time they are 6 years old.

Later in childhood reading skills are usually well developed, and what a child reads is largely influenced by the family. By 9 years of age, most children are self-motivated. They compete with themselves, and they like to plan in advance. By 12 years, they are motivated by inner drive rather than by competition with peers. They like to talk, to discuss different subjects, and to debate.

Moral Development

Some school-age children are at Kohlberg's stage 1 of the *preconventional level* (punishment and obedience), i.e., they

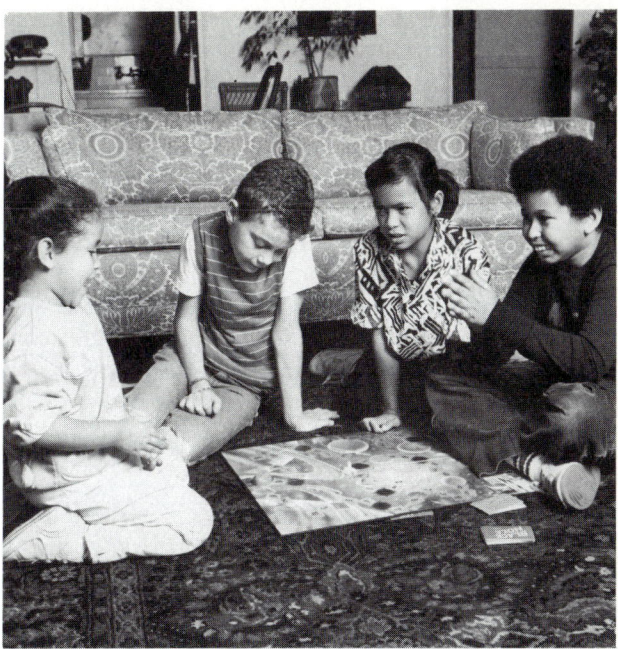

Figure 25–8 The expanding cognitive skills of school-age children enable cooperative interactions of an increasingly complex nature, as shown by the children playing this board game.

act to avoid being punished. Some school-age children, however, are at stage 2 (*instrumental-relativist orientation*). These children do things to benefit themselves. Fairness, i.e., everyone getting a fair share or chance, becomes important. Later in childhood, most children progress to the *conventional* level. This level has two stages: Stage 3 is the "good boy–nice girl" stage, and stage 4 is the *law and order orientation*. See Table 24–8 on page 594. Children usually reach the conventional level between the ages of 10 and 13. The child shifts from the concrete interests of individuals to the interests of groups. The motivation for moral action at this stage is to live up to what significant others think of the child (Hersh, Paolitto, and Reimer 1979, pp. 71–74).

Spiritual Development

According to Fowler, the school-age child is at stage 2 in spiritual development, the *mythical-literal stage*. Children learn to distinguish fantasy from fact. Spiritual facts are those beliefs that are accepted by a religious group, whereas fantasy is thoughts and images formed in the child's mind. Parents and the minister, rabbi, or priest help the child distinguish fact from fantasy. These people still influence the child more than peers in spiritual matters.

When children do not understand events such as the creation of the world, they use fantasy to explain them. The school-age child needs to have concepts such as prayer presented in concrete terms. For example, the child thinks of God as having human qualities, e.g., as a kind old man or a person who punishes when behavior does not meet his standards.

School-age children may ask many questions about God and religion in these years and will generally believe that God is good and always present to help. Just before puberty, children become aware that their prayers are not always answered and become disappointed. At this age, some children reject religion, while others continue to accept it. This decision is largely influenced by the parents. If a child continues religious training, the child is ready to apply reason rather than blind belief in most situations.

Health Promotion and Protection

During the assessment interview, the nurse responds to questions from the parent, gives appropriate feedback, and lends encouragement and support to the parent. The nurse also demonstrates interest in the child and enthusiasm for the child's strengths. Assessment activities are similar to those of the preschooler (see page 624). Assessment guidelines for growth and development of the school-age child are shown in the accompanying box.

Examples of wellness diagnoses (see Chapter 23) and NANDA nursing diagnoses and goals for the school-age child are shown in Table 25–12. *Outcome criteria* also need to be developed. The following are examples of criteria for the NANDA diagnosis **Potential for trauma** in Table 25–12:

- Within the next month, the child attends bicycle safety classes for a total of 4 hours.

- Within the next 2 months, the child learns safety in relation to skateboards and other equipment.

- The child passes a written test about safety issues in 6 months.

The school-age child can begin to take responsibility for self-care and be encouraged to utilize appropriate preventive measures, such as good nutrition and dental care. Most children in this age group still require adult supervision of their health maintenance activities. The following topics can be discussed with the parents and/or the child.

ASSESSMENT GUIDELINES
The School-Age Child

Does the school-age child:

- Indicate physical development within normal range?
- Possess coordinated motor skills?

By 12 years of age, is the child able to:

- Do tricks on a bike, climb a tree, shimmy up a rope?
- Participate in organized competitions?
- Read, print numbers and letters easily and correctly, and manipulate numbers?
- Throw and catch a small ball?
- Play musical instruments?
- Develop a concept of money and make change for small amounts of money?
- Express self in a logical manner and talk problems through?
- Enjoy riddles and read and understand newspaper comics?
- Invest in a hobby or collection?
- Make friends of the same sex and establish a peer group?
- Interact well with parents?
- Become less dependent on family and venture away from them?
- Control strong and impulsive feelings?
- Like to help others?
- Think of self as likeable and healthy?

Health Maintenance Visits and Immunization The school-age child should have health maintenance visits at 8 and 11 years of age as well as routine dental care. See the health maintenance schedule, Table 25–4, for specific information. Usually, children have received most of their immunizations prior to their entry into school. See Tables 25–5 and 25–6, earlier in this chapter.

TABLE 25–12 *Examples of Nursing Diagnoses and Goals for the School-Aged Child.*

	Diagnosis	Goal
Wellness diagnosis	**Positive self-concept** related to appropriate care and stimulation during infancy and childhood.	During the next year, the child continues to maintain a positive self-concept.
NANDA diagnosis	**Potential for injury** related to improper use of bicycles and sports equipment	During the next year, the child is free from accidents related to bicycles and sports equipment.

Regular dental checkups are required during these years. Permanent teeth begin to appear at about 7 years and are usually all in place except for the third molars (wisdom teeth) by 12 years of age. Nurses may need to teach children and their parents about regular dental checkups and dental hygiene. See Chapter 22 for additional information.

Safety   By the time children attend school, they are learning to think before they act. They often prefer adult equipment to toys. They want to be active with other children in such activities as bicycling, hiking, swimming, and boating. Although sensitive to peer pressure, the school-age child responds to rules. Children of this age engage in fantasy and magical thinking. They often imitate actions of parents and superheroes with whom they identify.

Accidents are the leading cause of death in school-age children. The most frequent case of fatalities, in descending order, are motor vehicle accidents, drownings, fires, and firearms. School-age children are also involved in many minor accidents, frequently resulting from outdoor activities and recreational equipment such as swings, bicycles, skateboards, and swimming pools. Potential hazards and preventive measures for the school-age child are listed in Table 25–13.

Nutrition   Nutrition continues to be a high priority for growing children. School-age children require a balanced diet including 2400 kcal per day. School-age children eat three meals a day and one or two nutritious snacks. Children need a protein-rich food at breakfast to sustain the prolonged physical and mental effort required at school. Studies have shown that children who skip breakfast become inattentive and restless by late morning and have decreased problem-solving ability (Baker and Henry 1987, p. 116). Undernourished children become fatigued easily and face a greater risk of infection, resulting in frequent absences from school.

The average healthy 8-year-old weighing 30 kg (66 lb) requires about 1750 ml of fluid per day (James and Mott 1988, p. 638). Many school-age children have only one meal a day with their family, at dinner. Mealtime should be a social time enjoyed by all, and parents should refrain from discussing a child's poor eating habits at this time. Parents should be aware that children learn many of their food habits by observing their parents. Eating a balanced diet should be the norm for both parent and child.

The school-age child generally eats lunch at school. The child may bring lunch from home or buy lunch at the school cafeteria. Many dietary problems stem from this independence in food choices. The children may trade their food, not eat lunch at all, or buy sweets or junk food with their lunch money. Parents should discuss with the child the foods that they should eat and continue to provide a balanced diet in the home setting. For additional information see Chapter 39.

TABLE 25–13 *Potential Hazards and Preventive Measures for School-Age Children (6 to 12 Years)*

Potential Hazards	Preventive Measures
Sports injuries	Teach the child safety rules for swimming, boating, ice skating and other recreations, e.g., "Never swim or skate alone. Always wear a life jacket when you are in a boat and do not skate unless the ice is proven safe or without my consent."
	Teach them to wear protective helmets, knee pads and elbow pads when appropriate.
	Carefully supervise any sport (e.g., archery) in which the child aims at a target, and place targets in isolated areas against walls.
	Teach the child not to throw objects at people or moving vehicles.
Traffic accidents	Teach the child traffic rules for bicycling.
	Caution the child to follow traffic safety rules while roller skating or skateboarding.
	Teach the child not to play or hide near cars.
	Make sure children wear seat belts at all times when they are in automobiles.
	Teach the child to wear light-colored clothing and reflective material when walking or cycling at night.
Tools and machinery	Teach the child safe ways to use the stove, garden tools, and other equipment.
	Supervise children when they use saws, electric appliances and tools, and other potentially dangerous equipment.
	Teach the child to avoid excavations, quarries, and vacant buildings and not to play around heavy machinery.
Firearms	Teach the child not to play with fireworks, gunpowder, and firearms.
	Keep firearms unloaded, locked up, and out of reach.
Substance abuse	Teach the child the effects of drugs and alcohol on judgment and coordination.

The result of poor eating habits may be obesity. Obesity in school-age children tends to result in decreased activity as well as psychosocial problems. Obese children may be ridiculed by their peers and discriminated against by peers and adults. Such behavior reinforces an already low self-esteem. Counseling should include

- Reviewing the child's eating habits, including snacks
- Altering meal content
- Using rewards other than food
- Regular exercise

Elimination   The school-age child's elimination system reaches maturity during this period. The kidneys double in size between ages 5 and 10. During this period, the child urinates six to eight times a day and averages one to two bowel movements per day. **Enuresis,** which is defined as the involuntary passing of urine when control should be established, can be a problem for some school-age children. About 10% of all 6-year-olds experience difficulty controlling the bladder. **Nocturnal enuresis,** or bedwetting, is the involuntary passing of urine during sleep. Bed-wetting should not be considered a problem until after the age of 6. The incidence of nocturnal enuresis declines as the child matures. About 75% of the children with bed-wetting problems experience this problem because of a small bladder capacity (Castiglia 1987b, pp. 280–282).

Bed-wetting can be a very stressful situation for both parents and children. Parents need information and emotional support from the nurse to help them deal effectively with this problem. The nurse can offer the following general guidelines concerning enuresis:

- Children should not be punished for bed-wetting; they are not doing it on purpose.
- Parents should not feel that bed-wetting is their fault.
- The child should maintain proper daily hygiene and have a supply of clothes and linen available.
- The parents and child should come to an agreement on how to handle the laundry problem; children should have a role in this process.
- Any discussion of the problem should be limited to the parents and the child involved; the privacy and self-esteem of the child should always be an important consideration.
- The child may be helped by limiting fluids after supper and urinating prior to bedtime.

Rest/Sleep   The school-age child sleeps between 8 and 12 hours a night without daytime naps. The 8-year-old requires at least 10 hours of sleep each night. As the child approaches 11 or 12 years of age, less sleep is required and bedtime may be as late as 10 P.M. Although some children still experience night awakenings due to nightmares, this problem continues to decrease with age. Most school-age children have less resistance to bedtime and enjoy a quiet,

private period of reading or listening to the radio before falling asleep.

Activity/Exercise   Most school-age children are very active physically. During this period, motor skills increase. Children enjoy a variety of group activities, such as baseball and hockey, and individual activities, such as bicycle riding, ice-skating, and dancing. These activities help the child to develop coordination, balance, and strength and enhance social, cognitive, and personal development. Parents can support and promote growth and development by being aware of the activities in the community and by encouraging their children's participation. Children also enjoy having parents and siblings attend their games or activities. Parental supervision may sometimes be required to ascertain that children's pursuits coincide with their abilities and developmental level. In this regard, parents need to have realistic expectations about their children's abilities.

The skills, attitudes, and habits developed by girls and boys during childhood, particularly during school-age, often set the groundwork for activities pursued as adults. Participation in a variety of activities during the early school-age period may help children to find one or more activities of special interest or in which they have a particular skill.

Children who learn, enjoy, and develop confidence in individual and group activities often pursue these interests throughout their college years and into adulthood. Parents should also be aware that they serve as role models for their child. Children may benefit from observing their parents' involvement in outdoor exercise and other healthy activities.

Sense of Self   The schoolchild's self-concept continues to mature. Children recognize similarities and differences between themselves and others. School-age children compare themselves with others and obtain feedback from teachers and peers. Children who are successful and receive recognition for their efforts feel competent and in control of themselves and of the environment. Children who feel unaccepted by their peers or who receive negative feedback and little recognition can feel inferior and worthless.

Although the focus of interest for this age group has moved to school, peers, and other activities, the home remains the crucial place for the child's development of high self-esteem.

Parents and caregivers can assist school-age children to develop psychosocially by

- Recognizing success and providing praise for achievements
- Guiding children to perform tasks in which they are likely to succeed
- Guiding the child to complete the task
- Teaching the child how to get along with peers by collaborating, compromising, cooperating, and competing
- Teaching the child how to get along with adults

Sexuality   By the age of 6, the child usually has a strong identification with the parent of the same sex. During the period from 6 to 12 years of age, children must learn the role and concepts of their gender as part of the total self-concept. In recent years, the stereotypical roles and behaviors for both sexes have changed. Many more women in North America now enter the fields of business, law, and medicine. In general, men have not entered the traditional women's professions such as nursing and teaching to the same extent. More men, however, are involved with child care and household tasks.

Beginning at about 8 or 9 years, children become very concerned about specific sex roles and often approach their parents with very explicit concerns about sexuality and reproduction. If parents cannot answer these questions, children will attempt to obtain the information from peers. To promote healthy development, the nurse should provide parents and children with opportunities to express their concerns and ask questions regarding sex. All questions should be answered by the nurse with factual data and perhaps followed up with appropriate books and other material. Parents should be advised to discuss basic information regarding sexual intercourse, menstruation, and reproduction with their children at about 10 years of age. Many parents may find it helpful to give children reading material and then discuss this material with them. Some parents may find it difficult to discuss sexual issues with their children and avoid doing so. Parents should be aware that if they do not provide such information, their children will seek answers from their peers and that the answers they obtain will frequently be incorrect or incomplete.

Social Interactions

Socially, children want to be accepted by their peers and enjoy having a best friend. School-age children often ridicule those whom they perceive as different from themselves, such as children with glasses or physical defects or those who have different clothes, skills, skin color, or religion. Parents can assist school-age children in their development by teaching and reinforcing the fact they should not be cruel to children or adults that are different from themselves. Parents can also act as role models in this regard.

The school-age child has an understanding of right and wrong. Eight-year-olds know that breaking rules can result in punishment from their parents or teachers. To avoid facing that danger, they often tell the story from their perspective. A parent who understands the normal moral behavior of the age level can deal with the child by calmly reviewing the rules and their importance and also explaining the importance of telling the truth. As children mature throughout the school-age period, they develop a better understanding of the need to tell the truth.

An issue of recent importance in some communities is whether children with AIDS should be allowed to attend public schools. Schools may handle this problem in a variety of ways. In some situations, the student with AIDS has

RESEARCH NOTE

Why Do Some Children Drink Alcohol?

Many factors play a role in a person's decision to consume alcoholic beverages. The purpose of this study was to determine if children's attitudes about alcohol consumption changed as they grew older and if others had a role in influencing their decision to drink. Five hundred children from a metropolitan school district, who were between 8 and 15 years of age, were asked to fill out a three-part questionnaire. The questionnaire asked for their responses to: (a) demographic questions about themselves, (b) alcohol-related decision-making situations that required a yes or no answer, and (c) the rationale for their decisions, based on a choice of six reasons. The six reasons, or rationale, for the decisions were based on Kohlberg's six stages of moral development.

The results of this study suggested that age was a factor in a child's attitude toward alcohol consumption. Older children, ages 14 to 15, were more favorably disposed toward drinking than were younger children. In one of the situations, the children were asked if they would take a sip of wine if a bottle was passed around at a party. Less than 25% of the children under 14 years of age said they would take a drink. Of the children over 14 years of age, 50% responded positively. This was a common pattern regardless of the situation that was described.

With respect to the question concerning what influence others had on a child's decision to drink alcohol, the data from this study indicated that parents' attitudes about drinking had a significant impact on their children's decision-making behavior. The authors plan to conduct further research on these children to determine whether their attitudes, and the factors that influence them, change over time.

Implications: In light of this research, it is suggested that parents reinforce their teaching about the effects of alcohol when their child reaches the age of 12 or 13. Parental guidance and reinforcement at this time could be a valuable resource in decreasing the trend toward alcohol consumption at a young age.

P. T. Castiglia, A. M. Glenister, B. P. Haughey, and G. W. Kanski. Influences on children's attitudes toward alcohol consumption, *Pediatric Nursing*, May/June 1989, 3:263–68.

been taught at home; in other situations, only a few people are informed of the child's diagnosis. Although no casual spread of AIDS has been reported, children and their parents often face severe discrimination and harassment from frightened families.

The nurse is in a key position to assist families, and to protect the child, as well as to teach the community the facts about AIDS. The entire community can benefit from learning about this disease. Knowledge and discussion helps to decrease fears, abolish myths, and deal with necessary issues using a rational approach. The nurse should also serve as an advocate for the child and the family and facilitate decisions that will enable the child to attain optimum physical, emotional, and cognitive development.

Cognitive Stimulation   The school-age child learns a variety of concepts and ideas through academic subjects such as mathematics, science, and reading and through play activities such as collections, hobbies, games, and field trips. Language skills continue to expand, and memory capabilities increase. To promote proper development of cognitive abilities, the nurse should screen the child for any vision or hearing problems. Parents can promote cognitive development by encouraging reading, showing interest in the child's work, and providing a home environment in which the child can complete home assignments. School-age children enjoy watching TV and playing video games, and parents may have to set time limits on these activities. Parents should also be aware of the child's progress in school, have realistic expectations of their child's abilities, and be encouraged to report any concerns to the teacher or to the school nurse.

School nurses play an important role in working with families to assess for learning difficulties. A nurse usually interviews the parents in the home to gather information about the family history, including learning difficulties, speech problems, or environmental problems. Nurses also interpret test results and provide ongoing counseling and support to the parent.

CHAPTER HIGHLIGHTS

▶ A sense of trust and security in the newborn is essential for subsequent development; the infant derives this sense from parental love, warmth, and prompt attention to physical needs.

▶ An essential nursing function is assessment of the newborn's physical status by the Apgar scoring system.

▶ Measurements of length, weight, head and chest circumferences, fontanelle size and status, reflex abilities, and motor development are important indicators of the newborn's growth and health.

▶ Infants from 1 month to 1 year reveal marked growth in size and stature with appropriate nutrition and care: birth weight is doubled by 5 months and tripled by 12 months.

▶ During infancy, motor development is notable: At 3 months, infants can raise their heads from the prone position; at 6 months, they can sit unsupported; and at 12 months, they can stand momentarily and walk with help.

▶ To develop cognitively, the infant needs a variety of sensory and motor stimuli.

▶ The nurse can assess the psychosocial and motor development of infants by using the Denver Developmental Screening Test and similar tests.

▶ Early childhood spans the period from 1 to 6 years and is subdivided into two groups: the toddler group, ages 1 to 3, and the preschool group, ages 4 and 5.

▶ During childhood, dramatic changes occur in physical, psychologic, and cognitive development; the child moves from being a dependent person to becoming an independent person entering school.

▶ As the nervous system develops, body systems mature to the point where the child can control the body, achieve finer muscle control, and perform all the activities of daily living, such as washing and dressing.

▶ The child also develops a unique personality and way of behaving.

▶ Critical to psychosocial development during childhood is the development of a sense of autonomy and initiative.

▶ By the end of early childhood, the child has reached the phase of intuitive thought in cognitive development, has developed some internal moral controls, and is at the undifferentiated level of spiritual development.

▶ The school-age period of development begins at age 6 and ends with the onset of puberty.

▶ School-age children perfect their muscular skills and coordination and develop a sense of competence, perseverance, and self-worth.

▶ During emotional development, school-age children face the conflict of industry versus inferiority.

▶ Peers are very important to school-age children; same sex-friendships develop.

▶ School-age children begin to understand relationships and change from being egocentric to having cooperative interactions; according to Piaget, they are in the concrete operations phase of cognitive development.

- Most school-age children progress to the conventional level of moral development and to the mythical-literal stage of spiritual development.

- The health promotion of a child is affected by sex, racial, social, and economic factors as well as the type of family environment provided.

- The nurse assists parents in health promotion by providing information and support related to the developmental level of the child.

- Attachment between the mother and the newborn is crucial for the optimum physical and emotional development of the infant.

- Assessment activities for health promotion are related to the specific developmental stage of the child.

- During the assessment, the nurse observes the interactions of the child and the parent and listens for areas of concern or questions that the parent may have.

- Intervention for health promotion includes parent teaching in regard to the importance of regular health maintenance visits, immunizations according to suggested schedule, and screening for early detection of disorders such as tuberculosis.

- Accidents are the leading cause of death in toddlers, preschool, and school-age children. Parents need specific teaching at each developmental level in relation to the potential safety hazards of the age group.

- The nurse should teach parents specific play activities for each developmental stage that promote healthy language, sensory, and cognitive development.

- Good nutritional habits begin in infancy. The nurse should provide parents with appropriate information on the nutritional needs of the child at each developmental stage.

- The problem of obesity may begin in infancy because of the myth that "fat babies are healthy babies."

- Toddlers engage in endless activity. The types of toddler play include onlooker play, such as watching TV; solitary play, such as independent activities; parallel play, such as sitting beside other children while playing; and associative play, which is engaging in activity with others.

- During the toddler stage, parents should be instructed to read labels and be aware that the use of table foods provides more variety and is less expensive and more nutritious than prepared toddler foods.

- Estimates are that 80% of preschool children have some tooth decay. Parents should provide instruction in dental care and limit the intake of sugary snacks.

- As children reach school age, they can begin to take more responsibility for self-care and utilize appropriate preventive measures such as good nutrition and dental care.

- During the school-age period, children engage in a variety of group and individual activities that help to develop coordination, balance, and strength, as well as enhance social, cognitive, and personal development.

- During the school-age period, parents need to be aware of the child's progress in school and have realistic expectations of their child's abilities.

READINGS AND REFERENCES

SUGGESTED READINGS

Castiglia, P. September/October 1987. Nocturnal enuresis. *Journal of Pediatric Health Care* 1:280–83.
  This author reviews the problem of nocturnal enuresis (bedwetting) in children. The incidence, predisposing factors, and common causes of bed-wetting are discussed and common methods of treatment presented. A multitreatment approach to nocturnal enuresis is considered most effective and may include drug therapy and/or the use of urine-sensitive alarms. The parents and the child need to be involved in the treatment plan and reassured that the problem will be resolved.

Smith, J. April 1988. Big differences in little people. *American Journal of Nursing* 88:459–62.
  This author provides a guided tour through an infant's major organ systems and explains the differences between the pulmonary, cardiovascular, and gastrointestinal systems of the child and those of the adult. Guidelines for assessing the normal development of each major system of the 8-month-old infant are presented. Common symptoms experienced by the baby are explained in light of the infant's physiologic stage of development.

Winkelstein, M. L. May/June 1989. Fostering positive self-concept in the school-age child. *Pediatric Nursing* 15:229–33.
  A healthy self-concept is an important component of the normal development of the school-age child. Pediatric nurses in schools and hospitals have frequent contacts with children and can be influential in fostering their positive self-concept during these years. This author describes a self-concept program comprised of three major sections and several learning objectives. A chart provides details about learning experiences and instructional materials for each objective. These interventions can be used to assess the child's self-concept, provide opportunities for positive growth, and create opportunities for parental discussion.

RELATED RESEARCH

Alexander, M. A., and Blank, J. J. Summer 1988. Factors related to obesity in Mexican-American children. *Image: Journal of Nursing Scholarship* 20:79–82.

Castiglia, P. T., Glenister, A. M., Haughey, B. P. and Kanski, G. W. May/June 1989. Influences on children's attitudes toward alcohol consumption. *Pediatric Nursing* 3:263–68

Holden, G. W., and Klingner, A. M. January 1988. Learning from experience: Differences in how novice vs. expert nurses diagnose why an infant is crying. *Journal of Nursing Education* 27:24–29.

Schraeder, B. D.; Rappaport, J.; and Courtwright, L. Winter 1987. Preschool development of very low birthweight infants. *Image: Journal of Nursing Scholarship* 19:174–78.

SELECTED REFERENCES

Baker, S., and Henry, R. 1987. *Parents' guide to nutrition.* Menlo Park, Calif.: Addison-Wesley Publishing Co.

Behrman, R. E., and Vaughan, V. C., III. 1983. In Nelson, W. E., editor. *Nelson textbook of pediatrics.* 12th ed. Philadelphia: W. B. Saunders Co.

Castiglia, P. T. May/June 1987a. Speech-language development. *Journal of Pediatric Health Care* 1:165–67.

———. September/October 1987b. Nocturnal enuresis. *Journal of Pediatric Health Care* 1:280–83.

Edelman, C., and Mandle, C. L. 1986. *Health promotion throughout the life span.* St. Louis: C. V. Mosby Co.

Engel, G. L. 1962. *Psychological development in health and disease.* Philadelphia: W. B. Saunders Co.

Erikson, E. H. 1963. *Childhood and society.* 2d ed. New York: W. W. Norton and Co.

Guyton, A. C., 1986. *Textbook of medical physiology.* 7th ed. Philadelphia: W. B. Saunders Co.

Hall, C. S., and Lindzey, G. 1970. *Theories of personality.* 2d ed. New York: John Wiley and Sons.

Hersh, R. H.; Paolitto, D. P.; and Reimer, J. 1979. *Promoting moral growth from Piaget to Kohlberg.* New York: Longman.

James, S. R., and Mott, S. R. 1988. *Child health nursing: Essential care of children and families.* Menlo Park, Calif.: Addison-Wesley Publishing Co.

Koniak-Griffin, D. April 1987. Developmental assessment with the Denver Developmental Screening Test: An effective approach for clinical instruction and performance evaluation. *Journal of Pediatric Nursing* 2:102–12.

Lippe, B. November/December 1987. Short stature in children: Evaluation and management. *Journal of Pediatric Health Care* 1:313–22.

Murray, R., and Zenter, J. 1989. *Nursing assessment and health promotion through the life span.* 4th ed. Englewood Cliffs, N.J.: Prentice-Hall.

Olds, S.; London, M.; and Ladewig, P. 1988. *Maternal newborn nursing.* 3d ed. Menlo Park, Calif.: Addison-Wesley Publishing Co.

Ryan, N. M. October 1988. The stress-coping process in school age children: Gaps in the knowledge needed for health promotion. *Advances in Nursing Science* 11:1–12.

Sande, D. R., and Billingsley, C. S. September 1985. Language development in infants and toddlers. *Nurse Practitioner* 10:39–41, 44, 47.

Schulman, M., and Mekler, E. 1985. *Bringing up a moral child: A new approach for teaching your child to be kind, just, and responsible.* Reading, Mass.: Addison-Wesley Publishing Co.

Schuster, C. S., and Ashburn, S. S. 1986. *The process of human development: A holistic approach.* 2d ed. Boston: Little, Brown and Co.

Sugarman, L. 1986. *Life-span development: Concepts, theories and interventions.* New York: Methuen & Co.

Yoos, L. January/February 1987. Chronic childhood illnesses: Developmental issues. *Pediatric Nursing* 13:25–28.

CHAPTER

26

Adolescence through Middle Adulthood

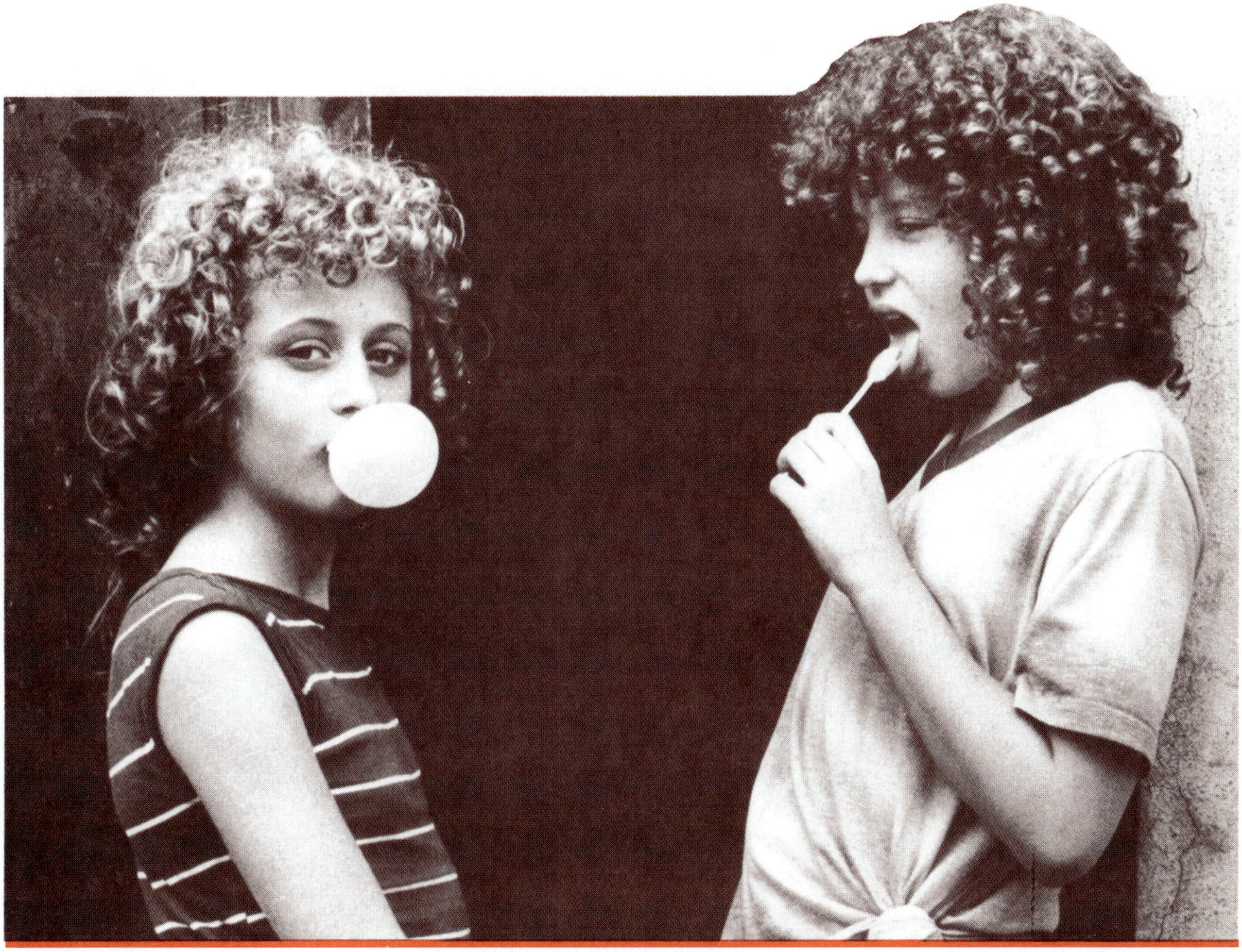

CONTENTS

OBJECTIVES

- Explain the essential changes in physical development from adolescence through middle adulthood.
- Explain psychosocial development of adolescents, young adults, and middle-aged adults according to Erikson.
- Explain the essential changes in cognitive development from adoles-

cence through middle adulthood as postulated by Piaget.

▶ Describe moral development of adolescents, young adults, and middle-

aged adults according to Kohlberg.

▶ Discuss spiritual development of adolescents, young adults, and middle-aged adults according to Fowler.

▶ Identify common health hazards and concerns of adolescents, young adults, and middle-aged adults.

▶ Discuss nursing implications related to common health concerns.

ADOLESCENCE

Adolescence is a critical period in development. Its length is culturally determined to some extent. In North America, adolescence is longer than in some cultures, extending to 18 to 20 years of age. **Adolescence** is the period during which the person becomes physically and psychologically mature and acquires a personal identity. At the end of adolescence, the person is ready to enter adulthood and assume its responsibilities.

Puberty is the first stage of adolescence in which sexual organs begin to grow and mature. **Menarche** (onset of menstruation) begins in girls. **Ejaculation** (expulsion of semen) occurs in boys. For girls, puberty normally starts between 10 and 14 years; for boys, between 12 and 16 years. The adolescent period is often subdivided into three stages: early adolescence lasts from ages 12 to 13; middle adolescence extends from 14 to 16 years; and late adolescence extends from 17 to 18 or 20 years. Late adolescence is a more stable stage than the other two. In the late period, adolescents are involved mostly with planning their future and economic independence.

Physical Development

During puberty, growth is markedly accelerated compared to the slow, steady growth of the child. This period, marked by sudden and dramatic physical changes, is referred to as the adolescent growth spurt. In boys, the growth spurt usually begins between ages 12 and 16; in girls, it begins earlier, usually between ages 10 and 14. Because the growth spurt begins earlier in girls, many girls surpass boys in height at this time.

Physical growth continues throughout adolescence. Growth is fastest for boys at about 14 years, and the maximum height is often reached at about 18 or 19 years. Some men add another 1 or 2 cm to their height during their 20s, as the vertebral column gradually continues to grow. During the period of 10 to 18 years of age, the average American male doubles his weight, gaining about 32 kg (72 lb), and grows about 41 cm (16 in) (James and Mott 1988, pp. 1244–45). The fastest rate of growth in girls occurs at about age 12; they reach their maximum height at about 15 to 16 years. During ages 10 to 18, the average American female

gains about 25 kg (55 lb) and grows about 24 cm (9 in) (James and Mott 1988, pp. 1241–42).

Physical growth during adolescence is greatly influenced by a number of factors. Some of these are heredity, nutrition, medical care, illness, physical and emotional environment, family size, and culture. Generally, people in the United States have grown taller in recent years. This increase in average height is thought to be due to many of the above factors.

Growth is noted first in the musculoskeletal system. This growth follows a sequential pattern: The head, hands, and feet are the first to grow to adult status. Next, the extremities reach their adult size. Because the extremities grow before the trunk, the adolescent looks leggy, awkward, and uncoordinated. After the trunk grows to full size, the shoulders, chest, and hips grow. Skull and facial bones also change proportions: The forehead becomes more prominent, and the jawbones develop.

Poor posture is a common problem during adolescence. The risk for postural problems increases among this age group because weight gains may precede a corresponding strengthening of postural muscles.

The eccrine and apocrine glands increase their secretions and become fully functional during puberty. The **eccrine glands,** found over most of the body, produce sweat. The **aprocine glands** develop in the axillae, anal and genital areas, external auditory canals and around the umbilicus and the areola of the breasts. Apocrine sweat is released onto the skin in response to emotional stimuli only.

Sebaceous glands also become active under the influence of androgens to both males and females. The sebaceous glands, which secrete **sebum,** become most active on the face, neck, shoulder, upper back, chest, and genitals. When these glands become plugged and inflamed, the result is **acne,** a condition common in adolescence. Noninflammatory acne appears as open and closed **comedones** (whiteheads and blackheads). Inflammatory acne appears as inflamed skin together with pustules and papules. A **pustule** is a visible collection of pus within the epidermis. A **papule** is a superficial, circumscribed elevation of the skin. Inflammatory acne may cause scarring.

During puberty, both primary and secondary sex characteristics develop. **Primary sexual characteristics** relate to the organs necessary for reproduction, such as the testes, penis, vagina, and uterus. **Secondary sexual characteristics** differentiate the male from the female but do not relate directly to reproduction. Examples are pubic hair growth, breast development, and voice changes.

The first noticeable sign that puberty has begun in males is the appearance of pubic hair. The milestone of male puberty is considered to be the first ejaculation, which commonly occurs at about 14 years of age. Fertility follows several months later. Sexual maturity is achieved by age 18.

Often the first noticeable sign of puberty in females is the appearance of the **breast bud,** although the appearance of hair along the labia may precede this. The milestone of female puberty is the menarche, which occurs about 2 years after the breast bud appears. At first, menstrual periods are scanty and irregular and may occur without ovulation. Ovulation is usually established 1 to 2 years after menarche. Female internal reproductive organs reach adult size about age 18 to 20.

Psychosocial Development

According to Erikson (1963, p. 261), the adolescent seeks answers to "Who am I?" and "What am I to be?" The psychosocial task of the adolescent is the *establishment of identity.* The danger of this stage is role confusion. The inability to settle on an occupational identity commonly disturbs the adolescent. Less commonly, doubts about sexual identity arise. Because of the adolescent's dramatic body changes, the development of a stable identity is difficult. Erikson says that adolescents help one another through this identity crisis by forming cliques and a separate youth culture. These cliques often exclude all those who are "different" in skin color, cultural background, aspects of dress, gestures, and tastes.

Adolescents are usually concerned about their bodies, their appearances, and their physical abilities. Hair styling, skin care, and clothes become very important. In-groupers of an adolescent clique can be excessively clanish and cruel in excluding out-groupers; this intolerance is a temporary defense against identity confusion (Erikson 1963, p. 236).

In their search for a new identity, adolescents have to refight the battles of many of the previous stages of development. The task of developing trust in self and others is again encountered when adolescents look for ideal persons whom they can trust and with whom they can prove trustworthy. Development of autonomy is restaged in their search for ways to express their right to choose freely. The search for an occupational role that allows expression of an autonomous, freely chosen direction is one example. Free choice and autonomy present conflicts to the adolescent. Conflict arises between behaving well in the eyes of the parents and behaving in a manner that may expose them to the ridicule of their peers. The sense of initiative is also restaged. The adolescent has unlimited imagination and ambition and aspires to great accomplishments. The sense of industry is

reenacted when the adolescent chooses a career. The extent to which these tasks were achieved earlier influences the adolescent's ability to achieve a healthy self-concept and self-identity.

The adolescent needs to establish a **self-concept** that accepts both personal strengths and weaknesses. Adolescents need to learn to build on their strengths and not be preoccupied by such defects as acne. They gain self-concepts largely from the impressions that others have of them. If others accept defects—e.g., a lost finger—adolescents accept those defects more readily.

Although sexual **identification** begins at about 3 or 4 years of age, it is a significant part of adolescence. The adolescent male strives to achieve a masculine sexual identity; the adolescent female, a feminine sexual identity. Because sex roles are becoming less defined in North American society, adopting masculine and feminine roles is increasingly confusing to today's adolescent. Job and family roles are less traditional and sex-specific. In forming a sexual identity, adolescents first fantasize the male or female role and then enact various aspects of that imagined role. In response to their own feelings and that of others, aspects of the role are either adopted or rejected. Later, adolescents begin to establish intimacy with a partner or partners. This intimacy lays the groundwork for the commitments of adulthood. Sexual experimentation is not part of true intimacy, but once intimacy is achieved, sexual activity is included.

Adolescents are sexually active and may engage in masturbation as well as heterosexual and homosexual activity. Homosexual activity during adolescence is not necessarily an indicator of sexual preference, since both gay and nongay adolescents may experiment sexually with persons of the same and opposite sex.

About the age of 15 years, many adolescents gradually draw away from the family and gain independence. This *need for independence* and the need for family support sometimes creates conflict within the adolescent and between the adolescent and the family. The young person may appear hostile or depressed at times during this painful process. At this age, adolescents prefer to be with their peers rather than their parents and may seek advice from adults other than their parents. Parents sometimes are bewildered by this stage of development; instead of reducing controls, they increase them, causing the adolescent to rebel.

Adolescents also have to resolve their ambivalent feelings toward the parent of the opposite sex. As part of the resolution, adolescents may develop brief crushes on adults outside the family—teachers or neighbors, for example. Adolescents sometimes adopt some of the attributes of the adults with whom they are infatuated. This modeling can be helpful in the maturing process.

Some of the discord in the family at this time is due to the generation gap. The values of the adolescent may differ from those of the parents. This difference may be difficult for the parents to understand and to accept. Adolescents still need guidance from their parents, although they appear neither to want it nor to need it. However, adolescents need to know that their parents care about them and that their parents still want to help them. Restrictions and guidance need to be presented in a manner that makes adolescents feel loved. They need consistency in guidance and fewer restrictions than previously. They should have the independence they can handle yet know that their parents will assist them when they need help.

During adolescence, **peer groups** assume great importance. See Figure 26–1. The peer group has a number of functions. It provides a sense of belonging, pride, social learning, and sexual roles. Most peer groups have well-defined, sex-specific modes of acceptable behavior. In adolescence, the peer groups change with age. They start as single-sex groups, evolve to mixed groups, and finally narrow to couples who share activities.

Dating helps prepare adolescents for marriage by teaching them how to act with members of the opposite sex. In the United States, dating starts early, often by 11 years for girls and later, perhaps 15, for boys, although dating ages vary with culture, social class, and pressures from society. Some adolescents initially date in groups of couples and eventually progress to going on dates alone.

Not all adolescents, however, are heterosexual. For homosexuals, adolescence is a difficult time. Because peer acceptance is crucial to self-acceptance, lesbian and gay adolescents usually conform to the heterosexual codes and behaviors of their peer groups even though these do not feel natural or correct. Conforming may exact a great personal cost. Adolescents who choose to be openly gay or

lesbian face not only the ostracism of their peers but also the misunderstanding and hostility of parents, teachers, and other important adults.

Cognitive Development

Cognitive abilities mature during adolescence. Between the ages of 11 and 15, the adolescent begins Piaget's *formal operations stage* of cognitive development. The main feature of this stage is that people can think beyond the present and beyond the world of reality. Adolescents are highly imaginative and idealistic. They consider things that do not exist but that might be and consider ways things could be or ought to be. This type of thinking requires logic, organization, and consistency.

The adolescent becomes more informed about the world and environment. Adolescents use new information to solve everyday problems and can communicate with adults on most subjects. The adolescent's capacity to absorb and use knowledge is great. Adolescents usually select their own areas for learning; they explore interests from which they may evolve a career plan. Study habits and learning skills developed in adolescence are used throughout life.

Moral Development

According to Kohlberg, the young adolescent is usually at the *conventional level* of moral development. Most still accept the Golden Rule and want to abide by social order and existing laws. Adolescents examine their values, standards, and morals. They may discard the values they have adopted from parents in favor of values they consider more suitable.

When adolescents move into the *postconventional* or *principled level,* they start to question the rules and laws of society. Right thinking and right action become a matter of personal values and opinions, which may conflict with societal laws. Adolescents consider the possibility of rationally changing the law and emphasize individual rights. Not all adolescents or even adults proceed to this postconventional level. See Kohlberg's stages of moral development in Table 24–8 on page 594.

Spiritual Development

According to Fowler, the adolescent or young adult reaches the synthetic-conventional stage of spiritual development (see Table 24–9 on page 597). As adolescents encounter different groups in society, they are exposed to a wide variety of opinions, beliefs, and behaviors regarding religious matters. The adolescent may reconcile the differences in one of the following ways:

- Deciding any differences are wrong
- Compartmentalizing the differences (For example, a friend may not be able to go to dances on Friday evenings because of religious observances, but the friend can share activities on other days.)

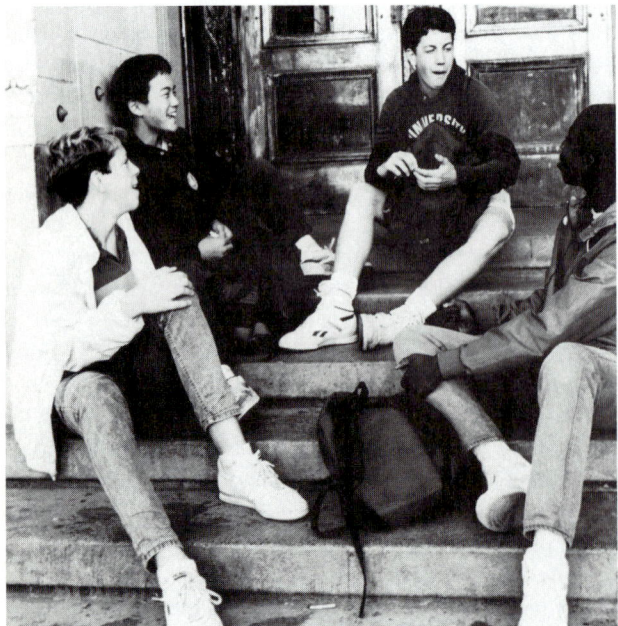

Figure 26–1 Adolescent peer group relationships enhance a sense of belonging, self-esteem, and self-identity.

- Obtaining advice from a significant other, e.g., a parent or a minister

Often the adolescent believes that various religious beliefs and practices have more similarities than differences. At this stage, the adolescent's focus is on interpersonal rather than conceptual matters.

Nursing activities relative to this stage of spiritual development include

- Presenting an open, accepting attitude to adolescent's questions and statements regarding spiritual matters and their implications to health.
- Arranging for adolescents to see a member of their religious faith if this is desired. Adolescents may want to talk with members of their church peer group for support.
- Providing a comfortable environment in which adolescents can practice the rituals of their faith.

Health Promotion and Protection

Assessment guidelines for growth and development of the adolescent are shown in the accompanying box. Assessment activities may include measurement of height and weight, measurement of vital signs (see Chapter 18), observation of the skin for acne, discussion of personal hygiene needs, and questions about the following: (a) goals and desires for the future, (b) recreational activities with family and friends, (c) knowledge of physical development, menstruation, and reproduction, (d) perception of family and peer relationships, (e) usual eating, exercise, and sleep patterns.

Examples of wellness diagnoses (see Chapter 23) and NANDA nursing diagnoses and goals for the adolescent are shown in Table 26–1. *Outcome criteria* also need to be developed. The following are examples of these criteria for the NANDA diagnosis **Potential for ineffective individual coping** in Table 26–1:

- The adolescent attends monthly classes related to pregnancy.
- The adolescent attends weekly support group for pregnant teenagers.
- The adolescent receives support from family and friends and professionals during the pregnancy.

Adolescents are usually self-directed in meeting their health needs. Because of maturation changes, however, they need teaching and guidance in the several health care areas that follow.

Health Maintenance Visits and Immunization
The adolescent should receive routine health assessments, appropriate laboratory screening, and periodic dental care. See the health maintenance schedule, Table 25–4, on page 609. If immunizations required for other age periods have not been received, they should be given at this time. For adolescents who have received the appropri-

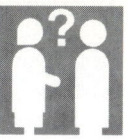

ASSESSMENT GUIDELINES
The Adolescent

Does the adolescent:

- Indicate physical and sexual development consistent with standards?
- Interact well with parents, peers, siblings, and persons in authority?
- Like self?
- Think and plan for the future, such as college or a career?
- Choose a life-style and interests that fit own identity?
- Determine own beliefs and values?
- Begin to establish a sense of identity in the family?
- Seek help from appropriate persons about problems?
- Exhibit healthy life-style practices?

ate immunizations, the combined tetanus and diphtheria toxoids (adult-type Td) should be given at about 14 to 16 years of age. Influenza virus vaccine, pneumococcal polysaccharide vaccine, and hepatitis B vaccine should be given to adolescents in selected high-risk groups (Murray and Zenter 1989, p. 356). Rubella (German measles) vaccine is recommended for female adolescents and women of childbearing age who are not protected against the disease. Rubella contracted during the first trimester of pregnancy may cause birth defects of the eyes, heart, and brain.

TABLE 26–1 *Examples of Nursing Diagnoses and Goals for Adolescents*

	Diagnosis	Goal
Wellness diagnosis	**Satisfying social interactions** related to ability to form and maintain positive relationships	During the next year, the adolescent continues to maintain healthy social relationships.
NANDA diagnoses	**Potential for injury:** poisoning related to ingestion of drugs and alcohol	During the next year, the adolescent does not ingest drugs or alcohol.
	Potential for **Ineffective individual coping** related to unplanned pregnancy	During the pregnancy, the adolescent is able to cope effectively.

Safety The adolescent needs to be safeguarded from accidents and injury. Accidents are the leading cause of death and injury among adolescents. Motor-vehicle accidents (automobiles, motorcycles, minibikes, and snowmobiles) and sports injuries are the most common accidents. Obtaining a driver's license is an important event in the life of an adolescent in the United States and Canada, but the privilege is not always wisely handled. Head injuries and fractures are frequent outcomes of automobile and motorcycle accidents. Adolescents need appropriate instruction about the safe handling of motor vehicles. Parents often need guidance in setting limits on the use of motor vehicles by their teenage children. Limits should be negotiated by the parents and the teenager and periodically reviewed and revised according to the teenager's safety record. Teenagers may use driving as an outlet for stress, as a way to assert independence, or as a way to impress peers. When setting limits on automobile use, parents need to assess the teenager's level of responsibility, common sense, and ability to resist peer pressure. The age of the teenager alone does not determine readiness to handle this responsibility.

Adolescents are at risk for sports injuries because their coordination skills are not fully developed. However, sports activities are important to the adolescent's self-esteem and overall development. In addition to providing beneficial exercise, sports activities enhance social and personal development. They help the adolescent experience competition, teamwork, and conflict resolution. The nurse and parents can help adolescents prevent sports injuries by encouraging

- The use of proper safety equipment
- Appropriate physical examinations before participating in sports
- Enforcement of regulations that prevent an injured player from further participation in sports activities until a physician advises it

See Table 26–2 for a list of potential hazards and preventive measures for adolescents.

Skin Care Adolescents need teaching and guidance to help them deal with the changing needs of their bodies. Secretions from newly active sweat glands react with bacteria on the skin, causing a pungent odor. Teenagers need to practice good hygiene to be sure that clothes smell fresh and clean.

A frequent skin problem of the adolescent is acne. The severity of acne varies widely from a few comedones to an intense inflammatory reaction. By the end of the teenage years, it is estimated that about 70% of adolescents will have had acne (Novotny 1989, p. 247).

The nurse should respond with support, guidance, and information to prevent the physical and emotional scarring that can occur with this problem. Problems such as acne may cause teenagers to feel depressed and frustrated at a

TABLE 26–2 *Potential Hazards and Preventive Measures for Adolescents (12 to 18 Years)*

Potential Hazards	Preventive Actions
Vehicle accidents	Have adolescents complete a driver's education course, and take practice drives with them in various kinds of weather.
	Reinforce the importance of wearing seat belts when driving and when riding as a passenger.
	Teach them to wear safety helmets when riding motorcycles, scooters, and the like.
	Set firm limits on automobile use, e.g., "Never drive after drinking or taking mind-altering drugs, and never ride with a driver who has done so."
	Encourage them to call home for a ride if they have been drinking by assuring them that they can do so without a reprimand.
Recreational accidents no longer under parental supervision	Encourage the adolescent to swim, jog, or go boating in groups so that others can obtain help in case of an accident.
	Reinforce water safety rules.
Firearms	Teach rules for hunting and proper use and care of firearms.
	Keep firearms unloaded and locked up.
Substance abuse	Inform the adolescent of the dangers of drugs and alcohol.
	Be alert to changes in the adolescent's mood and behavior.
	Listen to and maintain open communication with the adolescent. Open communication between parents and children is a powerful preventive measure.
	Set a good example of behavior that the adolescent can follow.

time when they are already insecure. To treat this problem, the teenagers should wash the affected area thoroughly but gently three times a day. Greasy ointments and make-up should be avoided, and the lesions should not be picked or squeezed. The role of diet and life-style in causing acne has not been determined, but the adolescent should be encouraged to eat a balanced diet and get adequate rest. A variety of oral and topical preparations, such as *tetracycline* and isotretinoin (*Accutane*), may be prescribed to treat acne. Accutane, introduced in 1982, is a very potent oral medication that is considered the wonder drug for the treatment of acne (Novotny 1989, p. 247). However, Accutane is a potent *teratogen,* an agent that causes the production of physical defects in developing embryos. The nurse who works with adolescents needs to be familiar with current therapies and their possible side-effects. Teenagers should be assured that scarring can usually be prevented if acne is treated promptly and follow-up care provided.

Nutrition   The adolescent's need for nutrients and calories increases, particularly during the growth spurt. The need for protein, calcium, vitamin D, iron, and B vitamins increases during adolescence. An adequate diet for an adolescent is 1 quart of milk per day as well as appropriate amounts of meat, vegetables, fruits, breads, and cereals.

Many parents may observe that teenagers, particularly boys, seem to be eating all the time. Teenagers have active life-styles and irregular eating patterns. They tend to snack frequently, often eating high-calorie foods such as doughnuts, soft drinks, ice cream, and fast foods. Parents and nurses can promote better lifelong eating habits by encouraging teenagers to eat healthy snacks. Parents can provide healthy snacks such as fruits and cheese and at the same time limit the amount of "junk food" available in the home. The teenager's food choices relate to physical, social, and emotional factors and impulses and may not be influenced by teaching. Nurses need to advise parents that adolescents must take responsibility for their decisions in many areas of life, and parents should avoid conflicts that relate to food.

Common problems related to nutrition and self-esteem among adolescents include obesity, anorexia nervosa, and bulimia. **Obesity** is a common problem of the preadolescent period and continues to be a problem in the adolescent period. It is estimated that 10% to 16% of people between the ages of 10 and 19 years are obese. Obese adolescents are frequently discriminated against in many ways. They are usually rejected by their peers, badgered by their parents, and ridiculed on television and in the movies. Many feel ugly and socially unacceptable. Depression is not unusual among obese adolescents. Treatment of obesity in this age group includes education on nutrition as well as assessment of psychosocial problems that may produce overeating.

Under social pressure to be slim, some adolescents severely limit their food intake to a level significantly below that required to meet the demands of normal growth. **Anorexia nervosa,** a severe psychophysiologic condition usually seen in adolescent girls and young women, is characterized by a prolonged inability or refusal to eat and rapid weight loss in persons who believe they are fat even though they are emaciated. Anorexics may also induce vomiting and use laxatives and diuretics to remain thin. This illness is most effectively treated in the early stages by psychotherapy that also involves the parents. Hospitalization may

be necessary when the effects of starvation become life-threatening.

An increasing problem among teenagers, **bulimia** is an uncontrollable compulsion to consume enormous amounts of food and then expel it by self-induced vomiting or by taking laxatives. For example, the afflicted person may consume a whole cake, a dozen doughnuts, and a half dozen apple turnovers before inducing vomiting. After prolonged periods of alternately gorging and vomiting, the person no longer needs to induce vomiting; it becomes an uncontrollable reflex. Voluntary organizations are established in some regions to assist individuals with bulimia.

Rest/Sleep   Most adolescents require 8 to 10 hours of sleep each night to prevent undue fatigue and susceptibility to infections. A change in sleep pattern is common in adolescence. Children who once were early risers begin to sleep late in the mornings and occasionally take afternoon naps. The reason for daytime sleeping is not fully understood, but it is possibly a result of physical maturity and reduced nocturnal sleep.

During adolescence boys begin to experience **nocturnal emissions** (orgasm and emission of semen during sleep), known as "wet dreams," several times each month. Boys need to be informed about this normal development to prevent embarrassment and fear.

Activity/Exercise   Many teenagers engage in a variety of physical activities. In the past, boys were active in team sports, whereas girls took up dancing, ice-skating, and the like. Currently, more girls and young women are participating in team sports and, in some cases, try out for the boys' teams and succeed. The experience of working with a team provides physical activity, prevents obesity related to inactivity, and promotes peer group involvement. The experiences of winning and losing and accepting and working with a variety of people prepare teenagers for the team approach of the work force. Nurses and parents should encourage both sexes to develop interests that balance sedentary activity with team involvement. Girls need encouragement at an early age to gain exposure and confidence in team sports that they can pursue during their high school years. Teenagers should have regular health maintenance check-ups to ascertain that they can physically cope with the demands of the program. They should also be taught strengthening and conditioning exercises to prevent sports injuries.

Feminine Hygiene   Girls need to be taught about the menstrual cycle and the necessary self-care responsibilities. Initially, teenagers have irregular menstruation, which may lead to embarrassment because of stained clothing. Teenagers can be taught to be aware of more subtle signs of impending menstruation, such as a tender breast, water retention or bloating, or the appearance of skin eruptions or pimples. Girls also should be counseled regarding the variety of feminine hygiene products available, such as sanitary pads and tampons, so that intelligent choices can be made. Recently, the incidence of **toxic shock syndrome** (TSS) has drawn attention to the use of tampons for women of all ages. Toxic shock syndrome is a serious, sometimes fatal illness that has been associated with tampon use. Parents and nurses should advise teenagers to wash their hands thoroughly before inserting a tampon, to change tampons frequently, to decrease their use by alternating them with sanitary pads, and to use pads at night. These measures will help to decrease local infection with *Staphylococcus aureus,* a possible antecedent of toxic shock syndrome. Thorough cleaning of the genital area and wiping from front to back will also decrease infection and prevent odors.

Menstrual Difficulties

Dysmenorrhea (painful menstruation) is prevalent among adolescent females and causes much short-term absenteeism. Cramping, lower abdominal pain radiating to the back and upper thighs, nausea, vomiting, diarrhea, and headaches may occur for a few hours up to 3 days. Dysmenorrhea results from powerful uterine contractions, which cause ischemia and in turn cramping pain. Dysmenorrhea is associated with the release of prostaglandins through the activity of progesterone. Traditional treatments for the symptoms of dysmenorrhea have been bed rest, administration of simple analgesics such as aspirin, application of heat to the abdomen, and certain exercises. Today, treatment with antiprostaglandins such as ibuprofen (Motrin or Advil) and naproxen (Naprosyn) helps many. These drugs, however, should be administered under medical supervision; they have potentially toxic effects. Aspirin itself is a mild antiprostaglandin. More recent, nondrug approaches, such as biofeedback, are being used. See Chapter 33 for further information about biofeedback.

Sex Education

Adolescents want to know about sex but are often uneasy about discussing these concerns with their parents. Nurses, the schools, and the family need to provide accurate information. Parents who have established open communication regarding sexual changes and reproduction during the school-age period are more likely to be asked questions and have discussions with their teenagers regarding sexual issues. Parents and nurses need to recognize all aspects of adolescent development in planning and discussing sex education. During the nursing assessment, teenagers should be asked directly what they know about sex, contraception, and reproduction. Sometimes a lot of the teenager's information is based on popular myths and little, if any, fact. Although sex education programs for high school students are discussed in the literature, only a small percentage of teens has the opportunity to attend these sessions. The nurse should discuss factual information about sex, sexual actions and their consequences, the individual's right to make a decision regarding ways to express oneself sexually, and the responsibilities of each person with respect to sexual activity.

An important role of the nurse working with teenagers is to provide information regarding birth control. The nurse should inform the teenager about the various methods of birth control: pills, diaphragms, intrauterine devices (IUDs), the rhythm method, and condoms (see Chapter 30).

Sexually transmitted diseases (STDs) are the most common bacterial infections among adolescents. STDs include syphilis, gonorrhea, genital warts, genital herpes virus type 2, chlamydial urethritis or nongonococcal urethritis (NGU), *Trichomonas* and *Candida* infections, and acquired immune deficiency syndrome (AIDS). *Trichomonas* and *Candida* infections can also be acquired nonsexually. Increases in these diseases are due to two factors: changing sexual mores of the young, which permit increased sexual activity, and an increase in the number of sexual partners. Because the term *sexually transmitted disease* elicits feelings of guilt, shame, and fear, adolescents frequently do not seek medical help as early as they should. Adolescents need education about these diseases, preventive measures, and early treatment. Table 26–3 lists common signs of STDs for which teenagers should seek medical care.

Unplanned Pregnancy

Adolescent pregnancy is reported by 1 out of 10 U.S. women each year. Annually, 500,000 American adolescents obtain legal abortions (Gilchrist and Schinke 1987, pp. 424–25). The pregnant teenager is under a tremendous amount of stress and requires expert support and counseling. The teenager should be encouraged to tell her parents and her partner about the pregnancy as soon as possible. The nurse should provide information about the available options for continuing or terminating the pregnancy and refer her to appropriate and competent practitioners. Many teens choose to have abortions.

Young women who choose to continue the pregnancy have a variety of special needs. Adolescents are high-risk mothers and require sensitive and expert care both physically and emotionally. Adolescent parents require continued support and teaching from the nurse. Teens who decide to give up their baby for adoption should be referred to the appropriate agencies and be provided with follow-up care and emotional support.

Self-Concept

Faced with dramatic changes in body structure and function and greater expectations to assume responsibilities, many adolescents experience temporary difficulty in developing a positive self-image. Adolescents who are accepted, loved, and valued by family and peers generally tend to gain confidence and feel good about themselves. Adolescents who have difficulty forming relationships or who are perceived by peers as too different and not included in adolescent cliques may develop less favorable self-images and have low self-esteem. Teenagers with physical handicaps or illnesses are particularly vul-

TABLE 26–3 *Clinical Signs of Sexually Transmitted Diseases*

Disease	Male	Female
Gonorrhea	Painful urination; urethritis with watery white discharge, which may become purulent.	May be asymptomatic; or vaginal discharge, pain, and urinary frequency.
Syphilis	Chancre, usually on glans penis, which is painless and heals in 4 to 6 weeks; secondary symptoms—skin eruptions, low-grade fever, inflammation of lymph glands—in 6 weeks to 6 months after chancre heals.	Chancre on cervix or other genital areas, which heals in 4 to 6 weeks; symptoms same as for male.
Genital warts (condyloma acuminatum)	Single lesions or clusters of lesions growing beneath or on the foreskin, at external meatus, or on the glans penis. On dry skin areas, lesions are hard and yellow-gray. On moist areas, lesions are pink or red and soft with a cauliflowerlike appearance.	Lesions appear at the bottom part of the vaginal opening, on the perineum, the vaginal lips, inner walls of the vagina, and the cervix.
Herpes genitalis (*Herpes simplex* of the genitals)	Primary herpes involves the presence of painful sores or large, discrete vesicles that last for weeks; vesicles rupture. Recurrent herpes is itchy rather than painful; it lasts for a few hours to 10 days.	Same as for males.
Chlamydial urethritis	Urinary frequency; watery, mucoid urethral discharge.	Commonly a carrier; vaginal discharge, dysuria, urinary frequency.
Trichomonas vaginalis	Slight itching; moisture on tip of penis; slight, early morning urethral discharge. Many males are asymptomatic.	Itching and redness of vulva and skin inside thighs; copious watery, frothy vaginal discharge.
Candida albicans	Itching, irritation, discharge, plaque of cheesy material under foreskin.	Red and excoriated vulva; intense itching of vaginal and vulvar tissues; thick, white, cheesy or curdlike discharge.
Acquired Immune Deficiency Syndrome (AIDS)	Symptoms can appear anytime from several months to several years after acquiring the virus. The person has reduced immunity to other diseases. Symptoms include any of the following for which there is no other explanation: persistent heavy night sweats; extreme fatigue; severe weight loss; enlarged lymph glands in neck, axillae, or groin; persistent diarrhea; skin rashes; blurred vision or chronic headache; harsh, dry cough; thick gray-white coating on tongue or throat.	

nerable to peer rejection. Nurses and educators can promote peer understanding and acceptance by discussing the individual's specific problems with the peer group. Establishing groups of peers who have similar problems can provide an opportunity for the individual to develop close relationships with others and feel valued and accepted.

Common teenage problems related to self-esteem and self-concept include drug abuse, suicide, and homicide, although they can also be considered protection needs.

Drug and substance abuse, including alcohol abuse, is on the rise among teenagers, especially among those with emotional problems. Many adolescents take drugs to have a new experience, to feel they belong to the group and thus relieve loneliness, or to prove they are courageous. This experimental use of drugs is a one-time or infrequent occurrence. Some teenagers, however, use drugs regularly. Compulsive users become dependent on drugs. Some drugs abused by teenagers are alcohol, glue and similar substances, barbiturates and amphetamines, hallucinogens, marijuana, cocaine, and crack.

Teenagers who use drugs habitually create problems for themselves and for the people with whom they associate. These teenagers may need help from nurses, physicians, and other professionals, such as psychiatrists specializing in adolescent problems.

Adolescent health promotion programs provided by nurses should include the following information:

- The underlying reasons for drug use and more positive coping mechanisms to deal with stress
- The hazards of drug misuse and abuse
- Responsible ways to make decisions about drug use before experimentation and ways to handle peer pressure

The nurse should also be alert for signs that a teenager is misusing drugs. Some of these are a drop in school achievement, mood swings, sleepiness or fatigue, and personality changes, such as withdrawal or boisterous behavior.

Adolescents also need to be informed that *nicotine* causes many harmful physiologic effects and is a precursor to lung cancer and coronary artery disease. It is also habit forming. Some teenagers who erroneously think that *smokeless* tobacco or *chewing* tobacco is less harmful than smoking tobacco need to be informed about the potential effects of smokeless tobacco (e.g., cancer of the mouth and tongue).

Suicide and *homicide* are two of the leading causes of death among teenagers. Adolescent males are more likely to commit suicide than adolescent females, and blacks are more likely to commit homicide than whites. Suicides by firearms, drugs, and automobile exhaust gases are the most common.

Most suicidal persons give verbal or behavioral warnings prior to suicide, and certain tendencies or behaviors are suspect. For example, most people who commit suicide have made previous attempts, are severely depressed, and are at odds with themselves and those close to them. Such individuals need to be referred to professional help.

Homicide is more common among the poor than other economic classes, and both killers and their victims are more likely to be men than women. Often homicide is associated with alcohol abuse and occurs most frequently at night and on weekends. Factors influencing the high homicide rate include economic deprivation, family breakup, and the availability of firearms, which are the most frequently used weapons. Cutting or stabbing tools are the next most frequently used weapons.

Health promotion programs for adolescents need to include information about suicide, alternatives to suicide, and ways to deal with a peer who might be suicidal.

ADULTHOOD AND MATURITY

The age at which a person is considered an adult depends on how adulthood is described. Legally, a person in the United States can vote at 18 years. The legal age for alcohol consumption outside the home varies among states from 18 to 21 years. Another criterion of adulthood is financial independence, which is also highly variable. Some adolescents support themselves as early as 16 years of age, usually because of family circumstances. By contrast, some adults are financially dependent on their families for many years, as for example, during prolonged education.

Adulthood may also be indicated by moving away from home and establishing one's own living arrangements. Yet this independence is also highly variable. Some adolescents leave home perhaps because of family problems. In recent years, however, an increasing number of young adults have been choosing to remain at home. In addition, many adults under 30 have returned to their parents' home to live. The factors contributing to this trend include high housing costs, high divorce rates, high unemployment rates, and the many problems resulting from drug abuse. Some young people who are employed full time receive only minimum wages and are unable to earn enough money to be totally self supporting.

Maturity is the state of maximal function and integration, or the state of being fully developed. Many other characteristics are generally recognized as representative of maturity. Mature individuals are guided by an underlying philosophy of life. They take many perspectives into account and are tolerant of the views of others. A comprehensive philosophy allows a person to make sense out of life and thus helps that person maintain a sense of purpose and hope in the face of human tragedies. Mature persons are open to new experiences and continued growth; they can tolerate ambiguity, are flexible, and can adapt to change. In addition, mature people have the quality of self-acceptance; they are able to be reflective and insightful about life and to see themselves as others see them. Mature persons also assume responsibility for themselves and expect others to do the same. The tasks of life are confronted in a realistic and mature manner; decisions are made and responsibility for those decisions accepted (Schuster and Ashburn 1986, pp. 577–78).

YOUNG ADULTS

The adult phase of development encompasses the years from the end of adolescence to death. Because the developmental tasks of young adults differ from those of older adults, adulthood is often divided into three phases: young adulthood, middle adulthood, and late adulthood. In this book young adults are defined as people 20 to 40 years old; middle-aged adults, as 40 to 65; and elderly adults, over 65.

During young adulthood, people become independent of their families, establish careers, often establish a close relationship with a significant other, and decide whether to have children. The young adult is typically a busy person who faces many challenges.

Physical Development

Persons in their early twenties are in their prime years physically. The musculoskeletal system is well developed and coordinated. This is the period when athletic endeavors reach their peak. Indeed, after 40 years, most athletes are considered old. All other systems of the body (e.g., circulatory and reproductive) are also functioning at peak efficiency. Although physical change during young adulthood is minimal, psychosocial development, by contrast, is great.

Psychosocial Development

According to Erikson, the central task of the young adult is *intimacy versus isolation*. Young adults are viewed as developing an intimate, lasting relationship with another person or a cause, institution, or creative effort (Erikson 1963, p. 263). The basic strength that evolves from this relationship is love; the outcome of negative resolution is exclusivity (Erikson 1982, p. 33).

Does Motherhood Make a Difference?

Many changes occur during the life cycle of a woman. The purpose of this study was to record and explore the life cycle of 80 women to determine if the experience of motherhood made a difference in development. The authors interviewed 50 mothers and 30 nonmothers, ages 60–95 years. All the participants were alert and active and able to maintain activities of daily living. The women were asked to share their life histories, from their earliest recollection, including events in the community, people and role models important to them, and transitions and turning points in their lives. (A transition is a turning point that results in new roles and new relationships. During a transition, new concepts of self may develop.) Each subject was specifically asked about the transition from childhood to adulthood.

The overall results showed that turning points or transitions over the life cycle did not differ significantly among mothers and nonmothers. Mothers, however, reported more turning points. The increase in the number of turning points for mothers was due to the increased complexity of family life and the mothers' involvement with graduations, weddings, grandchildren, and so on.

Other life experiences also differed in the two groups. Many of the mothers (30%) reported that they did not experience a normal childhood and were adults before age 15, in contrast to one (3%) of the nonmothers. The mothers had moved into marriage and motherhood earlier in life, whereas nonmothers completed their education and prepared for careers. As a result, nonmothers experienced greater stability in career paths. Later in life, some mothers were able to achieve their dreams of career and self-fulfillment. Many of the mothers began work roles at age 30, and some even later at age 40.

Implications: Although motherhood was an important factor in the mothers' lives, it was not found to be a significant influence in the achievement of integrity in later life. These researchers speculate that other factors such as events in society, family environment, individual development, and influence of birth order all seem to be related to early patterns of adult life and may influence life satisfaction during later life.

Source: R. Mercer, E. Nichols, and G. Doyle. Transitions over the life cycle: A comparison of mothers and nonmothers, *Nursing Research,* May/June 1988, 37:144–50.

Young adults face a number of new experiences and changes in life-style as they progress toward maturity. They must make decisions for themselves, and many of the decisions made now influence the person's life-style in years to come. The expectations of the young adult are often taken for granted, since they are well defined in most cultures. Choices must be made about education and employment, about whether to marry or remain single, about starting a home, and about rearing children. Social responsibilities include forming new friendships and assuming some community activities.

Occupational choice and education are largely inseparable. Education influences occupational opportunities; conversely, an occupation, once chosen, can determine the education needed and sought. Education enhances employment opportunities, enriches leisure time, and ensures economic survival. In the past, more young men than young women were encouraged to pursue advanced education, particularly college education. Education was deemed unnecessary for women who traditionally assumed the roles of wife and mother. This notion has changed as the role of women has changed. Many women now choose to assume active careers and civic roles in society in addition to their roles as mothers and/or wives.

Many women reenter the work force in their late thirties. This shift in family role may be met by the husband with support and flexibility or with open hostility. The husband may feel threatened by his wife's new role or by having to perform domestic chores he considers "feminine." The woman may also experience conflicts due to the change in roles. She may feel guilty because she is no longer home to nurture the family and, at the same time, anxious about the skills she may need as she enters the work force. Women reentering the job market experience considerable wage discrimination, despite current legislation and social trends that support equality.

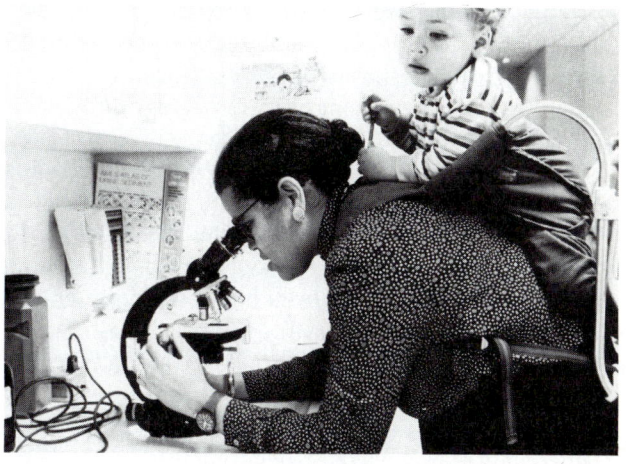

Figure 26–2 Many young women combine active careers with motherhood.

Remaining single is becoming the life-style of more and more young adults. Many people choose to remain single, perhaps to pursue an education and then to have the freedom to pursue their chosen vocations. Some unmarried individuals choose to live with another person of the opposite or same sex and share living arrangements and certain expenses. Some unmarried people are gay or lesbian and live with or are involved with a partner to whom they are committed.

Nurses should not assume that an unmarried person has no partner. Discreet, sensitive, and unprejudiced questioning of a client can often elicit information about a friend or support person who is especially significant to the client. Because single adults may live alone or with other adults who are employed, problems can arise when single persons are ill. Finding someone to drive them to a hospital or to help with shopping and meals during recuperation can be major challenges. A support system for a single adult may take more organization than the support system of a married person.

Deciding on a life partner is a difficult task. It is in many ways more complex and confusing than other tasks required of the young adult. In North America, there is emphasis on falling in love as a basis for mate selection. However, the multiple aspects of love make it difficult for some people to recognize and to know the meaning of love. Numerous definitions of love are available in literature, but the one important aspect of love is that it is lasting. *Love* survives times of frustration, strained relationships, and sadness, as well as times of happiness and achievement. It evolves out of interaction and requires adjustments and readjustments of the personalities of the people involved. There is a desire to do all one can to make the other person's life meaningful. In contrast, *infatuation* is sexually stimulating and exciting but is too shallow to nurture total personal growth of either partner and lasts only a short time.

Cognitive Development

Piaget believes that cognitive structures are complete during the *formal operations period,* from roughly 11 to 15 years. From that time, formal operations (for example, generating hypotheses) characterize thinking throughout adulthood and are applied to more areas. Egocentrism continues to decline; however, according to Piaget, these changes do not involve a change in the structure of thought, only a change in its content and stability (Miller 1983, pp. 62–65).

Recently, researchers in the field of psychology have suggested that a fifth and qualitatively higher stage of cognitive development may follow formal operations (Rybash, Hoyer, and Roodin 1986, p. 38). In addition to the adolescent ability to think in abstract terms, **post-formal operations thinkers** possess an understanding of the temporary or relative nature of knowledge. They are able to comprehend the contradictions that exist in both personal and physical reality. For instance, in a personal realm, an individual may understand that feelings toward another are not simply love or hate, but that these contrasting feelings may exist together in a relationship. Future research is needed to determine the existence of a fifth stage of cognitive development.

In recent years, cognitive psychologists have proposed an information-processing view of intelligence that seeks to explain the mental processes involved in solving a problem. **Information processing** has been described as the step-by-step mental operation that we use to solve problems. The steps of this approach include the following:

1. Encoding the items involved with a problem. This includes identifying all of the parts of a problem and determining what is already known about these parts.

2. Inferring relationships among the parts. This includes generating all of the possible links that may exist among the parts that might be helpful in solving the problem.

3. Applying relationships and justifying solutions to the problem. This involves both checking relationships and validating the information used.

4. Responding with the answer (Vander-Zanden 1985, pp. 430–32).

Individuals differ in their ability to carry out the various stages or components of this process. The best problem solvers are not necessarily the quickest. Experts often spend more time encoding a problem than do beginners, and they are often rewarded with the correct solution. According to Schuster and Ashburn (1986, p. 559), young adulthood is the time when people are most capable of forming new concepts and shifting their thinking in order to solve problems. However, other factors, such as motivation, education, memory, and maturity, also contribute to the problem-solving process.

Moral Development

Young adults who have mastered the previous stages of Kohlberg's theory of moral development now enter the *postconventional level.* See Table 24–8 on page 594. At this time, the person is able to separate self from the expectations and rules of others and to define morality in terms of personal principles. When individuals perceive a conflict with society's rules or laws, they judge according to their own principles. For example, a person may intentionally break the law and join a protest group to stop hunters from killing wild animals, believing that the principle of conservation of wildlife justifies the protest action. This type of reasoning is called **principled reasoning.** See also Gilligan's *ethic of care,* page 596. Gilligan argues that as individuals approach young adulthood, men and women tend to define moral problems somewhat differently. Men use an "ethic of justice" and define moral problems in terms of rules and rights. Women, by contrast, define moral problems in terms of obligation to care and to avoid hurt.

Spiritual Development

According to Fowler, the individual enters the *individuating-reflective period* sometime after 18 years of age. During this period, the individual focuses on reality. A 27-year-old adult may ask philosophic questions regarding spirituality and may be self-conscious about spiritual matters. The religious teaching that the young adult had as a child may now be accepted or redefined.

Health Promotion and Protection

Assessment guidelines for the growth and development of the young adult are shown in the accompanying box. Assessment activities may include measurement of height, weight, and vital signs (see Chapter 18) and questions about the following:

- History related to high blood pressure and heart disease.
- Vision and hearing, e.g., whether eyeglasses or contact lenses are prescribed
- Menstrual cycle and any problems
- Exposure to sexually transmitted diseases
- Stressors such as job or relationship problems and ways of coping with them
- Social activities and interests
- Usual patterns of nutrition, exercise, and rest/sleep

Examples of wellness diagnoses (see Chapter 23) and NANDA nursing diagnoses and goals for the young adult are shown in Table 26–4. *Outcome criteria* also need to be developed. The following are examples of outcome criteria for the NANDA diagnosis **Altered family process** in Table 26–4:

- The young adult attends job counseling sessions weekly for exploration and/or retraining opportunities.
- The young adult finds a job within 6 weeks.
- Family members discuss and determine temporary measures to cope with financial difficulties.
- Family members provide support and encouragement to one another during the period of unemployment.

Young adults are usually interested in meeting their health needs. However, because of the many stresses and changes throughout this 20-year period, the nurse will need to offer teaching and guidance in several health care areas. The nurse may wish to discuss some, or all, of the following topics with the young adult client.

Health Maintenance Visits and Immunizations Although many physicians may not recommend complete annual physical examinations, the nurse should encourage young adults to request a specific health maintenance schedule from their physicians. Some physicians

TABLE 26–4 *Examples of Nursing Diagnoses and Goals for Young Adults*

	Diagnosis	Goal
Wellness diagnosis	**Appropriate exercise level** related to integration of exercise regimen with life-style	During the next 3 months, the young adult continues to maintain exercise status.
NANDA diagnoses	Potential **Ineffective individual coping** related to new role as parent	Within 1 month, the young adult demonstrates appropriate coping strategies.
	Potential **Decisional conflict** related to career path	Within 1 month, the young adult chooses the best career option.
	Altered family process related to loss of employment	Family adjusts and copes with temporary lack of employment.

recommend a health risk appraisal at age 20, regular audiometry tests if the person is at risk, visual examinations every 2 to 4 years, yearly dental assessments, yearly Papanicolaou (Pap) tests for high-risk females, and a prostate examination every 5 years for males. If appropriate immunizations have not been received as recommended, they should be given at this time. Most colleges require that students show documentation of immunizations as a prerequisite to registration. Adults should receive a diphtheria and tetanus booster every 10 years and be vaccinated against influenza and hepatitis B if they are at risk of exposure. Young adults with no history of mumps should be vaccinated. Recently, public health authorities have reported an increase in the incidence of rubella among young adults due to the fact that they did not have the disease as children, were not vaccinated, or were vaccinated improperly. The nurse should assess whether the young adult is at risk for rubella. A rubella titer can be done to determine if immunity is low. A low immunity means that the client is susceptible to the disease, in which case immunization should be considered. Young women of childbearing age should be advised that rubella can cause severe complications during pregnancy. Therefore, the rubella vaccination should be given prior to pregnancy (preferably during childhood), and the client should be warned that serious side-effects could result if pregnancy occurs during the first 2 or 3 months after the rubella vaccine is administered.

Young adult women and men need to be informed about self-examination techniques that allow for possible early detection of cancers. For women, the focus is on breast self-examination; for men, on testicular examination.

Of all cancers among women, cancer of the breast is the most frequent cause of death. The peak incidence of breast cancer is during middle age. However, the young woman needs to form the habit of examining the breasts regularly. The effectiveness of treatment increases significantly the earlier a breast lump is discovered.

Breast self-examination (BSE) should be conducted once a month. A regular time is best—such as immediately following menstrual flow when breast tenderness and fullness caused by fluid retention have subsided—or on the first day of the month. Women who examine themselves regularly become familiar with the shape and texture of their breasts. Any changes must be reported immediately to a physician for accurate diagnosis. Before beginning to teach BSE to a client, the nurse needs to identify the client's attitudes toward this procedure. Some women are reluctant to conduct BSE because they fear what they might find. The nurse needs to explore these fears with the client. Women often offer these reasons for avoiding BSE: "I don't have time" and "I just don't think of doing it." The nurse also needs to explore these reasons with the client with particular reference to her self-esteem (see Chapter 29) and her need to spend time on herself.

BSE has three stages: the first takes place in the bath or shower; the second takes place while the client sits in front of a mirror; and the third takes place while the client lies down. During the *first stage* in a bath or shower, the woman checks for any lumps or thickenings by moving flat fingers over every part of each breast. Fingers glide easily over wet skin. The right hand is used to examine the left breast, and the left hand is used to examine the right breast.

In the *second stage,* the woman sits before a mirror with hands first at the sides and then clasped over the head. Each breast is observed in both positions for

- Indentations, rippling, puckering, or dimpling
- Asymmetry of the nipples; e.g., a nipple pulled to one side
- Discoloration
- Discharge from the nipple
- Any change in the size or shape of the breasts

Dimpling can be caused by scar tissue formation or a lesion. See Figure 19–73 on page 413. Show the client how to accentuate any retraction by raising her arms above her head, pushing her hands together with elbows flexed or pressing her hands down on her hips (see Figures 19–74 and 19–75 on page 413).

The client conducts the last part of the examination while lying in bed and palpating the breasts. Instruct the client to palpate the breast using the guidelines shown in the accompanying box.

Testicular cancer accounts for approximately 1% of all the cancer in men and often occurs in men in their early thirties (Crooks and Baur 1983, p. 129). It is most commonly found on the anterior and lateral surfaces of the testes. See Figure 26–3. This cancer is often serious and requires extensive surgery if discovered in the later stages. In the early stages, the cancer is asymptomatic except for a mass within the testicle. The lump often feels hard and bumpy and can usually be differentiated from tissue around it. The client may also experience a feeling of heaviness in the scrotum.

Testicular self-examination should be conducted monthly. The client can examine the testicles while he sits, stands, or lies down. A good time for this exploration is after a hot bath or shower since the heat causes the scrotal skin to relax and the testes to descend. Instructions for testicular self-examination are shown in the accompanying box.

Young adult females should also be screened for cervical cancer by having a routine Papanicolaou (Pap) test. A **Pap test** is done by obtaining and examining cells from the uterine cervical os. The cells are obtained during a pelvic examination. For more information on the pelvic exam, see Chapter 19. The nurse should also screen for high-risk factors for cervical cancer: sexual activity at an early age, multiple sexual partners, or a history of syphilis, herpes genitalis, or *Trichomonas* vaginitis. Many young adults are reluctant to have these examinations and screenings. Therefore, it is important for nurses to explain the purpose

CLIENT TEACHING
Breast Self-Examination

Instruct the woman to:

1. Examine the right breast by placing a pillow or folded towel under the right shoulder and the right hand behind the head. This position distributes breast tissue more evenly on the breast.

2. With the left hand:
   - Press the palmar surfaces of the middle three fingers on the skin surface, starting in the upper lateral quadrant, i.e., the outermost top of the breast.
   - Use a gentle rotating motion to press the breast tissue against the chest wall.
   - Palpate from the periphery to the areola.
   - Move the peripheral starting point around the breast clockwise.
   - Finally, squeeze the nipple of each breast gently between the thumb and index finger. Note any clear or bloody discharge.

3. Repeat the above for the left breast with a pillow under the left shoulder and the left hand behind the head.

4. Report a lump or nipple discharge to the physician immediately. A ridge of firm tissue in the curve of each breast is normal.

CLIENT TEACHING
Testicular Self-Examination

Instruct the man to:

1. Examine the testicles monthly, one at a time.

2. Use the fingertips to probe the surface gently, as if examining an egg for imperfections. The surface should be smooth and fairly firm.

3. Use the thumb and the index and middle fingers for examination, with the thumbs on top and the fingers on the underside of the scrotum.

4. Roll the testicles between the thumbs and fingers. The normal testicle is about 1½ to 2 inches long and feels rubbery, smooth, and firm, but not hard. It should be free of lumps.

5. Then palpate the epididymis, the storage tube found at the top of the testicle and extending behind it. It should feel soft, spongy, and slightly tender.

6. Last, locate the spermatic cord, which extends from the bottom of the epididymis and up into the pelvis. It normally feels firm and smooth (Malasanos et al. 1990, p. 543).

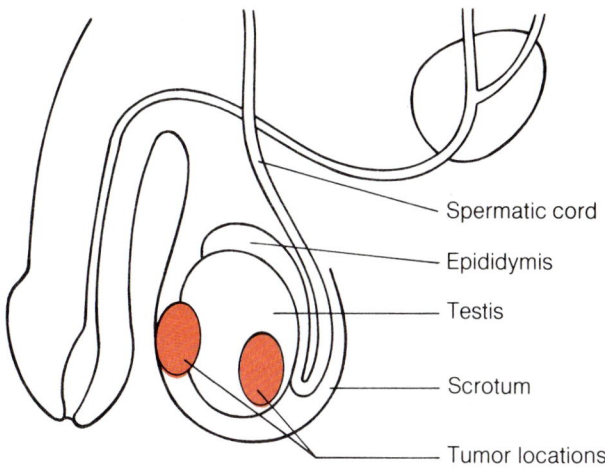

Figure 26–3 Common tumor locations of the testes.

of the test and to encourage all young women to begin this preventive measure by age 20. See Cancer Screening Guidelines in Chapter 19, page 362.

Safety Accident prevention is an important health promotion consideration during young adulthood. Among persons 15 to 24 years old, accidents are responsible for more deaths than all other causes combined (Hales 1989, p. 474). Motor vehicle accidents are, by far, the leading cause of mortality; other causes of accidental death for young adults include drowning, fires, burns, and firearms.

The nurse should provide the client with appropriate materials on motor vehicle safety and discuss driving attitudes and habits. Driving defensively and being alert for possible dangers are basic rules of safe driving. The client should be warned of the dangers of driving under the influence of alcohol or other drugs and encouraged to appoint a "designated driver" if the social activity involves consumption of alcohol. Seat belts and shoulder belts should be worn at all times, and approved car seats should be provided to protect infants and children. All drivers should maintain the safety of their automobiles by routinely checking the brakes and tires.

Young adults also need to be reminded of potential safety hazards both at home and at work. Fire hazards, such as faulty electrical wiring, should be repaired, and recreation areas with backyard pools should be supervised and properly maintained. Knowing the depth of a pool before diving into the water head first is an essential precaution. Diving into shallow pools is a leading cause of spinal cord injuries.

In the young male population, industrial accidents rank high as a major cause of death. Young adults should be educated about the potential for injury or death in various occupations before they decide on a lifelong career. Clients working in high-risk jobs should be encouraged to participate actively in programs to reduce occupational hazards. Nurses can provide young adults with the information, education, resources, and support needed to maintain a safe working environment and help prevent needless deaths and injuries.

Another safety hazard for many young adults is exposure to natural radiation from sunbathing. Many young men and women spend long hours in the sun during outdoor activities. Others sunbathe to obtain a tan. Exposure to the sun is directly related to skin cancer. Young adults should be cautioned to (a) avoid excessive sun exposure, particularly during midday, (b) use sun-blocking agents, such as para-aminobenzoic acid (PABA), which can be chosen according to skin type, and (c) avoid skin-tanning salons. The nurse should also provide information regarding skin changes that may indicate cancer. Many young adults regard a tan as "healthy" or looking "terrific." It is the nurse's role to reinforce the negative aspects and long-term risks of sun exposure.

Nutrition The nutritional habits established during young adulthood often lay the foundation for the patterns maintained throughout a person's life. Many young adults are aware of the four food groups but may not be knowledgeable about how many servings of each group they need or how much constitutes a serving. The nurse should pro-vide the young adult client with resources such as a chart or list that contains the foods and the amounts needed in each category. (See Chapter 39 for more detailed information on dietary requirements).

Young adult females need to increase their intake of vitamin C and also maintain an adequate iron intake. Approximately one-third of all women between the ages of 10 and 55 are anemic and receive only one-third of their daily iron requirements (Murray and Zentner 1989, p. 396). **Anemia** is defined as a condition characterized by a decrease in circulating red blood cells. To prevent anemia, females from ages 10 to 55 should ingest 18 mg of iron daily. The nurse should instruct the female client to include iron-rich foods, such as organ meats (liver and kidneys), eggs, fish, poultry, leafy vegetables, and dried fruits, in her daily diet.

The problems of obesity and hypertension may begin during young adulthood. Obesity may occur during the young adult years as the active teen becomes the sedentary adult but does not decrease caloric intake. The overweight or obese young adult is at risk for hypertension, a major health problem for this age group.

In the United States, 13% to 17% of whites and 26% to 28% of blacks age 20 and over have both high blood pres-

TABLE 26–5 *Criteria for Distinguishing the Physically Fit and the Physically Unfit Person*

Criterion	Physically Fit Person	Physically Unfit Person
1. Cardiorespiratory endurance	Decreased resting heart rate	Increased resting heart rate
	Increased resting stroke volume	Decreased resting stroke volume
	Can safely exceed baseline resting heart rate two or three times during strenuous exercise	No cardiorespiratory reserve with exercise; may overtax heart; danger of irregular heart rate with exercise
		Shortness of breath, chest pain, and skeletal muscle pain indicate inadequate perfusion of heart muscle and working skeletal muscle
2. Muscle strength and endurance	Firm muscle with increased tone	Flabby muscle with decreased tone
	Increased muscle size	Tone or muscle too tightly contracted, tight ligaments; decreased muscle size
	Increased muscle strength	Decreased muscle strength
	Increased muscle endurance	Decreased muscle endurance
3. Joint flexibility	Increased ROM of joints (as measured in degrees of movement)	Decreased ROM of joints (as measured in degrees of movement)
4. Body weight and composition	Ratio of weight to height is within normal limits	Ratio of weight to height is above normal limits (overweight)
	Percent of body fat is less than 15% in men, 25% in women	Percent of body fat is more than 16% in men, 26% in women
5. Motor skill performance	Performance demonstrates increased balance, power, agility, speed, reaction time, and coordination	Performance demonstrates decreased balance, power, agility, speed, reaction time, and coordination

sure (hypertension) and weight problems (Edelman and Mandle 1986, p. 491). Hypertension and obesity are 2 of more than 40 risk factors that have been identified in the development of cardiovascular (CV) disease. **Risk factors** are characteristics associated with an increased chance of developing a given health problem. Preventing these risk factors and lowering the risk of CV disease are critical. Current estimates show that CV and related diseases account for approximately 40% of the deaths in the United States each year (Christian and Greger 1988, p. 150). Low fat and/ or low cholesterol diets play a significant role in both the prevention and treatment of CV disease.

Exercise   All young adults need sufficient physical exercise to maintain their physical fitness. The actual amount of exercise that each person needs is highly individual, since each person develops a personal idea of "fitness." Some people think that fitness is the ability to finish a marathon; others see fitness as a lean or muscular body. In general, an individual who is physically fit has the ability to meet routine physical demands with sufficient reserve to meet a sudden challenge and is able to live an active life with minimum risk of injury or disability.

To assess the physical fitness of the young adult, the nurse may use the following five criteria: (1) cardiorespiratory endurance, (2) muscle strength and endurance, (3) joint flexibility, (4) body weight and fat composition, and (5) motor skill. Table 26–5 describes the criteria for distinguishing the physically fit and physically unfit person.

Exercise to attain an optimal cardiorespiratory system is called aerobic exercise. **Aerobic exercise** is any activity, such as brisk walking or swimming, in which the amount of oxygen taken into the body is slightly more than, or equal to, the amount of oxygen used by the body (Hales 1989, p. 146). In other words, the exercise is strenuous but does not leave the person breathless. The objective of an aerobic exercise program is to increase the maximum amount of oxygen that the body can process in a given time. These exercises also increase muscle fitness, flexibility, and endurance and provide a variety of other physical and psychosocial benefits. Table 26–6 lists the benefits of physical exercise. To obtain maximum effect from an aerobic exer-

TABLE 26–6   *Benefits of Physical Exercise*

Musculoskeletal System

Increased muscle strength

Increased muscle tone

Muscle hypertrophy (increased muscle mass)

Increased muscular endurance

Increased muscular coordination and balance

Overall increase in lean muscle tissue

Increased joint mobility/flexibility

Bone density maintained or increased

Cardiovascular System

Decreased heart rate during rest and during exertion

Faster recovery of heart rate following exertion

Increased size of heart muscle, especially of left ventricle

Increased strength of heart muscle contraction

Increased stroke volume with each heartbeat

Increased collateral blood supply to heart muscle

Decreased systolic and diastolic blood pressure, especially if previously elevated

Increased efficiency of peripheral circulation, especially venous

Decreased potential for cardiac arrythmia

Respiratory System

Increased vital capacity and functional capacity at rest and with exertion

Increased diffusion of oxygen and carbon dioxide

Increased maximal oxygen consumption (increased effectiveness of muscle tissue in extracting oxygen from the blood)

Metabolism and Nutrition

Decreased serum triglyceride levels

Decreased serum cholesterol levels

Increased glucose tolerance

Improved perfusion of nutrients into body tissues and removal of metabolic wastes from body tissues

Overall decrease in body fat and improved long-term control of body fat

Bowel Elimination

Increased motility of gastrointestinal tract, decreasing the potential for constipation

Social, Emotional, and Intellectual

Decreased nervous tension related to psychologic stress

Increased ability to cope with stress

Improved self-concept and sense of well-being

Increased energy levels

Decreased tendency toward depression and anxiety reactions

Improved work performance

Improved quality of sleep

Source: Adapted from N. J. Pender, *Health promotion in nursing practice* (Norwalk, Conn.: Appleton-Century-Crofts, 1982), pp. 234–35, and R. C. Cantu, editor, *Health maintenance through physical conditioning* (Littleton, Mass.: PSG Publishing Co., 1981), pp. 24–26.

cise program, the young adult should observe the following guidelines:

1. Follow sensible rules when preparing for exercise. See Table 26–7.

2. Begin the exercise period with 10 minutes of warming up and stretching, and end with 10 minutes of cooling down.

3. During exercise, increase the heart rate to 70% of the maximum rate. This is known as the target rate. Target rates should be achieved and maintained for about 15 to 20 minutes. Table 26–8 lists the target and maximum heart rates by age.

4. Make exercise a regular part of daily life. Exercises should be performed for 30 to 60 minutes, 3 to 4 days a week.

Young adults tend to ignore the idea of fitness for many reasons. Most individuals in this age group feel healthy, have busy lives with families, careers, and social activities, and in general tend to take their health for granted. It is important for the nurse to provide the young adult with information regarding fitness, explain the criteria for fitness, and discuss the need and benefits of regular exercise. In addition, the nurse should provide ongoing support and encouragement for clients about their fitness activities.

Sexual Concerns   Young adult men and women are often concerned about normal sexual response, both for themselves and their partners. Many problems arise in relationships because of basic differences in the male and female

TABLE 26–7   *Preparations for Exercise*

Preparation	Reason
Wear comfortable support shoes and well-fitting socks.	Proper footgear prevents blisters and injury.
Avoid running or walking on hard surfaces or in hilly areas.	Running on hard surfaces can jar the joints.
Avoid exercising on the hottest or most humid days.	Body temperature may become overly elevated.
Wait 1½ to 2½ hours after a meal.	Blood flow will be directed to the muscles rather than the alimentary tract.
Ingest increased amounts of glucose 1½ or 2½ hours before exercising.	Glucose provides energy for exercise.
Ingest adequate salt and potassium before exercising.	Salt and potassium prevent muscle cramps during exercise.
Drink ample fluid before exercising.	Adequate intake prevents dehydration due to fluid lost as perspiration.

TABLE 26–8   *Target and Maximum Heart Rates*

Age	Target Heart rate	Maximum Heart rate
20	120–150	200
25	117–146	195
30	114–142	190
35	111–138	185
40	108–135	180
45	105–131	175
50	102–127	170
55	99–123	165
60	96–120	160
65	93–116	155
70	90–113	150

Source: The American Heart Association, *Exercise diary* (Dallas: The Association, 1989), p. 3. Reproduced with permission.

sexual response patterns. Couples need to communicate their needs to one another early in their courtship so that a successful intimate relationship can develop and grow. Young adults should also be aware that because sexual needs and responses may change, each partner should listen and respond to the needs of the other. To promote a healthy sexual relationship, both partners should focus on being patient with one another and avoid the need to "perform." The nurse should encourage the young adult couple, or individual, to discuss sexual concerns and should provide information and resources that will promote ongoing growth and understanding in this developmental area.

Sexually transmitted diseases (STDs) such as genital herpes, AIDS, syphilis, and gonorrhea are common infections in young adults. Nursing functions are largely educational. The use of condoms greatly reduces the transfer of infectious microorganisms from one partner to another. Knowledge about the symptoms of these diseases can help the client obtain early treatment. In dealing with clients with STD, the nurse must be nonjudgmental and accepting of the client's life-style and treat any information obtained as confidential.

Work and Career Stress   During the young adult years, both men and women make career choices that they hope will give them a sense of accomplishment and help them to attain their personal goals. The job or workplace is also where young adults socialize and make new friends. However, some young adults have difficulty finding a job that is challenging and rewarding or in their area of preparation. Young women have the added burden of balancing career goals with childbearing responsibilities. Some women return to the work force a few months after having a child and find that they experience added stress due to the emotional strain and guilt of separation. Nurses need to be aware of work-related difficulties and the resulting stress and anxiety for the young adult. Some suggestions to promote health in the area of career and work life follow:

- Encourage the young adult to discuss the problems and stresses related to the work role.
- Discuss long-term work goals, and identify specific strategies to meet those goals.
- Assist young parents in obtaining professional child care, and discuss the concept of quality time for parents and children.
- Assess the young adult for problems of work stress or potential burnout.

Divorce and Separation

More than 40% of all marriages end in divorce. Divorce separates more than a million children from their families each year. The divorce rates of young adult women are rising with the result that many young women are now heads of households. In 1982, 29% of all households were headed by women (Edelman and Mandle 1986, p. 511). Divorce is an emotional stressor that may leave the young adult feeling angry, alone, betrayed, anxious, or depressed. These feelings may arise in the person initiating the divorce as well as the other partner. The nurse interviewing the young adult must be aware of the physical and emotional loss experienced as a result of divorce and separation. These individuals may need support and understanding from the nurse to deal with the crisis and grief. The nurse may suggest reading materials, support groups, or other resources. In addition, counseling on an ongoing basis may be suggested.

Battered or Abused Women

The problem of battering or abuse of women affects families at all socioeconomic levels. The attention directed to this problem by the media in recent years has resulted in more women coming forward and seeking help and protection from the abusive spouse or male companion. The legal system and law enforcement agencies have also become more aware of the pervasiveness of the problem and have developed systems to protect women against the threat of violent behavior. Stresses that predispose to abuse may include financial problems, separation from family and community support, and physical as well as social isolation. In working with women, the nurse should (a) have open communication that will encourage them to share their problems; (b) help them to develop self-esteem that will enable them to have the courage to leave the violent situation; (c) provide information and resources, such as welfare and shelters, that will allow them to begin an alternative life-style; and (d) continue to support and educate the young women so that they can understand the causes and results of abusive and violent behavior.

Substance Abuse

Drug abuse is a major threat to the health of young adults. Alcohol, marijuana, amphetamines, crack, and cocaine, for example, can bring about feelings of well-being that may be highly valued by people with adjustment problems. Prolonged use can lead to physical and psychologic dependency and subsequent health problems. For example, drug abuse during pregnancy can lead to fetal damage. Prolonged use of alcohol can lead to such diseases as cirrhosis of the liver and cancer of the esophagus.

Nursing strategies related to drug abuse include teaching about the complications of their use, changing individual attitudes toward drug abuse, and counseling regarding problems that lead to drug abuse.

Smoking is another type of drug abuse that can lead to diseases such as lung cancer and cardiovascular disease. The nurse's role regarding smoking is to (a) serve as a role model by not smoking; (b) provide educational information regarding the dangers of smoking; (c) help make smoking socially unacceptable, e.g., by posting "no smoking" signs in client lounges and offices; and (d) suggest resources, e.g., hypnosis, life-style training, and behavior modification, to clients who desire to stop smoking.

Suicide

Suicide is a leading cause of death in young adults. Many suicides may actually be mistaken for accidental death (automobile accidents, alcohol intoxication, and drug overdose). Suicide may result from problems with close relationships, such as those with marriage partners or parents, or from depression related to perceived occupational, academic, or financial failure. In general, suicide results from the young adult's inability to cope with the pressures, responsibilities, and expectations of adulthood.

The nurse's role in the prevention of suicide includes identifying behaviors that may indicate potential problems: depression; a variety of physical complaints, including weight loss, sleep disturbances, and digestive disorders; and decreased interest in social and work roles along with an increase in isolation. A young adult identified as at risk for suicide should be referred to a mental health professional or a crisis center. Nurses can also reduce the incidence of suicide by participating in educational programs that provide information about the early signs of suicide.

MIDDLE-AGED ADULTS

The middle years, from 40 to 65, have been called the years of stability and consolidation. For most people, it is a time when children have grown and moved away or are moving away from home. Thus, partners generally have more time for and with each other and time to pursue interests they may have deferred for years. See Figure 26–4.

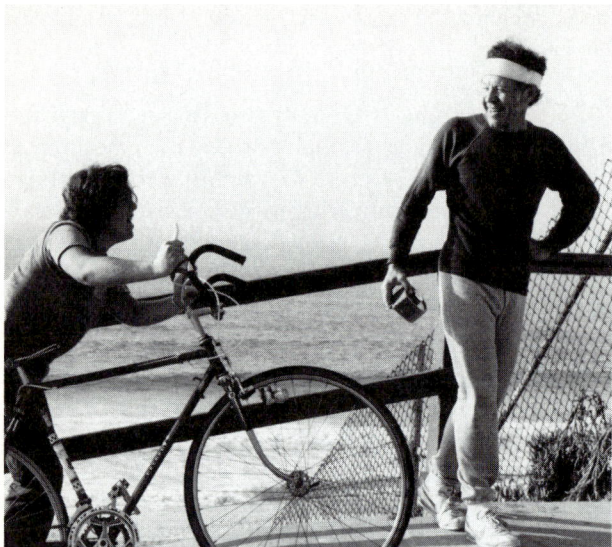

Figure 26–4 Middle-aged adults have time to pursue interests that were previously put aside for child care.

Physical Development

A number of changes take place during the middle years. At 40, most adults can function as effectively as they did in their twenties. However, during ages 40 to 65, many physical changes take place. See Table 26–9 for a summary of the physical changes of the middle-aged adult.

Both men and women experience decreasing hormonal production during the middle years. The **menopause** refers to the so-called change of life in women, when menstruation ceases. It is said to have occurred when a woman has not had a menstrual period within a year. The **climacteric** (andropause) refers to the change of life in men, when sexual activity decreases. The menopause usually occurs anywhere between ages 40 and 55. The average is about 47 years. At this time, the ovaries decrease in activity until ovulation ceases. A number of menstrual patterns can signal the menopause. Four of these are

1. Periods remain regular, but menstrual flow decreases.
2. Periods occur irregularly, and some periods are missed.
3. Menstrual flow ceases abruptly.
4. Menstrual flow occurs irregularly, with irregular amount of menses.

During menopause, the ovaries decrease in size, and the uterus becomes smaller and firmer. Progesterone is not produced, and the estrogen levels fall. Although the pituitary gland continues to produce the luteinizing hormone (LH) and the follicle-stimulating hormone (FSH), the ovaries do not respond. As a result of the lack of feedback, the pituitary gland increases the production of the gonadotro-

TABLE 26–9 *Physical Changes of the Middle-Aged Adult*

Category	Description
Appearance	Hair begins to thin, and gray hair appears. Skin turgor and moisture decrease, subcutaneous fat decreases, and wrinkling occurs. Fatty tissue is redistributed, resulting in fat deposits in the abdominal area.
Musculoskeletal system	Skeletal muscle bulk decreases at about age 60. Thinning of the intervertebral disks causes a decrease in height of about 1 inch. Calcium loss from bone tissue is more common among postmenopausal women. Muscle growth continues in proportion to use.
Cardiovascular system	Blood vessels lose elasticity and become thicker.
Sensory Perception	Visual acuity declines, often by the late forties, especially for near vision (presbyopia). Auditory acuity for high-frequency sounds (presbycusis) also decreases, particularly in men. Taste sensations also diminish.
Metabolism	Metabolism slows, resulting in weight gain.
Gastrointestinal system	Gradual decrease in tone of large intestine may predispose the individual to constipation.
Urinary system	Nephron units are lost during this time, and glomerular filtration rate decreases.
Sexuality	Hormonal changes take place in both men and women.

pins, in particular FSH. This disturbed endocrine balance accounts for some of the symptoms of the menopause. Common symptoms are hot flashes, chilliness, a tendency of the breasts to become smaller and flabby, and a tendency to become obese. Insomnia and headaches also occur with relative frequency. Psychologically, the menopause can be an anxiety-producing time, especially if the ability to bear children is an integral part of the woman's self-concept.

In men, there is no change comparable to the menopause in women. Androgen levels decrease very slowly; however, men can father children even in late life. The psychologic problems that men experience are generally related to the fear of getting old and to retirement, boredom, and finances.

Psychosocial Development

Until recently, the developmental tasks of middle-aged adults have received little attention. Erik Erikson (1963, p. 266) viewed the developmental choice of the middle-aged adult as *generativity versus stagnation*. **Generativity** is defined as the concern for establishing and guiding the next generation. In other words, there is concern about providing for the welfare of humankind that is equal to the concern of providing for self. People in their twenties and thirties tend to be self- and family-centered. In middle age, the self seems more altruistic, and concepts of service to others and love and compassion gain prominence. These concepts motivate charitable and altruistic actions, such as church work, social work, political work, community fund-raising drives, and cultural endeavors. Marriage partners have more time for companionship and recreation; thus, marriage can be more satisfying in the middle years of life. There is time to work together in volunteer activities. There is time for one partner to go out for lunch and for the other to go fishing. Generative middle-aged persons are able to feel a sense of comfort in their life-style and receive gratification from charitable endeavors.

Erikson believes that persons who are unable to expand their interests at this time and who do not assume the responsibility of middle age suffer a sense of boredom and impoverishment, i.e., stagnation. These persons have difficulty accepting their aging bodies and become withdrawn and isolated. They are preoccupied with self and unable to give to others. Some may regress to younger patterns of behavior, e.g., adolescent behavior.

Robert Peck (1968) believes that although physical capabilities and functions decrease with age, mental and social capacities tend to increase in the latter part of life. Peck recognizes four sets of developmental tasks that can be dealt with simultaneously during middle age. See the accompanying box.

Middle-aged adults usually face a number of adjustments in relation to their relationships and activities. Husbands and wives generally have more time for leisure activities. Relationships with families change. Children move away and marry and have children of their own. Parents are elderly and often have additional needs. Thus people in their forties and fifties often find themselves grandparents, enjoying their grandchildren but having few responsibilities for them, and at the same time assisting with the care of their own elderly parents. At this time people often face the death of a parent and as a result come to terms with their own aging and inevitable death.

For career-oriented adults, the middle adult years often represent the peak professional and occupational performance. Adults have many experiences behind them, which, together with intellectual skills, permit them to be effective in many areas, such as financial and career endeavors.

Retirement plans are also essential for middle-aged people. It is important that feelings about retirement be considered and that thought be given to ways in which increased leisure time is used. Middle-aged people who plan ahead for the financial needs of retirement and establish new ways to keep active often adapt to the retirement situation more effectively than those who do not.

The middle-aged person looks older and feels older. People usually accept the fact that they are aging; however, a few try to defy the years by their dress and even their actions. Some men and women have extramarital affairs and marry younger partners. A new freedom to be independent and follow one's individual interests arises. Prior to this period, the marriage partner or lover and other persons were crucial to a definition of self. Now the middle-aged person does not make comparisons with others, no longer fears aging or death, relaxes the sense of competitiveness, and enjoys

---

Peck's Tasks of Middle Age

- Valuing wisdom vs. physical power and attractiveness. As individuals approach middle age, physical strength and attractiveness decline. It then becomes necessary to gain satisfaction and ego strength through mental and intellectual abilities. Middle-aged persons must learn to rely more on their wisdom and accumulated experiences than on their physical powers.

- Socializing vs. sexualizing. In middle age, people should begin to redefine their interpersonal relationships. It is no longer appropriate to relate to the opposite sex in terms of physical attractiveness; other criteria such as friendship, warmth, and understanding should be adopted.

- Emotional flexibility vs. emotional rigidity. This task concerns the ability to become flexible, such as being able to shift emotional investment from one person to another and from one task to another. During this phase of life, the children often leave home, and parents may die. Middle-aged adults must be able to develop new roles, socially and emotionally, or they may find themselves isolated.

- Mental flexibility vs. mental rigidity. Individuals often become set in their ways as they approach middle age. They may not seek new ideas or accept the novel solutions of others. To cope most effectively, however, middle-aged adults should strive to remain flexible in their thinking. The solutions of the past may not solve today's problems. New ideas and perspectives should be considered.

Source: R. Peck, Psychological development in the second half of life, in B. L. Neugarten, editor, *Middle age and aging* (Chicago: University of Chicago Press, 1968), page 89.

the independence and freedom of middle age. Other people's opinions become less important, and the earlier habit of trying to please everyone is overcome. The person establishes ethical and moral standards that are independent of the standards of others. The focus shifts from inner self and being to outer self and doing. Religious and philosophical concerns become important.

In middle age, the interests set aside in favor of family and career can be renewed and developed. Hobbies such as photography, collecting antiques, or painting may develop into serious work. Some people who deferred education now pursue it or take refresher and other courses to keep abreast of changes. Some women enter the work force. Many middle-aged people feel a mixture of excitement and fear about these new undertakings.

Gail Sheehy (1977) suggests that the transition into middle life is as critical as adolescence. She outlines characteristics of the **midlife crisis** and calls the decade between the ages of 35 to 45 the "deadline decade." According to Sheehy, most women pass through the midlife crisis between 35 and 40; most men, between 40 and 45. This crisis occurs when individuals recognize that they have reached the halfway mark of life. Although people of these ages are reaching their prime, there is a beginning recognition that time is at a premium and that life is finite. Youthfulness and physical strength can no longer be taken for granted. Some characteristics of the midlife crisis include the following:

- Feeling bored, burdened, restless, and unappreciated
- Dissatisfaction with the way one's life has developed
- Ambivalence and uncertainty about the future
- Dismay about signs of aging
- Fear that time will be insufficient to accomplish goals
- Feelings of self-doubt
- Need to search for self, i.e., establish a true identity
- Worry about health
- Feelings of sadness, loneliness, or depression

Sheehy (1977, p. 44) describes this midlife crisis as an "inner crossroads" or "footbridge" leading to the second half of life. It is an "authenticity" crisis in which people face the discrepancy between their youthful ambitions and their actual attainment. To overcome this crisis, people need to reexamine their purposes and reevaluate ways to use their abilities and energies from now on. In Sheehy's words, it is a time when people ask, "Why am I doing all this? What do I really believe in? Is this all there is?" The parts of self that have been previously suppressed now need to be expressed. Both men and women in midlife crises sense a feeling of urgency and perhaps despair when they look at those options they have set aside and realize that aging and ill health may soon hinder such opportunities.

Women often respond to a midlife crisis by entering the job market or attending college. Men may respond by seeking second careers, by seeking promotions into manage-

ment, by departing from well-established baselines (such as marriage), or by becoming more interested in developing themselves personally. Some people become self-destructive. When people confront the midlife crisis constructively, they can feel revitalized; the middle years of life can be the happiest years of one's life. When people do not make changes through this transition stage, they experience a sense of staleness and feelings of resignation.

Midlife is a time when many events tend to occur simultaneously. For some, the transition precipitates a crisis; for others it does not. Vallient (1977, pp. 222–23) followed adults over a 40-year period and found that although change was characteristic of the midlife period, the presence of midlife crisis was more the exception than the rule.

Hultsch and Deutsch (1981) suggest that it is not the events themselves that make midlife a crisis, but an individual's response to these life events. How will an individual respond? According to Hultsch and Deutsch, the resources of the person, the ability to use effective coping strategies, and the life stage at which an event occurs will influence any changes in behavior. Internal and external resources include physical health, family income, the social support system, intelligence, and personality (p. 293). Thus, the crisis or transitions of midlife are not just within the individual but, rather, between the individual and the individual's world (pp. 216–18).

Cognitive Development

The middle-aged adult's cognitive and intellectual abilities change very little. Cognitive processes include reaction time, memory, perception, learning, problem solving, and creativity. Reaction time during the middle years stays much the same or diminishes during the later part of the middle years. Memory and problem solving are maintained through middle adulthood. Learning continues and can be enhanced by increased motivation at this time in life.

Middle-aged adults are able to carry out all the strategies described in Piaget's phase of *formal operations* (see Table 24–6, page 591). Some may use post-formal operations strategies to assist them in understanding the contradictions that exist in both personal and physical aspects of reality (see the discussion on cognitive development of the young adult, page 648). The experiences of the professional, social, and personal life of middle-aged persons will be reflected in their cognitive performance. Thus, approaches to problem solving and task completion will be considerably varied in a middle-age group. The middle-aged adult can "reflect on the past and current experience and can imagine, anticipate, plan and hope" (Murray and Zentner 1989, pp. 476–77).

Moral Development

According to Kohlberg, the adult can move beyond the *conventional level* to the *postconventional level*. Kohlberg believes that extensive experience of personal moral choice and responsibility is required before people can reach the postconventional level. Kohlberg found that few of his subjects achieved the highest level of moral reasoning. To move from stage 4, *a law and order orientation,* to stage 5, *a social contract orientation,* requires that the individual move to a stage in which rights of others take precedence. People in stage 5 take steps to support another's rights.

Spiritual Development

Not all adults progress through Fowler's stages to the fifth, called the *paradoxical-consolidative stage.* At this stage, the individual can view "truth" from a number of viewpoints. Fowler's fifth stage corresponds to Kohlberg's fifth stage of moral development. Fowler believes that only some individuals after the age of 30 years reach this stage.

In middle age, people tend to be less dogmatic about religious beliefs, and religion often offers more comfort to the middle-aged person than it did previously. People in this age group often rely on spiritual beliefs to help them deal with illness, death, and tragedy.

Health Promotion and Protection

Assessment guidelines for the growth and development of the middle-aged adult are shown in the accompanying box. Assessment activities may include measurements of weight, height, and vital signs (see Chapter 18), and questions about the following:

- Visual and hearing changes
- Cessation of menstruation
- Satisfaction with work
- Social activities
- Children and family relationships
- Usual patterns and any changes in eating, elimination, exercise

Examples of wellness diagnoses (see Chapter 23) and NANDA nursing diagnoses and goals for the middle-aged adult are shown in Table 26–10. *Outcome criteria* also need to be developed. The following are examples of criteria for the NANDA diagnosis **Diversional activity deficit** in Table 26–10:

- The middle-aged adult chooses three activities of interest within 2 weeks.
- The middle-aged adult participates in one of the three activities within 1 month.
- The middle-aged adult maintains a weekly schedule of at least one activity per week within 6 weeks.
- The middle-aged adult continues the schedule for 6 weeks.

Middle-aged adults usually take care of their health needs and are interested in maintaining health and preventing the

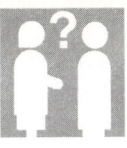

acceleration of the aging process. The nurse may wish to discuss some of the following topics with the middle-aged client and offer teaching, guidance, and support in accordance with the client's needs.

Health Maintenance Visits and Protection
Middle-aged adults should be encouraged to request a specific health maintenance schedule from their physicians.

TABLE 26–10 *Examples of Nursing Diagnoses and Goals for Middle-Aged Adults*

	Diagnosis	Goal
Wellness diagnosis	**Positive body image** related to acceptance of maturational changes	During the next year, the middle-aged adult continues to maintain a positive body image.
NANDA diagnoses	**Diversional activity deficit** related to life changes	The middle-aged adult increases diversional activities and opportunities within 3 months.
	Altered nutrition: More than body requirements related to change in activity and sedentary behavior	The middle-aged adult develops healthy nutritional habits.

Some physicians may recommend a yearly physical examination, audiometry if the individual is in a high-risk group, yearly visual examinations, yearly dental assessments, yearly mammogram, yearly Pap test if in high-risk group or every 3 years if not, and yearly prostate and testicular examination.

Middle-aged clients require a tetanus booster every 10 years, as well as influenza and pneumococcal vaccinations if they are in major high-risk groups, such as those with chronic lung disease or coronary artery disease.

To maintain health, middle-aged adults should learn to recognize the signs and symptoms of cancer. Cancer accounts for considerable mortality and morbidity in both men and women. It is the second leading cause of death among people between the ages of 25 and 64 in the United States. The patterns of cancer types and incidences for men and women have changed over the past several decades. Over one-third of the deaths due to cancer occur between the ages of 35 to 64. Men have a high incidence of cancer of the lung and bladder. In women, breast cancer is highest in incidence, followed by cancer of the colon and rectum, uterus, and lung. The incidence of lung cancer is increasing in women.

Female clients may need to be reminded to perform monthly breast self-examinations and male clients to perform monthly testicular self-examination in order to detect growths. See breast and testicular examination, earlier in this chapter. Postmenopausal women should report any vaginal bleeding. For information on sexually transmitted diseases, see the section on infections earlier in this chapter.

Safety   Changing physiologic factors, as well as concern over personal and work-related responsibilities, may contribute to the accident rate of middle-aged persons. Motor vehicle accidents are the most common cause of accidental death in this age group. Other accidental causes of death for middle-aged adults include falls, fires, burns, poisonings, and drownings (Hales 1989, p. 474). Occupational accidents continue to be a significant safety hazard during the middle years.

It is important that the middle-aged adult be aware of basic safety, such as using seat belts and driving within the speed limit. Physiologic changes also affect driving behavior. For example, decreased visual acuity may make night driving difficult, and a decrease in reaction time may make the middle-aged adult more prone to accidents. The middle-aged couple should make their home as safe as possible to prevent falls and other accidents. Stairways should be well lighted and uncluttered, and bathrooms should be equipped with hand grasps and nonskid bath mats. Fire alarms should be tested regularly and all machines and tools kept in good working condition.

Nutrition   The middle-aged adult should continue to eat a healthy diet, following the recommended portions of the four food groups, with special attention to protein, calcium, and limiting cholesterol and caloric intake. See Chapter 39 for further information. There is no evidence that vitamins or other supplements are needed unless specifically prescribed by a physician because of signs of nutritional deficiency or because of an insufficient diet (Murray and Zentner 1989, p. 47). Two or three liters of fluid should be included in the daily diet. Postmenopausal women need to ingest sufficient calcium and vitamin D to prevent **osteoporosis** (a decrease in bone density). See Chapter 27, pages 667 and 675.

Middle-aged adults who gain weight may not be aware of some common facts about this age period. Decreased metabolic activity and decreased physical activity mean a decrease in caloric need. For each decade after 25 years, there should be a 7.5% reduction in total calories consumed (Williams 1981, p. 474). The nurse's role in nutritional health promotion is to counsel clients to prevent obesity by reducing caloric intake and participating in regular exercise. Clients should also be warned that being overweight is a risk factor for many chronic diseases, such as diabetes and hypertension, and for problems of mobility such as arthritis.

For the client who requires additional management resources, a variety of programs are frequently available. Programs may be found at hospitals, clinics, universities, industries, and in the community. Most programs use behavior modification techniques and group support to assist clients in reaching their goals. Clients should seek medical advice before considering any major changes in their diets.

During the late middle-age period, there is a gradual decrease in gastric juice secretions and free acid. As a result, some individuals may complain of "heartburn" (acid indigestion) or an increase in belching. They may determine that certain foods disagree with them. Clients should be advised to develop sensible eating habits and avoid fried or fatty foods.

Exercise   Exercise is a key factor in delaying the aging process. Nevertheless, many middle-aged adults may not include exercise in their life-style. Many of the activities or routine chores that provided exercise in the past have been streamlined by modern devices that save time and require little if any energy, such as gas and electric lawn mowers. To promote health in relation to exercise, the nurse must assess the client's current level of activity and the client's physical fitness (see Table 26–5). Any exercise program for the middle-aged adult should (a) begin gradually, (b) increase to a moderately strenuous level, (c) be consistent, and (d) avoid overexertion. **Overexertion** is characterized by trembling, nausea, chest pain, extreme shortness of breath, or sudden headache (Diekelmann 1977, p. 98). Clients should stop exercising immediately if any of the symptoms of overexertion are experienced.

The exercise program for the person over 40 should focus on sports that require skill and coordination rather than speed or endurance. Persons over 50 should exercise additional caution by avoiding activities that require sudden stops and starts, and any situations or activities where they may fall. The overall objective of exercise for the middle-aged client is to increase the efficiency of the cardiovascular and respiratory system. To accomplish this objective, individuals should engage in continuous, rhythmic exercises maintained for about 30 minutes, 3 times per week. Walking briskly, jogging, and swimming are all highly recommended forms of exercise. For the middle-aged adult to obtain maximum benefit from an exercise program, the nurse should explain the importance of proper preparation for exercise (see Table 26–7), the concept of target heart rate (see Table 26–8), and the need for a warm-up and cool-down period. For additional information, see the general guidelines for aerobic exercise discussed in the young adult section.

Menopause   **Hot flashes,** reported by 50% of women, refer to a cluster of symptoms: heat rising on the chest, spreading to the neck and face (caused by vasodilation), sweating (mild to drenching), sleep disturbances, and occasional chills. Flashes may occur 20 to 30 times a day, lasting 3 to 5 minutes (Olds, London, and Ladewig 1988, pp. 148–49). Because a rise in body temperature may trigger a flash, women should be advised to consider the following measures:

- Maintain a comfortable environment. Use fans, light blankets, and air conditioning if possible.

- Use measures to cool body temperature. Increase the intake of cold fluids, and take cool showers or sponge baths. Dress lightly and loosely in cotton or other natural fibers.

- Avoid food that may trigger a flash. Chocolate, red wine, and cheeses contain tyramine, an amino acid that causes the release of norepinephrine in the hypothalamus, which resets the body's thermostat and triggers a flash (McKeon 1989, p. 56).

In the past, other maladies have been blamed on "the change": psychologic dysfunctions, weight gain, and anxiety attacks. However, recent studies have shown that psychologic problems such as anxiety and depression are far less common than previously believed and are not directly related to declining hormone levels (McKeon 1989, p. 52).

One of the myths of menopause is that women lose their interest in sexual activity. In fact, some middle-aged women experience a sense of relief from the fear of pregnancy and may find an increased pleasure from sexual intimacy. The level of sexual interest during midlife depends on the woman's self image, her previous sexual activity and expression, and the availability of a sexual partner. To promote sexual health, the nurse should teach women what to expect during menopause and suggest strategies to assist them through the midlife transition.

A few years after menopause begins, the middle-aged woman may complain of pain during intercourse, as well as symptoms of itching, burning, and vaginal discharge. These symptoms are due to **atrophic vaginitis,** or vaginal atrophy, which is characterized by a thinning and drying of the vaginal wall and a loss of elasticity and lubrication. Women should be advised that sexual activity helps to prevent the shrinkage of the vaginal mucosa and maintain an adequate vaginal outlet. The nurse can suggest that a water-soluble lubricant be used if intercourse becomes painful. To prevent vaginal itching, women should avoid tight clothing, such as girdles and pantyhose, that prevents air circulation. The middle-aged woman should be advised that even though menstrual periods are decreased or skipped, pregnancy may still occur up until age 50, and precautionary measures should be taken.

Women with severe menopausal symptoms should be referred to the physician for evaluation. Until recently, these symptoms were primarily treated with supplementary therapy. At present, the use of estrogen replacement therapy is controversial for long-term use because it has been found to predispose women to malignancy of the reproductive organs. Currently, low-dose estrogen therapy is prescribed for extensive troublesome hot flashes, and vaginal estrogen creams for vaginal atrophy (Olds, London, and Ladewig 1988, p. 149).

Male Climacteric   The male climacteric is difficult to evaluate, since few men discuss these changes with their doctors. Although the amount of sperm produced decreases, the male maintains the capacity for fathering children throughout life. Middle-aged men are more prone to sexual dysfunction than females. They may experience a decrease in virility and a decrease in the ability to perform sexually. As a result of aging, the male may take longer to attain an erection. However, he should retain his facility for erection (Schuster and Ashburn 1986, p. 749). To promote sexual health for the male client, the nurse should encourage him to discuss any concerns regarding changes in sexual ability or activity. The nurse should also assess the client for health risks associated with impotence: diabetes, alterations in nerves or blood supply, and medications such as antihypertensives and muscle relaxants.

Self-Concept   The midlife crisis may result in a decrease in self-concept for some middle-aged adults. To promote psychosocial health during midlife, the nurse should help the individual to work through the developmental changes of the period. The following can be used as guidelines.

1. Encourage both men and women to do some of the things they never had time to do previously. These may include taking up a sport such as golf, taking a cross-country trip, starting a business, joining a community or professional group, or taking a course and starting a new career.

2. Support middle-aged adults in accepting the changes of the period and adjusting to them. Discuss some of the things they can do to highlight their personal assets and make them feel attractive. For instance, they may be able to purchase some new clothes or make a change in hairstyle.

3. Assist middle-aged adults in discussing their changing role as parents. Some middle-aged parents experience

emotional changes when their children leave home. They may attempt to compensate for lost opportunities or perceived failures by becoming more involved in their children's daily lives and activities. Teenagers and adult children need to have independence and be given the freedom to make their own choices. The parents' role at this time is to offer love, encouragement, and emotional support while adult children determine their own path of life.

4. Emphasize the positive outcomes of maintaining old friendships and seeking new ones. Enlarging the circle of friends and activities helps the middle-aged adult to share life experiences with others and provide positive feedback that will enhance their self-esteem.

5. Discuss the middle-aged adult's role in the care of aging parents. Allow the individual to discuss the frustrations and concerns inherent in this role reversal. Present options related to the extended care of aging parents, and allow the client to weigh the benefits and problems of each choice.

6. Review the individual's plan for retirement. Individuals and couples should be encouraged to prepare financially as well as socially for the years ahead. Proper financial arrangements require careful planning that should begin during middle adulthood. Hobbies, leisure, and travel also require planning and discussion.

Divorce   Divorce is a major stressor and a potential cause of mental health alterations during middle adulthood. The negative impact of separation or divorce for middle-aged adults appears to be greater than for either the young or the older age group (Schuster and Ashburn 1986, p. 770), perhaps because the life of the middle-aged adult often revolves around family activities and structures. The

first year of divorce is often considered the most stressful, and money is often the major source of disruption.

A divorce affects each member of a family differently. Women often suffer more than men with respect to emotional stress, economic status, and role loss. Men, by contrast, have more difficulties with the daily tasks involved in self-care and maintaining a comfortable living environment. The children in this situation, usually teenagers or young adults, also suffer emotionally and need support and counseling. For some couples, divorce, although difficult, provides a sense of relief from the stress and pain of living in an unhappy marital situation. The nurse can provide support by assisting each member of the family in assessing life-style and determining changes that will need to be made under the new financial structures. All family members would benefit from support groups or individual therapy to help them cope with the feelings of loss and adjust to long-term changes.

Substance Abuse   The excessive use of alcohol is a multifaceted problem for the individual and society. Use of the drug is part of the life-style of many Americans and Canadians. Excessive use can result in unemployment, disrupted homes, accidents, and diseases. It is estimated that four million people in the United States are dependent on alcohol and can be considered alcoholics. Nurses can help clients by providing information about the dangers of excessive alcohol use, by helping the individual clarify values about health, and by referring the client to special groups such as Alcoholics Anonymous.

Heavy smoking increases the risk of pulmonary cancer, cardiovascular disease, and chronic obstructive lung disease. See the discussion of drug abuse earlier in the chapter for additional information.

CHAPTER HIGHLIGHTS

▶ Adolescence is a critical period of development extending from the onset of puberty to age 18 or 20.

▶ Rapid growth in height, development of secondary sexual characteristics, sexual maturity, and increasing independence from the family are major landmarks of adolescence.

▶ The dramatic physical changes of early adolescence require major adjustments in body image.

▶ Peer groups assume great importance during adolescence; they provide a sense of belonging and self-esteem and facilitate the development of a positive self-concept.

▶ Late adolescence is a more stable stage, during which the adolescent is mostly involved with planning a future and economic independence.

▶ Adolescents between the ages of 11 to 15 begin the formal operations stage of cognitive development; they are able to think logically, rationally, and futuristically and can conceptualize things as they could be rather than as they are.

▶ The adolescent is at Kohlberg's conventional level of moral development, and some proceed to the postconventional or principled level.

- Adolescents are at Fowler's synthetic-conventional stage of spiritual development.

- During the adolescent period, health promotion activities are focused on preventive interventions for the potential problems of obesity, sexually transmitted and other communicable diseases, bulimia, anorexia nervosa, unplanned pregnancy, motor vehicle accidents, sports injuries, drug abuse, and suicide.

- Maturity is the state of maximal function or the state of being fully developed. Mature persons take responsibility for their own behavior and do not expect others to make their decisions.

- The young adult is essentially in a stable period physically but psychosocial change is great.

- Cognitive development continues throughout adulthood.

- Some young adults enter Kohlberg's postconventional level of moral development and develop principled reasoning.

- Spiritual development of young adults continues into Fowler's paradoxical-consolidative stage; young adults often feel self-conscious about spiritual matters.

- Hazards to the health of young adults include accidents, sexually transmitted diseases, suicide and homicide, substance abuse, obesity, and hypertension. Nurses can assist clients to decrease the impact of these hazards.

- The middle-aged adult needs to adjust to an aging body, the increasing dependence of parents, and the increasing independence of children; however, new independent interests can be pursued.

- Both middle-aged men and women enter a midlife crisis in which they need to reexamine their purpose and reevaluate ways to use their energies and abilities.

- Common health hazards of middle-aged adults include obesity, cardiovascular diseases, substance abuse, and cancer.

- Positive health practices can protect and promote health.

READINGS AND REFERENCES

SUGGESTED READINGS

Gillis, A. January/February 1988. Promoting health among teenagers. *International Nursing Review* 35:10–12.

A number of problems face many of today's teens: drug addiction, suicide, abortion, delinquency, and alcoholism. According to Gillis, nurses need to respond to these problems by increasing access to nursing care and by offering health promotion programs that respond to the needs of the teenagers. Gillis presents a model and offers suggestions for practical applications.

Szydlo, V. L. November 1988. Approaching an adolescent about a pelvic exam. *American Journal of Nursing* 88:1502–6.

This author provides an overview about how to deal effectively with an adolescent who requires a pelvic exam. A pelvic exam may be necessary for an adolescent if she suspects pregnancy or STD (sexually transmitted disease). Usually, teenagers are reluctant to discuss any details of intimate sexual problems and may at first deny that they are sexually active. In this article, Szydlo focuses on several topics to consider when dealing with teenagers considering their first pelvic exam, including (a) trust, (b) control, (c) self-consciousness, and (d) fear of pain. Brief case examples are also presented.

RELATED RESEARCH

Campion, V. Summer 1989. Effect of knowledge, teaching method, confidence and social influence on breast self-examination. *Image: Journal of Nursing Scholarship* 21:76–80.

Duffy, M. November/December 1988. Determinants of health promotion in midlife women. *Nursing Research* 37:358–62.

Gillett, P. January/February 1988. Self-reported factors influencing exercise adherence in overweight women. *Nursing Research* 37:25–29.

Jordan-Marsh, M. September 1988. Measuring occupational health nurses' counseling on health promotion. *Public Health Nursing* 5:177–85.

Kulbok, P. P.; Earls, F. J.; and Montgomery, A. C. October 1988. Lifestyle and patterns of health and social behavior in high-risk adolescents. *Advances in Nursing Science* 11:221–35.

Mercer, R.; Nichols, E.; and Doyle, G. May/June 1988. Transitions over the life cycle: A comparison of mothers and nonmothers. *Nursing Research* 37:144–50.

SELECTED REFERENCES

American Heart Association. 1989. *Exercise diary.* Dallas, Texas: The Association.

Caliandro, G., and Judkins, B. 1988. *Primary nursing practice.* Glenview, Ill.: Scott, Foresman & Co.

———. Cantu, R. C., editor. 1981. *Health maintenance through physical conditioning.* Littleton, Mass.: PSG Publishing Co.

Carpenito, L. J. 1989. Nursing Diagnosis. *Application to Clinical Practice 3rd ed.* Philadelphia: J. B. Lippincott Co.

Christian, J. L., and Greger, J. L. 1988. *Nutrition for living.* Menlo Park, Calif.: Benjamin/Cummings Publishing Co.

Church, J. L., and Baer, K. J. March/April 1987. Examination of the adolescent: A practical guide. *Journal of Pediatric Health Care* 1:65–72.

Crooks, R., and Baur, K. 1983. *Our Sexuality.* 2d ed. Menlo Park, Calif.: Benjamin/Cummings Publishing Co.

Diekelmann, N. 1977. *Primary health care of the well adult.* New York: McGraw-Hill.

Disparti, J. 1988. Nutrition and self-care. In Caliandro, G. and Judkins, B., editors. pp. 134–50. *Primary nursing practice.* Glenview, Ill.: Scott, Foresman & Co.

Edelman, C., and Mandle, C. L. 1986. *Health promotion throughout the life span.* St. Louis: C. V. Mosby Co.

Erikson, E. H. 1963. *Childhood and society.* 2d ed. New York: W. W. Norton and Co.

————. 1982. *The life cycle completed: A review.* New York: W. W. Norton and Co.

Fowler, J., and Keen, S. 1978, 1985. *Life maps: Conversations in the journey of faith.* Waco, Texas: Word Books.

Fowler, J. W. 1981. *Stages of faith: The psychology of human development and the quest for meaning.* New York: Harper and Row.

Gilchrist, L., and Schinke, S. 1987. Adolescent pregnancy and marriage. In Van Hasselt, V. B., and Hersen, M., editors. *Handbook of adolescent psychology.* New York: Pergamon Press.

Gilligan, C. 1982. *In a different voice: Psychological theory and women's development.* Cambridge, Mass.: Harvard University Press.

Gillis, A. January/February 1988. Promoting health among teenagers. *International Nursing Review* 35:42–43.

Hales, D. 1989. *An invitation to health.* 4th ed. Redwood City, Calif.: Benjamin/Cummings Publishing Co.

Heywood, V. H. 1984. *Designs for fitness.* Minneapolis: Burgess Publishing Co.

Houldin, A., Saltstein, S., Ganley, K. 1987. *Nursing Diagnoses for Wellness.* Philadelphia: J.B. Lippincott.

Hultsch, D. F., and Deutsch, F. 1981. *Adult development and aging.* New York: McGraw-Hill.

Ireland, D. F. November 1988. Reading, writing and reasons for health. *American Journal of Nursing* 88:1506.

James, S., and Mott, S. 1988. *Child health nursing: Essential care of children and families.* Menlo Park, Calif.: Addison-Wesley Publishing Co.

Kohlberg, L. 1971. *Recent research in moral development.* New York: Holt, Rinehart and Winston.

Malasanos, L., Barkauskas, V. and Stoltenberg-Allen, K. 1990. *Health assessment.* St. Louis: C.V. Mosby Co.

McKeon, V. A. June 1989. Cruel myths and clinical facts about menopause. *RN:* 52:52–6, 58–9.

Marley, W. P. 1982. *Health and physical fitness.* Philadelphia: Saunders College Publishing.

Miller, P. H. 1983. *Theories of developmental psychology.* San Francisco: W. H. Freeman and Co.

Montoye, H.; Christian, J.; Nagle, F.; and Levin, S. 1988. *Living fit.* Menlo Park, Calif.: Benjamin/Cummings Publishing Co.

Murray, B. L. S., and Wilcox, L. J. December 1978. Testicular self-examination. *American Journal of Nursing.* 78:2074–75.

Murray, R., and Zentner, J. 1989. *Nursing assessment and health promotion strategies through the life span.* 4th ed. Norwalk, Conn.: Appleton & Lange.

NANDA approved nursing diagnostic categories for clinical use and testing. Summer 1988. *Nursing Diagnosis Newsletter* 15(1):1–3.

Nelms, B. C. January/February 1988. Promoting emotional health: Role of the nurse practitioner. *Journal of Pediatric Health Care* 2:1–2.

Novotny, J. May/June 1989. Adolescents, acne, and the side effects of Accutane. *Pediatric Nursing* 15:247–48.

Olds, S.; London, M.; and Ladewig, P. 1988. *Maternal newborn nursing.* 3d ed. Menlo Park, Calif.: Addison-Wesley Publishing Co.

Peck, R. 1968. Psychological development in the second half of life. In Neugarten, B. L., editor. *Middle age and aging.* Chicago: University of Chicago Press.

Pender, N. J. 1987. Health promotion and nursing practice. 2d ed. Norwalk, Conn.: Appleton & Lange.

Rubin, L. B. 1979. *Women of a certain age: The midlife search for self.* New York: Harper and Row.

Rybash, J., Hoyer, W., and Roodin, P. 1986. *Adult cognition and aging.* New York: Pergamon Press.

Sheehy, G. 1977. *Passages: Predictable crises of adult life.* New York: E. P. Dutton and Co.

Schuster, C. S., and Ashburn, S. S. 1986. *The process of human development: A holistic approach.* 2d ed. Boston: Little, Brown and Co.

Sugarman, L. 1986. *Life-span development: Concepts, theories and interventions.* New York: Methuen and Co.

Tzirides, E. April 1988. Health outreach program: Marketing the "Health Way." *Nursing Management* 19:557.

United States Department of Health and Human Services. August 1985. *Charting the nation's health trends since 1960.* DHHS Pub. no. (PHS) 85–1251. Hyattsville, Md.: Public Health Service.

Vallient, G. 1977. *Adaptation to life.* Boston: Little, Brown and Co.

Vander-Zanden, J. 1985. *Human development.* 3d ed. New York: Alfred A. Knopf.

Van Hasselt, V., and Hersen, M., editors. 1987. *Handbook of adolescent psychology.* New York: Pergamon Press.

Williams, S. R. 1981. *Nutrition and diet therapy.* 4th ed. St. Louis: C. V. Mosby Co.

Late Adulthood

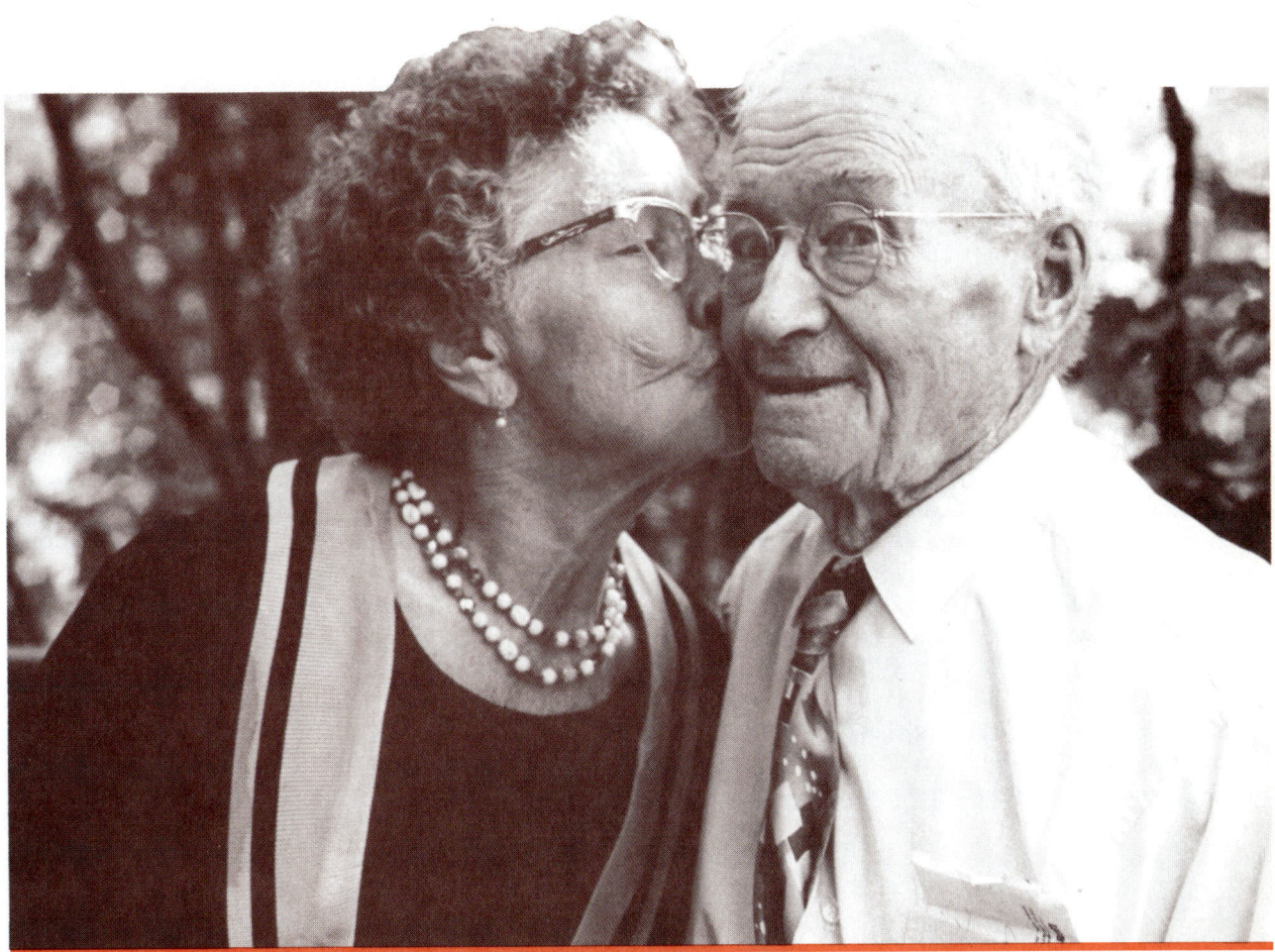

CONTENTS

OBJECTIVES

▶ Describe the physical changes that take place during late adulthood.

▶ Explain essential aspects of psychosocial changes.

▶ Describe essential aspects of cognitive changes.

▶ Explain essential aspects of moral development.

▶ Explain essential aspects of spiritual development.

▶ Identify common health concerns and hazards of older adults.

▶ Discuss nursing implications of the common health concerns and hazards identified.

LATE ADULTHOOD

Late adulthood, for the purposes of this book, is the years after 65. Sometimes it is referred to as **senescence,** or old age. Because of advances in medical and related sciences and health promotion and protection, an increasing number of people are living to an advanced age. In 1960, life expectancy at birth was about 70 years; i.e., the average person born in 1960 could expect to live about 70 years. By 1987, life expectancy had increased to 71.5 years for males and 78.3 years for females (U.S. Bureau of the Census 1989 p. 71). Because of increasing life expectancy, it may be helpful to divide late adulthood into three periods: 65–74 years, the "young-old," 75–84 years, the "middle-old"; and 85 years and older, the "old-old."

Gerontology is the study of all aspects of the aging process, including biologic, psychologic, and sociologic factors. **Nursing gerontology** refers to the scientific study of the nursing care of the elderly (Yurick, Spier, Robb, and Ebert 1989, p. 5). **Geriatrics** is the term for the medical specialty that addresses the diagnosis and treatment of the physical problems of the elderly person. Nursing care of the elderly may be called **geriatric, gerontologic,** or **gerontic** nursing. Nursing practice that focuses on the care of the elderly requires basic nursing knowledge and skills combined with specialized knowledge of the diverse needs of the aging population.

In the past decade, workers in the field of gerontology have dedicated themselves with renewed enthusiasm to answering the question "Why do we age?" According to Hayflick (1988, p. 87), little progress has been made in providing an answer to this question. Hayflick suggests that "perhaps aging simply means that we are running short on reserve capacity" (1988, p. 77). More theories about the aging process have proliferated. Table 27–1 lists some of these well-known theories. Biologic theories of aging are either intrinsic or extrinsic. **Extrinsic** theory encompasses factors in the environment; **intrinsic** theory addresses factors within the body.

Physical Changes

As the person ages, a number of physical changes occur; some are visible, some are not. See the accompanying box for a summary of the normal physiologic changes associated with aging.

Appearance   Obvious changes occur in the **integument** (skin, hair, nails) with age. A decrease in sebaceous gland activity, combined with the inability of the aged skin to retain fluid, results in dryness of the skin. Itching may increase because of dryness and the deterioration of nerve fibers and sensory endings. **Lentigo senilus** (brown "age spots") commonly appear on the hands and arms and, in some instances, on the face. These are the result of the clustering of **melanocytes** (pigment-producing cells). The skin also becomes paler and blotchy and loses its elasticity. Baldness and hair loss is thought to be due to the destruction of the tissue layer that produces hair follicles (Murray and Zentner 1989, p. 505). The loss of hair color is due to a decrease in the number of functioning pigment-producing cells. Fingernails and toenails become thickened and brittle, and in women over 60, facial hair increases.

The ways people respond to these changes vary among individuals and cultures. For example, one person may feel distinguished with gray hair, while another may feel embarrassed by it. Most women dislike their facial hair because hirsute women do not conform to the feminine cultural ideal of North Americans.

TABLE 27–1   *Biologic Theories of Aging*

Biologic Theory	Description
Genetic theory	Aging results from biochemical changes programmed into the DNA molecule in each cell.
Immunologic slow virus theory	The immune system becomes less effective with age, and viruses that have incubated in the body become able to damage body organs.
Autoimmune theory	The production of autoimmune antibodies increases, and they attack the body cells.
Cross-link theory	As cells age, chemical reactions create strong bonds, especially in collagen tissues. These bonds cause loss of elasticity, stiffness, and eventual loss of function.
Stress theory	Aging results from cellular loss due to wear and tear on the body. Regeneration of body tissues eventually cannot keep pace with wear and tear, and the body is unable to maintain a stable internal environment.
Free-radical theory	Unstable free radicals (groups of atoms) result from the oxidation of organic materials, such as carbohydrates and proteins. These radicals cause biochemical changes in the cells, and the cells cannot regenerate themselves.
Program theory	The organism is capable of a predetermined number of cell divisions, after which the cells die.

These integumentary changes accompany progressive losses of underlying adipose and muscle tissue, muscle atrophy, and loss of elastic fiber, creating a wrinkled and wasted appearance. Bony prominences become visible, a double chin develops, and lower eyelids appear puffy. In elderly women, the breasts become smaller and may sag; if large and pendulous, they may cause chafing where the skin surfaces touch. Loss of subcutaneous fat also decreases the elderly person's tolerance of cold.

Body Temperature

Body temperature is lower in the elderly adult because of a decrease in the metabolic rate. It is not uncommon for an elderly adult to have a temperature of 35 C (95 F), particularly in the early morning when the body's metabolism is low. Therefore, a temperature of 37.5 C (99.5 F) can represent a marked fever in some elderly people, although it represents only a mild fever in most young adults. It is important that the normal temperature of each individual person be known as a baseline for assessing changes.

One of the body's normal compensating reactions to a fall in heat production is the contraction of the surface blood vessels and shivering. Because elderly adults have a diminished shivering reflex and do not produce as much body heat from metabolic processes, they tolerate prolonged exposure to cold poorly. At the other extreme, the body compensates for higher temperatures by slowing down muscular activity to produce less heat and by dilating surface blood vessels and sweating to increase losses of body heat. Older people, however, often have sluggish sweating and circulatory mechanisms and therefore cannot cope with heat as well as younger people. For example, they do not tolerate working in moderately high temperatures for prolonged periods. It is therefore important for the elderly adult to have a constant, comfortable environmental temperature. Many elderly persons who feel cold in rooms with a "normal" temperature wear extra clothes.

Neuromusculoskeletal Changes

With aging there is *gradual reduction in the speed and power of skeletal or voluntary muscle contractions.* The capacity for sustained muscular effort is also decreased. Great individual differences in muscular efficiency are apparent throughout life. Exercise can strengthen weakened muscles, and up to about age 50 the skeletal muscles can increase in bulk and density. After that time, there is a steady decrease in muscle fibers, ultimately leading to the typical wasted appearance of the very old person. Thus, elderly adults often complain about their lack of strength and how quickly they tire. Activities can still be carried out, but at a slower pace. Often balance is impaired with age. Prolonged muscular efforts may be sustained by older people provided they take judicious rest pauses and avoid capacity or peak performance.

The person's **reaction time** is slowed with age because of the diminished conduction speed of nerve fibers. Reaction time can be delayed further by decreased muscle tone as a result of diminished physical activity. Elderly people compensate for this reaction difference by being exceptionally cautious, for instance, in their driving habits, which exasperate some impatient young drivers.

Slight loss in overall stature occurs with age due to atrophy of the discs between the spinal vertebrae. This can be exaggerated by muscular weakness resulting in a stooping posture and **kyphosis** (humpback of the upper spine). **Osteoporosis,** a decrease in bone density, along with increased brittleness of bone, makes the elderly adult prone to serious fractures, some of which are spontaneous. Since the incidence of osteoporosis is higher in elderly women, the effects of the menopause on the skeleton are being investigated. Causes of osteoporosis are thought to be lack of activity and inadequate calcium intake or inability to metabolize calcium.

Some degenerative joint changes occur, which make movement stiffer and more restricted. Stiffness is aggravated by inactivity; for example, if persons sit too long, their joints become stiff and they have difficulty standing and walking. A continuous program of physical activity and proper nutrition will slow bone density loss and decrease muscle atrophy and stiffness.

Cardiopulmonary Changes   **Respiratory efficiency** is reduced with age. The person inhales a smaller volume of air because of the musculoskeletal changes in the chest wall that reduce the size of the chest. There is a greater volume of residual air left in the lungs after expiration and a decreased capacity to cough efficiently because of weaker expiratory muscles. Mucous secretions tend to collect more readily in the respiratory tree because of decreased ciliary activity. Thus, susceptibility to respiratory infections is notable in elderly adults.

Dyspnea (difficult breathing) occurs frequently with increased activity, such as running for a bus or carrying heavy parcels up stairs. This dyspnea occurs in response to an oxygen debt in the muscles. Intense exercise is followed by short, heavy, rapid breathing, which is an attempt to repay this oxygen debt in the muscles. Although this response is normal, it occurs more quickly in the aged because delivery and diffusion of oxygen to tissues is often diminished by changes in both respiratory and vascular tissues.

Blood pressure measurements often indicate a significant increase in systolic and a slight increase in diastolic pressures. This is a result of the inelasticity of the systemic arteries and an increase in peripheral resistance. There are no changes with age in the heart rate at normal rest. However, the heart rate of the aged person is slow to respond to stress and slow to return to normal after periods of physical activity.

The *working capacity of the heart* is diminished with age. This is particularly evident when increased demands are made on the heart muscles, such as during periods of exercise or emotional stress. The valves of the heart tend to become harder and less pliable, resulting in reduced filling and emptying abilities. In addition, the pumping action of the heart is reduced due to changes in the coronary (cardiac) arteries, which supply progressively smaller amounts of blood to the heart muscle. These changes are evidenced by shortness of breath on exertion and pooling of blood in the systemic veins.

Changes in the *arteries* occur concurrently. The elasticity of smaller arteries is reduced by the thickening of their walls and increased calcium deposits in the muscular layer. Reduced arterial elasticity often results in diminished blood supply to, for instance, the legs and the brain, resulting in pain on exertion in the calf muscles and dizziness, respectively.

Sensory/Perceptual Changes   Changes in *vision* associated with aging include the obvious changes around the eye, such as the shrunken appearance of the eyes due to loss of orbital fat, the slowed blink reflex, and the looseness of the eyelids, particularly the lower lid, due to poorer muscle tone. Other changes result in loss of visual acuity, less power of adaptation to darkness and dim light, decrease in accommodation to near and far objects, loss of peripheral vision, and difficulty in discriminating similar colors. The degenerative changes in the eyes beginning in middle age lead to the relative inflexibility of the lens, called **presbyopia.**

As the lens of the eye ages, it becomes more opaque and less elastic. By the age of 80 all elderly people have some lens opacity (**cataracts**) that reduces visual acuity and causes glare to be a problem. Surgical removal of cataracts is common at this age. Accompanying this are changes in the ciliary muscles, which control the shape of the lens. These changes reduce the power of the lens to adjust to near and far vision. The diameter of the pupil is reduced, and the amount of light entering the eye is thereby restricted. This slows the reaction time to decreases in light or illumination, a problem compounded at night with driving. Reduced blood supply due to arteriosclerosis can diminish retinal function. Reduced peripheral vision also is thought to be a result of arteriosclerosis.

The loss of *hearing* due to senescent change is called **presbycusis.** These changes begin in middle adulthood and continue through later life. Up to 40% of those over 65 years of age and up to 90% of those over 80 are hearing impaired (Lichtenstein, Bess, and Logan 1988, pp. 2875–78). Presbycusis comes about through changes in the structure of the inner ear: changes in nerve tissues in the inner ear and a thickening of the eardrum. Gradual loss of hearing is more common among men than women, perhaps because men are more frequently in noisy work environments. Hearing loss is usually greater in the left ear than the right and greater in the higher frequencies than the lower. Thus, older adults with hearing loss usually hear speakers with low, distinct voices best. Older adults may have more difficulty compensating for hearing loss than the young, who pay closer attention to the lip movements of the speaker.

Older persons have a poorer sense of *taste and smell* and are less stimulated by food than the young. The number of taste buds in the tongue decreases, and the olfactory bulb (responsible for smell perception) at the base of the brain atrophies.

Loss of skin receptors takes place gradually, producing an increased threshold for *sensations of pain and touch.* The elderly person may not be able to distinguish hot from cold or the intensity of heat. Stimuli causing severe pain in a younger person may cause only minor sensation or pressure in the elderly.

Changes in Digestion   The digestive system is significantly less impaired by aging than are other body systems. Gradual decreases in digestive enzymes occur; examples are ptyalin in salivary secretions, which converts starch; pepsin and trypsin, which digest protein; and lipase, a fat-splitting enzyme.

There is also a decrease in the number of absorbing cells in the intestinal tract and a rise in gastric pH. These factors lower the absorption rate, slowing the absorption of nutrients and drugs. The muscle tone of the intestines also decreases, causing a decrease in peristalsis and elimination. These changes in muscle tone, digestive juices, and intestinal activity may lead to **indigestion** and **constipation** in the older adult.

Changes in Urinary Elimination

The excretory function of the kidney diminishes with age, but usually not significantly below normal levels unless a disease process intervenes. Blood flow can be reduced by arteriosclerotic changes, impairing renal function. With age, the number of functioning nephrons (the basic functional units of the kidney) decreases to some degree, thus impairing the kidney's filtering abilities.

More noticeable changes are those related to the bladder. Complaints of **urinary urgency** and **frequency** are common. In men, these changes are often due to an enlarged prostate gland and in women to weakened muscles supporting the bladder or weakness of the urethral sphincter. The capacity of the bladder and its ability to empty completely diminish with age. This explains the need for elderly adults to arise during the night to void (**nocturnal frequency**) and the **retention** of residual urine, predisposing the elderly adult to bladder infections.

Changes in Sexual Activity and Reproductive Organs

Sexual drives persist into the seventies, eighties, and nineties, provided that health is good and an interested partner is available. Interest in sexual activity in old age depends, in large measure, on interest in sexual activity earlier in life (Thienhaus 1988, p. 63). That is, people who are active in young and middle adulthood will remain active during their later years. However, sexual activity does become less frequent. Many factors may play a role in the ability of the elderly person to engage in sexual activity. For example, society does not look favorably on sexual feelings in the elderly. Physical problems such as diabetes, arthritis, and heart and respiratory conditions may also affect the elderly person's energy or physical ability to participate in sexual activity. In addition, several medications are known to impair sexual ability in men.

Degenerative changes in the gonads are very gradual in men. The testes can produce sperm well into old age, although there is a gradual decrease in the number of sperm produced. In women, the degenerative changes in the ovaries are noticed by the abrupt cessation of menses in middle age, during the menopause.

Changes in the gonads of elderly women result from diminished secretion of the ovarian hormones. Some changes, such as the shrinking of the uterus and ovaries, go unnoticed. Other changes are obvious. The breasts atrophy, and lubricating vaginal secretions are reduced. Reduced natural lubrication is the cause of painful intercourse, which often necessitates the use of lubricating jellies.

Psychosocial Development

A number of theories explain psychosocial aging. According to **disengagement theory,** aging involves mutual withdrawal (disengagement) between the older person and others in the elderly person's environment. This withdrawal relieves the elderly person of some of society's pressures and gradually reduces the number of people with whom the elderly person interacts. According to **activity theory,** the best way to age is to stay active physically and mentally, and according to **continuity theory,** people maintain their values, habits, and behavior in old age. A person who is accustomed to having people around will continue to do so, and the person who prefers not to be involved with others will more likely disengage. This theory accounts for the great variety of behavior seen in elderly people.

According to Erikson, the developmental task at this time is *ego integrity versus self-despair.* See Table 24–5 on page 588. People who attain ego integrity view life with a sense of wholeness and derive satisfaction from past accomplishments. They view death as an acceptable completion of life. According to Erikson, people who develop integrity accept "one's one and only life cycle" (Erikson 1963, p. 263). By contrast, people who despair often believe they have made poor choices during life and wish they could live life over. Robert Butler sees integrity as bringing serenity and wisdom, and despair as resulting in the inability to accept one's fate. Despair gives rise to feelings of frustration, discouragement, and a sense that one's life has been worthless (Butler 1963, p. 65).

Acknowledging that the "young-old" and the "old-old" differ not only in physical characteristics but also in psychosocial responses, many people have difficulty with Erikson's singular developmental task. Peck (1968) proposes three developmental tasks of the older adult in contrast to Erikson's task of ego integrity versus despair. See Chapter 24, page 590. Kart, Metress, and Metress (1978, p. 180) further clarify these three tasks and suggest how they should be achieved. First, elderly people must establish new activities so that the loss of accustomed roles is less keenly felt. Second, they must select activities compatible with the physical limitations of old age. Third, individuals may make contributions that extend beyond their own lifetimes, thereby providing a meaning for life.

Retirement

Today, a majority of the people over 65 are unemployed. Most industries and professions make retirement mandatory, although this policy is currently being questioned. Some who are self-employed continue to work as long as they are healthy. Work offers these people a better income, a sense of self-worth, and the chance to continue long-established routines. Some need to work for economic reasons.

Retirement can be a time when projects or recreational activities deferred for a long time can be pursued. Retired people are no longer governed by an alarm clock and can get up when they please. The enjoyment of staying up later is another luxury. Few elderly people, however, spend much time resting or sleeping. Being accustomed to activity most

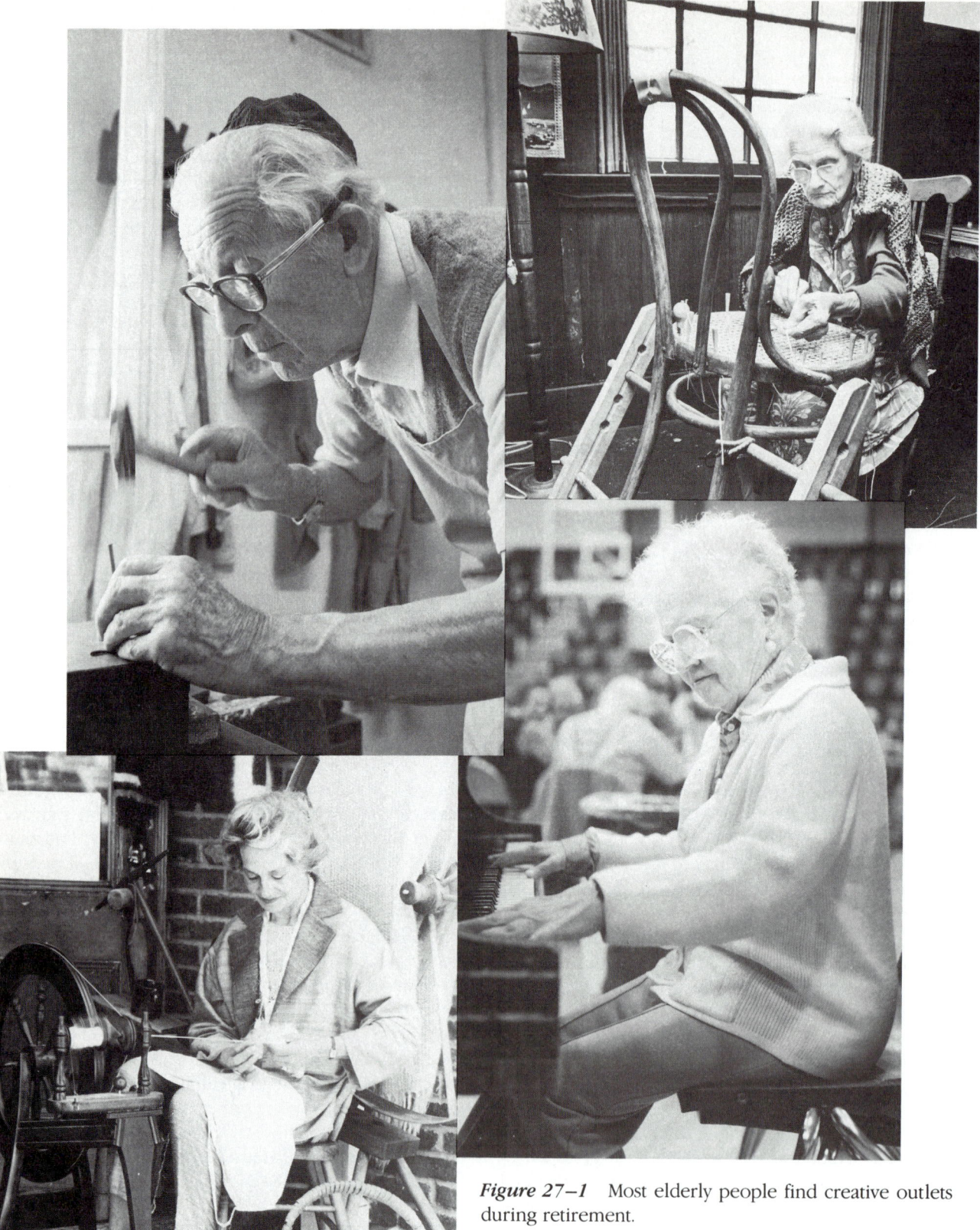

Figure 27–1 Most elderly people find creative outlets during retirement.

of their lives, most elderly find many outlets, jobs, community projects, volunteer services, intellectual or recreational pursuits, or hobbies such as stamp collecting or fishing. Travel opportunities are expanding.

The life-style of later years is to a large degree formulated in youth. This fact was recognized by Robert Browning: "Grow old along with me! / The best is yet to be, / The last of life, for which the first was made." People who attempt suddenly to refocus and enrich their lives at retirement usually have difficulty. Those who learned early in life to live well-balanced and fulfilling lives are generally more successful in retirement. The woman who has been concerned only with the accomplishments of her children or the man who has been concerned only with the paycheck and his job status can be left with a feeling of emptiness when children leave and the job no longer exists. The later years can foster a sense of integrity and continuity, or they can be years of despair.

Economic Change
The financial needs of elderly people vary considerably. Though most need less money for clothing, entertainment, and work, and although some own their homes outright, costs continue to rise, making it difficult for some to manage. Food and medical costs alone are often a financial burden. When older people speak about their greatest need, often it is not happiness or health, but money. Money allows them to be independent and look after themselves.

Problems with income are often related to low retirement benefits, lack of pension plans for many workers, and the increased length of the retirement years. Elderly members of minority groups have greater financial problems than elderly whites. Elderly women of all ages have lower incomes than men, and the oldest women are the poorest. Women, as a group, receive less from pensions, less from income, and less from government sources (Yurick, Spier, Robb, and Ebert 1989, p. 304–5).

Nurses should be aware of the costs of health care. For example, while assisting a client to plan a diet, the nurse must consider which foods the client can afford to buy. The nurse or the client can request the physician to order lower-priced medications. In addition, the supplies used in a client's care should be as economical as possible.

Relocation
During late adulthood, many people experience relocation. A variety of factors may lead to this decision. The house or apartment may be too large or too expensive. The work involved in maintaining the house may become burdensome or impossible for the aged person or couple. Some elderly persons with decreased mobility want living arrangements that are all on one floor or need more accessible bathroom facilities.

Making the decision to move is often a very stressful one. The elderly person may be moving to an apartment, which may mean leaving the comfort of the family home and the neighbors and friends of several decades. Some need to move nearer to their children for general support and supervision. For many, this decision is difficult and stressful. For others, relocation is voluntary. The person may be seeking a more moderate climate with better recreational facilities geared to a more leisurely life-style. Adjustment will be much easier for the elderly person making a voluntary move.

A small percentage of the elderly, between 5% and 7%, must relocate to long-term care facilities or nursing homes. The decision to enter a nursing home is frequently made when elderly persons can no longer care for themselves, often because of problems of mobility and memory impairment. An increasing number of nursing home residents are in the very old age group (85 years and over), and most are women (Fulmer 1988, p. 544).

The facilities in nursing homes differ in many ways and offer varying degrees of independence to the residents. All provide meals but vary in giving other services, such as assistance with hygiene and dressing, physical therapy or exercise, recreational activities, transportation services, and medical and nursing supervision.

Nurses in hospitals should find out whether a client is being discharged to a nursing home or to home. Many nursing homes provide nursing services to clients and require appropriate information to provide for continuity of care. Clients returning home, however, may require the assistance of a home care nurse.

Facing Death and Grieving
Well-adjusted aging couples usually thrive on companionship. Many couples rely increasingly on their mates for this company and may have few outside friends. Great bonds of affection and closeness can develop during this period of aging together and nurturing each other. When a mate dies, the remaining partner inevitably experiences feelings of loss, emptiness, and loneliness. Many are capable and manage to live alone; however, reliance on younger family members increases as age advances and ill health occurs. Some widows and widowers remarry, particularly the latter, because widowers are less inclined than widows to maintain a household.

Women face bereavement and solitude more often than men, since women usually live longer. The brevity of life is constantly reinforced by the death of friends. It is a time when one's life is reviewed with happiness or regret. Feelings of serenity or guilt and inadequacy can arise. Independence established prior to loss of a mate makes this adjustment period easier. A person who has some meaningful friendships, economic security, ongoing interests in the community, or private hobbies and a peaceful philosophy of life copes more easily with bereavement. Successful relationships with children and grandchildren are also of inestimable value. Facing death is discussed in Chapter 34.

Nurses can sometimes help clients who are alone a great deal to adjust their living arrangements or life-style so that they have more companionship. Moving to a retirement home that has other people in similar circumstances and organized social activities is one example. Many communities provide social centers for the elderly, for example, drop-in centers or community centers that offer day trips for seniors. Nurses can refer clients to services and encourage them to obtain companionship.

Cognitive Development

Piaget's phases of cognitive development end with the formal operations phase. However, considerable research on cognitive abilities and aging is currently being conducted. Researchers generally believe that there is minimal change in intellectual capacity of the healthy aging person (Murray and Zentner 1989, p. 519).

Intellectual capacity includes perception, cognitive agility, memory, and learning. **Perception,** or the ability to interpret the environment, depends on the acuteness of the senses. If the aging person's senses are impaired, the ability to perceive the environment and react appropriately is diminished. Perceptual capacity may be affected by changes in the nervous system as well. Cognitive ability, or the ability to know, is related to perceptual ability. An older man, for example, may know that he will be retiring next year but be unable to plan for retirement. He cannot accept the knowledge psychologically because his work provides his sense of worth, self-esteem, and identity.

Changes in cognitive structures occur as a person ages. It is believed that there is progressive loss of neurons. In addition, blood flow to the brain decreases, the meninges appear to thicken, and brain metabolism slows. Experts do not agree whether the brain decreases in weight with age, although it is thought that the brain loses about 7% of its mass by 80 years of age (Murray and Zentner 1989, p. 505). As yet, little is known about the effect of these physical changes on the cognitive functioning of the older adult. Neurofibrillary tangles have also been found in the hippocampal cortex, the area of the brain concerned with memory. A **neurofibrillary tangle** is an abnormal mass of fibrillar material found in the cytoplasm. Neuritic plaques are also found in the aging brain. A **neuritic plaque** is a structure composed of amyloid material surrounded by abnormal neural structures. Neurofibrillary tangles and neuritic plaques could account for some of the functional changes found in normal aging people.

Memory, or the ability to retain information, is also a component of intellectual capacity and is closely related to learning. The three-stage memory model divides memory into the sensory, primary, and secondary stages. **Sensory memory** is the momentary perception of stimuli by the senses. Information from the senses is then stored temporarily in the memory stores (e.g., visual information is stored in visual memory). Some of this information is then passed into primary memory. **Primary memory,** or short-term memory, is what one has in mind at a given moment. For information to be retained, it must enter secondary mem-

ory. **Secondary memory,** or long-term memory, contains all the information one knows, from minutes to years.

Research regarding the effects of aging on human memory has been carried out over the last several decades. These studies generally agree that despite age-related changes in the sensory organs, visual or auditory memory does not substantially decline with age (Ciocon and Potter 1988, p. 43). It is believed, however, that the elderly are able to remember information better when it is presented visually. Primary memory, which includes the ability both to retain and to retrieve information, is also considered to remain substantially unchanged with age. Secondary memory, however, is reported to decline with age. Older people have some impairment in their ability to enter new information into secondary memory; once it has been entered into secondary memory, moreover, they have some difficulty in bringing the information out of memory stores [Ciocon and Potter 1988, p. 45).

Older people need additional time for learning, largely because of the problem of retrieving information. Motivation is also important. Older adults have more difficulty than younger ones in learning information they do not consider meaningful. It is suggested that the older person remain mentally active to maintain cognitive ability at the highest possible level. Lifelong mental activity, particularly verbal activity, helps the older person retain a high level of cognitive function and may help maintain long-term memory. Cognitive impairment that interferes with normal life is not considered part of normal aging. A decline in intellectual abilities that interferes with social or occupational functions should always be regarded as abnormal. Family members should be advised to seek prompt medical evaluation.

Dementia
Dementia is a decline in memory and other cognitive abilities, in comparison to the individual's performance in the past. The onset of dementia is slow and is often denied or hidden by the client and family members. Some dementias, such as those caused by depression, infection, or thyroid disturbance, are reversible if treated promptly. The return of cognitive function for the person with a reversible dementia depends on prompt diagnosis and treatment. The large majority of older persons diagnosed with dementia will be found to have irreversible brain disease. The most common type of irreversible dementia in old age is *Alzheimer's disease* (AD), which accounts for 60% to 70% of all the cases. Other common types include multi-infarct dementia (10%), caused by repeated strokes, and Parkinson's disease (5%) (Rowe and Besdine 1988, pp. 377–81).

Dementia is recognized as a major public health problem in the United States, affecting approximately 5% of the population from 65 to 74 years of age, and more than 30% of those over age 80. Of the elderly residing in the community, 10% experience intellectual impairment; in the nursing home population, between 50% and 75% of the clients are affected with cognitive impairment that is thought to be dementia of the Alzheimer type (Rowe and Besdine 1988, pp. 377–81).

Alzheimer's disease affects about 3 million people in the United States. By the year 2030, that number is expected to rise to nearly 5 million. The monetary cost of care for AD clients is estimated at $30 billion annually in the United States. The symptoms of AD have been grouped into three or four stages and may vary somewhat from client to client. The most prominent symptoms are cognitive dysfunctions, including decline in memory, learning, attention, judgment, orientation, and language skills. The symptoms are progressive, and all victims experience a steady decline in cognitive and physical abilities, lasting between 7 and 15 years and ending in death. In the last stage, the client requires total assistance, is unable to communicate, is incontinent, and may be unable to walk.

Although several theories are being investigated, the cause of AD is not known. Some of the causative theories include accumulation of aluminum deposits in the neurons, changes in the immune system, active and latent viruses, and defects in the neurotransmitter system. Currently, definite diagnosis can be made only on autopsy, where the physical changes specific to AD can be validated. Scanning techniques, such as PET (positron emission tomography) and MRI (magnetic resonance imaging) are currently aiding physicians in following the clinical progression of AD. Recently, a protein designated A68 has been detected in the brain of AD victims and from the spinal fluid of AD clients. In addition, A68 is also associated with neurofibrillary tangles. If the results of further studies on A68 support these initial findings, a routine laboratory test could be developed that makes early and accurate diagnosis of AD possible.

There is no cure or specific treatment for AD. Several drugs have been developed, but none has been shown consistently to retard or reverse the progression of the disease. It is hoped that one experimental drug, tetrahydroaminocridine (THA), will allow the brain cells to function more efficiently, thereby improving cognitive function. Research is currently under way.

It is estimated that about one million people with AD are cared for in the home. The burden of care is frequently on women—wives and daughters—who are themselves aging. It has frequently been observed that "Alzheimer's causes more damage to the family than any other disease" (Burggraf and Stanley 1989, pp. 332–33). The nurse's responsibility is to provide supportive nursing care, accurate information, and referral assistance, if placement in a nursing care facility becomes necessary.

Moral Development

According to Kohlberg, moral development is completed in the early adult years. Most old people stay at Kohlberg's conventional level of moral development (see Table 24–8 on page 594), and some are at the preconventional level.

An elderly person at the preconventional level obeys rules to avoid pain and the displeasure of others. At stage 1, a person defines good and bad in relation to self, whereas older persons at stage 2 may act to meet another's needs as well as their own. Elderly people at the conventional level follow society's rules of conduct in response to the expectations of others. They value conformity, loyalty, and social order (Edelman and Mandle 1986, p. 548).

Rybash, Roodin, and Hoyer studied the kinds of moral problems elderly people face. These researchers found that the moral concerns of the elderly are more interpersonal than social or legalistic. For example, an elderly man is more likely to be concerned with the moral problems involving a member of his family than with the moral problems posed by his occupation or a friend's extramarital affair (Rybash, Roodin, and Hoyer 1983, p. 253).

Spiritual Development

Murray and Zentner (1989, p. 525) write that the elderly person with a mature religious outlook strives to incorporate views of theology and religious action into thinking. Elderly people can contemplate new religious and philosophical views and try to understand ideas missed previously or interpreted differently. The elderly person also derives a sense of worth by sharing experiences or views. In contrast, the elderly person who has not matured spiritually may feel impoverishment or despair as the drive for economic and professional success wanes.

The older person's knowledge becomes wisdom, an inner resource for dealing with both positive and negative life experiences. Many elderly persons have strong religious convictions and continue to attend church services. Involvement in religion often helps the elderly person to resolve issues related to the meaning of life, to adversity, or to good fortune (Yurick, Spier, Robb, and Ebert 1989, p. 207). The "old-old" person who cannot attend formal services often continues religious participation in a more private manner. Many elderly persons watch television evangelists and some, being vulnerable to fund raising ventures, send money that they can ill afford to spare to these organizations.

According to Fowler and Keen (1985), some people enter the sixth stage of spiritual development, *universalizing*. See Table 24–9 on page 597. People whose spiritual development reaches this level think and act in a way that exemplifies love and justice.

HEALTH PROMOTION AND PROTECTION

Guidelines for assessment of growth and development of the older adult are shown in the box on the following page. Assessment activities may include measurement of weight,

ASSESSMENT GUIDELINES
The Older Adult

Does the older adult:

- Adjust to the physiologic changes related to aging?

- Manage retirement years in a satisfying manner?

- Have satisfactory living arrangements and income to meet changing needs?

- Participate in social and leisure activities?

- Have a social network of friends and support persons?

- View life as worthwhile?

- Have high self-esteem?

- Have the abilities to care for self or to secure appropriate help?

- Gain support from value system or spiritual philosophy?

- Adapt life-style to diminishing energy and ability?

- Accept and adjust to the death of significant others?

TABLE 27–2 *Examples of Nursing Diagnoses and Goals for Older Adults*

	Diagnosis	Goal
Wellness diagnosis	**Adequate accident prevention** related to awareness of home safety	During the next year, the older adult continues to maintain a safe home environment
NANDA diagnoses	**Social isolation** related to inadequate individual resources	The older adult expands personal resources within three months.
	Spiritual distress related to relocation and inability to attend religious services	The older adult regains adequate spiritual support.

height, and vital signs (see Chapter 18); observation of the skin for hydration status or presence of lesions; examination of visual acuity using the Snellen chart; examination of hearing acuity using the whisper, Weber, and Rinne tests (see Chapter 19) and questions about the following:

- Usual dietary pattern

- Any problems with bowel or urinary elimination

- Activity/exercise and sleep/rest patterns

- Family and social activities and interests

- Any problems with reading, writing, or problem solving

- Adjustment to retirement or loss of partner

Examples of wellness diagnoses (see Chapter 23) and NANDA nursing diagnoses for the older adult are shown in Table 27–2. *Outcome criteria* also need to be developed. The following are examples of criteria for the NANDA diagnosis **Social isolation** in Table 27–2:

- Within 1 week, the older adult lists five interests or activities.

- Within 3 weeks, the older adult agrees on two activities that the person can pursue in the community.

- Within 1 month, the older adult pursues one activity per week.

- Within 3 months, the older adult establishes weekly community interests.

According to recent research, much of the decline in health that was previously considered to be due to "old age" is due to chronic illnesses resulting from unhealthy life-styles and poor health habits rather than aging itself (Smith 1988, p. 48). To retard the aging process, the older person must learn self-care techniques related to health promotion and disease prevention. Studies indicate that older persons are concerned about their health and are interested in information and behavioral strategies directed toward improving it (Smith 1988, p. 48). To assist the older adult in promoting health, the nurse may wish to discuss some or all of the following topics.

Health Maintenance Visits and Immunization The older adult should have routine health assessments that may involve a yearly physical examination including a urinalysis and stool test for occult blood, yearly visual examination, audiometry if hearing ability is at risk, yearly dental assessment, yearly mammogram, Pap test every year if in high-risk group or every 3 years if not, and yearly testicular and prostate examination. Some physicians may also recommend a sigmoidoscopy every 5 years and certain blood tests (e.g., blood lipids) on a regular basis.

The older adult should receive a diphtheria and tetanus booster every 10 years; for those at risk for hepatitis, hepatitis B vaccine is also recommended. Clients with a history of chronic respiratory or cardiac disease are usually encouraged to receive immunizations against pneumococcal pneumonia and influenza.

Safety Accident prevention is a major concern for elderly people. Because vision is limited, reflexes are slowed, and bones are brittle, climbing stairs, driving a car, and even walking require caution. Driving, particularly night driving, requires caution because accommodation of the eye to light is impaired and peripheral vision is diminished. Older persons need to learn to turn the head before changing lanes and should not rely on side vision, for example, when crossing a street. Driving in fog or other hazardous conditions should be avoided.

Fires are a hazard for the elderly person with a failing memory. The older person may forget that the iron or stove is left on or may not extinguish a cigarette completely. Because of reduced sensitivity to pain and heat, care must be taken to prevent burns when the person bathes or uses heating devices.

Many elderly persons suffer and die each year from hypothermia. **Hypothermia** is a body temperature below normal. A lowered metabolism and loss of normal insulation from thinning subcutaneous tissue decrease the elderly client's ability to retain heat. Health promotion should focus on teaching the elderly client to

- Dress warmly with layered clothing and protect head and hands when going outdoors in cold weather
- Use extra blankets at night and keep feet warm with woolen socks, which are safer than hot-water bottles.
- Eat a balanced diet, including high-energy foods such as fats and carbohydrates
- Learn to monitor the household thermostat and be sure that adequate home heating fuel is available

Because older clients who take analgesics or sedatives may become lethargic or confused, they should be monitored regularly and closely. Other measures to induce sleep should be used whenever possible. Nurses can help elderly clients make the home environment safe. Specific hazards can be identified and corrected; e.g., hand rails can be installed on staircases. The nurse teaches the importance of taking only prescribed medications and contacting a health professional at the first indication of intolerance to them.

Guidelines for accident prevention for the older adult are detailed in the box on the following page.

Nutrition   The older adult requires the same basic nutrition as the younger adult. However, fewer calories are needed by the older adult because of the lower metabolic rate and the decrease in physical activity. The older adult should consume about 1200 calories per day. This figure may vary for each person according to the level of individual activity.

A major problem of the elderly is tooth decay and the loss of teeth due to poor dental care or changes in gingival tissue. Poorly fitting dentures may also be a concern. These factors coupled with a decrease in salivation may cause difficulty in chewing and limit the type of food the older person can eat. As a result, the older person may avoid foods that require extensive chewing, such as meats or fresh fruits, and nutritional deficiencies may result.

A decrease in the thirst sensation, combined with a self-imposed limitation of fluids to compensate for incontinence, may result in an inadequate intake of fluids in elderly clients. The nurse should instruct the older adult that about 8 glasses of water a day is needed to maintain kidney function, soften stools, prevent dehydration, and moisturize skin.

Common problems related to diet include undernutrition and overnutrition. **Undernutrition** may result from a variety of physical and psychosocial factors. The elderly client may be eating empty calories rather than nutritious food, eating alone, or suffering from chronic diseases that affect food intake and metabolism, such as malignant disorders, alcoholism, or depression. Elderly clients frequently have dietary deficiencies of vitamins A, B, and C and iron. In the United States, 40% of the people over 60 years of age suffer from iron deficiency anemia from insufficient iron intake and poor absorption and utilization of iron (Schuster and Ashburn 1986, p. 808). The nurse should assess the dietary habits of the elderly client and ascertain that intake of foods rich in these vitamins is adequate (see Chapter 39 for appropriate food sources).

Decreased exposure to sunlight and changes in the intestines and liver that interfere with metabolism are thought to contribute to vitamin D deficiency and bone disorders. **Osteomalacia** is marked by "softening of the bones," which become bent and deformed. **Osteoporosis** causes bones to become porous and less dense, resulting in an increased susceptibility to fracture and collapse (Andreasen and Conley 1987, p. 176). To prevent these problems, the nurse must take special care to ensure that older adults ingest sufficient amounts of vitamin D and calcium. Outdoor activities should also be encouraged to increase exposure to sunlight, a natural source of vitamin D, as well as to enhance overall well-being.

Overnutrition may result from lifelong eating patterns coupled with a lack of exercise. Retirement from work or problems with mobility due to chronic disease may also compound the problem. Other reasons cited for overeating include past habits, occupation, anxiety or nervousness, difficult life situations, mental illness, glandular imbalance, and grief or loss (Saxon and Etten 1987, pp. 195–96). Overeating may lead to chronic illness such as heart disease, high blood pressure, arteriosclerosis, and diabetes.

Guidelines for promoting nutritional health of older adults include the following:

- Encourage regular visits to the dentist to have dentures repaired or replaced to ensure chewing ability.
- Advise having several small meals per day and smaller portions of all foods.
- Encourage use of leaner cuts of meat and broiling or baking foods instead of frying them.
- Advise substituting fruit for rich pastry and using low-fat milk and cheese.
- Encourage the client to take an interest in food preparation and serving for themselves or their spouses.

Preventing falls:

- Make sure all rooms, hallways, and stairwells are adequately lit.
- Have an easily accessible light switch next to the bed.
- Leave a night light on in the hallway or bathroom.
- Get out of bed slowly, i.e., sit before standing and stand briefly before walking, to prevent dizziness from orthostatic hypotension.
- Install grab bars in the bathroom near the toilet and tub.
- Make sure rugs and carpets are firmly attached to floors and stairs.
- Make sure that electrical cords are secured against baseboards to prevent tripping.
- Keep indoor and outdoor walkways and stairs in good repair.
- Install sturdy slip-resistant hand railings along stairs.

Preventing burns:

- Check the temperature of bath water and heating pads. Run cold water before hot water.
- Lower thermostats of water heaters to provide warm rather than very hot water.
- Avoid smoking in bed or when sleepy.
- Install smoke alarms.
- Place a hand fire extinguisher in a convenient area of the home, e.g., the kitchen.
- Smother kitchen grease fires with a large lid or baking soda.
- Avoid wearing loose-fitting clothing when cooking.
- Do not overload electric circuits and keep electrical appliances in good repair.
- Keep passageways to outside doors unobstructed.

Preventing pedestrian accidents:

- Wear reflective or light-colored clothing at night.

- Cross streets at intersections with cross walks and traffic lights when possible; do not cross major streets in the middle of the block.
- Be sure to look both ways before stepping from the curb.

Preventing automobile accidents:

- Have regular eye examinations to assess vision, acquire appropriate refractive corrections, and detect other problems early.
- Wear good-quality gray or green sunglasses during daytime driving to reduce glare.
- Keep car windows clean and windshield wipers in good condition.
- Place mirrors on both sides of the car and always check rearview and side mirrors before changing lanes.
- Always look behind your vehicle for people or obstacles before backing up.
- Avoid smoking when driving, especially at night. Smoke can reduce visibility.
- Follow your physician's restrictions, if any, about when and where to drive.
- Learn the effects of prescribed medications on driving ability.
- Do not drink and drive.
- Stop periodically to stretch your muscles and rest your eyes.
- Leave car windows partially open and set the radio and fans low so that you can hear sirens and horns.
- Have your ability to drive periodically reevaluated.
- Keep your automobile in good repair and keep headlights, tail lights, and turn signals clean so they are visible to others.

- Review diet restrictions, and find ways to make meals appealing within these guidelines.
- Discuss the food budget of the elderly client, and suggest more economical and nutritious choices, if appropriate.
- If food preparation is not possible for the older client, suggest community resources such as Meals on Wheels.

Elimination   **Constipation** is a common problem in the elderly population. Many elderly believe that "regular-

ity" means a bowel movement every day. Those who do not meet this criterion often seek over-the-counter preparations to relieve what they believe to be constipation. Elderly clients should be advised that normal patterns of bowel elimination vary considerably. Normal for some may be every other day, for others twice a day. Adequate roughage in the diet, adequate exercise, and 6 to 8 glasses of fluid daily are essential preventive measures for constipation. A cup of hot water or tea at a regular time in the morning is helpful for some. Responding to the gastrocolic reflex is also an important consideration.

The older adult should be warned that consistent use of over-the-counter preparations is thought to cause rather than cure constipation. In a few cases, moreover, they can cause serious problems such as appendicitis. Laxatives may also interfere with the body's electrolyte balance and decrease the absorption of certain vitamins. The reasons for constipation can range from life-style habits to serious malignant disorders. The nurse should evaluate any complaints of constipation carefully for each individual. A change in bowel habits over several weeks with or without weight loss, pain, or fever should be referred to a physician for a complete medical evaluation.

A decline in bladder capacity, plus weaker muscle tone, results in an increase in frequency as well as urgency in many older persons. The nurse should be aware of these changes and teach the elderly person appropriate strategies to prevent embarrassment due to incontinence. Toilet facilities should be accessible, and elderly persons should be instructed to give themselves enough time to get to the bathroom and remove their clothing. Bladder training exercises (see Chapter 43) as well as a regular toilet schedule may also be helpful adjuncts.

Many older people learn to deal with nocturnal frequency by restricting their fluid intake in the latter part of the evening, particularly those fluids that stimulate voiding, such as coffee or alcohol. Eventually most men require prostatic surgery to relieve increasing urinary frequency throughout the day, and some women require vaginal surgery for cystoceles or rectoceles. A **cystocele** is a protrusion of the urinary bladder through the vaginal wall. A **rectocele** is the protrusion of part of the rectum through the vaginal wall. Both of these conditions produce pressure and reduce bladder capacity, thereby creating urinary urgency and frequency.

Weakness in muscle tone in the ureters and bladder also increases the elderly person's risk for urinary tract infections (UTI). Preventive measures, such as increasing fluid intake, including juices that produce an acid ash such as cranberry juice, and preventing contamination of the urinary tract should be included in the teaching plan. Elderly clients should seek medical evaluation for any of the symptoms of UTI (e.g., burning on urination, frequency, and sometimes fever).

Activity and Exercise   A regular program of moderate exercise is recommended for elderly adults. Walking, golfing, gardening, bowling, and bicycling are common activities. These can be performed at a leisurely pace. It is important that exercise not be too strenuous and that rest periods be taken as needed. Rapid breathing and accelerated heartbeat should disappear within a few minutes after exercise; exercise should refresh rather than fatigue. People who are too disabled to engage in active exercise can

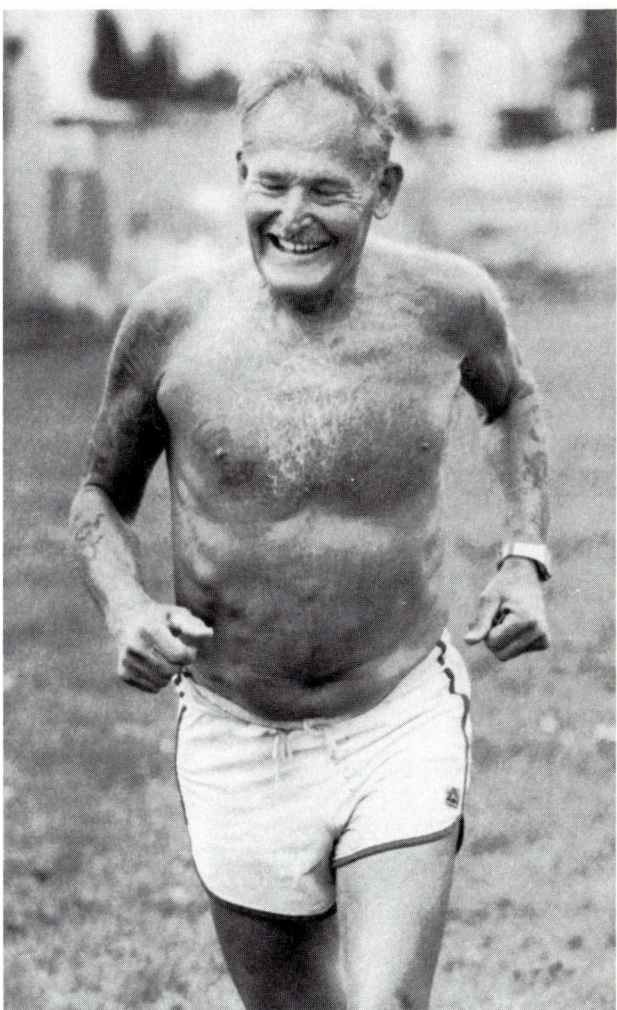

Figure 27–2   A regular program of exercise is important for maintenance of joint mobility and muscle tone.

implement a program of isometric exercises to maintain joint mobility and muscle tone.

Perhaps the most significant physical benefit of regular exercise for the older adult is a decrease in the risk for cardiovascular disease. In addition, exercise maintains bone calcification, helps to maintain muscle tone throughout the body, and reduces muscle tension and muscle pain.

The nurse should suggest some safety precautions for the elderly client beginning an exercise program. These include (1) wearing proper shoes with nonstick soles; (2) avoiding slick surfaces; (3) exercising or walking in safe, well-lighted areas; (4) being aware of adverse symptoms of exercise, such as dizziness, shortness of breath, or irregular heartbeat; and (5) beginning any exercise program slowly to allow the body time to adjust. See Tables 26–7 and 26–8 on page 654 for suggested preparations for exercise and target and maximum heart rates by age. Some physicians may recommend an exercise **stress test** to determine the type and intensity of exercise program that is best for the

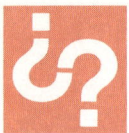

RESEARCH NOTE

Does Walking Reduce Fatigue?

The researchers involved in this study wanted to determine whether a short outdoor walk would be beneficial to the ambulatory nursing home resident. Although the answer would at first seem obvious, the authors found that some ambulatory elderly individuals living in nursing homes walk less frequently than their counterparts of comparable age and health status living in retirement villages. In fact, an alarming 81% of the sample surveyed reported that they had never walked outside. Most of the nursing home residents who went outside sat in rockers on the porch.

Thirty-two ambulatory and mentally alert individuals 60 to 93 years of age participated in the study. Subjects in Group A (16 patients) were residents of a nursing home. Group B comprised 16 individuals of similar age and health state residing in a retirement village nearby. Within each group, some subjects were assigned a walking protocol, while others simply continued their normal routines.

The findings revealed several significant differences between the groups. The nursing home residents who participated in the walking regimen reported significantly lower fatigue scores at the end of three weeks. The nursing home residents in the nonwalking group actually reported an increased feeling of fatigue. The fatigue scores of the walking and nonwalking groups at the retirement village were not very different, since daily outdoor walking was already a part of their usual routine.

The researchers acknowledge that the sample size was small. Yet, they feel it is conclusive that the nursing home residents who participated in the three-week walking regimen felt significantly less fatigued than both their counterparts in the retirement village and those in the groups that did not walk.

Implications: When health status and safety conditions permit, regular outdoor walking should be instituted as a standard intervention for all nursing home residents who are ambulatory, even if walkers or canes are necessary.

S. H. Gueldner and J. Spradley. Outdoor walking lowers fatigue, *Journal of Gerontological Nursing,* October 1988, 14:6–12.

individual client. During a stress test, blood pressure and heart rhythm are continuously monitored while the client exercises, either on a treadmill or on a bicycle.

Rest and Sleep

The aging process affects the length of sleep, distribution of sleep throughout a 24-hour period, and the sleep stage patterns (Schuster and Ashburn 1986, p. 510). Elderly adults tend to take somewhat longer to get to sleep, wake up frequently during the night, stay in bed longer to make up for missed sleep, and wake up feeling tired. The amount of deep sleep (Stage IV), as well as REM sleep, also decreases, compounding feelings of fatigue. The amount of sleep needed by the elderly client varies. In general, most healthy older adults require about the same amount of sleep as they did during the middle adult years. Measures to promote rest are discussed in Chapter 37. Moderate exercise often helps the client to sleep at night.

Maintaining Independence and Self-Esteem

Most elderly people thrive on independence. It is important to them to be able to look after themselves even if they have to struggle to do so. Although it may be difficult for younger family members to watch the elder completing tasks in a slow, determined way, aging persons need this sense of accomplishment. Children might notice that the aging father or mother with failing vision cannot keep the kitchen as clean as before. The aging father and mother may be slower and less meticulous in carpentry tasks or gardening. To maintain the elderly adult's sense of self-respect, nurses and family members need to encourage them to do as much as possible for themselves, provided that safety is maintained. Many young people err in thinking that they are helpful to older people when they take over for them and do the job much faster and more efficiently. See Figure 27–3.

Aging people need to be recognized for their unique individual characteristics. It can be difficult to recognize these differences, since elderly people have less energy than the young to show how they are different. Perhaps this is one reason elderly people tend to talk about past accomplishments, jobs, deeds, and experiences.

Nurses need to acknowledge the elderly client's ability to think, reason, and make decisions. Most elderly people are willing to listen to suggestions and advice, but they do not want to be ordered around. The nurse can support a decision by an elderly client even if eventually the decision is reversed because of failing health.

Older people appreciate thoughtfulness, consideration, and acceptance of their waning abilities. For example, having dinner out in a well-lighted restaurant or not expecting grandmother to babysit for too many hours, if at all, are actions that recognize the diminished vision and energy of older people. The values and standards held by older people need to be accepted, whether they are related to ethical, religious, or household matters. For example, it is wise to respect an older person's decision to hang the laundry outside rather than to use a dryer, or to cook on a wood stove.

Elder Abuse

Older adults who are unable to care for themselves are often cared for by family members, usually a daughter or spouse. Caring for a spouse or a parent often causes a great deal of strain and frustration in a relationship and may lead to violence and abuse. It is estimated that over one million elderly Americans are abused annually. The victims of abuse are likely to be white, female, and over

70 years of age. In addition, most victims of abuse are afflicted with substantial mental or physical impairments.

The types of abuse used against the elder include (1) psychologic abuse, such as yelling and screaming; (2) physical abuse, such as hitting, slapping, or restraining for long periods of time; (3) financial abuse, such as taking the older adults' money or forcing them to sign over their assets; and (4) neglect, such as withholding food, medication, or basic care.

The perpetrator of abuse is usually the spouse or the child of the victim. Caregivers who abuse their elderly family members are often middle-aged or older or have emotional problems such as alcoholism; in some cases, three or four generations may be sharing living quarters. Caregivers are often placed in the stressful situation of administering care to parents who treat them like children. Many elderly people use guilt to control their children's lives and do not give them the privacy and respect that they need. The cost of medical care may also be a burden for the caregiver, as well as the stress involved in 24-hour responsibility for another person.

To prevent abuse, the nurse should spend time counseling families prior to their making the decision to care for their elderly parent. The nurse should also be aware that ongoing support is needed for the caregiver as well as for the elderly client. Frequent visits should be made to the home of an elderly client to assess the home situation for factors that may lead to an abusive situation. The elderly in general are unwilling and/or often unable to report abuse. They may feel guilty that they have raised a child who has mistreated them, or they may feel that they have no other place to go. In some cases, the abused persons may be cognitively impaired and unable to advocate in their own behalf.

The nurse who suspects an abusive situation has an obligation to report it. Nurses should be familiar with the laws of their particular state regarding reporting of suspected or known abuse. The legally competent adult cannot be forced, however, to leave the abusive situation and in many cases may decide to stay. If the elderly client is not legally competent, court proceedings to attain guardianship can be initiated.

Drug Use and Misuse

When those who are now elderly were growing up, few pills or other cures were available to treat physical or emotional problems. In the past several decades, however, major progress has been made in the pharmaceutical industry. As a result, hundreds of prescription and nonprescription drugs are available to the public. Elderly adults frequently suffer from one or more chronic diseases that often require medication. Episodes of acute illness may require additional medications. The complexities involved in the self-administration of medication may lead to a variety of misuse situations, including taking too much or too little medication, combining alcohol and medication, combining prescribed medications with over-the-counter drugs, taking medications at the wrong

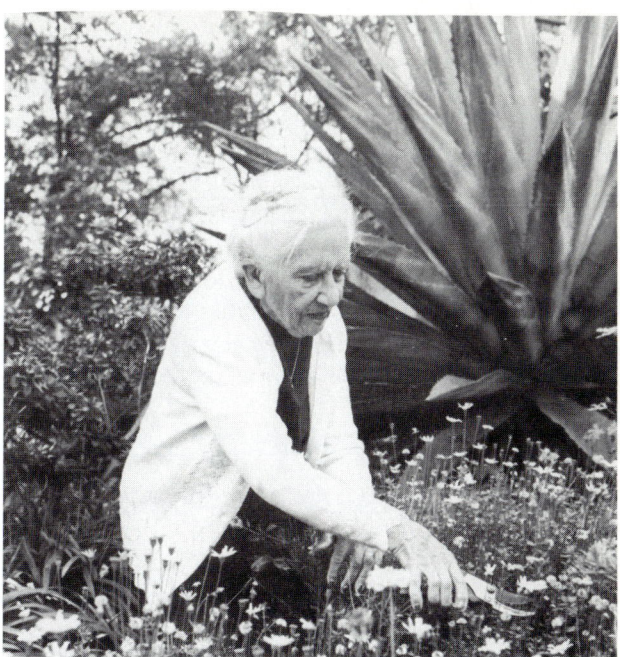

Figure 27–3 Independence fosters self-respect.

time, or taking someone else's medication. Other potential misuse situations occur when elderly people have more than one physician prescribing medications and fail to tell each doctor what has been previously prescribed.

To prevent drug misuse, the nurse should assess the drug history of the elderly person carefully and determine a realistic teaching plan. Elderly clients should be given written instructions, in large print and in language that they can understand. In addition, the side effects of each drug should be listed and reviewed with the client. In simple terms, elderly clients should be taught the importance of maintaining a schedule for important medications (e.g., digitoxin, insulin) and the risks involved in skipping a dose or "running out" of pills. Forgetful persons may need to use a pill organizer to ensure accurate medication ingestion. The nurse should also discuss any over-the-counter drugs the elderly client may use and explain potential risk and side effects of self-medication and multiple medications. In some cases, the nurse can offer conservative measures, such as relaxation techniques or soothing baths, to replace tranquilizers or pain medications. Health promotion activities, such as diet and exercise, may also be helpful adjuncts to reduce the need for medications for chronic disease.

Alcoholism

The estimates of alcohol abuse among elderly Americans vary from 5% to 20% of the population (Burnside 1988, p. 1009). In general, people tend to consume less alcohol as they get older. Elderly alcoholics include those who began drinking alcohol in their youth and those who began excessive alcohol use later in life. Alcoholics who begin drinking later in life do so to help them cope with the changes and problem of their older years. Many late-onset alcoholics are widowers.

Chronic drinking has major effects on all body systems, causes progressive liver and kidney damage, damages the stomach and related organs, and slows mental response, frequently leading to accidents and death. Alcohol interacts with various drugs, altering the normal effect of the medication on the body. Some medications have an increased effect when taken with alcohol (such as anticoagulants and narcotics), whereas the action of other medications (such as antibiotics) is inhibited. For the elderly person who has a chronic illness and takes many medications, the combination of drugs and alcohol can lead to serious drug overdose.

Elderly alcoholic clients should not be stereotyped or prejudged by the nurse. Rather, they should be accepted, listened to, and offered help. The nurse should assess the number and type of alcoholic beverages consumed as well as the pattern and frequency of consumption. It is important that the nurse discuss any medications the client is taking and review the side effects and interaction effects of alcohol and medication. The role of the nurse is to act as a client advocate and facilitate the treatment of the drinking problem and the prevention of complications.

CHAPTER HIGHLIGHTS

▶ The life expectancy of North Americans is increasing, so that late adulthood is now divided by some into three periods: "young-old" (65–74 years); "middle-old" (75–84 years); and "old-old" (85 years and over).

▶ A number of theories strive to account for the biologic aging process: genetic, immunologic slow virus, autoimmune, cross-link, stress, free-radical, and program theories.

▶ Psychosocial theories about aging include the disengagement, activity, and continuity theories.

▶ A number of physical changes occur with aging and involve most body systems: the integument, body temperature, and the neuromusculoskeletal, cardiopulmonary, sensory/perceptual, digestive, urinary, and reproductive systems.

▶ The older adult usually has to adjust to many psychosocial changes. Included are retirement (which necessitates financial and social adjustments), relocation, increasing dependence on others, and coping with death and grief.

▶ There is minimal change in the intellectual abilities of the healthy elderly person. Of the three types of memory (sensory, primary, and secondary), secondary memory has been found to decline with aging.

▶ A decline in memory and cognitive abilities (dementia) caused by such factors as depression, infection, and thyroid disorder are reversible if prompt diagnosis and treatment are obtained. Dementia caused by Alzheimer's disease, repeated strokes, and Parkinson's disease are irreversible at this time.

▶ The moral concerns of elderly people tend to be interpersonal rather than social or legalistic.

▶ Spiritual maturity can provide the elderly person with inner resources for dealing with life experiences.

▶ Much of the decline in health during late adulthood is due to chronic illnesses resulting from unhealthy lifestyles and poor health habits, rather than the aging process itself.

▶ Health promotion and protection activities of the older adult focus on regular health maintenance visits and immunization; accident prevention; ensuring adequate nutrition; prevention of elimination problems; encouraging appropriate exercise, rest, and sleep; and maintaining the person's self-esteem and independence to the maximum potential.

▶ Elder abuse, drug use and misuse, and alcoholism are situations that require sensitive assessment and counseling by the nurse.

READINGS AND REFERENCES

SUGGESTED READINGS

Andresen, G. P. June 1989. A fresh look at assessing the elderly. *RN* 52:28–40.
  Physiologic changes in the elderly are related to genetic inheritance, health history, life-style, environment, and social factors. Because of these factors, the elderly population will have great diversity in what is considered "normal aging." The author presents a review of each body system in both text and charts, including clinical assessment, cause, and related nursing interventions. Andresen also provides laboratory values for the elderly

client but cautions that findings must be interpreted carefully and always in light of the client's total health profile.

Nesbitt, B. July 1988. Nursing diagnosis in age-related changes. *Journal of Gerontological Nursing* 14:6–12.

Elderly individuals living at home should be assessed for any potential problems so that early intervention and support can be provided. Nurses need a format for documenting potential problems to demonstrate the "cognitive services" nursing provides. The NANDA list is offered as an appropriate structure for monitoring these problems. Nesbitt presents several nursing diagnoses and discusses defining characteristics and contributing factors.

Resnick, B. M. May/June 1989. Care for life ... even if a life care community is utopia, the move can be a dramatic change. Here's how to smooth the transition. *Geriatric Nursing* 10:130–32.

More than 150,000 elders live in over 600 life-care communities in the United States. A life-care community offers its residents the convenience of a comfortable, independent living situation with the guarantee of a nursing home bed when needed. Although the move is planned by the older adult, nursing care is needed to help ease the transition. The author suggests several strategies such as (1) initial nursing assessment to determine potential problems, (2) group support to allow the residents to build on each other's strengths, and (3) teaching the older adult the symptoms of stress they might experience.

Simon, J. M. August 1988. The therapeutic value of humor in aging adults. *Journal of Gerontologial Nursing* 14:8–13.

The author suggests that humor serves multiple functions in the health care setting. These functions include social, psychologic, physiologic, and communication aspects. Humor is described as a coping mechanism that helps to lessen tension and anxiety. The author suggests that structured humorous activities be planned, such as games, shows, and movies, and discusses the nursing implications.

Smith, D. L. September/October 1988. Health promotion for older adults. *Health Values* 12:46–51.

This article reviews recent health promotion programs focusing on the elderly population. These programs typically offer a combination of health education, fitness training, and preventive health screenings. The author proposes that health promotion for elderly adults must be taken seriously to prevent the disability as well as the costs incurred by the increases in chronic illness.

RELATED RESEARCH

Gueldner, S. H., and Spradley, J. October 1988. Outdoor walking lowers fatigue. *Journal of Gerontological Nursing* 14:6–12.

Ruffing-Rahal, M. January/February 1989. Ecological well-being: A study of community dwelling older adults. *Health Values.* 13:10–19.

Scura, K. W. October 1988. Audiological assessment program. *Journal of Gerontological Nursing* 14:19–25.

Steinke, E. Summer, 1988. Older adults' knowledge and attitudes about sexuality and aging. *Image: Journal of Nursing Scholarship* 20:93–5.

Thomas, B. December 1988. Self esteem and life satisfaction. *Journal of Gerontological Nursing* 14:25–30.

SELECTED REFERENCES

Andreasen, M. E. and Conley, D. M. July/August 1987. Let the sun shine in. *Geriatric Nursing* 8:174–77.

Burggraf, V., and Stanley, M. 1989. *Nursing the elderly: A care plan approach.* Philadelphia: J.B. Lippincott Co.

Burnside, I. M. 1988. *Nursing and the aged: A self-care approach.* 3d ed. New York: McGraw-Hill.

Butler, R. 1963. The life review: An interpretation of reminiscence in the aged. *Psychiatry* 26:65.

Caliandro, G., and Judkins, B. 1988. *Primary nursing practice.* Glenview, Ill.: Scott, Foresman & Co.

Carpenito, L. J. 1989. Nursing Diagnosis. *Application to Clinical Practice 3d ed.* Philadelphia: J.B. Lippincott Co.

Christian, J. L. and Greger, J. L. 1988. Nutrition for living. Menlo Park, Calif: Benjamin/Cummings.

Ciocon, J., and Potter, J. October 1988. Age related changes in human memory: Normal and abnormal. *Geriatrics* 43:43–48.

Disparti, J. 1988. Nutrition and self-care. In Caliandro, G., and Judkins, B., editors. pp. 134–50. *Primary nursing practice.* Glenview, Ill.: Scott, Foresman & Co.

Edelman, C., and Mandle, C. L. 1986. *Health promotion throughout the life span.* St. Louis: C. V. Mosby Co.

Erikson, E. H. 1963. *Childhood and society.* 2d ed. New York: W. W. Norton and Co.

———. 1982. *The life cycle completed: A review.* New York: W. W. Norton and Co.

Fowler, J., and Keen, S. 1985. *Life maps: Conversations in the journey of faith.* Waco, Texas: Word Books.

Fulmer, T. 1988. The older adult. In Caliandro, G., and Judkins, B., editors. pp. 543–57. *Primary nursing practice.* Glenview, Ill.: Scott, Foresman & Co.

Gioiella, E. C., and Bevil, C. W. 1985. *Nursing care of the aging client: Promoting healthy adaptation.* Norwalk, Conn.: Appleton-Century-Crofts.

Hales, D. 1989. *An invitation to health.* 4th ed. Menlo Park: Benjamin/Cummings.

Hawkins, W. E.; Duncan, D. F.; and McDermott, R. J. May 1988. A health assessment of older Americans: Some multidimensional measures. *Preventive Medicine* 17:344–56.

Hayflick, L. October 1988. Why do we live so long? *Geriatrics* 43:77–87.

Hogstel, M.; and Kashka, M. January/February 1989. Staying healthy after 85. *Geriatric Nursing.* 19:16–18.

Houldin, A., Saltstein, S., Ganley, K. 1987. *Nursing Diagnoses for Wellness.* Philadelphia: J.B. Lippincott.

Job, S., and Anema, M. December 1988. Elder care: Ethical dimensions. *Journal of Gerontological Nursing* 14:16–19.

Kart, C. S.; Metress, E. S.; and Metress, J. F. 1978. *Aging and health: Biologic and social perspectives.* Menlo Park, Calif.: Addison-Wesley Publishing Co.

Kohlberg, L. 1971. *Recent research in moral development.* New York: Holt, Rinehart and Winston.

Lenihan, A. A. July/August 1988. Identification of self care behaviors in the elderly: A nursing assessment tool. *Journal of Professional Nursing* 4:285–88.

Lichtenstein, M.; Bess, F.; and Logan, S. May 1988. Validation of screening tools for identifying hearing impaired elderly in primary care. *Journal of the American Medical Association* 259:2875–78.

Lyles, D. C.; Larisey, M. M.; and Morrill, L. S. May/June 1988. Health promotion for the elderly: A student experience. *Nurse Educator* 13:23–26.

McCracken, A. L. October 1988. Sexual practice by elders: The forgotten aspect of functional health. *Journal of Gerontological Nursing* 14:13–18.

Murray, R. B., and Zentner, J. P. 1989. *Nursing assessment and health promotion strategies through the life span.* 4th ed. Norwalk, Conn.: Appleton & Lange.

Nesbitt, B. July 1988. Nursing Diagnosis: Age related changes. *Journal of Gerontological Nursing* 14:6–12.

Peck, R. 1955. Psychological developments in the second half of life. In Anderson, J., editor. *Psychological aspects of aging.* Washington, D.C.: American Psychological Association.

———. 1968. Psychological development in the second half of life. In Neugarten, B. L., editor. *Middle age and aging.* Chicago: University of Chicago Press.

Pender, N. J. 1987. Health promotion and nursing practice. 2d ed. Norwalk, Conn.: Appleton & Lange.

Reed, A. T., and Birge, S. J. July 1988. Screening for osteoporosis. *Journal of Gerontological Nursing* 14:18–20.

Rowe, J., and Besdine, R. 1988. *Geriatric Medicine.* 2d ed. Boston: Little, Brown and Co.

Rybash, J.; Hoyer, W.; and Roodin, P. 1986. *Adult cognition and aging.* New York: Pergamon Press.

Rybash, J. M.; Roodin, P. A.; and Hoyer, W. J. 1983. Expressions of moral thought in later adulthood. *Gerontologist* 23:254–59.

Saxon, S. V., and Etten, M. J. 1987. *Physical change and aging: A guide for the helping professions.* 2d ed. New York: Tiresias Press.

Schuster, C. S., and Ashburn, S. S. 1986. *The process of human development: A holistic approach.* 2d ed. Boston: Little, Brown and Co.

Scura, K. W. October 1988. Audiological assessment program. *Journal of Gerontological Nursing* 14:19–25.

Smith, D. L. September/October 1988. Health promotion for older adults. *Health Values* 12:46–51.

Thienhaus, O. J. August 1988. Practical overview of sexual function and advancing age. *Geriatrics* 43:63–67.

Tzirides, E. April 1988. Health outreach program: Marketing the "Health Way." *Nursing Management* 19:557.

U.S. Bureau of the Census. 1989. *Statistical abstract of the United States,* 109th ed. U.S. Government Printing Office, Washington, D.C.

Utley, Q. E.; Hawkins, J. E.; Igou, J. F.; and Johnson, F. F. June 1988. Giving and getting support at the wellness center. *Journal of Gerontological Nursing* 14:23–25.

Vander-Zanden, J. 1985. *Human development.* 3d ed. New York: Alfred A. Knopf.

Webster, J. A. December 1988. Key to healthy aging: Exercise. *Journal of Gerontological Nursing* 14:8–15.

Yurick, A.; Spier, B.; Robb, S.; and Ebert, N. 1989. *The aged person and the nursing process.* Norwalk, Conn.: Appleton & Lange.

CHAPTER

28

Family Health

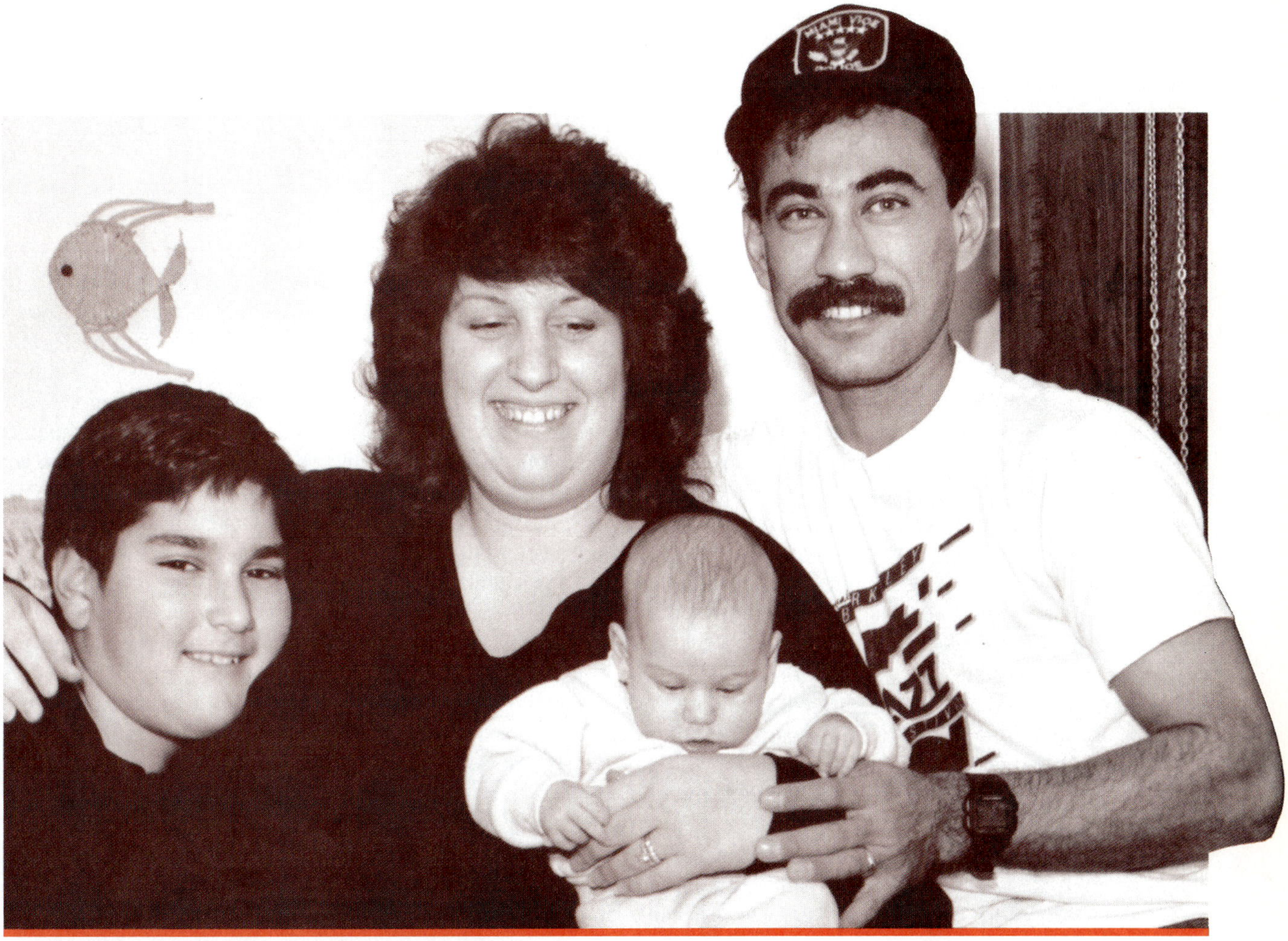

CONTENTS

OBJECTIVES

- Explain family-centered nursing.
- Describe different kinds of families.

- Describe the roles and functions of the family.
- Identify three frameworks for studying the family.
- Describe selected forms of families in society today.
- Identify the components of a family health assessment.

- Identify common risk factors to family health.
- Develop nursing diagnoses pertaining to family functioning.
- Develop outcome criteria for specific nursing diagnoses related to family functioning.

- Explain the common causes of a family health crisis.
- Discuss coping strategies used by families.
- Explain the nurse's function in family health promotion.

ROLES AND FUNCTIONS OF THE FAMILY

Considerable evidence underscores the importance of the family. Definitions of *family* are as numerous and different as the many forms of family seen in today's society. There has been a resurgence of interest in the family unit and its impact on the health, values, and productivity of individual family members. In the nursing profession, this interest in the family as a unit has been expressed by the emergence of **family-centered nursing:** nursing that considers the health of the family as a unit in addition to the health of individual family members.

Membership in a family has a tremendous influence on the individual through genetic endowment, ethnicity, and the development of personal, social, moral, and cultural values. Nurses must consider the family's influence on the individual as they assess, diagnose, plan, implement, and evaluate nursing care.

When one envisions a family, usually the first image that comes to mind is a mother and father—the husband and wife—and their children, usually a boy and a girl. A family of parents and their offspring is known as the **nuclear family**. The relatives of nuclear families, such as grandparents or aunts and uncles, comprise the **extended family.** In some families, members of the extended family live with the nuclear family. Such multigenerational families were more common during the last century but are still seen today in many cultures as well as in many North American homes. Although members of the extended family may live in different areas, they are a frequent source of support and companionship for the family.

The **family** is frequently defined as two or more persons who are related through marriage, blood, birth, or adoption (Duvall 1977). Although this definition characterizes a large number of families, it does not adequately describe the membership of many families today. In many family groups, there are no legal or blood relationships among members. As the structure of the family has become more diverse, it has been necessary to define the family more broadly to encompass the wide variety of family forms seen in today's society. To provide flexibility in the study of families, Friedman (1981, p. 8) defines the family as follows: "A family is composed of people (two or more) who are emotionally involved with each other and live in close geographical proximity." Emotional involvement is demonstrated through caring and a commitment to a common purpose.

The family is the basic unit of society. Its major roles are to protect and socialize its members. Among the many functions it serves, of prime importance is the role the family plays in providing emotional support and security to its members through love, acceptance, concern, and nurturing. This affective (emotional) component holds families together, gives family members a sense of belonging, and develops a sense of kinship.

In addition to providing an emotionally safe environment for members to thrive and grow, the family is also a basic unit of physical protection and safety. This is accomplished by meeting the basic needs of its members: food, clothing, and shelter. Provision of a physically safe environment requires knowledge, skills, and economic resources.

In modern society, the economic resources needed by the family are secured by adult members through employment or government programs. The family also protects the physical health of its members by providing adequate nutrition and health care services. Nutritional and life-style practices of the family not only influence the health of family members but also directly affect the developing health attitudes and life-style practices of children.

In addition to providing an environment conducive to physical growth and health, the family creates an atmosphere that influences the cognitive and psychosocial growth of its members. Children and adults in healthy, functional families receive support, understanding, and encouragement as they progress through predictable developmental stages, as they move in or out of the family unit, and as they establish new family units. In families where members are physically and emotionally nurtured, individuals are challenged to achieve their potential in the family unit. As individual needs are met, family members are able to reach out to others in the family and the community, and to society.

The family is a major educator of its members. Parents are often called a child's first teachers. This early learning plays an influential part in the development of a child's attitudes about family, education, health work, and recreation. These attitudes persist throughout their lives. In addition, families play a major role in the transmission of religious, cultural, and societal values. As the family socializes its new members to the expectations of home, community, and society, it provides a place of warmth, acceptance, and nurturing that insulates its members from the demands of society.

The family is a place of roots, refuge, and rejuvenation. It is a small network where members communicate and work together, delegating roles and responsibilities with a shared purpose: the protection and growth of its members. Through the experiences of family life, the individual learns to participate in and contribute productively to society.

FRAMEWORKS FOR STUDYING THE FAMILY

According to **systems theory,** a system is a unit composed of parts that are interdependent. (See Chapter 4 for systems theory.) The family unit can be viewed as a system. Its members are interdependent, working toward specific purposes and goals. Many families are described as *open systems,* for they are continually interacting and influenced by other systems in the community. Boundaries regulate the input from other systems that interact with the family system; they also regulate output from the family system to the community or to society. Boundaries protect the family from the demands and influences of other systems. Open families are likely to welcome input from without, encouraging individual members to adapt beliefs and practices to meet the changing demands of society. Such families are more likely to seek out health care information and use community resources. These families are adaptable and therefore better prepared to cope with changes in life-style needed to restore, maintain, or promote health.

Family systems also can be described as *closed systems.* Closed families are self-contained units resistant to outside interaction or influence. Such families may be suspicious of others and are content with the status quo. They are less likely to change values and practices; they tend to exert more control over the lives of their members and distrust recommendations made by nonfamily members. It is more difficult for closed family systems to use community resources that may be helpful in dealing with a family health crisis or to incorporate new behaviors that may promote a healthier family. The boundaries of most families, however,

are permeable and flexible, regulating input and output according to family needs, values, and developmental stage.

The **structural-functional theory,** as the name implies, focuses on family structure and function. The structural component of the theory addresses the membership of the family and the relationships among family members. Intrafamily relationships are complex because of the numerous relationships that exist within the family structure—mother-daughter, brother-sister. husband-wife, and so on. These relationships are constantly evolving as children mature and leave the family nest and adults age and become more dependent on others to meet their daily needs.

The functional aspect of the theory examines the effects of intrafamily relationships on the family system, as well as their effects on other systems. Some of the main functions of the family include developing a sense of family purpose and affiliation, adding and socializing new members, and providing and distributing care and services to members. A healthy family organizes its members and resources in meeting family goals; it functions in harmony, working toward shared goals.

Developmental theory views families as ever-changing and growing. Crucial, yet predictable, tasks occur at each level or stage of development. Achievement of tasks appropriate at one level is a prerequisite for successfully achieving the tasks expected at the next level. A major task of the family, from a developmental perspective, is to create an environment where the family can master critical developmental tasks. This ensures orderly progression through the stages of the family life cycle.

THE FAMILY IN TODAY'S SOCIETY

It is difficult to describe the family of today except as uniquely diverse. Improvements in health care have led to healthier people living longer and more productive lives. The development of reliable contraceptives and the legalization of abortion have resulted in greater control in the planning of families. Today's economic realities, coupled with liberation ideology, have moved many women out of the home and into the workplace, changing traditional family roles. Higher divorce rates and the acceptance of children born to unmarried mothers have led to a dramatic increase in the number of single-parent families. Individuals are also grouping together to form new family units based on sexual preference or economic need.

Traditional Families

The **traditional family** is often viewed as an autonomous unit in which both parents reside in the home with their children, the mother assuming the nurturing role and the father providing the necessary economic resources. The traditional family is still very much a part of North American culture, but it is no longer the predominant family form. Although members of the extended family are not likely to live with traditional nuclear families, they remain an important source of information, support, and security. Contact with members of the extended family is vital to mobile families in times of stress or crisis because contact gives a sense of stability in a complex, impersonal society.

In the modern family, changes are occurring in traditional role patterns. Today's fathers are more involved with their children and family life. Many attend prenatal classes and witness the birth of their infants. In addition, fathers are more involved with household chores as role stereotypes are challenged, even though wives continue to perform a large portion of the housework. Likewise, females are less bound by traditional role patterns in today's society.

Two-Career Families

In **two-career,** or **dual-career, families**, both the husband and wife are employed. Such families have been steadily increasing since the 1960s. The reasons for this trend are many, including the increased educational and career opportunities available to women, a desired increase in standard of living, and economic necessity. Many two-career families are young couples without children who desire to complete and use their education. Other working couples postpone childbearing until they are financially secure, have paid debts, and have purchased some of life's extras. Two-career families may also be parents who have launched their children and find they have many healthy, productive years to spend in the marketplace prior to retirement.

It is estimated that 60% to 70% of working women have children in the home, many of whom are preschoolers. When both parents work, the roles each partner plays are variable. Many husbands become more involved in the care of children and the management of household chores. Time and personal energy constraints also may lead to reevaluation of family activities and goals. Attention must be given to maintaining the husband-wife relationship and individual interests amidst the pressures of juggling family and career commitments.

The increased number of working parents has created a need for quality, affordable child care. Finding such child care is one of the greatest stresses faced by today's working parents. Many children spend part of each working day in daycare homes or child-care centers that may expose them at a young age to a host of people with a wide range of ideas and values.

Once children reach school age, parents find that few resources for after-school child care are available. Many school-age children come home to empty houses or apartments to care for themselves. These **latchkey children,** as they are called because they carry their own house key,

may become bored or frightened as they wait for the parents to return from work (McClellan 1984). Parents and professionals are realizing the importance of preparing these children with information about safety and household management to reduce their anxiety and help them make the most of these hours alone. Children of working parents are growing up with new family role models, which will no doubt have an effect on the families of tomorrow.

Single-Parent Families

Today it is estimated that over 50% of North American children live in a **single-parent family**—a home headed by one parent—sometime during their childhood. There are many reasons for single parenthood, including death of a spouse, separation, divorce, birth of a child to an unmarried woman, or adoption of a child by a single man or woman. Single parents frequently express concern about child care, adequate financial resources, social isolation, and lack of adult companionship. Single parents who work outside the home experience fatigue and role overload in managing growing children, household tasks, and a job. At times, these concerns seem to occupy their entire lives, leaving little time for personal or recreational activities.

Nearly 90% of single-parent families are headed by a female. Because these women are often young and poorly prepared for the job market, many single-parent families live with financial strain or poverty. In homes where a divorce has occurred, there is frequently a drop in the standard of living. Child support payments may dwindle after the first year and in many cases are never received. When families live with inadequate financial resources, the health of the family is likely to suffer from substandard living conditions, poor nutrition, stress, and inadequate health care services. The self-esteem of the family is impaired because members, particularly the head of the household, find it difficult to raise their standard of living due to stigma or lack of skills, time, and energy. Depression and despair are common among women struggling to raise a family (Duffy 1982); these feelings not only affect the woman but also influence the outlook of growing family members, who learn to view society as hostile, not as a place full of challenges and hope for the future.

Single-parent families need to identify a support system. Members of the extended family or friends who are supportive provide an opportunity for mutual caring and sharing of concerns. Such support networks reduce social isolation and provide opportunities for relaxation and recreation. A support system helps the single parent cope with and reduce stress; in addition, it gives the individual a chance to have fun and regain self-esteem. Referral to appropriate community resources helps the single parent locate child care, take advantage of financial or social programs, and develop job skills through education or job-training programs.

Blended Families

Existing family units who join together to form new family units are known as **blended** or **reconsitututed families.** Families with children living with a birth parent and a non-birth parent are commonly called step families. The blending of two families presents a unique set of challenges to the individuals involved. The joining of two families is often met with hope and anticipation. Each family brings its own history and expectations to the new family constellation. Often expectations for instantaneous adaptation and affection are too high. Children, depending on their ages and past experiences, usually adjust slowly to new patterns of communication and family authority. Family reintegration requires time and effort. Stress occurs as blended families get to know each other, respect differences, and establish new patterns of behavior (Reutter and Strang 1986).

The greatest success in blending families comes when each family member enters the new relationship with realistic expectations and plans to take the time to make the new family unit succeed. Successful parents get along with and enjoy each other, enjoy life, and bring a sense of humor to the challenge of blending the life-styles and values of two families into one.

Adolescent Parents

A disturbing trend is the growing proportion of infants born each year to **adolescent parents.** These young parents, who are still mastering the developmental tasks of childhood, are physically, emotionally, and financially ill prepared to undertake the responsibilities of parenthood. Over 600,000 infants in America are born each year to adolescent mothers (*The Adolescent Family* 1984, p.1). An increasing number of these mothers are 15 years and younger. A disproportionate number of adolescent births are to members of minority racial or ethnic groups.

Pregnant adolescents are at greater risk for health problems during pregnancy because of poor nutritional status, physiologic immaturity, and lack of prenatal care. They are more likely to deliver premature infants who are, in turn, at greater risk for subsequent health and developmental problems. In addition, adolescent mothers are more likely to give birth to another infant while still in their teens. Today there is a greater acceptance of unmarried parenthood, and fewer pregnant teens feel pressured to marry the father of the infant or to relinquish the infant for adoption.

Adolescent pregnancy frequently interrupts education and may necessitate changes in life goals of many young women. The newly formed family unit is often dependent upon others for physical, emotional, and financial assistance. Support systems are crucial to its success. Parenting skills need to be developed, and the completion of at least a high school education should be encouraged. While helping the new mother understand the needs of her growing infant is an important intervention for nurses, so is assisting the young mother progress through the developmental tasks of adolescence into adulthood.

The children of adolescent parents are at greater risk for health and social problems as they grow up. These children experience more accidents during their preschool years than their peers, are frequently behind in receiving their childhood immunizations, and are more prone to exhibit learning and behavior problems when they enter school. Often raised in poverty, children of adolescent mothers may have few role models to help them break out of the cycle of poverty and subsequent adolescent parenthood.

Cohabiting Families

A current and growing trend in alternate family forms is unrelated individuals or families cohabiting or living under one roof, forming new family units called **cohabiting** or **communal families**. Some individuals join together out of a need for companionship; for example, two widowed adults who share common interests found that living together eliminated previously lonely hours during the evening. Others cohabit to achieve a sense of family or belonging. Many unmarried couples choose to cohabit; some have no desire for a long-term commitment, others wish to test a relationship prior to marriage.

Financial need often leads to the formation of cohabiting families. In these situations, individuals or families share living expenses as well as the responsibilities of household management. Others may cohabit to share services. For example, a single mother moved in with an elderly man who desired to remain in his home but needed help with cooking and cleaning. The single mother was able to provide these services, and she benefited because she and her daughter were now regularly sitting down to nutritious meals, something they rarely experienced previously. An added bonus was the close friendship the elderly man established with her 6-year-old daughter. The formation of cohabiting families illustrates the flexibility and creativity of the family unit in adapting to meet individual challenges and responding to changing societal demands.

Gay and Lesbian Families

Of recent interest is the awareness of the number of homosexual adults in today's society who have formed **gay** and **lesbian families** based on the same goals of caring and commitment seen in heterosexual relationships. While homosexual relationships have been stereotyped as short term and casual, many gay and lesbian relationships are based on long-term mutuality. As the society becomes more educated about homosexuality, it will better understand the complex emotional attachments and affiliation of many homosexual couples and will provide a more accepting atmosphere for these relationships.

Although homosexual marriages are not legally recognized, many homosexual relationships are the basis of new family units. Lesbian women are more likely to live together or cohabit than gay men. Lesbians have fewer sexual partners, are more likely to spend time with their partner, and place a higher value on sexual fidelity than their male counterparts (Williamson 1986). Lesbian women are also more likely to bring children from previous marriages into their partnerships than gay men are. Although many are concerned about the effects of parental homosexuality on the growing child, studies have shown that these children develop sex-role orientations and behaviors similar to children in the general population (Hoeffer 1981). The greatest danger to children reared in gay and lesbian families is the prejudice and ridicule expressed by others in society. For this reason, many homosexual parents keep their sexual preference private to spare their children pain during early childhood, choosing to explain their sexual preference when the children are able to understand homosexuality and emotionally ready to deal with its implications.

Families from Different Cultures

Families from different cultures are an integral part of North America's rich heritage. Each family has values and beliefs (**cultural heritage**) that are unique to their culture of origin and that shape the family's structure, methods of interaction, health care practices, and coping mechanisms. These factors interact to influence the health of families. Families from different cultures may cluster to form mutual support systems and to preserve their heritage; however, this practice may isolate them from the larger society.

Children in cultural clusters often have greater contact with the world around them than adults; through school, children become more proficient in language and more comfortable with new customs and behaviors. Sometimes children create conflict in the family when they bring home new ideas and values. They want to become part of the culture in which they live and incorporate new practices into existing family customs. In the process, they may reject previously cherished cultural traditions.

Becoming acculturated is a slow, stressful process of learning the language and customs of a new country. Chapter 31 presents information that helps the nurse understand the family traditions, beliefs, and practices of different cultures. This information helps the nurse to provide nursing care that is sensitive to the unique needs of families from different cultural heritages.

Single Adults Living Alone

Although individuals living alone, by definition, are not considered a family unit, in today's society many individuals live by themselves. When society is studied from a family perspective, these individuals are frequently overlooked, yet they represent a significant proportion of the popula-

tion. Singles may include young, newly emancipated adults who have left the nuclear family and achieved independence. These young adults may have completed their education and entered the job market, becoming self-sufficient and self-supporting. As young adults postpone marriage or choose singleness, living alone is becoming a more prevalent life-style.

On the other end of the age spectrum is the older adult living alone. Having launched their families, many older adults find themselves single through divorce, separation, or death of a spouse. Some older adults remain in their homes, while others find an apartment more suitable to their changing needs. As they age, and depending on their health status and financial resources, some single adults relocate into retirement homes or extended care facilities. Although many older adults live alone, they may have frequent contacts with other family members, especially adult children and grandchildren. As they enter the golden years, their sense of family becomes stronger, and they seek to communicate the history and values of the family to the new generation.

ASSESSING THE HEALTH OF FAMILIES

The importance of family assessment cannot be overemphasized. The information gathered during assessment is the basis for planning and delivering nursing care to family members or to the family as a whole. Numerous family assessment tools are available. The nurse must consider a number of factors in selecting a family assessment tool or in developing a tool that meets the demands of the families served in a particular practice setting. The home care nurse, for instance, may develop a tool to assess the unique needs and problems of a family who has a member with diabetes.

A family assessment tool should be holistic, eliciting information about a wide variety of family characteristics, beliefs, and behaviors. The tool should be understandable and acceptable to both the family and the nurse (Speer and Sachs 1985). In other words, the nurse must use terminology comprehensible to a wide range of clients, and the tool should be quickly and easily administered. The instrument should also yield clinically relevant data about the family—information useful in formulating nursing diagnoses and planning nursing interventions that promote the health of families.

Overall Family Assessment

The purpose of family assessment is to determine the level of family functioning, to clarify family interaction patterns, to identify family strengths and weaknesses, and to describe the health status of the family and its individual members (Logan & Dawkins, 1986, p. 185).

An overall assessment of the family includes:

- Identification of family members
- Description of the living environment
- Health status of family members
- Financial status, including health insurance and patterns of health care utilization
- Health beliefs and goals of the family
- Occupation of family members
- Education level and aspirations of the family
- Social and community agencies utilized by the family
- Social patterns of the family

Also important are family living patterns, including communication, child rearing, coping strategies, and health practices. An overall family assessment gives an overview of the family process and helps the nurse identify areas that need further assessment. Nurses carry out a more detailed assessment in specific target areas as they become more acquainted with the family and begin to understand family needs and strengths more fully. In planning interventions, nurses need to focus not only on problems but also on family strengths and resources as part of the nursing care plan.

The family APGAR is a screening tool that reveals how family members perceive the level of functioning of the family unit as a whole (Smilkstein 1978) (see Figure 28–1). Open-ended questions assess family functioning in the areas of adaptation, partnership, growth, affection, and resolve. The nurse then elicits information on family satisfaction with each of the functional components of family functioning (see Table 28-1). The information gained provides basic data about the level of family functioning and gives the nurse an idea about which areas need more detailed assessment and intervention and about family strengths that can be mobilized in solving other family problems.

Health Appraisal

The **health appraisal** begins with a complete health history. The nurse focuses first on the family unit and then on

Family APGAR Questionnaire

	Almost always	Some of the time	Hardly ever
I am satisfied with the help that I receive from my family* when something is troubling me.	_____	_____	_____
I am satisfied with the way my family* discusses items of common interest and shares problem solving with me.	_____	_____	_____
I find that my family* accepts my wishes to take on new activities or make changes in my lifestyle.	_____	_____	_____
I am satisfied with the way my family* expresses affection and responds to my feelings, such as anger, sorrow, and love.	_____	_____	_____
I am satisfied with the amount of time my family* and I spend together.	_____	_____	_____

Scoring: The patient checks one of three choices, which are scored as follows: "Almost always" (2 points), "Some of the time" (1 point), or "Hardly ever" (0). The scores for each of the five questions are then totaled. A score of 7 to 10 suggests a highly functional family. A score of 4 to 6 suggests a moderately dysfunctional family. A score of 0 to 3 suggests a severely dysfunctional family.

* According to which member of the family is being interviewed, the interviewer may substitute for the word "family" either spouse, significant other, parents or children.

Figure 28–1 Family APGAR questionnaire. *Source:* G. Smilkstein, Assessment of family function, *Journal of Family Practice,* 1978, 6:1231–39. Reprinted with permission.

TABLE 28–1 *Family APGAR*

Component	Definition	Assessment questions
Adaptation	Use of intra- and extrafamilial resources for problem solving when family equilibrium is under stress	"How have family members aided each other in time of need?"
		"In what way have family members received help or assistance from friends and community agencies?"
Partnership	Sharing of decision-making and nurturing responsibilities by family members	"How do family members communicate with each other about such matters as vacations, finances, medical care, large purchases, and personal problems?"
Growth	Physical and emotional maturation and self-fulfillment achieved by family members through mutual support and guidance	"How have family members changed during the past years?"
		"How has this change been accepted by family members?"
		"In what ways have family members aided each other in growing or developing independent life-styles?"
		"How have family members reacted to your desires for change?"
Affection	Caring or loving relationship among family members	"How have members of your family responded to emotional expressions such as affection, love, sorrow, or anger?"
Resolve	Commitment to devote time to other members of the family for physical and emotional nurturing; also usually involves a decision to share wealth and space	"How do members of your family share time, space, and money?"

Source: S. R. Mott, N. F. Fazekas, and S. R. James, *Nursing care of children and families: A holistic approach* (Menlo Park, Calif.: Addison-Wesley Publishing Co., 1985), p. 571. Reproduced with permission.

the individuals in that family. The health history is one of the most effective ways of identifying existing or potential health problems. The history is followed by physical assessment of family members. If further evaluation is indicated, referral is made to the appropriate health care professional. Frequently the physical examination focuses on identifying disease conditions or the potential for them rather than on appraisal of health. When the focus is on health, the appraisal includes information on life-style behaviors and health beliefs. The nurse uses data from the health appraisal to formulate a health profile. The health profile provides the data necessary to establish a nursing diagnosis and to plan appropriate nursing interventions to promote optimal health through life-style modification.

Health Beliefs

To promote health, the nurse must understand the health beliefs of individuals and families and use this information in planning and delivering nursing care. Health beliefs may reflect a lack of information or misinformation about health or disease. They may also include folklore and practices from different cultures. Because of the many advances in medicine and health care during the last few decades, many clients have out-dated information about health, illness, treatment, and prevention. The nurse is frequently in a

position to give information or correct misconceptions about health. This function is an important component of the nursing care plan. For additional information on health beliefs, see Chapter 23.

Family Communication Patterns

The effectiveness of family communication determines its ability to function as a cooperative, growth-producing unit. Messages are constantly being communicated among family members, both verbally and nonverbally. The information transmitted influences how members work together, fulfill their assigned roles in the family, incorporate family values, and develop skills to function in society. **Intrafamily communication** plays a significant role in the development of self-esteem, which is necessary for the growth of personality.

Families who communicate effectively transmit messages clearly. Members are free to express their feelings without fear of jeopardizing their standing in the family. Family members support one another and have the ability to listen, empathize, and reach out to one another in times of crisis. When the needs of family members are met, they are more able to reach out to meet the needs of others in society.

When patterns of communication among family members are dysfunctional, messages are often communicated unclearly. Verbal communication may be incongruent with nonverbal messages. Power struggles may be evidenced by hostility, anger, or silence. Members may be cautious in expressing their feelings because they cannot predict how others in the family will respond. Many things remain unsaid to preserve family unity and tranquility. When family communication is impaired, the growth of individual members is stunted. Members often turn to other systems to seek personal validation and gratification.

The nurse needs to observe intrafamily communication patterns closely. Nurses should pay special attention to who does the talking for the family, which members are silent, how disagreements are handled, and how well the members listen to one another and encourage the participation of others. Nonverbal communication is important because it gives valuable clues about what people are feeling.

Family Coping Mechanisms

Family coping mechanisms are the behaviors families use to deal with stress or changes. Coping mechanisms can be viewed as an active method of problem solving developed to meet life's challenges. The coping mechanisms families and individuals develop reflect their individual resourcefulness. Friedman (1981, p. 249) states that families may use the same coping patterns rather consistently over time or may change their coping strategies when new demands are made on the family. Coping is a basic function that helps the family meet demands imposed both from within and without. The success of a family depends on how well it copes with the stresses it experiences.

Nurses working with families realize the importance of assessing coping mechanisms as a way of determining how families relate to stress. Also important are the resources available to the family. Internal resources, such as knowledge, skills, effective communication patterns, and a sense of mutuality and purpose within the family, assist in the problem-solving process. In addition, external support systems promote coping and adaptation. These external systems may be extended family, friends, religious affiliations, health care professionals, or social services. The development of social support systems is particularly valuable today, when many families, due to stress, mobility, or poverty, are isolated from resources that would help them cope.

Identifying Families at Risk for Health Problems

Risk assessment helps the nurse identify individuals and groups at higher risk than the general population of developing specific health problems, such as stroke, diabetes, and lung cancer. Risk may be related to genetic factors; for example, persons who have a family history of diabetes are at greater risk of developing diabetes than persons with no family history of diabetes. Certain practices also increase

the risk of health problems; for instance, cigarette smokers are at greater risk of developing lung cancer than non-smokers. Environmental factors, such as air pollution or exposure to toxic chemicals, increase the risk of certain health problems.

Risk reduction among individuals and groups identified as at risk poses a special challenge to health care professionals. Once the individuals or groups are identified, the nurse's role is to plan and implement interventions to reduce health risks when possible or to optimize the current health status of those individuals or groups when risks cannot be reduced. The vulnerability of family units to health problems may be based on family developmental level, age of family members, heredity or genetic factors, sociologic factors, and life-style practices. The goal of the nurse is to promote optimal family health and functioning.

Developmental Factors
Families at both ends of the age continuum are at risk of developing health problems. Newly formed families entering the childbearing and childrearing phases of development experience many changes in roles, responsibilities, and expectations. These changes occur when adult family members are attempting to establish financial security. The many, often-conflicting demands on the young family cause stress and fatigue, which may impede growth of family members and the functioning of the group as a unit.

Adolescent mothers, because of their developmental level and lack of knowledge about parenthood, and single-parent families, because of role overload experienced by the head of the household, are more likely to develop health problems. Moreover, the elderly are at risk of developing degenerative and chronic health problems. Because of the emphasis on youth in today's society, many elderly persons feel a lack of purpose and decreased self-esteem. These feelings in turn reduce their motivation to engage in health-promoting behaviors, such as exercise or community and family involvement.

Hereditary Factors
Persons born into families with a history of certain diseases, such as diabetes or cardiovascular disease, are at greater risk of developing these conditions. A detailed family health history, including genetically transmitted disorders, is crucial to the identification of persons and families at risk. These data are used not only to monitor the health of individual family members but also to recommend modifications in health practices that potentially reduce the risk, minimize the consequences, or postpone the development of genetically related conditions.

Other family units or family members may be at risk of developing a disease by reason of sex or race. Males, for example, are at greater risk of having cardiovascular disease at an earlier age than females, and females are at greater risk of developing osteoporosis, particularly after menopause. While at times it is difficult to separate genetic factors from cultural factors, certain risk factors seem to be related to race. Some diseases are more prevalent among whites than blacks, and vice versa. Sickle-cell anemia, for example, is a hereditary disease limited to blacks of African descent (McFarlane 1977). Native Americans and Asians seem more susceptible to certain diseases and less susceptible to others than the general population.

Life-Style Factors   As the understanding of health and illness increases, it has become clear that many diseases are preventable, the effects of some diseases can be minimized, or the onset of disease can be delayed through life-style modification. Cancer, cardiovascular disease, adult-onset diabetes, and tooth decay are among the life-style diseases. The incidence of lung cancer, for example, would be greatly reduced if people stopped smoking. Proper nutrition, good dental hygiene, and use of fluoride—in the water supply, in toothpaste, as a topical application, or as supplements—have been shown to reduce dental decay or caries, one of America's most prevalent health problems. Automobile accidents, the leading cause of death among adolescents and young adults, are frequently associated with alcohol consumption and increased risk taking.

In addition to health practices and nutrition, other important life-style considerations are exercise, stress management, and rest. Today, health professionals have the knowledge to prevent or minimize the effects of some of the main causes of disease, disability, and death. Too often, there is little consideration of health until sickness occurs. The challenge is to disseminate information about prevention and to motivate families to make life-style changes prior to the onset of illness. Many demands are made on today's family. An important question is: Will people take the time to be responsible for their own health?

Sociologic Factors   **Poverty** is a major problem that affects not only the family but also the community and society. Over 35 million people, or nearly one out of every six Americans, live in poverty (Moccia and Mason 1986, p. 20). A disproportionate number of today's poor belong to ethnic or racial minority groups. Poverty is a real concern among the rising number of one-parent families headed by a female, and, as the number of these families increases, poverty will affect a large number of growing children.

Because many poor families do not possess the skills or support systems necessary to break out of the cycle of poverty, it is likely that poverty will continue to escalate rapidly in the future. When ill, the poor are likely to put off seeking services until the illness reaches an advanced state and requires longer or more complex treatment. Even though the Surgeon General has reported that the health of the American people has never been better (U.S. DHEW 1979), it is clear that this progress has not benefited all segments of society, particularly the poor.

DIAGNOSING AND PLANNING

Data gathered during a family assessment may lead to the nursing diagnoses: **Altered family processes,** the state in which a normally supportive family experiences a stressor that affects its functioning; **Family coping: potential for growth,** the state in which a family member exhibits a desire and readiness for enhanced health and growth; **Ineffective family coping: disabling,** the state in which a family demonstrates destructive behavior or adapts detrimentally to a stressor; **Ineffective family coping: compromised,** a state similar to *altered family processes;* **Altered parenting,** the state in which one or more caregivers is unable to create an environment that promotes the optimal growth and development of a child or children; and **Impaired home maintenance management,** the state in which an individual or family is unable to independently maintain a safe, growth-promoting immediate environment. Examples of contributing factors for these diagnoses are shown below.

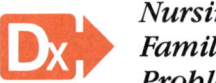 *Nursing Diagnoses Families at Risk for Health Problems*

Altered family processes related to:
- Illness of family member
- Loss of family member
- Gain of new family member
- Economic crises (e.g., unemployment)
- Change in family role (e.g., working mother)
- Retirement
- Divorce

Family coping: potential for growth related to:
- Role changes (e.g., marriage, parenthood)
- See also contributing factors for *Health seeking behaviors*

Ineffective family coping: disabling related to:
- Alcoholic parent
- Drug-addicted family member
- Dependent elderly parent
- Emotionally disturbed parent or child
- Terminally ill parent or child

Ineffective family coping: compromised related to:
- See *Altered family processes*

Altered parenting related to:
- Impaired parental infant attachment

- Mental or physical illness

Impaired home maintenance management related to:

- Chronic debilitating disease
- Injury to family member
- Parent with cognitive, motor, or sensory deficit

Planned nursing interventions need to focus on assisting the family to plan realistic strategies that enhance family functioning, such as improving communication skills, identifying and utilizing support systems, developing and rehearsing parenting skills, and becoming involved in community activities. For families who are functioning well, anticipatory guidance may assist families in preparing for predictable developmental transitions that occur in the life of families (Denehy 1990).

Examples of outcome criteria to evaluate the achievement of client goals and the effectiveness of nursing interventions are listed below.

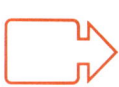

Outcome Criteria
Families at Risk for Health Problems

The client or family:

- Expresses feelings freely and appropriately
- Participates in problem-solving process directed at appropriate solutions for the crisis
- Participates in care of the ill family member
- Encourages ill family member to handle situation in own way, progressing toward independence
- Seeks appropriate external resources as needed
- States an intent to use positive coping mechanisms and constructive stress management
- Expresses more realistic understanding and acceptance of the family member demonstrating destructive or maladaptive behavior
- Seeks assistance for abusive behavior
- Verbalizes realistic expectations of parenting role
- Demonstrates appropriate parenting behaviors, e.g., attachment
- Identifies own needs as well as strengths and resources to meet needs
- Begins to verbalize positive feelings about infant
- Identifies factors that restrict self-care and home management
- Demonstrates ability to perform skills necessary for individual or home care

HEALTH PROMOTION IN THE FAMILY

Today's families are concerned about living healthy, productive, fulfilling lives. The media regularly inform the public that many personal behaviors endanger life and health, yet at the same time they accept advertising revenues from products that do not promote health. Much has been learned about the effects of diet, stress, and exercise on health, but changing long-established preferences and practices is difficult. Substance abuse, particularly of tobacco and alcohol, as well as personal and environmental safety hazards have

RESEARCH NOTE

Health Promotion in the Family

Duffy reviewed current research in health promotion for the family and suggests directives for future research. Four nursing journals—*Nursing Research, Research in Nursing and Health, Western Journal of Nursing Research,* and *International Journal of Nursing Studies*—were reviewed to identify the number of studies related to health promotion in the family published between January 1980 and June 1986. The review revealed a dearth of nursing research in family health promotion. Of the 105 issues reviewed, only five articles (4.8%) addressed health promotion activities in the family.

Duffy used the findings from these studies, as well as other research literature, to develop future directives, or areas for study. These directives address both the internal and external environment of the family. Areas related to the *internal environment* of the family include (a) family definitions of health and health promotion, (b) descriptions of current family health promotion behaviors and those practiced over time, (c) decision-making, (d) influence of parenting, (e) influence of fathering, and (f) methods of intervention most effective in encouraging health promotion in the family. Research of the *external* environment includes (a) the societal norms that facilitate or impede health promotion behaviors, (b) societal interventions, such as those that decrease the impact of poverty in families, and (c) the effects of social institutions on the practice of health.

Implications: Without further nursing research on health promotion in the family, nurses will not have a sufficient body of knowledge to influence public and health policies and to work with individuals and families in the promotion of their health.

Duffy, M. E. January 1988. Health promotion in the family: Current findings and directives for nursing research. *Journal of Advanced Nursing* 13:109–17.

needlessly decreased the productivity and shortened the lives of many persons.

To make changes that improve its own well-being, the family must be aware of potential health problems and their relationship to life-style practices. Information on how to reduce risks within the context of the family's value system is crucial. Support and encouragement of life-style changes help ensure that these changes are not temporary but become an important health value that influences lifelong health practices. The role of health education is to inform, motivate, and facilitate adoption of healthful life-style practices—activities the promote the well-being of individuals and families.

One of the major goals of health promotion is to help families take responsibility for their own health through self-care. **Self-care** is defined as activities individuals perform in their own behalf to maintain health and well-being (Orem 1980). Effective self-care requires knowledge and skills relating to health and illness. It includes knowing how to solve health problems of the family, as well as knowing when to seek outside guidance in meeting health problems. Self-care also encompasses health promotion for the family. Through health promotion, families can realize higher levels of wellness, productivity, self-awareness, and personal growth. For a more comprehensive discussion of health promotion, see Chapter 23.

THE FAMILY EXPERIENCING A HEALTH CRISIS

Illness of a Family Member

Illness of a family member is a crisis that affects the entire family system. The family is disrupted as members abandon their usual activities and focus their energy on restoring family equilibrium. Roles and responsibilities previously assumed by the ill person are delegated to other family members, or those functions may remain undone during the duration of the illness. The family experiences anxiety because members are concerned about the sick person and the resolution of the illness. This anxiety is compounded by additional responsibilities when there is less time or motivation to complete the normal tasks of daily living.

Many factors determine the impact of illness on the family unit. Among these are:

- The nature of the illness, which can range from minor to life-threatening.
- The duration of the illness, which ranges from short term to long term.
- The residual effects of the illness, including none to permanent disability.
- The meaning of the illness to the family and its significance to family systems.

- The financial impact of the illness, which is influenced by factors such as insurance and ability of the ill member to return to work.
- The effect of the illness on future family functioning. For instance, previous patterns may be restored or new patterns may be established.

The family's ability to deal with the stress of illness depends on the members' coping skills. Families with good communication skills are better able to discuss how they feel about the illness and how it affects family functioning. They can plan for the future and are flexible in adapting these plans as the situation changes. An established **social support network** provides strength, encouragement, and services to the family during the illness. During health crises, families need to realize that it is a strength, not a sign of weakness, to turn to others for support. Nurses can be part of the support system for families, or they can identify other sources of support in the community.

During a crisis, families are often drawn together by a common purpose. In this time of closeness, family members have the opportunity to reaffirm personal and family values and their commitment to one another. Indeed, illness may provide a unique opportunity for family growth.

Intervening in Families Experiencing Illness

Nurses committed to family-centered care involve both the ailing individual and the family in the nursing process. Through their interaction with families, nurses can give support and information. Nurses make sure that not only the individual but also each family member understands the disease, its management, and the effect of these two factors on family functioning. The nurse also assesses the family's readiness and ability to provide continued care and supervision at home when warranted. After carefully planned instruction and practice, families are given an opportunity to demonstrate their ability to provide care under the supportive guidance of the nurse. When the care indicated is beyond the capability of the family, nurses work with families to identify available resources that are socially and financially acceptable (McClelland et al. 1985).

In helping families to reintegrate the ill person into the home, nurses use data gathered during family assessment to identify family resources and deficits. By formulating mutually acceptable goals for reintegration, nurses help families cope with the realities of the illness and the changes it may have brought about, which may include new roles and functions of family members or the need to provide continued medical care to the ill or recovering person. Working together, nurses and families can create environments that restore or reorganize family functioning during illness and throughout the recovery process.

Death of a Family Member

The death of a family member has a profound effect on the family. The structure of the family is altered, and this change may in turn affect how it functions as a unit. Individual members experience a sense of loss. They grieve for the lost person, and they grieve for the family that once was. (See Chapter 34 for a discussion of loss and grieving.) Some of the early stages of grief accompany family disorganization. However, as the family begins to recover, a new sense of normalcy develops, the family reintegrates its roles and functions, and it comes to grips with the reality of the situation. This painful blow takes time to heal. After the death of a member, families may need counseling to deal with their feelings and to talk about the person who died. They may also want to talk about their fears about and hopes for the future. At this time, families often derive comfort from their religious beliefs and their spiritual adviser. Support groups are also available for families experiencing the pain of death. It is often difficult for nurses to deal with grieving families because the nurses also feel the loss and feel inadequate in knowing what to say or do. By understanding the effect death has on families, nurses can help families resolve their grief and move ahead with life.

CHAPTER HIGHLIGHTS

▸ The family is the basic unit of society.

▸ The family plays an important role in forming the health beliefs and practices of its members.

▸ Family-centered nursing addresses the health of the family as a unit, as well as the health of family members.

▸ Through family assessment, the nurse identifies health beliefs and practices that influence the wellness of the family.

▸ In working with the wide variety of family forms in today's society, the nurse must be aware of many factors that affect the health of families.

▸ Nurses must examine their own values about family, health, illness, and death to be effective in supporting families in crisis.

▸ Nurses can help families realize their potential and their dreams for health and happiness by promoting healthy family functioning.

READINGS AND REFERENCES

SUGGESTED READINGS

Friedman, M. M. 1981. *Family nursing theory and assessment.* Norwalk, Conn.: Appleton-Century-Crofts.
  A section discussing concepts and approaches to the family introduces this text. Discussions of family health assessment, family communication patterns, family power structure, and health care function follow.

Johnson, S. H. 1986. *Nursing assessment and strategies for the family at high risk: High risk parenting.* 2d ed. Philadelphia: J. B. Lippincott Co.
  Identification of and intervention in families at risk are essential to reduce the potential health care problems of these groups.

Logan, B. B., and Dawkins, C. E. 1986. *Family-centered nursing in the community.* Menlo Park, Calif.: Addison-Wesley.
  The authors integrate the areas of family and community health into a family-focused community-health nursing text, reflecting contemporary trends and changes in the family, communities, and health policies, and demonstrating the impact of these changes on community health nursing. Contemporary issues discussed include adolescent pregnancy, substance abuse, chronic mental illness, and family violence.

Ludder, P., et al. March/April 1983. Caring for children of divorced families. *The American Journal of Maternal Child Nursing* 8:120–30.
  By identifying and counseling the child at risk and providing guidance to the parents, nurses can ease the emotional problems caused by divorce.

Wright, L. M., and Leahey, M. 1984. *Nurses and families: A guide to family assessment and intervention.* Philadelphia: F. A. Davis.
  This book illustrates how family theory can be applied to clinical practice and emphasizes the development of interviewing skills with families.

RELATED RESEARCH

Gilliss, C. 1984. Reducing family stress during and after bypass surgery. *Nursing Clinics of North America* 19:103–12.

Jarrett, G. E. March/April 1982. Research: Childrearing patterns of young mothers. *The American Journal of Maternal Child Nursing* 7:119–24.

Lasky, P., Buckwalter, K. C.; Whall, A., Lederman, R.; Speer, J.; McLane, A.; King, J. M.; and White, M. A. February 1985. Developing an instrument in the assessment of family dynamics. *Western Journal of Nursing Research* 7:40–57.

Sund, K., and Oswald, S. K. November/December 1985. Dual-earner families' stress levels and personal and life-style-related variables. *Nursing Research* 34:357–61.

SELECTED REFERENCES

The adolescent family. 1984. Columbus, Ohio: Ross Laboratories.

Bradley, R., and Caldwell, B. M. 1977. Home environment, social status, and mental test performance. *Journal of Educational Psychology* 69:697–701.

Denehy, J. A. 1990. Anticipatory guidance. In Craft, M. J., and Denehy, J. A., editors. pp. 53–67. *Nursing Interventions for Infants and Children*. Philadelphia: W. B. Saunders Co.

Duffy, M. A. September/October 1982. When a woman heads a household. *Nursing Outlook* 30:468–73.

Duvall, E. M. 1977. *Marriage and family development*. 5th ed. Philadelphia: J. B. Lippincott Co.

Feetham, S. L., and Humenick, S. S. 1982. The Feetham family functioning survey. In Humenick, S. S. pp. 259–68. *Analysis of current assessment strategies in the health care of young children and childbearing families*. Norwalk, Conn.: Appleton-Century-Crofts.

Friedman, M. 1981. *Family nursing: Theory and assessment*. Norwalk, Conn.: Appleton-Century-Crofts.

Hoeffer, B. 1981. Childrens' acquisition of sex-role behavior in lesbian-mother families. *American Journal of Orthopsychiatry* 51:536.

Logan, B. B., and Dawkins, C. E. 1986. *Family-centered nursing in the community*. Menlo Park, Calif.: Addison-Wesley Publishing Co.

McClelland, M. A. May/June 1984. On their own: Latchkey children. *Pediatric Nursing* 10:198–204.

McFarlane, J. December 1977. Sickle cell disorders. *American Journal of Nursing* 77:1948–54.

Moccia, P. and Mason, D. J. January/February 1986. Poverty trends: Implications for nursing. *Nursing Outlook* 34:20–24.

Mott, S. R., James, S. R., and Sperhac, A. M. 1990. *Nursing care of children and families*. 2d ed. Redwood City, Calif.: Addison-Wesley Nursing.

Orem, D. E. 1980. *Nursing concepts of practice*. 2nd ed. New York: McGraw-Hill Book Company.

Pender, N. J. 1987. *Health promotion in nursing practice*. 2d ed. Norwalk, Conn.: Appleton & Lange.

Reutter, L. Strang, V. July/August 1985. Yours, mine and ours: Stepparents and their children. *The American Journal of Maternal/Child Nursing* 2:264–66.

Smilkstein, G. 1978. The Family APGAR: A proposal for a family function test and its use by physicians. *The Journal of Family Practice* 6:1231–39.

Speer, J. J., and Sachs, B. September/October 1985. Selecting the appropriate family assessment tool. *Pediatric Nursing* 11:349–55.

U. S. Department of Health, Education, and Welfare. 1979. *Healthy people: The Surgeon General's report on health promotion and disease prevention*. DHEW Pub. no. 79–555071. Washington, D. C.: U. S. Department of Health, Education, and Welfare.

Williamson, M. 1986. Lesbians. In Griffith-Kinney, J., Editor. pp. 278–96. *Contemporary women's health: A nursing advocacy approach*. Menlo Park, Calif.: Addison-Wesley Publishing Co.

Wright, L. M., Leahey, M. February 1990. Trends in nursing of families. *Journal of Advanced Nursing* 15:148–54.

SUPPORTING PSYCHOSOCIAL HEALTH PATTERNS

Self-Concept and Role Relationships

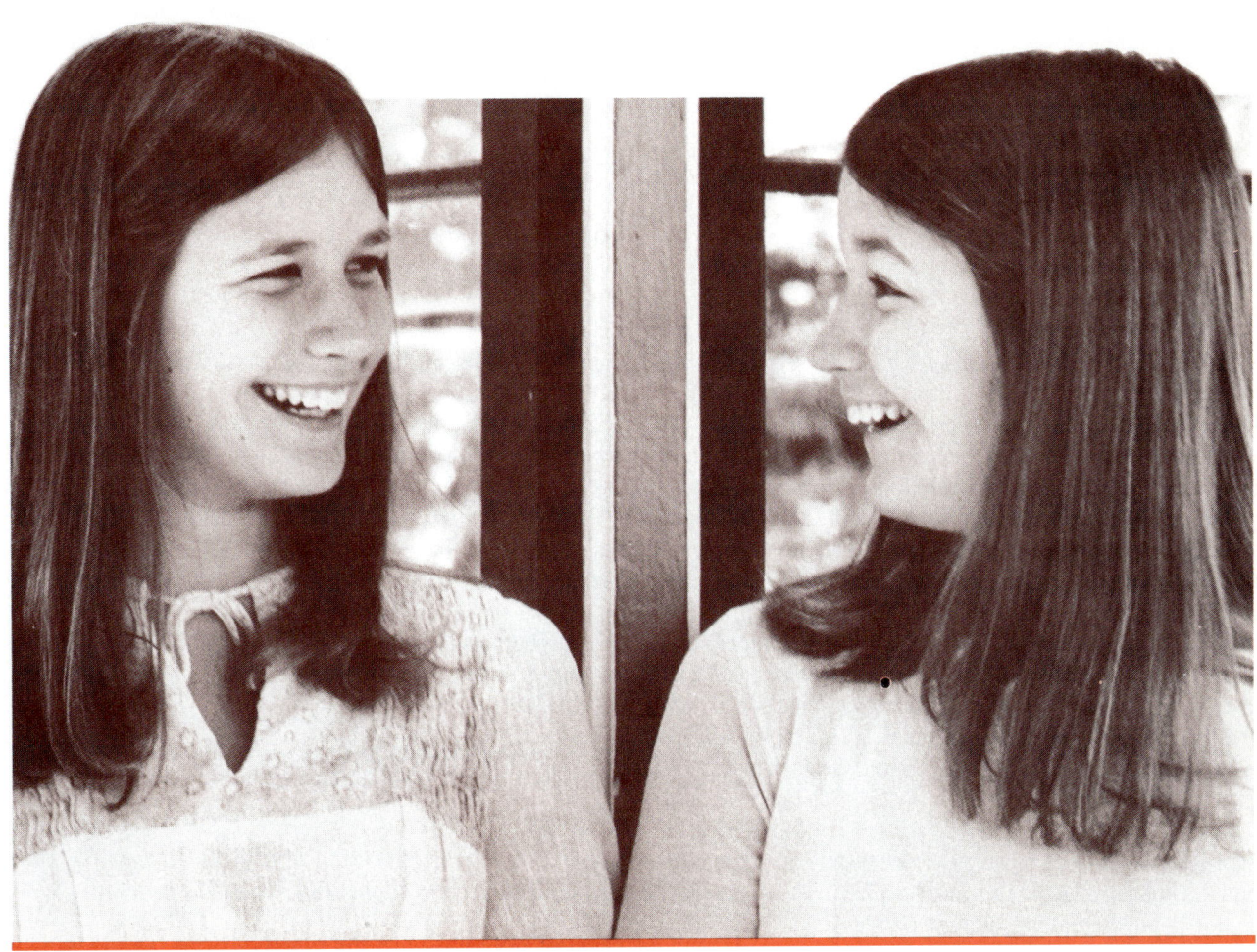

OBJECTIVES

▶ Differentiate *self-concept* from *self-esteem*.

▶ Describe the components of self-concept.

OBJECTIVES *(continued)*

▶ Give Erikson's explanation of the effects of psychosocial crises on self-concept and self-esteem.

▶ Describe the effects of communication/coping styles on self-esteem.

▶ Identify four areas involved in the nursing assessment of self-concept.

▶ Describe key data to be included when assessing self-perception.

▶ Describe the essential aspects of assessing role relationships.

▶ List important assessment data to be included when identifying clients' stressors and coping strategies.

▶ Identify common stressors affecting self-concept and self-esteem.

▶ List behaviors that could indicate altered self-concept.

▶ Identify nursing diagnoses concerning altered self-concept.

▶ Select appropriate goals for clients with altered self-concept.

▶ Describe nursing actions designed to implement identified goals for clients with altered self-concept.

▶ Describe ways to enhance the self-esteem of older adults.

▶ Identify outcome criteria that permit evaluation of clients with altered self-concept.

IMPORTANCE OF A HEALTHY SELF-CONCEPT

Self-concept, self-esteem, and *self-image* are essential to a person's mental and physical health. Individuals with a positive self-concept or high self-esteem are better able to develop and maintain warm interpersonal relationships and resist psychologic and physical illness. A healthy self-concept enables a person to find happiness in life and to cope with life's disappointments and changes. Failure to achieve a positive self-image presents major obstacles in the treatment of common disorders such as depression, eating disorders, postvictimization syndrome (abuse or rape), and crisis reactions. One of the nurse's major responsibilities is to identify persons with a negative self-concept or low self-esteem and to assist them in developing a more positive view of themselves. People who do not have a healthy self-concept are less able to live as fully or be as happy as they might be. People with an unhealthy self-concept generally express feelings of worthlessness, self-dislike or self-hatred, and, on some occasions, hatred for others. They often feel sad or hopeless and are drained of energy.

Self-concept or self-esteem influences a person in these ways (Sanford and Donovan 1984, p. 3):

■ It affects everything one thinks, says, or does.

■ It affects how others in the world see and treat one.

■ It affects the choices one makes, such as who one will be involved with and what to do with one's life.

■ It affects one's ability to give and receive love.

■ It affects one's ability to take action to change things that need to be changed.

The nurse's own self-concept is also important. Nurses who have difficulty meeting their own needs have difficulty meeting the needs of clients. Nurses who feel positive about themselves are better equipped to meet the needs of others. Such nurses feel good, look good, are effective and productive, and respond to people (including themselves) in healthy and positive ways.

CONCEPT OF SELF AND SELF-ESTEEM

The terms *self-concept, self-image, self-esteem, self-worth, sense of self-worth, self-respect,* and *self-love* are often used interchangeably. *Self-concept* has been referred to as the *cognitive* component of the self system, and *self-esteem* as the *affective* component (Hamachek 1978). In other words, **self-concept** is "how I *see* myself," and **self-esteem** is "how I *feel about* myself." Stanwyck (1983, p. 11), however, maintains that these two constructs are inseparable, since self-esteem is based on self-concept. To Stanwyck, self-esteem is "how I feel about how I see myself," even though most researchers use the terms interchangeably.

Three positions of self-concept have been delineated (Burns 1979, p. 50):

1. *Cognized self,* or self as known to the individual: "How I am," or, "How I perceive me."

2. *Other self,* or social self: "How I perceive others perceiving me."

3. *Ideal self:* "How I would like to be."

People who value most "how I perceive me" can be termed "me-centered." They try hard to live up to their own expectations and compete only with themselves, not others. In contrast, "other-centered" people have a high need for approval from others and try hard to live up to the expectations of others, constantly comparing, competing, and evaluating themselves in relation to others. They tend to avoid personal shortcomings, are unable to assert themselves, and continually fear disapproval. The healthy self-concept, therefore, is me-centered and is formed without reference to other persons.

Global and Specific Self-Concept

The term **global self** refers to the aggregate beliefs and images one holds about oneself. It is the most complete description that individuals can give of themselves at any one time. It is also a person's frame of reference for experiencing and viewing the world. Some of these beliefs and images represent statements of fact, for example, "I am a woman"; "I am a mother"; "I am black"; "I am short"; "I am a student"; "I am poor." Others refer to less tangible aspects of self, for instance, "I am stupid"; "I am competent"; "I am clumsy"; "I am lovable"; "I am no good"; "I am shy"; "I am strong"; "I am outgoing."

Each separate image and belief one holds about oneself has a bearing on self-concept. However, self-concept is not simply a sum of its parts, for the various images and beliefs persons hold about themselves are not given equal weight and prominence (Sanford and Donovan 1984, p. 9). Each person's self-concept is like a collage. At the center of the collage are the beliefs and images that are most vital to the person's identity and self-esteem. They constitute **core self-concept.** For example: "I am competent/incompetent"; "I am pretty/ugly"; "I am rich/poor"; "I am male/female." Images and beliefs that are less important to the person are on the periphery. For example: "I am left-/right-handed"; "I am athletic/unathletic"; "I am a good/poor cook"; "I have brown/blue eyes."

According to Goldin (1985, p. 33), people base their self-concept on how they perceive and evaluate themselves in these areas:

- Vocational performance
- Intellectual functioning
- Personal appearance and physical attractiveness
- Sexual attractiveness and performance
- Being liked by others
- Ability to cope with and resolve problems
- Independence
- Particular talents

Self-esteem categories for children include the following (Stanwyck 1983, p. 12):

- School performance
- Peer relationships
- Family relationships
- Emotional well-being
- Physical self-perception

A person's self-perception in any of these areas becomes a self-fulfilling prophecy: Individuals actually behave as they perceive themselves (Goldin 1985, p. 34).

Components of Self-Concept

The North American Nursing Diagnosis Association suggests four components of self-concept: body image, role performance, personal identity, and self-esteem (Kim, McFarland, and McLane 1989, p. 47).

Body Image   The image of physical self, or **body image,** is how a person perceives the size, appearance, and functioning of the body and its parts. It includes clothing, make-up, hairstyle, jewelry, and other things intimately connected to the person, e.g., artificial limb or wheelchair. A person's body image develops partly from others' attitudes and responses to that person's body. Cultural and societal values also influence a person's body image. For instance, Western societies value beauty, youth, and wholeness. Generally, a person has developed a stable body image over a long time; thus, actual or potential threats to alterations in body image can create considerable anxiety.

Role Performance   Throughout life people undergo numerous role changes. A **role** is a set of expectations about how the person occupying one position behaves toward a person occupying another position (Roy 1984, p. 285). Expectations, or standards of behavior, are set by society or the smaller group to which the person belongs. Each person usually has several roles, e.g., husband, parent, brother, son, employee, friend, golf club member. Some roles are assumed for only limited periods, e.g., client/nurse, student/instructor, and the sick role.

To act appropriately, people need to know who they are in relation to others and what society expects for the positions they hold. When there is **role ambiguity,** expectations are unclear, and people do not know what to do or how to do it and are unable to predict the reactions of others to their behavior. This creates confusion and stress. To relate or interact appropriately with others, people also need to know the role positions that others occupy.

Role performance relates what a person does in a particular role in relation to the behaviors expected of that role. **Role mastery** means that the person's behaviors meet social expectations. Failure to master a role creates frustration and feelings of inadequacy, often with consequent lowered self-esteem.

Self-concept is also affected by role strain and role conflicts. Persons undergoing **role strain** are frustrated because they feel or are made to feel inadequate or unsuited to a role. Role strain often is associated with sex role stereotypes. For example, women in occupations traditionally held by men may be thought less knowledgeable and less competent than men in the same roles. As a result, these women feel the need to surpass the level expected for role mastery by male counterparts.

Role conflicts arise from opposing or incompatible expectations. In an *interpersonal conflict,* different people have different expectations about a particular role. For example, a mother's parents may have different expectations about how the mother should care for her children. In an *interrole conflict,* one person's or group's role expectations differ from the expectations of another person or group. For example, a woman who works in an office 8 hours a day may have a role conflict if her husband expects her to be home with the children. In a **person-role con-**

flict, role expectations violate the beliefs or values of the role occupant. For example, a woman who values her right to choose abortion will have a conflict if this right is denied.

Personal Identity   A person's personal or **self-identity** is the conscious sense of individuality and uniqueness that is continually evolving throughout life. People often view their identity in terms of name, sex, age, race, ethnic origin or culture, occupation or roles, talents, and other situational characteristics (e.g., marital status and education). People usually first identify themselves by name and occupation or roles. When interactions progress beyond the superficial, other characteristics may be revealed, e.g., special talents or interests. Self-identity also includes a person's beliefs and values, personality, and character. For instance, is the person outgoing, friendly, reserved, generous, kind, honest, ruthless, selfish? Self-identity, thus, encompasses both the tangible and factual, such as name and sex, and the intangible, such as values and beliefs. In brief: Identity is what distinguishes self from others.

Self-Esteem   The way one perceives and structures one's self-concept can result in either positive or negative self-esteem. There are two types of self-esteem: global and specific (Sanford and Donovan 1984, p. 9). **Global self-esteem** is how much the person likes his or her perceived self as a whole. **Specific self-esteem** is how much a person approves of a certain part of himself or herself (Sanford and Donovan 1984, p. 9). Global self-esteem is influenced by specific self-esteem. For example, if a man values his looks, then how he looks will strongly affect his global self-esteem. By contrast, if a man places little value on his cooking skills, then how well or badly he cooks will have little influence on his global self-esteem.

Maintenance and Evaluation of Self-Esteem

By the time people reach adulthood, their *basic* self-concept and *basic* level of self-esteem are relatively well established, and they already have some idea about their **perceived self,** i.e., how they see themselves and how they are seen by others. In addition, they have an idea about their **ideal self,** i.e., how they should be or would prefer to be. Sometimes this ideal self is realistic; sometimes it is not. When perceived self is close to ideal self, people do not wish to be much different from what they believe they already are. When there is a discrepancy between ideal self and perceived self, this can be an incentive to self-improvement. However, when the discrepancy is large, low self-esteem can result.

Basic self-esteem refers to the foundation for self-esteem that is established during early life experiences, usually within the family. However, an adult's functional level of overall self-esteem may change markedly from day to day and moment to moment. *Functional self-esteem* is a result of the person's ongoing evaluation of interactions with people and objects. Functional self-esteem can exceed basic self-esteem, or it can regress to a level below that of basic self-esteem. Severe stress—for example, prolonged illness or unemployment—can substantially lower a person's basic self-esteem.

Perceptions of self (both as is and as desired) generally arise from self-evaluation in accordance with certain criteria. Four basic criteria by which people judge themselves are

1. *Power*—the ability to influence significant others and control events that are personally important

2. *Significance*—the acceptance, attention, and affection of others who communicate to the person a clear sense of being valued and cared about as a worthwhile human being

3. *Competence*—successfully meeting demands for achievement, particularly personally important goals

4. *Virtue*—adherence to moral and ethical standards

Self-evaluation is usually a covert mental process. Frequently, people label themselves negatively or project failures into the future. Positive self-credit is usually less frequent.

DEVELOPMENT OF SELF-ESTEEM

Four elements of experience that are pertinent to the development of self-esteem are (a) significant others, (b) social role expectations, (c) crises of psychosocial development, and (d) communication/coping style (Stanwyck 1983, p. 13).

Significant Others   The crucial role of social interaction in the development of self-esteem is recognized by most social psychologists. Because some people exert more influence than others on the development of an individual's self-esteem, Sullivan's term *significant other* has been generally accepted (Sullivan 1950). A **significant other** is an individual or group that takes on special importance for the development of self-esteem during a particular life stage. Significant others may include parents, siblings, peers, teachers, and the like. During various stages of development one or several significant others may be identified. Through social interaction with significant others and the resultant interpreted feedback on the perceptions of others, one develops attitudes toward oneself. Put more simply, "as a person is judged by others, so he comes to judge himself" (Burns 1979, p. 184). Many components of a person's self-evaluation are established early in life under the influence of significant others. These values often get so strongly reinforced that they are difficult to change later, even though it may benefit the person to do so.

Social Role Expectations

At the various stages of life, people are strongly influenced by general societal expectations regarding role-specific behavior. The larger society and smaller societal groups have expectations that differ in clarity and are communicated with varying degrees of force. Expectations differ by age, sex, socioeconomic status, ethnicity, and career identification. Smaller societal groups such as the family, school, armed forces, work groups, and recreational groups also expect certain behaviors and performance levels of people. Success in meeting such expectations has profound implications for self-esteem.

Because North American society is highly achievement oriented, everything a person does is evaluated, e.g., earning capacity, social skills, performance at school, athletic performance, and sexual performance. A high level of performance is rewarded; poor performance is belittled. As a result people tend to focus on their failures and shortcomings rather than on their strengths. In many instances a person's actual performance is superior to the person's *perception* of that performance. Compliance with the social expectations for role-specific behavior therefore leads to judgments of personal worth; noncompliance often leads to judgments of personal worthlessness.

Crises of Psychosocial Development

Throughout life people face certain developmental tasks that, if not successfully achieved, may lead to problems with self, self-concept, and self-esteem. Several developmental theories are discussed in Chapter 24. The eight psychosocial stages described by Erikson (1963) provide a convenient and familiar theoretic framework with obvious implications for self-esteem. The success with which a person copes with these developmental crises largely determines the development of self-concept. Inability to cope results in self-concept problems, at the time and often later in life. See Table 29–1 for behaviors indicating successful and unsuccessful resolution of these developmental crises.

Communication/Coping Styles

A person's choice of strategies to cope with a stress-producing situation is important in determining how successfully a person adapts to that situation and whether self-esteem is maintained, enhanced, or decreased. Reactions to stressful situations that threaten self-esteem include problem-solving reactions, assertive reactions, and defensive reactions.

Problem-solving reactions

Problem solving is a conscious, action-oriented response in which the person uses cognitive skills to deal with a stressor. First the person cognitively appraises the threatening situation by asking questions such as these:

- What is the exact nature of the threatening situation?
- What unfavorable consequences can I expect from the situation should it occur?
- What courses of action can I use to cope with the threat?
- What courses of action are most likely to succeed, i.e., cause the least personal loss or problem?

TABLE 29–1 *Examples of Behaviors Associated with Erikson's Stages of Psychosocial Development*

Stage: Developmental Crisis	Behaviors Indicating Positive Resolution	Behaviors Indicating Negative Resolution
Infancy: Trust vs mistrust	Requesting assistance and expecting to receive it	Restricting conversation to superficialities
	Expressing belief of another person	Refusing to provide a person with information
	Sharing time, opinions, and experiences	Being unable to accept assistance
Toddlerhood: Autonomy vs shame and doubt	Accepting the rules of a group but also expressing disagreement when it is felt	Failing to express needs
	Expressing one's own opinion	Not expressing one's own opinion when opposed
	Easily accepting deferment of a wish fulfillment	Overconcern about being clean
Early childhood: Initiative vs guilt	Starting projects eagerly	Imitating others rather than developing independent ideas
	Expressing curiosity about many things	Apologizing and being very embarrassed over small mistakes
	Demonstrating original thought	Verbalizing fear about starting a new project
Early school years: Industry vs inferiority	Completing a task once it has been started	Not completing tasks started
	Working well with others	Not assisting with the work of others
	Using time effectively	Not organizing work

TABLE 29–1 *Examples of Behaviors Associated with Erikson's Stages of Psychosocial Development (continued)*

Stage: Developmental Crisis	Behaviors Indicating Positive Resolution	Behaviors Indicating Negative Resolution
Adolescence: Identity vs role confusion	Asserting independence Planning realistically for future roles Establishing close interpersonal relationships	Failing to assume responsibility for directing one's own behavior Accepting the values of others without question Failing to set goals in life
Early adulthood: Intimacy vs isolation	Establishing a close, intense relationship with another person Accepting sexual behavior as desirable Making a commitment to that relationship, even in times of stress and sacrifice	Remaining alone Avoiding close interpersonal relationships
Middle-aged adults: Generativity vs stagnation	Being willing to share with another person Guiding others Establishing a priority of needs, recognizing both self and others	Talking about oneself instead of listening to others Showing concern for oneself in spite of the needs of others Being unable to accept interdependence
Elderly adults: Integrity vs despair	Using past experience to assist others Maintaining productivity in some areas Accepting limitations	Crying and being apathetic Not accepting changes Demanding unnecessary assistance and attention from others

After a realistic appraisal, the person chooses the most effective course of action, e.g., talking to a friend, calling a crisis center, doing nothing, or seeking out professional help.

Assertive reactions   Everyday interpersonal interactions can produce stress. In such situations, assertive behavior is useful. **Assertiveness** involves expressing oneself openly and directly without hurting others. It provides feelings of control and self-confidence for the communicator and is based on the belief that each person is important. Assertive people are able to present their feelings and values, stand up for themselves, and claim their rights. Assertiveness is prerequisite to building self-esteem. Because it enables the person to cope with a stressful event actively, it enhances self-esteem.

Assertiveness with individuals and groups facilitates

- Prompt coping with problems
- Achievement of group goals
- Communication of power within oneself
- Communication of competence and self-confidence
- Reduction of anxiety or tenseness in key situations

Assertive behavior can be described as falling between nonassertiveness and aggressive behavior on a continuum. Nonassertive or passive persons appear hesitant and unsure of themselves. Their feelings are hidden, for fear of hurting others or being hurt. Because nonassertive persons do not ask or know how to ask, they often do not obtain what they want and thus become frustrated. After a time, this frustration often results in explosively aggressive behavior, which helps the person feel better, but only briefly. Through **aggressiveness,** at the other extreme, people can make their feelings known, but often at others' expense. Although this behavior can result in change, it can be harmful to the individual eventually, as others respond negatively to the aggressive behavior.

Nurses, too, can benefit from using assertive responses. The example that follows illustrates the different types of responses in a typical nursing situation.

Situation
Charge nurse: Miss Eammons, why can't you ever take your blood pressures on time? This is the fourth day this week that they have not been taken.

Aggressive response
Nurse: It's not my fault they are late. You're always interrupting my work with extra duties.

Nonassertive response
Nurse: Yes, I'm sorry. We've been short staffed, and I have a very heavy load.

Assertive response
Nurse: I didn't know that all the blood pressures were late. I'd like to check that further. Could we discuss this in your office before you leave today?

The assertive techniques shown in the box below can help the nurse.

Three assertive methods of coping with criticism are fogging, negative assertion, and negative inquiry (Smith 1975, pp. 104–32). *Fogging* is agreeing in principle to a statement made by another. In this technique, the nurse listens carefully to the criticism and accepts it without becoming defensive or anxious.

Client: You can't do anything right.

Nurse: You're not satisfied with my work, Mr. Milos.

Negative assertion is the assertive expression of those attributes that are negative about oneself:

Client: You didn't give that injection well.

Nurse: I didn't give it very smoothly.

Negative inquiry asks for additional information about the critical statements:

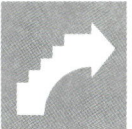

CLINICAL GUIDELINES
Assertive Techniques

- Include positive and negative information in a statement: "I like your plan, but...."

- Start the statement with "I," and avoid generalizations such as "we all believe" or "it seems like a good idea."

- Express your own beliefs and rights: "I believe that...."

- Express your thoughts and feelings directly to reinforce your identity: "I feel you are..." or "I want you to...."

- When replying negatively, state, "I won't..." not "I can't...." The latter implies lack of power, whereas the former communicates assumption of responsibility.

- Make assertive statements:
  a. Simple assertive: "I think...."
  b. Empathic assertive: "I realize you are very tired, but...."
  c. Confrontive assertive: "You said you could bathe Mr. Greene, but you didn't...."
  d. Soft assertive: "I am very grateful you did that for me, and I think...."
  e. Persuasive assertive: "I agree with most of what you said, but I also think...."

When an individual says something that the nurse perceives as negative or a "put-down," the following assertive responses can be given to provide time:

- "I need to think about this for a few minutes."

- "It seems to me that..." and a clear statement of personal feelings.

- Silence as an answer, giving no verbal response.

Charge nurse: You look messy today.

Nurse: What do you mean?

Charge nurse: You look untidy.

Nurse: Do you mean my uniform is wrinkled?

To learn assertiveness, nurses can take workshops or study articles on the subject.

Defensive reactions Defensive responses are generally used when other responses have been unsuccessful in adapting to the stressful event and anxiety or other feelings remain high. Specific defensive coping behaviors are called ego-defense mechanisms. These are discussed in Chapter 33, page 802.

ASSESSING

Assessing problems related to self-concept is normally indicated if (a) the client or support persons present cues that could reflect problems or (b) the client's illness is one often associated with self-concept problems. Problems with self-concept and self-esteem are frequently manifested by expressions of anxiety, fear, anger, hostility, guilt, and/or powerlessness. Behaviors reflecting excessive role conflict may also indicate the need for meaningful intervention by nurses.

A trusting client-nurse relationship is essential for an effective assessment of self-concept. Clients tend not to share personal feelings unless the nurse has established an empathetic, nonjudgmental relationship. Potential disclosure of personal data can be threatening. Some people, particularly those with low self-esteem, may fear that the nurse will not accept or like them if they reveal their true performance capabilities, thoughts, and feelings.

The nursing assessment involves four areas: (a) self-perception or self-awareness, (b) role performance and relationships, (c) major stressors and coping strategies, (d) behaviors suggestive of low self-esteem.

Self-Perception

Assessment of self-perception involves (a) determining the client's perceptions of physical and personal self and (b) observing for nonverbal cues that reflect the client's self-perception.

To determine the client's perception of *physical self,* or body image, the nurse either listens to comments the client makes about the physical self or asks the client the questions shown in the accompanying box. Responses such as "I feel ugly," "I'm awkward and clumsy," "I can't do anything now," "No one will like me now," and "I'm afraid my husband won't love me any more" indicate that the client's self-esteem is threatened or low. The client is focusing on par-

Physical Self

- How do you feel about your personal appearance (or physical features)?

- What do others say about your personal appearance (or physical features)?

- How would you describe your physical movements?

- What changes in your body do you expect as a result of this illness (or surgery, or treatment)?

- What changes have you noticed in how your body looks (or functions)?

- How have important persons in your life (e.g., spouse, parent, partner) reacted to changes in your body?

- How do you think the important people in your life will react to the anticipated change in your body?

Personal Self

- How would you describe your personal characteristics? or, How do you see yourself as a person?

- What do you like about yourself?

- How do others describe you as a person?

- What do you do well?

- What are your personal strengths, talents, and abilities?

- What would you change about yourself if you could?

- Does it bother you a great deal if you think someone doesn't like you?

- Is it difficult for you to say no when you want to say no?

- How do you feel about your educational accomplishments?

- Do you ever feel inadequate with certain people? Who?

- How easily can you express your opinion when it differs from that of others?

- Do you make friends easily?

- Generally, do you feel liked by your peers and coworkers?

- How do you feel about your occupation?

- Do you feel appreciated by your employer?

no good." For other clients, the nurse may consider asking some of the questions shown in the box in the left column.

Nonverbal behaviors—such as body posture, movements, gestures, tone of voice, speech pattern, and general appearance—tend to be more spontaneous than verbal messages and can provide important clues to the person's self-concept. Nonverbal cues that can indicate low self-esteem include stooped shoulders, lack of attention to hygiene or grooming, avoiding eye contact, hesitant speech, and withdrawing from social interaction. Nonverbal cues can help the nurse confirm the reliability of the client's verbal messages.

Role Relationships

The nurse assesses the client's satisfactions and dissatisfactions associated with role responsibilities and relationships: family roles, work roles, student roles, social roles. Family roles are especially important to clients, since family relationships are particularly close. Relationships can be supportive and growth-producing or, at the opposite extreme, highly stressful if violence and abuse permeate relationships. Assessment of family role relationships may begin with structural aspects such as number in the family group, ages, and residence location. For more information on the family, see Chapter 28. To obtain data related to the client's family relationships and satisfaction or dissatisfaction with work roles and social roles, the nurse might ask some of the questions shown in the box in the left column on the opposite page, keeping in mind, however, that questions need to be tailored to the individuals and their age and situation.

Major Stressors and Coping Strategies

The nurse needs to identify stressors that challenge the client's self-worth. Most people face numerous stress-producing events simultaneously. Illness and hospitalization can compound the effects. Common stressors that influence a client's self-concept and self-esteem are shown in the box on the opposite page.

When stressors are identified, the nurse needs to determine how the client perceives the stressor. A positive, growth-oriented perception of stressful events reinforces self-worth; a negative, hopeless, defeatist perception leads to decreased self-esteem. The nurse also should identify the client's coping style and determine whether or not this style is effective by asking the client such questions as these:

- When you have a problem or face a stressful situation, how do you usually deal with it?

- Do these methods work?

Behaviors Suggesting Low Self-Esteem

Some of the verbal and nonverbal behaviors that can indicate altered self-concept or low self-esteem were discussed

ticular disabilities or shortcomings and blocking out accurate perception of the total self.

In regard to *personal self,* some people may volunteer clearly self-deprecating or over-critical comments indicating low self-esteem—e.g., "People don't like me," or "I'm

Family Relationships

■ Tell me about your family.

■ What is home like?

■ Who are you closest to in the family?

■ Who are you most distant from in the family?

■ What are your relationships like with your other relatives?

■ What are your responsibilities in the family?

■ How well do you feel you accomplish what is expected of you?

■ What about your role or responsibilities would you like changed?

■ Do you see yourself as frequently getting the short end of things and coming out second best?

■ Are you proud of your family members?

■ Do you feel your family members are proud of you?

■ Tell me how you spend your time each day.

Work Roles and Social Roles

■ Do you like your work?

■ How do you get along at work?

■ What about your work would you like to change if you could?

■ How do you spend your free time?

■ Are you involved in any community groups?

■ Are you most comfortable alone, with one other person, or in a group?

■ Who is most important to you?

■ Whom do you seek out for help?

Stressors Affecting Self-Concept and Self-Esteem

Body-Image Stressors

■ Loss of body parts, e.g., amputation, mastectomy, hysterectomy

■ Loss of body functions, e.g., from heart disease, renal disease, spinal cord injury, cerebrovascular accident, neuromuscular disease, arthritis, declining mental or sensory abilities

■ Disfigurement, e.g., through pregnancy, severe burns, facial blemishes, colostomy, ileostomy, tracheostomy, laryngectomy

Role Stressors

■ Loss of parent, spouse, child, or close friend

■ Change or loss of job

■ Retirement

■ Divorce or separation

■ Illness

■ Hospitalization

■ Ambiguous role expectations

■ Conflicting role expectations

■ Inability to meet role expectations

Identity Stressors

■ Change in physical appearance

■ Declining physical, mental, or sensory abilities

■ Inability to achieve goals

■ Relationship concerns

■ Sexuality concerns

■ Unrealistic ideal self

■ Membership in a minority group

---

earlier in this section. Other behaviors associated with low self-esteem are listed in the box on the following page.

People with low self-esteem generally exhibit illogical and *distorted thinking.* Some cognitive therapists (Ellis and Harper 1975, p. 100; Beck 1979, p. 54) assert that illogical and distorted thinking causes or perpetuates low self-esteem. Common types of irrational, illogical, or muddled thinking include the following (Crouch and Straub 1983, p. 72).

■ *Catastrophizing,* the tendency to think the worst. For example, the person says, "If something bad can happen it will," or, "Things are bad now, but they will get worse."

■ *Minimizing and maximizing,* the tendency to minimize the positive, to overlook partial successes, to magnify the significance or meaning of the negative, and to emphasize mistakes.

■ *Black-and-white thinking,* the tendency to attribute things to one of two extremes. Things are either perfect or no good. Activities must be performed without mistake or the performance is a failure.

■ *Overgeneralization,* the tendency to believe that something that applied in one situation or that happened once will apply in all situations.

■ *Self-reference,* the tendency to believe that what others are thinking, saying, or doing relates to self. The person believes that others are highly concerned with that person's thoughts and actions and are particularly aware of the person's shortcomings and mistakes.

Behaviors Associated with Low Self-Esteem

The client:

- Avoids eye contact
- Stoops in posture and moves slowly
- Is poorly groomed and has an unkempt appearance
- Is hesitant or halting in speech
- Is overly critical of self, e.g., "I'm no good," "I'm ugly," or "People don't like me."
- May be overly critical of others
- Is unable to accept positive remarks about self
- Encourages reprimands from others, to punish self
- Apologizes frequently
- Verbalizes feelings of hopelessness, helplessness, and powerlessness, such as "I really don't care what happens," "I'll do whatever anyone wants," "Whatever is destined will happen."
- Verbalizes feelings of worthlessness, such as "Nobody cares about me," "I'm just a burden to everyone," "I'm not worth all that trouble."
- Verbalizes feelings of guilt, such as "It's all my fault," "I am to blame."
- Withdraws from or changes social involvements or relationships
- Fails to complete or follow through with activities
- Avoids initiating conversation or interaction with others
- Exhibits self-destructive behavior, such as excessive use of alcohol, drugs
- Has negative feelings about own body, e.g., avoids looking at or touching body part, or hides body part; emphasizes previous appearance or function; talks excessively about loss or change
- Is indecisive, e.g., "I can't make up my mind what to do," "I don't understand what's happening."
- Cannot solve problems effectively and does not ask for help
- Displays overdependence, e.g., asks for assistance unnecessarily, seeks attention by speaking loudly, asks irrelevant questions, seeks approval and praise
- Displays lack of energy, e.g., "I feel tired all the time."
- Verbalizes inability to cope
- Expresses or manifests anxiety, fear, anger
- Does not meet role expectations

- *Filtering,* the tendency to support beliefs or conclusions by selectively pulling certain details out of context and neglecting other facts. Usually, it is the negative details that are selected while positive facts are neglected.

DIAGNOSING

Nursing diagnoses for clients with problems related to self-concept include **Body image disturbance,** the state in which one experiences or is at risk of experiencing a disruption in the way one perceives one's body image; **Personal identity disturbance,** the inability to distinguish self from nonself; **Altered role performance,** the disruption in the way one perceives one's role performance; and **Self-esteem disturbance,** the state in which one experiences or is at risk of experiencing negative feelings or self-evaluation about oneself or one's capabilities.

The diagnosis of **Self-esteem disturbance** is subcategorized into **Chronic low self-esteem** and **Situational low self-esteem. Chronic low self-esteem** applies to clients with long-standing negative self-evaluation or feelings about self or their own capabilities. **Situational low self-esteem** applies to clients who previously had a positive self-evaluation but have developed negative self-evaluation or feelings about self in response to a loss or change.

Because the diagnosis of **Personal identity disturbance** requires further development and research, it is recommended that the student use other diagnoses at this time.

Other diagnoses that relate to self-concept include **Ineffective individual coping, Social isolation, Powerlessness, Sexual dysfunction, Anticipatory grieving,** and **Dysfunctional grieving.** These diagnoses are discussed in other chapters of this book.

Examples of contributing factors for selected diagnoses are shown below. Examples of assessment data clusters and related nursing diagnoses are shown in Table 29–2.

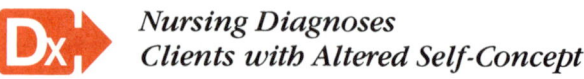

Nursing Diagnoses
Clients with Altered Self-Concept

Body image disturbance related to:

- Loss of body part (e.g., amputation, mastectomy)
- Loss of body function (e.g., from heart disease, spinal cord injury, neuromuscular disease)
- Disfigurement (e.g., pregnancy, severe burns, colostomy)
- Delayed development of secondary characteristics
- Extreme thinness or obesity

Altered role performance related to:

- Change in physical or mental capacity

- Newly assumed work and family roles
- Multiple life stressors

Chronic low self-esteem related to:

- Loss of body function
- Infant or childhood deprivation
- Unrealistic parental expectations
- Unrealistic personal expectations

Situational low self-esteem related to:

- Loss of body part or function
- Divorce
- Loss of job
- Termination of relationship

Powerlessness related to:

- Inability to perform activities of daily living secondary to neuromuscular disease
- Inability to perform role responsibilities secondary to progressive debilitating disease

Ineffective individual coping related to:

- Death of parent
- Inadequate personal resources and social support
- Divorce and change in financial status
- Need for mutilating surgery

PLANNING

The nurse's focus when planning is to assist the client to set goals that reflect a positive resolution of the problem or stressors identified in the nursing diagnosis. Goals should emphasize strengths rather than weaknesses or impairments. Broadly speaking, goals may be stated as follows. The client:

- Increases awareness of strengths and weaknesses.
- Improves feelings of self-worth.
- Perceives and responds to stressors in a constructive manner.
- Improves interpersonal relationships.

Two types of self-image goals can be considered: tangible and personality (Goldin 1985, p. 35). Tangible goals are those that can be measured by objective means, for example, to improve personal appearance, educational level, and fund of information. Personality goals are more subjective in nature, for example, to increase assertiveness, to enhance ability to reach out for new friendships, to become more independent and self-sufficient, to develop self-pride. Once

TABLE 29–2 *Examples of Assessment Data Clusters and Related Nursing Diagnoses*

Data Cluster	Nursing Diagnosis
Frank Sawyers had a permanent colostomy 7 days ago for cancer of the sigmoid colon. When the nurse was changing the colostomy appliance, Frank said, "My wife will be repulsed by this." He avoided looking at the stoma and put his arm over his eyes.	**Body image disturbance** related to disfigurement
Mary Gilbert, who lived with her boyfriend for six years, is distressed about an abrupt ending to their relationship. She says Brian had a full-time job and was taking a computer course at night school. "I guess I'm to blame for the breakup; it's all my fault. I got angry when he never had time to spend with me. Maybe I'm just not smart enough for him."	**Situational low self-esteem** related to termination of intimate relationship; associate with feelings of guilt and feeling unloved
George Kawazi, a first-year college student is studying liberal arts and the sciences. George states that even though he attends all his classes and studies every day and on weekends, his grades do not please his father, who expects straight A's. "I've always had trouble measuring up to Father's expectations. He never thought I was as good as my older brother."	**Chronic low self-esteem** related to unrealistic parental expectations
Sofie Ferraro, a 73-year-old with right-sided (dominant) hemiplegia, says, "Although the Rehabilitation Centre taught me so much about how to manage in my home, my poor husband has to do a lot to help me with cooking meals and cleaning the house."	**Altered role performance** related to change in physical capacity

goals for changing self-image are set, the process of modifying self-image begins.

Nursing strategies to help clients meet goals related to self-concept may include helping clients to (a) identify areas of strength, (b) learn to communicate more clearly, and (c) develop more positive thoughts and images about themselves. Planning also involves establishing outcome criteria by which to measure goal achievement. Examples of outcome criteria are shown on the following page.

The client with **Body image disturbance:**

- Describes changes in thoughts and feelings about self.
- Verbalizes acceptance of changes that have occurred.
- Looks at, touches, and discusses changed body part.
- Continues preexisting socialization pattern.
- Engages in appropriate role functions.
- Engages in recreational activities appropriate to limitations.
- Maximizes use of remaining strengths.
- Uses all available resources to improve functioning (or appearance) of body part.
- Accepts offers of help.

The client with a **Self-esteem disturbance:**

- Demonstrates an improvement in personal appearance.
- Verbalizes realistic perceptions of self.
- Identifies at least five positive personal attributes.
- Shares feelings about self with significant others.
- Compares ideal self and perceived self.
- Uses appropriate assertive and communication skills.
- Demonstrates use of active rather than passive language pattern (e.g., says, "I choose to" or "I choose not to").
- Demonstrates increased social contacts and friendship networks.
- Expresses satisfaction with own achievements.
- Engages in positive talk about self.
- Analyzes own behavior and its consequences.
- Discusses options and alternatives when trying to solve problems.
- Identifies ways of exerting control and influencing outcomes.

The client with **Altered role performance:**

- Verbalizes realistic perception and positive acceptance of self in changed role.
- Verbalizes understanding of role expectations and obligations associated with role.
- Develops realistic plans for adapting to new role or role changes.

IMPLEMENTING

Assisting people with self-concept disturbances requires skills in communicating and in developing helping relationships (see Chapter 15). Helping clients with self-concept distur-

bances is akin to promoting health, as discussed in Chapter 23. The client assumes responsibility for implementing the plans. The nurse provides information, education, and ongoing support; suggests strategies to encourage behavioral change; and implements techniques that help the client gain a realistic and acceptable view of self. Selected interventions to help clients with self-concept disturbances follow. Numerous community self-improvement programs are also available, many of which emphasize the need for individuals to take charge of their lives, to take responsibility for their actions, to think positively rather than negatively, and to become more assertive.

It is important for both the nurse and the client to realize that changes in self-concept require an extended period of time. Although varying from person to person, this may take several months or years. It is essential for the client to learn that self-concept or self-image is not etched in stone; it can change and improve in progressive small steps, particularly if the client desires such change.

Identifying Areas of Strength

Healthy people often perceive their problems and weaknesses more clearly than their assets and strengths. Average well-functioning persons with some college education, when asked to write down their strengths, are able to list only five or six; however, the same persons can list three to four times as many problems or areas of weakness (Otto 1965, p. 34).

Because people with low self-esteem tend to focus on their limitations, they may list even fewer strengths and many more problems. When a client has difficulty identifying personality strengths and assets, the nurse must provide the client with a framework to follow. Interests, abilities, and past accomplishments and experiences need to be included. An abbreviated framework for identifying personality strengths has been developed at the University of Utah. It is shown in the accompanying box. Such an inventory has the following advantages.

- It can result in a more well-rounded self-concept and more positive self-esteem.
- It can help mobilize health and regenerative processes.
- It can help the person to become more aware of the strengths of others and thus facilitate relationships. The person begins to see others' previously unrecognized strengths or "good side."

Developing Behavior Specificity

Many people overgeneralize and think in unspecific ways. The nurse can assist clients to think more clearly and to become more behavior specific in language and thought. Crouch and Straub (1983, p. 71) offer the following strategies for developing behavior specificity.

Framework for Identifying Personality Strengths

- *Spectator sports and similar activities.* The rationale here is that the client's current interest or participation in spectator sports, as well as past interests which he recalls with pleasure, constitutes a vital spark, is evidence of his creative engagement with life, and, in most instances, presages a movement in the direction of health.

- *Sports and activities.* Taking part in a program of bodybuilding, conditioning, or rehabilitative exercises or similar physical regimens, including an interest (and anticipated future participation) in sports and outdoor activities.

- *Hobbies and crafts.* Participating, or having participated in, some hobby or craft activity, and having the desire to start or resume a hobby, craft, or similar pursuit.

- *Expressive arts.* Past or current interest in writing, painting, sketching, or music appreciation with a desire to participate in one of the expressive arts.

- *Health status.* Desire to maintain or regain his health, as well as having an interest or ability to carry through with regimens and treatments designed to foster and facilitate health.

- *Education, training, and related areas.* Any education is seen as a personality asset—vocational trade or technical training, scholastic honors, self-education or a desire to obtain further education or training.

- *Work, vocation, job, or position.* Successful on-the-job performance or enjoyment in his work, a sense of pride in work or duties, earned seniority or recognition for work performed.

- *Special aptitudes or resources.* Included here are such diverse factors as sales ability, aptitude for mathematics or some other subject, ability to fix mechanical things, a "green thumb," ability to construct or teach, knowing how to make a good impression on people.

- *Strengths through family and others.* Such sources of strengths as a spouse or children, relationships with parents, in-laws, or relatives who give love and understanding.

- *Intellectual strengths.* Ability to apply reason to problem solving, do original, creative, and critical thinking, accept new ideas, work on broadening his mind through reading, conversation, and sharing ideas; the capacity to learn and enjoy learning.

- *Aesthetic strengths.* Recognizing and enjoying beauty, and being able to use the sense of beauty to enhance the physical environment.

- *Organizational strengths.* Capacity for systematic planning, developing sound short- and long-range goals, and organizing resources, energy, and time to achieve such goals; the ability to assign and carry out priorities and to coordinate or lead the efforts and labor of others in relation to specific tasks.

- *Imaginative and creative strengths.* Such characteristics as creativity, imagination, and inventiveness for the development of new and different ideas in connection with his home, family, work, or social relationships.

- *Relationship strengths.* Ability to make people feel comfortable and the capacity to enjoy being with people, being aware of people's needs and feelings, being able to listen, and being patient with children as well as with adults.

- *Spiritual strengths.* Religious faith or love of God, membership and participation in church and related activities, and the capacity to express moral and religious values in living, that is, "living what one believes."

- *Emotional strengths.* Capacity to give and receive warmth, affection, and love; ability to "take" anger and to feel and express a wide range of emotions; capacity for empathy.

- *Other strengths.* Included here are the ability to use humor, to "laugh" at oneself and take "kidding"; having a liking for adventure or pioneering; having sticktoitiveness, perseverance, and the drive or will needed to get things done.

Source: H. A. Otto, The human potentialities of nurses and patients, *Nursing Outlook,* August 1965, 13:32–35. Reprinted with permission.

1. *Define goals clearly.* For example, in response to the question "How would you like to feel differently about yourself?" the client may give an unspecific, subjective, and unmeasurable answer such as "better," "happier," or "not so uptight." To help the client, the nurse needs to bring unspecific answers into focus. This can be done by inquiring, for example, "How will you know you are better?" or "What do you mean by 'uptight'?" or "If I were to observe you now in your usual activities and then after you had made these changes, how could I tell you had achieved them?" Open-ended questions that probe into the who, what, how much, when, where, and

how of thought and behavior help the client and the nurse develop a clearer understanding of the individual, the problem, and the goals.

When formulating goals, and strategies for achieving them, and nurse needs to assess the client's ideal self and perceived self, along with the amount of discrepancy between them. Teaching clients about perceived self and ideal self can assist them in exploring areas in which they may be unduly biased. It is also of value for subsequent exploration and assessment. For example, if clients express discouragement about their behavior in a situation, the nurse could say, "Ideally, how do you think you should have acted or reacted?" and then "How do you perceive you actually acted?" Some situations involve complications that are beyond the person's control; such questioning will help clarify that for the client.

2. *Help the client think clearly.* Clients with low self-esteem tend to think negatively and irrationally. For example, a client with low self-esteem who has followed through on homework for three out of seven days might say, "There was no excuse; I failed," or "I didn't follow through; I can't do anything right." When responding, the nurse should avoid contradicting the client but need not accept the client's evaluation as accurate. The nurse might ask, "What exactly did you not follow through with?" or "How does not doing the homework perfectly mean you can't do anything right?"

Changing Language Patterns

Helping clients to change language patterns from passive phrases to more active phrases can help them assume greater responsibility for their power. Examples of passive phrases and alternate active phrases follow:

It makes me . . . (passive)
I choose to . . . *or* I do. (active)

I have to . . . (passive)
I want to . . . (active)

I can't . . . (passive)
I won't . . . *or* I choose not to . . . (active)

Changing language patterns does not alter a person's beliefs, but the process of recognizing and modifying language helps the person consider habitual as well as alternate ways of thinking and believing. To encourage the use of more active language, the nurse may have the client initially listen for passive language without modifying it and then deliberately notice passive language and modify it. It is also important for clients to gain awareness of their overall feeling states when using passive or active language.

Encouraging Positive Self-Evaluation

Persons with high self-esteem express positive self-evaluation more frequently than negative self-evaluation. Persons with low self-esteem, by contrast, frequently make negative self-evaluations and rarely give themselves positive feedback. Therefore, clients with low self-esteem need help in developing more positive thoughts and images about themselves. Strategies include modeling, praise or recognition, positive self-feedback, and visualization.

Modeling The nurse can model positive self-statements for the client by saying such things as "I did a good job painting my recreation room last weekend," or "I am improving my cooking," or "I am proud of the produce I'm getting from my vegetable garden."

Praise To help the client make the transition to self-recognition, the nurse provides honest, positive feedback. For example, the nurse might say, "I think you did a really fine job," or "It sounds like you worked very hard and have done well."

Positive Self-Feedback To help clients begin making positive self-statements, the nurse may implement some of the following strategies.

1. Ask the client: "Tell me some things you have done recently that you feel good about," or "Tell me some things you like about yourself."

2. Ask clients to develop a list of accomplishments they feel good about and a list of characteristics they like about themselves. Accomplishments, behaviors, and characteristics that hold high significance for the person are preferred, since they incorporate a sense of competence, virtue, and power. Frequent reference to this list or to one attribute on the list is encouraged.

3. Reduce negative self-feedback through thought-stopping techniques. For example, every time the client begins to think negatively about self, ask the client to say mentally, "Stop," or "No," or "Think about now," and then attend to the details of the present experience.

Visualization Because strong positive images or expectations often become self-fulfilling, visualization, or imagery procedures, can be used to enhance self-esteem. Positive images of desired changes are consciously imagined. This can be a powerful tool for achieving goals and gaining a positive self-concept. To strengthen goals with visualization, the client:

1. Sets a positive goal or image, such as "I am talking with someone at a party" or "I am saying to my family that I need some help from them to be able to manage work and home responsibilities."

2. Relaxes and slowly repeats the goal-phrase several times.

3. Closes the eyes and visualizes the goal-phrase on a written page.

4. Envisions self as having accomplished the goal.

Because a person's receptivity to positive suggestions is greater when that person is deeply relaxed, deep-breathing exercises, progressive relaxation techniques, meditation, and self-hypnosis are often introduced before imagery techniques are used in individual and group self-involvement programs. The nurse may refer clients to specific community programs.

Enhancing Self-Esteem in Children and Adolescents

The roles of parents and teachers are of great significance in determining children's self-concept. Children are able to grow in self-confidence, personal competence, and independence if they can develop five basic attitudes, involving (a) security and trust, (b) identity, (c) belonging, (d) purpose, and (e) personal competence (Reasoner 1983, p. 55). Parents and teachers have specific roles and responsibilities in helping children develop these five basic attitudes. The nurse can be instrumental in helping parents learn their supportive role.

Security and Trust
This first step in the development of self-esteem can be achieved by providing the child with well-defined limits, i.e., what is expected in terms of behavior and what has to be done to get approval. Limits need to be enforced consistently by all involved adults. Inconsistency tends to create anxiety and weakens feelings of security. Rules or standards need to be reasonable and broad enough to serve as general guidelines in new situations, such as in a neighbor's house, a friend's yard, or school classroom. Standards needs to be established for the treatment of others, respect for the property of others, the value of honesty, and routines such as getting ready for school in the morning, doing homework, completing chores, and going to bed at night.

Systems such as checklists, charts, and calendars can serve as reminders of what is expected and also enable children to monitor their own performance. Conforming to expectations builds positive self-esteem. Self-monitoring builds a sense of pride and provides opportunities for positive recognition as opposed to only negative feedback for uncompleted chores.

Preparing the child for what to expect if standards are *not* met is also effective in encouraging desired behavior and discouraging misbehavior. Restricting privileges tends to be more effective than scolding or lecturing and helps children learn the consequences of their behavior.

To feel secure, children also need to believe that the adults responsible for them are dependable and can be counted on. Adults, therefore, must serve as role models for appropriate behavior.

Identity
The second step in developing self-esteem is a strong sense of identity. Children need to feel they are unique. A child's identity is strengthened when the child is given positive feedback, recognition of strengths, love and acceptance, and help in assessing strengths and shortcomings.

Children need positive feedback from the people of greatest significance to them: parents, grandparents, older siblings, teachers, and close friends. The kind of feedback given can be more significant than the child's actual level of performance. Positive feedback enhances a child's sense of identity and self-concept. No feedback is likely to make a child hesitant and unsure in new situations. Predominantly negative feedback can give a child a negative self-image.

Adults foster a strong self-concept by recognizing a child's strengths. Parents and teachers who focus on the child's shortcomings and devote extra time to only those areas considered weak contribute to the child's negative feelings. Adults need to point out the child's special talents and qualities, such as an attractive smile, skill at playing games, desire to help others, and a strong sense of right and wrong.

Before they can accept themselves, children need to feel loved and accepted. Adults can demonstrate this by taking time to be with the child, to listen, to read, to play, or to just be there. Physical contact—a hand on the shoulder, or a hug—usually conveys warmth and caring more tellingly than words.

Children need to learn to assess their own level of performance and to build confidence in their own judgment. Even though positive feedback from others is always important, children also need to learn to rely on their own judgment. They can be encouraged to evaluate their performance through test results, grades, or other objective measures.

Belonging
Feeling socially accepted is important to children. Just as children need to feel unique, so do they need to feel just like everyone else. They need to dress the same, talk the same, and be in the same club. A sense of belonging can be developed through a family that is united. The family unit enables children to learn how to function as group members, to learn that they cannot always be first or have their way, and to learn that they need to handle their own share of responsibilities. In the family unit and in groups, children learn sensitivity and concern for others. Parents and group leaders can foster this concern by encouraging children to express empathy for others and to find ways to help others. Learning how to be of service to others and how to be a friend builds a sense of belonging and reduces feelings of alienation.

Purpose
Children need a sense of purpose to provide direction to their lives and a basis for success, fulfillment, and, therefore, a positive self-concept. Adults can help a child develop a sense of purpose by setting reasonable expectations, by helping the child set realistic goals, by conveying faith and confidence in the child's ability to achieve

the goals, and by helping the child expand interests, talents, and abilities.

Children tend to work toward expectations that are set for them by parents or teachers, especially if the goals are within their capabilities and the adults are confident the children can achieve them. If expectations are too high or too low, motivation is reduced. Expectations that are long-term and relatively general put less pressure on the child and tend to enhance motivation (Reasoner 1983, p. 60). For example, expecting a child to improve general math skills is more motivating and less stressful than expecting an A on the next math test. To encourage children to try new challenges and reach new levels of performance, adults can expose children to new experiences. For instance, watching a demonstration on how to cook Chinese food, observing a highly skilled gymnast's performance, or talking with a fireman can help children identify their own goals. The more opportunities children have, the more likely they will be motivated to learn and to acquire new skills.

Children need to help to be specific in defining what they want to learn or how to solve a problem. Parents can help by assisting children to identify the sequence of steps needed to achieve a goal or solve a problem. When a child sets a goal, involved adults should convey faith in the child's ability to achieve the goal. Children who sense a parent's or teacher's confidence in them tend to increase their efforts toward, and their chances for, success.

Personal Competence   A sense of personal competence grows out of a sequence of successes. This gives the child a feeling of being able to cope with problems or meet goals. Children with a sense of personal competence have a positive approach to solving problems, tend to achieve success, and feel responsible for their own actions. Children who lack a sense of personal competence are overwhelmed by problems and may attribute lack of success to fate or being victimized. Parents can foster a feeling of competence by helping the child achieve the goals. To do this, the parent needs to do the following:

1. Develop a plan of action by having the child list the steps to be taken or review alternatives for achieving the goals. Parents should avoid prescribing what to do. Directing tends to foster dependency rather than independence. The child needs the freedom to make final decisions on how a plan should proceed.

2. Provide encouragement and support while monitoring the child's progress. From time to time, the parent needs to check on the child's progress, helping assess what might still need to be done, fostering consideration of other resources, or—most important—praising the child's efforts and achievement.

3. Provide feedback that will help the child determine whether the goal has been achieved. This should include

more sharing of the joy of accomplishment and factual comparative information than judgment or praise, although some children value an extrinsic reward more highly. However, children need to learn to become less dependent on extrinsic or tangible rewards. Excessive praise also can make some children more dependent rather than less dependent (Reasoner 1983, p. 62).

Enhancing Self-Esteem in Older Adults

There is a wide variation in the way older adults perceive themselves; most, however, benefit from having their independence fostered. Low self-esteem is often associated with the dependence that accompanies the declining physical and mental capacities related to aging. The nurse can foster the older adult's independence and a more positive self-concept by doing the following (Hirst and Metcalf 1984, p. 76):

1. Encourage clients to participate in planning their care, and involve them in decision making. For example, encourage clients to choose what to wear or what activities to participate in, and consult them about food preferences.

2. Encourage clients to collect numerous objects around them. These establish one's territory or physical space as one's own.

3. Ask permission before putting the client's clothing (e.g., dressing gown, nightclothes) or other objects into the

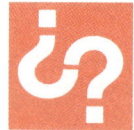

RESEARCH NOTE

Can the Elderly Increase Their Life Satisfaction and Self-Esteem?

The purpose of this study was to investigate whether elderly black females could be provided with a means for improving their perceptions of life satisfaction and self-esteem through regular practice of meditation/relaxation skills. The results of study indicated that the group who participated did report greater life satisfaction and self-esteem than the group that did not participate.

Implications: Nurses can help elderly clients improve their life satisfaction and self-esteem.

B. L. Thomas, Self-esteem and life satisfaction, *Journal of Gerontological Nursing,* December 1988, 14:25–30, 35–36.

client's locker or closet. To do so without permission would deny the existence of the client's personal space and can be perceived as disrespectful.

4. Listen to what the client is saying. Elderly people need to know their comments are valued.

5. Allow the client sufficient time to complete an interaction or activity. Older adults are often slow to respond. Attempts to hurry their responses can create anxiety and embarrassment and can lower self-esteem.

6. Receive contributions of thanks or appreciation (e.g., candy or fruit) graciously and sincerely. Having something to contribute helps older adults maintain or enhance their self-esteem.

EVALUATING

To evaluate the achievement of client goals, the nurse obtains data relevant to the outcome criteria established in the planning phase. To elicit such data, the nurse requires communication and interviewing skills such as listening attentively and asking open-ended questions. Observation skills are also essential for evaluating changes in behavior and appearance.

Examples of evaluative statements are "Client verbalized feelings of anger about his paralysis," "Client listed five of her strengths," and "Client described three situations in which he used active language rather than passive language this past week."

NURSING CARE PLAN FOR DAVID GINSBERG

ASSESSMENT DATA

Nursing Assessment

Mr. David Ginsberg is a 30-year-old married lawyer who has been treated for ulcerative colitis for the past few years. Recently, his symptoms have become exacerbated, and it was determined that surgery (an ileostomy) needed to be performed. Since his surgery, Mr. Ginsberg has been embarrassed and angry about his ostomy and refuses to see any of his friends and colleagues. He has refused to look at his stoma and has not permitted his wife to see it. He has not actively participated in self-care activities. On his fourth post-operative day, his newly assigned nurse, Judy Wright, enters his room and introduces herself. Mr. Ginsberg replies, "If you're here to give me my morning care, I want to pass on it today. What's the use of all this? The pouch will get filled up in a short time anyway. I don't particularly feel up to looking at it this morning, and I don't want you or anyone else to see it, either. It's disgusting. Please leave me alone."

Physical Examination

Height: 182.9 cm (6′)
Weight: 76 kg (165 lb)
Temperature: 37 C (98.6 F)
Pulse rate: 76 BPM
Respirations: 20 per minute
Blood pressure: 126/80 mm Hg
Skin warm, dry, and pale
Ileostomy stoma 2.5 cm midline; skin of lower abdomen pink and intact

Diagnostic Data

RBC: 3.4 ml/μL
Hgb: 10.2 grams/L
Hematocrit: 34%
Urine: Negative
Colon x-ray film: Diffuse lesions left colon

CARE PLAN

Nursing Diagnosis	Client Goals and Outcome Criteria	Nursing Interventions and Rationales	Evaluation
Body image disturbance related to ileostomy (fecal diversion) resulting in refusal to touch or look at body part, refusal to participate	Client Goal: Accept altered body image Outcome Criteria: Client views stoma by day 3.	Establish a trusting relationship with client. *Rationale:* Trust in the caregiver will encourage the client to express the way he feels, thinks, or views himself. Encourage client and significant others to verbalize their feelings about an ostomy.	He voiced his concern regarding his wife's reaction to his stoma and fecal diversion. He feared she may find him unattractive and per-

Nursing Diagnosis	Client Goals and Outcome Criteria	Nursing Interventions and Rationales	Evaluation
in self-care, withdrawal from social contacts and signs of grieving.	Begins to participate in stoma care by day 5. Participates in self-care activities like bathing and shaving by day 4. Verbalizes feelings about body changes by day 2.	*Rationale:* Feelings must be recognized before they can be dealt with effectively. Listen to client and significant others and show interest and concern rather than giving advice. *Rationale:* People generally clarify problems and solutions if they are permitted to express their thoughts and feelings. Allow the client to respond to loss of body function and changed body image with denial, shock, anger, depression, and other grieving behaviors. *Rationale:* These are normal reactions in the grieving process. Support client's strengths and assist him to look at himself in totality. *Rationale:* Focuses attention away from limitations and increases awareness of strengths. Encourage and provide opportunities for self-care of ostomy. *Rationale:* Independence in self-care increases self-esteem. Provide for opportunity for client to meet with other ostomates. *Rationale:* Provides a good support system and reinforcement.	haps repulsive. He also felt he would not be socially acceptable to his friends, colleagues and his profession with his ileostomy bag, possible odors, etc. He started looking at his stoma when Miss Wright changed his pouch on day 3. On day 5 he empties his pouch whenever necessary and he is beginning to participate in his stoma care. He showers and shaves each morning.
Ineffective individual coping related to depression in response to body image change resulting in verbalization of inability to cope; inability to ask for help; insomnia, lack of grooming, lack of social contact, and anger.	Client Goal: Identify problem and become involved in problem solving. Outcome Criteria: Verbalizes feelings of anger and sadness by day 2. Focuses attention on things that must be done, e.g., stoma care, by day 3. Expresses feelings about body changes by day 2. Shares feelings with wife by day 5.	Assess for causes of depression. *Rationale:* Identification of causes allows for more effective interventions. Assess client's coping status. *Rationale:* Will aid in determining whether coping behaviors are effective or ineffective in client's problem-solving process. Use active listening. *Rationale:* Aids in identifying client's needs and problems. Provide a nonthreatening environment. *Rationale:* Client will be less fearful of verbalizing concerns. Determine support persons and resources available to client and the responses of support persons. *Rationale:* These responses influence the client's acceptance of his altered appearance and behavior. Allow for client's input regarding sequence of care.	Client has begun to verbalize his feelings about his altered physical state with his wife, the nurses, and the social worker. He now participates in the care of his ostomy. He has accepted social visits from a few close friends. He states, "I think this condition is manageable. I'll just have to work at it." Client meets with ostomal therapist and ostomate from ostomy association on day 4.

Nursing Diagnosis	Client Goals and Outcome Criteria	Nursing Interventions and Rationales	Evaluation
		Rationale: Gives client sense of control and decreases sense of helplessness.	
		Be supportive of client's effective coping behaviors.	
		Rationale: Will assist client with maintaining self-concept and his relationship with others.	
		Discuss appropriate resources and initiate referrals as necessary.	
		Rationale: Will provide support system and aid client in coping.	

CHAPTER HIGHLIGHTS

► A healthy self-concept, or positive self-esteem, is essential to a person's physical and psychologic well-being.

► Self-concept is sometimes referred to as the cognitive component of the self system and self-esteem as the affective component.

► Self-concept and self-esteem are closely related, since self-esteem is "how I feel about how I see myself."

► Components of self-concept include body image, role performance, personal identity, and self-esteem.

► A person's self-perception can differ from the person's perception of how others see the person and from how the person would like to be.

► From the hour of birth, interactions with significant others create the conditions that influence self-esteem throughout life.

► When individuals are able to conceptualize the self, they begin a lifelong process of deciding whether and to what extent they are valuable and worthy.

► Individuals who grow up in families whose members value each other are likely to feel good about themselves.

► Most individuals feel good about themselves in some ways and bad about themselves in other ways.

► The development of self-esteem can be seen as a process of establishing a sense of security, a sense of identity, and a sense of belonging.

► When children feel secure and accepted, they can be encouraged to set goals for themselves.

► If adults help children to accomplish goals that are important to them, children begin to develop a sense of personal competence and independence.

► Four elements of experience that affect the development of self-esteem are significant others, social role expectations, psychosocial development crises, and communication/coping styles.

► Adults base their self-concept on how they perceive and evaluate their performance in the areas of work, intellect, appearance, sexual attractiveness, particular talents, ability to cope and to resolve problems, independence, and interpersonal interactions.

► An individual's functional level of overall self-esteem may change markedly from day to day and moment to moment.

► Because a healthy self-concept is basic to health, one of the nurse's major responsibilities is to assist clients whose self-concept is disturbed to develop a more positive and realistic image of themselves.

► A trusting client-nurse relationship is essential for the effective assessment of a client's self-concept, for providing help and support, and for motivating client behavior change.

READINGS AND REFERENCES

SUGGESTED READINGS

Meissner, J. E. February 1980. Semantic differential scales for assessing patients' feelings. *Nursing 80* 10:70–71.

This article presents a semantic differential scale on which clients are asked to check the boxes that most closely describe their feelings, e.g., "lonely," "nervous," "indifferent," "calm," and "dejected."

Self-esteem and health. August 1983. *Family and Community Health* 6: entire issue.

Articles in this issue deal with self-esteem and physical health, self-esteem throughout the lifespan, the evaluation of self-esteem, and the enhancement of self-esteem in children, adolescents, and adults.

RELATED RESEARCH

Baird, S. E. January/February 1985. Development of a nursing assessment tool to diagnose altered body image in immobilized patients. *Orthopedic Nursing* 4:47–54.

Thomas, B. L. December 1988. Self-esteem and life satisfaction. *Journal of Gerontological Nursing* 14:25–30, 35–36.

Volden, C.; Langemo, D.; Adamson, M.; Oechsle, L. February 1990. The relationship of age, gender, and exercise practices to measures of health, life-style and self-esteem. *Applied Nursing Research* 3:20–26.

SELECTED REFERENCES

Barry, P. D. 1989. *Psychosocial nursing assessment and intervention: Care of the physically ill person.* 2d ed. Philadelphia: J. B. Lippincott Co.

Beck, A. T. 1979. *Cognitive theory of depression.* New York: The Guilford Press.

Burns, R. B. 1979. *The self concept in theory, measurement, development, and behavior.* London: Longman Group Ltd.

Carpenito, L. J. 1989. *Nursing diagnosis: Application to clinical practice.* 3d ed. Philadelphia: J. B. Lippincott Co.

Crosby, R. September 1982. Self-concept development. *The Journal of School Health* 52:432–36.

Crouch, M. A., and Straub, V. August 1983. Enhancement of self-esteem in adults. *Family and Community Health* 6:65–78.

Ellis, A., and Harper, R. A. 1975. *A new guide to rational living.* North Hollywood, Calif.: Wilshire Book Co.

Erikson, E. H. 1963. *Childhood and society.* 2d ed. New York: W. W. Norton and Co.

Gillies, D. A. September/October 1984. Body image changes following illness and injury. *Journal of Enterostomal Therapy* 11:186–89.

Goldin, J. November/December 1985. The influence of self-image upon the performance of nursing home staff. *Nursing Homes* 34:33–38.

Hamachek, D. E. 1978. *Encounters with self.* 2d ed. New York: Holt, Rinehart and Winston.

Hirst, S. P., and Metcalf, B. J. February 1984. Promoting self-esteem. *Journal of Gerontological Nursing* 2:72–77.

Husted, G. L., Miller, M. C., Wilczynski, E. M. May 1990. 5 ways to build your self-esteem. *Nursing 90* 20:152, 154.

Kim, M. J.; McFarland, G. K.; and McLane, A. M. 1989. *Pocket guide to nursing diagnoses.* 3d ed. St. Louis: C. V. Mosby Co.

Mixson, K. November/December 1989. How to enhance our self-esteem. *Advanced Clinical Nursing* 4:12–14.

Muhlenkamp, A. F., and Sayles, J. A. November/December 1986. Self-esteem, social support, and positive health practices. *Nursing Research* 35:334–38.

Nelson, P. B. February 1990. Intrinsic/extrinsic religious orientation of the elderly: Relationship to depression and self-esteem. *Journal of Gerontological Nursing* 16:29–37.

Norris, J., and Kunes-Connell, M. December 1985. Self-esteem disturbance. *Nursing Clinics of North America* 20:745–61.

Oldaker, S. M. December 1985. Identity confusion. Nursing diagnoses for adolescents. *Nursing Clinics of North America* 20:763–73.

Otto, H. A. August 1965. The human potentialities of nurses and patients. *Nursing Outlook* 13:32–35.

Reasoner, R. W. August 1983. Enhancing self-esteem in children and adolescents. *Family and Community Health* 6:51–64.

Roy, S. C. 1984. *Introduction to nursing. An adaptation model.* 2d ed. Englewood Cliffs, N.J.: Prentice-Hall, Inc.

Sanford, L. T., and Donovan, M. E. 1984. *Women and self-esteem.* New York: Penguin Books.

Smith, M. J. 1975. *When I say no, I feel guilty.* New York: Bantam Books.

Stanwyck, D. J. August 1983. Self-esteem through the life span. *Family and Community Health* 6:11–28.

Sullivan, H. S. 1950. *The interpersonal theory of psychiatry.* New York: W. W. Norton and Co.

Sundeen, S. J.; Stuart, G. W.; Rankin, E. A. D.; and Cohen, S. A. 1989. *Nurse-client interaction.* 4th ed. St. Louis: C. V. Mosby Co.

Sexuality

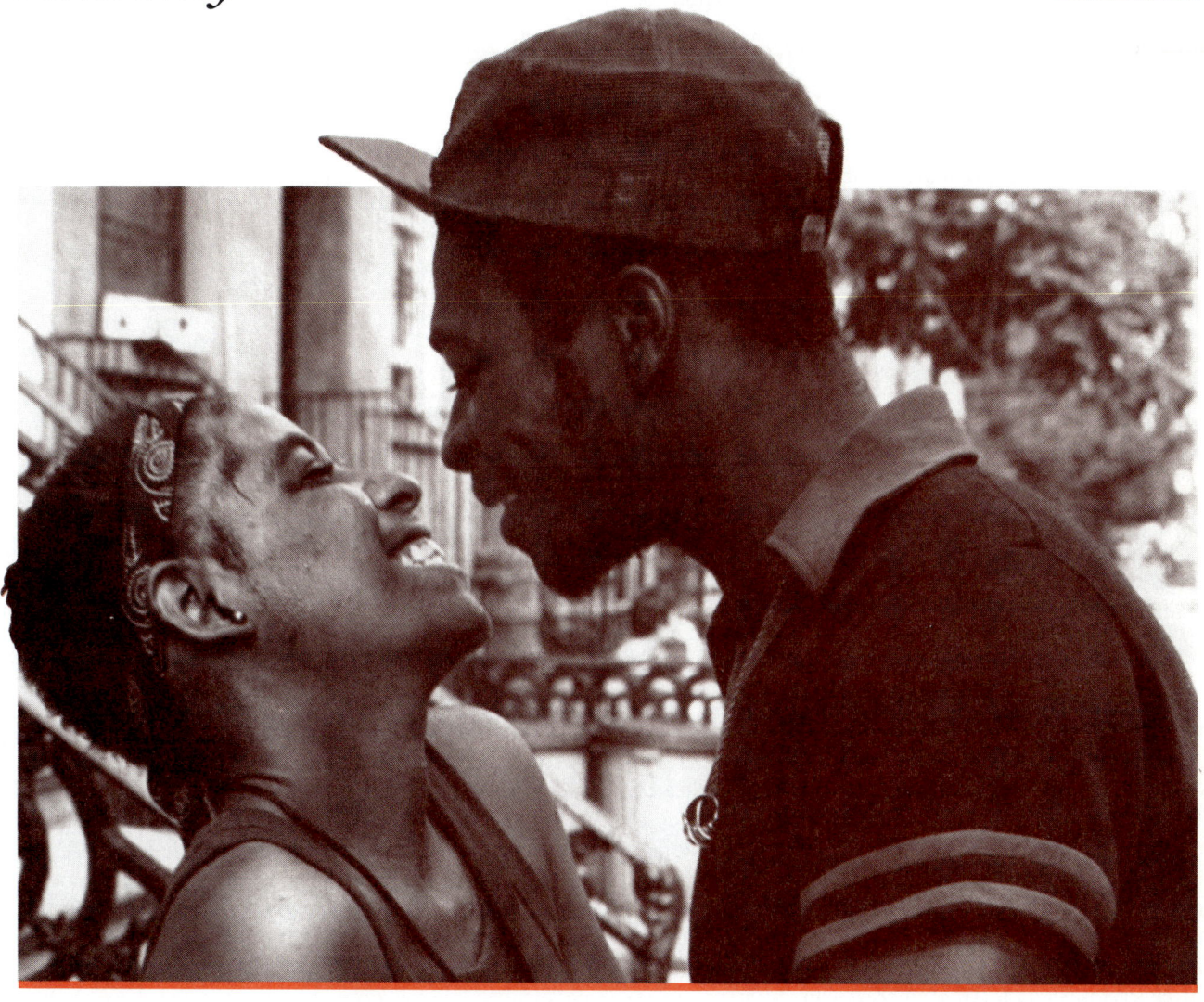

CONTENTS

OBJECTIVES

- Describe selected aspects of sexuality.

- Identify key aspects of the development of sexuality from the prenatal period to late adulthood.

- Compare selected physical and psychologic sexual stimulation patterns.

- Identify physiologic changes occurring in males and females during each phase of the sexual response as described by Masters and Johnson.

- List factors that affect an individual's sexual attitudes and behaviors.

- Give examples of how to obtain data about sexual functioning when conducting a health history.

- Identify factors contributing to sexual dysfunction.

- List factors that increase and decrease sexual motivation.

- Describe common problems of genital sexuality and possible causes.

- Identify common illnesses affecting sexuality.

- Compare selected intervention models for sexual counseling.

- Describe key points about breast and testicular self-examinations to include in health teaching.

- Identify essential aspects about selected contraceptive methods to include in health teaching.

- Describe guidelines for the prevention of sexually transmitted diseases.

- Describe essential outcome criteria that permit evaluation of client progress toward meeting planned goals.

SEX AND SEXUALITY

Sexuality is an integral characteristic of every human being. We are all born with the capacity to function as sexual beings. Clients do not leave their sexuality behind when they enter the health care system—their sexuality comes along as part of the whole person. Professional nurses, as health care providers focusing on the holistic nature of care, have a responsibility to provide effective sexual health care for their clients.

A holistic approach to client health care needs indicates that all aspects of being interact. Thus, sexuality influences and is influenced by the biologic, psychologic, sociologic, and spiritual aspects of being. The need to acknowledge and deal with issues of sexuality in health care practice cannot be overemphasized. Until fairly recently, health care has treated sexuality with benign neglect or has actively discouraged it as a focus of interest. Nursing has been as slow as the other health professions to identify sexuality as significant to health care. The difficulty of dealing with sexual issues continues today (Douglas, Kalman, and Kalman 1985). The evidence reinforces the need for improving nurses' ability to deal with sexual issues.

For nurses practicing in North America today, sexuality is a much more complex issue than it was for nurses in the past. Changes in beliefs, attitudes, and behaviors (and the resulting conflicts) have produced uncertainty and a need to assess nurses' understanding of and attitudes toward the many variations of sexuality. The multicultural nature of North American society has also been a major influence on sexuality, as has the vast increase in mass communication. The impact of such influence groups and movements as the women's movement, gay liberation, handicapped groups, and the "moral majority" has been powerful and is still creating change. To help clients deal with issues of sexual health, nurses must be aware of these multiple factors and must integrate them into effective sexual health care plans.

The words *sex* and *sexuality* are used interchangeably, and often incorrectly, to define different aspects of sexual being. **Sex** is the term most commonly used to denote biologic male or female status, but it is also used to describe specific sexual behavior, such as sexual intercourse. Examples of such usage include the labeled boxes on questionnaire forms to indicate male or female (M☐, F☐) and the question "How many partners have you had sex with since your last visit?" asked in a sexually transmitted disease clinic.

The more appropriate and descriptive term when dealing with sexual issues is **sexuality,** which "includes all of those aspects of the human being that relate specifically to being boy or girl, woman or man, and is an entity subject to lifelong dynamic change. Sexuality reflects our human character, not solely our genital nature. As a function of the total personality, it is concerned with the biological, psychological, sociological, spiritual, and cultural variables of life, which, by their effect on personality development and interpersonal relations, can in turn offer social structure" (Sex Information and Education Council of the United States 1980, p. 8). Although sexuality is an integral part of the whole human being, it can also be categorized and studied according to three separate aspects: (a) biologic sex, (b) gender identity, and (c) gender role.

Biologic sex includes all of the human being's genetically determined anatomy and physiology, which is also influenced by intrauterine conditions. The result of genetic plus other prenatal factors usually is clearly developed primary sex characteristics or variations of these characteristics, called ambiguous sex.

Gender identity is the individual's persisting inner sense of being male or female, masculine or feminine. Its development is based on biologic sex and sociocultural reinforcement, which begins at birth with identification of the baby as male or female. Ultimate congruence between biologic sex and learned sense of sexual self is the most common outcome of this developmental process. Variations of this congruence are common, principally at periods of significant change in the life span (e.g., adolescence, menopause, climacteric, old age). The term **sexual identity** is sometimes equivalent to **gender identity** but is more commonly used to indicate sexual orientation (e.g., **heterosexual, bisexual, homosexual**).

Gender role includes all behaviors reflecting the individual's learned sense of masculinity and femininity, sex behavior, sexual relationships, and sexual dimorphism. The discerning of a person's gender role is based on observation of the person's behavior. The conceptual distinction between gender identity and gender is for descriptive purposes only; in reality, the two are "opposite sides of the same coin."

THE CONTEXT OF SEXUALITY

Sexuality and the way we respond to it are influenced by a variety of factors. A review of historical, ethnocultural, religious-ethical, and contemporary perspectives on sexuality will help us see sexuality in the context of the broader human experience.

Historical Perspectives

Sexuality, as a part of the human condition, has been with us since the beginning of time. Humankind's understanding of sexuality has evolved over time, changing to adapt to changes in knowledge, beliefs, and values. The earliest clear knowledge of sexuality comes from writings, statues, and paintings as old as 10,000 years. Though some of the earlier paintings and sculptures indicate an awareness of sexuality, they give us no clues as to sexual beliefs or practices. The writings, paintings, and sculptures from 5000 B.C. onward, however, do provide clear information about sexual beliefs, values, laws, and practices; they demonstrate the existence of circumcision, heterosexual genital intercourse, fellatio, anal intercourse, homosexuality, prostitution (male and female), and many other sexual practices.

Historical records from the period after the birth of Christ are even clearer and reveal a great deal about the development of attitudes, beliefs, and laws relating to sexuality. The historical records from Europe (influenced by the Judeo-Christian tradition), the Middle East (predominantly Muslim), India (Hindu), and China (Buddhist and Confucian) show a wide variation in approaches to sexuality. The important message of history is that contemporary approaches to sexuality are part of an ever-evolving process.

Ethnocultural Perspectives

North America is a multicultural, ethnically mixed society. Although the majority of the population traces its roots to Europe, increasingly larger proportions of the population in both the United States and Canada come from non-European roots. Citizenship ceremonies in both countries commonly have participants from up to 50 or more different countries. Native American Indians, African-Americans, Latin Americans, Chinese, East Indians (including Muslim, Hindu, and Sikh), Japanese, and Southeast Asians exemplify the ethnic groups that make up significant portions of our society.

All of these groups have their own ethnic and cultural traditions that influence the ways they view the world and interact with society. Included in these traditions are rules, practices, and values relating to sexuality. Much anthropologic and ethnocultural research indicates that the predominant North American societal approaches to sexuality based on Judeo-Christian traditions are not universal: Many North Americans have strong negative attitudes about homosexuality; in a number of subcultures, however, homosexual behavior is tolerated, and in some instances it has become an integral part of rituals such as coming of age.

Different groups hold diverse attitudes about appropriate sexual behavior, husband/wife roles, childhood sexuality, and nudity. Because clients (and, often, colleagues) may differ in their approaches to sexuality, nurses must be aware of and consider ethnocultural factors when approaching sexual issues in health care. As simple a practice as giving a bed bath can have sexual implications, depending on the cultural traditions of the client and/or nurse.

Religious-Ethical Perspectives

Probably the most obvious influences on the approach to sexuality are religion and ethics. People's dealings with sexuality are affected by beliefs and values derived from either religious traditions or some other value system. One function of religion is to provide guidelines for the conduct of human affairs. These guidelines always include sexuality. The most common approach is for a particular religious group or organization to outline acceptable sexual behavior and acceptable circumstances for the behavior, as well as prohibited sexual behavior and the consequences of breaking the sexual rules. The guidelines or rules may be detailed and rigid or broad and flexible. Within the predominant Judeo-Christian value system in North America, there are variations that, along with beliefs and values from other religious traditions, produce the potential for ongoing societal strain as people attempt to integrate all the differing rules and values.

Although ethics is integral to religion, ethical thought and ethical approaches to sexuality can be viewed separately. Many people and groups have developed written or unwritten codes of conduct based on ethical principles. These principles draw from ethical theories that often cut across religious designations while incorporating important principles from different religious traditions. Again, the crucial issue in religious-ethical matters is understanding, respecting, and working with the person's own religious-ethical value system.

Contemporary Perspectives

The ever-evolving knowledge, beliefs, values, and attitudes about sexuality cause continuing societal stress. Currently, a major influence on sexual issues is exerted by certain Christian sects. There is increasing pressure to reinforce strict guidelines for sexual behavior based on their particular view of Christian values. These efforts have been aimed not only at the members of those religious sects but also at the law, the media, health care agencies, and groups viewed unfavorably. This has created great controversy, since others in the society are comfortable with and eager to maintain the more flexible values developed over the last few decades (often labeled the "sexual revolution"). Conflict has arisen because many people accept premarital sex, unwed motherhood, homosexuality, and abortion. These conflicts appear destined to continue in the future.

Another major influence on contemporary sexuality is the information explosion. The media (TV, print, movies, video, computer networks) provide continuous output that has major impact on our views of sexuality. Media stars become the role models for acceptable male or female behavior, at the same time creating potential conflicts. The media also reflect changes in society's attitudes toward sexuality. For instance, at one time (the 1950s and 1960s), television shows always portrayed heterosexual couples as married and sleeping in twin beds. Currently they show same-sex, unmarried, and married couples, often in bed together, and—in soap operas—in varying stages of undress.

People respond emotionally to certain issues related to sexuality (e.g., teenage sexuality, contraception, homosexuality, AIDS and other sexually transmitted diseases, abortion, pornography, and sexual abuse). These issues do not have simple solutions, and nurses will certainly confront these issues in their practice. Nurses have a responsibility to be aware of the factors that contribute to possible emotional conflicts and to use this awareness in helping clients develop sexual health on their own terms.

DEVELOPMENT OF SEXUALITY

The development of sexuality in the human begins with conception and is influenced continuously by many factors throughout the life span. A variety of theories try to explain the development of sexuality, including the interaction of biologic and psychosocial factors. The one currently accepted common understanding is that sexuality as a human experience is complex and multiply influenced. Thus, the psy-

chosocial components described here are to be understood as commonly accepted ways of looking at the interactions that influence the development of sexuality. Every society develops expectations about acceptable ways to be sexual. The components outlined in this section also reflect those societal influences and are organized according to previously identified developmental stages, including Erikson's widely accepted model of human development (see Table 24–5).

Prenatal Period and Infancy

Biologic Components   All cells of the body have 23 pairs of **chromosomes,** referred to as the **diploid number.** These cells multiply by dividing in half and producing two new cells, each of which contains 23 pairs of chromosomes. Such cell division is called **mitosis.** However, **sperm** cells (*male gametes,* or male reproductive cells) and egg cells (*ova,* or *female gametes,* or female reproductive cells) have only 23 single chromosomes, referred to as the **haploid number,** the result of specialized cell division called **meiosis.** Thus, when a sperm cell fertilizes an egg cell, the cell produced by their union has the required 23 pairs of chromosomes—23 single chromosomes from the female and 23 single chromosomes from the male.

In the developing human fetus, two of these chromosomes make up the **sex chromosome pair,** which determines whether the gonads will develop as testes or ovaries. The female has two identical sex chromosomes, referred to as XX. The male has two different chromosomes, designated XY; thus one chromosome is the same as the female's (X) but the other is different (Y). Sperm are of two types: an X-bearing sperm, called a **gynosperm,** and a Y-bearing sperm, called an **androsperm.** If a gynosperm fertilizes the egg, the fetus develops into a female, but if an androsperm fertilizes the egg, the fetus will be male.

Androsperm are smaller, have longer tails, move or swim faster, and are more susceptible to vaginal pH and other changes in the environment than are gynosperm. It is believed that for a male to be conceived, intercourse must occur very near or at the time of **ovulation** (the discharge of an ovum from an **ovary,** the organ where it is produced), when androsperm move toward the egg more quickly than gynosperm. A female is thought to be conceived if intercourse occurs a few days before the egg is ready to be fertilized, at which time gynosperm are thought to move more slowly and withstand the relatively acid vaginal fluids secreted, and then to unite with the egg once it is produced.

The most common outcome of the sex-chromosome influence is an infant with a clearly defined male or female anatomy and physiology. The neurologic, vascular, and other tissues are developed well enough at birth to allow the sexual organs to respond to stimulation. This can produce penile **erection** in infant boys and vaginal lubrication in infant girls. The infant's behavior in response to stimulation of the genitals (either by the infant or during washing, etc.)

indicates pleasure on the part of the infant. It is important to be aware that these small responses are reflexogenic and are not to be confused with postpubertal sexual responses. For the infant, this is just another pleasurable feeling.

Psychosocial Components   Much of our understanding of infant development is based on assumptions about the behavior we see. Infants behave in ways that indicate a focus on such basic needs as safety, security, comfort, nutrition, and pleasure. This is the period for development of trust, according to Erikson's model. It is during this period, in response to interactions with parenting figures and others, that infants begin to learn about gender role. From the moment of birth, the approaches and reactions to infants are based, in general terms, on society's guidelines for male and female gender roles. Little boys are talked to differently, handled differently, and expected to react differently than little girls. These adult behaviors are based on what our society believes about male or female gender roles.

There is also evidence, based on observations of behavior, that male and female infants demonstrate **sexual differentiation** in a variety of areas. These include motor activity, musculature, attention span, preference for stimuli, and interactions with parent figures. The origins of these differences are not clearly understood, but their existence demonstrates the complex interaction between biologic and psychosocial components of sexual development.

Early and Late Childhood

Biologic Components   In contrast to the rapid physical growth in other body systems, the anatomic and physiologic components of the sexual self change very little prior to puberty. Structurally, male and female children appear very similar in early childhood, with the genitals being the only obvious difference. Some changes become evident as late childhood progresses, with physical growth occurring fairly rapidly. Boys begin to develop a more solid musculature, and girls generally develop a slighter structure. It also becomes easier to distinguish boys' faces from girls' faces.

Psychosocial Components   The establishment of gender identity is one of the major issues in early childhood. By the age of 4 or 5 years, the combination of biologic and psychosocial factors has usually produced in the child a clear sense of being male or female. At age 3, children are usually able to identify themselves as either boy or girl. This understanding stems from the frequent use of the terms *boy, he, girl,* and *she* in describing the child. At the same time, the child is learning a sense of self through interaction with parent figures. This sense of self usually solidifies at about the same age as the sense of being a boy or a girl, 3 years. Other factors influencing the establishment of gender identity include interaction with parent figures, which provides feedback about gender-appropriate behavior, and

imitation, which allows the child to mimic and receive reinforcement for same-sex parent behaviors. As with infants, parents and other adults interact differently with boys and girls. Physical as well as interpersonal interactions differ, adding to the development of gender identity.

The development of gender role, another major focus during early and late childhood, is accomplished through some of the same mechanisms by which gender identity develops. The developmental task of this period is the acquisition of **sex-typed behaviors,** or **gender-appropriate behaviors,** behaviors that also are reinforced by positive responses from parents and later from others in the wider interpersonal world. These gender-appropriate behaviors can include what clothes are worn, games played, playmates chosen, toys played with, and manner of speech, among many others. The nurse needs to be aware that there is in present-day North America a wide variation in sex-typed or gender-appropriate behaviors. Many children will develop a repertoire of behaviors as part of their gender role, including both gender-appropriate and gender-inappropriate behaviors. It is important *not* to label children on the basis of these variations. Only when there is evidence of problems in gender role or gender identity is there a potential for intervention. Such extremes are termed as **gender dysphoria.**

As development progresses, children continue to be curious about their own and others' bodies. Preschool children express this curiosity during bathing, toileting, swimming, and playing. Such curiosity is an important part of learning and should be responded to with factual information in a matter-of-fact manner. As the child learns more socially acceptable ways of expressing curiosity, usually during the early school years, the need for information is expressed as questions. School-age children ask many questions about sex, which again are best responded to with factual answers. Their questions arise from observing adults interacting, from reading, from sharing stories with peers, and from fantasies. Children develop the capacity for fantasy after the age of 4 or 5.

School-age children also express curiosity about their own and others' bodies. This takes place in individual exploration, in mutual exploration (playing "doctor" or "house"), and by watching adults whenever possible. Mutual exploration involves members of the opposite sex and, because of the sexual separation that occurs in the prepubertal period, members of the same sex. Matter-of-fact, nonjudgmental responses to such behaviors are important in order to avoid children's adopting negative feelings about their own bodies or sexual interaction.

Puberty and Adolescence

Biologic Components   Changes in sexual anatomy and physiology are more profound during puberty than at any other comparable developmental period. These changes are discussed in Chapter 26. **Puberty** refers to the period of physiologic maturation, and **adolescence** refers to the period of psychosocial maturation.

Psychosocial Components

Changes in the psychosocial component of sexuality during adolescence are also profound. They include dealing with altered body image, dealing with changes in the body's functioning, consolidating gender identity, adjusting gender-role behavior, and learning new social-role behaviors.

Physiologic changes during puberty are relatively rapid and dramatic. The adolescent must deal with a body that is larger and proportioned differently and that requires new skills of coordination. In addition, the growth of secondary sexual characteristics and the development of physiologic functioning associated with these changes produce intense psychologic response. Conflicting emotions related to pride, embarrassment, shame, and discomfort require much adult understanding and explanation. Boys react to the comparison of their own changing body to the idealized male bodies in our culture. Height, weight, muscular development, body hair, and size of penis and testicles are all sources of anxiety as the boy compares himself to the ideal. Analogously for girls, height, weight, body shape, breast size, and menstrual cycles are all influenced by idealized norms. Adolescents need to know that there is a wide variation in healthy anatomy and physiology. This reassurance is particularly needed in response to media depictions of idealized male and female bodies. (Media stars never seem to have pimples, body odor, menstrual cramps, or spontaneous erections.)

The activation of sexual response potential during puberty puts a tremendous strain on the adolescent. Because of the hormonal triggers at work, the male body and female body become susceptible to a wide variety of sexually exciting stimuli. Adolescents respond to this new source of pleasurable sensations by engaging in erotic play, either alone through fantasy and masturbation or with others. Erotic play with a partner may include embracing, kissing, petting, and various methods of genital sexual activity.

Such sexual activity may involve partners of the same sex or the opposite sex. For the majority of adolescents, same-sex erotic play is experimental or exploratory. However, adolescents with a homosexual orientation require acknowledgment of and support for their sexual identity, to avoid anxiety, guilt, and negative self-image. Heterosexual and homosexual adolescents alike need both factual information about their bodies and support and reassurance about emotional and other psychosocial responses to their changing bodies and body functions. All adolescents are engaged in developing a clear sense of when and how to respond to intense sexual impulses.

As well as adapting to a changing body, the adolescent has opportunities to consolidate gender identity through psychosocial interactions. It is important during this period for the adolescent to understand that gender identity allows

RESEARCH NOTE

How Can Nurses Assist Gay Clients?

Nurses must meet the challenge of attending to whatever special health care needs their homosexual clients may have; indeed, the alarming rise in the incidence of AIDS brings nurses into increasing contact with the sensitivities, as well as some unusual medical needs, of gay clients.

This study asks and partially answers two questions: (1) How do gay men and lesbians learn they are gay and come to accept their gayness as a positive aspect of self? (2) What health care concerns arise in relation to "coming out" as a homosexual? The study found distinct differences between gay men and gay women in terms of their childhood upbringing and behavior patterns; the genesis of the homosexual orientation for either sex remained obscure, however. The study also found that coming out has four distinct stages: (1) identification of self as gay, (2) cognitive changes in previously held negative notions, (3) acceptance of self, and (4) action.

Implications: Kus asserts that nurses cannot provide adequate care to gay clients unless they understand this process. Nurses who do understand this process can perhaps help gay people to accept their homosexuality as a positive aspect of self.

R. Kus, Stages of coming out: An ethnographic approach. *Western Journal of Nursing Research,* May 1985, 7:177–98.

for wide variation in what constitutes male or female. The distinction between gender identity (maleness/femaleness) and sexual orientation (heterosexual/bisexual/homosexual) must be clarified for the adolescent, particularly in view of the complex signals being received. Gender-role-behavior development also is a source of stress, with frequently conflicting signals about what is gender-appropriate and what is not. There is, as well, an increased expectation for different social-role interactions on the part of the adolescent. The complexity of the influences related to psychosocial development of sexuality makes adolescence a very stressful period of growth and development. All adolescents require a factual, comprehensive knowledge base about biologic and psychosocial factors involved in the development of healthy adult sexuality.

Adulthood and Middle Years

Adulthood is the period when most developmental changes have reached maturity. The adult is both biologically and psychosocially prepared to engage in intimate psychosocial and sexual relationships. Typically, adulthood is seen as a time for developing intimacy with one partner, marrying, and parenting. Currently, a variety of alternatives to this traditional pattern is gaining wider acceptance. Regardless of the pattern of adult interpersonal relationships, sexuality is frequently a crucial component. Society continues to approve the capacity to become involved in a stable, heterosexual relationship as the ideal for adulthood.

Biologic Components Between the ages of approximately 18 and 30 years, the young adult reaches full anatomic and physiologic maturity. Height, weight, body condition, and secondary sexual characteristics are all at their peak. These years are, for the majority of adults, the prime childbearing and child-rearing years. The earlier, unpredictable intensity of sexual feelings experienced during adolescence evens out and becomes more predictable.

Development leading to the middle years includes changes in hormone levels in both men and women. For women, development culminates in the cessation of the menstrual cycle and a decrease in estrogens, leading to such changes as the beginning atrophy of breast and vaginal tissue, delay and decrease in vaginal lubrication during sexual arousal, and loss of elasticity of skin and other tissue. For men the changes involve delay in attaining erection, decrease in size and firmness of erection, decrease in expulsive force of ejaculation, and decrease in volume of semen.

Psychosocial Components Society's expectations for sexual development in adulthood include establishing a permanent intimate relationship with a partner of the opposite sex and bearing and raising children. This expectation may produce stress for many people as individual expectations increasingly differ from this societal "norm." The number of unmarried couples, both heterosexual and homosexual, has increased, as has the number of childless couples. Single parents are becoming more numerous, both as a result of relationship breakups and by choice. These changes in adult role relationships are not universally accepted but must be assessed by the nurse in terms of the overall health of the individual and the relationship.

The establishment of intimate adult relationships produces change in gender-role expectations. Adding to already existing role components are such expectations as partner (husband, wife, spouse), parent, and lover. These new role components require adjusting to patterns of behavior that are still developing. In addition, individual needs and preferences may encourage individuals to develop roles and role behaviors that are not congruent with broader societal expectations, for example, the househusband, woman as primary breadwinner, and commuting spouses.

Sexual interaction in adulthood is a major component of being, whether as part of a stable, intimate relationship or as part of a single life-style. The capacity to interact in sexually satisfying ways is influenced by a number of factors. A good knowledge of one's own body and its capabilities,

as well as knowledge of the partner, is an essential prerequisite. Open communication about sexuality between partners is also an important factor. Knowledge and communication are frequently described as the most crucial factors determining the health of any sexual relationship. Other factors, such as parenting, role changes, and differences in sexual responsiveness, have less influence when knowledge and communication are effective. Sexuality, like any other part of interpersonal relationships, consists of learned beliefs, attitudes, and behaviors. This learning is best accomplished when it is shared by the partners in a relationship.

Late Adulthood

Biologic Components The major biologic changes in the older female include a continued atrophy of vaginal and breast tissue (including loss of elasticity), decrease and slowing of vaginal lubrication during arousal, decreased vaginal expansion, diminished orgasmic intensity, and a more rapid resolution. (See the discussions of sexual stimulation and response patterns, later in the chapter.) Older women do retain the capacity for multiple orgasms.

Sexual changes in the older male include lowered sperm production, reduction in the size and firmness of the testicles, delay in achieving erection, greater ejaculatory control, less myotonia, reduced orgasmic intensity, more rapid resolution, and longer refractory period.

Psychosocial Components Major issues influencing sexual development in late adulthood include adjusting to changing body image, adjusting to changes in family or marital status, retirement, change in body function, and decrease in mobility. Despite all these adjustments, the older adult has the capacity to continue with satisfying interpersonal and sexual relationships indefinitely.

Our society places a high value on youth and youthful beauty. The aging person is unable to match such standards and may respond to changes in body image with lowered self-esteem. Widowhood or widowerhood, loss of contact with grown children, and loss of friends have the potential for creating loneliness and depression.

Lowered self-esteem and loneliness, combined with reduced body function and loss of mobility, can lead to social isolation and loss of interaction opportunities. Society has also made it difficult for older adults to interact sexually because of negative attitudes about sexual activity among the aging. The majority of older adults retain the interest and capacity to engage in satisfying sexual relationships, whose nature is frequently more nurturing and caring and less sexually intense than in earlier years. The greatest predictor of sexual interest and activity in the later years is the pattern of sexual activity and interest throughout life, true for married adults, widowed adults, and single adults—whether heterosexual or homosexual.

PATTERNS OF SEXUAL FUNCTIONING

The interaction of contextual and developmental factors results in people's capacity to function in reciprocal ways as sexual beings. As noted earlier, biologic sex, gender identity, and gender role are the major components of individual sexuality. With a basic understanding of these components, nurses are better able to comprehend sexual functioning.

Gender-Role Behavior

Gender-role behavior is the outward expression of a person's sense of maleness or femaleness as well as the expression of what is perceived as gender-appropriate behavior. Even newborns are influenced by expectations regarding gender-appropriate role behavior, and this influence continues throughout life. Each society or culture establishes boundaries for acceptable gender-role behavior. Congruence between an individual's gender identity and expression of role behavior is the ideal, but this ideal is not always easy to achieve.

Physical structure, variations in the internal sense of what is male or female, family values, and cultural values all influence gender-role behavior. As a result, the limits of appropriate gender-role behavior are fairly flexible in North America. Expected adult male roles include breadwinner, heterosexual lover, father, and athlete. Expected male behaviors include wearing trousers, demonstrating physical strength, and expressing feelings in a controlled fashion. Women are expected to express their emotions more freely and to be more gentle in their physical responses; they also have a broader choice of clothing than men.

These descriptions represent the kinds of gender-role behaviors that are reinforced in our society. However, many individuals today express themselves with gender-role behaviors that do not conform to these stereotypes. This stretching of the boundaries can create stress for the individual and for society. Though there has been more variation in gender roles and gender-role behavior in recent years, these variations frequently are still portrayed as aberrant, humorous, or wrong.

In actuality, however, many people are challenging these stereotypes. Men sport long hair, earrings, and cosmetics. Women wear construction boots, jeans, and men's suits. Men make loving and sensitive single fathers. Women are capably functioning as competitive and assertive executives. Openly gay male and lesbian relationships are on the increase. Sexual activity in older adults is common. Such gender-role behaviors are legitimate expressions of the self as a sexual being. All individuals need sanction of and support for those gender-role behaviors that validate their sense of self. Labeling these behaviors as aberrant and intervening for change should rightly occur only when the behaviors create significant problems for individuals and their relationship with the world.

Sexual Stimulation

The sexually functional human is capable of responding to a wide variety of physical and psychologic stimuli. These stimuli, often called **erotic,** may be real or symbolic. In the right circumstances, imagination, sight, hearing, smell, and touch can all invoke sexual arousal.

Physical Stimulation

Physical stimulation involves touch and/or pressure to parts of the body and may be applied by one's self, by another's body contact or by inanimate objects. Examples include kissing, stroking, hugging, squeezing, breast stimulation, manual stimulation of the genitals, oral-genital stimulation, and anal stimulation. Any of these may be engaged in for sexual pleasure on their own or—as is most common in North America—as prelude to genital intercourse. Physical stimulation used as a prelude to intercourse is called **foreplay** or **precoital stimulation.** Physical stimulation used for sexual pleasure is called **sex play.** Wide variations exist in the amount and types of physical stimulation used by North Americans.

Certain parts of the body are richly supplied with nerve endings and give sexual pleasure when stimulated. These areas are called **erogenous zones.** There is also a psychologic component that involves the linking of particular stimuli to a sexual context. The most common erogenous zones are, of course, the genitals of both sexes. Other areas include the breasts, the mouth, thighs, buttocks, earlobes, neck, and anus; however, stimulation of any body area can become sexually arousing. Erogenous zones adapt rapidly to continuous stimulation by becoming decreasingly responsive. Because touch and pressure receptors respond better to *changes* in stimulation, sexual arousal can be increased by alternating sites of stimulation rather than stimulating one or two areas continuously.

Kissing, which involves the senses of touch, taste, and smell, is unique to humans as a source of erotic stimulation. This type of sexual stimulation ranges from lip-to-lip kissing to deep tongue kissing. Stroking, hugging, and squeezing are behaviors that vary according to the preferences of the individuals involved, extending from light, gentle hugging and stroking, through firm, energetic hugging and stroking, to hard squeezing, pinching, biting, and scratching. These last examples involve some pain, which can be erotically stimulating when engaged in *voluntarily* by sexual partners.

Oral or manual stimulation of the female breasts can produce sexual pleasure. Stimulation of the breasts causes the release of the pituitary hormone oxytocin, which stimulates milk secretion and may cause smooth muscle contractions in the uterus and related structures. Breast stimulation thus can produce pleasurable contractions in the pelvic region. These sensations can be a source of sexual satisfaction on their own and may lead to orgasm, or breast stimulation may be used as an adjunct to other sexual interaction. Nursing mothers may also experience these contractions, and some mothers need reassurance that this is a healthy phenomenon. Stimulation of men's nipples may also produce erotic responses.

Manual stimulation of the genitals may be used to produce **orgasm** (climax of sexual excitement) or as a prelude to sexual intercourse. Manual self-stimulation is called **masturbation.** Reciprocal manual stimulation is called **mutual masturbation.** Stimulation of the penis generally produces a more erotic response than stimulation of the scrotum. The most common form of male masturbation is firm gripping and stroking of the shaft and glans of the penis. Light rubbing or tugging at the **frenulum** (the fold of tissue that connects the lower surface of the glans to the prepuce) can also produce sexual excitement. Whatever method is used, as sexual excitement increases, manipulation often becomes more rapid and intense, until **ejaculation** occurs. After ejaculation, the glans penis is often hypersensitive to touch.

Stimulation of the **clitoris** is usually a major erotic focus for females. This highly sensitive area rarely requires direct stimulation. Rubbing pressure on the **mons pubis (mons veneris),** pulling or rubbing the clitoral hood (prepuce), or pulling on the labia stimulate the clitoral shaft and produce intensely erotic responses. Some women use external manipulation as well as insertion of fingers into the vagina to produce sexual excitement.

Masturbation in itself is neither physically nor mentally harmful. More than 85% of males and 60% of females practice masturbation, ranging in frequency from several times a day to only occasionally. Most men begin to masturbate earlier in life (often before the age of 20 years) than women. Some individuals use sexual implements when masturbating, including vibrators, artificial penises, and other genital substitutes.

There are three forms of oral-genital stimulation: cunnilingus, fellatio, and soixante-neuf. **Cunnilingus** is oral stimulation (kissing, licking, or sucking) of the female genitals, including the mons pubis, vulva, clitoris, labia, and vagina. **Fellatio** is oral stimulation of the penis by licking and sucking. **Soixante-neuf** ("69") is simultaneous oral-genital stimulation by two persons. These practices, like other physical stimulation, may be engaged in for the pleasure they give, including orgasm, or as a prelude to genital intercourse. As with masturbation, there is no evidence that oral-genital contact is harmful. However, some people hold strong negative feelings about these behaviors.

Anal stimulation can be a source of sexual pleasure, since the anus is richly innervated. Oral-anal stimulation is called **anilingus.** Stimulation may also be applied by hands or by sex aids such as vibrators. Because the anus is associated with feces, many people do not include anal stimulation in their sexual repertoire.

Psychologic Stimulation   Although the excitatory process involves physiology, erotic stimulation through smell, taste, hearing, sight, or fantasy is considered psychologic because the responses relate to thought processes and feel-ings. The stimuli evoke pleasant past experiences or hopes and desires. Certain odors (e.g., body odors, perfumes, leather, flowers) can produce erotic responses in sexual situations.

Because of their specific associations, certain sights can also produce erotic responses. The more obvious sights include naked bodies and pictures of naked bodies and sexual acts. Other less obvious sights include romantic photographs, decor, lighting, and colors.

Sexual excitement is often enhanced by sound. The spoken word and music are frequent adjuncts to sexual activity. "Whispering sweet nothings" and "talking dirty" are examples. Music is frequently associated with specific sexual situations.

Most people engage in **sexual fantasy.** The fantasizing usually involves idealized sexual situations but may also include so-called forbidden fantasies: mental imagery of unusual or risqué activities that are out of bounds in real life. People engage in fantasy both during masturbation and when with a partner.

Sexual Response Patterns

Physiologic responses to sexual stimulation are basically the same for all individuals, male or female. However, such responses are highly variable, with differences occurring between males and females, among members of the same sex, and in the same person at different times. The most common form of sexual activity with a partner is heterosexual **genital intercourse,** also known as **coitus** or **copulation.** Penile-vaginal intercourse can be both physically and emotionally satisfying. There are a variety of positions for this kind of intercourse; the most common is lying face to face (with female or male on top). Side-lying, standing, sitting, and rear-entry positions are also used. Side-lying, female-on-top, and rear-entry positions facilitate clitoral stimulation, either by penile contact or manual contact. The choice of intercourse positions and activities depends on physical comfort and beliefs, values, and attitudes about different practices.

The other form of genital intercourse is **anal intercourse,** during which the penis is inserted into the anus and rectum of the partner. Anal intercourse is most commonly practiced by gay men, but some heterosexual couples engage in it as well. Positions for anal intercourse are similar to those for penile-vaginal intercourse, with minor differences due to the position of the anus.

Current practice dictates the use of a condom in both forms of intercourse to prevent the transmission of disease. Because anorectal tissue is not self-lubricating, a lubricant must be used on the condom. Also, since normal bacterial flora from the bowel can produce infection in other parts of the body, the used condom should be removed and another applied before inserting the penis into other body orifices. (Condoms are used for contraception as well as for preventing sexually transmitted diseases. See the discussion of sexual health teaching, later in this chapter.)

Lesbians and gay men engage in a variety of sexual activities that collectively can be labeled intercourse. Oral sex, manual sex, frottage (body rubbing), and the use of sex aids are among these. There is no evidence that this type of sexual interaction is less satisfying than heterosexual penile-vaginal intercourse.

The Sexual Response Cycle

Two primary physiologic changes occur during sexual arousal: **Vasocongestion** (congestion of the blood vessels) and **myotonia** (increased muscle tension). Physiologic changes have been identified in one model of physiologic response that fall into four phases: excitement, plateau, orgasm, and resolution (Masters and Johnson 1966, p. 4). Table 30–1 summarizes the physiologic changes associated with each of the phases of the sexual response cycle in both males and females. It is important to remember that many individual variations in this cycle fall within the norm.

During the **excitement phase,** erotic stimuli cause a gradual increase in the level of sexual arousal. This phase may last minutes to hours. The **plateau phase,** the period during which sexual tension increases to levels nearing orgasm, may last from 30 seconds to 3 minutes. The **orgasmic phase** is the involuntary climax of sexual tension, accompanied by physiologic and psychologic release. This phase is considered the measurable peak of the sexual experience. Although the entire body is involved, the major focus of the orgasm is felt in the pelvic region. The orgasmic phase is short, lasting 3 to 10 seconds. The **resolution phase,** the period of return to the unaroused state, may last 10 to 15 minutes after orgasm, or longer if there is no orgasm.

TABLE 30–1 *Physiologic Changes Associated with the Sexual Response Cycle*

Phase of the Sexual Response Cycle	Signs Present in Both Sexes	Signs Present in Males Only	Signs Present in Females Only
Excitement	Increased muscle tension Moderate increase in heart rate, respirations, and blood pressure Sex flush (less prevalent in men than in women; present in 75% of women) Nipple erection (60% of men and most women)	Penile erection Tensing, thickening, and elevation of the scrotum Partial elevation and increase in size of testicles	Enlargement of the clitoral glans Vaginal lubrication Widening and lengthening of vaginal barrel Separation and flattening of the labia majora Reddening of the labia minora and vaginal wall Breast tumescence and enlarged areolae
Plateau	Increased voluntary and involuntary myotonia Abdominal, intercostal, anal, and facial muscle contraction Accelerated heart rate and respiratory rate, and increased blood pressure Sex flush (appearance in some men late in the phase; spread over the entire body in women)	Increase in penile circumference, at the coronal ridge, and deepening of color 50% increase in testicular size, and elevation close to the perineum Appearance of a few drops of mucoid secretions from the bulbourethral glands	Retraction of the clitoris under the hood Appearance of the orgasmic platform, increase in the size of the outer one-third of the vagina and the labia minora Slight increase in the width and depth of the inner two-thirds of the vagina Further reddening of the labia minora Appearance of a few drops of mucoid secretion from the Bartholin's glands Further increase in breast size and areolar enlargement

Phase of the Sexual Response Cycle	Signs Present in Both Sexes	Signs Present in Males Only	Signs Present in Females Only
Orgasmic	Involuntary spasms of muscle groups throughout the body Diminished sensory awareness Involuntary contractions of the anal sphincter Peak heart rate, respiratory rate, and blood pressure	Rhythmic, expulsive contractions of the penis at 0.8-second intervals Emission of seminal fluid into the prostatic urethra from contraction of the vas deferens and accessory organs (stage 1 of the expulsive process) Ejaculation of semen through the penile urethra and expulsion from the urethral meatus. The force of ejaculation varies from man to man and at different times but diminishes after the first two to three contractions (stage 2 of the expulsive process)	Approximately 5 to 12 contractions in the orgasmic platform at 0.8-second intervals Contraction of the muscles of the pelvic floor and the uterine muscles Varied pattern of orgasms, including minor surges and contractions, multiple orgasms, or a simple intense orgasm similar to that of the male
Resolution	Reversal of vasocongestion; disappearance of all signs of myotonia within 5 minutes Genitals and breasts return to their preexcitement states Sex flush disappears in reverse order of appearance Heart rate, respiratory rate, and blood pressure return to normal Other reactions include sleepiness, relaxation, and emotional outbursts such as crying or laughing	A **refractory period** during which the body will not respond to sexual stimulation; varies, depending on age and other factors, from a few moments to hours or days	

ASSESSING SEXUAL HEALTH

Information about a client's sexual health status should always be an integral part of a nursing assessment. The amount and kind of data collected depend on the context of the assessment, that is, the client's reason for seeking health care and how the client's sexuality interacts with other problems. The nurse's professional preparation is another factor that influences the level of sexual health assessment.

Characteristics of Sexual Health

Lion (1982, pp. 9–10) has described the following characteristics of sexually healthy people:

- Expression of a positive body image
- Cognitive knowledge about human sexuality
- Congruence between biologic sex, gender identity, and gender-role behavior
- Behavior consistent with self-concept
- Awareness of own sexual feelings and attributes
- Capacity for physical and psychosexual responsiveness, which is enhancing to self and others
- Comfort with a range of sexual behavior and life-styles
- Acceptance of responsibility for pleasure and reproduction
- Ability to create effective interpersonal relationships with both sexes
- Value system that is developing and usable

These characteristics reflect the integral, holistic nature of sexuality as part of the human experience, and they provide a useful guide for measuring sexual health.

Integrating Sexuality into the Nursing History

Physiologic assessment should be included in any review of systems, including information on the functioning of the neurologic, cardiovascular, endocrine, and genitourinary systems. Data collected should include not only information about direct sexual functioning but also physiologic information that may relate to sexuality. For example, it is certainly important to collect data about erectile functioning in a diabetic male (cardiovascular, neurologic, and genitourinary systems), but it may also be important to note baldness (integumentary system) as a physiologic influence on sexual self-image.

Collecting such physiologic data for the nursing history does not require extensive or detailed questioning. The screening process of the systems review allows the nurse and client to identify problem areas. For example, answers to the question "Do you have any concerns about the amount or regularity of your menstrual flow?" can give clues to the presence of problems not otherwise identified. Also, questions asked about the functioning of systems directly related to sexuality often provide clients with an opportunity to give clues to sexual concerns or problems. Informing the client of the need for and use of the data reduces the reluctance of the client to talk about sexual issues. The thoroughness of the sexual assessment is directly related to the potential impact of sexuality on the health problem, or vice versa.

Psychosexual assessment should also be a part of the nursing history. Important influences include development, culture, religion, attitudes, and values. Again, specific, detailed questions about psychosexual issues are not necessary in the usual nursing history unless there are clues that potential or actual problems exist. A useful approach to psychosexual assessment is a review of sexual self-concept (see Table 30–2). Manner of dress, tone of voice, and comments about self and relationships with others can all give the nurse opportunities to explore issues of sexual self-concept more fully. Because illnesses and other health concerns can have a strong influence on sexual concept, assessment of these areas often provides the first clues to client concerns.

Watts (1979, p. 1570) outlines four levels of sexual assessment, each of which requires varying degrees of professional competence:

Level 1 focuses on screening for sexual function and dysfunction. It is conducted by the professional nurse during a health history.

Level 2 is a sexual history conducted by a professional nurse who has postgraduate education in sex education and counseling.

Level 3 is a sexual problem history conducted by qualified sex therapists.

TABLE 30–2 *Assessment of Sexual Self-Concept*

Aspect of Self	Assessment Criteria
Sense of being (identity)	Demonstrates a clear sense of self as male or female.
	Demonstrates comfort with own identity.
Physical self (body image)	Demonstrates a realistic perception of own body.
	Demonstrates comfort with own body image.
Social self (role behavior)	Demonstrates congruence between identity and behavior.
	Demonstrates comfort with own role behavior.
Knowledge (self-awareness)	Demonstrates accurate cognitive sexual knowledge.
	Demonstrates realistic sense of self-congruence with others' view.
	Demonstrates comfort with self in relation to others.
Expectations (ideal self)	Demonstrates realistic expectations of sexual being congruent with what is possible.
	Demonstrates comfort with ideal self.
Evaluation (self-esteem)	Demonstrates realistic appraisal of sexual self.
	Demonstrates growth based on realistic evaluation.
	Demonstrates overall positive sense of self.

Level 4 is a psychiatric and psychosexual history conducted by professionals who are specialized in sex therapy.

For the beginner, a basic assessment interview (as part of the health history) is shown in the box on the facing page. Notice that lead-in questions are asked before the questions about sexuality.

Factors Influencing Alterations in Sexual Functioning

To ensure that the assessment data base is complete, the nurse needs to gather information about factors known to alter sexual functioning. The following are some of the factors contributing to sexual dysfunction (Hurley 1986, p. 540):

- Ineffectual or absent role models
- Altered body structure or function due to disease or trauma, drugs, pregnancy or recent childbirth, or anatomic abnormalities of the genitals
- Lack of knowledge or misinformation about sexuality
- Physical abuse (e.g., sexual assault)
- Psychosocial abuse
- Value conflict
- Loss or lack of partner
- Vulnerability

When gathering a data base, the nurse also needs to be aware of common illnesses affecting sexual functioning, changes in sexual motivation, and genital sexual problems.

Common Medical and Surgical Conditions Affecting Sexuality

Heart disease and diabetes mellitus are two common illnesses that frequently influence sexual functioning. Clients with heart disease, particularly those experiencing or at risk for myocardial infarction, are often anxious about or afraid of sexual activity. Concerns about the effect of sexual activity on the heart cause people to restrict or avoid sexual activity. Many men with long-term diabetes mellitus develop erectile dysfunction related to neurologic changes secondary to the disease process.

Spinal cord injury also creates special problems. Because the level of the injury to the spinal cord determines the extent of effects on sexual functioning, individuals may be capable of erection and ejaculation and be fertile, may have psychogenic or reflexogenic genital arousal, or may have no physiologic genital responses.

Any surgical procedure has the potential to alter a person's body image, especially when the surgery involves mutilating, removing, or altering parts of the body. Examples include amputation of a leg, radical neck surgery, excision of large portions of the lower jaw, and ostomies. Impact is even greater when the surgery alters or removes body parts linked directly with sexual functioning, for instance, mastectomy, hysterectomy, and vaginal excision in women; orchiectomy (removal of the testicles), and penectomy in men. Feelings of ugliness and loss of masculinity or femininity are common after these surgeries.

Changes in Sexual Motivation

The urge or desire for sexuality activity is called **libido** (sexual motivation, sex drive). Libido fluctuates within each person and varies from person to person. The range of fluctuation in each individual is broad and is considered a problem only when the client (or those interacting with the client) identifies it as interfering with the ability to have satisfying sexual interactions.

Factors that may contribute to *decreased* sexual motivation include the following:

- *Drugs.* The following decrease sexual drive: all central nervous system depressants (e.g., alcohol, barbiturates, sedatives, morphine, heroin, and methadone), estrogens and adrenal steroids in large doses, certain psychotropic drugs, and some antihypertensive agents, e.g., reserpine (Serpasil) and methyldopa (Aldomet).
- *Depression.* This condition slows all body functions and lowers libido. It can affect both the depressed and nondepressed partner.
- *Disease.* Libido diminishes with general ill health and chronic diseases that cause debility or pain. Any disorder that causes dyspareunia (e.g., vaginitis, genital herpes, and **imperforate hymen**) also lowers libido.
- *Pregnancy.* Pregnancy affects sexuality if it is associated with physical discomfort, fear of injury to the fetus, or

perceived loss of attractiveness. For about 4 weeks following delivery, libido is often reduced due to decreased vaginal lubrication, thinner vaginal walls, and a slower response to stimulation.

■ *Aging.* Older people vary greatly in their sexual motivation. Psychosocial factors such as beliefs and attitudes about sexual functioning play an important role in this variation. Physical factors such as energy levels, pain, and immobility also have an effect.

Sexual motivation may also be enhanced by a number of various conditions and circumstances. This may or may not be a problem for the individual. Factors contributing to *increased* sexual motivation include the following:

■ *Puberty and adolescence.* Both males and females experience increased sexual motivation during puberty and adolescence as a result of hormonal and body changes. This population is at risk of pregnancy and sexually transmitted disease if they do not receive appropriate sex education.

■ *Drugs.* Amphetamines and cocaine enhance sexual motivation for some people for short periods. Lysergic acid diethylamide (LSD) and marijuana increase libido in some but inhibit it in others.

Problems with Genital Functioning

The ability to engage in genital intercourse is of great importance to most people. Many people experience transient problems with their ability to respond to sexual stimulation or to maintain the response. Common concerns for the male are being able to achieve and maintain an erection and to develop orgasmic timing with the partner. For women, common concerns relate to their ability to become and stay aroused and their ability to achieve orgasm.

The inability to achieve or maintain an erection sufficient for sexual satisfaction for the self and/or partner is called **erectile dysfunction.** Many believe that the term **impotence,** also commonly used, is inappropriate, because for many clients it has negative connotations. All men have transient interferences with the ability to attain and maintain erection.

Erectile dysfunction becomes a problem when it interferes significantly with the client's ability to satisfy himself or his partner. Such interference may occur consistently in all sexual situations, with or without a partner, or it may occur only in certain situations, such as with one partner but not with others, or with masturbation.

Erectile dysfunction is classified as primary or secondary. A man with primary erectile dysfunction has never been able to achieve an erection sufficient for intercourse. A man with secondary erectile dysfunction has functioned adequately for some time before developing erectile dysfunction. Both types of erectile dysfunction can be caused by physiologic or psychologic factors, but primary erectile

dysfunction is more often associated with psychologic factors. Physiologic factors include the following:

■ Neurologic disorders created by spinal cord injuries, injury to the genitals or perineal nerves, extensive surgery such as abdominal-perineal bowel resections, radical perineal prostatectomy, and diabetes mellitus

■ Prolonged use of drugs such as sedatives, heroin, antidepressants, and antipsychotics (phenothiazines)

■ Vascular diseases such as sickle-cell anemia and leukemia

■ Endocrine disorders such as hypothyroidism and Addison's disease

Psychologic factors may include the following:

■ Doubts about one's ability to perform or about one's masculinity

■ Fatigue, anger, or stress caused by problems at work, in the family, or in interpersonal relationships

■ Traumatic early sexual experiences (e.g., rejection)

■ Pain, fear, or guilt associated with erection

■ Boredom associated with a specific partner

The treatment for erectile dysfunction depends largely on the cause. Penile implants have been used to treat physiologic erectile dysfunction. Erectile dysfunction of psychologic origin often requires a change in both partners' views of sexuality. Awareness of the cause of the condition and exercises designed to increase sensations are also used.

Premature ejaculation occurs when a man is unable to delay ejaculation long enough to satisfy his partner. This usually means that ejaculation occurs after only very limited stimulation of the penis. Often the ejaculation occurs either during penetration (of the vagina, mouth, or anus) or immediately following. The condition may relate to conditioning regarding the need for rapid orgasm or performance demands.

Treatment advocated for couples by many sex therapists includes increased sexual communication and responsiveness as well as decreased performance demands. The couple together practice sensate exercises (learning to enjoy the sensation of touch) and then work together to establish satisfying coitus.

Orgasmic dysfunction, the inability of a woman to achieve orgasm, is of two types: primary and situational. A woman with primary orgasmic dysfunction has never been able to achieve orgasm. A woman with situational dysfunction has experienced at least one orgasm but is at that time nonorgasmic. Orgasmic dysfunction can be caused by drugs, alcohol, aging, and anatomic abnormalities of the genitals. However, most cases have psychologic causes, including hostility between partners, fear or guilt about enjoying the sexual act, and concern about performance.

Therapy usually involves helping both partners to establish new attitudes about sex. Pelvic muscle exercises (Kegel's exercises) can also increase the capacity of women to achieve orgasm by increasing the strength of the pubococcygeal muscle.

Vaginismus is the irregular and involuntary contraction of the muscles around the outer third of the vagina when coitus is attempted—that is, the vagina closes before penetration. Its causes can be severe sexual inhibition, often associated with early learning. Other causes can be rape, incest, and painful intercourse.

Treatment often involves sensate focus exercises and therapy to bring about psychologic changes. In some instances graduated vaginal dilators are used.

Dyspareunia describes the pain experienced by a woman during intercourse, a result of inadequate lubrication, scarring, vaginal infection, or hormonal imbalance. Treatment—such as supplying additional lubrication before intercourse—corrects the underlying cause.

DIAGNOSING SEXUALITY PROBLEMS

Nursing diagnoses for clients with problems related to sexuality are categorized as **Altered sexuality patterns.** This is a broad category that includes sexual identity, sexuality, and sexual function (Carpenito 1989, p. 666). It is defined as the state in which one expresses concern regarding one's sexuality or experiences or is at risk of experiencing a change in sexual health (Kim, McFarland, and McLane 1989, p. 57; Carpenito 1989, p. 666). **Sexual dysfunction,** the other NANDA diagnosis pertaining to sexuality, is defined as a perceived problem in achieving desired sexual satisfaction.

Examples of these nursing diagnoses and their contributing factors are shown below. Examples of assessment data clusters and related nursing diagnoses are shown in Table 30–3.

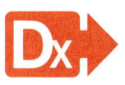 **Nursing Diagnoses**
Clients with Sexual/Sexuality
Problems

Altered sexuality patterns related to:

- Fear of pregnancy
- Fear of acquiring sexually transmitted disease
- Fear of effects of coitus following heart attack
- Impaired relationship with partner
- Body image disturbance secondary to trauma or radical surgery
- Current stressor (e.g., job problems, financial worries)
- Altered body function secondary to pregnancy, drugs, medications, surgery, disease process, trauma, radiation, or age (e.g., dyspareunia)
- Sexual trauma (e.g., rape or sexual exploitation)
- Unrealistic expectations of self and others

TABLE 30–3 *Examples of Assessment Data Clusters and Related Nursing Diagnoses for Clients with Sexuality Problems*

Data Cluster	Nursing Diagnosis
Marsha Ogilvy, 55 years old, reports vaginal burning and pain whenever she and her husband make love. Her last menses was 14 months ago. She says her husband is concerned about the lack of her usual response to lovemaking.	**Sexual dysfunction** related to painful intercourse from inadequate vaginal lubrication
Georgina Honey, 49 years old, had a total mastectomy 2 weeks ago. She says, "I'm sure not going to be sexually appealing to my husband anymore. How on earth will he ever want to make love to me again? I feel like a lopsided oddity."	**Altered sexuality pattern** related to body image disturbance secondary to mastectomy
Larry Stogryn, 52 years old, has a history of hypertension for which he has been taking an antihypertensive (reserpine [Serpasil]). He says he has lost interest in sex in the past few months, and when he does have sex, he has trouble keeping an erection.	**Altered sexuality pattern** related to altered body function secondary to use of antihypertensive medication

Sexual dysfunction related to:

- Excessive use of alcohol
- Painful intercourse from inadequate vaginal lubrication
- Misinformation or lack of knowledge
- Neurologic changes secondary to diabetes mellitus or spinal cord injury

Knowledge deficit (e.g., about conception or sexually transmitted diseases, contraception, or normal age-related sexual changes)

PLANNING

The overall client goals for persons with sexual problems is to maintain, restore, or improve sexual health. Outcome criteria to evaluate the achievement of client goals and the effectiveness of nursing interventions depend on the nursing diagnoses. Some suggested criteria follow.

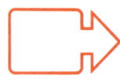

Outcome Criteria
Clients with Sexual/Sexuality Problems

The client:

- Verbalizes understanding of sexual anatomy and function.
- Verbalizes understanding of ways to avoid sexually transmitted disease.
- Identifies personal stressors that contribute to the dysfunction.
- Identifies attitudes restrictive to sexual behavior and sense of pleasure.
- Identifies alternative ways of dealing with sexual expression.
- Implements adaptive behaviors to accommodate altered body function, illness, or medical therapy.
- Expresses positive statements about alternative modes of sexual behavior.
- Verbalizes concerns about body image, sex role, or desirability as sexual partner.
- Expresses positive statements about gender, sex role, and/or sexual orientation.
- Reports diminished concern over sexual functioning.
- Verbalizes satisfactory/acceptable sexual practices to partner.
- States that desired sexual satisfaction has been achieved.
- Reports sense of pleasure (e.g., increased sense of erotic sensations) and gratification in sexual response.

IMPLEMENTING

Nursing responsibilities for clients with sexual problems include the following:

- Developing awareness of one's own sexual attitudes, beliefs, and knowledge
- Selecting appropriate interventions
- Providing accurate sexual information and education to clients
- Enhancing the client's body image and self-esteem (see Chapter 29).

Developing Self-Awareness

To be effective in helping clients with sexual problems, nurses must first have accurate information about sexuality, identify and accept their own sexual values and behaviors and those of others, and be comfortable acquiring and disseminating information about sexuality. Results of a study conducted at the School of Nursing, University of Wisconsin at Madison, revealed considerable misinformation and lack of information about sexual matters among graduate and undergraduate nursing students (Mims and Swenson 1978, p. 122). The following *misconceptions,* and their incidence, were reported:

- Impotence in men over 70 is nearly universal (35%).
- Certain mental and emotional instabilities are caused by masturbation (10%).
- Women are not able to respond to further stimulation for a period of time following orgasm (24%).
- A woman's chances to conceive are greatly enhanced if she has experienced orgasm (16%).
- Most homosexuals have a distinguishing body build (27%).
- Exhibitionists are latent homosexuals (32%).

Nurses who hold such misconceptions may be unable to give clients appropriate advice and assistance. Nurses need to become informed about the anatomy and physiology of sexual organs, psychosocial development of sexuality, psychosocial behaviors, sexual variations among people, and diseases and therapies that can alter sexual behavior.

Awareness of one's own attitudes (feelings, values, and beliefs) about sexuality is also essential. Before nurses can understand clients' sexuality, they must develop an awareness and tolerance of their own sexuality. This kind of self-awareness can be acquired via values clarification exercises and discussions. Nurses need to consider their feelings about matters such as masturbation, unwanted pregnancy and abortion, contraception, homosexuality and other sexual variations, nudity, and sterilization. When nurses clarify their own attitudes, they gain a greater understanding and tolerance of sexuality in others.

Selecting Appropriate Interventions

Interventions for sexual health problems are many and varied. Major components of any intervention strategy include counseling, education, and referral. Two models of intervention are presented as examples to guide nurses in selecting appropriate interventions.

Frank (1981, p. 64) suggests a three-part program for each sexual counseling session: (a) assessment, (b) information-sharing, and (c) discussion. The *assessment phase* involves asking the client questions and evaluating the answers. Frank suggests that before asking the questions of the client, the nurse should answer this question: "If I were in this client's place, what questions would I ask?" This exercise helps the nurse devise a list of questions and ways to ask them. For example, the nurse might ask a client recuperating from a heart attack the following questions:

"Now that you're recuperating and you've had some time to sort out your feelings, have you thought about how your heart attack might alter your sex life?"

"Have you and your partner discussed how you both feel about it?"

Information-sharing and discussion should follow each question. In this example, *sharing information* means the nurse informs the client about how his heart attack might affect his sex life, including the following:

"Your heart attack will not alter your capacity for sexual response. Most people can resume intercourse in 4 to 6 weeks, but this should be confirmed by your doctor."

"Many postcoronary clients fear sexual intercourse because of increased heart and respiratory rates associated with it. However, your prescribed program of progressive physical activity will also increase your tolerance for sexual activity."

After sharing information, the nurse should encourage discussion. If the nurse cannot answer the client's questions, the nurse refers the client to someone who can. The nurse may offer helpful suggestions during *discussion,* for example:

"Many people express concern about the stress of certain positions for intercourse, but you may use whatever position is comfortable for you and your partner."

Another model to help nurses deliver sexual health care, developed by Mims and Swenson (1978, p. 123), outlines three levels of nursing intervention, all of which require use of the nursing process and communication skills. At the *basic level,* the nurse helps the client develop awareness of sexuality, which involves knowledge, attitudes, and perceptions. Mims and Swenson believe that all nurses, regardless of educational preparation, should function at this level.

The *intermediate level* includes giving permission and giving information. This level presupposes teaching skills by the nurse. *Giving permission* means that the nurse by attitude or word lets the client know that sexual thoughts, fantasies, and behaviors between informed, consenting adults are sanctioned. Giving permission begins when the nurse acknowledges the client's verbal and nonverbal sexual concerns. For example, an older male with a reduced libido may feel that he cannot discuss sex with the nurse unless the nurse broaches the subject. Other clients may need acknowledgment to feel comfortable about their virginity, homosexual activities, oral-genital sex, or masturbation. Often, many sexual concerns are alleviated when the client receives permission from the nurse to engage or not engage in certain sexual behaviors. Permission giving can be detrimental unless at the same time the nurse provides accurate information. *Giving information* should include

1. General information about sexuality, including:
   a. Anatomy and physiology of sexual organs
   b. Stages of sexual development
   c. Sexual response cycles
   d. Coital positions
2. Information specific to the client's needs, which may include:

a. Alterations in sexuality made necessary by certain disease processes, medication, surgery, or therapies
b. Alternative modes of sexual expression
c. Contraception
d. Sexually transmitted diseases
e. Pregnancy
f. Abortion
g. Infertility

The *advanced level* of nursing intervention includes *giving suggestions,* which involves sexual therapy, educational programs, and research projects. For this level of functioning, the nurse requires specialized knowledge and skill.

For the client with **Sexual dysfunction** related to neurologic changes secondary to diabetes mellitus, implementation might involve teaching about etiology, supportive counseling related to self-image, teaching about continued ability to ejaculate, and providing information about options such as penile prostheses. Clients with **Sexual dysfunction** related to neurologic deficits secondary to spinal cord injury may need special rehabilitation programs, a good example of a third level of implementation.

Sexual Health Teaching

Providing education for sexual health is an important component of nursing implementation. Many sexual problems exist as a result of sexual ignorance; many others can be prevented with effective sexual health teaching. Examples of important areas of teaching include breast and testicular self-examination (see Chapter 26), prevention of sexually transmitted diseases, and contraception.

Sexually Transmitted Diseases Human immunodeficiency virus (HIV) infection, or acquired immune deficiency syndrome (AIDS), is a health problem of increasing severity. By mid-1990, 157,730 cases of AIDS had been diagnosed in the United States, Canada, and Mexico. This growing health problem has implications for nurses in health teaching as well as in providing direct care to individuals with AIDS and related conditions. Important issues noted earlier in this chapter, such as nonjudgmental attitudes and the need for accurate information, are vital to the proper understanding and care of individuals with HIV infection. AIDS is an extremely complex and sensitive issue. Information about the specifics of AIDS is available in and best sought from specialty publications, many of which are written specifically for nurses.

Common signs of sexually transmitted diseases for which people should seek medical care are shown in Chapter 26, page 645. The use of condoms is strongly advocated as a protective device against sexually transmitted diseases for homosexual and heterosexual couples (see page 736). Specific strategies to prevent AIDS are shown in the box on page 736.

abstain from heterosexual genital intercourse during that time.

Coitus interruptus is another method that does not employ chemical or mechanical barriers. The man withdraws his penis from his partner's vagina prior to ejaculation. While this is one of the oldest methods of birth control, it has certain disadvantages: It requires considerable self-control, the required constraint may decrease sexual gratification, and some semen may escape into the vagina prior to ejaculation.

Mechanical contraceptive methods (using a condom, diaphragm, or sponge) are also current popular choices. The **intrauterine device** (IUD), a preferred mechanical contraceptive method of the 1970s, is now used less frequently because of complications associated with its use and numerous lawsuits against its manufacturers. The **condom** (see Figure 30–1) is a covering sheath placed over the penis prior to intercourse. Since the ejaculate is deposited in the condom rather than in the vagina, the condom should be inspected for holes prior to application. The man or his partner places the condom on the erect penis, leaving a small space at the end of the condom for the ejaculate and rolling down the sheath from the tip to the end of the shaft. For maximum effectiveness, the penis should be carefully withdrawn after intercourse while still erect, with the rim of the condom held to prevent spillage. Should the penis become flaccid, the man should hold the edge of the condom while withdrawing from the vagina to prevent the condom from slipping off and spilling semen.

The **vaginal diaphragm** is a round rubber cup inserted into the vagina and placed over the cervix. It offers greater contraceptive protection than condoms, especially when used with **spermicides** (jellies or creams), but requires proper fitting (including refitting after the birth of a child or a change in body weight of twenty pounds) by trained personnel and yearly replacement. The diaphragm can be inserted by the woman or her partner up to 2 hours before intercourse. Longer time spans require additional applica-

Contraception **Contraception** is the voluntary prevention of conception or **impregnation** (fertilizing or making pregnant). Contraceptive methods include fertility awareness, mechanical and chemical contraception, and surgical procedures. Most people use several methods during their lives, so they need to be familiar with the various methods available. Increasingly, people are choosing methods that do not employ the use of artificial substances within the body. So-called natural methods have long been preferred by people whose religious beliefs conflict with artificial birth-control methods.

Fertility awareness methods depend upon identification of the days of the month when conception could take place and abstinence during that time. The nurse providing instruction describes the signs of ovulation (see the accompanying box) to the client and explains that, since conception is possible when a woman is ovulating, she should

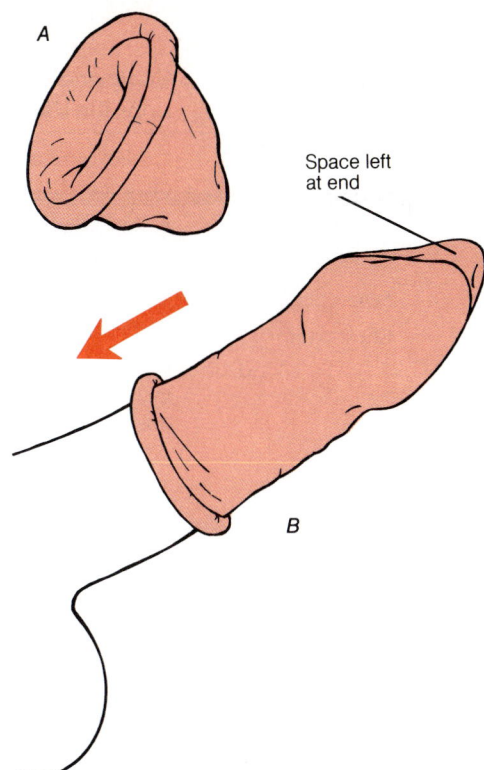

Figure 30–1 *A,* Condom. *B,* Condom applied to penis. Note space left at end to allow collection of ejaculate.

tion of spermicides. For maximum effectiveness, the diaphragm should be left in place for 6 hours following intercourse to ensure that the spermicide has killed all sperm in the vaginal folds. The nurse should instruct the client to hold the diaphragm up to a light periodically and inspect it for holes.

To insert the diaphragm, the woman is instructed to

1. Apply a tablespoon of spermicidal jelly into the cup of the diaphragm and around the rim that will face the cervix.

2. Cup the diaphragm between the thumb and fingers and insert it, cream side up, into the vagina, over the cervix.

3. Push the anterior rim of the diaphragm up under the symphysis pubis. (Some women report a popping sensation.)

4. Check its placement by touching the diaphragm with the index finger and feeling the cervix beneath. The **cervix** is a small rounded structure that feels somewhat like the

tip of the nose. The diaphragm should be centered over the cervix. See Figure 30–2 on page 738.

The **vaginal sponge** is a modification of the diaphragm, easier to use and requiring no professional fitting, but less effective as a contraceptive device. It is shaped like a mushroom cap, is saturated with spermicide, and fits into the upper vagina. It is moistened with water and inserted so that the concave surface is over the cervix. Some people express that using a diaphragm or sponge inhibits the spontaneity of intercourse; others report finding the genital manipulation necessary for insertion and removal offensive. Many people are successful in incorporating this procedure into their lovemaking experience.

Chemical contraception includes the use of synthetic **estrogen** and **progesterone** (birth-control pills or *oral contraceptives*) and inserting spermicidal foams, jellies, creams, or suppositories into the vagina prior to intercourse. The effectiveness of *spermicides* increases substantially when combined with the use of a condom or diaphragm. *Douching* after intercourse is *not* an effective contraceptive. The client who reports using douching for contraception should be informed that she may actually be increasing her chances for impregnation, as douching may assist the sperm in moving up toward the uterus (Olds, London, and Ladewig 1988, p. 162).

Oral contraceptives are preferred by many North American women. The increased estrogen levels suppress ovulation, and increased progesterone levels change the characteristics of the cervical mucus, interfering with the passage of sperm through the cervix. The woman choosing to use birth-control pills should be instructed to follow the specific instructions included with her prescription. The nurse should also inform the woman of possible side-effects and indications for contacting the primary care provider (i.e., the prescribing nurse practitioner or physician). Table 30–4 lists minor and major side-effects of oral contraceptives, as well as conditions contraindicating the use of oral contraceptives. Women using oral contraceptives should be instructed to contact the primary care provider if minor side-effects persist. Major side-effects are warnings of potentially serious problems and require a physician's immediate attention.

Surgical contraceptive methods include tubal ligation and vasectomy. While other surgical procedures involving reproductive organs (e.g., hysterectomy or bilateral orchiectomy) produce infertility, they are not performed for contraceptive purposes. A **tubal ligation** is the tying of a woman's fallopian tubes to interrupt tubal continuity. A small abdominal incision is made below the umbilicus under local or general anesthesia. Pregnancies following tubal ligation are about 4 out of 10,000 per year.

A **vasectomy** is the ligation and cutting of the man's vas deferens on either side of the scrotum. The procedure is usually performed under local anesthesia. Sperm are not

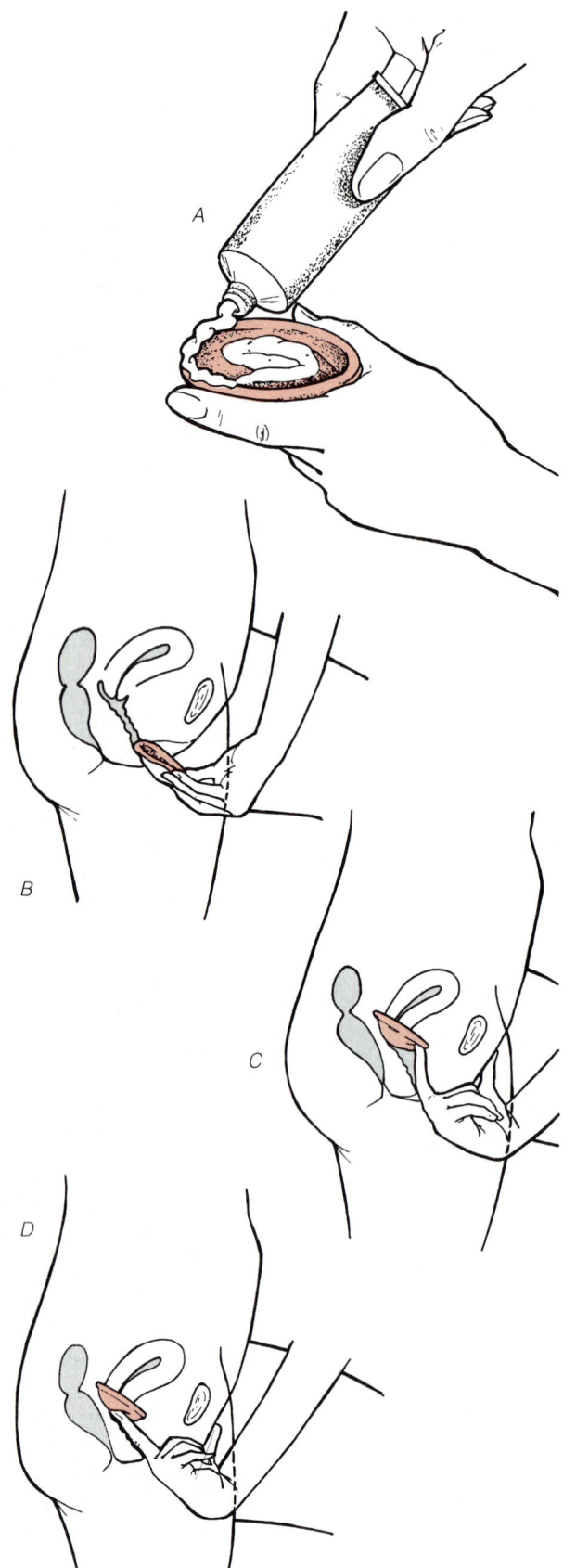

TABLE 30–4 *Using Oral Contraceptives*

Minor Side-Effects	Major Side-Effects	Contraindications for Use
Nausea	Severe headaches	Cardiovascular disorders
Weight gain	Severe abdominal pain	Severe migraine headaches
Breast tenderness		
Headaches	Blurred vision	Liver disease
Decreased menstrual flow	Severe leg pain	Diabetes mellitus
Spotting	Chest pain	Known or increased risk of breast cancer
Missed periods		
Vaginal itching		
Yeast infections		
Transient depression		

cleared from the genitourinary system for 4 to 6 weeks (approximately 6 to 36 ejaculations) after a vasectomy. The client should be instructed to use other contraceptive methods during that time span.

EVALUATING

Evaluation of goal achievement generally includes similar data collection activities implemented in the assessment phase; however, the focus is now on the expected outcomes developed in the planning phase. Evaluative activities may include (a) questioning the clients about their understanding of conception, sexual development, safer sex practices, signs of sexually transmitted diseases, and contraception; (b) asking the client about altered sexual practices; (c) observing the client demonstrate use of a condom or other contraceptive device on a model; (d) listening during an interview to the client's comments about level of sexual satisfaction and gratification of self and partner or about perception of self as being sexually acceptable.

◀ *Figure 30–2* *A,* Applying jelly to the rim and center of the diaphragm. *B,* Inserting the diaphragm. *C,* Pushing the rim of the diaphragm under the symphysis pubis. *D,* Checking placement of the diaphragm. Cervix should be felt through the diaphragm. *Source:* S. B. Olds, M. L. London, and P. L. Ladewig, *Maternal-newborn nursing,* 3d ed. (Menlo Park, Calif.: Addison-Wesley Publishing Co., 1988), p. 164. Reprinted with permission.

ASSESSMENT DATA

Nursing Assessment

Ellen Hopkins is an 18-year-old high school senior who delivered a healthy baby boy yesterday. She is not married and is not sure that she wants to marry the baby's father. She and her newborn will be going home to live with her parents in 2 days. Ellen wants to finish high school and go on to college to become a teacher. She tells the nurse that she doesn't want to get pregnant again until she is married and that this pregnancy was an accident. She doesn't know how it happened; she thought she was "safe." Ellen is lying in a semi-Fowler's position nursing her baby. She and the baby appear comfortable.

Physical Examination

Height: 165.1 cm (5′5″)
Weight: 52 kg (114 lb)
Temperature: 37 C (98.6 F)
Pulse: 74 BPM
Respirations: 18 per minute
Blood pressure: 106/80 mm Hg
Lochia clear
Breasts engorged

CARE PLAN

Nursing Diagnosis	Client Goals and Outcome Criteria	Nursing Interventions and Rationales	Evaluation
Knowledge deficit about contraception as verbalized by client and manifested by unplanned pregnancy.	Client Goal: Select appropriate method of contraception. Outcome Criteria: Client describes the physiology of conception by day 1. Describes the menstrual cycle and its relationship to conception by day 1. Requests information about alternative methods of contraception by day 2.	Establish a good rapport with client by being supportive and empathetic. *Rationale:* Encourages the client to ask questions and to seek assistance. Assess the client's knowledge about the physiology of menstruation and pregnancy. *Rationale:* Knowing the client's level of understanding enables the nurse to clarify misinformation and to plan appropriate instruction. Adapt teaching to client's abilities. *Rationale:* Learning will be more meaningful. Instruct client regarding the menstrual cycle and conception. *Rationale:* Knowledge establishes a basis for information about methods of contraception. Instruct client regarding alternative methods of contraception. *Rationale:* Client can better select a method consistent with her needs. Provide written instructional material regarding pregnancy and contraception. *Rationale:* Verbal instruction can be reinforced by visual materials that can be reviewed after the learning session.	Client was able to verbalize understanding of conception by day 1. She requested more specific written information about birth control pills and intrauterine devices as methods of contraception on day 2. She stated she would follow up on the information at her postpartum checkup visit to her doctor.

CHAPTER HIGHLIGHTS

▸ Sexuality is important in developing self-identity, interpersonal relationships, intimacy, and love.

▸ In its broad sense, sexuality involves physical, emotional, social, and ethical aspects of being and behaving. It has learned and inherited components.

▸ An understanding of the structure and function of the male and female genitals is essential for nurses.

▸ The components that contribute to the development of sexuality are numerous; both biologic and psychologic components exist at all ages.

▸ Biologic differences in the sexes are apparent at birth, but many behavioral differences are also notable throughout infancy and childhood.

▸ The establishment of sexual self-identity and gender role are critical between the ages of 18 months and 4 years.

▸ The learning of sex-typed behaviors depends on communication from parents and on imitation of parental behavior. Learning appropriate sex-typed behaviors takes several years.

▸ Adolescents may have problems establishing sexual self-identity.

▸ Adults also often experience sexual problems. A major task of the adult is to develop an intimate relationship with a partner.

▸ During the middle and later years, there are physical changes in the genitals. However, the desire and ability to maintain satisfying sexual relationships can remain.

▸ Assessing actual or potential sexual problems is conducted at four levels. The professional nurse assesses at only the first level. Assessment should be carried out when clients or support persons present cues that problems exist or when an illness could cause sexual problems.

▸ Nurses assess attitudes toward sexuality, including factors that affect attitudes and behaviors.

▸ An understanding of sexual stimuli and response patterns can help individuals have satisfying sexual relationships. This understanding is also vital for nurses wishing to help clients with psychologic problems, such as feelings of inadequacy, or medical problems, such as spinal cord injuries or myocardial infarctions.

▸ Common sexual problems of healthy adults are changes in libido, erectile dysfunction, premature ejaculation, orgasmic dysfunction, vaginismus, and dyspareunia.

▸ Illnesses that commonly affect sexuality include myocardial infarction and diabetes mellitus. Many surgical procedures also affect sexual abilities and sexual self-image, including mastectomy, hysterectomy, orchiectomy, and enterostomy.

▸ Nursing diagnoses for clients with sexual problems are related to many contributing factors, including altered body structure or function, lack of knowledge or misinformation about sexual matters, physical or psychologic abuse, value conflicts, and loss or lack of a partner.

▸ Before assisting clients with sexual problems, nurses must acquire accurate information about sexuality, identify and accept their own sexual values and behaviors as well as those of others, and be comfortable acquiring and disseminating information about sexuality.

▸ Nursing interventions include helping clients develop awareness of sexuality, giving permission, giving information, and, at an advanced level, giving suggestions.

READINGS AND REFERENCES

SUGGESTED READINGS

Chekryn, J. September 1989. Families of people with AIDS. *Canadian Nurse* 65:30–32.
    In a report on a research project to identify and understand the needs of families of clients with AIDS, Chekryn identifies factors that influence nursing care decisions.

Dickerson, J. October 1983. The pill: A close look. *American Journal of Nursing* 83:1392–98.
    Dickerson provides an extensive review of the risks and benefits of the various hormonal contraceptives available in the U.S.A.

Divasto, P. February 1985. Measuring the aftermath of rape. *Journal of Psychosocial Nursing and Mental Health Services* 23:33–35.

Divasto describes an interview scale for measuring the severity of postrape symptoms and outlines symptoms and use of the data to guide client care.

Irish, A. August 1983. Straight talk about gay patients. *American Journal of Nursing* 83:1168–70.

Irish discusses homophobia among nurses and the need to be nonjudgmental about sexual orientation in their professional role, with suggestions for effective ways to avoid judgmental responses.

Lutz, R. March 1986. Stopping the spread of sexually transmitted diseases. *Nursing* 16:47–50.

Lutz provides an overview of the most common STDs and outlines nursing activities in dealing with clients who have an STD and techniques to decrease the spread.

Simmons, K. N. March 1983. Sexuality and the female ostomate. *American Journal of Nursing* 83:409–11.

In an excellent overview, by an ostomate, of issues and concerns following ostomies, the author provides guidelines for dealing with problems.

Steinke, E. E., and Berger, M. B. June 1986. Sexuality and aging. *Journal of Gerontological Nursing* 12:6–10.

The article discusses stereotypes of aging and sexuality, emphasizing the need for nurses to examine their own stereotypes to provide effective care to promote sexual health in the elderly. The authors stress comprehensive assessment and intervention.

RELATED RESEARCH

Bullough, B.; Bullough, V.; and Smith, R. W. August 1985. Masculinity and femininity in transvestite, transsexual and gay males. *Western Journal of Nursing Research* 7:317–27.

Kus, R. May 1985. Stages of coming out: An ethnographic approach. *Western Journal of Nursing Research* 7:177–98.

Sachs, B. 1985. Contraceptive decision-making in urban, black, female adolescents: Its relationship to cognitive development. *International Journal of Nursing Studies* 22(2):116–17.

Sheehan, M. K.; Ostwald, S. K.; and Rothenberger, J. January/February 1986. Perceptions of sexual responsibility: Do young men and women agree? *Pediatric Nursing.* 12:17–21.

Webb, C. October 1987. Nurses' knowledge and attitudes about sexuality: Report of a study. *Nursing Education Today* 7:209–14.

SELECTED REFERENCES

Andrist, L. C. December 1988. Taking a sex history and educating clients about safe sex. *Nursing Clinics of North America* 23:959–73.

Benson, C. H. January/March 1988. Arthritis and sexuality. *Journal of Urological Nursing* 7:370–72.

Burke, P. J. 1987. Adolescents' motivation for sexual activity and pregnancy prevention. *Issues in Comprehensive Pediatric Nursing.* 10(3):161–71.

Carolan, C. September 26–October 2, 1984a. Handicap—less important than loving. Part 1. *Nursing Times* 80:28–30.

———. October 3–9, 1984b. Sex and disability: Bridging the gap. Part 3. *Nursing Times* 80:49–50.

Carpenito, L. J. 1989. *Nursing diagnosis: Application to clinical practice.* 3d ed. Philadelphia: J. B. Lippincott Co.

Crooks, R., and Baur, K. 1987. *Our sexuality.* 3d ed. Menlo Park, Calif.: Benjamin/Cummings.

Dolan, M. B. January 1985. An eternal flame . . . The elderly and sex. *Nursing* (Springhouse) 15:104.

Douglas, C. J.; Kalman, C. M.; and Kalman, T. P. December 1985. Homophobia among physicians and nurses. *Hospital and Community Psychiatry* 36:1309–11.

Flaskerud, J. H. 1989. *AIDS/HIV infection: A resource guide for nursing professionals.* Philadelphia: W. B. Saunders Co.

Frank, D. I. January 1981. You don't have to be an expert to give sexual counseling to a mastectomy patient. *Nursing 81* 11:64–67.

Glover, J. January 16, 1985. Family planning and sexual counseling . . . The nurse's role. *Nursing Mirror* 160:28–29.

Hogan, R. September 1982. Influences of culture on sexuality. *Nursing Clinics of North America* 17:365–76.

———. 1984. *Human sexuality, a nursing perspective.* 2d ed. New York: Appleton-Century-Crofts.

Howe, C. L. February 1986. Developmental theory and adolescent sexual behavior. *Nurse Practitioner* 11:65,68,71.

Hurley, M. E. (ed.) 1986. *Classification of Nursing Diagnoses: Proceedings of the Sixth National Conferences.* St. Louis: C. V. Mosby Co.

Kim, M. J.; McFarland, G. K.; and McLane, A. M. 1989. *Pocket guide to nursing diagnoses.* 3d ed. St. Louis: C. V. Mosby Co.

Kus, R. May 1985. Stages of coming out: An ethnographic approach. *Western Journal of Nursing Research* 7:177–98.

Lion, E. M., editor. 1982. *Human sexuality in nursing process.* New York: John Wiley and Sons.

McAndrew, T. January 1990. Elderly sexuality examined. *Pennsylvania Nurse* 45:16.

McCracken, A. L. October 1988. Sexuality practice by elders: The forgotten aspect of functional health. *Journal of Gerontological Nursing* 14:13–18.

Masters, W. H., and Johnson, V. E. 1966. *Human sexual response.* Boston: Little, Brown and Co.

———. 1970. *Human sexual inadequacy.* New York: Bantam Books.

———. 1979. *Homosexuality in perspective.* Boston: Little, Brown and Co.

Mims, F. H. September 1982. Sexual stress: Coping and adaptation. *Nursing Clinics of North America.* 17:395–405.

Mims, F. H., and Swenson, M. February 1978. A model to promote sexual health care. *Nursing Outlook* 26:121–25.

———. 1980. *Sexuality: A nursing perspective.* New York: McGraw-Hill.

Money, J. 1980. *Love and love sickness: The science of sex, gender difference and pair bonding.* Baltimore: Johns Hopkins University Press.

Moses, A. E., and Hawkins, R. O. 1982. *Counselling lesbian women and gay men.* St. Louis: C. V. Mosby Co.

Olds, S. B.; London, M. L.; and Ladewig, P. A. 1988. *Maternal-newborn nursing.* 3d ed. Menlo Park, Calif.: Addison-Wesley Publishing Co.

Osis, M. January/February 1986. Sexuality: An interactional perspective . . . Drugs and healthy aging. *Gerontion.* 1:6–8.

Penninger, J. A. April 1985. After the ostomy: Helping the patient reclaim his sexuality . . . a male ostomy patient. *RN* 48:46–50.

Pervin-Dixon, L. April 1988. Sexuality and the spinal cord injured. *Journal of Psychosocial Nursing and Mental Health Services* 26:31–35, 37.

Rosenberg, M. J. March 1990. Sexually transmitted diseases and the primary care provider. *Primary Care* 17:1–27.

Rothman, B., Sebastian, H. May 1990. Intimacy and cognitively impaired elders. *Canadian Nurse* 86:32, 34.

Sex Information and Education Council of the United States. 1980. The Siecus/New York University/Uppsala principles basic to education for sexuality. *Seicus Report* 8:8–9.

Slevin, A. P., and Marvin, C. L. 1987. Safe sex and pregnancy prevention: A guide for health practitioners working with adolescents. *Journal of Community Health Nursing* 4:234–35.

Telashek, M. L., Tichy, A. M., Epping, H. April 1990. Sexually transmitted diseases in the elderly: Issues and recommendations. *Journal of Gerontological Nursing* 16:33–42.

Watts, R. September 1979. Dimensions of sexual health. *American Journal of Nursing* 79:1568–72.

Wright, D. July 31, 1985. Sex and the elderly. *Nursing Mirror* 161:18–19.

Young, E. 1984. Patient's plea: Tell us about our sexuality. *Journal of Sex Education and Therapy.* 10:53–56.

Ethnic and Cultural Values

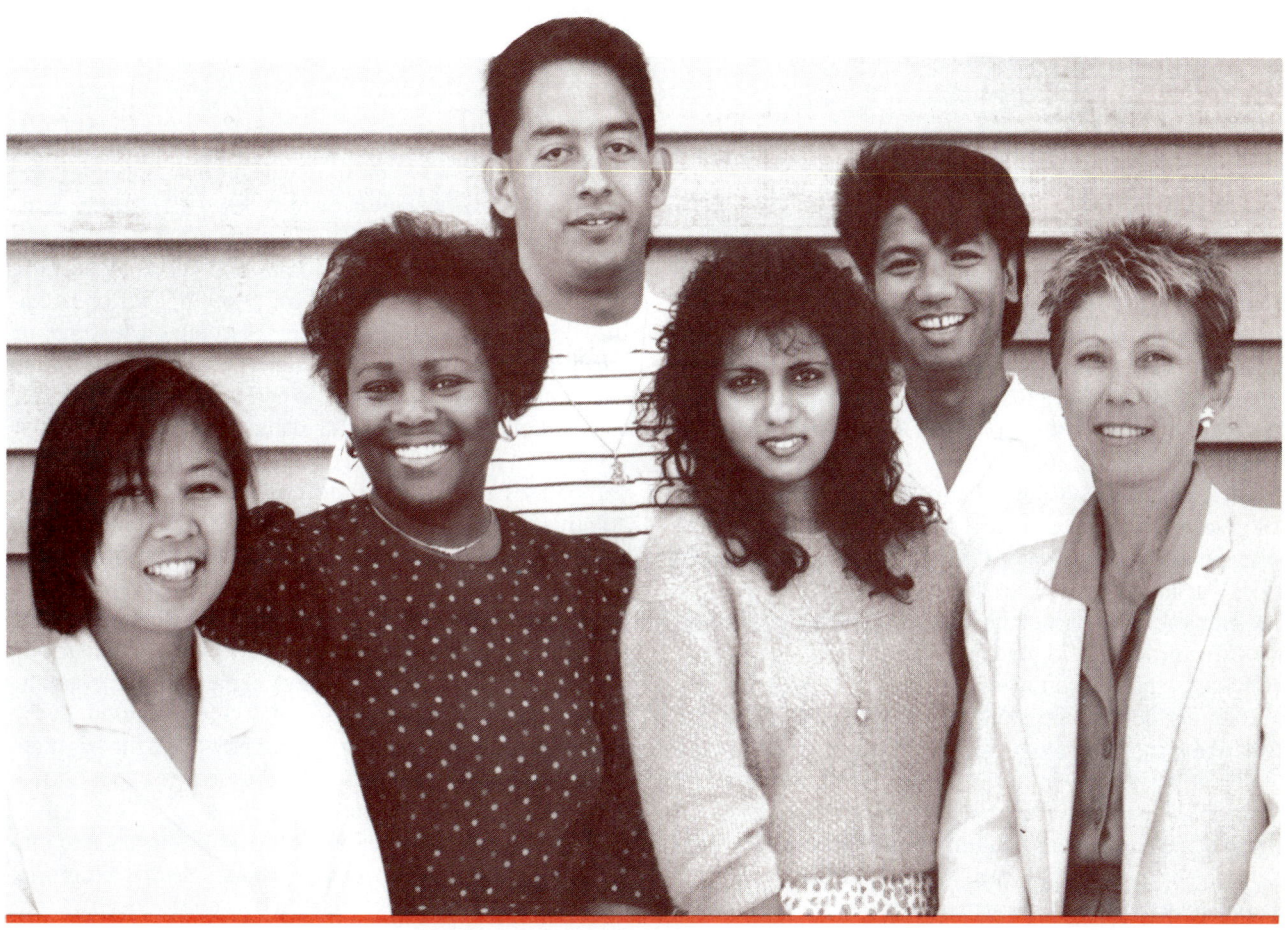

CONTENTS

OBJECTIVES

▶ Describe the concept of culture.
▶ Identify characteristics and universal attributes of culture.

▶ Identify social characteristics common to all ethnic/cultural groups that health care providers must consider.

▶ Identify problems unique to ethnic minorities in the provision and use of health care services.

▶ Relate the incidence of specific diseases to certain ethnic or cultural groups.

▶ Identify specific characteristics and values of selected cultural groups that may influence nursing assessment and intervention.

▶ Relate health-related beliefs and practices to economic status.

▶ Contrast the values of the health care culture and selected minority ethnic cultures.

CONCEPTS OF ETHNICITY AND CULTURE

Definitions

Ethnicity is the condition of belonging to a specific ethnic group. An **ethnic group** is a set of individuals who share a unique cultural and social heritage passed on from one generation to another (Henderson and Primeaux 1981, p. xx). Ethnicity thus differs from race. **Race** denotes a system of classifying humans into subgroups according to specific physical characteristics, including skin pigmentation, stature, facial features, texture of body hair, and head form (Henderson and Primeaux 1981, p. xix). The three racial types that are commonly recognized are Caucasoid, Negroid, and Mongoloid. However, because of the mixture of races, the three groups meld together, and there are many commonalities among groups.

Culture should not be confused with race or ethnic group. **Culture** is the beliefs and practices that are shared by people and passed down from generation to generation. Anthropologists have traditionally divided it into material culture and nonmaterial culture. **Material culture** consists of objects (such as dress, art, religious artifacts, or eating utensils) and the ways these are used. **Nonmaterial culture** consists of beliefs, customs, languages, and social institutions. Races have different ethnic groups, and the ethnic groups have different cultures. It is therefore important to understand that not all white or black people have the same culture. North America is inhabited by people of many different ethnic groups and cultures. Their cultural beliefs and practices can affect health and illness and thus become an important consideration for nurses.

Large cultural groups often have cultural subgroups or subsystems. A subculture is usually composed of people who have a distinct identity and yet are also related to a larger cultural group. A subcultural group generally has ethnicity, occupation, or physical characteristics in common with the larger cultural group. Examples of cultural subgroups are occupational groups (e.g., nurses), societal groups (e.g., feminists), and ethnic groups (e.g., Cajuns, who may be black, French, or German but who share French Acadian heritage and customs). A **bicultural group** is a group of people who embrace two cultures, life-styles, and sets of values (Chen-Louie 1980, p. 4).

Culture as a concept is a universal experience, but no two cultures are exactly alike. Two important terms identify the differences and similarities among peoples of different cultures. **Culture universals** are the common features or attributes of behavior or life pattern that are similar among different cultures. **Culture specifics** are the practices, values, beliefs, and behavior patterns that are special or unique to a given culture. For example, most cultures have ceremonies to celebrate the passage from childhood to adulthood; this practice is a culture universal. However, different cultural groups celebrate this important life event in very different ways. In Latin cultures, the "quince" party, which celebrates a girl's fifteenth birthday, signifies that the young girl has now become a woman. In some African tribes, ritual circumcision is performed as part of the ceremony that marks the passage from boyhood to manhood. In the Jewish culture, the bar mitzvah (for boys) and the bas mitzvah (for girls) are celebrations of the passage to adulthood. These are examples of culture specifics.

Two other terms commonly used with reference to ethnicity and culture are *dominant group* and *minority group*. A **dominant group** is "a collectivity within a society which has a preeminent authority to function as guardians and sustainers of the controlling value system and as prime allocators of rewards in the society" (Schermerhorn 1970, p. 13). A **minority group** or minority is a "group of people who, because of their physical or cultural characteristics, are singled out from the others in the society in which they live for differential and unequal treatment, and who therefore regard themselves as objects of collective discrimination" (Wirth 1945, p. 347). A dominant group is often the largest group in a society, for example, the white middle-class of the United States. However, the dominant group is not always the largest; for example, white South Africans are the dominant group and black South Africans are the minority group, yet the blacks far outnumber the whites.

Not uncommonly, people of a minority group often lose the cultural characteristics that distinguish them from the dominant group. This process is referred to as **cultural assimilation** or **acculturation.** Sometimes mutual cultural assimilation occurs, e.g., Chinese people coming to a North American community learn to speak English, and the people in the community learn to cook Chinese dishes.

Ethnocentrism is the belief that one's own culture is superior to all others. This can be seen in the comparison of the values and behavior of other cultures to those of one's own culture, using one's own culture as the standard. Although all people are subject to ethnocentrism, it is important for nurses to be consciously aware of ethnic and cultural differences and to accept these as appropriate. These differences should not be viewed as good or bad. Many immigrants to the United States and Canada maintain their ethnic and cultural identities in terms of their dress, language, customs, and rituals; accepting these is basic to accepting the client as an individual.

Stereotyping is assuming that all members of a culture or ethnic group are alike. For example, one may assume that all Italians express pain volubly or that all Chinese people like rice. Stereotyping may be based on generalizations founded in research, or it may be unrelated to reality. For example, research indicates that Italians are likely to express pain verbally; however, a particular Italian client may not verbalize pain. Stereotyping that is unrelated to reality may be positive or negative and is frequently an outcome of racism. **Racism** is the assumption of inherent racial superiority or inferiority and the consequent discrimination against certain races. An example of positive stereotyping is "All Jewish people are very clever." An example of negative stereotyping is "All Native Americans are alcoholics." Stereotyping can cause problems in nursing practice, especially if the nurse plans care based on stereotyping rather than on individual assessment of the client.

Ethnoscience is "the systematic study of the way of life of a designated cultural group with the purpose of obtaining an accurate account of the people's behavior and how they perceive and interpret their universe" (Leininger 1970, p. 168). Ethnoscientists attempt to provide an inside view of a culture from the way the people of the culture talk about it. They study and classify data about a cultural or subcultural group so that their report is meaningful to both people within the culture and people outside the culture who try to understand it. Emphasis is placed on the person's point of view, the person's vision, and the person's world.

Nurses can apply much of the knowledge gained by ethnoscientists, specifically about the health-illness behavior systems of people from cultural backgrounds different from their own. In the past decade or more, the client's personal view of illness has received recognition and emphasis. Nurses have, as a result, implemented methods to discover how well clients understand their illnesses, how clients perceive they can be helped by health personnel, and how illness has affected them and their families. In recent years, cultural views affecting health practices and beliefs have been receiving greater recognition. The fact that health beliefs and practices vary among cultures and the implications of this fact for nursing have also received greater attention. To provide effective nursing services to clients, nurses need data about the client's personal and cultural views regarding health and illness. When developing care plans, nurses need to consider the client's world and daily experiences. To make valid assessments, nurses need to try to see and hear the world as their clients do. Specific cultural data can provide scientific generalizations about health and illness behavior in different cultures. Clients' needs and behaviors can be better understood when particular health norms are identified.

Characteristics of Culture

- *Culture is learned.* It is not instinctive or innate. It is learned through life experiences after birth.

- *Culture is taught.* It is transmitted from parents to children over successive generations. All animals can learn, but only humans can pass culture along. Language is the chief vehicle of culture.

- *Culture is social.* It originates and develops through the interactions of people.

- *Culture is adaptive.* Customs, beliefs, and practices change slowly, but they do adapt to the social environment and to the biologic and psychologic needs of people. As life conditions change, some traditional forms in a culture may cease to provide satisfaction and are eliminated. For example, if it has been customary for family members of different generations to live together (extended family), yet education and employment may require children to leave their parents and move to other parts of the country, the extended family norm then changes.

- *Culture is integrative.* The elements in a culture tend to form a consistent and integrated system. For example, religious beliefs and practices influence and are influenced by family organization, economic values, and health practices.

- *Culture is ideational.* Ideational means forming images or objects in the mind. The group habits that are part of culture are to a considerable extent ideal norms or patterns of behavior. People do not always follow those norms. The norms of their culture may in fact be different from the norms of society as a whole.

- *Culture is satisfying.* Cultural habits persist only as long as they satisfy people's needs. Gratification strengthens habits and beliefs. Once they no longer bring gratification, they may disappear.

DIVERSITY OF NORTH AMERICAN SOCIETY

The populations of the United States and Canada are a mixture of many ethnic groups and cultures. In the United States, white Americans make up 79% of the total population; minority groups, 16.8%. The minority population can be further broken down as shown in Figure 31–1. In Canada, British Canadians make up 25.3% of the total population; French Canadians, 24.4%. See Figure 31–1.

The provision of quality nursing care to all North Americans is a desired goal. Because of the multicultural, multiethnic nature of American society, it is essential that consideration be given to the unique needs of ethnic and cultural groups. The following general considerations can help nurses develop an awareness and sensitivity to some of these specific needs.

Male-Female Roles

Most cultures are patriarchal; i.e., the man is the dominant figure. The degree of dominance of men is variable; when men are highly dominant, women are usually passive. An example of a patriarchal society is the Islamic culture of Iran, where women must be veiled in public and all important decisions are left to the men.

In contrast, the Native American culture is matriarchal, i.e., the woman is the dominant person in the family. Knowing who the decision maker or dominant person in a family is helps nurses understand the meaning of illness to a family and its decision-making process relative to health care. In Mexican American families, the father generally holds the primary power, whereas in Jewish American families, the mother is generally "the power behind the throne" (Friedman 1981, p. 271).

Language and Communication Patterns

People of an ethnic or cultural group may speak the language of their group fluently and not the language of the country. This is particularly true of certain women who, because they stay in the home, have limited interaction with people outside the family. Even the mother of a family who has been in the United States for 30 years may know very little English. This is also true of elderly immigrants or refugees, who may have little or no interaction with people

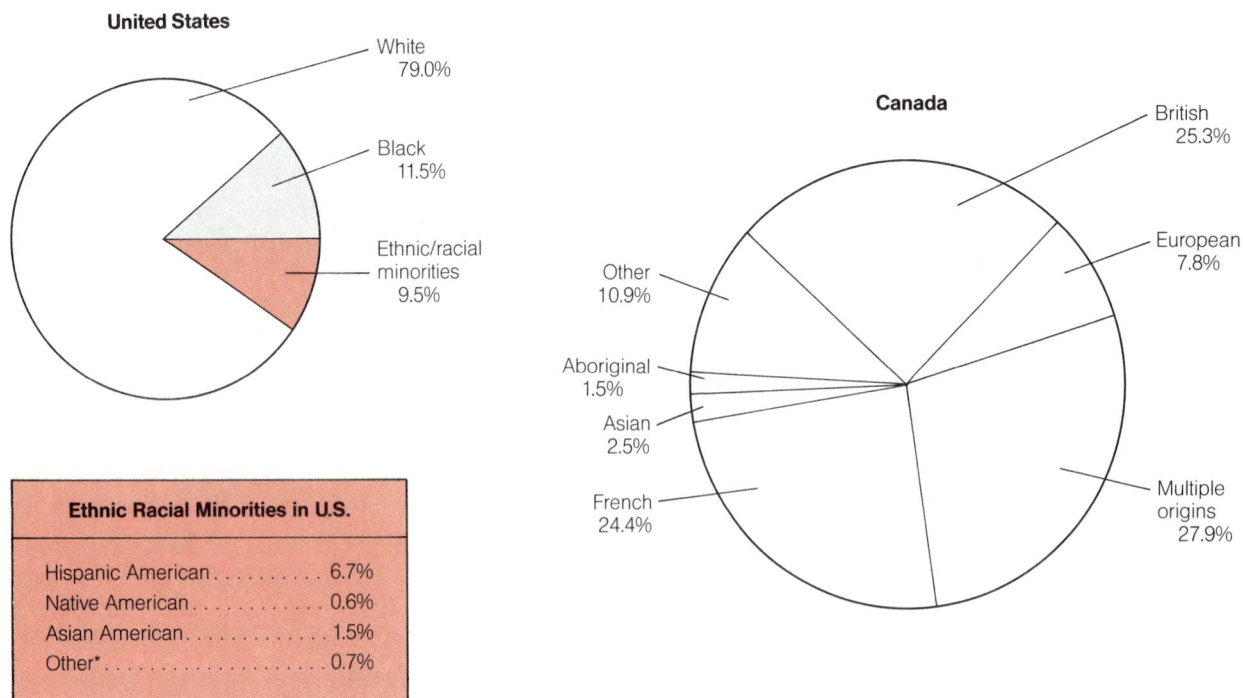

Figure 31–1 Estimates of the distribution of population by ethnic/racial origin based on statistical abstract of the United States (1989) and the Canadian 1990 census. **Sources** U.S. Department of Commerce, Bureau of the Census, *Statistical abstract of the United States,* 109th ed (Washington, D.C.: Government Printing Office, 1989), pp. 4–11, 15–57. Statistics Canada, January 1990, Census of Canada, Focus on Ethnic Diversity in Canada, Catalog 98-132, Minister of Supplies and Services, Ottawa, Canada.

of the dominant culture until they become ill. The degree to which people learn the language of a new country is highly variable. Some people may become fluent in English very quickly, while others may learn only enough English to get along in their daily activities. When people in the latter group become ill, they are frequently unable to describe their symptoms or answer a health questionnaire. Even if they have learned the language of their new home, they may have difficulty remembering or using the new language when under the stress of illness. If nurses do not establish that there is a language barrier, a client's needs may not be met. Most health agencies have interpreters to help nurses and clients.

Language barriers can be particularly frustrating and anxiety-producing when a person is ill and can neither state problems nor understand instructions. It is most difficult for people to convey their emotions about threatening situations in a second language, a crucial factor in cases of emotional and psychiatric illness. Language barriers also arise between people using the same language. The idiomatic English of a regional or cultural group may not be readily understood outside the group. For example, *belly* can mean the abdomen or the entire cavity from the nipple line to the pubic area.

Communication patterns also differ among subcultures. For example, Native Americans commonly do not say goodbye before they leave. Swedish people talk more freely over shared food, and most cultures talk more slowly than the dominant American culture (Wold 1981, p. 143).

An additional aspect of communication is body language. Facial gestures, eye contact, hand gestures, and body positioning are all part of communication. Different cultures place different meaning on these aspects of body language. For example, the Anglo-American usually places high value on maintaining eye contact. The Anglo-American may interpret a person's failure to maintain eye contact to mean that the individual is not trustworthy, is lying, or is trying to hide something. Conversely, the Native American may consider continuous eye contact insulting or disrespectful. "Staring into the eyes of a person is likened to controlling the person's spirit" (Wilson 1983, p. 278).

Territoriality and Personal Space

Both territoriality and personal space are influenced by an individual's culture and ethnicity. **Territoriality** is the pattern of behavior arising from an individual's feeling that certain spaces and objects belong to that person. **Personal space** is the distance a person prefers to maintain from others when interacting with them. In general, people of Arabic, Southern European, and African origins frequently sit or stand relatively close to each other when talking, whereas people of Asian, North European, and North American countries are comfortable talking farther apart. For additional information about territoriality and personal space, see Chapter 15, page 252.

Time Orientation

The middle-class in the United States and in Canada tends to be oriented to the future. People plan for the future, establish long-term goals, and are increasingly concerned about preventing future illness, e.g., by taking calcium to prevent osteoporosis in old age. In daily life, people are oriented to the time of day; meals are taken at a specified time, and clients have appointment times with many health care professionals. The nurse is also highly attuned to time; medications are given at specific times, and work begins and ends at specified times.

However, not all cultures are future oriented. People of other cultures, e.g., Asians, may be oriented to the past. This orientation is illustrated by ancestor worship and the influence of ancient beliefs such as Confucianism on the present. Other cultures, such as the Native American, are very much oriented to the present. Many Native American homes do not have clocks, and the people live one day at a time with little concern for the future. Hispanic Americans often value relationships with others and the present more than the future.

Family

The minority client's concept of family can differ from that of white middle-class culture. The minority group family may include the extended family (the nuclear family plus uncles, aunts, grandparents, cousins, and godparents). An associated concept is that family members are most important and must be helped at all costs. When health care is offered to such persons, it is important to consider the needs of the whole family. Sometimes, priorities in such families are detrimental to the health of one of its members. For example, a mother may not think that purchasing elastic stockings for her own ankle edema is as important as purchasing food for an unemployed relative. The home health care nurse in this instance may have to see that the relative's food needs are met before dealing with the mother's health needs.

Cultures that value the needs of the extended family as much as personal needs may also hold the belief that personal and family information must stay within the family. Some cultural groups, e.g., the traditional Chinese family, are very reluctant to disclose family information to outsiders, including physicians and nurses. This attitude can present difficulties for psychiatrists and mental health workers who view family interaction patterns as the locus of emotional problems.

Food and Nutritional Practices

The food people eat and the customs associated with food vary widely among subcultures and ethnic groups. For example, the staple food of Asians is rice; of Italians, pasta; and of Eastern Europeans, wheat bread. Even families who have been in the United States or Canada for several generations often continue to eat the food of their country (Christian and Greger 1985, p. 213).

Hospitalized clients often have very little choice about the food they are served. The nurse can encourage family members to bring in special meals if the client's health allows. Instructions about meal planning for clients requiring special diets at home may have to be given to younger family members who are fluent in English or given by a health worker of the same culture who can act as an interpreter.

When clients are learning about a special diet, nurses must be sensitive to the cultural meanings of food and to the foods a client is accustomed to. For example, it is unwise to recommend a service such as Meals on Wheels if the service is unable to supply the foods to which the client is accustomed, e.g., bean sprouts and vegetables for the Japanese client and fish and rice for the Chinese client.

SUSCEPTIBILITY TO DISEASE

Because of genetic and life-style influences, some ethnic and cultural groups in American society are more susceptible to certain diseases than the general population. Generally, bicultural groups in a lower socioeconomic area have a higher incidence of acquired diseases, such as infections. The following diseases are more prevalent in certain groups than in the general population:

- *Sickle-cell* disease affects approximately 50,000 Americans of African and Mediterranean descent. It affects both males and females equally. It is estimated that between 8% and 10% of the black population in the United States has the sickling trait. The inherited recessive trait is a defect in the hemoglobin molecule. Both parents must have the gene for sickling hemoglobin for their children to be affected clinically. In people with sickle-cell disease, the red blood cells have a 20-day life, in contrast to the normal 120-day life. The symptoms and severity of the disease are variable, depending on the syndrome. Some people are very ill and have a series of crises, while others live fairly long and normal lives (Richardson and Milne 1983, p. 417).
- *Hypertension* is more prevalent among black and other nonwhite Americans than white Americans, and the incidence is highest in Taiwan and Japan, two highly industrialized nations. It is also more common in recent immigrants to the United States. The pattern of incidence suggests that stress, obesity, and salt intake are implicated in hypertension (Overfield 1985, p. 114).
- *Diabetes mellitus* is a major health problem of Native Americans. It occurs at an early age, i.e., teens, and the rate of death from diabetes is 3 to 4 times higher among Native Americans than the general population. The inci-

dence may be related to a diet high in refined carbohydrate and fats and low in traditional foods, as well as a sedentary life-style (Overfield 1985, p. 153).

- A number of *cancers* vary racially in their incidence; however, diet and some other environmental factors appear to be better predictors of cancer than race (Overfield 1985, p. 91). In the United States, white women have a higher incidence of breast cancer than black women. Skin cancers of all types are less common among blacks than whites; this is thought to be due to the added protection dark pigmentation provides against the sun's rays. Although digestive tract cancers show high and low incidences relative to specific geographic areas and racial groups, diet rather than genetic factors are probably the cause (Overfield 1985, pp. 91–93).
- Differences among races have been found in *alcohol metabolism*. Many Asians and Native Americans convert alcohol into acetaldehyde more rapidly and convert acetaldehyde to acetic acid more slowly than the general population does. Therefore, these Asians and Native Americans experience a rapid onset of and prolonged exposure to high blood acetaldehyde levels, which cause many of the symptoms of alcohol intoxication (Overfield 1985, pp. 83–84).
- Certain *dermatologic conditions* are more common among blacks than whites. Keloid formation, an exaggerated wound healing process of the skin, is commonly found in blacks. Keloids develop following skin trauma, e.g., surgical incision and burns (Block 1976, p. 28).

FOLK HEALING AND TRADITIONAL WESTERN MEDICINE

People of many cultures use **folk medicine** as an alternative to traditional Western health care. The student may recall special teas or "cures" that were used by older family members to prevent or treat colds, fevers, indigestion, and other common health problems. People continue to use chicken soup as a treatment for "flu." Health care professionals are often unaware of the practices of folk medicine in their community because clients are embarrassed or afraid to relate the methods they use to prevent or treat illness. An additional concern about the use of such methods is the possible delay in treating a major health problem.

An important component of folk healing is the identification of the cause of illness. Many cultures attribute the cause of illness to evil spirits or evil curses. It therefore becomes the healer's role to cast out the evil spirits or to remove the curse. It is important to note that cultural healers often base their practices in religious or other spiritual belief systems. Examples of folk healing beliefs and practices are voodoo, root medicine, and "laying on of hands."

Why do individuals use these nontraditional folk healing methods? Folk medicine, in contrast to traditional health care, is thought to be more humanistic. The consultation and treatment take place in the community of the recipient, frequently in the home of the healer. It is less expensive than traditional health care, as the health problem is identified primarily through conversation with the client and the family. The healer often prepares the treatments, e.g., teas to be ingested, poultices to be applied, or charms or amulets to be worn. A frequent component of treatment is some ritual practice on the part of the healer or the recipient to cause healing to occur. Because folk healing is more culturally based, it is often more comfortable and less frightening for the client. Table 31–1 presents a comparison of the characteristics of folk medicine and traditional health care.

When folk healing practices have failed, the client may turn to traditional Western medicine for treatment. It is important for nurses to determine what folk treatments clients have used and what benefits were obtained without demeaning the clients or their health beliefs. The client may still be wearing a healing charm or amulet or wish to continue the folk treatment while accepting traditional treatment. Nurses should determine whether there are any medical contraindications to continuing their healing practices. If there are no contraindications, permiting the clients to maintain their practices may promote their well-being.

Some folk healing practices that were previously dismissed by practitioners of traditional Western medicine are gaining more interest as their effectiveness is recognized. Acupuncture, for example, is gaining more acceptance as its contributions to pain management are being demonstrated. This encourages continued research into other folk healing practices to determine their possible use in traditional Western health care.

TABLE 31–1   Characteristics of Folk Medicine versus Traditional Western Health Care

Folk Medicine	Traditional Health Care
Humanistic	Scientific
Familiar, practical, concrete	Unfamiliar, abstract
Holistic	Fragmented
Caring	Curing
Socioculturally based	Technologically based
Prevention oriented	Treatment oriented
Occurs in the home	Occurs in institutions/hospitals
Inexpensive	Expensive

CULTURAL AND ETHNIC GROUPS IN NORTH AMERICA

This section outlines some selected cultural and ethnic characteristics of significance to nurses. It is important to remember, however, that many people in ethnic and cultural subgroups do not conform to all the practices of their group. This is especially true of second- and third-generation family members, who may be assimilated into the dominant cultural group. Table 31–2 on the following pages presents a summary of the impact of culture on health and illness.

Native Americans

In the United States and Canada, the responsibility for health services for Native Americans rests with the federal government. There are, however, differences in health care practices in various geographic locations in the United States. For example, Native Americans living in the eastern states and in most urban areas are not covered by the services of the Indian Health Service, whereas Native Americans living on reservations in the western states are eligible for such services (Spector 1985, pp. 190–91).

Because about 200 different tribes of Native Americans exist in the United States, each with its own language, folkways, religion, mores, and patterns of interpersonal relationships, caution needs to be taken in generalizing about Native American culture. In terms of health care, this variability needs to be considered. For example, the Native American who lives in isolation on a reservation may hold to traditional beliefs of cure provided by the tribal medicine man, while the urban Native American who lives away from the reservation may respond more to the values of modern medicine provided by the majority culture. It is not uncommon for Native Americans to accept both kinds of health practices concurrently.

Various tribal groups differ in their traditional values and beliefs. Henderson and Primeaux (1981, pp. 73–74) list the following characteristics, which apply in general to traditional Native Americans:

- *Orientation to present.* Native Americans tend to live in the present and are not concerned about the future, whereas non-Native Americans tend to be future oriented.
- *Major concern with finishing a task.* Native Americans are more concerned about finishing a task rather than about being punctual. In the past, many Native American tribes had no word for time.
- *Giving.* The Native American who gives to others is highly respected. In some tribes, accumulating goods and saving money are not approved.
- *Respect for age.* Leadership positions are often given to the elderly rather than the young.

(continued on page 754)

TABLE 31-2 Comparison of Health-Related Factors and Subcultures

	Definition of Health	Cause of Illness—Is Prevention Possible; If so, How?	Name of Healer, Healing Practices	Problems of Entry to Health Care System	Communication Patterns	Sexuality and Family Life	Beliefs about Death
Navajo (Native American)	Harmony between individual, earth, and supernatural, as well as the ability to survive difficult circumstances[1,2]	Disease is disharmony and can be caused by violating taboo or attack by witch; illness prevented through elaborate religious rituals; do not believe in germ theory[1,2]	Medicine man, who is more than average human being, is therefore influential figure; medicine man diagnoses and treats problem; treatments include yucca root, massage, herbs, and chanting; his chant states person will get well, and person believes him[1,2]	Language; will first visit medicine man; general beliefs are not compatible with health care system and structure; problems also include money and past experiences of disrespect; fear of spirits of dead may influence decision to leave hospital early[1,2]	Time of silence after each speaker to show respect and reflection on what they said; little eye contact; time orientation not very strict; recording of conversation invasion of privacy[1,2]	Family, extended family, and tribal ties strong; cooperation emphasized; consider children as individuals as soon as they can talk, therefore can make own decisions[1,2]	Fear of spirits of dead; children and family should be with dying person[1]
Hispanic American	Gift from God, also good luck; can tell healthy person by robust appearance and report of feeling well[1,3,4]	Illness is punishment from God for wrongdoing, to be suffered; it can be prevented by eating well, praying, being good, and working; wearing medals may help; physical illness is an imbalance between "hot" and "cold" properties of body[1,3,4]	Healer called *curandero;* cures hot illness with cold medicine and reverse; classification of hot and cold diseases varies; penicillin is hot medicine; massages and cleanings are common[4]	Language; will first go to woman for advice, then if needed, to "señora," then to curandero, then to physician; many migrant workers are Hispanic, and frequent moves may make access to medical care difficult; belief that hospital is place	Confidentiality and modesty important; too many questions are insulting; it is more acceptable to make tentative statement to which they can respond; time orientation not strict; politeness essential[1,3–5]	High degree of modesty, may prefer home births for this reason; men are breadwinners, women homemakers; women are healers, men make all decisions[1,3–5]	Afterlife of heaven and hell exists

Traditional black	Harmony with nature, no separation of mind and body[4]	Disease is disharmony caused by spirits and demons; it can be prevented through good diet, rest, cleanliness, and laxatives to clean out system; some use of copper and silver bracelets for prevention	Some belief in voodoo still prevalent; religious healing practiced[4,6]	to go to die causes under-use of system; modesty may result in woman bringing friend to physician with her[1,3,4] May seek folk or religious healer first; money and type of service affect decision; emergency room frequent entry point; black women have high "noncompliance" rate[4,6]	Racism toward blacks still prevalent; common names for symptoms should be known by health worker; time orientation not strict	Matriarchy prevalent; almost 30% of black families have woman head of household; therefore women make decisions[4,6]	Death is passage from evils of this world to another state; blacks have shorter life expectancy than national average[6]
Chinese American	Balance of yin and yang (negative and positive energy forces); healthy body is gift from parents and ancestors[4,7,8]	Illness caused by imbalance of yin and yang, which may be due to overexertion or prolonged sitting; disease is prevented through better adaptation to nature[4,7]	Acupuncture and moxibustion (which is a therapeutic application of heat to skin) restore balance of yin and yang; herbal remedies such as ginseng used for many illnesses; healer is called physician[4,7]	Language; traditional Chinese physicians were paid to keep their clients well and cared for sick without fees because illness indicated they had failed in their job; Chinese physicians are available in community and may encourage clients to use Western physician; family spokesman may accompany	Open expression of emotions not acceptable; therefore might not complain about pain or symptoms; client may smile when they do not understand[4,7]	Women subservient to men; patriarchal family; ancestor worship and respect for obedience for parents observed; divorce considered disgrace[1,4,5]	Reincarnation[7]

TABLE 31–2 Comparison of Health-Related Factors and Subcultures *(continued)*

	Definition of Health	Cause of Illness—Is Prevention Possible; If so, How?	Name of Healer, Healing Practices	Problems of Entry to Health Care System	Communication Patterns	Sexuality and Family Life	Beliefs about Death
				client to Western physician[4,7]			Depends on culture and religion
Culture of poverty	Functional definition; if you can work, you are healthy[5,9]	Belief that illness is not preventable; fatalism common; future orientation minimal because present problems are too great[1,5,9]	Will often rely on folk healers and remedies because of belief and problems gaining access to health care system[5]	Use of public funding may limit access and type of care; present time orientation and beliefs about prevention may cause delay in obtaining care; inability to afford health insurance; may lose day's pay to go to physician[5,9]	May use slang and language of subculture; may view providers as authoritarian; time orientation not strict[5]	Many single-parent families with woman head of household[9]	
Health care culture	Optimal level of functioning; more than absence of disease; physical, emotional, social, and mental health included[5]	Scientific approach to cause of illness; prevention involves periodic physical examinations, laboratory studies, inoculations, as well as avoiding smoking and overeating[4]	Healing done by physician, usually takes place in office or hospital; treatments based on scientific knowledge and are frequently embarrassing or uncomfortable; often emotional component of disease is ignored[4]	Physician is main access to system; focus is basically curing illness rather than prevention; encouragement given to population to seek care as soon as symptoms appear; consider health care system as only provider	Widespread use of jargon and specialized language; large percentage of workers from middle class; often expect gratitude for care given; time orientation strict; written records kept[4]	Hierarchy, with physicians making decisions	Death usually means workers have failed to do their job; elaborate means are used to keep people alive; ethical and legal questions are being discussed and tested

[1] Data from A. T. Brownlee, *Community, culture, and care: A cross-cultural guide for health workers* (St. Louis: C. V. Mosby Co., 1978).

[2] Data from R. Wood, The American Indian and health. In *Ethnicity and health care* (NLN pub. no. 14–1625, 1976), pp. 29–35.

[3] Data from H. Gonzales, Health care needs of the Mexican American family. In *Ethnicity and health care*. (NLN pub. no. 14–1625, 1976), pp. 21–28.

[4] Data from R. Spector, *Cultural diversity in health and illness* (New York: Appleton-Century-Crofts, 1985).

[5] Data from R. Murray and J. Zentner, *Nursing assessment and health promotion through the life span* (Englewood Cliffs, N.J.: Prentice-Hall, 1975).

[6] Data from B. Martin, Ethnicity and health care: Afro-Americans. In *Ethnicity and health care* (NLN pub. no. 14–1625, 1976), pp. 47–55.

[7] Data from R. Wang, Chinese Americans and health care. In *Ethnicity and health care* (NLN pub. no. 14–1625, 1976). pp. 9–18.

[8] Data from G. Channing, What is a Christian Scientist? In Rosten, L., editor: *A guide to religions of America* (New York: Simon & Schuster, 1955).

[9] Data from M. Fromer, Community health care and the nursing process (St. Louis: C. V. Mosby Co., 1979).

Source Adapted from Joanne Gingrich-Crass, Structural variables: Factors affecting adaptation, in S. J. Wold, *School nursing: A framework for practice* (St. Louis: C. V. Mosby Co.) pp. 136–41. Copyright 1981 by Susan Wold, RN, MPH. Reprinted by permission of the author.

- *Cooperation.* A high value is placed upon working together rather than on competition.
- *Harmony with nature.* Native Americans believe in living in harmony with nature and taking from it only what one needs to live.
- *Integration into the extended family.* The Native American extended family may include three generations in one household and includes other households of relatives. The elderly are often the official and symbolic leaders.

Native Americans are sometimes assumed to be inattentive because they may not make direct eye contact when speaking with another person. This practice is based on their respect for the other person's privacy and the other person's soul. Some Native Americans believe that direct eye contact is disrespectful, intrudes on individual privacy, and may even take the other's soul away.

Associated with this belief is the Native American's commitment to autonomy. Each person has the right to speak only for himself or herself, and each person's actions should be self-initiated. Thus, the nurse may have difficulty obtaining a client's history from close family members. Family members may believe they have no right to give personal information about another; they do not mean to be uncooperative but are following an unwritten ethical code.

Native Americans accept that they will die as part of the life cycle and do not worry about how or when or why. They know they will join another world of long-ago ancestors when the Spirit intends. Funerals generally take place in the home and are associated with a large feast and gifts for relatives of the deceased. Burial rituals according to tribal tradition are important to many Native Americans.

Associated with burial is the belief of wholeness. Thus, some Native Americans may want to reclaim amputated limbs and retain them for burial when the person dies. Native Americans also fear the spirits of the dead. It is important to the dying Native American client and family that people, e.g., relatives, be present at the death.

Family   During illness, the client is comforted by visits from relatives and friends. Visits convey caring and enduring bonds of support. Being present is generally more important than talking, and it is not uncommon for large numbers of people to congregate. Most often, one person likes to remain near the client for long periods. The Native American's kinship system can be confusing to nurses of other cultures. A child, for example, may have several mothers or several sets of brothers or sisters who are not direct relatives but are considered such. These people are all-important to the ill client. The aged, particularly, are looked upon for counsel and wisdom. Friendship ties are strong and can be as meaningful as those of the family or extended family in sustaining the client's recuperative powers.

Health Beliefs   Native Americans believe that a state of health exists when a person is in total harmony with nature. Each rock, tree, animal, flower, and person is equally respected, and all are seen to coexist in harmony. The earth is considered a living organism that has a will and desire to be well, but, just as human beings, may be healthy or not. It is believed that when people harm the earth they harm themselves, and vice versa. Thus, Native Americans believe they should treat the body and the earth with respect.

Many Native Americans view illness not as an altered physiologic state but as an imbalance between the person who is ill and the natural or supernatural forces around the person. Causes of illness relate to this concept. Native Americans believe that if one interferes with this harmony by abusing or offending another person or thing, one may become ill. Even bad thoughts or wishes, such as jealousy or anger, may cause illness. In addition, supernatural or spiritual forces may be involved. In the Papago tribe of southern Arizona, for example, many persons believe that ghosts of the dead, returning as owls or other animals of night, bring sickness. All animals are believed to have supernatural powers, which they can use to send sickness (Winn 1976, p. 281).

Native Americans do not relate disease causation to germ theory. A survey of Native American registered nurses from 23 tribes revealed that none of these tribes had a word for *germ* (Henderson and Primeaux 1981, p. 243). This trait makes it difficult for Native Americans to understand the cause of tuberculosis, for example. Some Navajo Native Americans believed that the signs and symptoms caused by tuberculosis were the result of lightning. Using the wood of a tree struck by lightening for firewood or other purposes would cause abscesses to develop in the lungs (Wauneka 1976, p. 236).

Health Practices   Various curative and preventive rituals may be conducted to restore balance when illness occurs. Some of these may be carried out by medicine men, others by family members. Sacred foods, such as cornmeal, may be sprinkled on people's shoulders before they enter a home to prevent disease from entering the home. This sacred food or other substance, such as tobacco or feathers, may be sprinkled around an ill person's bed. It is important for nurses to provide privacy for such ceremonies and to inquire about how long the substance is to be left in place, how to dispose of it, and, if it must be disturbed, exactly how and where the nurse may do so. Items such as herbs or mixtures are frequently placed near the client on the bedside stand or on the bed; some may be worn by the client. Nurses need to acquire permission from the client, family, or medicine man, if these have to be removed.

Healing ceremonies, sometimes referred to as *sings* or *prayers,* may be requested. These vary in length from 30 minutes to 9 days. Space and privacy need to be provided for such ceremonies. In the hospital, the sing usually lasts less than 1 hour. A medicine man may also be requested to perform curative rituals, which vary with the signs and symptoms of the client.

Health Problems   The leading causes of death in the Native American population are accidents, suicide, diabetes, alcoholism, and homicide (Primeaux 1977, pp. 58–59). At least one-third of the Native American population is poverty-stricken. Associated with this income level are poor living conditions, malnutrition, tuberculosis, and high maternal and infant death rates. Native Americans have the highest infant mortality rate in the United States, even though their birth rate is almost twice that of the general population. This mortality rate is attributed to the high incidence of diarrhea in young babies and the harsh environment in which they live (Spector 1985, p. 187).

Nursing Implications   When caring for Native American clients, nurses need to consider the following:

- Although most Native Americans recognize the value of Anglo-Western health care, many continue to use traditional medicine and cures either independently or in conjunction with such care.
- Native Indian medicine and religion cannot be separated. Native Americans make no distinction between physical and mental illness or the mind and the body. They live the concept of wholeness.
- Tribal healing ceremonies and practices are highly ritualistic, religious ways to deal with sickness and death.
- Tribal rituals that include extended "family" members are the way that Native Americans share all aspects of life.
- Each tribe assigns symbolic meanings to foods or other substances.
- Such characteristics as not looking others in the eye should not be interpreted as disrespect, inattention, lack of interest, or avoidance.
- Nurses attempting communication with Native Americans need to be aware of the following factors:
  a. It is the custom for the person to speak only for himself or herself.
  b. Use of extensive questions during history taking may be construed as an intrusion on individual privacy. The history taker may need to rely on observation techniques and make declarative statements to elicit information from the client, such as, "You have an obvious cough that keeps you awake at night."
  c. Note taking may pose a barrier to communication, since Native Americans tend to value conversation, story telling, and listening.
  d. Native Americans often use a very low tone of voice, and the listener is expected to pay attention.

Black Americans

Black culture in America is a composite of the cultures of many black groups, all of which trace their roots to Africa. With the arrival of the first African slaves in Jamestown, Virginia, in 1619, a history of deprivation for blacks on this continent began. Even after slavery was abolished, black people endured severe economic and social deprivation. The struggles to overcome these deprivations continue today. More recently, black immigrants have come to the United States from Jamaica, Haiti, and other islands of the Caribbean, fleeing oppression and seeking economic opportunity. Black American culture is more similar to white American culture now than it was 300 years ago.

There is a large black middle class and a large black lower class. There are strong kinship bonds in both low-income and more prosperous black families. These families provide financial support, assist with child care, and serve as buffers against racism and discrimination during children's growing years. A black family may show much cohesion and sharing, particularly in times of trouble.

Often a significant member of a black family must be consulted before important decisions are made. This person may be a father, mother, aunt, son, or grandparent. Nurses need to be sensitive to the fact that a decision may not be made until this person is consulted.

When black Americans who are not familiar with the health care system enter it, they may show defensive behaviors such as hostility and suspicion. These attitudes are often adopted in expectation of being demeaned in some manner. It is important for nurses to recognize the reasons for these responses and learn to relate to all clients as worthy human beings.

Family   Middle-class black households tend to have two parents, and often both parents work to maintain a middle-class life-style. Children of middle-class black families often feel the need to achieve. Many plan to attend college to maintain or advance their position in the community.

Lower-income blacks often live in extended families, i.e., grandparents, aunts, uncles live in the house with the parents and children. Single-parent families in financial difficulty may depend on government programs for income. Black families frequently have extended support systems. LaFargue (1980, p. 1637) states that part of the survival strategy of blacks in the urban north is to immerse themselves in a domestic circle of kinfolk who will help them.

Health Beliefs   Black Americans may believe traditionally that health is maintained by proper diet, which includes a hot breakfast. Some believe that laxatives are important to keep the system running and open (Spector 1985, p. 147). A person who is a practicing Black Muslim does not eat pork or pork products.

It is important for nurses to understand the values held by a black client and that person's definition of health. Traditional definitions in black culture stem from the African view of life as a process rather than a state. All things, whether living or dead, were believed to influence each other (Spector 1985, p. 142). Health meant being in harmony with nature; illness was a state of disharmony. Therefore, illness could be treated in a number of ways, including reliance on the power of a "healer." These beliefs and practices may or may not apply to a particular black client. However, nurses should be aware of any cultural differences and take these into consideration when planning care. See also Table 31–2. In LaFargue's study, blacks defined illness as "feeling bad" or "inhibition of physical activity" (LaFargue 1972, p. 54).

Health Practices   The poor black client may not seek help until a health problem is serious for many reasons, e.g., "finances, child care problems, fear of hospitals, possibility of becoming a 'guinea pig,' and fear of death" (White 1977, p. 30), reasons often cited by poor clients regardless of ethnicity. Many black families in rural areas of the South continue to use folk health practices (Henderson and Primeaux 1981, p. 210) and home remedies. Voodoo and witchcraft are practiced to a minor extent. (Disease, for instance, may be attributed to a hex.) Spiritualists or sorcerers may sometimes be consulted, or clients may vacillate between Western physicians and witch doctors or spiritualists who can remove spells. Historically, churches have been a bulwark of support for blacks, hence religious practices and Bible reading often continue during hospitalization. Often the black clergy can help bridge the gap between the black client and health professionals because they have "the understanding of the rituals, folkways, and mores" of black culture (Smith 1976, p. 12). See Figure 31–2.

Health Problems   The major health problems of blacks in the United States are hypertension, sickle-cell disease, and cancers of the lungs, oral cavity, larynx, pharynx, esophagus, and urinary bladder. The increase in cancer in these areas is thought to be largely due to the increase in smoking (Orque et al. 1983, p. 106). Poverty among blacks leads to relatively high morbidity and mortality rates among infants and mothers, even though these rates have declined since 1960 (National Center for Health Statistics 1985, p. 2).

Obesity is a greater problem among black women than white women. Approximately 60% of black females 45 to 75 years were overweight in 1975 to 1980 (National Center for Health Statistics 1985, p. 9). Although hypertension is a problem among black adults, the incidence of hypertension decreased from 33.9% in 1971–74 to 28.6% in 1976–80 (National Center for Health Statistics 1985, p. 18).

Nursing Implications   Nursing implications relative to the care of the black client include: skin and hair care, assessing skin color, communication, and food preferences. Skin and hair care are discussed in Chapter 22, page 512 and page 538.

Many black people are very much aware of any signs of racial discrimination. A sensitive nurse should be alert to actions or behavior that may be interpreted as discriminatory and intervene as the client's advocate.

Some black clients speak black English, a highly rhythmic and stylized speech. It differs from standard English in its pronunciation and syntax and in the connotations of some words. Black English has also been called black dialect, black Creole, soul talk, Afro-American speech, Ebonics, and Afro (Orque et al. 1983, p. 86). Refugees from Haiti speak Creole, French and African dialect. Because this language is primarily spoken rather than written, communication with this group can be difficult.

Black clients may favor a traditional rural Southern diet, an urban middle-class diet, or a combination of the two. Soul food is the traditional diet of the Southern black. Pork is the chief meat. Hominy grits, black-eyed peas, and mustard and collard greens are also consumed. To these are often added cabbage, rice, white potatoes, okra, macaroni, and noodles (Orque et al. 1983, pp. 95–96). Nurses can often assist blacks who are accustomed to eating soul food to adapt special diets to their tastes.

Asian Americans

The term *Asian American* refers to four primary ethnic groups: Chinese, Japanese, Koreans, and Vietnamese. Recently, the term *Pacific Asian* has been used to include people originally from the Pacific islands, such as the Philippines, Samoa, and Guam, as well as the other Asian countries.

It is difficult to classify many Asians because they are of mixed national parentage. For example, the person's parents may be Chinese and Korean or Japanese and Filipino. In addition, most Asians view themselves as belonging to particular subgroups and ethnic groups and generally dislike being viewed as a member of another group. For example, the Chinese Americans and Japanese Americans in Hawaii consider themselves different from the "mainlanders," i.e., those in the United States.

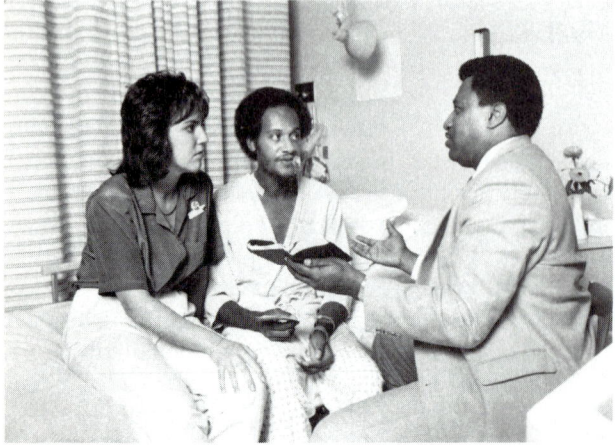

Figure 31–2   Black clergy can often help bridge the gap between the black culture and other cultures, such as the health care culture.

Because of the wide diversity of groups of Asians, full coverage of their views is beyond the scope of this book. This section focuses primarily on Chinese health beliefs and practices, since the traditions of many other Asians derive in part from them. The health beliefs and practices of Japanese Americans, Vietnamese Americans, and Filipino Americans will be considered briefly in separate sections. First, however, some general, traditional Asian values and behaviors are outlined, but the student must recognize that a wide range of behaviors exists among and within groups.

General Traditional Asian Values and Beliefs

Chang (1981, pp. 260–75) outlines the following general Asian values and behaviors:

- Traditionally, the Asian household consisted of the extended kinship family, in which grandparents, parents, siblings, uncles, aunts, and cousins lived together. Although such households are rare in North America today, members of traditional families often maintain strong emotional bonds. It is not unusual, therefore, for hospitalized Asians to have many family members visit them.

- The traditional Asian family is male dominated. Elderly persons who live with the family are usually the husband's parents. Asian women historically occupied an inferior position to men, and sons were more welcome in a family than daughters. Even in modern families, sons may receive preferential treatment. It is wise, therefore, for nurses to ascertain the opinion of the father, or in his absence the eldest son, on health care issues requiring decision making.

- Traditionally, there is unquestioning respect for and deference to authority. It is expected that each individual will maintain filial piety (devotion and loyalty to family authority). Asian families are considered a continuum from past to future. Membership includes not only the present generation but also the ancestors and the unborn. Failure to comply with familial authority, duty, and obligations, to pay obedience to the family, and to engage in behavior that gives the family and the ethnic group a good name results in feelings of shame and guilt.

- Interactions in the Asian family tend to be less verbal than those of the white middle-class family, and praise of self or of members of one's own family is considered bad manners. This behavior of Asians is often misconstrued as lack of self-esteem or as belittling of family members. This does not imply that nurses should not offer appropriate praise; but they should accept a self-deprecating response as a cultural variant.

- Asians strongly emphasize harmony and avoidance of conflict in groups. In contrast to the behavior of whites, who may consider the individual most important, the behavior of Asians may be best not for the individual but for the situation and for others in the group. Often, behavior is quiet, obedient, unassertive, reticent, agreeable, and reserved. For example, an individual may remain quiet or simply nod the head, often to avoid conflicts in ambiguous, embarrassing, or anxiety-producing situations. This behavior may be more apparent in Asian women because of their socialization. Asians avoid direct confrontations in which one of the parties must lose face; to do so, they may blame themselves for a mistake even when facts indicate that it was the other person's error.

- Asian respect for those in positions of authority such as doctors, teachers, and nurses, often evokes a yes response that is different from the American connotation of the word. Asians tend to answer yes to be polite and to mean, "I don't want to cause embarrassment." For example, in response to a nurse's question, "Is that clear?" an Asian may say yes because it is considered impolite to say "No, it is not clear"; that response may imply that the nurse is either confused or unable to communicate. It is wise, therefore, for nurses to ask questions that require more than a yes-or-no answer.

- Outward signs of feelings are discouraged. Asians are taught patterns of self-control and bravery even in situations of emotional conflict, hardship, and pain. Nurses must be aware of these attitudes when assessing pain and assisting Asians during emotional crises. Often, Asians express feelings of caring by their physical presence and attendance in times of illness rather than by an outward verbal expression of feelings.

- Asians characteristically avoid attracting special attention to themselves. This inconspicuousness is related to their culture, which emphasizes harmony, consideration of others' rights and feelings, avoidance of behavior that would dishonor the family, and respect for and obedience to those in authority.

Chinese Americans

The Chinese in the United States and Canada are largely concentrated on the west coasts of the countries, on the east coast of the United States, and in large cities such as New York and Chicago. The Chinese population can be considered in three groups: immigrants from rural China who arrived in North America 40 to 50 years ago (who still are largely oriented to Chinese folk medicine), new immigrants from several Asian countries and Hong Kong (who often practice a mixture of Chinese folk and Western medicine), and native North American descendants of nineteenth-century Chinese immigrants (who are oriented to Western medical practices but still may be influenced by their elders in regard to health care).

Family

Prior to the revolution in China, the Chinese family was patriarchal and patrilineal (tracing descent through the paternal line). Respect for ancestors and parents and obedience to the family were important. The Chinese family was frequently an extended one, with several generations living in one household. Family clans formed of people of the same bloodline with the same surnames were strong social organizations. People who came to North America 40 to 50 years ago set up the same traditional families.

Following the revolution, traditional family practices and superstitions became less evident in China and among immigrants. Although family ties continue to be strong, the nuclear family is now more common than the extended family in Chinese-American society. In many Asian families, at least two people are employed full time; they often use their income to support the extended family (Wang 1976, pp. 33–41).

Health beliefs Chinese folk medicine originated with Taoist philosophy. It proposes that the universe and health are regulated by two forces, the *yin* and the *yang*. The yin is a negative, female force; some of its characteristics are darkness, cold, and emptiness. The yang represents the positive, maleness, light, warmth, an fullness. When these two energy forces are in balance, health exists. A person with too much yin is nervous and predisposed to digestive disorders. Too much yang, on the other hand, causes dehydration, fever, and irritability.

The Chinese do not consider their bodies to be personal property. The body is viewed as a gift provided by parents and ancestors, and it thus must be cared for. Various parts of the body are controlled by yin and yang. The inside, the front part of the body, and five solid organs (*ts'ang*) that collect and store secretions—i.e., the liver, heart, spleen, lungs, and kidneys—are controlled by yin. The outside, the back part of the body, and five hollow organs (*fu*) that excrete—i.e., the gallbladder, stomach, large and small intestines, and bladder—are controlled by yang. Yin stores the vital strength of life; yang protects the body from outside forces. A person who does not balance yin and yang properly will have a short life. Illness occurs when an imbalance of yin and yang exists. The sole cause of disease is considered to be disrupted harmony.

Chinese staples are tofu and polished rice. In addition vegetables such as *bok choy, gai lan,* spinach, Chinese cabbage, and mustard greens are favored. Many Chinese do not tolerate milk or cheese well.

Health practices Some Chinese-American clients follow both Western and Chinese medical advice at the same time. This can produce problems if the therapies are not correlated. For example, a client may be receiving two forms of the same drug, one from an herbalist and one from the Western physician, thus taking a double dose. Chinese clients should be encouraged to tell a doctor whether they are taking or receiving other therapy.

Pregnant women often observe folk medicine practices (e.g., the use of soy sauce may be restricted so that the baby's skin will not be very dark). In Chinese folk medicine, herbs and acupuncture are used. A folk medicine diagnosis is made chiefly by observing, questioning, listening to the body, and taking the pulse. The prescription is a combination of herbs, which are obtained from a Chinese pharmacy.

Acupuncture is used chiefly to treat muscular and skeletal disorders and diseases characterized by excessive yang. Needles are inserted into the body at specific points along certain internal channels, which are called meridians. The internal organs are believed to be connected to the skin points and to the meridians; the acupuncture helps to balance the energy that flows within them.

The concept of yin and yang also applies to the balance of a meal. Yin is cold and includes fruits, vegetables, cold drinks, and hot (in temperature) melon soup. Yang is hot and includes, for example, soups containing ginger and scrambled eggs. In Chinese culture, the concepts of hot and cold have nothing to do with the temperature of the food. A Chinese client who is ill with a hot disease, such as an eye infection, may wish to eat cold foods rather than hot foods in order to get well.

Chinese people of the older generations may also believe that their blood is not replaceable. Therefore, they are often very reluctant to give blood even for a blood test. Like many other people, the elderly Chinese often believe that a hospital is a place to go to die rather than to get well.

Following are some differences between Western practice and Chinese folk medicine (see also Table 31–2 on page 750):

- One dose of an herbal medicine is thought to cure a person or make the person feel better. Thus, the Chinese client may be puzzled by a multiplicity of medicines prescribed in multiple doses.

- Herbs are generally boiled in water for a prescribed time before being ingested rather than prepared as capsules or pills.

- Chinese clients may change physicians during an illness in order to find the best cure. When they do so, they may not tell the former doctor because they do not want the doctor to lose face.

- Some Chinese do not understand or react well to painful diagnostic procedures. They believe that a physician should be able to make a diagnosis solely on the basis of a physical examination. Many may leave the Western health care system to avoid distasteful procedures.

- Most Chinese believe that it is best to die with the body intact. This belief originates with Confucius, who taught that only those who at the end of their lives return their physical bodies whole and sound shall be truly revered. As a result, Chinese clients may refuse surgery and donation of organs after death.

- Ginseng is a highly valued herb used as a general strength tonic for the pregnant woman (Chung 1977, p. 71).

Health problems Specific health problems more prevalent among the Chinese than the general population are eye problems, tuberculosis, dental caries, malnutrition, and mental illness. Some of these are directly related to the poor environmental conditions of North American China-towns rather than to an inherited predisposition.

Because of the stress of adjusting to American culture and the lack of family support, mental health problems among aged male Chinese have increased. Emotional problems are also related to the bicultural conflict between the individual values of freedom, egalitarianism, and individualism and the Chinese values of filial piety, loyalty, and authoritarianism (Orque et al. 1983, p. 196).

Nursing implications   Implications relative to the care of Chinese clients include the following:

1. Nurses should always convey respect by addressing the client and family members by their given names.
2. Nurses should try to provide Chinese clients with the food to which they are accustomed. Some communities have hospitals that provide special food for their Chinese clients.
3. Chinese clients are often reluctant to be admitted to hospitals. They believe hospitals are unclean places where people go to die. They may require supportive nursing intervention for reassurance.

Japanese Americans   Japanese Americans often maintain a number of their cultural values while at the same time acculturating to the larger society. Four values of the Japanese are gaman, haji, enryo, and koko. *Gaman* means self-control. A Japanese person who is stoic when experiencing pain is probably practicing gaman. The client will not verbalize the pain and may try to deal with it. Japanese who carry on in spite of adversity are considered strong (Orque et al. 1986, p. 223).

Haji, or shame, is an important cultural concept. Japanese children are taught not to bring shame on themselves or their families by unacceptable behavior. *Enryo* is a type of behavior that encompasses politeness, respect, deference, reserve, and humility. The opposite of enryo is aggressive, boisterous, loud, rude behavior (Orque et al. 1983, p. 224). For example, a Japanese man might not turn on his signal light because he does not want to bother the nurses. *Koko* is filial piety. The Japanese perceive dependence as natural for the elderly and young children. An elderly person who is dependent and has reduced authority still maintains self-esteem. This attitude contrasts to the North American view of dependence as a sign of weakness (Kalish 1967, pp. 65–69).

Japanese Americans consider time valuable and like to use it well. They will usually follow medication schedules precisely.

Vietnamese Americans   Thousands of Vietnamese came to the United States following the Vietnamese war. Another, smaller, group came later. South Vietnamese have a family-centered culture in which the children are taught to value the family's interests over their own (Orque et al. 1983, p. 250). Vietnamese value propriety over time and

indirectness over confrontation in a disagreement in order to preserve harmony. A Vietnamese client who is embarrassed at a nurse's question may say yes or laugh to lessen the embarrassment.

Filipino Americans   The Filipino culture is diverse. However, its central cultural values are shaped by a fatalistic view that God's will and supernatural forces determine what happens. Filipino culture is family centered, stressing interdependence among members of the family. Filipinos also emphasize achievement and social acceptance. A Filipino client is likely to avoid a disagreement with a nurse and speak evasively. By contrast, the white middle-class American may value an open expression of feelings and honest expression of thoughts. Because of their fatalistic view, Filipinos often show great patience and endurance when faced with illness.

Hispanic Americans

Hispanic Americans have their origins in a number of Spanish-speaking countries. The greatest numbers of Hispanic Americans in the United States come from Mexico, Puerto Rico, and Cuba, in that order. In recent years, increasing numbers of immigrants have come to the United States from Nicaragua, El Salvador, and other strife-torn countries of Central and South America. While the primary language of the Hispanic American is Spanish, it is important for the caregiver to know that there are differences in dialect and word usage among the different countries of origin.

There are many similarities and some differences among Hispanic Americans. Because a full discussion of each Hispanic American culture and its health care implications is beyond the scope of this book, the following pages focus on identified Mexican-American and Cuban-American beliefs and practices, many of which are common to other Hispanic cultures.

Traditional Mexican-American foods are beans and tortillas. Traditional foods for the Cuban American are beans and rice. For clients requiring a special diet, traditional foods can present problems. This situation requires special planning in consultation with dietitians. For example, Hispanics generally prefer rice to potatoes. The manner of preparing the rice is important; it differs from the Asian method, and even among Hispanic cultures there are differences in preparation. The diet of many low-income Hispanic Americans often contains a high proportion of starches: tortillas, rice, beans, corn, plantains, and so on. It is usually possible to plan diets to meet clients' preferences and thus increase the chances that the food will be eaten.

Family   Hispanic Americans have extended families that play an important part in their lives. The family is usually large, and life revolves around the home. Often the family's needs take precedence over the individual's needs. At a time of illness, the family will give a great deal of support.

In the Hispanic-American family, the woman is the primary caregiver, and often she decides when medical assistance should be sought.

Health Beliefs

Many Mexican Americans entered the United States during the early 1900s and brought with them the values, beliefs, and practices of rural Mexico; others are more recent immigrants. Cuban Americans started entering the United States in large numbers in the 1960s, escaping political and economic oppression in their homeland. Folk concepts of health and illness continue to affect the thinking of some second- and third-generation Mexican Americans and Cuban Americans today. See also Table 31–2 on page 750.

Mexican Americans may hold the following health-related beliefs to varying degrees:

- Certain foods promote good health, while others can produce poor health. An example of the former is tea made from fresh orange leaves; examples of the latter are rice and coffee, which should not be taken during an evening meal.

- A person must be in tune with God to maintain good health. Thus, a person who is chronically ill is believed to have offended God and is being punished.

- Health means being free of pain and being robust, even obese, rather than thin.

In addition, health is perceived as the ability to maintain a high level of normal physical activity and illness as a state of discomfort. Some Mexican Americans also believe that certain people can use magical powers to make others ill (Abril 1977, pp. 169–70). Some Mexican Americans believe that illness is due to life-style. They often have precise ideas about the types of rest, activity, recreation, and nutrition that lead to poor and good health (Gonzalez-Swafford and Gutierrez 1983, p. 29). Illness is seen as an imbalance in the individual's body or as a punishment for wrongdoing. The causes of illness can be grouped into four categories (Spector 1985, pp. 161–63):

1. *Imbalance between "hot" and "cold" or "wet" and "dry."* The four humors, or body fluids, that must be in balance are: blood (hot and wet), phlegm (cold and wet), yellow bile (hot and dry), and black bile (cold and dry). When these fluids are not in balance, illness results. Treatment in hospitals can be based on the principles of hot and cold. For example, illnesses that are classified as hot are treated with food, drugs, and drinks that are classified as cold.

2. *Magic or supernatural forces. Mal de ojo* (evil eye) is disease caused by forces outside the body, such as a person's admiration of part of another person's body, e.g., the hair. The victim can lose the admired part or fall ill. In some places, mal de ojo is thought to be prevented by having the admirer touch the admired person while complimenting him or her, and it is believed to be cured with eggs in a ritual. The symptoms of mal de ojo include headaches, fever, fatigue, and prostration.

3. *"Dislocation" of body parts.* One example of a disease of "dislocation" is *empacho,* a disease primarily seen in children that produces swelling of the abdomen as a result of intestinal blockage. It is thought to be caused by overeating foods such as soft bread and bananas.

4. *Strong emotional states. Susto,* a disease of emotional origin, is fright caused by natural phenomena such as lightning or loud noises. The symptoms have been described as insomnia, restlessness, and nervousness. It is a common folk disease that is difficult to cure but can be treated with herbal tea. *Espanto* is a disease with symptoms similar to susto. Its origin is fright caused by seeing supernatural spirits or events and can be likened to being "spooked" in American slang. *Caraje* is a rage, a response to a particular situation. The victim may continually scream, cry, or yell and display hyperactivity.

Many Mexican and Cuban Americans, when they are ill, may believe a folk medicine diagnosis rather than a Western diagnosis, even though they may also seek help from a Western physician. Healers within the Mexican American community can be either male (a *curandero*) or female (a *curandera*). Healers consulted by Cuban Americans are called *espíritos.* They offer a number of treatments; one of the most frequently used is herb tea. Both Cuban Americans and Mexican Americans have a personal relationship with their healers in contrast to the relations in a hospital.

Puerto Rican beliefs about health and illness are not unlike those of Mexican Americans. Their diseases are also classified as hot and cold; however, food and medications are classified as hot *(caliente),* cold *(frio),* and cool *(fresco)* (Spector 1985, p. 167).

Hispanic Americans consider the appearance of blood and the presence of pain as indicators that an illness is severe. If it is "natural" for a condition to occur, it is considered harmless. When it is unnatural and folk methods fail, most Mexican Americans seek medical assistance from Western practitioners.

Health Practices

Mexican Americans are generally proud people. Those who are socially and economically deprived may well have low self-esteem and be reluctant to accept care for which they cannot pay. Therefore, Mexican American clients in the hospital may not ask for help when they have pain; a young Mexican-American male may react with hostility rather than passivity in response to nursing intervention to uphold his self-image.

As do people of diverse ethnic backgrounds, many Mexican Americans look upon the hospital as a place to die. Thus, they may avoid hospitals when they can and enter only with great fear, feeling that death is imminent. Illness is generally regarded not as a personal affair but as a family affair. Therefore, when a person is ill, many relatives generally gather around and visit. Restricting visitors can cause mistrust; nurses need to deal with such a requirement in the context of illness and discuss the matter with the entire family. See Figure 31–3.

As a cultural group, Mexican Americans are very modest. Usually they consider bathing, defecating, and urinating to be very personal matters, yet they may be shy about asking a nurse to leave at such times. The sensitive nurse will provide complete privacy when possible.

Hispanic Americans encounter a number of barriers to health care: language, poverty, and time orientation. To many Hispanic Americans, time is relative; the exact time is not a primary consideration. This attitude hinders effective use of a health care system that values promptness for appointments and mandates specific intervals between doses of medications. Language is another major barrier for many Hispanic Americans seeking help from the health care delivery system. Some do not speak English, and communication is difficult and embarrassing in a system where the English language predominates. In addition, some Hispanic Americans live in the poverty line. They may not have knowledge of available health resources in the community or the money to use them.

Health Problems   Drug addiction is a major health problem among Puerto Ricans. Mexican Americans who are economically deprived may be poorly nourished, e.g., have protein and vitamin deficiencies.

Nursing Implications   Not all Hispanic Americans identify with their ethnic groups; many identify with white middle-class Americans.

- The nurse should not stereotype the Hispanic-American client. There are diverse beliefs and practices among various Hispanic-American groups. For example, the majority of Hispanic Americans, though not all, are Roman Catholic (Orque et al. 1983, p. 121).
- Hispanic Americans value modesty and privacy. The nurse should provide privacy when they must undress for an examination. The male client may find it especially difficult for a young, female nurse to provide personal care.
- The man in a Hispanic-American family may find it difficult to depend on other family members or even a nurse to do things for him. He expects to decide when and how things should be done and should be involved in decisions if health permits.

Appalachians

The 24 million Appalachians in the United States, 6 million of whom live in the Southern Appalachian region, are a subculture in American society (Tripp-Reimer and Freidl 1977, p. 4). A family-oriented group, Appalachians include upper, middle, and poor working classes. The upper and middle classes tend to share many values with the rest of

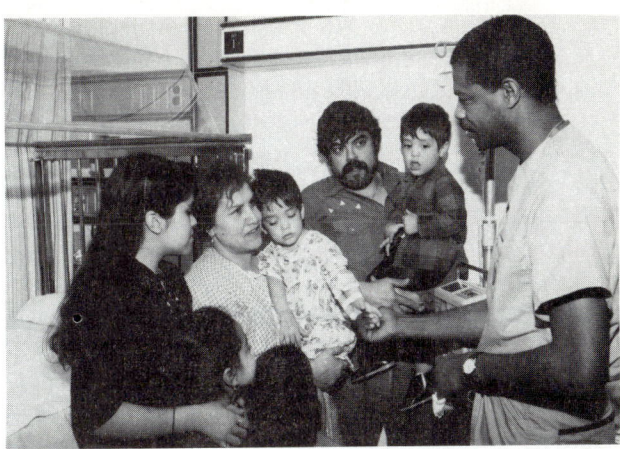

Figure 31–3   Illness is a matter of concern for an entire Hispanic family.

the United States, just as the poverty group does with other poverty groups in America. Much of Appalachia is rural, encompassing parts of the states of New York, Pennsylvania, Ohio, Maryland, West Virginia, Virginia, Kentucky, Tennessee, North Carolina, South Carolina, Georgia, and Alabama (Tripp-Reimer and Freidl 1977, p. 43).

Tripp-Reimer (1982, p. 185) found that

- Appalachians tend to have large families.
- Migrants tend to move between urban areas and "the hills."
- Migrants tend to quit school at an early age.
- Many Appalachians use welfare services.
- Appalachian migrants tend to be oriented to the present.

The religion of the Appalachians tends to be fundamentalist and fatalistic. Sometimes this fatalism prevents clients from seeking help when they are ill (Lewis et al. 1985, p. 24).

Family   Appalachians value family greatly. The family provides its members with a sense of belonging and a sense of identity. Appalachians value family privacy, a situation that has created some social and cultural isolation. Often many family members accompany a client to a health appointment, and they may wish to stay with the client if he or she is hospitalized. For many Appalachians, socialization begins and ends within the family.

The family is generally large and patriarchal. There are definite divisions between the work of men and women. Family ties are strong, and antagonism against another family may be intense. Time orientation is to the present, and the pressure of finances makes it difficult to plan ahead. Education is usually not high priority.

Health Beliefs   Appalachians tend to define an individual as ill only when the person feels ill. They have a general distrust of health organizations and fear surgery.

Health Practices When Appalachians feel ill, they tend to try home remedies, e.g., herb teas and tonics. If these cures are not effective, they may seek the advice of a lay practitioner, e.g., "granny midwife," a herbalist, or a faith healer. In an emergency or during childbirth, an Appalachian may seek "orthodox" medical or nursing help.

Health Problems The health problems of the Appalachians are largely related to their economic circumstances and to their occupations. Nutritional problems are frequently due to the fact that they cannot afford to buy much meat, and the diet may be deficient in protein and iron. Some Appalachians work in coal mines, and prolonged exposure to coal dust can cause sarcoidosis, a disease of the lungs.

Nursing Implications The nurse caring for an Appalachian client can be guided by the following (Hicks 1976):

- Appalachians consider direct eye contact to be staring, which is impolite. Nurses should be aware that Appalachians use direct eye contact to express anger or aggression.
- Nurses should also understand that Appalachians follow the "ethic of neutrality."
  a. A person must not be assertive or aggressive.
  b. People should mind their own business unless asked to do otherwise.
  c. A person should not assume authority over others.
  d. Appalachians avoid argument and seek agreement.

Arab Americans

There are approximately three million Arabs in the United States, including people who are in America temporarily (Meleis 1981, p. 1181). These include citizens of Egypt, Lebanon, Saudi Arabia, Kuwait, and many other Arab nations. Most Arabs have a common language and share symbols, mores, and beliefs. Arabs are traditionally future oriented and value the use of time to achieve future goals.

Family The Arab family is traditionally patriarchal and extended. The male of the household is responsible for earning the living outside the home and for making the decisions; women usually remain at home. Arabs have a need to affiliate with others and use an extensive social network to cope with daily stress (Meleis 1981, p. 1181).

Food plays an important part in Arab family life. When family members assemble, it is often around elaborate meals. Love and care are interwoven with food (Meleis 1981, p. 1182). Christian Arabs consume pork and alcohol, whereas Muslims consume neither. Sometimes Arab Americans find hospital food too bland and prefer to have food brought from home.

Health Beliefs Arabs believe that injury or disease affects the whole person. Often Arabs provide a vague description of their illness rather than precise symptoms because they do not have a framework for signs and symptoms. Arabs usually do not refute the germ theory, but they do believe in disease-causing entities such as the evil eye. Arabs also believe that being deprived of food can cause illness.

Health Practices Arabs do not believe in sharing a problem or asking for advice until help is offered. The person offering assistance should be able to assess the need without verifying the problem. If a nurse offers an Arab client a choice in care, the client is likely to say "No, thank you." If the nurse accepts this refusal, the client believes the nurse is not interested.

Arabs dislike disclosing information about themselves to strangers and will provide as little information as possible. Nurses must be sensitive to an Arab's dislike of revealing personal information. Sometimes Arabs will defer dealing with a matter until they feel more comfortable sharing information and may rely upon others, i.e., the social network, to give advice at times of stress. Arabs generally respect Western health care. Intrusive procedures are often highly regarded and thought to offer the greatest chance of cure.

Many Arabs regard health care as their right, and some may view health care professionals as their employees. Arab Americans respect expertise, which they regard as knowing about problems, making decisions for others, and being accountable for those decisions (Meleis 1981, p. 1182). Arab Americans may not question caregivers openly because of their respect for authority. Some Arabs wear amulets for protection. Even to say the number "five" is believed to increase protection. Deaths are believed to be the result of the will of God and the inadequacy of equipment and medicine.

Health Problems One health problem that Arabs have in common with people in the Middle East is thalassemia, a genetic condition that results in anemia. It occurs in 7% to 15% of the population in the Middle East (Overfield 1985, p. 85).

Culture of Poverty

The status of being poor is often referred to as the "culture of poverty," a phrase coined by anthropologist Oscar Lewis in the 1960s. Lewis (1966, p. 19) defined the culture of poverty as a subculture of Western society with its own values and behaviors that differ from those of the nonpoor and are passed on from generation to generation. This subculture transcends ethnic and regional boundaries. Characteristics of the poor include the following (Lewis 1966, pp. 19–25):

- Lack of participation in the larger society
- Hostility toward and mistrust of bureaucratic institutions
- Inadequate use of health services
- Long periods of unemployment
- Use of public assistance

Lewis's portrayal of the poor as a subculture is challenged by other researchers, who believe this cultural viewpoint is negative, makes no attempt to question why these features exist, and fails to recognize the role of the larger society in perpetuating poverty. Some research has shown, for example, that the poor have the same values as the rest of society and that the traits Lewis identified may not be cultural but rather responses to situational circumstances. For example, the negative work behaviors associated with the lower class are not culturally derived but situationally induced. It has been shown that the poor have a strong work ethic, want to work, and do work when given equal opportunity (Mason 1981, p. 83). Lack of societal incentives prevents the poor from obtaining and holding a job. Situational theorists believe, therefore, that if society were rid of poverty, the former poor would demonstrate middle-class attitudes and behaviors.

Still other researchers suggest that all members of a society share general, abstract values but that specific, concrete values differ among subgroups and social classes. This viewpoint combines the cultural and situational perspectives of poverty into an adaptational perspective. In other words, the poor are considered a special subgroup of society in response to social structures that make it impossible for them to actualize the values and behavior forms of the dominant society.

Health Considerations
Low-income families often define health in terms of work; if people can work they are healthy. They tend to be fatalistic and believe that illness is not preventable. Because their present problems are so great and all efforts are exerted toward survival, an orientation to the future may be lacking. Most low-income people do not have regular preventive medical checkups, because they cannot afford them. It is more important to them to work than to lose a day's pay visiting a physician. Reliance on public assistance and inability to afford health care insurance limit both the low-income person's access to health care and the type of care available.

The environmental conditions of poverty-stricken areas also have a bearing on overall health. Slum neighborhoods are overcrowded and in a state of deterioration. Neglect and disorder are common. Sanitation services tend to be inadequate. Many streets are strewn with garbage, and alleys are overrun by rats. Fires and crime are constant threats. Recreational facilities are almost nonexistent, forcing children to play in streets and alleys. Parents who can work usually work long hours and earn barely enough for sub-

sistence. They are often too tired to spend much time with their children, even though they love them. As a result, preschool children often come and go as they please, and older siblings assume the role of parent for younger children. With all of these problems confronting the poverty-stricken, it is little wonder that frustration tolerance levels are low, physical abuse is used as the form of discipline, and value is placed on children seeking employment rather than completing their educations.

Recently attention has been focused on a subculture within the poor, the *homeless*. No longer considered derelicts, bums, or drifters, there are an estimated 250,000 to 3 million people who are homeless in the United States, including families, children, military veterans, and persons with serious and persistent alcohol, drug abuse, and mental health disorders (ANA 1987, p. 26). Recognizing that the existing health care system is not accessible to the homeless, the 1987 ANA House of Delegates adopted an emergency resolution on housing and health care for people who are homeless. In this resolution, the delegates pledged to work to ensure that funding is available to provide needed services.

The poor have the same needs and feelings as other people. They are sensitive, concerned, and easily embarrassed. When admitted to health care agencies, they are sometimes treated in humiliating, condescending, and prejudicial ways by professional caregivers. Because prejudice is usually based on fear of the unknown, and because fear is based on insecurity, it is important for nurses to examine their own values and attitudes. Nurses need to become culturally sensitive and to accept and respect the differences in the life-styles of others.

HEALTH CARE SYSTEM AS A SUBCULTURE

Nurses should remember that the health care system is also a subculture. This system has rules, customs, and a language of its own.

When obtaining an education in health care, individuals become acculturated into the system. But clients who enter the system may experience culture shock.

For example, the health care culture values cleanliness; thus, nurses wash their hands often and expect their clients to wash daily. This value may not be shared by all clients, and the practice of washing daily may be new for some people.

The health care culture has its own definition of health; often it is defined as "an optimal level of functioning." See Chapter 5 for additional information. Diagnosis and prescription are usually carried out by physicians, often in offices, clinics, or hospitals. Healing practices are based on scientific knowledge. Treatment procedures are frequently embarrassing or uncomfortable. The emotional component of disease is often ignored (Wold 1981, p. 140).

Jargon is widely used in the system and tends to make clients and support persons feel more like outsiders. Many health care workers are from the middle class; they often expect gratitude for the care they give. Strict time orientation is adhered to and highly valued. This orientation may conflict with the client's. By keeping written records, caregivers may create conflict with clients' cultural beliefs.

Traditionally, health care workers interpreted the death of a client as failure. This belief is currently being reconsidered. Measures were often taken to preserve the lives of clients but seldom to facilitate death. Currently, clinical nurse specialists called *thanatology nurses* work with families and clients coping with a terminal illness.

By recognizing that they have been acculturated into the health care system, nurses can often identify the values of the system they have adopted. It is then easier to recognize how a client's values differ from those of the system. These differing values may be a source of anxiety or frustration to clients and their support persons.

CULTURE SHOCK

Culture shock is the reaction of many people to an unfamiliar situation where former patterns of behavior are ineffective. Culture shock can occur when members of one culture are abruptly moved to another culture or setting, for example, when people of Asian background and upbringing suddenly move to the United States, or when clients are abruptly thrust into the health care subculture. When this occurs, a number of stressors impinge on the individual.

Brink and Saunders (1976, pp. 129–30) describe four phases of culture shock:

1. *Phase one.* The initial phase is identified as one of excitement and is called the *honeymoon phase*. People are stimulated by being in a new environment. Behavior that indicates this feeling varies with the ethnic origin of the person and the individual personality. Some clients, for example, may express their excitement outwardly, while others are quiet. People try to learn the norms of behavior appropriate for the new environment and often ask questions.

2. *Phase two.* Once the individual feels somewhat comfortable in the new environment, phase two begins. Phase two is the realization of having to exist in the new environment. This awareness is often accompanied by feelings of frustration and embarrassment because of errors the individual makes. Accompanying this may be feelings of inadequacy, which can diminish the individual's self-concept and self-esteem. To these feelings is added loneliness. Although many people may be around, there

may be no one who enhances the individual's feelings of self-worth. Feelings of anxiety and inadequacy may be expressed through periods of withdrawal or anger.

3. *Phase three.* During the third stage, the individual seeks new patterns of behavior appropriate to the environment. The individual makes friends and can often give newcomers advice. Current friendships take on importance and occupy much of the individual's conversation. At this time, ties to the old culture become weaker.

4. *Phase four.* In the fourth phase, the individual functions comfortably and effectively. A person who returns to the former culture during this phase may experience reverse culture shock.

Nurses can assist clients and their families who are experiencing culture shock in a number of ways:

- If there is a language barrier, an interpreter can help with explanations and provide the nurse with information to incorporate into the client's care plan. The interpreter should be a trained professional. If a professional interpreter is unavailable, the nurse should obtain the services of a neutral person. The nurse should avoid having children or other family members translate for the client because the client may not wish the family to know about the health problems and because children may not understand the problem sufficiently to provide an accurate translation.

- Nurses can support clients' customs; for example, the nurse can encourage a Sikh to wear his turban in the hospital, unless this is contraindicated for health reasons. In addition, nurses can offer explanations to other health personnel about values, beliefs, and customs important to the client.

- Nurses must convey respect for a client's values, beliefs, and customs. The client will interpret an attitude of disdain or amusement as a lack of respect.

Where there is a conflict between, for example, the client's beliefs and the health care system, nurses can try to help the client find a common ground. When the client tries new behavior patterns, nurses can support the client's efforts and provide positive reinforcement. If the client experiences inadequacy or anxiety during culture shock, nurses can help by openly accepting the client and the values, beliefs, and customs.

APPLYING THE NURSING PROCESS

To provide meaningful nursing care, nurses must be aware of a client's ethnic and cultural values, beliefs, and practices as they relate to the client's health and health care. Tripp-

Reimer et al. (1984) state, "A thorough cultural assessment is not necessary;" however, basic cultural data are required.

Initially, nurses must be aware of their own ethnic and cultural values, attitudes, and practices and of the relation of these beliefs to nursing practice. As the client's culture and the nurse's culture come together in the client-nurse relationship, a unique cross-cultural environment is created (see Figure 31–4) that can either improve or impair the client's outcome. Self-awareness of personal biases can enable nurses to develop modifying behaviors or (if unable to do so) to remove themselves from situations where care may be compromised. Cultural awareness can be attained by using a values clarification approach discussed in Chapter 7.

Assessing

A structured assessment guide can help nurses gather ethnic cultural data. See Table 31–3. The purpose of an ethnic-cultural assessment is "to identify deviations in cultural parameters with the goal of modifying the client's system or modifying the health care professional's system in order to increase congruence between them" (Tripp-Reimer et al. 1984, p. 81).

A general assessment of the client identifies significant characteristics and points out areas for in-depth assessment. At this stage, the nurse makes no conclusions but obtains information from the client. The data should be both subjective, preferably in the client's words, and objective. An example of subjective data is this client statement: "I think it is very important to be healthy." An example of objective data is "Spanish speaking, born in Cuba."

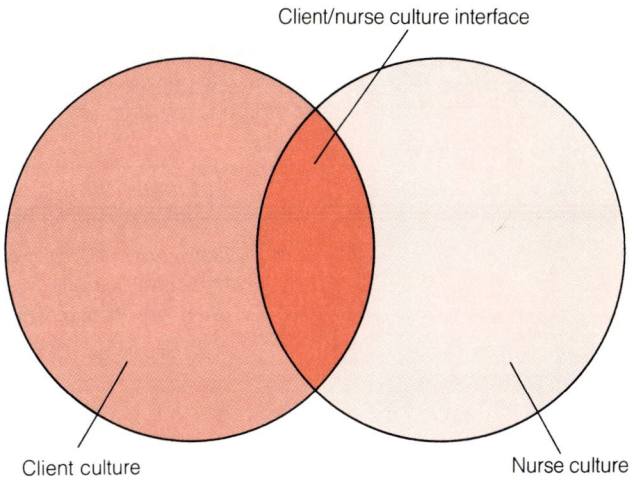

Figure 31–4 When the client culture and the nurse culture come together, a new and unique cultural environment is created.

Basic cultural data that should be obtained as part of the health assessment include some information about each of the following parameters:

- *Ethnicity.* Knowledge about the client's ethnic affiliation can enable the nurse to better understand the client's needs. It is also helpful to know if the client is a recent immigrant or refugee or if the client is the child or grandchild of immigrants. The longer the client and family have lived in North America, the more acculturated they will be to their new homeland.

(continued on page 769)

TABLE 31–3 *Bloch's Ethnic/Cultural Assessment Guide*

Data Categories	Guideline Questions/Instructions
Cultural	
Ethnic origin	Does the patient identify with a particular ethnic group (e.g., Puerto Rican, African)?
Race	What is the patient's racial background (e.g., Black, Filipino, American Indian)?
Place of birth	Where was the patient born?
Relocations	Where has the patient lived (country, city)? During what years did patient live there and for how long? Has patient moved recently?
Habits, customs, values, and beliefs	Describe habits, customs, values, and beliefs patient holds or practices that affect attitudes toward birth, life, death, health and illness, time orientation, and health care system and health care providers. What is degree of belief and adherence by patients to the overall cultural system?
Behaviors valued by culture	How does patient value privacy, courtesy, respect for elders, behaviors related to family roles and sex roles, and work ethics?

TABLE 31–3   *Bloch's Ethnic/Cultural Assessment Guide (continued)*

Data Categories	Guideline Questions/Instructions
Cultural, continued	
Cultural sanctions and restrictions	*Sanctions*—What is accepted behavior by patient's cultural group regarding expression of emotions and feelings, religious expressions, and response to illness and death?
	Restrictions—Does patient have any restrictions related to sexual matters, exposure of body parts, certain types of surgery (e.g., hysterectomy), discussion of dead relatives, and discussion of fears related to the unknown?
Language and communication processes	What are some overall cultural characteristics of patient's language and communication process?
Language(s) and/or dialect(s) spoken	Which language(s) and/or dialect(s) does patient speak most frequently? Where? At home or at work?
Language barriers	Which language does patient predominantly use in thinking? Does patient need bilingual interpreter in nurse-patient interactions? Is patient non-English-speaking or limited-English-speaking? Is patient able to read and/or write in English?
Communication process	What are rules (linguistics) and modes (style) of communication process (e.g., "honorific" concept of showing "respect or deference" to others using words only common to specific ethnic/cultural group)?
	Is there need for variation in technique of communicating and interviewing to accommodate patient's cultural background (e.g., tempo of conversation, eye-body contact, topic restrictions, norms of confidentiality, and style of explanation)?
	Are there any conflicts in verbal and nonverbal interactions between patient and nurse?
	How does patient's nonverbal communication process compare with other ethnic/cultural groups, and how does it affect patient's response to nursing and medical care?
	Are there any variations between patient's interethnic and interracial communication process or intracultural and intraracial communication process (e.g., ethnic minority patient and white middle-class nurse, ethnic minority patient and ethnic minority nurse; beliefs, attitudes, values, role variations, stereotyping [perception and prejudice])?
Healing beliefs and practices	
Cultural healing system	What cultural healing system does the patient predominantly adhere to (e.g., Asian healing system, Raza/Latina curanderismo)? What religious healing system does the patient predominantly adhere to (e.g., Seventh Day Adventist, West African voodoo, Fundamentalist sect, Pentacostal)?
Cultural health beliefs	Is illness explained by the germ theory or cause-effect relationship, presence of evil spirits, imbalance between "hot" and "cold" (yin and yang in Chinese culture), or disequilibrium between nature and man?
	Is good health related to success, ability to work or fulfill roles, reward from God, or balance with nature?
Cultural health practices	What types of cultural healing practices does person from ethnic/cultural group adhere to? Does he use healing remedies to cure *natural* illnesses caused by the external environment (e.g., massage to cure *empacho* [a ball of food clinging to stomach wall], wearing of talismans or charms for protection against illness)?
Cultural healers	Does patient rely on cultural healers (e.g., medicine men for American Indian, curandero for Raza/Latina, Chinese herbalist, hougan [voodoo priest], spiritualist, or minister for black American)?
Nutritional variables or factors	What nutritional variables or factors are influenced by the patient's ethnic/cultural background?

TABLE 31–3 *(continued)*

Data Categories	Guideline Questions/Instructions
Cultural, continued	
Characteristics of food preparation and consumption	What types of food preferences and restrictions, meaning of foods, style of food preparation and consumption, frequency of eating, time of eating, and eating utensils are culturally determined for patient? Are there any religious influences on food preparation and consumption?
Influences from external environment	What modifications if any did the ethnic group patient identifies with have to make in its food practices in white dominant American society? Are there any adaptations of food customs and beliefs from rural setting to urban setting?
Patient education needs	What are some implications of diet planning and teaching to patient who adheres to cultural practices concerning foods?
Sociologic	
Economic status	Who is principal wage earner in patient's family? What is total annual income (approximately) of family? What impact does economic status have on life-style, place of residence, living conditions, and ability to obtain health services?
Educational status	What is highest educational level obtained? Does patient's educational background influence ability to understand how to seek health services, literature on health care, patient teaching experiences, and any written material patient is exposed to in health care setting (e.g., admission forms, patient care forms, teaching literature, and lab test forms)?
	Does patient's educational background cause the patient to feel inferior or superior to health care personnel in health care setting?
Social network	What is patient's social network (kinship, peer, and cultural healing networks)? How do they influence health or illness status of patient?
Family as supportive group	Does patient's family feel the need for continuous presence in patient's clinical setting (is this an ethnic/cultural characteristic)? How is family valued during illness or death?
	How does family participate in patient's nursing care process (e.g., giving baths, feeding, using touch as support [cultural meaning], supportive presence)?
	How does ethnic/cultural family structure influence patient response to health or illness (e.g., roles, beliefs, strengths, weaknesses, and social class)?
	Are there any key family roles characteristic of a specific ethnic/cultural group (e.g., grandmother in black and some American Indian families), and can these key persons be a resource for health personnel?
	What role does family play in health promotion or cause of illness (e.g., would family be intermediary group in patient interactions with health personnel and making decisions regarding care)?
Supportive institutions in ethnic/cultural community	What influence do ethnic/cultural institutions have on patient receiving health services (i.e., institutions such as Organization of Migrant Workers, NAACP, Black Political Caucus, churches, school, Urban League, community clinics)?
Institutional racism	How does institutional racism in health facilities influence patient's response to receiving health care?
Psychologic	
Self-concept (identity)	Does patient show strong racial/cultural identity? How does this compare to that of other racial/cultural groups or to members of dominant society?
	What factors in patient's development helped to shape self-concept (e.g., family, peers, society labels, external environment, institutions, racism)?
	How does patient deal with stereotypic behavior from health professionals?

TABLE 31–3 *Bloch's Ethnic/Cultural Assessment Guide (continued)*

Data Categories	Guideline Questions/Instructions
Psychologic, continued	
	What is impact of racism on patient from distinct ethnic/cultural group (e.g., social anxiety, noncompliance to health care process in clinical settings, avoidance of utilizing or participating in health care institutions)?
	Does ethnic/cultural background have impact on how patient relates to body image change resulting from illness or surgery (e.g., importance of appearance and roles in cultural group)?
	Any adherence or identification with ethnic/cultural "group identity" (e.g., solidarity, "we" concept)?
Mental and behavioral processes and characteristics of ethnic/cultural group	How does patient relate to external environment in clinical setting (e.g., fears, stress, and adaptive mechanisms characteristic of a specific ethnic/cultural group)? Any variations based on the life span?
	What is patient's ability to relate to persons outside of ethnic/cultural group (health personnel)? Is patient withdrawn, verbally or nonverbally expressive, negative or positive, feeling mentally or physically inferior or superior?
	How does patient deal with feelings of loss of dignity and respect in clinical setting?
Religious influences on psychologic effects of health/illness	Does patient's religion have a strong impact on how patient relates to health/illness influences or outcomes (e.g., death/chronic illness, cause and effect of illness, or adherence to nursing/medical practices)?
	Do religious beliefs, sacred practices, and talismans play a role in treatment of disease?
	What is role of significant religious persons during health/illness (e.g., black ministers, Catholic priests, Buddhist monks, Islamic imams)?
Psychologic/cultural response to stress and discomfort of illness	Based on ethnic/cultural background, does patient exhibit any variations in psychologic response to pain or physical disability of disease processes?
Biologic/Physiologic (consideration of *norms* for different ethnic/cultural groups)	
Racial-anatomic characteristics	Does patient have any distinct racial characteristics (e.g., skin color, hair texture and color, color of mucous membranes)? Does patient have any variations in anatomic characteristics (e.g., body structure [height and weight] more prevalent for ethnic/cultural group, skeletal formation [pelvic shape, especially for obstetric evaluation], facial shape and structure [nose, eye shape, facial contour], upper and lower extremities)?
	How do patient's racial and anatomic characteristics affect self-concept and the way others relate to patient?
	Does variation in racial-anatomic characteristics affect physical evaluations and physical care, skin assessment based on color, and variations in hair care and hygienic practices?
Growth and development patterns	Are there any distinct growth and development characteristics that vary with patient's ethnic/cultural background (e.g., bone density, fatfolds, motor ability)? What factors are important for nutritional assessment, neurologic and motor assessment, assessment of bone deterioration in disease process or injury, evaluation of newborns, evaluation of intellectual status, or capacity in relationship to motor/sensory development in children? How do these differ in ethnic/cultural groups?
Variations in body systems	Are there any variations in body systems for patient from distinct ethnic/cultural group (e.g., gastrointestinal disturbance with lactose intolerance in blacks, nutritional intake of cultural foods causing adverse effects on gastrointestinal tract and fluid and electrolyte system, and variations in chemical and hematologic systems [certain blood types prevalent in particular ethnic/cultural groups])?

▶

TABLE 31–3 *(continued)*

Data Categories	Guideline Questions/Instructions
Biologic/Physiologic, continued	
Skin and hair physiology, mucous membranes	How does skin color variation influence assessment of skin color changes (e.g., jaundice, cyanosis, ecchymosis, erythema, and its relationship to disease processes)?
	What are methods of assessing skin color changes (comparing variations and similarities between different ethnic groups)?
	Are there conditions of hypopigmentation and hyperpigmentation (e.g., vitiligo, mongolian spots, albinism, discoloration caused by trauma)? Why would these be more striking in some ethnic groups?
	Are there any skin conditions more prevalent in a distinct ethnic group (e.g., keloids in blacks)?
	Is there any correlation between oral and skin pigmentation and their variations among distinct racial groups when doing assessment of oral cavity (e.g., leukoedema is normal occurrence in blacks)?
	What are variations in hair texture and color among racially different groups? Ask patient about preferred hair care methods or any racial/cultural restrictions (e.g., not washing "hot combed" hair while in clinical setting, not cutting very long hair of Raza/Latina patients).
	Are there any variations in skin care methods (e.g., Using Vaseline on black skin)?
Diseases more prevalent among ethnic/cultural group	Are there any specific diseases or conditions that are more prevalent for a specific ethnic/cultural group (e.g., hypertension, sickle cell anemia, lactose intolerance)?
	Does patient have any socioenvironment diseases common among ethnic/cultural groups (e.g., lead paint poisoning, poor nutrition, overcrowding [prone to tuberculosis], alcoholism resulting from psychologic despair and alienation from dominant society, rat bites, poor sanitation)?
Diseases ethnic/cultural group has increased resistance to	Are there any diseases that patient has increased resistance to because of racial/cultural background (e.g., skin cancer in blacks)?

Source From M. S. Orque, B. Bloch, and L. S. A. Monrroy, *Ethnic nursing care: A multicultural approach* (St. Louis: C. V. Mosby Co., 1983), pp. 63–69. Used by permission.

■ *Language.* The primary language should be identified, even if the client speaks English fluently. When under the stress of illness, the client often finds it difficult to communicate in English and reverts back to the primary language. Additionally, the nurse should be sure that the client understands instructions or descriptions of procedures and treatments. Sometimes, the client exhibits behaviors of understanding, e.g., nodding the head affirmatively while instructions are given. Nurses should assess understanding by having clients repeat the instructions in their own words. If the nurse feels that the client does not understand such instructions when given in English, the nurse should obtain an appropriate interpreter.

■ *Religious or spiritual requirements.* An understanding of the client's religious or spiritual beliefs is necessary for providing culture-specific care. Although the nurse is usually aware of the requirements of the religions most commonly practiced in the United States and Canada (see Chapter 32), less common religious or spiritual practices may also affect the health needs of the client. The client may wish to have a cultural healer present to conduct prayers or ritual practices. The client may be wearing protective charms or amulets. Knowing the nature of these requirements can enable the nurse to be supportive of the client's spiritual needs.

■ *Family patterns.* The nurse should identify family roles and patterns and ascertain which family member is the primary decision maker. Female clients from cultures where the husband or father assumes this role may refuse to make decisions. The nurse should recognize the significance of statements such as, "I can't make a decision until I talk to my husband," or "Ask my husband; he knows best." Another factor to determine is the client's need for the presence of family members and loved ones, especially if the client is dying.

- *Food preferences and patterns.* Beliefs about food can have great impact on the health of the client. The nurse needs to identify the foods that are forbidden in the client's culture; for example, Muslims are forbidden to eat pork products, and Orthodox Jews will not mix meat and dairy products at the same meal. At the same time, the nurses should ask the client about any food preferences that are believed to have healing qualities. Additionally, the nurse should assess the client's eating behaviors to differentiate cultural from physical manifestations; the client who does not eat, for instance, may believe that fasting will cleanse the body of impurities or atone for God's punishment.

- *Health beliefs and practices.* The nurse should assess the client's beliefs about the cause of the illness. Does the client believe that illness is caused by germs or life-style risks, or does the client believe that illness is a punishment, a curse, or an imbalance with nature? What remedies has the client already tried, and how effective have they been?

The general assessment is then followed by an assessment that is specific to the health care area of concern, e.g., preschool immunizations, diabetic teaching, home care. At this time, the nurse obtains information about the client's own reason for seeking out health care, ideas about the current problem and any previous problems, and the treatment the client anticipates. For example, the client may say, I came to the center because I feel ill; the world is moving around me. This happened once before. The doctor gave me some pills, and it went away."

Some questions that may elicit this information are:

- What do you think caused your problem?
- What treatment do you think you need now?
- What are the chief problems your sickness has caused you? (Kleinman et al. 1978, p. 254).

Diagnosing

The nursing diagnoses for a client who has special ethnic or cultural needs can relate to any number of factors, such as language and diet. See examples and possible contributing factors, below.

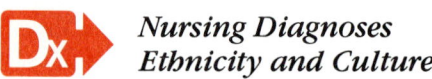

Nursing Diagnoses Ethnicity and Culture

Impaired verbal communication related to language barrier

Ineffective individual coping related to change in environment

Ineffective family coping related to absence of extended family

Powerlessness related to inability to communicate verbally

Social isolation related to language barrier

Impaired verbal communication is the "state in which the individual experiences, or could experience, a decreased ability to speak but can understand others" (Carpenito 1989, p. 238). Among the defining characteristics of this nursing diagnosis are the inability to speak the dominant language and difficulty in finding the correct words when speaking, both of which the person of a minority ethnic group or culture might display. In addition to the listed etiologic factor (language barrier), this diagnosis may also be related to fear, shyness, lack of privacy, or lack of a support system (all possible etiologic or contributing factors for minority group clients) as well as pathophysiologic and situational conditions.

Ineffective individual and **family coping** are discussed in Chapter 33. **Powerlessness** is the "state in which an individual perceives a lack of personal control over certain events or situations" (Carpenito 1989, p. 591). Its characteristics include expressing dissatisfaction over inability to control what is happening, refusing or being reluctant to participate in decision making, apathy, depression, or resignation to the situation. As discussed earlier in this chapter, people from some cultures are fatalistic about the meaning of illness and the purpose of hospitalization. It would be incorrect for the nurse to make this nursing diagnosis if the client values such a belief.

Social isolation is the "state in which the individual experiences a need or desire for contact with others but is unable to make that contact" (Carpenito 1989, p. 695). This is a difficult diagnosis to describe. Carpenito comments: "Since social isolation is a subjective state, all inferences made regarding a person's feelings of aloneness must be validated. Because the causes vary and people show their aloneness in different ways, there are no absolute clues to this diagnosis" (1989, p. 695). This diagnosis is most likely for the client whose family or support persons are not nearby during the hospitalization.

Planning

When planning nursing goals, the nurse needs to include appropriate cultural factors relative to the client. According to Tripp-Reimer et al. (1984, p. 81), this stage "is directed at cultural factors that may influence nursing intervention." For example, nurses can ask a client:

- What would you normally eat while you have this condition?
- What will your family do?
- Is there something I haven't mentioned that you think would be helpful?

After obtaining this information, a nurse must organize the data. According to Tripp-Reimer et al. (1984, p. 81), "the nurse is interested in the extent to which the client's beliefs, values, and customs are congruent with a trifold set of standards:

- Standards of the client's identified culture or ethnic group
- Standards of the nurse's own culture
- Standards of the health care facility that serves as the setting for the interaction"

A nurse may find that the data among the three standards are not congruent. For example, a client always eats rice as a major part of each meal. The nurse (a) learns that this practice is standard for the client's ethnic group, (b) recognizes that this practice differs from the nurse's own, and (c) realizes that the health care facility cannot provide rice for each meal. Next, the nurse relates this information by determining whether the treatment plan accommodates the client's eating practices. If not, then the nurse can find ways of integrating the client's practice into the nursing care plan, e.g., the client's family might bring cooked rice to the hospital. If, however, rice is contraindicated because of the client's condition, the nurse must establish ways to help the client change if the client is amenable to change or ways to understand the client if the client will not change (Tripp-Reimer et al. 1984, p. 81).

It is often important to include the client's family in the planning of nursing care, particularly if the client is a member of an extended family and if the family is a major support for the client. When planning care strategies, nurses should consider language barriers and assess the need for an interpreter. Sometimes ethnic clients require information to avoid confusion or embarrassment. For example, an ethnic client who is extremely modest may require considerable preparation and support before having an enema.

Possible client goals for the nursing diagnoses discussed earlier in this chapter are to:

- Reduce or resolve impaired communication.
- Establish effective verbal and nonverbal communication to indicate basic needs.
- Adapt to the change in environment necessitated by hospitalization.

- Maintain social contact with family, other visitors, and staff.

A goal for the family might be to establish effective coping mechanisms for dealing with the client's hospitalization.

Specific outcome criteria that make these goals measurable are provided below.

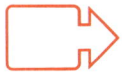

Outcome Criteria
Ethnicity and Culture

The client:
- Relates feelings, concerns, requests through interpreter.
- Uses an effective method of communication with verbal and nonverbal cues.
- Participates in the decision-making process regarding planned care.
- Uses family/friends and unit staff to assist with adaptation to changes in the environment.
- Indicates feelings of greater control over the illness and therapy.
- Interacts with staff through an interpreter or by using nonverbal cues.

The client's family:
- Uses available resources to adapt to the client's hospitalization.
- Employs effective alternative strategies for meeting those needs usually met by the extended family.

Implementing

Successful nursing interventions for clients of different cultures require supportive communication by nurses and respect for the client's values, beliefs, and practices. White (1977) stresses the importance of being culturally sensitive. Cultural sensitivity includes respecting individuals, recognizing the diversity of cultural beliefs and practices, acting on behalf of the ethnic client who is being denied safe, quality care, and modifying the care plan by incorporating those client beliefs and practices that are not life-threatening (Bello 1976, pp. 36–38, 45). Suggested guidelines for nurses are shown in the box on the following page.

Evaluating

To evaluate the effectiveness of nursing care of clients in special ethnic and cultural groups, the nurse determines the extent to which the goals have been met by comparing the client's current status with predetermined outcome or evaluation criteria.

Nurses must also evaluate their own competence in this area by asking themselves questions such as these: "How well did I communicate?" "How well did I include the client and the family in the nursing process?" "How well do I understand the client's values, beliefs, and customs?" "How well did I communicate respect for these?" "Was I able to incorporate any of the client's values, beliefs, and customs into the plan of care?" "How well did I communicate my acceptance of values, beliefs, and customs that differ from mine?" "Am I aware of my values, beliefs, and customs?"

RESEARCH NOTE

Are Community Health Nurses Confident in Caring for the Culturally Different Client?

Community health nurses responded to a 30-item Likert-type cultural self-efficacy scale to determine their degree of confidence in caring for three culturally distinct ethnic groups: blacks, Puerto Ricans, and Southeast Asians. The highest confidence scores were reported in the evaluation of care of the black population; the care of Southeast Asians received the lowest ratings, while scores rating the care of Puerto Ricans fell between the other two groups. Low scores were noted on items that involved knowledge of health beliefs and practices and views about respect, authority, and modesty. Higher scores were observed when an interpreter was used correctly. In no instance did ratings reach even moderate levels of confidence. Results suggest that nurses do not feel confident about caring for any of the three major ethnic groups in American communities.

Implications: Nurses need to receive adequate education and preparation in cross-cultural concepts to be able to serve ethnically diverse populations.

H. Bernal and R. Froman. The confidence of community health nurses in caring for ethnically diverse populations, *Image: Journal of Nursing Scholarship,* Winter 1987 19:201–203.

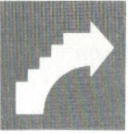

CLINICAL GUIDELINES
Interacting with Clients of Differing Culture or Ethnicity

- Convey respect for the individual and respect for the individual's values, beliefs, and cultural and ethnic practices.

- Learn about the major ethnic or cultural groups with whom you are likely to have contact.

- Analyze your own communication, e.g., facial expression and body language, and how it may be interpreted. See Chapter 15 for additional information.

- Recognize differences in ways clients communicate, and do not assume the meaning of a specific behavior, e.g., lack of eye contact, without considering the client's ethnic and cultural background.

- Understand your own biases, prejudices, and stereotypes.

- Relate clients' different cultural beliefs, e.g., the cause of swollen feet, to your own. In this way, you convey interest and respect for the clients' beliefs.

- Recognize that cultural symbols and practices can often bring a client comfort.

- Support the client's practices and incorporate them into nursing practice whenever possible and not contraindicated for health reasons; for example, provide hot tea to a client who drinks hot tea and never drinks cold water.

- Don't impose a cultural practice on a client without knowing whether it is acceptable; for example, Puerto Rican clients prefer not to be touched unnecessarily (Shubin 1980, p. 29).

- Remember that the color of a client's skin does not always determine the client's culture.

- Learn how a client views health, illness, grieving, and the health care system.

- Review your own attitudes and beliefs about health and objectively examine the logic of those attitudes and beliefs and their origins.

- Increase your knowledge about different beliefs and values and learn not to be threatened when they differ from your own.

- Remember that during illness clients may return to preferred cultural practices; for example, the client who has learned English as a second language may revert to the primary language.

CHAPTER HIGHLIGHTS

▶ North Americans come from a variety of ethnic and cultural backgrounds, and many North Americans retain at least some of their traditional values, beliefs, and practices.

- Many minority groups in North America are bicultural, i.e., they embrace two cultures: their original ethnic culture and a North American culture.

- An individual's ethnic and cultural background can influence beliefs, values, and customs.

- Through acculturation, most ethnic and cultural minority groups in North America modify some of their traditional cultural characteristics.

- Individual factors frequently modify an individual's cultural values, beliefs, and customs.

- Stereotyping individuals can lead to incorrect assumptions.

- When assessing a client's culture, the nurse considers values, beliefs, and customs related to health and health care.

- Some health problems are more prevalent in certain ethnic groups than in the general population.

- Nurses must understand their own cultural values, beliefs, and customs in order to provide meaningful nursing care.

- An ethnic and cultural assessment guide can help the nurse gather data about a client.

- People can experience culture shock when they enter an unfamiliar environment where previous patterns of behavior are ineffective.

READINGS AND REFERENCES

SUGGESTED READINGS

Kwok, A. W. H. March 1982. Culture conflict: A study of the problems of Chinese immigrant adolescents in Canada. *Canadian Nurse* 78:32–34.

This author interviewed one Chinese and two Vietnamese adolescents about the conflicts they encounter not only as adolescents but also as individuals having to deal with two cultures. The values of one culture often conflict with those of the other.

Powers, B. A. April 1982. The use of orthodox and black American folk medicine. *Advances in Nursing Science* 4:35–47.

Powers describes the function of healers in black folk culture, including their characteristics and functions. The beliefs and practices of the black folk medical system are explained. The implications for nursing practice include the possible reluctance of clients to admit using folk practices, the need for mutual respect between the nurse and client, and the use of culture brokers.

Tripp-Reimer, T., Brink, P. J., and Saunders, J. M. March/April 1984. Cultural assessment: Content and process. *Nursing Outlook* 32:78–82.

The authors present a process for assessment of a client's ethnic/cultural values, beliefs, and customs. Included is a table comparing the content of nine cultural assessment guides.

White, E. H. March 1977. Giving health care to minority clients. *Nursing Clinics of North America* 12:27–40.

White discusses black, Spanish-speaking, Native American, and Asian clients in this article. Topics covered include life-styles, health problems, health practices, and nursing implications.

RELATED RESEARCH

Aroian, K. J., Patsdaughter, C. A. Summer 1989. Multiple-method, cross-cultural assessment of psychological distress. *Image: Journal of Nursing Scholarship* 21:90–3.

Bernal, H., Froman, R. Winter 1987. The confidence of community health nurses in caring for ethnically diverse populations. *Image: Journal of Nursing Scholarship* 19:201–3.

Cameron, E., Badger, F., Evers, H. May 1989. District nursing, the disabled and the elderly: Who are the Black patients? *Journal of Advanced Nursing* 14:376–82.

SELECTED REFERENCES

Abril, I. F. May/June 1977. Mexican-American folk beliefs: How they affect health care. *The Journal of Maternal Child Nursing* 2:168–73.

American Journal of Nursing. June 1979. Black skin problems. *American Journal of Nursing* 79:1092–94.

American Nurses Association. 1987a. *1987–88 Health Legislation Fact Sheets*. Kansas City, Mo.: ANA.

American Nurses Association. 1987b. *1987 House of Delegates Summary of Proceedings*. Kansas City, Mo.: ANA.

Anderson, A. B., and Frideres, J. S. 1981. *Ethnicity in Canada: Theoretical perspectives*. Toronto: Butterworths.

Backup, R. W. February 1980. Health care of the American Indian patient. *Critical Care Update* 7:16 + .

Bannerman, R. H., Burton, J., and Wen-Chieh, C., editors. 1983. *Traditional medicine and health-care coverage: A reader for health administrators and practitioners*. Geneva: World Health Organization.

Bello, T. A. February 1976. The third dimension: Cultural sensitivity in nursing practice. *Imprint* 23:36–38, 45.

Bigham, G. D. September 1964. To communicate with Negro patients. *American Journal of Nursing* 64:113–5.

Bloch, B. 1976. Nursing intervention in black patient care. In Luckraft, D., editor. *Black awareness: Implications for black patient care*. New York: American Journal of Nursing Co.

Boyle, J. S., and Andrews, M. M. 1989. *Transcultural concepts in nursing care*. Boston: Scott, Foresman & Co.

Brink, P. J., editor. 1976. *Transcultural nursing. A book of readings*. Englewood Cliffs, N.J.: Prentice-Hall.

Brink, P. J., and Saunders, J. M. 1976. Culture shock: Theoretical and applied in Brink, P. J., editor. pp. 126–38. *Transcultural nursing: A book of readings*. Englewood Cliffs, N.J.: Prentice-Hall.

Calhoun, M. A. September 1986. Providing health care to Vietnamese in America: what practitioners need to know. *Home Healthcare Nurse* 4:14–19.

Campbell, T., and Chang, T. April 1973. Health care of the Chinese in America. *Nursing Outlook* 21:245–49.

———. 1981. Health care of the Chinese in America. In Henderson, G., and Primeaux, M., editors. *Transcultural health care*. Menlo Park, Calif.: Addison-Wesley Publishing Co.

Carpenito, L. J. 1989. Nursing diagnosis. *Application to clinical practice*. 3d ed. Philadelphia: J. B. Lippincott Co.

Chae, M. November 1987. Older Asians. *Journal of Gerontological Nursing* 13:10–17.

Chang, B. 1981. Asian-American patient care. In Henderson, G., and Primeaux, M., editors. *Transcultural health care*. Menlo Park, Calif.: Addison-Wesley Publishing Co.

Chen-Louie, T. T. 1980. Bicultural experiences, social interactions, and health care implications. In Reinhardt, A. M., and Quinn, M. D. *Family-centered community nursing: A sociocultural framework*. St. Louis: C. V. Mosby Co.

Christian, J. L., and Greger, J. L. 1985. *Nutrition for living*. Menlo Park, Calif.: Benjamin/Cummings Publishing Co.

Chung, H. J. March 1977. Understanding the Oriental maternity patient. *Nursing Clinics of North America* 12:67–75.

Davis, M., and Yoshida, M. March 1981. A model for cultural assessment of the new immigrant. *Canadian Nurse* 77:22–23.

DeSantis, L. October 1989. A profile of cultural diversity in nursing practice. *Florida Nurse* 37:15.

Drakwlic, L., and Tanaka, W. March 1981. The East Indian family in Canada. *Canadian Nurse* 77:24–26.

Friedman, M. M. 1981. *Family nursing theory and assessment*. Norwalk, Conn.: Appleton-Century-Crofts.

Giger, J. N., Davidhizar, R. January/February 1990. Transcultural nursing assessment: A method for advancing nursing practice. *International Nursing Review.* 37(1):199–202.

Gonzalez-Swafford, M. J., and Gutierrez, M. G. November/December 1983. Ethno-medical beliefs and practices of Mexican-Americans. *Nurse Practitioner* 8:29–30, 32, 34.

Gordon, V. C.; Matousek, I. M.; and Lang, T. A. November 1980. Southeast Asian refugees: Life in America. *American Journal of Nursing* 80:2031–36.

Grasska, M. A., and McFarland, T. September 1982. Overcoming the language barrier: Problems and solutions. *American Journal of Nursing* 82:1376–79.

Henderson, G., and Primeaux, M. editors. 1981. *Transcultural health care*. Menlo Park, Calif.: Addison-Wesley Publishing Co.

Hicks, G. 1976. *Appalachian valley*. New York: Holt, Rinehart and Winston.

Holleran, C. March/April 1988. Nursing beyond national boundaries: The 21st century. *Nursing Outlook* 36:72–75.

Kalish, R. A. 1967. Of children and grandfather: A speculative essay on dependency. *Gerontologist* 7:65–69.

Kim, M. J.; McFarland, G. K.; and McLane, A. M. 1989. *Pocket guide to nursing diagnoses*. 3d ed. St. Louis: C. V. Mosby Co.

Kleinman, A. et al. February 1978. Culture, illness, and care: Clinical lessons from anthropologic and cross-cultural research. *Annals of Internal Medicine* 88:251–58.

LaFargue, J. P. 1972. Role of prejudice in rejection of health care. *Nursing Research* 2:53–58.

———. September 1980. A survival strategy: Kinship network. *American Journal of Nursing* 80:1636–40.

Leininger, M. 1970. *Nursing and anthropology: Two worlds to blend*. New York: John Wiley and Sons.

———. 1974. Humanism, health, and cultural values. In Leininger, M., editor. *Health care dimensions*. Philadelphia: F. A. Davis Co.

———. November 1987. Transcultural eating patterns and nutrition: Transcultural nursing and anthropological perspectives. *Holistic Nursing Practice* 3:16–25.

Lewis, O. October 1966. The culture of poverty. *Scientific American* 215:19–25.

Lewis, S.; Messner, R.; and McDowel, W. August 1985. An unchanging culture: Caring for Appalachian patients and their families. *Journal of Gerontological Nursing* 11:20–24, 26.

MacDonald, J. September 1987. Preparing to work in a multicultural society. *Canadian Nurse* 83:31–32.

Martin, B. J. W. Ethnicity and health care: Afro-Americans. In *Ethnicity and health care*. 1976. New York: National League for Nursing.

Martinelli, A. M. August 1987. Pain and ethnicity: How people of different cultures experience pain. *AORN Journal* 46:273–74, 276, 278.

Mason, D. J. October 1981. Perspectives on poverty. *Image* 13:82–85.

Meleis, A. I. June 1981. The Arab American in the health care system. *American Journal of Nursing* 81:1180–83.

Murillo-Rhode, I. May 1980. Health care for the Hispanic patient. *Critical Care Update* 7:29–36.

North American Nursing Diagnosis Association. Approved nursing diagnostic categories for clinical use and testing. Summer 1988. *Nursing Diagnosis Newsletter* 15:1–3.

National Center for Health Statistics. August 1985. *Charting the nation's health trends since 1960*. DHHS pub no. (PHS) 85-1251. U.S. Department of Health and Human Services, Hyattsville, Md.: Public Health Service.

Ohlson, V. M., and Franklin, M. 1985. *An international perspective on nursing practice*. Pub. No. NP-68F. Kansas City, Mo.: American Nurses' Association.

Orque, M. S.; Bloch, B.; and Monrroy, L. S. A. 1983. *Ethnic nursing care: A multicultural approach*. St. Louis: C. V. Mosby Co.

Overfield, T. 1985. *Biologic variation in health and illness*. Menlo Park, Calif.: Addison-Wesley Publishing Co.

Powers, B. A. April 1982. The use of orthodox and black American folk medicine. *Advances in Nursing Science* 4:35–47.

Primeaux, M. H. March 1977. American Indian Health care practices. *Nursing Clinics of North America* 12:55–65.

Rempusheski, V. F. September 1989. The role of ethnicity in elder care. *Nursing Clinics of North America* 24:717–24.

Richardson, E. A. W., and Milne, L. S. November/December 1983. Sickle-cell disease and the childbearing family: An update. *American Journal of Maternal/Child Nursing* 8:417–22.

Roberson, M. H. B. January 1987. Home remedies: A cultural study. *Home Healthcare Nurse.* 5:35–40.

Rothenburger, R. L. May 1987. Understanding cultural differences is the key to transcultural nursing. *AORN Journal* 45:1203, 1205–6, 1208.

———. May 1990. Transcultural nursing: Overcoming obstacles to effective communication. *AORN Journal* 51:1349–50.

Schermerhorn, R. A. 1970. *Comparative ethnic relations: A framework for theory and research*. New York: Random House.

Shubin, S. June 1980. Nursing patients from different cultures. *Nursing 80* 10:78–81. Canadian edition 10:26–29.

Smith, J. A. 1976. The role of the black clergy as allied health care professionals in working with black patients. In Luckraft, D., editor. *Black awareness: Implications for black patient care*. New York: American Journal of Nursing Co.

Spector, R. E. 1985. *Cultural diversity in health and illness.* 2d ed. New York: Appleton-Century-Crofts.

Statistics Canada. June 1989. *Census Canada* 1986. Cat. no. 93-109. Ottawa: Minister of Supplies and Services.

Tripp-Reimer, T. Spring 1982. Barriers to health care: Variations in interpretation of Appalachian client behavior by Appalachian and non-Appalachian health professionals. *Western Journal of Nursing Research* 4:179–91.

Tripp-Reimer, T. Afifi, L. A. September 1989. Cross-cultural perspectives on patient teaching. *Nursing Clinics of North America* 24:613–9.

Tripp-Reimer, T., and Freidl, M. March 1977. Appalachians: A neglected minority. *Nursing Clinics of North America* 12:41–54.

Tripp-Reimer, T.; Brink, P. J.; and Saunders, J. M. March/April 1984. Cultural assessment: Content and process. *Nursing Outlook* 32:78–82.

U.S. Department of Commerce, Bureau of the Census. April 1984. *Census of Population, General Population Characteristics United States Survey.* Washington, D.C.: Government Printing Office.

———. 1989. *Statistical abstract of the United States.* 109th ed. pp. 4–11, 15–57. Washington, D.C.: Government Printing Office.

Wang, R. M. 1976. Chinese Americans and health care. In *Ethnicity and health care.* New York: National League for Nursing.

Wauneka, A. D. 1976. Helping a people to understand. In Brink, P. R., editor. *Transcultural nursing: A book of readings.* Englewood Cliffs, N.J.: Prentice-Hall.

White, E. H. March 1977. Giving health care to minority patients. *Nursing Clinics of North America* 12:27–40.

Wilson, U. M. 1983. Nursing care of American Indian patients. In Orque, M. S.; Bloch, B.; and Monrroy, L. S. A. *Ethnic nursing care: A multicultural approach.* St. Louis: C. V. Mosby Co.

Winn, M. C. 1976. A proposed tuberculosis program for Papago Indians. In Brink, P. J., editor. *Transcultural nursing: A book of readings.* Englewood Cliffs, N.J.: Prentice-Hall.

Wirth, L. 1945. The problem of minority groups. In Linton, R. *The science of man in the world crisis:* New York: Columbia University Press.

Wold, S. J. 1981. *School nursing: A framework for practice.* St. Louis: C. V. Mosby Co.

Wood, R. 1976. The American Indian and health. In *Ethnicity and health care.* New York: National League for Nursing.

Spiritual and Religious Beliefs

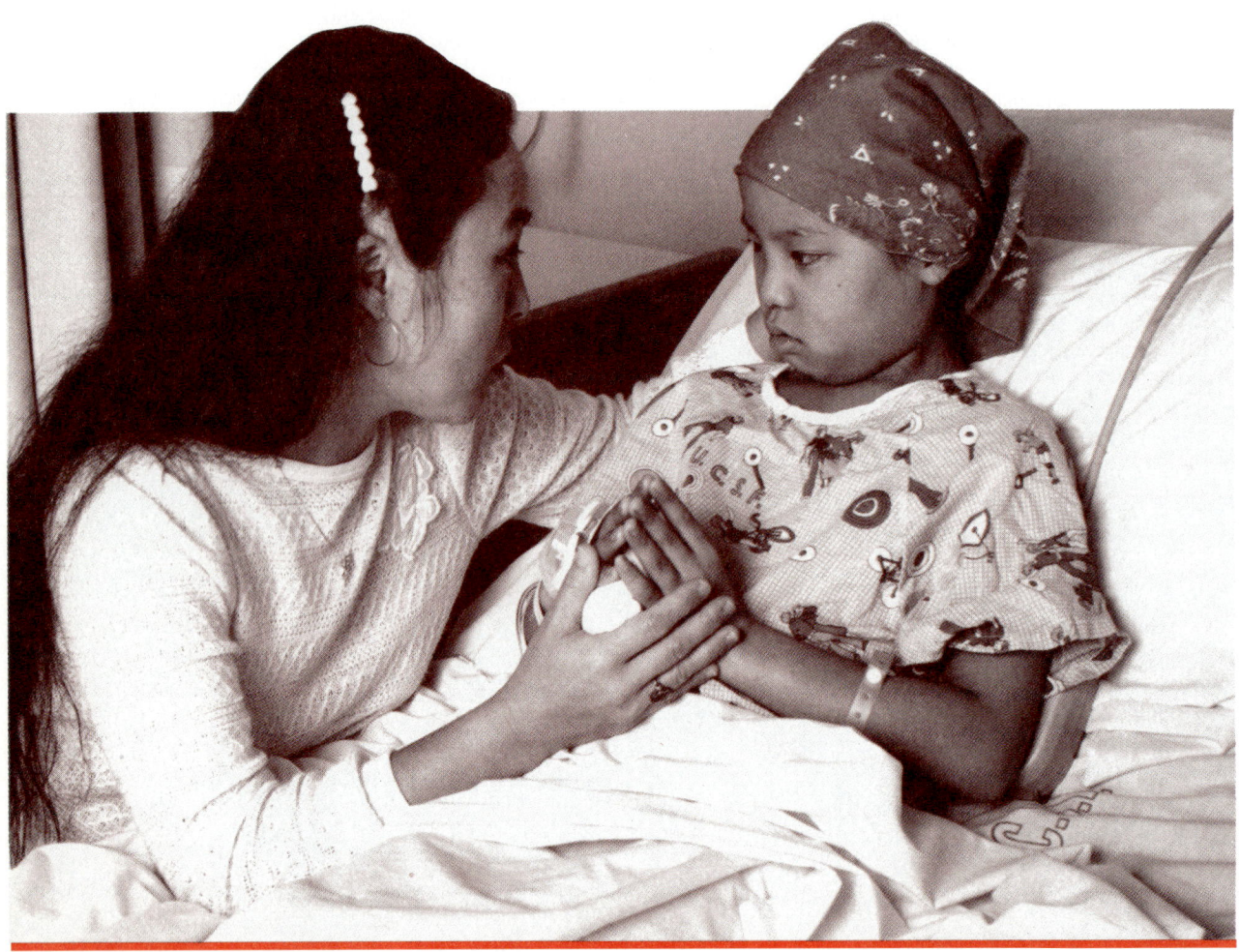

CONTENTS

OBJECTIVES

▶ List essential facts about spiritual beliefs and religious practices as they relate to health care.

▶ Describe essential facts about the spiritual development of different age groups.

▶ List expressions of spiritual well-being.

▶ Identify categories of information to obtain through the nursing history and clinical assessment.

▶ List essential aspects of nursing diagnosis related to spiritual care.

▶ Explain facts about nursing interventions to support clients' spiritual beliefs and religious practices.

▶ State outcome criteria essential for evaluating the clients' progress.

SPIRITUALITY, FAITH, AND RELIGION

Spirituality, faith, and religion are separate entities, yet some people use the words interchangeably. **Spirituality** or spiritual belief is a belief in or relationship with some higher power, creative force, divine being, or infinite source of energy. For example, a person may believe in "God," in "Allah," or in a "higher power." "The spiritual dimension tries to be in harmony with the universe, strives for answers about the infinite and especially comes into focus or sustaining power when the person faces emotional stress, physical illness, or death. It goes outside a person's own power" (Murray and Zentner 1989, p. 78).

Stoll (1989, p. 7) describes spirituality as a two-dimensional concept: the vertical dimension is the relationship with the transcendent/God or whatever supreme values guide the person's life; the horizontal dimension is the person's relationship with self, others, and the environment. There is a continuous interrelationship between and among the two dimensions. A *spiritual need* is a person's need to maintain, increase, or restore beliefs and faith and to fulfill religious obligations. It is often the nurse who identifies a need for spiritual assistance and obtains the desired help. According to Shelly and Fish, certain spiritual needs underlie all religions: (a) the need for meaning and purpose, (b) the need for love and relatedness, and (c) the need for forgiveness (1988, pp. 40–53). Some people believe that these needs are common to all humanity.

Faith, according to Fowler and Keen (1985, p. 18), is a universal—a feature of living, acting, and self-understanding. To have faith is to believe in or be committed to something or someone. In a general sense, religion or spiritual beliefs are an individual's attempt to understand one's place in the universe, i.e., how that person sees the self in relation to the total environment. For additional information about Fowler's stages of spiritual development, see Chapter 24, page 596.

Religion is an organized system of worship. Religions have central beliefs, rituals, and practices usually related to death, marriage, and salvation. They also often have rules of conduct applicable to daily life. Many people satisfy their spiritual needs through a specific religion or religious framework.

Religious development of an individual refers to the acceptance of specific beliefs, values, rules of conduct, and rituals. Religious development may or may not parallel spiritual development. For example, a person may follow certain religious practices and yet not internalize the symbolic meaning behind the practices.

RELIGION AND ILLNESS

Spiritual and religious beliefs are important in many people's lives. They can influence life-style, attitudes, and feelings about illness and death. Some organized religions specify practices about diet, birth control, and appropriate medical therapy. Some religious groups condemn modern science because of "false teachings," such as evolution. Other groups support medical therapy in general but object to specific practices; e.g., the Seventh Day Adventist Church urges its members to avoid all drugs unless they are exceedingly ill.

Spiritual beliefs may assume greater importance at a time of illness than at any other time in a person's life, helping some people accept illness and explaining illness for others. Some clients may look upon illness as a test of faith; i.e., "If I have enough faith I will get well." Viewed from this perspective, illness is usually accepted by the client and the client's support persons and does not shake their religious beliefs.

Other people may look upon illness as punishment and think, "What have I done to deserve this?" These people associate disease with immoral behavior and believe their illness is punishment for past sins. They may believe that through prayer, promises, and perhaps penance, the cause of the disease will disappear. Such people may believe that health professionals treat only the symptoms of disease and that they will become well if they are forgiven. If such an individual does not get well, then the support persons either accept the "punishment" or view the "punishment" as unfair.

Usually, spiritual beliefs help people to accept illness and to plan for the future. Religion can help people prepare for death and strengthen them during life. It can provide a meaning to life and to death; a haven of strength, serenity, and faith at a time of crisis; a sense of security; and a tangible network of social support.

Certain spiritual beliefs are in conflict with accepted medical practice. When a person's faith leads the person to reject certain medical treatment, life may be threatened. For example, many practicing Jehovah's Witnesses will not accept blood transfusions because of religious doctrine.

SPIRITUAL DEVELOPMENT

Table 32–1 summarizes human spiritual development from infancy to adulthood.

James Fowler describes the development of faith in people. Fowler believes that faith, or the spiritual dimension, is a force that gives meaning to a person's life. Fowler uses the term *faith* as a form of knowing, a way of being in relation to "an ultimate environment" (Fowler and Keen 1985, p.21). To Fowler, **faith** is a relational phenomenon; it is "an

active 'mode-of-being-in-relation' to another or others in which we invest commitment, belief, love, risk and hope" (Fowler and Keen 1985, pp. 21–23). Fowler's stages in the development of faith are given in Table 24–9, page 597.

RELIGIOUS BELIEFS RELATED TO HEALTH CARE

Meeting the spiritual needs of clients and their support persons is part of the function of nurses as well as designated chaplains and other clergy. The term **clergy** refers to priests, rabbis, ministers, church elders, deacons, and other spiritual advisers. Some religious groups, such as the Church of Latter-Day Saints and the Christian Scientists, do not have ordained clergy; they usually do have people whose role it is to minister to the ill, and these people must be recognized by nurses as having appropriate functions. In Chris-

TABLE 32–1 *Summary of Spiritual Development*

Developmental Stage	Characteristics	Developmental Stage	Characteristics
Infants and toddlers	Both infants and toddlers have no sense of right or wrong, spiritual beliefs, or convictions to guide activities.		because they understand it but because it is part of daily life.
	Toddlers may follow rituals (e.g., saying prayers at bedtime) in imitation of their parents.		Five-year-olds often make up prayers themselves.
	Toddlers may attend a church nursery school, but emphasis is on enhancing their positive self-image.		They believe that God or human beings are responsible for such natural events as rain and wind. They may reason, "The rain is God crying; the wind is God blowing air out of His mouth."
Preschoolers	Parental attitudes toward moral codes and religion convey to children what is considered good and bad.		Many go to church school and participate in religious holidays. They ask many questions about the meaning of the holidays and need explanations about them. However, they are more occupied with such rituals as Santa Claus coming at Christmas than with the reason behind the holiday. When children begin to question such myths as the Easter Bunny, they are ready for a more sophisticated explanation about Easter.
	Preschoolers copy what they see rather than what they are told. If what they see and what they are told are contradictory, problems arise.		
	They often ask questions about morality and religion (e.g., "Why is [some action or word] wrong?" and "What is heaven?"). They believe that their parents, like God, are omnipotent.	School-age children	Young school-age children expect that their prayers will be answered, good rewarded, and bad punished.
	Two methods of spiritual education are used with preschool children: indoctrinating them and letting them choose their own way.		During the prepuberty stage, children become aware of spiritual disappointments. They realize that their prayers
	Preschoolers follow a religion not		

tian Science, the role of ministering to the sick is carried out by a practitioner (reader).

Although nurses cannot expect to be well versed about the practices of all the religious groups in North America, it is important to be familiar with the major religious groups of the community. Representatives of a religion will usually give nurses information required in the care of clients. Some of the larger religious groups are discussed briefly here. Other reference texts can supply greater detail and information not included in this summary.

The major religions of North America are Protestantism, Catholicism, and Judaism. There are many Protestant denominations, e.g., Episcopalians, Methodists, and Baptists. The denominations share some doctrines, but each denomination has its own interpretation of scripture and its own religious practices. Catholicism also encompasses several groups, e.g., the Roman Catholic Church, the Greek Orthodox Church, and the Russian Orthodox Church. See the accompanying box for a summary of the major beliefs of Protestantism, Catholicism and Judaism.

Major religions, denominations, and some spiritual groups are listed alphabetically below. Selected facts about each group are included, but no attempt has been made to discuss broad philosophical beliefs or issues.

Agnosticism and Atheism

An **agnostic** is a person who doubts the existence of God or a supreme being or believes the existence of God has not been proved. An **atheist** denies the existence of God. **Theism** is the belief in the existence of a god or gods. **Monotheism** is the belief in the existence of one God. The moral and ethical codes of agnostics and atheists are not derived from theistic beliefs.

American Muslim Mission (Black Muslim)

The American Muslim Mission is not the same as Islam, although their beliefs are similar. Members emphasize black

TABLE 32–1 *Summary of Spiritual Development* (continued)

Developmental Stage	Characteristics	Developmental Stage	Characteristics
	are not always answered on their own terms, and they begin to reason rather than accept a faith blindly.	Adults	Young adults who need to answer the religious questions of their own children may find that the teachings of their own early childhood are more acceptable to them now than during adolescence.
	Some children drop or modify certain religious practices (e.g., praying for tangible benefits); others continue to follow religious practices because of dependence on their parents.		During the middle years, adults often find that they have more time for religious activities because their children are older.
	During adolescence, children compare the standards of their parents with others and determine which ones they want to incorporate into their own behavior.		Older adults who have developed religious values often endeavor to broaden them and to understand the newer values of younger people.
	Adolescents also compare the scientific viewpoint with the religious viewpoint and try to bring the two together.		Elderly adults who do not have mature religious beliefs may experience a feeling of deprivation as they become less active, e.g., because of retirement.
	By 16 years, many adolescents have decided whether to accept the family religion. They may experience personal religious awakenings, such as being saved or converted, either suddenly or gradually.		During these years, people face death (their own, their spouses', and their friends'). This recognition may make them despondent. The development of a mature religious philosophy can often help older people face reality, participate in life, have feelings of self-worth, and accept death as inevitable.
	Adolescents with parents of different faiths may choose one faith over the other or no faith.		
	For some, a firm faith provides strength during these turbulent years.		

independence and are encouraged to obtain health care provided by the black community.

Black Muslims have a special procedure for washing and shrouding the dead and special funeral rites. Dietary considerations include prohibitions against alcoholic beverages and pork. Because the use of tobacco is forbidden, clients who are sharing a room require nonsmoking roommates.

Baptist

Baptists believe in the possibility of cure of illness by the "laying on of hands." Although some believe in faith healing to the exclusion of medical therapy, most seek competent medical help. Some Baptists do not drink coffee or tea, and many Baptists do not take alcohol. Birth control, sterilization, and abortion (therapeutic or demand) are left to indi-

vidual choice. When clients are clearly terminally ill, artificial prolongation of life is discouraged. Full-term stillborn babies are buried; less than full-term fetuses are not. Infant baptism is not practiced.

Buddhism

The doctrine of avoidance of extremes is practiced by Buddhists and applied to the use of drugs, blood, or vaccines. Buddhism does not condone the taking of lives in any form, but, if a client is beyond recovery and can no longer strive toward "enlightenment," euthanasia *may* be permitted. Likewise, certain circumstances may warrant abortion. Buddhists approve of either burial or cremation. Last rite chanting is frequently practiced at the bedside of the deceased. Cleanliness is very important.

Buddhists generally do not practice any dietary restrictions, although members of some sects are strict vegetarians. Many Buddhists do not use tobacco, alcohol, or drugs. Buddhists have special holy days: January 1, February 15, March 21, April 8, May 21, July 15, September 1 and 23, and December 8 and 31. Buddhist clients may need to be asked how they feel about tests and treatments on those days.

Church of Christ, Scientist (Christian Science)

Members of the Church of Christ, Scientist, oppose human intervention to cure illness, seeing it as God's will. Sickness and sin are errors of the human mind and can be changed by altering thoughts rather than by medicine. People who strictly follow this religion will not accept a physician's consultation or medical treatment and rarely, if ever, enter a hospital. Christian Scientists do not permit psychotherapy, because in this process the mind is altered by others. A Christian Science "practitioner" can be called to minister to the sick, and spiritual healing is practiced. Physicians and midwives may be used during childbirth, however.

Drugs and blood transfusions are not used, and biopsies and physical examinations are not sought. Tobacco and alcohol are considered drugs and not used. Tea and coffee are often refused. Vaccines are accepted only as required by law. Christian Scientists do not have strictly defined policies about birth control, sterilization, or abortion. Autopsy is discouraged but accepted in sudden deaths, and Christian Scientists are unlikely to seek or donate organs for transplant. Whether a person wishes to rely completely upon Christian Science is up to the individual. In some areas, the church operates nursing homes in which there is complete reliance on church doctrine.

Eastern Orthodoxy

There are a number of Eastern Orthodox denominations, including Greek, Armenian, Ukrainian, Bulgarian, and Syrian. Most believe in infant baptism by immersion 8 to 40 days after birth. The last rites may be obligatory if death is impending. Dietary restrictions depend on the particular sect. During Lent, abstinence from meat and dairy products is carried out unless this is harmful to health. Eastern Orthodox beliefs and practices generally do not restrict medical science; however, the Russian Orthodox church discourages autopsy as well as donation of body parts.

The Greek Orthodox church opposes abortion. The church advocates confession at least yearly. The last rites include administration of **Holy Communion** (also referred to as the *Eucharist* or the *Lord's Supper*), a memorial sacrament in which the worshipper receives consecrated bread (or a thin wafer) representing the body of Jesus Christ, and wine or grape juice representing the blood of Jesus. The church encourages prolonging life, even for terminally ill clients.

Episcopalian (Anglican)

The Episcopal or Anglican religion places no restrictions on the use of drugs, blood, or vaccines; biopsies, or amputations or transplants for saving life. It permits birth control and sterilization, autopsy, therapeutic abortion as a life-saving measure, burial or cremation, and genetic counseling. Abortion on demand, however, is regarded as unacceptable. Episcopalians celebrate Holy Communion. Some members of this church fast before receiving Communion and abstain from meat on Fridays. The church advocates confession. The rite for anointing of the sick may be performed but is not mandatory.

Hinduism

Hindus have many dietary variations, and these vary according to the particular sect. Some do not eat veal and beef and their derivatives. Some are strict vegetarians. Alcohol may be consumed at Western social functions. Most Hindus accept modern medical practices; artificial insemination is rejected, however, because sterility reflects divine will. When giving a Hindu medications, the nurse avoids touching the client's lips, if possible.

Hindus practice special rites at death. Death is considered rebirth. The priest pours water into the mouth of the corpse and ties a thread around the wrist or neck to indicate blessing. This thread must not be removed. The body undergoes cremation, and the ashes are disposed of in holy rivers. Some injuries, such as loss of a limb, are considered signs of wrongdoing in a previous life, although the afflicted person is not an outcast from society. Hindus do believe there is a natural division among people, so that little mixing occurs among castes (hereditary social classes).

Jehovah's Witness

Jehovah's Witnesses are opposed to blood transfusions and organ transplants, although some individuals do agree to them in a crisis. Nonblood plasma expanders and autologous transfusions may be accepted. When parents refuse to have an infant transfused, a court order may be sought transferring custody to the courts or to an official of the hospital.

Members of the church eat meat that has been drained of blood. The use of alcohol and tobacco is discouraged. Some oppose modern medicine. Infant baptism is not practiced.

Jehovah's Witnesses generally have a neutral attitude toward birth control, believing it is a matter of individual conscience. Both therapeutic and demand abortions are forbidden. Burial and cremation are approved. Autopsy is approved only as required by law, and no parts of the body are to be removed. This restriction has implications for donor transplants.

Judaism

There are the three main Jewish groups: the Orthodox is the most strict; the Conservative and Reform groups are less so. Jewish law demands that Jews seek competent medical care. Jews allow the use of drugs, blood, and vaccines; biopsies and amputations are also permitted. Some Orthodox Jews believe that the entire God-given body must be returned to the earth, and they require any body tissue to be buried. Donor transplants may therefore not be acceptable to Orthodox Jews. The nurse must ensure that amputated limbs or organs are made available to such Orthodox families for burial. Cremation is discouraged. Autopsy may be permitted in less strict groups, provided that parts of the body are not removed. Bodies, even those of fetuses, are washed by the ritual burial society and buried as soon as possible after death.

Therapeutic abortion is permissible if the woman's physical or psychologic health is threatened. Demand abortion is prohibited. Vasectomy is not permitted.

Orthodox and Conservative Jews observe kosher dietary laws, which prohibit pork, shellfish, and other foods and the eating of milk products and meat products at the same meal. Reform Jews usually do not observe kosher dietary regulations.

Circumcision is performed by Orthodox and Conservative Jews on the eighth day of a male baby's life, although it may be delayed if medically contraindicated. The rabbi and male synagogue members may be present, and a Jewish physician or *mohel* (ritual circumciser acquainted with Jewish law and hygienic medical technique) performs the circumcision. Special arrangements generally need to be made for the ceremony and the physician's approval obtained.

Orthodox and some Conservative Jews observe the Sabbath from sunset Friday to sunset Saturday and may resist hospital admission or medical procedures during that period or during major Jewish festivals, unless the treatment is necessary to preserve life. Rosh Hashanah is the first day of the Jewish new year, which occurs in September. Ten days later, Yom Kippur marks the end of the time devoted to reflecting upon life.

Lutheran

The Lutheran church imposes no restrictions on medical procedures, including autopsies and therapeutic abortions, and no dietary restrictions. Abortion on demand is not approved, however. Marriage and procreation are discouraged when offspring are likely to inherit severe physical or mental deficits. Birth control and sterilization are left to the individual's conscience. Members are baptized 6 to 8 weeks after birth, and those who wish may be anointed and blessed before death. Burial rites are generally performed on infants who die after 6 to 7 months' gestation.

Mennonite

Members of the Mennonite church are baptized in their middle teens. The church advocates no special dietary restrictions, although some congregations require abstinence from alcohol. No restrictions are placed on medical procedures, although demand abortion is not approved in some sects of the church; in others, it is left to individual conscience. Some mennonites oppose the laying on of hands.

Mormon (Church of Jesus Christ of Latter-Day Saints)

Some Mormons believe in healing by the power of God through authorized priesthood holders. However, there is no prohibition on medical therapy—in fact, the church operates health facilities. Alcohol, tobacco, tea, coffee, and other drinks with caffeine (e.g., cola) are prohibited, and meat is eaten sparingly. Some members of the church wear a special undergarment. Mormon clients in the hospital may request the Sacrament of the Lord's Supper by a church priesthood holder. Abortion is opposed unless the life of the woman is in danger.

Muslim/Moslem (Islam)

Islam is a major religion of North Africa and the Near East. There are over 70 sects of the Islamic faith. It emphasizes strict rituals and prayers.

All pork products are prohibited, and some oppose alcoholic beverages. There is a fasting period in the ninth month of the Mohammedan year (Ramadan), but people who are ill are exempt from it. Circumcision is practiced, and cleanliness is very important.

If a fetus is aborted 130 days or more after conception, it is treated as a fully developed human being. Before that time, it is looked upon as discarded tissue. Abortion is forbidden.

The dying person must confess sins and beg forgiveness. Only relatives and family can touch the body after death. They wash and prepare it and turn it toward Mecca. Islam encourages prolonging life, even for the terminally ill.

Pentecostal (Assemblies of God)

The Pentecostal church has no doctrine against modern medical science, including blood transfusions. Members are encouraged to abstain from use of alcohol, tobacco, and illegal drugs. Some members do not eat pork. Members may pray for divine healing, and in some congregations anointing with oil is practiced.

Roman Catholicism

It is a Catholic belief that an infant has a soul from the moment of conception; therefore, a fetus must be baptized unless it is obviously dead, as must all babies whose health or life is endangered. Baptism may be performed by any person (e.g., a physician or nurse in the absence of a priest) who does what the church requires. A valid baptism requires pouring water on the baby's head while repeating the prescribed Trinitarian invocation: "I baptize thee in the name of the Father, of the Son, and of the Holy Spirit." When performed by a nurse or physician, the baptism should be recorded on the infant's chart and the family and priest informed.

The Roman Catholic church encourages anointing of the sick. The **sacrament of the sick** is now considered both a source of strength or healing and a preparation for death. The priest anoints several areas of the body with oil. Catholics can now be anointed more than once. Many older Catholics, however, may respond to this sacrament with fear or dread, considering it a sign of imminent death. Thus, before a reluctant client is anointed, the nurse or priest should interpret its current meaning to the client, to minimize apprehension. Anointing of the sick may be preceded by confession and Holy Communion. These sacraments are also performed by a priest or other commissioned person.

The Roman Catholic belief in the "principle of totality" underlies a general acceptance of medical procedures. A donor transplant is accepted as long as loss of the organ does not deprive the donor of life or functional integrity of the body. Biopsies and amputations are accepted in the same light. Autopsy is also accepted; again, all major parts of the body (those retaining human quality) must be given an appropriate burial or cremation.

Strict laws govern birth control, sterilization, and abortion. The only approved method of birth control is abstinence; artificial means are illicit. Sterilization is forbidden unless there is a sound medical indication for it. Both demand

and therapeutic abortions are prohibited, even to save the mother's life.

Some Catholics observe certain dietary and fasting practices but are excused from otherwise obligatory fasting or abstaining from meat on Ash Wednesday and Good Friday. Sunday is the day of worship, although church services are held in some churches other days of the week as well.

Salvation Army

The Salvation Army places no restrictions on medical procedures, including transplants and autopsies. Birth control and sterilization are acceptable within marriage. Demand abortions are opposed, but therapeutic ones are approved. The Army has many hospitals and social centers for people, e.g., hostels for the indigent.

Seventh-Day Adventist (Church of God, Advent Christian Church)

The Adventist church does not practice infant baptism but conducts baptism of adults by immersion. In dietary matters, it prohibits alcohol, tobacco, tea, coffee, and the use of illegal drugs, and some members advocate ovolacto-vegetarian diets. Some sects practice divine healing and anointing with oil. Saturday is considered the Sabbath by some.

Adventists are encouraged to avoid drugs, but they recognize that blood transfusions, vaccines, and drugs are sometimes necessary. Birth control and sterilization are left to individual conscience. Abortion is approved if the mother's life is endangered or if pregnancy is due to rape or incest. The use of hypnotism is opposed.

Unitarian Universalist Association

Unitarian Universalists emphasize reason, knowledge, individual responsibility, and personally established values. There are no dietary restrictions or official sacraments in the church, and no medical practices are prohibited. The Unitarian Universalist church encourages its members to donate parts of their bodies to research and to medical banks. Cremation is often preferred to burial.

United Church of Canada

The United Church of Canada is the largest Protestant denomination in Canada. It was formed in 1925 by the amalgamation of the Methodist, Presbyterian, and Congregationalist Churches. It operates some hospitals in underserviced areas of Canada. There are no restrictions about the use of blood or vaccines. Burial and cremation are approved.

SPIRITUAL HEALTH AND THE NURSING PROCESS

Assessing

Spiritual health, or **spiritual well-being,** is a feeling of being "generally alive, purposeful, and fulfilled" (Ellison 1983, p. 332). According to Pilch (1988, p. 31), spiritual wellness is "a way of living, a lifestyle that views and lives life as purposeful and pleasurable, that seeks out life-sustaining and life-enriching options to be chosen freely at every opportunity, and that sinks its roots deeply into spiritual values and/or specific religious beliefs."

Ellison and Paloutzian (1982) designed a spiritual well-being scale that includes specific questions for a client (see Table 32–2 for sample statements). They found that people who scored high on the scale tended to be less lonely, more socially skilled, and higher in self-esteem; furthermore, their religious commitment was more intrinsic to their personalities.

Nursing History   Nurses may elicit data about a client's spiritual beliefs as part of the general history. Often the information elicited is limited to the client's religious affiliation. Nurses should never assume, however, that a client follows all the practices of the client's stated religion.

Stoll (1979, p. 1574) suggests a spiritual history guide to elicit information in four areas: (a) the person's concept of God or deity, (b) the person's source of hope and strength,

TABLE 32–2   *Spiritual Well-Being*

Religious component

I believe that God loves me and cares about me.

I have a personal and meaningful relationship with God.

I believe God is concerned about my problem.

My relationship with God helps me not to feel lonely.

I feel most fulfilled when I am in close communion with God.

My relationship with God contributes to my sense of well being.

Meaning and purpose in life

I feel that life is a positive experience.

I feel very fulfilled and satisfied with life.

I feel a sense of well-being about the direction my life is headed in.

I feel good about my future.

I believe there is some real purpose in life.

Source: Sample statements from a scale on religious meaning and purpose of life. © Spiritual Well-Being Scale. 1982 by Craig W. Ellison and Raymond F. Paloutzian. All rights reserved.

ASSESSMENT INTERVIEW
Spirituality

- Are any particular religious practices important to you? If so, could you please tell me about them?

- Will being here interfere with your religious practices?

- Do you feel your faith is helpful to you? In what ways is it important to you right now?

- In what ways can I help you to carry out your faith? For example, would you like me to read your prayer book to you?

- Would you like a visit from your spiritual counselor or the hospital chaplain?

- What are your hopes and your sources of strength right now?

(c) the significance of religious practices and rituals to the person, and (d) the relationship the person perceives between the individual's spiritual beliefs and state of health. Stoll further cautions that all people have a right to their own values and beliefs and that they have a right not to discuss or reveal these beliefs to others. The spiritual assessment is best taken at the end of the assessment process or following the psychosocial assessment, once the nurse has developed a relationship with the client and/or support person and feels that it is appropriate to discuss spiritual matters. The questions provided in the box above may be suitable.

Clinical Assessment   **Spiritual distress** may be revealed by one or more of the following:

1. *Affect and attitude.* Does the client appear lonely, depressed, angry, anxious, agitated, apathetic, or preoccupied?

2. *Behavior.* Does the client appear to pray before meals or at other times? Does the client read religious literature? Does the client complain frequently, need unusually high doses of sedation, pace the halls at night, joke inappropriately, have nightmares and sleep disturbances, or express anger at religious representatives or a deity?

3. *Verbalization.* Does the client mention God, prayer, faith, the church, or religious topics (even briefly)? Does the client ask about a visit from the clergy? Does the client express fear of death, concern with the meaning of life, inner conflict about religious beliefs, concern about a

relationship with the deity, questions about the meaning of existence, the meaning of suffering, or the moral/ethical implications of therapy?

4. *Interpersonal relationships.* Who visits? How does the client respond to visitors? Does a minister come? How does the client relate to other clients and nursing personnel?

5. *Environment.* Does the client have a Bible, prayer book, devotional literature, religious medals, a rosary, or religious get-well cards in the room? Does a church send altar flowers or Sunday bulletins? (Shelley and Fish 1988, pp. 61–62).

Signs of spiritual health are given in Table 32–3.

Diagnosing

The nursing diagnosis that relates to problems with spirituality is **Spiritual distress,** defined as "a disruption in the life principle that pervades a person's entire being and that integrates and transcends one's biologic and psychological nature" (Kim, McFarland, and McLane 1989, p. 62) *or* "the state in which the individual experiences or is at risk of experiencing a disturbance in the belief or value system which provides strength, hope, and meaning to life" (Carpenito 1989, p. 710).

O'Brien (1982, p. 81) subcategorizes spiritual distress as follows:

- Spiritual *pain,* i.e., difficulty accepting the loss of a loved one or intense suffering (physical or emotional)

- Spiritual *alienation,* i.e., separation from religious or faith community

- Spiritual *anxiety,* i.e., challenge to beliefs and value systems (e.g., by moral/ethical nature of therapy such as abortion, blood transfusion, surgery, etc.)

- Spiritual *guilt,* i.e., failure to abide by religious rules

- Spiritual *anger,* i.e., difficulty accepting illness, loss, or suffering.

- Spiritual *loss,* i.e., difficulty finding comfort in religion

- Spiritual *despair,* i.e., feeling that no one cares

Carpenito (1989, p. 710) provides the following etiologies, i.e, contributing factors, for the NANDA diagnosis **Spiritual distress.**

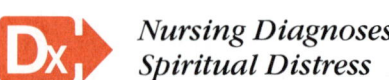

Nursing Diagnoses
Spiritual Distress

Spiritual distress related to:

- Crisis of illness/suffering/death (e.g., terminal illness, debilitating disease, chronic pain, or death or illness of significant other)

- Inability to practice spiritual beliefs
- Conflict between religious or spiritual belief and prescribed health regimen (e.g., blood transfusion, dietary restrictions, amputation, or medications)

Spiritual distress may also be the etiology of several other diagnoses such as **Sleep pattern disturbance, Hopelessness, Powerlessness, Self-esteem disturbance, Impaired adjustment, Ineffective coping,** and **Dysfunctional grieving.**

Planning

Nursing interventions are identified to help the client achieve the overall goals of spiritual strength, serenity, and satisfaction.

Planning in relation to spiritual distress should be designed to meet one or more of the following needs:

- To help the client fulfill religious obligations
- To help the client draw on and use inner resources more effectively to meet the present situation
- To help the client maintain or establish a dynamic, personal relationship with a supreme being in the face of unpleasant circumstances
- To help the client find meaning in existence and the present situation
- To promote a sense of hope
- To provide spiritual resources otherwise unavailable

Sometimes clients ask directly for a visit from the hospital chaplain or their own clergyman. Others may discuss their concerns with the nurse and ask about the nurse's beliefs as a way of seeking an empathic listener. Some people are embarrassed to ask for spiritual counsel but may hint at their concern in such statements as, "I've been wondering what will happen to me when I die," or "Do you go to a church?"

Any client or support person may desire spiritual assistance. The client facing death may have accepted it, but the family and support persons may not. Often relatives are grateful for spiritual support by a nurse or pastor. Assisting them may indirectly assist the client. Among those who may desire spiritual assistance are:

- Clients who appear lonely and have few visitors
- Clients who express fear and anxiety
- Clients about to have surgery
- Clients whose illness is related to the emotions or whose illness has religious or social implications

TABLE 32–3 *Signs of Spiritual Health*

Need	Behavior or Condition
Need for meaning and purpose in life	Expresses that he has lived in accordance with his value system in the past
	Expresses desire to participate in religious rituals
	Lives in accordance with value system at present
	Expresses contentment with life
	Expresses hope in the future
Need to receive love	Expresses hope in life after death
	Expresses confidence in the health care team
	Expresses feelings of being loved by others/God
	Expresses feelings of forgiveness by others/God
	Expresses desire to perform religious rituals leading to salvation
	Trusts others/God with the outcome of a situation in which he feels he has no control
Need to give love	Expresses love for others through actions
	Seeks the good of others
Need for hope and creativity	Asks for information about his condition realistically
	Talks about his condition realistically
	Sets realistic personal health goals
	Uses time during illness/hospitalization constructively
	Values his inner self more than his physical self

Source: From M. F. Highfield and C. Carson, Spiritual needs of patients: Are they recognized? *Cancer Nursing,* June 1983, 6:187–192. Reprinted with permission.

- Clients who must change their life-style as a result of illness or injury
- Clients preoccupied about the relationship of their religion and health
- Clients whose pastor is unable to visit

It is important to ask the individual before obtaining assistance. Some people profess no religious beliefs and may be angered if the nurse makes arrangements for a chaplain to visit. The nurse needs to respect the client's wishes and not make a judgment of right or wrong, good or bad. Planning also involves establishing outcome criteria. Examples of relevant outcome criteria are listed below.

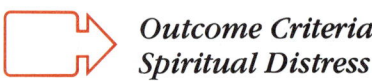

Outcome Criteria
Spiritual Distress

The client:

- Expresses comfort with spiritual beliefs
- Continues spiritual practices appropriate to health status
- Expresses decreased feelings of guilt
- States acceptance of moral decision
- Displays positive affect
- Expresses finding positive meaning in the present situation and in own existence
- Verbalizes relief from or acceptance of suffering
- Verbalizes relief of anger toward transcendent being, self, and others
- Verbalizes a closeness with God
- Experiences a sense of forgiveness

Implementing

Once spiritual distress has been identified as a relevant nursing diagnosis and specific strategies have been planned, the nurse is ready to implement the plan. To be effective when intervening, nurses should have already examined and clarified their own spiritual beliefs and values (see Chapter 7). A nurse who feels uncomfortable assisting the client spiritually (e.g., reading devotional material or praying with the client on request) should verbalize this discomfort and offer to obtain assistance for the client. It is important to respect the client's beliefs and maintain a supportive relationship. It is equally important for the nurse not to feel guilty about her or his discomfort.

To decrease spiritual distress, nurses should focus attention on the client's perception of his or her spiritual needs rather than on the practices or beliefs of the client's religious affiliation. Individual spiritual beliefs may vary greatly among members of a given religion. People join religious groups for many reasons (e.g., to have a place of worship, to find an avenue for social action such as helping the poor or homeless, to gain friends for recreational purposes, or to have a place for important life events such as weddings and funerals). Similarly, nurses should not assume that a

RESEARCH NOTE

What Are Nurses' Attitudes About Providing Spiritual Care?

The research focused on one major explanation for the lack of spiritual care given to patients: Many nurses lack the spiritual resources and spiritual well-being to meet clients' needs effectively in this regard. Graduate students and undergraduate students in their senior year were surveyed using tools; one measured their religious and existential welfare, and the other measured attitudes regarding the role of care providers in patients' spiritual care. The study confirmed that a strong relationship existed between a nurse's spiritual well-being and the nurse's views about the provision of spiritual care by health professionals. The authors believe that an individual with a high degree of spiritual well-being has a motivating sense of direction and order that can be used to assist another. Such harmony with the self is necessary before the nurse can assist the client spiritually.

Implications: Nurses who have a high degree of spiritual well-being are most effective in helping clients spiritually.

K. L. Soeken and V. J. Carson, Study measures nurses' attitudes about providing spiritual care, *Health Progress,* April 1986, 67:52–55.

client has no spiritual needs because the record states no religious affiliation or specifies atheist or agnostic.

To further individualize care, the nurse determines the meaning the client attaches to the situation. Such meanings can influence the client's response to an illness or condition and may either hinder nursing intervention or provide hope, courage, and strength. For example, a person who believes that illness is God's punishment may feel powerless and demonstrate little interest in therapy designed to prevent illness.

When orienting clients to the nursing unit, the nurse can provide information about hospital services to help clients meet spiritual needs and arrange for clients to participate in these as they are able. Many large hospitals have full-time chaplains who assist clients, support persons, and staff with spiritual needs. For smaller hospitals that do not have chaplains, clergy in the community usually provide this service. Many nursing units have a list of clergy who are on call when needed.

Some agencies have a chapel where religious services are regularly held for clients, support persons, and staff. Most hospitals also have quiet rooms that can be used for meditation, counsel, and even worship services. Sometimes a client prefers to meet the chaplain in a quiet, private room, particularly when the client shares his or her hospital room. A hospital may hold nondenominational religious services or several services for different denominations. If a client expresses a desire to attend services, the nurse needs to help organize the client's care so that attendance is possible if health permits.

The nurse sometimes determines that there is a true conflict between spiritual beliefs and medical therapy. In this case, the nurse encourages the client and physician to discuss the conflict and consider alternative methods of therapy. The nurse always supports the client's right to make an informed decision. If the beliefs of the nurse and client conflict, the nurse should discuss this conflict with the nurse in charge and her or his own spiritual leader. It may be preferable for the client to receive care from a nurse with compatible views. The nurse may also wish to discuss her or his feelings with other health professionals, e.g., other nurses on the team.

See the accompanying box for a nurse's prayer.

Evaluating

To evaluate whether or not the client achieved the goals established during the planning phase, the nurse collects data pertaining to the outcome criteria established. Skill in observation, helping relationships, and communication are required. The nurse needs to observe the client when alone and when interacting with others and listen to what the client says and does not say. See Table 32–2, earlier.

Caring

Lord of love, guide me as I begin a new day of caring for clients and their dear ones using my knowledge, skills, talents and self in grateful service to those in need. Thank you for my daily blessings and gifts to share. Thank you for a place in life to do my part.

Lord, grant me the strength, courage and grace to meet their needs and direct my vision and judgment in their behalf. I will see You in every distraught, frightened, disabled, comatose and dying person I gently touch. To lessen the burden and sorrow, I will tend to all the little things that count and bring joy to life.

Lord, stay close to me today and every day as I minister to individuals of all ages, races, colors and religious denominations placed in my trust. Fill me with your presence as I stumble and rise again. Assist me in sharing my humanness, my spirituality and my love with all communicants. Be my beacon of light on this journey.

Lord, this prayer I offer for their well-being and healing and ask that you grant me the same. You are my help and hope and in your love I dwell. I place my hand in Yours, Lord to begin a new day.

Sarah Marie Cimino

NURSING CARE PLAN FOR SALLY HORTON

ASSESSMENT DATA

Nursing Assessment

Mrs. Sally Horton is a 60-year-old hospitalized homemaker who is recovering from a right radical mastectomy. Yesterday, she was told by her physician that due to widespread metastases of the cancer, her prognosis is poor. This morning Marilyn Fleener, her primary nurse, finds her to be tearful and obviously upset and depressed. She asks Miss Fleener, "Why has God done this to me? Perhaps it's because I have sinned in my life. I've not gone to church or spoken to a minister in a number of years. Is there a chapel in the hospital where I could go and maybe pray? I'm terribly afraid of dying and what awaits me."

Physical Examination
Height: 165.1 cm (5′5″)

Weight: 54.0 kg (119 lb)
Temperature: 36.6 C (98 F)
Pulse rate: 88 BPM
Respirations: 22 per minute
Blood pressure: 146/86 mm Hg
Large surgical dressing to right chest wall and axillary region dry and intact
Slight edema of right hand and arm

Diagnostic Data
RBC: 3.5 ml/uL
Hgb: 10.5 grams/L
Hematocrit: 35%
Mammography reveals large right breast mass in upper outer quadrant

CARE PLAN

Nursing Diagnosis	Client Goals and Outcome Criteria	Nursing Interventions and Rationales	Evaluation
Spiritual distress related to separation from religious rituals resulting in questioning credibility of beliefs, depression, expressions of fear of death and relationship to deity.	Client Goal: Express sense of spiritual satisfaction. Outcome Criteria: Expresses comfort with relationship with deity by day 4. Visits with clergyman by day 2. Displays absence of feelings of guilt by day 5.	Assess for factors contributing to spiritual distress. *Rationale:* Enables the nurse to deal more effectively with problem when client's needs are known. Acknowledge and respond to client's verbal and nonverbal cues about spiritual needs. *Rationale:* Demonstrates interest in the client's religious concerns. Determine the meaning the client attributes to physical/spiritual situation. *Rationale:* Spiritual care may directly influence a client's recovery. Provide for the client's meeting of spiritual obligations. *Rationale:* This will aid in reducing spiritual distress. Inform client of spiritual services provided by the institution to assist her to meet her spiritual needs. *Rationale:* Permits client to choose to avail herself of these spiritual services. Encourage and provide for client's preferred spiritual rituals. *Rationale:* All people have basic spiritual dimensions, and spiritual practices assist in meeting their spiritual needs.	Client has been visited on several occasions by her clergyman. She reads scripture each day and has found consolation, especially in reading the Book of Psalms. She states, "God is merciful and will help me bear my suffering."
Fear related to terminal illness and dying resulting in feeling of loss of control; increased pulse, respirations, and blood pressure; and increased questioning.	Client Goal: Experience greater psychologic and physiologic comfort. Outcome Criteria: Clearly identifies actual source of fear by day 2. Distinguishes between ineffective and effective coping behaviors by day 5. Identifies individual coping response by day 5.	Acknowledge client's fear. *Rationale:* Feelings are real, and discussing them may assist in resolving them. Reduce or eliminate factors contributing to fear. *Rationale:* Will reduce intensity and/or incidence of fear. Encourage normal coping mechanisms. *Rationale:* Enhances control and diffuses fear. Be available and provide a nonthreatening atmosphere. *Rationale:* Establishes rapport and permits client to voice her feelings.	Client talked about her fear of dying and her concern for her husband, who is disabled with Parkinson's disease and cannot care for himself. She feels her coping response is her spiritual renewal and her visits with her clergyman. Clergyman has arranged for client's husband to be admitted to the Presbyterian Nursing Home.

CHAPTER HIGHLIGHTS

▶ The spiritual needs of clients and support persons often come into focus at a time of illness.

▶ Nurses must respect the rights of people to hold their own spiritual beliefs and to communicate or not communicate these to others.

▶ Spiritual beliefs and practices are highly personal.

▶ Spiritual and religious beliefs can influence life-style, attitudes, and feelings about illness and death.

▶ Spiritual beliefs often help people accept illness and plan for the future.

▶ A spiritual assessment is best obtained after the nurse has developed a relationship with the client. Information about a client's concept of God or deity, the client's source of hope and strength, the significance of religious practices and rituals, and the relationship the client perceives between health and spiritual beliefs should be obtained.

▶ Spiritual distress may be reflected in a number of behaviors, including depression, anxiety, and verbalizations of fear of death.

▶ Nurses should be aware of their own spiritual beliefs in order to be comfortable assisting others.

▶ Nurses and clergy may intervene directly to help clients and support persons meet spiritual needs.

READINGS AND REFERENCES

SUGGESTED READINGS

Carson, V. January/February 1980. Meeting the spiritual needs of hospitalized psychiatric patients. *Perspectives in Psychiatric Care* 18:17–20.
Carson describes how a prayer group for psychiatric clients promoted such benefits as increased support among members for each other.

Granstrom, S. L. April 1985. Spiritual care for oncology patients. *Topics in Clinical Nursing* 7:39–45.
Granstrom discusses how oncology nurses can help their clients clarify their experiences of suffering, doubt, and fear within a framework of faith, hope and love that brings meaning and purpose (i.e., self-actualizing), not in spite of the illness and crisis but because of it.

Henderson, K. J. May 1989. Dying, God, and anger. *Journal of Psychosocial Nursing* 27:17–21.
Henderson describes how reading psalms from the Bible permits the release of emotional and spiritual pain for the chronically ill and dying. The train of thought in psalms of lament parallels the stages of dying as Kübler-Ross has described them.

Ruffing-Rahal, M. A. March/April 1984. The spiritual dimension of well-being: Implications for the elderly. *Home Healthcare Nurse* 2:12–13, 16.
Ruffing-Rahal introduces the concept of holistic health care and the spiritual dimension. The losses of the elderly are briefly outlined together with an explanation of holistic well-being. Religion and spirituality are defined as separate entities. Ruffing-Rahal then describes the nurse's role in hospital and home care. The author discusses how to assess and assist clients.

RELATED RESEARCH

Highfield, M. F., and Cason, C. June 1983. Spiritual needs of patients: Are they recognized? *Cancer Nursing* 6:187–192.

Sodestrom, K. E., and Martinson, I. M. February 1987. Patient's spiritual coping strategies: A study of nurse and patient perspectives. *Cancer Nursing* 14:41–45.

Soeken, K. L., and Carson, V. J. April 1986. Study measures nurses' attitudes about providing spiritual care. *Health Progress* 67:52–55.

SELECTED REFERENCES

Berkowitz, P., and Berkowitz, N. S. November 1967. The Jewish patient in the hospital. *American Journal of Nursing,* 67:2335–37.

Brooke, V. July/August 1987. The spiritual well-being of the elderly. *Geriatric Nursing* 8:194–95.

Burkhardt, M. A., and Nagai-Jacobson, M. G. April 1985. Dealing with spiritual concerns of clients in the community. *Journal of Community Health Nursing* 2:191–98.

Burnard, P. May 1987. Spiritual distress and the nursing response: Theoretical considerations and counselling skills. *Journal of Advanced Nursing* 12:377–82.

Carpenito, L. J. 1989. Nursing diagnosis. *Application to Clinical Practice.* 3d ed. Philadelphia: J. B. Lippincott Co.

Carson, V. B. 1989. *Spiritual dimensions of nursing practice.* Philadelphia: W. B. Saunders Co.

Cook, T. C. 1980. Preface. In Thorson, J. A., and Cook, T. C., editors. *Spiritual well-being of the elderly.* Springfield, Ill.: Charles C. Thomas.

Dickinson, C. October 1975. The search for spiritual meaning. *American Journal of Nursing.* 75:1789–93.

Ellison, C. W. April 1983. Spiritual well-being: Conceptualization and measurement. *Journal of Psychology and Theology* 11:330–40.

Fehring, R. J., and McLane, A. M. 1989. Value belief: Spiritual distress (distress of the human spirit). In Thompson, J. M.; McFarland, G. K.; Hirsch, J. E.; Tucker, S. M.; and Bowers, A. C., editors. pp. 1821–25. *Mosby's manual of clinical nursing* 2d ed. St. Louis: C. V. Mosby.

Forbis, P. A. May/June 1988. Meeting patients' spiritual needs: Helping patients to fulfill their spiritual needs is part of the nursing process. *Geriatric Nursing* 9:158–59.

Fowler, J. W., and Keen, S. 1985. *Life maps: Conversation on the journey of faith,* Waco, Texas: Word Books.

Harmon, Y. May/June 1985. The relationship between religiosity and health. *Health values: Achieving high level wellness* 9:23–25.

Highfield, M. F., and Cason, C. June 1983. Spiritual needs of patients: Are they recognized? *Cancer Nursing* 6:187–92.

Kim, M. J.; McFarland, G. K.; and McLane, A. M., editors. 1984. *Classification of nursing diagnoses* St. Louis: C. V. Mosby Co.

———. 1989. *Pocket guide to nursing diagnoses.* 3d ed. St. Louis: C. V. Mosby Co.

Labun, E. May 1988. Spiritual care: An element in nursing care planning. *Journal of Advanced Nursing* 13:314–20.

Lyon, J. L., and Nelson, S. May/June 1988. Mormon health. *Health Values* 12:37–44.

Moberg, D. 1979. The development of social indicators of spiritual well-being for quality of life research. In Moberg D., editor. *Spiritual well-being: sociological perspectives* Washington, DC: University Press of America.

Murray, R. B., and Zentner, J. B. 1989. *Nursing assessment and health promotion strategies through the life span.* 4th ed. Norwalk, Conn.: Appleton & Lange.

Nagai-Jacobson, M. G., and Burkhardt, M. A. May 1989. Spirituality: Cornerstone of holistic nursing practice. *Holistic Nursing Practice* 3:18–26.

Naiman, H. L. November 1970. Nursing in Jewish Law. *American Journal of Nursing* 70:2378–79.

NANDA approved nursing diagnostic categories for clinical use and testing. Summer 1988. *Nursing Diagnosis Newsletter* 15:1–3.

O'Brien, M. E. 1982. The need for spiritual integrity. In Yura, H., and Walsh, M., editors. pp. 81–115. *Human needs 2 and the nursing process.* Norwalk, Conn.: Appleton-Century-Crofts.

Paloutzian, R. T., and Ellison, C. W. 1982. Loneliness, spiritual well-being, and the quality of life. In Peplau, L. A., and Perlman, D., editors. *Loneliness: A sourcebook of current theory, research and therapy.* New York: John Wiley and Sons.

Pilch, J. J. May/June 1988. Wellness spirituality. *Health Values* 12:28–31.

Piles, C. L. January/February 1990. Providing spiritual care. *Nurse Education Today* 15:36–41.

Pumphrey, J. B. December 1977. Recognizing your patient's spiritual needs. *Nursing 77* 7:64–69.

Saylor, D. February 1990. Pastoral care: The chaplain's perspective. *Journal of Nursing Administration* 20:15–19.

Shelly, J. A., and Fish, S. 1988. *Spiritual care: The nurse's role.* 3d ed. Downers Grove, Ill.: Inter Varsity Press.

Stoll, R. T. September 1979. Guidelines for spiritual assessment. *American Journal of Nursing* 79:1574–77.

———. 1989. The essence of spirituality. In Carson, V. B., editor. *Spiritual dimensions of nursing practice.* Philadelphia: W. B. Saunders Co.

Stress, Tolerance, and Coping

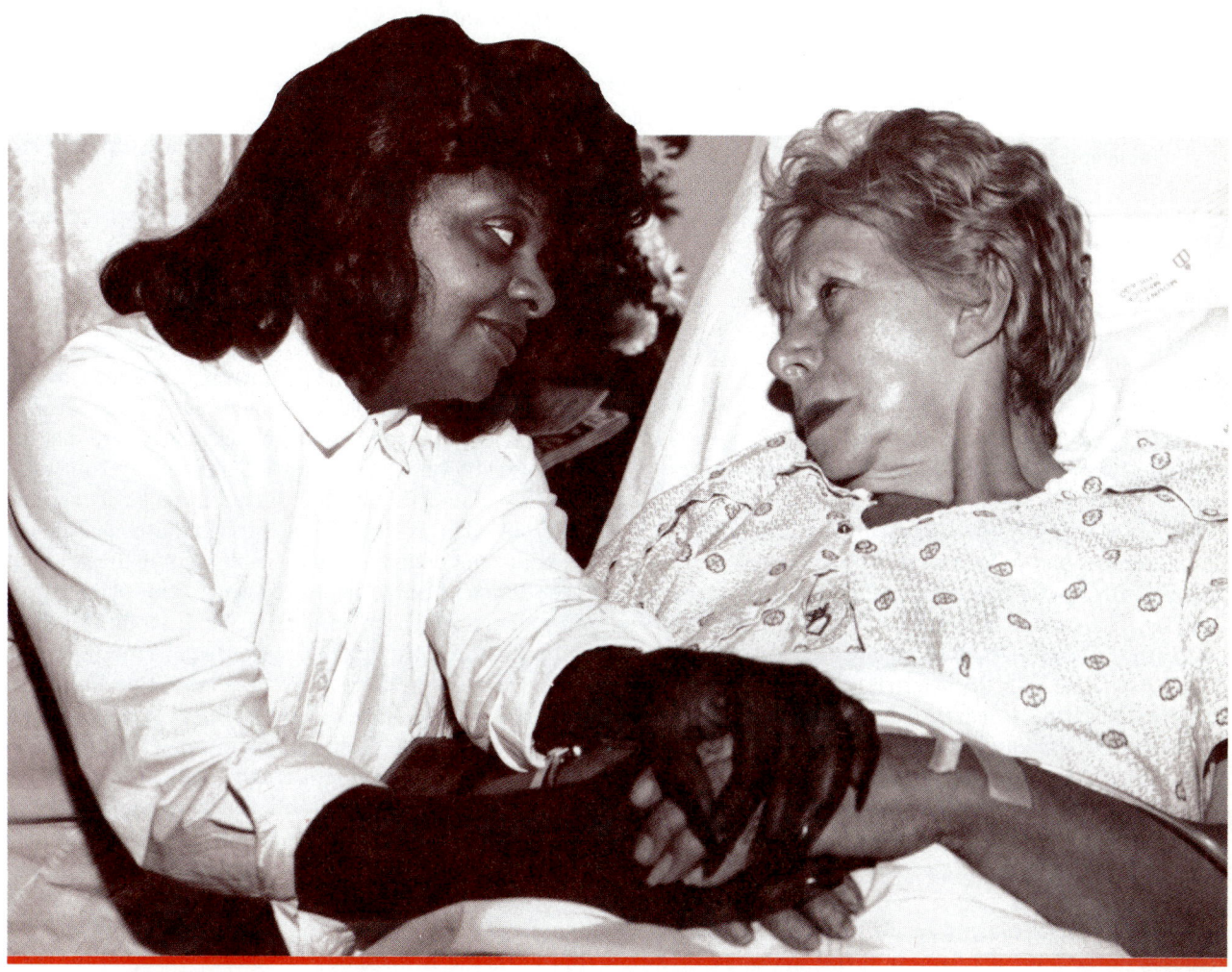

CONTENTS

OBJECTIVES

▶ Give four main characteristics of
homeostatic mechanisms.

▶ Explain how the autonomic nervous
system and the endocrine system
regulate homeostasis. ▶

▶ Describe how the respiratory, cardiovascular, renal, and gastrointestinal systems interact to maintain homeostasis.

▶ Differentiate the concepts of stress as a stimulus, as a response, and as a transaction.

▶ Identify Selye's definition of stress.

▶ Describe the three stages of Selye's general adaptation syndrome.

▶ Describe essential aspects of the Lazarus stress model.

▶ Identify physiologic and psychologic (cognitive, verbal, and motor) manifestations of stress.

▶ Identify behaviors related to specific ego defense mechanisms.

▶ Differentiate four levels of anxiety.

▶ Describe the relationship of anger to anxiety.

▶ Give examples of constructive and destructive anger.

▶ Give examples of three modes of adaptation.

▶ Identify characteristics of adaptive responses.

▶ Identify examples of nursing diagnoses related to stress.

▶ Identify general guidelines to minimize a client's anxiety and stress.

▶ Identify interventions to help clients cope with stress.

▶ Describe outcome criteria that can be used to evaluate whether a client is effectively coping with a stressful problem.

▶ Identify sources of stress in the nurse.

HOMEOSTASIS

The concept of homeostasis was first introduced by W. B. Cannon (1939) to describe the relative constancy of the internal processes of the body, such as blood oxygen and carbon dioxide levels, blood pressure, body temperature, blood glucose, and fluid and electrolyte balance. To Cannon, the word *homeostasis* did not imply something stagnant, set, or immobile; it meant a condition that might vary but remained relatively constant. Cannon viewed the human being as separate from the external environment and constantly endeavoring to maintain physiologic **equilibrium,** or balance, through adaptation to that environment. **Homeostasis,** then, is the tendency of the body to maintain a state of balance or equilibrium while continually changing.

Physiologic Homeostasis

Physiologic homeostasis means that the internal environment of the body is relatively stable and constant. All cells of the body require a relatively constant environment to function; thus, the body's internal environment must be maintained within narrow limits. Homeostatic mechanisms have four main characteristics:

1. They are self-regulating.
2. They are compensatory.
3. They tend to be regulated by negative feedback systems.
4. They may require several feedback mechanisms to correct only one physiologic imbalance.

Self-regulation means that homeostatic mechanisms come into play automatically in the healthy person. However, if a person is ill, or if a respiratory organ such as a lung is injured, the homeostatic mechanisms may not be able to respond to the stimulus as they would normally. Homeostatic mechanisms are **compensatory** (counterbal-ancing), because they tend to counteract conditions that are abnormal for the person. An example is a sudden drop in temperature. The compensatory mechanisms are that the peripheral blood vessels constrict, thereby diverting most of the blood internally; and increased muscular activity and shivering occur to create heat. Through these mechanisms the body temperature remains stable despite the cold.

Feedback is the mechanism by which some of the output of a system is "fed back" into the system as input. This input influences the behavior of the system and its future output. **Negative feedback** inhibits change; **positive feedback** stimulates change. Most biologic systems are controlled by negative feedback to bring the system back to stability. This type of feedback system senses and counteracts any deviations from normal. The deviations may be greater or less than the normal level or range. Negative feedback is a common control mechanism for hormone levels. For example, an increase in the production of parathyroid hormone is stimulated by a drop in blood calcium, but, when parathyroid hormone is increased and raises the level of blood calcium, its production is then inhibited. Several negative feedback systems may be required to correct one physiologic imbalance. For example, with hypoxia (shortage of oxygen), the concentration of red blood cells increases and the heart rate becomes faster to transport the blood and available oxygen around the body adequately.

The two major homeostatic regulators are the autonomic nervous system and the endocrine system. In addition, the cardiovascular system, the renal system, the respiratory system, and the gastrointestinal system are important in maintaining homeostasis. See Figure 33–1.

Autonomic Nervous System
The **autonomic nervous system** operates without conscious control to regulate visceral activities. The *parasymphathetic* or *craniosacral division* functions under normal everyday conditions and when the body is at rest, serving as the main

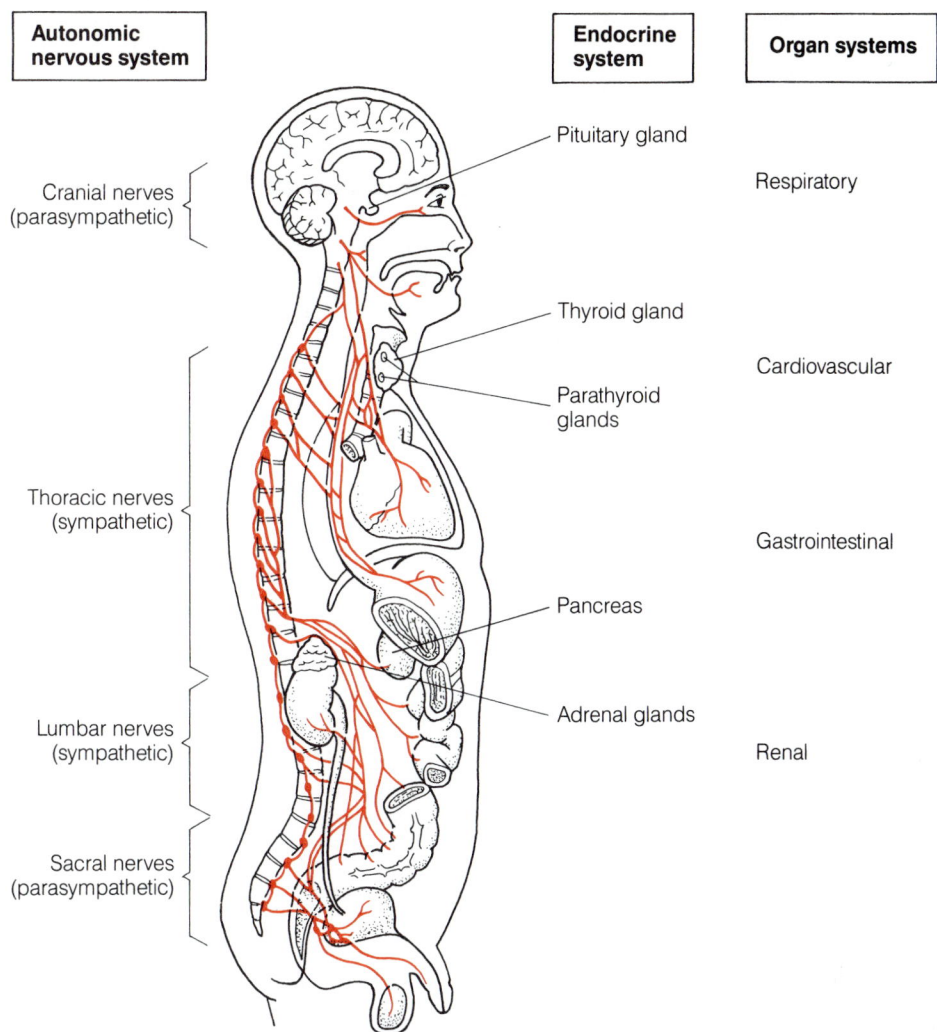

| Autonomic nervous system | | Endocrine system | Organ systems |

Cranial nerves (parasympathetic)

Thoracic nerves (sympathetic)

Lumbar nerves (sympathetic)

Sacral nerves (parasympathetic)

Pituitary gland

Thyroid gland

Parathyroid glands

Pancreas

Adrenal glands

Respiratory

Cardiovascular

Gastrointestinal

Renal

Figure 33–1   The homeostatic regulators of the body: autonomic nervous system, endocrine system, and specific organ systems.

regulator of the heart, stimulating the secretion of digestive juices and insulin, and increasing peristalsis by stimulating the smooth muscle of the digestive tract. The *sympathetic* and *thoracolumbar division* functions chiefly as an emergency system that, under stress conditions, produces a group of responses commonly known as the *fight-or-flight response* for maximum energy expenditure. These responses include a faster, stronger heartbeat, dilated blood vessels in skeletal muscles, dilated bronchi, and increased blood sugar level.

Endocrine System   The **endocrine system** regulates homeostasis through the islands of Langerhans in the pancreas and the pituitary, adrenal, thyroid, and parathyroid glands. The *pituitary gland* (hypophysis), although only the size of the tip of the little finger, releases several hormones in response to the body's needs. Two major hormones secreted from the anterior pituitary are *adrenocor-*

ticotropic hormone (ACTH), which stimulates the adrenal cortex to produce steroids, and *thyrotropic* (or *thyroid-stimulating) hormone (TSH),* which stimulates the secretion of thyroxin from the thyroid gland to control the body's rate of metabolism. The homeostatic hormone stored in and released from the posterior pituitary gland is *antidiuretic hormone (ADH),* which controls water reabsorption in the kidney tubules and thus prevents the body fluids from becoming too concentrated. An increase in the amount of water in the bloodstream causes the blood pressure to rise; thus ADH is sometimes referred to as a **vasopressor** drug when it is given therapeutically.

The *adrenal glands* secrete homeostatic hormones in two different areas of each gland. The medulla produces *epinephrine (adrenaline)* and *norepinephrine (noradrenaline).* Although the adrenal medulla is not essential for life, these hormones help the person meet certain emergency situations and support the sympathetic nervous system in the *fight-or-flight response*.

The outer part of the adrenal glands, the cortex, secretes two types of homeostatic hormones: *mineralocorticoids* and *glucocorticoids*. The most abundant mineralocorticoid is *aldosterone,* which induces sodium chloride retention, potassium excretion, and water reabsorption by the kidneys. It is therefore an important hormone in regulating the body's fluid and electrolyte levels (see Chapter 40).

Glucocorticoids, the most abundant of which is *cortisol hydrocortisone,* influence the metabolism of glucose, protein, and fat, and thus the production of energy for the body. The term *glucocorticoid* refers to the ability of these hormones to raise the blood sugar by mobilizing protein and fat from their storage areas and converting them into glucose. Glucocorticoids keep the blood glucose concentration high even during starvation periods and provide essential nutrients for nerve cells, which can use only glucose for energy. Another major function of the glucocorticoids is to increase a person's resistance to such physical stresses as injury, cold, pain, or fright.

The *thyroid gland,* located in the neck below the larynx, consists of two fairly large lateral lobes that are joined by a connecting portion called the isthmus. This gland stores and secretes two homeostatic hormones: *thyroid hormone (thyroxine and triiodothyronine, TH)* and *calcitonin*. The primary physiologic actions of thyroid hormone are to regulate the body's metabolic rate and the processes of growth. Calcitonin decreases the blood's calcium concentration either by promoting the deposit of calcium into bone or by inhibiting bone breakdown, which would release calcium into the blood.

The four *parathyroid glands* located behind the thyroid gland secrete *parathyroid hormone (parathormone, PTH),* which raises plasma calcium levels and lowers plasma phosphate levels. Although knowledge about this hormone and its relationship to calcium and phosphorus metabolism is still incomplete, PTH is considered important for the body's homeostasis since calcium and phosphorus are necessary for healthy bones and teeth. Calcium is also necessary for blood coagulation and for proper transmission of nerve impulses. A dramatic example of low calcium levels is *tetany,* a condition in which the body's skeletal muscles are hyperirritable and in spasm. When spasm of the laryngeal muscles occurs, respiratory obstruction and death can ensue.

The *islands of Langerhans* are clusters of endocrine-secreting cells located in the pancreas. The islands contain two types of cells: alpha cells, which secrete glucagon, and beta cells, which secrete insulin. *Insulin* accelerates the movement of sugar (glucose), protein (amino acids), and fats (fatty acids) out of the blood and into the tissue cells. Insulin, therefore, is a key regulator, since it lowers the blood concentration of these nutrients and promotes their metabolism and use by the cells. *Glucagon,* by contrast, tends to increase blood glucose concentration by stimulating the breakdown of liver glycogen.

Other Regulatory Systems   The *kidneys* are responsible for excretion and absorption of many by-products of metabolism. Their role in maintaining homeostasis of the body's fluids, electrolyte levels, and acid-base balance is vital. The *cardiovascular system* is the transport system that provides and removes essential elements for all body cells. The *respiratory system* regulates intake of oxygen and exhalation of carbon dioxide. Oxygen is essential for metabolism and hence the production of energy. Elimination of carbon dioxide is also essential to maintain the body's acid-base balance, which is a very precise regulatory mechanism. For further discussion, see Chapter 40. The *gastrointestinal system* is normally the only route for intake of fluids and electrolytes.

Psychologic Homeostasis

The term **psychologic homeostasis** refers to emotional or psychologic balance or a state of mental well-being. It is maintained by a variety of mechanisms. Each person has certain psychologic needs, such as the need for love, security, and self-esteem, that must be met to maintain psychologic homeostasis. When one or more of these needs is not met or is threatened, certain coping mechanisms are activated to protect the person and provide psychologic homeostasis.

Psychologic homeostasis is acquired or learned through the experience of living and interacting with others. In addition, societal norms and culture influence behavior. Some prerequisites for a person to develop psychologic homeostasis can be summarized:

- A stable physical environment in which the person feels safe and secure. For example, the basic needs for food, shelter, and clothing must be met consistently from birth onward.

- A stable psychologic environment from infancy onward, so that feelings of trust and love develop. Growing children and adolescents also need kind but firm and consistent discipline, encouragement, and support to be their own unique selves.

- A social environment that includes adults who are healthy role models. Children learn the customs and values of society from these individuals.

- A life experience that provides satisfactions. Throughout life, people encounter many frustrations. People deal with these better if enough satisfying experiences have occurred to counterbalance the frustrating ones.

CONCEPT OF STRESS

In recent years, **stress** has become a household word. Parents refer to the stress of raising children; working people talk of the stress of their jobs. Stress is a universal phenomenon. All people experience it. The concept of stress is important because it provides a way of understanding the person as a unified being who responds in totality (mind and body) to a variety of changes that take place in daily life.

Stress can have physical, emotional, intellectual, social, and spiritual consequences. Usually, the effects are mixed because stress affects the whole person. Physically, stress can threaten a person's physiologic homeostasis. Emotionally, stress can produce negative or nonconstructive feelings about self. Intellectually, stress can alter a person's perceptual and problem-solving abilities. Socially, stress can alter a person's relationships with others. Spiritually, stress can change a person's general outlook on life. Many illnesses, including hypertension, duodenal ulcers, bronchial asthma, and coronary heart disease, have been linked to stress.

Stress as a Stimulus

Stress may be defined as a **stimulus,** a life event (sometimes called a "life change") or set of circumstances causing a disrupted response (Lyon and Werner 1987) that increases the individual's vulnerability to illness. Holmes and Rahe (1967) assigned a numerical value to 43 life changes or events. The scale of stressful life events is used to document a person's relatively recent experiences, such as divorce, pregnancy, and retirement. In this view, both positive and negative events are considered stressful.

Since 1967, similar scales have been developed. Burgess and Lazare (1976, p. 58) caution people in the use of such scales. They emphasize that the degree of stress the event presents can be highly individual. For example, a divorce may be highly traumatic to one person and cause relatively little anxiety to another. What is important is that research has shown that people who have a high level of stress are often more prone to illness and have lowered ability to cope with illness and subsequent stress.

Stress as a Response

Stress may also be defined as a **response,** the disruption caused by a noxious stimulus or stressor (Lyon and Werner 1987). In this definition of stress, reactions rather than events are the focus. The response view was developed by Hans Selye (1956, 1976). He defined stress as "the nonspecific response of the body to any kind of demand made upon it" (1976, p. 1). Regardless of the cause, situation, or psychologic interpretation of a demanding situation, Selye's stress response is characterized by the same chain or pattern of physiologic events. This nonspecific response was called the **general adaptation syndrome (GAS)** or **stress syndrome.**

To differentiate the cause of stress from the response to stress, Selye created the term **stressor** (1976, p. 51) to denote any factor that produces stress and disturbs the body's equi-

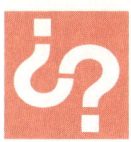

RESEARCH NOTE

Can Ethical Dilemmas of Nursing Practice Contribute to Stress and Burnout?

Martin surveyed 75 nurses who were primary caregivers of persons with AIDS. The instruments used in this study were the AIDS Ethical Dilemma Scale, the Maslach Burnout Inventory (MBI), and the COPE Inventory. The focus of the study was to relate the ethical dilemmas experienced by nurses caring for AIDS patients to burnout and coping mechanisms. The findings suggest that ethical dilemmas posed in caring for AIDS patients are stressful. Fifty percent of the nurses surveyed reported a high degree of emotional exhaustion on the MBI. The findings also suggest that nurses who had more nursing experience were able to use more effective coping mechanisms in stressful situations.

Implications: Nurses facing ethical dilemmas in practice need to identify what issues are presenting the dilemma. They also need to identify their positive coping strategies and use them when confronting stressful situations. Nurses working in care areas that have a high degree of ethical dilemmas should form support groups to deal effectively with those issues and prevent harmful stress and burnout.

D. Martin. Effects of ethical dilemmas on stress felt by nurses providing care to AIDS patients. *Critical Care Nursing Quarterly,* 12:4 March 1, 1990, 53–57.

librium. Because stress is a state of the body, it can be observed only by the changes it produces in the body. This response of the body, the stress syndrome or general adaptation syndrome, occurs with the release of certain adaptive hormones and subsequent changes in the structure and chemical composition of the body. Body organs affected by stress are the gastrointestinal tract, the adrenals, and the lymphatic structures. With prolonged stress, the adrenals enlarge considerably; the lymphatic structures, such as the thymus, spleen, and lymph nodes, atrophy (shrink) and deep ulcers appear in the lining of the stomach. In addition to adapting globally, the body can also react locally, i.e., one organ or a part of the body reacts alone. This is referred to as the **local adaptation syndrome,** or **LAS.** One example of the LAS is inflammation. See the section on the inflammatory response in Chapter 20. Selye proposed that both the GAS and the LAS have three stages (1976, p. 38): alarm reaction, resistance, and exhaustion. See Figure 33–2.

Alarm Reaction (AR)
The initial reaction of the body is the alarm reaction, which alerts the body's defenses against the stressor, whether the stressor is heat, bacteria, or a verbal or physical attack from someone. Selye divided

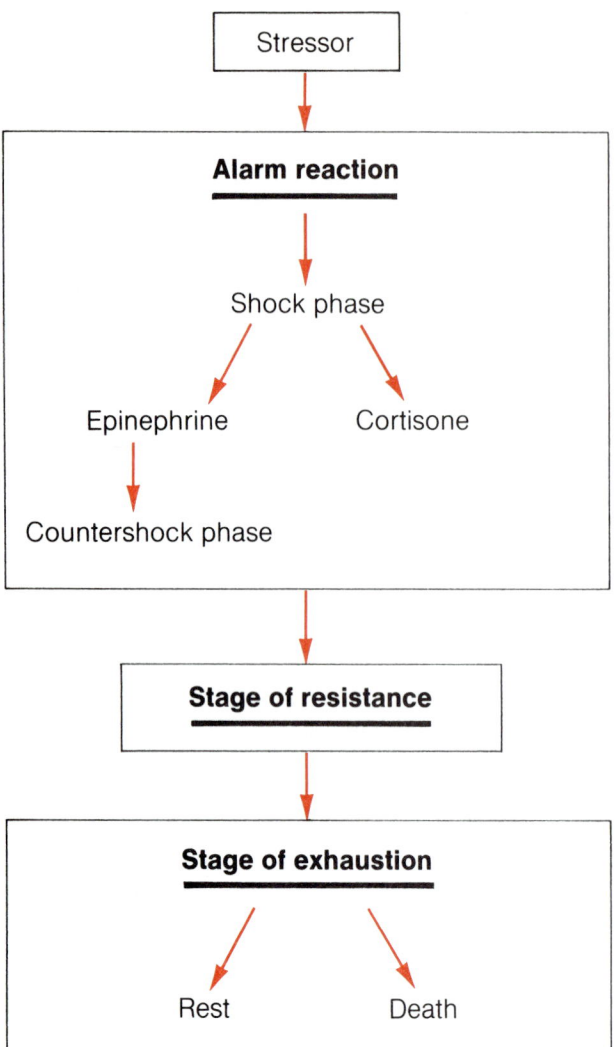

Figure 33–2 The three stages of adaptation to stress: the alarm reaction, the stage of resistance, and the stage of exhaustion.

this stage into two parts: the shock phase and the counter-shock phase.

During the **shock phase,** the stressor may be perceived consciously or unconsciously by the person. In any case, the autonomic nervous system reacts, and large amounts of epinephrine (adrenaline) and cortisone are released into the body. The person is then ready for fight or flight. This primary response is short lived, lasting from 1 minute to 24 hours.

The second part of the alarm reaction is called the **countershock phase.** During this time, the body changes produced during the shock phase are reversed. It is, therefore, during the shock phase of the alarm reaction that a person is best mobilized to react.

Stage of Resistance (SR)   During the second stage in the GAS and LAS syndromes, the body's adaptation takes place. In other words, the body attempts to cope with the stressor and to limit the stressor to the smallest area of the body that can deal with it.

Stage of Exhaustion (SE)   During the third stage, the adaptation that the body made during the second stage cannot be maintained. This means that the ways used to cope with the stressor have been exhausted. If adaptation has not overcome the stressor, the stress effects may spread to the entire body. At the end of this stage, the body may either rest and return to normal, or death may be the ultimate consequence. The end of this stage depends largely on the adaptive energy resources of the individual, the severity of the stressor, and the external adaptive resources that are provided, such as oxygen.

Selye's general adaptation syndrome encompasses a range of *physiologic* responses to stressors in the body as a whole. See Figure 33–3. Stressors stimulate the sympathetic nervous system, which in turn stimulates the hypothalamus. The hypothalamus releases corticotropin-releasing hormone (CRH), which stimulates the anterior pituitary gland to release adrenocorticotropin (ACTH). During stress, the adrenal medulla, which is functionally related to the sympathetic nervous system, secretes epinephrine and norepinephrine in response to sympathetic stimulation. Significant body responses to epinephrine include the following:

1. Increased myocardial contractility, which increases cardiac output and blood flow to active muscles
2. Bronchial dilation, which allows increased oxygen intake
3. Increased blood clotting
4. Increased cellular metabolism
5. Increased fat mobilization to make energy available and to synthesize other compounds needed by the body

The principal effect of norepinephrine is decreased blood to the kidneys and increased secretion of renin. *Renin* is an enzyme that hydrolyzes one of the blood proteins to produce *angiotensin*. Angiotensin tends to increase the blood pressure by constricting arterioles. The sum of all these adrenal hormonal effects permits the person to perform far more strenuous physical activity than would otherwise be possible.

Stress as a Transaction

Lazarus's Model   Transactional theories of stress are based on the work of Lazarus (1966), who states that the stimulus theory and the response theory do not consider individual differences. Neither explains which factors lead some persons and not others to respond effectively nor interprets why some persons are able to adapt over longer periods than others. According to Lazarus, "Stimulus definitions focus on events in the environment such as natural disasters, illness, or termination of employment. This approach assumes that certain situations are normatively stressful but does not allow for individual differences in

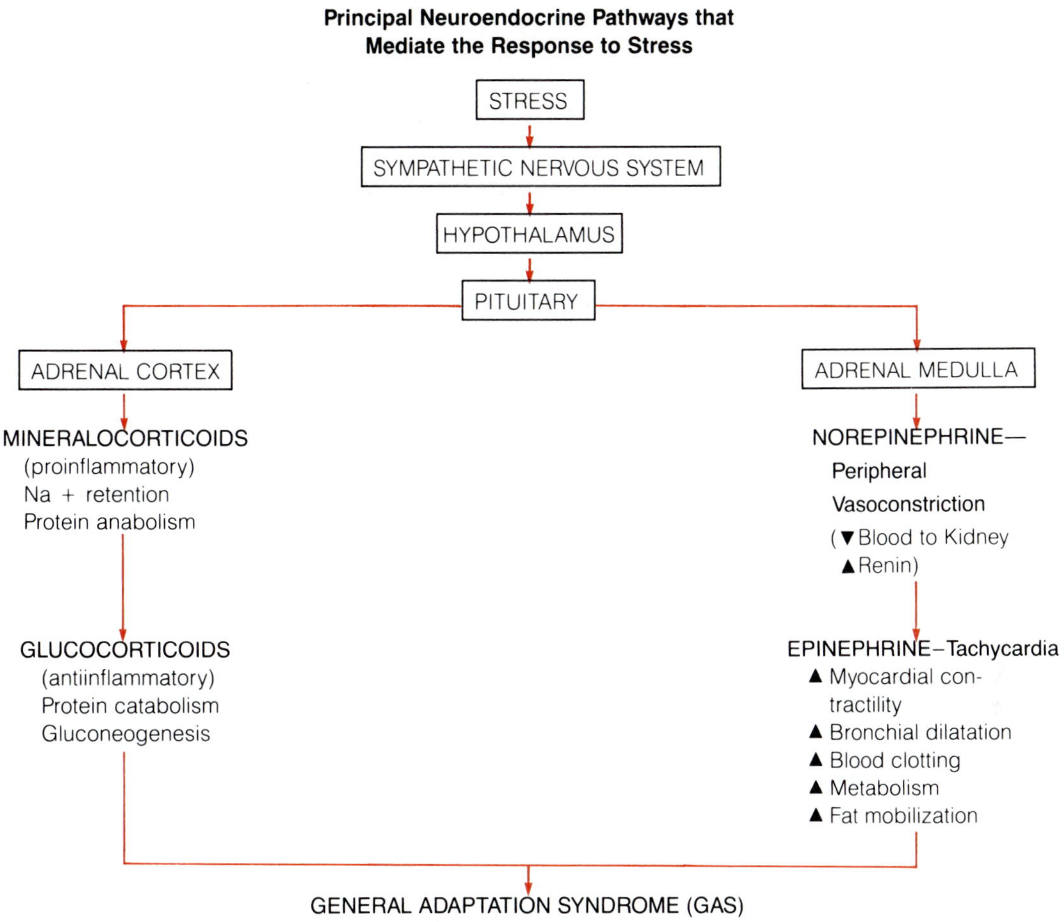

Principal Neuroendocrine Pathways that Mediate the Response to Stress

```
                    ┌─────────────┐
                    │   STRESS    │
                    └─────────────┘
                           │
          ┌────────────────────────────────────┐
          │   SYMPATHETIC NERVOUS SYSTEM        │
          └────────────────────────────────────┘
                           │
                  ┌──────────────────┐
                  │   HYPOTHALAMUS   │
                  └──────────────────┘
                           │
                    ┌──────────────┐
                    │   PITUITARY  │
                    └──────────────┘
```

ADRENAL CORTEX	ADRENAL MEDULLA

MINERALOCORTICOIDS
(proinflammatory)
Na + retention
Protein anabolism

NOREPINEPHRINE—
Peripheral
Vasoconstriction
(▼Blood to Kidney
▲Renin)

GLUCOCORTICOIDS
(antiinflammatory)
Protein catabolism
Gluconeogenesis

EPINEPHRINE–Tachycardia
▲ Myocardial con-
  tractility
▲ Bronchial dilatation
▲ Blood clotting
▲ Metabolism
▲ Fat mobilization

GENERAL ADAPTATION SYNDROME (GAS)

Stage 1. **ALARM REACTION**
Enlargement of adrenal cortex
Enlargement of lymphatic system
Increase in hormone levels

Stage 2. **RESISTANCE**
Shrinkage of adrenal cortex
Lymph nodes closer to normal size
Hormone levels sustained

Stage 3. **EXHAUSTION**
Enlargement/dysfunction of
  lymphatic structures
Increase in hormone levels
Depletion of adaptive hormones

A stress syndrome, termed the General Adaption Syndrome (GAS) by Hans Selye, evolves in three stages. Stages 1 and 2 are continuously repeated throughout a lifetime cycle. If resistance cannot be sustained, exhaustion (Stage 3), with its altered psycho-physiological functioning, occurs.

Figure 33–3 Physiologic response to stress: general adaptation syndrome. ***Source:*** Physiologic responses of the general adaptation syndrome. From M. J. Smith and H. Selye, Stress: Reducing the negative effects of stress, *American Journal of Nursing,* November 1979, 79:1954. Used by permission.

the evaluation of events. Response definitions refer to a state of stress; the person is spoken of as reacting with stress, being under stress, and so on. Stimulus and response definitions have limited utility, because a stimulus gets defined as stressful only in terms of a stress response" (Lazarus and Folkman 1984, p. 21).

Although Lazarus recognizes that certain environmental demands and pressures produce stress in substantial numbers of people, he emphasizes that people and groups differ in their sensitivity and vulnerability to certain types of events, as well as in their interpretations and reactions. For example, in terms of illness, one person may respond with denial, another with anxiety, and still another with depression. To explain variations among individuals under comparable conditions, the Lazarus model takes into account cognitive processes that intervene between the encounter and the reaction, and the factors that affect the nature of this process. In contrast to Selye, who focuses on physiologic responses, Lazarus includes mental and psychologic components or responses as part of his concept of stress.

The Lazarus **transactional stress theory** encompasses a set of cognitive, affective, and adaptive (coping) responses that arise out of person-environment transactions. The person and the environment are inseparable; each affects and is affected by the other. **Stress** is defined as a particular relationship between the person and the environment that is appraised by the person as taxing or exceeding the person's resources and endangering well-being (Lazarus and Folkman 1984, p. 19). The individual responds to perceived environmental changes by adaptive or coping responses. **Cognitive appraisal** is an evaluative process that determines why and to what extent a particular transaction or series of transactions between the person and the environment is stressful. Coping is the process through which the individual manages the demands of the person-environment relationship that are appraised as stressful and the emotions they generate (Lazarus and Folkman 1984, p. 19).

Nuernberger's Model   Nuernberger (1981, p. 69) believes that there is an adaptive pattern of responding beyond the arousal mechanism of the sympathetic nervous system. This other response, based on stimulation of the parasympathetic nervous system, is one of inhibition. He calls this response the **general inhibition syndrome** or **possum response.** To Nuernberger (1981, p. 71), healthy nonstress functioning is represented by a balance between the two parts of the autonomic nervous system: sympathetic and parasympathetic branches. Stress is a state of internal imbalance reflecting the unrelieved dominance of either arousal by the sympathetic nervous system (fight-or-flight response) or inhibition by the parasympathetic nervous system (possum response). The effects of excessive stimulation of or dominance by either of these systems are evinced as a localized response in a specific organ or as a general-

ized response pattern. Both responses are designed for self-protection.

Nuernberger maintains that the presence of either arousal or inhibition does not in itself constitute stress. Stress occurs only when arousal is not balanced by relaxation or when relaxation (inhibition) is not balanced by activity. Prolonged or intense parasympathetic imbalances are associated with such diseases as asthma or depression. Prolonged sympathetic imbalances are associated with, for example, cardiovascular disease.

Nuernberger (1981, p. 81) writes that the primary source of stress is not the external environment; it is a person's internal state of mind; it is the emotional and perceptual factors that form a person's basic personality. The greatest source of hypothalamic arousal is the cerebral cortex in response to repetitive thought patterns and apprehensions about unresolved past, present, or future events that people associate with potentially painful or negative consequences in their lives.

Nuernberger defines emotional stress as the result of a mental process: It is a state of autonomic imbalance generated as a reaction to the perception of some kind of threat, pain or discomfort. This perception involves an interpretation of selected sensory stimuli, which is colored, or structured, by memories of past pain. It is also involved with the anticipation that this pain will occur in the future as a consequence of present sensory stimuli and environmental conditions. It is sustained by indecisiveness, the inability to resolve the threat" (Nuernberger 1981, p. 86).

MANIFESTATIONS OF STRESS

Manifestations of the stress experience, both physiologic and psychologic, may be considered coping strategies or mechanisms. **Coping** is the immediate response of a person to a threatening situation. In contrast, **adaptation** is the final response or change that occurs. According to Lazarus and Folkman (1984, p. 141), coping refers to constantly changing cognitive and behavioral efforts to manage specific external and/or internal demands that are appraised as taxing or exceeding the resources of a person.

Coping may be described as dealing with problems and situations, or contending with them successfully. A **coping strategy** (*coping mechanism*) is an innate or acquired way of responding to a changing environment or specific problem or situation. In nursing literature, effective and ineffective coping are often differentiated. *Effective coping* results in adaptation; *ineffective coping* results in maladaptation. Although coping behavior may not always seem appropriate, the nurse needs to remember that coping is always purposeful.

Coping strategies vary among individuals and are often related to the individual's perception of the stressful event.

A person's coping strategies often change with a reappraisal of a situation. There is never only one way to cope. Some people choose avoidance; others confront a situation as a means of coping. Still others seek information or rely on religious beliefs as a means of coping. Bell (1977, p. 137) places coping strategies into two groups: long term and short term. Long-term coping strategies can be constructive and realistic. For example, in certain situations talking with others about the problem and trying to find out more about the situation are long-term strategies.

Short-term coping strategies can reduce stress to a tolerable limit temporarily but are in the long run ineffective ways to deal with reality. They may even have a destructive or detrimental effect on the person (Bell 1977, p. 137). Examples of short-term strategies are using alcoholic beverages or drugs, daydreaming and fantasizing, and relying on the belief that everything will work out.

Physiologic Manifestations

Physiologic manifestations may or may not occur in clients experiencing stress, depending on the way the client perceives the stressful event and on the effectiveness of his or her coping strategies. There is considerable evidence that a person's cognitive coping strategies mediate blood pressure and heart rates. For example, when a person cognitively attends to the stressor or threat, there is a decrease in heart rate. Specific physiologic manifestations are presented in the accompanying box.

Psychologic Manifestations

Psychologic manifestations include anxiety, anger, cognitive behaviors, verbal and motor responses, and unconscious ego defense mechanisms. Some of these coping patterns are helpful; others are a hindrance, depending on the situation and the length of time they are used or experienced. Indeed, anxiety is often considered to be a response to a stressful event rather than a coping mechanism, since it may impede action to remove the stressor.

Anxiety, a common reaction to stress, is a state of mental uneasiness, apprehension, dread, or foreboding or a feeling of helplessness related to an impending or anticipated unidentified threat to self or significant relationships. Anxiety can be experienced at the conscious, subconscious, or unconscious levels. It differs from fear in four ways:

1. Its source is not identifiable; the source of fear is identifiable.
2. It is related to the future, i.e., an anticipated event. Fear is related to the present.
3. It is vague, whereas fear is definite.
4. It is the result of psychologic or emotional conflict; fear is the result of a discrete physical or psychologic entity.

---

*Physiologic Manifestations of Stress**

- Pupils dilate to increase visual perception when serious threats to the body arise.
- Sweat production (diaphoresis) is increased to control elevated body heat due to increased metabolism.
- The heart rate increases, which leads to an increased pulse rate to transport nutrients and by-products of metabolism more efficiently.
- Skin is pallid due to constriction of peripheral blood vessels, an effect of norepinephrine.
- Blood pressure is elevated, due to
    a. constriction of vessels in blood reservoirs, such as the skin, kidneys, and most large interior organs.
    b. increased secretion of renin, an effect of norepinephrine.
    c. increased sodium and water retention due to release of mineralocorticoids, which results in increased blood volume.
    d. increased cardiac output.
- The rate and depth of respirations increase due to dilation of the bronchioles, promoting hyperventilation.
- Urinary output is decreased.
- The mouth may be dry.
- Peristalsis of the intestines is decreased, resulting in possible constipation and flatus.
- Mental alertness is improved for serious threats.
- Muscle tension is increased to prepare for rapid motor activity or defense.
- Blood sugar is increased due to release of glucocorticoids and gluconeogenesis.
- Lethargy, mental lassitude, inactivity (parasympathetic dominance) may ensue.
- There may be decreased physiologic functioning and loss of skeletal muscle tone (parasympathetic dominance).

*All signs are the result of increased activity of the sympathetic nervous system unless indicated otherwise.

All people experience anxiety to some degree most of the time. Mild or moderate anxiety is needed to accomplish developmental tasks and motivate goal-directed behavior. In this sense, anxiety is an effective coping strategy. For example, mild anxiety motivates students to study. Excessive anxiety, however, often has destructive effects.

Anxiety may be manifested on four different levels:

1. *Mild anxiety,* which produces a slight arousal state that enhances perception, learning, and productive abilities. Most healthy persons experience mild anxiety, perhaps as a feeling of mild restlessness that prompts a person to seek information and ask questions.

2. *Moderate anxiety,* which increases the client's arousal state to a point where the person expresses feelings of tension, nervousness, or concern. Perceptual abilities are narrowed. Attention is focused more on a particular aspect of a situation than on peripheral activities.

3. *Severe anxiety,* which consumes most of the person's energies and requires intervention. Perception is further decreased. The person, unable to focus on what is really happening, focuses on only one specific detail of the situation generating the anxiety.

4. *Panic,* which is an overpowering, frightening level of anxiety causing the person to lose control. It is less frequently experienced than other levels of anxiety. The perception of a panicked person can be altered to the point where the person distorts events. See Table 33–1 for signs of these levels.

Anger is an emotional state consisting of a subjective feeling of animosity or strong displeasure. Many people feel guilty when they feel anger, because they have learned that to feel angry is wrong. In fact, anger, hostility, violence, and aggression differ. Anger can be expressed in a nonalienating verbal manner; it is then considered a positive emotion and a sign of emotional maturity, since growth and beneficial interactions result from it.

Anger is commonly manifested in altered voice tone as a communication to desist from some action or other. Verbal expression of anger can therefore be considered a signal to others of one's internal psychologic discomfort and a call for assistance to deal with perceived stress. In contrast, *hostility* is usually marked by overt antagonism and harmful or destructive behavior; *aggression* is an unprovoked attack or a hostile, injurious, or destructive action or outlook; and *violence* is the exertion of physical force to injure or abuse. Verbally expressed anger differs from hostility, aggression, and violence, but it can lead to destructiveness and violence if the anger persists unabated.

Clearly expressed verbal communication of anger, when the angry person tells the other person about the anger and carefully identifies the source, is constructive. This clarity of communication gets the anger out into the open so that the other person can deal with it and help to alleviate it. The angry person "gets it off his chest" and prevents an emotional buildup. Constructive expressions of anger have three elements (Duldt 1981, p. 516):

1. *Alerting,* the act of engaging another's attention
2. *Describing,* the process of delineating the source of the

angry person's feelings, i.e., what has happened here and now
3. *Identifying,* the act of seeking a response and support from others

The following are examples of constructive anger:

- "Darn! (Alerting) This electric drill won't work. (Describing) What am I doing wrong?" (Identifying)
- "Robert! (Alerting) Your going to the football game this afternoon infuriates me. You said yesterday you'd clean the car for me before I have to drive my friends to the church social tonight. (Describing) Now what am I going to do?" (Identifying)

Unclear communication of anger is destructive. It is similar to constructive expressions only in the alerting behavior. Then the person fails to describe the source of the feelings adequately and denies any responsibility for the anger by blaming others or by generalizing to other people or past situations. Thus, those in the presence of the angry person are unable to respond helpfully. The following examples of unclearly expressed anger:

- "Darn it! (Alerting) A woman can never win." (Generalizing)
- "You weasel! (Alerting) You're always leaving me in the lurch." (Generalizing, blaming)

Cognitive Manifestations

Cognitive manifestations of stress are thinking responses that include problem solving, structuring, self-control or self-discipline, suppression, fantasy, and prayer. *Problem solving* involves thinking through the threatening situation, using specific steps, similar to those of the nursing process, to arrive at a solution. The person assesses the situation or problem, analyzes or defines it, chooses alternatives, carries out the selected alternative, and evaluates whether the solution was successful.

Structuring is the arrangement or manipulation of a situation so that threatening events do not occur. For example, a nurse can structure or control an interview with a client by asking only direct, closed questions. This strategy avoids information or questions that may be threatening to the nurse's knowledge or values. Structuring, however, can be productive in certain situations. A person who schedules a dental examination semiannually to prevent severe dental disease is using productive structuring.

Self-control (discipline) is assuming a manner and facial expression that convey a sense of being in control or in charge, no matter what the situation is. When self-control prevents panic and harmful or nonproductive actions in a threatening situation, it is a helpful response that conveys strength. Self-control carried to an extreme, however, can delay problem solving and prevent a person from receiving

TABLE 33–1 *Signs of Mild, Moderate, and Severe Anxiety*

Sign	Mild	Moderate	Severe (Panic)
Verbalization changes	Expresses feelings of increased arousal and concern Increased questioning or information seeking	Expresses feelings of tension, apprehension, nervousness, or concern Verbalized expectation of danger Voice tremors and pitch changes Increased rate and quantity of verbalization	Expresses feelings of severe dread, apprehension, nervousness, concern, helplessness, and isolation Absence of verbalization Inappropriate verbalization, e.g., false cheerfulness or laughing while discussing a serious subject
Motor activity changes	Mild restlessness	Pacing Hand tremor or shakiness Increased muscle tension	Immobilization Purposeless activity Increased muscle tension Rigid posture Fixed or scattered perceptual focus
Perception and attention changes	Increased awareness Increased attending Ability to focus on most of what is really happening	Narrowed focus of attention Ability to focus on most of what is really happening	Intellectualizing about a subject, e.g., explaining the pathophysiology of leukemia rather than describing own feelings Intent and fearful watching of everything going on Inability to focus on what is really happening Inability to focus on reality, e.g., denial, saying "I don't want to talk about it"
Respiratory and circulatory changes	Nil	Rapid pulse Increased respiratory rate	Tachycardia Palpitations Hyperventilation
Other changes	Nil	Diaphoresis Sleep or eating disturbances, e.g., insomnia, somnolence, overeating, or anorexia Irritability	Diaphoresis Dilated pupils Pallor Clammy hands and skin Dry mouth Sullenness, withdrawal

Sources: Compiled from M. Gordon, *Manual of nursing diagnosis* (New York: McGraw-Hill, 1982), pp. 153–60; and Anxiety: recognition and intervention (programmed instruction) *American Journal of Nursing* September 1965, 65:129–52. Copyright © 1965 The American Journal of Nursing Company; M. J. Kim, G. K. McFarland, and A. M. McLane, *Pocket guide to nursing diagnoses,* 3d ed. (St. Louis: C. V. Mosby Co., 1989), p. 4; and L. J. Carpenito, *Nursing diagnosis: Application to clinical practice,* 3d ed. (Philadelphia: J. B. Lippincott Co., 1989).

the support of others, who may perceive the person as handling the situation well, as cold, or as unconcerned.

Suppression is consciously and willfully putting a thought or feeling out of mind: "I won't deal with that today. I'll do it tomorrow." This response relieves stress temporarily but does not solve the problem. A man who keeps ignoring a toothache, pushing it out of his mind because he fears the pain of having a filling, will not relieve his symptoms or find the solution.

Fantasy or daydreaming is likened to make-believe. Unfulfilled wishes and desires are imagined as fulfilled, or a threatening experience is reworked or replayed so that it ends differently from reality. Experiences can be relived, everyday problems solved, and plans for the future made. The outcome of current problems may also be fantasized. For example, a client who is awaiting the results of a breast biopsy may fantasize the surgeon as saying, "You do not have cancer." Fantasy responses can be helpful if they lead to problem solving. For example, the client awaiting breast biopsy results might say to herself, "Even if the doctor doesn't say 'You do not have cancer,' as long as he says I won't need mutilating surgery, I can accept that." Fantasies can be destructive and nonproductive if a person uses them to excess and retreats from reality.

Prayer often involves identifying and describing the problem, suggesting solutions, and reaching out for support and help. For example, a young woman may pray: "Please help me. The doctor says I have headaches and hypertension because I'm overweight (describing problem). What I need is to discipline myself to exercise more and go on a diet" (suggesting solutions). If these first two problem-solving steps lead to action, prayer can be a constructive response, aside from the support and meaning the person derives from it.

Verbal and Motor Manifestations

Verbal or motor manifestations of stress may be the first responses evident. Among these responses are crying, verbal abuse, laughing, screaming, hitting and kicking, and holding and touching. *Crying* releases tension in situations perceived as painful, joyful, or sad and when the situation cannot yet be managed cognitively. As a response, crying tends to be more socially acceptable in women and in certain cultures, for instance, among Hispanics or Mediterranean people. People often cry when they perceive that others care. Crying is beneficial as a release of tension and if it is followed by problem solving. It is not helpful without problem solving.

Verbal abuse is another release mechanism most often expressed toward stress-producing objects and events, such as nonfunctional equipment, misplaced or lost items, and rainy weather. *Laughing* is also an anxiety-reducing response that can lead to constructive problem solving. People may laugh at small incidents and at the way they handled a situation. For example, a preoccupied, stressed man whose wife has had an accident may laugh at having put on one black shoe and one brown shoe before rushing to the emergency room.

Screaming is a response to fear or intense frustration and anger. One may scream in response to a person appearing suddenly out of the dark or in response to a family member who keeps planning other activities to avoid cleaning the garage. Screaming, like other verbal responses, reduces tension but can be harmful if the person is unable to control it and becomes hysterical. The hysterical, frightened person needs to be moved to a quiet place and assured that the threat is over. The hysterical, frustrated person needs assistance to deal with the situation with a more effective coping strategy, e.g., problem solving.

Hitting and kicking are spontaneous responses to physical threats. Adults who are socialized to control such responses toward people may direct them toward objects by pounding a table with a fist or kicking a wastebasket. Preschoolers, however, have not matured enough to develop control and may, for example, hit or kick a nurse who is administering an injection. Hitting or kicking can be helpful in reducing tension provided the person or object is not damaged and provided they lead toward cognitive coping techniques.

Holding and touching are often responses to joyful, painful, or sad events. Holding or touching another is a gesture of support and comfort. Holding and touching responses vary considerably, however, among cultures and among individuals in a culture. Verbal communication can also convey caring. "Crisis lines" or close friends often provide meaningful and supportive verbal communication that conveys caring over the telephone or in person.

Unconscious Ego Defense Mechanisms

Unconscious **ego defense mechanisms** are psychologic defensive (adaptive) mechanisms or, in the words of Sigmund Freud (1946), mental mechanisms, which develop as the personality attempts to defend itself, establish compromises among conflicting impulses, and allay inner tensions. Defense mechanisms are the working of the unconscious mind to protect the person from anxiety. They can be considered precursors to conscious cognitive coping mechanisms that will ultimately solve the problem. Like some verbal and motor responses, defense mechanisms release tension. Table 33–2 describes these mechanisms and lists examples of their adaptive and maladaptive use.

TABLE 33–2 *Unconscious Ego Defense Mechanisms*

Mechanism	Description	Adaptive Use	Maladaptive Use
Denial	Blocking painful or anxiety-producing aspects of reality out of consciousness. Reality is either completely disregarded or transformed so that it is no longer threatening.	A man does not acknowledge that he has cancer even though the physician has told him the results of the biopsy. A child insists his mother is not dead, just "out of town for a few days."	A woman who has had a heart attack refuses to acknowledge illness and does not follow prescribed therapy.

TABLE 33–2 *Unconscious Ego Defense Mechanisms (continued)*

Mechanism	Description	Adaptive Use	Maladaptive Use
Rationalization	Often referred to as the "sour-grapes" or "half-truth" mechanism. Good reasons, acceptable to the conscious mind, are given for behavior or circumstances instead of the real reason. The person often disparages some goal that in reality the person would like to attain.	A student who fails an examination because she doesn't understand the material says that the teacher did not clarify the material sufficiently or she did not prepare adequately. A client whose work is interrupted by illness prematurely gives up the work and says he wouldn't have been successful in that field anyway.	A man always gives reasons for not attaining his goals and refuses to accept self-responsibility for not achieving them.
Compensation	Substituting an activity for one that the person really would like to do or cannot do.	A short man shows aggressive, dominating traits to suggest strength and authority that his stature does not convey. A boy who cannot participate in athletics studies hard and attains high grades.	A woman abuses alcohol and drugs to make up for feelings of inadequacy.
Repression	Excluding from consciousness desires, impulses, thoughts, memories, and strivings that conflict with self-image or that involve guilt, shame, or lowering of self-esteem. The painful events cannot be recalled or recognized. Repression is the underlying basis of all defense mechanisms.	A woman forgets a repugnant work assignment. A young woman who was raped and was brought to the outpatient clinic by her roommate says she feels very anxious but cannot remember the events of the past few hours.	A woman excludes a number of events from memory (amnesia).
Regression	Adopting behavior that was comforting earlier in life to overcome the discomfort and insecurity of the present situation.	A toilet-trained preschooler begins bed-wetting after his mother returns home with a new baby. A hospitalized elderly woman becomes more dependent on the nurse than is physically warranted.	A teenager assumes the fetal position for prolonged periods or plays with the genitals.
Sublimation	Redirecting libidinal drives (sexual and aggressive) into socially acceptable channels.	A person channels, to a limited degree, a sex drive into athletic activity, work, poetry, or music. A man who is fired goes to the gym and punches a punching bag to express rage at his boss.	A person has extreme difficulty in communicating with others.
Identification	Assuming the attitudes, ideas, and behavior patterns of another person or persons; it is an important growth mechanism for children. It is unconscious and differs from imitation, which is conscious.	A teenager changes her hairstyle to that of an idolized movie star. After having surgery, a young boy decides to become a doctor.	A man imitates socially unacceptable or harmful behavior.
Projection	Attributing to others characteristics and feelings that one does not want to admit are one's own.	A woman criticizes a neighbor for being a terrible gossip when in fact the woman herself gossips.	A person fails to take any responsibility for own behavior.

TABLE 33–2 *Unconscious Ego Defense Mechanisms* (continued)

Mechanism	Description	Adaptive Use	Maladaptive Use
Conversion	Transforming a mental conflict into a physical symptom.	A wife with illicit sexual wishes claims that all husbands are unfaithful and not to be trusted. Before taking a math exam, a young girl develops a headache. A woman develops a "lump in her throat" at a sad event.	A man experiences paralysis of his punching arm to avoid letting his anger get out of control and punching his boss. A girl develops an inability to speak in the context of protecting a sexually abusive father. A pregnant woman develops pathologic vomiting to express the forbidden desire not to have the baby.
Displacement	Transferring an emotion or feeling from the actual object to a less dangerous or threatening substitute.	A child directs hostility toward a parent to a teacher. A woman who has had an unpleasant experience with a man with red hair reacts strongly against all men with red hair.	A man is verbally or physically aggressive toward all authority or oppressive figures.
Reaction formation	Acting oppositely to what the person truly feels.	A woman shows great interest and concern for her mother-in-law, whom she dislikes. A man strongly criticizes pornographic literature when he has a desire to read it.	A young woman is always unnaturally sweet and loving and is unable to consider the possibility of being angry. A person with strong sadistic tendencies becomes an ardent opponent of surgical research on animals.

Source: Adapted with permission from P. Solomon and V. I. Patch. *Handbook of Psychiatry* 3d ed. (Los Altos, Calif.: Lange Medical Publications, 1974), pp. 500–505. Copyright © Lange Medical Publications.

FACTORS INFLUENCING THE MANIFESTATIONS OF STRESS

The degree to which a stressor affects an individual depends on the nature of the stressor, perception of the stressor, number of simultaneous stressors, duration of exposure to the stressor, experiences with a comparable stressor (Byrne and Thompson 1978, p. 3), age, and support people available. The *nature of the stressor* refers to its magnitude. Obviously, a fall from the roof of a building is more stressful than a fall from a chair. Similarly, angry remarks from a loved one are more stressful than those from a stranger.

Perception of the stressor (what the stressor means to the person) can be as important as the actual magnitude of the stressor. Because perception is a subjective phenomenon, there are wide differences in how people regard a stressor. Being late can create a greater stress response in a punctual person than a nonpunctual person. Some clients associate hospitals solely with dying friends and relatives. To such clients, the act of entering the hospital is particularly stressful, because they worry about whether they will die.

The *number of stressors* a person is experiencing at one time can greatly affect the responses. This often explains why a stressor that the nurse considers small can elicit a disproportionate response. For example, a hospitalized client who is coping with separation from her family, the unknown outcome of her illness, and financial problems can react angrily when the nurse brings her the wrong fruit juice. Normally, this woman would not be upset whichever juice was served; however, she is using up her coping energies on the other problems and has little left to adapt to this incident.

The *duration of exposure to the stressor* can also influence the manifestations of stress. If the duration of the stressor extends a person's stage of resistance beyond the person's coping powers, the person becomes exhausted and can eventually die. An example is a man admitted to a hospital with a fractured femur. The client survives the surgery and is healing well but develops an acute pain in the gallbladder, necessitating another operation. By this time, the client's energy reserves have been used up, and, although the operation is successful, the client develops an infection that delays his return home.

Previous *experience with a comparable stressor* can be useful both in predicting how the person will react and in reducing stress in the current situation. A person who has successfully adjusted to a situation once before is more likely to do so again in a similar situation than a person who is adjusting to the situation for the first time. Such people are strengthened by knowledge that they handled the situation successfully before. A client who has had an unsuccessful interaction with a physician and other health care personnel once before is more likely to experience stress during a second interaction. Determining what a particular event means to a person can help the nurse plan care.

The *age* of the individual affects response and adaptation to stressors. Infants, for example, have poorly developed immune mechanisms and cannot tolerate large fluid losses. Elderly people may have declining physical and mental resources to cope with increased stressors. *Support people* can assist a person coping with stress to maintain psychologic and physical integrity. They provide emotional support, often help in decision making, and, by sharing the experience, can relieve the intensity of the stress response.

Friedman and Rosenman (1974) identify two *personality types:* type A and type B. They point out that type A personalities are very prone to cardiovascular disease, whereas type B personalities do not usually develop it. The most pervasive cardiovascular disease is hypertension: the higher a person's blood pressure, the higher the risk of developing hardening of the arteries, which results in heart attacks and strokes. See the accompanying box for behavior patterns typical of both personality types.

Type A personalities are under constant pressure to perform and are hurried, impatient, and sometimes hostile. Type B personalities are relaxed, free from the urgencies of time, and able to enjoy work or play. Nuernberger (1981, p. 12) identifies another personality type, called type C, the coping personality. This personality sustains considerable stress but has learned to cope with it. Nuernberger believes many people are type C, since most people share some of the characteristics of types A and B.

ADAPTATION

Adaptation is the basis of homeostasis and resistance to stress. To adapt is to modify to meet new, changing, or different conditions. Because it is a phenomenon of all living things, adaptation is studied in many disciplines, such as

---

Characteristic Behavior Patterns of Type A and Type B Personalities

Type A Behaviors

- Hurried speech
- Constant, rapid movement/eating
- Aggression, ambition, and competitive spirit
- Inability to delegate authority
- Preoccupation with deadlines
- Chronic sense of time urgency
- Impatience with the rate at which things occur and the way others operate
- Career orientation, lack of hobbies
- Little satisfaction with accomplishments
- Restlessness and feelings of guilt during periods of relaxation
- Tendency to think and perform several things at once
- Obsession with money and numbers
- Tendency to dominate conversation, determine topics
- Preoccupation with own thoughts when others are talking
- Overconcern with getting things worth having, less concern with becoming things worth being
- Facade of self-assurance and confidence to hide insecurity about status
- Tendency to measure self-worth by number of achievements
- Nervous gestures: tics, clenched fist or jaw, tooth grinding

Type B Behaviors

- Freedom from all type A traits
- No sense of time urgency
- Ability to relax without guilt
- Ability to work without agitation
- Belief that the purpose of play is fun and relaxation, not to demonstrate superiority
- Tendency to discuss achievements and accomplishments only when situation demands it

Sources: Adapted from M. Friedman and R. Rosenman, *Type A behavior and your heart* © 1974 by Meyor Friedman. Reprinted by permission of Alfred A. Knopf, Inc. and P. Nuernberger, *Freedom from stress: A holistic approach* (Honesdale, Penn.: The Himalayan International Institute of Yoga Science and Philosophy, 1981).

plant biology, physics, psychology, education (personality adaptation), biochemistry, psychiatry, and ecology. In all disciplines, adaptation denotes interaction and change. The change is viewed as positive, for the better, or healthy.

Modes of Adaptation

Human adaptation occurs in three interrelated modes: physiologic, psychologic, and sociocultural.

Physiologic Mode
Physiologic or **biologic adaptation** occurs in response to increased or altered demands placed on the body and results in compensatory physical changes (e.g., increased muscle size and strength following prolonged exercise, increased capacity of the heart and lungs after prolonged exercise, and immunity to a specific disease following the invasion of a specific microorganism).

Psychologic and Sociocultural Modes
Psychologic adaptation involves a change in attitude and behavior, e.g., coping strategies, toward emotionally stressful situations. Examples include changing a life-style pattern (such as eating a balanced diet, exercising regularly, or balancing leisure time with work), using problem solving in decision making instead of anger or other nonconstructive responses, and stopping smoking.

Adaptation in the psychologic mode may also be maladaptive. For example, abusing alcohol and constantly giving in to others to avoid their anger are maladaptive.

Sociocultural adaptation involves changes in the person's behavior in accordance with the norms, conventions, and beliefs of various groups, such as family, society, ethnic group, religious group, professional group, and economic group (e.g., becoming socialized into a profession or military group, or living in a new country and learning to speak the language).

Characteristics of Adaptive Responses

All adaptive responses, whether physiologic, psychologic, or sociocultural, have common characteristics:

1. All adaptive responses are attempts to maintain homeostasis.

2. Adaptation is a whole body or total organism response.

3. Adaptive responses have limits. Physiologic adaptive responses are more limited than psychologic or social responses.

4. Adaptation requires time. A person adapts to an inadequate cardiac output that occurs gradually because the heart increases its pumping rate and the size of the ventricles. In the psychologic realm, people are able to think

more rationally in controlled or expected situations than in emergencies.

5. Adaptability varies from person to person. The person who is physically healthy has greater resources to adapt. The person who is flexible, responds readily to change, and uses a wide range of coping strategies is more likely to adapt than the person who does not tolerate change and responds in a limited way.

6. Adaptive responses may be inadequate or excessive. For example, the inflammatory response to bacterial invasion may not be sufficient to overcome an infection without antibiotic therapy. Inflammation in response to allergies can be excessive and create other problems.

7. Adaptive responses are egocentric and tiring because they require body energy and tax physical and psychologic resources. Adapting can consume a person's energy to the point that the person overlooks the needs of others and fails to give the support they require.

ASSESSING

How a person perceives and responds to stressors is highly individual. Vulnerability to stressors is largely related to previous learning, stage of development, life events, health, and coping methods. The nurse can help the client recognize stress and support effective coping strategies or teach the client new and more effective ways of handling stress.

Assessment relative to a client's stress and coping patterns includes (a) a stress and coping pattern history and (b) clinical examination of the client for indicators of stress. Questions to elicit data bout the client's stress and coping patterns are shown in the accompanying box. In addition, the nurse should be aware of expected developmental transitions (predictable tasks that must be accomplished if the person is to grow psychologically as well as physically; see Chapter 24.) This knowledge helps the nurse identify additional stressors that are present and the client's response to them. Table 33–3 provides an overview of these developmental stressors.

Indicators of stress were discussed earlier in this chapter. See the box entitled "Physiologic Manifestations of Stress" and Table 33–1 for descriptions of levels of anxiety. Observe the client also for verbal, motor, and cognitive manifestations. Remember, however, that clinical signs and symptoms may not occur when cognitive coping is effective.

DIAGNOSING

Several nursing diagnoses may apply to clients who are experiencing stress and having difficulties in coping with that stress. According to the NANDA definition, the nursing

- On a scale of one to ten, how would you rate the stress you are experiencing in the following areas?
  a. Home
  b. Work or school
  c. Finance
  d. Recent illness or loss of loved one
  e. Your health
  f. Family responsibilities
  g. Ethnic or cultural group
  h. Religion
  i. Relationships with friends
  j. Relationship with parents or children
  k. Relationship with partner
  l. Recent hospitalization
  m. Other (specify)
- How long have you been dealing with the above stressor(s)?
- How do you usually handle stressful situations?
  a. Cry?
  b. Get angry?
  c. Become verbally abusive?
  d. Talk to someone (who)?
  e. Withdraw from the situation?
  f. Structure and control others or situation?
  g. Go for a walk or physical exercise?
  h. Try to arrive at a solution?
  i. Pray for wisdom and courage?
  j. Other (specify)?
- How does your usual coping strategy work?

TABLE 33–3 *Selected Stressors Associated with Developmental Stages*

Developmental Stage	Stressors
Child	Resolving conflict between independence and dependence
	Beginning school
	Establishing peer relationships and adjustments
	Coping with peer competition
Adolescent	Accepting changing body physique
	Developing heterosexual or other relationships
	Achieving independence
	Choosing a career
Young adult	Getting married
	Leaving home
	Managing a home
	Getting started in an occupation
	Continuing one's education
	Rearing children
Middle adult	Accepting physical changes of aging
	Maintaining social status and standard of living
	Helping teenage children to become independent
	Adjusting to aging parents
Older adult	Accepting decreasing physical abilities and health
	Accepting changes in residence
	Adjusting to retirement and reduced income
	Adjusting to death of spouse and friends

diagnosis **Anxiety** is a "state in which the individual experiences feelings of uneasiness (apprehension) and activation of the autonomic nervous system in response to a vague, nonspecific threat" (Carpenito 1989, p. 128). When the nurse assesses that the client manifests physiologic symptoms of anxiety (e.g., increased heart rate, diaphoresis, trembling), emotional symptoms (e.g., apprehension, nervousness, tension), and cognitive symptoms (e.g., inability to concentrate, forgetfulness, lack of awareness of surroundings), the nurse can be reasonably sure that the client is anxious.

Fear is "a state in which an individual or group experiences a feeling of physiological or emotional disruption related to an identifiable source that is perceived as dangerous" (Carpenito 1989, p. 324). Unlike the anxious person, the fearful person can identify the specific threat. According to Carpenito (1989, p. 324), **Fear** and **Anxiety** often coexist in clinical practice.

Ineffective individual coping is a "state in which the individual experiences or is at risk of experiencing an ina-

bility to manage internal or environmental stressors adequately because of inadequate resources (physical, psychological, or behavioral)" (Carpenito 1989, p. 242). This diagnosis is appropriate when the nurse assesses that the client is not meeting role expectations, is using defense mechanisms inappropriately, or verbalizes an inability to cope. As with most nursing diagnoses, the etiology may be physiologic, psychologic, situational, or maturational. **Ineffective family coping** is discussed in Chapter 28.

Decisional conflict is the "state in which an individual or group experiences uncertainty about a course of action when the choice involves risk, loss, or challenge" (Carpenito 1989, p. 277). This diagnosis applies when the client verbalizes uncertainty about choices or undesired consequences of alternative actions being considered and vacillates between choices or delays decision making.

Examples of these diagnoses and possible contributing factors are shown below. Examples of assessment data clusters and related nursing diagnoses are shown in Table 33–4.

Dx **Nursing Diagnoses**
Clients Experiencing Stress and Difficulties Coping with Stress

Anxiety related to:

- Perceived threat to self-concept
- Threat of dying
- Change in health status
- Actual or perceived loss of loved one
- Maturational crisis (e.g., parenting, career development, retirement)
- Change in environment (e.g., hospital, nursing home)
- Change in socioeconomic status
- Conflict about essential values

Fear related to:

- Perceived changes in body integrity (e.g., loss of body part, disfigurement)
- Separation from family or other support persons
- Language barrier
- Pain and perceived inability to cope

Ineffective individual coping related to:

- Changes in body (e.g., loss of body part)
- Inadequate support system
- Unrealistic perceptions
- Inadequate coping method
- Work overload
- Impairment of nervous system
- Chronic pain

Decisional conflict (specify) related to:

- Knowledge deficit
- Conflict with personal values/beliefs
- Unclear values/beliefs
- Ethical dilemma
- Disagreement with significant others

PLANNING

The nurse develops plans in collaboration with the client and significant support persons when possible, according to the client's state of health (e.g., ability to return to work),

TABLE 33–4 *Examples of Assessment Data Clusters and Related Nursing Diagnoses: Stress and Coping Abilities*

Assessment Data Cluster	Nursing Diagnosis
LaMar Johnson, a 47-year-old accountant, was admitted to the emergency ward with a heart attack. He says, "I'm sacred about this. My dad died 2 months ago with the same thing." He appears restless, watches everything that goes on, and is hyperventilating.	**Anxiety** related to change in health status and threat of dying
Maria Panetti, an 85-year-old widow, says she feels "jittery and frightened" since entering the nursing home. "I've always had my daughter around to help me since Wilf died. I can't seem to concentrate on anything anymore." P, 98; R, 22; BP, 160/90. Appears wide-eyed and tense.	**Fear** related to separation from family
Sonia Park, a 33-year-old mother of three, returned to nursing after taking a refresher course. She says, "I'm so tired since I started work. I'm not keeping up with housekeeping the way I should, and I'm not spending as much time with the kids. I'm too tired to shop and go to my son's basketball game. Tom and all the kids are helping out and not complaining, but I just keep thinking they wish I still baked cookies and played more with them. I'm sure not sleeping well and am having awful headaches."	**Ineffective individual coping** related to work overload and unrealistic perceptions
Amit Singh, a 52-year-old woman, had a biopsy for a breast lump that was diagnosed as malignant. Her doctor says she can choose either a lumpectomy or a total mastectomy. She says, "My husband thinks I should have the lumpectomy, but I wonder if the total mastectomy is better for removing all the cancer. I just don't know what to do!"	**Decisional conflict** related to lack of information and disagreement with husband

level of anxiety, support resources, coping mechanisms, and sociocultural and religious affiliation. The nurse with little experience intervening with clients undergoing stress may wish to consult with a clinical specialist or more experienced nurse to develop effective plans. Nurse and client set goals to change the existing client responses to the stressor or stressors. Examples of possible goal statements for some of the sample nursing diagnoses are shown in the accompanying box.

Nursing interventions for achieving the goals planned may include

- Minimizing anxiety or mediating anger
- Identifying the coping mechanisms most useful to the client
- Identifying meaningful support persons who can help the client
- Planning stress reduction measures, such as physical exercise, rest periods, or time management, or providing referral for advanced stress reduction techniques, such as yoga.

Examples of outcome criteria to measure goal achievement and the effectiveness of nursing interventions are shown below.

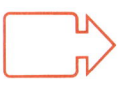

**Outcome Criteria
Clients Experiencing Stress and
Difficulties Coping with Stress**

The client experiencing **Anxiety:**

- Verbalizes awareness of feelings of anxiety.
- Keeps a log of incidents that arouse anxiety, frustration, or time urgency.
- Reports an increase in psychologic and physiologic comfort.
- Experiences a reduction in the manifestations of anxiety (specify).
- Uses adaptive coping methods to reduce anxiety (e.g., relaxation techniques; time management strategies; direct, open discussion; problem-solving skills).
- Avoids blaming others and expecting others to change.

The client experiencing **Fear:**

- Discusses fears.
- Reports an increase in psychologic and physiologic comfort.
- Experiences reduction in manifestations indicative of fear (e.g., tension, apprehension, panic).
- Has blood pressure and heart rate within normal range, relaxed muscles, and normal pupil size.
- Describes effective and ineffective coping patterns.
- Identifies own coping resources.

The client with **Ineffective individual coping:**

- Identifies ineffective coping behaviors and consequences.
- Verbalizes awareness of own coping.
- Identifies personal strengths (skills, knowledge, abilities) to cope with threats.
- Seeks new knowledge and skills to resolve stressful event(s).
- Reports decrease in emotional responsiveness.
- Demonstrates increased objectivity, ability to solve problems, and assertiveness.
- Uses appropriate coping resources (e.g., support systems, problem-solving and decision-making skills, professional help, spiritual values).
- Performs usual family, social, and work roles.

The client with **Decisional conflict:**

- Verbalizes fears and concerns regarding choices and responses of others.
- Identifies and assesses available alternatives.
- Recognizes consequences of available alternatives.
- Makes decisions compatible with personal values and lifestyle.
- Seeks support as needed for decision making.

IMPLEMENTING

Although stress accompanies every disease and illness, it is also highly individual; a situation that to one person is a major stressor may not affect another. Some methods to help reduce stress will be effective for one person; other methods will be appropriate for a different person. A nurse who is sensitive to clients' needs and reactions can choose those methods of intervention that will be most effective for each individual.

Minimizing Anxiety One way to reduce or perhaps eliminate anxiety is for the nurse and client to establish goals that are attainable. Clients must first recognize that they are anxious. This recognition is best brought about in an atmosphere of warmth and trust. Sometimes anxious clients react negatively to nurses because of personal frustration. It is important for nurses to understand this response and react to the behavior in a calm, accepting, and confident manner.

After clients realize that they are anxious, it is important to discuss all the possible reasons for their anxiety. Perley (1984, p. 362) categorizes three underlying states of mind associated with anxiety: *helplessness,* such as that in the person who has recently had a stroke and is unable to perform previous functions; *isolation,* such as that in an adolescent who fears rejection because of a sexually transmitted disease; and *insecurity,* such as that in a person who is worried about being unable to earn a living or pay medical bills. When clients can identify the cause of their anxiety, they may find it helpful to explore the cause with the objective of learning better coping strategies. General nursing guidelines to minimize the client's anxiety and stress follow:

1. *Support the client and family at a time of illness.* By conveying caring and understanding, the nurse can help clients reduce their stress. Feeling that someone else cares is a source of support to stressed people. Often families require time to talk about their worries and anxieties before they can feel assured and less stressed.

2. *Orient the client to the hospital or agency.* The nurse helps the client adjust to the role change from, for example, independent wage earner to relatively dependent client. The nurse can help family members by giving information, for instance, about visiting hours and specific unit policies.

3. *Give the client in a hospital some way of maintaining identity.* A person's name and clothes are important parts of the person's uniqueness as an individual. Nurses can help clients maintain identity by addressing them by the name they prefer and by assisting them to wear their own clothes in a hospital setting, when this is possible.

4. *Provide information when the client has insufficient information.* Fear of the unknown and incorrect information can frequently cause stress. Stressed clients often misunderstand facts related by health personnel. Additional information or clarification can allay stress.

5. *Repeat information when the client has difficulty remembering.* Nurses can assist clients by repeating information when it is requested and assisting people to apply it when they so desire. This problem is particularly prevalent among elderly people who are stressed by a change of setting as well as by their illness.

6. *Encourage the client to participate in the plan of care.* Loss of the right to determine their own destiny can be very stressful to some people, particularly adults who function independently or who assume responsibility for others in their daily lives.

7. *Give the client time to express feelings and thoughts.* Allow time for clients to describe their feelings and worries if they wish. Nurses should be sensitive to clients' needs and neither probe with prying questions nor be too busy to listen.

8. *Ensure that expectations are within the client's capabilities.* Whatever the activity, whether an exercise or recreation, the nurse should make sure that it is possible for the client to accomplish it. If an activity is beyond the client's ability, the client is likely to be more stressed by not achieving the goal.

9. *Be sensitive to specific situations and experiences that increase anxiety and stress for clients.* For example, a man might appear highly stressed each time he receives an intramuscular injection. A careful remark by the nurse about the stress may elicit information that the nurse can use to assist the client.

10. *Assist a client to make a correct appraisal of a situation.* Sometimes, through a lack of knowledge or misinterpretation of a sequence of events, people draw incorrect conclusions. Having valid information might relieve the client's stress.

11. *Provide an environment in which a person can function independently to some degree without assistance.* It may be difficult and stressful for an adult to assume the dependent client role even for a short time. By restoring some degree of independent functioning, such as by adapting eating utensils so that clients can feed themselves, nurses can lower clients' stress levels.

12. *Reinforce positive environmental factors and recognize negative ones to help reduce stress.* Dwelling on problems and difficulties increases stress, but focusing on what can be accomplished positively usually decreases stress.

13. *Arrange for other clients with similar experiences to visit.* Clients with colostomies or similar conditions may be highly stressed and feel that they will never be able to live a normal life again. Meeting another person who has successfully adjusted to a colostomy can lower the stress greatly.

14. *Bring clients and their support persons into contact with people in community agencies who can help them make valid plans.* Social workers are familiar with discharge planning and arrangements that a client may need to make. Often people are stressed needlessly because they do not know what help is available to them in the community.

15. *Communicate competence, understanding, and empathy rather than stress and anxiety.* When a nurse conveys stress or anxiety, the client and support persons may be concerned about the nurse's ability to function where the client's health and life are involved. To reduce a client's stress, nurses need to know themselves well and be able to function in a nondefensive manner that conveys competence and empathy.

Mediating Anger Often nurses find clients' anger difficult to handle. Caring for the client who is angry is difficult for two reasons (Gluck 1981, p. 9):

1. Clients rarely state "I feel angry or frustrated" and rarely indicate the reason for their anger. Instead, they may refuse treatment, become verbally abusive or demanding, may threaten violence, or become overly critical. Their complaints rarely reflect the cause of their anger.

2. Anger from clients can elicit fear and anger in the nurse, who may respond in a manner that intensifies the client's anger even to the point of violence. The majority of nurses respond in a way that reduces their own stress rather than the client's stress (Gluck 1981, p. 11).

Responses whose major purpose is to reduce the nurse's stress include defending, providing reassurance, offering advice or persuading, and retaliating aggressively. For example, this response to a client's demands is defensive: "I can't take care of everyone at once! We've been very busy this evening." This response does not recognize the client's problem and increases the client's tension and anger. A reassuring response, such as "You'll feel better as soon as you are up and about," is a way to recognize the problem and calm the client; however, it does not encourage the person to talk about the problem. Responses meant to offer advice or persuade often begin with the words "Yes, but, . . ." By offering advice or persuading, nurses focus on their own values and ideas, thus increasing the client's sense of powerlessness. Aggressive responses indicate disapproval of the client's behavior. For example, a nurse might say, "You're spoiled. You could do that yourself." Or a nurse might say, "What do *you* want *now*? Some people here are a lot sicker than you and need my help."

Responses that reduce the client's anger and stress include offering help, apologizing, asking relevant questions, and conveying understanding. For example, the nurse might respond by saying, "I guess it's pretty frustrating being alone and having to wait for others to do things for you." Gluck (1981, p. 10) suggests that nurses wishing to provide understanding responses to clients follow these guidelines:

1. Focus on the feeling words of the client.
2. Note the general content of the message.
3. Restate the feeling and content of what the client has communicated.
4. Observe the client's body language.
5. Ask yourself, "If I were in the client's shoes, what would I be feeling?"

In addition to these general guidelines for minimizing stress, several health promotion strategies (see Chapter 23) are often appropriate as interventions for clients with stress-related nursing diagnoses. Among these are physical exercise, optimal nutrition, adequate rest and sleep, time management, and relaxation techniques.

EVALUATING

To evaluate the achievement of client goals, the nurse collects data in accordance with the outcome criteria established earlier. Evaluation activities may include the following:

- Observing the client for absence or reduction of manifestations of fear and/or anxiety
- Measuring blood pressure and pulse rate
- Listening to the client's reports of increased physiologic or psychologic comfort, decreased emotional responsiveness, or verbalizations of fears and concerns
- Asking the client about personal strengths or coping resources identified
- Questioning the client about effective and ineffective coping responses and consequences
- Discussing situations in which the client has used specific adaptive coping methods and the client's perception of their effectiveness
- Asking the client about specific resources used, including support persons

Examples of evaluative statements indicating goal achievement are "The client identified four personal strengths as requested to cope with threats to self," "The client cited two examples in which problem solving and assertiveness were used in a stressful situation rather than her usual emotional reaction of anger," and "The client attended a time-management seminar on July 20, 1991 and stated it was valuable."

STRESS MANAGEMENT FOR NURSES

Nurses, like clients, are susceptible to experiencing anxiety and crises. In recent years, more attention has been given to the occupational stress nurses experience. Nursing practice involves many stressors related to both clients and the work environment. Kinzel (1982, p. 55) devised a 20-item, 24-hour scale to help nurses measure their stress levels. All 20 items fall into five main categories: inadequate knowledge, inadequate support from peers and supervisors, dealing with death, poor communication, and salary and staffing problems. The purpose of such a scale is to make nurses aware of the source of negative feelings and frustration on the job, to help them make adjustments, and to support colleagues.

Nurses can manage stress by using all of the techniques discussed for clients. In addition, Hamilton (1984), Scully (1980), and Wilson (1986) suggest the following:

1. First recognize that you are stressed. Become attuned to feelings of being overwhelmed, fatigue, angry outbursts,

and physical illness. Also be aware of increases in smoking, drinking coffee, or other substance abuse and determine whether you are distancing yourself from client interaction.

2. When attuned to your reactions to stress, determine when the reactions occur.

3. When attuned to your stress and when it occurs, determine alternative actions to deal with it constructively. Some suggestions follow:
   a. Plan a daily relaxation program with meaningful quiet times to reduce tension.
   b. Establish an activity program to direct energy outward.
   c. Become more assertive to overcome feelings of powerlessness in relationships with others. Learn to say no.
   d. Manage time better by delegating to others and combining tasks.
   e. Take a course in biofeedback, yoga, meditation, or some other advanced relaxation technique.
   f. Learn to accept failures and learn from them.
   g. Learn to ask for help, and share your feelings with colleagues.
   h. Learn to support your colleagues in times of need. Give them a chance to "ventilate" feelings and listen to their concerns.
   i. Learn to handle problems constructively instead of defensively.
   j. Accept what cannot be changed. There are certain limitations in every situation.
   k. If working in an intensive care or similar unit (ICU), establish a structured emotional support group. These groups are identified by various names: ventilation groups, discussion forums, or regular staff meetings for the purpose of dealing with feelings and anxieties generated in the work setting.

CHAPTER HIGHLIGHTS

▶ Homeostasis is the tendency of the body to maintain a state of relative balance or constancy in response to a changing internal and external environment.

▶ Physiologic homeostasis is maintained by coordinated functioning of the autonomic nervous, endocrine, respiratory, cardiovascular, renal, and gastrointestinal systems.

▶ Homeostatic mechanisms regulate hormone secretion, fluid and electrolyte levels, the functions of body viscera, and metabolic processes that provide energy for the body.

▶ Psychologic homeostasis, or emotional well-being, is acquired or learned through the experience of living and interacting with others.

▶ Stress is a state of physiologic or psychologic tension that affects the whole person—physically, emotionally, intellectually, socially, and spiritually.

▶ A person's response to stressors varies according to the way the stressor is perceived, its intensity and duration, the number of stressors, previous experience, coping mechanisms used, support people available, and age.

▶ A common psychologic response to stress is anxiety, which is manifested in a variety of cognitive, verbal, and motor responses that reduce tension.

▶ Unconscious psychologic defense mechanisms, such as denial, rationalization, compensation, and sublimation, also protect the individual from tension.

▶ Both physiologic and psychologic responses to stressors can be adaptive or maladaptive.

▶ Adaptation is a process of change that occurs in response to stress. It occurs in three interrelated modes: physiologic, psychologic, and sociocultural.

▶ Coping is a more immediate response to stress than adaptation.

▶ Coping strategies can be either effective or ineffective and result in adaptation or maladaptation, respectively.

▶ The nurse can help clients recognize stress and support clients' effective coping mechanisms.

▶ Nursing interventions for stress are aimed at reducing anxiety, at promoting clients' physical and mental well-being so that they handle stress more effectively, and at helping clients learn more effective coping mechanisms.

▶ The nurse, too, is prone to occupational stress and needs to learn effective stress-management techniques.

READINGS AND REFERENCES

SUGGESTED READINGS

Leidy, N. K. October 1989. A physiologic analysis of stress and chronic illness. *Journal of Advanced Nursing* 14:868–76.

    The author briefly reviews the history of stress research, explains the general adaptation syndrome (GAS) and relates it to nursing practice. In summary, Leidy writes that "Selye's principles of stress adaptation and GAS provide a useful framework for understanding the physiologic processes involved in the stress-illness relationship."

Wilson, L. K. December 1989. Professional growth section. High-gear nursing: How it can run you down and what you can do about it. *Nursing 89* 19:81–2, 84, 86, 88.

    The author points out that the nurse's reaction to stress can cause burnout. The warning signs of stress mentioned include feeling overwhelmed, fatigue, angry outbursts and depression, forgetfulness and disorganization, guilt, and self-sacrifice. The ways to cope with stress include developing a "can do" attitude, becoming more assertive, managing time better, and nurturing oneself and each other.

RELATED RESEARCH

Biggers, J.; Zimmerman, R. S.; and Alpert, G. November 1988. Nursing, nursing education, and anxiety. *Journal of Nursing Education* 27:411–17.

Dewe, P. J. April 1989. Stressor frequency, tension, tiredness and coping: Some measurement issues and a comparison across nursing groups. *Journal of Advanced Nursing* 14:308–20.

McGrath, A.; Reid, N.; and Boore, J. 1989. Occupational stress in nursing. *International Journal of Nursing Studies* 26(4):343–58.

Martin, D. March 1, 1990. Effects of ethical dilemmas on stress felt by nurses providing care to AIDS patients. *Critical Care Nursing Quarterly,* 12:53–57.

Pollock, S. E. June 1989. Adaptive responses to diabetes mellitus. *Western Journal of Nursing Research* 11:265–75.

Van Os, D.; Clark, C.; Turner, C.; and Herbst, J. August 1985. Life stress and cystic fibrosis. *Western Journal of Nursing Research* 7:301–15.

SELECTED REFERENCES

Bell, J. M. March/April 1977. Stressful life events and coping methods in mental-illness and wellness behaviors. *Nursing Research* 26:136–40.

Breakwell, G. M. August 1990. Are you stressed out? *American Journal of Nursing* 90:31–33.

Burgess, A. W., and Lazare, A. 1976. *Community mental health: Target populations.* Englewood Cliffs, N.J.: Prentice-Hall.

Byrne, M. L., and Thompson, L. F. 1978. *Key concepts for the study and practice of nursing.* St. Louis: C. V. Mosby Co.

Cannon, W. B. 1939. *The wisdom of the body.* 2d ed. New York: Norton Publishing Co.

Caplan, G. February 1990. Loss, stress, and mental health. *Community Mental Health Journal* 26:27–48.

Caroselli-Dervan, C. September 1989. Modifying stress in cardiovascular patients: Nursing intervention. *Journal of Advanced Medical-Surgical Nursing* 1:11–20.

Carpenito, L. J. 1989. *Nursing diagnosis: Application to clinical practice.* 3d ed. Philadelphia: J. B. Lippincott Co.

Detherage, K. S., and Johnson, S. S. 1986. Primary prevention in stress and crisis. In Edelman, C., and Mandle, C. L., editors. *Health promotion throughout the life span.* St. Louis: C. V. Mosby Co.

Dugan, D. O. 1987–1988. Essays on the art of caring in nursing: The human spirit in stress management. *Nursing Forum* 23(3):108–17.

Duldt, B. W. September 1981. Anger: An occupational hazard for nurses. *Nursing Outlook* 29:510–18.

Freud, S. 1946. *The ego and the mechanisms of defense.* New York: International Universities Press.

Friedman, M., and Rosenman, R. 1974. *Type A behavior and your heart.* Greenwich, Conn.: Fawcett Publications.

Gluck, M. March 1981. Learning a therapeutic verbal response to anger. *Journal of Psychiatric Nursing and Mental Health Services* 19:9–12.

Graydon, J. E. Summer 1984. Measuring patient coping. *Nursing Papers* 16:3–12.

Guyton, A. C. 1986. *Textbook of medical physiology.* 7th ed. Philadelphia: W. B. Saunders Co.

Hamilton, J. M. July/August 1984. Effective ways to relieve stress. *Nursing Life* 4:24–27.

Holmes, T. H., and Rahe, R. H. August 1967. The social readjustment rating scale. *Journal of Psychosomatic Research* 11:213–18.

Johnson, J. E., and Lauver, D. R. January 1989. Alternative explanations of coping with stressful experiences associated with physical illness. *Advances in Nursing Science* 11:39–52.

Kaseman, D. F., and Young, S. H. September/October 1988. Stress: An added incapacitator. *Geriatric Nursing* 9:274–77.

Kim, M. J.; McFarland, G. K.; and McLane, A. M. 1989. *Pocket guide to nursing diagnoses.* 3d ed. St. Louis: C. V. Mosby Co.

Kinzel, S. L. March/April 1982. What's your stress level? *Nursing Life* 2:54–55.

Lazarus, R. S. 1966. *Psychological stress and the coping process.* New York: McGraw-Hill.

Lazarus, R. S., and Folkman, S. 1984. *Stress, appraisal, and coping.* New York: Springer Publishing Co.

Lederer, J. R.; Marculescu, G. L.; Mocnik, B.; and Seaby, N. 1990. *Care Planning Pocket Guide.* 3d ed. Redwood City, Calif.: Addison-Wesley Nursing.

Lyon, B. L., and Werner, J. 1987. Stress. In Fitzpatrick, J. J. and Taunton, R. L., editors. *Annual Review of Nursing Research.* New York: Springer Publishing Co. vol 5, pp. 3–22.

Monat, A., and Lazarus, R. S. (editors). 1985. *Stress and coping: An anthology.* 2d ed. New York: Columbia University Press.

NANDA approved nursing diagnostic categories for clinical use and testing. Summer 1988. *Nursing Diagnosis Newsletter* 15:1–3.

Nuernberger, P. 1981. *Freedom from stress.* Honesdale, Pa.: The Himalayan International Institute of Yoga Science and Philosophy.

Perley, N. Z. 1984. Problems in self-consistency: Anxiety. In Roy, C., editor. *Introduction to nursing: An adaptation model.* Englewood Cliffs, N.J.: Prentice-Hall.

Roberts, S. L. 1987–1988. A framework for coping with stress and its application in patient care. *Nursing Forum* 23(3):101–107.

Scully, R. May 1980. Stress in the nurse. *American Journal of Nursing* 80:912–14.

Selye, H. 1956. *The stress of life.* New York: McGraw-Hill.

———. 1976. *The stress of life.* Rev. ed. New York: McGraw-Hill.

Smith, M. J. T., and Selye, H. November 1979. Stress: Reducing the negative effects of stress. *American Journal of Nursing* 79:1953–55.

Taché, J., and Selye, J. 1985. On stress and coping mechanisms. *Issues in Mental Health Nursing* 7:3–24.

Wilson, L. K. December 1989. Professional Growth Section: High-gear nursing: How it can run you down and what you can do about it. *Nursing 89* 19:81–2, 84, 86, 88.

Coping with Loss, Grieving, and Death

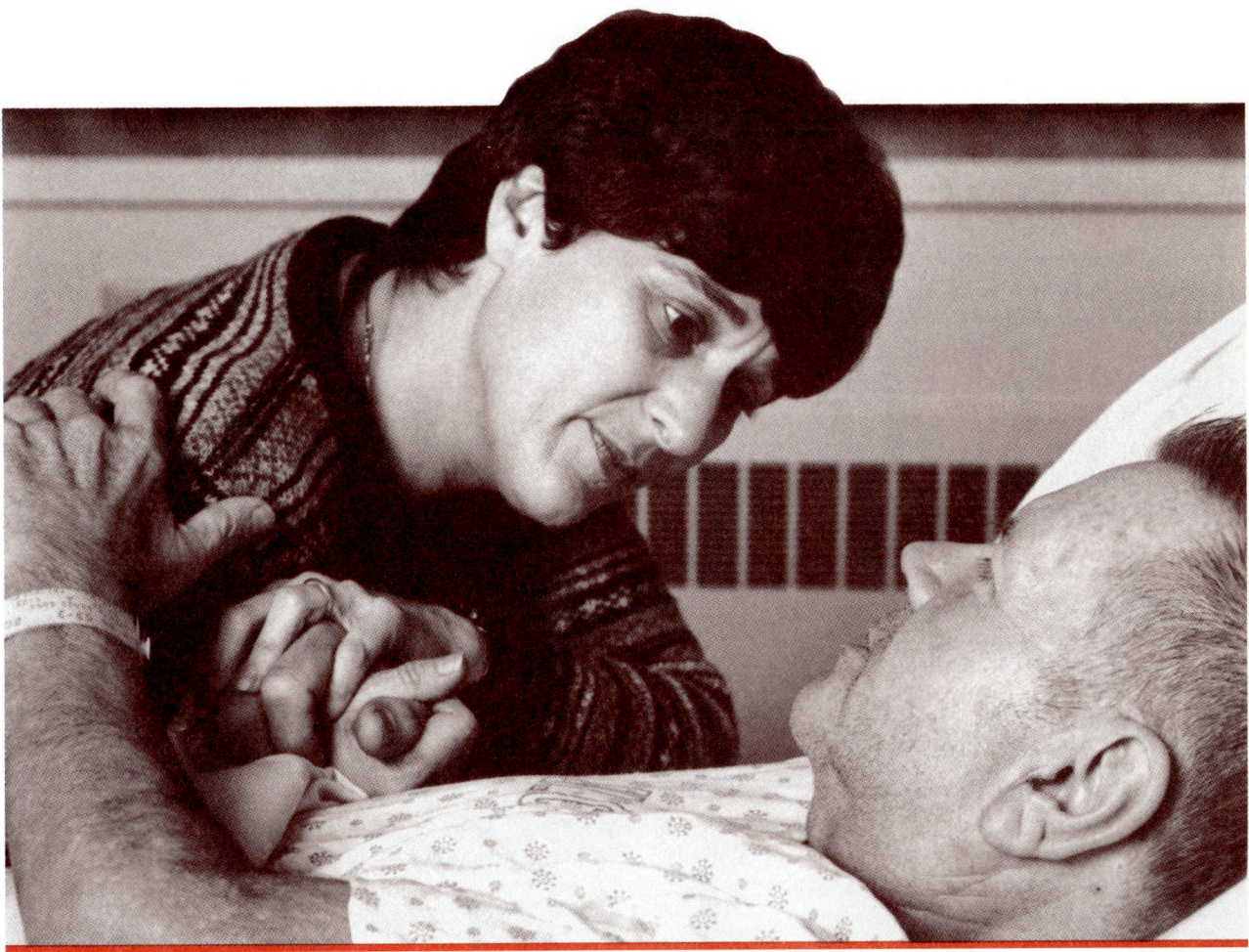

CONTENTS

OBJECTIVES

▶ Recognize selected frameworks for identifying stages of grieving.

▶ Identify clinical symptoms of grief.

▶ Discuss factors affecting a loss reaction.

▶ Recognize common fears associated with dying.

▶ Identify factors contributing to unresolved grief.

OBJECTIVES (continued)

▶ Describe guidelines for helping clients to die with dignity.

▶ Identify measures that facilitate the grieving process.

▶ List clinical signs of impending and imminent death and of death itself.

▶ List changes that occur in the body after death.

▶ Describe nursing measures for care of the body after death.

LOSS

Loss is an actual or potential situation in which a valued object, person, or the like is inaccessible or changed so that it is no longer perceived as valuable. People can experience the loss of body image, a significant other, a sense of well-being, a job, personal possessions, beliefs, a sense of self, and so on. Illness and hospitalization often produce losses.

Death is a fundamental loss, both for the dying person and for those who survive. Although death is inevitable for everyone, it is a lonely experience that each person ultimately faces alone. Yet even death, like loss, can stimulate people to grow in perception of both themselves and others. Death can be viewed not simply as loss of life, but as the dying person's final opportunity to experience life in ways that bring meaning and fulfillment.

Types and Sources of Loss

There are two general types of loss, actual and perceived. Both actual losses and perceived losses can be anticipatory. An **actual loss** can be identified by others and can arise either in response to or in anticipation of a situation. For example, a woman whose husband is dying may experience actual loss in anticipation of his death. A **perceived loss** is experienced by one person but cannot be verified by others. Psychologic losses are often perceived losses, in that they are not directly verifiable. For example, a woman who leaves her employment to care for her children at home may perceive a loss of independence and freedom. An **anticipatory loss** is experienced before the loss really occurs.

There are many sources of loss: (a) loss of an aspect of oneself—a body part, a physiologic function, or a psychologic attribute, (b) loss of an object external to oneself, (c) separation from an accustomed environment, and (d) loss of a loved or valued person.

Aspect of Self

The loss of an aspect of self changes a person's body image, even though the loss may not be obvious to others. A face scarred from a burn is generally obvious to people; loss of part of the stomach or loss of ability to feel emotion may not be as obvious. The degree to which these losses affect a person largely depends on the integrity of the person's body image (part of self-concept). Sometimes changes in self-image affect a person's social roles, such as employee, father, and husband. Any change that the person perceives as negative in the way the person relates to the environment can be considered a loss of self.

Losses such as divorce can have considerable impact. A divorce may mean loss of financial security, a home, and daily routines. Therefore, even when the divorce was desired, the sense of loss can last for some time afterward.

During old age, dramatic changes occur in physical and mental capabilities. Again the self-image is vulnerable, and support and reassurance are important. Old age is when people usually experience many losses: of employment, of usual activities, of independence, of health, of friends, and of family.

External Objects

Loss of external objects includes (a) loss of inanimate objects that have importance to the person, such as the loss of money for a person without financial means, or the burning down of a family's house, and (b) loss of animate objects such as pets that provide love and companionship.

Accustomed Environment

Separation from an environment and people who provide security can result in a sense of loss. The 6-year-old sheltered by home and family is likely to feel loss when first attending school and relating to more people. The university student who moves away from home for the first time also experiences a sense of loss.

Loved Ones

The loss of a loved one or valued person through illness, separation, or death can be very disturbing. In illness such as brain damage from viral infection or stroke, a person may undergo personality changes that make friends and family feel they have lost that person.

The death of a loved one is a permanent and complete loss. In primitive societies, death was considered a normal, natural event, and life was seldom long. The death of a young man brought greater grief than the deaths of women, children, or elderly people. In contemporary North American society, death is considered unacceptable and usually occurs in private, unless there is an accident. Death often happens in a hospital or in a home in the presence of immediate family. There is a tendency to prolong and preserve life. The culture reveres youthfulness; although people expect to live to old age, this is not considered as attractive as youth.

Loss as Crisis

Loss, especially loss of life or a loved one, can be viewed as either a situational or developmental crisis. The loss of a job or the loss of a young child, for example, is usually an unexpected situational crisis. On the other hand, losses incurred in the process of normal development—such as the departure of grown children from the home, retirement from a career, and the death of aged parents—are developmental crises that can be anticipated and, to some extent, prepared for.

How individuals deal with loss is closely related to their stage of development, personal resources, and social support systems. In dealing with loss of life, the nurse needs to consider the influence of these factors on the dying person and the surviving loved ones. As with all people in crisis, the experience of a dying person cannot be properly understood apart from the social context (Hoff 1984). In crisis situations, including the crisis of death, it is important for the nurse to consider the entire family as the client of care.

Bereavement and Grief

Bereavement is the subjective response to a loss through the death of a person with whom there has been a significant relationship. **Grief** is the total response to the emotional experience of the loss and is manifested in thoughts, feelings, and behaviors (Martocchio 1985, p. 327). **Mourning** is the behavioral process through which grief is eventually resolved or altered; it is often influenced by culture and custom.

Bereavement and grief cannot be viewed as a single crisis but rather are a series of crises that constitute a "life transition period" (Demi and Miles 1986). To view death as a single crisis can mislead caregivers into believing that short-term crisis intervention will bring positive resolution of the grief experience. In fact, normal bereavement can last as long as a year or more. Dealing with death loss is complex and intensely emotional and should not be oversimplified.

Age and the Impact of Loss

Age affects a person's understanding of and reaction to loss. With experience, people usually increase their understanding and acceptance of life, loss, and death. As in other aspects of human development, children show more rapid and dramatic variation and changes in their understanding of death. Their understanding is susceptible to influence by outside events, such as life-threatening illness, which usually deepens the child's understanding of death and makes it more like that of an adult (Fetsch 1984). Table 34–1 outlines the development of the concept of death through the life span.

People do not usually experience the loss of life or loved ones at regular intervals. As a result, preparation for these experiences is difficult. Coping with other of life's losses, such as the loss of a pet, the loss of a friend, and the loss of youth or a job, can help people anticipate the more severe loss of death by teaching them successful coping strategies.

Childhood   Children differ from adults not only in their understanding of loss and death, but also in how they are

TABLE 34–1 *Development of the Concept of Death*

Age	Beliefs/Attitudes
Infancy to 5 years	Does not understand concept of death
	Infant's sense of separation forms basis for later understanding of loss and death
	Believes death is reversible, a temporary departure, or sleep
	Emphasizes immobility and inactivity as attributes of death
5 to 9 years	Understands that death is final
	Believes own death can be avoided
	Associates death with aggression or violence
	Believes wishes or unrelated actions can be responsible for death
9 to 12 years	Understands death as the inevitable end of life
	Begins to understand own mortality, expressed as interest in afterlife or as fear of death
	Expresses ideas about death gathered from parents and other adults
12 to 18 years	Fears a lingering death
	May fantasize that death can be defied, acting out defiance through reckless behaviors, e.g., dangerous driving, substance abuse
	Seldom thinks about death, but views it in religious and philosophic terms
	May seem to reach "adult" perception of death but be emotionally unable to accept it
	May still hold concepts from previous developmental stages
18 to 45 years	Has attitude toward death influenced by religious and cultural beliefs
45 to 65 years	Accepts own mortality
	Encounters death of parents and some peers
	Experiences peaks of death anxiety
	Death anxiety diminishes with emotional well-being
65 years +	Fears prolonged illness
	Encounters death of family members and peers
	Sees death as having multiple meanings, e.g., freedom from pain, reunion with already deceased family members

affected by the loss of others. The child's patterns progress rapidly; adult patterns of growth and development are generally stable. The loss of a parent or other significant person can threaten the child's ability to develop, and regression sometimes results. Assisting the child with the grief experience includes helping the child regain the normal continuity and pace of emotional development.

Adults often assume that children do not have the same need as an adult to grieve the loss of others. In situations of crisis and loss, children are sometimes pushed aside or protected from the pain. They can feel afraid, abandoned, and lonely. Careful work with bereaved children is especially necessary, because experiencing a loss in childhood can have serious effects later in life. Research suggests a connection between early loss of a parent through death or divorce and increased risk of depression or suicide in adulthood (Taylor 1983–84).

Early and Middle Adulthood

As people grow, loss comes to be experienced as part of normal development. By middle age, for example, the loss of a parent through death seems a normal occurrence compared to the death of a younger person. Coping with the death of an aged parent has even been viewed as a necessary developmental task of the middle-aged adult. Society does not support intense or prolonged mourning for such a normal event (Moss and Moss 1983–84).

For the middle-aged adult, the loss of a parent can signal the disintegration of the family of origin. It is also a forceful reminder that the adult child is part of the older generation and therefore closer to death. The challenge of this developmental crisis for adult children is to assess the psychologic legacy of the parent, integrating what is valuable into their own identity. If the relationship with the parent was full of conflict, the parent's death can help release the child's energy for more productive use.

Late Adulthood

For older adults, the loss through death of a long-time mate is profound. Though individuals differ in their ability to deal with such a loss, research suggests an increase in health problems for widows and widowers during the first year following (Richter 1984). Because the majority of deaths occur among the elderly, and because the number of elderly is increasing in North America, nurses will need to be especially alert to the potential problems of older grieving adults.

Educating the Nurse About Loss

People in North America are socialized to think of death as the worst occurrence in life. They therefore do their best to avoid thinking or talking about death—especially their own. Death is thought about rarely, and almost exclusively in negative terms. Nurses are not immune to such attitudes. They need to take time to analyze their own feelings about death before they can effectively help others with a terminal illness. Nurses who are unconsciously uncomfortable with dying clients tend to impede the clients' attempts to discuss dying and death in these ways:

- Changing the subject, e.g., "Let's think of something more cheerful," or "You shouldn't say things like that."
- Offering reassurance, e.g., "You are doing very well."
- Denying what is happening, e.g., "You don't really mean that," or "You're going to live until you are a hundred."
- Being fatalistic, e.g., "Everyone dies sooner or later," or "God will take you when He wants you."
- Blocking discussion, e.g., "I don't think things are really that bad," conveying an attitude that stops further discussion of the subject
- Being aloof and distant or avoiding the client
- "Managing" the client's care and making the client feel increasingly dependent and powerless

The curricula of many nursing schools include education about death. Agencies and associations sponsor continuing education programs aimed at reducing death anxiety among nursing staff. Other programs help nurses explore the specific problems of direct contact with terminally ill clients and around-the-clock responsibility for their care. In all such programs nurses learn not only their own attitudes and concerns but also ways to support and comfort each other when they experience anger and frustration in the grief that follows the death of clients whom they not only cared for but also cared about.

Caring for the dying and the bereaved is one of the nurse's most complex and challenging responsibilities, bringing into play all the skills needed for holistic physiologic and psychosocial care. To be effective, nurses must come to grips with their own attitudes toward loss, death, and dying, because these attitudes will directly affect their ability to provide care. No single textbook chapter can give nursing students all the information and guidance needed to prepare them to care for dying clients and their families. Each nurse is personally responsible for actively engaging in a career-long process of education through reading, listening, and self-examination.

GRIEF

Grieving, the normal subjective emotional response to loss, is essential for good mental and physical health. It permits the individual to cope with the loss gradually and to accept it as part of reality. Grief is a social process; it is best shared and carried out with the assistance of others.

Grief work is important, because bereavement has been shown to have potentially devastating effects on health. Among the symptoms that can accompany grief are anxiety, depression, weight loss, difficulties in swallowing, vomiting, fatigue, headaches, dizziness, fainting, blurred vision, skin rashes, excessive sweating, menstrual disturbances, palpitations, chest pain, dyspnea, and infection (Gonda and Ruark 1984). The bereaved may also experience alterations in libido, concentration, and patterns of eating, sleeping, activity, and communication.

Although bereavement can threaten health, a positive resolution of the grieving process can enrich the individual with new insights, values, challenges, openness, and sensitivity. This applies to both the dying person and surviving loved ones, for the dying person is also living. If the quality of life permits, the dying person also should have the opportunity to grow emotionally and spiritually in the time that remains.

Stages of Grieving

Many authors have described stages or phases of grieving, perhaps the most famous of them being Kübler-Ross, who has described five stages: denial, anger, bargaining, depression, and acceptance (Kübler-Ross 1969, pp. 38–137). See Table 34–2. Engel (1964, pp. 94–96) has identified six stages of grieving: shock and disbelief, developing awareness, restitution, resolving the loss, idealization, and outcome. See Table 34–3 on page 820.

Nurses also have begun to write about the components of grief. Clark (1984) describes a three-phase course through which the bereaved progresses, lasting 6 months to 2 years. Martocchio (1985) discusses five clusters of grief and maintains that there is no single correct way, nor a correct timetable, by which a person progresses through the grief process. Whether a person can succeed in integrating the loss, and how this is accomplished, is related to that person's individual development and personal makeup. And individuals responding to the very same loss cannot be expected to follow the same pattern or schedule in resolving their grief, even while they support each other. Martocchio's five clusters of grief include the following:

1. *Shock and disbelief.* A feeling of numbness is a common response immediately following the death of a loved

TABLE 34–2 *Kübler-Ross's Stages of Grieving*

Stage	Behavioral Responses	Nursing Implications
Denial	Refuses to believe that loss is happening Is unready to deal with practical problems, such as prosthesis after loss of leg May assume artificial cheerfulness to prolong denial	Verbally support client's denial for its protective function. Examine your own behavior to ensure that you do not share in client's denial.
Anger	Client or family may direct anger at nurse or hospital staff, about matters that normally would not bother them	Help client understand that anger is a normal response to feelings of loss and powerlessness. Avoid withdrawal or retaliation with anger; do not take anger personally. Deal with needs underlying any angry reaction. Provide structure and continuity to promote feelings of security. Allow clients as much control as possible over their lives.
Bargaining	Seeks to bargain to avoid loss May express feelings of guilt or fear of punishment for past sins, real or imagined	Listen attentively, and encourage client to talk to relieve guilt and irrational fears. If appropriate, offer spiritual support.
Depression	Grieves over what has happened and what cannot be May talk freely (e.g., reviewing past losses such as money or job), or may withdraw	Allow client to express sadness. Communicate nonverbally by sitting quietly without expecting conversation. Convey caring by touch. Help support persons understand importance of being with the client in silence.
Acceptance	Comes to terms with loss May have decreased interest in surroundings and support persons May wish to begin making plans, e.g., will, prosthesis, altered living arrangements	Help family and friends understand client's decreased need to socialize and need for short, quiet visits. Encourage client to participate as much as possible in the treatment program.

TABLE 34-3   *Engel's Stages of Grieving*

Stage	Behavioral Responses
Shock and disbelief	Refusal to accept loss
	Stunned feelings
	Intellectual acceptance but emotional denial
Developing awareness	Reality of loss begins to penetrate consciousness
	Anger may be directed at hospital, nurses, etc.
	Crying and self-blame
Restitution	Rituals of mourning, e.g., funeral
Resolving the loss	Attempts to deal with painful void
	Still unable to accept new love object to replace lost person
	May accept more dependent relationship with support person
	Thinks over and talks about memories of the dead person
Idealization	Produces image of dead person that is almost devoid of undesirable features
	Represses all negative and hostile feelings toward deceased
	May feel guilty and remorseful about past inconsiderate or unkind acts to deceased
	Unconsciously internalizes admired qualities of deceased
	Reminders of deceased evoke fewer feelings of sadness
	Reinvests feelings in others
Outcome	Behavior influenced by several factors: importance of lost object as source of support, degree of dependence on relationship, degree of ambivalence toward deceased, number and nature of other relationships, and number and nature of previous grief experiences (which tend to be cumulative)

Source: G. L. Engel, Grief and grieving. *American Journal of Nursing,* September 1964, 64:93–98. Used by permission.

one. The bereaved may feel depressed, angry, guilty, and sad. Disbelief or denial may persist even though the loss has been accepted intellectually.

2. *Yearning and protest.* The anger that the bereaved feel may be directed at the deceased for having died, at God, at others whose loved ones are still alive, or at the caregivers. The bereaved may begin to fear their own mental deterioration and withdraw from sharing their thoughts and feelings with others.

3. *Anguish, disorganization, and despair.* When the reality of the loss is genuinely admitted, depression can set in. Weeping is common at this time. The bereaved lose interest and motivation in pursuing the future, are unable to make decisions, and lack confidence and purpose. Activities that were once enjoyed with the deceased are now without attraction. Coping strategies such as excessive drinking may compromise health.

4. *Identification in bereavement.* The bereaved may take on the behavior, personal traits, habits, and ambitions of the deceased. Sometimes they may also experience the same symptoms of physical illness.

5. *Reorganization and restitution.* Achieving stability and a sense of reintegration can take a period of time that ranges widely, from less than a year to several years. Although the bereaved are able to experience a sense of well-being and can resume most normal patterns of functioning, the feelings of grief do not simply cease. For many the pain of loss, though diminished, recurs for the rest of their lives.

A normal grief reaction may be abbreviated or anticipatory. *Abbreviated grief* is brief but genuinely felt. The lost object may not have been sufficiently important to the grieving person or may have been replaced immediately by another, equally esteemed object. *Anticipatory grief* is experienced in advance of the event. The wife who grieves before her ailing husband dies is anticipating the loss. A beauty queen may grieve in advance of an operation that will leave a scar on her body. Because many of the normal symptoms of grief will have already been expressed in anticipation, the reaction when the loss actually occurs may be quite abbreviated.

Unhealthy grief—that is, *pathologic* or *dysfunctional grief*—may be unresolved or inhibited. Both normal and unhealthy grief may be delayed. Many factors can contribute to dysfunctional grief, including a prior traumatic loss in childhood and the circumstances of the present loss. For instance, the sudden, untimely death of an adolescent or young adult can complicate the expression and resolution of grief. Other influences include family or cultural barriers to the emotional expression of grief.

Unresolved grief is extended in length and severity. The same signs are expressed as with normal grief, but the bereaved may also have difficulty expressing the grief, may deny the loss, or may grieve beyond the expected time. With *inhibited grief,* many of the normal symptoms of grief are suppressed, and other effects, including somatic, are experienced instead.

Burgess and Lazare (1976, p. 100) state that dysfunctional grief may be inferred from the following data or observations:

- The client fails to grieve following the death of a loved one; e.g., a husband does not cry at, or absents himself from, his wife's funeral.

- The client becomes recurrently symptomatic on the anniversary of a loss or during holidays (especially Thanksgiving and Christmas).
- The client avoids visiting the grave and refuses to participate in religious memorial services of a loved one, even though these practices are a part of the client's culture.
- The client develops persistent guilt and lowered self-esteem.
- Even after a prolonged period, the client continues to search for the lost person. Some make the search while in fugue states. Others may wander from town to town or act as if they were expecting the deceased to return. Some may consider suicide to effect reunion.
- A relatively minor event triggers symptoms of grief.
- Even after a period of time, the client is unable to discuss the deceased with equanimity, e.g., the client's voice cracks and quivers, eyes become moist.
- An interview of the client is characterized by themes of loss.
- After the normal period of grief, the client experiences physical symptoms similar to those of the person who died.
- The client's relationships with friends and relatives worsen following the death.

Many factors contribute to *unresolved grief* (Burgess and Lazare 1976, pp. 97–100):

- Ambivalence (intense feelings of both love and hate) toward the lost person. The bereaved is often afraid to grieve for fear of discovering unacceptable negative feelings.
- A perceived need to be brave and in control; fear of losing control in front of others.
- Endurance of multiple losses, such as the loss of an entire family, which the bereaved finds too overwhelming to contemplate.
- Extremely high emotional value (overcathexis) invested in the dead person. Failure to grieve in this instance helps the bereaved avoid the reality of the loss.
- Uncertainty about the loss—for example, when a loved one is "missing in action."
- Lack of support persons.
- Subjection to socially unacceptable loss that cannot be spoken about, e.g., suicide, abortion, or giving a child up for adoption.

Assessing Loss and Grieving

To gather a complete database that allows accurate analysis and identification of appropriate nursing diagnoses for clients experiencing losses and grieving, the nurse first needs to recognize the state of awareness the client and family manifest, the symptoms of grief, and the factors influencing a loss reaction.

States of Awareness　　In cases of terminal illness, the state of awareness shared by the dying person and the family affects the nurse's ability to communicate freely with clients and other health care team members and to assist in the grieving process. Three types of awareness that have been described are closed awareness, mutual pretense, and open awareness (Strauss and Glaser 1970, p. 300).

In **closed awareness,** the client and family are unaware of impending death. They may not completely understand why the client is ill, and they believe the client will recover. The physician may believe it is best not to communicate a diagnosis or prognosis to the client or family. Nursing personnel are confronted with an ethical problem in this situation, and they have several choices. One course is to answer questions evasively or falsely. But ultimately the client and family will know the truth, and when they do they may recognize that information given them earlier was false. See Chapter 7 for further information on ethical dilemmas.

With **mutual pretense,** the client, family, and health personnel know that the prognosis is terminal but do not talk about it and make an effort not to raise the subject. Sometimes the client refrains from discussing death to protect the family from distress. The client may also sense discomfort on the part of health personnel and therefore not bring up the subject. Mutual pretense permits the client a degree of privacy and dignity, but it places a heavy burden on the dying person, who then has no one in whom to confide fears.

With **open awareness,** the client and people around know about the impending death and feel comfortable about discussing it, even though it is difficult. This awareness provides the client an opportunity to finalize affairs and even participate in planning funeral arrangements. One study indicates that nurses prefer the state of open awareness and prefer to become emotionally involved with their clients, since it "allows them to fully implement their ideal of nursing care" (Field 1984, p. 67).

Not all people can handle open awareness. For example, a 45-year-old man who knows he is dying may be unable to discuss his forthcoming death without becoming angry at people around him. Whether to inform dying clients that their condition is terminal is a difficult issue for physicians. Some authorities believe that terminal clients acquire knowledge of their condition even if they are not directly informed. Others believe that many clients remain unaware of their condition until the end. It is difficult, however, to distinguish what clients know from what they are willing to accept. A study by Cappon (1970) asked groups of healthy persons, physically ill clients, psychiatric clients, and dying clients whether they would like to know if a serious illness was terminal. The majority responded yes; however, of the four groups, the dying least desired this information (33% did not want to be told). Cappon concluded that physicians should be cautious and not give more information than the client wants.

Symptoms of Grief

The nurse assesses the grieving client and/or family members following a loss to determine the phase or stage of grieving. The following clinical symptoms of grief are described by Schulz (1978, pp. 142–43):

- Repeated somatic distress
- Tightness in the chest
- Choking or shortness of breath
- Sighing
- Empty feeling in the abdomen
- Loss of muscular power
- Intense subjective distress

Physiologically, the body responds to a current or anticipated loss with a stress reaction. The nurse can assess the clinical signs of this response. See Chapter 33. See also coping mechanisms and responses in Chapter 33.

Factors Influencing a Loss Reaction

The influence of age and developmental level on a person's reaction to loss has already been discussed. Other factors include the personal significance of the loss, culture, spiritual beliefs, sex role, and socioeconomic status.

Significance of the loss   The significance of a loss depends on the perceptions of the individual experiencing the loss. One person may experience a great sense of loss over a divorce; another may find it only mildly disrupting. A number of factors affect the significance of the loss:

- Age of the person
- Value placed on the lost person, body part, and so on
- Degree of change required because of the loss
- The person's beliefs and values

Expectations can also greatly affect significance. For elderly people who have already encountered many losses (e.g., family, health, independence), an anticipated loss such as their own death may not be important; they may be apathetic about it instead of reactive. More than fearing death, some may fear loss of control or becoming a burden (Charmaz 1980, p. 77).

Culture   Culture influences an individual's reaction to loss. How grief is expressed is often determined by the customs of the culture. It has been suggested that the Protestant ethic—individualism, self-reliance, independence, and hard work—leads to the practice of handling grief only with significant others, not a larger community (Charmaz 1980, p. 284). In the United States and Canada, unless an extended family structure exists, grief is handled by the nuclear family, which, because of its small size, emphasizes self-reliance and independence.

Many Americans appear to have internalized the belief that grief is a private matter to be endured internally. Therefore, feelings tend to be repressed and may remain unidentified. People who have been socialized to "be strong" and "make the best of the situation" may not express deep feelings or personal concerns when they experience a serious loss.

Some cultural groups value social support and the expression of loss. In certain black churches, the expression of emotion plays a prominent part. In Hispanic American groups where strong kinship ties are maintained, support and assistance are provided by family members, and the free expression of grief is encouraged.

Spiritual beliefs   Spiritual beliefs and practices greatly influence both a person's reaction to loss and subsequent behavior. Most religious groups have practices related to dying, which are often important to the client and support persons. For additional information, see Chapter 32. To provide support at a time of death, nurses need to understand the client's particular beliefs and practices.

Sex role   The sex roles into which many people are socialized in the United States and Canada affect their reactions at times of loss. Men are frequently expected to "be strong" and show very little emotion during grief, whereas it is acceptable for women to show grief by crying. Often when a wife dies, the husband, who is the chief mourner, is expected to repress his own emotions and to comfort sons and daughters in their grieving.

Sex roles also affect the significance of body image changes to clients. A man might consider a facial scar to be "macho," but a woman might consider it ugly. Thus, the woman, but not the man, would see it as a loss.

Socioeconomic status   The socioeconomic status of an individual often affects the support system available at the time of a loss. A pension plan or insurance, for example, can offer a widowed or disabled person choices of ways to deal with a loss: A woman who loses a hand and can no longer do her previous work may be able to pursue vocational reeducation; a man whose wife has died can afford to take a cruise or visit relatives in Europe. Conversely, a person who is confronted with both severe loss and economic hardship may not be able to cope with either.

Diagnosing

Many of the NANDA nursing diagnoses apply to grieving clients, depending on the information obtained from individual assessment. Some diagnoses that may be applicable are **Anticipatory grieving, Dysfunctional grieving, Impaired adjustment,** and **Social isolation. Anticipatory grieving** is often a healthy response. It is used as a diagnosis when the client expresses sorrow, anger, or guilt

What Responses Can Nurses Expect of the Bereaved?

The purpose of this study was to identify themes associated with bereavement. An analysis of 30 narrative accounts revealed nine themes: five core themes, three meta-themes, and one contextual theme. The *core themes* are *being stopped* (the interruption of life's usual flow following the death of a loved one, characterized by varying degrees of inability, frequently stated in terms of "I can't"); *hurting* (cluster of intensely painful emotions); *missing* (acute awareness of all that has been lost); *holding* (desire to maintain all, particularly that which was good, from the loved one's lost existence); and *seeking* (a search for help).

The *meta-themes* are *change* (the dynamic, change-inducing character, or wavelike quality, of bereavement); *expectations* (a sense of "rightness" or "oughtness" that hovers over bereavement); and *inexpressibility* (inadequacy of words to describe the experience).

The one *contextual theme, personal history,* is the theme in which the five core themes are embedded and is the one essential to understanding the quality of bereavement. These themes were compared with three theoretical perspectives on bereavement by Freud, Kübler-Ross, and one existential-phenomenological perspective. Features of bereavement that are dissimilar or unaddressed by the theoretical perspectives are (a) the quality of grief's changing character, (b) holding, (c) expectations of how the bereaved should overlay the experience, and (d) how the personal history affects the quality and meaning of the loss.

Implications: Using these themes as a guide, nurses can expect a broad range of unique responses from the bereaved. In particular, nurses need to understand the changing character of grief that may be triggered years after the death. Obtaining a personal history is critically important in determining the quality and meaning of the person's bereavement.

S. L. Carter, Themes of grief, *Nursing Research,* November/December 1989, 38:354–58.

about the potential loss and experiences changes in eating habits, sleep patterns, activity levels, and communication.

Dysfunctional grieving is the state in which an individual or group experiences prolonged unresolved grief and engages in detrimental activities (Carpenito 1989, p. 364). This diagnosis is not appropriate until several months or a year after the loss. It is appropriate when the nurse assesses that the client is not performing usual expected roles, denies the loss, has continued difficulty in expressing the loss, has continued alterations in sleep patterns, and

fails to develop new relationships or interests. See also the manifestations described earlier.

Impaired adjustment may be the diagnosis for clients with loss of a body part or physiologic function. It is the "state in which the individual is unable to modify his/her behavior or lifestyle in a manner consistent with a change in health status" (Kim et al. 1989, p. 2). Such clients may verbalize nonacceptance of the change in health status, lack movement toward independence, or be unable to limit expectations of self. This diagnosis can be applied either to the person suffering the loss or to a significant other. For instance, the husband of a woman hospitalized with a life-threatening illness may feel unable to assume unaccustomed domestic duties, such as child care, and he may feel resentment because the disease has removed the person who maintained the stability of family life. The athlete who suffers a sudden heart attack might also be diagnosed with **Impaired adjustment.** The reduced capacity for physical exertion that the condition imposes may threaten self-image and self-esteem.

Social isolation occurs when the painful nature of grief causes those experiencing it to withdraw from their normal social support systems. These clients may have a sad, dull affect, be uncommunicative and withdrawn, express feelings of loneliness, and lack supportive others. Some people feel the need to display mastery of the situation or wish not to burden friends. They may be afraid to test the strength of friendships. A new widow, for example, might feel awkward maintaining a social relationship in the circle of married couples she had participated in with her husband.

Social support is a major positive influence on the successful resolution of grief (Richter 1984). **Social isolation,** as a nursing diagnosis, can therefore be useful in directing nursing interventions that help the client to build the necessary support network.

Altered family processes occur when a family that normally functions effectively experiences a dysfunction. See the discussion about this diagnosis in Chapter 28.

Examples of these diagnoses and contributing factors are shown below. Examples of assessment data clusters and related nursing diagnoses are shown in Table 34–4, later in this chapter.

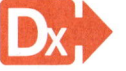 *Nursing Diagnoses Clients with Grief and Loss*

Anticipatory grieving related to:

- Perceived potential loss of loved one
- Perceived potential loss of body part or function
- Perceived potential loss of physiopsychosocial well-being
- Perceived potential loss of personal possessions
- Perceived potential loss of social role
- Perceived impending death of self

Dysfunctional grieving related to:

- Multiple past or current losses
- Lack of resolution of previous grieving response
- Unresolved guilt related to the deceased
- Lack of adequate social supports
- Unconscious gain from others to maintain grieving
- Difficulty or inability to express feelings freely

Impaired adjustment related to:

- Disability requiring change in life-style
- Inadequate or unavailable support systems
- Impaired cognition
- Ineffective denial

Social isolation related to:

- Inability to engage in satisfying personal relationships
- Inadequate personal resources
- Alterations in physical appearance
- Altered state of wellness

Assisting Clients with Their Grief

- Provide opportunity for the persons involved to "tell their story."
- Recognize and accept the varied emotions that people express in relation to a significant loss.
- Provide support for the expression of difficult feelings, such as anger and sadness, recognizing that people must do this in their own way and at their own pace.
- Include children in the grieving process.
- Encourage the bereaved to maintain established relationships.
- Acknowledge the usefulness of mutual-help groups.
- Encourage self-care by family members—in particular, the primary caregiver.
- Acknowledge the usefulness of counseling for especially difficult problems.

Source: J. Q. Benoliel, Loss and terminal illness, *Nursing Clinics of North America,* June 1985, 20:445.

Planning

The goals of grieving are to be able to remember the lost object or person without intense pain and to be able to redirect emotional energy into one's own life and regain the capacity to love. More specifically, the client needs to (a) feel free from emotional bondage to the deceased person, (b) be able to adjust to the changed environment, (c) be capable of developing new relationships and renewing old ones, and (d) feel comfortable with both positive and negative memories of the deceased (Martocchio 1985).

Examples of outcome criteria for grieving clients are shown below.

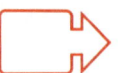

Outcome Criteria
Clients with Grief and Loss

The client:

- Verbalizes feelings of sorrow (or anger or loss).
- Shares thoughts and feelings with significant others.
- Uses appropriate resources (e.g., friends, clergy, support groups).
- Resumes usual activities (e.g., activities of daily living, work, recreation).
- Maintains constructive interpersonal relationships.
- Establishes new relationships.
- Verbalizes sense of progress toward resolution of the grief.
- Identifies alternative plans for meeting goals that were important before the loss.

Implementing

The skills most relevant to situations of loss and grief are attentive listening, silence, open and closed questioning, paraphrasing, clarifying and reflecting feelings, and summarizing. Less helpful to clients are responses that give advice and evaluation, those that interpret and analyze, and those that give unwarranted reassurance (Martocchio 1985). To ensure effective communication, the nurse must make an accurate assessment of what is appropriate for the client.

Communication with grieving clients needs to be relevant to their stage of grief. Whether the client is angry or depressed affects how the client hears messages and how the nurse interprets the client's statements. Implications for nurse-client communication are related to Kübler-Ross's five stages in Table 34–2, earlier.

The guidelines in the box above can assist nurses in helping the bereaved.

Evaluating

Evaluating the effectiveness of nursing care of the grieving client is difficult because of the long-term nature of the life transition. Criteria for evaluation must be based on goals set by the client and family, and not on an arbitrary standard of success (Benoliel 1985). A follow-up visit to the surviving family members may be an appropriate nursing measure not only to obtain information for evaluation but also to assist nurses in working through their own grief by expressing their continuing concern for the family.

CARE OF THE DYING CLIENT

Assessing

Nursing care and support for the dying client and family include making an accurate assessment of the physiologic signs of approaching death. In addition to signs related to the client's specific disease, certain other physical signs are indicative of impending death. The four main characteristic changes are loss of muscle tone, slowing of the circulation, changes in vital signs, and sensory impairment. See the box below for indications of impending clinical death.

Signs of Impending Clinical Death

Loss of muscle tone

- Relaxation of the facial muscles (e.g., the jaw may sag)
- Difficulty speaking
- Difficulty swallowing and gradual loss of the gag reflex
- Decreased activity of the gastrointestinal tract, with subsequent nausea, accumulation of flatus, abdominal distention, and retention of feces, especially if narcotics or tranquilizers are being administered
- Possible urinary and rectal incontinence due to decreased sphincter control
- Diminished body movement

Slowing of the circulation

- Diminished sensation
- Mottling and cyanosis of the extremities
- Cold skin, first in the feet and later in the hands, ears, and nose (the client, however, may feel warm due to elevated temperature)

Changes in vital signs

- Decelerated and weaker pulse
- Decreased blood pressure
- Rapid, shallow, irregular, or abnormally slow respirations; Cheyne-Stokes respirations; noisy breathing, referred to as the *death rattle,* due to collection of mucus in the throat; mouth breathing, which leads to dry oral mucous membranes.

Sensory impairment

- Blurred vision
- Impaired senses of taste and smell

Various consciousness levels occur just before death. Some clients are alert, whereas others are drowsy, stuporous, or comatose. Hearing is thought to be the last sense lost.

The traditional *clinical signs of death* were cessation of the apical pulse, respirations, and blood pressure. However, since the advent of artificial means to maintain respirations and blood circulation, identifying death is more difficult. In 1968, the World Medical Assembly adopted the following guidelines for physicians as indications of death (Benton 1978, p. 18):

- Total lack of response to external stimuli
- No muscular movement, especially breathing
- No reflexes
- Flat encephalogram

In instances of artificial support, absence of electric currents from the brain (measured by an electroencephalogram) for at least 24 hours is an indication of death. Only a physician can pronounce death, and only after this pronouncement can life-support systems be shut off.

Another definition of death is **cerebral death,** which occurs when the higher brain center, the cerebral cortex, is irreversibly destroyed. The client may still be able to breathe but is irreversibly unconscious. People who support this definition of death believe the cerebral cortex, which holds the capacity for thought, voluntary action, and movement, *is* the individual (Schulz 1978, p. 92).

Diagnosing

The full range of nursing diagnoses, addressing both physiologic and psychosocial needs, can be applied to the dying client, depending on the assessment data. Three diagnoses that may be particularly appropriate are **Fear, Hopelessness,** and **Powerlessness.**

Fear　　The diagnosis of **Fear** was discussed in detail in Chapter 33. Many fears are associated with death, and the nurse needs to determine a client's specific fears. Gonda and Ruark (1984, pp. 31–32) discuss three objects of the dying person's fear: the process of dying, nonexistence, and what comes after death. The nurse is usually better able to assist a client with the complex process of dying than with the spiritual fears of nonexistence and the hereafter.

Schulz (1978, p. 27) outlines the following fears related to a person's own death: pain, body misfunction, humiliation, rejection or abandonment, nonbeing, punishment, interruption of goals, and negative impact on survivors (e.g., psychologic suffering, economic hardship).

Sheehy (1981, pp. 27–62), in his discussion about common fears of dying, includes fear of pain, loneliness, dependence, the moment of death, and annihilation. Although there is no pain at the moment of death and the transition from life to death seems easy, many people fear this moment. Sheehy believes that fear of the moment of death is the result of the emotional sting and pain experienced during the death of a parent. People remember this previous pain and, therefore, believe that dying is painful. Fear of annihilation, or being reduced to nothingness after death, and questions about immortality need to be faced. Does immortality rest in what the individual achieved in this life, or does the soul survive after death? Whatever a person believes about life after death, both body and mind may be viewed as reentering the universe and becoming part of it as some form of energy.

Hopelessness   The very nature of a terminal illness or any other dying process can lead to a client's loss of hope. The nurse can identify this subjective state by noting some of the following behaviors: (a) passivity, (b) decreased verbalization, (c) decreased affect, (d) verbal cues (sighing, "I can't," or "Why bother?"), (e) lack of initiative, and (f) decreased response to stimuli. Feelings of hopelessness often follow an awareness of the reality of the loss and may be expressed in the despair phase of mourning (Gonda and Ruark 1984, p. 38). Real or perceived abandonment can also mean a diagnosis of **Hopelessness.** A loss of belief in religious and spiritual values or powers may be related to the development of hopelessness. The return of realistic hope can be facilitated by the nurse through assisting the client and/or family to focus on the outcomes of specific, short-term goals (Gonda and Ruark 1984, pp. 89–90).

Powerlessness   The dying client or the family may express a lack of control over the situation. **Powerlessness** is a likely diagnosis when the impending death is sudden and unexpected or when the dying client is a child. However, this diagnosis is not limited to such situations. Dying clients who have confronted chronic debilitating diseases may perceive that they can no longer control their conditions. The nurse can identify powerlessness by observing the following behaviors: (a) verbal expression of having no control or influence over the situation or outcome, (b) frustration about inability to perform previously mastered activities, (c) aggressive behavior when goals are not achieved, (d) lack of participation in decision making, and (e) feelings of depression or resentment.

Examples of these nursing diagnoses and possible contributing factors are shown below. Examples of assessment data clusters and related nursing diagnoses are shown in Table 34–4.

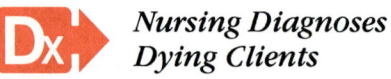

Nursing Diagnoses
Dying Clients

Fear related to:

- Knowledge deficit (concern about pain and inability to cope)
- Lack of social support in threatening situation

TABLE 34–4 *Examples of Assessment Data Clusters and Related Nursing Diagnoses for Clients Who Are Grieving or Dying*

Data Cluster	Nursing Diagnosis
Teresa Jimenez's son Ramon, age 15, has cystic fibrosis of the lung. Mother and son are waiting for an appropriate donor for a heart-lung transplant. She says, "We've been called to the transplant unit twice, but things didn't work out. Ramon gets his hopes all geared up, and then he's deflated. I'm worried that they won't get the right donor in time. I can't eat or sleep worrying. I don't know what I'll do if he doesn't get that transplant. He's all I've got since my husband left us 6 years ago."	**Anticipatory grieving** related to perceived potential loss of loved one.
Tom Bauer's wife died 14 months ago of a ruptured aortic aneurysm at age 59. He lives alone, has no children, and refuses to see friends. He reports frequent headaches, inability to concentrate at work, little interest in food, and early morning insomnia. These symptoms increase at the time of his wife's birthday and their anniversary. He says, "I still can't find it in myself to visit her grave. There are times when I'd just like to die and be with her."	**Dysfunctional grieving** related to lack of adequate social support
John Yee, age 63, has metastatic carcinoma of the bowel. He has noticed a rapid deterioration in energy in the past week and feels bloated and nauseated. He has become increasingly jaundiced and says, "I know I haven't long to live. Why can't they just give me a big dose of morphine and get it over with?"	**Powerlessness** related to terminal illness and inability to terminate life
Keisha Washington, who has multiple sclerosis and is paralyzed from the neck down, has appealed for someone to help her commit suicide. Her mind and speaking ability are unimpaired. She states, "I dread the same fate as my sister, who also had multiple sclerosis and before death had pain and became blind and mute."	**Hopelessness** related to deteriorating physiologic condition

- Negative impact on survivors

Hopelessness related to:

- Prolonged restriction of activity resulting in isolation
- Deteriorating physiologic condition
- Terminal illness
- Long-term stress (e.g., chronic pain)
- Perceived significant loss of loved one, youth, influence, opportunity

Powerlessness related to:

- Chronic debilitating disease
- Terminal illness
- Institutional environment
- Interpersonal behavior of others

Planning

Major goals of dying clients are (a) maintaining physiologic and psychologic comfort and (b) achieving a dignified and peaceful death. When planning care with these clients, the Dying Person's Bill of Rights can be a useful guide (see the accompanying box). Outcome criteria for clients with diagnoses of **Fear, Hopelessness,** and **Powerlessness** are shown below.

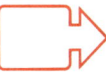

Outcome Criteria
Dying Clients

The client:

- Is free of pain.
- Participates in self-care activities in accordance with health status.
- Makes choices related to care and treatment.
- Verbalizes feelings of anger, sorrow, or loss.
- Maintains open relationship with support persons and staff.
- Identifies areas of personal control.
- Expresses sense of control over the present situation.
- Expresses feelings of optimism about the present and future.
- Expresses positive feelings about relationships with significant others.
- Shares values and personal meaning of life.
- Reminisces and reviews personal life positively.
- Accepts limitations and seeks help as needed.

Implementing

The major nursing responsibility for clients who are dying is to assist the client to a peaceful death. More specific responsibilities are:

1. To provide relief from loneliness, fear, and depression
2. To maintain the client's sense of security, self-confidence, dignity, and self-worth
3. To maintain hope

4. To help the client accept his or her losses

5. To provide physical comfort

People facing death need help facing the fact that they will have to depend on others. Some dying clients require only minimal care and can be cared for at home; others need continuous attention and the services of a hospital and its staff. People need help, well in advance of death, in planning for the period of dependence. They need to consider what will happen and how and where they would like to die.

Helping Clients Die with Dignity

Dignity may be defined as the ability to function as a significant and integrated person (Sheehy 1981, p. 56). True dignity comes from within. Generally, dependence on others and loss of control over oneself and interactions with the environment are associated with loss of dignity. Dying clients often feel they have lost control over their lives and over life itself. By introducing options available to the client and significant others, nurses can restore and support feelings of control. Some choices that clients can make are the location of care, e.g., hospital, home, or hospice; times of appointments with health professionals; activity schedule; use of health resources; and times of visits from relatives and friends.

Most clients interviewed about dying indicate that they want to be able to manage the events preceding death so they can die peacefully. Nurses can help clients to find meaning and completeness and to determine their own physical, psychologic, and social priorities. Dying people often strive for self-fulfillment more than self-preservation, and they need to find meaning in continuing to live while suffering. Part of the nurse's challenge, then, is to help maintain, day to day, the client's will and hope.

Salter (1982, p. 21) believes it is important for nurses and clients to focus not on the end, but on three stages of living fully until death:

1. *Developing and growing.* In this stage, the client can be assisted to paint, sculpt, go to a library, visit an art gallery, etc. An occupational therapist can help clients do what they still can do and what is pleasurable.

2. *Lying fallow.* In this stage, physiotherapy measures, such as breathing exercises and passive exercises, help the client to relax and enhance self-esteem.

3. *Letting go and becoming dependent.* In this stage, nursing intervention is usually required to meet both physical and psychologic needs.

Hospice and Home Care

Hospice care, palliative care, and home care focus on support and care of the dying person and family, with the goal of facilitating a peaceful and dignified death. **Hospice care** is based on holistic concepts that emphasize care rather than cure. Its goals are

- Control and relief of pain and symptoms of the illness

- Provision of physical comfort for the terminally ill

- Provision of social, emotional, and spiritual comfort for the client, family, and friends throughout the final stage of illness, at the time of death, and during the bereavement period of the survivors

The principles of hospice care can be carried out in a variety of settings, the most common being the autonomous hospice and the hospital-based **palliative-care** unit. Palliative care is special care that is challenging and requires skillful interpersonal relationships and compassion (see Suggested Readings at the end of this chapter). Services range from fully comprehensive to a focus on selected areas, such as symptom control and pain management, in some palliative care units. Home care services for the dying client maintain the client in the natural home environment until that is no longer possible or until death. Hospice care is always provided by a team of both health professionals and nonprofessionals to ensure a full range of care services. In the United States these services have been delivered primarily through autonomous, community-based hospices. In Canada most hospice programs are hospital-based. This difference may be a function of different methods for funding health care (Corless 1983, pp. 336–39). Both countries have established standards and guidelines for the development and operation of hospice programs (Health and Welfare Canada 1981; National Hospice Organization 1981).

Meeting Physiologic Needs of the Dying Client

The physiologic needs of the dying are related to a slowing of body processes and to homeostatic imbalances. Interventions include personal hygiene measures; pain control; relief of respiratory difficulties; assistance with movement, nutrition, hydration, and elimination; and measures related to sensory changes. See also Table 34–5.

Pain control is essential to enable clients to maintain quality life activities, including eating, moving, and sleeping. Many drugs have been used to control the pain associated with terminal illness: morphine, heroin, methadone, alcohol, marijuana, and LSD. In hospitals the most frequently used agents are morphine, methadone, and alcohol. Usually the physician determines the dosage, but the client's opinion should be considered; the client is the one ultimately aware of personal pain tolerance and fluctuations of internal states. Because of decreased blood circulation, analgesics may be administered by intravenous infusion rather than subcutaneously or intramuscularly.

Spiritual Support

Spiritual support is of great importance in dealing with death. Although not all clients identify with a specific religious faith or belief, the majority have a need for meaning in their lives, particularly as they experience a terminal illness. Conrad (1985, pp. 417–19) has categorized the spiritual needs of the dying as follows:

TABLE 34–5 *Physiologic Needs of Dying Persons*

Problem	Nursing Interventions
Ineffective airway clearance	Fowler's position: conscious clients
	Throat suctioning: conscious clients
	Low-Fowler's position: unconscious clients
	Oxygen therapy as needed
Potential self-care deficit: Bathing/ hygiene	Frequent baths and linen changes if diaphoretic
	Encourage wearing of daytime clothes
	Clean eyelids with absorbent cotton and saline if secretions gather in eyelids
	Mouth care as needed for dry mouth
Impaired physical mobility	Assist client out of bed periodically, if client able
	Regularly change bedridden clients' position
	Support client's position with rolls of blankets or towels as needed
	Lateral position in bed, to decrease aspiration of saliva
	Elevate client's legs when sitting up, to prevent pooling of blood
Altered nutrition: Less than body requirements	Antiemetics or alcoholic beverages to stimulate appetite
	High-calorie, high-vitamin diet
Fluid volume deficit, actual or potential	Semisolid, soft, or liquid foods because of decreased gag reflex
	Continuing assessment of gag reflex
Constipation	Laxatives as needed to prevent constipation
Altered pattern of urinary elimination	Skin care because of incontinence of urine or feces
	Bedpan, urinal, or commode chair within easy reach
	Call light within reach for assistance onto bedpan or commode
	Absorbent pads placed under incontinent client; linen changed as often as needed
	Catheterization in some cases
	Keep room as clean and odor-free as possible
Sensory/perceptual alteration: Visual tactile	Clients prefer a light room
	Hearing is *not* diminished; speak clearly and do not whisper
	Touch is diminished, but client will feel pressure of touch

1. Search for meaning
2. Sense of forgiveness
3. Need for love
4. Need for hope

The nurse has a responsibility to ensure that the client's spiritual needs are attended to, either through direct intervention or by arranging access to individuals who can provide spiritual care. Nurses need to be aware of their own comfort with spiritual issues and be clear about their own ability to interact supportively with the client. Nurses have a responsibility to not impose their own religious/spiritual beliefs on a client, but to respond to the client in relation to the client's own background and needs. Communication skills are most important in helping the client articulate needs and in developing a sense of caring and trust.

Specific interventions may include facilitating expressions of feeling, prayer, meditation, reading, and discussion with appropriate clergy/spiritual advisor. It is important for nurses to establish an effective interdisciplinary relationship with spiritual support specialists. For a further discussion of spiritual issues, see Chapter 32. Death-related beliefs and practices of selected religious groups are shown in Table 34–6 on page 830.

Evaluating

Examples of outcome criteria are listed on page 827.

TABLE 34-6 Death-Related Beliefs and Practices of Selected Religious Groups

Group	Afterlife	Rituals/Funerals	Autopsy	Organ Donation	Cremation	Prolonging Life
American Indian	Beliefs vary	Practices vary; most want family present	Prohibited		Practices vary	
Black Muslim		Special procedures for washing and shrouding the dead; special funeral rites				
Buddhist in America	Reincarnation; after reaching state of enlightenment, may attain nirvana	Last rite; chanting at bedside	No restriction		No restriction	Permit euthanasia in hopeless illness
Church of Christ Scientist	Yes	No last rites	Only in sudden death	No	Individual decision	
Church of Jesus Christ of Latter Day Saints (Mormon)	Yes	Baptism of dead essential; may preach gospel to the dead	No restriction	No restriction	Discouraged	
Eastern Orthodox (Greek and Russian Orthodox)	Yes	Last rites (administration of Holy Communion obligatory for some)	Discouraged		Discouraged	Encouraged
Episcopal (Anglican)	Yes	Last rites not mandatory	No restriction	No restriction	No restriction	
Hindu	Reincarnation; after leading a perfect life, may join Brahma	Priest pours water into mouth of corpse and ties string around wrist or neck as sign of blessing; string must not be removed; family washes body	No restriction	No restriction	Preferred; ashes cast in holy river	
Islam (Moslem, Muslim)	May join Allah by being a good Moslem and observing rituals daily	Dying person must confess sins and ask forgiveness in presence of family; family washes and prepares body (female body cannot be washed by male) and turns body toward Mecca	May oppose	Prohibited	Prohibited	Encouraged

▶

TABLE 34–6 *(continued)*

Group	Afterlife	Rituals/ Funerals	Autopsy	Organ Donation	Cremation	Prolonging Life
Jehovah's Witness			Prohibited unless required by law. No body parts may be removed	Prohibited	No restriction	
Judaism	Dead will be resurrected with coming of Messiah; man lives on through survival of memory	Body ritually washed by members of Ritual Burial Society; burial as soon as possible after death; dead not left unattended; five stages of mourning extending over a year; no embalming; no flowers at funeral because flowers are a symbol of life	Orthodox prohibit; some liberals permit; no body parts removed	Beliefs vary	Largely prohibited; beliefs vary	Generally oppose after irreversible brain damage
Lutheran	Yes	Last rites optional	No restriction	No restriction	No restriction	
Roman Catholicism	Yes; resurrection with second coming of Christ	Rites for anointing the sick not mandatory; receiving Holy Communion mandatory	Permitted, but all body parts must be given appropriate burial	No restriction	No restriction	Discouraged
Seventh Day Adventist	Dead are asleep until return of Christ, when final rewards and punishments will be given					
Unitarian	Beliefs vary		No restriction	No restriction	Encouraged	Support for death with dignity and self-determination in dying

Sources: H. M. Ross, Societal/cultural views regarding death and dying, *Topics in Clinical Nursing,* 1981, 3(3):1–16; H. M. Ross and J. B. Pumphrey (consultant), Recognizing your patient's spiritual needs, *Nursing 77,* December 1977, 7:64–70; and L. J. Carpenito, *Nursing diagnosis: Application to clinical practice.* 3d ed. (Philadelphia: J. B. Lippincott Co., 1989), pp. 713–19.

CARE OF THE BODY AFTER DEATH

Body Changes

Rigor mortis is the stiffening of the body that occurs about 2 to 4 hours after death. It results from a lack of adenosine triphosphate (ATP), which is not synthesized because of a lack of glycogen in the body. ATP is necessary for muscle fiber relaxation. Its lack causes the muscles to contract, which in turn immobilizes the joints. Rigor mortis starts in the involuntary muscles (heart, bladder, and so on) then progresses to the head, neck, and trunk, and finally reaches the extremities.

Because the deceased's family often wants to view the body, and because it is important that the deceased appear natural and comfortable, nurses need to position the body, place dentures in the mouth, and close the eyes and mouth *before* rigor mortis sets in. Rigor mortis usually leaves the body about 96 hours after death.

Algor mortis is the gradual decrease of the body's temperature after death. When blood circulation terminates and the hypothalamus ceases to function, body temperature falls about 1 C (1.8 F) per hour until it reaches room temperature. Simultaneously, the skin loses its elasticity and can easily be broken when removing dressings and adhesive tape.

After blood circulation has ceased, the skin becomes discolored. The red blood cells break down, releasing hemoglobin, which discolors the surrounding tissues. This discoloration, referred to as **livor mortis,** appears in the lowermost or dependent areas of the body.

Tissues after death become soft and eventually liquefied by bacterial fermentation. The hotter the temperature, the more rapid the change. Therefore, bodies are often stored in cool places to delay this process. Embalming reverses the process through injection of chemicals into the body to destroy the bacteria.

Legal Aspects of Death

Of the many legal ramifications of human death, the most basic for the nurse is that death must be certified by a physician. In circumstances of unusual death, an **autopsy (postmortem examination)** may be required. Nurses have a responsibility to be aware of the legal ramifications of death in the jurisdiction in which they practice. Chapter 8 provides legal information about death certificates, labeling the deceased, autopsy, organ donation, and inquest. Wills, euthanasia, and the right to die (living wills) are also discussed in Chapter 8.

Nursing Intervention

Nursing personnel may be responsible for care of a body after death. If the deceased's family or friends wish to view the body, it is important to make the environment as clean and pleasant as possible and to make the body appear natural and comfortable. All equipment and supplies should be removed from the bedside. Some agencies require that all tubes in the body be clamped and remain in place; in other agencies, tubes may be cut to within 2.5 cm (1 in) of the skin and taped in place. Soiled linen is removed so that the room is free from odors.

The body is normally placed in a supine position with the arms either at the sides, palms down, or across the abdomen. The wristband is left on unless it is too tight. One pillow is placed under the head and shoulders to prevent blood from discoloring the face by settling in it. The eyelids are closed and held in place for a few seconds so they remain closed. If they will not stay closed, a moistened cotton fluff will hold them in place. Dentures are usually inserted to help give the face a natural appearance. The mouth is then closed; a rolled towel under the chin will hold it closed.

Soiled areas of the body are washed; however, a complete bath is not necessary, since the body will be washed by the **mortician** (also referred to as an **undertaker**), a person trained in care of the dead. Absorbent pads are placed under the buttocks to take up any feces and urine released because of relaxation of the sphincter muscles. A clean gown is placed on the client and the hair is brushed and combed. All jewelry is removed, except a wedding band in some instances, which is taped to the finger. The top bed linens are adjusted neatly to cover the client to the shoulders. Soft lighting and chairs are provided for the family. All the client's valuables, including clothing, are listed and placed in a safe storage area for the family to take away.

After the body has been viewed by the family, additional identification tags are applied, one to the ankle and one to the wrist if the client's wrist identification band was not left in place. The body is wrapped in a **shroud,** a large rectangular or square piece of plastic or cotton material used to enclose a body after death. Another identification band is then applied to the outside of the shroud. The body is taken to the morgue for cooling, if arrangements have not been made to have a mortician pick it up from the client's room. Agencies vary in their policies about transporting bodies. Some close all room doors before transporting a deceased client through corridors, and service elevators are often used.

NURSING CARE PLAN FOR STEPHANIE SMITH

ASSESSMENT DATA

Nursing Assessment

Stephanie Smith is a 58-year-old widow whose husband died of a heart attack 6 months ago. Her children are grown and either are pursuing careers in other cities or are away at school. Mrs. Smith's husband was a prominent physician who served on the faculties of a number of medical schools. As his wife, she was largely responsible for the rearing of the children. She was always perceived as a strong person who made the best of most situations. Mrs. Smith's interests were focused primarily on her husband's work and career and her family. Immediately after his death, she continued to be a source of strength to her children and close friends. Now, 6 months later, her daughter comes home to find her mother depressed, withdrawn, and tearful. She complains of being ill and on occasion having headaches, backaches, chest pains, and gastrointestinal disturbances. She states that she has not been able to socialize with her friends because of her poor health and constant fatigue. She spends her days alone, reading her husband's papers or looking through photo albums. Her daughter insists that Mrs. Smith seek medical attention.

Physical Examination
Height: 167.6 cm (5'6")
Weight: 50.3 kg (111 lb)
Temperature: 37 C (98.6 F)
Pulse rate: 78 BPM
Blood pressure: 112/72 mm Hg
Skin warm, dry, and pale

Diagnostic Data
Urine: Negative
Chest x-ray film: Negative
Electrocardiogram: Normal
Gastrointestinal series: Essentially negative

CARE PLAN

Nursing Diagnosis	Client Goals and Outcome Criteria	Nursing Interventions and Rationales	Evaluation
Dysfunctional grieving related to death of spouse, resulting in crying, depression, withdrawn behavior, and somatic complaints.	Client Goal: Experience a resolution of grief. Outcome Criteria: Expresses her grief by day 2. Verbalizes understanding of feelings experienced by day 3. Resumes usual activities by day 14.	Assess for factors that prolong grieving. *Rationale:* Identification of such factors will assist in determining appropriate intervention. Provide a safe, secure environment. *Rationale:* Less threatening to client and allows client to ventilate feelings. Establish a trusting relationship with client. *Rationale:* Client will feel more secure in discussing her grief. Encourage client to express her sorrow, sense of loss, and feelings of guilt. *Rationale:* Promotes the work of grieving. Ensure that the bereaved client has support persons. *Rationale:* Support persons are essential in assisting the bereaved client with the work of grieving. Encourage client to seek spiritual assistance from clergy. *Rationale:* During the grieving process, spiritual assistance aids the client in dealing with her sorrow. Encourage the client to continue in familiar roles and to accept new ones. *Rationale:* Will increase client's self-esteem and decrease incidence of unresolved grief.	Client has cried and expressed her sorrow and pain over the death of her husband to her children and her caregivers. Her children have provided loving support and have requested that she spend time visiting each of them for extended periods. She is considering the possibility of rejoining her bridge club.

Nursing Diagnosis	Client Goals and Outcome Criteria	Nursing Interventions and Rationales	Evaluation
Social isolation related to death of spouse, resulting in increased signs of illness, underactivity, failing to interact with others.	Client Goal: Reestablish old contacts and participate in usual activities. Outcome Criteria: Identifies causes of feelings of isolation by day 3. Identifies means of increasing social contacts by day 3. Identifies 1 or 2 diversional activities of interest by day 5.	Identify factors that contribute to social isolation. *Rationale:* Appropriate interventions can be taken when causative factors are identified. Enlist aid of family members and significant others. *Rationale:* Promotes social interaction and decreases sense of isolation. Encourage participation in outside activities of interest to client, e.g., golf and bridge club. *Rationale:* Activity increases sense of well-being and self-esteem. Initiate referrals as needed. *Rationale:* Socially isolated clients are not always able to initiate or undertake social activities on their own.	Client states that she has been depressed since her husband's death, and she didn't want to burden her friends or family with her sorrow and pain. She now acknowledges this has only increased her grief and grieving. She has accepted visits from several good friends, who have urged her to rejoin their bridge club. She hopes to get a new puppy for companionship.

CHAPTER HIGHLIGHTS

▶ Nurses help clients deal with all kinds of losses, including loss of body image, loss of a loved one, loss of a sense of well-being, and loss of a job.

▶ Loss, especially loss of a loved one or a valued body part, can be viewed as a crisis event, either situational or developmental, and either actual or perceived (both of which can be anticipatory).

▶ How an individual deals with loss is closely related to the individual's stage of development, personal resources, and social support systems.

▶ Caring for the dying and the bereaved is one of the nurse's most complex and challenging responsibilities.

▶ Nurses' attitudes about death and dying directly affect their ability to provide care.

▶ Nurses must consider the entire family as the client of care in situations involving loss, especially the crisis of death.

▶ Grieving is a normal, subjective emotional response to loss; it is essential for mental and physical health. Grieving allows the bereaved person to cope with loss gradually and to accept it as part of reality.

▶ Knowledge of different stages or phases of grieving and factors that influence the loss reaction can help the nurse understand the responses and needs of clients.

▶ Nurses caring for clients who are suffering loss or dying need effective communication skills.

▶ Dying clients require physical help and emotional support to ensure a peaceful and dignified death.

SUGGESTED READINGS

Bennett, J. December 1988. Helping people with AIDS live well at home. *Nursing Clinics of North America* 23:731–48.

Over two-thirds of those living with AIDS are not in a hospital or hospice situation, i.e., they are neither acutely ill nor dying. Bennett discusses nursing care goals for the person with AIDS, the challenge of living with AIDS, assessment, recurrent problems, and needs. Individual decision making is encouraged; physical comfort and symptom relief is emphasized.

Benoliel, J. Q. June 1985. Loss and terminal illness. *Nursing Clinics of North America* 20:439–48.

This leading nurse-scholar writing on loss and grief presents a succinct overview of loss and the implications for the individual, the family, and nursing care.

Campbell, A. June 21–27, 1989. Hospices are for living . . . from patient profiles. *Nursing Times* 85:39–41.

With four patient profiles, Campbell illustrates how patients are allowed to be home as much as possible and how families treat the hospice as an extension of their own homes. Campbell emphasizes the importance of liaison between the hospice home care team, the general practitioner, and the community nurse.

Gifford, B. J., and Cleary, B. B. February 1990. Supporting the bereaved. *American Journal of Nursing* 90:48–55.

The authors present four stages related to grieving and how the nurse can help the grieving person deal effectively with each stage. They suggest specific actions for nurses to help grieving people. Following the article are multiple-choice questions to test the reader's understanding of the article.

RELATED RESEARCH

Carter, S. L. November/December 1989. Themes of grief. *Nursing Research* 38:354–58.

Kirschling, J. M., and McBride, A. B. April 1989. Effects of age and sex on the experience of widowhood. *Western Journal of Nursing Research* 11:207–18.

Masters, M., and Shontz, F. C. August 1989. Implications of problems and strengths of the hospice client by clients, caregivers, and nurses: Implications for nursing. *Cancer Nursing* 12:226–35.

Pfost, K. S.; Stevens, M. J., and Wessels, A. B. 1989. Relationship of purpose in life to grief experiences in response to the death of a significant other. *Death Studies* 13(4):371–78.

SELECTED REFERENCES

Alexander, J., and Kiely, J. March/April 1986. Working with the bereaved. *Geriatric Nursing* 7:85–86.

Benoliel, J. Q. June 1985. Loss and terminal illness. *Nursing Clinics of North America* 20:439–48.

Benton, R. E. 1978. *Death and dying: Principles and practices in patient care.* New York: D. Van Nostrand Co.

Betz, C. L., and Poster, E. C. June 1984. Children's concepts of death: Implications for pediatric practice. *Nursing Clinics of North America* 19:341–49.

Burgess, A. W., and Lazare, A. 1976. *Community mental health: Target populations.* Englewood Cliffs, N.J.: Prentice-Hall.

Cantor, R. C. 1978. *And a time to live.* New York: Harper and Row.

Cappon, D. February 1970. Attitudes towards death. *Coast Graduate Medicine* 47:257.

Carpenito, L. J. 1989. *Nursing diagnosis: Application to clinical practice.* 3d ed. Philadelphia: J. B. Lippincott Co.

Clark, C.; Curley, A.; and Hughes, A. December 1988. Hospice care: A model for caring for the person with AIDS. *Nursing Clinics of North America* 23:851–62.

Clark, M. D. December 1984. Healthy and unhealthy grief behaviors. *Occupational Health Nursing* 32:633–35.

Conrad, N. L. June 1985. Spiritual support for the dying. *Nursing Clinics of North America* 20:415–26.

Corless, I. B. 1983. The hospice movement in North America. In Corr, C. A., and Corr, D. M. (editors). *Hospice care: Principles and practice.* New York: Springer Publishing Co.

Demi, A. S., and Miles, M. S. 1986. Bereavement. *Annual Review of Nursing Research* 4:105–23.

Dobratz, M. C. April 1990. Hospice nursing: Present perspectives and future directives. *Cancer Nursing* 13:116–22.

Engel, G. L. September 1964. Grief and grieving. *American Journal of Nursing* 64:93–98.

Enlow, P. M. July 1986. Coping with anticipatory grief. *Journal of Gerontological Nursing* 12:36–37.

Fetsch, S. H. November/December 1984. The 7- to 10-year-old child's conceptualization of death. *Oncology Nurses' Forum* 11:52–56.

Field, D. January 1984. "We didn't want him to die on his own"—Nurses' accounts of nursing dying patients. *Journal of Advanced Nursing* 1:59–70.

Gabriel, R. M., and Kirschling, J. M. 1989. Assessing grief among the bereaved elderly: A review of existing measures. *Hospice Journal* 5:29–54.

Gifford, B. J., and Cleary, B. B. February 1990. Supporting the bereaved. *American Journal of Nursing* 90:48–55.

Gonda, T. A., and Ruark, J. E. 1984. *Dying dignified: The health professional's guide to care.* Menlo Park, Calif.: Addison-Wesley.

Health and Welfare Canada. 1981. Palliative care services in hospitals: Guidelines. Ottawa: Ministry of National Health and Welfare.

Hoff, L. A. 1984. *People in crisis.* Menlo Park, Calif.: Addison-Wesley.

Kennedy, S. R. January/February 1985. Sharing, caring, living, dying. *Geriatric Nursing* 6:12–17.

Kim, M. J.; McFarland, G. K., and McLane, A. M. 1989. *Pocket guide to nursing diagnoses,* 3d ed. St. Louis: C. V. Mosby.

Kübler-Ross, E. 1969. *On death and dying.* New York: Macmillan Publishing Co.

———. 1974. *Questions and answers on death and dying.* New York: Macmillan Publishing Co.

———. 1975. *Death: The final stage of growth.* Englewood Cliffs, N.J.: Prentice-Hall.

———. 1978. *To live until we say good-bye.* Englewood Cliffs, N.J.: Prentice-Hall.

Martocchio, B. C. June 1985. Grief and bereavement: Healing through hurt. *Nursing Clinics of North America* 20:327–41.

Masson, V. September/October 1989. On hearing the news of a patient's death. *Nursing Outlook* 37:245.

Morris, E. October 19–25, 1988. A pain of separation . . . How can nurses best assist the dying and the bereaved? *Nursing Times* 84:54–56.

Moss, M. S., and Moss, S. Z. 1983–84. The impact of parental death on middle-aged children. *Omega* 14(1):65–75.

National Hospice Organization. 1981. Standards of a hospice program of care. Arlington, Va.: National Hospice Organization.

Peterson, E. A. October 1985. The physical . . . The spiritual . . . Can you meet all of your patients' needs? *Journal of Gerontological Nursing* 11:23–27.

Richter, J. M. July 1984. Crisis of mate loss in the elderly. *American Nursing Society* 6(4):45–54.

Salter, R. March 1982. The art of dying. *Canadian Nurse* 78:20–21.

Schulz, R. 1978. *The psychology of death, dying and bereavement.* Reading, Mass.: Addison-Wesley Publishing Co.

Sheehy, P. F. 1981. *On dying with dignity.* New York: Pinnacle Books.

Strauss, A. L., and Glaser, B. G. 1970. Awareness of dying. In Schoenberg, B., Carr, A. C., Peretz, D., and Kutcher, A. H., editors. *Loss and grief.* New York: Columbia University Press.

Taylor, D. A. 1983–84. View of death from sufferers of early loss. *Omega* 14(1):77–82.

Tschudin, V. March 21–27, 1990. Essentials of management: Support yourself. *Nursing Times* 86:40–2.

Walker, M. J. April 1990. Attitudes are contagious: What are you spreading around? *Today's OR Nurse* 12:9–12, 31–3.

SUPPORTING PHYSIOLOGIC HEALTH PATTERNS

Mobility and Immobility

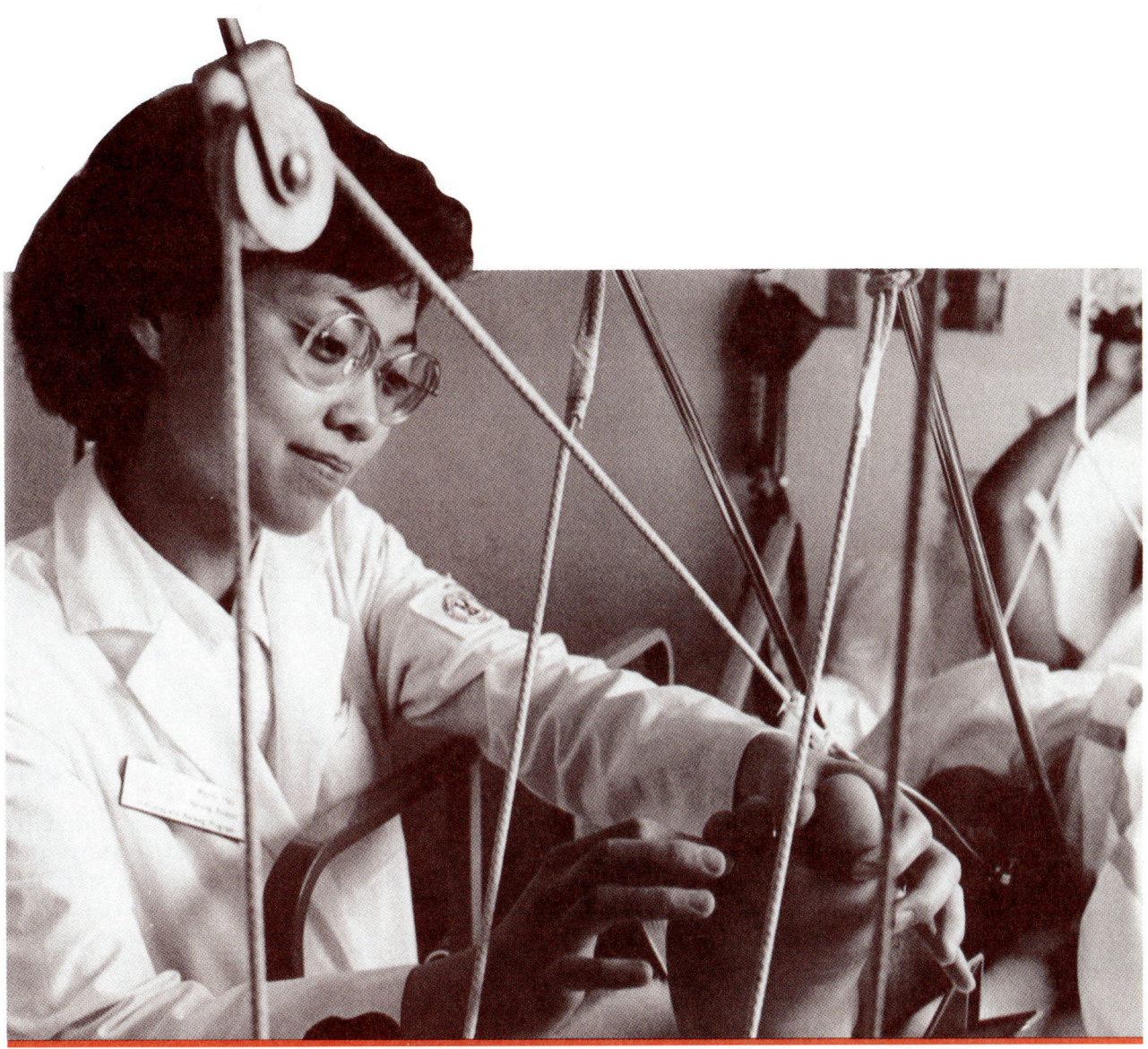

CONTENTS

OBJECTIVES

▶ Describe the concepts of mobility and immobility.

▶ Identify factors that affect a person's mobility.

▶ Identify physiologic responses to immobility.

▶ Describe psychosocial responses to immobility.

▶ Describe the etiology and pathogenesis of pressure sores.

▶ Identify essential data required to assess a client's mobility status.

▶ Identify clients at risk of developing pressure sores.

▶ Develop nursing diagnoses related to the client's mobility problems.

▶ Develop goals and outcome criteria for specific diagnoses.

▶ Plan and implement nursing interventions that prevent the problems of immobility.

PHYSICAL MOBILITY AND IMMOBILITY

The ability to move freely, easily, rhythmically, and purposefully in the environment is an essential part of living. People must move to obtain food and water, to protect themselves from trauma, and to meet other basic needs. Mobility is vital to independence; a fully immobilized person is as vulnerable and dependent as an infant.

People often define their health and physical fitness by their ability to move, since mental well-being and the effectiveness of body functioning depend largely on their mobility status. For example, when a person is upright, the lungs expand more easily, intestinal activity (peristalsis) is more effective, and the kidneys are able to empty completely. In addition, motion is essential for proper functioning of bones and muscles.

The ability to move also influences a person's self-esteem and body image, both components of self-concept. For most people, self-esteem depends on a sense of independence and a feeling of usefulness or being needed. People with mobility impairments may feel helpless and burdensome to others. Body image can be altered by paralysis, amputations, or any motor impairment. The reaction of others to impaired mobility can also alter self-esteem and body image significantly.

Joint Mobility

A *joint* is the functional unit of the musculoskeletal system. The bones of the skeleton articulate at the joints. Most of the skeletal muscles attach to the two bones at the joint. These muscles are categorized according to the type of joint movement they produce upon contraction. Muscles are therefore called flexors, extensors, internal rotators, and the like. The flexor muscles are stronger than the extensor muscles. Thus, when a person is inactive, the joints are pulled into a flexed (bent) position. If this tendency is not counteracted with exercise and position changes, the muscles

are permanently shortened, and the joint becomes fixed in a flexed position.

Range of Motion   The *range of motion* of a joint is the maximum movement that is possible for that joint. Joint range of motion varies from individual to individual and is determined by genetic makeup, developmental patterns, the presence or absence of disease, and the amount of physical activity in which the person normally engages.

Types of Synovial Joints   A **synovial joint** is freely movable and characteristically has a cavity enclosed by a capsule. Within this capsule is a lining of synovial membrane, which secretes synovial fluid to lubricate the joint. Cartilage provides a smooth surface on which the bone glides during movement. Thick bands of collagenous fibers extending from one bone to another are called **ligaments.** Ligaments strengthen the joint, and they are usually stretched taut when the joint is in the position of greatest stability. The muscles surrounding the joint provide the most stability for the joint. The primary functions of synovial joints are to bear weight and to allow movement. There are six types of synovial joints (see Table 35–1), and only certain movements are normally possible for each type. For information about the synovial joint movements, see Table 35–2 on page 842.

Factors Affecting Mobility

A person's mobility depends to a large degree on habits developed throughout life and on the importance the individual attaches to activity by life-style, primary disability, individual energy level, and age.

Life-Style   People learn early in life, often from their families, the value of activity in relation to health. Some children are encouraged to play out of doors, while others spend much of their time watching television. Some people

TABLE 35–1 *Types of Synovial Joints*

Type	Description	Examples	Movement
Ball-and-socket	The ball-shaped head of one bone fits into the concave socket of another bone.	The hip and shoulder joints	Movement in three planes. Greatest range of all joints: flexion and extension; abduction and adduction; rotation.
Hinge	The convex, spool-shaped end of one bone fits into the concave surface of another bone.	The elbow, knee, ankle, finger, and toe joints	Movement in one plane. Flexion and extension.
Pivot	An arch-shaped surface rotates in a rounded or longitudinal axis.	The axis and atlas joints of the vertebral column, the joints between the radius and the ulna	Movement in one plane. Rotation only.
Condyloid (ovoid)	The oval-shaped part of one bone fits into an elliptical cavity.	The wrist joints	Movement in two planes at right angles to each other. Flexion and extension; abduction and adduction.
Saddle	Two bones have opposite concave-convex surfaces that fit together.	The base of the thumb only	Same movements as for condyloid joints but freer.
Gliding	Two flat bone surfaces glide over each other.	The carpal bones, the tarsal bones, the medial end of the clavicle with the sternum, the ribs with the bodies of the vertebrae, the sacrum and the ilia, the fibula with the tibia	Gliding only.

participate in physical activity regularly in an effort to maintain or improve their health.

Some cultures value physical activity more than others do. The boy who lives in a small town in France walks to and from school each day, while the North American boy living in a middle-class suburb rides to and from school. Adults in North America often watch sports activities, while adults in less industrialized nations often participate in such activities.

Disability   A **disability** is a persistent mental or physical dysfunction or weakness that prevents a person from carrying out the normal activities of life and work. Disabilities are of two types:

1. Primary disabilities, e.g., paralysis due to a spinal cord injury, are a direct result of disease or trauma.
2. Secondary disabilities, e.g., muscle weakness and bedsores, do not exist at the onset of the primary disability but develop later as a result of the disorder causing the primary disability.

Disuse syndrome is often used as a synonym for secondary disability due to immobility. Disuse syndromes are physiologic and psychologic dysfunctions that occur in all body organs and systems as a result of immobility and lack of use. Each of these pathologic changes begins with the onset of immobility. Primary disabilities, such as multiple sclerosis and injuries to the spinal cord, can seriously restrict an individual's mobility.

Mobility can also be limited because of fear and/or pain. A client recovering from surgery may be reluctant to move for fear of opening the incision or because of the pain experienced with movement.

A person with a disease or injury is often restricted in activity. Bed rest is commonly advised in illness. It usually has two purposes: (a) to conserve energy so that a diseased or injured part of the body will heal, and (b) to prevent further damage to a body part. A person who has had a myocardial infarction usually requires bed rest for both purposes. A person with a fractured hip may be confined to bed with the leg in traction while healing takes place. See the accompanying box for the major reasons for client immobility.

Major Reasons for Client Immobility

- Severe pain
- Impairment of the musculoskeletal or nervous systems
- Generalized weakness
- Psychosocial problems, e.g., depression
- Infectious processes

TABLE 35–2 *Types of Synovial Joint Movements*

Movement	Action	Movement	Action
Flexion	Decreasing the angle of the joint (e.g., bending the elbow)	Eversion	Turning the sole of the foot outward by moving the ankle joint
Extension	Increasing the angle of the joint (e.g., straightening the arm at the elbow)	Inversion	Turning the sole of the foot inward by moving the ankle joint
Hyperextension	Further extension or straightening of a joint (e.g., bending the head backward)	Pronation	Moving the bones of the forearm so that the palm of the hand faces downward when held in front of the body
Abduction	Movement of the bone away from the midline of the body	Supination	Moving the bones of the forearm so that the palm of the hand faces upward when held in front of the body
Adduction	Movement of the bone toward the midline of the body	Protraction	Moving a part of the body forward in the same plane parallel to the ground
Rotation	Movement of the bone around its central axis	Retraction	Moving a part of the body backward in the same plane parallel to the ground
Circumduction	Movement of the distal part of the bone in a circle while the proximal end remains fixed		

Energy Level   Energy levels vary greatly among individuals. Also, one individual demonstrates different energy levels at different times. Sometimes people voluntarily restrict activity without always knowing why or without feeling ill. The reason is generally that the person needs to withdraw from physical and psychologic stressors to maintain physical and psychologic equilibrium. After final examinations, a student may want only to go to bed and sleep, to regain energy and stability.

Age   Age greatly affects activity levels. Generally, people slow down as they grow older.

Degrees of Immobility

There are varying degrees of immobility. The unconscious client is often completely immobilized. Immobility is sometimes partial, as in a client with a fractured leg. In addition, some clients restrict activity for health reasons. For example, a client who is short of breath may be advised not to walk up stairs.

Nurses use the term **bed rest** to describe a client's degree of immobility. The term has different meanings in different nursing settings. For example, in some settings, "complete bed rest" means that the client never moves from the bed and does not go to the bathroom or sit in a chair. "Bed rest,"

in contrast, may mean that the client stays in bed except when he or she uses a bedside commode or goes to the bathroom. Nurses should be familiar with the meaning of such terms in their practice setting. See the accompanying box for some of the common benefits of bed rest.

Whether bed rest causes any problems often depends on the duration of the bed rest, the client's health, and the client's sensory awareness. When confined to bed, many clients are aware of pressure on their bodies and can change position slightly to relieve this pressure. Such clients are less susceptible than others to decubitus ulcers and other problems. Clients on bed rest, like clients immobilized in other ways, must be continually assessed for problems.

Benefits of Bed Rest

- Reduces the needs of the body cells for oxygen because of reduced metabolism secondary to reduced activity

- Directs energy resources toward the healing process rather than toward activity.

- Reduces pain in some instances, thereby decreasing the need for analgesics

---

PHYSIOLOGIC RESPONSES TO IMMOBILITY

Many body systems respond physiologically to immobility. The degree of change depends largely on the risk factors mentioned earlier.

Musculoskeletal System

The most obvious signs of prolonged immobility are often manifested in the musculoskeletal system. The client experiences a significant decrease in muscular strength whenever he or she does not maintain a moderate amount of physical activity. The studies of Hettinger and Mueller demonstrate that as much as 20% of muscle strength may be lost after 1 week of bed rest, and as much as another 20% may be lost with each succeeding week of bed rest (Hettinger and Mueller 1953, pp. 111–26). A decrease in physical endurance is a direct result of decreased muscle strength and occurs at a similar rate (Kottke et al. 1990, p. 1115). A decrease in the muscle mass, or muscle **atrophy,** occurs when the muscle fibers do not contract as much as they would during normal physical activity. Muscle atrophy is the cause of decreased muscle strength and endurance.

Muscular dysfunction due to immobility is, in turn, the primary cause of skeletal dysfunction. In a mobile person, there is a balance between the forming and breaking down of bone tissue. This balance is brought about primarily by the daily stresses of the tendons pulling on the bones and of gravity pulling on the weight-bearing structures as the client stands and moves. Prolonged immobilization in a horizontal position causes dramatic changes in the bones and joints.

Disuse osteoporosis is a result of lack of weight-bearing, decreased muscular activity, and complex endocrine and metabolic disturbances that accompany bed rest. During immobility, increased amounts of calcium are extracted from the bone, resulting in a significant decrease in bone mass. Studies demonstrate that bone **demineralization** starts in the second or third day of immobilization; there is measurable calcium loss from bone after 2 weeks of bed rest (Mitchell and Laustau 1981, p. 355). The bone becomes porous and brittle and can fracture easily. Demineralization occurs regardless of the amount of calcium in the person's diet.

Bone demineralization in turn affects other body systems, primarily because the excessive amounts of calcium extracted from the bones produce slight hypercalcemia, significant hypercalcuria, and frequently deposition of calcium in injured soft tissues (Kottke et al. 1990, p. 1122). Taking dietary supplements of calcium increases this problem.

Fibrosis (an increase in the amount of fibrous connective tissue) and **ankylosis** (fixation) of joining structures occur whenever joints are not moved normally. The flexor muscles of an immobilized person, because they are strong, often remain contracted for long periods, and the weaker extensors are not used. In turn, the fibrous muscle tissue that covers the joint is gradually replaced by connective tissue, and the joint becomes increasingly stiff and painful. The problem may be exacerbated by the deposition of excessive amounts of calcium in the soft tissues around the joint. In time, the joint may become irreversibly deformed and ankylosed, and the muscles that cover the joint may permanently shorten into a **contracture.** The most common are flexion contractures of the lower extremities: hips, knees, and the plantar flexors of the ankles. The position that the client most consistently assumes in bed and wheelchair is mirrored when the person eventually is able to stand and walk. The result is a stooped "wheelchair" posture: The client's heels cannot rest flat on the floor, making ambulation difficult or impossible.

Muscle atrophy, decreased muscle strength, and limited endurance can impair muscle coordination in both upper and lower extremities. Lack of coordination hinders the client's ability to perform normal daily activities and impairs balance and ability to stand and walk.

Cardiovascular System

Prolonged immobility weakens the cardiovascular system, which cannot fully meet the demands placed on it. Decreased mobility creates an imbalance in the autonomic nervous system, resulting in a preponderance of sympathetic activity over cholinergic activity that increases heart rate. Resting heart rate increases approximately 0.5 beats/minute per each day of immobilization (Kottke et al. 1990, p. 1124).

In a mobile, active person with a slow heart rate, the diastolic phase of the cardiac cycle is longer than the systolic phase. Since blood flow through coronary vessels occurs primarily during the diastolic phase, there is sufficient time for adequate blood flow through the coronary arteries. During immobility, however, the rapid heart rate reduces diastolic pressure, coronary blood flow, and the capacity of the heart to respond to any metabolic demands above basal levels. Due to this diminished cardiac reserve, the immobilized person may experience tachycardia and angina with even minimal exertion. Bedfast clients tend to use the **Valsalva maneuver,** during which the person takes a deep breath and strains against a closed glottis while moving. The Valsalva maneuver markedly increases intrathoracic pressure, which is followed by a marked increase in the volume of blood within the heart and possible arrhythmias when the glottis is again opened. When the heart has marginal reserves, the client may have difficulty coping with this additional stress.

Orthostatic (postural) hypotension is a common sequel of immobilization. Due to sympathetic nervous system activity, automatic vasoconstriction normally occurs in the blood vessels in the lower half of the body when a mobile person changes from a horizontal to a vertical pos-

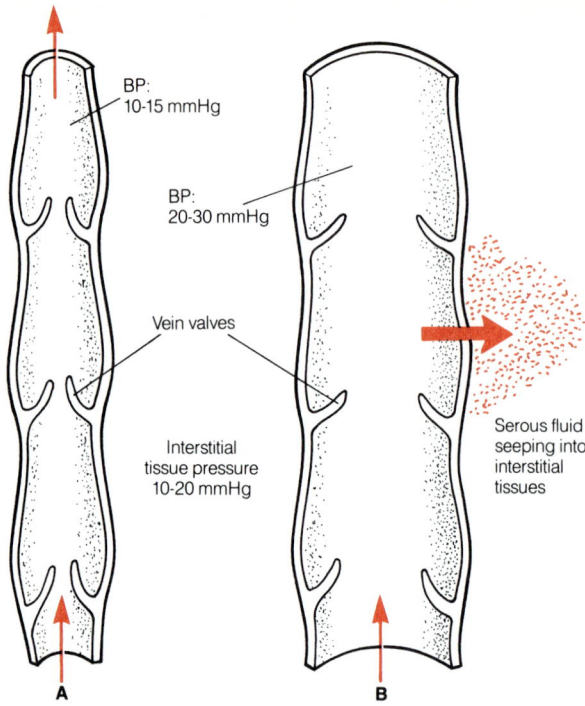

BP:
10-15 mmHg

BP:
20-30 mmHg

Vein valves

Interstitial
tissue pressure
10-20 mmHg

Serous fluid
seeping into
interstitial
tissues

A

B

Figure 35–1 Leg veins: **A**, in a mobile person, and **B**, in an immobilized person.

ture. Vasoconstriction prevents pooling of the blood in the legs and effectively maintains central blood pressure to ensure adequate perfusion of the heart and brain. During prolonged immobility, this reflex becomes dormant. When the immobilized person attempts to sit or stand, this reconstricting mechanism fails to function properly in spite of increased adrenalin output. The blood pools in the lower extremities, and central blood pressure drops. Cerebral perfusion is seriously compromised, and the person feels dizzy or lightheaded and may even faint. This sequence is usually accompanied by a sudden and marked increase in heart rate, the body's effort to protect the brain from an inadequate blood supply.

The skeletal muscles of an active person contract with each movement, compressing the blood vessels in those muscles and helping to pump the blood back to the heart against gravity. The tiny valves in the leg veins, which remain constricted, aid in venous return to the heart by preventing backward flow of blood and pooling. In an immobilized person, the skeletal muscles do not contract sufficiently, and the muscles atrophy. The skeletal muscles can no longer assist in pumping blood back to the heart against gravity. Blood pools in the leg veins, causing vasodilation and engorgement. The valves in the veins can no longer work effectively to prevent backward flow of blood and pooling (see Figure 35–1). This phenomenon is known as **incompetent valves.** As the blood continues to pool in the veins, its greater volume increases venous blood pressure, which can become much higher than that exerted by

the tissues surrounding the vessel. When the venous pressure is sufficiently great, some of the serous part of the blood is forced out of the blood vessel into the interstitial spaces surrounding the vessel, causing edema. Edema is most common in parts of the body positioned below heart level and maintained in that position. Dependent edema is most likely to occur around the sacrum or heels of a client who sits up in bed or in the feet and lower legs of a client who sits on the side of the bed. Edema further impedes venous return of blood to the heart, causing more pooling and more edema. Edematous tissue is uncomfortable and more susceptible to injury than normal tissue.

Three factors, known as **Virchow's triad,** collectively predispose a client to the formation of a **thrombophlebitis** (a clot that is loosely attached to an inflamed vein wall). These are impaired venous return to the heart, hypercoagulability of the blood, and injury to a vessel wall.

Although prolonged immobility has not clearly been shown to slow venous return in most persons, it can be a significant factor in the immobile elderly who are paralyzed, have heart disease, or have had recent surgery (Kottke et al. 1990, p. 1124; Patrick et al. 1986. p. 623). Hypercoagulability due to a disturbance in the clotting mechanism or to decreased blood volume may be a factor in immobilized persons as it is in postoperative clients. Injury to vein walls can occur as a result of (a) atherosclerotic plaque formation often associated with aging or (b) sustained pressure against a leg due to improper body alignment and immobility.

A thrombus is particularly dangerous if it breaks loose from the vein wall to enter the general circulation as an **embolus.** At least 15% of deep vein thrombi do migrate (Fahey 1984, p. 36). Large emboli that enter the pulmonary circulation may occlude the vessels that nourish the lungs to cause an infarcted (dead) area of the lung. If the infarcted area is large, pulmonary function may be seriously compromised, or death may ensue. Emboli travelling to the coronary vessels or brain can produce a similarly dangerous outcome.

Respiratory System

An upright, mobile person has no impediments against the chest wall to restrict respiratory movement. During normal activity, the person periodically sighs, maximally inhaling or forcefully exhaling to expand the alveoli fully and allow effective gaseous exchange. Mucus, normally present in the respiratory tract, is loosened by movement and removed from the bronchi by ciliary action and coughing.

In a recumbent, immobilized client, ventilation of the lungs is passively altered. The rigid bed presses against the body and curtails chest movement. The abdominal organs push against the diaphragm, further restricting chest movement and making it difficult to expand the lungs fully. An immobilized, recumbent person rarely sighs, partly because overall muscle atrophy also affects the respiratory muscles and partly because there is no need to do so without the stimulus of activity. Without these periodic stretching movements, the cartilaginous intercostal joints may become fixed in an expiratory phase of respiration, further restricting the potential for maximal ventilation. These changes produce shallow respirations and reduce vital capacity significantly. An immobilized, paralyzed client can lose as much as 25% to 50% of normal vital capacity (Kottke et al. 1990, p. 1128).

Blood flow through the lungs is also passively altered by the client's horizontal position, due primarily to the effects of gravity. The dependent parts of the lung, tightly pressed against the bed with the body's weight on top, expand less effectively with each respiration. These dependent areas are least effectively ventilated, yet blood tends to pool there. See Figure 35–2. The result is reduced gaseous exchange. Poor oxygenation and retention of carbon dioxide in the blood can, if allowed to continue, predispose the person to respiratory acidosis, a potentially lethal disorder.

Mucous secretions are affected by gravity and inactivity. The secretions tend to accumulate in the dependent areas of the alveoli. In immobilized persons, these secretions become more viscous and stick to the lining of the respiratory tract. Due to weakened thoracic muscles, the inability to inhale maximally, and decreased ciliary movement, the coughing mechanism is impaired and the client cannot effectively clear the bronchi of the mucus.

When ventilation is decreased, these secretions may accumulate in a dependent area of a bronchiole and effectively block it. Due to changes in regional blood flow, bed rest decreases the amount of surfactants produced. (Surfactants enable the alveoli to remain open.) The combination of decreased surfactants and blockage of a bronchiole with mucus can cause **atelectasis** (the collapse of a lobe or of an entire lung) distal to the mucous blockage. Immobilized, elderly, postoperative clients are at greatest risk of atelectasis.

Static mucus is an excellent medium for bacterial growth. Under these conditions, a minor upper respiratory infection can evolve rapidly into a severe infection of the lower respiratory tract. **Hypostatic pneumonia** caused by static respiratory secretions can severely impair oxygen-carbon dioxide exchange in the alveoli and is a fairly common cause of death among weakened, immobilized individuals, especially those who are heavy smokers.

Metabolic and Nutritional Systems

In immobilized clients, the basal metabolic rate decreases as the energy requirements of the body decrease. Gastrointestinal motility and secretions of various digestive glands are also reduced.

In an active person, there is a balance between protein synthesis (**anabolism**) and protein breakdown (**catabolism**). Immobility creates a marked imbalance, and the catabolic processes exceed the anabolic processes. Over time, more nitrogen is excreted than is ingested, producing

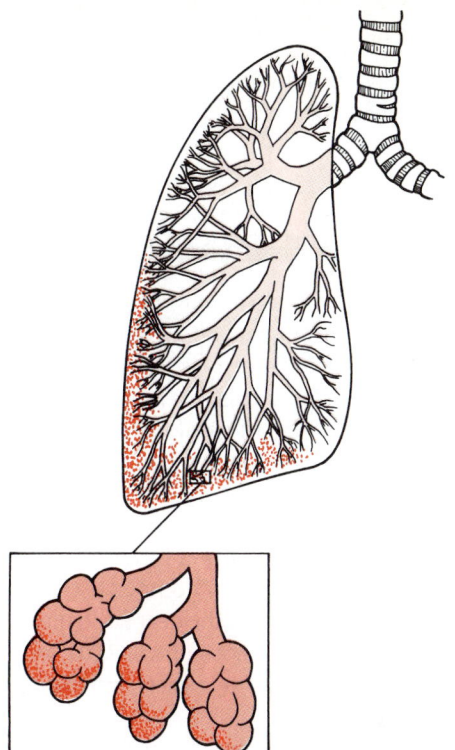

Figure 35–2 Pooling of secretions in the lungs of an immobilized person.

a negative nitrogen balance. Catabolized muscle mass is the source of this excreted nitrogen. Excessive amounts are excreted in the urine, reaching peak levels at about the sixth to tenth day of immobilization (Kottke et al. 1990, p. 1125). The negative nitrogen balance represents a depletion of protein stores that are essential for building muscle tissue and for wound healing. The problem is further compounded by **anorexia** (lack of appetite), common among immobilized persons. The anorexic client may reduce his or her intake of protein and calories. If protein intake is reduced, the nitrogen imbalance may become more pronounced, sometimes so severely, that malnutrition ensues. Reduced caloric intake is usually a response to the decreased energy requirements of the inactive person. See Chapter 39 for more information on negative nitrogen balance.

Hypoproteinemia (abnormally small amounts of protein in the circulating blood plasma), if severe, can alter fluid pressures in the body, causing fluid to shift from the vascular to the interstitial compartments. The result is edema in dependent parts of the body.

A negative calcium balance occurs as a direct result of immobility. Greater amounts of calcium are extracted from bone than can be replaced. The absence of weight-bearing and of stress on the musculoskeletal structures is the direct cause of the calcium loss from bones. Weight-bearing and stress, absent during immobility, are also required for calcium to be replaced in bone. A similar process occurs with the body's stores of phosphate to cause a negative phosphate balance during immobility.

Urinary and Endocrine Systems

Primarily in the early stages of immobility, **diuresis** (increased excretion of urine) occurs. This is due to a temporary increase in the circulating blood volume and the renal blood flow, resulting in an inhibition of antidiuretic hormone (ADH). This diuresis is accompanied by a temporary **natriuresis** (increased excretion of sodium in the urine), the body's attempt to maintain plasma concentrations at a normal level. Later, urine production usually decreases, and the urine is more concentrated. This condition is probably partly due to the stress of immobility and partly to the disease or condition for which the person is immobilized. Decreased urinary output also is an attempt by the body to compensate for the decreased blood volume. As a result, fluid-retaining hormones—ADH, aldosterone, and cortisol—may be secreted in excessive amounts (Kottke et al. 1990, p. 1127).

Gravity plays an important role in the emptying of the kidneys and the bladder in mobile persons. The shape and position of the kidneys and active kidney contractions are important in completely emptying the urine from the calyces, renal pelvis, and ureters. See Figure 35–3, A. The shape and position of the urinary bladder (the detrusor muscle), and active bladder contractions are also important in achieving complete emptying. See Figure 35–4, A.

When the person remains in a horizontal position, gravity impedes the emptying of urine from the kidneys and the urinary bladder. To urinate, the person who is supine (in a back-lying position) must push upward, against gravity. See Figures 35–3, B and 35–4, B. The renal pelvis may fill with urine before it is pushed into the ureters. Emptying is not as complete, and **urinary stasis** (stagnation) occurs after a few days of bed rest. Due to the overall decrease in muscle tone during immobilization, including the tone of the detrusor muscle, bladder emptying is further compromised.

In a mobile person, calcium in the urine remains dissolved due to a balance of calcium and citric acid in an appropriately acid urine. With immobility and the resulting excessive amounts of calcium (and phosphate) in the urine, this balance is no longer maintained. The urine becomes more alkaline, and the calcium salts precipitate out as crystals to form **renal calculi** (stones) (Mitchell and Laustau 1981, p. 364). In an immobile person in a horizontal position, the renal pelvis filled with stagnant, alkaline urine is an ideal location for calculi to form. The stones usually develop in the renal pelvis and pass through the ureters into the bladder. As the stones pass along the long, narrow ureters, they cause extreme pain and bleeding and can sometimes obstruct the urinary tract. Some researchers suggest that 15% to 30% of persons who have been immobilized for prolonged periods develop renal stones (Mitchell and Laustau 1981, p. 365).

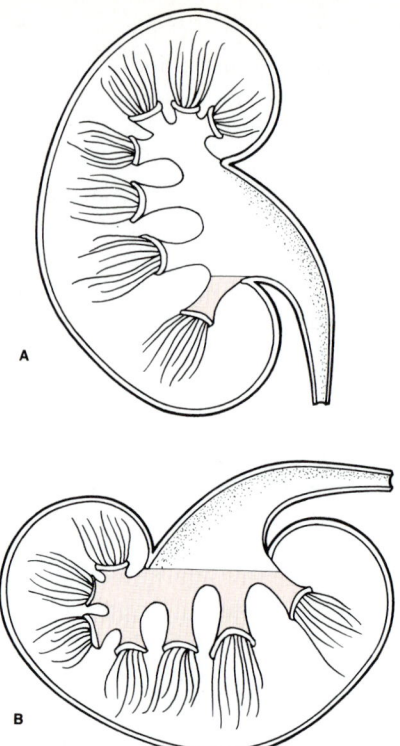

Figure 35–3 Pooling of urine in the kidney: **A,** The client is in an upright position; and **B,** the client is in a back-lying position.

The immobile person may suffer from urinary retention, bladder distention, and occasionally urinary **incontinence** (involuntary urination). The decreased muscle tone of the urinary bladder inhibits its ability to empty completely, and the immobilized person is unable to relax the perineal muscles sufficiently to urinate. The discomfort of using a bedpan or urinal, the embarrassment and lack of privacy associated with this function, and the unnatural position for urination combine to make it difficult for the client to relax the perineal muscles sufficiently to urinate while lying in bed.

When urination is not possible, the bladder gradually becomes distended with urine. The bladder may stretch excessively, eventually inhibiting the urge to void. When bladder distention is considerable, some involuntary urinary "dribbling" may occur (**retention with overflow**). This does not relieve the urinary distention because most of the stagnant urine remains in the bladder.

Static urine provides an excellent medium for bacterial growth. The flushing action of normal, frequent urination is absent, and urinary distention often causes minute tears in the bladder mucosa, allowing infectious organisms to enter. The increased alkalinity of the urine caused by the hypercalcuria supports bacterial growth.

The organism most commonly causing urinary tract infections is *Escherichia coli,* which normally resides in the colon. See Chapter 20 for additional information. The nor-

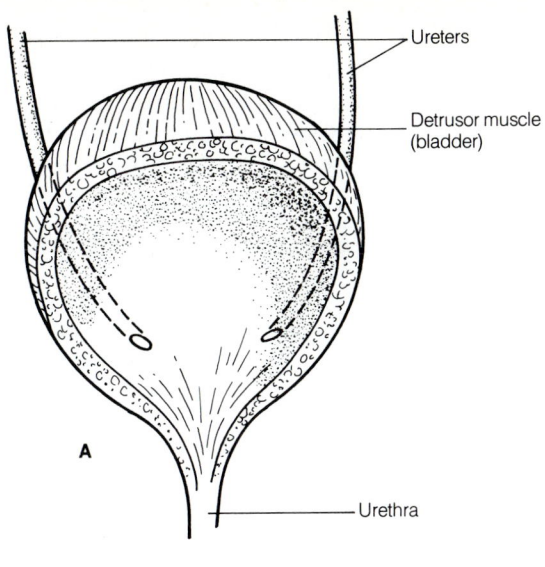

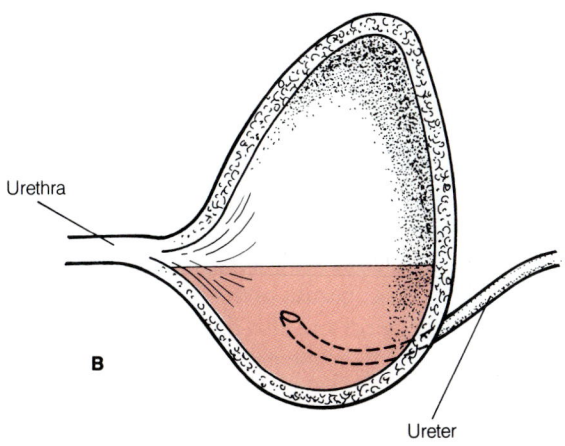

Figure 35–4 Pooling of urine in the urinary bladder; **A**, the client is in an upright position; **B**, the client is in a back-lying position.

mally sterile urinary tract may be contaminated by improper perineal care, the use of an indwelling urinary catheter, or occasionally **urinary reflux** (backward flow). During reflux, contaminated urine from an overly distended bladder backs up into the renal pelvis to contaminate the kidney pelvis as well.

Fecal Elimination

Constipation is a frequent problem for immobilized persons. Due to increased adrenalin production, peristalsis and colon motility are decreased, and the sphincters are more tightly constricted (Kottke et al. 1990, p. 1128). The overall skeletal muscle weakness affects the abdominal and perineal muscles used in defecation. When the stool becomes very hard, more strength is required to expel it. The immobilized person may lack this strength.

The bedfast person's unnatural and uncomfortable posi-

tion on the bedpan does not facilitate elimination. The backward-leaning posture does not promote effective use of the muscles used in defecation. Some persons are reluctant to use the bedpan in the presence of others. The embarrassment, lack of privacy, dependence on others to assist with the bedpan, and disruption of normal bowel habits may cause the individual to postpone or ignore the urge for elimination. Repeated postponement eventually suppresses the urge and weakens the defecation reflex.

The longer the fecal mass remains in the colon, the more water is extracted from it, making the stool increasingly hard, dry, and difficult to expel. The situation may be exacerbated by a decreased intake of food, including fibrous foods. If the person also decreases his or her intake of fluid or is dehydrated, the body may compensate by extracting more fluid from the colon. Severe constipation is often accompanied by headache, abdominal distention and discomfort, malaise, nausea, and dizziness, all of which further decrease appetite. Some persons may make excessive use of the Valsalva maneuver by straining at stool in an attempt to expel the hard stool, dangerously increasing intraabdominal and intrathoracic pressures and placing undue stress on the heart and circulatory system.

When repeated attempts to evacuate the hard stool are unsuccessful, a fecal impaction may develop. The rock-hard stool is pushed distally as the newer, softer stool collects behind it, to create a partial or complete mechanical colon obstruction. The intraluminal pressures created by colonic contractions can be so great that the fluid part of the softer stool may be forced around the hard, unyielding stool and be expelled from the body in a ribbon of diarrhea or as a fecal-colored smear. This type of diarrhea is symptomatic of a fecal impaction, which can be very painful and embarrassing to have removed. If severe, the fecal impaction can further depress colon function and predispose the client to fluid and electrolyte imbalances. See Chapter 42 for more information on fecal impaction.

Integumentary System

The skin can atrophy as a result of prolonged immobility. Shifts in body fluids between the fluid compartments can affect the consistency and health of the dermis and subcutaneous tissues in dependent parts of the body, eventually causing a gradual loss in skin **turgor** (elasticity). Another common but not inevitable consequence of prolonged immobility is decubitus ulcer formation. See the section later in this chapter.

Neurosensory System

Prolonged immobilization causes some disturbances in the central and the autonomic nervous systems. The central nervous system is the primary regulator and coordinator of movement; the decrease in motor activity and the hyperactive state of sympathetic stimulation produce several effects, including the increased heart rate often seen in immobilized persons.

Immobility can further impoverish an already unstimulating environment. The inability to change position restricts sensory input severely. When tendons, muscles, and other structures are not moved to stimulate the proprioceptors, and tactile senses are stimulated only by the bed and its linens, sensory deprivation may be particularly acute. Alterations in the sensations of immobilized clients have been reported as feelings of disembodiment (Downs 1974, p. 436). Other responses include restlessness, drowsiness, irritability, unrealistic perceptions, and confusion (Patrick et al. 1986, p. 105).

PSYCHOSOCIAL RESPONSES TO IMMOBILITY

The social, emotional, and intellectual changes brought on by immobility are gradual and subtle. Most of these are due to either a decrease in the quality and quantity of sensory input or to the client's increasing awareness of the limitations of immobility. These two factors are the primary contributors to the depression-anxiety syndrome frequently seen in immobilized persons.

The lack of sensory input and the new and strange environment can be a frightening and anxiety-producing experience for the client. Significant changes in self-concept and role perception often occur as the person becomes aware of a new dependence on others and observes the effect on the family. Financial and work concerns often cause considerable worry and anxiety. The client may have unwarranted feelings of personal worthlessness, hopelessness, and emptiness, which the client may express as hostility, beligerence, confusion, withdrawal, apathy, or anxiety. Clients often have, but seldom express, concerns about perceived changes in sexuality.

Intellectual capabilities often decline in the person who experiences prolonged immobility. Problem-solving and decision-making abilities often deteriorate, probably as a result of a lack of intellectual stimulation and the stress of

Changes in Mental Function

- Decreased motivation to learn and solve problems
- Decreased perception of time and space
- Increased sense of powerlessness
- Diminished ability to make decisions, concentrate, or cope
- Inability to sleep

the illness and immobility. This decline is often accompanied by diminished ability to concentrate, exaggeration of the person's usual defense mechanisms, and decreased ability to cope with problems effectively. Changes in mental function are summarized in the accompanying box.

Immobility affects children, especially those not yet of school age, and the elderly most significantly. Immobilization can slow the intellectual and social development of young children and retard the development of motor skills. Immobilization of the elderly can increase their dependence on others.

ETIOLOGY AND PATHOGENESIS OF PRESSURE SORES

Pressure sores, also called decubitus ulcers, pressure ulcers, bedsores, or distortion sores, are reddened areas, sores, or ulcers of the skin occurring over bony prominences. They are due to interruption of the blood circulation to the tissue, resulting in a localized ischemia. The tissue is caught between two hard surfaces, usually the surface of the bed and the bony skeleton. The localized ischemia means that the cells are deprived of oxygen and nutrients, and the waste products of metabolism accumulate in the cells. The tissue dies because of the resulting anoxia. Prolonged, unrelieved pressure also damages the small blood vessels. This appears to be the most significant injury caused by pressure (Torrance 1981a).

Causes of Pressure Sores

Shannon (1984) describes three causes of pressure sores: pressure, friction, and shearing force. Usually, two causes must be present before a pressure sore develops.

Pressure Pressure is the perpendicular force exerted on the skin by gravity. Lindan et al. (1965) found that for a person of ideal weight, the points of highest pressure in the supine position are the sacrum, buttocks, and heels. These areas support pressure of 40 to 60 mm Hg. Clients in the prone position have fewer areas of high pressure and more areas of low pressure than clients in the supine position do. The knees were found to support pressures up to 50 mm Hg. Clients in the sitting position experience the greatest pressure over the ischial tuberosities. These pressures range up to 75 mm Hg (Lindan et al. 1965). Husian (1953) found that evenly distributed pressure over a larger area is less injurious than localized pressure to a very small area and that low pressure over a long period is more damaging than high pressure for a short period. Because the normal hydrostatic pressure of blood in the capillaries is 32 mm Hg at the arteriole end and 15 mm Hg at the venous end, the pressure placed on the skin exceeds these pressures, obstructing the capillaries.

After the skin has been compressed, it appears white, as if the blood had been squeezed out of it. A white person's skin loses its pink color in the affected area, and a black person's skin is also less pink, although the change is more difficult to see.

When pressure is relieved, the skin takes on a bright red flush, called **reactive hyperemia,** which is the body's mechanism for preventing pressure ulcers. The flush is due to vasodilation; extra blood floods to the area to compensate for the preceding period of impeded blood flow. The blood carries oxygen and removes the accumulated metabolic wastes. Reactive hyperemia is effective only if the pressure is relieved before irreversible changes occur in the tissues and blood vessels. The hyperemia is also thought to reduce the risk of microvascular thrombosis (Smith 1978) and to increase the sensitivity of the nerve endings in the area so that further injury to the area can be avoided or reduced (Lowthian 1982).

Reactive hyperemia usually lasts one half to three quarters as long as the duration of impeded blood flow to the area (Shannon and Miller 1988). If the redness disappears in that time, no tissue damage can be anticipated. If, however, the redness does not disappear, then tissue damage has occurred.

Friction　Friction is a force acting parallel to the skin. For example, when a client pulls up in bed, the skin rubbing against the sheet creates friction. Friction can abrade the skin, i.e., remove the superficial layers, making it more prone to breakdown.

Shearing Force　Shearing force is a combination of friction and pressure. It occurs commonly when a client assumes a Fowler's position in bed. In this position, the body tends to slide downward toward the foot of the bed. This downward movement is transmitted to the sacral bone and the deep tissues. At the same time, the skin over the sacrum tends not to move because of the friction between the skin and the bedsheets. The skin and superficial tissues are thus relatively unmoving in relation to the bed surface, whereas the deeper tissues are firmly attached to the skeleton and move downward. This causes a shearing force in the area where the deeper tissues and the superficial tissues meet. The force damages the blood vessels and tissues in this area.

Categories and Stages of Pressure Sores

Pressure sores can be categorized as superficial or deep (Ahmed 1980). **Superficial ulcers,** which most often result from friction, start at the skin with excoriation. If left untreated, they can penetrate to deeper tissue layers. **Deep ulcers,** most often the result of shearing forces and pressure, start in underlying tissues over a bony prominence and extend upward to the surface. Initially, deep ulcers may not be obvious except as a dusky redness, even though the

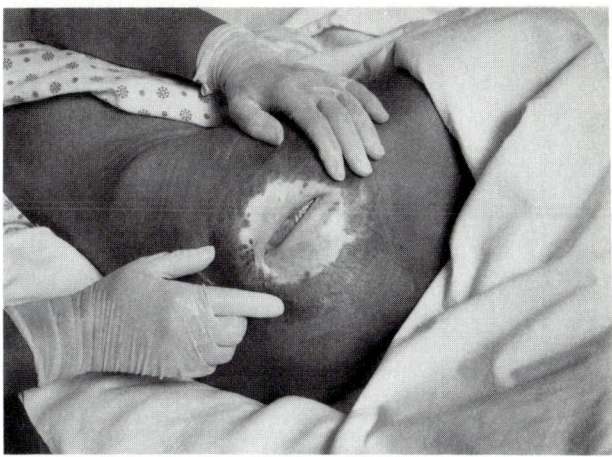

Figure 35–5　Decubitus ulcers most commonly form on the skin over bony prominences: shoulder blades, elbows, sacrum, hips (as in photo), knees, ankles, and heels.

destruction of underlying tissue may be extensive. It may take several days before the pressure is apparent (Norton 1975). See Figure 35–5.

Guttmann (1955) proposes six stages in the development of *superficial* pressure sores.

1. Transient circulatory disturbance. This stage is reversible: the skin reddens when the pressure is relieved. See the discussion of reactive hyperemia in the section "Causes of Pressure Sores."

2. Permanent damage to superficial blood vessels and tissue. Redness and congestion of the area do not disappear with relief of the pressure. The superficial skin layers may be blistered or excoriated. If the deeper tissues are involved, superficial necrosis and ulcers may result.

3. Deep penetrating necrosis. Destruction extends to subcutaneous tissue, including fascia, muscle, and bone. This stage usually develops over the sacrum and trochanters.

4. Infection of the pressure sore. Mixed infections are common with microorganisms such as *Staphylococcus aureus,* β-hemolytic *Streptococcus, Proteus,* and *Escherichia coli.*

5. Closed ischial bursa. The skin over the bursa becomes ischemic and necrotic, and a sinus sore develops.

6. Cancerous degeneration of the sore. This is a rare complication of a pressure sore.

Of Guttmann's six stages, the last three are in effect complications of a pressure sore.

Byrne and Feld (1984) define four stages of *superficial* decubitus ulcers:

1. Pinkish-red mottled skin that does not return to normal color after the pressure is relieved

2. Cracked, blistered, broken skin; shallow to full-thickness skin injury

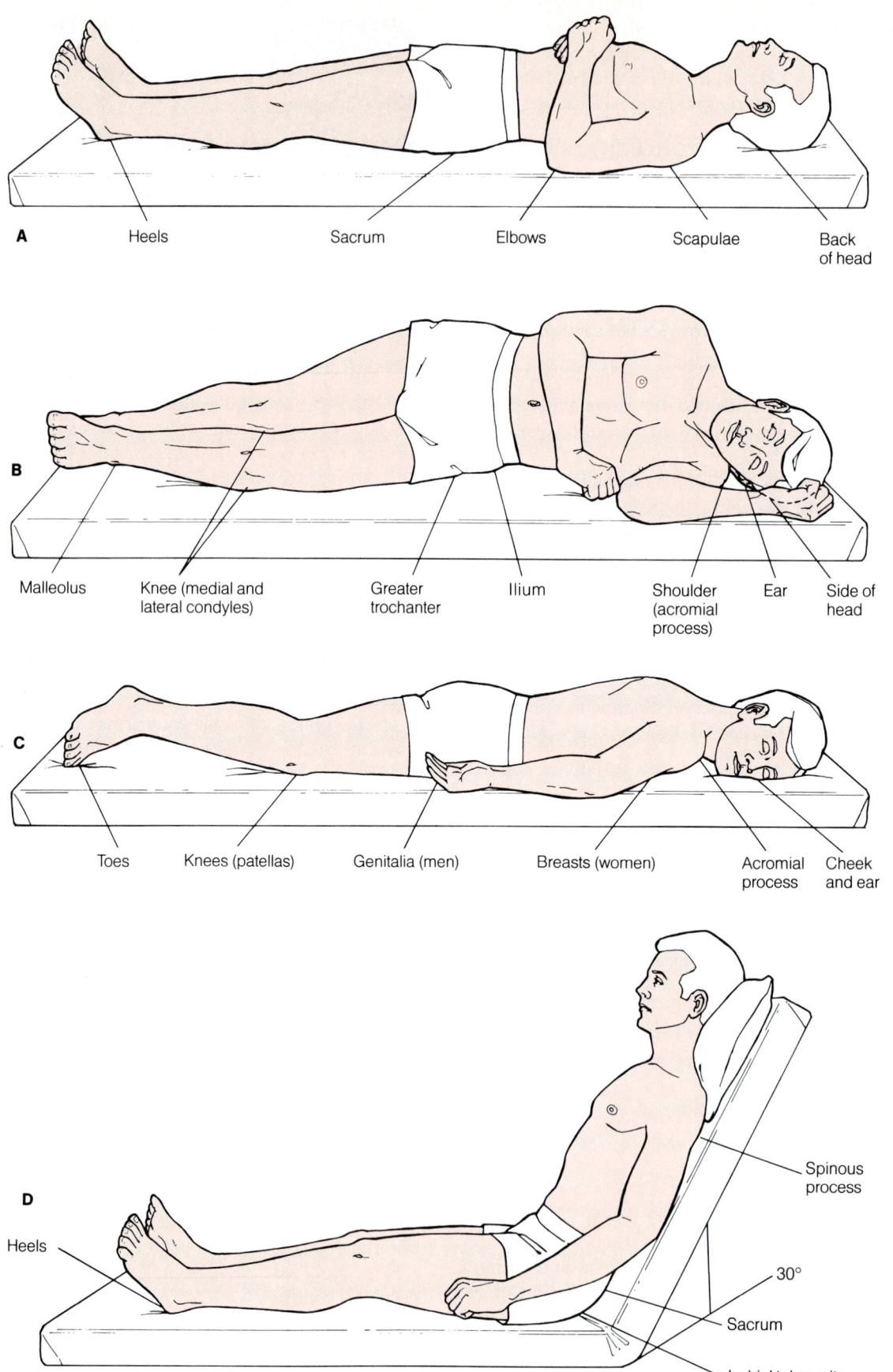

Figure 35–6 Body pressure areas in **A**, supine position; **B**, lateral position; **C**, prone position; **D**, Fowler's position.

3. Broken skin with tissue involvement, exudate (usually), and a distinct ulcer

4. Extensive ulceration with penetration to the muscle and bone; necrotic tissue and profuse drainage usually present

Color illustrations of decubitus ulcers may be found at the end of the "Skin Lesions" color section in Chapter 19, following page 402.

Factors Affecting the Formation of Pressure Sores

Six factors affect the formation of decubitus ulcers: moisture, hygiene, nutrition, body heat, anemia, and mobility.

Moisture   Moisture due to urine, feces, drainage, and perspiration reduces the resistance of the skin to other forces, such as friction. The presence of moisture, e.g., due to incontinence, was found to be the single most reliable indicator of future development of a pressure sore (Exton-Smith et al. 1963).

Hygiene   Good hygiene reduces the number of microorganisms present on the skin. Bacteria localize in ischemic tissue, which is a good medium for their growth, and the presence of bacteria increases the severity of the sore and its rate of development.

Nutrition   Nutritional factors are crucial in the development of decubitus ulcers. Generally, prolonged inadequate nutrition causes weight loss, muscle atrophy, and the loss of subcutaneous tissue. These three reduce the amount of padding between the skin and the bones, thus increasing the risk of pressure sore development. More specifically, hypoproteinemia (abnormally low protein content in the blood), either due to inadequate intake or abnormal loss, results in negative nitrogen balance, which predisposes the client to dependent edema. The presence of edema makes skin more prone to injury by decreasing its elasticity, resilience, and vitality. Edema also slows the diffusion of oxygen to the tissue cells and metabolites away from the cells because of the increased distance between the capillaries and the cells. Vitamin C is essential for healing tissue damage due to pressure.

Body Heat   Body heat is a factor in the development of pressure sores. **Pyrexia** (elevated body temperature) increases the body's metabolic rate, thus increasing the need of the cells for oxygen. This increased need is reflected in the cells of the area under pressure, which is already oxygen deficient. Therefore, severe infections with accompanying elevated body temperatures can affect the body's ability to deal with the effects of tissue compression.

Anemia   Anemia or anoxemia results in the decreased delivery of oxygen to the body cells. This is due to a decrease in the amount of hemoglobin present in the blood, since hemoglobin carries oxygen to the cells. Therefore, decreased hemoglobin exacerbates the oxygen deficiency already present in the tissues because of tissue compression.

Mobility   Normally, people move when they experience discomfort due to pressure on an area of the body. Healthy people rarely exceed their tolerance to pressure. However, paralysis, sensory disturbances, extreme weakness, apathy, and clouding of consciousness may diminish the ill person's response to tissue compression.

Other factors contributing to the formation of pressure sores are poor lifting techniques, incorrect positioning, repeated injections in the same area, hard support surfaces, and incorrect application of pressure-relieving devices. See Figure 35–6 for pressure areas in selected positions.

ASSESSING MOBILITY AND IMMOBILITY

It is extremely important to obtain and record baseline assessment data soon after the client is first immobilized. These baseline data serve as the standard against which all data collected throughout the period of immobilization are compared. As with any assessment, it is just as important to obtain and record normal as abnormal data, in order to analyze the changes and progress of the client accurately.

To obtain data about a client's mobility and immobility problems, the nurse assesses or determines the client's joint range of motion, the presence of complications of immobility, the client's risk for immobility complications (including the presence of pressure areas), the client's ability to perform the activities of daily living, and the client's activity tolerance.

Joint Range of Motion

When assessing joint movement, ask the client to move selected body parts as shown in Table 35–3. The amount of movement can be measured by a goniometer, a device that measures the angle of the joint in degrees. See Figure 19–94 on page 427.

When the client moves a joint, the nurse should assess:

1. The degree of movement of the joint

2. Any discomfort reported by the client

3. Any joint swelling or redness, which could indicate the presence of an injury or an inflammation

4. The muscle development associated with each joint and the relative size and symmetry of the muscles on each side of the body

5. The client's tolerance of the movement

Assessment of joint range of motion can usually be carried out while the client is in either a standing or supine position with heels parallel and arms placed along the sides. When
(continued on page 858)

TABLE 35-3   *Joint Movements*

Movement	Major Muscle(s)	Normal Range	Illustration
Tempromandibular Joint (TMJ)			
TMJ opening. Open mouth.		3 to 6 cm (1 to 2.3 in)	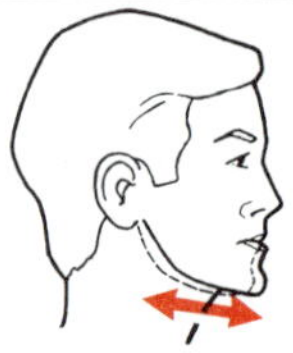 Figure 1
TMJ closure. Close mouth.	Masseter and temporalis	Complete closure	
Protrusion. Jut chin out. See Figure 1.	Pterygoideus lateralis		
Retrusion. Tuck chin in. See Figure 1.			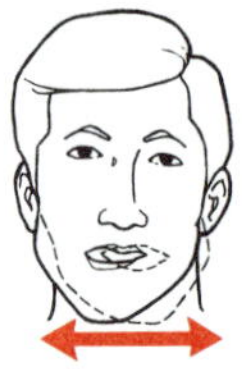 Figure 2
Lateral motion. Move jaw from side to side. See Figure 2.	Pterygoideus lateralis and pterygoideus medialis	1 to 2 cm (0.3 to 0.7 in) from midline	
Neck—Pivot Joint			
Flexion. Move the head from the upright midline position forward, so that the chin rests on the chest. See Figure 3.	Sternocleidomastoideus	45° from midline	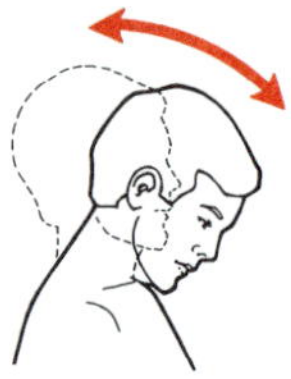 Figure 3
Extension. Move the head from the flexed position to the upright position. See Figure 3.	Trapezius	45° from midline	
Hyperextension. Move the head from the upright position back as far as possible.	Trapezius	10°	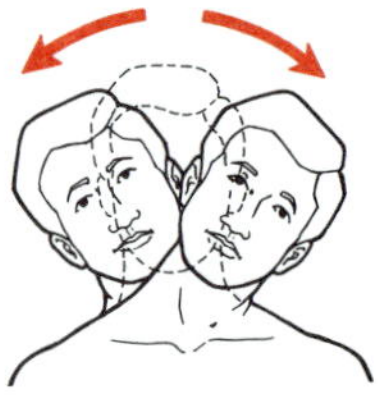 Figure 4
Lateral flexion. Move the head laterally to the right and left shoulders, while facing front. See Figure 4.	Sternocleidomastoideus	40° from midline	
Rotation. Turn the face as far as possible to the right and left. See Figure 5.	Sternocleidomastoideus and trapezius	70° from midline	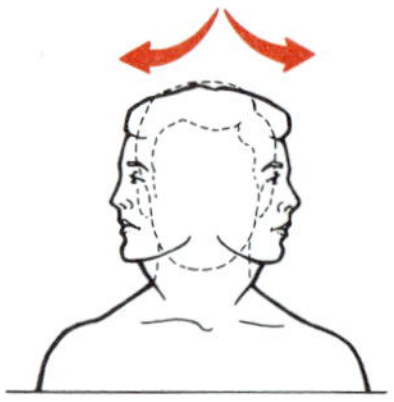 Figure 5
Shoulder—Ball-and-Socket Joint			
Flexion. Raise each arm from a position by the side forward and upward to a position beside the head. See Figure 6.	Pectoralis major, coracobrachialis, and deltoideus	180° from the side	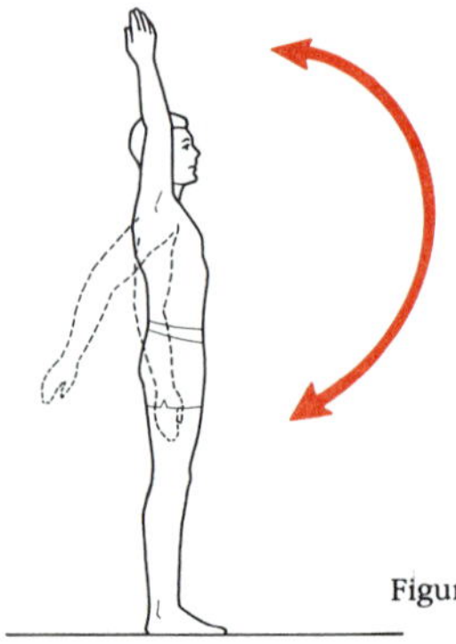 Figure 6
Extension. Move each arm from a vertical position beside the head forward and down to a resting position at the side of the body. See Figure 6.	Latissimus dorsi, deltoideus, and teres major	180° from vertical position beside the head	
Hyperextension. Move each arm from a resting side position to behind the body. See Figure 6.	Latissimus dorsi, deltoideus, and teres major	50° from side position	

TABLE 35-3 (continued)

Movement	Major Muscle(s)	Normal Range	Illustration
Shoulder—Ball-and-Socket Joint			
Abduction. Move each arm laterally from a resting position at the sides to a side position above the head, palm of the hand away from the head. See Figure 7.	Deltoideus and supraspinatus	180°	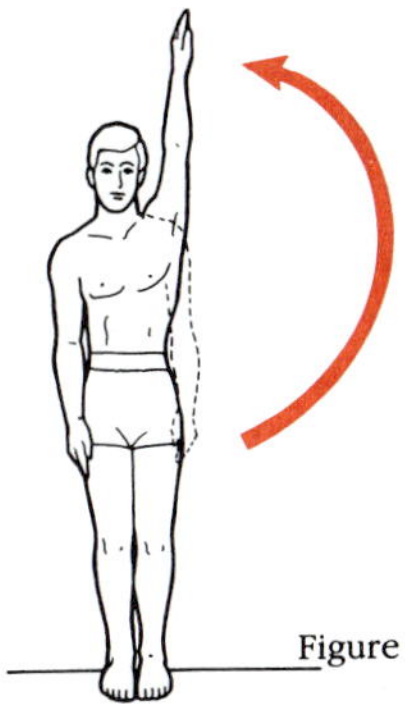
Adduction (anterior). Move each arm from a position beside the head downward laterally and across the front of the body as far as possible. See Figure 8.	Pectoralis major and teres major	230°	Figure 7
Adduction (posterior). Move each arm from a position beside the head downward laterally and across behind the body as far as possible.	Latissimus dorsi and teres major	230°	
Horizontal flexion. Extend each arm laterally at shoulder height and move it through a horizontal plane across the front of the body as far as possible. See Figure 9.	Pectoralis major and coracobrachialis	130° to 135°	Figure 8
Horizontal extension. Extend each arm laterally at shoulder height and move it through a horizontal plane as far behind the body as possible. See Figure 9.	Latissimus dorsi, teres major, and deltoideus	45°	
Circumduction. Move each arm forward, up, back, and down in a full circle. See Figure 10.	Deltoideus, coracobrachialis, latissimus dorsi, and teres major	360°	Figure 9
External rotation. With each arm held out to the side at the shoulder level and the elbow bent to a right angle, fingers pointing down, move the arm upward so that the fingers point up. See Figure 11.	Infraspinatus and teres minor	90°	Figure 10
Internal rotation. With each arm held out to the side at shoulder level and the elbow bent to a right angle, fingers pointing up, bring the arm forward and down so that the fingers point down. See Figure 11.	Subscapularis, pectoralis major, latissimus dorsi, and teres major	90°	Figure 11

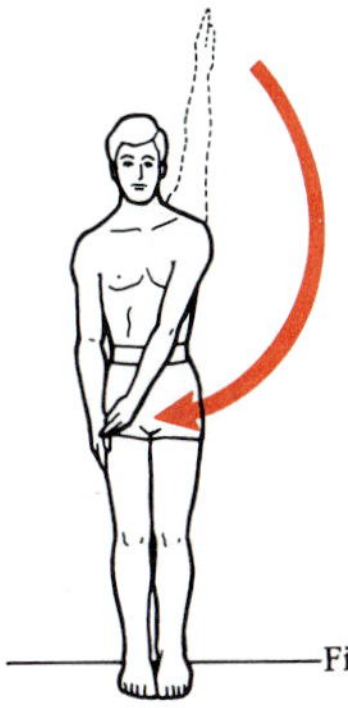

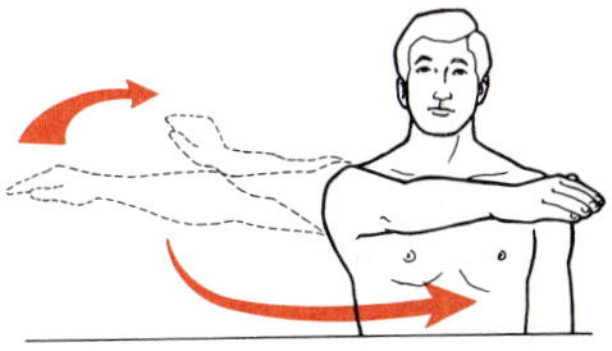

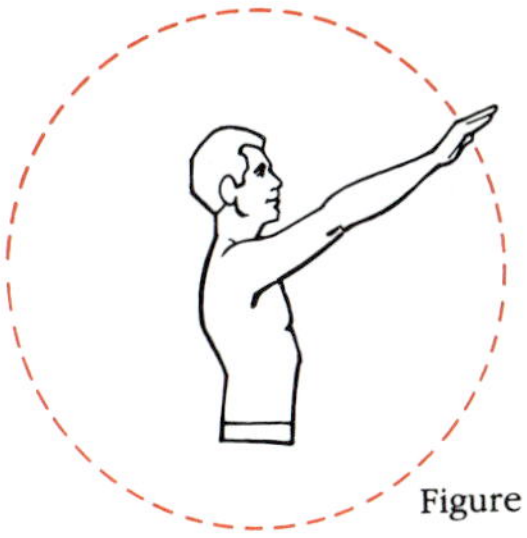

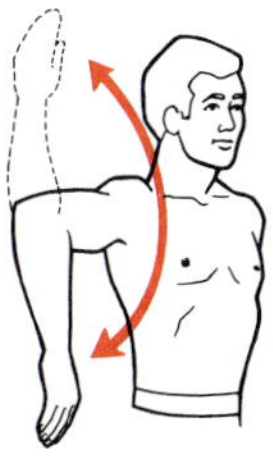

TABLE 35–3 *Joint Movements* (continued)

Movement	Major Muscle(s)	Normal Range	Illustration
Elbow—Hinge Joint			
Flexion. Bring each lower arm forward and upward so that the hand is at the shoulder. See Figure 12.	Biceps brachii, brachialis, and brachioradialis	150°	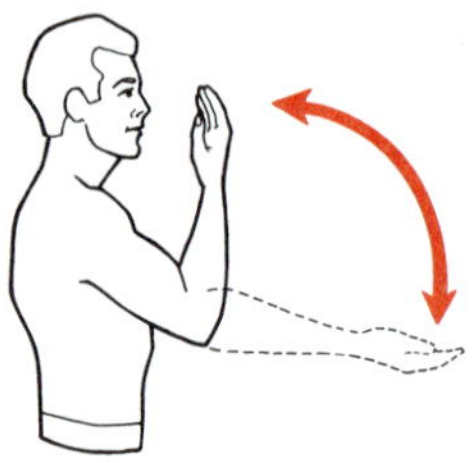
Extension. Bring each lower arm forward and downward, straightening the arm. See Figure 12.	Triceps brachii	150°	Figure 12
Rotation for supination. Turn each hand and forearm so that the palm is facing upward. See Figure 13.	Biceps brachii and supinator	70° to 90°	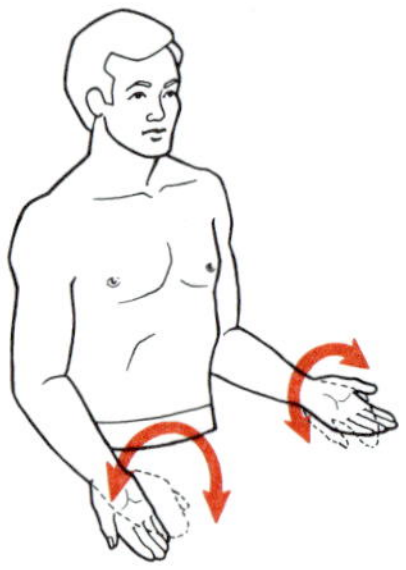
Rotation for pronation. Turn each hand and forearm so that the palm is facing downward. See Figure 13.	Pronator teres and pronator quadratus	70° to 90°	Figure 13
Wrist—Condyloid Joint			
Flexion. Bring the fingers of each hand toward the inner aspect of the forearm. See Figure 14.	Flexor carpi radialis and flexor carpi ulnaris	80° to 90°	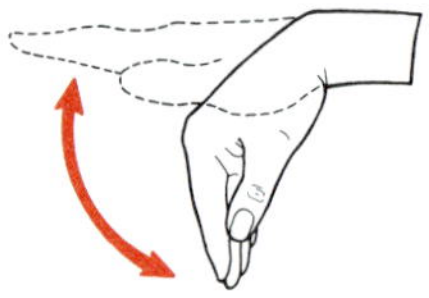
Extension. Straighten each hand to the same plane as the arm. See Figure 14.	Extensor carpi radialis longus	80° to 90°	Figure 14
Hyperextension. Bend the fingers of each hand back as far as possible. See Figure 15.	Extensor carpi radialis longus extensor, carpi radialis brevis, and extensor carpi ulnaris	70° to 90°	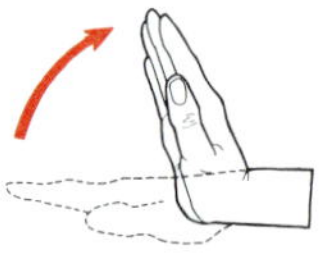
Radial flexion. (abduction). Bend each wrist laterally toward the thumb side with hand supinated. See Figure 16.	Extensor carpi radialis longus	0 to 20°	Figure 15
Ulnar flexion (adduction). Bend each wrist laterally toward the fifth finger with the hand supinated.	Extensor carpi ulnaris	30° to 50°	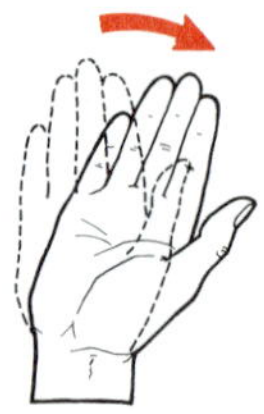 Figure 16
Hand and Fingers: Metacarpophalangeal Joints—Condyloid; Interphalangeal Joints—Hinge			
Flexion: Make a fist with each hand. See Figure 17.	Interossei dorsales manus and flexor digitorum superficialis	90°	
Extension. Straighten the fingers of each hand. See Figure 17.	Extensor indicis and extensor digiti minimi	90°	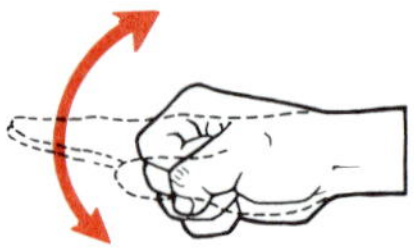
Hyperextension. Bend the fingers of each hand back as far as possible.	Extensor indicis and extensor digiti minimi	30°	Figure 17

TABLE 35–3   *(continued)*

Movement	Major Muscle(s)	Normal Range	Illustration
Hand and Fingers: Metacarpophalangeal Joints—Condyloid; Interphalangeal Joints—Hinge (continued)			
Abduction: Spread the fingers of each hand apart. See Figure 18.	Interossei dorsales manus, abductor digiti minimi manus, and opponens digiti minimi	20°	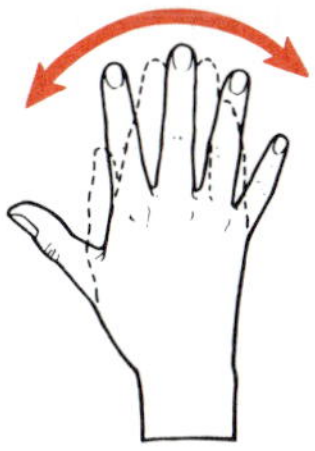
Adduction. Bring the fingers of each hand together. See Figure 18.	Interrossei palmares.	20°	Figure 18
Thumb—Saddle Joint			
Flexion. Move each thumb across the palmar surface of the hand toward the fifth finger. See Figure 19.	Flexor pollicis brevis and opponens pollicis	90°	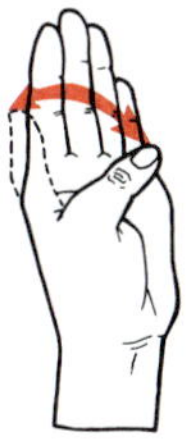
Extension. Move each thumb away from the hand.	Extensor pollicis brevis and extensor pollicis longus	90°	
Abduction. Extend each thumb laterally. See Figure 20.	Abductor pollicis brevis and abductor pollicis longus	30°	Figure 19
Adduction. Move each thumb back to the hand. See Figure 20.	Adductor pollicis	30°	Figure 20
Opposition. Touch each thumb to the tip of each finger of the same hand. The thumb joint movements involved are abduction, rotation, and flexion. See Figure 21.	Opponens pollicis and flexor pollicis brevis		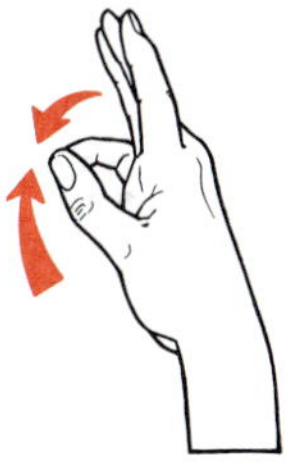 Figure 21
Hip—Ball-and-Socket Joint			
Flexion. Move each leg forward and upward. The knee may be extended or flexed. See Figure 22.	Psoas major and iliacus	Knee extended, 90°; knee flexed, 120°	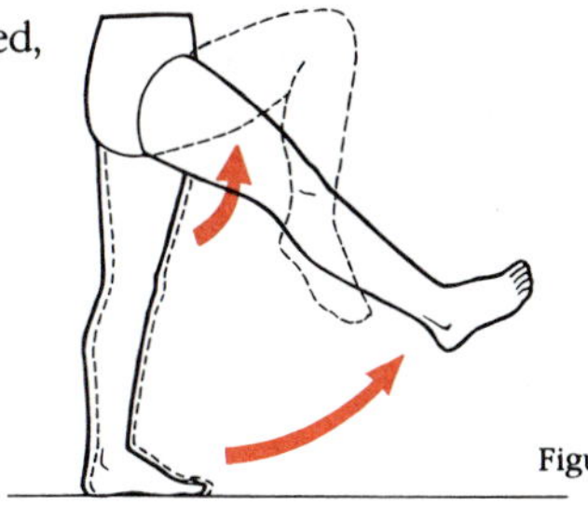
Extension. Move each leg back beside the other leg. See Figure 23.	Gluteus maximus, adductor magnus, semitendinosus, and semimembranosus	90° to 120°	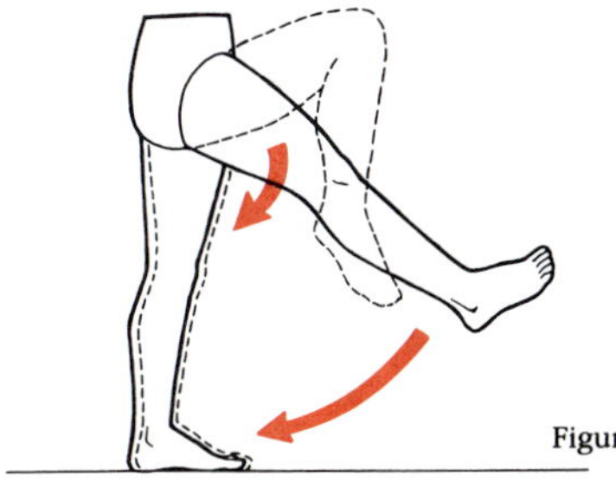
Hyperextension. Move each leg back behind the body.	Gluteus maximus semitendinosus, and semimembranosus	30° to 50°	Figure 22
			Figure 23

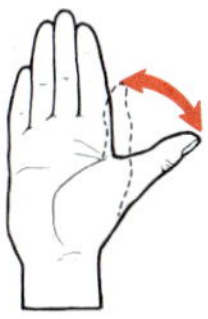

TABLE 35–3 *Joint Movements* (continued)

Movement	Major Muscle(s)	Normal Range	Illustration
Hip—Ball-and-Socket Joint (continued)			
Abduction. Move each leg out to the side. Side Figure 24.	Gluteus medius and gluteus minimus	45° to 50°	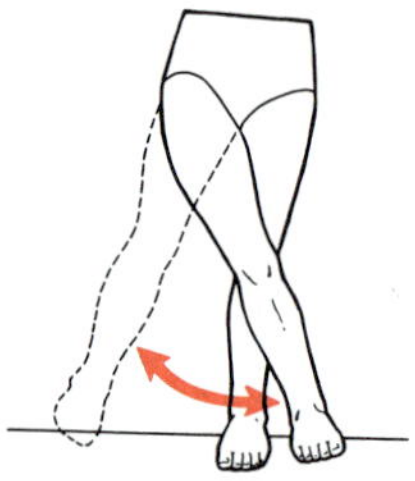
Adduction. Move each leg back to the other leg and beyond in front of it. See Figure 24.	Adductor magnus, adductor brevis, and adductor longus	20° to 30° beyond other leg	Figure 24
Circumduction. Move each leg backward, up, to the side, and down in a circle. See Figure 25.	Psoas major, gluteus maximus, gluteus medius, and adductor magnus	360°	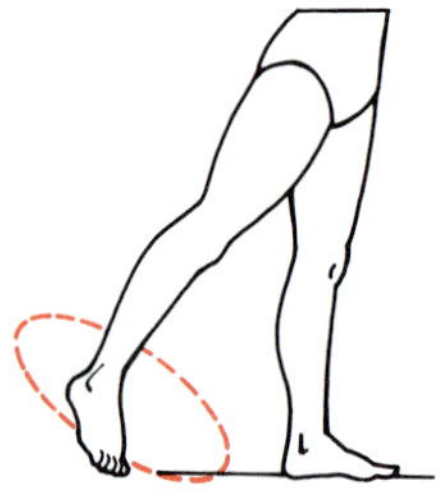 Figure 25
Internal rotation. Turn each foot and leg inward so that the toes point as far as possible toward the other leg. See Figure 26.	Gluteus minimus and tensor fasciae latae	90°	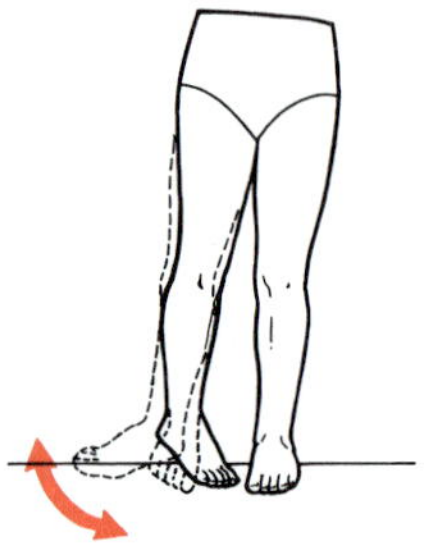
External rotation. Turn each foot and leg outward so that the toes point as far as possible away from the other leg. See Figure 26.	Obturator externus, obturator internus, and quadratus femoris	90°	Figure 26
Knee—Hinge Joint			
Flexion. Bend each leg bringing the heel toward the back of the thigh. See Figure 27.	Biceps femoris, semitendinosus, and semimembranosus	120° to 130°	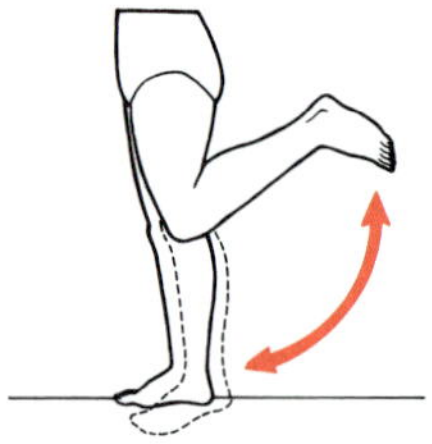
Extension. Straighten each leg, returning the foot to its position beside the other foot. See Figure 27.	Rectus femoris, vastus lateralis, vastus medialis, and vastus intermedius	120° to 130°	Figure 27
Ankle—Hinge Joint			
Extension (plantar flexion). Point the toes of each foot downward. See Figure 28.	Gastrocnemius and soleus	45° to 50°	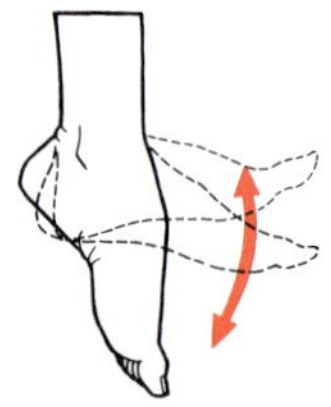
Flexion (dorsiflexion). Point the toes of each foot upward. See Figure 28.	Peroneus tertius and tibialis anterior	20°	Figure 28

TABLE 35-3   *(continued)*

Movement	Major Muscle(s)	Normal Range	Illustration
Foot and Toes: Interphalangeal Joint—Hinge; Metatarsophalangeal Joint—Hinge; Intertarsal Joint—Gliding			
Eversion. Turn the sole of each foot laterally. See Figure 29.	Peroneus longus and peroneus brevis	5°	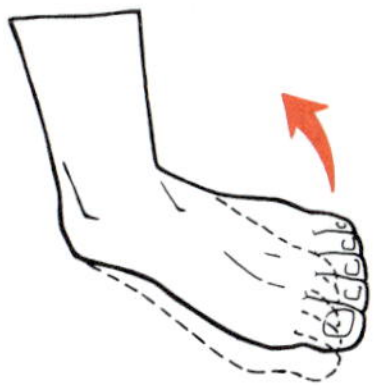
Inversion. Turn the sole of each foot medially.	Tibialis posterior and tibialis anterior	5°	
Flexion. Curve the toe joints of each foot downward. See Figure 30.	Flexor hallucis brevis, lumbricales pedis, and flexor digitorum brevis	35° to 60°	
Extension. Straighten the toes of each foot. See Figure 30.	Extensor digitorum longus, extensor digitorum brevis and extensor hallucis longus	35° to 60°	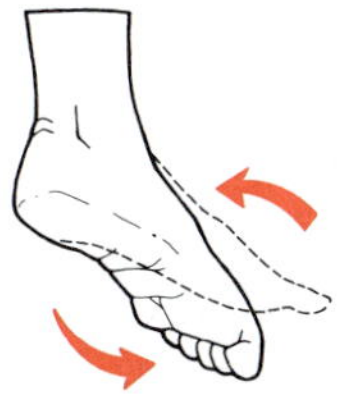
Abduction. Spread the toes of each foot apart.	Interossei dorsales pedis and abductor hallucis	0° to 15°	
Adduction. Bring the toes of each foot together.	Adductor hallucis and interossei plantares	0° to 15°	
Trunk—Gliding Joint			
Flexion. Bend the trunk toward the toes. See Figure 31.	Rectus abdominis, psoas major, and psoas minor	70° to 90°	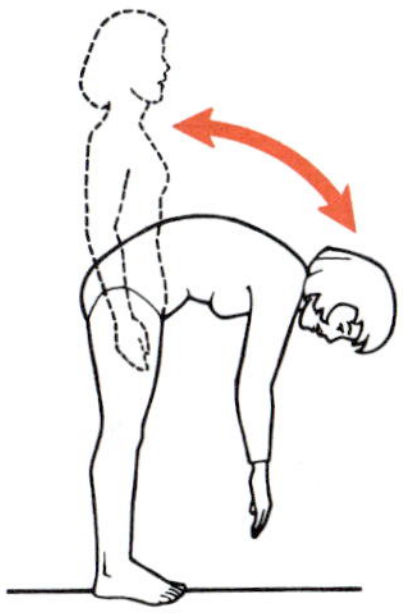
Extension. Straighten the trunk from a flexed position. See Figure 31.	Longissimus thoracis, iliocostalis thoracis, iliocostalis lumborum, erector spinae, and longissimus cervicis	70° to 90°	
Hyperextension. Bend the trunk backward.	Longissimus thoracis, iliocostalis thoracis, iliocostalis lumborum, erector spinae, and longissimus cervicis	20° to 30°	
Lateral flexion. Bend the trunk to the right and to the left. See Figure 32.	Quadratus lumborum	35° on each side	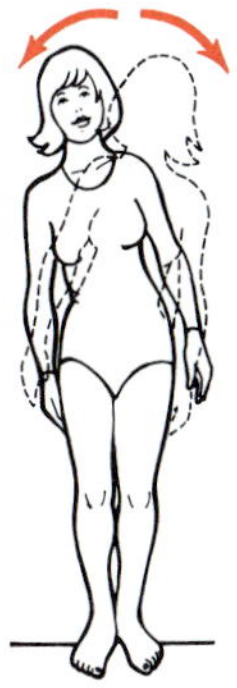
Rotation. Turn the upper part of the body from side to side. See Figure 33.	Erector spinae	30° to 45°	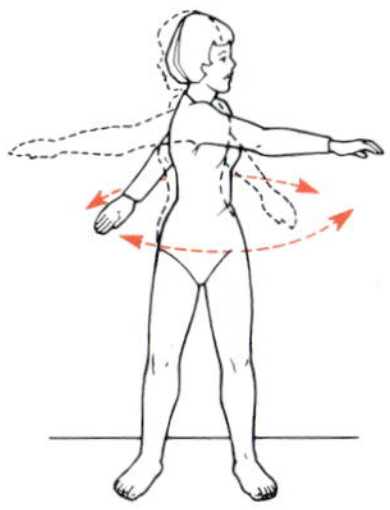

Figure 29

Figure 30

Figure 31

Figure 32

Figure 33

the client is lying down, the prone or lateral position is required for hyperextension of the neck, hips, and shoulders.

Make sure that the client is not wearing clothing that restricts movement or conceals the joint.

Assessment of range of motion should not be unduly fatiguing, and the joint movements need to be performed smoothly, slowly, and rhythmically. No joint should be forced. Uneven, jerky movement and forcing can injure the joint and its surrounding muscles and ligaments. Table 35–3 shows the various joint movements and the normal ranges of motion.

Problems of Immobility

When collecting data pertaining to the problems of immo-bility, the nurse uses the assessment methods of inspection, palpation, and auscultation; checks results of laboratory tests; and takes measurements, including body weight, fluid intake, and fluid output.

Specific techniques for assessing immobility problems and abnormal assessment findings related to the complications of immobility are summarized in Table 35–4.

Because a major nursing responsibility is to prevent the complications of immobility, the nurse needs to identify clients at risk of developing such complications before problems arise. Clients at risk include those who (a) are poorly nourished; (b) have decreased sensitivity to pain, temperature, or pressure; (c) have existing cardiovascular, pulmonary, or neuromuscular problems; and (d) are unconscious.

TABLE 35–4 *Assessing the Complications of Immobility*

Assessment Technique	Abnormal Findings Related to Immobility
Musculoskeletal system	
Measure arm and leg circumferences	Decreased circumference
Observe lab tests	Decreased serum protein levels
	Increased serum calcium and phosphate levels
	Increased urine calcium and phosphate levels
Palpate, observe	Stiffness or pain in joints
	Painful calcium deposits in soft tissue around joints
Take goniometric measurements of joint ROM	Inability to extend joints, especially of lower extremities, fully
	Decreased ROM of joints
Observe	Poorly coordinated movements of upper and lower extremities
Cardiovascular system	
Auscultate	Increased resting heart rate
	Increased heart rate with chest pain after minimal exertion
Auscultate, palpate	Narrow pulse pressure
Auscultate	Presence of a third heart sound at heart apex
Palpate, observe	Peripheral dependent edema at sacrum, legs, feet
Auscultate, palpate, observe	Sudden decrease in blood pressure, sudden increase in heart rate, dizziness upon change from supine to vertical position
Palpate, observe	Increased peripheral vein engorgement, dilation, and edema that make palpation of peripheral pulses difficult.
Palpate	Cold feet and hands
Observe, palpate	Thigh or calf tenderness, edema in affected leg, pain with movement, pain when area quickly squeezed front to back or side to side
Measure thigh and calf circumferences	Increased circumference of thigh or calf
Respiratory system	
Observe	Shallow respirations
Auscultate	Diminished breath sounds in any portion of lung

TABLE 35–4   *(continued)*

Assessment Technique	Abnormal Findings Related to Immobility
Respiratory System (continued)	
Observe lab tests	Increased Pco_2 level and decreased Po_2 level in blood
Auscultate	Moist lung sounds or wheezes
Observe	Asymmetrical chest wall movement with full inspiration and expiration
	Moist, productive cough with thick, sticky greenish-yellow mucus
	Pain with respirations, labored respirations
Measure body temperature	Fever
Metabolism and nutrition	
Measure height and weight	Weight loss due to decreased food intake and muscle atrophy
Observe	Decreased intake of protein and calories
Observe lab tests	Decreased serum protein levels
	Increased blood urea nitrogen (BUN)
Observe, palpate	Peripheral dependent edema
Observe	Slow wound healing
Observe lab test	Increased serum calcium and phosphate
Urinary and endocrine systems	
Measure 24-hour input and output	Dehydration
Measure body weight	Weight loss due to dehydration
Observe lab tests	Increased specific gravity of urine, increased BUN, increased serum hematocrit
Observe, palpate	Restlessness; decreased urinary output; lower abdominal discomfort; or hard, distended bladder: urine retention
	Voiding very small amounts of urine or "dribbling" urine: retention with overflow or incontinence
Observe lab tests	Increased serum calcium and phosphate and significantly increased urine calcium and phosphate levels
	Increased urine pH (alkalinity)
	Increased white blood cell count
	Increased urine cloudiness, turbidity
	Urine specimen with more than 100,000 colonies of bacteria per ml urine (unsterile specimen); positive urine culture for *E. coli* or other organisms
Observe	Restlessness, frequent urination of small amounts, burning with urination, fever, malaise
Observe	Abdominal cramping or pain, blood or stones in urine
Fecal elimination	
Measure 24-hour input and output	Dehydration
Observe	Decreased dietary intake and decreased intake of high-fiber foods
	More time elapsed since last bowel movement than usual
	Stool is unusually hard, dry, small, or difficult or painful to expel
	Lower abdominal discomfort, abdominal distention, nausea, malaise, headache, dizziness
	Increased use of Valsalva maneuver to expel stool
Observe, palpate	Rock-hard mass felt in lower abdomen; fecal-colored smear or ribbon of diarrhea (impaction)
Ausultate	Decreased bowel sounds

TABLE 35-4 *(continued)*

Assessment Technique	Abnormal Findings Related to Immobility
Integumentary system	
Measure 24-hour input and output	Dehydration
Observe lab tests	Increased specific gravity of urine, increased BUN, increased hematocrit
Observe	Dependent, peripheral edema in sacrum, legs, feet
Palpate, observe	More than 5 seconds for skin to return to position after a gentle pinch: decreased skin turgor, reactive hyperemia
Neurosensory system	
Observe	Overall decrease in motor activity
	Comments about unrealistic perceptions, including feelings of disembodiment
	Restlessness, drowsiness, irritability, or confusion
Social, emotional, and intellectual considerations	
Observe	Behaviors that suggest anxiety, hostility, belligerence, or confusion
	Behaviors that suggest depression: unwarranted feelings of personal worthlessness, hopelessness, emptiness, apathy, or withdrawal
	Behaviors that suggest alterations in self-concept, independent-dependent status, role in family or work group
	Concerns about finances
	Concerns about sexuality
	Behaviors that suggest diminished ability to concentrate, make decisions, or cope

Pressure Areas

Physical Assessment
Assessment includes inspection and palpation of common pressure sites (e.g., those over bony prominences) and identification of clients at risk for development of pressure sores. The accompanying box outlines guidelines for assessing pressure areas.

Clients at Risk
Clients at risk include:

- Those with paralysis from either brain or spinal cord injury. Incidence rates for these people are as high as 80%, due to their extensive loss of sensory and motor function.

- Those with a reduced level of awareness, e.g., unconscious or heavily sedated clients (those taking analgesics, barbiturates, or tranquilizers). In these clients, the usual perceptions stimulating changes of position are reduced or absent.

- Those who are malnourished and whose diet is insufficient in protein and vitamin C. Good nutrition promotes normal tissue maintenance and healing.

- Those who are over age 85. These clients more often have problems with mobility and incontinence and are generally lean. The circulatory system of aging clients is less able to carry essential nutrients to the skin.

- Those who are confined to bed or to a wheelchair, particularly if they are dependent on others for movement.

Several guides for assessing risk for breakdown have been developed. These guides should be used weekly or whenever there is a change in the client's condition or situation.

A guide by Norton et al. (1962) includes five categories: physical condition, mental condition, activity, mobility, and incontinence. See Table 35–5. Their study showed that only 5% of clients in good general condition developed pressure sores. Among clients with a score of 12 and below, almost 50% developed pressure sores (Norton 1975). In 1987, Norton revised her guide to include medications and concluded that scores of 15 or 16 should be viewed as indicators, not predictors, of risk (Anthony, 1987, p. 6).

Kerr et al. (1981, p. 27) adapted Norton's assessment scale slightly. They added brief descriptions to the rating scale category and changed the continence levels to none, minimal, occasional, and total.

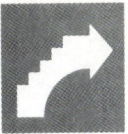

CLINICAL GUIDELINES
Assessing Pressure Areas

- Be sure there is good lighting, preferably natural or fluorescent, since incandescent lights can create a transilluminating effect.

- Regulate the environment prior to beginning assessment so that the room is neither too hot nor too cold. Heat can cause the skin to flush; cold can cause the skin to blanch or become cyanotic.

- Inspect pressure areas (see Figure 35–6, earlier) for any whitish or reddened spots; discoloration can be caused by impaired blood circulation to the area. It should disappear in a few minutes when rubbing restores circulation.

- Inspect pressure areas for abrasions and excoriations. An **abrasion** (wearing away of the skin) can occur when skin rubs against a sheet, e.g., when the client is pulled. **Excoriations** (loss of superficial layers of the skin) can occur when the skin has prolonged contact with body secretions or excretions or with dampness in skin folds.

- Inspect pressure sores for amount, color, consistency, and odor of drainage. If a sore is infected, the drainage may be abnormal, e.g., thick white drainage with a putrid odor.

- Palpate the surface temperature of the skin over the pressure areas (warm the hands first). Normally, the temperature is the same as that of the surrounding skin. Increased temperature is abnormal and may be due to inflammation or blood trapped in the area.

- Palpate over bony prominences and dependent body areas for the presence of edema, which feels spongy.

Shannon (1984) published a scoring system for identifying clients at risk. This form has eight categories. See Table 35–6 on the following page. Clients with a score of 16 or less are at significant risk of developing pressure sores.

Waterlow (1985) developed a risk assessment card that includes six categories: build (weight for height), visual

skin type, continence, mobility, sex and age, and appetite. Further research indicates that nutritional status is an important factor in pressure sore development (Osborne 1987, p. 75).

In 1987, Bergstrom et al. published the Braden Scale for predicting pressure sore risk. Their scale consists of six subscales: sensory perception, activity, mobility, moisture, friction, and nutrition. Five of the six subscales are rated from 1 (least favorable) to 4 (most favorable). The friction subscale is rated from 1 to 3. A total of 23 points is possible. The research indicates that this tool is promising as a predictor of pressure sore risk. Three studies of reliability and two studies of validity were conducted. The scale has proved a highly reliable instrument when used by RNs, primary nurses, and graduate students.

Activities of Daily Living

Activities of daily living (ADLs) are the tasks of daily life, e.g., feeding oneself, bathing, and dressing oneself. Several different rating scales help the nurse to assess a client's capabilities and define the degree of the client's current functional abilities in each of ten areas:

- Eating
- Dressing
- Bathing
- Toileting
- Achieving urinary continence
- Achieving bowel continence
- Ambulating
- Using a wheelchair
- Transferring:
  From bed to chair
  In and out of bath
  In and out of car
- Communicating

A rating scale applied to these areas may include dependency ratings (independent, partially dependent, and totally

TABLE 35–5 *Breakdown of Pressure Areas: Risk Assessment Form (Scoring System)*

A General Physical Condition		B Mental State		C Activity		D Mobility		E Incontinence	
Good	4	Alert	4	Ambulatory	4	Full	4	Absent	4
Fair	3	Apathetic	3	Walks with help	3	Slightly limited	3	Occasional	3
Poor	2	Confused	2	Chairbound	2	Very limited	2	Usually urinary	2
Very bad	1	Stuporous	1	Bedfast	1	Immobile	1	Double	1

Source: D. Norton, R. McLaren, and A. N. Exton-Smith, *An investigation of geriatric nursing problems in hospital* (Edinburgh: Churchill Livingstone, 1962). Reissued, 1975. Used by permission.

TABLE 35–6 *Determining Clients at Risk of Developing Pressure Sores**

	Mental Status	Continence	Mobility	Activity	Nutrition	Circulation	Temperature	Medications
4	Alert	Continent	Fully mobile	Ambulatory	Good	Immediate capillary refill	36.6–37.2 C (98–99 F)	No analgesics, tranquilizers, or steroids
3	Apathetic	Incontinent of urine (without catheter)	Slightly limited	Walks with assistance	Fair	Delayed capillary refill	37.2–37.7 C (99–100 F)	One of the above
2	Confused	Incontinent of feces	Very limited	Confined to wheelchair	Poor	Mild edema	37.7–38.3 C (100–101 F)	Two of the above
1	Stuporous or comatose	Incontinent of urine and feces	Immobile	Bedridden	Cachectic	Moderate to severe edema	>38.3 C (>101 F)	All of the above

*Evaluate clients for each of the above categories, then assign appropriate score. Clients with a score of 16 or less on this assessment scale are at significant risk of developing pressure sores.

Source: Reprinted, with permission, from M. L. Shannon EdD, RN, Five famous fallacies about pressure sores, *Nursing 84,* October 1984, 14:37, Copyright © 1984, Springhouse Corp. All rights reserved.

dependent) and an indication of how the ADL is achieved (by family, friend, agency, or through use of specialized equipment). Where problems exist, the nurse needs to determine the exact nature of help required and its frequency.

Activity Tolerance

By determining an appropriate activity level for a client, the nurse can predict whether a client has the strength and endurance to participate in activities that require similar expenditures of energy. This assessment is useful in encouraging increasing independence in a disabled person and is especially important for the client who has a cardiovascular or respiratory disability or who has been completely immobilized for a prolonged period.

The most useful measures in predicting activity tolerance are heart rate, strength, and rhythm, particularly for those clients with heart problems. Blood pressure readings are also useful. Assessment data are collected by measuring heart rate:

1. Before the activity starts (baseline data)
2. During the activity
3. Immediately after the activity stops, and
4. At intervals of 3, 5, and 10 minutes after the activity has stopped (Gordon 1976, p. 73)

The activity should be stopped immediately if any of the following changes occur (Ibid, p. 73):

1. The heart rate exceeds 20 beats per minute above baseline levels (cardiac client only).

2. The heart rhythm changes from regular to irregular.

3. The pulse weakens.

4. Chest pain occurs.

These warning signals indicate that the activity is too stren-

TABLE 35–7 *Energy Costs of Activities of Daily Living*

Activity	Number of Calories used per Minute
Resting, back-lying bed position	1.0
Sitting	1.2
Standing, relaxed	1.4
Eating	1.4
Conversing	1.4
Dressing/undressing	2.3
Washing hands and face	2.5
Using bedside commode	3.6
Walking 2.5 mph	3.6
Showering	4.2
Using bedpan	4.7
Walking downstairs	5.2
Walking 3.75 mph	5.6

Source: Adapted from M. A. Levin, Bed exercises for acute cardiac patients, *American Journal of Nursing,* July 1973, 73:1227.

uous or prolonged for the client and that the client's health status needs to be reassessed before any other activity.

If, however, the client tolerates the activity well, and if the client's heart rate returns to baseline levels within 5 minutes after the activity ceases, the activity is considered safe. This activity, then, can serve as a standard for predicting the client's tolerance for similar activities.

The most useful measures in predicting the activity tolerance of clients with respiratory problems are measurements of respiratory rate, depth, and rhythm, at 3-, 5-, and 10-minute intervals. **Dyspnea** (difficult breathing), a decreased respiratory rate, or an irregular respiratory rhythm during the activity indicate that the activity should be stopped immediately. If the client's respiratory rate returns to baseline levels within 3 or 4 minutes after the activity ceases, the activity is considered to be within safe limits.

Other more subjective measures of activity tolerance are useful when combined with the measures described. The nurse may need to determine whether client complaints of fatigue during activity are due to decreased activity tolerance, anxiety, or decreased motivation (Gordon 1976, p. 75).

Accomplishment of ADLs places demands on the client's tolerance for activity. The energy costs of some common ADLs are shown in Table 35–7. Note especially the greater energy levels required to get onto and off a bedpan in bed than to use a bedside commode.

DIAGNOSING

Numerous nursing diagnoses pertain to clients with actual or potential problems associated with immobility. **Potential for disuse syndrome** is the diagnosis given to clients at risk for deterioration of body systems as a result of prescribed or unavoidable musculoskeletal inactivity. Other diagnoses and possible contributing factors are categorized and listed below. Examples of assessment data clusters and related nursing diagnoses are shown in Table 35–8.

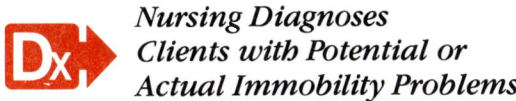

Nursing Diagnoses Clients with Potential or Actual Immobility Problems

Potential for disuse syndrome related to:

- Paralysis
- Prescribed bed rest
- Altered level of consciousness
- Skeletal traction

Musculoskeletal System

Potential for injury (falling when ambulated) related to:

- Limited endurance associated with immobility
- Decreased muscle size and strength associated with immobility
- Joint stiffness and pain associated with immobility
- Orthostatic hypotension associated with immobility

Cardiovascular System

Activity intolerance related to:

- Prolonged bed rest

Altered tissue perfusion (peripheral) related to:

- Interrupted venous flow secondary to deep vein thrombosis associated with pressure and prolonged immobilization
- Dependent edema

Respiratory System

Ineffective breathing pattern related to:

- Decreased lung expansion associated with (horizontal bed position, or painful abdominal or chest surgery)
- Chest muscle atrophy associated with prolonged bed rest
- Respiratory depressant agents (analgesic, sedative, anesthetic)

Impaired gas exchange (O_2:CO_2 ratio) related to:

- Stasis of respiratory secretions associated with immobility
- Decreased lung expansion associated with horizontal bed position

TABLE 35–8 *Example of Assessment Data Clusters and Related Nursing Diagnoses*

Data Cluster	Nursing Diagnosis
Florence Grayson was admitted to hospital with a cerebrovascular accident 2 days ago. She weighs 46 kg, is stuporous, is anorexic and malnourished, has flaccid paralysis of her left arm and leg, and is incontinent of urine. Is unable to move without help.	**Potential for disuse syndrome** related to neuromuscular impairment (hemiplegia), altered level of consciousness, and inactivity.
Fred Brown, recently diagnosed with AIDS, expresses feelings of aloneness and lack of contact with people since his friend died 3 months ago and since his diagnosis was confirmed. Expresses feelings of rejection and doubts about ability to survive. Appears anxious.	**Social isolation** related to altered state of wellness and fear by others about catching disease.

Ineffective airway clearance related to:

- Inability to inhale maximally and cough effectively secondary to painful surgery or weakened thoracic muscles
- Respiratory depressant medication
- Stasis of pulmonary secretions

Potential for aspiration related to:

- Depressed cough and gag reflexes associated with unconsciousness or anesthetic agent

Metabolic/Nutritional Systems

Altered nutrition: less than body requirements related to:

- Anorexia secondary to social isolation
- Negative nitrogen balance associated with immobility and catabolized muscle mass

Altered nutrition: potential for more than body requirements related to:

- Imbalance of intake versus activity expenditures

Urinary System

Potential for infection related to:

- Stasis of urine
- Obstruction of urinary flow (renal calculi)

Fecal Elimination

Altered bowel elimination (constipation) related to:

- Reduced physical activity
- Lack of privacy
- Less than adequate dietary intake and bulk

Integumentary System

Potential (or actual) impaired skin integrity related to:

- Physical immobilization and pressure
- Shearing forces

Psychosocial Aspects

Diversional activity deficit related to:

- Long-term hospitalization
- Monotonous environment

Powerlessness related to:

- Inability to perform activities of daily living
- Inability to perform role responsibilities
- Altered personal territory
- Social isolation

Social isolation related to:

- Altered state of wellness
- Physical handicap

PLANNING

Depending on which nursing diagnoses have been identified, the nurse and client establish relevant goals and nursing interventions to achieve them. The overall client goal for all immobilized clients is to be free of any complications associated with immobility.

When planning nursing interventions, the nurse considers two aspects of care: prevention strategies and strategies to treat existing complications (e.g., pressure sores). Interventions may include: encouraging weight-bearing activities (early ambulation if possible); scheduling deep-breathing and coughing exercises; positioning and turning the client according to a schedule; providing an exercise program (isotonic, isometric, or passive exercises) to maintain muscle strength and joint mobility; encouraging independence in performing the activities of daily living; ensuring an appropriate diet and fluid intake; keeping the client's skin clean and dry; providing mechanical devices (e.g., special mattresses) to cushion bony prominences; and planning stimulating activities.

The following section lists outcome criteria to evaluate the achievement of client goals and the effectiveness of nursing interventions.

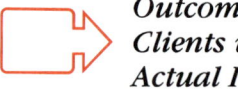

Outcome Criteria
Clients with Potential or Actual Immobility Problems

The client:

Maintains normal musculoskeletal function

- Demonstrates usual range of motion in all body joints
- Performs isotonic (and/or isometric) exercises as taught every 4 hours to specified body joints
- Retains baseline muscle mass and strength
- Participates actively in self-care activities without fatigue
- Moves safely from a lying position to a sitting or standing position without adverse effects
- Stands at the bedside for 3 minutes twice a day

Has minimum cardiovascular alterations

- Maintains baseline vital signs
- Indicates signs of adequate venous blood flow (absence of edema, calf pain, inflammation, venous distention, skin changes)

Maintains normal respiratory function

- Takes five deep breaths and coughs every waking hour
- Has normal breath sounds during auscultation
- Retains normal chest expansion
- Experiences no chest pain, fever, or other respiratory signs indicative of pulmonary infection, emboli, or atelectasis

Maintains appropriate nutritional and fluid pattern

- Maintains baseline weight
- Has normal serum protein values
- Has adequate tissue turgor
- Has a balanced fluid intake and output

Maintains normal elimination pattern

- Voids at least 1500 mL per day
- Has an acidic urine
- Is free of signs of urinary retention, infection, and renal calculi
- Passes a formed semisolid stool at least every 2 or 3 days
- Remains free of signs of fecal impaction

Maintains intact integument

- Has a clean, intact, well-hydrated skin
- Is free of pressure signs (pallor, redness, increased warmth or tenderness) over pressure areas

Maintains normal psychosocial function

- Participates actively in decisions about care
- Develops ways to overcome boredom
- Verbalizes concerns and feelings
- Accepts help from others

IMPLEMENTING

Preventing Problems from Immobility

Musculoskeletal Problems   The following interventions help to prevent the musculoskeletal complications of immobility or to restore musculoskeletal function following a period of disabling immobility:

1. Body repositioning
2. Weight-bearing activity
3. Independence in ADLs
4. Isotonic and isometric exercises
5. Range-of-motion (ROM) exercises

These activities are most useful when initiated as soon as possible after the client is immobilized.

Body repositioning   Correct body alignment in each position is essential. Interventions to promote correct body

alignment in standing, sitting, and bed-lying positions are outlined in Chapter 36. Improper body positioning can exacerbate many of the complications of immobility. The nurse and client should plan daily and full extensions of the hips and knees, which are especially vulnerable to flexion contractures.

Normally, an individual changes position automatically every few minutes in response to increasing pressure sensed in a body area. The immobilized person unable to sense this pressure or to move is highly vulnerable to deterioration of the musculoskeletal and other systems. A schedule for position changes, at least every 2 hours and preferably every hour, should be planned with the client and posted in the nursing care plan or in the client's room. If possible, standing, sitting, and all bed-lying positions should be included.

Nurses should teach clients to shift, adjust, or change their positions frequently. Clients can learn to use their feet and legs to turn and position themselves in bed and to use the side rails or an overhead trapeze to become more independent in these activities. Clients in wheelchairs should be taught to shift their weight from one ischial tuberosity to the other every 15 minutes or so to relieve pressure. The top bed linens over the foot of the bed should be loose so that they do not restrict leg and foot movement, and unnecessary pillows or other encumbrances on the bed should be removed, as they may restrict movement.

Weight-bearing activity   Interventions for assisting clients to ambulate are outlined in Chapter 36. Early ambulation is practiced almost universally today. In other words, the client is helped to get out of bed and assisted to walk as soon as possible after surgery or any period of immobility. First the client sits up in bed, then on the side of the bed. Then the client is assisted out of bed to stand and move into a chair. Finally, the client is made to walk with assistance. Distances are gradually increased. Many postoperative clients are ambulatory on the day of surgery or the day after surgery.

Standing and walking not only fully extend the hip and knee joints but also produce the stress of weight-bearing to halt calcium loss from bone. Clients who do not have the strength or balance to stand and walk can be assisted to achieve passive weight-bearing through the use of a tilt table or CircOlectric bed. Clients are strapped into these special beds, which are then tilted to a vertical position, allowing the client to stand and bear weight.

Independence in activities of daily living   Clients need to be encouraged to become as independent as possible as soon as possible without being made to face the frustration of attempting ADLs they cannot yet handle successfully.

Carefully assessing for activity intolerance during the client's performance of ADLs is useful for encouraging steady progress toward greater independence. Nurses need to teach clients to monitor their heart rates before, during, and after an activity. The client should be taught the signs and symptoms of activity intolerance (fatigue, dizziness, chest pain, shortness of breath, or profuse perspiration) and be warned to stop activity if these signs and symptoms occur.

Isotonic and isometric exercises **Isotonic** (dynamic) **exercises** are those in which muscle tension is constant and the muscle shortens to produce muscle contraction and movement. Most physical conditioning exercises—running, walking, swimming, cycling, and other activities—are isotonic, as are ADLs and active ROM exercises. Examples of isotonic bed exercises are pushing or pulling against a stationary object, pressing the feet against a footboard, using a trapeze to lift the body off the bed, lifting the buttocks off the bed by pushing with the hands against the mattress, and pushing the body to a sitting position.

Isotonic exercises increase muscle strength and endurance and can improve cardiorespiratory function. During isotonic exercise, both heart rate and cardiac output quicken to increase blood flow to all parts of the body. Little or no change in blood pressure occurs.

Isometric (static or setting) **exercises** are those in which there is a change in muscle tension but no change in muscle length. No muscle or joint movement occurs. These exercises are useful for strengthening abdominal, gluteal, and quadriceps muscles used in ambulation but are not useful in preventing joint contraction since joint movement is absent. When an immobilized client's leg is confined in a cast or traction, isometric exercises may help to maintain muscle strength in the affected limb. Isometric exercises may be useful for strengthening arm muscles in preparation for crutch-walking. These exercises are most effective in increasing muscle strength when five maximal tensions are achieved in succession, each lasting 5 seconds with 2 minutes rest in between (Brower and Hicks 1972, p. 1252). Although isotonic exercise is the basis of most physical conditioning programs, many programs also include some isometric exercises as well.

Isometric exercises produce a moderate increase in heart rate and cardiac output, but no appreciable increase in blood flow to other parts of the body. A marked increase in blood pressure occurs with isometric exercise, and use of the Valsalva maneuver is essentially unavoidable. This combination can pose real danger for any cardiac client, who should be taught to *exhale* when performing these exercises.

Active and passive range-of-motion exercises
Active ROM exercises are isotonic exercises in which the client moves each joint in the body through its complete range of movement, maximally stretching all muscle groups within each plane, over the joint. These exercises maintain or increase muscle strength and endurance and help to maintain cardiorespiratory function in an immobilized client. They also prevent deterioration of joint capsules, ankylosis, and contractures.

Full ROM does not occur spontaneously in the immobi-

lized individual who independently achieves ADLs, independently moves about in bed, independently transfers between bed and wheelchair or chair, or independently ambulates a short distance, since only a few muscle groups are maximally stretched during these activities. Although the client may successfully achieve some active ROM movements of the upper extremities while combing the hair, bathing, and dressing, the immobilized client is very unlikely to achieve any active ROM movements of the lower extremities when these are not used in their normal functions of standing and walking about. For this reason, most wheelchair and many ambulatory clients need active ROM exercises until they regain their normal activity levels. An automatic passive ROM machine is occasionally used for clients recovering from knee surgery. The machine provides continuous exercise and is set to move the knee to a prescribed degree over a prescribed time.

A physician's order for ROM exercises is usually required if a client has an abnormal or injured musculoskeletal part or if the client's overall condition could be compromised by exercise. A nursing order is expected before a client with an otherwise normal musculoskeletal system but suffering from the consequences of immobility begins preventive exercises.

The nurse encourages the client to perform each ROM exercise to the point of slight resistance, but not beyond, and never to the point of discomfort. The client should perform the movements systematically, using the same sequence during each session.

At first, the nurse may need to help the client perform the needed ROM exercises; eventually, the client may be able to accomplish these independently, with only periodic guidance from the nurse.

During **passive ROM exercises,** another person moves each of the client's joints through their complete range of movement, maximally stretching all muscle groups within each plane over each joint. Since the client does not contract the muscle, passive ROM exercises are of no value in maintaining muscle strength but are useful in maintaining joint flexibility. For this reason, passive ROM exercises should be performed only when the client is unable to accomplish the movements actively.

Passive ROM exercises should be accomplished for each movement of the arms, legs, and neck that the client is unable to achieve actively. As with active ROM exercises, passive ROM exercises should be accomplished to the point of slight resistance, but not beyond, and never to the point of discomfort. The movements should be systematic, and the same sequence should be followed during each exercise session. Each exercise should consist of three repetitions, and the series of exercises should be done twice daily (Kottke 1990, p. 444). Performing one series of exercises along with the bath is helpful. Passive ROM exercises should be incorporated into the plan of care.

Passive ROM exercises are accomplished most effectively when the client lies on his or her back in bed. Procedure

35–1 on the following page explains how to perform the exercises. General guidelines for providing passive exercises follow.

- Ensure that the client understands the reason for doing ROM exercises.
- If there is a possibility of hand swelling, make sure rings are removed.
- Clothe the client in a loose gown and cover the body with a bath blanket.
- Use correct body mechanics when providing ROM exercises to avoid muscle strain or injury to both yourself and the client.
- Position the bed at an appropriate height.
- Expose only the limb being exercised, to avoid embarrassing the client.
- Support the client's limbs above and below the joint as needed to prevent muscle strain or injury (see Figure 35–7). This may also be done by cupping joints in the palm of the hand or cradling limbs along the nurses forearm (see Figure 35–8). If a joint is painful (e.g., arthritic), support the limb in the muscular areas above and below the joint.
- Use a firm, comfortable grip when handling the limb.
- Move the body parts smoothly, slowly, and rhythmically. Jerky movements cause discomfort and, possibly, injury. Fast movements can cause spasticity or rigidity.
- Avoid moving or forcing a body part beyond the existing range of motion. Muscle strain, pain, and injury can result. This is particularly important for people with flaccid (limp) paralysis, whose muscles can be stretched and joints dislocated without their awareness.
- If muscle spasticity occurs during movement, stop the movement temporarily but continue to apply slow, gentle pressure on the part until the muscle relaxes; then proceed with the motion.
- If a contracture is present, apply slow firm pressure without causing pain, to stretch the muscle fibers.
- If rigidity occurs, apply pressure against the rigidity, and continue the exercise slowly.

Considerations for the elderly   For elderly clients it is not essential to achieve full range of motion in all joints. Instead, emphasize achieving a sufficient range of motion to carry out ADLs such as walking, dressing, combing hair, showering, and preparing a meal.

Neck hyperextension movements should be avoided in the immobilized elderly client, because such movements can cause painful nerve damage (Hogan and Beland 1976, p. 1106).

Active-assistive range-of-motion exercises   During **active-assistive ROM exercises,** the client uses a stronger, opposite arm or leg to move each of the joints of

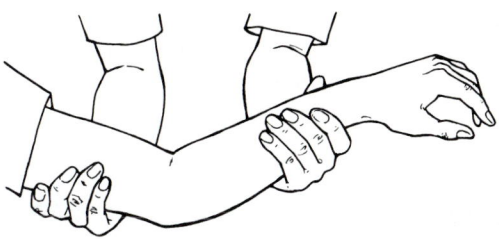

Figure 35–7   Supporting a limb above and below the joint for passive exercise.

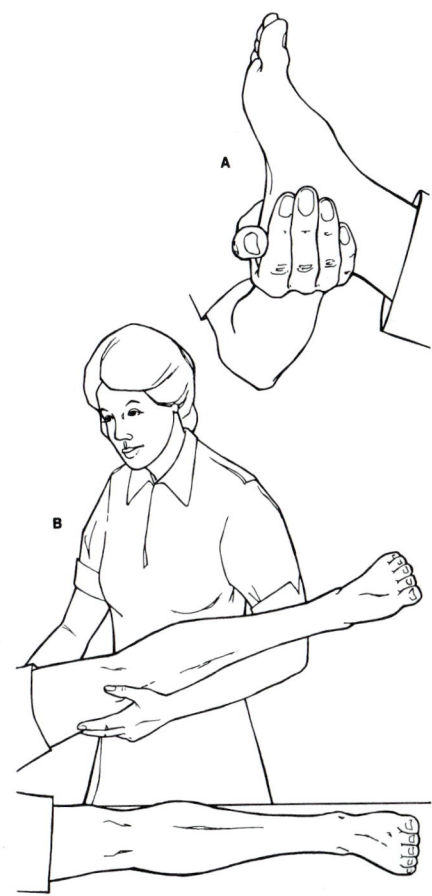

Figure 35–8   Holding limbs for support during passive exercise: **A,** cupping; **B,** cradling.

a limb incapable of active motion. The client learns to support and move the weak arm or leg with the strong arm or leg as far as possible. Then the nurse continues the movement passively to its maximal degree. This activity increases active movement on the strong side of the client's body and maintains joint flexibility on the weak side. Such exercise is especially useful for stroke victims who are hemiplegic (paralyzed on one half of the body). Some clients who begin with passive ROM exercises after a disability progressively
(continued on p. 872)

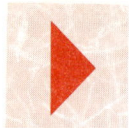

PROCEDURE 35–1

PROVIDING PASSIVE RANGE-OF-MOTION EXERCISES

Intervention

1. **Assist the client to a supine position near the nurse, and expose the body parts requiring exercise.**

- Place the client's feet together, place the arms at the sides, and leave space around the head and the feet. *Positioning the client close to the nurse prevents excessive reaching.*

2. **Return to the starting position after each motion. Repeat each motion three times.**

3. **Throughout the exercises assess**

a. ability to tolerate the exercise
b. range of motion of an affected joint

Shoulder and Elbow Movement

Begin each exercise with the client's arm at the client's side. Grasp the arm beneath the elbow with one hand and beneath the wrist with the other hand, unless otherwise indicated. See Figure 35–9.

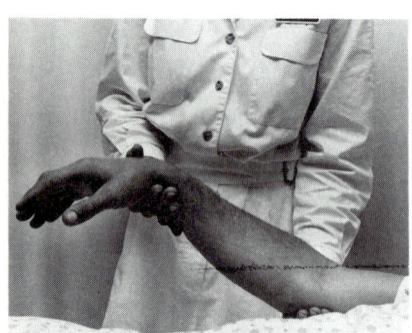

Figure 35–9 Supporting the client's arm.

4. **Flex, externally rotate, and extend the shoulder.**

- Move the arm up to the ceiling and toward the head of the bed. See Figure 35–10. The elbow may need to be flexed if the headboard is in the way.

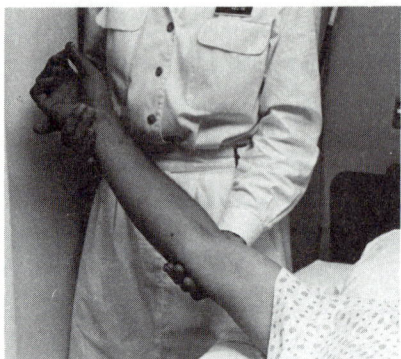

Figure 35–10 Flexing and extending the shoulder

5. **Abduct and externally rotate the shoulder.**

- Move the arm away from the body (see Figure 35–11) and toward the client's head until the hand is under the head (see Figure 35–12).

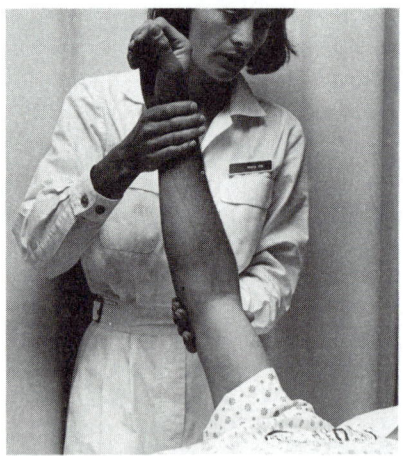

Figure 35–11 Abducting the shoulder.

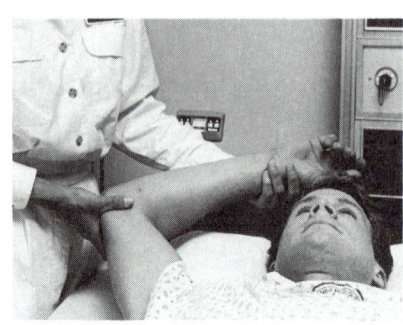

Figure 35–12 Externally rotating the shoulder.

6. **Adduct the shoulder.**

- Move the arm over the body (see Figure 35–13) until the hand touches the client's other hand.

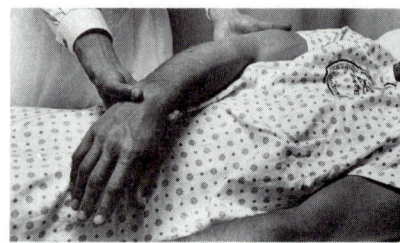

Figure 35–13 Adducting the shoulder.

7. **Rotate the shoulder internally and externally.**

- Place the arm out to the side at shoulder level (90° abduction), and bend the elbow so that the forearm is at a right angle to the mattress. See Figure 35–14.

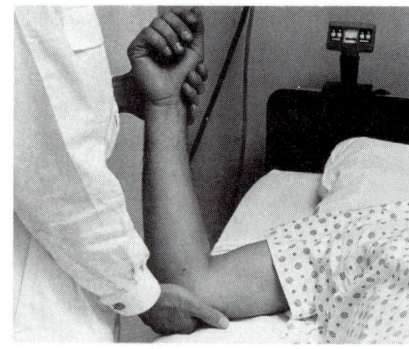

Figure 35–14 Position before rotating the shoulder.

- Move the forearm down until the palm touches the mattress and then up until the back of the hand touches the bed (see Figure 35–15).

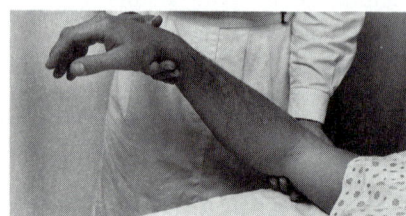

Figure 35–15 Rotating the shoulder.

8. **Flex and extend the elbow.**

■ Bend the elbow until the fingers touch the chin, then straighten the arm. See Figure 35–16.

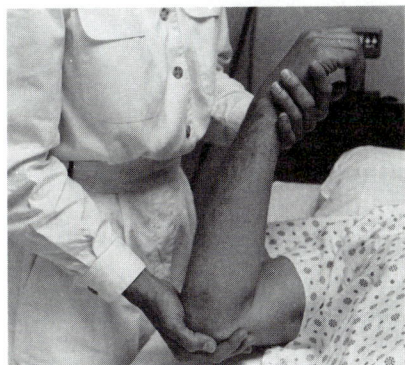

Figure 35–16 Flexing and extending the elbow.

9. **Pronate and supinate the forearm.**

■ Grasp the client's hand as for a handshake and turn the palm downward (see Figure 35–17) and upward (see Figure 35–18), ensuring that only the forearm (not the shoulder) moves.

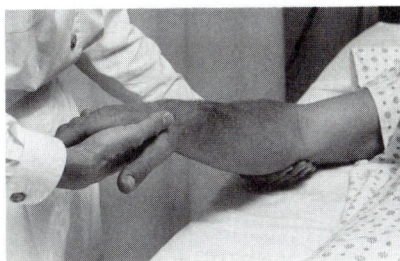

Figure 35–17 Pronating the forearm.

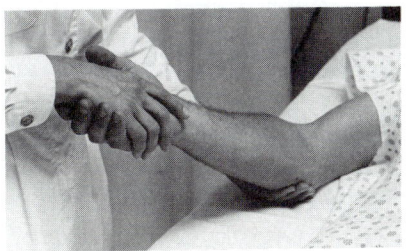

Figure 35–18 Supinating the forearm.

Wrist and Hand Movement

For wrist and hand exercises, flex the client's arm at the elbow until the forearm is at a right angle to the mattress. Support the wrist joint with one hand while your other hand manipulates the joint and the fingers. See Figure 35–19.

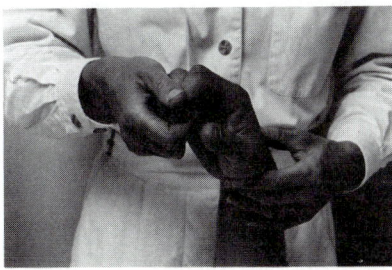

Figure 35–19 Position for wrist and hand movements.

10. **Hyperextend the wrist and flex the fingers.**

■ Bend the wrist backward and at the same time flex the fingers, moving the tips of the fingers to the palm of the hand. See Figure 35–20.

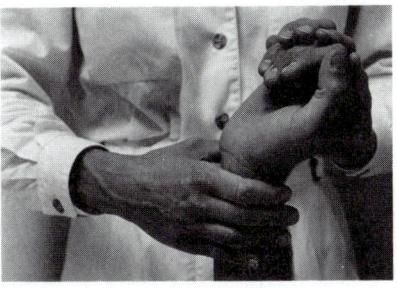

Figure 35–20 Hyperextending the wrist and flexing the fingers.

■ Align the wrist in a straight line with the arm and place your fingers over the client's fingers to make a fist.

11. **Flex the wrist and extend the fingers.**

■ Bend the wrist forward and at the same time extend the fingers. See Figure 35–21.

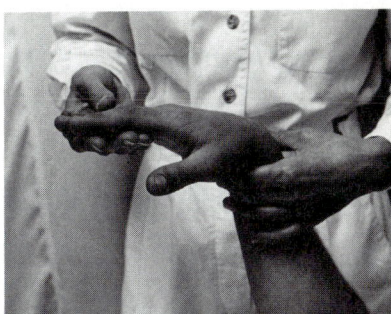

Figure 35–21 Flexing the wrist and extending the fingers.

12. **Abduct and oppose the thumb.**

■ Move the thumb away from the fingers and then across the hand toward the base of the little finger. See Figure 35–22.

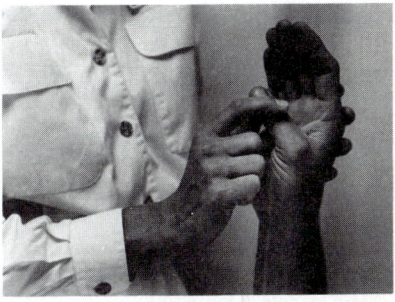

Figure 35–22 Abducting the thumb.

Leg and Hip Movement

To carry out leg and hip exercises, place one hand under the client's knee and the other under the ankle. See Figure 35–23.

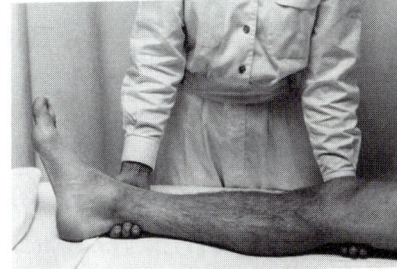

Figure 35–23 Position for knee and hip movements.

13. Flex and extend the knee and hip.

- Lift the leg and bend the knee, moving the knee up toward the chest as far as possible. Bring the leg down, straighten the knee, and lower the leg to the bed. See Figure 35–24.

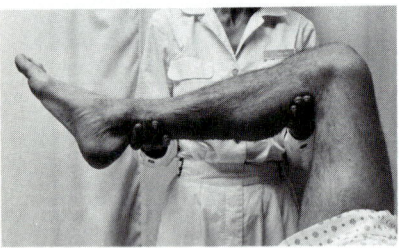

Figure 35–24   Flexing the knee and the hip.

14. Abduct and adduct the leg.

- Move the leg to the side, away from the client (see Figure 35–25) and back across in front of the other leg (see Figure 35–26).

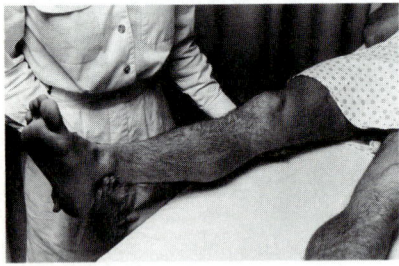

Figure 35–25   Abducting the leg.

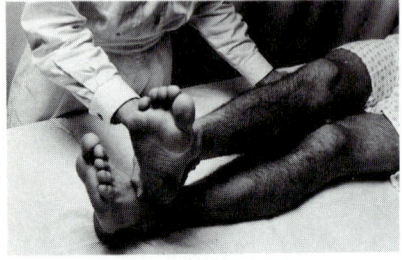

Figure 35–26   Adducting the leg.

15. Rotate the hip internally and externally.

- Roll the leg inward (see Figure 35–27), then outward (see Figure 35–28).

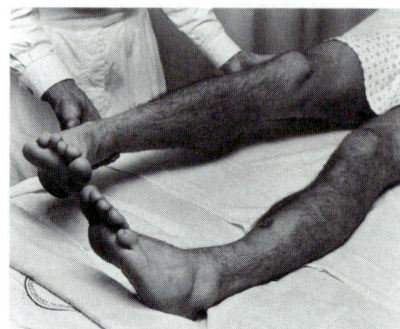

Figure 35–27   Internally rotating the hip.

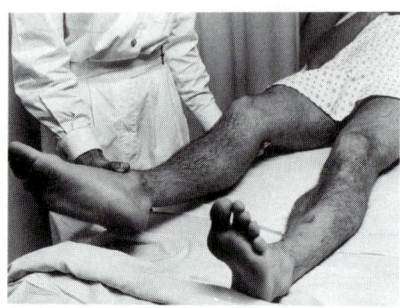

Figure 35–28   Externally rotating the hip.

Ankle and Foot Movement

For ankle and foot exercises, place your hands in the positions described, depending on the motion to be achieved.

16. Dorsiflex the foot and stretch the Achilles tendon (heel cord).

- Place one hand under the client's heel, resting your inner forearm against the bottom of the client's foot.
- Place the other hand under the knee to support it.
- Press your forearm against the foot to move it upward toward the leg. See Figure 35–29.

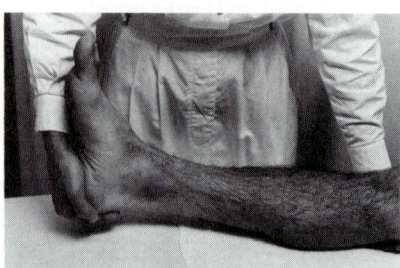

Figure 35–29   Dorsiflexing the foot.

17. Invert and evert the foot.

- Place one hand under the client's ankle and the other over the arch of the foot.
- Turn the whole foot inward (see Figure 35–30), then turn it outward (see Figure 35–31).

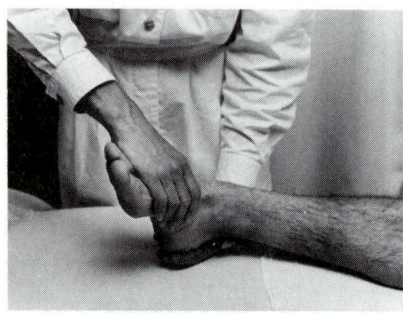

Figure 35–30   Inverting the foot.

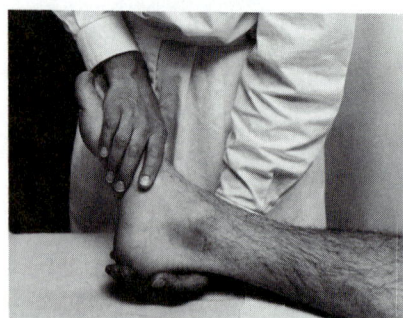

Figure 35–31   Everting the foot.

18. Plantar flex the foot and extend and flex the toes.

- Place one hand over the arch of the foot to push the foot away from the leg.

- Place the fingers of the other hand under the toes, to bend the toes upward (see Figure 35–32), and then over the toes, to push the toes downward (see Figure 35–33).

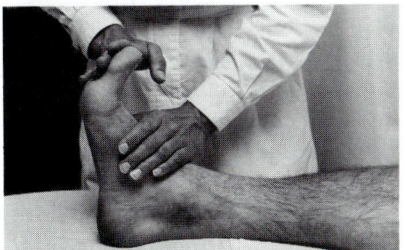

Figure 35–32 Extending the toes.

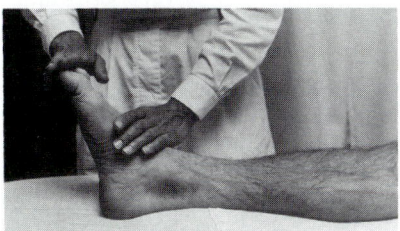

Figure 35–33 Plantar flexing the foot and flexing the toes.

Neck Movement

Remove the client's pillow.

19. **Flex and extend the neck.**

- Place the palm of one hand under the client's head and the palm of the other hand on the client's chin.
- Move the head forward until the chin rests on the chest, then back to the resting supine position without the head pillow. See Figure 35–34.

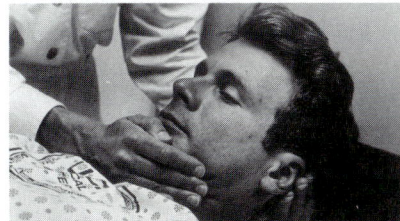

Figure 35–34 Flexing the neck.

20. **Laterally flex the neck.**

- Place the heels of the hands on each side of the client's cheeks.
- Move the top of the head to the right and to the left. See Figure 35–35.

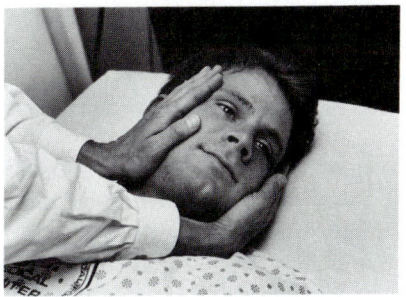

Figure 35–35 Laterally flexing the neck.

Hyperextension Movements

21. **Assist the client to a prone or lateral position on the side of the bed nearest the nurse but facing away from the nurse.**

22. **Hyperextend the shoulder.**

- Place one hand on the shoulder to keep it from lifting off the bed and the other under the client's elbow.
- Pull the upper arm up and backward. See Figure 35–36.

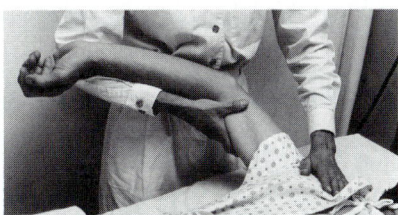

Figure 35–36 Hyperextending the shoulder.

23. **Hyperextend the hip.**

- Place one hand on the hip to stabilize it and keep it from lifting off the bed. With the other arm and hand, cradle the lower leg in the forearm, and cup the knee joint with the hand.

- Move the leg backward from the hip joint. See Figure 35–37.

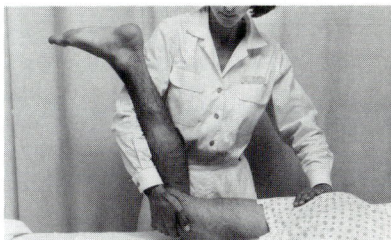

Figure 35–37 Hyperextending the hip.

24. **Hyperextend the neck.**

- Remove the pillow. With the client's face down, place one hand on the forehead and the other on the back of the skull.
- Move the head backward. See Figure 35–38.

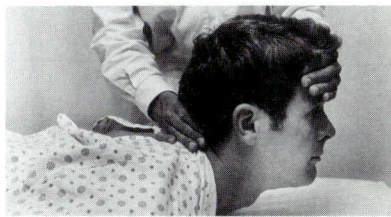

Figure 35–38 Hyperextending the neck.

Following the Exercises

25. **Assess the client's pulse and endurance of the exercise.**

26. **Report to the nurse in charge any unexpected problems or notable changes in the client's movements, e.g., rigidity or contractures.**

27. **Document the exercises and your assessments.**

Sample Recording

Date: 6-14-91	Time: 1100

Passive exercises provided to R leg and foot for 5 minutes with no pain. Full ROM in hip, knee, and ankle.
—Sally S. Ames, SN

improve to use active-assistive ROM exercises, and finally active ROM exercises.

Resistive exercises   **Resistive exercises** are a form of either isotonic or isometric exercise during which the client moves (isotonic) or tenses (isometric) against resistance. Resistive exercise is used in physical conditioning. Helping clients to push their feet against a footboard placed in the bed, lift weights, or use an overhead trapeze to lift themselves up toward the head of the bed are examples.

Cardiovascular Problems

Nursing interventions to prevent cardiovascular complications due to immobility or to restore cardiovascular function are multiple.

Movement and exercise   Some of the most effective interventions to prevent the cardiovascular complications of immobility are described previously under interventions to prevent musculoskeletal complications. Movements and exercises of all kinds—early ambulation, active exercises of any kind (especially those involving the legs), independence in ADLs, and turning and moving in bed—are valuable. These activities slow heart rate and improve cardiac reserve, stimulate the sympathetic nervous system to restore peripheral vasoconstriction with postural changes, improve muscle tone and thus prevent or reduce dependent edema, and prevent thrombus and embolus formation.

Discouraging use of the Valsalva maneuver   The Valsalva maneuver increases the stress placed on the heart of the immobilized client. The nurse should teach the client to avoid taking a deep breath and holding it prior to turning, moving, or lifting in bed. For instance, the nurse might suggest that the client count or even sing during these activities to avoid holding the breath, thus preventing use of the Valsalva maneuver. Preventing constipation reduces straining at stool and decreases the potential for use of the Valsalva maneuver.

Regaining peripheral vasoconstriction with vertical postures   The period of immobility gives the nurse an opportunity to promote the recovery of the sympathetic nervous system and to assess its recovery before the client gets out of bed for the first time. Gradually increasing the height of the head of the bed for longer periods of time stimulates the peripheral vasoconstrictors. Meanwhile, the nurse carefully assesses for a decrease in blood pressure, a sudden or marked increase in heart rate, or client complaints of dizziness or lightheadedness, all of which indicate that the sympathetic nervous system has not yet fully regained its function. If these occur, the head of the bed should be lowered until dizziness and other symptoms subside. During all position changes, it is important to remind and teach the client to move slowly so that the sympathetic nervous system can adjust to the new posture.

Before the client gets out of bed the first time after a period of immobility, and while the client is still lying flat in bed, the nurse should measure and record baseline blood pressure and heart rate. These should again be measured after the client has been slowly moved into a high Fowler's position, after the client sits in the "dangle" position, and after assisting the client to stand at the bedside. If the client's heart rate and blood pressure remain stable when compared with baseline levels, and if the client does not complain of dizziness or lightheadedness in this position, the nurse assists the client to ambulate under close supervision. The nurse must be prepared to take quick action if the client becomes lightheaded or dizzy. (See *Ambulation Guidelines* in Chapter 36, p. 924.) The nurse and client together should determine the duration and distance of this first ambulation.

When the client completes the ambulation and returns to bed, the nurse again measures heart rate and blood pressure and compares them to baseline levels. This measurement helps the nurse assess activity tolerance. These data are the basis for determining the duration and distance of the client's next ambulatory session.

Elastic stockings   Elastic stockings (antiemboli stockings) or elastic bandages help to prevent orthostatic hypotension, pooling of blood in the leg veins causing vein dilation and engorgement, incompetent valves in the leg veins, and dependent edema and thrombus formation while improving venous return of blood to the heart. See Chapter 47, page 1361. The custom-fitted stockings are available in toe-to-knee length and in toe-to-mid-thigh length. They should be put on the legs after the client has been lying flat in bed with legs slightly elevated for 20 minutes. The stockings are removed twice daily for 20 to 30 minutes while skin care is given.

Automatic "pulsating" (pneumatic compression) stockings are occasionally used for very high-risk immobilized clients following certain kinds of surgery. The stockings exert continuous pressure against the leg, and a motor creates an additional pulsating, compressing movement that stimulates the leg muscles to contract, thus increasing venous return to the heart.

Protective leg positioning   Proper alignment in standing, sitting, and bed-lying positions is described in Chapter 36. It is important to prevent undue pressure to the intimal lining of the veins since this pressure may cause injury, and thrombi often begin at the roughened, inflamed, and healing sites where injury has occurred. Improper positioning can create the pressure that causes intimal damage. Examples are positioning one leg directly on top of the other in the lateral (side-lying) position, placing undue pressure at the popliteal space behind the knee or intense point pressure anywhere along the calf, or sitting in one position or with the legs crossed for a prolonged time. Improper positioning can also impede venous circulation in the legs and impair venous return to the heart. The client should be taught to avoid garters or knee-high socks for similar reasons.

Immobilized persons should be encouraged to elevate their legs several times each day for 20 minutes and to do five or six full ROM exercises of the ankles every hour to improve peripheral venous circulation. They should also be warned not to massage their calves. If a thrombus is present, massaging could dislodge it.

A thrombus suspected in a client's leg must be reported immediately. The client's leg should be elevated and the client prevented from ambulating, exercising, or massaging the leg. These activities could dislodge the thrombus, enabling it to migrate upward in the circulation, for example to the heart or lungs.

Respiratory Problems

Nursing interventions for the respiratory system focus on increasing alveolar expansion, preventing stasis of respiratory secretions, maintaining a patent airway, and promoting adequate exchange of gases in the alveoli.

Deep-breathing and coughing exercises Performing deep-breathing and coughing exercises is an effective way to achieve all four goals for the respiratory system. See Chapter 41. A *fluid intake* of at least 2,000 ml per day is essential for liquifying lung secretions and making them easier to expectorate.

Diaphragmatic-abdominal breathing exercises Diaphragmatic-abdominal breathing exercises help decrease the amount of trapped, stagnant air in the alveoli and reduce the effort of breathing. While lying on the back, the client watches the abdomen, rather than the chest, rise with deep inspirations, and fall with slow, forceful contractions of the abdominal muscles. For additional information, see Chapter 41.

Turning, positioning, and exercise Changing the client's position allows previously dependent lung areas to expand and to drain by gravity. Pulmonary secretions in the alveoli, bronchi, and trachea are moved along the respiratory tract to a point where coughing can effectively expel them, reducing the potential for bacterial growth and hypostatic pneumonia. In addition, blood that has pooled in the dependent part of the lung can circulate after the client changes position, reducing the potential for vascular complications. To achieve these results, the client should change position every 1 to 2 hours. Any exercise that moves the chest from one position to another enhances these effects.

Postural drainage, a technique in which the client assumes a variety of postures to promote drainage by gravity from each lobe of each lung, promotes the drainage of respiratory secretions. In addition, the techniques of chest percussion and vibration, which require special skills, may be performed while the client assumes the positions for postural drainage. These techniques help to dislodge respiratory secretions and move them along the respiratory tract to a point where they can be removed by coughing. See Chapter 41.

Metabolic and Nutritional Problems

Diet The immobilized client needs a diet that is high in protein, calories, and fiber. Protein is necessary to replace depleted body protein stores and to repair damaged tissue. Calories provide the fuel needed for energy and tissue repair; energy stores have been depleted by anorexia and by immobility itself. Fiber is needed to prevent or correct the constipation that often accompanies immobility.

Encouraging an anorexic client to eat is a challenge for the nurse. It is important to include (a) easily chewed and swallowed foods so that eating will not tire the client and (b) foods that the client especially enjoys. Favorite items prepared by family members or friends may improve both food intake and morale. Flavorful high-protein, high-calorie dietary supplements between meals are often useful.

Vitamin and mineral supplements Due to the decrease in overall food intake, the immobilized client often has reduced vitamin and mineral stores. The client needs mineral and vitamin supplements, especially those containing vitamin C, to help replace protein stores. It is important not to include excess calcium (and phosphate) because the body will not use this mineral to replace calcium lost from bone unless weight-bearing occurs. Instead, the excess calcium circulates in the blood and is excreted in the urine, increasing the complications caused by calcium loss from bone. Sources of vitamins and minerals include food given at meals, dietary supplements (many high-protein, high-calorie dietary supplements are also high in vitamins and minerals), and multivitamin with mineral tablets ordered by the physician.

Weight-bearing and exercise Weight-bearing is essential for replacing calcium and phosphate in bone. If possible, the nursing plan should include some weight-bearing activity for a few minutes each day. Any form of exercise helps to prevent muscle atrophy and protein loss.

Parenteral and enteral dietary supplements When the client is unable to eat, total parenteral nutrition (TPN), in which nutritional supplements are delivered through a central intravenous catheter, or nasogastric tube feeding, in which nutritional supplements are delivered directly into the gastrointestinal tract, may be necessary to prevent further debilitation and to restore energy levels so that the client can again eat.

Urinary and Endocrine Problems

Turning, repositioning, and exercise Frequent turning and repositioning reduce the amount of stagnant urine in the kidneys and bladder and help to achieve complete kidney and bladder emptying with each urination. Assisting the client to assume an upright sitting or, if possible, standing position several times each day is especially important to counteract the urinary stagnation and incomplete emptying. Exercise enhances this process and strengthens the muscles that control urination.

Improving hydration   Improved hydration is especially important in preventing or reducing the effects of immobility on the urinary tract. Unless the client has a disease process that could be exacerbated by increased fluid intake, he or she should be encouraged to drink 2000 ml or more of fluid each day. Adequate intake increases the volume of urine flushing through the kidneys and bladder, reduces urinary stagnation, and lessens the risk of renal calculi formation and urinary tract infections.

Increased fluid intake, however, can increase the possibility of urinary retention and bladder distention. It is prudent to measure fluid intake and urinary output as well as the frequency and amount of urinations to assess for this potential complication.

If the immobilized client is incontinent, increased intake can make incontinent episodes more frequent. This, in turn, can increase the possibility for skin breakdown in the perineal area. If the client is incontinent, meticulous perineal care is essential to prevent skin breakdown and decubitus ulcer formation.

Perineal hygiene   In any immobilized client, careful perineal hygiene is important in preventing urinary tract infections. Careful cleaning of the perineal area from front to back after each urination and scrupulous personal hygiene with soap and water at least twice daily reduce the likelihood of bladder infection.

Acidifying the urine   Acidifying the urine reduces the potential for both renal calculi formation and urinary tract infections. One can lower urine pH by eating meat, eggs, cheese, whole grains, cranberries, prunes, and plums. Cranberry juice, readily available in most agencies, is effective in lowering urine pH. Foods that increase urine pH, such as carbonated drinks, foods containing baking powder or soda, and fruit juices, should be avoided. The physician may prescribe high doses of ascorbic acid, ammonium chloride, or aspirin to lower urine pH.

Position and relaxation for urination   Nursing measures to facilitate urination, prevent urinary retention and bladder distention, and prevent urinary reflux from a distended bladder are essential in reducing the potential for urinary tract infections. An upright, natural posture during urination is especially important in achieving a normal urination pattern and complete bladder emptying. Enhancing relaxation and providing privacy during urination are also important.

Urinary catheterization   When normal urination is not possible and the client's bladder is distended, catheterization is necessary before distention becomes so pronounced that bladder injury occurs. See Chapter 43.

Preventing urinary incontinence   Urinary incontinence often occurs in immobilized, elderly clients who are dependent on others for assistance with toileting. Incontinence is more likely among clients who do not receive sufficient assistance with urination at sufficiently frequent intervals. Immobilized clients are more likely to be incontinent at night, when they are drowsy and haven't urinated for 4 or 5 hours. Providing sufficient fluid throughout the day so that fluids can be somewhat restricted after the evening meal helps reduce clients' need to urinate at night. Scheduling times for assistance with toileting every 2 hours (somewhat less frequently at night) reduces the incidence of incontinence.

Fecal Elimination Problems   Some of the nursing interventions effective in facilitating urinary elimination are also effective in facilitating fecal elimination.

Movement and exercise   Movement and exercise improve the tone and strength of the abdominal and perineal muscles used in defecation. Movement and exercise improve smooth muscle tone and enhance peristalsis. See Chapter 42 for further interventions to promote bowel evacuation.

Integumentary Problems   See the following section on pressure sores.

Neurosensory Problems

Turning, repositioning, and exercise   All movement increases motor activity and stimulates the proprioceptive sense organs.

Increasing tactile stimuli   Any activity that increases stimulation and use of the tactile sensory organs is useful in preventing sensory deterioration or reducing its severity. Increasing client independence in ADLs and encouraging recreational and social activities that provide tactile stimulation are especially useful.

Social, Emotional, Intellectual, and Developmental Problems   The social, emotional, intellectual, and developmental problems associated with immobility usually occur gradually and subtly. The skills of a perceptive, sensitive, knowledgeable, and caring nurse are needed to prevent or minimize their consequences.

Social   Social stimulation and interaction help to prevent withdrawal of the immobilized client. If possible, an immobilized client should share a room with a mobile, active person who has a similar life-style and values. If possible, the same group of nurses should care for the client throughout the hospital stay. Nurses and roommates who are honestly interested in the client as a person foster positive social interaction.

It is important, however, to promote positive relationships with family members, friends, coworkers, or others whose social contact the client values. The nurse encourages visits by the client's clergy or employer and, when possible, by the client's children or pets. Such visits are reassuring and reinforce a positive perception of the client's role in the family and work group. When visitors arrive, it is important to make them feel welcome. Chairs and privacy should be graciously provided. The nurse may also supply a telephone and letter-writing materials.

Emotional Assisting an immobilized client to maintain a self-image as a worthwhile, independent, and productive individual is important. When possible, clients should be encouraged to attend to their own hygiene and wear their house clothes rather than institutional clothing or night clothes, which foster a dependent, sick-role image. Attention to appearance—e.g., dentures, shaving, or wearing cosmetics—enhances self-image. It is especially important to encourage the client to become as independent in ADLs as possible. Placing toilet and personal items within easy reach increases the client's sense of independence. Demonstrating respect for the client's privacy and belongings helps to promote the client's self-image as a worthwhile person.

Helping the immobilized client to set realistic short- and long-term goals for recovery and to make rational plans for working toward these goals is a useful way to bolster the client's self-image and feelings of personal worth. The nurse should provide opportunities for clients to make choices and decisions about their own care and to solve problems and make plans for their own future during recovery.

Frequent interruptions in normal sleep patterns are tiring and predispose the immobilized client to anxiety, depression, or disorientation. It is important to plan nursing activities to minimize the interruption of sleep during the night.

When the client provides cues of potential problems, the nurse should, in a nonjudgmental, accepting, and supportive manner, encourage the client to express feelings and concerns about immobility, disease, dependent status, finances, work, family, and sexuality. The nurse must be a good listener. The nurse should also encourage the client to discuss these feelings with family members, close friends, or others whose judgment the client values. If cues suggest that the client is experiencing difficulty in coping, outside professional assistance and referral may be needed.

Intellectual Magazines, newspapers, books, television, and radio help immobile clients maintain intellectual capabilities. A project from home or work not only stimulates

intellectual activity but also helps the client to achieve worthwhile, productive tasks that foster independence and feelings of self-worth.

Nurses strive to maintain client orientation and prevent disorientation, especially when the immobilized client is elderly. A clock with a large dial, a calendar marked so that the client can immediately determine the correct day, and a daily newspaper are useful in preventing disorientation related to time, day, or date. To prevent disorientation of person or place, the nurse frequently addresses the client by name, consistently reorients the client to the names of staff, and provides explanations about impending nursing activities, meal times, and other activities. Encouraging the client to wear a hearing aid, glasses, or contact lenses, if needed, helps to reduce sensory distortions.

Developmental It is probably unrealistic to expect anyone of any age to continue making progress toward their developmental tasks during a period of immobility.

With children, it is especially important to stimulate social and intellectual development so that they will not lose ground in achievements made prior to the period of immobility. When possible, the nurse should place the immobilized child with more active children of the same age or provide opportunities to socialize with other children. Play activities sharpen fine motor and intellectual skills. Family members can help by providing favorite games, toys, and books. The nurse can encourage visits from the child's teacher or friends, and, if the child's health permits, the teacher can assign schoolwork. Of course, every opportunity for visits from the child's parents must be provided. Involving children in decisions about their own care also fosters intellectual development.

Preventing and Treating Pressure Sores

Prevention Preventive measures to reduce the risks of pressure sore development include manipulation of the environment, ongoing assessment, proper positioning and nutrition, meticulous hygiene, and instruction in preventing pressure sores. The nurse manipulates the environment when making the client's bed, providing a smooth, firm, wrinkle-free foundation on which the client can lie. Some clients may require a special mattress, such as an alternating pressure, egg crate, or flotation mattress (available for beds and wheelchairs), to decrease pressure on body parts. See Table 35–9.

Using foam rubber pads and artificial sheepskins under pressure areas, such as the sacrum and heels, and elevating the heels above the bed surface decrease the likelihood that pressure sores will develop. Urine passes through artificial sheepskins, whereas real sheepskins retain urine. Thus, artificial sheepskins are preferred, especially for incontinent clients.

The nurse can reduce friction by applying a thin layer of cornstarch to the bedsheet or wheel chair seat cover. Shear-

TABLE 35–9 *Mechanical Devices for Preventing and Treating Pressure Sores*

Device	Description/Comments
Alternating pressure mattress	Composed of a number of cells in which the pressure alternately increases and decreases; utilizes a pump
Foam mattress	Foam molds to the body
Air-fluidized bed	Provides uniform support; controls temperature and humidity
Low air loss (LAL) bed	Supports the client and reduces amount of air required; utilizes a pump; provides very low pressure; controls temperature
Water bed	Special mattress filled with water; controls temperature of water
Egg crate mattress	Polyurethane foam mattress resembling an egg crate; some types are flammable
Gel flotation pads	Polyvinyl, silicone, or Silastic pads filled with a gelatinous substance similar to fat
Sheepskins (natural and artificial)	Some manufacturers produce mixed natural and synthetic pads; artificial pads are less likely to be damaged by washing but are more likely to make the client hot than natural skins
Air or foam rings	Limit blood supply to the area
Cushions (foam, gel and air, foam and fluid)	Some have cutouts for the pressure points
Heel protectors (sheepskin boots, padded splints, foam wedges)	Limit pressure on heels when client is in bed

ing force can be reduced by elevating the head of the bed of bedfast clients no more than 30° if this position is not contraindicated by the client's condition (e.g., clients with respiratory disorders may find it easier to breathe in a Fowler's position).

Ongoing assessment is essential in preventing pressure sores. Every interaction with a client is an opportunity to assess developing problems. The nurse needs to be alert to early symptoms of pressure sores, particularly over bony prominences. See Figure 35–6. These symptoms include localized redness or pallor, tenderness, an unpleasant sensation frequently described as burning, coldness, and localized edema. See the assessment guidelines on page 861.

The bedfast client's position should be changed at least every 15 minutes to 2 hours, depending on the client's need, even when a special support mattress is used, so that another body surface bears the weight. Six body positions can usually be used: prone, supine, right and left lateral (side-lying), and right and left Sims's positions. See Chapter 36. Good nutrition, particularly a diet high in protein and vitamin C, is an important preventive measure. Elderly people have increased protein requirements (up to 0.6 g per kg of body weight) to maintain proper nitrogen balance (Kerr et al. 1981, p. 26).

Meticulous nursing attention to client hygiene is another strategy for decreasing the incidence of pressure sores. The client's skin should be kept clean and dry. Damaged skin should be protected from irritation and maceration by urine, feces, sweat, incomplete drying after a bath, soap, and alcohol. Powders (rather than astringents, such as alcohol or witch hazel) are applied to tissues with limited blood flow. Astringents constrict the blood vessels and thus inhibit the supply of blood and essential nutrients to the skin. Powder should be applied sparingly since excessive accumulations may retain moisture, cause clumping and aggravate the problem.

When bathing the client, the nurse avoids massaging bony prominences with soap. The alkalis in soap cause the skin to swell, dry, and lose its natural oils. In addition, prolonged exposure to soap alters the pH of the skin, one of its natural defense barriers (Kerr et al. 1981, p. 25). Superfatted soaps and oils may be used. Vigorous massage over bony prominences should be avoided, since it increases tissue damage in deep ulcers that are not apparent to the eye (Kerr et al. 1981, p. 24). Pressure areas are massaged gently and only if there is no evidence of underlying tissue damage. After a bath dry skin areas are lubricated to prevent cracking.

Client teaching is another effective strategy in preventing pressure sores. The nurse teaches clients to be aware of discolored areas and of sensations such as tingling, which can indicate pressure, and to report changes in color or sensation promptly. The client needs to know that frequent shifts in position, even if only slight, effectively change the pressure point. The nurse encourages the client to change

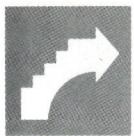

CLINICAL GUIDELINES
Treating Pressure Sores

- Clean the pressure sore daily, preferably in a whirlpool bath. The warmth and mechanical action of the whirlpool promotes circulation, decreases pressure on soft tissues, and helps debride the ulcer.

- Clean and dress the sore using surgical asepsis. Refrain from using antiseptics, such as alcohol, which are vasoconstrictors and reduce blood flow to the area.

- If the pressure sore **is not infected, cover it** with an occlusive dressing, e.g., Opsite, and leave the wound undisturbed for several days. Covering the sore with an occlusive-dressing prevents microorganisms from entering it, and leaving the sore undisturbed promotes healing.

- If the pressure sore **is infected, obtain a sample** of the drainage for culture and sensitivity to antiseptic agents.

- Minimize direct pressure on the sore. Reposition the client at least every 2 hours. Make a schedule and record position changes on the client's chart.

- Reduce friction by applying a small amount of cornstarch to the bedsheet.

- Reduce shearing force by keeping the head of the bed flat or elevated to a maximum of 30° unless contraindicated by the client's condition.

- If the client cannot keep weight off the pressure sore, **use a special mattress** or pad. See Table 35–9.

- Teach the client to move, if only slightly, to relieve pressure.

- Encourage ambulation or sitting in a wheelchair if the client's condition permits. See Chapter 36.

- Provide range-of-motion exercises as the client's condition permits.

- Application of topical agents to promote healing and control infection, or both. Examples of these are *Debrisan beads* (small, sterile, porous spheres that readily absorb moisture and exudate), vitamin A and D ointments, and antibiotic ointments such as neomycin (Neosporin) and zinc bacitracin (Polysporin). These agents, however, do not penetrate hard eschar.

- Application of occlusive dressings such as Opsite or a hydrocolloid dressing such as DuoDerm. These dressings maintain high humidity at the wound–dressing interface to enhance healing and provide protection against secondary infection. See the Research Note below.

- **Debridement** of necrotic tissue by surgery, or chemically by an enzymatic agent such as collagenase (Santyl), fibrinolysin, and desoxyribonuclease (Elase), and sutilains (Travase). Use of enzymes requires a physician's order. Because enzymes do not penetrate thick, hard eschar,

RESEARCH NOTE

Is Opsite an Effective Treatment for Decubitus Ulcers?

A comparative study was conducted at Stanford University Medical Center for 1 year to determine a standardized nursing care plan for the treatment of decubitus ulcers. This plan focused on client comfort, rapid healing of the decubitus ulcer, and cost containment.

Two nursing care plans—one using Opsite and the other a traditional method of decubitus care—were devised. Opsite is a self-adhesive transparent polyurethane dressing that seals in the body's normal leukocytes, plasma, and fibrin to promote natural healing. Although the Opsite did not improve healing time, it did significantly reduce the average nursing time required to care for decubitus ulcers and was found to be cost effective.

Implications: Decubitus ulcers are a major problem for both clients and nursing staff because they are painful and time consuming to care for. Preventive measures such as egg crate mattresses, frequent position changes, massage, and adequate nutrition are mandatory for clients confined to bed. When decubitus ulcers occur, these measures, along with Opsite, maintain client comfort and promote healing.

Howard-Kurzuk, G.; Simpson, L.; Palmeri, A. 1985. Decubitus ulcer care: A comparative study. *Western Journal of Nursing Research* 7(1):58–79.

positions often, and, whenever possible, to exercise or ambulate to stimulate blood circulation.

 Treatment Pressure sores are a challenge for nurses because of the number of variables involved (e.g., risk factors, types of ulcers, and degrees of impairment) and because numerous treatment measures are advocated. Existing and potential infection are the most serious complications of pressure sores. Suggested guidelines for treating existing pressure sores are included in the box above.

Treatments of decubitus ulcers may include:

- Irrigations to clean the ulcer. Isotonic saline irrigations are most commonly used and preferred, but in some situations other solutions such as hydrogen peroxide, aluminum acetate (Burow's solution), and acetic acid may be used.

either the eschar is softened for several days or weeks with continuous saline soaks or the eschar is surgically scored or crosshatched to permit the enzyme to penetrate. Once the eschar is softened, it is removed with forceps and scissors. Before applying enzymes, the nurse cleans the ulcer with normal saline to remove old ointment and digested material. The enzyme ointment is applied to only the ulcerated area, since it can irritate normal skin and damage new granulation tissue. Surrounding skin may be protected with zinc oxide, karaya paste, or petroleum jelly. Generally, a moist gauze dressing is applied over the area and covered with a waterproof (e.g., plastic) pad. Ahmed (1980, p. 114) cautions that antiseptics or detergents containing metal ions or acidic substances should not be used in conjunction with enzymes. When debridement is complete (i.e., the wound appears clean), the enzyme ointment is discontinued and other measures are initiated.

■ Stimulation of circulation with massage or specialized equipment such as a whirlpool bath, warm, moist packs, and ultraviolet light.

Treatment of decubitus ulcers is a complex matter, requiring strict surgical asepsis. Very superficial ulcers may heal within a few days; deep, necrotic ulcers may take several months. The nurse must set specific outcome criteria to evaluate the effects of therapy. If after a specified period (e.g., 14 or 21 days) the criteria have not been met, the therapy must be reevaluated.

EVALUATING

At designated intervals, the nurse determines whether the client has achieved the goals and outcome criteria established during the planning phase. To evaluate whether client goals have been achieved, the nurse collects data relevant to the outcome criteria previously established. For instance, the nurse may ask the client to demonstrate specific exercises, measure muscle size, observe the client's activity tolerance when performing self-care activities, measure vital signs before and after exercise and ambulation, auscultate the lungs for absence of adventitious breath sounds, palpate extremities for temperature and edema, ask the client about any discomfort, observe times of fecal elimination, and check fluid balance and laboratory records.

Here are three examples of evaluative statements indicating goal achievement: "The client's thigh muscle is the same size as baseline measurement." "The client's blood pressure remained the same when rising from a lying position to a standing position." "The client's lungs are clear on auscultation."

NURSING CARE PLAN FOR KEVIN ANDREWS

ASSESSMENT DATA

Nursing Assessment
Several weeks ago, Kevin Andrews, a 17-year-old high school gymnast, fell from the parallel bars and fractured his left femur. Kevin has been on bed rest in skeletal traction since the accident. He is quite depressed and bored with the hospital routine of care. Because of painful muscle spasms, he often refuses to be turned or to move voluntarily. His appetite is poor, and he often refuses his hospital meals. He needs encouragement from the nursing staff to cough and deep breathe.

Physical Examination
Height: 175.3 cm (5'9")
Weight: 70 kg (155 lb) on admission
Temperature: 37 C (98.6 F)
Pulse rate: 80 BPM
Respirations: 16 per minute
Blood pressure: 114/70 mm Hg

Diagnostic Data
Chest x-ray film: Negative
Urine: Negative
Hemoglobin: 12.2
Hematocrit: 37%

CARE PLAN

Nursing Diagnosis	Client Goals and Outcome Criteria	Nursing Interventions and Rationales	Evaluation
Impaired physical mobility related to left fractured femur/skeletal traction resulting in decreased muscle strength, weakness, pain, and limitations in range of motion.	Client Goal: Client will regain use and strength of upper and lower limb musculature. Outcome Criteria: ROM exercises of upper limbs and unaffected lower limb are performed by client 3 × daily. Overhead trapeze is used q3 hrs to strengthen muscles in upper limbs by day 3. Supplemental feedings, e.g., milk shakes and eggnogs, are taken 1 × daily. Performs activities of daily living within limitation of skeletal traction.	Assist client with full range of motion to all unaffected joints of extremities 3 or 4 × daily. *Rationale:* ROM exercises help maintain muscle tone and mobility. Teach the client isometric exercises for left lower limb. *Rationale:* Isometric exercises cause muscles to contract without involving joints and help maintain muscle strength and mass. Encourage client to participate in activities of daily living as much as possible. *Rationale:* Independence enhances client's self-esteem and increases muscular activity and strength. Offer client supplemental feedings high in protein and vitamins. *Rationale:* Proteins and vitamins are necessary for bone healing and positive nitrogen balance.	Performs active ROM exercises of upper limbs and unaffected lower limb daily before breakfast, lunch, and dinner. Uses overhead trapeze to strengthen upper limbs at least 5 × daily. Drinks 4 oz of milkshake or eggnog each day after lunch or at bedtime. Participates in his bath each morning and feeds himself 3 × a day.
Potential for injury, infection, thrombus formation, and nerve damage related to skeletal traction and immobility resulting in odors, redness, pain, numbness, and elevated temperature and WBC.	Client Goal: Infection and thrombophlebitis do not occur. Outcome Criteria: Temperature remains normal. Traction site remains free of drainage and odor. Homans' sign remains negative.	Inspect pin insertion site for signs of inflammation. *Rationale:* Skin infection may lead to bone infection. Instruct client not to touch pin insertion sites. *Rationale:* Reduces chance of infection. Use sterile technique when doing site care. *Rationale:* Reduces chance of infection to skin and/or bone. Assess for Homans' sign frequently. *Rationale:* A positive Homans' sign is an indicator of thrombophlebitis. Encourage ROM and involvement with ADLs. *Rationale:* Exercise prevents complications of immobility.	Temperature remains at 37 C. Skin surrounding pin insertion site remains odorless, dry, and intact. Homans' sign is negative.

READINGS AND REFERENCES

SUGGESTED READINGS

Exton-Smith, N. October 1987. The patient's not for turning. *Nursing Times* 83:42–44.

Exton-Smith reviews some studies on pressure sore development. He sees sustained pressure on the tissues as the single most important factor in the development of pressure sores. The first step in prevention is recognizing which patients are at risk. An important aspect of prevention is the provision of support systems, such as the alternating pressure mattress.

Rameizl, P. November/December 1983. CADET: A self-care assessment tool. *Geriatric Nursing* 4:377–78.

CADET, a self-care assessment tool, is an acronym for communication, ambulation, daily activities, excretion, and transfer functions. A technique for scoring each category is included.

Shannon, M. L. October 1984. Five famous fallacies about pressure sores. *Nursing 84* 14:34–41.

Shannon discusses common misconceptions nurses have about pressure sores and gives facts and realistic interventions. Two tables are included: one about determining clients at risk and the other about the effects of nursing interventions on the causes of pressure sores.

Shannon, M. L., and Miller, B. M. May/June 1988. Pressure sore treatment: A case in point. *Geriatric Nursing* 9:154–57.

The authors describe the treatment of pressure sores using hydrocolloid dressing. They describe the advantages and actions of these dressings. A case study illustrates their healing properties.

RELATED RESEARCH

Bergstrom, N.; Braden, B. J.; Laguzza, A.; and Holman, V. July/August 1987. The Braden Scale for predicting pressure sore risk. *Nursing Research* 36:205–210.

Clarke, M., and Kadhom, H. M. May 1988. The nursing prevention of pressure sores in hospital and community patients. *Journal of Advanced Nursing* 13:365–373.

Diekmann, J. M. September/October 1984. Use of a dental irrigating device in treatment of decubitus ulcers. *Nursing Research* 33:303–5.

Goldstone, L. A., and Goldstone, J. September 1982. The Norton score: An early warning of pressure sores? *Journal of Advanced Nursing* 7:419–426.

Howard-Kurzuk, G., Simpson, L. and Palmeri, A. 1985. Decubitus ulcer care: A comparative study. *Western Journal of Nursing Research* 7(1):58–79.

SELECTED REFERENCES

Ahmed, M. C. December 1980. Special report: Choosing the best method to manage pressure ulcers. *Nurses' Drug Alert* 4(15):113–20.

Anthony, D. August 26, 1987. Norton revises risk scores. *Nursing Times* 83:6.

Anthony, D., and Dunn, A. September 1987. Keeping up-to-date on treatments. *Nursing Times* 83:42–44.

Arnell, I. June 1983. Treating decubitus ulcers: Two methods that work. *Nursing 83* 13:50–55.

Baum, L. March 1985. Heed the early warning signs of peripheral vascular disease. *Nursing 85* 15:50–58.

Beller, L. C., and Neunaber, K. L. April 1986. The "simple" Valsalva. *American Journal of Nursing* 86:398–99.

Bergstrom, N.; Braden, B. J.; Laguzza, A.; and Holman, V. July/August 1987. The Braden Scale for predicting pressure sore risk. *Nursing Research* 36:205–210.

Blom, M. F. March/April 1985. Dramatic decrease in decubitus ulcers. *Geriatric Nursing* 6:84–87.

Braden, B. J., Bryant, R. August 1990. Innovations to prevent and treat pressure sores. *Geriatric Nursing* 11:182–86.

Brower, P., and Hicks, D. July 1972. Maintaining muscle function in patients on bedrest. *American Journal of Nursing* 72:1250–53.

Byrne, C. J.; Saxton, D. F.; Pelikan, P. K.; and Nugent, P. M. 1986, *Laboratory tests: Implications for nursing care* 2d ed. Menlo Park, Calif.: Addison-Wesley Publishing Co.

Byrne, N., and Feld, M. April 1984. Preventing and treating decubitus ulcers. *Nursing 84* 14:55–57.

Carpenito, L. J. 1987. Nursing Diagnosis. *Application to Clinical Practice 3d ed.* Philadelphia: J. B. Lippincott Co.

Clarke, M., and Kadhom, H. M. May 1988. The nursing prevention of pressure sores in hospital and community patients. *Journal of Advanced Nursing* 13:365–373.

De Witt, P. E. March 17, 1986. Extra years for extra effort. *Time*, p. 66.

Dimant, J., and Francis, M. E. August 1988. Pressure sore prevention and management. *Journal of Gerontological Nursing* 14:18–25.

Doenges, M. E., Moorhouse, M. F. 1988. *Nurse's Pocket Guide: Nursing Diagnoses with Interventions, 2d ed.* Philadelphia: F. A. Davis Co.

Downs, F. March 1974. Bed rest and sensory disturbances. *American Journal of Nursing* 74:434–38.

Exton-Smith, N. October 21, 1987. The patient's not for turning. *Nursing Times.* 83:42–44.

Exton-Smith, A. N., et al. 1963. A study of factors concerned in the production of pressure sores and their prevention. In *Investigation of geriatric nursing problems in hospitals.* London: The National Corporation for Care of Old People.

Fahey, V. March 1984. An in-depth look at deep-vein thrombosis. *Nursing 84* 14:35–41.

Goldstone, L. A., and Goldstone, J. September 1982. The Norton score: An early warning of pressure sores? *Journal of Advanced Nursing* 7:419–426.

Gordon, M. January 1976. Assessing activity tolerance. *American Journal of Nursing* 76:72–75.

Guttmann, L. 1955. The problem of treatment of pressure sores in patients with spinal paraplegia. *British Journal of Plastic Surgery* 8:196.

Guyton, A. C. 1986. *Textbook of medical physiology:* 7th ed. Philadelphia: W. B. Saunders Co.

Hettinger, T., and Mueller, S. A. 1953. Muskelleistung und Muskeltraining. *Arbeitsphysiologie* 15:111–26.

Hogan, L., and Beland, I. July 1976. Cervical neck syndrome. *American Journal of Nursing* 76:1104–7.

Husian, T. 1953. An experimental study of some pressure effects on tissues, with references to the bed-sore problem. *Journal of Pathology and Bacteriology* 66:347–58.

Kerr, J. C.; Stinson, S. M.; and Shannon, M. L. July/August 1981. Pressure sores: Distinguishing fact from fiction. *Canadian Nurse* 77:23–28.

Kim, M. J., McFarland, G. K., and McLane, A. M. 1989. *Pocket guide to nursing diagnoses,* 3d ed. St. Louis: C. V. Mosby Co.

Kottke, F. J.; and Lehmann, J. F., editors. 1990. *Krusen's handbook of physical medicine and rehabilitation.* 4th ed. Philadelphia: W. B. Saunders Co.

Lederer, J. R., Marculescu, G. L., Mocnik, B., and Seaby, N. 1990. *Care Planning Pocket Guide 3d ed.* Redwood City, Calif.: Addison-Wesley Nursing.

Lindan, O.; Greenway, R. M.; and Piazza, J. M. 1965. Pressure distribution on the surface of the human body, evaluation in lying and sitting positions using a bed of springs and nails. *Archives of Physical Medicine and Rehabilitation* 46:378–85.

Low, A. W. March/April 1990. Prevention of pressure sores in patients with cancer. *Onocology Nursing Forum* 17:179–84.

Lowthian, P. January 20, 1982. A review of pressure sore pathogenesis. *Nursing Times* 78:117–21.

McConnell, E. A. July 1990. Placing your patient in the lateral position. *Nursing 90* 20:65.

Meissner, J. E. September 1980. Evaluate your patient's level of independence. *Nursing 80* 10:72–73.

Milde, F. K. March 1988. Impaired physical mobility. *Journal of Gerontological Nursing* 14:20–24.

Mitchell, P. H., and Laustau, A. 1981. *Concepts basic to nursing.* 3d ed. New York: McGraw-Hill Book Co.

Morley, M. H. July/August 1981. Sixteen steps to better decubitus ulcer care. *Canadian Nurse* 77:29–31.

NANDA approved nursing diagnostic categories for clinical use and testing. Summer 1988, *Nursing Diagnosis Newsletter* 15(1): 1–3.

Norton, D. February 13, 1975. Research and the problem of pressure sores. *Nursing Mirror* 140:65–67.

Norton, D.; McLaren, R.; and Exton-Smith, A. N. 1962. An investigation of geriatric nursing problems in hospital. Edinburgh: Churchill and Livingstone.

Olson, E. V., Johnson, B. J. Thompson, L. F. March 1990. The hazards of immobility. *American Journal of Nursing* 90:43–44, 46–48.

Osborne, S. February 18–24, 1987. A quality circle . . . reducing the incidence of pressure sores. Investigation. *Nursing Times* 83:73, 75–76.

Patrick, M. I., et al., editors. 1986. *Medical-surgical nursing: Pathophysiological concepts.* Philadelphia: J. B. Lippincott Co.

Pieper, B., Mikols, C., Mance, B. et al. February 1990. Nurses' documentation about pressure ulcers. *Decubitus* 3:32–4.

Robertson, D., and Robertson, R. February 1985. Orthostatic hypotension: Diagnosis and therapy. *Modern concepts of cardiovascular disease* 54:1–14.

Shannon, M. L., and Miller, B. M. May/June 1988. Pressure sore treatment: A case in point. *Geriatric Nursing* 9:154–157.

Shea, J. D. October 1975. Pressure sores: Classification and management. *Clinical Orthopedics* 112:89–100.

Smith, B. April 20, 1983. Danger: Points under pressure. *Nursing Mirror* 156:24–27.

Smith, S. E. 1978. Prostaglandins. *Nursing Times* 74(6):231–33.

Spenceley, P. August 10, 1988. Norton V. Waterlow. *Nursing Times* 84:52–53.

Torrance, C. January 15, 1981a. Pressure sores. Part 1. Pathogenesis. *Nursing Times* 77: center pages.

———. February 19, 1981b. Pressure sores. Part 2. Predisposing factors: The "at-risk" patient. *Nursing Times* 77:5–8.

———. March 19, 1981c. Pressure sores. Part 3. Medical management and surgical intervention. *Nursing Times* 77:9–12.

———. April 16, 1981d. Pressure sores. Part 4. Mechanical devices. *Nursing Times* 77:13–16.

———. May 7, 1981e. Pressure sores. Part 5. Topical applications and wound agents. *Nursing Times* 77:17–20.

———. June 18, 1981f. Pressure sores. Part 6. Physical methods. *Nursing Times* 77:21–24.

Tyler, M. L. May 1984. The respiratory effects of body positioning and immobilization. *Respiratory Care* 29:472–83.

Waterlow, J. November 27, 1985. A risk assessment card. *Nursing Times* 81:49, 51, 55.

Watson, R. April 1990. The benefits of excellence: A cost-effective treatment programme for pressure sores. *Professional Nurse.* 5:356, 358, 360+.

Winslow, E. H., and Weber, T. M. March 1980. Progressive exercises to combat the hazards of bedrest. *American Journal of Nursing* 80:440–45.

CHAPTER

36 Activity and Exercise

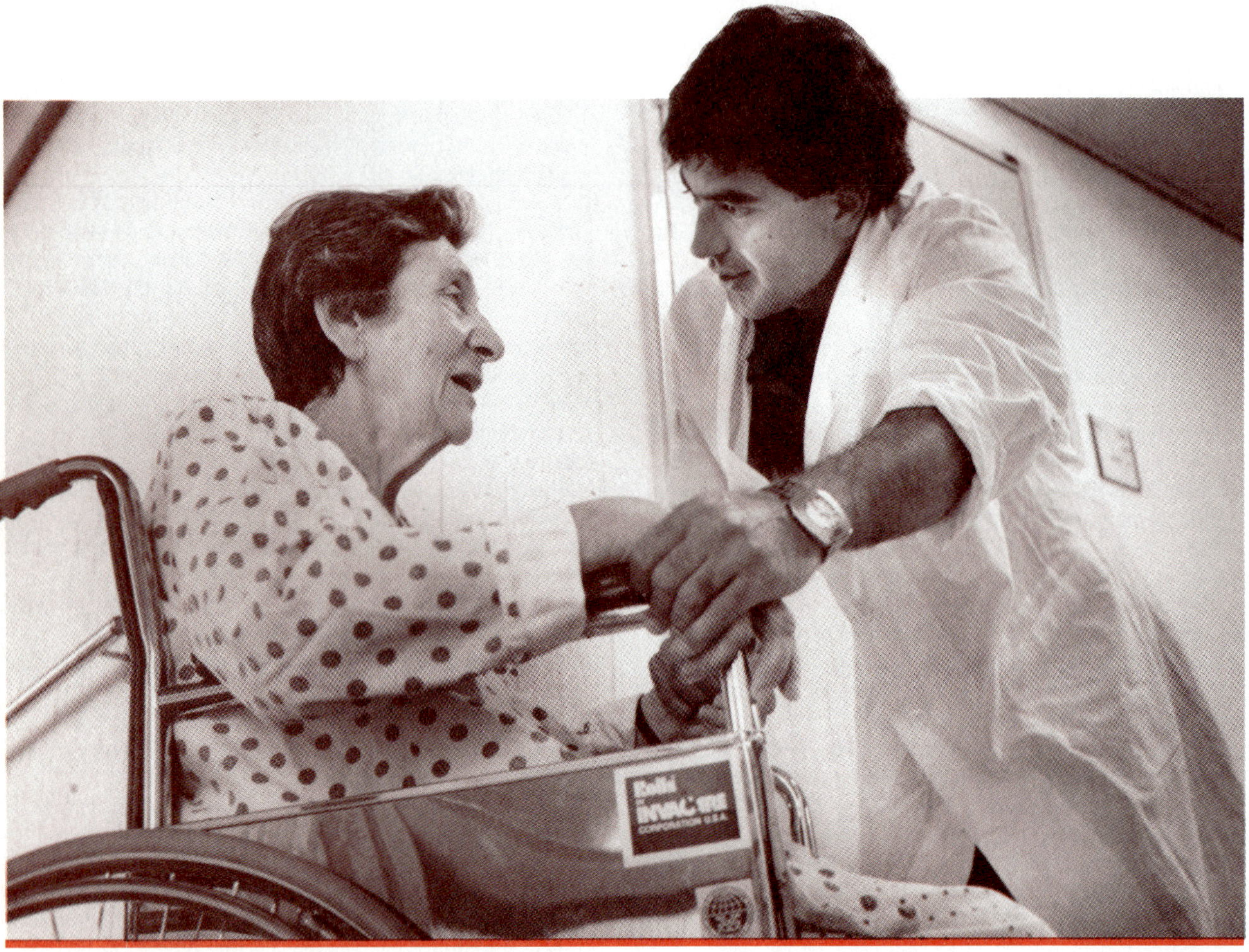

CONTENTS

OBJECTIVES

▸ Identify the importance for both clients and nurses of using good body mechanics.

▸ Describe the importance of good body alignment for clients and nurses.

▸ Describe how musculoskeletal function and voluntary and involuntary muscle and reflex activity affect movement.

▸ Identify factors that influence body mechanics, ambulation, and alignment.

▸ Identify occupational groups at risk of back injury.

▸ Describe ways to prevent back injury.

▸ Identify structural abnormalities that affect body mechanics and ambulation.

▸ Identify ways to determine the client's capabilities and limitations for movement.

▸ Identify criteria used to assess a client's gait.

▸ Describe assessment criteria for the alignment of adults in standing, sitting, and various bed-lying positions.

▸ State nursing diagnoses for clients with alignment and ambulation problems.

▸ State outcome criteria for evaluating client responses to nursing interventions.

▸ Describe nursing interventions to maintain, promote, or restore normal body mechanics, alignment, and ambulation.

▸ Describe how to move and turn a client in bed and to transfer a client between a bed, a chair, or a stretcher.

BODY MECHANICS

Good **body mechanics** is the efficient, coordinated, and safe use of the body to produce motion and maintain balance during activity. Proper movement promotes body musculoskeletal functioning, reduces the energy required to move and maintain balance, therefore reducing fatigue, and decreasing the risk of injury.

The major purpose of proper body mechanics is to facilitate safe and efficient use of appropriate groups of muscles. Good body mechanics is essential to both clients and nurses to prevent strain, injury, and fatigue.

Body mechanics involves three basic elements: Body alignment (posture), balance (stability), and coordinated body movement.

Body Alignment

Body alignment is the geometric arrangement of body parts in relation to each other. Good alignment promotes optimal balance and maximal body function in whatever position the client assumes: standing, sitting, or lying down. Good body alignment and good **posture** are synonymous terms. When the body is well aligned, balance is achieved without undue strain on the joints, muscles, tendons, or ligaments. Muscles are usually in a state of slight tension (**tonus**) when the body is healthy and well aligned. This state requires minimal muscular force and yet supports the internal framework and organs.

Proper body alignment enhances lung expansion and promotes efficient circulatory, renal, and gastrointestinal functions. Conversely, poor body alignment detracts from a pleasing appearance and affects an individual's health adversely. A person's posture is one criterion for assessing general health, physical fitness, and attractiveness. Posture reflects the mood, self-esteem, and personality of an individual.

Balance

Balance is a state of equipoise (equilibrium) in which opposing forces counteract each other. Good body alignment is essential to body balance. It is difficult to differentiate balance from body alignment, although balance is the result of proper alignment. A person maintains balance as long as the **line of gravity** (an imaginary vertical line drawn through an object's center of gravity) passes through the **center of gravity** (the point at which all of the mass of an object is centered) and the **base of support** (the foundation on which an object rests).

The center of gravity of a well-aligned standing adult is located slightly anterior to the upper part of the sacrum.

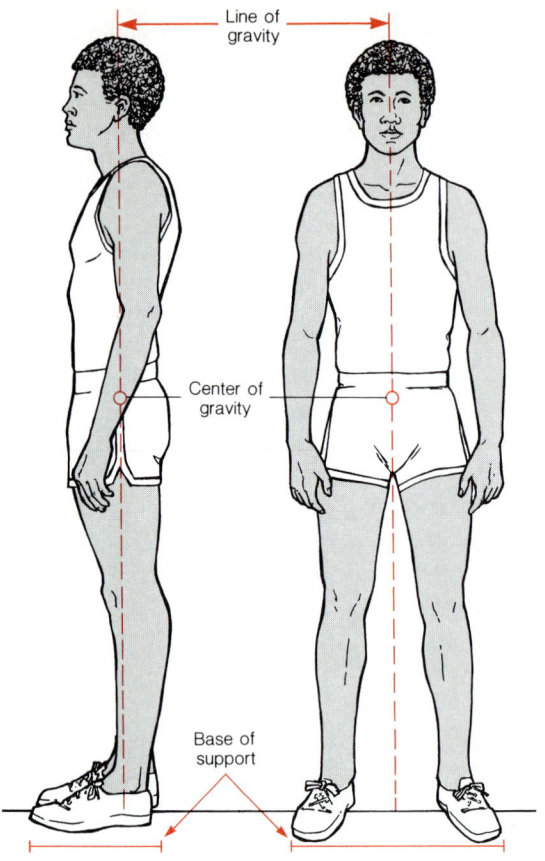

Figure 36–1 The center of gravity and the line of gravity influence standing alignment.

See Figure 36–1. Standing posture can be unstable because of a narrow base of support, a high center of gravity, and a constantly shifting line of gravity. For greatest balance and stability, a standing adult must center body weight symmetrically along the line of gravity.

In a well-aligned standing person, the center of gravity remains fairly stable. When the person moves, however, the center of gravity shifts continuously in the direction of the moving body parts. Balance depends on the interrelationship of the center of gravity, the line of gravity, and the base of support. When a person moves, the closer the line of gravity is to the center of the base of support, the greater his or her stability. See Figure 36–2, A. Conversely, the closer the line of gravity is to the edge of the base of support, the more precarious the balance. See Figure 36–2, B. If the line of gravity falls outside the base of support, the person falls. See Figure 36–2, C.

The broader the base of support and the lower the center of gravity, the greater the stability and balance. Body balance, therefore, can be greatly enhanced by (a) widening the base of support and (b) lowering the center of gravity, bringing it closer to the base of support. The base of support is easily widened by spreading the feet farther apart. The center of gravity is readily lowered by flexing the hips and knees until a squatting position is achieved. The importance of these alterations cannot be overemphasized for nurses.

When a person rests in a chair or bed, the feet of the chair or bed form a considerably wider base of support. The cen-

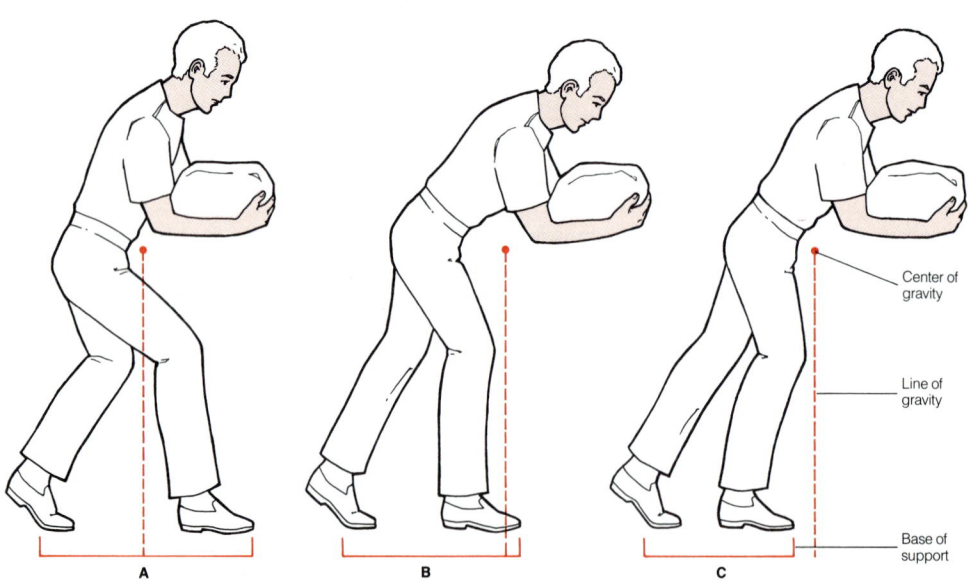

Figure 36–2 A, Balance is maintained when the line of gravity falls close to the base of support. B, Balance is precarious when the line of gravity falls at the edge of the base of support. C, Balance cannot be maintained when the line of gravity falls outside the base of support.

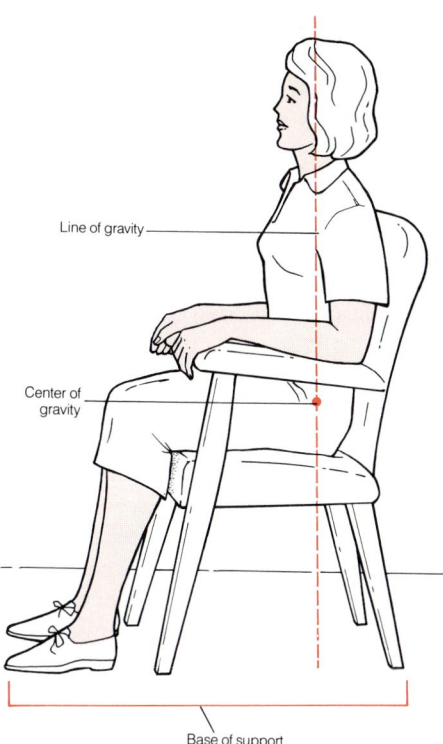

Figure 36–3 A sitting position provides stability through a wide base of support and low center of gravity.

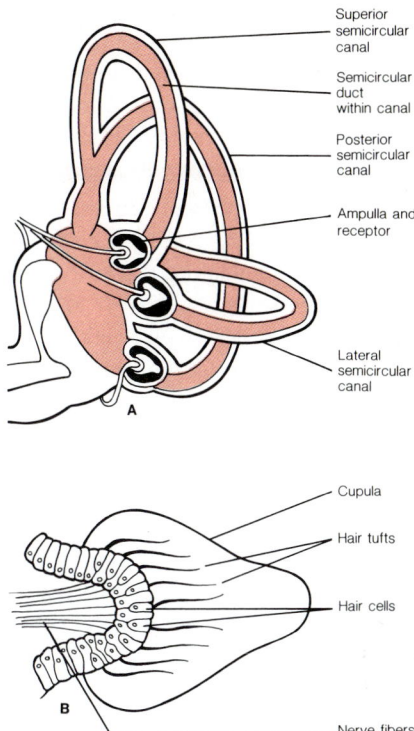

Figure 36–4 The inner ear: A, semicircular canals; B, cupula.

ter of gravity is lower, and the line of gravity is less mobile. Thus, a person has greater stability and balance in a sitting or lying position than in a standing position. See Figure 36–3.

Coordinated Body Movement

Body mechanics involves the integrated functioning of the musculoskeletal and nervous systems. Muscle tone, the neuromuscular reflexes (including the visual and proprioceptive reflexes), and the coordinated movements of opposing voluntary muscle groups (the antagonistic, synergistic, and antigravity muscles) play important roles in producing balanced, smooth, purposeful movement.

Postural Reflexes and Opposing Muscle Groups Continuous action of postural muscles sustains humans in an upright position against the force of gravity. The extensor muscles, often referred to as the antigravity muscles, carry the major load. Sustained contraction of the muscles supporting this upright position is called **postural tonus.** Numerous postural or **righting reflexes** stimulate and maintain postural tonus:

1. *Labyrinthine sense.* Sensory organs of the inner ear stimulate postural tonus through impulses that arise when the head is moved. To maintain balance, the body responds to changes of head position through information received by the cerebellum from receptors in the ampullae of the three semicircular ducts of the inner ear. Each duct contains endolymph, and the three are arranged at right angles to one another. Any body movement is relayed by the endolymph in these ducts to sensory hair cells embedded in a gelatinous, dome-shaped structure called the **cupula.** Stimulation of the hair cells produces nerve impulses that flow along the nerve fibers of the vestibular division of the vestibulocochlear nerve to the brain. See Figure 36–4.

2. *Tonic neck-righting reflexes.* Movement of the head from side to side affects tonic neck reflexes as well as labyrinthine reflexes. Tonus of the neck muscles seems most affected when the head is thrown backward.

3. *Visual or optic reflexes.* Visual impressions are important in maintaining erect posture. Visual sensations help the person establish spatial relationships to objects in the environment.

4. *Proprioceptor or kinesthetic sense.* The kinesthetic sense, sometimes referred to as the sixth sense, is activated when nerve endings in muscles, tendons, and fascia are stimulated by movements of joints. Individuals become aware of their position when the brain is informed of the location of a limb or body part at any given moment.

5. *Extensor or antigravity (stretch) reflexes.* One of the basic elements of posture is the so-called stretch reflex. This reflex is best developed in the extensor muscles, which counteract the tendency of the body to flex at the hip and the knees because of its own weight. If, for example, the knees begin to buckle under the influence of gravity, the extensor muscles of the knee joint are stretched, and their muscle spindles are stimulated. Stimulation results in a reflex contraction of the extensor muscles, which straightens the knee joint and maintains upright posture. Extensor muscles involved in posture include the extensors of the lower extremities, the abdominal muscles, the adductors of the scapulae, and the extensors of the spinal column. Extensors of the spinal column are the site of the spinal stretch reflex.

6. *Plantar reflexes.* Pressure against the sole of the foot by the ground elicits a reflexive contraction of the extensor muscles of the lower legs.

Structures in the cerebral cortex, midbrain, brain stem, cerebellum, and spinal cord regulate and control these reflexes. Postural reflexes enable opposing muscle groups to work together automatically to coordinate the delicate muscle movements required to maintain upright posture, body alignment, and balance. When the flexors contract to bend a joint, the extensors relax; when the extensors contract to straighten a joint, the flexors relax.

Whenever the line of gravity moves away from the center of the base of support, muscles on the side of the body opposite the direction of movement contract to bring the body back into alignment. Whenever the line of gravity shifts away from the center of the base of support, the energy required to maintain balance is increased. Constant muscle activity to maintain balance and to prevent instability and falling contributes to increased energy expenditure and muscle fatigue. Good posture reduces the number of muscle contractions needed to maintain balance by dividing the work evenly among opposing muscle groups.

Voluntary Muscle Activity

The cerebellum coordinates all voluntary muscle activity, especially that involved in the complex movements. Skeletal muscle activity is initiated in the cerebral cortex. Most motor nerves descend and cross over in the area of the medulla to the spinal cord, traveling through efferent (outward) pathways to the muscles, where purposeful movement is produced.

Most skeletal muscle movement is a combination of isotonic and isometric contraction (see Chapter 35). At the initiation of movement, an isometric contraction occurs. When enough tension is achieved, an isotonic contraction occurs to produce movement. The preparatory isometric contraction, during which muscle tension is greatly increased, is especially important prior to lifting. The greater this preparatory isometric tensing, the less the energy required to lift an object.

The larger muscles of the lower extremities and the muscles of the abdomen and back all produce movement by leverage and synchronized action. The flexors of the legs, and to a lesser degree the leg extensors, are the largest and strongest muscles in the body.

PRINCIPLES OF BODY MECHANICS

The concepts of center of gravity, line of gravity, and base of support were discussed earlier in relation to body alignment and balance. In addition to these concepts, the nurse needs to consider the concepts of **leverage, force, friction,** and **inertia** when moving clients or objects. These concepts are defined and discussed in Tables 36–1 and 36–2.

Two movements to avoid because of their potential for causing back injury are twisting (rotation) of the thoracolumbar spine and acute flexion of the back with hips and knees straight (stooping). Undesirable twisting of the back can be prevented by squarely facing the direction of movement, whether pushing, pulling, or sliding, and moving the object directly toward or away from one's center of gravity.

Lifting

When a person lifts or carries an object, the weight of the object becomes part of the person's body weight. This weight affects the location of the person's center of gravity, which
(continued on page 888)

TABLE 36–1 *Concepts Applicable to Moving Clients*

Concept	Definition
Friction	Force that opposes the motion of an object as it is slid across the surface of another object.
Force	The energy or power required to accomplish movement.
Inertia	The tendency of an object at rest to remain at rest and an object in motion to remain in motion.
Fulcrum	A fixed point (e.g., elbow) about which a lever moves.
Lever (first class)	A rigid piece that transmits or modifies motion or force. When force (energy) is applied to the rigid arm with a fixed point (fulcrum), an object at the other end of the rigid arm can be lifted more easily.

TABLE 36–2 *Summary of Principles and Guidelines Related to Body Mechanics*

Principles	Guidelines
Balance is maintained and muscle strain is avoided as long as the line of gravity passes through the base of support.	Start any body movement with proper alignment.
	Stand as close as possible to the object to be moved.
	Avoid stretching, reaching, and twisting, which may place the line of gravity outside the base of support.
The wider the base of support and the lower the center of gravity, the greater the stability.	Before moving objects, increase your stability by widening your stance and flexing your knees, hips, and ankles.
Objects that are close to the center of gravity are moved with the least effort.	Adjust the working area to waist level, and keep the body close to the area.
	Elevate adjustable beds and overbed tables or lower the side rails of beds to prevent stretching and reaching.
Balance is maintained with minimal effort when the base of support is enlarged in the direction in which the movement will occur.	When *pushing* an object, enlarge the base of support by moving the front foot forward.
	When *pulling* an object, enlarge the base of support by either moving the rear leg back if facing the object or moving the front foot forward if facing away from the object.
The greater the preparatory isometric tensing, or contraction of muscles, before moving an object, the less the energy required to move it, and the less the likelihood of musculoskeletal strain and injury.	Before moving objects, contract your gluteal, abdominal, leg, and arm muscles to prepare them for action.
The synchronized use of as many large muscle groups as possible during an activity increases overall strength and prevents muscle fatigue and injury.	To move objects below your center of gravity, begin with the back and knees flexed. Use your gluteal and leg muscles rather than the sacrospinal muscles of your back to exert an upward thrust when lifting the weight.
	Distribute the work load between both arms and legs to prevent back strain.
	Always face the direction of the movement to prevent twisting of the spine and ineffective use of major muscle groups.
The closer the line of gravity to the *center* of the base of support, the greater the stability.	When moving or carrying objects, hold them as close as possible to your center of gravity.
	Pull an object toward you whenever possible rather than pushing it away to control its movement and keep it close to your center of gravity.
The greater the friction against the surface beneath an object, the greater the force required to move the object.	Provide a firm, smooth, dry bed foundation before moving a client in bed.
Pulling creates less friction than pushing.	Pull clients rather than push them whenever possible.
The heavier an object, the greater the force needed to move an object.	Encourage clients to assist as much as possible by pushing or pulling themselves to reduce the muscular effort of the nurse.
	Use arms as levers whenever possible to increase lifting power.
	Use own body weight to counteract the weight of the object. For example, lean forward when pushing an object, and rock your body weight backward when pulling an object or client toward you.
	Obtain the assistance of other persons or use mechanical devices to move objects that are too heavy.
Moving an object along a level surface requires less energy than moving an object up an inclined surface or lifting it against the force of gravity.	Avoid working against gravity.
	Pull, push, roll, or turn objects instead of lifting them.
	Lower the head of the client's bed before moving the client up in bed.
Continuous muscle exertion can result in muscle strain and injury.	Alternate rest periods with periods of muscle use to help prevent fatigue.

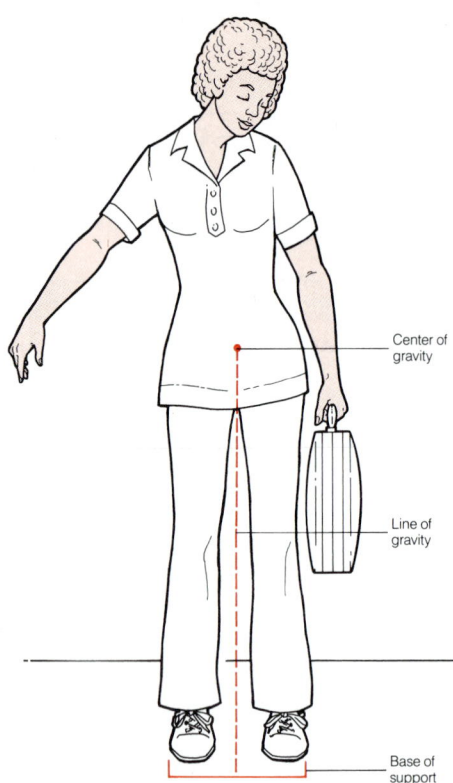

Figure 36–5 Body parts move in the direction opposite the weight to compensate for it and maintain the center of gravity over the base of support.

is displaced in the direction of the added weight. To counteract this potential imbalance, body parts move in a direction away from the weight. In this way, the center of gravity is maintained over the same point in the base of support. See Figure 36–5. By holding the center of gravity of the lifted object as close as possible to the body's center of gravity, the lifter avoids undue displacement of the center of gravity and achieves greater stability.

Although there are three types of levers, the type nurses use most frequently in lifting is the third class lever. See Figure 36–6, *A*. In the body the joints are the fulcrums and the bones of the skeleton act as levers. The force, or effort, provided by muscle contraction is applied where a muscle attaches to bone. When the nurse lifts objects, the resisting force or weight is held in the hands or on the forearms, the fulcrum is the elbow, and the force is applied by contraction of the flexor muscles of the forearm. See Figure 36–6, *B*. The lifting power is increased when the elbow (fulcrum) is supported on a bed surface or a countertop. People can lift more weight when they use this lever than when they do not. Use of the arms as levers is often applied in clinical practice when the nurse needs to raise the head or buttocks of a client in bed, e.g., to assist the client onto a bedpan or to give back care to a client in traction. Figure 36–7 illustrates this lifting technique.

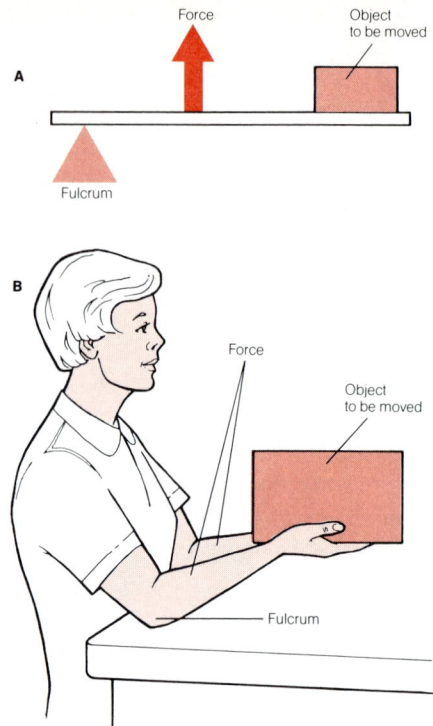

Figure 36–6 A, A third-class lever; B, Using the arm as a lever.

Because lifting involves movement against gravity, the nurse must use major muscle groups of the thighs, knees, upper and lower arms, abdomen, and pelvis to prevent back strain. The nurse can increase overall muscle strength by synchronized use of as many muscle groups as possible during an activity. For instance, when the arms are used in an activity, dividing the work between the arms and legs helps to prevent back strain. Lifting power is further enhanced by using the nurse's body weight to counteract the client's weight. The nurse increases hip and knee flexion to lower the center of gravity. As the nurse does so, the forearms and hands supporting the client automatically rise. See Figure 36–7, *C* and *D*.

Nursing personnel often lift objects from the floor and assume a bending position, e.g., when helping persons to put on slippers, placing foot pedals down on wheelchairs, picking up laundry and isolation bags, picking up toddlers, and lifting supplies from the bottom shelves of carts. The ordinary person can lift only about 20 pounds of weight without danger of back strain when a lever is not used. When the weight to be lifted exceeds 35% of body weight, the lifter must use mechanical devices or seek the assistance of other persons (Owen 1980, p. 896).

Three commonly used lifting techniques are described by Davies (1978, p. 176):

1. The *kinetic method,* which entails almost full flexion of the hips and knees with the feet parallel and not necessarily apart

(continued on page 890)

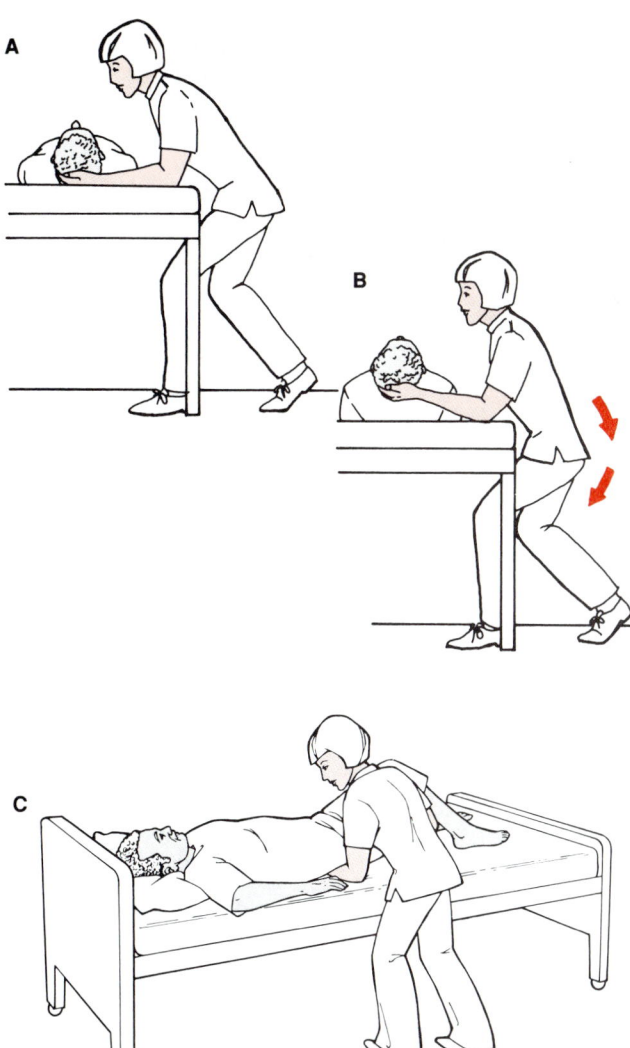

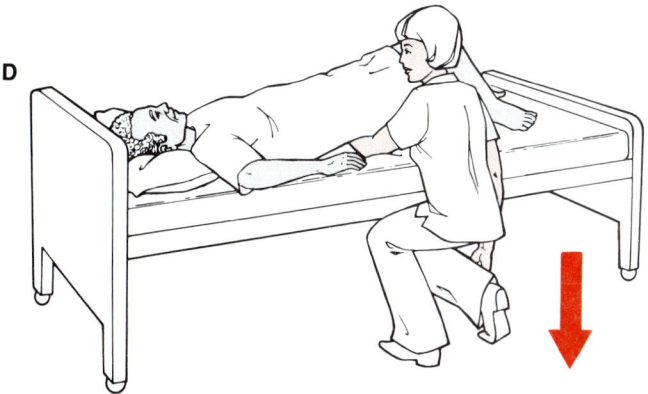

Figure 36–7 This nurse uses her arms as levers and employs her body weight to lift a client. A, Position before lifting; B, Position after lifting; C and D, The nurse uses positions A and B to lift a client's buttocks.

RESEARCH NOTE

What Lifting Method Is Desirable?

Owens conducted a study to discover the relationship of selected aspects of the lifting process to the occurrence of back injury in hospital nursing personnel. The sample consisted of 64 nurses divided into two groups: the group with back injuries (B1) and the group without back injuries (NB1), each group consisting of 21 registered nurses and 11 nursing assistants. Ages ranged from 21 to 64 years.

The subjects were asked to demonstrate their skill in lifting by picking up a 16-inch square, 15-pound box without handles from the floor and placing it on a table that stood about waist level approximately 6 feet away from the box. The lifting technique of each subject was recorded on camera, and the thirteen measurements relating to the lifting posture were taken (with the aid of a computer). Measurements taken as the box was being lifted from the floor included the *angle of flexion* (a) of the back, (b) between the abdomen and thigh, (c) of the knees, and (d) of each foot (if not flat on the floor); *three distances* (a) how far the feet were apart, (b) how far one foot was in front of each other, and (c) how far the box was from the body; and the *location of the hands* on the box. Measurements taken while the box was at knee level included the angle of flexion of (a) the back, (b) the feet, and (c) the knees and the distance of the box from the body.

Significant differences were found between the B1 and NB1 groups in (a) the distance the feet were apart during the lift (more NB1 subjects stood with feet further apart then the B1 group); (b) the distance of the load from the body when the box was lifted to the knee level (NB1 subjects pulled the load in closer to their bodies); (c) the angle of back flexion when the box was at floor level (no subjects lifted with a completely straight vertical back; fewer NB1 subjects, however, used the bent-over technique, and more used a variation between the straight back, flexed knees, and bent-over technique); and (d) the distance one foot was in front of the other during the lift (NB1 subjects stood with one foot slightly farther in front of the other than the B1 group).

Implications: This study shows that some lifting techniques are important in preventing back injury and that the position for lifting that has been advocated for decades (straight back and acutely flexed knees) may not even be achievable or desirable.

B. D. Owen, The lifting process and back injury in hospital nursing personnel, *Western Journal of Nursing Research*, November 1985, 7:445–49.

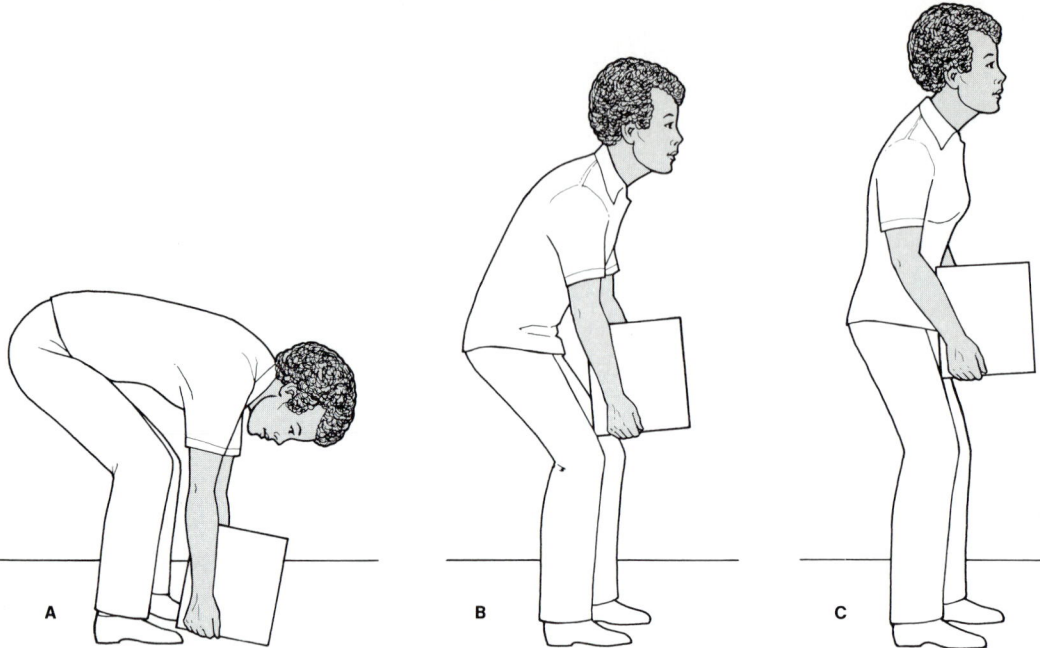

A   B   C

Figure 36–8 Stages in lifting an object to the waist: A, Move close to the object, and begin with the back and knees flexed to grasp the object. B, Start the lift by keeping the back flexed while the knees begin to straighten so that the leg muscles can exert an upward thrust. C, Keep the back and knees in a less flexed but not straight position (Owen 1980, p. 895).

2. The *straight-back and bent-knees* method, which involves squatting and lifting with the total burden on the leg and thigh muscle groups while the back is straight and vertical

3. The *bend-over* or *freestyle* lift, in which the back is stooped and hyperflexed and the knees are only slightly flexed

Traditionally, nurses have been taught the straight-back and bent-knees method as the proper lifting technique to avoid any exertion on the lumbar muscle groups. However, this method ignores the principle of balance, since the only way balance could be maintained was to straighten the legs and flex the back or lose balance and fall. In addition, with consistent use of this method, back muscles became weakened from little use; consequently, simple tasks such as bending over to remove something from a drawer or bending over the sink to brush the teeth could cause strain on the lumbar muscles.

A newer technique based on the principle of leverage is now being recommended. In this technique, the back and knees are flexed until the load is at thigh level, at which point the knees are flexed more to provide thrust as the back begins to straighten (Owen 1980, p. 895). See Figure 36–8. This technique provides for better balance, leverage, and synchronized use of muscles, which help to avoid back pain and injury. When one lifts an object to knee level, the shoulder and arm muscles pull, the abdominal and lumbar muscles contract for leverage and pull, and the thigh and leg muscles exert the upward thrust to bring the object off

the floor. When one lifts an object from mid-thigh to waist level, force is provided essentially by the leg and thigh muscle groups, but the back and lumbar muscles remain contracted.

In all positions, it is important to maintain a distance of at least 30 cm (12 in) between the feet and to keep the load close to the body, especially when it is at knee level (Owen 1985, p. 457). Before attempting the lift, the nurse must ensure that there are no hazards on the floor, that there is a clear path for moving the object, and that the nurse's base of support is secure.

Pulling and Pushing

When pulling or pushing an object, a person maintains balance with least effort when the base of support is enlarged in the direction in which the movement is to be produced or opposed. For example, when pushing an object, a person can enlarge the base of support by moving the front foot forward. When pulling an object, a person can enlarge the base of support by (a) moving the rear leg back if the person is facing the object; or (b) moving the front foot forward if the person is facing away from the object. It is easier and safer to pull an object toward one's own center of gravity than to push it away, as the person can exert more control of the object's movement when pulling it.

Friction can be reduced by sliding the object on a smooth, clean, dry, firm surface, in contrast to a rough, wet, or soiled surface. To reduce friction when moving (sliding) a client up in bed, for example, the nurse provides a smooth, dry, firm bed foundation. It is preferable to pull rather than push a client along the surface of a bed because pushing compresses the client's vertebrae and creates discomfort. Also, pulling creates less friction than pushing, since the nurse must pull at an upward angle that reduces friction between the client and the bed. Friction can be further avoided by rolling, rather than pushing or pulling, the person. Because of inertia, the nurse must use more force to put an object into motion than to keep it in motion. The heavier the object, the greater the force required to put it into motion. To move an object efficiently, the nurse applies force directly toward or against the object's center of gravity and in the direction in which the movement is to occur. Use of the nurse's body weight in a rocking motion applies additional force or leverage. This counteracts the object's inertia and reduces the energy required to start the pulling, pushing, or lifting movement.

Proper use of body mechanics to pull objects is shown in Figure 36–9.

Pivoting

Pivoting is a technique in which the body is turned in a way that avoids twisting of the spine. To pivot, place one foot ahead of the other, raise the heels very slightly, and put the body weight on the balls of the feet. When the weight is off the heels, the frictional surface is decreased and the knees are not twisted when turning. Keeping the body aligned, turn (pivot) about 90° in the desired direction. The foot that was forward will now be behind.

FACTORS THAT INFLUENCE BODY MECHANICS AND AMBULATION

General health, nutrition, emotions, situational factors, habits, life-style, attitudes, values, level of understanding, and neuromusculoskeletal impairments are some of the factors that influence body mechanics, body alignment, and ambulation.

General Health   The client's general health status is reflected in how the individual usually moves about. Illness, disability, immobility, inactivity, poor physical fitness, and chronic fatigue have unfavorable effects on musculoskeletal function.

Nutrition   Adequate nutrition supplies vitamins and minerals essential for normal bone and muscle function. It also supplies glucose that powers muscle. Poor nutrition may cause muscle weakness and fatigue. An inadequate calcium intake increases an older woman's risk of painful compression fractures of the vertebrae. Obesity distorts movement, and the obese person must expend extra energy to move and maintain balance.

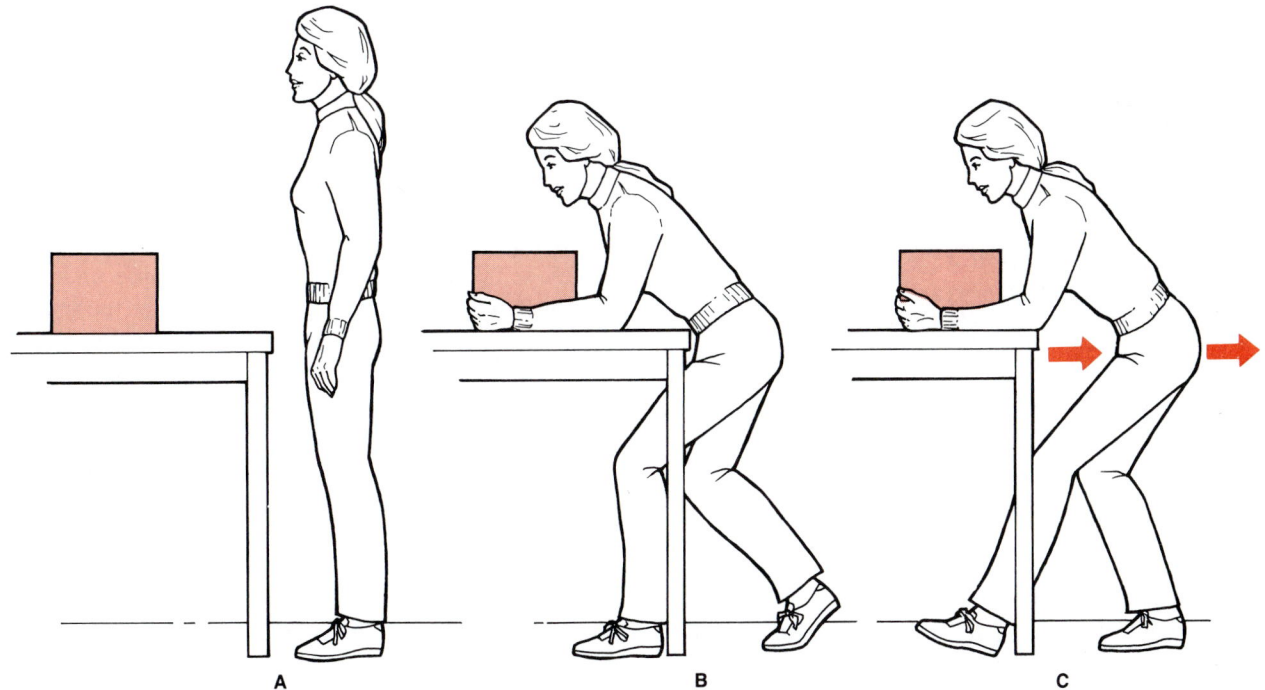

Figure 36–9   Schematic of proper body mechanics applied to pulling. A, Load to be pulled rests on a surface about as high as the person's center of gravity. B, The base of support is enlarged, the body is flexed, and the muscles are tensed for action. C, The weight is shifted toward the rear leg as the load is pulled toward the person.

Emotions   The client's emotional state may influence posture and ways of moving about. Security, joy, confidence, and self-esteem are reflected in the use of good body mechanics and gait. Worry, discouragement, insecurity, and poor self-esteem are often reflected in the use of poor body mechanics.

Situational Factors or Habits   People can develop poor body mechanics and gait from situational factors or habits, such as the following:

- Frequent twisting of the back in work or daily activities, such as driving a truck or loading or unloading a dishwasher
- Frequent lifting of heavy loads in work or daily activities, such as stocking shelves or carrying small children
- Frequent stooping in work or daily activities, such as housework or gardening
- Frequent pulling or pushing of heavy loads in work or daily activities, such as moving furniture
- Frequent moving of items stored in low or high areas to waist-level work areas
- Walking on slick or uneven surfaces, which predispose the person to falls
- Wearing tight clothing that restricts freedom of movement
- Wearing shoes with uneven or slick soles or high heels, which predispose the wearer to falls

People can also develop poor posture due to situational causes, such as the following:

- Soft beds with sagging springs, which disrupt the appropriate distribution of weight
- Chairs not adjusted to body height and build or tables, desks, and working equipment placed so that the person must strain to work at them
- Shoes that are worn down at the heels and tilt the body out of line and/or constant wearing of high-heeled shoes, which exaggerate the forward tilt of the body
- Bifocal eyeglasses, because the person may need to make abnormal adjustments in head alignment to see clearly.

Life-Style   An individual's life-style can affect posture and mobility. Postures repeatedly assumed during work can result in permanent postural defects; for example, a mail carrier may walk for years leaning to one side from carrying a heavy bag, or an assembly line worker may sit for hours hunched over a bench. Repeated physical activity, e.g., by a weight lifter, can produce muscle hypertrophy and concomitant alignment changes to accommodate the hypertrophy. Continual inactivity and resulting poor physical fitness can produce muscle atrophy and concomitant alignment changes to accommodate the atrophy, possibly resulting in back injuries. Repeatedly performed movements, especially twisting or bending of the back, can result in permanent disability. Repeatedly walking on slippery or uneven surfaces can result in disabling falls. The person who leads an overly busy, stressful, and active life can become careless and is at risk of injury.

Personal Values   Personal values about body alignment and the use of good body mechanics are important influences. Tall adolescents may slouch because they do not value being taller than peers. Some people value good posture and intentionally try to maintain body alignment for reasons of health or appearance. Persons who value their appearance and health are more likely to practice good body mechanics and gait to protect their backs and prevent falls.

Level of Understanding About Body Mechanics   An understanding of the elements of good alignment is conducive to good posture. An understanding of the elements of good body mechanics usually encourages its use. Unfortunately, many individuals either have no opportunity to learn correct habits, are misinformed, or have forgotten what they once learned.

Neuromuscular and Skeletal Impairments
Diseases and injuries that affect the neuromuscular or skeletal systems can severely hinder movement. Genetically transmitted muscle-wasting diseases, disorders causing sensory or motor impairment, inflammatory conditions, injuries, and pain can severely impair movement. Damage from injury or disease to any part of the neuromuscular or skeletal systems increases the risk of potential or actual impairment of movement. Many disorders produce pain, often severe, that further limits movement.

Osteoporosis, a condition in which the bones become brittle and fragile due to calcium depletion, is common in older women and primarily affects the weight-bearing joints of the lower extremities and the back. Weaknesses of the vertebrae may cause one vertebra to collapse under the weight of the upper body and crush down upon the anterior surface of the vertebra below it. This *compression fracture* of the vertebrae produces pain and nerve damage. When this type of fracture occurs, the spine bends sharply forward, producing a **kyphosis** (humpback) and an overall reduction in the person's height. Fractures of bones or joints in any part of the body can severely limt movement.

Degenerative arthritis (**osteoarthritis**) is another common cause of damage to the skeletal system. This disorder, common among the elderly, also affects the weight-bearing joints of the lower extremities and the back. Frequently, the knee and hip joints degenerate or develop bony spurs that cause pain upon movement. In the back, degeneration of the vertebrae may produce painful narrowing of disc spaces or bony spurs on the edges of a vertebra.

Many foot problems severely hamper movement due to pain. Corns, bunions, hammer toes, and overgrown, horny toenails are common among the elderly. A number of disorders of the muscles and related structures can impair movement. Immobility can decrease muscle strength and mass markedly, often causing profound generalized muscle weakness. Muscle **atrophy** (a reduction in the size of a muscle) and joint stiffness can readily occur with disuse. Less frequently, strains and sprains, damage to cartilage, joint dislocations, or damage as a result of injury can impair movement. Muscle-wasting diseases, such as muscular dystrophy, can also take their toll.

Disorders of the nervous system that impair movement occur less frequently but are often more serious. Inner ear infections and dizziness can impair balance with movement. Parkinson's disease, multiple sclerosis, central nervous system tumors, cerebral vascular accidents (strokes), and spinal cord injuries can leave muscle groups weakened, paralyzed, **spastic** (with too much muscle tone), or **flaccid** (without muscle tone).

CONSEQUENCES OF POOR BODY MECHANICS

An awareness of the consequences of *not* using good body mechanics may motivate both nurses and clients to learn good habits. The consequences of poor body alignment are multiple. The musculoskeletal system is particularly affected by poor alignment. Fatigue and muscle strain occur when the work of maintaining balance is not evenly divided among opposing muscle groups. Contractures brought about by using poor alignment over a prolonged time may eventually develop into permanent disabilities. Muscles, ligaments, and joint structures in the back may be weakened and permanently damaged when not aligned correctly over time. Poor posture also contributes to problems with balance, which may predispose the person to accidents.

Poor alignment can affect the function of other body systems as well. Poor alignment can reduce chest expansion. Undue or prolonged pressure brought about by improper body alignment may impede blood flow, damage superficial nerves, and contribute to the formation of decubitus ulcers. When the abdominal muscles are weakened and the spinal column is not properly aligned, gastrointestinal function can be compromised, predisposing the person to a variety of problems, including constipation. All of these consequences of poor body alignment can be prevented.

Falls

Falls are, by far, the most common serious consequence of improper body mechanics and ambulatory problems. The elderly are most susceptible to falls, and the consequences of falling are far more serious for the elderly than for younger persons.

About 6% of all falls among the elderly result in a fractured bone, and as many as 17% of those with broken bones die as a result of complications of the fracture (Hogue 1982, pp. 185–86). There are many reasons for the elderly person's susceptibility to falls. Most are associated with the normal processes of aging. The most significant are poor vision, dizziness, and sudden loss of muscle tone in the legs ("drop attacks").

There is a high incidence of dizziness among elderly persons, and some clouding of the ocular lenses occurs in almost everyone by age 65. Drop attacks occur without warning but with no loss of consciousness. Several hours may elapse before the person regains muscle tone and can get up alone or with assistance. While the cause is unknown, drop attacks seem to occur exclusively among the elderly and account for about 25% of falls among this group (Hogue 1982, p. 185). Other factors include declining postural and movement reflexes resulting in unstable posture and gait, increased body sway with gait, and increased difficulty regaining balance when it becomes unstable.

When an elderly person is hospitalized, additional factors increase the potential for a fall:

- Unfamiliarity with the surroundings
- Strangeness of the diagnostic tests and surgery
- Immobilization and the weakness it causes
- Pain
- Loss of independence and control over one's own activities
- Drugs that contribute to dizziness, sedation, and confusion, especially diazepam (Valium), furosemide (Lasix), and antidepressants
- Elimination dysfunction, which often intensifies with hospitalization
- Confusion

After surgery, the elderly person is often more likely to be confused than a younger person and may attempt to get out of bed without help. Primarily due to the effects of osteoporosis, an older person is much more likely to fracture a bone during a fall than a younger person is. The most common fractures in elderly people who fall are hip fractures, Colles's (wrist) fractures, and compression fractures of vertebrae. When an elderly person breaks a bone, the complications of immobility may be more dangerous than the fracture itself.

Physical Stresses to the Back

The spine supports over one half of the body's weight (chest, arms, shoulders, and head) (Donaldson and Hoover 1982, p. 42). In a person with good standing alignment, the lumbar spine is somewhat curved. In a person with poor standing alignment, the lumbar curvature is exaggerated and the spine cannot support the weight that a well-aligned column can support.

The muscles of the lumbar spine support and protect the

spinal vertebrae, which in turn protect the delicate spinal cord. The abdominal muscles also support the back structures. Lumbar muscles are not strong enough, by themselves, to lift the upper body against gravity when it is bent forward with a load. A person can lift such a load only if the lumbar muscles are strong and if they work in synchrony with other strong muscle groups.

When a person bends forward only 20 degrees with knees extended, pressure on the lower back is 50% greater than in a person standing erect. If, in addition, the forward-leaning person is carrying a 44-pound load, the pressure on the lower back is more than 100% greater than in a person standing erect. Bending forward while keeping the knees straight to lift a load, and twisting the spine is the worst possible combination of events predisposing to back injury (Donaldson and Hoover 1982, pp. 142–44).

Long-Term Effects

A strong and healthy back, undamaged by disease or previous injury, can usually handle the sequence of events just described. Not all backs, however, are strong and healthy. Most lower back problems are the result of a series of minor injuries and strains over many years. Each additional insult further damages the vertebrae and discs or the muscles and ligaments that support them. These minor injuries have a cumulative effect and often lead to more serious and painful disease or injury of the back. Most of these back problems occur in the lower back, just below the waist, at lumbar vertebrae 4 and 5 (L4-L5).

Lower back problems usually first occur in the young adult and persist for years, flaring up from time to time and just as spontaneously subsiding. Most frequently the cause is a **strain** (an overstretching of a muscle or ligament often due to overexertion) or, less frequently, a **sprain** (a partial tearing of a muscle or ligament usually due to injury).

These injuries usually become more serious with each additional insult to the back. The discomfort usually reaches a peak during middle age (30 to 55 years), and the person seeks medical advice. The most effective treatment for long-term back problems is prevention: taking care of the back all one's life.

Occupational Groups at Risk of Back Injury

Studies demonstrate that in all occupational groups backaches are second only to upper respiratory infections as a cause of absence from work. Most back problems are a result of lifting a heavy load from floor or knee level to waist level (Owen 1980, p. 894). A significant proportion of all compensation paid for disability injuries in recent years has been for back injuries. Workers who lift and transfer heavy loads, especially furniture movers, warehouse and storeroom workers, truck drivers, housekeepers, mothers of small children who lift and carry them about, and nurses and other caregivers, are at risk of back injury.

Harber et al. (1985) list the five most common causes of work-related back injury among hospital nurses:

- Lifting a client in bed (48%)
- Helping a client out of bed (30%)
- Moving the bed itself (27%)
- Lifting a client to a stretcher (22%)
- Carrying equipment weighing more than 30 pounds (10%)

Fifty-two percent of the nurses in this study experienced work-related back pain within a 6-month period (Harber et al. 1985). Another study of nurses, 80% of whom experienced occasional back problems, indicates that most had lax postural, exercise, and activity habits (Drapeau 1975, p. 63). A third study suggests that most of the nurses who experienced back problems did not remember how to use the pelvic tilt or proper lifting techniques that they learned in their nursing programs and were not using these in their work (Hoover 1973, p. 2079). Some hospitals have developed programs to reduce back injuries among staff (Gates 1988, p. 657).

Many factors increase the potential for lower back injuries. A major contributor is habitually poor standing and sitting posture, which produces an exaggerated lumbar lordosis. Overweight individuals who carry their extra weight over their abdomen, pregnant women, and women who consistently wear high-heeled shoes are at risk because of the exaggerated lumbar curvature these situations produce. Sedentary persons are at greater risk because of weak back and abdominal muscles.

Lower back injuries are preventable. Guidelines to prevent back injuries are summarized in the accompanying box.

ASSESSING

Assessment of the client's problems related to immobility, joint range of motion and activities of daily living, and activity tolerance is discussed in Chapter 35. A discussion of assessment of body alignment, ambulation, and ability to move follows.

To assess the client's body alignment, ability to move, and ambulation, the nurse collects information from the client, from other nurses, and from the client's records. The physician's physical examination and history are important sources of information about disabilities affecting the musculoskeletal system, e.g., contractures, edema, pain in the extremities, or generalized fatigue, that affect the planning of nursing interventions for that client. A review of the recent nurses' notes is also useful.

Diagnostic tests chiefly used to assess the integrity of the musculoskeletal and neuromuscular systems involve roentgenography (x-ray examination) to determine the size and shape of bones or areas of variable density. Blood tests for serum calcium levels can detect some types of bone pathol-

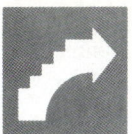

CLINICAL GUIDELINES
Preventing Back Injuries

- Become consciously aware of your posture and body mechanics.

- Make a conscious effort to improve your posture and body mechanics. Seek assistance if you need it.

- Minimize lumbar lordosis as much as possible:
  - When standing for a period of time, periodically flex one hip and knee and rest your foot on an object if possible.
  - When sitting, keep your knees slightly higher than your hips.
  - Unless you have a pillow or other support beneath your abdomen, avoid sleeping in the prone position.

- Use a firm mattress that provides good body support at natural body curvatures.

- Exercise regularly to maintain overall physical condition; include exercises that strengthen the pelvic, abdominal, and lumbar muscles.

- Avoid exercises that cause pain or require spinal flexion with straight legs (e.g., toe-touching and sit-ups) or spinal rotation (twisting).

- Avoid activities that require an excessive arching of the spine (e.g., hockey) and spinal rotation (e.g., golf or tennis) unless you are physically fit.

- Apply principles of body mechanics continuously in your work and daily life. For example:
  - Rearrange storage areas so that frequently used items are at least 2 feet above the floor. (Lifting from this height to waist level minimizes back strain.)
  - Avoid lifting above waist level when possible. Lifting a load above this level places strain on the lower back.
  - Avoid catching a heavy, falling object.
  - Avoid lifting more than 20 pounds of weight alone. A load that exceeds 35% of body weight is considered excessively heavy.

- Coordinate your efforts and use smooth, rhythmic movements when lifting a load with another person. Choose a leader so that you can lift simultaneously.

- Plan ahead how you will move a load and where you will move it. Make sure the area is free of obstructions.

- Wear clothing that allows you to use good body mechanics and comfortable low-heeled shoes that provide good foot support and will not cause you to slip, stumble, or turn your ankle.

ogy. Calcium excess, (**hypercalcemia**) may indicate demineralization of bones. Calcium deficiency (**hypocalcemia**) resulting from insufficient intake can lead to **rickets** (decalcification of bone) in children and **osteomalacia** in adults.

Serum phosphate and inorganic phosphorus have a function in maintaining serum calcium concentrations. Phosphate is needed for the generation of bone. Phosphate levels are always in inverse proportion to calcium levels in the blood. Increased phosphorus levels (**hyperphosphatemia**) are often found in clients with kidney dysfunction. They are also associated with bone tumors. Phosphorus deficiency (**hypophosphatemia**) is found in clients with rickets and osteomalacia.

Assessing Body Alignment

Assessment of body alignment includes an inspection of the client while standing, sitting, or lying. The purpose of body alignment assessment is to identify the following:

- Normal changes resulting from growth and development
- Poor posture and learning needs to maintain good posture
- Factors contributing to poor posture, such as fatigue or low self-esteem
- Muscle weakness or other motor impairments

To assess **stance** (the manner in which a person stands), the nurse views the client from anterior, lateral, and posterior perspectives:

- *Normally, when viewed anteriorly:* A vertical line from the body's center of gravity (located on the midline halfway between the umbilicus and the symphysis pubis) falls between the feet (the body's base of support) and extends upward through the middle of the forehead. The shoulders are level. The arms are relaxed at the sides, and the elbows are slightly flexed. A line drawn through the patella and the middle of the ankle ends at the second or third toe. The toes point forward. See Figure 36–1, earlier in the chapter.

- *Normally, when viewed laterally:* The pelvis is well aligned, i.e., "tucked under" (see Figure 36–10, *A*), and the lumbar spine is elongated. Proper alignment flattens the abdomen and prevents an exaggerated lumbar curvature of the spine. This tensed trunk alignment in which the pelvis is tucked under is referred to as the **pelvic tilt,** using a *long midriff,* or putting on an *internal girdle.* The pelvic tilt is absent when alignment is poor.

The "slumped" posture (see Figure 36–10, *B*) is the most common problem that occurs when people stand. The neck is flexed far forward, the abdomen protrudes, the pelvis is thrust forward to create an exaggerated curvature of the lumbar spine (**lordosis**), and the knees are markedly hyperextended. Lower back pain and fatigue occur quickly in people with poor posture. When one

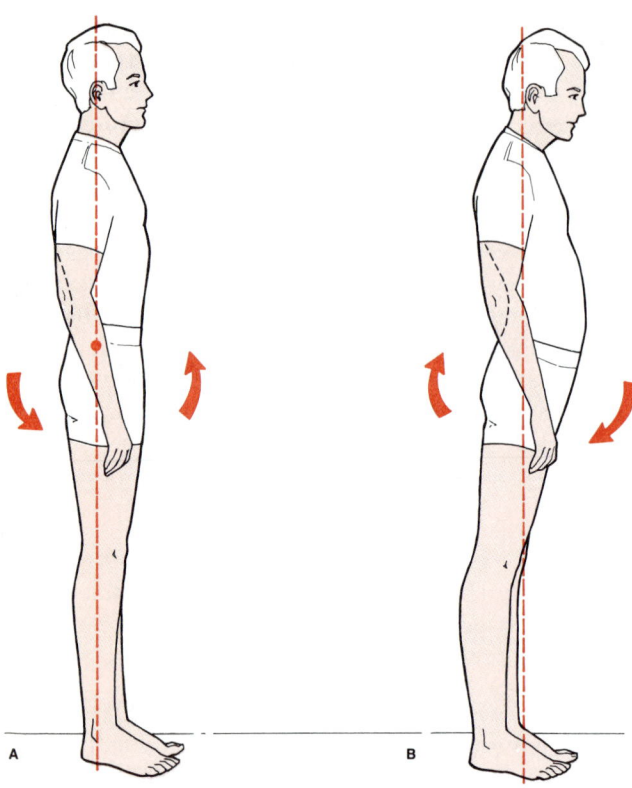

Figure 36–10 A standing person with: A, good trunk alignment; B, poor trunk alignment. The arrows indicate the direction in which the pelvis is tilted.

segment of the body deviates from proper alignment, compensatory deviations occur in other body segments; the result is strain and damage to the malaligned ligaments and joint structures supporting body weight.

■ *Normally, when viewed posteriorly:* The shoulders are level. The hips are level. The spine is straight, not curved to either side. The main body weight is borne well forward on the outer sides of the feet.

To assess sitting alignment, the nurse views the client from the lateral perspective. Normally, the head and trunk are the same as in the standing position, but the lumbar curve is less anteriorly convex because of hip flexion. The weight of the body is centered on the buttocks and thighs. The thighs are horizontal to the trunk. Both feet are on the floor (one foot may be in front of the other), and the forearms are supported to prevent upward or downward pulling of the shoulder girdle. See Figure 36–3, earlier in the chapter. The popliteal spaces should be at least 2.5 cm (1 in) away from the edge of the chair to avoid pressure on the blood circulation and the nerves of the legs.

Sitting with one leg crossed over the other creates a C shape, or postural **scoliosis,** of the lumbar-thoracic spine. It may be relaxing to assume this position for short periods, but care must be taken not to exert undue pressure against the delicate nerves and blood vessels in the popliteal area. Persons who have peripheral vascular problems should avoid crossing the legs for this reason. Habitually sitting with the same leg crossed over the other can eventually contribute to permanent postural scoliosis. Slouching while sitting may be relaxing for short periods, but habitual slouching can contribute to permanent postural abnormalities.

TABLE 36–3 *Common Structural Abnormalities that Affect Alignment*

Deviation	Description	Cause	Treatment
Scoliosis	Lateral curvature of the spine, which increases during active growth periods	May be secondary to other deformities, such as a discrepancy in leg lengths, or defects of spinal supporting tissues (a functional scoliosis); the most common cause of structural scoliosis is heredity, which produces an idiopathic structural scoliosis, a condition occurring five times more often in females than males, between the ages of 8 and 15	Treatment of underlying cause or application of a brace or cast from occiput to pelvis; surgical fusion of the spinal vertebrae may be necessary
Kyphosis (roundback or humpback)	A fixed flexion deformity of the thoracic spine	Congenital—rickets, tuberculosis of spine	Exercises to extend the thoracic spine; sleeping without a pillow; occasionally, bracing or spinal fusion may be required
Lordosis (swayback)	A fixed hyperextension deformity of the lumbar spine	Congenital, most often secondary to other abnormalities such as kyphosis or muscular dystrophy	Treatment of the underlying disease

TABLE 36–4 *Developmental Variations in Body Alignment*

Age Group	Characteristics	Implications
Newborns	Usual posture is horizontal rather than upright; the spine is straight and lacks the anteroposterior curves of the adult but can be flexed; the abdomen is rounded and prominent; all extremities are generally flexed but can be passively moved through a full range of motion; the feet are usually **inverted** (toes point inward) but can be passively **everted** (toes point outward).	The congenital condition **metatarsus adductus** may be present if inversion of feet occurs in early infancy, especially if the lower legs are straight. Inversion is normally the result of internal **tibial torsion,** or inward rotation of the lower legs.
Infants (1 year)	Usually stands with legs slightly bowed, feet far apart, toes turned outward, and knees hyperextended; the head and upper part of the trunk are carried forward, and the arms are abducted to enhance balance; has an exaggerated lumbar curvature and a "pot belly."	Balance is precarious as the infant learns to stand and walk; may fall backward.
Toddlers	Marked lumbar lordosis and protruding abdomen; slight outward rotation of hips and eversion of feet.	Child commonly widely abducts arms for balance. Growth should produce inward rotation of hips and correct foot eversions.
Preschoolers	Protrusion of abdomen less exaggerated; extremities more proportionate to trunk.	Developing coordination and refining gross motor skills.
School-age children	Legs have straightened and toes point straight ahead; appear more steady and evenly balanced on the feet. Scoliosis screening should be performed.	Usually has excellent posture, often best during lifetime.
Adolescents	Posture is highly individual and determined to a large extent by the person's self-image and the significant changes in body proportions and contour; postural problems are common at this age.	Growth spurts may result in awkwardness, which may be manifested in posture. Postural habits formed during adolescence often persist into adulthood.
Older Adults	Tend to have some contractures of flexor muscles; may show kyphosis with disappearance of earlier lumbar lordosis; osteoporosis common among older women and may cause compression fractures of the vertebrae, resulting in a forward-leaning, stooped posture, sometimes called **dowager's hump.**	Deterioration of postural reflexes may require conscious widening of base of support to maintain balance; use of bifocals may result in hyperextension of cervical spine and may cause injury to nearby ligaments and joints.

Structural Abnormalities Affecting Alignment Structural impairments in body alignment are usually caused by congenital abnormalities, developmental abnormalities, or abnormal intrauterine positions before birth. Several common abnormalities are listed in Table 36–3. Of course, functional abnormalities, such as poor posture during the growing years or improper alignment during illness, can also cause these abnormalities.

Developmental Variations in Body Alignment Body alignment or posture changes significantly during growth and with age. An understanding of the normal variations is helpful for the nurse in promoting good posture, in assessing postural faults, and in helping others correct them. Normal developmental posture variations are shown in Table 36–4.

Assessing Capabilities and Limitations for Movement

The nurse needs to obtain data that may indicate hindrances or restrictions to the client's movement, including the following:

- *How does the client's illness influence the ability to move?* Unconscious clients and those with generalized muscular weakness, loss of or injury to one or both lower extremities, acute spinal cord injury, paralysis of one or both lower extremities, or paralysis of one or both upper extremities need assistance by one, two, or more nurses.

Clients with severe cardiac or respiratory impairments often cannot tolerate what would be minor exertion to most people. Certain activities and positions may be contraindicated. The client who has a pathologic respiratory condition may require a high elevation of the head of the bed (see Fowler's Position later in this chapter) to breathe satisfactorily; this client may not be able to tolerate lying flat on the back even for a few minutes.

- *Is the client's movement hampered by pain, obesity, age, or poor vision?* Clients who experience severe discomfort when moving, such as those with painful burns, acute inflammatory disease of the joints (e.g., arthritis), or recent surgery, require more help. These clients may require an analgesic at least 30 minutes before they are moved to help them relax and move with minimal discomfort. Obese or elderly clients may require physical assistance to move. Clients whose visual activity is limited may not be able to detect environmental hazards and prevent falls.

- *What encumbrances to the client's movement are there?* For example, does the client have an intravenous hookup in place or a heavy cast on one leg?

- *How mentally alert and able to comprehend and follow instructions is the client?* Obviously, unconscious clients are unable to participate or to assist the nurse. Clients who have experienced brain changes associated with age or disease may be too lethargic or mentally impaired to understand instructions. Other clients who are generally mentally alert may be receiving medications that hinder ability to walk safely; for example, narcotics, sedatives, tranquilizers, and antihistamines cause drowsiness, dizziness, weakness, and orthostatic hypotension.

To determine the client's specific capabilities and limitations for movement, the nurse assesses the client:

- Rising from a lying position to a sitting position on the edge of the bed. The client can normally rise without support from the arms; however, a client with muscle weakness may roll to the side and push with the arms or pull with the arms on side rails or nearby furniture to rise.

- Rising from a chair to a standing position. Normally this can be done without pushing with the arms; however, a person with weak muscles may use the arms to push upward and may thrust the upper body forward before rising.

- Moving in the bed, the nurse specifically observes the amount of assistance required for turning:
  a. From a supine position to a lateral position
  b. From a lateral position on one side to a lateral position on the other
  c. From a supine position to a prone position
  d. From a supine position to a sitting position in bed

In addition, the nurse assesses or determines the client's

- Range of motion of joints needed to ambulate or to complete transfer movements. The nurse asks the client to perform range-of-motion exercises for the arms, ankles, knees, and hips. While the client performs the range-of-motion exercises, the nurse assesses

a. The degree of movement of the joint
b. Any discomfort experienced by the client
c. Any joint swelling or redness, which could indicate the presence of an injury or an inflammation
d. Any contractures

- Strength in lower extremities by
  a. Inspecting muscles of the thigh and calf for size. Compare the muscle on one side of the body to the same muscle on the other side. If there appears to be a discrepancy between the sides, measure the muscle with tape.
  b. Testing for muscle strength. Compare the right side with the left side. Note whether there is paralysis or normal movement against gravity and minimal or full resistance.
  Hip muscles: While the client is supine with both legs extended, ask the client to raise one leg at a time while you attempt to hold it down.
  Hamstrings: While the client is supine with both knees bent, ask the client to resist while you attempt to straighten them.
  Quadriceps: While the client is supine with knees partially extended, ask the client to resist while you attempt to flex the knee.
  Muscles of the feet and ankles: Ask the client to resist while you attempt to dorsiflex the foot and then plantar flex the foot.

- Assistive devices used, such as a cane, walker, crutches, braces. If assistive devices are used, the nurse specifically determines the strength of the upper extremities:
  Flexor muscles: While the client fully extends each arm, ask the client to flex the arm while you attempt to hold it in extension.
  Extensor muscles: While the client flexes each arm, ask the client to extend the arm while you attempt to keep it flexed.

Assessing Ambulation (Gait)

There are two distinct phases in walking: the weight-bearing phase and the swing phase. Each leg alternates between these two phases to produce a smooth, rhythmic motion. The **weight-bearing, double-stance,** or **support phase** is initiated when the heel strikes the ground. This slows the forward momentum of the body slightly. The body weight is spread over this supporting foot until the weight reaches the toes. At this point, the ball of the foot and the extended toes, now behind the body, push off with force to propel the body forward. See Figure 36–11, *A*.

The **swing phase** is initiated as the hip joint flexes to lift the toes from the ground. Then the knee and ankle flex as the leg and foot are swung forward. As the leg begins to swing in front of the body, the hip begins to extend. The swing phase is ended as the heel strikes the ground to initiate the weight-bearing phase. See Figure 36–11, *B*.

Like standing stability, walking stability is directly related

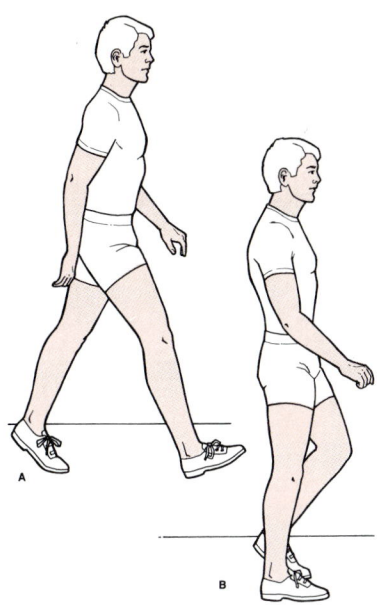

Figure 36–11 Phases in walking: A, weight-bearing phase; B, beginning of swing phase.

to the size of the base of support. When a person walks, the base of support shifts from side to side, and the center of gravity shifts to a position above the supporting foot with each step. This shifting of weight produces a slight swaying motion with each step. Foot position is important in walking. As a person walks, the inner borders of the feet should move along a path where the line of gravity would naturally fall. The toes should point straight ahead. This pattern of ambulation produces minimal body sway from side to side and directs the force of movement straight ahead.

As a person walks, the arms should swing in opposition to the leg movements to counteract the tendency of the body to rotate as a result of the off-center application of force with each step. The reflexive arm swing helps to propel the body forward without wasted energy.

Normal **gait** (the characteristic pattern of a person's walk) and common abnormalities of gait are described in Table 36–5. Gait can be assessed not only by observing a person walk but also by observing the pattern of wear on the soles and heels of the shoes.

To assess the client's gait, the nurse asks the client to walk down a corridor and observes whether the client's:

TABLE 36–5 *Assessing Gait*

Normal Fidings	Abnormal Findings	Some Associated Conditions
Head is erect, and vetebral column is straight.	Body is rigid and bent forward.	Parkinsonism
Gaze is straight ahead.	Gaze is toward ground.	Fear of falling
Toes point forward.	Toes are everted.	Flat-footedness
Kneecaps point forward.	Legs are knock-kneed with feet apart (normal until age 3 or 4).	Rickets; congenital bone disorders
	Legs are bowlegged with feet together (normal until age 2 or 2½).	Rickets; congenital bone disorders
Elbows are slightly flexed.	One elbow is flexed and held close to body.	Hemiplegia
Foot is dorsiflexed in swing phase.	One foot is plantar flexed and drags.	Hemiplegia
Arm opposite swing-through foot moves forward at same time.	Arms swing forward and do not swing with steps.	Parkinsonism
Steps are smooth, coordinated, and rhythmic.	Steps are weaving, uncoordinated, and uneven.	Alcohol or barbiturate intoxication; cerebellar disorder
	Steps are short, shuffling, and often on tiptoe.	Parkinsonism
	Gait starts slowly, gradually increases, and may be difficult to stop.	Parkinsonism
	Steps are stiff, jerking, and uncoordinated, with legs held stiffly together.	Spastic paraplegia; multiple sclerosis; spinal cord tumor
	Exaggerated lateral leaning accompanies steps.	Hip disorder

- Trunk is steady and upright
- Arms swing appropriately
- Gait is free and easy or unsteady
- Legs follow through in the swing phase
- Steps are appropriate or too small
- Instep falls along the line of gravity or whether the feet are spread apart
- Feet are dorsiflexed in the swing phase
- Gait starts and stops with ease

Pace is the number of steps taken per minute. A normal walking pace is 70 to 100 steps per minute. A fast pace is 120 steps per minute. The pace of an elderly person may slow to about 40 steps per minute. A person can increase pace by moving the center of gravity slightly forward, lengthening the stride, and increasing the pushing force of the toes at the end of each weight-bearing phase of a step.

DIAGNOSING

Depending on the assessment data obtained, numerous nursing diagnoses (actual and potential) that pertain to the client's mobility status may be derived. These may be derived from *Pattern VI: Moving* in the NANDA nursing diagnosis taxonomy and include **Impaired physical mobility; Activity intolerance (actual or potential); bathing/ hygiene, dressing/grooming, toileting self-care deficits; Impaired home maintenance management;** and **Altered health maintenance.** Because mobility affects many areas of human functioning, the diagnoses of **Impaired physical mobility** and **Activity intolerance** may themselves be the etiology of other diagnoses, e.g., **Self-care deficit, Impaired home maintenance management,** and **Altered health maintenance.** Other diagnoses that may pertain to mobility status include **Potential for injury,** and **Fear** of falling. Examples of these nursing diagnoses are shown below. Examples of data clusters and related nursing diagnoses are shown in Table 36–6.

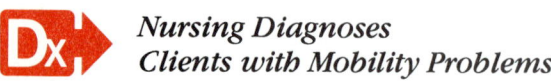

Nursing Diagnoses
Clients with Mobility Problems

Impaired physical mobility related to:

- Neuromuscular impairment
- Musculoskeletal impairment
- Trauma or surgical procedure
- Decreased motor agility and muscle weakness associated with advanced age
- Pain and discomfort

- External device (cast, intravenous tubing)
- Intolerance to activity
- Bed rest

Activity intolerance related to:
- Prolonged bed rest or decreased mobility
- Generalized weakness, fatigue
- Sedentary lifestyle

Potential activity intolerance related to:
- Sedentary lifestyle
- Fatigue/weakness
- Prolonged inactivity
- Presence of chronic or progressive disease (e.g., chronic obstructive pulmonary disease)

(Bathing/hygiene; dressing/grooming; feeding; toileting) self-care deficit related to:
- Impaired mobility status
- Intolerance to activity
- Decreased strength and endurance
- Neuromuscular impairment
- Musculoskeletal impairment
- Perceptual or cognitive impairment
- Impaired transfer ability for bathing and toileting
- Pain or discomfort

Impaired home maintenance management related to:
- Chronic debilitating disease
- Lack of equipment or aids for home care
- Lack of adaptation of home structure or furnishings
- Lack of community professional home care services
- Lack of familiarity with neighborhood resources
- Inadequate support systems
- Injury or surgery (fractured limb)

Altered health maintenance related to:
- Complete or partial lack of gross and/or fine motor skills

Potential for injury related to:
- Unsteady gait associated with advanced age
- Musculoskeletal disability
- Incoordination associated with neuromuscular impairment
- Decreased muscle strength and endurance
- Improper use of body mechanics
- Improper transfer techniques

Fear of falling related to:

- Loss or injury to body part
- Disabling musculoskeletal or neuromuscular illness
- Muscle weakness and fatigue

- Stands erect when walking
- Uses a walker to move independently from the bed to the nursing station three times a day
- Demonstrates correct use of four-point (or three-point) crutch gait
- Demonstrates correct methods of getting into and out of a chair and ascending and descending stairs with crutches

PLANNING

The nurse uses assessment data and nursing diagnoses to identify goals for care and design an individualized plan of nursing interventions. The overall *client goals* for persons with potential or actual problems related to body alignment or mobility include the following:

- Maintain proper body alignment
- In persons who have poor body alignment:
  a. Restore body alignment to an optimal level
  b. Prevent muscle shortening (contractures), reduced chest expansion, and other complications of poor alignment
- Improve use of body mechanics in work and in daily life
- Restore or improve ambulatory capability
- Prevent back injuries and falls

Planning also involves specifying outcome criteria (as shown below) for individual nursing diagnoses.

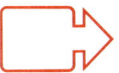

Outcome Criteria
Clients with Mobility Problems

The client

- Demonstrates use of good body mechanics when lifting and pulling objects, by
  - Using a wide base of support when moving objects
  - Enlarging the base of support by placing feet appropriately in the direction in which the movement occurs
  - Keeping objects to be moved close to the body (center of gravity)
  - Pushing, pulling, rolling, or sliding objects rather than lifting them whenever possible
  - Avoiding twisting the spine by pushing or pulling objects directly away from or toward the body and squarely facing the direction of movement
  - Squatting rather than stooping to pick up heavy objects from the floor and using large muscle groups of the body
  - Using the body's weight to counteract the weight of the object when pushing or pulling objects
  - Tensing stabilizing muscles before moving objects
  - Maintaining muscle mass and strength through exercise
- Identifies factors contributing to back strain
- Experiences no back pain or muscle fatigue

As part of planning, the nurse is responsible for identifying those clients who need assistance with body alignment and determining the degree of assistance they need. The nurse must be sensitive to the client's need to function

TABLE 36–6 *Examples of Data Clusters and Related Nursing Diagnoses*

Data Cluster	Nursing Diagnoses
Peter Brown, a 22-year-old truck driver, loads and unloads furniture for a major retail store. States he has "had back pain on occasion" but prides himself in his physical condition and in being able to lift heavy loads with little assistance. Has had minor back injuries and strain over the years, but these flare-ups subside spontaneously.	**Potential for injury** related to improper body mechanics
Mrs. Ivy Snowfield, a frail-appearing 82-year-old, has an unsteady gait and increasing difficulty maintaining her balance. Pace is slow (20 steps per minute). Posture is stooped. Leg and arm muscle strength is symmetric but weak. Has difficulty rising from a sitting to a standing position. No mechanical assistive devices are used.	**Impaired physical mobility** related to decreased motor agility and muscle weakness associated with advanced age
Mr. Tim Cherry, a 93-year-old widower, has chronic obstructive lung disease. States, "I can't breathe properly when I move about. I cannot maintain the house the way my wife did. All I can do is feed myself. Luckily, I have a nice neighbor who shops for me every week."	**Impaired home maintenance management** related to chronic debilitating disease, activity intolerance, and lack of familiarity with neighborhood resources

as independently as possible yet provide assistance when the client needs it. Clients who are not very mobile and can help themselves only minimally may also have low energy levels. They are at high risk of developing permanent shortening of muscles and other complications of immobility outlined in Chapter 35. These persons are totally dependent on caregivers and must be instructed to achieve and maintain correct body alignment.

Most clients require some nursing guidance and assistance to learn about, achieve, and maintain proper body mechanics, including alignment. All nurses have the responsibility to use proper body mechanics to prevent back injury to themselves and their clients. A serious back injury could prevent a nurse from participating in the full range of nursing activities. As role models, nurses continuously teach clients through the body mechanics they use. The nurse is expected to protect the client from harm, anticipating safety risks and protecting the client from unsafe practices. The more vulnerable the client, the greater the nurse's responsibility to protect the client from harm.

The nurse should also plan to teach clients applicable skills. For example, a postoperative cataract client needs to learn to squat rather than stoop to avoid increased intraocular pressure. Similarly, a client with a back injury needs to learn how to get out of bed safely and comfortably; a client with an injured leg needs to learn how to transfer from bed to wheelchair safely; and a client with a newly acquired walker needs to learn how to use it safely. Nurses often teach family members or caregivers in the home safe moving, lifting, and transfer techniques. Nurses who practice in hospitals and nursing homes have a responsibility to teach nursing assistants how to protect their backs from injury as they move, lift, and transfer clients.

Positioning, transferring, and ambulating clients are almost always independent nursing functions. Although certain activity orders are medically prescribed, the physician rarely writes specific directions to indicate how the order is to be accomplished. The physician usually orders specific body positions only after surgery, anesthesia, or trauma involving the nervous and musculoskeletal systems. The client's current "activity order" contains data essential for planning nursing interventions for body alignment. All clients should have an activity order written by their physician when they are admitted to the agency for care. Examples of common activity orders are shown in the accompanying box.

IMPLEMENTING

Postural Problems

As noted earlier, many problems concerning alignment, body mechanics, and ambulation are preventable and/or treatable. General exercise promotes good *standing alignment*. Walking and swimming, which maintain overall muscle tone, are especially useful. Conscientious and continuous awareness of and effort to improve posture in everyday activities are important in achieving and maintaining good posture. To put forth this effort, the client must be motivated; motivation is in turn usually dependent on self-image. The nurse who practices good postural habits can be a significant role model and motivator. No amount of verbal instruction and encouragement will influence clients to use good posture as strongly as the example of nurses who "practice what they preach."

Exercises to strengthen and protect the back muscles that support the lumbar spine and the abdominal muscles help prevent or reduce postural lordosis. Conscientious use of the pelvic tilt, shown in Figure 36–10, *A*, flattens the abdomen and prevents lordosis of the lumbar spine. Persons with a history of back problems should follow an exercise program prescribed by a physician. Any program of exercise should be started slowly and intensified gradually.

Clients should avoid prolonged standing. When prolonged standing is unavoidable, the client should elevate one foot onto a support to straighten the spine. Periodically changing the foot that is elevated prevents undue strain to one side of the spinal column at the expense of the other. Flexion of the hip and knee straightens the lumbar spine and reduces lordosis.

Nusing interventions to promote good *sitting alignment* apply whether the client is sitting in a chair, in a wheelchair, or on the side of the bed. When the client is sitting, alignment problems frequently affect not only the back but also the top extremities. Alignment problems are often due to the size and shape of the object on which the person is sitting (e.g., the chair or wheelchair may simply not fit the person).

A chair seat that is too high creates undue pressure against the thighs, especially in the popliteal area behind the knees, since the lower legs and feet are unsupported. Prolonged pressure can damage the delicate nerves and blood vessels in the popliteal area. Fatigue and discomfort can ensue rapidly. A firm footrest of an appropriate height improves alignment and comfort.

A chair seat that is too low causes no alignment problems of the back but, unless the thighs are supported, exerts undue pressure on the ischial tuberosities, because of the narrow base of support for the trunk. If too low, the seat may be difficult to get into and, especially, out of. Pillows placed on the chair seat support the thighs and improve alignment.

A chair seat that is too deep produces undue flexion of the thoracolumbar spine. The weight of the body does not rest on the ischial tuberosities, and the lower back is not supported properly by the chair back. This position can be quite uncomfortable. Pillows placed between the chair back and the person's back improve alignment.

If the chair back is too low or if there is no chair back, there is no effect on alignment, but most persons find that a higher chair back supports the spinal column and prevents fatigue.

In all instances, proper alignment in the sitting client is best promoted by a chair seat that allows the knees to be slightly higher than the hips and supports the full length of the thighs (see Figure 36-3, earlier in the chapter) and by a chair back that supports the entire back.

For certain individuals (e.g., those who have musculoskeletal impairments of the arm and shoulder), support of the arm is essential. If the armrests of a chair are too high, the person's shoulder girdle may be forced upward into an uncomfortable position. In this case, placing pillows on the chair seat to elevate the body improves alignment. When the armrests of the chair are too low, the person's shoulder girdle is pulled downward, causing the shoulders and back to slump when the person attempts to rest the arms on the chair armrests. Padding to raise the level of the armrests improves alignment.

Positioning Clients in Bed

Many clients depend on nurses for assistance in body alignment when lying in various positions in bed. Clients often evaluate the quality of the nursing care they receive by how comfortable they feel, and proper alignment is crucial to comfort.

Any position, correct or incorrect, can be detrimental if maintained for a prolonged period. Frequent change of position helps to prevent muscle discomfort, undue pressure resulting in decubitus ulcers, damage to superficial nerves and blood vessels, and **contractures** (permanent shortening of a muscle). Position changes also maintain muscle tone and stimulate postural reflexes. Principles of positioning clients are outlined in the accompanying box.

 When the client is not able to move independently or assist with moving, the *preferred method is to use two or more nurses to move or turn the client*. The risk of muscle strain and body injury, to both the client and nurse is lowered when appropriate assistance is provided.

When positioning clients in bed, there are a number of things the nurse can do to ensure proper alignment and promote client comfort and safety:

- Prior to placing the client in bed, make sure the mattress is firm and level yet has enough give to fill in and support natural body curvatures. A sagging mattress, a mattress that is too soft, or an underfilled water bed, when used over a prolonged period, can contribute to the development of hip flexion contractures and low back strain and pain. Bed boards made of plywood and placed beneath a

---

Principles of Positioning Clients

- The lower the degree of mobility, the capacity for self-care, and the energy level, the greater the need for careful alignment.

- Postural lordosis, kyphosis, and scoliosis created by malpositioning contribute to back and neck pain and to the development of contractures.

- When poor body alignment is prolonged, temporary postural contractures may develop into permanent contractures.

- In the immobilized client, the most frequently occurring contractures are flexion contractures of the hips, knees, and plantar flexors of the ankles. Flexion contractures of the cervical spine and shoulders are also common.

- Body parts aligned in a functional position of comfort, as close to anatomic position as possible, ensure the least stress on muscles and joints and the greatest comfort for the client.

- Gravity pulls unsupported body parts downward. Support devices (e.g., bedboards, pillows, trochanter rolls, sandbags, footboards, and hand-wrist splints) counteract the pull of gravity.

- Supportive devices that provide a broad base of support pose the least risk of focal pressure areas. Devices with a narrow base of support can cause discomfort to the area and undue pressure against tissues, blood vessels, and nerves.

- Use of too many pillows beneath the head of a client lying in bed promotes flexion contractures of the neck.

- Dorsiflexor muscles of the ankle deteriorate rapidly when not used for standing and walking. Plantar flexor muscles of the ankles are stronger than dorsiflexor muscles.

Source Adapted from M. K. Memmer, *Posture and alignment* (Los Angeles: The Intercampus Nursing Project, California State University and College System, 1974), pp. 21–23.

sagging mattress are increasingly recommended for clients who have back problems or are prone to them.

■ Ensure that the bed is kept clean and dry. Wrinkled or damp sheets increase the risk of decubitus ulcer formation. Make sure extremities can move freely whenever possible. For example, the top bedclothes need to be loose enough for the client to move the feet.

■ Place support devices (e.g., pillows, rolled towels, foam rubber supports) in specified areas according to the client's position. See Procedures 36–1 to 36–6. Use only those support devices needed to maintain alignment and to prevent stress on the client's muscles and joints. If the person is capable of movement, too many devices limit mobility and increase potential for muscle weakness and atrophy. Common alignment problems that can be corrected with support devices include the following:

a. Flexion of the neck
b. Internal rotation of the shoulder
c. Adduction of the shoulder
d. Flexion of the wrist
e. Anterior convexity of the lumbar spine
f. External rotation of the hips
g. Hyperextension of the knees
h. Plantar flexion of the ankle

■ Avoid placing one body part, particularly one with bony prominences, directly on top of another body part. Excessive pressure can damage veins and predispose the client to thrombus formation. Pressure against the popliteal space may damage nerves and blood vessels in this area.

■ Plan a *systematic 24-hour schedule* for position changes. See the box below. Frequent position changes are essential to prevent decubitus ulcers in immobilized clients (see Chapter 35). Such clients should be repositioned every 2 hours throughout the day and night and more frequently when there is concern about skin breakdown. This schedule is usually outlined on the client's nursing care plan. Schedule periods throughout the day during which the client assumes positions that provide full extension of the neck, hips, and knees to prevent flexion contractures of these joints.

■ Always elicit information from the client to determine which position is most comfortable and appropriate. Seeking information from the client about what feels best is a useful guide when aligning persons and is an essential aspect of evaluating the effectiveness of an alignment intervention. Sometimes a person who appears well-aligned may be experiencing real discomfort. Both appearance, in relation to alignment criteria, and comfort are important in achieving effective alignment. To promote comfort, the nurse may administer prescribed analgesics approximately 30 minutes before moving or ambulating the client. Table 36–7 outlines criteria to assess alignment of clients in the various bed positions.

Fowler's Position　**Fowler's position,** or semisitting position, is a bed position in which the head and trunk are raised 45° to 90°. See Figure 36–12 and Procedure 36–1 on page 906. In **low-Fowler's,** or **semi-Fowler's,** position, the head and trunk are raised 15° to 45°; in **high-Fowler's position,** the head and trunk are raised 90°. In this position, the knees may or may not be flexed. Nurses need to clarify the meaning of the term *Fowler's position* in a particular agency. In some hospitals, *Fowler's position* refers to elevation of the upper part of the body without knee flexion, and the term *semi-Fowler's* is used to refer to the sitting position with knee flexion.

Fowler's position is the position of choice for people who have difficulty breathing and for some people with heart problems. When the client is in this position, gravity pulls the diaphragm downward, allowing greater lung expansion. Clients confined to bed but capable of eating, reading, watching television, or visiting find this position comfortable.

One of the devices nurses use to support clients in Fowler's position is the **trochanter roll,** a roll of cloth, frequently a towel, placed against the greater trochanter of the femur to prevent external rotation of the hip. The greater trochanter is palpated and the middle of the roll is placed against it. Trochanter rolls need not extend more than 8 to 10 inches on either side of the trochanter, since leg rotation occurs at the hip joint. Firm support by the trochanter roll

---

Sample Schedule for Position Changes

Time		Position	Time		Position
10:00 A.M.	(1000 hr)	Left lateral	10:00 P.M.	(2200 hr)	Left Sims's
Noon	(1200 hr)	Fowler's or chair	Midnight	(2400 hr)	Supine
2:00 P.M.	(1400 hr)	Right lateral	2:00 A.M.	(0200 hr)	Right lateral
4:00 P.M.	(1600 hr)	Right Sims's	4:00 A.M.	(0400 hr)	Right Sims's
6:00 P.M.	(1800 hr)	Fowler's or chair	6:00 A.M.	(0600 hr)	Supine
8:00 P.M.	(2000 hr)	Left lateral	8:00 A.M.	(0800 hr)	Fowler's

TABLE 36–7 *Criteria to Assess Clients in Bed Positions*

Body Region	Frontal View (From Foot of Bed)	Lateral View (From Side of Bed)
Head and neck	Head is midline to the trunk and erect in all positions except the prone and Sims's positions, where it is rotated to one side.	Head is neither hyperextended nor flexed except in lateral and Sims's positions, where it may be slightly flexed.
		Chin is at a 90° angle to the body.
Shoulders and arms	Shoulders are level in all positions.	
	Shoulder girdle is relaxed, neither pulled upward or downward.	Shoulder girdle is relaxed, pulled neither forward nor backward.
	Shoulders are slightly abducted from body except in the lateral position, where only the upper shoulder is abducted.	In lateral and Sims's positions, the upper shoulder and arm are slightly flexed.
		In lateral position, the lower shoulder and elbow are flexed in front of the body.
		In Sims's position, the lower shoulder is extended, and the same elbow is flexed behind the body.
	Arms are relaxed at sides with: hands in lap (Fowler's position), hands on abdomen or above head (dorsal recumbent position), one or both hands near head (prone position).	
Wrists and hands	Wrists are extended, and fingers are flexed in all positions.	
Trunk	Trunk is straight and not curved to either side in all positions.	Slight lumbar curvature occurs in all positions.
Hips and legs	Hips are level in all bed positions.	Hips are in the same plane as the shoulders.
		Hips are flexed in varying degrees in all positions except the prone position, where they are extended.
	Hips are slightly abducted from each other.	The upper hip and knee are more acutely flexed than the lower leg in lateral and Sims's positions.
		In the lateral position, the upper knee and ankle are in a horizontal plane with the hip and parallel to the bed.
		Knees are slightly flexed in all positions.
	Patellae face: upward in Fowler's and dorsal recumbent positions, downward in prone position, and laterally in lateral position. In Sims's position, the patellae lie at a point halfway between lateral and downward.	
Ankles and feet	Toes point: upward in Fowler's and dorsal recumbent positions, downward in prone position, laterally in lateral position, and halfway between the lateral and downward plane in Sims's position.	Ankles are dorsiflexed as much as possible in all positions.
		Toes and heels are kept off the bed surface in prone, dorsal recumbent, and Fowler's positions.

inhibits outward rotation. Trochanter rolls are made commercially or can be constructed as described in Figure 36–13 on page 907. A commercial roll needs only to be covered before it is used. Covered sandbags are commonly used.

A common error nurses make when aligning clients in Fowler's position is placing an overly large pillow or more than one pillow behind the client's head. These errors promote the development of neck flexion contractures. If a client desires several head pillows, the nurse should encourage the client to rest without a pillow for several hours each day to extend the neck fully and counteract the effects of poor neck alignment.

Malalignments associated with an *unsupported* Fowler's position are

- Hyperextension or flexion of the neck
- Flexion of the lumbar curvature
- Hyperextension of the knees

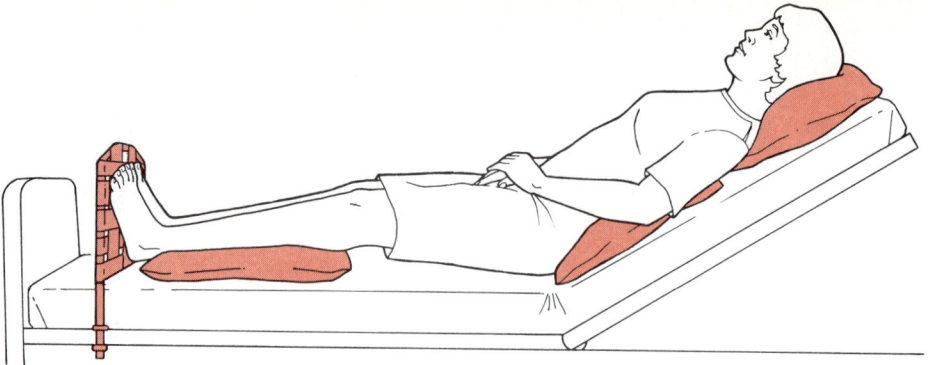

Figure 36–12   Fowler's position (supported).

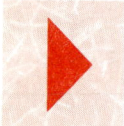

PROCEDURE 36–1

SUPPORTING A CLIENT IN FOWLER'S POSITION

Equipment ☑

One to six small pillows, depending on client need

One or two trochanter rolls (optional)

Footboard

Intervention

 1. **Assess pressure areas of particular concern in the Fowler's position** (see Figure 35–6, *D* on page 850):

- Heels
- Spinous process
- Sacrum
- Ischial tuberosities
- Scapulae

2. **Position the client.**

- Have the client flex the knees slightly before raising the head of the bed. *Slight knee flexion prevents the person from sliding toward the foot of the bed as the bed is raised.* Be certain the client's hips are positioned directly over the point where the bed will bend when the head is raised. *An appropriate hip position ensures that the client will be sitting on the ischial tuberosities when the head of the bed is raised.*

- Raise the head of the bed to 30°, 45°, or the angle required by or ordered for the client.

3. **Provide supportive devices to align the client appropriately.**

- Place a small pillow or roll under the lumbar region of the back if you feel a space in the lumbar curvature. *The pillow supports the natural lumbar curvature and prevents flexion of the lumbar spine.*

- Place a small pillow under the client's head. *The pillow supports the cervical curvature of the vertebral column.* Alternatively, have the client rest the head against the mattress. *Too many pillows beneath the head can cause neck flexion contracture.*

- Place one or two pillows under the lower legs from below the knees to the ankles. *The pillows provide a broad base of support that is soft and flexible, prevent uncomfortable hyperextension of the knees, and reduce pressure on the heels.* Make sure that no pressure is exerted on the popliteal space and that the knees are flexed. *Pressure against the popliteal space can damage nerves and vein walls, predisposing the client to thrombus formation. Keeping the knees slightly flexed also prevents the person from sliding down in the bed.*

- Avoid using the knee gatch of a hospital bed to flex the client's knees. *The position of the knee*

gatch rarely coincides with the position of the client's knees. Even when the knee gatch does bend at the client's knees, considerable pressure (due to the narrow base of support beneath the knees and the firm, unyielding mattress) can be exerted against the popliteal space and beneath the client's calves.

- Put a trochanter roll lateral to each femur (optional). *This prevents external rotation of the hips.*

- Support the client's feet with a footboard. *This prevents plantar flexion.* The footboard should protrude several inches above the toes. *This protects the toes from pressure exerted by the top bedding.* The footboard should be placed 1 inch away from the heels. *This prevents undue pull on the Achilles tendon and discomfort.*

- Place pillows to support both arms and hands if the client does not have normal use of them. *These pillows prevent shoulder and muscle strain from the effects of downward gravitational pull, dislocation of the shoulder in paralyzed persons, edema of the hands and arms, and flexion contracture of the wrist.* Arrange the pillows to support only the forearms and hands, up to the elbow. In this way, the pillows support the shoulder girdle.

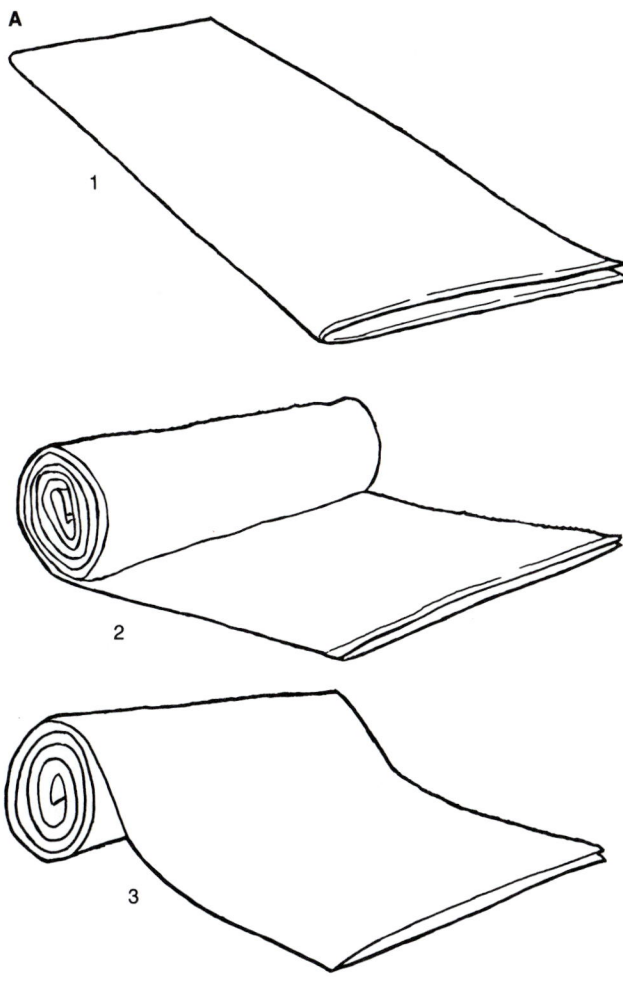

- External rotation of the legs
- Plantar flexion

In clients who lack arm movement, shoulder muscle strain, edema of the hands and arms, and wrist flexion are added problems.

Orthopneic position   An adaptation of high-Fowler's position is the **orthopneic position.** The client sits either in bed or on the side of the bed with an overbed table across the lap. See Figure 36–14. This position facilitates respiration by allowing maximum chest expansion. It is particularly helpful to clients who have problems exhaling, because they can press the lower part of the chest against the overbed table.

Dorsal Recumbent Position   In the **dorsal recumbent (back-lying) position,** the client's head and shoulders are slightly elevated on a small pillow. See Figure 36–15 and Procedure 36–2 on the following page. Although in some agencies the terms *dorsal recumbent* and *supine* are used interchangeably, strictly speaking, in the **supine** or **dorsal position** the head and shoulders are not elevated. In both positions, the client's forearms may be elevated on pillows or placed at the client's sides. Supports are similar in both positions, except for the head pillow.

Malalignments associated with an *unsupported* dorsal recumbent position are

- Hyperextension or flexion of the neck
- Flexion of the lumbar curvature
- External rotation of the legs
- Hyperextension of the knees
- Plantar flexion

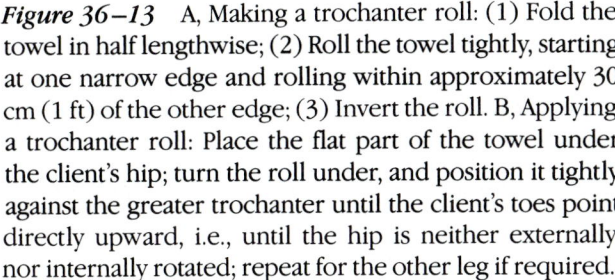

Figure 36–13   A, Making a trochanter roll: (1) Fold the towel in half lengthwise; (2) Roll the towel tightly, starting at one narrow edge and rolling within approximately 30 cm (1 ft) of the other edge; (3) Invert the roll. B, Applying a trochanter roll: Place the flat part of the towel under the client's hip; turn the roll under, and position it tightly against the greater trochanter until the client's toes point directly upward, i.e., until the hip is neither externally nor internally rotated; repeat for the other leg if required.

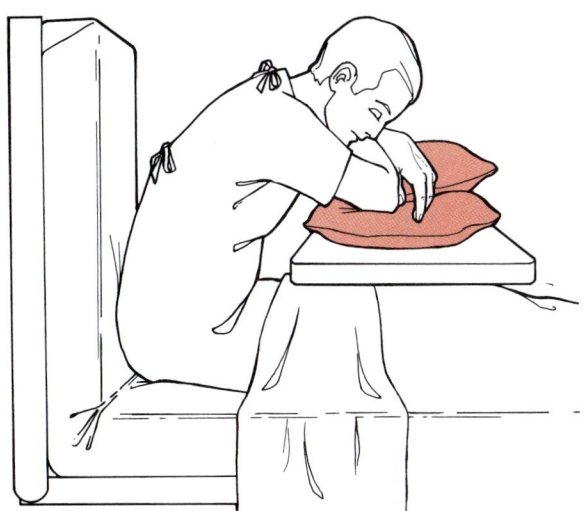

Figure 36–14   Orthopneic position.

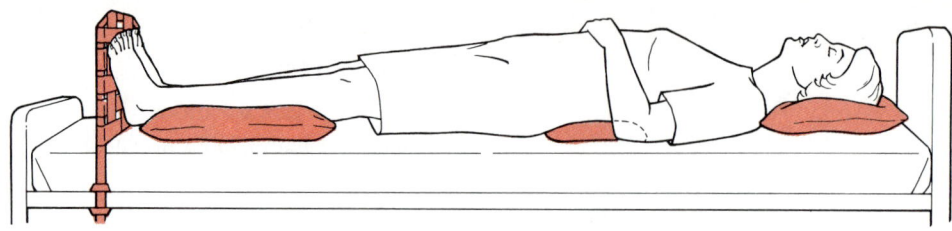

Figure 36–15 Dorsal recumbent position (supported).

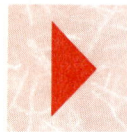

PROCEDURE 36–2

SUPPORTING A CLIENT IN DORSAL RECUMBENT POSITION

Equipment ☑

Up to six small pillows, depending on client need

Two trochanter rolls (optional)

Footboard

Handrolls or wrist splints, if needed

Intervention

 1. **Assess pressure areas of particular concern in the dorsal recumbent position** (see Figure 35–6, *A* on page 850):

- Heels
- Sacrum
- Elbows
- Scapulae
- Back of head

2. **Assist the client to a supine position.**

3. **Provide supportive devices to align the client appropriately.**

- Place a pillow of suitable thickness under the client's head and shoulders as needed. *This prevents hyperextension of the neck. Too many pillows beneath the head may cause or worsen neck flexion contracture.*

- Place a pillow under the lower legs from below the knees to the ankles. *This prevents hyperextension of the knees, keeps the heels off the bed, and reduces lumbar lordosis.*

- Place trochanter rolls laterally against the femurs (optional). *These prevent external rotation of the hips.*

- Place a rolled towel or small pillow under the lumbar curvature if you feel a space between the lumbar area and the bed. *This pillow supports the lumbar curvature and prevents flexion of the lumbar spine.*

- Put a footboard or rolled pillow on the bed to support the feet. *This prevents plantar flexion (foot drop).*

- If the client is unconscious or has paralysis of the upper extremities, elevate the forearms and hands (*not* the upper arm) on pillows. *This position promotes comfort and prevents edema. Pillows are not placed under the upper arms because they can cause shoulder flexion.*

- If the client has actual or potential finger and wrist flexion deformities, use handrolls or wrist/hand splints. *This prevents flexion contractures of the fingers.* Handrolls, having a circumference of 13–15 cm (5–6 in) exert even pressure over the entire flexor surface of the palm and fingers. Evidence suggests that a firm, unyielding handroll made of cardboard is more useful in preventing contractures than a soft, pliable roll (Dayhoff 1975, p. 1143).

Prone Position   In the **prone position,** the client lies on the abdomen with the head turned to one side. The hips are not flexed. Both chidren and adults sleep in this position, sometimes with one or both arms flexed over their heads. See Figure 36–16 and Procedure 36–3. This position has several advantages. It is the only bed position that allows full extension of the hip and knee joints. When used periodically, the prone position helps to prevent flexion contractures of the hips and knees, thereby counteracting a problem caused by all other bed positions. The prone position also promotes drainage from the mouth and is especially useful for clients recovering from surgery of the mouth or throat.

The prone position poses some distinct disadvantages. The pull of gravity on the trunk produces a marked lordosis in most persons, and the neck is rotated laterally to a significant degree. For this reason, physicians may not recommend this position, especially for persons with problems of the cervical or lumbar spine. This position also causes plantar flexion. Some clients with cardiac or respiratory problems find the prone position confining and suffocating, because chest expansion is inhibited during respirations. The prone position should be used only when the client's back is properly aligned, only for short periods, and only for persons with no evidence of spinal abnormalities.

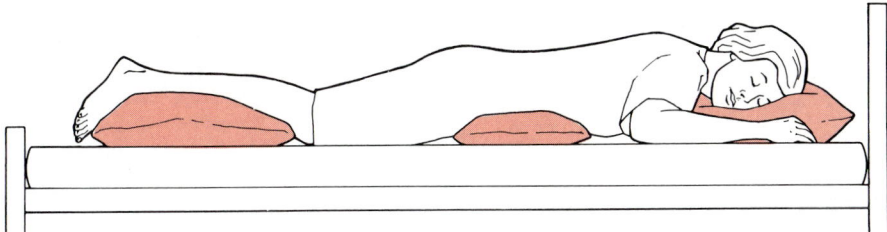

Figure 36–16 Prone position (supported).

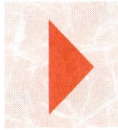

PROCEDURE 36–3

SUPPORTING A CLIENT IN PRONE POSITION

Equipment ☑

Three pillows

Intervention

 1. **Assess pressure areas of particular concern in the prone position** (see Figure 35–6, *C* on page 850).

- Toes
- Knees
- Genitals (men)
- Breasts (women)
- Acromial process of shoulders
- Cheek and ear

2. **Assist the client to a prone position.**

3. **Provide supportive devices to position the client appropriately.**

- Turn the client's head to one side, and either omit the pillow entirely if drainage from the mouth is being encouraged, or place a small pillow under the head to align the head with the trunk. *This prevents flexion of the neck laterally.* Avoid placing the pillow under the shoulders. *A pillow placed under the shoulders increases lumbar lordosis.*

- Place a small pillow or roll under the abdomen in the space between the diaphragm (or the breasts of a woman) and the iliac crests. *The pillow prevents hyperextension of the lumbar curvature, difficulty breathing, and pressure on some women's breasts. Supports placed too low can increase lumbar lordosis and pressure on bony prominences.*

- Place a pillow under the lower legs from below the knees to just above the ankles. *This raises the toes off the bed surface and reduces plantar flexion. This pillow also flexes the knees slightly for comfort and prevents excessive pressure on the patellae.*

  or

Position the client on the bed so that the feet are extended in a normal anatomic position over the lower edge of the mattress. There should be no pressure on the toes.

Malalignments and other problems associated with an *unsupported* prone position are

- Acute flexion or hyperextension of the neck
- Hyperextension of the lumbar curvature
- Plantar flexion
- Pressure on a woman's breasts
- Inhibited chest expansion

Lateral Position   In the **lateral** or **side-lying position,** the person lies on one side of the body. See Figure 36–17 and Procedure 36–4 on the following page. By having the client flex the top hip and knee and placing this leg in front of the body, a wider, triangular base of support is created, and greater stability is achieved. The greater the flexion on the top hip and knee, the greater the stability

and balance in this position. This flexion reduces lordosis and promotes good back alignment. For this reason, the lateral position is good for resting and sleeping clients. The lateral position helps to relieve pressure on the sacrum and heels in persons who sit for much of the day or who are confined to bed and rest in Fowler's or dorsal recumbant positions much of the time. In the lateral position, most of the body's weight is borne by the lateral aspect of the lower scapula, the lateral aspect of the ilium, and the greater trochanter of the femur. Persons who have sensory or motor deficits on one side of the body usually find that lying on the uninvolved side is more comfortable.

Malalignments associated with the *unsupported* lateral position include

- Lateral flexion of the neck
- Internal shoulder rotation/adduction of the upper arm

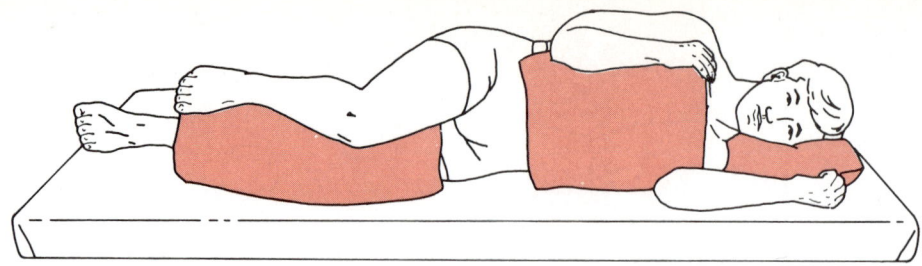

Figure 36–17 Lateral position (supported).

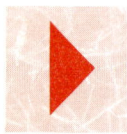

PROCEDURE 36–4

SUPPORTING A CLIENT IN LATERAL POSITION

Equipment ☑

Up to five small pillows

Folded towel (optional)

Intervention

 1. **Assess pressure areas of particular concern in the lateral position** (see Figure 35–6, *B* on page 850):

■ Lateral malleolus of lower ankle

■ Medial malleolus of upper ankle

■ Medial condyle of uppermost knee

■ Lateral condyle of lower knee

■ Greater trochanter of lower hip

■ Ischium of lower pelvis

■ Acromial process of lower clavicle

■ Lower ear and cheek

2. **Assist the client to a lateral position.**

3. **Provide supportive devices to align the client appropriately.**

■ Place a pillow under the client's head so that the head and neck are aligned with the trunk. *The pillow prevents lateral flexion and discomfort of the major neck muscles, e.g. the sternocleidomastoid muscles.*

■ Have the client flex the lower shoulder and position it forward so that the body does not rest on it. Rotate it into any position of comfort. *In this way, circulation is not disrupted.*

■ Place a pillow under the upper arm. *This prevents internal rotation and adduction of the shoulder and downward pressure on the chest that could interfere with chest expansion during respiration.* If the client has respiratory difficulty, increase the shoulder flexion and position the upper arm in front of the body off the chest.

■ Place two or more pillows under the upper leg and thigh so that the extremity lies in a plane parallel to the surface of the bed. *A position parallel to the bed most closely approximates correct standing alignment and prevents internal rotation of the thigh and adduction of the leg. The pillow also prevents pressure caused by the weight of the top leg resting on the lower leg. Such pressure can damage the vein walls in the lower leg and predispose the client to thrombus formation.*

■ Ensure that the two shoulders are aligned in the same plane as the two hips. If they are not, pull one shoulder or hip forward or backward until all four joints are aligned in the same plane. *Proper alignment prevents twisting of the spine.*

■ Place a folded towel under the natural hollow at the waistline (optional). *This prevents postural scoliosis of the lumbar spine.* Take care to fill in only the space at the waistline. *A towel support that extends too high or too low creates undue pressure against the rib cage or iliac crests.*

■ Place a rolled pillow at the client's back to stabilize the position (optional). This pillow is not usually needed when the client's upper hip and knee are appropriately flexed.

■ Internal hip rotation/adduction of the upper leg

■ Tendency for the spine to curve laterally toward the bed at the waist (postural scoliosis)

■ Twisting of the lumbar spine

■ Plantar flexion

Sims's Position In **Sims's**, or the **semiprone position,** the client assumes a posture halfway between the lateral and the prone positions. See Figure 36–18 and Procedure 36–5. In Sims's position, the lower arm is positioned behind the client, and the upper arm is flexed at the shoulder and the elbow. Both legs are flexed in front of the client.

(continued on page 912)

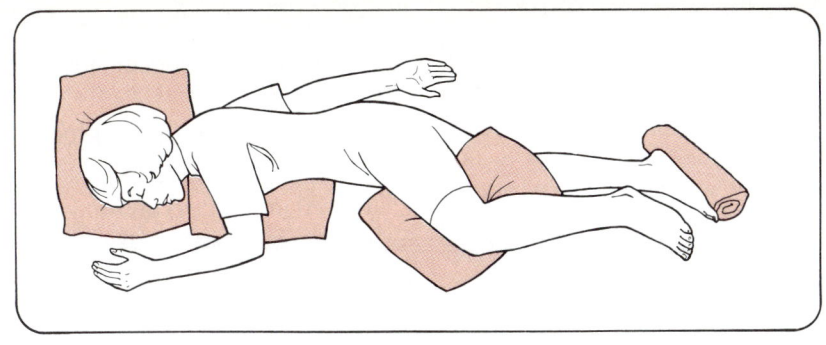

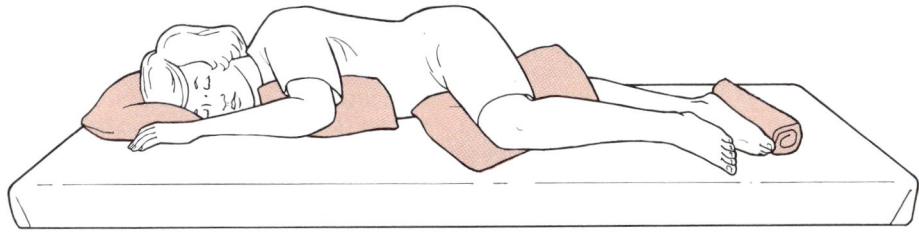

Figure 36–18   Sims's position (supported).

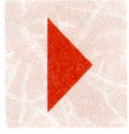

PROCEDURE 36–5

SUPPORTING A CLIENT IN SIMS'S POSITION

Equipment

Three small pillows
Sandbag or rolled towel

Intervention

1. Assess pressure areas of particular concern in the Sims's position:

- Side of the skull (temporal and parietal bones and the ear)
- Acromial process of lowermost clavicle
- Lowermost anterior superior iliac spine
- Lowermost greater trochanter of the femur
- Lateral aspect of undermost knee
- Medial aspect of uppermost knee
- Lateral malleolus of undermost ankle
- Medial malleolus of uppermost ankle
- Medial aspect (epicondyle) of uppermost elbow

2. Turn the client as for a prone position.

3. Provide supportive devices to align the client appropriately.

- Place a small pillow under the client's head, unless drainage from the mouth is being encouraged. *The pillow prevents lateral flexion of the neck and cushions the cranial and facial bones and the ear.* It is contraindicated if drainage of mucus is required. *Too large a pillow produces an uncomfortable lateral flexion of the neck.*

- Place the lower arm behind and away from the client's body in a position that is comfortable and does not disrupt circulation. *This position prevents damage to nerves and blood vessels in the axillae.*

- Position the upper shoulder so that it is abducted slightly from the body and the shoulder and elbow are flexed. Place a pillow in the space between the chest and abdomen and the upper arm and bed. *This position and support prevent internal shoulder rotation and adduction and maintain alignment of the upper trunk.*

- Place a pillow in the space between the abdomen and pelvis and the upper thigh and bed. *This position prevents internal rotation and adduction of the hip and also reduces lumbar lordosis.*

- Ensure that the two shoulders are aligned in the same plane as the two hips. If they are not, pull one shoulder or hip forward or backward until all four joints are aligned in the same plane. *This prevents twisting of the spine.*

- Place a support device, e.g., a sandbag or rolled towel, against the lower foot. *This device may prevent foot drop.* Efforts to correct plantar flexion in this position, however, are usually unsuccessful.

The upper leg is more acutely flexed at both the hip and the knee than the lower one is.

Sims's position is occasionally used for unconscious clients because it facilitates drainage from the mouth. It is also used for paralyzed (paraplegic or hemiplegic) clients because it reduces pressure over the sacrum and greater trochanter of the hip. It is often used for clients receiving enemas and occasionally for clients undergoing examinations or treatments of the perineal area. Many people, especially pregnant women, find Sims's position comfortable for sleeping. Persons with sensory or motor deficits on one side of the body usually find that lying on the uninvolved side is more comfortable.

Malalignments associated with the *unsupported* Sims's position include

- Lateral flexion of the neck

- Internal shoulder rotation and adduction of the upper arm
- Internal hip rotation and adduction of the upper leg
- Twisting of the thoracolumbar spine if the shoulders are rotated in one direction and the hips in another
- Lumbar lordosis
- Plantar flexion

Moving and Turning Clients in Bed

Although healthy people usually take for granted that they can change body position and go from one place to another with little effort, ill people may have difficulty moving even in bed. How much assistance clients require depends on

PROCEDURE 36–6

MOVING A CLIENT UP IN BED

Intervention

1. **Adjust the bed and the client's position.**

- Adjust the head of the bed to a flat position or as low as the client can tolerate. *Moving the client upward against gravity requires more force and can cause back strain.*

- Raise the bed to the height of your center of gravity.

- Lock the wheels on the bed and raise the rail on the side of the bed opposite you.

- Remove all pillows, then place one against the head of the bed. *This pillow protects the client's head from inadvertent injury against the top of the bed during the upward move.*

2. **Elicit the client's help in lessening your workload.**

- Ask the client to flex the hips and knees and position the feet so that they can be used effectively for pushing. *Flexing the hips and knees keeps the entire lower leg off the*

bed surface, preventing friction during movement, and ensures use of the large muscle groups in the client's legs when pushing, thus increasing the force of movement.

- Ask the client to
a. Grasp the head of the bed with both hands and pull during the move, *or*
b. Raise the upper part of the body on the elbows and push with the hands and forearms during the move, *or*
c. Grasp the overhead trapeze with both hands and lift and pull during the move.

Client assistance provides additional power to overcome friction during the move. These actions also keep the client's arms partially off the bed surface, reducing friction during movement, and make use of the large muscle groups of the client's arms to increase the force during movement.

3. **Position yourself appropriately and move the client.**

- Face the direction of the movement and assume a broad stance, with the foot nearest the bed behind the forward foot and weight on the forward foot. Incline your trunk forward from the hips. Flex hips, knees, and ankles.

- Place your near arm under the client's thighs. *This supports the heaviest part of the body (the buttocks).* Push down on the mattress with the far arm. See Figure 36–19. *The far arm acts as a lever during the move.*

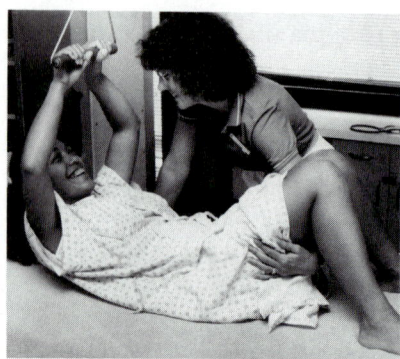

Figure 36–19 Moving a client up in bed.

- Tighten your gluteal, abdominal, leg, and arm muscles, and rock from the back leg to the front leg and back again. *Then* shift weight to the front leg as the client pushes with the heels and pulls with the arms, moving the client toward the head of the bed.

4. **Ensure client comfort.**

- Elevate the head of the bed and provide appropriate support devices for the client's new position.
- See the sections on positioning clients earlier in this chapter.

Variation: A Client Who Has Limited Strength of the Upper Extremities

Assist the client to flex the hips and knees as above. Place the client's arms across the chest. *This keeps them off the bed surface and minimizes friction during movement.* Ask the client to flex the neck during the move and keep the head off the bed surface. Position yourself properly (as above), and place one arm under the client's back and shoulders and the other arm under the client's thighs. *This placement of the arms distributes the client's weight and supports the heaviest part of the body (the buttocks).* The nurse shifts weight as above.

Variation: Pulling a Client Up in Bed

This method emphasizes pulling the client up toward the head of the bed rather than lifting the client. It is designed to create less back strain for the nurse than a method that utilizes lifting. The steps are as follows:

- After lowering the head of the bed and removing all pillows, move the client to the edge of the bed closest to your body. (Procedure 36–7 describes this action).
- Ask the client to assist (see step 2 above) or, if the client has limited strength of the upper extremities, place the client's arms across the chest and ask the client to flex the neck during the move.
- Stand toward the head of the bed and face the foot of the bed. Position yourself appropriately, and place both hands together beneath the client's coccyx. Align your body so that it is directly in line with your hands. The nurse's elbow closest to the client will be beneath the client's upper back. Both elbows should rest on the surface of the bed. This placement of the arms, beneath the heaviest part of the client's body, allows you to pull the client directly toward the center of gravity, preventing spinal twisting. Pulling from the client's center of gravity directly toward your own center of gravity requires less force than lifting and allows greater control over the movement.
- Coordinating your efforts with those of the client, rock backward and shift weight from the forward to the backward foot, pulling the client directly toward you while the client pushes with the heels and pulls with the arms. The hip closest to the bed should slide along the side of the mattress. Your elbows should slide along the bed surface.
- Raise the side rail and move to the opposite side of the bed. Move or pull the client as above, and move again to the opposite side of the bed. Move or pull the client back to the center of the bed. Raise the side rail.

---

their own ability to move and their health status. In general, nurses should be sensitive to both the need of people to function independently and their need for assistance to move.

 When a nurse assists a person to move, correct body mechanics need to be employed so that the nurse is not injured. Actions and rationales common to the lifting and moving procedures that follow are outlined in the box on the following page. Correct body alignment for the client must also be maintained so that undue stress is not placed on the musculoskeletal system.

Moving a Client Up in Bed
Clients who have slid down in bed from the Fowler's position or been pulled down by traction need assistance to move up in bed. See Procedure 36–6. The client should be encouraged to accomplish this movement independently whenever possible.

Two nurses using a hand-forearm interlock Two people are required to move clients who are unable to assist because of their condition or weight. Using the technique described in Procedure 36–6, with the second nurse on the opposite side of the bed, the two nurses interlock their forearms under the client's thighs and shoulders and lift the client up in bed. See Figure 36–20 on page 914.

Two nurses using a turn sheet Two nurses can use a turn sheet to move a client up in the bed. A turn sheet distributes the client's weight more evenly, decreases friction, and exerts a more even force on the client during the move. In addition, it prevents injury of the client's skin, since the friction created between two sheets when one is moved is less than that created by the client's body moving over the sheet.

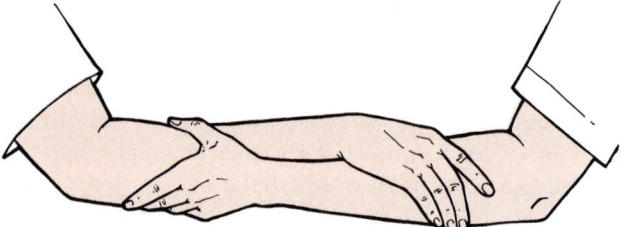

Figure 36–20 Two nurses using a hand-forearm interlock.

A drawsheet or a full sheet folded in half is placed under the client, extending from the shoulders to the thighs. Each nurse rolls up or fanfolds the turn sheet close to the client's body on either side. The nurses then grasp the sheet close to the shoulders and buttocks of the client. This draws the weight closer to the nurses' center of gravity, and increases the nurses' balance and stability, permitting a smoother movement. The method described for clients with limited strength in Procedure 36–6 is then used to move the client up in the bed.

Moving a Client to the Side of the Bed in Segments

This movement is used in preparation for moving the client onto a stretcher, in preparation for turning the client to the lateral (side-lying) position, or when changing the client's bed. See Procedure 36–7. Whenever capable of assisting with this movement, the client lifts the body by holding onto the raised side rail or by using the overhead trapeze. In this movement, the nurse's weight is used to counteract the client's weight; the nurse's arms serve as connecting bars between the client and the nurse.

Turning a Client to a Lateral or Prone Position in Bed

Movement to a lateral (side-lying) position may be necessary when placing a bedpan beneath the client, when changing the client's bed linen, or when repositioning the client. See Procedure 36–8.

Logrolling a Client

Logrolling is a technique used to turn a client whose body must at all times be kept in straight alignment (like a log). See Procedure 36–9 on page 916. An example is the client with a spinal injury. Considerable care must be taken to prevent additional injury. This technique requires two nurses or, if the client is large, three nurses. *For the client who has a cervical injury, one nurse must maintain the client's head and neck alignment.*

Assisting a Client to a Sitting Position in Bed

A client may need assistance to raise the head and shoulders while pillows are rearranged or for back care. If the client needs to rise to a sitting position in bed, the easiest method is simply to raise the head of the bed to the desired height. If the client is not in a hospital bed that can be raised mechanically, the nurse may need to assist the client. See Procedure 36–10 on page 918.

Moving a Client to a Sitting Position on the Edge of the Bed

The client assumes a sitting position on the edge of the bed before walking, moving to a chair or wheelchair, eating, or performing other activities. See Procedure 36–11 on page 918.

Transferring Clients

Many clients require some assistance in transferring between bed and chair or wheelchair, between wheelchair and toilet, and between bed and stretcher. Before transferring any client, however, the nurse must determine the client's physical and mental capabilities to participate in the transfer technique. Essential data include the following:

- Ability to follow instructions
- Activity tolerance
- Muscle strength
- Joint mobility

(continued on page 919)

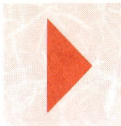

MOVING A CLIENT TO THE SIDE OF THE BED IN SEGMENTS

Intervention

1. Position yourself and the client appropriately before the move.

■ Stand as close as possible at the side of the bed toward which the client will be moved and opposite the client's chest. *This position lessens the client's fear of falling and places your center of gravity close to the client's center of gravity.*

■ Place the client's near arm across his or her chest. *This avoids friction and resistance to movement and prevents injury to the arm.*

■ Incline your trunk forward from the hips. Flex your hips, knees, and ankles. Assume a broad stance, with one foot forward and the weight placed upon this forward foot.

2. Move the client's head and trunk.

■ Place your arms and hands with palms facing upward close together beneath the client's scapulae. *This focuses the force for movement under the heaviest part of the upper trunk. Placing the arms close together reduces the friction of the client's body against the bed, making the pull easier.*

■ Flex your fingers around the client's far shoulder and rest your elbows on the surface of the bed. *This prevents inadvertent lifting.*

■ If the client cannot support the head during the movement, position your arm nearest the head of the bed so that it cradles the client's head.

■ Tighten your gluteal, abdominal, leg, and arm muscles, rock backward, and shift your weight from the forward to the backward foot, while pulling the client's shoulders directly toward you.

3. Move the client's buttocks.

■ Place your arms and hands close together beneath the client's buttocks, and pull the buttocks to the side of the bed as described above.

4. Move the client's legs and feet.

■ Place your hands close together beneath the client's ankles, and repeat the steps above, pulling the client's legs and feet to the side of the bed.

■ Elevate the side rail next to the client. *This prevents the client from falling off the bed.*

Variation: Using a Pull Sheet

Use a pull sheet beneath the client's trunk and thighs to pull the client to the side of the bed. Roll up the sheet as close as possible to the client's body and pull the client's shoulders, then the buttocks, to the side of the bed. Move the legs and feet as described above.

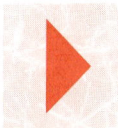

TURNING A CLIENT TO A LATERAL OR PRONE POSITION IN BED

Intervention

1. Position yourself and the client appropriately before the move.

■ Move the client closer to the side of the bed opposite the side the client will face when turned. See Procedure 36–7. *This ensures that the client will be positioned safely in the center of the bed after turning.*

■ While standing on the side of the bed nearest the client, place the client's near arm across the chest. Abduct the client's far shoulder slightly from the side of body. *Pulling the one arm forward facilitates the turning motion. Pulling the other arm away from the body prevents that arm from being caught beneath the client's body during the roll.*

■ Place the client's near ankle and foot across the far ankle and foot. *This facilitates the turning motion. Making these preparations on the side of the bed closest to the client helps the nurse prevent unnecessary reaching.*

■ Raise the side rail next to the client before going to the other side of the bed. *This ensures that the client, who is close to the edge of the mattress, will not fall.*

■ Position yourself on the side of the bed toward which the client will turn, directly in line with the client's waistline and as close to the bed as possible.

■ Incline your trunk forward from the hips. Flex your hips, knees, and ankles. Assume a broad stance with one foot forward and the weight placed upon this forward foot.

2. **Pull or roll the client to a lateral position.**

■ Place one hand on the client's far hip and the other hand on the client's far shoulder. See Figure 36–21 A. *This position of the hands supports the client at the two heaviest parts of the body, providing greater control in movement during the roll.*

■ Tighten your gluteal, abdominal, leg, and arm muscles; rock backward, shifting your weight from the forward to the backward foot; and roll the client onto the side of the body to face you. See Figure 36–21 B.

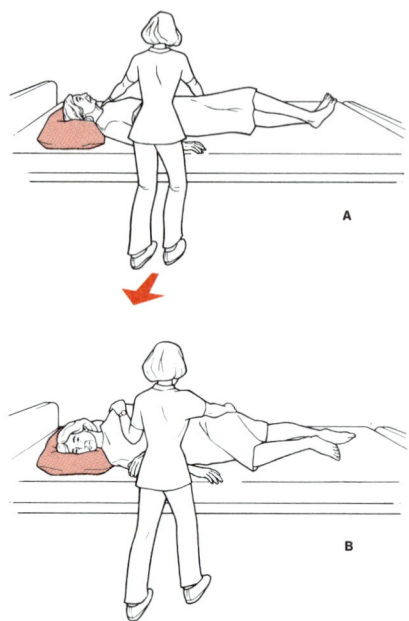

Figure 36–21 Moving a client to a lateral position.

Variation: Turning the Client to a Prone Position

To turn a client to the prone position, follow all of the above steps, with two exceptions:

■ Instead of abducting the far arm, keep the client's arm alongside the body for the client to roll over. *Keeping the arm alongside the body prevents it from being pinned under the client when the client is rolled.*

■ Roll the client completely onto the abdomen. *It is essential to move the client as close as possible to the bed edge before the turn so that the client will be lying in the center of the bed after rolling.* Never pull a client across the bed while the client is in the prone position. *Doing so can injure a woman's breasts or a man's genitals.*

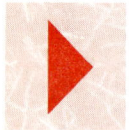

PROCEDURE 36–9

LOGROLLING A CLIENT

Intervention

1. **Position yourselves and the client appropriately before the move.**

■ Stand on the same side of the bed and assume a broad stance with one foot ahead of the other.

■ Place the client's arms across the chest. *Doing so ensures that they will not be injured or become trapped under the body when the body is turned.*

■ Incline your trunk and flex your hips, knees, and ankles.

■ Place your arms under the client as shown in Figure 36–22 or Figure 36–23, depending on the client's size. *Each nurse then has a major weight area of the client centered between the arms.*

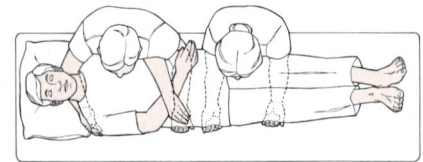

Figure 36–22 Proper arm placement for pulling the client to the side of the bed: two nurses.

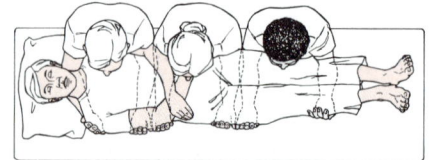

Figure 36–23 Proper arm placement for pulling the client to the side of the bed: three nurses.

■ Tighten your gluteal, abdominal, leg, and arm muscles.

2. Pull the client to the side of the bed.

■ One nurse counts, "one, two, three, go." Then, at the same time, all nurses pull the client to the side of the bed by shifting weight to the back foot. *Moving the client in unison maintains the client's body alignment.*

■ Elevate the side rail on this side of the bed. *This prevents the client from falling while lying so close to the edge of the bed.*

3. Move to the other side of the bed, and place supportive devices for the client when turned.

■ Place a pillow where it will support the client's head after the turn. *The pillow prevents lateral flexion of the neck and ensures alignment of the cervical spine.*

■ Place one or two pillows between the client's legs to support the upper leg when the client is turned. *This pillow prevents adduction of the upper leg and keeps the legs parallel and aligned.*

4. Roll and position the client in proper alignment.

■ All nurses flex the hips, knees, and ankles and assume a broad stance with one foot forward.

■ All nurses reach over the client and place hands as shown in Figure 36–24. *Doing so centers a major weight area of the client between each nurse's arms.*

■ One nurse counts, "one, two, three, go." Then, at the same time, all

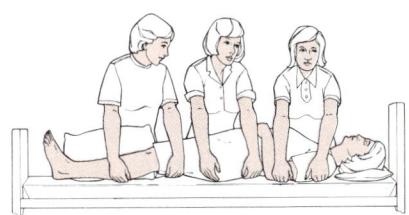

Figure 36–24 Proper hand placement in logrolling a client.

nurses roll the client to a lateral position.

■ Place pillows to maintain the client's lateral position. See the discussion of the lateral position on page 000.

Variation: Using a Turn Sheet

■ Use a turn sheet to facilitate logrolling. First, stand with another nurse on the same side of the bed. Assume a broad stance with one foot forward, and grasp half of the fanfolded or rolled edge of the turn sheet. On a signal, pull the client toward both of you. See Figure 36–25.

■ Before turning the client, place pillow supports for the head and legs, as described in step 3 of Procedure 36–9. This maintains the client's alignment when turning. Then go to the other side of the bed (farthest from the client) and assume a stable stance. Reaching over the client, grasp the far edges of the turn sheet, and roll the client toward you. See Figure 36–26. The second nurse (behind the client) helps turn the client and provides pillow supports to ensure good alignment in the lateral position.

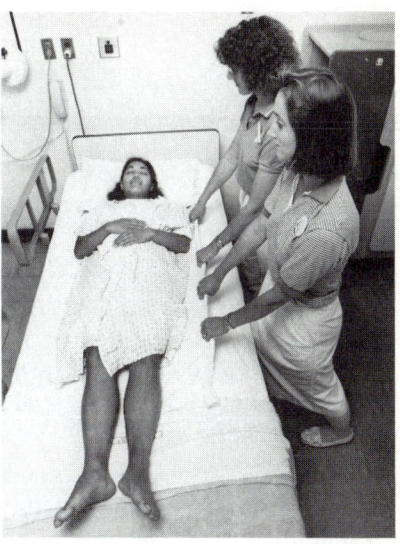

Figure 36–25 Using a turn sheet, the nurses pull the client toward them to the edge of the bed.

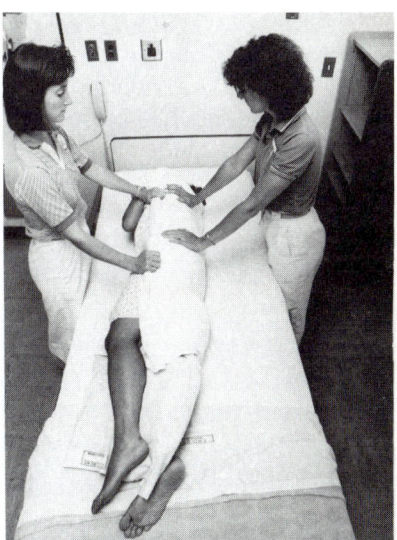

Figure 36–26 One nurse uses the far edge of the sheet to pull the client toward her, while the second nurse remains behind the client to assist.

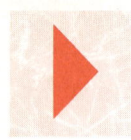

PROCEDURE 36–10

ASSISTING A CLIENT TO A SITTING POSITION IN BED

Intervention

1. **Position yourself and the client appropriately before the move.**

- Ask the client to place arms at the sides with the palms of the hands against the surface of the bed. *In this way, the client can push against the bed surface to provide additional power for the lift.*

- Face the head of the bed, and stand at the side of the bed beside the client's buttocks. Assume a broad stance with the foot farthest from the bed forward and body weight on this foot.

2. **Lift the client to a sitting position.**

- Place the hand nearest the client over the client's far shoulder to rest between the shoulder blades. *This hand position enables you to pull*

the client's upper body directly toward your center of gravity and prevents spinal twisting.

- Place the hand of your free arm on the edge of the surface of the bed near the client's shoulder, and use it to push during the lift. See Figure 36–27, A. *This provides balance and leverage.*

- Have the client lift with you simultaneously on your signal. Lift by pulling with the arm and hand over the client's shoulder, pushing on the bed surface with the other hand, and shifting your weight from the forward to the back foot in a rocking motion. See Figure 36–27, B. *Pushing with the muscles of one arm while pulling with the muscles of the other arm distributes the workload and increases lifting power.* The client simultaneously pushes with the hands and arms.

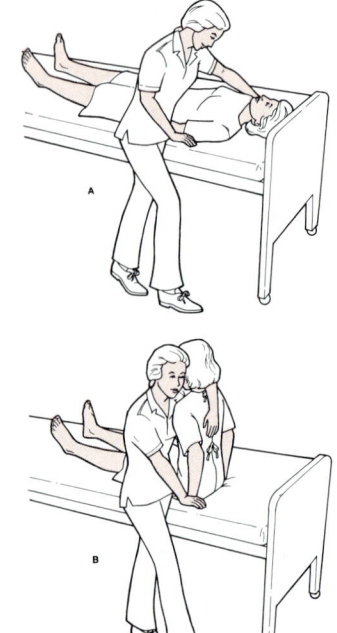

Figure 36–27 Assisting a client to a sitting position in bed.

PROCEDURE 36–11

MOVING A CLIENT TO A SITTING POSITION ON THE EDGE OF THE BED

Intervention

1. **Position yourself and the client appropriately before the move.**

- Assist the client to a lateral position facing you. See Procedure 36–8.

- Raise the head of the bed slowly as high as it will go. *This decreases the distance that the client needs to move to sit up on the side of the bed.*

- Position the client's feet and lower legs just over the edge of the bed.

This enables the client's feet to move easily off the bed during the movement, and the client is aided by gravity into a sitting position.

- Stand beside the client's hips and face the far corner of the bottom of the bed (the angle in which movement will occur). Assume a broad stance, placing the foot nearest the client forward. Incline your trunk forward from the hips. Flex your hips, knees, and ankles. See Figure 36–28 A.

2. **Move the client to a sitting position.**

- Place one arm around the client's shoulders and the other arm beneath both of the client's thighs near the knees. See Figure 36–28 A. *Supporting the client's shoulders prevents the client from falling backward during movement. Supporting the client's thighs reduces friction of the thighs against the bed surface during the move and increases the force of the movement.*

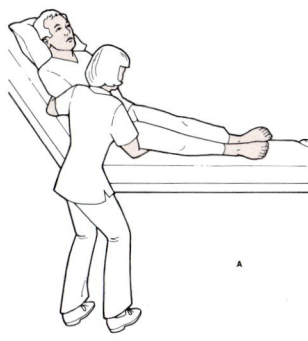

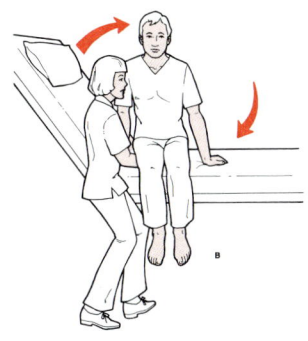

Figure 36–28 Assisting a client to a sitting position on the edge of the bed.

- Tighten your gluteal, abdominal, leg, and arm muscles.
- Lift the client's thighs slightly. *This reduces the friction of the client's*

thighs and your arm against the bed surface.

- Pivot on the balls of your feet in the desired direction facing the foot of the bed while pulling the client's feet and legs off the bed. See Figure 36–28 B. *Pivoting prevents twisting of your spine. The weight of the client's legs swinging downward increases downward movement of the lower body and helps make the client's upper body vertical.*
- Keep supporting the client until the client is balanced and comfortable. *This movement may cause some clients to faint.*

Variation: Teaching a Client How to Sit on the Side of the Bed Independently

A client who has had recent abdominal surgery or who is weak may have too much abdominal pain or too little strength to sit straight up in bed. This person can be taught to assume a "dangle" position without assistance. Instruct the client to

- Roll to the side and lift the far leg over the near leg. See Figure 36–29A.

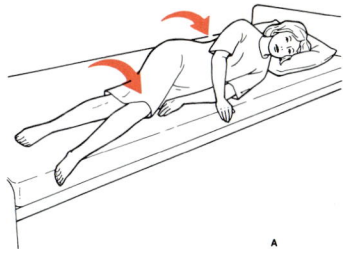

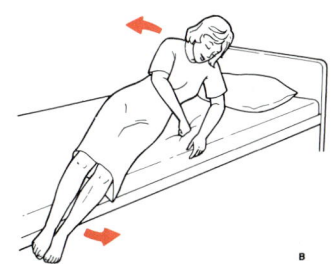

Figure 36–29 Moving to a sitting position independently.

- Grasp the mattress edge with the lower arm and push the fist of the upper arm into the mattress. See Figure 36–29B.
- Push up with the arms as the heels and legs slide over the mattress edge. See Figure 36–29B.
- Maintain sitting position by pushing both fists into the mattress behind and to the sides of the buttocks.

(continued from page 914)

- Presence of paralysis
- Level of comfort
- Presence of orthostatic hypotension

In addition, the nurse must mentally analyze and organize the activity. General guidelines for transfer techniques include the following:

- Planning what to do and how best to do it
- Obtaining essential equipment, e.g., transfer belt, sliding board, wheelchair, stretcher and checking them for function and safety
- Removing obstacles in the transfer area

- Informing the client about the transfer, enlisting the client's help, and explaining how the client can help
- Informing assitants of their roles and who will give directions (one person needs to be in charge)
- Always supporting or holding the client, not the equipment
- During the transfer, again informing the client step-by-step what the client is to do
- Making a written plan of the transfer so that all health care professionals can follow the same plan with the client (including how the client is to be returned to the original place)

Because wheelchairs and stretchers are unstable, they can predispose the client to falls and injury. Guidelines for the

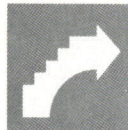

CLINICAL GUIDELINES
Wheelchair Safety

- Always lock the brakes on both wheels of the wheelchair when the client transfers in or out of it.
- Raise the footplates before transferring the client into the wheelchair.
- Lower the footplates after the transfer, and place the client's feet on them.
- Ensure the client is positioned well back in the seat of the wheelchair.
- Use seat belts that fasten behind the wheelchair to protect confused clients from falls.
- Back the wheelchair into or out of an elevator, rear large wheels first.
- Place your body between the wheelchair and the bottom of an incline.

CLINICAL GUIDELINES
Safe Use of Stretchers

- Lock the wheels of the bed and stretcher before the client transfers in or out of them.
- Fasten safety straps across the client on a stretcher, and raise the side rails.
- Never leave a client unattended on a stretcher unless the wheels are locked and the side rails are raised on both sides and/or the safety straps are securely fastened across the client.
- Always push a stretcher from the end where the client's head is positioned. This position protects the client's head in the event of a collision.
- If the stretcher has two swivel wheels and two stationary wheels:
  - Always position the client's head at the end with the stationary wheels
    and
  - Push the stretcher from the end with the stationary wheels. The stretcher is maneuvered more easily when pushed from this end.
- Maneuver the stretcher when entering the elevator so that the client's head goes in first.

safe use of wheelchairs and stretchers are shown in the accompanying boxes.

Transferring a Client between a Bed and a Wheelchair A client may need to be transferred between the bed and a wheelchair or chair, the bed and the commode, and a wheelchair and the toilet. There are numerous variations of this transfer technique; several are described in Procedure 36–12. Which variation the nurse selects depends on a number of factors: the client's disabilities and body size, the technique with which the client is familiar, the space in which the transfer is maneuvered (bathrooms, for instance, are usually cramped), the number of assistants (1 or 2) needed to accomplish the transfer safely, and the skill and strength of the nurse(s).

Transfer belts provide the greatest safety. See Figure 36–30. This belt has a handle that allows the nurse to control movement of the client during the transfer. An increasing number of hospitals and nursing homes are requiring that personnel use the transfer belt to transfer clients.

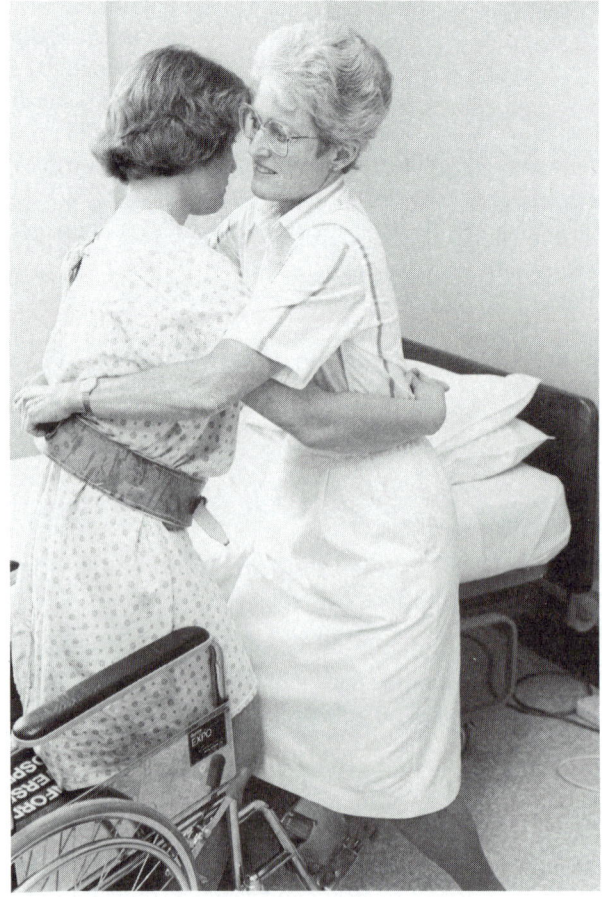

Figure 36–30 Using a transfer belt.

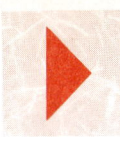

PROCEDURE 36–12

TRANSFERRING A CLIENT BETWEEN A BED AND A WHEELCHAIR

Intervention

1. Position the equipment appropriately.

- Lower the bed to its lowest position so that the client's feet will rest flat on the floor. Lock the wheels of the bed.

- Place the wheelchair parallel to the bed as close to the bed as possible, as shown in Figure 36–31. Lock the wheels of the wheelchair, and raise the footplate.

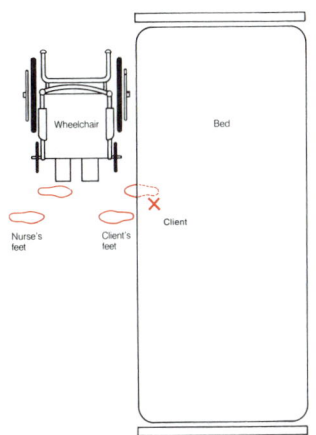

Figure 36–31 The wheelchair is placed parallel to the bed as close to the bed as possible. Note that the placement of the nurse's feet mirrors that of the client's feet.

2. Prepare and assess the client.

- Assist the client to a sitting position on the side of the bed. See Procedure 36–11.

- Assess the client for orthostatic hypotension before moving the client from the bed.

- Assist the client in putting on a bathrobe and nonskid slippers or shoes.

- Place a transfer belt snugly around the client's waist. Check to be certain that the belt is securely fastened.

3. Give explicit instructions to the client. Ask the client to

- Move forward and sit on the edge of the bed. *This brings the client's center of gravity closer to yours.*

- Lean forward slightly from the hips. *This brings the client's center of gravity more directly over the base of support and positions the head and trunk in the direction of the movement.*

- Place the foot of the stronger leg beneath the edge of the bed and put the other foot forward. *In this way, the client can use the stronger leg muscles to stand and power the movement. A broader base of support makes the client more stable during the transfer.*

- Place the hands on the bed surface or on your shoulders so that the client can push while standing. *This provides additional force for the movement and reduces the potential for strain on your back.* The client should not grasp your neck for support. *Doing so can injure the nurse.*

4. Position yourself appropriately.

- Stand directly in front of the client. Incline the trunk forward from the hips. Flex the hips, knees, and ankles. Assume a broad stance, placing one foot forward and one back. Mirror the placement of the client's feet, if possible (see Figure 36–31. *This helps prevent loss of balance during the transfer.*

- Encircle the client's waist with your arms, and grasp the transfer belt at the client's back with thumbs pointing downward. *The belt provides a secure handle for holding onto the client and controlling the movement. Downward placement of the thumbs prevents potential wrist injury as the nurse lifts* (Lein-

weber 1978). *By encircling the client in this manner, the nurse keeps the client from tilting backward during the transfer.*

- Tighten your gluteal, abdominal, leg, and arm muscles.

5. Assist the client to stand and then move together toward the wheelchair.

- On the count of three:
  a. Ask the client to push with the back foot, rock to the forward foot, extend (straighten) the joints of the lower extremities, and push or pull up with the hands, while
  b. You push with the forward foot, rock to the back foot, extend the joints of the lower extremities, and pull the client (directly toward your center of gravity) into a standing position.

- Support the client in an upright standing position for a few moments. *This allows you and the client to extend the joints and provides you with an opportunity to ensure that the client is all right before moving away from the bed.*

- Together, pivot or take a few steps toward the wheelchair.

6. Assist the client to sit.

- Ask the client to
  a. Back up to the wheelchair and place the legs against the seat. *Having the client place the legs against the wheelchair seat minimizes the risk of the client's falling when sitting down.*
  b. Place the foot of the stronger leg slightly behind the other. *This supports body weight during the movement.*
  c. Keep the other foot forward. *This provides a broad base of support.*
  d. Place both hands on the wheelchair arms or on your shoulders.

This increases stability and lessens the strain on you.

■ Stand directly in front of the client. Place one foot forward and one back.

■ Tighten your grasp on the transfer belt, and tighten your gluteal, abdominal, leg, and arm muscles.

■ On the count of three:

a. Have the client shift the body weight by rocking to the back foot, lower the body onto the edge of the wheelchair seat by flexing the joints of the legs and arms, and place some body weight on the arms, while

b. You shift your body weight by rocking to the forward foot and flex the hips and knees to lower and guide the client onto the wheelchair seat.

7. Ensure client safety.

■ Ask the client to push himself back into the wheelchair seat. *Sitting well back on the seat provides a broader base of support and greater stability and minimizes the risk of falling from the wheelchair. A wheelchair can topple forward when the client sits on the edge of the seat and leans far forward.*

■ Lower the footplates, and place the client's feet on them.

■ Apply a seat belt as required.

Variation: Angling the Wheelchair

For clients who have difficulty walking, place the wheelchair at a 45° angle to the bed. *This enables the client to pivot into the chair and lessens the amount of body rotation required.*

Variation: Transferring Without a Belt

For clients who need minimal assistance, place the hands against the sides

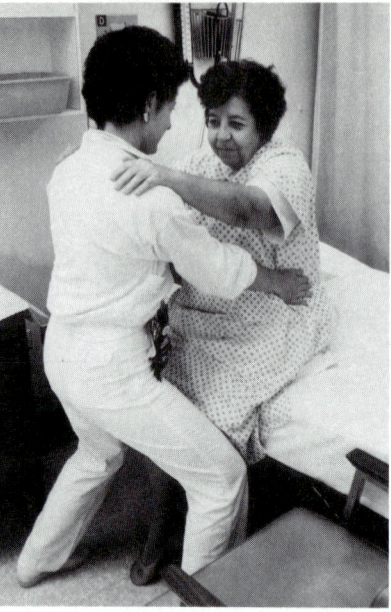

Figure 36–32   Transferring without a belt.

of the client's chest (not at the axillae) during the transfer. See Figure 36–32. For clients who require more assistance, reach through the client's axillae, and place the hands on the client's scapulae during the transfer. Avoid placing hands or pressure on the axillae, especially for clients who have upper extremity paralysis or paresis. The other steps are the same as described previously.

Variation: Transferring with a Belt and Two Nurses

When the client is able to stand, position yourselves on both sides of the client, facing the same direction as the client. Flex your hips, knees, and ankles; grasp the client's transfer belt with the hand closest to the client; and with the other hand support the client's elbows. Coordinating your efforts, all three of you stand simultaneously, pivot, and move to the

wheelchair where the process is reversed to lower the client onto the wheelchair seat.

Variation: Transferring a Client with an Injured Lower Extremity

When the client has an injured lower extremity, movement should always occur toward the client's unaffected (strong) side. For example, if the client's right leg is injured and the client is sitting on the edge of the bed preparing to transfer to a wheelchair, position the wheelchair on the client's left side. *In this way, the client can use the unaffected leg most effectively and safely.*

Variation: Using a Sliding Board

Have a client who cannot stand use a sliding board to move without nursing assistance. This method not only promotes the client's sense of independence but preserves your energy. See Figure 36–33.

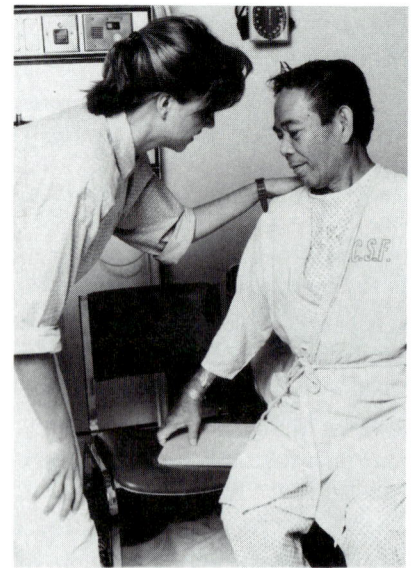

Figure 36–33   Using a sliding board.

Transferring a Client between a Bed and a Stretcher   The stretcher, or gurney, is used to transfer supine clients from one location to another. Whenever the client is capable of accomplishing the transfer from bed to stretcher independently, either by lifting onto it or by rolling onto it, the client should be encouraged to do so. If the client cannot move onto the stretcher independently, at least two nurses are needed to assist with the transfer; more are needed if the client is totally helpless or heavy. See Procedure 36–13.

Transferring a Client to a Chair Using a Mechanical Lifter   Mechanical lifters are used primarily for clients who cannot help themselves or who are too heavy for others to lift safely. Transfers may be made between the bed and a wheelchair, the bed and the bathtub, and the bed and a stretcher. Various types of mechanical lifters are used to lift and move clients. The lifter may have a one-piece or two-piece canvas seat. The one-piece seat stretches from the client's head to the knees. See Figure 36–34. The two-piece seat has one canvas strap to support

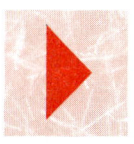

PROCEDURE 36–13

TRANSFERRING A CLIENT BETWEEN A BED AND A STRETCHER

Equipment

Stretcher
Roller bar (optional)

Intervention

1. **Adjust the client's bed in preparation for the transfer.**

- Lower the head of the bed until it is flat or as low as the client can tolerate.

- Raise the bed so that it is slightly higher than the surface of the stretcher. *It is easier and requires less effort for the client to move down an incline.*

- Ensure that the wheels on the bed are locked.

- Pull the drawsheet out from both sides of the bed.

2. **Move the client to the edge of the bed, and position the stretcher.**

- Roll the drawsheet as close to the client's side as possible.

- Pull the client to the edge of the bed, and cover the client with a sheet or bath blanket to maintain comfort.

- Place the stretcher parallel to the bed, next to the client, and lock its wheels.

- Fill the gap that exists between the bed and the stretcher loosely with bath blankets (optional).

3. **Transfer the client to the stretcher.**

- In unison with the other nurses, press your body tightly against the stretcher. *This prevents the stretcher's movement.*

- Roll the pull sheet tightly against the client. *This achieves better control over client movement.*

- Flex your hips, and pull the client on the pull sheet in unison directly toward you and onto the stretcher. *Pulling downward requires less force than pulling along a flat surface.*

- Ask the client to flex the neck during the move, if possible, and place arms across the chest. *This prevents injury to these body parts.*

4. **Ensure client comfort and safety.**

- Make the client comfortable, unlock the stretcher wheels, and move the stretcher away from the bed.

- Immediately raise the stretcher side rails and/or fasten the safety straps across the client. *Because the stretcher is high and narrow, the client is in danger of falling unless these safety precautions are taken.*

Variation: Using a Roller Bar During the Transfer

A roller bar is a metal frame covered with longitudinal rollers. Place the bar over the gap between the bed and the stretcher. Using a pull sheet, pull the client onto the roller bar, and roll the client easily onto the stretcher.

Variation: Using a Long Board

The long board, which may be referred to as the Smooth Mover or Easyglide, is a lacquered or smooth polyethylene board measuring 45–55 cm (18–22 in) by 182 cm (72 in) with handholds along its edges. This device may be used by one nurse alone or up to four nurses together. Turn the client to a lateral position away from you, position the board close to the client's back, and roll the client onto the board. Pull the client and board across the bed to the stretcher. Safety belts may be placed over the chest, abdomen, and legs.

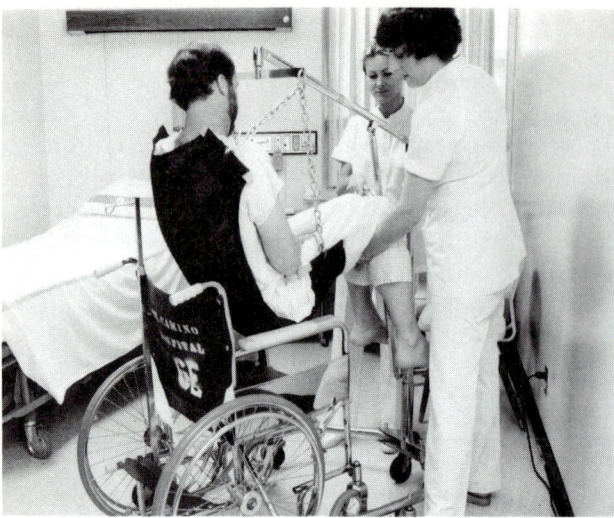

Figure 36–34 A one-piece seat mechanical lifter.

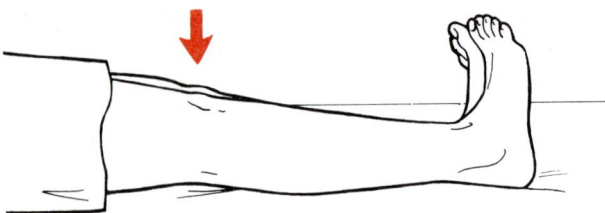

Figure 36–35 Tensing the quadriceps femoris muscles before ambulation.

the client's buttocks and thighs and a second strap to support the back, extending up to the axillae.

It is important that nurses be familiar with the model used and the practices that accompany use. Before using the lifter, the nurse ensures that it is in working order and that the hooks, chains, straps, and canvas seat are in good repair. Most agencies recommend that two nurses operate a lifter. Agency policy should be checked in this regard.

Before lifting the client, the nurse explains the procedure and demonstrates the lifter. Some clients are afraid of being lifted and will be reassured by a demonstration.

Assisting Clients to Ambulate

Even 1 or 2 days of bed rest can make a person feel weak, unsteady, and shaky when first getting out of bed. A client who has had surgery, is elderly, or has been immobilized for a longer time will feel more pronounced weakness. The potential problems of immobility (see Chapter 35) are far less likely to occur when clients become ambulatory as soon as possible. The nurse can assist clients to prepare for ambulation by helping them become as independent as possible while in bed. Nurses should encourage clients to perform activities of daily living, maintain good body alignment, perform orthostatic tension stimulating exercises, and carry out active range-of-motion exercises to the maximum degree possible yet within the limitations imposed by their illness and recovery program.

Preambulatory Exercises   Clients who have been in bed for long periods often need a plan of muscle tone exercises to strengthen the muscles used for walking before attempting to walk. One of the most important muscle groups is the quadriceps femoris, which extends the knee and flexes the thigh. This group is also important for elevating the

legs, e.g., for walking upstairs. To strengthen these muscles, the client consciously tenses them, drawing the kneecap upward and inward. The client pushes the popliteal space of the knee against the bed surface, relaxing the heels on the bed surface. See Figure 36–35. On the count of 1, the muscles are tensed; they are held during the counts of 2, 3, 4; and they are relaxed at the count of 5. The exercise should be done within the client's tolerance, i.e., without fatiguing the muscles. Carried out several times an hour during waking hours, this simple exercise significantly strengthens the muscles used for walking.

Ambulation Guidelines   When the client is ready to ambulate, the nurse follows the guidelines in the accompanying box to ensure client safety and facilitate ambulation.

Protecting a Client Who Begins to Fall While Ambulating   If a client begins to experience the signs and symptoms of orthostatic hypotension or extreme weakness, the client should be quickly assisted into a nearby wheelchair or other chair and helped to lower the head between the knees. The nurse must stay with the client. A client who faints while in this position could fall, head first, out of the chair. When the weakness subsides, the client can be assisted back to bed.

If a chair is not close by, the client should be assisted to a horizontal position on the floor before fainting occurs, since a vertical position may increase feelings of faintness. Clients who do faint or start to fall and cannot regain their strength or balance usually drop straight downward or pitch slightly forward due to the momentum of ambulating; thus, the head, hips, and knees are most vulnerable to injury. In this situation, a nurse assumes a broad stance with one foot in front of the other and brings the client backward so that the person is supported by the nurse's body. The nurse then allows the client to slide down the nurse's leg and lowers the person gently to the floor, making sure that the client's head does not hit any objects. See Figure 36–36. The nurse's broad stance widens the base of support for stability. Placing one foot behind the other allows the nurse to rock backward and use the femoral muscles when supporting the client's weight and lowering the center of gravity, thus preventing back strain. Bringing the client's weight backward

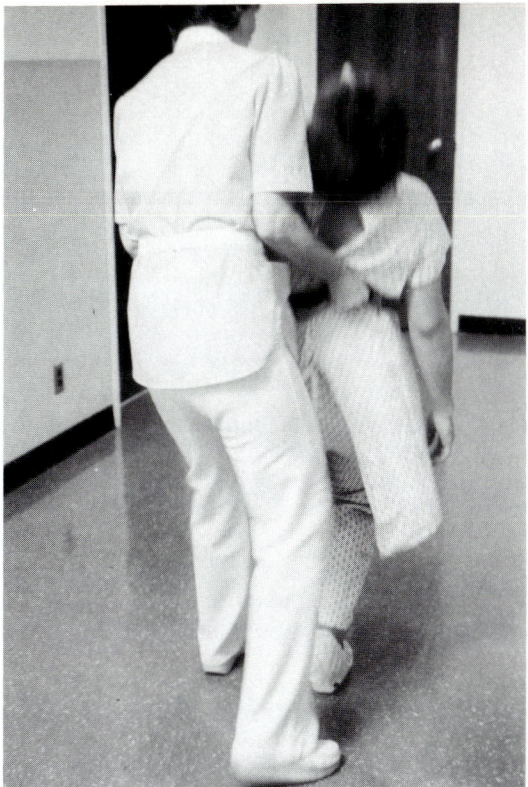

Figure 36–36 A client who has fainted is lowered to the floor.

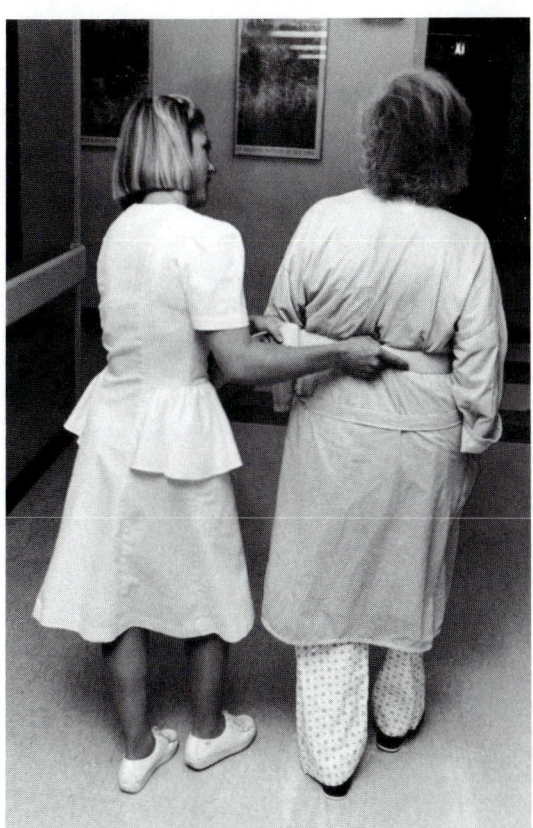

Figure 36–37 A walking belt.

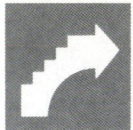

CLINICAL GUIDELINES
Ambulation

- Assess the client carefully for signs and symptoms of orthostatic hypotension (dizziness, lightheadedness, or a sudden increase in heart rate) prior to leaving the bedside and periodically during the ambulatory experience.

- Have the client wear comfortable shoes with nonskid soles.

- Remain physically close to the client in case assistance is needed.

- Encourage the client to ambulate independently if the client is able, but walk beside the client.

- Use a transfer or walking belt if the client is slightly weak and unstable. Make sure the belt is pulled snugly around the client's waist and fastened securely. Grasp the belt at the client's back and walk behind and slightly to one side of the client. See Figure 36–37.

- Have an assistant follow the nurse and client with a wheelchair in the event that it is needed quickly, if it is the client's first time out of bed following surgery, injury, or an extended period of immobility, or if the client is quite weak or unstable.

- Interlock your forearm with the client's closest forearm and walk on the client's weaker side if the client is moderately weak and unstable. Encourage the client to press the forearm against your hip or waist for stability if desired. In addition, have the client wear a transfer or walking belt so that you can quickly grab the belt and prevent a fall if the client feels faint.

- Place your near arm around the client's waist if the client is very weak and unstable, and with your other arm support the client's near arm at the elbow. Walk on the client's stronger side. Again, have the client wear a transfer or walking belt in case of an emergency.

- Encourage the client to assume a normal walking stance and gait as much as possible.

against the nurse's body allows gradual movement to the floor without injury to the client.

If the client who is ambulating with two nurses starts to fall, the two nurses slip their arms under the client's axillae, grasp the client's hands, and lower the client gently to the floor or to a nearby chair.

Teaching Clients to Use Mechanical Aids for Walking

Canes   Three types of canes are used today: the standard straight-legged cane; the tripod or crab cane, which

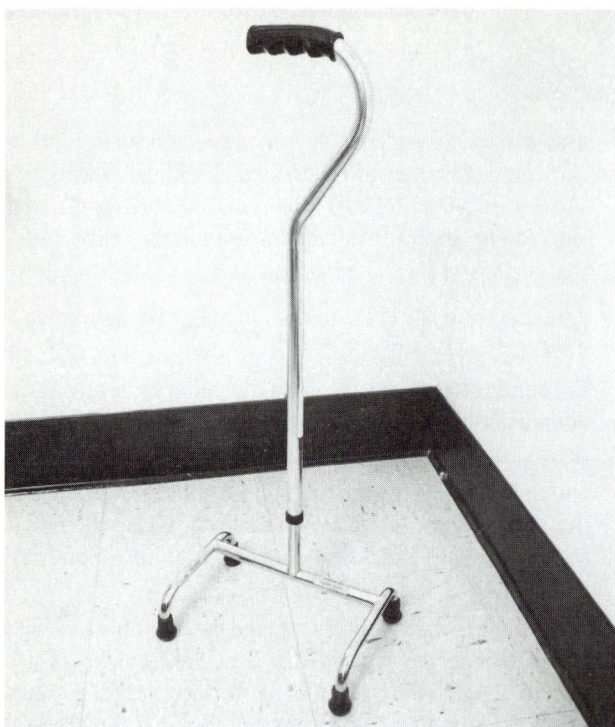

Figure 36–38 A quad cane.

- Hold the cane with the hand on the stronger side of the body to provide maximum support and appropriate body alignment when walking.
- Position the tip of a standard cane (and the nearest tip of other canes) about 15 cm (6 in) to the side and 15 cm (6 in) in front of the near foot, so that the elbow is slightly flexed.

When maximum support is required:
- Move the cane forward about 30 cm (1 ft), or a distance that is comfortable while the body weight is borne by both legs.
- Then, move the affected (weak) leg forward to the cane while the weight is borne by the cane and stronger leg.
- Next, move the unaffected (stronger) leg forward ahead of the cane and weak leg while the weight is borne by the cane and weak leg.
- Repeat above three steps. This pattern of moving provides at least two points of support on floor at all times.

As you become stronger and require less support:
- Move the cane and weak leg forward at the same time, while the weight is borne by the stronger leg.
- Move the stronger leg forward, while the weight is borne by the cane and the weak leg.

has three feet; and the quad cane, which has four feet and provides the most support. See Figure 36–38. Cane tips should have rubber caps to improve traction and prevent slipping. The standard cane is 91 cm (36 in) long; some aluminum canes can be adjusted from 56 to 97 cm (22 to 38 inches). Clients may use either one or two canes, depending on how much support they require. The accompanying box provides instructions for clients in the use of a cane.

Walkers Walkers are mechanical devices for ambulatory clients who need more support than a cane provides. There are many types of walkers of different shapes and sizes, with devices suited to individual needs. The standard type is made of polished aluminum. It has four legs with rubber tips and plastic hand grips. See Figure 36–39. Many walkers have adjustable legs.

The standard walker needs to be picked up to be used. The client therefore requires partial strength in both hands and wrists, strong elbow extensors, such as the triceps brachii, and strong shoulder depressors, such as the pectoralis minor. The client also needs the ability to bear at least partial weight on both legs.

Four-wheeled models of walkers (roller walkers) do not need to be picked up to be moved, but they are less stable than the standard walker. They are used by clients who are too weak or unstable to pick up and move the walker with each step. Some roller walkers have a seat at the back so the client can sit down to rest when desired. An adaptation

of the standard and four-wheeled walker is one that has two tips and two wheels. This type provides more stability than the four-wheeled model yet still permits the client to keep the walker in contact with the ground all the time. The client tilts the walker toward the body, lifting the tips while the wheels remain on the ground, then pushes the walker forward.

The nurse may need to adjust the height of a client's walker so that the hand bar is just below the client's waist and the client's elbows are slightly flexed. This position helps the client assume a more normal stance. A walker that is too low causes the client to stoop; one that is too high makes the client stretch and reach. The accompanying box provides instructions for clients in the use of a walker.

Crutches Crutches may be a temporary need for some people and a permanent one for others. Crutches should enable a person to ambulate independently; therefore, it is important to learn to use them properly.

There are several kinds of crutches. The most frequently used are the underarm or **axillary crutch** with hand bars and the **Lofstrand crutch,** which extends only to the forearm. The underarm crutch can be extended. It has dou-

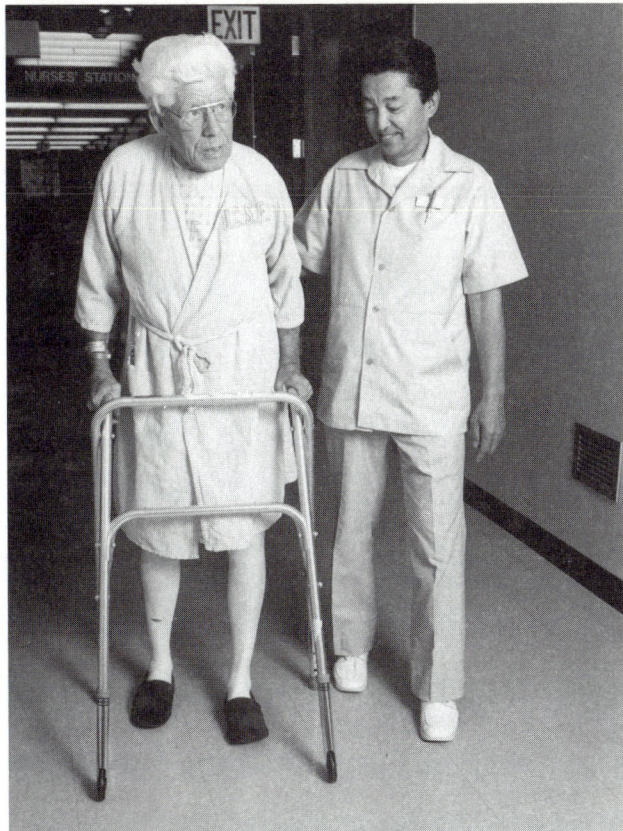

Figure 36–39 A standard walker.

CLIENT TEACHING
Using Walkers

When maximum support is required:

■ Move the walker ahead about 15 cm (6 in) while your body weight is borne by both legs.

■ Then, move the right foot up to the walker while your body weight is borne by the left leg and both arms.

■ Next, move the left foot up to the right foot while your body weight is borne by the right leg and both arms.

If one leg is weaker than the other:

■ Move the walker and the weak leg ahead together about 15 cm (6 in) while your weight is borne by the stronger leg.

■ Then, move the stronger leg ahead while your weight is borne by the affected leg and both arms.

ble uprights, an underarm bar, and a hand bar. See Figure 36–40, *A*. The Lofstrand crutch is a single adjustable tube of aluminum to which are attached a curved piece of steel, a rubber-covered hand bar, and a metal forearm cuff. See Figure 36–40, *B*. This type of crutch is most useful as a substitute for a cane. The metal cuff around the forearm and the metal bar stabilize the wrists and thus make walking safer and easier. The person can release the hand bar to use his or her hand, and the metal cuff will hold the crutch in place, while a cane would fall.

The **Canadian** or **elbow extensor crutch,** like the Lofstrand, is made of a single tube of aluminum with lateral attachments, a hand bar, and a cuff for the forearm, but it also has a cuff for the upper arm. See Figure 36–40, *C*. This crutch is usually used by clients who require support for weak extensor muscles of the arm (e.g., weak triceps brachii).

All crutches require suction tips, usually made of rubber, which help to prevent the crutches from slipping on a floor surface. Suggested instructions for using crutches are provided in the box on the following page.

Measuring clients for crutches When nurses measure clients for axillary crutches, it is most important to

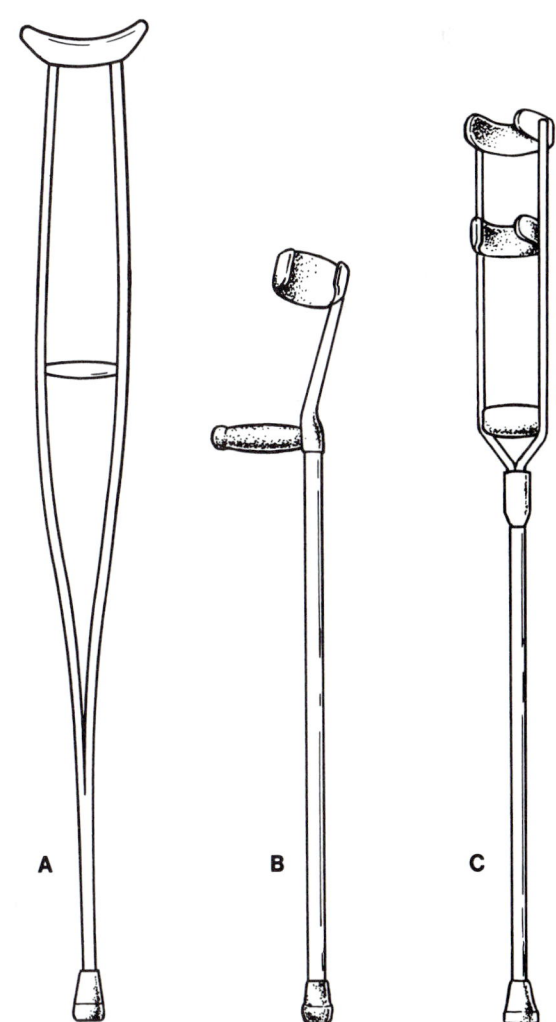

A   B   C

Figure 36–40 Three types of crutches: A, Axillary crutch; B, Lofstrand crutch; C, Canadian or elbow extensor crutch.

CLIENT TEACHING
Using Crutches

- Follow the plan of exercises developed for you to strengthen your arm muscles before beginning crutch walking.

- Have a health care professional establish the correct length for your crutches and the correct placement of the handpieces. Crutches that are too long force your shoulders upward and make it difficult for you to push your body off the ground. Crutches that are too short will make you hunch over and develop an improper body stance.

- The weight of your body should be borne by the arms rather than the axillae (armpits). Continual pressure on the axillae can injure the radial nerve and eventually cause crutch palsy, a **paresis** (weakness of the muscles) of the forearm, wrist, and hand.

- Maintain an erect posture as much as possible to prevent strain on muscles and joints and to maintain balance.

- Each step taken with crutches should be a comfortable distance for you. It is wise to start with a small rather than large step.

- Inspect the crutch tips regularly and replace them if worn.

- Keep the crutch tips dry to maintain their surface friction. If the tips become wet, dry them well before use.

30° elbow flexion

15 cm (6 in)

5 cm (2 in)

Figure 36–41 The standing position to measure the correct length of crutches.

obtain the correct length for the crutches and the correct placement of the hand piece. There are two methods of measuring crutch length:

1. The client lies in a supine position and the nurse measures from the anterior fold of the axilla to a point 10 cm (4 in) lateral from the heel of the foot.

2. The client stands erect and positions the crutch tips 5 cm (2 in) in front of and 15 cm (6 in) to the side of the feet. See Figure 36–41. The nurse makes sure the shoulder rest of the crutch is at least 3 finger widths, i.e., 2.5 to 5 cm (1 to 2 in), below the axilla.

To determine the correct placement of the hand bar:

1. The client stands upright and supports the body weight by the hand grips of the crutches.

2. The nurse measures the angle of elbow flexion. It should be about 30°. A goniometer (see Figure 19–94 on page 427) may be used to verify the correct angle.

Exercises for crutch walking   In crutch walking, the client's weight is borne by the muscles of the shoulder girdle and the upper extremities. Five major muscle groups used are shown in Table 36–8.

Before beginning crutch walking, the client should exercise to develop and strengthen these muscle groups. A plan of exercises should be developed for each client. The following exercises are recommended.

- Flexing and extending the arms in several directions

- Moving from a supine position to a sitting position by flexing the elbows and pushing the hands against the bed surface. See Figure 36–42. This exercise strengthens the flexor and extensor muscles of the arms and the muscles that dorsiflex the wrist.

- Lifting the body off the bed surface by pushing down with the hands and extending the elbows. See Figure 36–43. This exercise is particularly useful in strengthening the extensor muscles of the arms.

- Squeezing a rubber ball or a gripper with the hands. This exercise strengthens the flexor muscles of the fingers.

Crutch gaits   The crutch gait is the gait a person assumes on crutches by alternating body weight on one or both legs and the crutches. Five standard crutch gaits are the four-point gait, three-point gait, two-point gait, swing-to gait, and swing-through gait. The gait used depends on the following individual factors:

TABLE 36–8 *Major Muscle Groups Used in Crutch Walking*

Major Muscle Group	Examples	Action in Crutch Walking
Flexor muscles of the arms	Pectoralis major and brachialis	Move the crutches forward.
Extensor muscles of the forearms	Triceps brachii	Hold the elbows up at an angle while the body weight is raised off the ground.
Finger and thumb flexors	Flexor pollicis brevis	Allow the hands to grasp the hand bars.
Muscles that dorsiflex the wrists	Flexor carpi radialis	Maintain the hands in the correct position on the hand bars.
Shoulder girdle depressors and downward rotators	Pectoralis minor	Support the body weight off the floor.

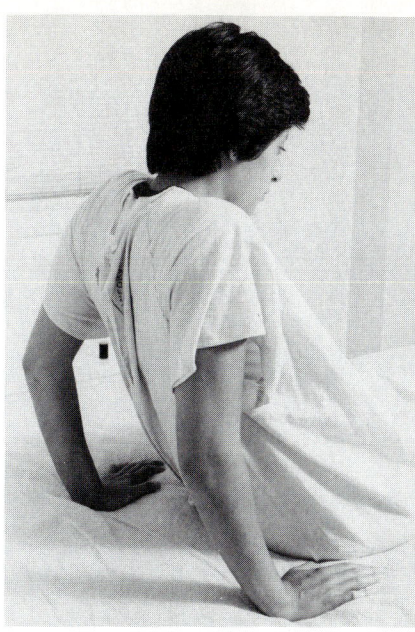

Figure 36–42 Strengthening the flexor and extensor muscles of the arms and the muscles that dorsiflex the wrists.

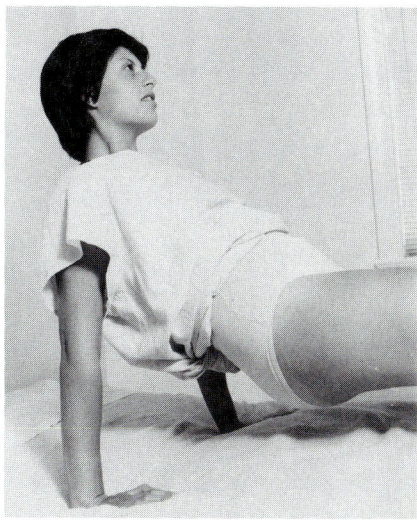

Figure 36–43 Strengthening the extensor muscles of the arms in preparation for crutch walking.

- Ability to take steps
- Ability to bear weight and keep balance in a standing position on both legs or only one
- Ability to hold the body erect

A physiotherapist or a physician usually decides which crutch gait is best for a particular client. Nurses are increasingly involved in these decisions, however. Often, a physiotherapist teaches the crutch gait initially, but nurses give follow-through lessons. In some instances, nurses alone teach the client the technique.

Clients also need instruction about how to get into and out of chairs and go up and down stairs safely. All of these crutch skills are best taught before the client is discharged and preferably before the client has surgery.

Crutch stance (tripod position) Before crutch walking is attempted, the client needs to learn facts about posture and balance. The proper standing position with crutches is called the **tripod (triangle) position.** See Figure 36–44. The crutches are placed about 15 cm (6 in) in front of the feet and out laterally about 15 cm (6 in), creating a wide base of support. The feet are slightly apart. A tall person requires a wider base than a short person. Hips and knees are

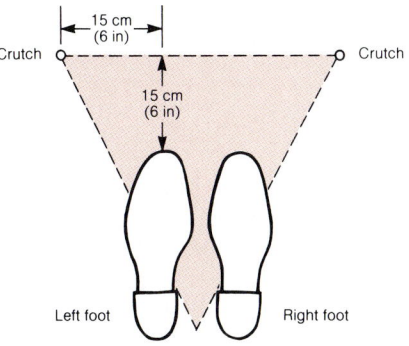

Figure 36–44 The tripod position.

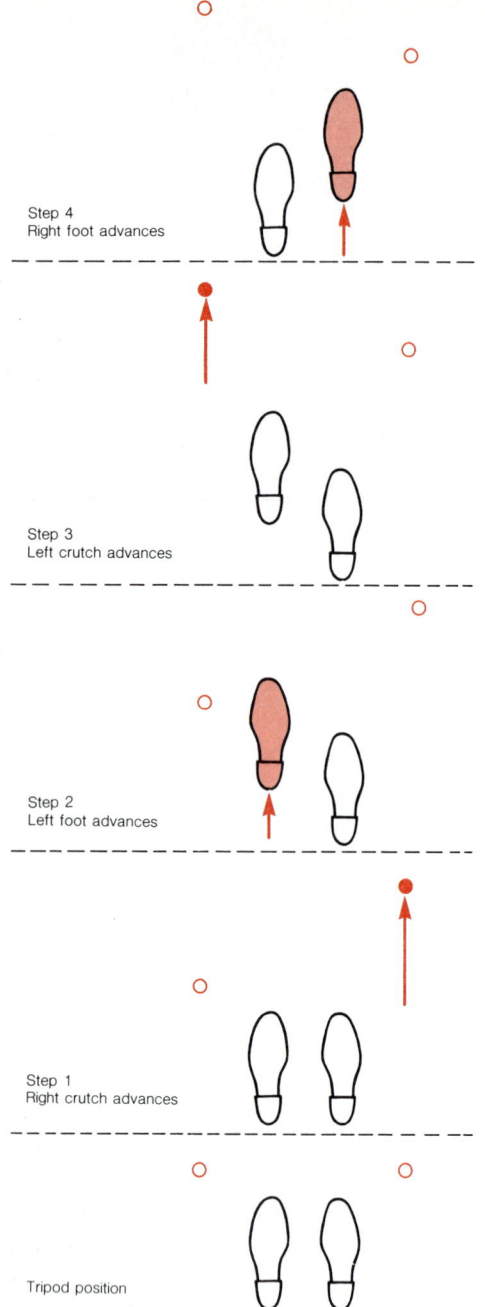

Step 4
Right foot advances

Step 3
Left crutch advances

Step 2
Left foot advances

Step 1
Right crutch advances

Tripod position

Figure 36–45   The four-point alternate crutch gait.

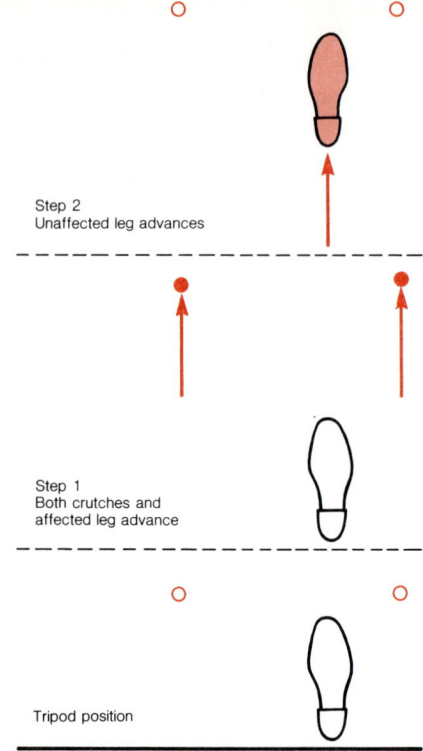

Step 2
Unaffected leg advances

Step 1
Both crutches and
affected leg advance

Tripod position

Figure 36–46   The three-point crutch gait.

crutch walking. Clients confined to bed are often unaware of weakness that becomes apparent when they try to stand or walk. Clients realize that they can no longer take balance for granted when they must cope with the weight of a heavy cast or a paralyzed limb. Frequently, progress may be slower than the client anticipated. Encouragement from the nurse and the setting of realistic goals are especially important.

Four-point alternate gait   This is the most elementary and safest gait, providing at least three points of support at each time, but it requires coordination. Clients can use it when walking in crowds because it does not require much space. To use this gait, the client needs to be able to bear weight on both legs. See Figure 36–45 (reading from bottom to top). The nurse asks the client to

1. Move the right crutch ahead a suitable distance, e.g., 10 to 15 cm (4 to 6 in)
2. Move the left front foot forward, preferably to the level of the left crutch
3. Move the left crutch forward
4. Move the right foot forward

Three-point gait   To use this gait, the client must be able to bear entire body weight on the unaffected leg. The two crutches and the unaffected leg bear weight alternately. See Figure 36–46 (reading from bottom to top). The nurse asks the client to

extended, the back is straight, and the head is held straight and high. There should be no hunch to the shoulders and thus no weight borne by the axillae. The elbows are extended sufficiently to allow weight bearing on the hands. If the client is unsteady, the nurse places a walking belt around the client's waist and grasps the belt from above, not from below. A fall can be prevented more effectively if the belt is held from above.

Sometimes clients are discouraged when they attempt

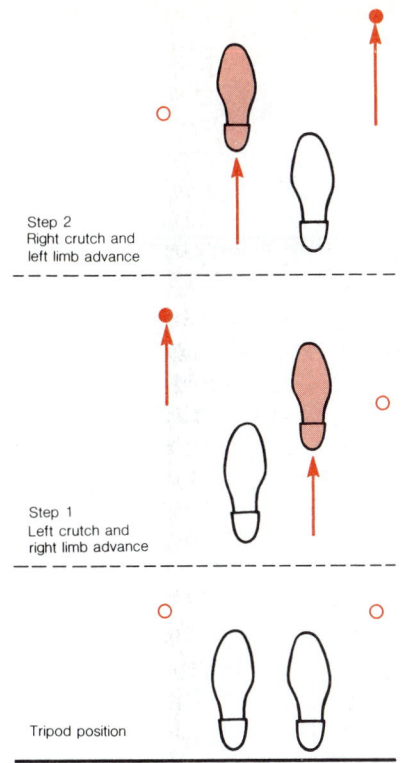

Figure 36–47   The two-point alternate crutch gait.

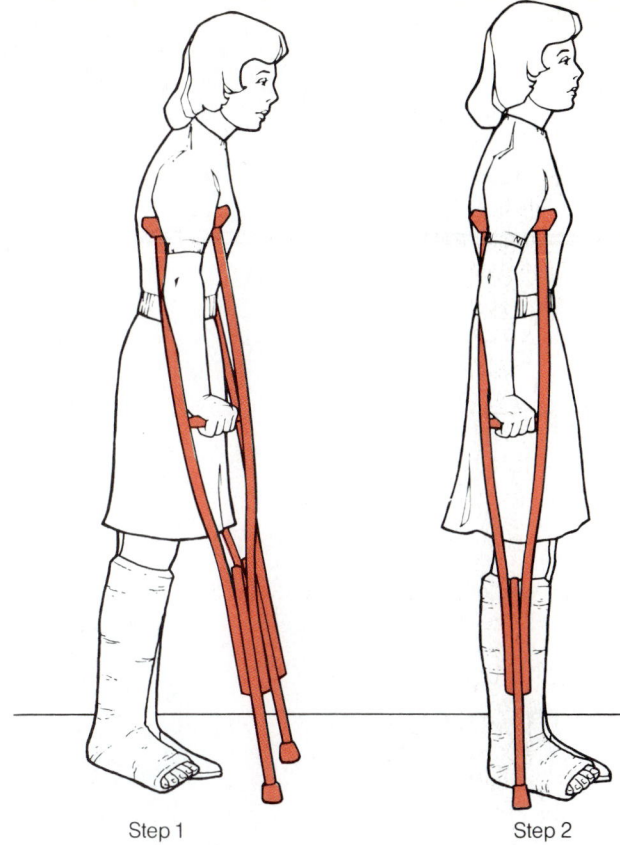

Step 1   Step 2

Figure 36–48   The swing-to crutch gait.

1. Move both crutches and the weaker leg forward
2. Move the stronger leg forward

Two-point alternate gait   This gait is faster than the four-point gait. It requires more balance, because only two points support the body at one time; it also requires at least partial weight bearing on each foot. In this gait, arm movements with the crutches are similar to the arm movements during normal walking. See Figure 36–47 (reading from bottom to top). The nurse asks the client to

1. Move the left crutch and the right foot forward together
2. Move the right crutch and the left foot ahead together

Swing-to gait   The swing gaits are used by clients with paralysis of the legs and hips. Prolonged use of these gaits results in atrophy of the unused muscles. The swing-to gait is the easier of these two gaits. See Figure 36–48. The nurse asks the client to

1. Move both crutches ahead together
2. Lift body weight by the arms and swing *to* the crutches

Swing-through gait   This gait requires considerable skill, strength, and coordination. See Figure 36–49. The nurse asks the client to

1. Move both crutches forward together
2. Lift body weight by the arms and swing *through and beyond* the crutch

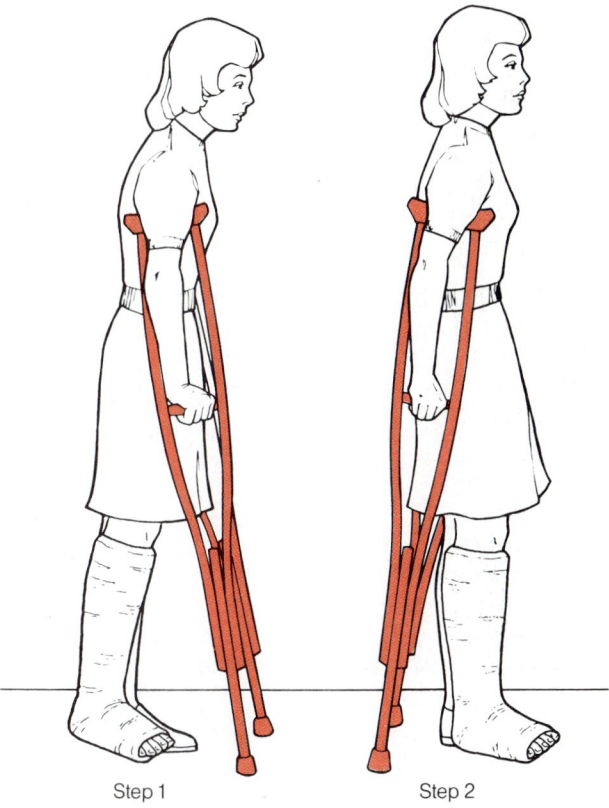

Step 1   Step 2

Figure 36–49   The swing-through crutch gait.

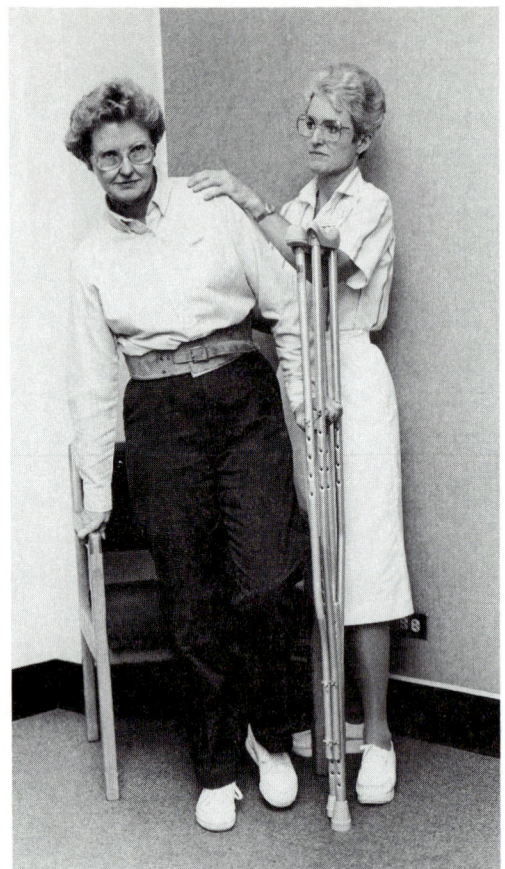

Figure 36–50   Client with crutches getting into a chair.

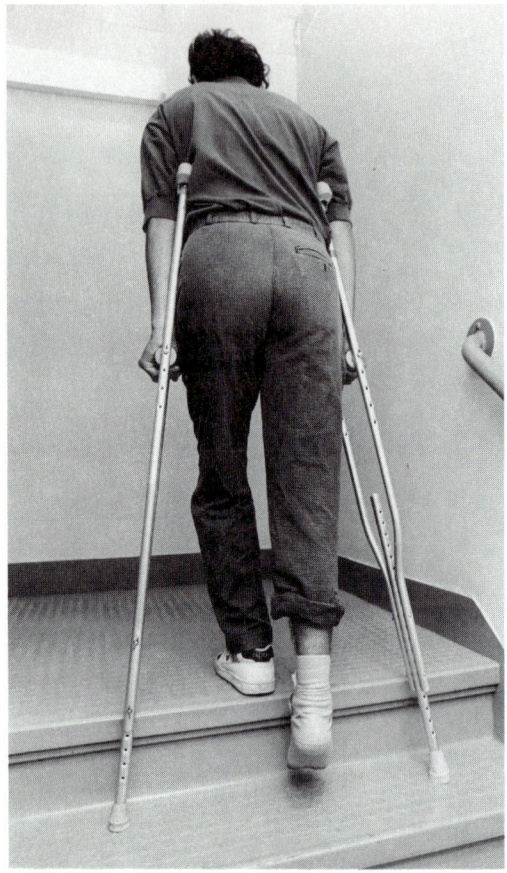

Figure 36–51   When climbing stairs, the client places weight on the crutches while first moving the unaffected leg onto a step.

Getting into a chair   Chairs that have armrests and are secure or braced against a wall are essential for clients using crutches. For this procedure the nurse instructs the client to

1. Stand with the back of the unaffected leg centered against the chair. The chair helps support the client during the next steps.

2. Transfer the crutches to the hand on the affected side and hold the crutches by the hand bars. The client grasps the arm of the chair with the hand on the unaffected side. See Figure 36–50. This allows the client to support the body weight on the arms and the unaffected leg.

3. Lean forward, flex the knees and hips, and lower into the chair.

Getting out of a chair   For this procedure, the nurse instructs the client to

1. Move forward to the edge of the chair and place the unaffected leg slightly under or at the edge of the chair. This position helps the client stand up from the chair

and achieve balance, since the unaffected leg is supported against the edge of the chair.

2. Grasp the crutches by the hand bars in the hand on the affected side, and grasp the arm of the chair by the hand on the unaffected side. The body weight is placed on the crutches and the hand on the armrest to support the unaffected leg when the client rises to stand.

3. Push down on the crutches and the chair armrest while elevating his or her body out of the chair.

4. Assume the tripod position before moving.

Going up stairs   For this procedure, the nurse stands behind the client and slightly to the affected side if needed. The nurse instructs the client to

1. Assume the tripod position at the bottom of the stairs.

2. Transfer the body weight to the crutches and move the unaffected leg onto the step. See Figure 36–51.

3. Transfer the body weight to the unaffected leg on the step and move the crutches and affected leg up to the step. The affected leg is always supported by the crutches.

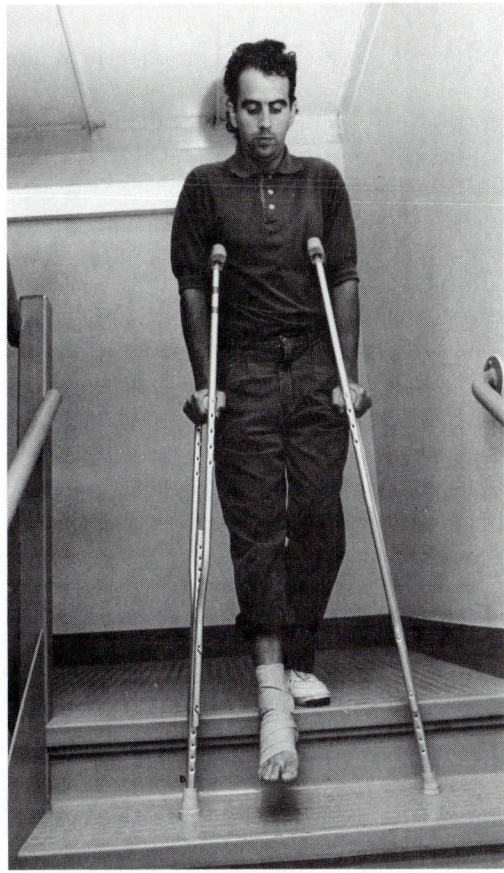

Figure 36–52 When descending stairs, the client first moves the crutches and affected leg down to the next step.

4. Repeat steps 2 and 3 until the client reaches the top of the stairs.

Going down stairs For this procedure, the nurse stands one step below the client on the affected side if needed. The nurse instructs the client to

1. Assume the tripod position at the top of the stairs.

2. Shift the body weight to the unaffected leg, and move the crutches and affected leg down onto the next step. See Figure 36–52.

3. Transfer the body weight to the crutches, and move the

unaffected leg to that step. The affected leg is always supported by the crutches.

4. Repeat steps 2 and 3 until the client reaches the bottom of the stairs.

EVALUATING

Body alignment can most easily be observed and evaluated by the following:

1. Standing directly in front of the person to evaluate the frontal plane of standing and sitting positions or by standing at the foot of the bed to evaluate the bed positions

2. Standing at the side of the person, chair, or bed to inspect the lateral view

3. Asking how comfortable the client feels in that position

Each body area—head and neck, shoulders, arms and hands, trunk, and finally hips, legs, and feet—is viewed from both frontal and lateral perspectives.

For examples of outcome criteria for evaluating standing and sitting body alignment, see the assessment section earlier in this chapter. Criteria for clients in well-aligned bed positions are shown in Table 36–7, earlier in this chapter.

The quality of the client's ambulation is evaluated according to how well the client achieves stability in gait without falling and whether preset goals have been achieved. Criteria for evaluating gait are shown earlier in Table 36–5. Examples of outcome criteria for measuring goal achievement are shown on page 900. For example, the nurse determines whether "the client walked independently with the aid of a walker from the bed to the nursing station three times a day" or whether "the client stood erect when walking" or whether "the client demonstrated correct use of a four-point crutch gait."

The quality of a client's body mechanics in daily activities can be evaluated only by observing how well the person conforms to the principles of body mechanics and prevents back injury. Proper use of body mechanics when moving objects is outlined on page 890.

The sample nursing care plan that follows indicates the evaluation of specific outcome criteria related to the nursing diagnoses for a specific client.

NURSING CARE PLAN FOR HARRIET LONG

ASSESSMENT DATA

Nursing Assessment

Ms. Harriet Long is a 69-year-old retired crossing guard. She suffers from osteoarthritis and has bilateral cataracts. As of late she has experienced "drop attacks." She uses a cane when walking. Ten days ago she suffered back strain when attempting to move an old trunk. She was admitted to the hospital for treatment of back strain. She has been on bed rest with a firm mattress for support and in Fowler's position with the knees flexed. She has B.R.P. She has been receiving pain medications for her back pain. On occasion, she becomes slightly disoriented and confused at night and has attempted to get out of bed unassisted.

Physical Examination

Height: 160 cm (5'3")
Weight: 61.3 kg (135 lb)
Temperature: 36.0 C (98.6 F)
Pulse rate: 82 BPM
Respirations: 20 per minute at rest
Blood pressure: 156/88 mm Hg
Heberden's nodes at distal interphalangeal joints of fingers

Diagnostic Data

Chest x-ray film: Negative
Knee x-ray film: Bony hypertrophy with spur formation
Spinal column x-ray film: Evidence of degenerative joint disease and spurs

---

CARE PLAN

Nursing Diagnosis	Client Goals and Outcome Criteria	Nursing Interventions and Rationales	Evaluation
Potential for injury related to impaired vision and limited movement possibly resulting in falls, fracture, contusions, and abrasions.	Client Goals: Ambulates independently without falling. Outcome Criteria: Uses call system before attempting to get out of bed during the night. Verbalizes helpfulness of night light and is oriented to placement of room furnishings.	Orient client to surroundings and system. *Rationale:* Provides for greater comfort and decreases disorientation. Encourage client to request assistance during the night by using call system. *Rationale:* Decreases chance of client falling while attempting to get out of bed without assistance. Keep bed in low position at all times. *Rationale:* Increases safety of client by decreasing chance of falling from a height. Turn on night light each night. *Rationale:* Decreases risk of falling. Observe for signs of disorientation in the evening. *Rationale:* Disorientation may occur in the evening, especially if client is sedated. Keep side rails up at all times. *Rationale:* Decreases risk of falling.	Client has attempted to get out of bed without assistance only once in 3 nights and has used call system appropriately on all other occasions. States night light is helpful to see where things are in this room: "I use one at home all the time."

Nursing Diagnosis	Client Goals and Outcome Criteria	Nursing Interventions and Rationales	Evaluation
Knowledge deficit of disease process and body mechanics resulting in questioning etiology of low back pain, need for proper body mechanics, and possibility of paralysis.	Client Goals: Uses good body mechanics. Outcome Criteria: Identifies cause of low back pain. Identifies proper body mechanics to be utilized when moving heavy objects by day 3. Identifies proper posture for standing and sitting by day 3. Identifies proper sleeping position by day 2.	Assess client's learning needs regarding etiology of low back pain. *Rationale:* Can build upon knowledge client already has regarding causes of back pain. Allow adequate time for discussing problem, giving and reinforcing information. *Rationale:* Adequate time is necessary to help the client develop understanding of disease and its treatment. Instruct client regarding sleep patterns, e.g., to avoid prone position and to sleep on side with knees flexed. *Rationale:* Understanding and then practicing proper sleep positions will decrease back strain. Discuss importance of proper body mechanics, e.g., keep the back straight and the knees bent when lifting and do not lift above the elbows. *Rationale:* Understanding and practicing good body mechanics will decrease chances of back pain. Instruct client about proper standing and sitting positions. *Rationale:* Knowledge of proper posture positions will help to decrease back strain.	Client is able to discuss but not demonstrate proper body mechanics for pulling, pushing, and lifting heavy objects. States, "I should not sleep on my stomach because it'll give me a backache." Knows to use footstool when sitting and watching TV. Client demonstrates proper standing and sitting positions.

CHAPTER HIGHLIGHTS

▶ Good body mechanics is the efficient, coordinated, and safe use of the body to produce motion and maintain balance during activity.

▶ Body mechanics involves three basic elements: body alignment, balance, and coordinated body movement.

▶ Maintaining good body alignment and using good body mechanics are essential for good body function and for preventing discomfort, fatigue, and injury to body structures.

▶ The nurse acts as a role model and teacher of good body alignment and body mechanics.

▶ A person maintains balance as long as the line of gravity passes through the center of gravity and the base of support.

▶ The broader the base of support and the lower the center of gravity, the greater the stability and balance achieved.

▶ Factors influencing body alignment and body mechanics include general health, nutrition, emotions, situational factors or habits, life-style, attitudes and values, level of understanding, and neuromuscular or skeletal impairments.

▶ When lifting, pushing, or pulling clients or objects, the nurse needs to consider the concepts of leverage, force, friction, and inertia.

▶ To prevent spinal twisting, the nurse faces the direction of movement and moves objects directly toward or away from the nurse's center of gravity.

▶ Squatting, in contrast to stooping or partially flexing the hips and knees, is essential when moving objects.

▶ Falls and back injuries are the most common and serious consequences of improper body mechanics.

▶ Assessment of body mechanics includes assessment of body alignment according to specific criteria for standing, sitting, and lying positions; identification of the client's capabilities and limitations in regard to movement; use of body mechanics; and gait.

▶ Postural variations occur among different age groups.

▶ Common structural abnormalities that affect alignment are scoliosis, kyphosis, and lordosis.

▶ Neuromusculoskeletal problems such as hemiplegia, Parkinson's disease, or arthritis can seriously affect a client's gait and ability to move.

▶ Nursing diagnoses related to a client's alignment and gait may include **Impaired physical mobility, Potential for injury, Fear, Self-care deficit,** and **Knowledge deficit.**

▶ The nurse uses assessment data and nursing diagnoses to identify goals for care and to design an individualized plan of nursing interventions.

▶ Overall client goals include maintenance or restoration of body alignment, prevention of contractures, improved use of proper body mechanics in work and in daily life, restored or improved ambulatory capability, and prevention of back injuries and falls.

▶ The principles of body alignment and the guidelines for positioning clients help the nurse to plan individualized interventions.

▶ Before positioning dependent clients, the nurse should plan a systematic 24-hour schedule for position changes, including positions that provide for full extension of the neck, hips, and knees.

▶ Before moving or turning a client, the nurse must consider the client's health and mental status, degree of exertion permitted, degree of discomfort, position required, and amount of force required.

▶ Assistance from others or the use of mechanical lifting aids is essential when clients are too heavy for the nurse to move or lift safely.

▶ Ambulating techniques that facilitate normal walking gait yet provide the support needed are most effective.

▶ The nurse can assist clients to prepare for ambulation by helping them become as independent as possible while in bed.

▶ Preambulatory exercises that strengthen the muscles for walking are essential for clients who have been immobilized for prolonged periods.

▶ Clients need specific instructions about appropriate use of canes, walkers, and crutches.

▶ Safety precautions and the use of appropriate body mechanics are essential whenever the nurse assists clients to move.

READINGS AND REFERENCES

SUGGESTED READINGS

Cushing, M. February 1985. First, anticipate the harm. *American Journal of Nursing* 85:137–38.
This nurse-attorney discusses some legal implications that client falls pose for nurses.

Drinker, P. A.; Phipps, M. A.; and Gannon, J. J. February 1985. Air bags: An uplifting idea. *American Journal of Nursing* 85:150–51.
Low-pressure air bags, widely used in industrial lifting, offer a simple, safe, and low-cost solution to the problem of lifting and turning immobilized clients, especially those who are obese or have troublesome musculoskeletal or skin conditions. Air bags can be useful in both the hospital and home care settings.

Hollis, M. 1985. *Safer lifting for patient care.* 2d ed. Oxford, England: Blackwell Scientific Publications.
This 150-page book outlines various lifts, including the Australian shoulder lift, the floor-to-wheelchair lift, and many others. Initial sections discuss friction, posture, bracing, and commands; the mechanics of stability and stances; ten different ways to grasp the client; the mechanics and performance of rocking maneuvers; and the use of blocks.

Mather, D., and Bennett, B. March 1987. How to move patients the easy way . . . and save your back. *Nursing 87* 17:55–57.
Use of a new device called the Smooth Mover reduces the risk of back injuries for the nurse moving clients between a bed and

a stretcher. Step-by-step, one-person and two-person transfers are illustrated with eight photographs in this article.

Thomas, D. F. November 1986. An ambulation assessment system you can count on. *Nursing 86* 16:58–59.

This ambulation assessment guide is designed to help the nurse assess the amount of help a client needs to get out of bed or to walk. A "1, 2, 3" rating scale is used to determine activity level, mobility, bilateral weakness, understanding, length of time in bed, attitude, time up in past, and energy.

Tinetti, M. E. February 1986. Performance-oriented assessment of mobility problems in elderly patients. *Journal of the American Geriatrics Society* 34:119–26.

Tinetti introduces a performance-oriented guide to assessing mobility of elderly clients. Three tables indicate specific maneuvers (e.g., rising from a chair, turning 360°, and bending down to pick up small objects) that may be used to assess balance and gait. The tables indicate normal, adaptive, and abnormal responses for each maneuver.

RELATED RESEARCH

Borello-France, D. F.; Burdett, R. G.; and Gee, Z. L. January 1988. Modification of sitting posture of patients with hemiplegia using seat boards and backboards. *Physical Therapy* 68:67–71.

Carlton, R. S. January 1987. The effects of body mechanics instruction on work performance. *American Journal of Occupational Therapy* 4:16–20.

Goldberg, W. G., and Fitzpatrick, J. J. November/December 1980. Movement with the aged. *Nursing Research* 29:339–46.

Owen, B. D. November 1985. The lifting process and back injury in hospital nursing personnel. *Western Journal of Nursing Research* 7:445–59.

Snook, S. H.; Camponelli, R. A.; and Harsh, J. W. July 1978. A study of three preventive approaches to low back injury. *Journal of Occupational Health Medicine* 20:478–81.

SELECTED REFERENCES

Bates, B. 1987. *A guide to physical examination and history taking.* 4th ed. Philadelphia: W. B. Saunders Co.

Cozen, L. N. January 1984. Walking aids: Select the right one, teach its use, and avoid damage elsewhere. *Consultant* 24:268–273, 276.

Davies, B. T. 1978. Training in manual handling and lifting. In Drury, C., editor. pp. 175–85. *Safety in manual material handling.* DHEW (NIOSH) Pub. no. 78–185, July. Cincinnati, Ohio: National Institute of Occupational Safety and Health.

Dayhoff, N. July 1975. Soft or hard devices to position hands? *American Journal of Nursing* 75:1142–44.

Dionne, K. E. January 1985. The no-strain approach to back-breaking work. *RN* 48:45–47.

Donaldson, W. F., and Hoover, N. W. 1982. *The American Medical Association book of back care.* New York: Random House.

Drapeau, J. September 1975. Getting back into good posture: How to ease your lumbar aches. *Nursing 75* 5:63–65.

Farmer, P. July 1987. Mechanical aids: Easyslide lifting aid. *Nursing Times* 83:36–37.

Freed, M. M.; Hofkosh, J.; Kaplan, L. I., and Neuhauser, C. October 1987a. Choosing ambulatory aids. *Patient Care* 21:20–23, 26–27, 30–32.

———. October 1987b. Using ambulatory aids. *Patient Care* 21:36–40, 42, 45–47.

Gates, S. May 1988. On-the-job back exercises. *American Journal of Nursing* 88:656–59.

Gates, S. J., and Starkey, R. D. February 1986. Back injury prevention: A holistic approach. *American Association of Occupational Health Nurses Journal* 34:58–62.

Goodwin, M. P., and Mohn, S. P. November/December 1987. Easy transfer with the long board. *Geriatric Nursing* 8:333.

Harber, P., et al. July 1985. Occupational low-back pain in hospital nurses. *Journal of Occupational Medicine* 27:518–24.

Hogue, C. March 1982. Injury in late life. Part I: Epidemiology. *American Geriatric Society* 30:183–89.

Hoover, S. December 1973. Job-related back injuries in a hospital. *American Journal of Nursing* 73:2078–79.

Kottke, F.; Stillwell, G.; and Lehmann, J., editors. 1990. *Krusen's handbook of physical medicine and rehabilitation.* 4th ed. Philadelphia: W. B. Saunders Co.

Leinweber, E. December 1978. Belts to make moves smoother. *American Journal of Nursing* 78:2080–81.

Love, C. July 1986. Do you roll or lift? Potential for back injury. *Nursing Times* 82:44–46.

Mandzak-McCarron, K., and Drayton-Hargrove, S. May/June 1987. Ambulation aids. *Rehabilitation Nursing* 12:139–41.

Marchette, L., and Marchette, B. November/December 1985. Back injury: A preventable occupational hazard. *Orthopedic Nursing* 4:25–29.

Marino, N. M. April 1985. After the fall: An analysis. *American Journal of Nursing* 95:362.

Memmer, M. K. 1974. *Posture and alignment.* Los Angeles: The Intercampus Nursing Project, California State University and College System.

Owen, B. D. May 1980. How to avoid that aching back. *American Journal of Nursing* 80:894–97.

———. November 1985. The lifting process and back injury in hospital nursing personnel. *Western Journal of Nursing Research* 7:445–59.

Walsh, R. August/September 1988. Human kinetics: On the move. *Nursing Times* 84:26–28, 30.

———. September 1988. Human kinetics: Good movement habits. *Nursing Times* 84:59–61.

Wightwick, S. June 1987. Canadian padded transfer board. *Physiotherapy* 73:309–10.

Williamson, K. M.; Turner, J. G.; Brown, K. C.; Neuman, K. D.; Sirles, A. T.; and Selleck, C. S. Fall 1988. Occupational health hazards for nurses. Part II. *Image* 20:162–68.

Rest and Sleep

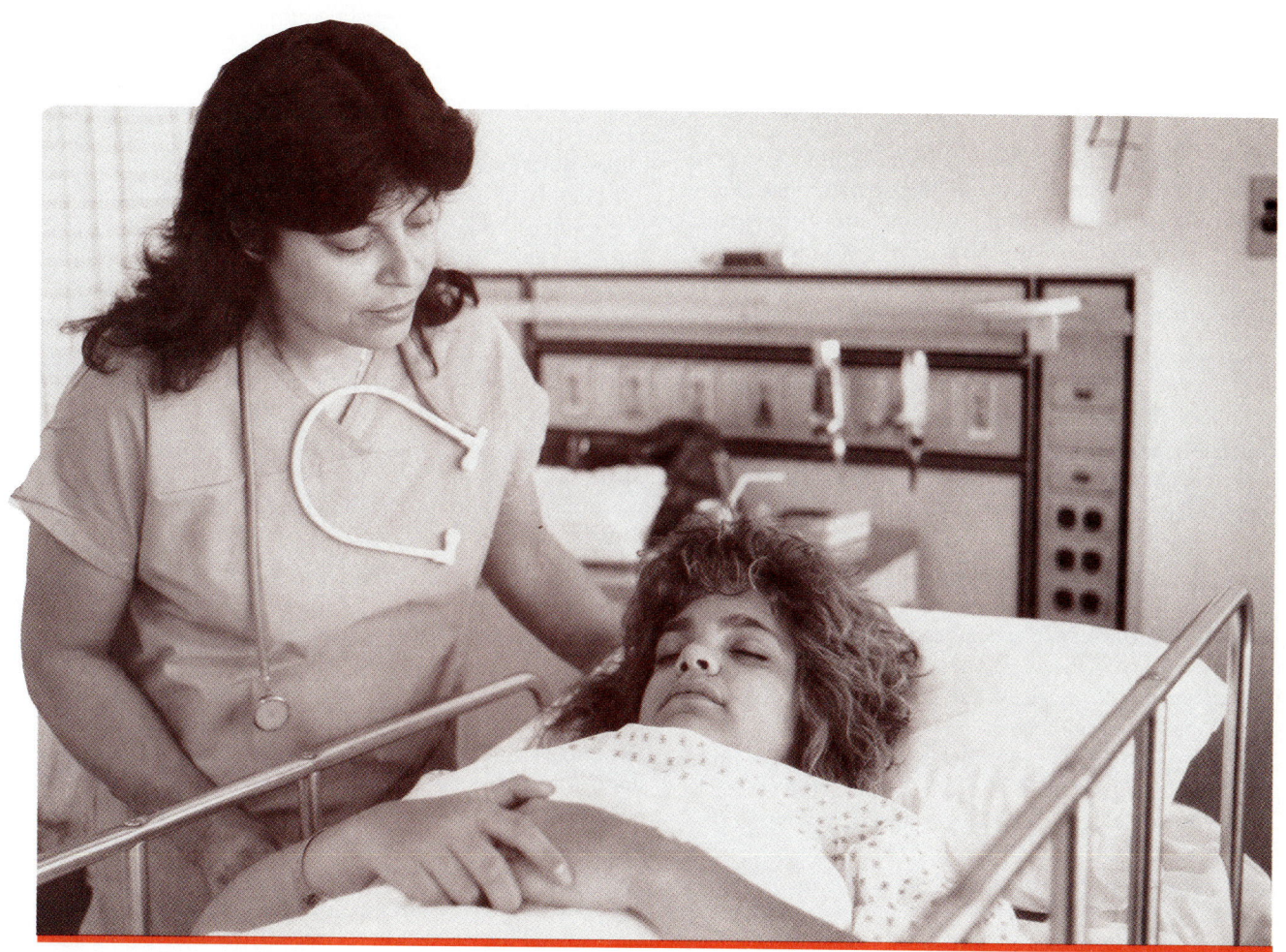

CONTENTS

OBJECTIVES

▶ Explain the physiologic basis of sleep.

▶ Identify the characteristics of NREM and REM sleep.

▶ Identify the four stages of NREM sleep.

▶ Identify the developmental variations in sleep patterns.

▶ Identify interventions that promote sleep at various ages.

▶ Identify factors that affect normal sleep.

▶ Define terms related to common sleep disorders.

▶ Identify the components of a sleep assessment.

▶ Identify interventions that promote normal sleep.

▶ Describe outcome criteria for evaluating a client's response to interventions employed to promote sleep.

REST AND SLEEP

Rest and sleep are essential for health. People who are ill frequently require more rest and sleep than normal. Often, debilitated people expend unusual amounts of energy just to regain health or maintain the activities of daily living. As a result, such people experience increased and frequent fatigue and thus need more rest and sleep than usual.

Rest The ill and injured need rest. Rest, however, is not mere inactivity, and distraught clients may find rest difficult. **Rest** implies calmness, relaxation without emotional stress, and freedom from anxiety. Therefore, rest does not always imply inactivity; in fact, some people find some activities restful. For example, a student studying for examinations may find it restful to walk in the fresh air. The meaning of rest and the need for rest vary among individuals. Providing a restful environment for clients is an important function of nurses. To assess the client's need for rest and to evaluate how effectively this need is met, nurses need to consider conditions that promote rest.

Narrow (1967, p. 169) outlines six characteristics most people associate with rest. These summarize the meaning of rest and guide the nurse in assessing and promoting rest for clients.

Most people can rest when they

1. Feel that things are under control
2. Feel accepted
3. Feel that they understand what is going on
4. Are free from irritation and discomfort
5. Have a satisfying amount of purposeful activity
6. Know they will receive help when it is needed

To rest, clients need to feel that their personal lives are under control and that they are receiving competent health care. By providing competent care, the nurse gives peace of mind and helps the client to relax. A nurse often can promote rest by listening carefully to clients' personal concerns and alleviating them when possible. For example, a man taken to an emergency ward may be unable to relax until a nurse telephones his wife to inform her.

Rest is impossible for clients who do not feel accepted. Clients need to feel acceptable to themselves and to others. Acceptance by the staff is important to the client. Accep-

tance can be conveyed, for instance, by recognizing both client limitations and client progress and recognizing individual differences.

A client's understanding of what is happening is another condition essential for rest. The unknown generates varying degrees of anxiety and interferes with rest. The nurse can help by offering explanations about diagnostic tests, surgery, agency policies or routines, and the client's progress. When information is given freely, clients do not feel the tension associated with having to ask questions.

Irritation and discomfort have both physical and emotional aspects. Generally, the nurse can easily detect physical discomforts, such as pain, insufficient supports for body positions, damp bedclothes, and loud noise. Emotional discomforts include having too many or too few visitors, feeling a lack of privacy, being hurried, having to wait long periods, being alone, or being concerned about the life problems of self or others.

Purposeful activity can be relaxing and often provides a sense of self-worth, e.g., the child who makes a toy puppet generally has a sense of contentment and accomplishment. Such activity often promotes rest throughout the day and undisturbed sleep at night.

The last prerequisite for rest is the security of knowing help is available when needed. The client who feels isolated and helpless cannot rest properly. Friends and family members can promote rest by helping the client with daily tasks and difficult decisions. Nurses can help by anticipating and meeting clients' needs. Knowing that the call bell will be answered, for example, can be exceedingly important to a client.

Sleep According to Maslow, sleep is a basic human need (Maslow 1970, p. 92); it is a universal process common to all people. In spite of considerable research, there is no commonly accepted definition of sleep. Historically, it was considered to be a state of unconsciousness. More recently, **sleep** has come to be considered a state of consciousness in which the individual's perception and reaction to the environment are decreased. Sleep is characterized by minimal physical activity, variable levels of consciousness, changes in the body's physiologic processes, and decreased responsiveness to external stimuli (Hayter 1980, p. 457). Some environmental stimuli, e.g., a smoke detector alarm, will awaken a sleeper, while other noises will not. It appears that individuals respond to meaningful stimuli while sleeping and selectively disregard unmeaningful stimuli.

PHYSIOLOGY OF SLEEP

Control of the cyclic nature of sleep is centered in two specialized areas of the brain stem: the reticular activating system (RAS) and the bulbar synchronizing region (BSR) in the medulla. The RAS consists of neurons in the medulla oblongata, pons, and midbrain. See Figure 37–1. These centers are involved in maintaining a state of wakefulness but also in mediating some stages of sleep. The physiologic changes in the body that occur during sleep are shown in the box below.

There are two theories about sleep, the passive theory and the active theory. The passive theory holds that the reticular activating system of the brain simply fatigues and therefore becomes inactive. The active theory, which is more widely accepted today, proposes some sort of center or centers that cause sleep by inhibiting other parts of the brain (Guyton 1986, p. 672).

The two systems, RAS and BSR, are thought to activate and then suppress the brain centers intermittently. The RAS is associated with the body's state of alertness and receives sensory input, i.e., auditory, visual, pain, and tactile stimuli. These sensory stimuli maintain a person's sense of wakefulness and alertness. During sleep the body sends fewer stimuli from the cerebral cortex or the peripheral sensory receptors to the RAS. The person awakens from sleep when there is an increase in such stimuli. There is less known about the BSR; however, it is known that its activity increases with sleep.

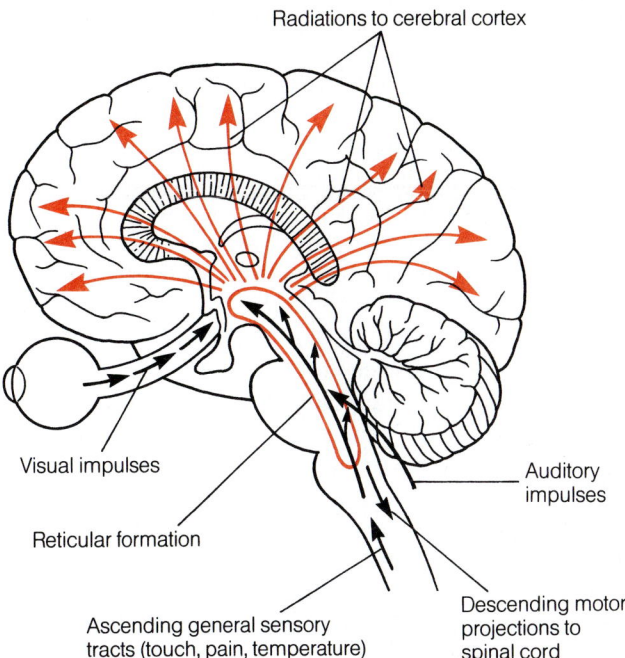

Figure 37–1 The reticular formation. The reticular formation extends the length of the brain stem. A portion of this formation, the reticular activating system (RAS), maintains alert wakefulness of the cerebral cortex. Ascending arrows on the diagram indicate input of sensory systems to the RAS and then output from the reticular formation to the cerebral cortex. Other reticular nuclei are involved in the coordination of muscle activity. Their output is indicated by the arrow descending the brain system. *Source:* Adapted from E. N. Marieb, *Human anatomy and physiology* (Redwood City, Calif.: Benjamin/Cummings, 1989) p. 397. Reproduced with permission.

Biorhythms

Biorhythmology, the study of the biologic rhythms of the body, is receiving increasing attention from biologists and health professionals. **Biorhythms** (rhythmic biologic clocks) exist in plants, animals, and humans. In humans, these are controlled from within the body and synchronized with environmental factors, such as light and darkness, gravity, and electromagnetic stimuli. Human rhythms are demonstrated biologically and behaviorally. Examples of biologic rhythms in humans are the repetitive rhythmic contractions of the heart muscle, the waking and sleeping cycles, and regular temperature fluctuations. Each biorhythmic cycle has peaks and troughs. These cycles vary somewhat among individuals. For example, most adults sleep at night, and most sleep about 8 hours. However, some people, referred to as "night owls," seem to be more alert during the late evening hours and retire late. Others, referred to as "early birds," prefer to retire early and perform well in the early hours of the morning. Some people need only 4 hours of sleep daily.

Biorhythms are classified according to the length of the cycle. The most common cycle is the **circadian rhythm,**

Physiologic Changes During Sleep

- Arterial blood pressure falls.
- Pulse rate decreases.
- Peripheral blood vessels dilate.
- Activity of the gastrointestinal tract occasionally increases.
- Skeletal muscles relax.
- Basal metabolic rate decreases 10% to 30%.

Source: A. C. Guyton, *Textbook of Medical Physiology* 7th ed. (Philadelphia: W. B. Saunders Co., 1986), p. 674.

a 1-day cycle. The term *circadian* is from the Lation *circa dies,* meaning "about a day." A second rhythm is the **infradian rhythm,** a monthly cycle. An example is the menstrual cycle. A third rhythm is the **ultradian rhythm,** consisting of cycles completed in minutes or hours. An example is the rapid eye movement (REM) cycle of sleep. Biorhythms are not altered by changes in the environment. They are *endogenous,* that is, arising from within the human body and persisting regardless of environmental influences (Deters 1980, p. 250).

Sleep is a complex biological rhythm. When a person's biological clock coincides with sleep-wake patterns, the person is said to be in **circadian synchronization,** i.e., the person is awake when the physiologic and psychologic rhythms are most active and is asleep when the physiologic and psychologic rhythms are most inactive.

Circadian regularity approaching that of adults begins by the 3rd week of life and may be inherited. Babies are awake most often in the early morning and the late afternoon. After 4 months of age, babies enter a 24-hour cycle in which they sleep mostly during the night. By the end of the 5th or 6th month, babies' sleep-wakefulness patterns are almost like those of adults.

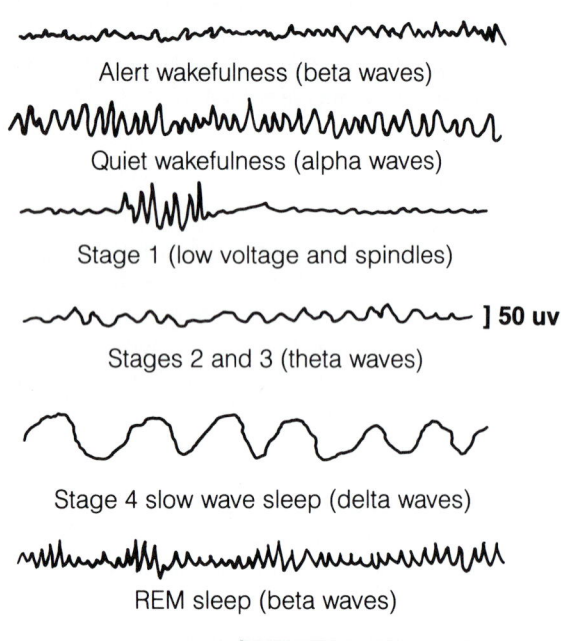

Alert wakefulness (beta waves)

Quiet wakefulness (alpha waves)

Stage 1 (low voltage and spindles)

] 50 uv

Stages 2 and 3 (theta waves)

Stage 4 slow wave sleep (delta waves)

REM sleep (beta waves)

1 sec

Figure 37–2 Characteristic brain waves during waking, the four stages of NREM sleep, and REM sleep. *Source:* A. C. Guyton, *Textbook of medical physiology,* 7th ed. (Philadelphia: W. B. Saunders Co., 1986), p. 671. Used by permission.

Stages of Sleep

The **electroencephalogram (EEG)** provides a good picture of what occurs during sleep. Electrodes are placed on various parts of the sleeper's scalp. The electrodes transmit electric energy from the cerebral cortex to pens that record the **brain waves** (fluctuations in energy) on graph paper. Each pen of the electroencephalogram corresponds to an electrode, moving up when the electric charge is negative and down when it is positive. Before sleeping, a person has high-frequency beta waves of alert wakefulness. This is followed by quiet wakefulness, when the alpha waves appear.

Two types of sleep have been identified: **NREM** (non-REM) sleep and **REM** (rapid eye movement) sleep. NREM sleep is also referred to as deep, restful sleep or slow-wave sleep, because the brain waves of a sleeper during NREM sleep are slower than the alpha and beta waves of a person who is awake or alert. See Figure 37–2. NREM sleep is divided into four stages.

Stage I is the stage of very light sleep. The brain waves are of low voltage, though broken periodically by *sleep spindles* (short, spindle-shaped bursts of alpha waves). During Stage I the person feels drowsy and relaxed, the eyes roll from side to side, and the heart and respiratory rates drop slightly. The sleeper can be readily awakened during this stage.

Stage II is the stage of light sleep during which body processes continue to slow down. The eyes are generally still, the heart and respiratory rates decrease slightly, and body temperature falls. The brain waves during stages II and III are theta waves. Stage II lasts only about 10 to 15 minutes.

During *stage III*, the heart and respiratory rates as well as other body processes slow further, due to domination of the parasympathetic nervous system. The sleeper becomes more difficult to arouse. The brain waves become more regular. Slow delta waves are added to the stage II theta wave pattern.

Stage IV signals deep sleep, during which delta waves predominate and become even slower. The sleeper's heart and respiratory rates drop 20% to 30% below those exhibited during waking hours. The sleeper is very relaxed, rarely moves, and is difficult to arouse. Stage IV is thought to physically restore the body. Physical exercise 2 hours before bedtime promotes stage IV sleep (Hayter 1980, p. 457). During this stage, the eye movements are usually rolling, and some dreaming occurs.

These four stages of NREM usually last about one hour in adults and are followed by NREM stage III, then II. Thereafter the first REM stage occurs, lasting about 10 minutes. This sequence completes the first sleep cycle. The usual sleeper experiences four to six cycles of sleep during 7 to 8 hours. Each cycle lasts about 70 minutes. See Figure 37–3. A sleeper passes from stage I NREM sleep through stages II and III to stage IV in about 20 to 30 minutes. Stage IV may last about 30 minutes. The process is then reversed, and the sleeper ascends through stages III and II, after which REM sleep occurs. REM sleep completes the first cycle, and the cycle then repeats. The sleeper who is awakened during any stage must begin anew at stage I NREM sleep and proceed through all the stages to REM sleep. See Figure 37–3. The characteristics of NREM sleep are given in Table 37–1. REM sleep, a relatively active state, is also referred to as *paradoxical sleep*. The main characteristics of REM sleep are listed in the box below.

The sympathetic nervous system dominates during REM sleep. REM sleep is thought to restore a person mentally— that is, for learning, psychologic adaptation, and memory (Hayter 1980, p. 458). During REM sleep, the sleeper reviews the day's events and processes and stores the information. The sleeper gains perspective on problems and may resolve some problems. Thus, there is wisdom in the traditional advice to "sleep on" a problem or big decision.

The duration of NREM stages and REM sleep varies throughout the 8-hour sleep period. As the night progresses, the sleeper becomes less tired and spends less time in stages III and IV of NREM sleep. REM sleep increases, and dreams tend to lengthen. If the sleeper is very tired, REM cycles are often short—for example, 5 minutes instead of 20—during the early portion of sleep. Before sleep ends, periods of near wakefulness occur, and stages I and II NREM sleep and REM sleep predominate.

The ratio of NREM to REM sleep varies with age. See Figure 37–4 on page 944.

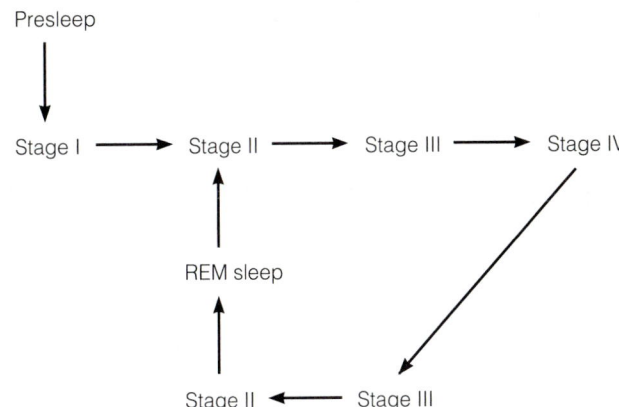

Figure 37–3   The adult sleep cycle.

Functions of Sleep

Theories about the functions of sleep can generally be placed in either of two categories: restorative-synthetic and behavioral. Traditionally, sleep was thought to be restorative. When people feel ill they tend to retire to bed often to assist the healing process. It has been suggested that sleep is a time for body and brain restoration. NREM sleep is directed toward body restoration and REM sleep toward increases in synthetic processes in the brain (Adam and Oswald 1977, p. 388).

Most research related to sleep and behavior involves changes in behavior as a result of sleep deprivation. The type of sleep lost appears to relate to the particular behavioral change; for example, loss of REM sleep leads to feel-

TABLE 37–1   *Characteristics of NREM Sleep*

Stage	Characteristics
Stage I	Relaxed and drowsy Profound restfulness Usually lasts only a few minutes Floating sensation Eyes roll from side to side
Stage II	Lightly asleep Easily aroused Constitutes 40–45% of total sleep time
Stage III	Less easily aroused Medium-depth sleep Muscles totally relaxed Blood pressure lowers Body temperature lowers
Stage IV	Deepest sleep stage Rarely moves Muscles completely relaxed Difficult to arouse Occurs 30 to 40 minutes following sleep onset

Characteristics of REM Sleep

- Active dreaming occurs.
- The sleeper is more difficult to arouse than during NREM (slow-wave) sleep.
- Muscle tone is depressed.
- Heart rate and respiratory rate often are irregular.
- A few irregular muscle movements occur—in particular, rapid eye movements.
- Metabolism increases.
- Body temperature increases.
- Respirations are irregular, and sleeper may have periods of apnea.
- Flow of stomach acid increases.

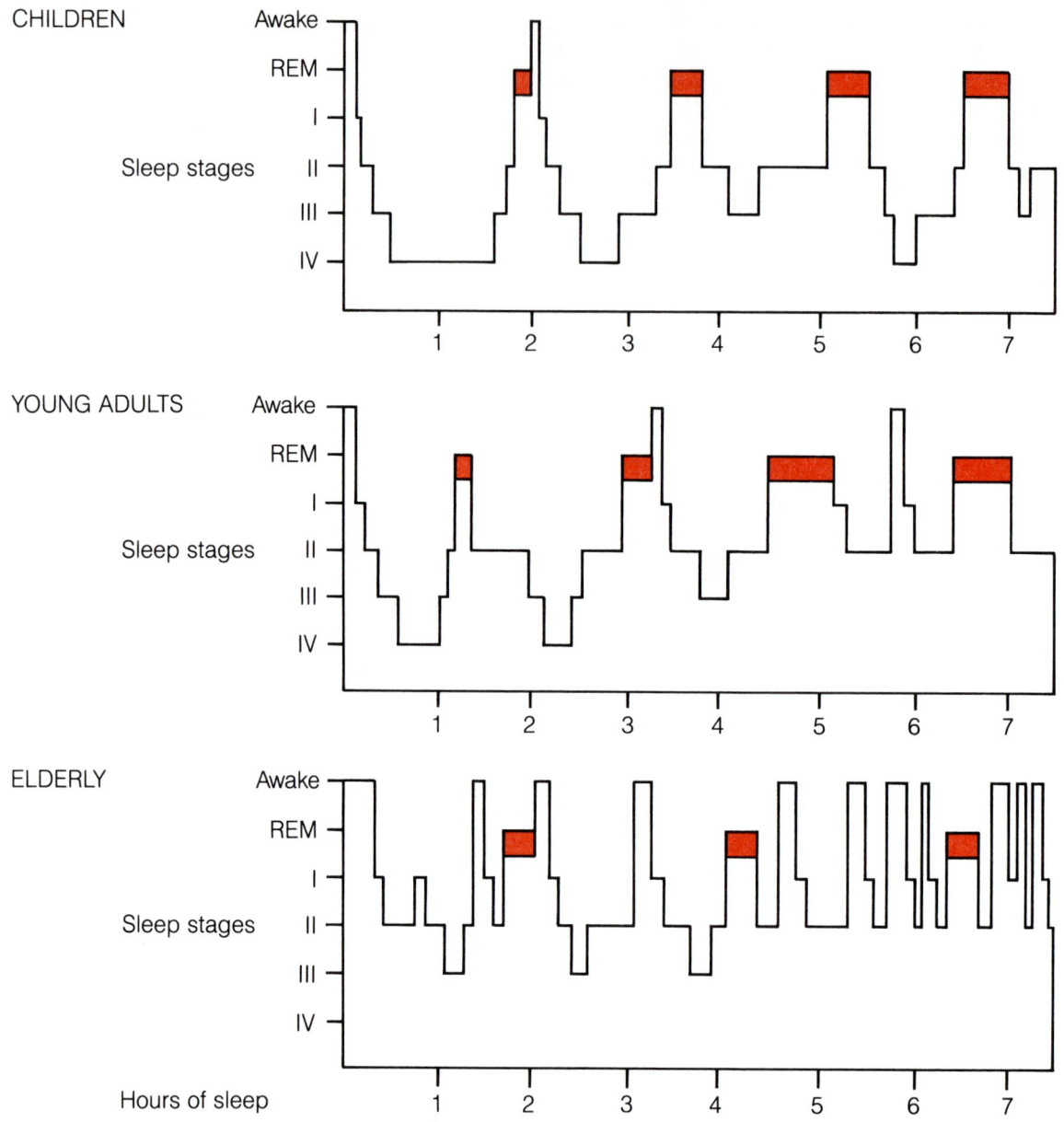

Figure 37–4 Normal sleep cycles of children, young adults, and elderly adults. The sleep of children and young adults shows early preponderance of NREM stages III and IV, progressive lengthening of the first three REM periods, and infrequent awakenings. In elderly adults, there is little or no NREM stage IV sleep, REM periods are fairly uniform in length, and awakenings are frequent and often lengthy. *Source:* A. Kales, Sleep and dreams: Recent research in clinical aspects, *Annals of Internal Medicine,* May 1968, 68:1078. Reprinted with permission.

ings of irritability, excitability, and restlessness, whereas loss of stage III and IV NREM sleep leads to physical discomfort and feeling withdrawn (Webster and Thompson 1986, p. 450). See Table 37–4, later in this chapter.

Generally, during REM sleep oxygen use by the brain is great and temperature, blood pressure, and heart rate

increase. It is thought that during REM sleep, the brain can analyze the day's activities and work through emotional problems in dream imagery (Marieb 1989, p. 478).

Sleep does not appear to be necessary to recharge energy lost during the day. If that were the case, the relative durations of wakefulness and sleep would remain constant, and they do not. For example, when people are deliberately kept awake for 3 to 10 days, they sleep for less than a day after the enforced wakefulness. Conversely, when people are immobilized for long periods, they still sleep and apparently need to. Sleep is also unnecessary for body organ function, although physiologic changes occur during sleep (Guyton 1986, p. 674).

SLEEP VARIATIONS ACCORDING TO AGE

Sleep patterns vary over the life cycle in accordance with age and growth rate. Decreases occur in the time spent in total sleep, in stage IV sleep, and in REM sleep. Table 37–2 and Chapters 25 through 27 detail people's need for sleep at different ages.

FACTORS AFFECTING NORMAL SLEEP

Both the quality and the quantity of sleep are affected by several factors (see Table 37–3 on page 946). *Quality of sleep* means the individual's ability to stay asleep and to get appropriate amounts of REM and NREM sleep. Sleep stages can be differentiated and measured only in a laboratory. *Quantity of sleep* is the total time the individual sleeps.

Illness   People who are ill require more sleep than normal, and the normal rhythm of sleep and wakefulness is also disturbed. People deprived of REM sleep subsequently spend more sleep time than normal in this stage. Pain also can affect sleep—either preventing sleep or awakening the sleeper.

Respiratory conditions can disturb an individual's sleep. Shortness of breath often makes sleep difficult, and people

TABLE 37–2   *Sleep Patterns According to Age*

Developmental Level	Normal Sleep Pattern	Developmental Level	Normal Sleep Pattern
Newborn	Sleeps 14 to 18 hours a day.		an afternoon nap or siesta is customary.
	50% REM sleep.	School-age child	Sleeps about 10 hours at night.
	Most remaining time spent in Stages III and IV NREM sleep.		18.5% REM sleep.
	Sleep cycles last 45 to 60 minutes each.		Sleep time remains relatively constant.
Infant	Sleeps 12 to 14 hours a day.	Adolescent	Sleeps about 8.5 hours a day.
	20 to 30% REM sleep.		20% REM sleep.
	Sleeps longer at night (8 to 10 hours) and has a scheduled pattern of naps.	Young adult	Most sleep 7 to 9 hours a day.
			20 to 25% REM sleep.
	At 12 months, naps once or twice a day.		5 to 10% Stage I sleep.
			50% Stage II sleep.
Toddler	Sleeps about 10 to 12 hours a day.		10 to 20% Stage III and IV.
	25% REM sleep.	Middle-aged adult	Sleeps about 7 hours a day.
	Most sleep during the night.		About 20% REM sleep.
	Midmorning naps decrease.		May have insomnia.
	Normal sleep-wake cycle is established by most at age 2 or 3 years.	Elderly adult	Sleeps about 6 hours a day.
			20 to 25% REM sleep.
Preschooler	Sleeps about 11 hours at night.		Stage IV sleep is markedly decreased and sometimes absent.
	20% REM sleep.		First REM period is longer.
	Second nap eliminated by most at age 3.		May awaken more often during the night.
	At age 5 daytime naps are relinquished, except in cultures where		

Sources: L. Malasanos, V. Barkauskas, M. Moss, and K. Stoltenberg-Allen, *Health assessment,* 3d ed. (St. Louis: C. V. Mosby Co., 1990), pp. 97–99; L. F. Whalley and D. L. Wong, *Essentials of pediatric nursing,* 3d ed. (St. Louis: C. V. Mosby Co., 1989), pp. 81–82, 292, 355, 381, 438, 460; and C. Hoch and C. Reynolds, Sleep disturbances and what to do about them, *Geriatric Nursing,* January/February 1986, 7:25.

TABLE 37–3 *Factors Affecting Sleep*

Factor	Effect
Liver failure	Day-night reversal
Encephalitis	Day-night reversal
Hypothyroidism	Decreases NREM Stage IV sleep
Antidepressant	Decreases REM sleep
Amphetamine	Decreases REM sleep
Alcohol	Speeds onset of sleep, but decreases REM sleep and disrupts other stages
Depression	Decreases or increases REM sleep
Sedative-hypnotic drug	Suppresses REM sleep and decreases NREM Stages III and IV. On withdrawal, causes rebound REM sleep with vivid dreams and increased awakening
Tranquilizer	Interferes with REM sleep
Bedtime snack of protein food	Induces and maintains sleep

RESEARCH NOTE

Do Sleep Patterns of Elderly People Change in a Long-Term Care Facility?

Clapin-French studied the sleep patterns of elderly clients (35 males and 67 females) in a long-term care facility. Their study focused on those factors involved in changes in the clients' sleep patterns. Records revealed that 71% received some type of sleep medication regularly, yet 77 clients said they did not take sleep medication at home. There were significant changes in the individuals' sleep patterns following admission to the agency. Clients napped frequently during the day, reported interrupted sleep twice as frequently, and indicated a preference for an earlier bedtime than at preadmission. Reports concerning difficulties falling asleep showed little change after admission, and their usual waking time showed little change. Nocturnal awakenings associated with elimination increased following admission. The proximity of other people and pain were major factors causing nocturnal awakenings; traffic noises were a less significant cause. The study also revealed that only 54% of the clients had a sleep history completed, suggesting that the nursing sleep history is underutilized.

Implications: A sleep history would help nurses understand and help clients obtain needed sleep.

E. Clapin-French, Sleep patterns of aged persons in long-term care facilities, *Journal of Advanced Nursing* January 1986, 11:57–66.

---

who have nasal congestion or sinus drainage may have trouble breathing and hence a difficult sleep. Recent research also indicates that hypoxia and hypercapnia may interfere with normal sleep (Closs 1988, p. 50).

People who have gastric or duodenal ulcers may find their sleep disturbed because of pain, often a result of the increased gastric secretions that occur during REM sleep. Certain endocrine disturbances can also affect sleep. Hyperthyroidism lengthens presleep time, often making it difficult for a client to fall asleep. Hypothyroidism, on the other hand, decreases stage IV sleep. Pain associated with certain diseases such as arthritis, asthma, and migraine can also affect normal sleep. Elevated body temperatures can cause some reduction in stages III and IV NREM sleep and REM sleep.

The need to urinate during the night (enuresis) also disrupts sleep, and people who awaken at night to urinate sometimes have difficulty getting back to sleep.

Environment Environment can promote or hinder sleep. Any change—e.g., in the noise level in the environment—can inhibit sleep. The absence of usual stimuli or the presence of unfamiliar stimuli can keep people from sleeping.

Life-Style It is thought that a person who is moderately fatigued usually has a restful sleep. Fatigue can also affect a person's sleep pattern. The more tired the person is, the shorter the first period of paradoxical (REM) sleep. As the person rests, the REM periods become longer.

Psychologic Stress Anxiety and depression frequently disturb sleep. A person preoccupied with personal problems may be unable to relax sufficiently to get to sleep. Anxiety increases the norepinephrine blood levels through stimulation of the sympathetic nervous system. This chemical change results in less stage IV NREM and REM sleep and more stage changes and awakenings (Closs 1988, p. 49).

Medications Medications, especially hypnotics and sedatives, affect the sleep pattern. Hypnotics and barbiturates decrease REM sleep, even though they may increase total sleep time. Amphetamines and antidepressants decrease REM sleep abnormally. A client withdrawing from any of these drugs gets much more REM sleep than usual and as a result may experience upsetting nightmares.

Alcohol and Stimulants People who drink an excessive amount of alcohol often find their sleep disturbed. Excessive alcohol disrupts REM sleep, although it may hasten the onset of sleep. While making up for lost

REM sleep after some of the effects of the alcohol have worn off, clients often experience nightmares. Tolerance to alcohol also affects sleep; the alcohol-tolerant person may be unable to sleep well and may become irritable as a result.

Caffeine-containing beverages act as stimulants of the central nervous system, thus interfering with sleep.

Diet Weight loss and weight gain have been found to affect sleep. Crisp and Stonehill (1976, p. 166) found that weight loss is associated with reduced total sleep time as well as broken sleep and earlier awakening. Weight gain, on the other hand, was associated with an increase in total sleep time, less broken sleep, and later waking.

The amino acid L-tryptophan is thought to affect sleep. Dietary L-tryptophan—found, for example, in cottage cheese, milk, beef, and canned tuna—may be sleep-inducing, a fact that might explain why warm milk helps some people get to sleep.

COMMON SLEEP DISORDERS

Knowledge about common sleep disorders assists the nurse to obtain and recognize pertinent data. Sleep disorders may be categorized as primary disorders, secondary disorders, and the parasomnias. **Primary sleep disorders** are those in which the person's sleep problem is the main disorder. Disorders include insomnia, hypersomnia, narcolepsy, sleep apnea, and parasomnias. **Secondary sleep disorders** are sleep disturbances caused by another clinical disorder, such as thyroid dysfunction, depression, or alcoholism.

Insomnia **Insomia,** the most common sleep disorder, is the inability to obtain an adequate amount or quality of sleep. People suffering from insomnia do not feel refreshed on arising. There are three types of insomnia:

1. Difficulty in falling asleep (initial insomnia)
2. Difficulty in staying asleep because of frequent or prolonged waking (intermittent or maintenance insomnia)
3. Early morning or premature awakening (terminal insomnia)

Some insomniacs have been observed to fall asleep and obtain more sleep than they say they do. This type of insomnia is referred to by some as subjective or imaginary insomnia. Such a condition is no less distressing than the above types of insomnia and may lead to increased wakefulness.

Insomnia can result from physical discomfort but more often is a result of mental overstimulation due to anxiety. People sometimes become anxious because they think they might not be able to sleep. People who become habituated to drugs or who drink large quantities of alcohol are likely to have insomnia.

Treatment for insomnia frequently requires the client to develop new behavior patterns that induce sleep. The usefulness of sleeping medications is questionable. Such medications do not deal with the cause of the problem, and their prolonged use creates drug dependencies.

Hypersomnia **Hypersomnia,** the opposite of insomnia, is excessive sleep, particularly in the daytime. The afflicted person often sleeps until noon and takes many naps during the day. Hypersomnia is generally related to psychophysiologic problems, such as psychiatric disorders (depression or anxiety), central nervous system damage, and certain kidney, liver, or metabolic disorders such as diabetic acidosis and hypothyroidism. In many instances, hypersomnia is used as a coping mechanism to avoid facing the responsibilities of the day.

Narcolepsy **Narcolepsy**—from the Greek *narco,* meaning "numbness," and *lepsis,* meaning "seizure"—is a sudden wave of overwhelming sleepiness that occurs during the day; thus it is referred to as a "sleep attack." Its cause is unknown, although it is believed to be a genetic defect of the central nervous system in which the REM period cannot be controlled. In narcoleptic attacks, sleep starts with the REM phase. Even though narcoleptics sleep well at night, they nod off several times a day even when conversing with someone or driving a car.

Many narcoleptics have bouts of **cataplexy,** that is, partial or complete muscle paralysis. Sometimes the person's jaw slackens or the head falls to the chest. These cataplectic bouts are often preceded by moments of exertion or strong emotion, such as laughing or crying.

Sleep Apnea **Sleep apnea** is the periodic cessation of breathing during sleep. This disorder needs to be assessed by a sleep expert, but it is often suspected when the person has loud snoring, frequent nocturnal awakenings, excessive daytime sleepiness, insomnia, morning headaches, intellectual deterioration, irritability or other personality changes, and physiologic changes such as hypertension and cardiac arrhythmias (Weaver and Millman 1986, p. 148). It is most frequent in men over 50 and in postmenopausal women.

The periods of apnea, which last from 10 seconds to 2 minutes, occur during REM or NREM sleep. Frequency of episodes ranges from 50 to 600 per night. These apneic episodes drain the person of energy and lead to excessive daytime sleepiness.

Sleep apnea profoundly affects a person's work or school performance. In addition, prolonged sleep apnea can cause a sharp rise in blood pressure and may also lead to cardiac arrest. Over time, apneic episodes can cause cardiac arrhythmias, pulmonary hypertension, and subsequent left-sided heart failure.

Parasomnias   **Parasomnias** refer to a cluster of waking behaviors that appear during sleep and interfere with sleep. Parasomnias include **somnambulism** (sleepwalking), **night terrors** (horrifying dreams), and **nocturnal enuresis** (bedwetting), talking in one's sleep, nocturnal erections, and **bruxism** (grinding of the teeth during sleep).

Somnambulism   About 1% to 6% of children, and more males than females between the ages of 5 and 12 years, walk in their sleep (Malasanos, Barkauskas, Moss, and Stoltenberg-Allen 1990, p.103). Sleepwalking occurs during the transition of sleep from stage IV to III of NREM sleep, is episodic, generally occurs 1 to 2 hours after falling asleep, and usually does not last longer than 10 minutes. It is normally outgrown without incident within 2 to 3 years. It tends to occur in children after a distressing experience, such as the loss of a parent or pet. Adults tend to sleepwalk after the death of a loved one or when in a new environment. Because sleepwalkers tend not to notice dangers such as open window and stairs, the main concern is to protect the sleepwalker from injury. Usually the sleepwalker can be awakened and quietly led back to bed.

Night terrors   are frightening to both parents and children. Children 6 and younger are most often afflicted. After having slept a few hours, the child bolts upright in bed, shakes and screams, appears pale and terrified, and is unable to tell the parent what is wrong. Night terrors tend to run in families and differ from nightmares in that the child is unable to recall any frightening thoughts or dreams associated with the awakening. This lack of recall is understandable because the night terror emerges from an arousal from stage IV slow-wave deep sleep rather than an arousal from REM sleep. Night terrors usually disappear without treatment.

Nocturnal enuresis   Bed-wetting is the most common sleep disorder occurring in children past the age of 3. More males than females are afflicted. Enuresis usually occurs 1 to 2 hours after falling asleep, when rousing from NREM stages III to IV, and is often associated with increased muscle tone, tachycardia, tachypnea, and erection in males. Immediately after micturition, the child may be difficult to waken and when wakened has no recall of the incident. The cause of nocturnal enuresis is unknown, although in preschool children bladder training that is too severe or too early may be responsible.

Sleeptalking   People of any age can talk in their sleep. Talking usually occurs before REM sleep. It rarely presents a sleep problem to the person unless it becomes troublesome to others.

Nocturnal erections   During adolescence boys begin to experience nocturnal erections and emissions (commonly referred to as "wet dreams") several times each month. They generally occur during REM sleep and do not present a sleep problem if the boy is informed that this is a normal development.

Bruxism   Clenching and grinding of the teeth generally occurs during stage II sleep. Because the person is often oblivious to this habit, a sleep disturbance may not be a problem. However, bruxism can eventually erode and diminish the height of dental crowns and cause the teeth to become loose. A dentist can make a splint to be worn over the teeth to prevent grinding movements.

SLEEP DEPRIVATION

A prolonged disturbance results in decreases in amount, quality, and consistency of sleep and can lead to a syndrome referred to as **sleep deprivation.** This is not a sleep disorder in itself but a result of sleep disturbances. It produces a variety of physiologic and behavioral symptoms, the severity of which depends on the degree of the deprivation. Two major types of sleep deprivation are REM deprivation, in which dreaming is absent, and NREM deprivation, in which slow-wave or delta sleep is significantly reduced. A combination of the two types increases the severity of symptoms. Table 37–4 shows the causes and signs/symptoms of each type.

ASSESSING

Assessment relative to a client's sleep includes a sleep history, a sleep diary, and clinical examination.

Sleep History

A general sleep history, which is usually part of the comprehensive nursing history form, is obtained for all clients entering a health care facility. This enables the nurse to incorporate the client's needs and preferences in the plan of care. A general sleep history often includes the following:

- Usual sleeping pattern, specifically sleeping and waking times; hours of undisturbed sleep; quality of sleep (e.g., effect on energy level for daily functioning); and time and duration of naps.

- Bedtime rituals performed to help the person fall asleep (e.g., a glass of hot milk, reading or other method of relaxing, and special equipment or positioning aids).

- Use of sleep medications. Sleep can be disturbed by a variety of drugs taken close to bedtime, e.g., stimulants and steroids. Hypnotics and sedating antidepressants may cause excessive daytime sleepiness.

TABLE 37–4 *Types, Causes, and Signs of Sleep Deprivation*

Type	Causes	Signs and Symptoms
REM deprivation	Alcohol, barbiturates, shift work, jet lag, extended ICU hospitalization, morphine, meperidine hydrochloride (Demerol)	■ Excitability, restlessness, irritability, and increased sensitivity to pain ■ Confusion and suspiciousness ■ Emotional lability
NREM deprivation	All of the above plus diazepam (Valium), flurazepam hydrochloride (Dalmane), hypothyroidism, depression, respiratory distress disorders, sleep apnea, and age (common in the elderly)	■ Withdrawal, apathy, hyporesponsiveness ■ Feeling physically uncomfortable ■ Lack of facial expression ■ Speech deterioration ■ Excessive sleepiness
Both REM and NREM deprivation	As above	■ Decreased reasoning ability (judgment) and ability to concentrate ■ Inattentiveness ■ Marked fatigue manifested by blurred vision, itchy eyes, nausea, headache ■ Difficulty performing activities of daily living ■ Lack of memory, mental confusion, visual or auditory hallucinations, and illusions

ASSESSMENT INTERVIEW
Sleep Disturbances

■ How would you describe your sleeping problem? What changes have occurred in your sleeping pattern? How often does this happen?

■ Do you have difficulty falling asleep?

■ Do you wake up often during the night? If so, how often?

■ Do you wake up earlier in the morning than you would like and have difficulty falling back to sleep?

■ How do you feel when you wake up in the morning?

■ Do you sleep more than usual? If so, how often do you sleep?

■ Do you have periods of overwhelming tiredness? If so, when does this happen?

■ Have you ever suddenly fallen asleep in the middle of a daytime activity? If so, has any muscle weakness or paralysis occurred?

■ Has anyone ever told you that you snore, walk in your sleep, talk in your sleep, or stop breathing for a while when sleeping?

■ What have you been doing to deal with this sleeping problem? Does it help?

■ What do you think might be causing this problem? Do you have any medical condition that might be causing you to sleep more (or less)? Are you receiving medications for an illness that might alter your sleeping pattern? Are you experiencing any stressful or upsetting events or conflicts that may be affecting your sleep?

■ How do you feel your sleeping problem is affecting you?

■ Sleep environment (e.g., dark room, cool or warm temperature, noise level, nightlight).

■ Recent changes in sleep patterns or difficulties in sleeping.

If the client indicates a recent pattern change or difficulties in sleeping, a more detailed history is required. This detailed history should explore the exact nature of the problem and its cause, when it first began and its frequency, how it affects daily living, what the client is doing to cope with the problem, and whether these methods have been effective. Questions the nurse might ask the client with a sleeping disturbance are shown in the box above.

Sleep Diary

Sometimes clients with a sleeping problem can provide more precise information if they keep a written record of their sleep pattern and the habits associated with it. Such a sleep diary or log can be kept by clients who are sleeping at home and should be maintained for at least 1 week. A sleep diary may include all of the following information or selected aspects of it that pertain to the client's specific problem.

■ Time of (a) Going to bed, (b) Trying to fall asleep, (c) Falling asleep (approximate), (d) Any awakening and duration, and (e) Awakening in the morning

- Activities performed before bedtime (type, duration, and time)
- Bedtime rituals (e.g., ingestion of food, fluid, or medication) before going to bed
- Presence of any worries that the client believes may affect sleep

Keeping such a diary may become stressful for some clients and further affect their sleep. The nurse needs to advise the client to obtain the assistance of a bed partner in keeping the diary or to discontinue the diary if it presents a problem. When a diary is completed, the nurse and client can develop flow charts or graphs that will assist in organizing the data and identifying the specific problem.

Physical Examination

Examination of the client includes observation of the client's facial appearance, behavior, and energy level. Darkened areas around the eyes, puffy eyelids, reddened conjunctiva, glazed or dull-appearing eyes, and limited facial expression are indicative of sleep insufficiency. Behaviors such as irritability, restlessness, inattentiveness, slowed speech, slumped posture, hand tremor, yawning, rubbing the eyes, withdrawal, confusion, and incoordination are also suggestive of sleep problems. Lack of energy may be noted by observing whether the client appears physically weak, lethargic, or fatigued.

In addition, the nurse assesses whether the client has a deviated nasal septum, enlarged neck, or is obese. These findings may be associated with obstructive sleep apnea and/or snoring.

Diagnostic Studies

Sleep is measured objectively in a sleep disorder laboratory by **polysomnography;** an electroencephalogram (EEG), electromyogram (EMG), and electro-oculogram (EOG) are recorded simultaneously. This simultaneous recording divides sleep into REM and NREM sleep. Electrodes are placed on the center of the scalp to record brain waves (EEG) (See Figure 37–2), on the outer canthus of each eye to record eye movement (EOG), and on the chin muscles to record the structural electromyogram (EMG). The following may also be monitored, depending on findings of the initial interview: respiratory effort and airflow, ECG, leg movements, and oxygen saturation. Oxygen saturation is determined by monitoring arterial blood or by an *oximeter,* a light-sensitive cell that attaches to the ear or a finger. Oxygen saturation and ECG assessments are of particular importance if sleep apnea is suspected. Through polysomnography, the client's activity (movements, struggling, noisy respirations) during sleep can be assessed. Such activity of which the client is unaware may be the cause of arousal during sleep.

Nocturnal myoclonus is a disorder requiring polysomnography for diagnosis unless a bed partner can verify its presence. Nocturnal myoclonus involves leg-kicking movements that may occur every 20 to 40 seconds and last 5 minutes to 2 hours. Both legs are involved.

DIAGNOSING

Sleep pattern disturbance is the nursing diagnosis given to clients with sleeping problems. It is defined as a disruption of sleep time that causes discomfort or interferes with desired life-style (Kim et al 1989, p. 60). After assessment data are grouped, patterns emerge that will enable the nurse to specify this diagnosis and perhaps provide an etiology. Sleep pattern disturbances may also be stated as the *etiology* of another diagnosis, in which case the nursing interventions are directed toward the sleep disturbance itself.

Examples of assessment data clusters and related nursing diagnoses for primary sleep disturbances are shown in Table 37–5. Examples of nursing diagnoses and contributing factors related to sleep problems are listed below.

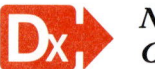 **Nursing Diagnoses Clients with Sleep Problems**

Sleep pattern disturbance related to:

- Worries about actual or anticipated loss of a loved one, loss of a job, loss of life due to serious disease process or worry about a family member's behavior or illness
- Frequent changes in sleep time due to shift work or overtime
- Specific illness that affects the sleep cycle, or pain and discomfort associated with a disease process
- Inability to cope with multiple stresses
- Changes in sleep environment or bedtime rituals (e.g., noise or overstimulation of hospital environment)
- Alcohol or other drug dependency
- Drug withdrawal
- Misuse of sedatives prescribed for insomnia

Potential for injury related to somnambulism

Self-esteem disturbance related to nocturnal enuresis

Ineffective individual coping related to sleep deprivation

Fatigue related to insomnia

Potential for impaired gas exchange related to sleep apnea

Knowledge deficit (nonprescription remedies for insomnia)

TABLE 37–5 *Examples of Assessment Data Clusters and Related Nursing Diagnoses for Clients with Sleep Problems*

Data Cluster	Nursing Diagnoses
51-year-old woman states she has a problem falling asleep since her mastectomy for breast cancer 2 months ago. Says fears of prognosis become prominent when she is not active and busy. Has tried reading or watching TV but neither make her sleepy or relaxed. Appears agitated and restless.	**Sleep pattern disturbance: insomnia (difficulty falling asleep)** related to fear of prognosis and difficulty relaxing
83-year-old man admitted to four-bed room in extended care unit 3 days ago. States he falls asleep about 10 P.M. but is awakened by room-mate's snoring. States, "At home I used to have a hot cup of Ovaltine whenever I awakened."	**Sleep pattern disturbance: insomnia (difficulty staying asleep)** related to change in sleep environment and sleep-time rituals.
Client states he was fired from his job because of alcohol abuse. Has joined Alcoholics Anonymous but has been unable to get any work for the past 2 years. States, "Every day I wake up at 4:00 A.M. (full of self-reproach and self-punitive thinking) and can't get back to sleep."	**Sleep pattern disturbance: insomnia (early morning awakening)** related to low self-esteem secondary to loss of job and inability to obtain employment
High school student's father and mother recently divorced, and her boyfriend broke up with her 2 weeks ago. States she doesn't have the energy to get up in the morning and just wants to sleep all the time. She has Grade 12 examinations next week.	**Sleep pattern disturbance** related to inability to cope with multiple stresses
Client states that recent shortage of fire fighters has resulted in extensive over-time work, often "double shifts" and frequent rotations from his usual 2 weekly 7–3 and 3–7 shifts. States, "All I want to do is sleep when I get home, but I can't get to sleep. I guess I'm too riled up."	**Sleep pattern disturbance: altered sleep-wake pattern** related to frequent shift changes and overtime

PLANNING

Overall client-goals and nursing interventions to achieve them are identified from the nursing diagnosis. The overall goal for clients with sleep disturbances is to maintain (or develop) a sleeping pattern that provides sufficient energy for daily activities. Specific nursing interventions are planned from the etiology of each nursing diagnosis. These may include reducing environmental distractions; promoting bedtime rituals; providing comfort measures; scheduling nursing care to provide for uninterrupted sleep periods; teaching stress reduction, relaxation techniques, or ways to develop good sleep habits; and promoting self-esteem. If the sleep disturbance is the etiology of the nursing diagnosis, the nurse plans specific strategies to relieve insomnia, deal with sleep deprivation, reduce the potential for injury, prevent nocturnal enuresis, and so on.

Examples of outcome criteria to evaluate the achievement of client goals and the effectiveness of nursing interventions are shown below.

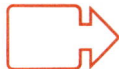 **Outcome Criteria**
Clients with Sleep Problems

The client:

- Falls asleep within 30 minutes after going to bed.
- Sleeps at least 6 hours without awakening.
- Awakens no more than twice during sleep and falls asleep within 15 minutes.
- Verbalizes feeling refreshed after awakening.
- Demonstrates decreased signs of sleep deprivation.
- Describes factors that prevent or inhibit sleep.
- Describes relaxation techniques that induce sleep.

IMPLEMENTING

For hospitalized clients, sleep problems are often related to the hospital environment or their illness. Assisting the client to sleep in such instances can be challenging to a nurse, often involving scheduling activities, administering analgesics, and providing a supportive environment. Explanations and a supportive relationship are essential for the fearful or anxious client.

Creating a Restful Environment

Environmental distractions are particularly troublesome for hospitalized clients. The noises are strange to most clients, and it is usually impossible to eliminate all sounds. Some of the interventions that may help are listed in the box above.

To reduce sleep interruptions, nurses can schedule activities so that the client has the fewest possible interruptions while resting or sleeping. For example, if a client requires an intramuscular injection during the night, other interventions may be carried out at the same time, such as assessing vital signs or changing a position. Nurses should also avoid waking a sleeping client for unnecessary care, such as to ask if the client wants a sleeping medication. Visits just prior to sleeping should be limited and perhaps rescheduled to another time.

The environment must also be safe so that the client can relax. People who are unaccustomed to narrow hospital beds may feel more secure with side rails. See the box below for additional safety measures.

Individuals vary in what they consider a comfortable environment for sleeping; for example, choices about room

temperature, ventilation, and number of pillows are individualistic. Whenever possible, nurses should provide the environment most conducive to sleep for the individual.

Supporting Bedtime Rituals

Most people are accustomed to bedtime rituals or presleep routines that are conducive to comfort and relaxation. Altering or eliminating such routines can affect a client's sleep. Common prebedtime activities of adults include an evening stroll, listening to music, taking a soothing bath, and praying. Children too are socialized into presleep routines such as a bedtime story, or holding on to a favorite toy or blanket. Sleep is also usually preceded by hygienic routines such as washing the face and hands (or bathing), brushing the teeth, and voiding.

In addition, many people take snacks of some sort before bedtime to allay hunger that may interfere with sleep. Some high-protein beverages and snacks such as a hot milky drink, cheese, or nuts are known to promote sleep when taken before bedtime. These promote sleep because they contain the amino acid L-tryptophan, a sleep inducer. Excessive fluid intake before retiring should also be avoided. This prevents the need to use the bathroom during sleeping hours.

People need to learn to avoid excessive physical exercise and excessive mental stimulation such as office work or dealing with family problems before bedtime. Such activity prolongs falling asleep. Exercise performed 2 hours before bedtime, however, can promote sleep because it contributes to physical fatigue and invites sleep. Adherence to a consistent time for sleep and getting up at the same time each morning is also important in establishing a healthy sleep pattern.

Promoting Comfort and Relaxation

Comfort measures are essential to help the client fall asleep and stay asleep, especially if the effects of the person's illness interfere with sleep. A concerned, caring attitude, along with the interventions described in the box on the opposite page, can significantly promote client comfort and sleep.

Emotional stress obviously interferes with a person's ability to relax, rest, and sleep; inability to sleep further aggravates feelings of tension. Sleep rarely occurs until a person is relaxed. Relaxation techniques can be encouraged as part of the nightly routine. Slow, deep breathing for a few minutes followed by slow, rhythmic contraction and relaxation of muscles can alleviate tension and induce calm. Imagery, meditation, and yoga can also be taught. See specialized stress reduction techniques in Chapter 33, page 810, and distraction techniques in Chapter 38, page 974.

Administering Sleep Medications

Sleep medications often prescribed on a p.r.n. basis for clients include sedative-hypnotics, which induce sleep, and antianxiety drugs or tranquilizers, which decrease anxiety and tension. Because a tolerance to the sleep-inducing properties develops after several weeks, clients may increase the dosage or complement the drug with alcohol.

Nurses need to teach clients about the action and side-effects of such drugs and the risks of overreliance and to caution clients about taking drugs with alcohol. The use of nonprescription sleeping medications should be discouraged. When administering prescribed drugs to clients in hospital, the nurse must be knowledgeable about expected side-effects and administer them only when indicated. Elderly clients, in particular, are prone to side-effects because of their altered rates of gastrointestinal absorption, decreased ability to metabolize and excrete drugs, and, in some cases, increased body fat. Whenever possible, nonpharmacologic interventions to induce and maintain sleep are preferred interventions.

Client Teaching

Many insomniacs or people suffering from sleep deprivation can benefit from instructions about good sleep habits and factors that interfere with sleep. Most people also need instruction about the proper use of sleep medications. Client teaching for promoting sleep is shown in the box below.

EVALUATING

To evaluate whether client goals have been achieved, the nurse may observe the duration of the client's sleep, observe the client for signs of REM and NREM sleep deprivation, ask how the client feels on awakening, or question the client about the effectiveness of specific interventions, e.g., use of relaxation techniques, adherence to a consistent sleep-wake cycle, or ingestion of milk products before bedtime.

Examples of evaluative statements indicating goal achievement are "The client stated, 'I fell asleep without any trouble every night for the past week.'" Remember to date and sign the evaluative statement when recording it.

NURSING CARE PLAN FOR JACK HARRIS

ASSESSMENT DATA

Nursing Assessment

Jack Harris is a 36-year-old police officer assigned to a high-crime police precinct. One week ago he received a surface bullet wound to his arm and has now come to the outpatient clinic to have his wound redressed. While speaking with the nurse, he mentions that he has recently been promoted to the rank of detective and has assumed new responsibilities. He states that since his promotion, he has experienced an increasing amount of difficulty falling asleep and sometimes staying asleep. Mr. Harris expressed considerable concern over the danger of his occupation and also his desire to do well in his new position. He complains of waking up feeling tired and of becoming quite irritable.

Physical Examination

Height: 185.4 cm (6'1")
Weight: 85.7 kg (189 lb)
Temperature: 37.0 C (98.6 F)
Pulse rate: 80 BPM
Respirations: 18 per minute at rest
Blood pressure: 144/88 mm Hg
Pale, drawn with dark circles under eyes

Diagnostic Data

CBC within normal range
X-ray film of left arm: Evidence of superficial soft tissue injury

CARE PLAN

Nursing Diagnosis	Client Goals and Outcome Criteria	Nursing Interventions and Rationales	Evaluation
Sleep pattern disturbance related to anxiety and overstimulation resulting in difficulty falling asleep and remaining asleep, fatigue, irritability, yawning, drawn appearance with dark circles under eyes.	Client Goal: Establishes a satisfactory sleep-rest pattern and awakens feeling rested. Outcome Criteria: Describes one or two factors that cause insomnia. Identifies two or three measures that induce sleep. Sleeps 7–8 hours a night by day 14. Demonstrates less irritability and a greater sense of well-being by day 21.	Assist client in identifying factors that cause or contribute to insomnia. *Rationale:* Knowledge of causative factors can enable client to begin to control these factors. Encourage client to establish and maintain a bedtime routine. *Routine:* A routine may assist in inducing sleep. Encourage client to utilize sleep aids such as reading, getting a back rub, or listening to soft music. *Rationale:* This promotes emotional and muscle relaxation. Instruct the client in use of soporifics, e.g., milk and protein foods at bedtime. *Rationale:* Milk and protein foods contain tryptophan, a precursor of serotonin which is thought to induce and maintain sleep. Instruct client in use of relaxation techniques. *Rationale:* Relaxation techniques provide distraction and comfort and induce sleep. Instruct client to avoid caffeine stimulants in the evening before bedtime. *Rationale:* Stimulants inhibit sleep.	Client is able to identify the stress and anxiety of his occupation and promotion as a source of his insomnia. He is practicing relaxation techniques each night at bedtime. Client drinks warm milk at bedtime. He sleeps 7 hours approximately 3–4 days a week and has experienced a greater sense of well-being.

► Care Plan for Jack Harris *(continued)*

Nursing Diagnosis	Client Goals and Outcome Criteria	Nursing Interventions and Rationales	Evaluation
Anxiety (mild) related to promotion and change in socio-economic status resulting in insomnia, elevated blood pressure, apprehension, and irritability.	Client Goal: Identify source of anxiety and cope effectively with the situation. Outcome Criteria: Recognizes his coping patterns by day 7. Experiences a decrease in insomnia by day 14. Uses effective coping mechanisms.	Assist client in identifying and acknowledging his anxiety/stressors. *Rationale:* Feelings are real, and it is best to bring them out in the open so that they may be worked through. Be available as a listener and provide reassurance and comfort. *Rationale:* Establishes a rapport and allows client to express himself Assist client with adaptive coping mechanisms, e.g., talking with wife or counselor about problem *Rationale:* Adaptive coping mechanisms will assist client in dealing effectively with his anxiety/stressors.	Client acknowledges his insomnia is a somatic expression of his anxiety over his new promotion and a fear of failing. Uses coping mechanism of talking with police department counselor when difficulties arise in the department.

CHAPTER HIGHLIGHTS

► Sleep is a conscious state in which a person's perception and reaction to the environment are decreased.

► The sleep cycle is controlled by the reticular activating system (RAS) and the bulbar synchronizing region (BSR) in the brain stem.

► During a normal night's sleep an adult has four to six sleep cycles, each with NREM sleep and REM sleep.

► NREM (slow-wave) sleep constitutes most of a sleep cycle.

► The ratio of NREM to REM sleep varies with age.

► Many factors can affect normal sleep, including illness, environment, life-style, psychologic stress, medications, alcohol, stimulants, and diet.

► Common sleep disorders include insomnia, hypersomnia, narcolepsy, sleep apnea, and parasomnias such as somnambulism, night terrors, and nocturnal enuresis.

► A sleep history helps the nurse plan interventions to assist clients to sleep.

► People usually develop their own bedtime rituals to help prepare them for sleep.

► Pain control and comfort are important for sleeping.

READINGS AND REFERENCES

SUGGESTED READINGS

Hoch, C., and Reynolds, III, C. January/February 1986. Sleep disturbances and what to do about them. *Geriatric Nursing* 7:24–27.
Hoch and Reynolds describe the normal sleep cycle and potential altered sleep-wake patterns. Included is how physical illness, psychologic factors, and medications can affect sleep. Sleep assessment is covered, as are nursing interventions that aid sleep. Specific reference is made to elderly clients.

McNeil, B. J.; Padrick, K. P.; and Wellman, J. January 1986. "I didn't sleep a wink." *American Journal of Nursing* 86:26–27.
These authors developed a sleep questionnaire to assess sleep patterns. Six items elicit responses about the client's perception of the sleep problem, fourteen items relate to the problems in falling asleep or frequent awakenings, and the remainder identify daytime and bedtime behaviors that induce or prevent sleep.

Weaver, T., and Millman, R. P. February 1986. Broken sleep. *American Journal of Nursing* 86:146–50.

The incidence, development, clinical manifestations, and current therapies of obstructive and central sleep apnea syndromes are included in this article. Sleep apnea is becoming recognized as a common problem among elderly people.

Webster, R. A., and Thompson, D. R. July 1986. Sleep in hospital. *Journal of Advanced Nursing* 11:447–57.

This comprehensive paper reviews sleep and its relationship to nursing practice. The authors discuss nursing interventions that are likely to ensure that adequate sleep is maintained.

RELATED RESEARCH

Clapin-French, E. January 1986. Sleep patterns of aged persons in long-term care facilities. *Journal of Advanced Nursing* 11:57–66.

Edgil, A. E.; Wood, K. R.; and Smith, D. P. March/April 1985. Sleep problems of older infants and preschool children. *Pediatric Nursing* 11:87–89.

Hayter, J. July/August 1983. Sleep behaviors of older persons. *Nursing Research* 32:242–46.

———. March/April 1985. To nap or not to nap? *Geriatric Nursing* 6:104–6.

Hoch, C. C.; Reynolds III, C. F.; and Houck, P. R. June 1988. Sleep patterns in Alzheimer, depressed and healthy elderly. *Western Journal of Nursing Research* 10:239–56.

Johnson, J. August 1985. Drug treatments for sleep disturbances: Does it really work? *Journal of Gerontological Nursing* 11:9–12.

SELECTED REFERENCES

Adam, K., and Oswald, I. 1977. Sleep is for tissue restoration. *Journal of the Royal College of Physicians* 11:376–88.

Biddle, C., Oaster, T. R. F. The nature of sleep. *AANA Journal* 58:36–44.

Bouton, J. December 10–16, 1986. Falling asleep. *Nursing Times* 82:36–37.

Closs, J. January 6–12 and 13–20, 1988. Patients' sleep-wake rhythms in hospital. Parts I and II *Nursing Times* 84:48–50; 54–55.

Crisp, A. N., and Stonehill, E. 1976. *Sleep, nutrition and mood.* New York: John Wiley and Sons.

Deters, G. E. July/August 1980. Circadian rhythm phenomenon. *Maternal Child Nursing* 5:249–51.

Grimes, J., and Burns, E. 1987. *Health assessment in nursing practice.* 2d ed. Boston: Jones and Bartlett Publishers, Inc.

Guyton, A. C. 1986. *Textbook of medical physiology.* 7th ed. Philadelphia: W. B. Saunders Co.

Hayter, J. March 1980. The rhythm of sleep. *American Journal of Nursing* 80:457–61.

Hoch, C., and Reynolds, C. January/February 1986. Sleep disturbances and what to do about them. *Geriatric Nursing* 7:24–27.

Horne, J. A. 1980. "Restitution" and sleep: Some qualifications. *Sleep Research* 9:19.

Kavey, N. B., and Anderson, D. December 1986. Why every patient needs a good night's sleep. *RN* 49:16–19.

Kim, M. J.; McFarland, G. K.; and McLane, A. M. 1989. *Pocket guide to nursing diagnoses.* St. Louis: C. V. Mosby Co.

Locsin, R. C. November/December 1988. Sleeplessness among the elderly. *Rehabilitation Nursing* 13:340–41.

Lukasiewicz-Ferland, P. November 1987. When your ICU patient can't sleep. *Nursing 87* 11:51–53.

Malasanos, L.; Barkauskas, V.; Moss, M.; and Stoltenberg-Allen, K. 1990. *Health assessment.* 4th ed. St. Louis: C. V. Mosby Co.

Maslow, A. 1970. *Motivation and personality.* New York: Harper and Row.

Marieb, E. N. 1989. *Human anatomy and physiology.* Redwood City, Ca.: Benjamin/Cummings.

Narrow, B. W. August 1967. Rest is . . . *American Journal of Nursing* 67:1646–49.

Roberts, A. March 14–20, 1990. Senior systems . . . older patients and their medication . . . sleep and sleep difficulties in later life, Part 46. *Nursing Times* 86:61–64.

Ross, M.; Hare, K.; and McPherson, M. October 1986. When sleep won't come: Helping our elderly clients. *Canadian Nurse* 82:14–18.

Walsleben, J. June 1982. Sleep disorders. *American Journal of Nursing* 82:936–40.

Weaver, T., and Millman, R. P. February 1986. Broken sleep. *American Journal of Nursing* 86:146–50.

Webster, R. A., and Thompson, D. R. July 1986. Sleep in hospital. *Journal of Advanced Nursing* 11:447–57.

Comfort and Pain

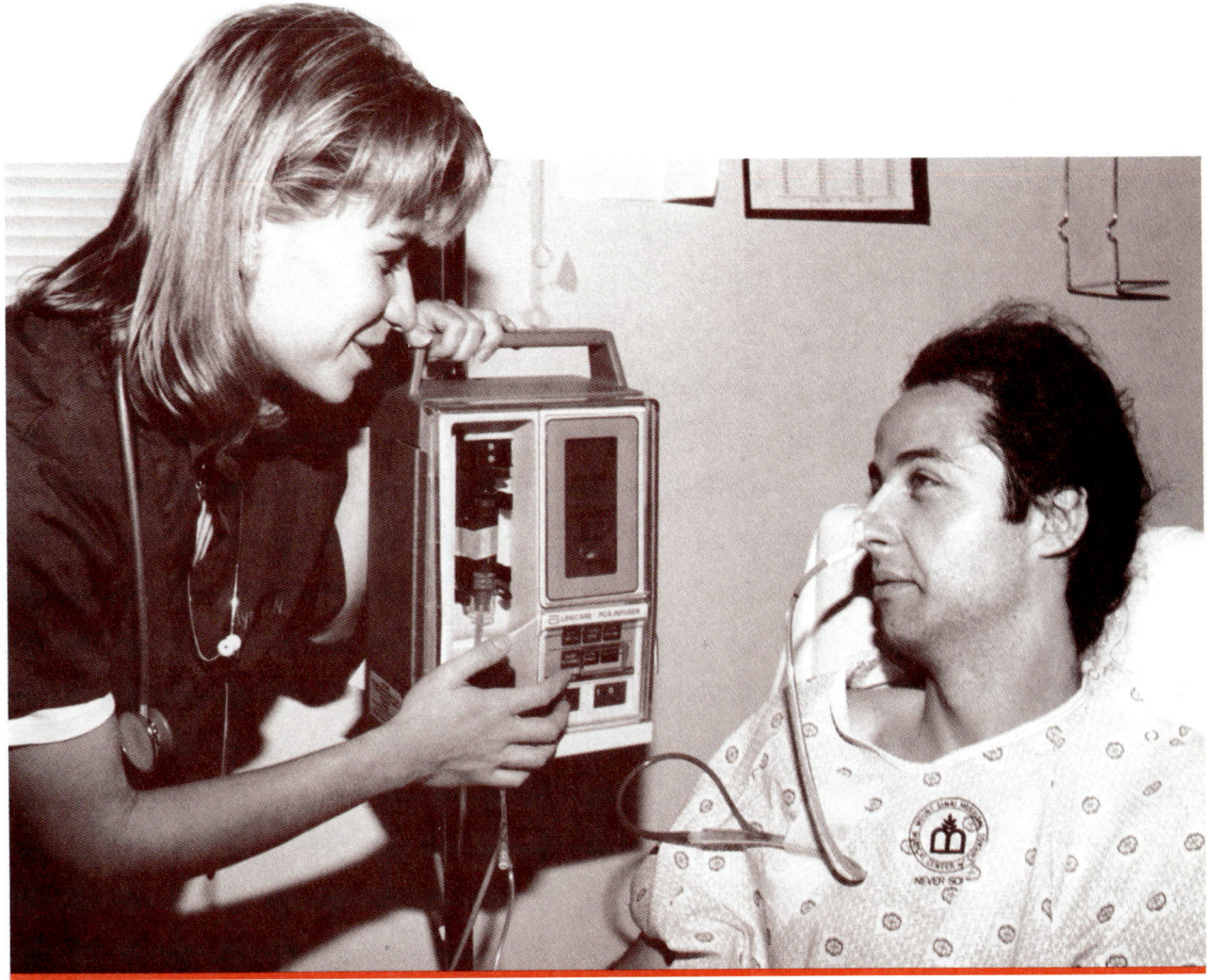

OBJECTIVES

▶ Identify various types of pain.

▶ Describe pain pathways to the brain.

▶ Identify physiologic manifestations of the response to pain.

OBJECTIVES *(continued)*

- Describe subjective and objective data to be collected and analyzed when assessing pain.
- Identify examples of possible nursing diagnoses for clients with pain.
- List ways of decreasing factors that amplify the pain experience.

- Explain methods used to reduce pain intensity.
- Identify situations in which relaxation techniques can relieve pain effectively.
- Describe selected skin stimulation techniques used to relieve pain.

- Identify methods used to control intractable pain.
- Describe selected medical interventions to control pain.
- State outcome criteria by which to evaluate a client's response to interventions for pain.

THE NATURE OF PAIN

Pain is a highly unpleasant and very personal sensation that cannot be shared with others. It can occupy all of one's thinking, direct one's activities, and change one's life. Pain often is an important sign that something is physiologically wrong, e.g., tissues are damaged. As such, pain is useful because it prompts the client to seek help for a health problem that might otherwise go unnoticed. Pain is usually accompanied by other bodily sensations, such as pressure, heat, or perhaps cold. Geach (1987, p. 12) defines pain as "the noxious stimulation of threatened or actual tissue damage."

McCaffery (1979, p. 11) defines pain as "whatever the experiencing person says it is, existing whenever he says it does." Basic to this definition is the caregiver's willingness to believe the client's pain. Cleeland, (1984, p. 2638) refers to the first and second levels of pain. First-level pain corresponds to Geach's description. Second-level pain in this definition incorporates how the individual thinks, feels, and acts in response to the stimulus.

TYPES OF PAIN

Pain can be described as either acute or chronic. **Acute pain** is intense and generally of relatively short duration (i.e., less than 6 months), such as the pain of a fracture or abdominal surgery. Clients may respond to acute pain by crying, moaning, or rubbing the painful area, although the absence of these behaviors does not mean a client is not experiencing pain. **Chronic pain** develops more slowly and lasts much longer than acute pain (more than 6 months). Sufferers may find it difficult to remember when such pain first started. Clients with chronic pain may present few if any clinical signs of pain. Some find a way to handle the pain or are so accustomed to it that their reaction is minimal. See Table 38–1 for differentiation of acute and chronic pain.

TABLE 38-1 *Common Differentiations of Acute and Chronic Pain**

Acute Pain	Chronic Pain
Localized	Diffuse
Sharp	Dull, aching
Sympathetic nervous system responses	Parasympathetic nervous system responses
Appears restless and anxious	Appears depressed and withdrawn
Well-defined onset pattern	Insidious onset pattern

*Acute pain lasts less than 6 months; chronic pain lasts more than 6 months.

Intractable pain is resistant to cure or relief. An example is the pain of arthritis, for which narcotic analgesics are contraindicated because of the long duration of the disease and the risk of addiction. Behavior modification is used in some cases of intractable pain. Behavior that is not pain-oriented is rewarded, and pain-oriented behavior is ignored. The aim of this technique is to change behavior so that the client can live more comfortably and productively.

Phantom pain is actual pain felt in a body part that is no longer present, such as an amputated foot. It can be distinguished from a **phantom sensation,** i.e., feeling that a missing body part is still present. Phantom pain is thought to result from stimulation of a severed dendrite rather than stimulation of the usual receptor. It occurs most frequently in clients who experienced pain before the removal of the body part, especially if that pain was dismissed as not significant.

Radiating pain is perceived at the source and extends to surrounding or nearby tissues. For example, cardiac pain may be felt radiating to the left shoulder and down the left arm, or the pain from an inflamed appendix may be felt throughout the abdomen.

There are two *physiologic sources* of pain, somatic and visceral. **Somatic pain** arises from the skin, muscles, or joints. It may be superficial or deep. *Superficial somatic pain* is often a sharp, prickling type of pain. It is usually readily localized and brief. It is transmitted along myelinated A delta nerve fibers. *Deep somatic pain* is most likely described as burning or aching. It is a result of stimulation of the pain receptors in the deeper skin layers, muscles, or joints. It is more diffuse than superficial somatic pain, lasts longer, and is transmitted along unmyelinated C nerve fibers (Marieb 1989, p. 468). It is possible to experience both types of pain as a result of a single trauma such as a severe burn. The individual first experiences a brief, severe, sharp pain followed by a burning pain that lasts much longer.

Visceral pain results from stimulation of pain receptors in the abdominal cavity and thorax. It is often accompanied by an autonomic nervous system response, e.g., sweating and accelerated pulse. Visceral pain tends to appear diffuse and often feels like deep somatic pain, i.e., burning, aching, or a feeling of pressure. Visceral pain is frequently caused by stretching of the tissues, ischemia, or muscle spasms. Visceral pain travels along the same nerve pathways and therefore may be perceived as somatic pain. This circumstance is called **referred pain.** For example, cardiac pain may radiate to the left shoulder and down the left arm, or the pain from an inflamed appendix may be felt throughout the abdomen. Figure 38–1 on page 960 shows the skin areas to which pain is commonly referred.

THE PAIN EXPERIENCE

The pain experience can be divided into three stages: reception, transmission/perception, and modulation.

Pain Reception

The skin and certain internal tissues such as the periosteum, the joint surfaces, and the arterial walls have many receptors, whereas most other deep tissues have few pain receptors. The alveoli of the lungs and the brain have no pain receptors.

A pain receptor, called a **nociceptor,** is stimulated either directly by damage to the receptor cell or secondarily by the release of chemicals such as bradykinin. Basically, there are three types of stimuli that excite corresponding types of nociceptors: mechanical, thermal, and chemical. See Table 38–2.

Recent research indicates that bradykinin is the universal pain stimulus. **Bradykinin** is an amino acid chain that causes powerful vasodilation and increased capillary permeability, constricts smooth muscle, and stimulates pain receptors. It is thought to be generated whenever there is tissue damage. Enzymes that release bradykinin from molecules present in the blood and tissues are activated at the site of injury. The bradykinin is also thought to bind to the pain receptor endings, thus causing them to produce pain impulses. In addition, bradykinin triggers the production of inflammatory chemicals such as histamine, which separates the cells in the capillary walls, permitting more fluid and leukocytes to move into the area. This movement causes the area to become reddened, swollen, and tender. Bradykinin also stimulates the release of prostaglandins. These are compounds derived from the breakdown of the fatty acid arachidonic acid; they sensitize the pain receptors and enhance the effects of bradykinin and histamine.

Although all nociceptors are structurally similar, they respond differently to noxious stimuli according to their body location. For example, a cutting injury in the skin causes acute pain, but a similar injury in the viscera does not. Similarly, moderate stretching produces visceral pain but not skin pain.

TABLE 38–2 *Types of Pain Stimuli*

Stimulus Type	Physiologic Basis
Mechanical	
1. Trauma to body tissues, e.g., surgery	Tissue damage; direct irritation of the pain receptors; inflammation
2. Alterations in body tissues, e.g., edema	Pressure on pain receptors
3. Blockage of a body duct	Distention of the lumen of the duct
4. Tumor	Pressure on pain receptors; irritation of nerve endings
5. Muscle spasm	Stimulation of pain receptors (also see *Chemical*)
Thermal	
Extreme heat or cold, e.g., burns	Tissue destruction; stimulation of thermosensitive pain receptors
Chemical	
1. Tissue ischemia, e.g., blocked coronary artery	Stimulation of pain receptors because of accumulated lactic acid (and possibly other chemicals, such as bradykinin) in tissues
2. Muscle spasm	Secondary to mechanical stimulation (see above), causing tissue ischemia

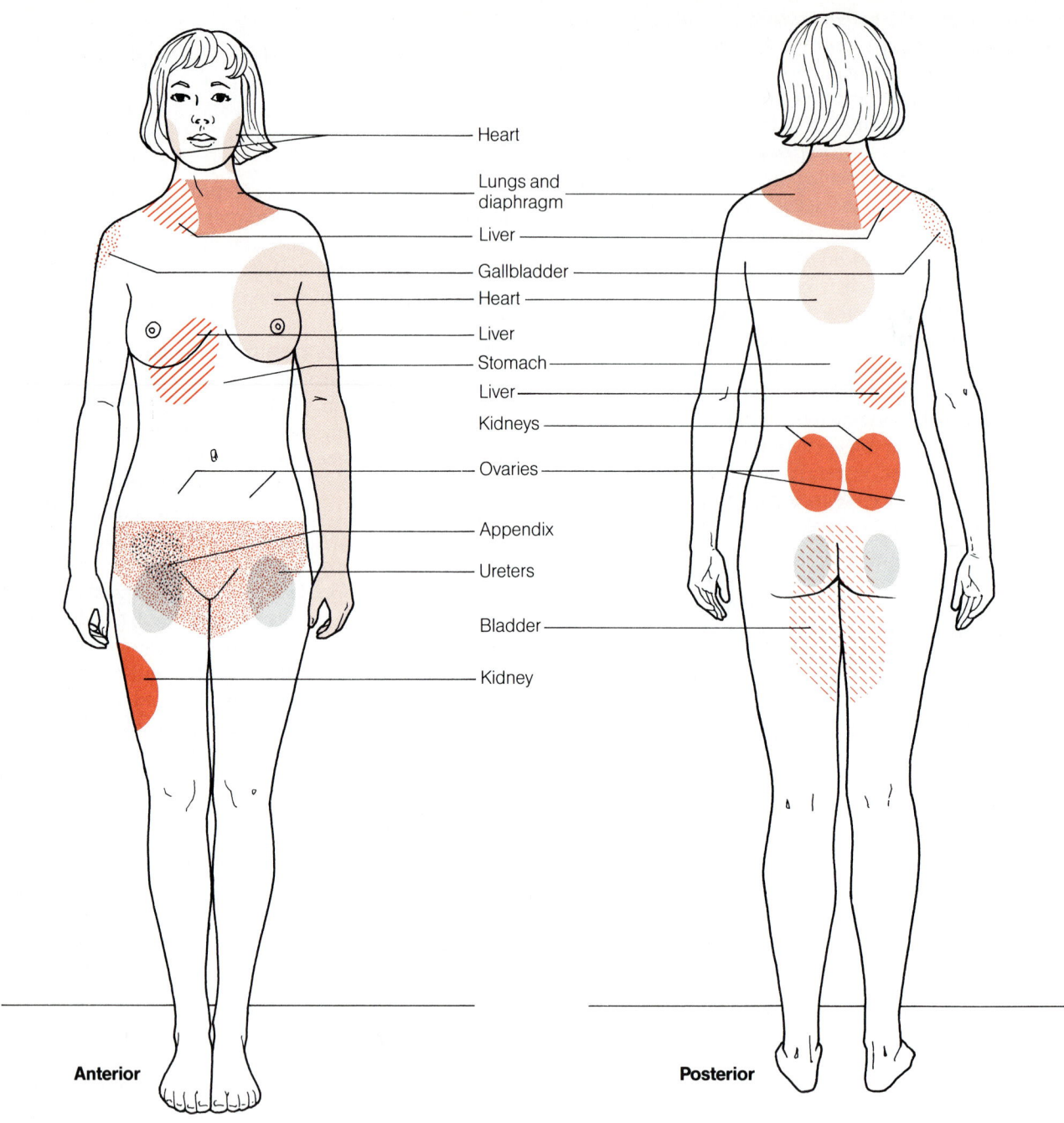

Heart
Lungs and diaphragm
Liver
Gallbladder
Heart
Liver
Stomach
Liver
Kidneys
Ovaries
Appendix
Ureters
Bladder
Kidney

Anterior

Posterior

Figure 38–1   Common referred pain sites from various body organs.

Pain does not necessarily result, however, when the nociceptors are stimulated. Pain occurs only when the pain message is relayed via the spinal cord to the brain, which then interprets the stimuli.

Transmission/Perception

An individual's **pain threshold** is the amount of pain stimulation a person requires before feeling pain. People's pain threshold is generally fairly uniform, although it can be dramatically altered by each person's state of consciousness. For instance, an anesthetized client feels no pain; an unconscious client may or may not react to suborbital pressure, that is, pain on the lower aspect of the eye. It is also possible for a person's pain threshold to change. For example, the same stimuli that once produced mild pain can produce intense pain. Such excessive sensitivity to pain is called **hyperalgesia**.

Two additional terms used in the context of pain are pain sensation and pain reaction. **Pain sensation** can be considered the same as pain threshold; **pain reaction** includes the autonomic nervous system and behavioral responses to pain. The autonomic nervous system response is the automatic reaction of the body that often protects the individual from further harm, for example, the automatic withdrawal of the hand from a hot stove. The behavioral response is a learned response used as a method of coping with the pain.

Pain tolerance is the maximum amount and duration of pain that an individual is willing to endure. Some clients are unable to tolerate even the slightest pain, whereas others are willing to endure severe pain rather than be treated for it. Thus, pain tolerance varies greatly among people and is widely influenced by psychologic and sociocultural factors. Pain tolerance appears to increase with age. Although the precise mechanism of pain transmission and perception is unknown, the following sequence of events is a widely accepted explanation. See also the discussion of pain theories in the next section.

Pain signals are transmitted along only two types of nerve fibers: myelinated type A fibers and unmyelinated type C fibers. Type A fibers are further subgrouped into alpha, beta, gamma, and delta fibers. The type A delta fibers conduct impulses quickly, from 12 to 80 meters per second (up to 250 feet per second). It is thought that they transmit sharp, prickling pain sensations associated with superficial somatic pain. Type C fibers, which are smaller in diameter, transmit signals more slowly, i.e. at a rate of 0.4 to 1 meter per second, or up to 3.5 feet per second. It is believed that they transmit dull, aching, and burning sensations of deep somatic and visceral pain. Pain transmitted by type C fibers is less localized but more persistent than that transmitted by Type A delta fibers.

Pain fibers enter the spinal cord through the dorsal horn (see Figure 38–2), where they synapse with second-order neurons. Transmission of pain impulses along the first-order neurons in the dorsal horn causes the release of **substance P,** a neurotransmitter that acts to enhance transmission of pain impulses into the synaptic cleft, across the synapse, and into the second-order nueron. It appears that axons of the second-order neurons then cross the spinal cord and enter the lateral spinothalmic tract, which ascends in the lateral area of the spinal cord's white matter to the thalamus in the brain. After reaching the thalamus, pain impulses travel to the somatosensory area in the cerebral cortex for interpretation. See Figure 38–3 on page 962.

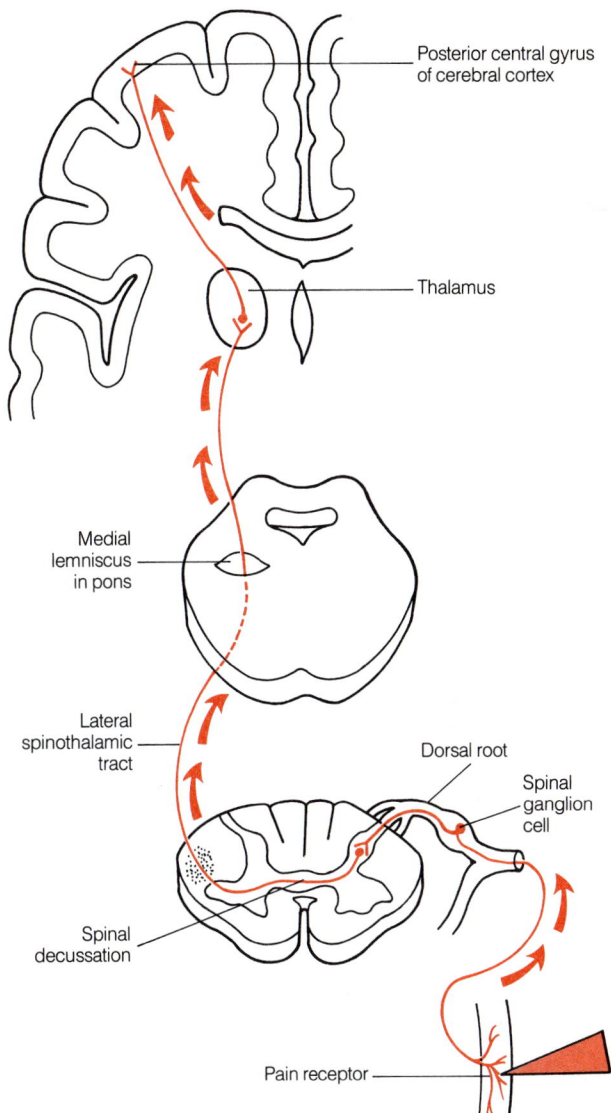

Figure 38–2 Acute pain pathway.

Because some second-order nerve fibers ascend directly to the ventrobasal nuclei in the thalamus, the sensory cortex is able to make a quick analysis of the pain location and intensity. Other fibers in the spinothalamic tract, however, make abundant synapses in the brain stem, hypothalamus, and limbic structures before reaching the thalamus. This slower pathway is believed to be involved in processes of mediating the pain and emotionally reacting to it. These two different pathways are associated with the two parallel subdivisions of the lateral spinothalamic tract: the neospinothalamic tract and the paleospinothalamic tract.

The *neospinothalamic tract* carries impulses transmitted initially by type A delta fibers to the ventrolateral and posterior portions of the thalamus. Because type A delta fibers are associated with quick transmission and sharp, well-localized pain, this tract permits quick perception of pain location and intensity and may trigger the fight-or-flight

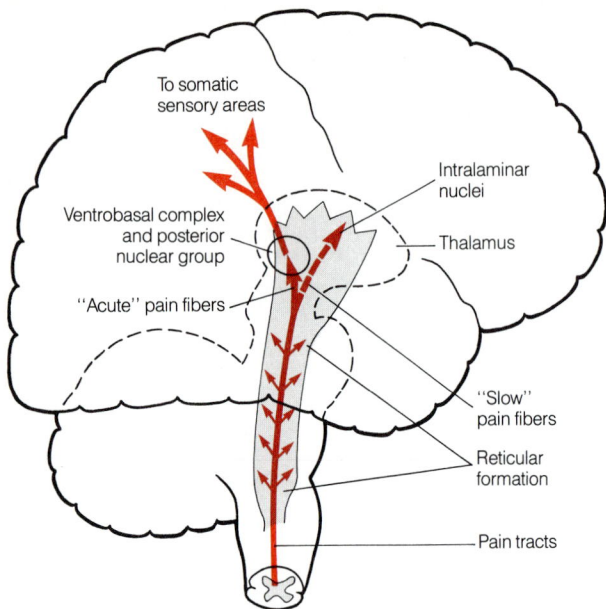

Figure 38–3 Transmission of pain signals to the higher brain centers.

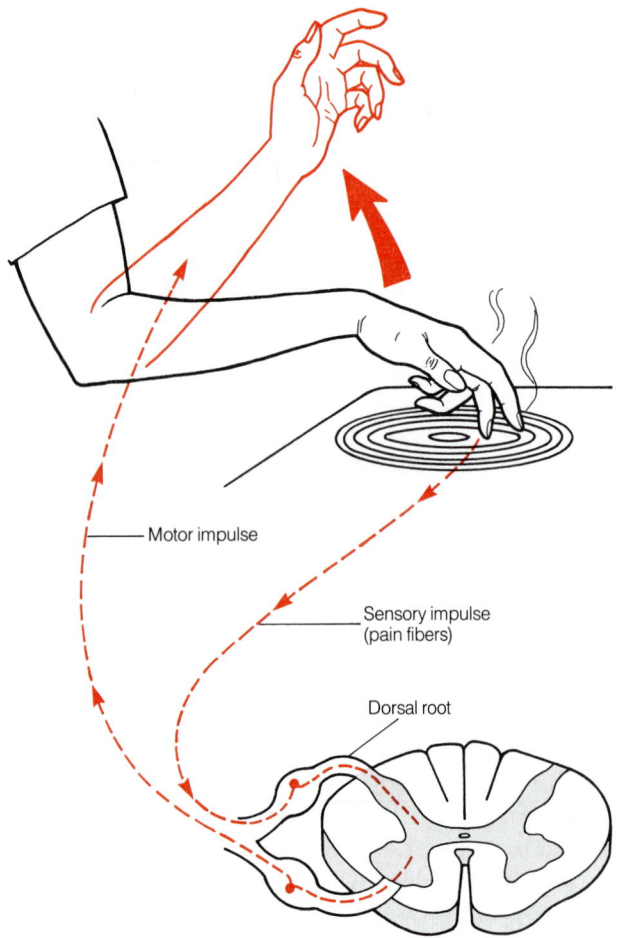

Figure 38–4 Proprioceptive pain reflex to a pain stimulus.

response. The *paleospinothalamic tract* transmits initial impulses from the type C fibers to various synaptic junctions such as the brain stem and hypothalamus before relaying them to the thalamus and sensory cortex. Because this tract transmits impulses more slowly, it is associated with aching, burning, dull, and poorly localized pain sensations. It may also be involved in emotional responses to pain, since it affects brain structures that control memory and recall (Nursing Now 1985, p. 13).

There is also a proprioceptive reflex that occurs with the stimulation of pain receptors. Impulses travel along sensory pain fibers to the spinal cord. There they synapse with motor neurons, and the impulses travel back via motor fibers to a muscle near the site of the pain. See Figure 38–4. The muscle then contracts in a protective action. For example, when a person touches a hot stove the hand reflexively draws back from the heat even before the person is aware of the pain.

Modulation

It appears that there are natural mechanisms within the body that modulate pain transmission and pain perception. **Endogenous opioids** are chemical regulators that may modify pain. They are thought to bind with opiate receptor sites throughout the body, particularly in the dorsal horn of the spinal cord, thereby inhibiting the production of substances that probably transmit pain impulses and that may also alter pain perception. Certain pain relief therapies, such as acupuncture, are thought to work by stimulating the release of endogenous opioids. Three groups of opioids have so far been identified: enkephalins, endorphins, and dynorphins.

Enkephalins   **Enkephalins** (meaning "in the head") are small polypeptides. They combine with opiate receptors in the dorsal horn of the spinal cord and apparently inhibit the release of substance P, defined earlier. Enkephalins are also found outside the spinal cord—in the brain stem, limbic system, hypothalamus, adrenal glands, and gastrointestinal tract. The two most prominent are leu-enkephalin and met-enkephalin.

Endorphins   **Endorphins** (meaning "morphine within") are larger polypeptides. They may be synthesized and stored by the pituitary gland. They are also found in the hypothalamus, midbrain, and limbic system of the central nervous system. There are several subgroups of endorphins, including beta-endorphins, which are highly concentrated in the hypothalamus and pituitary gland. The beta-endorphins have been found to be more potent than the enkephalins. It is suggested that they are increased with exercise (Whitaker and Warfield 1988, p. 160).

Dynorphins   **Dynorphins** only recently discovered, are compounds found in the pituitary gland, hypothalamus, and spinal cord. They seem to have an analgesic effect, one that is 50 times greater than that of the beta-endorphins.

PAIN THEORIES

A number of theories propose how pain is transmitted and perceived. Four of these are the specificity theory, the pattern theory, the gate-control theory, and the parallel processing model of pain.

Specificity Theory

The *specificity theory* originated about 200 years ago. This theory assumes that pain travels from a specific nociceptor to a pain center in the brain. Current knowledge sheds light on several limitations of this theory. Research has shown that the nerve fibers that carry pain impulses also carry pressure and temperature sensations (Nursing Now 1985, p. 16). Two other assumptions of this theory conflict with current research findings: it assumes a direct relationship between the intensity of the pain stimulus and the perceived intensity of pain; and it assumes that only one structure in the brain is involved in a pain response.

Pattern Theory

The *pattern theory,* which followed the specificity theory, includes several different theories, such as the peripheral pattern theory, the central summation theory, and the sensory interaction theory. The *peripheral pattern theory* assumes that peripheral nerve fibers are all essentially the same and that a given pattern of fiber stimulation is interpreted by the central nervous system as pain. The *central summation theory* focuses on the dorsal horn of the spinal cord. This theory proposes that stimulation of the peripheral sensory nerves in turn stimulates specific areas in the dorsal horn, which, when stimulated, are interpreted as pain. Input into the dorsal horn creates abnormal reverberatory activity in closed self-exciting neuron loops. Prolonged activity stimulates T cells, which then project impulses to the brain, where the pain is interpreted. This theory is helpful in explaining phantom limb pain and neuralgia. *Sensory interaction theory* proposes that there are two types of neurologic fibers involved in pain: small- and large-diameter fibers. The small fibers carry nerve impulse patterns that produce pain, and the large fibers inhibit the pain impulses. When the number of fibers that carry the pain impulses outnumber the inhibitory fibers, pain results.

Gate-Control Theory

In 1965, Melzack and Wall proposed the *gate-control theory* (Melzack and Wall 1982, p. 232). According to this theory, peripheral nerve fibers carrying pain to the spinal cord can have their input modified at the spinal cord level before transmission to the brain. Synapses in the dorsal horns act as gates that close to keep impulses from reaching the brain or open to permit impulses to ascend to the brain. Melzack and Wall further hypothesize that when there are a great number of impulses along the thick nerve fibers, which carry impulses of heat, cold, touch, and so on, the gates close to the pain impulses on the thinner fibers, thus blocking the pain. (Pain impulses are thought to travel along the thinner type A delta and type C fibers.) Only when the synaptic gates are open, as when impulses on the pain fibers predominate, does the person feel pain. This theory also suggests that "higher" central nervous system activities, such as anxiety, past experience, attention, and the meaning of the situation, can influence the opening or closing of the gate.

Parallel Processing Model

This model by Leventhal and Everhart (1979) integrates both the physiologic and cognitive-emotional aspects of pain. According to this theory, the physiologic or neurologic deciphering of the pain sensation and the cognitive-emotional properties of pain occur along *different* nerve fibers.

In this model, pain is thought to be processed at three levels. Level one involves autonomic neural coding of the pain stimulus along specific neural fibers. This process initiates awareness, meaning, and emotion relative to the pain stimulus and records the location, duration, and intensity of pain. Level two involves combining the neural encoding with past pain experience. As a result, the individual can add new data to the experience and adapt to it. Level three involves utilizing the individual's beliefs about pain that affect the person's needs and activities relative to the pain.

PAIN RESPONSES

The body's response to pain is a complex process rather than a specific action. The *pain response* can be studied by separating it into three stages: activation, rebound, and adaptation. The initial state, *activation,* begins with the perception of pain. The body assumes a fight-or-flight reaction, initiated by the sympathetic nervous system. See Table 38–3 and Chapter 33 for further information.

During the *rebound* stage, the pain experienced is intense but brief. It is at this stage that the parasympathetic nervous system takes over. Its effects, the opposite of the sympathetic system's, include decreased cardiac rate and decreased blood pressure. When pain is long-lasting, the physiologic response is *adaptation,* i.e., a decreased sympathetic response. Adaptation may be due to endorphins counteracting the pain. The body experiences a general adaptive reaction when the pain lasts for many hours or days. See

TABLE 38–3 *Responses to Pain*

Sympathoadrenal Responses	Parasympathetic Responses	Behavioral Responses	Affective (Feeling) Responses
Increased pulse rate	Decreased pulse rate	Immobility	Fear/fright
Increased systolic blood pressure	Decreased systolic blood pressure; syncope	Withdrawal	Anxiety
Increased respiratory rate		Rubbing body part	Depression
Diaphoresis	Nausea/vomiting	Grimacing	Anger
Increased muscle tension	Warm, dry skin	Restlessness	Hopelessness
Pallor	Prostration	Writhing	Powerlessness
Pupil dilation	Pupil constriction	Unusual postures	Fatigue/exhaustion
Rapid speech/elevated pitch	Slow, monotonous speech	Extreme quietness (stoicism)	Feeling of being punished
Increased alertness	Withdrawal	Groaning	
		Crying	

the section on the general adaptation syndrome, Chapter 33, for current concepts of physiologic reactions to stress.

Geach points out that the coping mechanisms used in response to pain may be more active, willed processes than adaptation and, therefore, may be a more appropriate view of an individual's response to pain. In this instance, coping consists of managing the situation without being overwhelmed by it (Geach 1987, p. 13). See also the discussion of coping resources, later in this chapter.

According to Kotarba (1983, p. 687), people with chronic pain either "give up" or "fight back." Those who give up tend to have limited resources and feel helpless and hopeless. People who fight back require encouragement and need strong cognitive resources in the form of a strong belief system.

FACTORS AFFECTING THE PAIN EXPERIENCE

Numerous factors can affect a person's perception and reaction to pain. These include the ethnic/cultural values, environment, emotions, expectations/presence of others, past experience, and age.

Ethnic/Cultural Values In many cultures based on the Judeo-Christian ethic, pain may be considered a punishment for bad deeds; the individual is, therefore, to tolerate without complaint in order to atone for sins. In some Middle Eastern and African cultures, self-infliction of pain is a sign of mourning or grief. In other groups, pain may be anticipated as a part of the ritualistic practices of passage ceremonies, and therefore tolerance of pain signifies strength and endurance. The meaning of pain will affect the individual's perception of pain, tolerance of painful stimuli, and the expression of or reaction to pain.

Chapman and Jones (1944), Zborowski (1952, 1969), Weisenberg (1975), and Flannery (1981) have studied the perception and manifestations of pain in different cultural groups. Responses to pain range from stoic denial or objective reporting to social withdrawal to emotional expressions of crying, screaming, writhing, and complaining. Individuals of some groups want to endure their pain privately, whereas others of different groups want the sympathy and support of family members, loved ones, and caregivers.

Environment An individual's environment affects pain perception and response. For instance, the woman entertaining coworkers at home may have decreased perceptions and responses to her pain while the guests are present; but later she may perceive the pain as more severe and respond more openly.

Emotions Emotions influence the perception of pain. Think of individuals so absorbed in playing football that they are unaware of the pain of an injury until after the game is over. By contrast, people who are bored or depressed are more likely to think about their pain and be more aware of it. Also, a highly anxious client is more likely to have a heightened perception of pain, and a less anxious person will tolerate pain more effectively.

Expectations/Presence of Others Expectations of significant others can affect a person's perceptions of and responses to pain. In some situations, for example, girls may be permitted to express pain more openly than boys. Family role can also affect how a person perceives or responds to pain. For instance, a single mother supporting three children may ignore pain because of her need to stay on the job. The presence of support persons often changes a client's reaction to pain. For example, toddlers often tolerate pain more readily when supportive parents or nurses are nearby.

Age Age also affects an individual's perception of pain. Hurley and Whelan relate children's cognitive development to their perception of pain. Using Piaget's stages as a frame of reference, they found that as children develop, their perceptions of the nature and experience of pain change (Hurley and Whelan 1988, p. 24). See Table 38–4.

ASSESSING

To assess a client's pain, the nurse obtains a pain history and conducts a physical examination that focuses on the client's physiologic and behavioral responses to the pain.

Pain History

Data that should be obtained in a pain history include pain location, intensity, quality, patterns, precipitating factors, alleviating factors, associated symptoms, effect on activities of daily living, past pain experiences, meaning of the pain to the person, coping resources, and affective responses. Questions to elicit this data are shown in the accompanying box.

While taking the pain histories, the nurse must provide an opportunity for clients to express in their own words how they view the pain and the situation. This will help the nurse understand what the pain means to the client and how the client is coping with it. Remember that each person's pain experience is unique and that the client is the best interpreter of the pain experience. This history should be geared to the specific client: for example, questions asked of an accident victim would be different from those asked of a postoperative client or one suffering from chronic pain.

Location Superficial pain usually can be located quite accurately by a client; however, pain arising from the viscera is perceived more generally. Nurses need to ascertain where the client experiences pain. The various body landmarks for describing abdominal pain location are shown in Chapter 19, page 417. In addition, the nurse needs to use such

ASSESSMENT INTERVIEW
Pain History

- *Location:* Where is your pain?
- *Intensity:* On a scale of one to ten (with one representing the least pain level), how would you rate the degree of discomfort you are having?
- *Quality:* Tell me what your pain feels like.
- *Pattern:*
  Time of onset: When did or does the pain start?
  Duration: How long have you had it or how long does it usually last?
  Constancy: Do you have pain-free periods? When? And for how long?
- *Precipitating factors:* What triggers the pain or makes it worse?
- *Alleviating factors:* What measures or methods have you found helpful in lessening or relieving the pain? What pain medications do you use?
- *Associated symptoms:* Do you have any other symptoms (e.g., nausea, dizziness, blurred vision, shortness of breath) before, during, or after your pain?
- *Effects on activities of daily living:* How does the pain affect your daily life (e.g., eating, working, sleeping, social/recreational activities)?
- *Past pain experiences:* Tell me about past pain experiences you have had and the effectiveness of pain relief measures.
- *Meaning of pain:* How do you interpret your pain? What outcomes (implications) do you anticipate from this pain? What do you fear most about your pain?
- *Coping resources:* What do you usually do to help cope with pain?
- *Affective response:* How does the pain make you feel? Anxious? Depressed? Frightened? Tired? Burdensome?

TABLE 38–4 *Cognitive Development, Response to Pain, and Nursing Interventions*

Developmental Stage (Piaget)	Pain Perception	Nursing Inteventions
Preoperational (2–7 years)	• Relates pain mainly as a physical experience • Tends to hold someone accountable • Feels sad • May consider pain a punishment	• Explore misconceptions about pain. Provide verbal reassurance. Hold the child to provide comfort. Provide play therapy with equipment e.g., syringe and doll or stuffed animal
Concrete-operational (7–12 years)	• Relates pain physically • Can specify location • Fears of harm and even death	• Provide support and nurturing. Teach ways to control pain. Teach significance of pain.

TABLE 38—4 (continued)

Developmental Stage (Piaget)	Pain Perception	Nursing Inteventions
Transitional-formal (10–12 years)	• May exhibit anxiety • May pretend comfort to appear brave	• Teach, using reasons such as "Keep your foot on the chair to have less pain and swelling." • Clarify exactly whether there is pain. Clarify any misunderstandings about suffering and denying pain.
Formal-operational (12 + years)	• May be embarassed about discussing pain • Is developing problem-solving skills	• Provide opportunities to discuss pain. Provide privacy. Present choices for dealing with pain.

Sources: J. Piaget, *Origins of intelligence in children* International Universities Press © 1966; A. Hurley and E. G. Whelan, Cognitive development and children's perception of pain, *Pediatric Nursing* January/February 1988, 14:21–24.

terms as *proximal, distal, medial,* and *lateral* when describing the location of pain. See Chapter 35. The term *diffuse pain* refers to pain perceived over a large area.

When assessing the location of a child's pain, the nurse needs to understand the child's vocabulary. For example, *tummy* might refer to the abdomen or part of the chest. It is wise for a nurse to ask a child to point to the pain rather than to rely on the child's description, which may be highly idiosyncratic. Parents can help nurses interpret the meaning of a child's words. Observing when a smaller child or baby cries in response to movement can help the nurse establish the location of a baby's pain.

Intensity   Although the intensity or severity of pain is subjective, it is also true that certain tissues are more sensitive than others. Several factors affect the perception of intensity. One is amount of distraction, or the client's concentration on another event; a second is the client's state of consciousness, and a third is the person's expectations.

Pain may be described as slight, mild, medium, severe, or excruciating. Two simple descriptive scales are shown in Figure 38–5. The client is asked to indicate the scale point that best represents the client's pain intensity. It is very important to note and report any change in intensity. For example, the abrupt cessation of acute abdominal pain may indicate a ruptured appendix.

A client's report of pain must be considered in relation to the client's ability and need to report. The elderly or confused client may distort the intensity of pain; a child may minimize pain to avoid unpleasant tests. The pain ruler shown in Figure 38–6 is designed to assist clients in describing the intensity of their pain.

Pain assessment tools to help nurses assess pain intensity are in the process of being developed. Gaston-Johansson and Asklund-Gustafsson's study to determine whether clients, nurses, and nursing students use the same word descriptions to describe painlike experiences is one example of the research being conducted to develop such a tool. Their findings confirm that clients, nurses, and students do agree on the differences in intensity among the words pain, ache, and hurt, since most used the same sensory and affective word descriptions to represent these concepts. See Table 38–5.

Quality   Descriptive adjectives help people communicate the quality of pain. A headache may be described as "hammerlike" or an abdominal pain as "piercing like a knife." Sometimes clients have difficulty describing pain because they have never experienced any sensation like it. This is particularly true of children, and of adults who have pain originating within the nervous system. Some of the terms used to describe pain are listed in the accompanying box.

Nurses need to record the exact words clients use to describe pain. A client's words are more accurate and descriptive than an interpretation in the nurse's words.

Pattern   The pattern of pain includes time of onset, duration, and persistence of or intervals without pain. The nurse therefore determines when the pain began; how long the pain lasts; whether it recurs and, if so, the length of the interval without pain; and when the pain last occurred.

The interval between pains can be very important. For example, the intervals between labor contractions help the maternity nurse assess the client's progress in labor. As birth becomes more imminent, labor pains become more frequent and more severe.

Two simple descriptive pain-intensity scales

0	1	2	3	4	5	6	7	8	9
No pain				Moderate pain				Severe pain	

No pain	Mild pain	Moderate pain	Severe pain	Unbearable pain

Figure 38–5   Two descriptive pain intensity scales.

TABLE 38-5 *Sensory and Affective Descriptors Which Discriminate Pain, Ache and Hurt from Each Other or at Least Two of These Concepts from the Other (54 Nursing Students)*

	Descriptors	
Concepts	**Sensory**	**Affective**
Pain	Crushing Sharp Tearing Cutting	Dreadful Torturing Killing
Pain and ache	Penetrating	Unbearable Terrifying Suffocating Exhausting
Ache	Gnawing Dull/aching Pulling	Unhappy
Ache and hurt	Grinding	Troublesome Annoying Irritating
Hurt	Sore Stinging Pricking Pinching	Fearful

Source: F. Gaston-Johansson and M. Asklund-Gustafsson. A baseline study for the development of an instrument for the assessment of pain, *Journal of Advanced Nursing* November 1985, 10:543. Used with permission from Blackwell Scientific Publications Limited.

Terms That Describe Pain Quality

- Aching
- Burning
- Constant
- Cramping
- Crushing
- Cutting
- Diffuse
- Dull
- Excruciating
- Gnawing
- Hammering
- Heavy
- Intermittent (spasmodic)
- Irritating
- Jabbing
- Knifelike
- Knotting
- Lancing
- Piercing
- Pinching
- Pounding
- Prickly
- Radiating
- Searing
- Sharp
- Shifting
- Squeezing
- Stabbing
- Tearing
- Throbbing
- Tingling
- Viselike

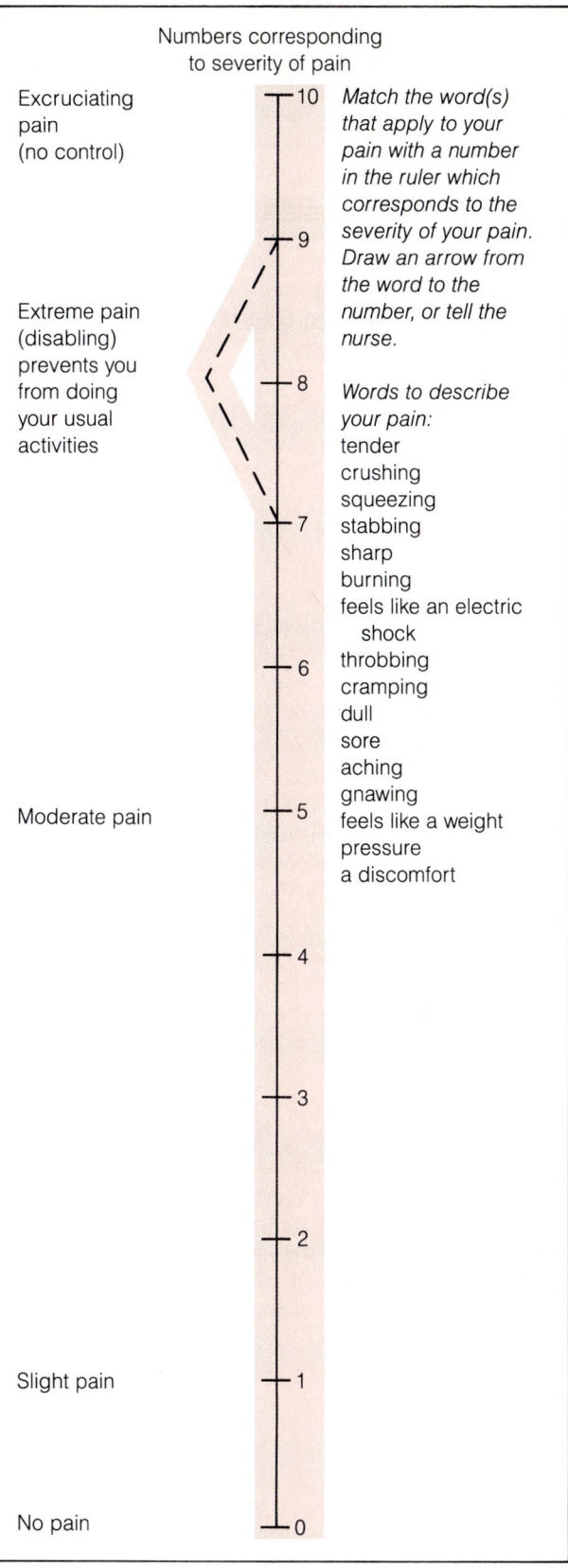

Numbers corresponding to severity of pain

Excruciating pain (no control) — 10

9

Extreme pain (disabling) prevents you from doing your usual activities — 8

7

6

Moderate pain — 5

4

3

2

Slight pain — 1

No pain — 0

Match the word(s) that apply to your pain with a number in the ruler which corresponds to the severity of your pain. Draw an arrow from the word to the number, or tell the nurse.

Words to describe your pain:
tender
crushing
squeezing
stabbing
sharp
burning
feels like an electric shock
throbbing
cramping
dull
sore
aching
gnawing
feels like a weight
pressure
a discomfort

Figure 38-6 The pain ruler. Clients match the words that describe their pain to a number that corresponds to the intensity of their pain. ***Source:*** F. Bourbonnais, Pain assessment: Development of a tool for the nurse and the patient, *Journal of Advanced Nursing* 1981, 6:280. Reprinted with permission of Blackwell Scientific Publications Ltd.

Precipitating Factors Certain activities sometimes precede pain; for example, physical exertion may precede chest pain, or abdominal pain may occur after eating. These observations can help prevent pain and determine its cause.

Environmental factors can increase pain in those who are well or ill. Extreme cold or heat and extremes of humidity can affect some types of pain. For example, sudden exercise on a hot day can cause muscle spasm.

Physical and emotional stressors can precipitate pain. Emotional tension frequently brings on a migraine headache. Intense fear or physical exertion can cause angina.

Alleviating Factors Included in this area of assessment are analgesics taken, rest, and applications of heat or cold. The nurse should also explore how long such measures were employed before relief was obtained and whether they had any effect at all or even made the pain worse.

Associated Symptoms Also included in the clinical appraisal of pain are any other associated symptoms, such as vomiting, dizziness, and constipation. Sometimes clients experience such a symptom immediately prior to the pain.

Effect on Activities of Daily Living Knowing how activities of daily living are affected by the pain helps the nurse understand the client's perspective on the pain's severity. A number of tools have been developed to assist the nurse with this assessment, including a scale measuring the effects of pain on daily life. See Table 38–6.

Past Pain Experiences Previous pain experiences alter a client's sensitivity to pain. People who have personally experienced pain or who have been exposed to the suffering of someone close are often more threatened by anticipated pain than people without a pain experience. In addition, the success or lack of success of pain relief measures influence a person's expectations for relief. For example, a person who has tried several pain relief measures without success may have little hope about the helpfulness of nursing interventions.

Meaning of Pain Some clients may accept pain more readily than others, depending on the circumstances and the client's interpretation of its significance. A client who associates the pain with a positive outcome may withstand the pain amazingly well. For example, a woman giving birth to a child or an athlete undergoing knee surgery to prolong his career may tolerate pain better because of the benefit associated with it. These clients may view the pain as a temporary inconvenience rather than a potential threat or disruption to daily life.

By contrast, clients with unrelenting chronic pain may suffer more intensely. They may respond with despair, anxiety, and depression, since they cannot attach a positive significance or purpose to the pain. In this situation, the pain may be looked upon as a threat to body image or lifestyle and as a sign of possible impending death.

Coping Resources Clients sometimes learn highly effective ways of coping with pain. These methods may modify the pain to such a degree that assessment of pain will be incomplete unless the nurse is aware of them. For example, Mr. Green may tell the nurse that his abdominal pain lasted only a few minutes and neglect to say that he took an antacid when the pain started.

People in pain often display coping strategies and styles learned in childhood. Although assessment of coping strategies does not help the nurse assess the client's pain, it does lead to an understanding of the person in pain.

Copp (1955, p. 69) sees a relationship between different types of copers, their self-image, and the way each type copes with pain. Copp classifies the self-image of a coper as victim, combatant, responder, reactor, or interactor. For example, clients who perceive the pain as all-powerful see themselves as victims. See Table 38–7 for corresponding descriptions of pain to the five self-image categories.

Affective Responses Affective responses vary according to the situation, the degree and duration of pain, the interpretation of it, and many other factors. The nurse needs to explore the client's feelings, e.g., anxiety, fear, exhaustion, depression, and a sense of failure. Because many people with chronic pain become depressed and potentially suicidal, it may also be necessary to assess the client's suicide risk. In such situations, the nurse needs to ask the client, "Do you ever feel so bad that you want to die? Do you feel that way now?" (Nursing Now 1985, p. 31).

TABLE 38–6 *Scale for Assessing the Effects of Pain on Daily Life*

On a scale of 0 (no pain) to 5 (maximum pain) the client should indicate the areas of life (listed below) currently affected and the severity of the interference. If the client's current level of pain is less than that usually felt, the client should be asked to rate the most pain ever experienced in these areas.

Sleep	Home activities
Appetite	Driving/walking
Concentration	Leisure activities
Work/school	Emotional status (mood, irritability, depression, anxiety)
Interpersonal relationships	
Marital relations/sex	

Source: E. Matassarin-Jacobs PhD, RN, OCN, unpublished presentation, "Pain Assessment," Chicago, Illinois, May 1981. Used by permission. As cited in Bellack, J. P., Bamford, P. A. 1984. *Nursing assessment: A multidimensional approach.* Monterey, Calif.: Wadsworth Health Sciences, p. 338.

TABLE 38-7 *Pain Perception and Coping Image and Methods*

Perception of the Pain	Categories of Coping (Self-image)	Coping Methods
Powerful	Victim (passive)	Skeptical of help
Invading	Combatant	Insistent on help
Reality	Responder	Withdraws from help to find own meaning
Cunning	Reactor	Expects vigilance from self and others
Demanding	Interactor	Creates rules for everyone

Adopted from Laurel Archer Copp PhD, University of North Carolina at Chapel Hill, Pain coping model and typology, *Image: Journal of Nursing Scholarship*, Summer 1985, 17:69–71. Used with permission.

The McGill-Melzack Pain Questionnaire Some pain centers ask clients to complete a pain questionnaire. The McGill-Melzack Pain Questionnaire shown in Figure 38-7 incorporates 20 categories of pain descriptors grouped into (a) sensory components, (b) affective components, (c) one evaluative component, and (d) miscellaneous terms. In addition, a present pain intensity (PPI) rating scale of 0 to 5 enables clients to indicate the degree of pain they experience. The anterior and posterior figures of the human body allow the client to mark the location of the pain.

RESEARCH NOTE

Does the Nurse's Personal Pain Experience Affect the Assessment of a Client's Pain?

Nurses must recognize factors that influence pain assessments because they must objectively determine the degree of pain and distress of a client before selecting appropriate nursing interventions. In this study, 135 registered nurses answered a personal pain history questionnaire and the Davitz and Davitz (1981) Standard Measure of Inferences of Suffering Questionnaire. The latter questionnaire investigates the nurse's perception of physical pain and psychologic distress. A major finding of this study was that the assessment of a patient's pain was significantly influenced by the intensity of a nurse's personal pain experience. Other variables, such as age, race, or sex of the patient, had little impact on pain assessment. It appears that nurses who have experienced intense pain are generally more sympathetic to the patient in pain.

Implications: Nurses need to be aware of their own personal biases in relation to assessing and helping clients in pain.

K. Holm, F. Cohen, S. Dudas, P. G. Medema, and B. L. Allen. Effect of personal pain experience on pain assessment, *Image: Journal of Nursing Scholarship*, Summer 1989, 21:72–75.

Physical Examination

To determine the client's physiologic and behavioral responses to pain, the nurse assesses the client's vital signs and observes the client for skin color changes, skin dryness, diaphoresis, facial expression, and body gestures that reflect pain, discomfort, or anxiety. These findings provide valuable information about the severity of pain and how the client is coping with it.

Physiologic Responses Physiologic responses vary according to whether the pain is acute or chronic. Acute pain stimulates the sympathetic nervous system, resulting in increased blood pressure, pulse rate, respiratory rate, pallor, diaphoresis, and pupil dilation. With prolonged severe chronic pain or visceral pain, signs of parasympathetic stimulation may be observed: lowered blood pressure, lower pulse rate, pupil constriction, and warm, dry skin.

Behavioral Responses The very young, the aphasic, and confused or disoriented persons often communicate their experience of pain only nonverbally. Facial expression is often the first indication of pain and may be the only one. Clenched teeth, tightly shut eyes, open somber eyes, biting of the lower lip, and other facial grimaces are indicative of pain.

Immobilization of the body or a part of the body may also indicate pain. The client with chest pain often holds the left arm across the chest. A person with abdominal pain may assume the position of greatest comfort, often with the knees and hips flexed, and moves reluctantly.

Purposeless body movements can also indicate pain—for example, tossing and turning in bed or flinging the arms about. Involuntary movements such as a reflexive jerking away from a needle inserted through the skin indicate pain. An adult may be able to control this reflex; however, a child may be unable or unwilling to do so.

Rhythmic body movements or rubbing may indicate pain. An adult or child may assume a fetal position and rock back and forth when experiencing abdominal pain. During labor a woman may massage her abdomen rhythmically with her hands.

Figure 38–7 *A,* McGill Pain Questionnaire. The descriptors fall into four major groups: *sensory*, 1 to 10; *affective*, 11 to 15; *evaluative*, 16; and *miscellaneous*, 17 to 20. The rank value of each descriptor is based on its position in the word set. The sum of the rank values is the pain rating index (PRI). The present pain intensity (PPI) is based on a scale of 0 to 5. *B,* Spatial display of pain descriptors based on intensity ratings by clients. The intensity scale values range from 1 (mild) to 5 (excruciating). *Source:* *A* and *B* reprinted with permission from R. Melzack, *Pain measurement and assessment* (New York: Raven, 1983).

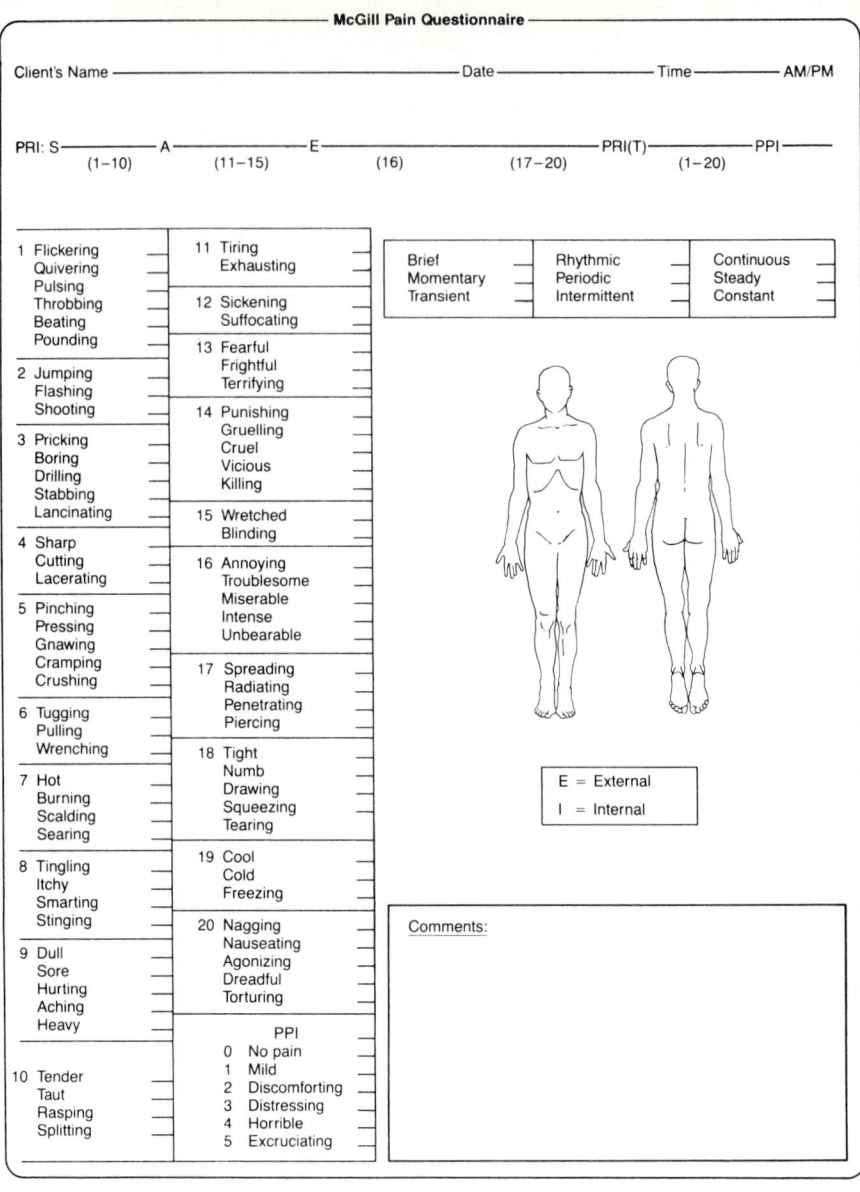

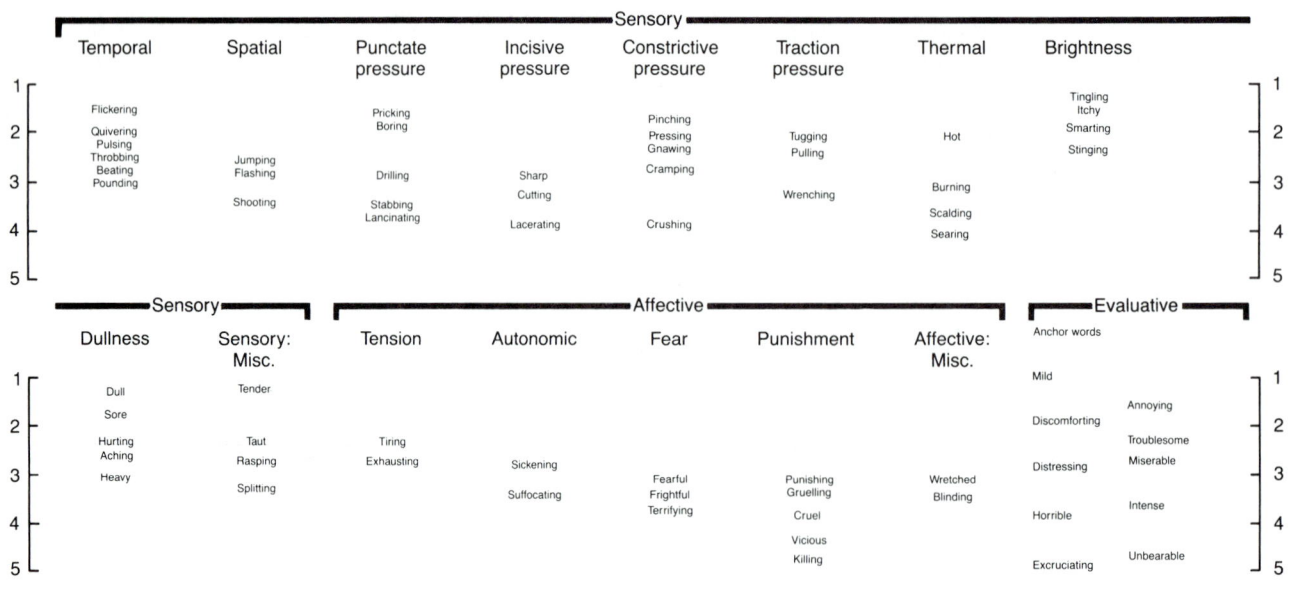

Speech and vocal pitch can help the nurse assess pain. Rapid speech and elevated pitch reflect anxiety, and slow speech and monotonous tone can signal intense pain.

DIAGNOSING

The nursing diagnoses given to clients experiencing pain are **Pain** (implying acute pain), and **Chronic pain**. When writing the diagnostic statement, the nurse may further specify the type or location of the pain (e.g., postoperative, chest, abdominal, back). Etiologic factors, when known, must be part of the diagnostic statement. These include the biologic, chemical, physical, or physiologic injuring agent. Biologic agents refer to disease, inflammation, and ischemia. Chemical agents include noxious agents, cytotoxic agents, electrolyte imbalance, and endocrine dysfunction. Physical agents refer to trauma and temperature extremes. Psychologic agents include anxiety, distress, fear, stress, and tension. Many other factors may contribute to **Chronic pain**. See contributing factors listed with the nursing diagnoses below.

Because the pain experience affects so many facets of human functioning, **Pain** itself may be the etiology of other nursing diagnoses. Example of such nursing diagnoses are also shown below. Examples of assessment data clusters and related nursing diagnoses are shown in Table 38–8.

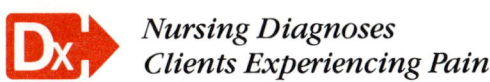

Nursing Diagnoses
Clients Experiencing Pain

Pain related to:

- Emotional stress
- Overactivity
- Ineffective pain management strategies

Chronic pain related to:

- Fear of addiction from prescribed drugs
- Knowledge deficit about pain control measures
- Disbelief of others that pain exists
- Fatigue
- Monotony
- Past experiences of poor pain control
- Feelings of hopelessness associated with the belief that the medication will gradually lose its effectiveness

Ineffective airway clearance related to postoperative incisional chest pain

Anxiety related to past experiences of poor control of pain and to anticipation of pain

---

TABLE 38–8 Examples of Assessment Data Clusters and Related Nursing Diagnoses

Data Cluster	Nursing Diagnoses
Mr. Rodriguez Sanchez, a 73-year-old widower, has joint stiffness, swelling, and tenderness of the feet, knees, and hips. States pain gets worse when he walks to do his shopping and works in the garden all day. Weight is 25% above norm for height. States he eats mostly fried foods.	**Chronic pain** related to overactivity, and excess weight secondary to rheumatoid arthritis
Mrs. Rene Laurent, a frail 84-year-old, has osteoporosis and kidney disease. She rates her hip and back pain as an 8 on a scale of 0 (least intense) to 10. Is unable to sleep at night. Has tried various analgesics (prescribed and over-the-counter drugs) but because of kidney disease is unable to tolerate side effects (dizziness and nausea).	**Chronic pain** related to fatigue, and ineffective pain management strategies secondary to osteoporosis
Mrs. Maria Domingo was diagnosed with breast cancer 3 years ago and had a metastatic lung tumor removed 4 months ago. Describes prolonged post thoracotomy pain as "unbearable." Sister says that although Maria loves sewing and needlepoint, Maria states she is too ill to perform previous hobbies.	**Chronic pain** related to fear of outcome, and inadequate coping method secondary to metastatic cancer
Mrs. Robin Wilson is the mother of 2 children recently separated from her husband. Works as bank clerk full time. Is worried about her finances and the responsibilities of her children. "Pounding" frontal headaches occur in the late afternoon and evening. At interview, held the palm of her hand across her forehead. Brow is furrowed and facial muscles tense.	**Pain**: recurrent headaches related to emotional stress

Ineffective breathing pattern related to postoperative abdominal pain

Ineffective individual coping related to prolonged continuous back pain, ineffective pain management, and inadequate support systems

Fear related to anticipated pain after surgery

Altered health maintenance related to chronic pain and fatigue

Hopelessness related to ineffective pain management strategies

Knowledge deficit about pain control measures related to lack of exposure to information resources

Impaired physical mobility related to arthritic pain in knee and ankle joints

Self care deficit: Bathing/hygiene, dressing/grooming, toileting related to pain in the joints

Sleep pattern disturbance related to increased pain perception at night

PLANNING

The nurse identifies nursing interventions that will assist the client in achieving the overall client goals of preventing, modifying, or eliminating pain so that the client is able partially or completely to resume usual daily activities and be able to cope more effectively with the pain experience. Examples of outcome criteria to evaluate the achievement of client goals and the effectiveness of nursing interventions are shown below.

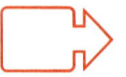

Outcome Criteria
Clients Experiencing Pain

The client:

- Verbalizes increased control over pain or increased feelings of comfort.
- Verbalizes reduction in fatigue.
- Identifies effective and ineffective pain strategies.
- Is free of nonverbal signs of pain (e.g., guarding, protective behavior).
- Resumes prepain activities.
- Modifies activities according to limitations inflicted by the pain experience.
- Resumes normal sleep pattern.
- Uses noninvasive pain control strategy to reduce anxiety (or depression) or to manage the pain.

- Develops effective coping strategy.
- Carries out deep-breathing exercises, coughs, and ambulates without severe pain postoperatively.

Scheduling measures to *prevent* pain is far more supportive of the client than trying to deal with pain when the client perceives it. Many postoperative clients need regularly administered analgesics as well as other nursing measures. In this way, the client's pain is anticipated and avoided, and recovery is often hastened.

When planning, nurses need to choose pain relief measures appropriate for the client. Nursing interventions may include one or more of the following strategies for either acute or chronic pain: exploring strategies that have been helpful in the past; helping the client identify activities that may augment or precipitate the pain; instructing the client about noninvasive strategies to reduce pain; helping the client identify measures to implement life-style modifications; using distraction, counterstimulation (pressure, massage, heat/cold), imagery, therapeutic touch, and relaxation techniques; immobilizing and resting a body part; and administering medication ordered by the physician.

IMPLEMENTING

Nursing management of pain consists of both independent and collaborative nursing actions. In general, noninvasive measures may be performed as an independent nursing function, whereas administration of analgesic medications requires a physician's order. However, the decision to administer the prescribed medication is frequently the nurse's, often requiring judgment as to the dose to be given and the time of administration.

Generally speaking, a combination of strategies is best for the client in pain. Sometimes strategies need to be tried and changed until the client obtains effective pain relief. See the accompanying box for individualizing care for clients with pain.

General Strategies for Pain

Acknowledging the Client's Pain   Basic to all strategies for reducing pain is that nurses convey to clients that they believe the client is having pain. Four ways of communicating this belief follow:

1. Verbally acknowledge the presence of the pain. "I understand your leg is very painful. How do you feel about the pain?"

2. Listen attentively to what the client says about the pain.

CLINICAL GUIDELINES
Individualizing Care for Clients with Pain

- Use a variety of pain relief measures. It is thought that more than one measure has an additive effect in relieving pain. Two measures that should always be part of a pain relief plan are (a) establishing a client-nurse relationship and (b) client teaching. Because a client's pain may vary throughout a 24-hour period, different types of pain relief are often indicated during that time.

- Provide measures to relieve pain before it becomes severe. For example, the provision of an analgesic before pain is expected is preferable to waiting for the client to complain of pain, when a larger dose may be required.

- Use pain-relieving measures that the client believes are effective. It has been recognized that clients are usually authorities about their own pain. Thus, incorporating the client's measures into a pain relief plan is sensible unless they are harmful.

- Consider the client's willingness to be an active participant in the use of pain relief measures.

- Base the choice of the pain relief measure on the client's behavior reflecting the severity of the pain. If a client reports mild pain, an analgesic such as aspirin may be indicated, whereas a client who reports severe pain often requires a more potent relief measure.

- If a pain relief measure is uneffective, encourage the client to try it once or twice more before leaving it. Anxiety may prevent a relief measure from being effective, and some approaches, such as distraction strategies, require practice before they are effective.

- Maintain an unbiased attitude about what may relieve the pain. New ways to relieve pain are being continually developed. It is not always possible to explain pain relief measures; however, measures should be supported unless they are harmful.

- Keep trying. Do *not* ignore a client because pain persists in spite of measures. In these circumstances, reassess the pain, and consider other relief measures.

- Prevent harm to the client. Pain therapy should not increase discomfort or harm the client. Some pain relief measures may have outward effects, such as fatigue, but they should not disable the client (McCaffery 1979, pp. 36–42).

3. Convey that you are assessing the client's pain to understand it better, *not* to determine if the pain is real, for example, "How does your pain feel now?" or "Tell me how it feels compared to an hour ago."

4. Attend to the client's needs promptly.

Assisting Support Persons   Support persons often need assistance to respond positively to the client experiencing pain. Nurses can help by giving them accurate information about the pain and providing opportunities for them to discuss their emotional reactions, which may include anger, fear, frustration, and feelings of inadequacy. Enlisting the aid of support persons in the provision of pain relief to the client, such as massaging the client's back, may diminish their feelings of helplessness and foster a more positive attitude toward the client's pain experience. Support persons also may need the nurse's verbal recognition of their concern and participation in the client's care.

Reducing Misconceptions About Pain   Reducing a client's misconceptions about the pain and its treatment will often avoid intensifying the pain. The nurse should explain to the client that pain is a highly individual experience and that it is only the client who really experiences the pain, although others can understand and empathize. Misconceptions are also dealt with when nurse and client discuss why the pain has increased or decreased at certain times. For example, a client whose pain increases in the evening may mistakenly think this is the result of eating dinner rather than fatigue.

Applying Heat and Cold   The nurse may need a physician's order before applying heat or cold. The use of heat and cold is known to affect the vascular and muscular systems of the body as well as the production of hormones. Heat is known to stimulate the production of serotonin, which in turn helps an individual feel secure, serene, and safe. Depleted serotonin levels, seen in clients with chronic pain, produce tension, agitation, anxiety, hypersensitivity, and a variety of sleep disorders (Booker 1982, p. 49). Heat can be applied as warm soaks, compresses, or pads. See Chapter 46 for more information. Cold stimulates the production of norepinephrine.

Changes in body chemistry due to pain influence a person's behavior. The secretion of excessive norepinephrine causes the individual to feel powerful, in control, confident, and excited. However, when norepinephrine is depleted (e.g., when the pain is prolonged), the individual may feel helpless, worthless, and lethargic (Booker 1982, p. 50). Clients with depleted levels of both norepinephrine and serotonin may demonstrate agitated depression. In addition, depression may be aggravated by narcotics, which block the norepinephrine and serotonin receptor sites in the central nervous system (Booker 1982, p. 49). See also the discussion of cutaneous stimulation later in this chapter.

Reducing Fear and Anxiety   It is important to help relieve the emotional component, i.e., anxiety or fear, associated with the pain. When clients have no opportunity to talk about their pain and associated fears, their reactions to the pain can be intensified. The client may become angry or complain about the nurse's care when the problem really is a belief that the pain is not being attended to. If the nurse is honest and sincere and promptly attends to the client's needs, the client is much more likely to know that the nurse does believe the client is in pain.

By providing accurate information, the nurse can also reduce many of the client's fears, such as a fear of addiction or a fear that the pain will always be present. It also helps many clients to have privacy when they are experiencing pain. It is always wise to encourage clients to share their fears and concerns about how they are handling the pain.

Specific Strategies for Pain

Using Distraction Techniques

Distraction draws the person's attention away from the pain and lessens the perception of pain. In some instances, distraction can make a client completely unaware of pain. For example, a client recovering from surgery may feel no pain while watching a football game on television, yet feel pain again when the game is over.

The effectiveness of distraction to decrease pain can be explained by the gate-control theory. In the spinal cord, the receptor cells receiving the peripheral pain stimuli are inhibited by stimuli from other peripheral nerve fibers carrying different stimuli. Because pain messages are slower than diversional messages, the spinal cord gate, which controls the amount of input to the brain, closes, and the client feels less pain (Cummings 1981, p. 62).

Distraction is most effective when pain is mild or moderate, but intense concentration on other subjects can also relieve acute pain. An example of the latter is an adolescent who feels pain from a fractured foot bone only after she finishes playing a basketball game. Certain distractions, however, (e.g., disturbing stimuli such as loud noises, bright lights, unpleasant odors, or an argumentative visitor), can increase pain perception. Therefore, the nurse needs to reduce disturbing stimuli. Guidelines for using selected distraction techniques are included in the accompanying box.

Using Relaxation Techniques

Relaxation techniques, a specific form of distraction, are effective primarily for chronic pain and thus provide many benefits. Using relaxation techniques enables the client to reduce anxiety related to pain or stress, ease muscle tension pain, dissociate himself or herself from pain, obtain maximum benefits from rest and sleep periods, enhance the effectiveness of other pain therapies, and relieve hopelessness and depression associated with pain. For many years, nurses or maternity units have encouraged women in labor to relax and breathe rhythmically. These techniques, however, can be useful for any client in pain.

Three requisites to relaxation are correct posture, a mind at rest, and a quiet environment. The client must be positioned comfortably, with all body parts supported, joints slightly flexed, and no strain or pull on muscles (e.g., arms

---

Distraction Techniques

- **Slow, rhythmic breathing.** Instruct the client to stare at an object and inhale slowly through the nose while counting from 1 to 4 and then exhale slowly through the mouth while counting to 4 again. Encourage the client to concentrate on the sensation of breathing and to picture a restful scene. Continue until a rhythmic pattern is established.

- **Massage and slow, rhythmic breathing.** Instruct the client to breathe rhythmically and at the same time massage a painful body part with stroking or circular movements.

- **Rhythmic singing and tapping.** Ask the client to select a well-liked song and concentrate attention on its words and rhythm. Encourage the client to mouth or sing the words and tap a finger or foot. Loud, fast songs are best for intense pain.

- **Active listening.** Have the client listen to music and concentrate on the rhythm by tapping a finger or foot.

- **Guided imagery.** Ask the client to close his or her eyes and imagine and describe something pleasurable. As the client describes the image, ask about the sights, sounds, and smells imagined, encouraging the client to provide details.

---

and legs should not be crossed). To rest the mind, the client is asked to gaze slowly around the room, e.g., across the ceiling, down the wall, along a window curtain, around the fabric pattern, and back up the wall. This exercise focuses the mind outside of the body (away from the pain) and creates a second center of concentration. To relax the face, the client is encouraged to smile slightly or let the lower jaw sag. Stewart (1976, p. 959) describes one relaxation technique:

1. The client takes a deep breath and fills the lungs with air.

2. The client slowly hisses out the air while letting the body go limp and concentrating on how good this feels.

3. The client breathes in natural rhythm a few times.

4. The client takes another deep breath and releases it slowly, this time letting only the legs and feet go limp. The nurse asks the client to concentrate on how each leg feels (e.g., loose, heavy, and warm).

5. The client repeats step 4, concentrating on the arms, abdomen, back, and other muscle groups.

6. After the client is relaxed, slow, rhythmic breathing is added. Either abdominal or chest breathing may be used. If pain becomes intense, the client can use a more rapid, shallow breathing pattern.

There are several relaxation methods. Some recommend that separate muscle groups (e.g., neck, shoulder, back, arm, leg) be first tensed and then relaxed. After all muscle groups are tensed and relaxed, the whole body is tensed and then relaxed. Others suggest a stretching form of relaxation. The client lies supine, points the toes toward the knees, presses the back of the knees against the mattress or floor, flattens the hollow of the back and neck as much as possible, holds this position for several minutes, and then relaxes completely for several minutes.

Conscious suggestion by the nurse can help relax an anxious, frightened client in pain. It involves skillful use of the voice, body language, and word choice. A calm, soft, but distinct voice makes the client listen and gives a sense of security. Bending near the client, establishing eye contact, and placing a hand on the client's shoulder communicate the nurse's concern and calmness to the client. Positive, affirmative words help to convey the suggestion of relaxation to the client.

Using Guided Imagery

Guided imagery involves the use of images or fantasy to achieve specific health-related goals. Imagery is "the formation of a mental representation of an object that is usually only perceived through the senses" (Sodergren 1985, p. 104). Images can have visual, auditory, olfactory, gustatory, or tactile-proprioceptive qualities. For examples of the different types of images see Table 38–9. Images are often made up of more than one sense. For example, the image of waves breaking upon a shore may combine the visual picture with the sound of the waves and the smell of the salt air. When a client concentrates upon an image, pain awareness decreases.

Providing Cutaneous Stimulation

Cutaneous stimulation of the skin can reduce pain intensity. Again, this is another refinement of distraction, using tactile stimulation to "distract" the client from the pain experience. Guidelines for using specific techniques for cutaneous stimulation are summarized in the accompanying box.

Using Therapeutic Touch

Therapeutic touch (TT) is a process by which energy is transmitted or transferred

TABLE 38–9 *Types of Images*

Type	Example
Visual	A valley scene with its many shades of greenery
Auditory	Ocean waves breaking rhythmically upon a beach
Olfactory	Freshly baked bread
Gustatory	A juicy hamburger
Tactile-proprioceptive	Stroking a soft, furry cat

CLINICAL GUIDELINES
Cutaneous Stimulation

- **Cold packs** slow the conduction of pain impulses to the brain and motor impulses to muscles in the painful area. They provide quicker and longer-lasting pain relief than hot packs (McCaffery 1980d, p. 57). Use cold packs to help relieve headaches, muscle strains, joint pain, muscle spasm, and back pain during childbirth.

- **Analgesic ointments** containing menthol relieve pain, but the analgesic mechanism is unknown. These ointments produce immediate sensations of warmth that last for several hours, and even longer if the body part is wrapped in plastic. They can be used to relieve joint or muscle pain. Moreover, menthol ointment rubbed into the neck, scalp, or forehead sometimes relieves tension headaches, and some cultures (e.g., Filipino) use it on the abdomen to relieve gas pains or on the abdomen or lower back to relieve the pain of labor or delivery (McCaffery 1980d, p. 57).

- **Counterirritants,** such as mustard plasters, flaxseed poultices, and liniments, may be used to relieve the aching joint pain of rheumatoid arthritis and osteoarthritis. Counterirritants are thought to relieve pain by increasing circulation to the painful area.

- **Contralateral stimulation** can be accomplished by stimulating the skin in an area opposite to the painful area (e.g., stimulating the left knee if the pain is in the right knee). The contralateral area may be scratched for itching, massaged for cramps, or treated with cold packs or analgesic ointments. This method is particularly useful when the painful area cannot be touched because it is hypersensitive, inaccessible by a cast or bandages, or when the pain is felt in a missing part (phantom pain). (McCaffery 1980d, p. 57).

from one person to another with the intent of potentiating the healing process of one who is ill or injured. It is derived from, but not the same as, the "laying on of hands" associated with Eastern, European, and religious philosophies. Delores Krieger (1979), who coined the term *therapeutic touch,* refers to TT as a healing meditation, since the primary act of the nurse (healer) is to "center" the self and to maintain that center (mental concentration and focusing) throughout the process.

Basic to therapeutic touch are the concepts that the human being has an energy field, or, more properly, *is* an energy field (human field) and that energy can be intentionally channeled from one person to another. The human field extends beyond the level of the skin and is perceptible to the trained sense (primarily touch) of a healer. This energy field can be most clearly "felt" within several feet of the body. An everyday experience that may demonstrate this field phenomenon is the feeling of having one's space invaded when someone stands too close in a crowded elevator, even though there is no physical contact.

The body and the environment are considered open systems and constantly exchange energy and matter. The pattern and organization of the human field are constantly affected by the flow of energy from the environment. In situations of disease, illness, or pain, the pattern and organization of the field are disrupted; there may be a loss of energy, a disruption in the flow, an accumulation, or a blockage (Wright 1987, p. 708).

Therapeutic touch is a complex process that requires special knowledge and skill but is an independent nursing function that can be used alone or in conjunction with other pain relief measures. TT can begin to ease pain in a few minutes, and its effects last for a few hours to several days (Egan 1985, p. 208).

Administering Analgesics
Analgesics alter perception and interpretation of pain by depressing the central nervous system at the thalamus and cerebral cortex. Analgesics are more effective before the client feels severe pain than when given after the pain is severe. For this reason, analgesics are given at regular intervals, such as every 4 hours (q4h) after surgery.

There are two major classifications of analgesics: narcotic (strong analgesics) and nonnarcotic (mild analgesics). **Narcotic analgesics** include opiate derivatives, such as morphine and codeine. Narcotics relieve pain largely by binding to opiate receptors and activating endogenous pain suppression in the central nervous system. Changes in mood and attitude and feelings of well-being make the person feel more comfortable even though the pain persists. **Nonnarcotic analgesics** include nonsteroidal anti-inflammatory drugs (NSAIDS), aspirin, and acetaminophen. Nonnarcotic analgesics relieve pain by acting on peripheral nerve endings at the injury site and interfering with the prostaglandin system (American Pain Society 1988, p. 817). In addition, several combinations of analgesic drugs are available, e.g., a narcotic and nonnarcotic such as Tylenol #3, which combines acetaminophen with codeine, 30 mg.

A newer type of injectable analgesic is the **narcotic agonist-antagonist.** This type has *agonistic* properties in that it acts like a narcotic and relieves severe pain, but it also has *antagonistic* properties in that it acts against a narcotic. When given to a client who has taken a pure narcotic, these drugs reverse its effects; when given to a narcotic-free client, they have a narcotic effect. Examples are butorphanol (Stadol), nalbuphine (Nubain), and pentazocine (Talwin, Fortal).

When administering analgesics, it is essential that the nurse review the side effects. For example, narcotic analgesics depress respiration and must be used cautiously in clients with respiratory problems. If the client experiences significant respiratory depression (e.g., a drop from 18 to 12) or is overly sedated, the dosage is excessive. *Before* adminis-

tering narcotics, the nurse needs to assess a client's respiratory rate and level of alertness, for baseline data. The nurse also needs to note other side effects, such as nausea and vomiting. Nonnarcotics such as aspirin may aggravate gastrointestinal bleeding and therefore are contraindicated in clients with peptic ulcers. *After* medicating the client, the nurse records the response. Some nurses use pain medication flow-sheets for this purpose. See Figure 38–8.

A **placebo** is any form of treatment, e.g., medication or nursing intervention, that produces an effect in the client because of its intent rather than its physical or chemical properties (McCaffery 1982, p. 22). A medication that contains no analgesic properties (e.g., sugar, normal saline, or water) but is intended to relieve pain is a placebo. Years ago, the client who claimed the placebo gave relief was assumed to be malingering or falsely claiming pain. These assumptions have been proved wrong. Placebos do provide pain relief. Thirty-six percent of subjects in a study of 446 clients with severe postoperative pain reported relief after taking a placebo (Goodwin et al. 1982, p. 25). Placebos may help clients return to health and do have a physiologic effect; in some instances they cause the body to release endorphins, which are powerful analgesics (McCaffery 1982, pp. 23–24). It has also been proposed that placebos relieve pain by relieving anxiety or by classic conditioning. In the latter instance the client is conditioned to pain relief and responds positively to the placebo (Nursing Now 1985, p. 95).

Before administering a placebo, nurses must have a physician's order. Just because there are no active chemical ingredients in a placebo does not mean that nurses can administer them independently. It is important that nurses know why a placebo is being given before they give it. Placebos should not be used to punish a "difficult" client. Nor can they be used to prove that a client does not really have pain.

Since it is legal to administer placebos, nurses must also examine their own values relative to the ethics of giving placebos. Nurses have a number of choices. They can deceive the client by giving the placebo and saying it is another medicine. They can refuse to give the placebo. They can inform the client about the placebo and obtain his or her consent to use it. They can set up a double-blind situation, explaining the double blind to the client and requesting his or her consent. Neither the nurse nor the client knows whether a placebo or an active drug is being administered, because both have been packaged identically by the pharmacist. Nurses need to clarify their own feelings about placebos before selecting an option for intervening.

MANAGING INTRACTABLE PAIN

The management of intractable pain presents a special challenge to nurses working closely with the physician and clin-

PAIN FLOW SHEET

DATE 5/31/91

PURPOSES:
1) Record the patient's pain levels.
2) Provide data to titrate the analgesic's dosage.
3) Evaluate adverse reactions to the analgesic.

Patient's pain rating goal: ___2 or less___

JOHN D. ELLIOT   Name
1000 ELM STREET   Address
ALBERT, MICHIGAN

RM. 301/DR. DIRK

DATE TIME INITIALS	ANALGESIC DOSE ROUTE	PAIN RATING 0 – 10 0 = No pain 10 = Unbearable pain	VITAL SIGNS			LEVEL OF AROUSAL/ ACTIVITY	MISCELLANEOUS: Adverse reactions, bowel function, other pain relief measures, care plan, and comments
			R	P	BP		
5/31 TJ. 2P	M.S. 10mg IM	8	14	90	130/80	Restless	Describes severe pain
TJ. 2⁴⁵P		6	14				
TJ. 4P		4					Describes moderate pain
RS 5p	M.S. 15mg. IM	8		84	126/80		Describes increased pain
RS 6¹⁵p		4	12		124/76		
RS 7p		1	12			Relaxed, dozing	
RS 8¹⁰p	M.S. 15mg. IM	5			130/80		
RS 9p		2					
RS 9⁴⁵p		1	12	84	120/80	Sitting up, reading	
RS 11p	M.S. 15mg. IM	2					
							pt. states pain
	continued on M.S.						just about gone

Figure 38–8 Pain flowsheet. *Source:* From T. McCormick-Vandenbosch, How to use a pain flowsheet effectively, *Nursing 88,* August 1988, 18:50. Used by permission from Springhouse Corporation, 1111 Bethlehem Pike, Springhouse, PA 19477. All rights reserved.

ical pharmacist. A physician's order is required to administer the prescribed medications, but the nurse implements the orders and evaluates the client's response. Thus, the client and the nurse assume much of the responsibility for controlling the pain. Drugs commonly used for intractable pain are methadone, Brompton's mixture, and continuous morphine infusion. Patient controlled analgesia (PCA) is gaining popularity as an effective method of pain control.

Methadone is advantageous because it is effective orally, has a long duration of action, has a cumulative effect that can maintain steady analgesic levels, and does not substantially alter mood (Maxwell 1980, p. 1606). **Brompton's**

mixture, developed in the 1930s at Brompton's Hospital, London, was originally used as an oral analgesic for post-operative clients. Several different preparations are called Brompton's mixture, since these mixtures are prepared in hospice and hospital pharmacies. The original mixture contained heroin (narcotic analgesic), cocaine (central nervous system stimulant to counteract the sedation and respiratory depression of the narcotic), alcohol (flavor enhancer), and syrup and chloroform water to improve the taste and texture (Gever 1980, p. 57). In many places in North America, morphine or methadone is substituted for heroin, and amphetamine is used in place of cocaine, since cocaine is poorly absorbed and its importation is curtailed. The alcohol component may be ethanol, gin, or brandy. Fruit-flavored syrups are used to improve the flavor. In some hospitals, an antiemetic is also added for its tranquilizing effect.

Continuous morphine infusion is used for clients with end-stage terminal illness who are suffering extreme pain, have built up a tolerance to other pain medication, have difficulty taking anything orally, and cannot tolerate repeated injections. This method of pain control provides continuous pain relief, allows the client limited functional capacity, and supports the client's desire to die with dignity (O'Donnell and Papciak 1981, pp. 69–71).

Patient-controlled analgesia (PCA) is a new method of pain control that is useful for clients with severe pain not readily controlled by usual methods of administering analgesics. It employs the use of a programmable intravenous infusion pump to administer intermittent boluses of medication. Its use is not limited to clients with terminal illness; it has been shown effective in controlling various types of pain. For example, one study demonstrated improved pain control in adolescents in sickle-cell crisis (Schechter et al. 1988, p. 719).

The client pushes a button attached to the infusion pump when he or she needs pain medication and a small preset dose of analgesic is administered. After each dose is administered, there is a programmable lockout interval (usually 10–15 minutes) during which the infusion pump cannot be reactivated, allowing time for the medication to take effect before the client receives another dose. There is also a mechanism for programming the maximum amount of medication to be administered within a given time interval (usually 4 hours). Thus, the client typically receives the same amount of medication that would be given on a p.r.n. or a.t.c. schedule (and frequently less), but the client, rather than the nurse, decides when the medication is actually administered.

As with more traditional methods of pain control, the nurse is responsible for frequent assessments of the client and for recording the medication administered. A flow sheet may be used (see Figure 38–8, earlier). The nurse is also responsible for setting up and maintaining the infusion pump system and for teaching the client how to operate the system.

RESEARCH NOTE

How Effective Is Patient-Controlled Analgesia (PCA) for Postoperative Pain?

In this research, two pumps (PA and PB) were used to administer patient-controlled analgesia. PA emitted a signal when the drug was administered into the intravenous line. PB emitted a signal when the client depressed the trigger button, thereby producing a placebo effect. Another patient group received conventional therapy. Patients in both pump groups used less analgesia and perceived less pain than those on conventional therapy. Statistically, less anxiety and greater pain relief and client and nurse satisfaction were reported with the PA group.

Implications: PCA is more effective than traditional methods and should be considered for clients requiring analgesics.

B. R. Hecker and L. Albert, Patient-controlled analgesia: A randomized prospective comparison between two commercially available PCA pumps and conventional analgesia therapy for postoperative pain, *Pain* October 1988, 35:115–20.

MEDICAL MANAGEMENT OF PAIN

In addition to pharmaceutical measures for pain, there are a number of other treatments for pain which the physician may prescribe. Nursing roles in these therapies vary according to legal standards, institutional policies, physician preferences, and the qualifications of the nurse. Among these therapies are nerve blocks, electric stimulation, acupuncture, hypnosis, surgery, and biofeedback.

A **nerve block** is a chemical interruption of a nerve pathway, effected by injecting a local anesthetic into the nerve. Nerve blocks are widely used during dental work: The injected drug blocks nerve pathways from the painful tooth, thus stopping the transmission of pain impulses to the brain. Nerve blocks are often used to relieve the pain of whiplash injury, low-back disorders, bursitis, and cancer. Sometimes alcohol blocks are used. These, however, destroy nerve fibers and as a result are generally used for peripheral blocks only, since peripheral nerve fibers regenerate.

Electric stimulation is sometimes used to combat certain intractable pain. There are several methods. In **transcutaneous electric stimulation**, electrodes are placed on the surface of the skin over the painful area and over peripheral nerve pathways. In **percutaneous electric stimulation**, needles are inserted near a major peripheral nerve (e.g., the sciatic nerve). In both methods, an electric charge blocks the pain impulse by stimulating the gate-control mechanism. The percutaneous method is used primarily to determine whether a client should consider having a permanent implant inserted.

Acupuncture has been practiced for centuries in China and is receiving increasing attention in North America. It is currently being used selectively in North America to treat chronic pain. The acupuncturist inserts long, slender needles into the body at various sites, which are not necessarily near the body parts to be treated. The needles can be heated, attached to a mild electric current, or twirled continuously with the hand. It is possible that the insertion of the acupuncture needle closes the gate mechanism to pain or stimulates sites near pain fibers leading to the brain, thereby blocking the perception of pain.

Pain conduction pathways can be interrupted surgically. Because this disruption is permanent, surgery is performed only as a last resort, generally for intractable pain. Several surgical procedures may be performed. A **cordotomy** obliterates pain and temperature sensation below the level of the spinothalamic portion of the anterolateral tract severed, and is usually done for pain in the legs and trunk. **Rhizotomy** interrupts the anterior or posterior nerve root between the ganglion and the cord. Interruption of anterior *motor* nerve roots stops spasmodic movements that accompany paraplegia. Interruption of posterior *sensory* nerve roots eliminates pain in areas innervated by that specific nerve root. Rhizotomies are generally performed on cervical nerve roots to alleviate pain of the head and neck from cancer or neuralgia.

In **neurectomy**, peripheral or cranial nerves are interrupted to alleviate localized pain, such as pain in the lower leg or foot arising from a vascular occlusion. In a **sympathectomy**, pathways of the sympathetic division of the autonomic nervous system are severed. This procedure eliminates vasospasm, improves peripheral blood supply, and thus is effective in treating painful vascular disorders such as angina and Raynaud's disease.

Hypnosis is an altered state of consciousness in which an individual's concentration is focused and distraction is minimized. Scientists do not understand exactly how hypnosis relieves pain; however, one theory is that it prevents pain stimuli in the brain from penetrating the conscious mind. Hypnosis requires a client's active participation; clients can even learn to invoke their own hypnotic state. Hypnosis does not take away a person's self-control; in fact, people under hypnosis cannot be made to do anything that they consider amoral or dangerous. In a hypnotic trance, the client does not fall asleep but does become so sharply focused that minor distractions are ignored. A number of hypnosis techniques are used for clients, depending on the type of pain, and the preference of the client and the therapist. One of the most commonly used is symptom suppression, in which the client's awareness of the pain is blocked and the client is distanced from the pain. The effectiveness of this type of hypnosis depends on the severity of the pain and the ability of the client to concentrate (Nursing Now 1985, p. 51).

EVALUATING

To evaluate whether client goals have been achieved, the nurse collects data pertaining to the outcome criteria established. Because pain is a subjective experience, most of the data collected are obtained by questioning the client about specific information taught; about level of comfort, level of energy, and sleep pattern; and whether modifications in activities or the use of noninvasive strategies were helpful. Some objective data may be obtained, particularly from clients with acute pain (e.g., vital signs, behavioral postures and gestures).

To assist in the evaluation process, flowsheet records or a client diary may be helpful. See Figure 38–8 for an example of a flowsheet to evaluate the effectiveness of an analgesic. A weekly log or diary can be structured in a similar fashion for the individual client. For example, columns including day, time, onset of pain, activity before pain, pain relief measure, and duration of pain can be devised to help the client and nurse determine the effectiveness of pain relief strategies. Examples of evaluative statements indicating goal achievement are "The client states his sleep pattern has returned to normal," "Client verbalizes increased control over pain," "Client rates his pain as 4 instead of 8 on the 0 (no pain) to 10 (severe pain) rating scale."

NURSING CARE PLAN FOR LEE CHIN

ASSESSMENT DATA

Nursing Assessment

Mr. Lee Chin is a 57-year-old Chinese businessman who was admitted yesterday morning to the surgical unit at the hospital for the treatment of a possible strangulated inguinal hernia. Yesterday afternoon he went to surgery, and a partial bowel resection was performed. This morning, Mr. Chin is NPO. He has an intravenous infusion in the left arm, a nasogastric tube attached to low intermittent suction, and a clear dermal dressing applied to his large abdominal incision. He is in a dorsal recumbent (supine) position and is attempting to draw up his legs. Mr. Chin appears to be somewhat restless and pale. He appears to be generally uncomfortable.

Physical Examination
Height: 188 cm (6′2″)
Weight: 90.9 kg (200 lb)
Temperature: 37 C (98.6 F)
Pulse rate: 90 BPM

Respirations: 24 per minute
Blood pressure: 158/82 mm Hg
Skin pale and moist
Midline abdominal incision—sutures dry and intact
Pupils dilated

Diagnostic Data
Chest x-ray film: Negative
WBC: 12,000
Urine: Negative

CARE PLAN

Nursing Diagnosis	Client Goals and Outcome Criteria	Nursing Interventions and Rationales	Evaluation
Pain due to surgical incision stimulation of mechanosensitive receptors, resulting in grimacing; pallor; restlessness; elevated pulse, respirations, and systolic blood pressure; and dilated pupils.	Client Goal: Experiences minimal abdominal pain and discomfort. Outcome Criteria: States that postoperative discomfort is relieved within 20–30 minutes of verbalization of pain. Practices one relaxation technique for relief of pain by end of first day. Practices one distraction technique for relief of pain by day 2. Requests medication for relief of pain before pain becomes severe. Turns, coughs, and deep breathes with a minimum amount of discomfort by day 2.	Assess and record the description, location, duration and characteristics of client's pain. *Rationale:* Pain is a personal experience, and the nurse will need to rely on the client's description of pain in order to treat it effectively. Maintain frequent contact with client and encourage verbalization of discomfort and pain. *Rationale:* Cultural beliefs about pain may result in a stoic attitude about the pain experience. Reduce or eliminate pain-producing factors, e.g., fear, anxiety, lack of knowledge, a wet dressing, improper positioning. *Rationale:* Eliminating precipitating factors decreases incidence of pain. Employ distraction techniques, e.g., slow rhythmic breathing and guided imagery, to provide pain relief. *Rationale:* Distraction draws the client's attention away from the pain and lessens the perception of pain. Provide cutaneous stimulation, e.g., back rub. *Rationale:* Cutaneous stimulation provides pain relief by blocking pain impulses along the thinner nerve fibers in the synapses in the dorsal horn (gate control theory). Administer prescribed analgesics. *Rationale:* Analgesics alter perception and interpretation of pain by depressing the central nervous system at the thalamus and cerebral cortex. Note response to medication. *Rationale:* The medication dose may not be adequate to raise the client's pain threshold, or side-effects, e.g., respiratory depression, may occur. Instruct client to request analgesic before pain becomes severe. *Rationale:* Severe pain is more difficult to control and increases client's anxiety and fatigue.	Client verbalizes pain and discomfort and requests analgesics at onset of pain. States, "Pain is practically gone" 20 minutes after administration of analgesic. Reads, watches TV, and listens to his favorite music frequently throughout the day. Practices rhythmic breathing q3 to 4 hrs during his waking hours by day 2. Requests analgesic 30 minutes before turning in bed and assuming new position. Coughs and deep breathes q1 to 2 hrs after analgesic is administered.

Nursing Diagnosis	Client Goals and Outcome Criteria	Nursing Interventions and Rationales	Evaluation
		Instruct client in relaxation techniques, e.g., tensing and relaxing muscle groups and rhythmic breathing. *Rationale:* Relaxation techniques enhance the effect of other pain therapies, reduce anxiety, and relieve depression.	
Impaired skin integrity due to surgical incision, resulting in disruption of skin layers.	Client Goal: Healed surgical wound without complications. Outcome Criteria: Edges of surgical wound remain approximated throughout healing phase (21 days). No evidence of reddened skin in immediate area of wound after day 7. Vital signs remain within normal range. Splints abdominal incision with hands and/or pillow when turning, coughing, and deep breathing first post-op day.	Monitor vital signs frequently, especially increased temperature/pulse and respirations. *Rationale:* Increased temperature may indicate wound infection, which will delay healing. Employ surgical asepsis in dressing changes. *Rationale:* Sterile technique will decrease chance of wound infection and subsequent delayed healing. Splint incision with hands and/or pillow during coughing and deep-breathing exercises. *Rationale:* Incisional support decreases stress on healing wound edges. Monitor laboratory data such as WBC. *Rationale:* An elevated leukocyte count may indicate infection and subsequent delayed wound healing. Encourage adequate protein and vitamin C intake. *Rationale:* Protein and vitamin C are essential for tissue repair.	Wound edges remain approximated and intact. There is no evidence of redness or swelling of the wound. Vital signs are within normal range. Client splints his abdomen with his pillow before making position changes. He supports his abdominal wall with his hands or a pillow when coughing.

CHAPTER HIGHLIGHTS

▶ Pain is a personal experience to which no two people respond in the same way.

▶ Pain is useful in that it warns the individual of tissue injury.

▶ Pain can be classified according to duration, origin, or physiologic source.

▶ The pain experience can be analyzed in three stages: pain reception, transmission/perception, and modulation.

▶ Nociceptors must initially be stimulated if pain is to be perceived. Three types of pain stimuli are mechanical, thermal, and chemical.

▶ The precise mechanism of pain transmission and perception is unknown. Myelinated A delta fibers are associated with superficial somatic pain; unmyelinated C fibers are associated with deep somatic and visceral pain.

▶ Pain threshold is similar in all people, but pain tolerance and response vary considerably.

▶ Natural mechanisms within the body modulate pain transmission and perception. These endogenous opioids include enkephalins, endorphins, and dynorphins, which are morphinelike in their actions.

▶ Four theories that propose how pain is transmitted

▶

and perceived are the specificity theory, pattern theory, gate-control theory, and the parallel processing model.

▶ The pain response has three stages: activation, rebound, and adaptation. However, a person's coping mechanisms in response to pain are more useful to nurses.

▶ Numerous factors influence a person's perception and reaction to pain: culture, environment, emotions, expectations of others, past experience, and age.

▶ Assessment of a client who is experiencing pain should include a comprehensive pain history and physical examination focusing on autonomic nervous system responses and behavioral responses. Because pain is a subjective phenomenon, pain assessment is a complex process; however, tools are being developed to assist the nurse in this matter.

▶ Although the nursing diagnosis given to clients suffering pain is **Pain** or **Chronic pain**, the pain itself may be the etiology of many other nursing diagnoses.

▶ Planning intervention for a client in pain must include reducing or eliminating factors that intensify pain.

Overall client goals include preventing, modifying, or eliminating pain.

▶ Nursing management of pain includes both independent and collaborative nursing actions. Noninvasive measures such as distraction, relaxation techniques, therapeutic touch, guided imagery, and certain cutaneous stimulation techniques, may be performed as independent nursing functions. The major collaborative action involves the administration of analgesics.

▶ Major nursing functions for all clients are to acknowledge and convey belief in the client's pain, assist support persons, and reduce misconceptions about pain.

▶ Management of terminal or intractable pain requires specialized nursing skills. Patient-controlled analgesia, a recent development, enables the client to exercise control and minimize feelings of helplessness.

▶ Evaluation of the client's pain therapy includes the response of the client, the changes in the pain, and the client's perceptions of the effectiveness of the therapy. Ongoing verbal or written feedback from the client and family is integral to this process.

READINGS AND REFERENCES

SUGGESTED READINGS

Copp, L. A. Summer 1985. Pain coping model and typology. *Image: Journal of Nursing Scholarship* 17:69–71.
    Copp relates the self-image of the person experiencing pain to the nature of that person's perception of the pain. Five types of self-image are described: victim, combatant, responder, reactor, interactor. Copp also presents a coping model that includes a guideline for assessing pain from the client's point of view. Copp also presents coping strategies used by each type.

DeCrosta, T. March/April 1984. Relieving pain: Four noninvasive ways you should know more about. *Nursing Life* 4:29–33.
    DeCrosta describes four noninvasive methods for pain relief: transcutaneous electric nerve stimulator (TENS), ice massage, myotherapy, and distraction. Each of these techniques is described in considerable detail. The author points out that noninvasive methods work best if implemented before pain becomes intense.

McCaffery, M. September 1980. Understanding your patient's pain. *Nursing 80* 10:26–31.
    The author defines pain and describes the signs of acute pain. The causes of pain are discussed together with descriptions of psychogenic and somatogenic pain. Duration, severity, and client tolerance are considered.

———. November 1980. How to relieve your patients' pain fast and effectively . . . with oral analgesics. *Nursing 80* 10:58–63.
    The author outlines guidelines that help nurses choose and administer oral analgesics effectively. Equianalgesic lists are provided for commonly used oral analgesics.

McCormick-Vandenbosch, T. August 1988. How to use a pain flow sheet effectively. *Nursing 88* 18:50–51.
    The author gives practical advice on using flowsheets to help the client's efforts to relieve pain and to help the nurse understand the client's pain. Recording pain levels and fine-tuning the dosage are among the subjects described. A sample pain flowsheet accompanies the article.

RELATED RESEARCH

Camp, L. D. August 1988. A comparison of nurses' recorded assessments of pain with perceptions of pain as described by cancer patients. *Cancer Nursing* 11:237–43.

Camp, L. D., and O'Sullivan, P. S. September 1987. Comparison of medical, surgical and oncology patients' descriptions of pain and nurses' documentation of pain assessments. *Journal of Advanced Nursing* 12:593–98.

Gaston-Johansson, F., and Asklund-Gustafsson, M. November 1985. A baseline study for the development of an instrument for the assessment of pain. *Journal of Advanced Nursing* 10:539–46.

Geden, E.; Beck, N.; Hauge, G.; and Pohlman, S. September/October 1984. Self-report and psychophysiological effects of five pain-coping strategies. *Nursing Research* 33:260–65.

Giuffre, M.; Keane, A.; Hatfield, S. M.; and Korevaar, W. July/August 1988. Patient-controlled analgesia in clinical pain research measurement. *Nursing Research* 37:254–55.

Guck, T. P.; Meilman, P. W.; and Skultety, F. M. Winter 1987. Pain assessment index: Evaluation following multidisciplinary pain treatment. *Journal of Pain Symptom Management* 2:23–27.

Hecker, B. R., and Albert, L. October 1988. Patient-controlled analgesia: A randomized, prospective comparison between two commercially available PCA pumps and conventional analgesic therapy for postoperative pain. *Pain* 35:115–20.

Holm, K.; Cohen, F.; Dudas, S.; Medema, P. G.; and Allen, B. L. Summer 1989. Effect of personal pain experience on pain assessment. *Image: Journal of Nursing Scholarship.* 21:72–75.

Panfilli, R.; Brunckhorst, L.; and Dundon, R. March/April 1988. Nursing implications of patient-controlled analgesia. *Journal of Intravenous Nursing* 11:75–77.

Taylor, A. G.; Skelton, J. A.; and Butcher, J. January/February 1984. Duration of pain condition and physical pathology as determinants of nurses' assessments of patients in pain. *Nursing Research* 33:4–8.

SELECTED REFERENCES

Blaylock, J. 1968. The psychological and cultural influences on the reaction to pain. A review of literature. *Nursing Forum* 7(3):262–74.

Booker, J. E. March 1982. Pain: It's all in your patient's head (or is it?) *Nursing 82* 12:46–51.

Carpenito, L. J. 1989 *Nursing diagnosis application to clinical practice* 3rd ed. Philadelphia: J. B. Lippincott, Co.

Chapman, W. P., and Jones, C. M. 1944. Variations on cutaneous and visceral pain sensitivity in normal subjects. *Journal of Clinical Investigation* 23:81–91.

Cleeland, C. S. 1984. The impact of pain on the patient with cancer. *Cancer* 54:2635–41.

Copp, L.A. Summer 1985. Pain coping model and typology. *Image: Journal of Nursing Scholarship.* 17:69–71.

———. August 1990. The spectrum of suffering. *American Journal of Nursing* 90:35–39.

Coyle, N. September 1987. Analgesics and pain: Current concepts. *Nursing Clinics of North America* 22:727–41.

Cummings, D. January 1981. Stopping chronic pain before it starts. *Nursing 81* 11:60–62.

Diamond, M. January/March 1987. Analgesia on demand. *Canadian Intravenous Nurses Association Journal* 3:16–18.

Dunwoody, C. J. September/October 1987. Patient-controlled analgesia: Rationale, attributes, and essential factors. *Orthopaedic Nursing* 6:31–36.

Egan, E. C. 1985. Therapeutic touch. In Snyder, M., editor. pp. 199–210. *Independent nursing interventions.* New York: John Wiley and Sons.

Engel, G. L. 1970. Pain. In MacBryde, C. M., and Blacklow, R. S. editors. *Signs and symptoms: Applied physiologic physiology and clinical interpretation.* 5th ed. Philadelphia: J. B. Lippincott Co.

Ferrell, B. R., Ferrell, B. A. July/August 1990. Easing the pain. *Geriatric Nursing* 11:175–178.

Flannery, R. et al. 1981. Ethnicity as a factor in the expression of pain. *Psychosomatics* 22:39–50.

Gaston-Johansson, F., and Asklund-Gustafsson, M. November 1985. A baseline study for the development of an instrument for the assessment of pain. *Journal of Advanced Nursing* 10:539–46.

Geach, B. Spring 1987. Pain and coping. *Image: Journal of Nursing Scholarship* 19:12–15.

Gedaly-Duff, V. October 1988. Pain theories and their relevance to nursing practices. *Nurse Practitioner* 13:66–68.

Gever, L. N. May 1980. Brompton's mixture. How it relieves pain of terminal cancer. *Nursing 80* 10:57.

Goodwin, J. S.; Goodwin, J. M.; and Vogel, A. V. February 1982. Placebo misuse. *Nursing 82* 12:24–25.

Holderby, R. A. May 1981. Conscious suggestion: Using talk to manage pain. Part 9. *Nursing 81* 11:44–46.

Hurley, A., and Whelan, E. G. January/February 1988. Cognitive development and children's perception of pain. *Pediatric Nursing* 14:21–24.

Kahn, D. L., and Steeves, R. H. November 1986. The experience of suffering: Conceptual clarification and theoretical definition. *Journal of Advanced Nursing* 11:623–31.

Kim, M. J.; McFarland, G. K., and McLane, A. M. 1987. *Pocket Guide to Nursing Diagnoses.* 2d ed. St. Louis: C. V. Mosby Co.

Kotarba, J. A. 1983. Perceptions of death, belief systems and the process of coping with pain. *Social Science Medicine* 17:681–89.

Kresl, J. S. September 1988. Patient-controlled analgesia: A new system for pain management. *AORN Journal* 48:481–82, 484, 486–87.

Krieger, D. May 1975. Therapeutic touch: The imprimature of nursing. *American Journal of Nursing* 75:784–87.

———. 1979. *The therapuetic touch: How to use your hands to help or heal.* Englewood Cliffs, N.J.: Prentice-Hall.

Leventhal, H., and Everhart, D. 1979. Emotion, pain and physical illness. In Izard, C. E., editor. *Emotions and psychopathology.* New York: Plenum Press.

Ludwig-Beymer, P. 1983. Transcultural aspects of pain. In Boyle, J. and Andrews, M. *Transcultural concepts in nursing care.* Boston: Little, Brown and Co.

McCaffery, M. 1979. *Nursing management of the patient with pain.* 2d ed. Philadelphia: J. B. Lippincott Co.

———. October 1980a. Patients shouldn't have to suffer. How to relieve pain with injectable narcotics. *Nursing 80* 10:34–39.

———. December 1980b. Relieving pain with noninvasive techniques. *Nursing 80* 10:55–57.

———. February 1982. Would you administer placebos for pain? These facts can help you decide. *Nursing 82* 12:22–27.

———. November 1987. Patient-controlled analgesia: More than a machine. *Nursing 87* 17:63–64.

McCaffery, M., Beebe, A. 1989. *Pain: Clinical manual for nusing practice.* St. Louis: C. V. Mosby.

McCaffery, M., Ferrell, B. June 1990. Do you know a narcotic when you see one? *Nursing 90* 20:62–63.

McCaffery, M., Ferrell, B., O'Neil-Page, E. et al. February 1990. Nurses' knowledge of opioid analgesic drugs and psychological dependence. *Cancer Nursing* 13:21–27.

Nolan, M. F. January/February 1990. Pain: The experience and its expression. *Clinical Management* 10:22–25.

Marieb, E. N. 1989. *Human anatomy and physiology.* Redwood City, Calif.: Benjamin/Cummings.

Maxwell, M. B. September 1980. How to use methadone for the cancer patient's pain. *American Journal of Nursing* 80:1606–9.

Meinhart, N. T., and McCaffery, M. 1983. *Pain: A nursing approach to assessment and analysis.* Norwalk, Conn: Appleton-Century-Crofts.

Meissner, J. E. January 1980. McGill-Melzack pain questionnaire. *Nursing 80* 10:50–51.

Melzack, R., and Wall, P. D. 19 November 1965. Pain mechanisms: A new theory. *Science* 150:971–79.

———. 1982. *The challenge of pain.* New York: Penguin Books.

Nursing Now. 1985. *Pain.* Hicksville, N.Y.: Nursing 85 Books, Spring House Corp.

O'Donnell, L., and Papciak, B. August 1981. When all else fails: Continuous morphine infusion for controlling intractable pain. *Nursing 81* 11:69–72.

Paice, J. A. September 1987. New delivery systems in pain management. *Nursing Clinics of North America* 22:715–26.

Sodergren, K. M. 1985. Guided imagery. In Snyder, M. pp. 103–24. *Independent nursing interventions.* New York: John Wiley and Sons.

Stewart, E. June 1976. To lessen pain: Relaxation and rhythmic breathing. *American Journal of Nursing* 76:958–59.

Taylor, A. G. May 1988. Chronic pain: A guide to nursing intervention. *Applied Nursing Research* 1:8–13.

Weisenberg, M. 1975. Cultural influences on pain perception. In *Pain: Clinical and experimental perspectives.* pp. 141–143. St. Louis: C. V. Mosby Co.

Whitaker, O. C., and Warfield, C. A. February 15, 1988. The measurement of pain. *Hospital Practice* 23:155–56, 159–62.

Wright, S. M. September 1987. The use of therapeutic touch in the management of pain. *Nursing Clinics of North America* 22:705–13.

Zborowski, M. 1952. Cultural components in responses to pain. *Journal of Social Issues* 8:16–30.

Zborowski, M. 1969. *People in pain.* San Francisco: Jossey-Bass.

Nutrition

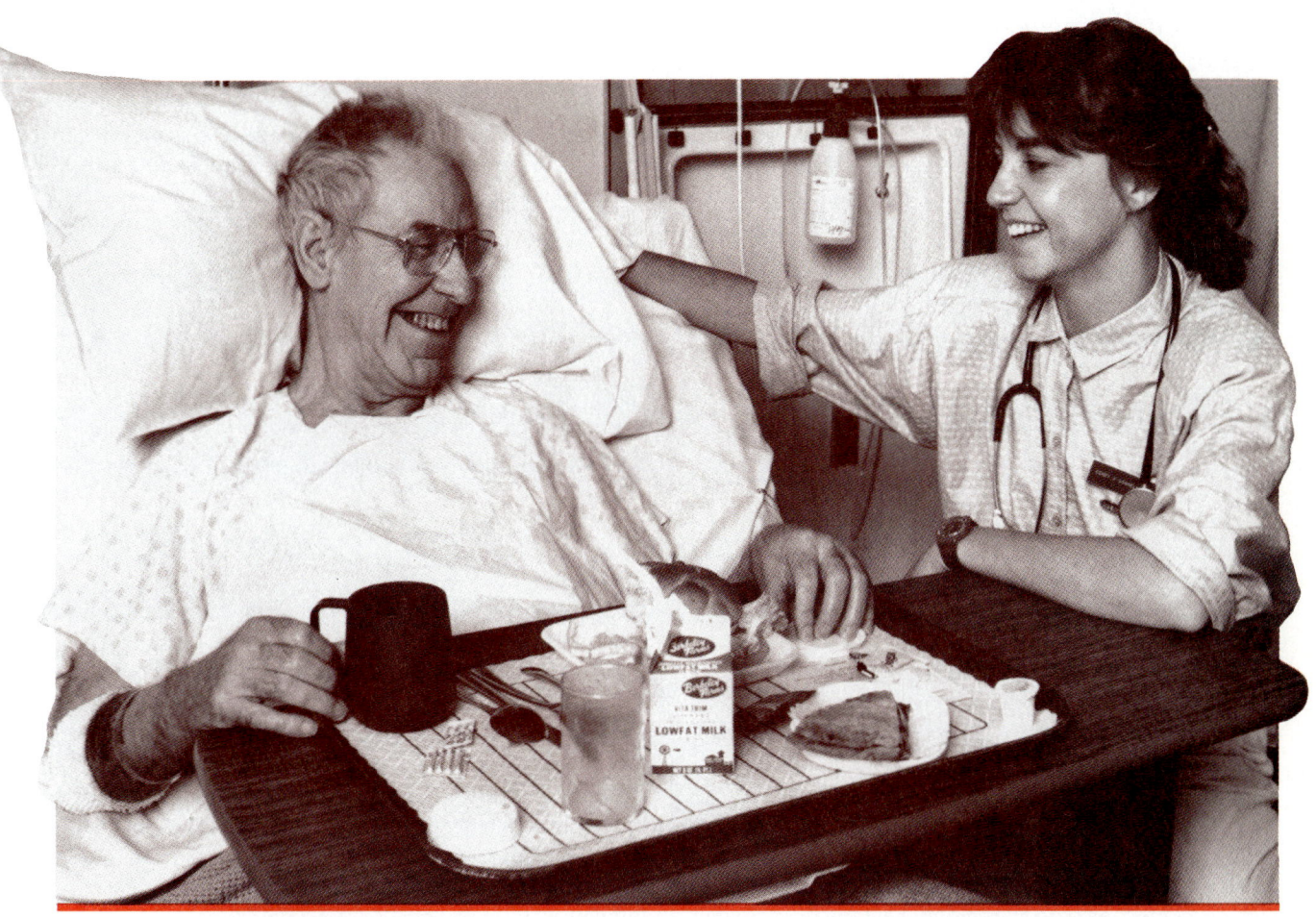

CONTENTS

OBJECTIVES

▸ Describe nutrition, metabolism, and energy requirements

▸ Identify functions and food sources of selected nutrients and some clinical signs of deficiency and excess.

▸ Describe the use of daily food group guides.

▸ Identify potential nutritional problems of vegetarians and suggest ways to avoid them.

▸ Describe necessary dietary modifications for older adults.

▸ Identify clinical signs of inadequate nutritional status.

▸ Describe a format for nutritional assessment.

▸ Identify factors that influence a person's eating patterns.

▸ Identify nursing diagnoses and factors contributing to the client's nutritional status.

▸ Identify interventions to stimulate a client's appetite.

▸ Describe ways to assist clients with meals.

▸ Describe some aids that enable self-feeding.

▸ Discuss some special nutritional services available for selected subgroups of the population.

▸ Recognize characteristics of commonly prescribed diets.

▸ Identify nursing responsibilities in administering enteral and parenteral nutrition.

NUTRITION AND METABOLISM

Nutrition

Nutrition is the sum of all the interactions between an organism and the food it consumes (Christian and Greger 1988, p. 4). In other words, nutrition is what a person eats and how the body uses it. People require food or essential nutrients for the growth and maintenance of all body tissues and the normal functioning of all body processes. **Nutrients** are the organic and inorganic chemicals found in foods and required for proper body functioning.

An adequate food intake consists of a balance of essential nutrients: water, carbohydrates, proteins, fats, vitamins, and minerals. Foods differ greatly in their **nutritive value** (the nutrient content of a specified amount of food), and no one food provides all essential nutrients. Nutrients have three major functions: providing energy for body processes and movement, providing structural material for body tissues, and regulating body processes.

The amount of energy that nutrients or foods supply to the body is their **caloric value. A calorie** is a unit of heat energy. A **small calorie** is the amount of heat required to raise the temperature of 1 g of water 1 degree C. A **large calorie (Calorie, kilocalorie [kcal])** is the amount of heat required to raise the temperature of 1 kg of water 1 degree C and is the unit used in nutrition. The energy liberated from each gram of carbohydrate and protein after it is metabolized is about 4 kcal; from each gram of fat, about 9 kcal are liberated through metabolism. The average North American receives approximately 45% of energy from carbohydrates, 40% from fat, and 15% from protein (Guyton 1986, p. 861). In most other parts of the world, people derive far more energy from carbohydrates than from fats and proteins.

Metabolism

Metabolism refers to all cellular chemical reactions that make it possible for body cells to continue living (Guyton 1986, p. 844). The energy in food maintains the basal metabolic rate of the body and provides energy for activities such as running and walking. Metabolic rate is normally expressed in terms of the rate of heat liberated during chemical reactions. The **basal metabolic rate (BMR)** is the rate at which the body metabolizes food to maintain the energy requirements of a person who is awake and at rest.

A person's energy requirements beyond the BMR are influenced by many factors, e.g., age, body size, activity, body temperature, environmental temperature, growth, sex, and emotional state. When energy requirements are completely met by calories taken in as food, people maintain their activity level without weight change. When caloric intake exceeds energy needs, the person gains weight. When caloric intake fails to meet energy requirements, the person burns body fat and muscle for energy and loses weight. Energy requirements vary from day to day. Illness often increases energy requirements because of increased metabolic rate and stress.

Some of the variables affecting an individual's caloric needs are discussed below.

Age and Growth

During periods of growth, the body uses more energy. Rapid growth during the first 2 years of life, adolescence, and pregnancy increase the need for calories. For example, an active adolescent body may need 3600 kcal, whereas a 70-year-old woman may require only 1800 kcal or less.

Gender Men usually have higher basal metabolic rates than women, a fact largely explained by the greater proportion of muscle in men's bodies. Pregnant women also have higher basal metabolic rates.

Climate Climate affects heat production. People in cold climates have a higher (about 20%, on average) metabolic rate than people in hot climates. This fact may be due to increased thyroxine levels in people who live in cold climates.

Sleep People need less energy during sleep, when the muscles are relaxed and physiologic processes are slowed. The metabolic rate drops about 10% to 15% during sleep.

Activity Muscular activity affects metabolic rate more than any other factor; the more strenuous the activity, the greater the stimulation. Mental activity, which requires only about 4 kcal per hour, provides very little stimulation.

ESSENTIAL NUTRIENTS

Essential nutrients include water, carbohydrates, proteins, fats, vitamins, and minerals. The most basic nutrient need is water. Because every cell requires a continuous supply of fuel, the body's most urgent nutritional need, after water, is for nutrients that provide fuel, or energy. The energy-providing nutrients are carbohydrates, fats, and proteins. Hunger impels people to eat enough energy-providing nutrients to satisfy their energy needs, but no clear-cut body signals lead a person to ingest certain vitamins or minerals, both of which are often referred to as **micronutrients.**

Carbohydrates

Carbohydrates are composed of the elements carbon, hydrogen, and oxygen and are of two basic kinds: sugars (simple carbohydrates) and starches (complex carbohydrates). The sugars may be **monosaccharides** (single molecules), which include glucose, fructose, and galactose, or **disaccharides** (double molecules), which include sucrose, or table sugar (a combination of glucose and fructose); maltose, or grain sugar (two glucose molecules); and lactose, or milk sugar (a combination of glucose and galactose). Starches are **polysaccharides;** they are composed of branched chains of dozens of molecules of glucose. Nearly all carbohydrates (with the exception of those in milk and milk products, which contain the disaccharide lactose) are derived from plants.

Carbohydrates are also categorized as natural (those found in foods as they come from the earth, e.g., fruits, vegetables, wheat) and refined or processed (those extracted from their natural sources and added to foods, e.g., cookies, candy, cakes, and pies). The natural carbohydrates supply vital nutrients such as protein, vitamins, and minerals and an important nonnutrient, dietary fiber. **Fiber,** a carbohydrate derived from plants, cannot be digested by humans but supplies roughage or bulk to the diet. This bulk not only satisfies appetite but also helps the digestive tract to function effectively and to eliminate wastes. Refined carbohydrates are relatively low in nutrients in relation to the large number of calories they contain and thus are often referred to as empty calories.

The desired end products of carbohydrate digestion are monosaccharides (glucose, fructose, and galactose). Some simple sugars, therefore, require no digestion. Of the three monosaccharides, glucose is by far the most abundant. Major enzymes of carbohydrate metabolism include ptyalin (salivary amylase), pancreatic amylase, and the disaccharidases: maltase, sucrase, and lactase. **Enzymes** are biologic catalysts that speed up chemical reactions. Digestive enzymes, which break down nutrients chemically into smaller compounds by hydrolysis, are categorized according to the types of nutrients on which they act. See Table 39–1 on page 988.

In healthy persons, essentially all digested carbohydrate is absorbed by the small intestine. Glucose transport through the cell membrane is augmented by insulin, a hormone secreted by the pancreas. In the absence of insulin, the amount of glucose that diffuses to the cell is far too little to supply normal requirements for energy (with the exception of the liver and brain cells). Glucose metabolism is therefore controlled by the rate at which insulin is available from the pancreas.

Storage Once in the cell, glucose is either used for immediate release of energy or stored in the form of **glycogen** (a large polymer of glucose). Although all cells of the body are capable of storing some glycogen, certain cells (liver and muscle) can store large amounts. The process of glycogen formation is called **glycogenesis,** and the breakdown of glycogen to re-form glucose is called **glycogenolysis.** Two hormones activate glycogenolysis: *glucagon* from the alpha cells of the pancreas, and *epinephrine* from the adrenal medulla. Glucagon is secreted when blood glucose concentrations fall to low levels; glucagon stimulates glycogenolysis mainly in the liver. The liver delivers large amounts of glucose into the bloodstream, thus elevating the blood glucose. Epinephrine is released whenever the sympathetic nervous system is stimulated. Epinephrine stimulates glycogenolysis in both liver and muscle cells, thereby releasing energy needed by the body for action during sympathetic stimulation.

When the body's stores of carbohydrates fall below normal, certain quantities of glucose are formed from protein (amino acids) and fat reserves by **gluconeogenesis,** a process that occurs in the liver. Up to 60% of the amino acids in the body's protein can be converted into glucose. Some types of amino acids cannot be converted. During periods of starvation, the body depletes first its fat and later its protein reserves.

TABLE 39–1 *Actions of Major Digestive Enzymes*

Name	Source	Site of Action	Agents Acted Upon	Resulting Products
Carbohydrate Enzymes				
Ptyalin (salivary amylase)	Saliva (secretions from parotid and submaxillary glands)	Mouth; some in body of stomach	Starch, e.g., grains, potatoes, legumes	Dextrins, maltose, glucose
Pancreatic amylase	Pancreatic secretions	Small intestine	Starch	As above
			Dextrins	Maltose, glucose
Disaccharidases	Small intestine	Brush border of small intestine	Disaccharides	Monosaccharides
a. Lactase			Lactose in milk	Glucose and galactose
b. Maltase			Maltose in corn syrup	Glucose
c. Sucrase			Sucrose in table sugar, fruits	Glucose and fructose
Protein Enzymes				
Pepsin	Peptic cells of stomach; inactive proenzyme pepsinogen is activated to pepsin by hydrochloric acid	Stomach	Large protein molecules	Proteoses, peptones, and large polypeptides
Rennin (in infants only)	Gastric mucosa	Stomach; calcium is necessary for activity	Casein in milk	Coagulated milk
Trypsin	Pancreatic cells; inactive proenzyme trypsinogen activated to trypsin by enterokinase (hormone produced in duodenal wall)	Lumen of small intestine	Whole and partially digested proteins, e.g., proteoses, peptones	Smaller polypeptides and dipeptides
Chymotrypsin	Pancreatic cells; inactive proenzyme chymotrypsinogen is activated to chymotrypsin by trypsin	Lumen of small intestine	Same as trypsin	Same as trypsin; also coagulates milk
Carboxypeptidase	Pancreatic cells; inactive proenzyme procarboxypeptidase is activated to carboxypeptidase by trypsin	Lumen of small intestine	Same as trypsin	Same as trypsin plus some amino acids
Aminopeptidase	Glands in intestinal wall	Brush border of small intestine	Polypeptides	Short chain peptides and amino acids
Dipeptidase	Glands in intestinal wall	Brush border of small intestine	Dipeptides	Amino acids
Fat Enzymes				
Pancreatic lipase	Pancreas	Small intestine	Triglycerides, diglycerides	Diglycerides, monoglycerides, fatty acids

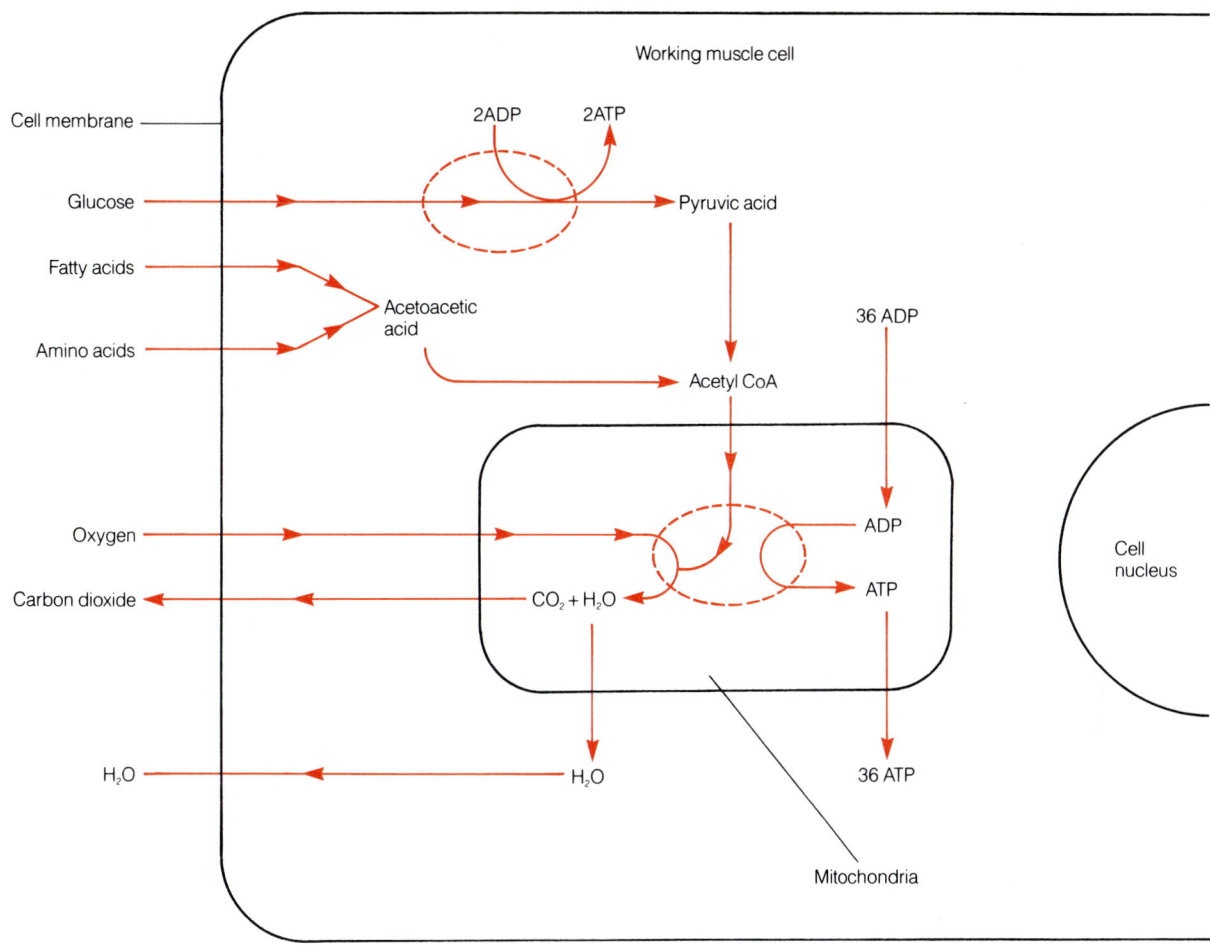

Working muscle cell

Cell membrane

2ADP 2ATP

Glucose — Pyruvic acid

Fatty acids

Acetoacetic
acid

Amino acids

Acetyl CoA

36 ADP

Oxygen

ADP

Carbon dioxide — $CO_2 + H_2O$

ATP

Cell
nucleus

H_2O — H_2O

36 ATP

Mitochondria

Figure 39–1   The Krebs cycle: The formation of adenosine triphosphate (ATP), the energy used to produce muscle work in aerobic exercise.   ***Source:***   Adapted from A. C. Guyton, *Textbook of medical physiology,* 7th ed. (Philadelphia: W. B. Saunders Co., 1986), p. 22.

Metabolism   Once in the cells, glucose undergoes a series of reactions to produce energy for the body's varied demands. There are two major pathways for breaking down glucose into the end products of carbon dioxide and water, thus producing energy:

1. Glycolysis and the formation of pyruvic acid (Embden-Meyerhof glycolytic pathway)

2. Citric acid cycle (Krebs cycle or tricarboxylic acid cycle)

Glycolysis is the release of energy through the **catabolism** (breaking down) of a glucose molecule into two molecules of pyruvic acid. This is a complex process involving 10 successive steps of chemical reactions, each of which is catalyzed by specific enzymes. During the process, the end-products of glycolysis are oxidized, and energy is released in small packets to form **adenosine triphosphate (ATP).** ATP is a compound with high-energy bonds

that stores the energy produced during glucose oxidation. Not all of the energy is stored, however. Some of it is lost in the form of heat. Because of the formation of ATP, the body's energy supply is conserved rather than dissipated all at once. The formation of pyruvic acid ends this glycolytic pathway; however, pyruvic acid provides the gateway to the next pathway, the citric acid cycle. The pyruvic acid is first broken down into two molecules of acetyl coenzyme A (acetyl-CoA).

The **citric acid cycle,** or the **Krebs cycle,** is a complex series of chemical reactions by which the acetyl portion of acetyl-CoA is broken down to carbon dioxide and hydrogen atoms. The hydrogen atoms are subsequently oxidized, thus releasing more energy to form ATP. In the initial stage of the citric acid cycle, acetyl-CoA combines with oxaloacetic acid to form citric acid, which gives this cycle its name. See Figure 39–1.

Proteins

Proteins are organic substances that upon hydrolysis or digestion yield amino acids. Like carbohydrates, proteins are composed of carbon, hydrogen, and oxygen, but proteins also contain nitrogen. Every cell in the body contains some protein, and about three-quarters of body solids are proteins. The only body substances normally lacking protein are urine and bile.

Proteins can be categorized by chemical structure as simple or compound. **Simple proteins** contain only amino acids or their derivatives, e.g., lactalbumin in milk, serum albumin in blood, keratin in hair and skin, ovoglobulin in egg, gluten in wheat. **Compound proteins** are composites of simple protein and another nonprotein group, e.g., hemoglobin, mucin found in mucous membrane secretions, and purines found in glandular tissue.

Amino acids are categorized as essential or nonessential. **Essential amino acids** are those that cannot be manufactured in the body and must be supplied in their final form as part of the protein ingested in the diet. They are essential for tissue growth and maintenance. Ten essential amino acids are threonine, leucine, isoleucine, valine, lysine, methionine, phenylalanine, tryptophan, histidine, and arginine. Histidine and arginine are necessary during growth but not during adulthood.

Nonessential amino acids are those that the body can manufacture. The body takes apart amino acids derived from the diet and reconstructs new ones from their basic elements (carbohydrates and nitrogen). Nonessential amino acids include glycine, alanine, aspartic acid, glutamic acid, proline, hydroxyproline, cystine, tyrosine, and serine.

Proteins may be complete or incomplete. **Complete proteins** contain all of the essential amino acids plus many nonessential ones. Most animal proteins, including meats, poultry, fish, dairy products, and eggs, are complete proteins. Some animal proteins, however, contain less than the required amount of one or more essential amino acids and therefore alone cannot support continued growth. These proteins are sometimes referred to as partially complete proteins. Examples are some fish, which have small amounts of methionine, and the milk protein casein, which has little arginine.

Incomplete proteins are deficient in one or more essential amino acids (most commonly deficient in lysine, methionine, or tryptophan) and are usually derived from vegetables. If, however, an appropriate mixture of plant proteins is provided in the diet, a balanced ration of essential amino acids can be created. Because protein is not stored, these mixtures must be eaten at the same meal. For example, a combination of corn (low in tryptophan and lysine) and beans (low in methionine) is a complete protein. Such combinations of two or more vegetables are called **complementary proteins.** Another way to take full advantage of vegetable proteins is to eat them with a small amount of animal protein. Examples are spaghetti with cheese, rice with pork, noodles with tuna, and cereal with milk.

Like carbohydrates, protein foods are altered physically by mechanical breakdown in the mouth and mixing with secretions in the stomach and intestine. Complete digestion of proteins to amino acids (the desired end products of protein digestion) could occur in the stomach if protein were held in the stomach longer. However, because the stomach normally empties in a relatively short time, only the beginning stages of protein breakdown are activated by pepsin, the main gastric enzyme specific for protein. Protein breaks down into successively smaller molecules in this sequence: proteins, proteoses, peptones, polypeptides, dipeptides, and finally amino acids.

Storage Amino acids are absorbed from the small intestine directly into the portal blood. They are transported into the cells only by active transport or facilitated diffusion through carrier mechanisms. Soon after entry into the cells, amino acids are converted by intracellular enzymes into cellular protein. Thus, amino acids are not stored in the cells as amino acids but as actual proteins.

Several hormones regulate the balance of amino acids in the cells (tissues) and the amino acid concentration of plasma. Insulin and growth hormone increase the formation of tissue proteins (anabolism); adrenocortical glucocorticoid hormones and thyroxine increase the concentration of plasma amino acids (catabolism).

The plasma proteins (albumin, globulin, and fibrinogen) are produced primarily in the liver and can be used for the rapid replacement of tissue proteins. Whole plasma proteins can be transferred (under the influence of the reticuloendothelial system) into the tissue cells, where they are split into amino acids, transported back into the blood, and used throughout the body to build cellular proteins. Plasma proteins, therefore, act as a labile protein storage medium.

Metabolism Metabolic activities of protein can be categorized into three broad divisions of **anabolism** (building tissue), catabolism (breakdown of tissue), and balance.

Anabolism Proteins are synthesized in all cells of the body, provided the appropriate amino acids are present. The types of proteins formed depend on the functional characteristics of each cell and are controlled basically by the genes of the cells.

Breakdown of tissue Because there is a limit to the amount of protein that can accumulate in a cell, additional amino acids are degraded and used for energy or stored as fat. This degradation occurs primarily in the liver and begins with the process of **deamination**—the removal of the amino (NH_2) groups by hydrolysis from the amino acids. Ammonia (NH_3) is a toxic byproduct of this process. Ammonia is removed from the blood almost entirely by the liver, which converts ammonia to urea. Urea is then excreted by the kidney.

After deamination, keto-acid products are released. These acids may be oxidized to release energy for metabolism. Because some of the deaminated amino acids are similar to the breakdown products of glucose and fat metabolism, they may also be converted to glucose or fatty acids. For example, deaminated alinine is pyruvic acid, which can be converted into glucose or glycogen (gluconeogenesis) or converted into acetyl-CoA. Acetyl-CoA can then be converted into fatty acids by a process called **ketogenesis.**

An obligatory loss of proteins occurs daily if a person eats no proteins. Certain proportions of body proteins (20 to 30 g) continue to be degraded into amino acids, then deaminated and oxidized. Thus, to prevent a net loss of protein, a person must ingest at least 20 to 30 g of protein each day (Guyton 1986, p. 833).

The state of protein nutrition is usually referred to as the state of **nitrogen balance,** since nitrogen is the element that distinguishes protein from carbohydrate and fat. Almost all nitrogen ingested is in the form of protein. However, most of the nitrogen lost from the body is in the form of nonprotein nitrogen compounds, i.e., the end products of protein catabolism. These end products include urea, creatinine, uric acid, and ammonia salts.

The state of nitrogen balance is the net result of intake and loss of nitrogen. When intake of nitrogen equals output, a state of nitrogen balance exists. People are usually in nitrogen balance when they appear ambulatory and healthy, are not growing or replenishing body tissue, and are consuming a diet adequate in essential amino acids, calories, and micronutrients.

Positive nitrogen balance exists when nitrogen input exceeds output; in other words, when the total anabolism of protein and other nitrogenous substances exceeds catabolism and loss. A state of positive nitrogen balance often exists under the following conditions:

- During periods of growth, such as
  a. Childhood and adolescence, when there are increases of height and lean body mass
  b. Pregnancy, when there are increases in maternal and fetal tissues
  c. Phases of physical exercise, when there are increases in muscle growth.
- During periods of tissue replacement, such as
  a. Convalescence from an illness that caused protein depletion, when body tissues are regenerated
  b. After fasting or inadequate intake of protein and calories, when body tissues are regenerated

Eating more protein than is necessary to meet body needs does *not* result in an increase in positive nitrogen balance or lean body mass in healthy adults. However, excess protein intake can lead to weight gain (positive caloric bal-

ance). Generally, a surplus of nitrogen intake is balanced by increased excretion of nitrogen as urea.

Negative nitrogen balance exists when nitrogen output exceeds intake (when catabolism exceeds anabolism). This state usually occurs when (a) a person consumes a diet inadequate in essential amino acids and calories, (b) is immobilized, or (c) is exposed to unusual stress as a result of trauma.

Fats

Fats are groups of organic substances (fats, oils, waxes, and related compounds) that are greasy and insoluble in water but soluble in alcohol or ether. These organic substances are **lipids.** Fats have the same elements (carbon, hydrogen, and oxygen) as carbohydrates, but the hydrogen content of fats is higher. Fats are actual or potential esters of fatty acids, which are used in metabolism. **Fatty acids** are the basic structural units of fats. **Esters** are compounds of an alcohol and an acid.

Fats can be classified as simple lipids or compound lipids. *Simple lipids,* or *neutral fats,* are known also as **triglycerides,** since they are esters of fatty acids with glycerol in the ratio of three fatty acids to each glycerol base. *Compound lipids* are various combinations of triglycerides with other components. Three compound lipids important in nutrition are:

1. Phospholipids, which are compounds of neutral fat, phosphoric acid, and a nitrogen base.
2. Glycolipids, which are compounds of fatty acids combined with carbohydrates and nitrogen. Because these are found mainly in brain tissue they are also referred to as cerebrosides.
3. Lipoproteins, which are compounds of various lipids with protein. They contain mixtures of triglycerides, phospholipids, cholesterol, and protein. There are three major classes of lipoproteins:
   a. Very-low-density lipoproteins contain high concentrations of triglycerides and moderate concentrations of phospholipids and cholesterol.
   b. Low-density lipoproteins contain few triglycerides but very high concentrations of cholesterol.
   c. High-density lipoproteins contain small concentrations of lipids but high concentrations of protein (about 50%).

Cholesterol is also classified as a lipid. Although cholesterol does not contain fatty acid, it does have many of the physical and chemical properties of other lipids and is capable of forming esters with fatty acids. **Cholesterol** is a fat-like steroid alcohol found in animal fats and oils, in bile, blood, brain tissue, milk, egg yolk, myelin sheaths of nerve fibers, the liver, the kidneys, and adrenal glands. Most of the body's cholesterol is synthesized in the liver. Some cholesterol is absorbed from the diet. Cholesterol is a precursor of bile acids and is important in the synthesis of steroid hormones. Large quantities of cholesterol and phospholipids are present in cell membranes and are essential for the structural elements of cells.

High blood levels of one or more of the lipids, particularly cholesterol or triglycerides, is called **hyperlipidemia.** Hyperlipidemia puts people at risk of coronary heart disease. The precise relationship between plasma cholesterol levels and cardiovascular disease, however, has not been established.

Fatty acids are described as saturated or unsaturated. The degree of saturation is determined by the relative number of hydrogen atoms in the fatty acid. **Saturated fatty acids** are those in which all carbon atoms are filled to capacity (i.e., saturated) with hydrogen. An example of a saturated fatty acid is butyric acid found in butter. **Unsaturated fatty acids** have less hydrogen attached to the available carbon atoms. When several carbon atoms in a fatty acid are not bonded to a hydrogen atom, the fatty acid is **polyunsaturated.** An example of a polyunsaturated fatty acid is linoleic acid found in vegetable oil.

Although chemical digestion of fats begins in the stomach, fats are digested mainly in the small intestine. Enzymes that break down fats include lipase, a pancreatic enzyme, and enteric lipase, an intestinal enzyme. Most chemical digestion is facilitated by pancreatic lipase. See Table 39–1, earlier. The desired end products of chemical digestion of fats are monoglycerides, fatty acids, and glycerol.

Some end products of fat digestion (e.g., glycerol and some free fatty acids) are absorbed into the portal blood system and carried to the liver. Other end products (e.g., monoglycerides and cholesterol) are absorbed into the abdominal lacteals and transported through the lymphatic system to the thoracic duct, where they enter the blood through the left subclavian vein. Large quantities of fat are stored in two major tissues: adipose tissue and the liver. Adipose tissue, referred to as the fat depot, stores triglycerides until they are needed for energy. Adipose tissue also has the subsidiary function of providing body insulation. The liver functions in lipid metabolism to degrade fatty acids into smaller compounds that can be used for energy, synthesize triglycerides from carbohydrates and proteins, and synthesize other lipids from fatty acids, such as cholesterol and phospholipids (Guyton 1986, p. 820).

Micronutrients

A **vitamin** is an organic compound that cannot be manufactured by the body and is needed in small quantities to catalyze metabolic processes. Thus, when vitamins are lacking in the diet, metabolic deficits result. Vitamins are generally classified as fat soluble or water soluble. **Fat-soluble vitamins** include A, D, E, and K. **Water-soluble vitamins** include C and the B-complex vitamins: B_1 (thiamine), B_2 (riboflavin), B_3 (niacin or nicotinic acid), B_6 (pyridoxine), B_9 (folic acid), B_{12} (cobalamin), pantothenic acid, and biotin. The body cannot store water-soluble vitamins; thus, people must get a daily supply in the diet. Water-soluble vitamins can be affected by food processing, storage, and preparation. The body can store fat-soluble vitamins, although there is a limit to the amounts of vitamins E and K the body can store. A daily supply of fat-soluble vitamins is therefore not absolutely necessary. Vitamin content is highest in fresh foods that are consumed as soon as possible after harvest. Table 39–2 indicates the usually recom-

(continued on page 995)

TABLE 39–2 *Key Information about Vitamins*

Vitamin	RDAs* for Healthy Adults (per day)	Major Food Sources	Major Functions	Signs of Severe Prolonged Deficiency	Signs of Extreme Excess
Water-Soluble					
C (ascorbic acid)	50 to 60 mg (100 mg for smokers)	Citrus fruits, cantaloupe, strawberries, tomatoes, potatoes, broccoli, green pepper, spinach	Still under intense study. Thought to aid in metabolism of certain amino acids, aid collagen formation for healing, enhance iron absorption, aid in formation of red blood cells, and maintain integrity of capillary walls.	Scurvy (bleeding gums, loose teeth, skin spots, and bruising); delayed wound healing; impaired immune response	Gastrointestinal upsets, poorer immune response, confounds certain lab tests

Vitamin	RDAs* for Healthy Adults (per day)	Major Food Sources	Major Functions	Signs of Severe Prolonged Deficiency	Signs of Extreme Excess
B$_1$ (thiamine)	Females: 1.2 to 1.3 mg Males: 1.2 to 1.5 mg	Pork, liver, whole grains, peas, eggs, milk, peanuts, oatmeal, pasta	Function as coenzymes in metabolism of carbohydrates, fats, amino acids, and alcohol.	Beriberi (nerve changes; sometimes edema, heart failure, muscle weakness)	Unknown
B$_2$ (riboflavin)	Females: 1.2 to 1.3 mg Males: 1.2 to 1.5 mg	Milk and milk products; eggs; cheddar cheese; organ meats (liver, heart, kidney); whole grains; green vegetables	As above for thiamine.	Skin lesions, e.g., inflammation and cracking at angles of mouth, dermatitis at angles of nares, keratitis of corneas	Unknown
B$_3$ (niacin or nicotinic acid)	Females: 13 to 15 NE (niacin equivalents) Males: 15 to 20 NE	Beef, pork, fish, liver, whole grains, peanuts, green vegetables, dairy products	As above for thiamine.	Pellagra (diarrhea, dermatitis, dementia)	Flushing of face, neck, hands; liver damage
B$_6$ (pyridoxine)	Females: 1.4 to 1.6 mg Males: 1.7 to 2 mg	High-protein foods (e.g., meat, liver, tuna, poultry, nuts); some vegetables (e.g., green beans, potatoes; bananas)	Protein metabolism, acts in transport of some amino acids across cell membranes, converts tryptophan to niacin.	Nervous and muscular problems, e.g., depression, confusion, weakness, convulsions	Unstable gait, numb feet, poor hand coordination, abnormal brain function
B$_9$ (folacin or folic acid)	Females: 150 to 180 μg (microgram) Males: 150 to 200 μg	Green leafy vegetables, broccoli, green beans, whole grains, nuts, orange juice, cottage cheese, peanuts	Maturation of red blood cells; acts as coenzyme in metabolism of certain amino acids and DNA and RNA; essential during growth periods.	Megaloblastic anemia (large, immature red blood cells), gastrointestinal disturbances	None known
B$_{12}$ (cobalamin)	2 μg	Animal products (meats, chicken, fish, eggs, liver, milk)	As above for folacin.	Megaloblastic anemia, pernicious anemia when due to inadequate intrinsic factor, nervous system damage	Unknown
Pantothenic acid	4 to 7 mg	Widely distributed in foods	Assists in metabolism of carbohydrates in fats.	Fatigue, sleep disturbances, nausea, poor coordination	Unknown
Biotin	100 to 200 μg	Widely distributed in foods	As above for pantothenic acid.	Fatigue, depression, muscular pain, dermatitis	Unknown

TABLE 39-2 *Key Information about Vitamins (continued)*

Vitamin	RDAs* for Healthy Adults (per day)	Major Food Sources	Major Functions	Signs of Severe Prolonged Deficiency	Signs of Extreme Excess
Fat-Soluble					
A (retinol, retinoic acid, carotene, palmitate)	Females: 800 RE (retinol equivalents), 4000 IU (international units) Males: 1000 RE, 5000 IU	Dark green and deep orange fruits and vegetables: apricots, broccoli, cantaloupe, carrots, pumpkin, winter squash, sweet potatoes, spinach and other dark leafy greens	Still under intense study: known to maintain health and normal functioning of cartilage, bone, and body coverings and linings (e.g., corneas, mucous membrane, skin); is a component of rhodopsin, a colored and light-sensitive substance in retina.	Keratinization of epithelial tissues, opacity of the cornea, night blindness, dry and scaling skin	Damage to liver, kidney, bone, headache, irritability, vomiting, hair loss, blurred vision, yellow skin from carotene
D (cholecalciferol, ergocalciferol)	5 μg or 200 IU	Fortified and full-fat dairy products, egg yolk; synthesized in the skin on exposure to sunlight	Increases calcium absorption from gastrointestinal tract; helps control calcium deposition in bones.	Rickets (bone deformities in children), osteomalacia (bone softening) in adults	Gastrointestinal upset; lethargy; cerebral, cardiovascular, and kidney damage; kidney stones
E (tocopherols: alpha, beta, gamma, and delta)	8 to 10 mg as alpha tocopherol equivalents	Vegetable oils and their products (e.g., salad dressings, many margarines); peanuts	Antioxidant, i.e., prevents oxygen from combining with other substances (vitamins A and C and polyunsaturated fatty acids) and damaging them; prevents cell membrane damage.	Possible anemia	In anemic children, blood abnormalities may develop
K (menadione, phylloquinone)	Females: 65 μg Males: 80 μg	Green leafy vegetables (e.g., lettuce, cabbage, spinach, peas, asparagus); meat	Necessary for formation of prothrombin in liver; prothrombin is essential for blood clotting.	Severe bleeding on injury; internal hemorrhage	Liver damage and anemia from high doses of synthetic forms

*RDAs are recommended daily allowances. The range reflects variables by age.

Sources: Adapted from National Research Council, Committee on Dietary Allowances, Food and Nutrition Board, *Recommended dietary allowances,* 10th ed. (Washington, D.C.: National Academy of Sciences, 1989) and J. L. Christian and J. L. Greger, *Nutrition for living,* 2d ed. (Menlo Park, Calif.: Benjamin/Cummings, 1988).

mended daily requirement of vitamins, food sources, functions, and signs of deficiencies and excesses.

Minerals are found in organic compounds, as inorganic compounds, and as free ions. Upon oxidation, minerals leave an ash, which can be acid or alkaline. Calcium and phosphorus make up 80% of all the mineral elements in the body. There are two categories of minerals: macrominerals and microminerals. **Macrominerals** are those that people require daily in amounts over 100 mg. They include calcium, phosphorus, sodium, potassium, magnesium, chloride, and sulfur. **Microminerals** are those that people require daily in amounts less than 100 mg. They include iron, zinc, manganese, iodine, fluoride, copper, cobalt, chromium, and selenium.

Common problems associated with the mineral nutrients are iron deficiency resulting in anemia, and osteoporosis resulting from loss of bone calcium. Key information about many essential minerals is shown in Table 39–3. Additional information about major minerals associated with the body's fluid and electrolyte balance is given in Chapter 40.

TABLE 39–3   *Key Information about Many Essential Minerals*

Mineral	RDA for Healthy Adults	Major Dietary Sources	Major Functions	Signs of Severe, Prolonged Deficiency	Signs of Extreme Excess
Major Minerals					
Calcium	800 to 1200 mg (1200 to age 25)	Milk, cheese, dark green vegetables, legumes	Bone and tooth formation; blood clotting; nerve transmission	Stunted growth; maybe bone loss	Depressed absorption of some other minerals
Phosphorus	800 to 1200 mg	Milk, cheese, meat, poultry, whole grains	Bone and tooth formation; acid-base balance; component of coenzymes	Weakness; demineralization of bone	Some forms depress absorption of some minerals
Magnesium	Females: 280 to 300 mg Males: 350 to 400 mg	Whole grains, green leafy vegetables	Component of enzymes	Neurologic disturbances	Neurologic disturbances
Sulfur	(Provided by sulfur amino acids)	Sulfur amino acids in dietary proteins	Component of cartilage, tendon, and proteins; acid-base balance	(Related to protein deficiency)	Excess sulfur amino acid intake leads to poor growth; liver damage
Sodium	1100 to 3300 mg*	Common salt, soy sauce, cured meats, pickles, canned soups, processed cheese	Body water balance; nerve function	Muscle cramps; reduced appetite	High blood pressure in genetically predisposed individuals
Potassium	1875 to 5625 mg*	Meats, milk, many fruits and vegetables, whole grains	Body water balance; nerve function	Muscular weakness; paralysis	Muscular weakness; cardiac arrest
Chloride	1700 to 5100 mg*	Common salt, many processed foods (as for sodium)	Plays a role in acid-base balance; formation of gastric juice	Muscle cramps; reduced appetite; poor growth	Vomiting

TABLE 39–3 *Key Information about Many Essential Minerals (continued)*

Mineral	RDA for Healthy Adults	Major Dietary Sources	Major Functions	Signs of Severe, Prolonged Deficiency	Signs of Extreme Excess
Trace Minerals					
Iron	Females: 10 to 15 mg Males: 10 to 12 mg	Meats, eggs, legumes, whole grains, green leafy vegetables	Component of hemoglobin and enzymes	Iron-deficiency anemia, weakness, impaired immune function	Acute: shock, death; chronic: liver damage, cardiac failure
Iodine	150 μg	Marine fish and shellfish; dairy products; iodized salt; some breads	Component of thyroid hormones	Goiter (enlarged thyroid)	Iodide goiter
Fluoride	1.5 to 4.0 mg*	Drinking water, tea, seafood	Maintenance of tooth (and maybe bone) structure	Higher frequency of tooth decay	Mottling of teeth; skeletal deformation
Zinc	12 to 15 μg	Meats, seafood, whole grains	Component of enzymes	Growth failure; reproductive failure; impaired immune function	Nausea; vomiting; diarrhea; adversely affects copper metabolism
Selenium	Females: 45 to 55 μg Males: 40 to 70 μg	Seafood, liver, whole grains	Component of enzymes; functions in close association with vitamin E; helps body disarm dangerous chemical oxidants	Muscle pain; maybe heart muscle deterioration	In animals: liver damage; depressed growth
Copper	1.5 to 3 mg*	Seafood, nuts, legumes, organ meats	Component of enzymes	Anemia; bone changes	Liver and neurologic damage
Chromium	50 to 200 μg	Brewers' yeast, liver, seafood, meat, some vegetables	Involved in glucose and energy metabolism	Impaired glucose metabolism	Lung, skin, and kidney damage (occupational) exposures)
Manganese	5.0 μg*	Nuts, whole grains, vegetables and fruits	Component of enzymes	Abnormal bone and cartilage	Neuromuscular effects
Molybdenum	75 to 250 μg*	Legumes, cereals, some vegetables	Component of enzymes	Disorder in nitrogen excretion	Inhibition of enzymes; adversely affects cobalt metabolism

*Estimated safe and adequate daily dietary intake.

Source: National Research Council, Committee on Dietary Allowances: Food and Nutrition Board, *Recommended dietary allowances,* 10th ed. (Washington, D.C.: National Academy of Sciences, 1989).

STANDARDS FOR A HEALTHY DIET

Daily Food Group Guides

Various daily food group guides have been developed to help healthy people meet the daily requirements of essential nutrients and to facilitate meal planning. Food group plans emphasize the general types or groups of foods eaten rather than the specific foods eaten, since related foods are similar in composition and often have similar nutrient values. For example, all grains, whether wheat, oats, or other grains, are significant sources of carbohydrate, iron, and the B vitamin thiamine. Although the exact amounts of each nutrient in each grain food are not identical, they are similar.

Daily food group plans that have been in use recently include the *Basic Four Food Guide,* the *Hassle-Free Guide to a Better Diet,* and the *Basic Food Guide.*

Basic Four Food Guide

The *Basic Four Food Guide* was introduced by the USDA in 1956. This plan is based on four basic food groups: milk and milk products; meats and alternates; breads and cereals; and fruits and vegetables. Foods selected from the guide generally supply 1000 to 1400 kcal daily. Numbers and sizes of servings are listed for each group. See Table 39–4 on page 998 and Appendix E.

Because individual needs vary with age, sex, and activity, additional calories to meet energy requirements can be obtained by increasing the number and size of servings from the various food groups and/or by adding other foods that are not listed in the food groups. Critics of the *Basic Four Food Guide* point out that it does not provide guidance on judicious choices of low-nutrient-density foods and beverages such as butter, margarine, and carbonated beverages. In addition, it does not provide guidelines about convenience foods such as hamburgers, milk shakes, and pizzas, which have become so much a part of the North American diet.

Another criticism is that the *Basic Four Food Guide* does not address fluid intake. A daily intake of 4 to 6 cups or more from any source is recommended. Iodized salt should be used. Unless there is an adequate supply in drinking water, fluoride, too, should be supplemented. Also, a person can follow this guide and still eat insufficient fiber, which is found in raw fruits, vegetables, and whole grains.

However, the four groups are easily remembered. Although the plan does not guarantee that a person will consume the recommended levels of essential nutrients, it suggests that people are likely to come close to recommended levels, especially if they eat more than the minimum amounts recommended.

The Hassle-Free Guide

In 1979, the USDA modified the *Basic Four Food Guide* and published the *Hassle-Free Guide,* or *Modified Food Guide.* This plan adds a fifth group to the basic four. The fifth group includes foods high in fats, sugar, and alcohol. Moderation in consumption of these foods is recommended. Critics of this plan say that people may misinterpret the purpose of the fifth group and believe that the foods in the fifth group are being recommended for regular consumption rather than being restricted.

The Basic Food Guide

The *Basic Food Guide,* developed by Christian and Greger (1988, p. 31), is an attempt to build on the strengths of previous guides and add other useful information. This guide recommends the same major food groups found in the *Basic Four Food Guide* and *Hassle-Free Guide* and the same numbers of daily minimum servings for an adult, but it has other unique aspects:

- *Limited extras.* The foods in this additional group are not needed for good nutrition, since they do not contain the essential nutrients in significant amounts. Therefore, they should be used as limited supplements rather than as mainstays of the diet. Many of these foods, e.g., fatty foods, sugary foods, alcoholic beverages, and unenriched baking goods, are high in calories. Examples are salad dressings, cream cheese, bacon, chocolate, sour cream, soy sauce, olives, ketchup, jam, jellies, and cakes. Overweight people should eat fewer of these foods. Other foods in this group are low both in calories and nutrients but contribute water. Examples are tea, coffee, broth, low-calorie soft drinks, and diet gelatin desserts.

- *Plant sources of protein.* The plant sources are richer in certain nutrients, e.g., magnesium and the B vitamin folacin, than meats are and should be substituted for meat sources several times each week. Plant sources include legumes (e.g., garbanzo, kidney, lima, navy, and pinto beans; soybeans; lentils; and split peas), nuts, seeds, and nut or seed butters.

- *Fat, sodium, and sugar content.* The guide indicates the relative content of fat, sodium, and added sugar of certain foods in each group, allowing the user to reduce the amounts of fat, sodium, and added sugar in the diet.

- *Combination foods.* Directions for including common combination foods, e.g., casseroles and sandwiches, are given. Each ingredient must be identified by group. For example:
  — 1 cup spaghetti with meatballs includes 1 serving meat (2 oz); 1 serving grain (3/4 cup spaghetti); and 1/2 serving vegetable (1/4 cup tomato sauce).
  — 1/4 of a 12-inch cheese pizza includes 1 1/2 servings milk (2 oz cheese); 3 servings grain (pizza dough); 1/2 serving vegetable (1/4 cup vegetables).

Recommended Dietary Allowances

The Committee on Dietary Allowances of the Food and Nutrition Board of the National Academy of Sciences in Washington D.C. publishes lists of recommended dietary

TABLE 39–4 *Basic Four Food Guide*

Food Groups and Servings	Foods and Sizes of Servings	Major Nutrients
Dairy Group		
Child, under 9: 2 to 3 Child, 9 to 12: 3 or more Teenager: 4 or more Adult: 2 or more Pregnant: 3 or more Lactating: 4 or more	One serving = 8 oz fluid milk: whole, low-fat, skim, buttermilk, or reconstituted dry milk or evaporated milk; 1⅓ oz hard cheese, 1⅓ cups cottage cheese, 1⅔ cups ice cream, 1 cup yogurt	Protein; fat; vitamins A and D; riboflavin; B_{12}; calcium; phosphorus
Protein Group		
2 or more servings	One serving = 2 to 3 oz beef, pork, lamb, veal, poultry, or fish. Substitutes for ½ serving of meat: 1 egg, ½ cup cooked dry beans or peas, or 2 tbsp peanut butter	Protein; carbohydrate in plant alternatives; fat, except in legumes; B_{12} in meat, fish, and poultry; niacin; iron; zinc
Vegetable-Fruit Group		
4 or more servings, including:	One serving = ½ cup vegetable or fruit or one piece fresh fruit	Carbohydrate; vitamin C in citrus fruits and tomatoes; vitamin A in dark green or deep yellow vegetables; folacin; iron; calcium; fiber
1 or 2 servings of good sources of vitamin C	Grapefruit or grapefruit juice, orange or orange juice, cantaloupe, raw strawberries, broccoli, Brussels sprouts, green pepper. Fair sources include melons, tangerines, asparagus, cabbage, cauliflower, collards, potatoes, spinach, tomatoes	
1 good source of vitamin A at least every other day	Apricots, broccoli, cantaloupe, carrots, chard, collards, kale, pumpkin, spinach, sweet potatoes, turnip greens, winter squash	
Grain Group		
4 or more servings	One serving = 1 slice whole grain or enriched bread, 1 oz ready-to-eat cereal, ½ cup of the following: cooked cereal, cornmeal, grits, spaghetti, macaroni, noodles, or rice	Carbohydrate; some protein; thiamine; niacin; iron; fiber
Other Foods		
Sweets, oil, butter, salad dressings, condiments, alcohol	Used to round out meals, provide flavor, and meet energy requirements	Fat; carbohydrate

Sources: Adapted from S. G. Dudek, *Nutrition handbook for nursing practice* (Philadelphia: J. B. Lippincott Co., 1987), pp. 177–78; D. E. Scholl, *Nutrition and diet therapy: A handbook for nurses* (Oradell, N.J.: Medical Economics Books, 1986), pp. 4–6; and Minister of Health and Welfare, Department of Health and Welfare, *Canada's food guide* (Ottawa: Department of Health and Welfare, 1983).

allowances (RDAs). RDAs are the levels of intake of essential nutrients that, to the best available scientific knowledge, adequately meet the known nutritional needs of most healthy persons (National Research Council 1989). About every 5 years, the findings of recent studies are reviewed, and daily nutrient intake recommendations are updated. The Canadian Department of National Health and Welfare also prepares standards, called the recommended daily nutrient intakes, which are published by the Committee for Revision of the Canadian Dietary Standard, Bureau of Nutritional Sciences, Health and Welfare. These Canadian standards provide nutrient intakes for 15 different age groups, for each trimester of pregnancy, and for lactating women.

Because a person's actual need for any given nutrient can be influenced by sex, body size, growth, and reproductive status, separate recommendations are made for various subgroups, defined by sex, age, pregnancy, and lactation. Recommended nutrient levels are usually set high enough to include the needs of 97.5% of the people in that group and to allow for some loss of the nutrient as it makes its way through the body. For example, the RDA allows for losses that occur during absorption or conversion from one chemical form to another, when some of the nutrient's activity may be decreased. Factors not taken into account in the RDAs are the effect of illness or injury (increasing the need for nutrients) and the variability among individuals within any given group.

Dietary Goals/Guidelines for Americans

In December 1977, the U.S. Senate Select Committee on Nutrition and Human Needs (1977, p. 4) released the second edition of *Dietary Goals for the United States,* which recommended *specific* reductions in fats, refined and processed sugars, cholesterol, and salt and suggested caloric intakes to achieve or maintain desirable body weight. Critics of these guidelines said that such specific restrictions were unnecessary for the general population. They thought such restrictions should be prescribed only for persons at risk for certain health problems and that the recommendations were difficult for people to incorporate into meal planning.

In 1980, the USDA and the Department of Health and Human Services jointly produced *Nutrition and Your Health: Dietary Guidelines for Americans.* These recommendations were based on the *Dietary Goals* but were less specific. Key points of the *Dietary Guidelines* follow:

- Eat a variety of foods.
- Maintain ideal body weight.
- Eat less fat, saturated fat, and cholesterol.
- Eat foods with adequate starch and fiber.
- Eat less sugar.

- Eat less sodium (including salt).
- If you drink alcohol, do so in moderation.

Vegetarian Diets

There are two basic vegetarian diets: those that allow only plant foods and those that include milk, eggs, and dairy products. Some people, not strictly vegetarians, eat fish and poultry but not beef, lamb, or pork; others eat only fresh fruit, juices, and nuts; and still others eat plant foods and dairy products but not eggs. See Table 39–5.

People may become vegetarians for economic, health, religious, ethical, and ecologic reasons. Increased meat prices during the last decade have forced some people to become vegetarians or eat meat infrequently. Some people avoid meat because they believe it is healthy to do so. They cite as evidence that vegetarians tend to be less obese than others and that blood cholesterol levels of vegetarians tend to be lower, two factors that reduce the probability of heart disease. Some people are vegetarians for ethical reasons: They object to the killing of animals or the way they are raised. People who follow vegetarian diets for ecologic reasons point out the wastefulness of eating animals that consume a large part of the world's supply of grain when this grain could be better used for people.

Nutritional Concerns   Vegetarian diets can be nutritionally sound if they include a wide variety of legumes, grains, fruits, vegetables, nuts, milk, and milk products and if proper protein complementation and vitamin-

TABLE 39–5 *Types of Vegetarian Diets*

Kind	Description
Vegans	Strict vegetarians, avoid all foods of animal origin
Lacto-ovo-vegetarians	Use dairy products and avoid eating flesh
Lacto-vegetarians	Use dairy products but avoid eating flesh and eggs
Ovo-vegetarians	Use eggs but avoid dairy products and flesh
Pesco-vegetarians	Use dairy products, eggs, and fish but avoid all other meat products
Partial vegetarians (semivegetarians)	Avoid selected meats, e.g., red meat
Fruitarians	Use only fresh (raw) fruits, juices, nuts, honey, and/or olive oil
Macrobiotic vegetarians	Progress through ten dietary stages from a widely inclusive selection to a restrictive selection

mineral supplementation is provided. Protein intake can be insufficient if complementary protein relationships are not understood and followed. The phenomenon of one food supplementing low levels of amino acids in another is called **protein complementing** or **mutual supplementation.** Generally, legumes (starchy beans, peas, lentils) have complementary relationships with grains and with nuts and seeds. Protein complementing is of particular importance for growing children and pregnant and lactating women, whose protein needs are high.

Because foods of animal origin provide vitamin B_{12}, vegans need to eat other sources of vitamin B_{12}: brewer's yeast, foods fortified with vitamin B_{12}, or a direct vitamin supplement. A person who eats no red meat may acquire iron deficiency because plant sources of iron are not absorbed efficiently. Vegans, therefore, are advised to consume iron-rich foods (e.g., green leafy vegetables, whole grains, raisins, and molasses), iron-enriched foods, and a vitamin-C-rich food with each meal to enhance iron absorption from plant sources. Calcium deficiency is a concern for strict vegetarians. It can be prevented by including soybean milk fortified with calcium, leafy green vegetables, and tofu (soybean curd) that has added calcium.

Vegetarian Food Guide   A food guide for vegetarians is shown in the box below. It includes specific vegetables that supplement any calcium, riboflavin, and

vitamin D deficiencies. Diets such as the fruitarian diet do not provide sufficient amounts of essential nutrients and are not recommended for long-term use.

Dietary Modifications for Older Adults

Metabolic rates decrease with age and physical activity usu-

TABLE 39–6   *Major Food Sources of Calcium*

Foods	Household Measure	Calcium (mg)
Dairy Products		
Milk, nonfat dry (reconstituted)	1 cup	240
Milk, skim (1% fat)	1 cup	296
Milk, whole	1 cup	288
Cheese, processed	1 oz (1 slice)	198
Cheese, cheddar	1 oz	213
Cheese, cottage, 4% milk fat	1 oz	27
Cheese, Swiss	1 oz	262
Custard	½ cup	148
Ice cream	½ cup	97
Yogurt	1 cup	295
Fish, Meat, and Poultry		
Salmon (canned)	1 oz	91
Sardines	1 oz	124
Shellfish	1 oz	35
Vegetables		
Broccoli (cooked)	1 medium stalk	158
Greens, Collards	½ cup	179
Beet greens	½ cup	72
Okra	10 pods	98
Fruits		
Orange	1 medium	54
Blackberries	1 cup	46
Dates	10	45
Rhubarb (sweetened)	½ cup	105

Sources: A. B. Natow and J. Heslin, *Nutritional care of the older adult* (New York: Macmillan Co., 1986), p. 212; and D. E. Scholl, *Nutrition and diet therapy: A handbook for nurses* (Oradell, N.J.: Medical Economics Books, 1986), p. 214.

Dietary Recommendations for Lacto-Vegetarians and Lacto-Ovo-Vegetarians

- Whole-grain bread and cereals, legumes, and nuts
- Calcium-rich foods (dark leafy vegetables, legumes, rutabaga)
- Riboflavin-rich foods (e.g., whole grains, dark leafy vegetables, broccoli, avocado)
- Vitamin-D-rich food (fortified soybean milk) and dietary supplements
- Four to six daily servings of complementary protein (each of the following constitutes 1 serving):
  - 1 egg
  - ½ to ¾ cup dried peas, beans, lentils
  - 2 tbsp peanut butter
  - ¼ to ½ cup nuts, seeds
  - ½ cup cottage cheese
  - 1 oz cheddar cheese

Adapted from S. G. Dudek, *Nutrition handbook for nursing practice* (Philadelphia: J. B. Lippincott Co., 1987), pp. 45–46; D. E. Scholl, *Nutrition and diet therapy* (Oradell, N.J.: Medical Economics Books, 1986), pp. 21–23; and S. R. Williams, B. S. Worthington-Roberts, E. D. Schlenker, P. Pipes, J. M. Rees, and L. K. Mahan (editors), *Nutrition throughout the life cycle.* St. Louis: Times Mirror/Mosby College Publishing, 1988), pp. 119–20.

ally slackens; therefore, elderly people require fewer calories than they required formerly. Some may have an increased need for carbohydrates for fiber and bulk, but most nutrient requirements remain relatively unchanged. Such physical changes as tooth loss and impaired sense of taste and smell may also affect eating habits. Other physical deficiencies that may affect eating habits and nutritional status are decreased bile/gastric juice secretion, peristalsis, and glucose tolerance; impaired circulation; and loss of bone density and lean body mass (Raab and Raab 1985, p. 24).

Psychosocial factors may also contribute to nutritional problems. Some elderly people who live alone do not want to cook for themselves or eat alone. As a result, the person may adopt poor dietary habits and be at risk of malnourishment. Loss of spouse, living alone, anxiety, depression, dependence on others, and lowered income all affect eating habits. Guidelines for the inclusion of high-nutrient foods that are compatible with the diminished chewing and swallowing abilities and other problems of older adults are summarized in the box below.

Nutrition for Older Adults

■ Reduce fat consumption by drinking low-fat milk, eating more poultry and fish rather than red meats, limiting meat portions to 4 to 6 oz per day, and limiting the intake of added fats, e.g., butter, margarine, and oil-based salad dressings.

■ Consume desserts such as fresh or canned fruit and puddings made with low-fat milk rather than pies, cookies, cakes, or ice cream.

■ Make sure that intake of meat, poultry, fish, eggs, and cheese is sufficient, since intakes of these foods are often decreased in the older population.

■ Because of a lowered glucose tolerance, consume more complex carbohydrates, e.g., breads, cereals, rice, pasta, potatoes, and legumes, rather than sugar-rich foods.

■ Ensure an intake of at least 800 mg of calcium to prevent bone loss. Milk and milk products, e.g., cheese, yogurt, cream soups, milk puddings, and frozen milk products, are principal sources of calcium. See Table 39–6 for additional calcium-rich foods.

■ Make sure that intake of vitamin D is sufficient. Vitamin D is essential to maintain calcium homeostasis. To meet vitamin D requirements, include some milk in the diet, since such dairy products as cheese, cottage cheese, and yogurt are not usually fortified with vitamin D. If milk or milk products cannot be tolerated due to a lactose deficiency, supplements should be taken.

■ Because sodium may be restricted for older adults who have hypertension or other cardiac problems, avoid such foods as canned soups; ketchup; mustard; and salted, smoked, cured, and pickled meats, poultry, and fish. No salt should be added during the cooking of foods.

■ Due to the increased incidence of gastrointestinal disturbances and chronic diarrhea, the regular aspirin use among some elderly women, and the possible reduction in meat intake, the need for iron may be increased. See Table 39–7 on the following page for iron-rich foods.

■ Difficulties with chewing raw fruits and vegetables may lead to a deficiency in vitamins A and C, minerals, and fiber. Adaptations in food preparation may be necessary. Chop fruits and vegetables finely, shred green leafy vegetables, and select ground meat, poultry, or fish rather than foods that are more difficult to chew.

■ Consume fiber-rich foods to prevent constipation and minimize use of laxatives. See Table 39–8 on the following page for examples of fiber-rich foods. Fiber-rich foods also provide bulk and a feeling of fullness. They are therefore useful in helping people control their appetites and lose weight.

■ Mealtime is commonly a social activity. When possible, make arrangements to promote appropriate social interaction at meals.

■ Eat essential foods first and follow with limited foods in moderation afterward.

■ Having the major meal at noon may decrease difficulty sleeping at night after a heavy meal. Avoid tea, coffee, or other stimulants in the evening.

TABLE 39–7 *Major Food Sources of Iron*

Foods	Household Measure	Iron (mg)
Meat, Fish, Poultry		
Beef (ground)	3 oz	3.2
Beef liver	3 oz	5.1
Beef heart	3½ oz	5.9
Beef kidneys	3½ oz	7.4
Chicken (breast)	3 oz	1.3
Oysters	5 to 8 medium	5.5
Scallops	3½ oz	3.0
Shrimp	3½ oz	3.1
Tuna (canned)	3 oz	1.5
Vegetables and Fruits		
Spinach		
raw	½ cup	2
cooked	½ cup	2.2
Beet greens	⅔ cup	1.9
Chick peas	½ cup	3
Kidney beans	½ cup	2.2
Soybeans	3½ oz	2.8
Dates (pitted)	½ cup	3
Prune juice	½ cup	4.1
Raisins	⅔ cup	3.5
Grain Products		
Bread		
white	1 slice	0.6
whole wheat	1 slice	0.8
Enriched pasta	½ cup	2.0
Cereal (bran flakes)	1 oz	5.3
Cereal (oat flakes)	1 oz	5.4
Spaghetti (enriched)	½ cup	0.3
Other		
Tofu (soybean curd)	½ cup	1.9
Eggs	2 medium	2.3
Peanuts	⅔ cup	2.1
Corn syrup	⅓ cup	4.1
Molasses	1 tbsp	0.9

Sources: J. L. Christian and J. L. Greger, *Nutrition for living,* 2d ed. (Menlo Park, Calif.: Benjamin/Cummings, 1988), pp. 348–49; A. B. Natow and J. Heslin, *Nutritional care of the older adult* (New York: Macmillan Publishing Co., 1986), p. 212; and S. G. Dudek, *Nutrition handbook for nursing practice* (Philadelphia: J. B. Lippincott Co., 1987), pp. 520–59.

TABLE 39–8 *Fiber-Rich Foods*

Food	Portion	Insoluble Dietary Fiber Content (g)
Fresh pear	1 medium	3.6
Blueberries, frozen	½ cup	1.5
Beans, green	½ cup	1.6
Bran Buds	⅓ cup	6.4
Bran Chex	⅔ cup	3.9
Wheat bran	½ cup	11.2
Lima beans	½ cup	3.3
Kidney beans	½ cup	3.9

Source: Adapted from Johnson, E. J. & Marlett, J. A. 1986. A simple method to estimate neutral detergent fiber content of typical daily menus. © American Journal of Clinical Nutrition 44:127-134. American Society for Clinical Nutrition.

FACTORS INFLUENCING DIET

Before attempting to assess a client's nutritional status, the nurse needs to recognize factors that affect an individual's eating habits, such as culture, religion, economic status, or personal preference. These factors frequently occur in combination.

Culture Ethnicity often determines food preferences. Traditional foods (e.g., rice for Orientals, pasta for Italians, curry for Indians) are eaten long after other customs are abandoned. Although food patterns vary from region to region and person to person, the examples in the accompanying box illustrate the diversity of food preferences among cultures.

Religion Religious practice also affects diet. Some Roman Catholics avoid meat on certain days, and some Protestant faiths prohibit tea, coffee, or alcohol. Both Orthodox Judaism and Islam prohibit pork. Orthodox Jews observe kosher customs, eating certain foods only if they are inspected by a rabbi and prepared according to dietary laws. The nurse must be sensitive to such religious dietary practices.

Economic Status What, how much, and how often a person eats are frequently affected by economic status. For example, people with limited income, including some elderly people, may not be able to afford beef and fresh vegetables. In contrast, people with higher incomes may purchase more proteins and fats and fewer complex carbohydrates. Regardless of economic status, people may not purchase foods containing essential nutrients. Many other factors, such as personal food preferences, are involved.

Peer Groups   Peer groups or other subgroups distinguished by age, sex, occupation, or other interests also influence a person's food choices. For example, certain foods may become "in" with teenagers. Members of any group may change their food choices to align themselves more closely with an influential group member. For example, when a financially successful member of a group of business executives shows a strong preference for decaffeinated coffee, some associates are likely to make similar choices. Sexism may also influence food choices. Some men, for example, may not choose a salad as an entree because they perceive such a choice as feminine.

Personal Preference and Uniqueness   What an individual likes and dislikes significantly affects eating habits. People often carry childhood preferences into adulthood. People develop likes and dislikes based on associations with a typical food. A child who loves to visit his grandparents may love pickled crabapples because they are served in the grandparents' home. Another child who dislikes a very strict aunt grows up to dislike the chicken casserole she often prepares.

Individual likes and dislikes can also be related to familiarity, particularly for children. Children often say they dislike a food before they sample it. Some adults are very adventuresome and eager to try new foods. Others prefer to eat the same foods over and over again. Preferences in the tastes, smells, flavors (blends of taste and smell), textures, temperatures, colors, shapes, and sizes of food influence a person's food choices uniquely. For example, some people may prefer sweet and sour tastes to bitter or salty tastes. Textures play a great role in food preferences. Some people prefer crisp food to limp food, firm to soft, tender to tough, smooth to lumpy, or dry to soggy. Many people like certain combinations of taste and textures.

Life-Style   Certain life-styles are linked to food-related behaviors. People who are always in a hurry probably buy convenience grocery items or eat restaurant meals. People who spend many hours at home may take time to prepare more meals "from scratch." Individual differences also influence life-style patterns. Is the person skilled in cooking? Is the person willing to learn to make new things? Does the person thrive on routine and familiarity? Does the person skip meals and eat whenever it is convenient? Is the person concerned about health foods and adequate exercise that enhance well-being?

Beliefs About Health Effects of Food   Beliefs about effects of foods on health and well-being can affect food choices. For example, a person who feels stomach pain after eating spicy foods may avoid these foods or eat them less often and in smaller amounts. Beliefs about effects of

Examples of Foods Preferred by Selected Ethnic Groups	
Chinese	Rice Green tea Mixtures of fish, pork, or chicken and vegetables (bamboo shoots, broccoli, cabbage, mushrooms, onions, and pea pods)
Italian	Pasta Crusty bread Cheese Pepperoni
Japanese	Rice Green tea Raw fish and soy sauce Abundance of vegetables
Mexican	Dried beans Tortillas made from wheat or corn flour instead of bread Tacos, burritos, enchiladas Chili peppers, especially in sauces
Polish	Highly salted and seasoned foods Sausages; smoked and cured meats Noodles, potatoes, dumplings Bread Coffee with sugar and cream
Puerto Rican	Rice and beans with spicy sauce Bananas, oranges, mango, papaya, acerola Coffee with hot milk
Southern black	Pork and chicken Dried peas, beans, squash, and greens cooked with fatback or salt pork Sweet potatoes

food on health often arise from what a person learns about nutrition through radio, television, magazines, newspapers, and books. For example, many people are reducing their intake of animal fats in response to published evidence that excessive consumption of animal fats is a major risk factor in cardiovascular disease.

Food fads that involve nontraditional food practices are relatively common. A **fad** is a widespread but short-lived interest or a practice followed with considerable zeal. Often the truth about a food is exaggerated or used out of context to support the rationale behind the fad. A fad may be based either on the belief that certain foods have special curative powers or on the notion that certain foods are harmful. Examples of some food fads are given in the box above.

Food fads typically appeal to the individual seeking a miracle cure for a disease or the person who desires superior health and wants to delay aging. Food fads also appeal to people who follow fashion and to people who distrust the medical profession. Persons in the latter group hope that the diet will allow them to avoid medical treatment. Some fad diets are harmless, but others are potentially dangerous. Determining what needs the fad diet fills for the client enables the nurse to both support these psychologic needs and suggest a more nutritious diet.

Advertising   Food producers try to persuade people to change from the product they currently use to the brand of the producer. Often popular actors and actresses are used to influence television viewers' or radio listeners' choices. Although more research is needed to determine whether and to what extent such messages affect people's food choices, advertising is thought to influence people's food choices and eating patterns to a certain extent. Of note is that such products as alcoholic beverages, cake and other dessert mixes, soups, tea, coffee, frozen dinners, and soft drinks are more heavily advertised than such products as milk, canned seafood, bread, cheese, poultry, vegetables, and fruits (Christian and Gregor 1988, p. 212).

Psychologic Factors   Anorexia and weight loss can indicate severe stress or depression. Although some people overeat when stressed, depressed, or lonely, others eat very little under the same conditions. Anorexia nervosa and bulimia are severe psychophysiologic conditions seen most frequently in female adolescents.

Health Status   An individual's health status greatly affects eating habits and nutritional status. The lack of teeth, ill-fitting teeth, or a sore mouth make the mastication of food difficult. Difficulty swallowing (dysphagia) due to a painfully inflamed throat or a stricture of the esophagus can discourage a person from obtaining adequate nourishment. Many disease processes and surgery of the gastrointestinal tract and related structures can affect digestion, absorption, metabolism, and excretion of essential nutrients. For example, inflammatory disease, tumors, or ulcers often impair digestion and absorption of nutrients. Gastrointestinal and other diseases also create anorexia, nausea, vomiting, and diarrhea, all of which adversely affect a person's eating habits and nutritional status. Gallstones, which can block the flow of bile, are a common cause of impaired digestion of fat.

Many other disease processes affect nutrition. Disease of the liver can impair metabolic processes. Disease of the kidney can impair excretion of the end products of metabolism. Disease of the pancreas can affect glucose metabolism or fat digestion. Malignancies anywhere in the body increase metabolic needs, since malignant cells compete with normal cells for nutrients. Disease of endocrine glands, e.g., thyroid, parathyroid, and adrenal glands, can result in severe hormonal imbalances that affect the client's nutritional status.

Therapies prescribed for certain diseases may also adversely affect eating patterns and nutrition. For example, cancer clients who receive chemotherapy and radiation are at risk of nutritional deficits. Normal tissue cells, e.g., those of the bone marrow and the gastrointestinal mucosa, are naturally very active and particularly susceptible to antineoplastic agents. Oral ulcers, intestinal bleeding, or diarrhea resulting from the toxicity of antineoplastics can diminish a person's nutritional status seriously.

The effects of radiotherapy depend on the area that is treated. For example, radiotherapy of the head and neck may cause decreased salivation, taste distortions, and swallowing difficulties; radiotherapy of the abdomen and pelvis may cause malabsorption, nausea, vomiting, and diarrhea. Many clients feel profound fatigue and anorexia.

Alcohol and Drugs   Excessive consumption of alcohol contributes to nutritional deficiencies if alcohol constitutes a large part of the person's food intake. Chronic consumption of alcohol often leads to deficiencies in protein, thiamine, folacin, niacin, and vitamin B_6 as a result of interruptions in the body's normal nutritional processes anywhere from ingestion through excretion.

The effects of drugs on nutrition vary considerably. They may alter appetite, disturb taste perception, or interfere with nutrient absorption or excretion. Nurses need to be aware of the nutritional effects of specific drugs when evaluating a client for nutritional problems. The nursing history interview should include questions about the medications the client is taking. Nutrients can also affect drug utilization. Some nutrients can decrease drug absorption; others enhance absorption. For example, the calcium in milk hinders absorption of the antibiotic tetracycline but enhances the absorption of the antibiotic erythromycin. Selected drug and nutrient interactions are shown in Table 39–9.

TABLE 39—9 *Selected Drug-Nutrient Interactions*

Drug	Effect on Nutrition
Acetylsalicylic acid (aspirin)	Decreases serum folate and folacin nutrition
	Increases excretion of vitamin C, thiamine, potassium, amino acids, and glucose
	May cause nausea and gastritis
Antacids containing aluminum or magnesium hydroxide (Maalox)	Decrease absorption of phosphate and vitamin A
	Inactivate thiamine
	May cause deficiency of calcium and vitamin D
Thiazide diuretics (Diuril, HydroDIURIL)	Increase excretion of sodium, potassium, chloride, calcium, magnesium, zinc, and riboflavin
	May cause anorexia, nausea, vomiting, diarrhea, or constipation
Potassium chloride (Kaochlor, K-Lor, Slow-K)	Decreases absorption of vitamin B_{12}
	May cause diarrhea, nausea, or vomiting
Digitalis	Increases excretion of potassium, magnesium, and calcium
	May cause anorexia, nausea, or vomiting
	Is incompatible with protein hydrolysates
Laxatives	May cause calcium and potassium depletion
	Mineral oil and phenolphthalein (Ex-lax) decrease absorption of vitamins A, D, E, and K.
Antihypertensives	Hydralazine (Apresoline) may cause anorexia, vomiting, nausea, and constipation
	Methyldopa (Aldomet) increases need for vitamin B_{12} and folate
	May cause dry mouth, nausea, vomiting, diarrhea, constipation
Antiinflammatory agents	Colchicine decreases absorption of vitamin B_{12}, carotene, fat, lactose, sodium, potassium, protein, and cholesterol
	Prednisone decreases absorption of calcium and phosphorus
Antidepressants	Amitriptyline (Elavil) increases food intake (large amounts may suppress intake)

Sources: A. B. Natow and J. Heslin, *Nutritional care of the older adult* (New York: Macmillan Publishing Co., 1986), pp. 252–255; and D. Raab and N. Raab, Nutrition and the aging: An overview, *Canadian Nurse,* March 1985, 81:3.

ASSESSING NUTRITIONAL STATUS

One method of assessing a client's nutritional status is to follow the "ABCD" approach:

A: Collecting *anthropometric measurements*

B: Looking at *biochemical data*

C: Examining the client for the *clinical signs* of nutritional status

D: Obtaining a *dietary history*

Anthropometric Measurements

Anthropometric measurements are measurements of the size and composition of the body. They include measurements of height, weight, body mass index, skinfolds (fat folds), and arm muscle circumference. Anthropometric measurements reflect the client's caloric-energy expenditure balance, muscle mass, body fat, and protein reserves.

Assessment of height and weight is discussed in Chapter 19. Ideal body weight (IBW) ranges by age, sex, and frame for adults are given in Table 19–6, page 369. An inadequately nourished person can be underweight, overweight, or obese: In every case caloric intake is not in balance with expenditure of energy. Clients whose weight is 20% greater than ideal or 10% less than ideal and those who have had an unintentional weight gain or loss of 10% are considered at risk for poor nutritional status.

The **body mass index (BMI)** indicates whether weight is appropriate for the person's height. To calculate the BMI, measure the height in meters and the weight in kilograms (e.g., 5 feet, 7 inches equals 1.7 meters, and 153 pounds equals 69 kilograms). Then multiply the height by itself (1.7 multiplied by 1.7 equals 2.89) and divide the weight by this

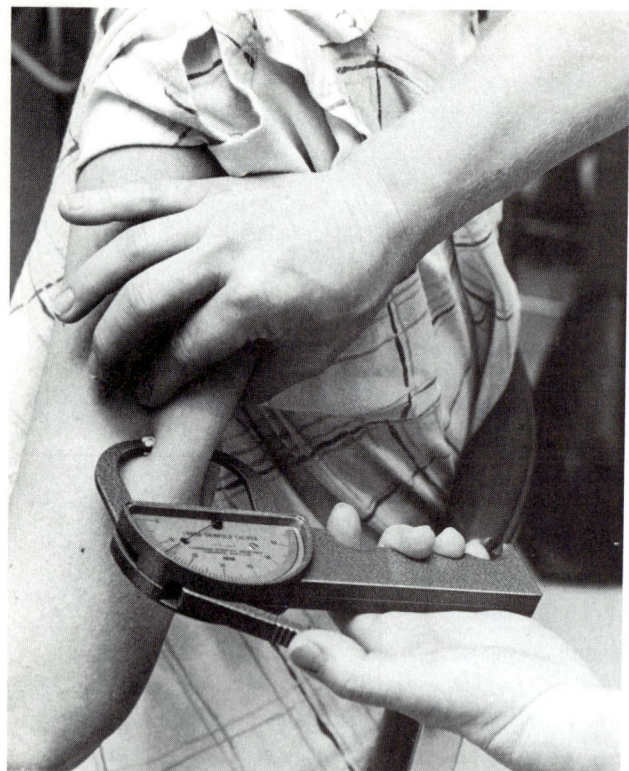

Figure 39–2 Measuring the triceps skinfold.

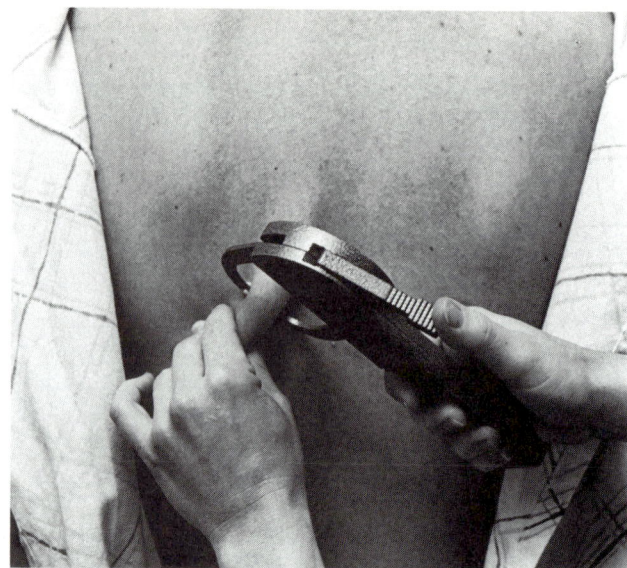

Figure 39–3 Measuring the subscapular skinfold.

total to obtain the BMI (69 divided by 2.89 equals 24). A BMI from 20 to 27 is generally considered healthy, although the risk of health problems (e.g., heart disease) increases with an index over 25.

A **skinfold measurement** indicates the amount of body fat, the main form of stored energy. The fold of skin includes the subcutaneous tissue but not the underlying muscle. This measurement can be considered an index of the body's energy stores. The triceps, subscapular, biceps, and supra-iliac skinfolds can be measured with special calipers. The site most commonly used is the triceps fold. This section describes only the triceps and subscapular skinfold measurements.

To measure the *triceps skinfold* (TSF), first locate the midpoint of the upper arm, then grasp the skin on the back of the upper arm along the long axis of the humerus. See Figure 39–2. Placing the calipers 1 cm (0.4 in) below the fingers, measure the thickness of the fold to the nearest millimeter. Average ranges for white adults over 25 years of age are 10 to 12 mm in men and 21 to 25 mm in women. However, wide variations occur (National Center for Health Statistics). To measure the *subscapular skinfold,* pick up the skin below the scapula. Three fingers should be on top of the fold just below the scapula, the thumb below the fold, and the forefinger at the lower tip of the scapula. The skinfold should be angled about 45° from the horizontal, upward medially and downward laterally. See Figure 39–3. Place

the calipers about 1 cm (0.4 in) above or below the fingers, and measure the skinfold.

Since muscle serves as the major protein reserve of the body, the **arm muscle circumference (AMC)** can be considered an index of the body's protein reserves. The arm muscle circumference is calculated from the triceps skinfold and mid-upper-arm circumference (MUAC). To measure the MUAC, make sure the client's upper arm hangs freely in a dependent position and the forearm is positioned horizontally. Locate the midpoint of the upper arm, i.e., halfway between the acromial process and the olecranon process. See Figure 39–4. Use a tape measure calibrated in millimeters to measure the circumference of the arm at the midpoint. Read the measurement to the nearest millimeter. Maintain the tape in a horizontal plane and avoid distortion of the skin surface. Average mid-upper arm circumferences for white adults over 25 years of age are 319 to 322 mm in men and 277 to 299 in women (Ibid).

Use the following formula to calculate the AMC in millimeters:

$$AMC = MUAC\ (mm) - [3.14 \times triceps\ skin\ fold\ (mm)]$$

Tables can be used instead. Average arm muscle circumferences for white adults over 25 years of age are 279 to 281 mm in men and 212 to 220 mm in women.

Biochemical Data

Biochemical measurements can be used to detect subclinical malnutrition. In contrast to anthropometric measures, which let the nurse assess observable changes in the body, laboratory tests help the nurse determine what is happening inside the body. Blood and urine samples are taken to

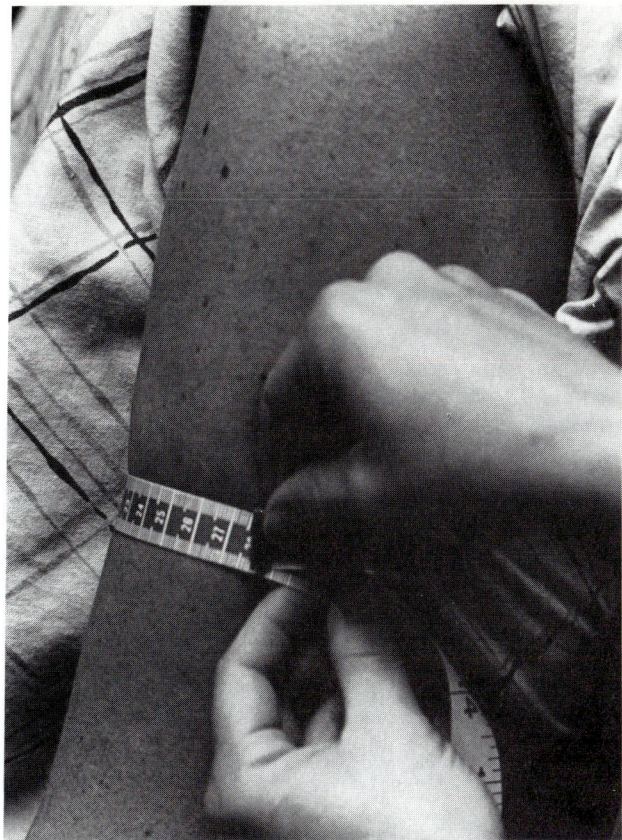

Figure 39–4 Measuring the mid-upper arm circumference.

measure a nutrient or a **metabolite** (end product or enzyme) that is affected by that nutrient. Blood tests are often ordered in packages referred to as SMAs (simultaneous multiple analysis) followed by a number, e.g., SMA-12 or SMA-18. Each package includes several biochemical measurements; the number following SMA indicates the number of tests that will be done.

The laboratory studies most commonly used today to assess nutrition include hemoglobin and hematocrit, total lymphocyte count, albumin, transferrin, nitrogen balance, and creatinine excretion tests. Although less commonly used, other laboratory tests can be performed to assess vitamins, minerals, and trace elements. Because many factors can influence these laboratory tests, no single test can confirm a nutritional problem.

Hemoglobin and Hematocrit Indices

A low hemoglobin level may be evidence of iron-deficiency anemia. **Hematocrit** (Hct), or packed cell volume, is a measure of the percentage of a given volume of whole blood occupied by red blood cells. Thus, a hematocrit of 45% indicates that 45 ml of each deciliter of peripheral blood is composed of red blood cells. An elevated hematocrit level is evidence of dehydration.

Serum Albumin

Albumin, which accounts for over 50% of the total serum proteins, helps to maintain fluid and electrolyte balance and to transport many nutrients, hormones, and drugs. Albumin synthesis depends on healthy, functioning liver cells and on an appropriate supply of amino acids. Albumin is a useful indicator of prolonged protein depletion. Because there is so much albumin in the body and because it is not broken down very quickly, albumin concentrations change slowly.

Many conditions besides malnutrition can depress albumin concentration, however. These include liver disease, advanced kidney disease, infection, cancer, and malabsorption disorders. Thus serum albumin level is used as only one indicator among several to determine protein status.

Transferrin

Transferrin is a blood protein that binds with iron and transports it throughout the body. Transferrin level is considered a more sensitive indicator of protein malnutrition than albumin level, because transferrin responds more promptly to changes in protein intake and has a smaller body pool.

Most transferrin is synthesized in the liver. Transferrin levels are high when iron stores are low and low when iron stores are excessive. Certain diseases, e.g., liver disease, advanced kidney disease, and burns, also cause decreases in transferrin levels.

Because some laboratories do not have the equipment required to determine transferrin levels directly, an estimate of a client's transferrin level is obtained by measuring the total iron-binding capacity (TIBC). The TIBC test is more widely available. The equation for converting the TIBC reading to a transferrin measurement is determined in each laboratory.

Total Lymphocyte Count

Certain nutrient deficiencies and forms of PCM (protein-calorie malnutrition) can depress the immune system. The total number of lymphocytes decreases as protein depletion occurs.

Nitrogen Balance

Nitrogen balance is discussed on page 991. Nitrogen balance studies are useful in estimating the degree to which protein is being depleted or replaced in the body. Tests to measure nitrogen balance include the blood urea nitrogen (BUN) and the urine urea nitrogen (UUN), which requires the collection of urine excreted by the client during a 24-hour period. Urea is the chief end product of protein and amino acid metabolism. It is formed from ammonia detoxified by the liver and transported to the kidneys for excretion in urine. Urea concentrations in the blood and urine, therefore, are directly influenced by the intake and breakdown of dietary protein, the rate of urea production in the liver, and the rate of urea removal by the kidneys. Elevated BUN levels may be caused by excessive protein intake, severe dehydration, or general ill health and malnutrition; however, the most common cause is inadequate excretion of urea due to kidney disease or urinary obstruction. Decreased BUN levels may be caused by a low-protein diet. Elevated BUN levels may occur with starvation.

Creatinine Excretion   Creatinine is the chief end product of the creatine produced when energy is released from phosphocreatine, an energy-storing compound, during skeletal muscle metabolism. The rate of creatinine formation is directly proportional to the total muscle mass. Creatinine is removed from the bloodstream by the kidneys and excreted in the urine at a rate that closely parallels its formation. Creatinine excretion, therefore, reflects a person's total muscle mass. As skeletal muscle atrophies during malnutrition, creatinine excretion decreases.

Measurement of urinary creatinine requires collection of urine excreted by the client during a 24-hour period. Standards for creatinine excretion are developed on the basis of sex and height. These standards are used with the creatinine measurement to determine the creatinine height index (CHI) expressed as a percentage. For example, a CHI of 70% means that the client's skeletal muscle mass is approximately 70% of that expected in a person of the same size.

Clinical Signs

Since nutrition affects most body systems, an assessment of these systems can reveal nutritional problems. Table 39–10 lists some of the data that can be collected to assist nursing personnel in determining a client's nutritional status. This list is not exhaustive; for more detailed information, consult nutrition and assessment texts. A thorough assessment is usually done with the initial physical examination when the client is admitted to a health care agency. The data obtained serve as baseline data for comparison with later findings during the client's stay.

Dietary History

A dietary history generally includes data about the client's usual eating patterns and habits, food preferences and restrictions, daily fluid intake, use of vitamin or mineral supplements, any dietary problems (e.g., difficulty chewing or swallowing), physical activity, health history, and concerns related to food buying and preparation. See Figure 39–5 for an abbreviated nutritional history tool for an adult.

To obtain data about eating patterns and habits, the nurse elicits a typical 24-hour diet history. More detailed records of the client's food intake can be kept over a 3-day period, including 1 weekend day. Such a record enables the nurse and the client to compare the data listed with recommended daily allowances or to determine whether the client is receiving a nutritionally balanced diet. The nurse also acquires the client's perspective of the nutritional status. Nurses must not judge differences from their own practices. A question about what foods the client considers harmful or helpful to health is beneficial in eliciting cultural data.

Data about the client's medication intake are also important, especially in relation to mealtimes. Many medications are to be taken only before or after meals, so variations

TABLE 39–10   *Clinical Signs Indicating Nutritional Status*

Body Part or System	Normal Signs	Abnormal Signs
Hair	Shiny, neither dry nor oily	Oily, dry, dull, patchy in growth
Skin	Smooth slightly moist, good turgor	Dry, oily, broken out in rash, scaly, rough, bruised
Eyes	Bright, clear	Dry, reddened
Tongue	Pink, moist	Reddened in patches, swollen
Mucous membranes	Reddish pink, moist	Reddened, dry, cracked
Cardiovascular	Heart rate and blood pressure within normal ranges, heart rhythm regular	Rapid heart rate, elevated blood pressure, irregular heart rhythm
Muscles	Firm, well developed	Poor in tone, soft, underdeveloped
Gastrointestinal	Appetite good, elimination regular and normal	Manifesting anorexia, indigestion, diarrhea, constipation
Neurologic	Reflexes normal, alert, good attention span, emotionally stable	Reflexes decreased, irritable, inattentive, confused, emotionally labile
Vitality	Vigorous, energetic, able to sleep well	Lacking energy, tired, apathetic, sleeping poorly
Weight	Normal for age, build, and height	Overweight, underweight

NUTRITIONAL HISTORY

Name _____

Age _____ Height _____

WEIGHT
Current weight _____

Weight history (obesity, onset, fluctuations) _____

Percentage of

Overweight _____

Underweight _____

OTHER ANTHROPOMETRIC DATA
Triceps skin fold measurement _____

Arm muscle circumference _____

EATING PATTERNS AND HABITS
1. Typical day's food intake

Time	Item	Portion
_____	_____	_____
_____	_____	_____
_____	_____	_____
_____	_____	_____
_____	_____	_____
_____	_____	_____
_____	_____	_____
_____	_____	_____
_____	_____	_____
_____	_____	_____
_____	_____	_____
_____	_____	_____
_____	_____	_____

2. Food likes _____

_____

3. Food dislikes _____

_____

4. Food allergies _____

_____

5. Foods considered harmful or beneficial to health

Harmful _____

_____

Beneficial _____

_____

6. Food restrictions

Special diet _____

Religious _____

Cultural _____

7. Fluid intake

Number of glasses of water per day _____

Number of cups of tea or coffee per day _____

Number of soft drinks per day _____

Amount of alcohol or wine per day _____

8. Use of vitamins

Kind _____

Frequency _____

9. Use of minerals (eg, calcium, iron)

Kind _____

Frequency _____

10. Perception of diet

Nutritionally balanced _____

Not nutritionally balanced _____

DIETARY PROBLEMS
1. Describe appetite (usual, increased, decreased) _____

_____

2. Foods causing indigestion, diarrhea, or gas _____

_____

3. Difficulty following special diet

Yes _____ No _____

If yes, how _____

4. Chewing difficulties

Number of teeth

Upper _____ Lower _____

Dentures

Partial _____

Complete _____

Fit of dentures _____

5. Swallowing difficulties _____

6. Usual bowel movements _____

HEALTH HISTORY
1. Physical activity

Type _____

Frequency _____

2. Medication intake

Name _____

Time _____

3. History of diseases, surgical procedures, or weight problems

	Yes	No
Diabetes	____	____
Heart problems	____	____
Surgery (specify) _____	____	____
Cancer	____	____
Kidney stones	____	____
Gallstones	____	____
Ulcers	____	____
Intestinal disorder	____	____
Allergies other than food (specify) _	____	____
_____		
Weight problems	____	____

4. Perception of general health

Good _____

Satisfactory _____

Poor _____

FOOD BUYING AND PREPARATION
1. Ingredients used

Salt _____

Soy _____

MSG _____

Other _____

2. Methods most used

Boil _____

Bake _____

Fry _____

Broil _____

Steam _____

Other _____

3. Shopping/cooking capabilities

Is able to shop _____

Relies on others _____

Is able to cook _____

Relies on others _____

4. Living situation

Number of family members _____

Lives alone _____

5. Do food costs affect diet?

Yes _____ No _____

How? _____

Figure 39–5 A sample adult nutritional history tool.

Diet History

- Chewing or swallowing difficulties (including ill-fitting dentures, dental caries, and missing teeth)
- Inadequate food intake
- Restricted or fad diets
- No intake for 10 or more days
- Intravenous fluids (other than total parenteral nutrition for 10 or more days)
- Inadequate food budget
- Inadequate food preparation facilities
- Inadequate food storage facilities
- Physical disabilities
- Elderly living and eating alone

Medical History

- Weight 20% greater than ideal
- Weight 10% less than ideal
- Unintentional weight loss or gain of 10% within 6 months
- Recent major illness
- Recent major surgery
- Surgery of the GI tract
- Anorexia
- Nausea
- Vomiting
- Diarrhea
- Alcoholism
- Cancer
- Liver disease
- Kidney disease
- Diabetes
- Thyroid or parathyroid disease
- Adrenal disease
- Mental disability
- Teenage pregnancy
- Multiple pregnancies
- Pancreatic insufficiency
- Radiation therapy

Medication History*

- Aspirin
- Antacid
- Antidepressants
- Antihypertensives
- Antiinflammatory agents
- Antineoplastic agents
- Digitalis
- Laxatives
- Diuretics (thiazides)
- Potassium chloride

*The potential effects of medications on nutrition are shown in Table 39–9.

from the usual breakfast-lunch-dinner mealtimes need to be documented.

Two commonly used approaches for analyzing the data obtained from the dietary history involve using daily food group guides and food composition tables. Using daily food group guides is a relatively workable approach for the nurse and provides a quick estimate of the client's nutritional balance. The nurse simply determines whether the client is receiving the daily recommended servings of the four basic food groups.

Dietary analyses using food composition tables provide more specific data about specific nutrient intake. This calculation method takes time. Fortunately, computerized nutrient data bases and diet analysis software have been developed.

Identifying Clients at Risk for Nutritional Problems

To identify clients at risk for nutritional problems, the nurse considers data from the client's dietary history, medication history, and medical history. Any person who has a condition that interferes with the ability to ingest, digest, absorb, and metabolize nutrients can be considered at risk (see *Health Status,* page 1004). Clients who have an increased demand for nutrients to meet metabolic needs may also be at risk, e.g., pregnant women, clients with hyperthyroidism, and those with cancer. Certain medical therapies place clients at risk. Surgery, for example, often interferes with food intake and, if performed on any part of the alimentary tract, may temporarily alter the ingestion, digestion, and absorption of nutrients. Clients undergoing radiation therapy may also experience nutritional problems (see *Health Status,* page 1004). Medications, as noted earlier, can alter the absorption and metabolism of nutrients. See Table 39–9, earlier. A summary of risk factors for nutritional problems is shown in the accompanying box.

DIAGNOSING

Nursing diagnoses that may apply to clients with or at risk for nutritional problems are broadly stated as **Altered nutrition** and further categorized as **Less than body requirements** (insufficient intake), **More than body requirements** (excessive intake), or **Potential for more than body requirements.** "Intake" here is a relative term that depends on the client's energy expenditures. For example, a person who eats an apparently balanced and adequate diet but who routinely performs rigorous physical activity may have a nutritional deficit. Similarly, a client may have what appears to be a "normal" intake that is, in fact, excessive in light of the person's minimal activity level.

Altered nutrition: Less than body requirements is the state in which the intake of one or more nutrients required to meet metabolic needs is insufficient. When possible, the nurse should state the specific deficit, e.g., inadequate intake of protein, iron, or vitamin C. Indications of nutritional deficits of specific vitamins are outlined in Table 39–2. A very severe protein deficit results in **kwashiorkor,** a disease of many Eastern undernourished populations. It is characterized by retarded growth and development; mental apathy; extreme muscular wasting, which may be masked by edema; depigmentation of the hair and skin; and scaly changes in skin texture.

Generalized nutritional deficits may be indicated by the following signs:

- Inadequate food intake less than the daily recommended dietary allowance (with or without weight loss)
- Body weight 10% to 20% below ideal for height and frame
- Body mass index below 20
- Triceps skinfold measurement, mid-arm circumference, and mid-arm muscle circumference less than 60% of the standard measurement
- Reported or evidence of lack of food
- Aversion to eating
- Perceived or actual inability to ingest food
- Muscular weakness and tenderness
- Reduced energy level
- Decreased hemoglobin, serum albumin, serum transferrin, and BUN levels

Altered nutrition: More than body requirements is the condition in which calorie intake exceeds metabolic need. People become obese by eating too much food or eating too many foods of high caloric density. **Caloric density** describes the number of kilocalories per unit weight of food. Fats and oils have the highest caloric density, whereas vegetables such as celery and lettuce have low densities. Energy expenditure is also a factor in weight control. By increasing activity, the individual increases energy expenditure and often decreases weight. **Obesity** is present when the weight is 20% greater than the ideal for height and frame. Currently one of the most prevalent health problems in North America, obesity is associated with hypertension, cardiovascular disease, and diabetes. **Overweight** refers to weight 10% greater than the ideal for height and frame. Excessive intake is also manifested when the triceps skinfold is greater than 15 mm in men and 25 mm in women (Carpenito 1989, p. 551).

Altered nutrition: Potential for more than body requirements is the state in which a person is at risk of consuming nutrients in excess of metabolic needs. Defining characteristics of this diagnosis are usually similar to the risk factors or etiology. Examples of these diagnoses with possible contributing factors are shown below. The etiology of **Altered nutrition: More than body requirements** is often complex, with psychologic, metabolic, and sociocultural implications. Because the focus of treatment is often

TABLE 39–11 *Examples of Assessment Data Clusters and Related Nursing Diagnoses*

Assessment Data Cluster	Nursing Diagnosis
Mark Malakoff, a 71-year-old Ukranian, has a history of COLD. He says, "I'm not interested in food. Even if I were, I don't have the energy to buy food. It's too much bother to fix meals for just me." (His wife died two years ago.) Height, 5'10"; weight, 61.2 kg; triceps skinfold measurement, 9.2 mm; arm muscle circumference, 20.4. Dietary assessment indicates insufficient daily intake of fruits and vegetables. Eats mostly bread, cereal, whole milk, and canned fish and meats.	**Altered nutrition: Less than body requirements** related to anorexia and physical and psychologic inability to procure and prepare food
Rose Rosenthal, a 27-year-old taxi dispatcher, says both her mother and father, who are pastry cooks, are "fat but jolly." "I love Dad's iced doughnuts and often bring a package to work to munch on through the day. I hate exercise, but at this rate, I'm going to have to do something, or I'll end up looking like mum and dad." Height, 5'4"; weight, 58.9 kg.	**Altered nutrition: Potential for more than body requirements** related to inappropriate eating patterns, familial disposition, and sedentary life-style

behavior modification and change in life-style, the diagnostic category **Altered health maintenance** related to excessive intake for metabolic requirements may be more relevant for some individuals (Carpenito 1989, p. 551). Examples of assessment data clusters and related nursing diagnoses are shown in Table 39–11.

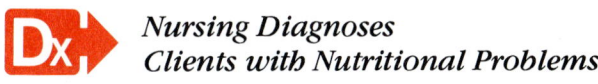 *Nursing Diagnoses Clients with Nutritional Problems*

Altered nutrition: Less than body requirements related to:

- Inability to ingest or digest food secondary to biologic or psychologic factors (e.g., anorexia, ill-fitting dentures, anxiety)
- Inability to absorb nutrients secondary to biologic or psychologic factors (e.g., malabsorption condition, severe stress and anxiety)

- Inability or difficulty to procure food secondary to economic, biologic, or physical factors (e.g., inadequate finances, lack of transportation, physical disability)
- Knowledge deficit about, for example, calcium requirements to prevent osteoporosis

Altered nutrition: More than body requirements related to:

- Excessive intake of foods high in caloric density or of supplements (vitamin and/or mineral) in relation to energy expenditure

Altered nutrition: Potential for more than body requirements related to:

- Reported or observed obesity in one or both parents
- Pattern of excessive food intake in early infancy and childhood
- Genetic predisposition
- Reported or observed use of food for comfort or reward
- Sedentary habits (low activity level)
- Inappropriate eating patterns (e.g., eating large amounts of carbohydrates and saturated fats or eating the largest meal at the end of the day)
- Frequent, closely spaced pregnancies
- Reported or observed higher baseline weight at the beginning of pregnancy

Because nutritional problems may affect other areas of human functioning, other NANDA nursing diagnoses may apply to certain individuals. In this case, the nutritional problem is the *etiology* of the diagnosis. Examples are **Activity intolerance** related to inadequate intake of iron-rich foods, resulting in iron deficiency anemia; **Constipation** related to inadequate fluid and fiber intake; **Diarrhea** related to excessive intake of alcohol, sugar, or fiber; **Knowledge deficit** related to inadequate nutritional information or misinterpretation of information; **Self-esteem disturbance** related to obesity; and **Potential impaired skin integrity** related to insufficient intake of tissue-building nutrients.

PLANNING

Overall client goals for persons with nutritional problems include maintaining, improving, or restoring nutritional status and preventing nutritional problems. Nursing interventions to achieve planned goals may include the following:

- Counseling clients to help them change eating habits
- Instructing clients about newly prescribed therapeutic diets

- Implementing measures to stimulate clients' appetites
- Feeding clients or assisting them to eat with self-feeding aids
- Providing increased numbers of feedings or high-calorie foods
- Helping clients choose healthy foods within their financial means
- Informing clients about appropriate community resources (e.g., adult education programs, nutritionist's services)
- Administering and/or teaching clients about alternative feeding methods via nasogastric tube or gastrostomy or jejunostomy stomas
- Monitoring food and fluid intake, daily calorie counts, weight and skinfold measurements

Examples of outcome criteria to evaluate the achievement of goals and the effectiveness of nursing interventions are shown below.

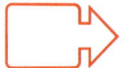

Outcome Criteria
Clients with Nutritional Problems

The client:

- Identifies factors contributing to inadequate (or excessive) nutritional intake.
- Explains necessary dietary alterations (foods to include and avoid).
- Keeps a log of foods ingested in a 7-day period.
- Has a triceps skinfold measurement, AMC, and BMI within predetermined ranges.
- Has a stable daily weight, or weight increase of 2 kg/week, or decrease of 1.5 kg/week.
- Feeds self independently using self-feeding aid.
- Plans a balanced meal using the diet information provided.
- Identifies foods high in specific nutrients (e.g., calcium, iron, potassium)
- Reports decrease (or absence of) signs of malnutrition cited in the defining characteristics.
- Demonstrates life-style changes to regain or maintain weight at satisfactory level for height and body build.

IMPLEMENTING

Teaching is an important aspect of nursing intervention for clients with nutritional problems. Depending on clients' learning needs, specific information concerning a prescribed diet or general counseling on nutrition may be planned. Clients with problems involving the actual intake of nutrients are assisted by nurses to attain the specific nutrients required.

Counseling about Nutrition

Nutrition counseling involves much more than simply providing information. The nurse must help clients integrate diet changes into their life-styles and provide strategies to motivate them to change their eating habits. Counseling can be likened to the teaching-learning process discussed in Chapter 16. First, the nurse assesses the client's nutritional status and nutrient intake thoroughly. Next, the nurse finds out what the client knows about nutrition. At this point, nurses must assess their own knowledge of the client's specific learning needs and, if necessary, obtain the appropriate information or refer the client to an expert on the subject. Then the client and nurse set goals or objectives for learning, plan strategies to achieve the goals, and establish criteria to evaluate achievement of the goals. Because it is the client's responsibility to make the necessary dietary changes and to change behavior, the nurse's role is to support and encourage the client.

Teaching about Special Diets

Assisting clients and support persons with special or therapeutic diets prescribed by the physician is a function shared by the dietitian and the nurse. The dietitian informs the client and support persons about the specific foods allowed and not allowed and assists the client with meal planning. The nurse reinforces this instruction, assists the client to make beneficial changes, and evaluates the client's response to the planned changes.

Physicians order special diets for clients who cannot eat the usual foods. A special or therapeutic diet is one in which the amount of food, the kind of food, or the frequency of eating is prescribed. Special diets are used to treat a disease process, e.g., a low-salt diet for high blood pressure; to prepare for a special examination or surgery; and to promote health, e.g., a low-calorie diet for an overweight client.

Some diets are temporary, observed perhaps for one meal or 1 week, but some clients must follow certain diets (e.g., the diabetic diet) for a lifetime. If the diet is long term, the client must not only understand the diet but also develop a healthy, positive attitude toward it. The client needs to know the consequences of choosing not to comply with the prescribed dietary regimen. Progressive hospital diets (e.g., postoperative dietary protocols) are often unique to institutions, and nurses need to be familiar with the diets prescribed in their agencies.

Clients who do not have special needs eat the **regular diet,** whose quantity and content are designed to meet the needs of most clients. In some agencies, the regular diet is referred to as the normal, house, or standard diet. Some hospitals offer clients a daily menu from which to select their meals for the next day. Other hospitals provide standard meals to each client on the general diet. Certain foods (e.g., cabbage, which tends to produce flatus, and highly seasoned and fried foods, which are difficult for some people to digest) are usually omitted from the regular diet.

A variation of the regular diet is the **light diet,** designed for postoperative and other clients who are not ready for the regular diet. Foods in the light diet are plainly cooked. Foods containing large amounts of fat are usually omitted, as are bran and foods containing a great deal of fiber. Not all agencies provide a light diet.

A **soft diet** is easily chewed and digested. It is often ordered for clients who have difficulty chewing and swallowing. It is a lightly seasoned, low-residue (low-fiber) diet. Examples of foods that can be included in a soft or semisoft diet are shown in the box below. The **pureed diet** is a modification of the soft diet. Liquid may be added to the food, which is then blended to a semisolid consistency.

Food Suggestions for a Soft Diet

Meats and Alternates

Any tender meat, fish, poultry (chopped or shredded)

Chopped meat in cream sauce

Omelet or scrambled egg

Spaghetti sauce with chopped meat over small shaped pasta

Cottage cheese

Vegetables

Rice in cream or cheese sauce

Mashed potatoes

Mashed sweet potatoes

Mashed squash

Mashed potatoes with chopped spinach

Vegetables in cream or cheese sauce

Vegetables pureed with diced vegetables (e.g., carrot or turnip puree with baby peas)

Avocado

Cauliflower

Asparagus tips

Spinach

Fruits

Chunky apple sauce

Ripe banana

Cooked, peeled fresh fruits

Canned fruits

Desserts

Pudding

Custard

Ice Cream

Yogurt

Pudding cake

Junket

Gelatin

Sherbet

Soft cake

Cereals and Breads

Cooked cereal

Crustless bread

Liquids

All allowed (except when restricted by physician)

A **full liquid diet** contains only liquids or foods that turn to liquid at room temperature, such as ice cream. Full liquid diets are eaten by clients who have gastrointestinal disturbances or are otherwise unable to tolerate solid or semisolid foods. Full fluid foods are free of cellulose, irritating condiments such as mustard or ketchup, and spices such as black pepper or chili powder. This diet is not recommended for long-term use. Its iron content, protein content, and caloric density are low, and its cholesterol content is high because of the amount of milk offered. Clients who must receive only liquids for longer periods are usually given a nutritionally balanced oral supplement, e.g., Sustacal. The full liquid diet is monotonous and difficult for clients to accept. Planning six or more feedings per day may encourage a more adequate intake.

The **clear liquid diet** is often limited to water, tea, coffee, clear broths, ginger ale or other carbonated beverages, apple juice, and plain gelatin. It does not permit milk. This diet provides the client with fluid and carbohydrate (in the form of sugar) but does not supply adequate protein, fat, vitamins, minerals, or calories. No more than 600 kcal/day are provided. It is usually a short-term diet (24 to 36 hours) provided for clients after certain surgery or for clients in the acute stages of infection, particularly of the gastrointestinal tract. The major objective of this diet is to relieve thirst, prevent dehydration, and minimize stimulation of the gastrointestinal tract. Clear fluids are offered throughout the day as tolerated by the client.

There are many other special diets, sometimes especially devised for individual clients. Details about these diets are provided in nutrition and medical/surgical nursing textbooks. Common special diets are reducing, diabetic, low-salt, and allergy diets.

Clients often need assistance in adapting special diets to their cultural, religious, ethnic, and economic patterns. Most diets in North America are devised for the Anglo-American taste and omit many otherwise acceptable ethnic foods. Such a diet may be unfamiliar or unpalatable to the ethnic client. Nutritionists and dietitians can often assist nurses to adapt a diet to suit a person's life-style. Another important aspect is adapting a diet to a person's economic status. Often, less costly foods can be substituted for recommended foods, such as powdered milk for fresh milk.

Motivation is highly important for success. Clients who do not accept the need for a diet will probably not adhere to it, and its therapeutic value will be lost. A client may understand that sugar in coffee is not allowed on a low-calorie diet but may not understand that bread also contains sugar and is also restricted. An elderly woman may understand that she is not to add salt to foods when cooking but salts her food at the table. This client does not really understand the importance of or the reason for salt restriction.

Stimulating Appetite

Because of accompanying physical illness, unfamiliar food or food the client finds unpalatable, environmental and psychologic factors, and physical discomfort or pain, many hospitalized clients have poor appetites. Lowered food intake of a few days' duration is not often a problem for adults; however, a prolonged decreased food intake leads to weight loss, decreased strength and stamina, and subsequent nutritional problems. Decreased food intake is often accompanied by decreased fluid intake, which may cause fluid and electrolyte problems. See Chapter 40 for further information.

Increasing a person's appetite requires determining the reason for the lack of appetite and then dealing with the problem. Some guidelines for interventions that may improve the client's appetite are summarized in the box in the left column.

Assisting Clients with Meals

Because clients are frequently confined to their beds, particularly in acute care settings, most hospitals must have meals brought to the client. Often the client receives a tray that has been assembled in a central hospital kitchen or a kitchen adjacent to the nursing unit. Nursing personnel may be responsible for giving out and collecting the trays; in some settings this is done by special dietary personnel. Some hospitals serve meals to ambulatory clients in a special dining area, and the clients are expected to go there to eat. Other agencies, e.g., day-care centers, have a coffee shop for food or machines from which clients can obtain sandwiches and beverages. Guidelines for providing meals to clients are summarized in the box on the opposite page.

Improving Appetite

- Relieve illness symptoms that deaden appetite prior to mealtime; e.g., give an analgesic for pain or an antipyretic for a fever or allow rest for fatigue.

- Provide familiar food that the person likes. Often the relatives of clients are pleased to bring food from home but may need some guidance about special diet requirements.

- Select small portions so as not to discourage the anorexic client.

- Avoid unpleasant or uncomfortable treatments immediately before or after a meal.

- A tidy, clean environment that is free of unpleasant sights and odors is important. A soiled dressing, a used bedpan, an uncovered irrigation set, or even used dishes can destroy appetite.

- Reduce psychologic stress. A lack of understanding of therapy, the anticipation of an operation, and fear of the unknown can cause anorexia. Often, the nurse can help by discussing feelings with the client, giving information and assistance, and allaying fears.

Providing Client Meals

- Check the client's chart or Kardex for the diet order and to determine whether the client is fasting for laboratory tests or surgery or whether the physician has ordered "nothing by mouth" (NPO). For clients who are fasting or on NPO, ensure that the appropriate signs are placed on either the room door or the client's bed, according to agency practice.

- If there is a change in the type of food the client is to receive, notify the dietary staff.

- Assist the client to the bathroom or onto a bedpan or commode if the client needs to urinate.

- Offer the client assistance in washing the hands prior to a meal. If the client has problems with oral hygiene, brushing the teeth or using a mouthwash can improve the taste in the mouth and hence the appetite.

- Assist the client to a comfortable position for eating. Most people sit during a meal; if it is permitted, assist the client to sit in bed (see Figure 39–6) or in a chair, whichever is appropriate.

- Clear the overbed table so that there is space for the tray. If the client must remain in a lying position in bed, arrange the overbed table close to the bedside, so that the client can see the food.

- Check each tray for the client's name, the type of diet, and completeness. If the diet does not seem to be correct, check it against the client's chart. Confirm the client's name by checking the wristband before leaving the tray. Do *not* leave an incorrect diet for a client to eat.

- Assist the client as required, e.g., to remove the food covers, butter the bread, pour the tea, and cut the meat.

- For a blind person, identify the placement of the food as you would describe the time on a clock. For instance, the nurse may say, "The potatoes are at eight o'clock; the beef steak at 12 o'clock; and the green beans at 4 o'clock." See Figure 39–7.

- After the client has completed the meal, replace the food covers, and note how much and what the client has eaten and the amount of fluid taken. Record fluid intake and calorie count as required.

- If the client is on a special diet or is having problems eating, record the amount of food eaten and any pain, fatigue, or nausea experienced.

- If the client is not eating, notify the nurse in charge so that the diet can be changed or other nursing measures can be taken, e.g., rescheduling the meals, providing smaller, more frequent meals, or obtaining special self-feeding aids.

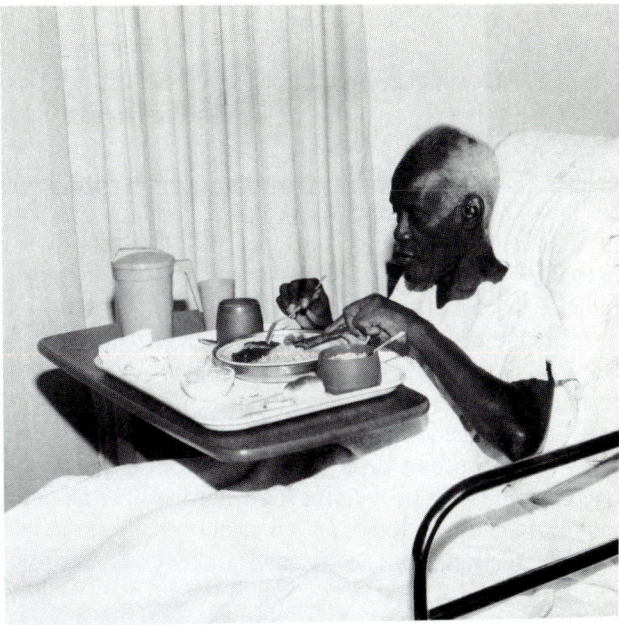

Figure 39–6 A supported sitting position contributes to a client's comfort while eating.

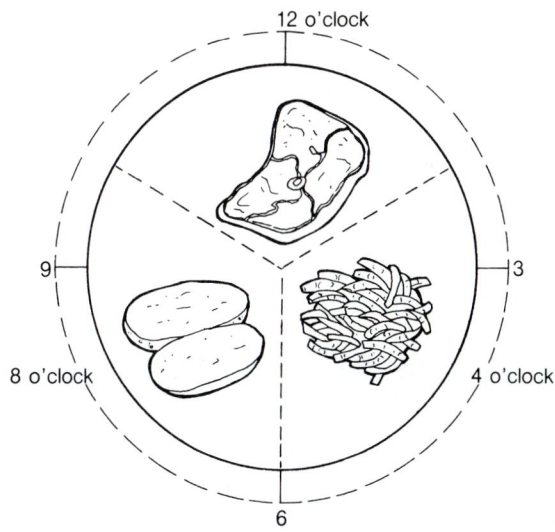

Figure 39–7 If the client is blind, the nurse can use the clock system to describe the location of food on the plate.

Assisting Clients with Feeding

The amount and kind of assistance a client needs with eating depend on the physical and mental limitations of the client. Two groups of people frequently require help: the elderly, who are weakened and quickly fatigued when they are ill; and the handicapped, e.g., blind clients, those who must remain in a back-lying position, or those who do not have use of their hands. The client's nursing care plan will indicate that assistance is required with meals.

The nurse must be sensitive to feelings of embarrassment, resentment, and loss of autonomy in clients who cannot feed themselves. Whenever possible, the nurse should help incapacitated clients feed themselves rather than feed them. Some clients become depressed because they require help and because they believe they are burdensome to busy nursing personnel. Nurses must not convey, either verbally or nonverbally, impatience or annoyance with clients who require assistance eating. Rather, they should appear unhurried and convey that they have ample time.

Although normal utensils should be used whenever possible, the nurse may need to use special utensils to assist a client to eat. Straws help many people who have difficulty drinking from a cup or glass. Straws often permit clients to obtain liquids with less effort and with less spillage, which can be embarrassing to many clients. Special drinking cups are also available. One model has a spout; another is specially designed to permit drinking with less tipping of the cup than is normally required. See Figure 39–8.

Before feeding clients, ask them in which order they desire to eat the food. Tell a client who cannot see which food you are giving. Always allow ample time for the client to chew and swallow the food before offering more. Provide clients with fluids as requested, or, if they are unable to tell you, offer fluids after every three or four mouthfuls of solid food. Make the time a pleasant one, choosing topics of conversation that are of interest to clients who want to talk.

Many adaptive feeding aids are available to help clients maintain independence. A standard eating utensil with a built-up or widened handle helps clients who cannot grasp objects easily. Utensils with wide handles can be purchased, or a regular eating utensil can be modified by taping foam around the handle. The foam increases friction and thus steadies the client's grasp. Handles may be bent or angled to compensate for limited motion. Collars or bands that prevent the utensil from being dropped can be attached to the end of the handle and fit over the client's hand.

Plates with rims and plastic or metal plate guards enable the client to pick up the food by first pushing it against this raised edge. A suction cup or damp sponge or cloth may be placed under the dish to keep it from moving while the client is eating. No-spill mugs and two-handled drinking cups are especially useful for persons with impaired hand coordination. Stretch terry cloth and knitted or crocheted glass covers enable the client to keep a secure grasp on a glass. Lidded tip-proof glasses are also available. Figures 39–9 and 39–10 show some of these eating aids.

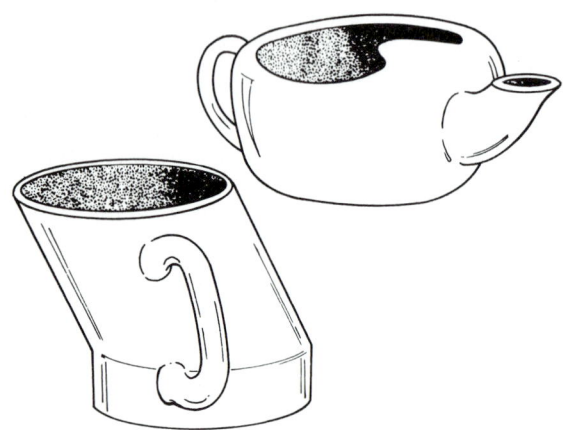

Figure 39–8   Two types of special drinking cups.

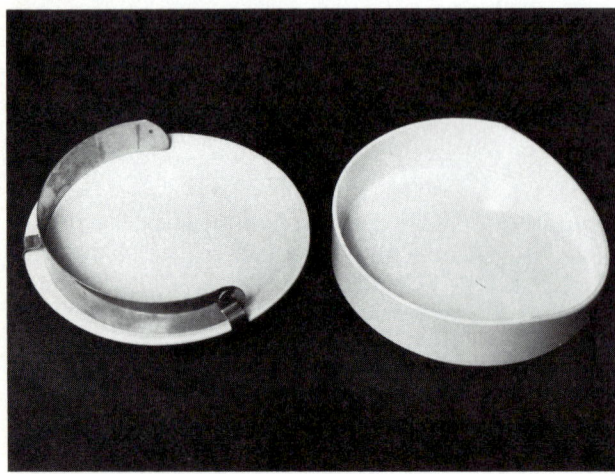

Figure 39–9   Left to right: *A,* dinner plate with guard attached; *B,* lipped plate.

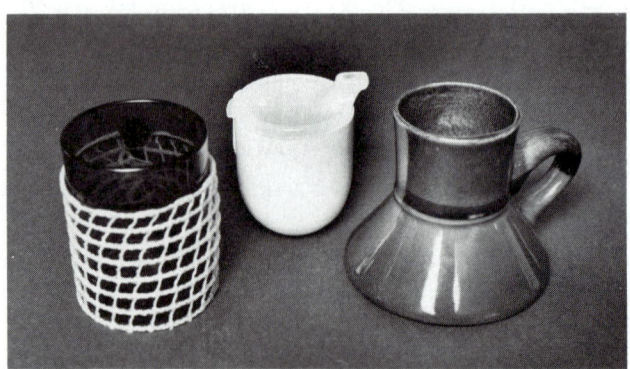

Figure 39–10   Left to right: *A,* stretch terry cloth or knitted glass cover; *B,* lidded, tip-proof glass; *C,* no-spill mug.

Special Community Nutritional Services

In many areas, community programs have been developed to help special subgroups of the population meet their nutritional needs. For the elderly who cannot prepare meals or leave their home, ready-to-eat meals or frozen dinners are delivered to the home by local organizations. Meals-on-Wheels is one such well-known organization. For people who can prepare meals but are physically handicapped and unable to shop for groceries, some organizations provide grocery delivery services.

The Nutrition Program for Older Americans, administered by the Department of Health and Human Services, provides community-based noon meals at an optional nominal fee for mobile people over age 60. This program is also referred to as Title III or congregate meals for the elderly. The Title III meals are designed to provide one-third of the RDAs. In addition to providing a nutritious meal, this program offers nutrition education and health and welfare counseling. An added benefit for the participants is regular social interaction with others.

For the impoverished, the U.S. Department of Agriculture funds a food stamp program. People with low incomes can use stamps to purchase food at any approved grocery store. The value of the food stamps provided depends on the size and income of the family.

Many industries have established health maintenance programs for their employees. These programs generally include exercise facilities, education, stress management, and nutritional counseling. In some companies, the food service departments make a special effort to adhere to the recommendations of the *Dietary Guidelines*. Such programs are thought to be cost effective; illness is reduced, less time is lost from work, and employee satisfaction increases work productivity.

Alternative Feeding Methods

Clients who are unable to ingest a sufficient amount of foods and fluids through oral intake may require alternative feeding methods to ensure maintenance of adequate nutrition. These methods include both enteral (through the gastrointestinal system) and parenteral (intravenous) methods. The more common enteral feedings are administered through nasogastric and small-bore feeding tubes or through gastrostomy or jejunostomy tubes. Total parenteral nutrition (TPN), administered through the intravenous route, is discussed in Chapter 40, page 1085.

Nasogastric/Nasointestinal Feedings   A **nasogastric feeding (gastric gavage)** or small intestine tube feeding is the instillation of specially prepared nutrients into the digestive tract through a tube that is inserted through one of the nostrils, down the nasopharynx, and into the alimentary tract. In some instances, the tube is passed through the mouth and pharynx, although this route may be more uncomfortable for the adult client and cause gagging. This approach is often used for infants who are obligatory nose breathers (who must breathe through the nose) and premature infants who have no gag reflex.

Traditional firm *large-bore* nasogastric tubes (i.e., those larger than 12 Fr. in diameter) are placed in the stomach. Examples are the *Levin tube,* a flexible, rubber or plastic, single-lumen tube with holes near the tip, or the *Salem sump tube,* with a double lumen. The larger tube of the Salem sump tube drains gastric contents; the smaller tube allows for an inflow of atmospheric air which prevents a vacuum if the gastric tube adheres to the wall of the stomach. Irritation of the gastric mucosa is thereby avoided. Newer, softer, more flexible and less irritating *small-bore* tubes (smaller than 12 Fr. in diameter) can be placed in either the stomach or the upper small intestine (i.e., duodenum or jejunum). Clients at risk for pulmonary aspiration (e.g., those with altered pharyngeal reflexes and/or unconsciousness) should be fed via the small intestine rather than the stomach (Metheny 1988, p. 324).

Generally, the position of small-bore pliable tubes is confirmed by radiography before introducing feedings. A major responsibility of the nurse, however, is to verify tube placement (i.e., gastrointestinal placement versus respiratory placement) before each intermittent feeding and at regular intervals (e.g., at least once per shift) when continuous feedings are being administered. Traditionally, placement of large-bore tubes has been verified by the following methods, none of which alone is any guarantee that the tube is correctly positioned. In addition, many methods do not apply to small-bore tubes.

1. *Aspirate gastrointestinal secretions.* Gastrointestinal secretions are aspirated more readily through large-bore tubes than through small-bore tubes. Failure to obtain aspirate even with large-bore tubes may or may not indicate that the tube is malpositioned. For example, the tubing parts may be obstructed by the stomach mucosa. Failure to obtain fluid from a small-bore tube may indicate that the walls of the tube collapsed on syringe application. Findings of one clinical study (Metheny, Spies, and Eisenberg 1988, p. 367), reveal that over 50% of the attempts to aspirate even small volumes of fluid through a small-bore feeding tube were unsuccessful. However, these same researchers found that more fluid was aspirated from small-bore polyurethane tubes and #10 and #12 Fr. tubes than from small-bore silicone tubes and #8 Fr. tubes (Metheny, Spies, and Eisenberg 1988, p. 375). Furthermore, several authors (Theodore, Frank, Ende, Snider, and Beer 1984; and Hand, Kempster, Levy, Rogol, and Spirn 1984) have reported instances in which pleural fluid was aspirated from small-bore tubes inadvertently placed in the pleural space or lung. This straw-colored, clear fluid closely resembles gastric fluid and can be erroneously mistaken for gastric fluid.

2. *Measure the pH of aspirated fluid.* An acidic pH generally indicates gastric fluid. Values within the acidic range may be as low as 0.8 (with hydrochloric acid secretion) and as high as 5 (Guyton 1986, p. 774). If the client is taking medication altering the pH, some secretions may even become alkaline. Intestinal fluids have a slightly alkaline pH in the range of 7.5 to 8.0 (Guyton 1986, p. 784). Because normal pleural fluid has a pH of 7.4 (Byrne, Saxton, Pelikan, and Nugent 1986, p. 468), this test to determine placement of small-bore intestinal tubes is not effective in differentiating intestinal from pleural fluid. However, it is effective in differentiating gastric from intestinal fluid.

3. *Inject 5 to 20 ml of air through the feeding tube while auscultating the epigastrum or left upper abdominal quadrant and listening for a whooshing, gurgling, or bubbling sound.* Because of the difficulty encountered in aspirating gastrointestinal secretions through small-bore tubes, many nurses in practice prefer and use this method to test tube placement. Air injected in the stomach should be heard immediately. However, it is difficult to differentiate esophageal, gastric, distal duodenal, and proximal jejunal placement because of the proximity of these sites. Several authors also report "pseudoconfirmatory gurgling" sounds heard when the tube is malpositioned in the pharynx, esophagus, and respiratory tract (Hand, Kempster, Levy, Rogol, and Spirn 1984; Miller, Tomlinson, and Sahn 1985; and Metheny, Spies, and Eisenberg 1988). Further research may indicate more precise differentiation of sounds using a Doppler stethoscope.

4. *Ask the client to speak or hum.* It is generally assumed that large-bore tubes placed in the trachea will interfere with the client's ability to speak. However, clients with small-bore tubes may be able to speak since the vocal cords may not be sufficiently separated to affect phonation. In one study, all clients with small-bore tubes were able to speak unless they were comatose, aphasic, or intubated (Metheny, Spies, and Eisenberg 1988, p. 376).

5. *Observe the client for coughing and choking.* Coughing and choking are likely to occur when large-bore tubes enter the respiratory tract but are less likely to occur with the use of small-bore tubes. These responses, however, may be absent with either type of tube in clients with decreased tracheal irritation and an altered level of consciousness.

Currently, the most effective method appears to be radiographic verification of tube placement. Repeated x rays, however, are not feasible in terms of cost and radiation risk. More research is required to devise effective alternatives, especially for placement of small-bore tubes. In the meantime, nurses should (a) ensure initial radiographic verification of small-bore tubes, (b) aspirate contents when possible and check their acidity, (c) auscultate air insufflation, (d) closely observe the client for signs of obvious distress, and (e) suspect tube dislodgement after episodes of coughing, sneezing, and vomiting.

Tube feedings are indicated for clients who cannot eat by mouth or swallow a sufficient diet without aspirating food or fluid into the lungs. Feedings may be given continuously over a 24-hour period or at prescribed intervals, e.g., four times per day. Liquid feeding mixtures are available commercially or may be prepared by the dietary department in accordance with the physician's orders. A standard formula provides 1 kcal per milliliter of solution with protein, fat, carbohydrate, minerals, and vitamins in specified proportions. See Table 39–12 for information about various for-

TABLE 39–12 *Commercially Available Formulas for Tube Feeding*

Classification	Product Names	kcal/ml	mOsm/kg water	Advantages	Disadvantages
Blenderized	Compleat B	1	405	Nutritionally complete*	High viscosity makes administration difficult through small bore tubes
	Compleat Modified	1	300	High residue makes them ideal for elderly or those who have altered bowel function	Most contain lactose
	Vitaneed	1	375		Not for oral consumption
					Relatively expensive

TABLE 39-12 *(continued)*

Classification	Product Names	kcal/ ml	mOsm/ kg water	Advantages	Disadvantages
Milk-based	Carnation Instant Breakfast	1	615 to 650	Palatable	High lactose content
				Good for clients who have increased protein and calorie requirements	High osmolality
	Meritene	1	505 to 690		
	Sustacal Powder	1	644		
	Sustagen	1.7	1110		
Lactose-free	Ensure	1	450	Nutritionally complete*	Protein quality not as high as blenderized or milk-based formulas
	Isocal	1	300	Relatively inexpensive	
	Osmolite HN	1	310	Free-flowing consistency	
	Nutri-Aid	1	300	May be used orally	
	Osmolite	1	300		
	Portagen	1	354		
	Renu	1	300		
	Sustacal Liquid	1	625		
	Travasorb	1	450		
High density lactose-free	Ensure Plus	1.5	600	Nutritionally complete*	Protein quality not as high as blenderized or milk-based formulas
	Isocal HCN	2	740	Relatively inexpensive	
	Magnacal	2	590	Free-flowing consistency	Must be diluted and advanced slowly
	Sustacal HC	1.5	650	Ideal for fluid-restricted clients	
Chemically defined	Citrotein	0.66	500	Require minimal digestion	High osmolality
	Criticare HN	1	650		Some are relatively unpalatable
	Isotein HN	1.2	300	Lactose-free	
	Precision Isotonic	1	300	Low viscosity, so easily administered through small bore tubes	Relatively expensive
	Precision HN	1	500		Some contain minimal amounts of long-chain fats
	Precision LR	1	525 to 545		
	Travasorb HN	1	560		
	Travasorb MCT	1 to 2	300 to 500		
	Travasorb Std	1	560		
	Vital HN	1	460		
Free amino acid	Vivonex HN	1	810		
	Vivonex Std	1	550		
Specialty formulas	Amin-Aid	1.9	1095	May be given by tube or mouth	High osmolality
	Hepatic-Aid	1.6	1158		High carbohydrate
	Travasorb Hepatic	1.1	690	Require minimal digestion	Some are nutritionally incomplete
	Travasorb Renal	1.35	590		Very expensive
	Trauma-Aid	1	800		Formulas designed for trauma do not meet currently accepted standards for nutritional requirements for increased stress
	Trauma-Cal	1.5	550		
	Vivonex Ten	1	630		
	Stresstein	1.2	910		

TABLE 39–12 *Formulas for Tube Feeding (continued)*

Classification	Product Names	kcal/ml	mOsm/kg water	Advantages	Disadvantages
Modules	*Carbohydrate*			Flexible—may be combined to yield specific formula	Takes longer to prepare
	Moducal	4 kcal/g 2 kcal/ml	(powder) 752		May alter taste and/or texture if added to food
	Polycose	4 kcal/g 2 kcal/ml	(powder) 850	May be added to food	
	Sumacal	4 kcal/g	(powder)		
	Fat				
	Lipomul	6 kcal/ml	Not applicable for fats		
	MCT (medium chain triglyceride)	7.7 kcal/ml			
	Microlipid	4.5 kcal/ml			
	Protein				
	Casec	4 kcal/g	24 g protein/30 ml		
	Promix	4 kcal/g	24 g protein/30 ml		
	Propac	4 kcal/g	23 g protein/30 ml		
	Nutrisource				

*Nutritionally complete when given in appropriate volumes.

Source: N. N. Konstantinides and E. Shronts, Tube feeding: Managing the basics. *American Journal of Nursing,* September 1983, 83:1316. Reprinted with permission.

mulas. The frequency of feedings and amounts to be administered are ordered by the physician. An adult often requires 300 to 500 ml of mixture per feeding.

Before administering a tube feeding, the nurse must determine any food allergies of the client and assess tolerance to previous feedings. See the accompanying box. The nurse checks the expiration date on a commercially prepared formula or the preparation date and time of agency-prepared solution, discarding any formula that has passed the expiration date or solution more than 24 hours old.

Feedings are usually administered at room temperature unless the order specifies otherwise. The specified amount of solution is warmed in a basin of warm water or left to stand for a while until it reaches room temperature. Continuous feeding should be kept cold; excessive heat coagulates feedings of milk and egg, and hot liquids can irritate the mucous membranes. However, excessively cold feedings can reduce the flow of digestive juices by causing vasoconstriction and may cause cramps. Commercially prepared feedings are available in cans and bottles ready for administration. Some containers are designed so that ice chips can be placed in an outer section to keep the formula cooled. Table 39–13 summarizes common problems of tube feeding.

A feeding pump can be used with a prefilled tube-feeding set to regulate the exact amount of feeding for the client. See Figure 39–11. The pump is often used to administer

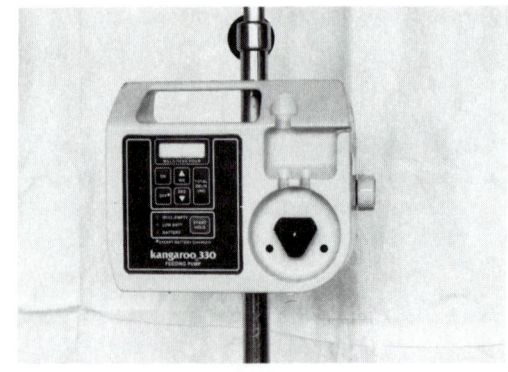

Figure 39–11 A feeding pump.

CLINICAL GUIDELINES
Tube Feedings

Assess the patient for the following:

- Allergies to any food in the feeding. Commonly included foods are milk, sugar, water, eggs, and vegetable oil.

- Bowel sounds prior to each feeding (or every 4 to 8 hours for continuous feedings) to determine intestinal activity.

- Abdominal distention at least daily. Measure the client's abdominal girth at the umbilicus. A distended abdomen may indicate intolerance to a previous feeding.

- Correct placement of the tube before feedings.

- Presence of regurgitation and feelings of fullness after feedings.

- Dumping syndrome. Jejunostomy clients may experience nausea, vomiting, diarrhea, cramps, pallor, sweating, heart palpitations, increased pulse rate, and fainting after a feeding. These are signs of dumping syndrome, which results when hypertonic foods and liquids suddenly distend the jejunum. To make the intestinal contents isotonic, body fluids shift rapidly from the client's vascular system. Smaller, more frequent feedings, slower feedings, and a longer adjustment period may relieve dumping.

- Presence of diarrhea, constipation, or flatulence. The lack of bulk in liquid feedings may cause constipation. The presence of concentrated ingredients may cause diarrhea and flatulence.

- Urine for sugar and acetone. Monitor the client's urine every 4 to 6 hours for the first 48 hours after initial feedings are begun.

- Hydration status. Measure the client's fluid intake and output, and note complaints of thirst. Additional water may need to be instilled between feedings.

Before administering the feeding:

- Check the expiration date of the feeding.

- Warm the feeding to room temperature.

- Confirm correct placement of the tube.

- Aspirate residual stomach contents, measure the amount, and check about reinstilling it or continuing the feeding.

- Remove air from the feeding tubes of feeding bag and prefilled bottles with drip chambers.

- Deliver the feeding over the desired length of time.

After the feeding:

- Rinse the nasogastric tube with water.

- Clamp the nasogastric tube before all of the rinse solution has run through.

- Have the client remain in a Fowler's or slightly elevated right lateral position for at least 30 minutes.

TABLE 39–13   *Common Problems of Tube Feedings*

Factors to Assess to Determine How Client Is Tolerating the Feeding	Possible Causes of Problems	Corrective Measures
Gastrointestinal Function		
Vomiting	Feeding too soon after intubation	Allow client to relax and rest after tube is inserted
	Improper location of tip of feeding tube	Repositioning of tube by qualified health professional
	Rapid rate of infusion	Administer slowly
	Excessive volume: (1) Air (2) Formula	Be sure tube feeding container does not run dry before feeding is completed Check with physician regarding number and size of feedings
	Position of client	Position on right side for ½ hr following feeding—reverse Trendelenburg or semi-Fowler's

TABLE 39–13 *Common Problems of Tube Feedings (continued)*

Factors to Assess to Determine How Client Is Tolerating the Feeding	Possible Causes of Problems	Corrective Measures
(Applies to both vomiting and diarrhea)	Food infection or poisoning	Check sanitation of formula and equipment
	Anxiety	Explain procedures; provide reassurance and other needed types of support; provide privacy
Diarrhea	Rapid rate of infusion	Administer slowly—very slowly if formula is cold
	High osmolality of formula or high concentration of formula	Adapt client to formula gradually
	Lactose intolerance	Contact physician regarding change of formula
Constipation	High content of milk in formula	Contact physician regarding:
	Lack of fiber	(1) Change in formula
	Inadequate fluid intake	(2) Laxatives
		(3) Increasing fluid

Fluid and Electrolyte Balance

Dehydration	Rapid infusion of carbohydrate → hyperglycemia → osmotic diuresis → dehydration	Administer slowly; exogenous insulin sometimes needed
	Excess protein and electrolytes in formula	Change formula and/or increase fluid according to physician's orders
	Inadequate fluid intake	
Edema	Excessive sodium in formula	Check with physician about change in formula

Nutritional Adequacy

Undernutrition (gradual weight loss)	Inadequate number of calories to meet energy requirements	Check to see if client is receiving prescribed amount of formula; estimate client's caloric intake
		Check with physician regarding increasing the volume, concentration, or number of feedings given
Overnutrition (gradual gain of undesirable weight)	Excessive caloric intake	Check with physician regarding decreasing the volume, concentration, or number of feedings given
Undernutrition (inadequate intake of protein and/or micronutrients leading to biochemical or clinical signs of deficiency)	Amount of standard formula needed to maintain weight is too low to meet requirements for essential nutrients	Check with physician regarding providing appropriate nutrient supplements

Source: C. W. Suitor and M. F. Hunter, *Nutrition: Principles and applications in health promotion,* 2d ed. Philadelphia: J. B. Lippincott Co., 1984. Reprinted with permission.

the feeding in instances when smaller-bore gastric tubes are used or when gravity flow is insufficient to instill the feeding. Because the feeding is administered over a long time period, a formula that is warmed can grow microorganisms. It should not hang longer than the manufacturer recommends, e.g., 3 to 4 hours. If it will hang longer, it should be kept cool with ice chips.

Although the focus of this chapter is nutrition, *nasogastric tubes* may be inserted for reasons other than providing a route for feeding the client. These include

1. To prevent nausea, vomiting, and gastric distention fol-

lowing surgery. In this case the tube is attached to a suction source.

2. To remove stomach contents for laboratory analysis.

3. To lavage (wash) the stomach in cases of poisoning or overdose of medications.

Procedure 39–1 provides guidelines for inserting a nasogastric or nasointestinal tube. Procedure 39–2 provides the essential steps involved in administering a tube feeding, and Procedure 39–3 indicates the steps involved in removing a nasogastric tube.

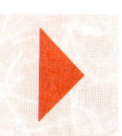

PROCEDURE 39–1

INSERTING A NASOGASTRIC TUBE

Equipment ☑

A large- or small-bore tube (plastic or rubber)

Solution basin filled with warm water or ice. Rubber tubes are placed on ice to stiffen them for easier insertion. Plastic tubes are placed in warm water to make them more flexible for insertion.

Water-soluble lubricant

20- to 50-ml syringe with an adapter

Basin

Nonallergenic adhesive tape, 2.5 cm (1 in) wide

Clamp (optional)

Suction apparatus if required

Gloves (optional)

Gauze square or plastic specimen bag and elastic band

Safety pin and elastic band

Bib or towel

Glass of water and drinking straw

Facial tissues

Stethoscope

Intervention

1. **Prepare the client.**

- Explain to the client what you plan to do. The passage of a gastric tube is not painful, but it is unpleasant because the gag reflex is activated during insertion.

- Assist the client to a high-Fowler's position if health permits, and support the head on a pillow. *It is often easier to swallow in this position, and gravity helps the passage of the tube.*

2. **Assess the client's nares.**

- Ask the client to hyperextend the head and using a flashlight observe the intactness of the tissues of the nostrils, including any irritations or abrasions.

- Examine the nares for any obstructions or deformities by asking the client to breathe through one nostril while occluding the other.

- Select the nostril that has the greatest airflow.

3. **Determine how far to insert the tube.**

- Use the tube to mark off the distance from the tip of the client's nose to the tip of the earlobe and then from the tip of the earlobe to the tip of the sternum. See Figure 39–12. *This length approximates the distance from the nares to the stomach. This distance varies among individuals.*

- Mark this length with adhesive tape if the tube does not have markings.

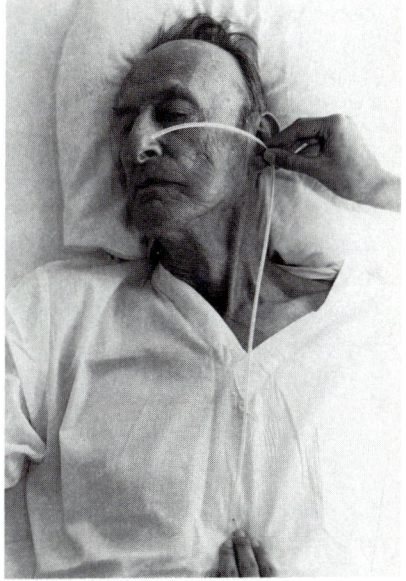

Figure 39–12 Measuring the appropriate length to insert a nasogastric tube.

■ For tubes that are to be placed into the duodenum or jejunum, add an additional 20 to 30 cm (Grant and Kennedy-Caldwell 1988, p. 126).

4. Insert the tube.

■ Lubricate the tip of the tube well with water-soluble lubricant to ease insertion. *A water-soluble lubricant dissolves if the tube accidentally enters the lungs. An oil-based lubricant, such as petroleum jelly, will not dissolve and could cause respiratory complications if it enters the lungs.*

■ Insert the tube, with its natural curve toward the client, into the selected nostril. Ask the client to hyperextend the neck, and gently advance the tube toward the nasopharynx. *Hyperextension reduces the curvature of the nasopharyngeal junction.*

■ Direct the tube along the floor of the nostril and toward the ear on that side. *Directing the tube along the floor avoids the projections (turbinates) along the lateral wall.*

■ Slight pressure is sometimes required to pass the tube into the nasopharynx, and some clients' eyes may water at this point. Tears are a natural body response. Provide the client with tissues as needed.

■ If the tube meets resistance, withdraw it, relubricate it, and insert it in the other nostril. *The tube should never be forced against resistance because of the danger of injury.*

■ Once the tube reaches the oropharynx (throat) the client will feel the tube in the throat and may gag and retch. Ask the client to tilt the head forward and encourage him or her to drink and swallow. *Tilting the head forward facilitates passage of the tube into the posterior pharynx and esophagus rather than into the larynx; swallowing*

moves the epiglottis over the opening to the larynx. See Figure 39–13.

■ If the client gags, stop passing the tube momentarily. Have the client rest, take a few breaths, and take sips of water to calm the gag reflex.

■ In cooperation with the client, pass the tube 5–10 cm (2–4 in) with each swallow, until the indicated length is inserted.

■ If the client continues to gag and the tube does not advance with each swallow, withdraw it slightly and inspect the throat by looking through the mouth. *The tube may be coiled in the throat.* If so, it is withdrawn until it is straight, and the nurse tries again to insert it.

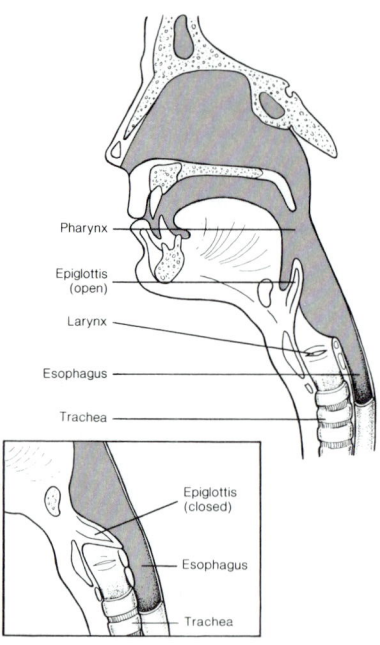

Pharynx

Epiglottis (open)

Larynx

Esophagus

Trachea

Epiglottis (closed)

Esophagus

Trachea

Figure 39–13 Swallowing closes the epiglottis.

5. Ascertain correct placement of the tube.

■ Aspirate stomach contents and check their acidity.

■ Auscultate air insufflation.

■ Use other methods in accordance with agency protocol (see page 1017 earlier).

■ If the signs do not indicate placement in the stomach, advance the tube 5 cm (2 in) and repeat the tests.

6. Secure the tube by taping it to the bridge of the client's nose.

■ If the client has oily skin, wipe the nose first with alcohol.

■ Cut 7.5 cm (3 in) of tape and split it lengthwise at one end, leaving a 2.5-cm (1 in) tab at the end.

■ Place the tape over the bridge of the client's nose, and bring the split ends under the tubing and back up over the nose. See Figure 39–14. *Taping in this manner prevents the tube from pressing against and irritating the edge of the nostril.*

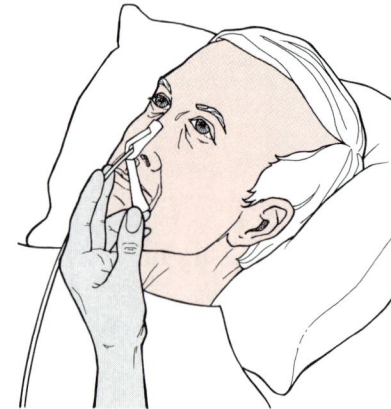

Figure 39–14 Taping a nasogastric tube to the bridge of the nose.

7. Attach the tube to a suction source or feeding apparatus as ordered or clamp the end of the tubing.

■ The tube, if inserted preoperatively, is usually clamped or it may be covered with a gauze square or plastic specimen bag and an elastic band.

▶

8. Secure the tube to the client's gown.

- Loop an elastic band around the end of the tubing and attach the elastic band to the gown with a safety pin.

    or

- Attach a piece of adhesive tape to the tube, and pin the tape to the gown. *The tube is attached to prevent it from dangling and pulling.*

9. Document relevant information.

- Document the insertion of the tube, means by which correct placement was determined, and assessments, e.g., discomfort, abdominal distention.

10. Establish a plan for providing daily nasogastric tube care.

- Inspect the nostril for discharge and irritation.
- Clean the nostril and tube with moistened, cotton-tipped applicators.
- Apply water-soluble lubricant to the nostril if it appears dry or encrusted.
- Change the adhesive tape as required.
- Give frequent mouth care, since the client may breathe through the mouth and cannot drink.

11. If suction is applied, ensure that the patency of both the nasogastric and suction tubes is maintained.

- Irrigations of the tube with 30 ml of normal saline may be required at regular intervals. In some agencies, irrigations must be ordered by the physician. Managing gastrointestinal suction and irrigating a nasogastric tube are discussed in Procedures 47–5 and 47–6.
- Keep accurate records of the client's fluid intake and output, and record the amount and characteristics of the drainage.

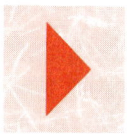

PROCEDURE 39–2

ADMINISTERING A TUBE FEEDING THROUGH AN ESTABLISHED FEEDING TUBE

Equipment ☑

Correct amount of feeding solution ordered by the physician

20- to 50-ml syringe with an adapter

Emesis basin

Bulb syringe (for an intermittent feeding)

or

Calibrated plastic feeding bag and a drip chamber, which can be attached to the tubing

or

Prefilled bottle with a drip chamber, tubing, and a flow-regulator clamp

Measuring container from which to pour the feeding (if using bulb syringe)

Water (60 ml unless otherwise specified) at room temperature

Feeding pump (optional)

Intervention

1. Assess and prepare the client.

- Assess the client for allergies (if not previously established), bowel sounds, and any problem that suggests lack of tolerance of previous feedings (e.g., abdominal distention). See the box on page 1021.

- Explain to the client that the feeding should not cause any discomfort but may cause a feeling of fullness. For an adult, the usual intermittent feeding takes about 30 minutes; the exact length of time depends largely on the volume of the feeding.

- Provide privacy for this procedure if the client desires it. *Nasogastric feedings are embarrassing to some people.*

- Assist the client to a Fowler's position in bed or a sitting position in a chair, the normal position for eating. If a sitting position is contraindicated, a slightly elevated right side-lying position is acceptable. *These positions enhance the grav-*

itational flow of the solution and prevent aspiration of fluid into the lungs.

2. Assess tube placement.

■ Attach the syringe to the open end of the tube, and aspirate alimentary secretions. Check the pH. See page 1018 for other methods.

3. Assess residual feeding contents.

■ Aspirate all the stomach contents, and measure the amount prior to administering the feeding. *This is done to evaluate absorption of the last feeding, i.e., whether undigested formula of a previous feeding remains.*

■ If 50 ml or more of undigested formula is withdrawn in adults, or 10 ml or more in infants, check with the nurse in charge before proceeding. The precise amount is usually determined by the physician's order or by agency policy. *At some agencies a feeding is withheld when the specified amount or more of formula remains in the stomach. In other agencies, the amount withdrawn is subtracted from the total feeding and that volume (less the undigested portion) is administered slowly.*

   or

Reinstill the gastric contents into the stomach if this is the agency or physician's practice. Remove the syringe bulb or plunger, and pour the gastric contents via the syringe into the nasogastric tube. *Removal of the contents could disturb the client's electrolyte balance.*

4. Administer the feeding.

When using a bulb syringe:

■ Remove the bulb from the syringe, and connect the syringe to a pinched or clamped nasogastric tube. *Pinching or clamping the tube prevents excess air from entering the stomach and causing distention.*

■ Add the feeding to the syringe barrel. See Figure 39–15.

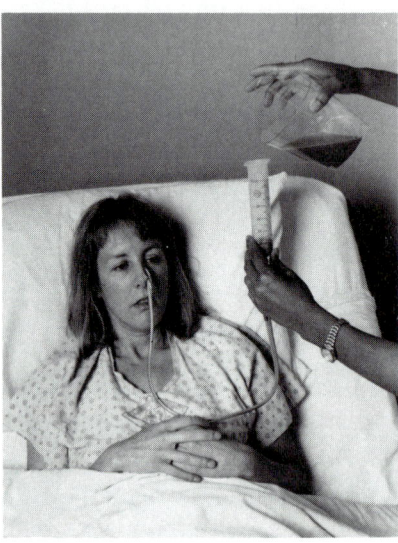

Figure 39–15   Using a bulb syringe to administer a tube feeding.

■ Permit the feeding to flow in slowly. Raise or lower the syringe to adjust the flow as needed. Pinch or clamp the tubing to stop the flow for a minute if the client experiences discomfort. *Quickly administered feedings can cause flatus, crampy pain, and/or reflux vomiting.*

When using a feeding bag:

■ Hang the bag from an infusion pole about 30 cm (12 in) above the tube's point of insertion into the client.

■ Clamp the tubing, and add the formula to the bag if it is not prefilled.

■ Open the clamp, run the formula through the tubing, and reclamp the tube. *The formula will displace the air in the tubing, thus preventing the instillation of excess air into the client's stomach or intestine.*

■ Attach the bag to the nasogastric tube (see Figure 39–16) and reg-

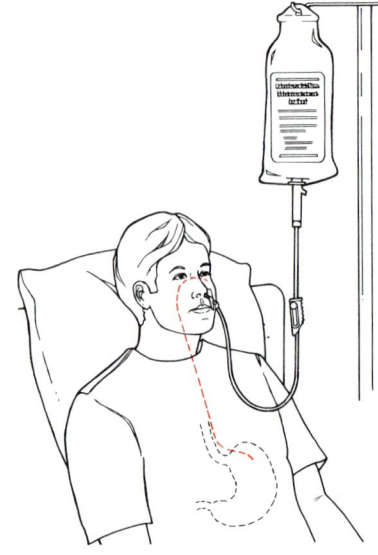

Figure 39–16   Using a calibrated plastic bag to administer a tube feeding.

ulate the drip by adjusting the clamp.

When using a prefilled bottle with drip chamber:

■ Remove the sealed cap from the container, and replace it with the screw-on cap to which the drip chamber and tubing are attached. See Figure 39–17.

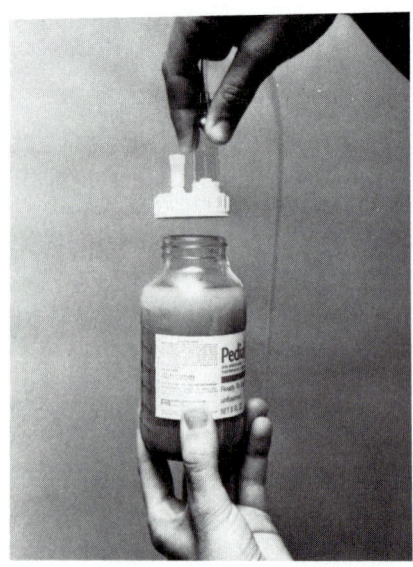

Figure 39–17   A prefilled bottle with drip chamber.

- Close the clamp on the tubing.

- Hang the container on an intravenous pole about 30 cm (12 in) above the tube's insertion point into the client. *At this height the formula should run at a safe rate into the stomach or intestine.*

- Squeeze the drip chamber to fill it to one-third to one-half of its capacity.

- Open the tubing clamp, run the formula through the tubing, and reclamp the tube. *The formula will displace the air in the tubing, thus preventing the instillation of excess air.*

- Attach the feeding set tubing to the feeding tube, and regulate the drip rate to deliver the feeding over the desired length of time. Some prefilled tube-feeding sets can be attached to a feeding pump.

5. Rinse the feeding tube immediately before all of the formula has run through the tubing.

- Instill 60 ml of water through the feeding tube. *Water cleans the lumen of the tube, preventing future blockage by sticky formula.*

- Be sure to add the water before the feeding solution has drained from the neck of a bulb syringe or from the tubing of an administration set. Before adding water to a feeding bag or prefilled tubing set, first clamp and disconnect both feeding and administration tubes. *Adding water before the syringe or tubing is empty prevents the instillation of air into the stomach or intestine, which causes unnecessary distention.*

6. Clamp and cover the feeding tube.

- Clamp the feeding tube before all of the water is instilled. *Clamping prevents leakage and air from entering the tube if done before water is instilled.*

- Cover the end of the feeding tube with gauze held by an elastic band. *Covering the tube end prevents leakage from it.*

7. Ensure client comfort and safety.

- Pin the tubing to the client's gown. *This minimizes pulling of the tube, thus preventing discomfort and dislodgement.*

- Ask the client to remain sitting upright in Fowler's position or in a slightly elevated right lateral position for at least 30 minutes. *These positions facilitate digestion and movement of the feeding from the stomach along the alimentary tract, and prevent potential aspiration of the feeding into the lungs.*

- Check the agency's policy on the frequency of changing the nasogastric tube and the use of smaller-lumen tubes if a large-bore tube is in place. *These measures prevent irritation and erosion of the pharyngeal and esophageal mucous membranes.*

8. Dispose of equipment appropriately.

- If the equipment is to be reused, wash it thoroughly with soap and water so that it is ready for reuse.

- Change equipment every 24 hours or according to agency policy.

9. Document relevant information.

- Document the feeding, including the amount and kind of solution taken, duration of the feeding, and assessments of the client. See sample below.

- Record the volume of the feeding and water administered on the client's intake and output record.

10. Monitor the client for possible problems.

- Carefully assess clients receiving tube feedings for possible problems. See Table 39–13, earlier.

- To prevent dehydration, give the client supplemental water in addition to the prescribed tube feeding.

Variation: Continuous-Drip Feeding

If the feeding is a continuous-drip tube feeding, discontinue the feeding at least every 6 hours, or as indicated by agency policy, and aspirate and measure the gastric contents. Then flush the tubing with 30 to 50 ml of water. Small-bore tubes should be flushed but not aspirated. *This ensures adequate absorption and verifies correct placement of the tube. If placement of a small bore tube is questionable, a repeat x ray should be done.*

Sample Recording

Date 6/9/91	Time 1210

350 ml Meritene feeding administered in 30 min. Eructed small amount of flatus. Tolerated feeding s̄ emesis. No discomfort noted.————Juan S. Ramirez, SN

REMOVING A NASOGASTRIC TUBE

Equipment ☑

Tissues
Plastic disposable bag
Clean disposable glove(s)
Disposable pad
50-ml syringe (optional)

Intervention

1. Confirm the physician's order to remove the tube.

2. Prepare the client.

- Explain that the procedure will cause no discomfort.

- Assist the client to a sitting position if health permits.

- Place the disposable pad across the client's chest to collect any spillage of mucous and gastric secretions from the tube.

- Provide tissues to the client to wipe the nose and mouth after tube removal.

3. Detach the tube.

- Disconnect the nasogastric tube from the suction apparatus if present.

- Unpin the tube from the client's gown.

- Remove the adhesive tape securing the tube to the nose.

4. Remove the tube.

- Put on disposable gloves.

- (Optional). Instill 50 ml of air into the tube. *This clears the tube of any contents such as feeding or gastric drainage.*

- Ask the client to take a deep breath and to hold it. *This closes the glottis, thereby preventing accidental aspiration of any gastric contents.*

- Pinch the tube with the gloved hand. *Pinching the tube prevents any contents inside the tube from draining into the client's throat.*

- Quickly and smoothly withdraw the tube.

- Place the tube in the plastic bag. *Placing the tube immediately into the bag prevents the transference of microorganisms from the tube to other articles or people.*

5. Ensure client comfort.

- Provide mouthwash if desired.

- Assist the client as required to blow the nose. *Excessive secretions may have accumulated in the nasal passages.*

6. Dispose of the equipment appropriately.

- Place the pad, bag with tube, and gloves in the receptacle designated by the agency. *Correct disposal prevents the transmission of microorganisms.*

7. Assess the nasogastric drainage if suction was used.

- Measure the amount of gastric drainage and record it on the client's fluid output record.

- Inspect the drainage for appearance and consistency.

8. Document relevant information.

- Record the removal of the tube, the amount and appearance of any drainage if connected to suction, and any relevant assessments of the client.

Gastrostomy or Jejunostomy Feeding   A **gastrostomy feeding** is the instillation of liquid nourishment through a tube that enters a surgical opening (called a gastrostomy) through the abdominal wall into the stomach. A **jejunostomy feeding** is the instillation of liquid nourishment through a tube that enters a surgical opening (a jejunostomy) through the abdominal wall into the jejunum. These feedings are usually temporary measures. When there is an obstruction in the esophagus, they may become permanent measures, for example, after removal of the esophagus.

Increasingly, **percutaneous endoscopic gastrostomy (PEG)** is being used. This procedure does not require general anesthesia or the use of an operating room. PEG is usually performed in the endoscopy suite but may also be done in the client's room. Using an endoscope to visualize the inside of the stomach, the physician makes a puncture through the skin and subcutaneous tissues of the abdomen into the stomach and inserts the PEG catheter through the puncture. The catheter has internal and external bumpers and an inflatable retention balloon to maintain placement. Once the opening has healed, replacement tubes can be inserted without the use of endoscopy.

Long-term use of PEG feedings is preferable to gastric or small intestine feedings; there are fewer risks of aspiration, and it is psychologically more acceptable. Clients initially receive feedings continuously but are advanced to intermittent feedings after a few days of uncomplicated continuous feedings. Thus, the feeding tube is not visible except when in use. PEG tubes often have smaller lumens than other types of feeding tubes (except for the small-intestine tubes), and care must be taken to avoid clogging the tube. Use liquid medications when possible. If liquid preparations are not available, finely crush tablets and dissolve with water before inserting; flush with water afterward.

For conventional gastrostomies and jejunostomies, a surgeon inserts a plastic or rubber tube or catheter into either the stomach or the jejunum. The surgical opening is sutured tightly around the tube or catheter to prevent leakage. Care of this opening before it heals requires surgical asepsis. When the incision heals (10 to 14 days), the tube or catheter

can be removed and reinserted for each feeding. Between feedings, a prosthesis may be used to close the ostomy opening. It consists of a shaft 3 to 5 cm (1 1/2 to 2 in) long, with internal and external flanges and a screw cap.

Gastrostomy and jejunostomy feedings allow clients greater mobility than gastric or duodenal tube feedings and enable clients to feed themselves. Similar principles for administration and assessment are appropriate. Procedure 39–4 provides the steps in administering a gastrostomy or jejunostomy feeding. The amount of solution is gradually increased with each feeding, from 200 to 800 ml. Commercially prepared formulas that are past the manufacturer's expiration date and agency-prepared solutions older than 24 hours must be discarded.

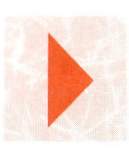

PROCEDURE 39 – 4

ADMINISTERING A GASTROSTOMY OR JEJUNOSTOMY FEEDING

Equipment ☑

Correct amount of feeding solution

Large bulb syringe

Graduated container to hold the feeding

Graduated container with 60 ml of water to flush the tubing

Graduated container to measure residual formula

For a tube sutured in place:

4 × 4 gauze squares to cover the end of the tube

Elastic band

For tube insertion:

Water-soluble lubricant

Clean disposable gloves

#18 Fr. whistle-tip catheter or other feeding tube

Tubing clamp

Moistureproof bag

For a prosthesis:

Water-soluble lubricant

#18 Fr. whistle-tip catheter or other feeding tube

For cleaning the peristomal skin and dressing the stoma:

Mild soap and water

Petrolatum, zinc oxide ointment, or other skin protectant

Precut 4 × 4 gauze squares

Uncut 4 × 4 gauze squares

Abdominal pads

Abdominal binder or Montgomery straps

Intervention

1. **Assess and prepare the client.**

■ See Procedure 39–1.

2. **Insert a feeding tube if one is not already in place.**

■ Wearing gloves, remove the ostomy dressing. If a prosthesis is in place, remove the screw cap on the prosthesis. Discard the dressing and gloves in the moistureproof bag.

■ Lubricate the end of the tube, and

insert it into the ostomy opening 10 to 15 cm (4 to 6 in).

3. **Check the patency of a tube sutured in place.**

■ Pour 15 to 30 ml of water into the syringe, remove the tube clamp, and allow the water to flow into the tube. *This determines the patency of the tube. If water flows freely, the tube is patent.*

■ If the water does not flow freely, notify the nurse in charge and/or physician.

4. **Check for residual formula.**

■ Attach the bulb to the syringe, and compress the bulb. *Compressing the bulb before the syringe is attached to the feeding tube prevents the instillation of air into the stomach or jejunum.*

■ Attach the syringe to the end of the feeding tube, and withdraw and measure the stomach or jejunal contents.

- Follow agency practice if there is no more than 50 ml of undigested formula. Hold the feeding if there is more than 150 ml, and recheck in 3 to 4 hours. Notify the physician if a large residual remains at that time.

- For continuous feedings, check the residual every 4 to 6 hours, and hold feedings if there is a 2-hour volume. Recheck in 2 hours, and restart unless the residual remains large; the physician should be notified if a large residual persists.

5. Administer the feeding.

- Hold the syringe 7 to 15 cm (3 to 6 in) above the ostomy opening.

- Slowly pour the solution into the syringe, and allow it to flow through the tube by gravity.

- Just before all the formula has run through and the syringe is empty, add 30 ml of water. *Water rinses the tube and preserves its patency.*

- If the tube is sutured in place, hold it upright, remove the syringe, and then clamp the tube to prevent leakage. Cover the end of the tube with a 4 × 4 gauze, and secure the gauze with a rubber band.

- If a catheter was inserted for the feeding, remove it. Apply the screw cap to a prosthesis if present.

6. Ensure client comfort and safety.

- After the feeding, ask the client to remain in the sitting position or a slightly elevated right lateral position for at least 30 minutes. *This minimizes the risk of aspiration.*

- Assess status of peristomal skin. *Gastric or jejunal drainage contains digestive enzymes that can irritate the skin.* Document any redness and broken skin areas.

- Check orders about cleaning the peristomal skin, applying a skin protectant, and applying appropriate dressings. Generally, the peristomal skin is washed with mild soap and water at least once daily.

Petrolatum, zinc oxide ointment, or other skin protectant may be applied around the stoma, and precut 4 × 4 gauze squares may be placed around the tube. The precut squares are then covered with regular 4 × 4 gauze squares, and the tube is coiled over them. The coiled tube is covered with abdominal pads and secured with either an abdominal binder or Montgomery straps.

- Observe for common complications of enteral feedings: aspiration, hyperglycemia, abdominal distention, diarrhea, and fecal impaction. Report findings to physician. Often a change in formula or rate of administration can correct problems.

- When appropriate, teach the client how to administer feedings and when to notify the physician or nurse practitioner concerning problems.

7. Document all assessments and interventions.

EVALUATING

Depending on the outcome criteria established in the planning phase, the nurse may perform the following evaluative activities: (a) taking anthropometric measurements, (b) observing the client for changes in signs of malnutrition, (c) questioning the client about dietary alterations required or listening to the client's reports of dietary alterations achieved, (d) reviewing and discussing a dietary log or plan of a balanced meal, and (e) checking laboratory data for desired changes. Examples of evaluative statements indicating goal achievement are "Client identified the five major food sources of calcium from a list of 20 items," "Client submitted a written balanced menu for 1 week that is low in fat and meets the criteria of the food guide provided," and "Client reports feeling more vigorous and energetic since diet initiated 2 weeks ago."

NURSING CARE PLAN FOR ROSE SANTINI

ASSESSMENT DATA

Nursing Assessment

Mrs. Rose Santini, a 59-year-old homemaker, attends a community-hospital–sponsored health fair. She approaches the nutrition information booth, and Miss Pamela Norris, the nurse-clinical specialist in nutritional support, gathers a nursing history of Mrs. Santini's nutritional problems. Mrs. Santini is very upset about her 9-kg (20-lb) weight gain. She relates to Miss Norris that since the death of her husband a month ago, she has lost interest in many of her usual physical and social activities. She no longer attends the YMCA exercise and swimming sessions and has all but lost contact with her couples bridge group at her church. She states that she is bored, depressed, and very unhappy about her appearance. She has a small frame and has always prided herself on her "girlish figure." Mrs. Santini says her eating habits have changed considerably. She tends to snack a great deal while watching TV and rarely prepares a complete meal.

Physical Examination

Height: 162.6 cm (5'4")
Weight: 63.6 kg (140 lb)
Temperature: 37 C (98.6 F)
Pulse rate: 76 BPM
Respirations: 16 per minute at rest
Blood pressure: 144/84 mm Hg
Triceps skin fold 27 mm
Small frame, weight in excess of 10% over ideal for height and frame

Diagnostic Studies

CBC: Normal
Urine: Negative
Chest x-ray film: Negative
Thyroid profile: Within normal limits

CARE PLAN

Nursing Diagnosis	Client Goals and Outcome Criteria	Nursing Interventions and Rationales	Evaluation
Altered nutrition: More than body requirements, related to excess intake and decreased activity expenditure, resulting in weight gain of 20 lbs, triceps skin fold greater than 25 mm, undesirable eating patterns.	Client Goal: Ideal body weight for height and frame. Outcome Criteria: Loses 2 kg (4 lbs) in 14 days. Plans 3 menus each day that result in a 500-calorie reduction in intake. Engages in physical exercise for 15 to 20 minutes by day 3. Identifies eating habits that lead to weight gain.	Assess for causes of excessive weight gain. *Rationale:* Excessive food intake is a complex problem with physical and psychosocial aspects. Encourage client to keep a 24-hour diet log. *Rationale:* Increases client's awareness of activities and foods that contribute to excessive intake. Encourage client to set realistic goals, e.g., decrease caloric intake by 500 calories each day. *Rationale:* A reduction of 500 calories per day will result in a 1 to 2 lb weight loss per week. Encourage client to knit or sew instead of eating snacks while watching TV. *Rationale:* Activity may distract the client from thinking about and taking snacks. Instruct client in behavior modification techniques, e.g., drink 8 oz of water before each meal, eat slowly and chew thoroughly. *Rationale:* Behavior modification may assist client in losing weight. Encourage client to increase physical exercise and/or to enroll in physical fitness program. *Rationale:* Exercise produces weight loss by increasing caloric requirements of the body	Client kept a dietary log for 5 days and as a result now plans balanced meals each day, resulting in a daily loss of 400 to 500 calories. She is aware that she eats excessively because she is bored and depressed, and is now attempting to reestablish some of her former social contacts and activities. She has purchased a stationary bicycle and exercises 15 to 30 minutes each day. This past week she has enrolled in a knitting class as well, and she hopes this will help to keep her hands busy while she is watching TV. She has lost 1½ lbs in the past week.

Nursing Diagnosis	Client Goals and Outcome Criteria	Nursing Interventions and Rationales	Evaluation
Body image disturbance related to excessive weight gain resulting in withdrawal from social contacts and expressions of disgust with bodily appearance.	Client Goal: Achieve realistic concept of body image. Outcome Criteria: Verbalizes a realistic self-concept by day 14. Begins to assume responsibility for weight loss by day 7. Expresses confidence in ability to change body image by losing weight by day 14.	Establish a good nurse/client rapport. *Rationale:* A good nurse/client rapport will allow client to vent her feelings about her self-concept. Encourage client to reestablish social contacts. *Rationale:* Social acceptance can increase self-esteem. Refer client to a weight-loss support group. *Rationale:* Support groups can provide companionship, increase motivation, and offer practical solutions to common problems. Discuss the client's view of being fat. *Rationale:* A mental image includes the ideal and is not always realistic.	Client states she hopes her old friends will accept her changed appearance. She has joined Weight Watchers and finds the persons in her group to be supportive and very helpful. She states that she knows she can lose weight if she "puts her mind to it," but that she may not be a size 8 by the end of 6 months.

CHAPTER HIGHLIGHTS

▶ Nutrition is the sum total of all interactions between an organism and the food it consumes.

▶ Although people are continually bombarded with information about what to eat and what not to eat, each person is responsible for selecting foods that provide essential nutrients.

▶ Nurses can assist people to evaluate the information they receive about nutrients.

▶ Essential nutrients are grouped into six categories: water, carbohydrates, fats, proteins, vitamins, and minerals.

▶ Nutrients serve three basic purposes: forming body structures (such as bones and blood), providing energy, and helping to regulate the body's biochemical reactions.

▶ Both inadequate and excessive intakes of nutrients result in malnutrition.

▶ The effects of malnutrition can be general or specific, depending on which nutrients and what level of deficiency or excess are involved.

▶ Some of the long-range effects of certain nutrient excesses are among the many factors involved in certain diseases, e.g., coronary artery disease and cancer.

▶ Nutritional needs vary considerably according to age, growth, and energy requirements.

▶ Adolescents have high energy requirements due to their rapid growth; a diet plentiful in milk, meats, green and yellow vegetables, and fresh fruits is required.

▶ Middle-aged adults and older adults often need to reduce their caloric intake because of decreases in metabolic rate and activity levels. Fats, sugary foods, and sodium must often be limited.

▶ To assess the nutritional status of a person, the nurse follows the ABCD approach: anthropometric measurements are taken, biochemical data are assessed, clinical signs of nutritional status are assessed, and a dietary history is obtained.

▶ During the assessment stage and when planning nursing interventions to help clients reach nutritional goals, nurses must consider the many factors that influence a person's dietary patterns.

▶ Nursing diagnoses for clients with nutritional problems are broadly stated as **Altered nutrition** and are further categorized as **Less than body requirements, More than body requirements,** or **Potential for more than body requirements.**

- Obesity is a common nutritional problem of North Americans. Nurses can assist obese clients by recommending increased activity and intake of foods that have a low caloric density.

- Counseling about nutrition can be likened to the teaching-learning process, which includes assessing specific learning needs, setting goals, planning strategies to meet goals, and establishing outcome criteria to evaluate goal achievement.

- Assisting clients and support persons with therapeutic diets is a function shared by the nurse and the dietitian. The nurse reinforces the dietitian's instructions, assists the client to make beneficial changes, and evaluates the client's response to planned changes.

- Because many hospitalized clients have poor appetites, a major responsibility of the nurse is to provide nursing interventions that stimulate their appetites.

- Whenever possible, the nurse should help incapacitated clients to feed themselves; a number of self-feeding aids help clients who have difficulty handling regular utensils.

- The nurse can refer clients to various community programs that help special subgroups of the population meet their nutritional needs.

- The administration of enteral and parenteral feedings to clients unable to ingest sufficient intake to maintain nutritional balance requires skill to prevent aspiration of the feeding.

READINGS AND REFERENCES

SELECTED READINGS

Curtas, S.; Chapman, G.; and Meguid, M. M. June 1989. Evaluation of nutritional status. *Nursing Clinics of North America* 24:301–13.
The article begins with an overview of the body composition, followed by a description of three types of malnutrition: marasmus, kwashiorkor, and mixed marasmus-kwashiorkor. The authors also discuss the nutritional history and related physical examination, including measurements of skinfold thickness and skeletal muscle mass; blood studies; and immunocompetence.

Iverson-Carpenter, M. S.; Haskin, D.; Maas, M.; Hardy, M.; and Button, M. April 1988. Fulfilling nutritional requirements. *Journal of Gerontological Nursing* 14:16–24, 46–47.
The authors explain the scope of a nutritional assessment and the factors underlying undernutrition, with special reference to the elderly. They provide a table listing the etiologies and defining characteristics for the diagnosis of **Altered nutrition: Less than body requirements.** The signs and symptoms resulting from undernutrition conclude the article. A case study is included.

Kohn, C. L., and Keithley, J. K. June 1989. Enteral nutrition: Potential complications and patient monitoring. *Nursing Clinics of North America* 24:339–53.
Kohn and Keithley describe the mechanical complications, including potential pulmonary complications, of tube feeding. The authors also discuss gastrointestinal complications and seven nursing interventions that should be taken to avoid them. Other topics addressed include hyperglycemia, tube-feeding syndrome, and hypercapnia. In summary, the authors caution that although gastrointestinal disturbances are the most frequently encountered complications, many of them can be prevented.

Stoy, D. B. December 1989. Controlling cholesterol with diet. *American Journal of Nursing* 89:1625–27.
According to Stoy, a person on the Step One diet can lower LDL cholesterol 10% to 15%. She describes how to reduce fat intake and provides a primer on dietary fat with explanatory illustrations.

RELATED RESEARCH

Dimant, J., and Solow, B. A. Summer 1988. Nutritional assessment in nursing home patients: Improving nutritional status. *The Journal of Long Term Care Administration* 16:7–9.

Ford, V. L., and Harris, M. B. February/March 1988. Planning a nutrition curriculum: Assessing availability, affordability, and cultural appropriateness of recommended foods. *Health Education* 19:26–30.

Jamison, M. T. May 1988. Nutrition in the elderly: A descriptive study. *Nutritional Support Services* 8:23–25.

Metheny, N. November/December 1988. Measures to test placement of nasogastric and nasointestinal feeding tubes: A review. *Nursing Research* 37:324–29.

Norberg, A.; Backstrom, A.; Athline, E.; and Norberg, B. July 1988. Food refusal amongst nursing home patients as conceptualized by nurses' aides and enrolled nurses: An interview study. *Journal of Advanced Nursing* 13:478–83.

SELECTED REFERENCES

Bunston, T., Breton, M. 1990. The eating patterns and problems of homeless women. *Women & Health* 16(1):43–62.

Byrne, C. J.; Saxton, D. F.; Pelikan, P. K.; and Nugent, P. M. 1986. *Laboratory tests: Implications for nursing care.* 2d ed. Menlo Park, Calif.: Addison-Wesley Publishing Co.

Carpenito, L. J. 1989. *Nursing diagnosis: Application to clinical practice.* 3d ed. Philadelphia: J. B. Lippincott Co.

Chernoff, R. February 1990. Physiologic aging and nutritional status. *Nutrition in Clinical Practice* 5:8–13.

Chicago Dietetic Association and South Suburban Dietetic Association of Cook Will County. 1981. *Manual of Clinical Dietetics.* 2d ed. Philadelphia: W. B. Saunders Co.

Christian, J. L., and Greger, J. L. 1988. *Nutrition for living.* 2d ed. Menlo Park, Calif.: Benjamin/Cummings.

Doenges, M. E., and Moorhouse, M. F. 1988. *Nurse's pocket guide: Nursing diagnoses with interventions.* 2d ed. Philadelphia: F. A. Davis Co.

Dudek, S. G. 1987. *Nutrition handbook for nursing practice.* Philadelphia: J. B. Lippincott Co.

Gordon, M. 1982. *Manual of nursing diagnosis.* New York: McGraw-Hill.

Grant, J. A., and Kennedy-Caldwell, C. 1988. *Nutritional support in nursing.* New York: Grune and Stratton.

Guyton, A. C. 1986. *Textbook of medical physiology.* 7th ed. Philadelphia: W. B. Saunders Co.

Hand, R.; Kempster, M.; Levy, J.; Rogol, R.; and Spirn, P. 1984. Inadvertent transbronchial insertion of narrow-bore feeding tubes. *Journal of the American Medical Association* 251:2396–97.

Heaney, R. P.; Gallger, J. C.; Johnson, C. C.; et al. 1982. Calcium nutrition and bone health in the elderly. *American Journal of Clinical Nutrition* 36:986–1013.

Howard, R. B., and Herbold, N. H. 1982. *Nutrition in clinical care.* 2d ed. New York: McGraw-Hill.

Kim, M. J.; McFarland, G. K.; and McLane, A. M. 1989. *Pocket guide to nursing diagnoses.* 3d ed. St. Louis: C. V. Mosby Co.

Kim, M. J., and Mortiz, D. A., editors. 1982. *Classification of nursing diagnoses: Proceedings of the third and fourth national conferences.* New York: McGraw-Hill.

Konstantinides, N. N., and Shronts, E. September 1983. Tube feeding: Managing the basics. *American Journal of Nursing* 83:1312–18.

Metheny, M. M. January 1985. 20 ways to prevent tube-feeding complications. *Nursing 85* 15:47–50.

Metheny, N. November/December 1988. Measures to test placement of nasogastric and nasointestinal feeding tubes: A review. *Nursing Research* 37:324–29.

Metheny, N. A.; Spies, M. A.; and Eisenberg, P. August 1988. Measures to test placement of nasoenteral feeding tubes. *Western Journal of Nursing Research* 10:367–83.

Mikan, K. J., Robuck, J. T. June 1990. Software for a healthy diet: Nutritionist 111. *American Journal of Nursing.* 90:111.

Miller, K.; Tomlinson, J.; and Sahn, S. August 1985. Pleuropulmonary complications of enteral tube feeding. *Chest* 88:230–33.

NANDA approved nursing diagnostic categories for clinical use and testing. Summer 1988. *Nursing Diagnosis Newsletter* 15:1–3.

National Center for Health Statistics. *Health and Nutrition Examination Survey of 1971 to 1974,* DHEW Pub. No. (PHS) 79–1310.

National Research Council, Committee on Dietary Allowances: Food and Nutrition Board. 1989. *Recommended dietary allowances.* 10th ed. Washington, D.C.: National Academy of Sciences.

Natow, A. B., and Heslin, J. 1986. *Nutritional care of the older adult.* New York: Macmillan Publishing Co.

Raab, D., and Raab, N. March 1985. Nutrition and the aging: An overview. *Canadian Nurse* 81:24–26.

Russell, R. M., and Naccarto, D. V. October 1982. Current perspectives on trace elements. *Drug Therapy* 7:115–18.

Scholl, D. E. 1986. *Nutrition and diet therapy: A handbook for nurses.* Oradell, N.J.: Medical Economics Books.

Suitor, C. W., and Hunter, M. F. 1984. *Nutrition: Principles and application in health promotion.* 2d ed. Philadelphia: J. B. Lippincott Co.

Theodore, A.; Frank, J.; Ende, J.; Snider, G.; and Beer, D. 1984. Errant placement of nasogastric feeding tubes: A hazard in obtunded patients. *Chest* 86:931–33.

U.S. Congress. Senate Select Committee on Nutrition and Human Needs. 1977. *Dietary goals for the United States.* 2d ed. Washington, D.C.: Government Printing Office.

U.S. Department of Agriculture. 1979. *The Hassle-free guide to a better diet.* Science and Education Administration Leaflet No. 567: U.S. Government Printing Office.

———. 1981. *Nutritive value of foods.* Home and Garden Bulletin No. 72: U.S. Government Printing Office.

U.S. Department of Agriculture and U.S. Department of Health and Human Services. 1980. *Nutrition and your health: Dietary guidelines for Americans.* Home and Garden Bulletin No. 232: U.S. Government Printing Office.

Vhymeister, I. B.; Register, U. D.; and Sonnenberg, L. M. February 1977. Safe vegetarian diets for children. *Pediatric Clinics of North America* 24(1):207.

Williams, S. R. 1981. *Nutrition and diet therapy.* 4th ed. St. Louis: C. V. Mosby Co.

Williams, S. R.; Worthington-Roberts, B. S.; Schlenker, E. D.; Pipes, P.; Rees, J. M.; and Mahan, L. K., editors. 1988. *Nutrition throughout the life cycle.* St. Louis: Times Mirror/Mosby College Publishing.

Fluid and Electrolytes

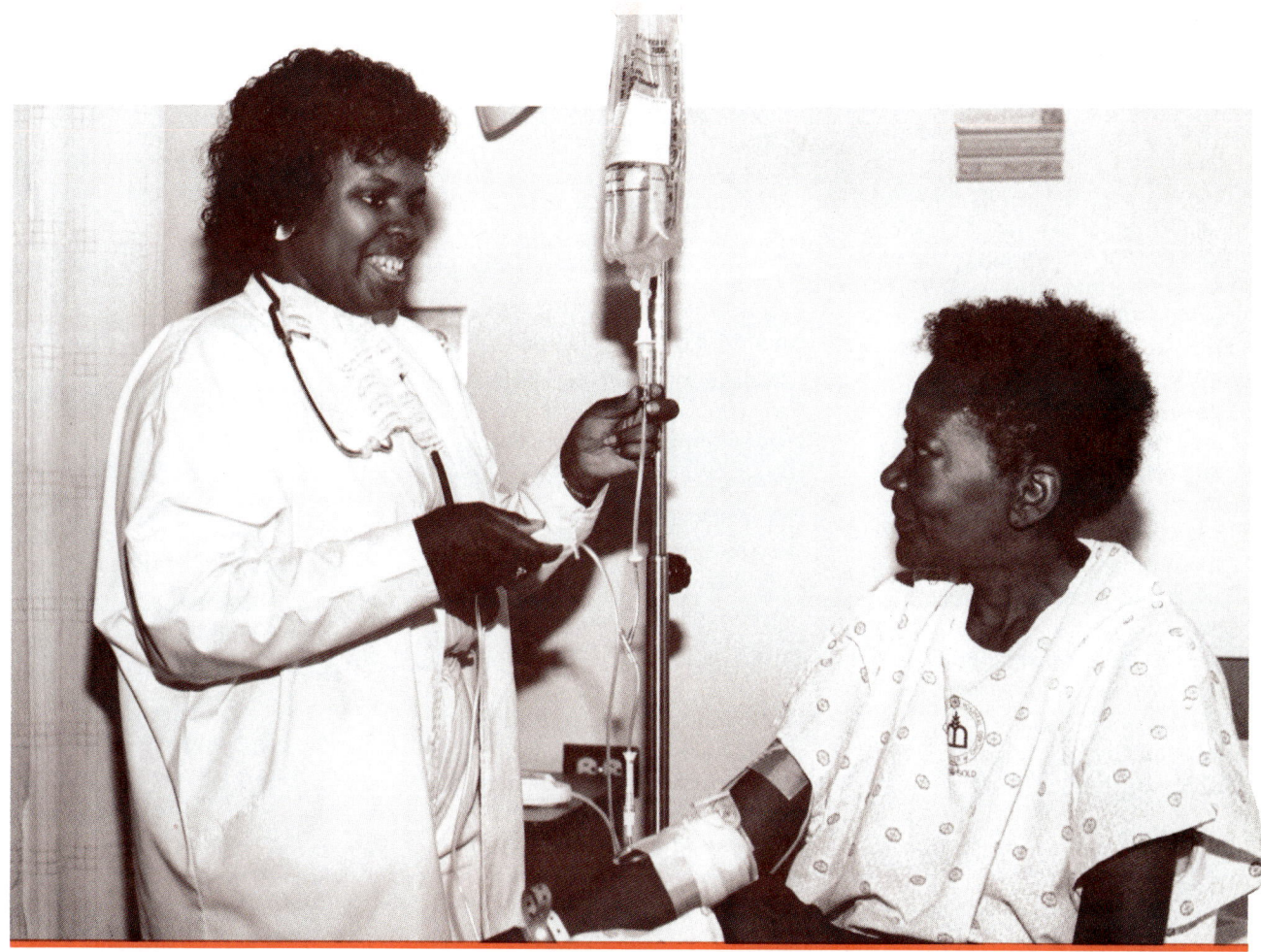

CONTENTS

OBJECTIVES

▶ Describe factors affecting the proportion of the body weight that is fluid.

▶ Identify the major electrolytes of the intracellular and extracellular fluid compartments and body secretions.

▶ Describe how fluids and electrolytes move through the body.

▶ Explain how the osmotic and hydrostatic pressures influence movement of fluid through membranes.

▶ List factors that influence fluid and electrolyte balance.

▶ Describe how body mechanisms regulate fluid and electrolyte balance.

▶ Describe the role of the lungs and kidneys in regulating acid-base balance.

▶ Identify information to obtain in a health history to assess fluid and electrolyte balance.

▶ Describe the significance of diagnostic tests used to monitor fluid, electrolyte, and acid-base balance.

▶ Identify the causes of selected fluid, electrolyte, and acid-base imbalances.

▶ Recognize clinical signs and laboratory findings of selected fluid and electrolyte imbalances.

▶ Describe four primary acid-base disturbances.

▶ List examples of nursing diagnoses related to fluid, electrolyte, and acid-base balance.

▶ State outcome criteria for evaluating the client's responses to strategies implemented to promote fluid and electrolyte balance.

▶ Assist clients to modify their fluid intake.

▶ Monitor and regulate intravenous infusions.

▶ Describe how to change intravenous containers and tubing.

▶ Give guidelines for discontinuing an intravenous infusion.

▶ Identify potential problems and risks of blood transfusions.

▶ Explain basic purposes of and sites used for total parenteral nutrition.

DISTRIBUTION OF BODY FLUID

Fluids and electrolytes are necessary to maintain good health, and their relative amounts in the body must be maintained within a narrow range. The balance of fluids and electrolytes in the body is a part of physiologic homeostasis. See Chapter 33.

A great deal has been learned about the roles of fluids and electrolytes in both health and disease. This delicate balance is maintained in health by the body's physiologic processes. Almost every illness, however, threatens the balance. Even in normal daily living, excessive temperatures or excessive activity can disturb the balance if adequate water or salt intake is not maintained. Some therapeutic measures for clients, such as the use of diuretics, can also disturb the body's homeostasis unless water and electrolytes are replaced.

The body's fluid is divided into two major reservoirs, intracellular and extracellular. The **intracellular fluid (ICF),** also referred to as the **cellular fluid,** is found within the cells of the body. It constitutes two-thirds to three-quarters of the total body fluid. The **extracellular fluid (ECF)** is found outside the cells; it is subdivided into two compartments, **intravascular** (plasma) and **interstitial. Plasma** is fluid found within the vascular system; **interstitial fluid** is fluid that surrounds the cells, and it includes lymph. Extracellular fluids constitute one-third to one-fourth of the total body fluid.

Extracellular fluid is in constant motion throughout the body. Although it is the smaller of the two compartments, it is the transport system that carries nutrients to and waste products from the cells. For example, plasma carries oxygen in the hemoglobin of red blood cells from the lungs and glucose from the gastrointestinal tract to the capillaries of the vascular system. From there, the oxygen and glucose move across the capillary membranes into the interstitial spaces and then across the cellular membranes into the cells. The opposite route is taken for waste products, such as carbon dioxide going from the cells to the lungs and metabolic acid wastes going eventually to the kidneys. Interstitial fluid transports wastes from the cells by way of the lymph system as well as directly into the blood plasma through capillaries. Lymph circulation ultimately enters the vascular circulation through the thoracic duct into the venous system.

Interstitial fluid comprises three-quarters of extracellular fluid. Normal body functioning requires that the volume of each fluid compartment remain relatively constant. Regulating mechanisms are discussed later in this chapter.

Secretions and excretions are also part of the body's total fluid volume and serve essential functions. They are part of the extracellular fluid. A **secretion** is the product of a gland, for example, the salivary glands. Examples are cerebrospinal fluid, synovial fluid, pericardial fluid, and alimentary secretions. An **excretion** is waste produced by the cells of the body. Just as balances exist between cellular and extracellular compartments, special balances exist between plasma and secretions and excretions. Alimentary secretions for an adult, for example, are estimated to be about 6700 ml per day. See Table 40–1.

PROPORTIONS OF BODY FLUID

The proportion of the human body composed of fluid is surprisingly large, considering that the external appearance suggests mostly solid tissue such as muscle and bone. Fluid constitutes about 57% of the average healthy adult man's weight. In health, this volume (about 40 liters) of body fluid remains relatively constant. In fact, a healthy person's weight varies less than 0.2 kg (0.5 lb) in 24 hours, regardless of the amount of fluid ingested. Some diseases cause serious excesses or deficiencies of body fluid. For example, a client with heart failure can retain fluid in the tissues and may suffer a fluid excess. A person with kidney disease may not be able to excrete the required amount of urine and also suffer a fluid excess. Another person with a mouth injury may not be able to drink and may suffer a fluid loss.

The percentage of total body fluid varies according to the individual's age, body fat, and sex. See Table 40–2. Infants have the highest proportion of fluid; as people grow older, the proportion decreases. Body fat is essentially free of fluid; therefore, the amount of fat a person has alters the proportion of body fluid to body weight. In other words, the less body fat present, the greater the proportion of body fluid. For example, a thin man's body may be 70% fluid, whereas an obese man's may be only 53%. This variable, body fat, also accounts for the difference in total body fluid between the sexes. After adolescence, women have proportionately more fat than men. Thus, they have a smaller percentage of fluid in relation to total body weight than do men.

Large volumes of fluid also carry dissolved waste materials through the kidneys and through the gastrointestinal tract. However, in both instances, most of this fluid is reabsorbed into the vascular spaces and reused by the body. For example, of 6700 ml produced in the alimentary tract, only 100 ml is usually excreted in the feces, just enough to keep the feces lubricated. Of 180 liters of glomerular filtrate that filters through the kidneys per day, only 1.4 liters are excreted from the body under normal conditions. See Table 40–3.

Nurses need to be aware of abnormal amounts of secretions and excretions. Excessive losses can seriously deplete first the extracellular fluid volume and then the intracellular fluid volume. Excessive or inadequate secretions interfere with a number of body processes, e.g., digestion and elimination.

TABLE 40–1 *Secretions of the Adult Alimentary Tract*

Secretion	Volume (ml/day)
Saliva	1000
Gastric secretion	1500
Pancreatic secretion	1000
Bile	1000
Small-intestine secretion	1800
Brunner's gland secretion	200
Large-intestine secretion	200
Total	6700

Source: Adapted from A.C. Guyton, *Textbook of medical physiology,* 7th ed. (Philadelphia: W. B. Saunders Co., 1986), p. 772. Reprinted with permission.

TABLE 40–2 *Fluid Percentage of Body Weight, by Age**

Developmental Stage	Percentage of Water (Approximate)
Newborn infant	75
Adult male	57
Adult female	55
Elderly adult	45

*Note: As age increases, proportion of body water decreases.

TABLE 40–3 *Average Daily Fluid Output for an Adult*

Route	Amount at Normal Temperature (ml)
Urine	1400
Insensible losses:	
Lungs	350
Skin	350
Sweat	100
Feces	100
Total	2300

Source: Adapted from A.C. Guyton, *Textbook of medical physiology,* 7th ed. (Philadelphia: W. B. Saunders Co., 1986), p. 383. Reprinted with permission.

BODY ELECTROLYTES

Extracellular and intracellular fluids are similar in their content of electrolytes and other substances. These fluids contain oxygen from the lungs; dissolved nutrients, from the gastrointestinal tract; excretory products of metabolism, of which carbon dioxide is the most abundant; and particles called **ions.**

Many salts dissociate in water, i.e., break up into electrically charged ions. The salt sodium chloride breaks up into one ion of sodium (Na^+) and one ion of chloride (Cl^-). These charged particles are called **electrolytes** because they are capable of conducting electricity. Ions that carry a positive charge are all **cations,** and ions carrying a negative charge are called **anions.** Examples of cations are sodium (Na^+), potassium (K^+), calcium (Ca^{2+}), and magnesium (Mg^{2+}). Anions include chloride (Cl^-), bicarbonate (HCO_3^-), monohydrogen phosphate (HPO_4^{2-}), and sulfate (SO_4^{2-}).

Electrolyte Composition of Body Fluids

The electrolyte composition of fluids varies from one compartment to another. Principal ions of extracellular fluid are sodium and chloride; principal ions of cellular fluid are potassium and phosphate. The ion composition of the two extracellular fluid reservoirs (intravascular and interstitial) is similar; the main difference is that intravascular fluid (plasma) has a greater quantity of protein than interstitial fluid does. This is because large particles of protein have difficulty passing through the vascular (capillary) membranes into the interstitial fluid. All other electrolytes move readily between these two extracellular compartments.

The higher quantity of protein in plasma plays a significant role in maintaining the intravascular fluid volume and blood pressure. When quantities of plasma protein are low in the body, the blood volume diminishes noticeably and results in a state of hypotension (low blood pressure). This is particularly manifest in people with diseases of the liver (the source of body plasma proteins), who are unable to produce sufficient quantities of plasma proteins.

Just as fluid volumes must be maintained within compartments, so must the electrolyte composition of the various compartments. Balances of electrolytes are maintained in proportion to the quantities of fluid in the compartments. Although the specific numbers of cations and anions may differ in the fluid compartments, in a state of homeostasis the total number of cations equals the number of anions within each compartment.

Body secretions and excretions also contain electrolytes. This is of particular concern when excretions are abnormally increased or decreased or when a secretion is lost from the body (for example, when gastric suction removes the gastric secretions). Fluid and electrolyte imbalance can result from prolonged loss through these routes. See Table 40–4 for the electrolyte composition of body secretions and excretions.

Measurement of Electrolytes

Electrolytes are measured in milliequivalents per liter of water (mEq/liter) or milligrams per 100 milliliters (mg/100 ml). The term **milliequivalent** means one thousandth of an equivalent; equivalent refers to the *chemical combining power* of a substance, or the capacity of cations to unite with anions to form molecules. This chemical combining activity is measured in relation to the chemical combining activity of the hydrogen ion (H^+). One mEq equals the chemical combining capacity of 1 mg of hydrogen. Thus, 1 mEq of any anion equals 1 mEq of any cation. For example, sodium and chloride ions are equivalent, since they combine equally: 1 mEq of Na^+ equals 1 mEq of Cl^-. However, these cations and anions are not equal in weight: 1 mg of Na^+ does not equal 1 mg of Cl^-; rather, 3 mg of Na^+ equals 2 mg of Cl^-

Clinically, the milliequivalent system is commonly used. However, nurses need to be aware of the different systems of measurement when interpreting laboratory results. It is also important to realize that a laboratory examination usually indicates the findings of blood plasma, since intracellular fluid is not easily accessible for examination. Examination of extracellular fluid (plasma) can frequently reflect the state of the intracellular fluid, though not always precisely.

MOVEMENT OF BODY FLUID AND ELECTROLYTES

Movement of fluid and transport of substances occur in three phases. First, blood plasma moves around the body within the circulatory system, and nutrients and fluids are picked

TABLE 40-4 Electrolyte Composition of Secretions and Excretions Compared to Plasma

Substance	Electrolyte (mEq/L)			
	Sodium (Na$^+$)	Potassium (K$^+$)	Chloride (Cl$^-$)	Bicarbonate (HCO$_3^-$)
Plasma (serum)	135–145	3.6–5.0	95–108	21–28
Gastric secretions	70	5+	140	5
Pancreatic juice	140+	5	35	115+
Hepatic duct bile	140+	5	100+	40
Jejunal secretions	140	5	135	30
Perspiration	80	5	85	—

up from the lungs and the gastrointestinal tract. Second, interstitial fluid and its components move between the blood capillaries and the cells. Third, fluid and substances then move from the interstitial fluid into the cells. In the reverse direction, fluid and its components move back from the cells to the interstitial spaces and then to the intravascular compartment. The intravascular fluid then flows to the kidneys, where the metabolic by-products of the cells are excreted.

Methods of Movement

The methods by which body fluids and electrolytes move are: diffusion, osmosis, and active transport.

Diffusion   **Diffusion** is the continual intermingling of molecules in liquids, gases, or solids brought about by the random movement of the molecules. For example, two gases become mixed by the incessant motion of their molecules. The process of diffusion occurs even when two substances are separated by a thin membrane. In the body, diffusion of water, electrolytes, and other substances occurs through the "slit pores" of capillary membranes.

The rate of diffusion of substances varies according to (a) size of the molecules, (b) concentration of the solution, and (c) temperature of the solution. Larger molecules move less quickly than smaller ones, since they require more energy to move about. Molecules move more rapidly from a solution of higher concentration to a solution of lower concentration. Increases in temperature increase the rate of motion of molecules and therefore the rate of diffusion.

Osmosis   **Osmosis** is the movement of water across cell membranes, from the less concentrated solution to the more concentrated solution. In other words, water moves toward the higher concentration of solute. **Solutes** may be **crystalloids** (salts that dissolve readily into true solutions) or **colloids** (substances such as large protein molecules that do not readily dissolve into true solutions). A **solvent**

is the component of a solution that can dissolve a solute. In a salt solution, water is the solvent, and sodium chloride (NaCl) is the solute. Osmosis is important in maintaining proper balance in the volumes of extracellular and intracellular fluid.

Osmolarity is a measure of the concentration of a solution, expressed in a unit called the osmol: 1 osmol is the number of particles in 1 gram molecular weight of dissociated solute. Osmolarity is expressed in osmols per liter of solution.

The principle of osmosis can be applied clinically in the administration of intravenous solutions. Usually, the solutions given are **isotonic,** having the same concentration (osmolarity) as blood plasma. This prevents sudden shifts of fluids and electrolytes. In some cases, however, hypertonic or hypotonic solutions are infused. **Hypertonic** solutions have a greater concentration of solutes than plasma does; **hypotonic** solutions have a lesser concentration of solutes. An example of hypertonic solution is 50% glucose, which may be given to reduce cerebral edema. The high concentration of glucose temporarily draws fluid from interstitial spaces in the brain into the blood compartment. Use of hypotonic solutions is rare.

Active Transport   Substances can move across cell membranes from a less concentrated solution to a more concentrated one by **active transport.** This process differs from diffusion and osmosis in that metabolic energy is expended. In active transport, the substance combines with a carrier on the outside surface of the cell membrane. The combined carrier and substance then move to the inside surface. Once inside, they separate, and the substance is released to the inside of the cell. A specific carrier is required for each substance, and enzymes are required for active transport.

This process is of particular importance in maintaining the differences in sodium and potassium ion concentrations of extracellular and intracellular fluid. Under normal conditions, sodium concentrations are higher in the extracellular fluid, while potassium concentrations are higher inside the cells. To maintain this balance, the active transport mechanism (the **sodium-potassium pump**) is activated, moving sodium from the cells and potassium into the cells.

Fluid Pressures

A number of pressures are exerted as part of the movement of fluid and electrolytes from one compartment to another. Two of these are osmotic pressure and hydrostatic pressure, each of which can cause a flow of fluid through the capillary membranes.

Osmotic and Oncotic Pressure
Osmotic pressure is the amount of fluid pressure required to completely stop or prevent the osmotic flow of water between two solutions. This pressure opposing osmosis occurs when the flow of water from an area of lesser concentration to an area of greater concentration causes the amount of water in the latter, concentrated solution to develop a pressure difference great enough to oppose the osmosis—even though a concentration gradient of solutes may still remain.

Oncotic pressure is the pulling force exerted by colloids (e.g., albumin in plasma) that help hold the water content of the blood in the intravascular space.

Hydrostatic Pressure
Hydrostatic pressure is the pressure exerted by a fluid within a closed system. The hydrostatic pressure of blood is the force exerted by blood against the vascular walls, e.g., the artery walls. It is also referred to as **filtration force.** The principle involved in hydrostatic pressure is that fluids move from the area of greater pressure to the area of less pressure. For this reason, fluid moves out of blood vessels.

The net movement of water from plasma to tissue spaces thus depends on which force is greater: hydrostatic pressure, which forces fluid out of the blood vessels, or oncotic pressure, which draws fluid into the blood vessels. Normally, fluid moves out of capillaries at the arterial end, where the intravascular hydrostatic pressure exceeds the oncotic pressure. At the venous end of the capillaries, where the oncotic pressure is greater, fluid is drawn from the interstitial compartment into the intravascular compartment.

Selective Permeability of Membranes

Capillary and cellular membranes in the body are described as selectively permeable because not all substances move with the same ease across the membranes. Compounds such as proteins and glycogen do not readily cross capillary and cellular membranes. Organic compounds such as glucose and amino acids move freely across capillary walls, although they often require active transport. Certain membranes, called **dialyzing membranes,** allow water molecules and particles in true solution (crystalloids), but not particles in colloid dispersion, to pass through. Most of the membranes that surround cells are dialyzing membranes.

Cellular (not capillary) membranes are particularly selective in regard to sodium and potassium ions. Movement of potassium across cell membranes depends on metabolic cellular activities. Administration of glucose or insulin accelerates the movement of potassium into the cells. Sodium enters in greater quantities when the cells lose potassium. Any factor that alters the properties of the cell membranes brings about changes in the distribution of sodium and potassium. Some of these factors are excitation of nerve and muscle cells, changes in pH, and anoxia.

REGULATING FLUID VOLUME

In a healthy person, the fluid volume and chemical composition of the fluid compartments stay within narrow safe limits. Normally, a person's fluid intake is counterbalanced by fluid loss. Illness can upset this balance so that the body has too little or too much fluid.

Fluid Intake

During periods of moderate activity at moderate temperature, the average adult drinks about 1500 ml per day but needs 2500 ml per day, an additional 1000 ml. This added volume is acquired from foods (referred to as preformed water) and from the oxidation of these foods during metabolic processes. Interestingly, the water content of food is relatively large, contributing about 750 ml per day. The water content of fresh vegetables is approximately 90%, of fresh fruits about 85%, and of lean meats around 60%.

Oxidative water, which is formed as a by-product of the body's oxidation of food, accounts for most of the remaining fluid volume required. This quantity ranges from 150 to 250 ml per day for the average adult (Guyton 1986, p. 382).

The primary regulator of fluid intake is the body's thirst mechanism. The thirst center is situated in the supraoptic nuclei in the lateral preoptic area of the hypothalamus. A number of stimuli trigger this center: intracellular dehydration, excess angiotensin II (a hormone released into the blood in response to very low blood pressure) in the body fluids, hemorrhage, and low cardiac output resulting in lowered blood volume. Angiotensin II is a potent vasoconstrictor. It forms largely in the small blood vessels in the lungs, in response to release of renin to the bloodstream from the kidneys.

Dryness of the mouth is often associated with thirst but can occur independently (for example, when a person's salivary glands do not secrete saliva). Thirst is normally relieved immediately after drinking a small amount of fluid, even before it is absorbed from the gastrointestinal tract. However, this relief is only temporary, and the thirst returns in about 15 minutes. The thirst is again temporarily relieved after the ingested fluid distends the upper gastrointestinal tract. These mechanisms protect the individual from drinking too much, because it takes from 30 minutes to 1 hour for the fluid to be absorbed and distributed throughout the body. If a person continued to drink during that time, the fluid ingested would overdilute the body fluids. See Table 40–5 for average water requirements.

Fluid Output

Fluid losses counterbalance the adult's 2500-ml daily intake of water. The main channel of excretion is the kidneys, which are responsible for an output of about 1500 ml per day in the adult. This approximates the amount of fluid an adult drinks per day. Oral intake and kidney output are frequently and easily measured in nursing practice.

The following are three other routes of fluid output:

1. Insensible loss through the skin as perspiration and through the lungs as water vapor in the expired air
2. Noticeable loss through the skin as sweat
3. Loss through the intestines in feces

See Table 40–3, earlier in the chapter for the average daily fluid output for an adult. The normal loss from skin and lungs accounts for about two-thirds of the urinary loss, whereas loss in the feces is minimal. It is important to remember that daily intake equals daily output.

Obligatory loss is the essential fluid loss required to maintain body functioning. Water lost as vapor in expired air and as vapor from the skin, a minimum volume of about 500 ml from the kidneys, and the fluid required to excrete the solid metabolic wastes produced daily are the obligatory losses, totaling about 1300 ml per day.

Since the vaporized losses are not readily measured, the measured obligatory kidney loss becomes of prime importance in critical illness. An adult hourly urine volume of less than 30 ml or daily volume under 500 ml is serious. Clients with inadequate output require immediate attention, and such a finding by the nurse must therefore be reported promptly. Although losses from the skin, lungs, and intestines in health account for approximately half of the daily loss, they can account for a much larger percentage of loss from a client who has a fever or accelerated respiration. Increases in respiratory rate, fever, **diaphoresis** (sweating), and diarrhea can magnify fluid loss from the normal routes immensely. Other routes of loss, such as from the stomach through emesis or suction or from abnormal body openings such as fistulas or surgically implanted drainage tubes, often account for significant losses, all of which require intake replacements.

In health, the output volumes shown in Table 40–3 may

TABLE 40–5 *Average Daily Fluid Requirements, by Age and Weight*

Age	Approximate Body Weight (kg)	ml/24 hours
3 days	3.3	300
1 year	10.0	1000
3 years	15.0	1250
5 years	20.0	1500
8 years	30.0	1750
13 years	60.0	2050
Adult	65.0	2500

Adapted from S. R. James and S. R. Mott, *Child health nursing. Essential care of children and families* (Menlo Park, Calif.: Addison-Wesley Publishing Co., 1988), p. 638; M. F. Hazinski, Nursing care of the critically ill child: A seven-point check. *Pediatric Nursing* November/December 1985 (11), p. 460 and John Plonk, M.D., chief pediatric resident, Vanderbilt University Hospital, December 1984.

vary noticeably from day to day and throughout the day. For example, sweat gland activity can increase when the environmental temperature increases. Urinary volume automatically increases as the amount of fluids ingested increases, e.g., on a hot summer day. If fluid loss from the skin is large, however, the urinary volume may decrease to maintain the fluid volumes in the body. Balance is maintained between the intake and output by the homeostatic mechanisms already discussed in this chapter.

Urine   The formation of urine by the kidneys and its subsequent excretion from the urinary bladder is the major avenue of fluid output. The two kidneys each contain about 2,400,000 nephrons (Guyton 1986, p. 393). The nephron is described in Chapter 43. The glomerulus filters glomerular fluid into a long tubule, where most of the fluid is reabsorbed into the bloodstream. The remainder of the fluid that is not absorbed becomes urine. The formation of urine and the control of that process are highly complex. One of the major controls of urine formation is blood volume. When the volume of circulating blood becomes excessive, the stretch receptors in the walls of the left and right atria are triggered to transmit impulses to the brain. The brain reacts by inhibiting sympathetic nervous impulses to the kidneys, reducing the secretion of antidiuretic hormone (ADH), and dilating the body's peripheral capillaries. As a result of these mechanisms, the rate of urine output is increased and excess blood volume filters temporarily into the tissue spaces.

Another control mechanism is the osmoreceptor of sodium and antidiuretic hormone system. This feedback system controls the concentration of sodium in the extracellular fluid, the fluid's osmolarity, and thus urine formation. An increase in the osmolarity (sodium concentration) of the extracellular fluid stimulates osmoreceptors, which are located in the supraoptic nuclei of the hypothalamus. These stimulate the production of antidiuretic hormone (ADH) by the hypothalamus and release of ADH by the posterior pituitary gland. ADH acts on the cells of the distal and collecting tubules of the glomeruli to make them more permeable to water. As a result, more fluid is reabsorbed into the bloodstream to dilute the sodium and other substances in the extracellular fluid, and less urine is formed. When the extracellular fluid becomes sufficiently diluted, the osmoreceptors respond to the decreased sodium concentration by reducing the production of ADH. Consequently, the antidiuretic effect ceases, and additional urine is produced.

Insensible Losses

Insensible fluid loss occurs through the skin and lungs. It is called *insensible* because it is usually not noticeable. The insensible loss through the skin is by diffusion. It is normally controlled by the outer layer of the epidermis, the stratum corneum. However, when the skin layers are destroyed by burns and abrasions, fluid loss can increase considerably.

Another type of insensible loss is the water in exhaled air. In an adult, this is normally 300 to 400 ml per day. When respiratory rate accelerates, e.g., due to exercise or an elevated body temperature, this loss can increase.

Sweat

Sweating occurs when the body becomes overheated. The sweat glands secrete large quantities of sweat onto the surface of the body to provide cooling by evaporation. Sweating occurs in response to stimulation of the preoptic area in the anterior hypothalamus. Impulses are transmitted to the spinal cord and via the sympathetic nervous system to the skin.

The rate of flow of sweat can vary from none in a cold environment to 1.5 to 2 liters per hour in an adult not acclimatized to a hot environment (Guyton 1986, p. 853).

Large amounts of sweat contain large amounts of sodium chloride, whereas small amounts of sweat contain lower concentrations of sodium chloride. Sweat also contains urea, lactic acid, and potassium ions. The concentrations of these substances can be very high when the rate of sweat secretion is low and are lower when the rate of sweat secretion is high (Guyton 1986, p. 852).

Feces

The chyme that passes from the small intestine into the large intestine is composed of water and electrolytes. The volume of chyme that passes through the ileocecal valve in an adult is normally about 1500 ml per day (Guyton 1986, p. 796). Of this amount, all but about 100 ml is reabsorbed in the proximal half of the large intestine. Sodium and chloride ions are also actively absorbed, and bicarbonate ions are secreted by the mucosa of the large intestine. The bicarbonate helps to neutralize the acidic end products of bacterial action in the colon. For further information about the composition of feces, see Chapter 42.

FACTORS AFFECTING FLUID AND ELECTROLYTE BALANCE

Age

Fluid intake requirements vary with age. Intake requirements have been determined for various ages in relation to body surface area, metabolic requirements, and body weight.

Infants and growing children have much greater fluid turnover than adults, i.e., greater water needs and greater water losses. This is due to their greater metabolic rate, which increases fluid loss through the kidneys. Because immature kidneys are less efficient than adult kidneys, infants lose more fluid through the kidneys. Infant losses from both the lungs and the skin are also greater in proportion to body weight, essentially because respirations are more rapid and the body surface area is proportionately greater. The more rapid turnover of fluid plus the losses produced by disease can create critical fluid imbalances in children much more rapidly than in adults. See Table 40–5 for approximate fluid requirements at different ages according to body weight.

In elderly people, fluid and electrolyte imbalances are often associated with kidney or cardiac problems. Because the kidneys are less able to concentrate urine, elderly persons may need to take in additional fluid to meet their fluid needs. Whereas water accounts for 60% of the body weight of young males, it accounts for only 52% of the body weight of elderly males and 46% of the body weight of elderly females (Metheny and Snively 1983, p. 371).

Environmental Temperature

Excessive heat stimulates the sympathetic nervous system and causes the person to sweat. When the person is not acclimatized to the heat, the sweat glands are strongly stimulated, and as much as 700 ml to 2 liters per hour can be lost through sweating. The sodium chloride (NaCl) in the sweat is also lost. An unacclimatized person can lose as much as 15 to 30 g of salt each day (Guyton 1986, p. 853).

Diet

A person's diet obviously affects the intake of fluids and electrolytes. When nutritional intake is inadequate or unbalanced, the body tries to preserve stored protein by breaking down glycogen and fat. Once these resources are gone, the body draws on protein stores, and the serum albumin level decreases. Serum albumin plays an important role in drawing fluid from the interstitial body compartment into the blood through osmosis. When fluid is not drawn normally into the bloodstream, it remains in the interstitial space, causing edema.

Stress

Stress affects a person's fluid and electrolyte balance. Stress can increase cellular metabolism, blood glucose concentration, and muscle glycolysis. These mechanisms can lead to sodium and water retention. In addition, stress can increase production of the antidiuretic hormone, which in turn decreases urine production. The overall response of the body to stress is to increase the blood volume. See Chapter 33, page 793, for additional information.

Illness Extensive surgical procedures can change a person's fluid and electrolyte balance through a number of mechanisms. The stress response mentioned above is one of these. In addition, tissue trauma can cause the loss of fluid and electrolytes from within the damaged cells. An example of such trauma is severe burns. The burned person loses plasma and interstitial fluid as exudate. (An **exudate** is material that has escaped from the blood vessels and is deposited in the tissues or on the tissue surfaces.) Also, water vapor is lost from the burn site, blood leaks from damaged capillaries, and water and sodium move into the tissue cells.

Cardiac and renal disorders also affect the body's fluid and electrolyte balance. For example, impaired heart function can decrease blood flow to the kidneys and thus hinder the elimination of the waste products of metabolism. When urine output decreases, the body retains sodium, and circulatory overload (hypervolemia) can result. Fluid retention can also lead to pulmonary edema (fluid in the lungs).

DISTURBANCES IN FLUID AND ELECTROLYTE BALANCE

Extracellular Fluid (ECF) Deficit

An extracellular fluid deficit is also called a *fluid volume deficit* (FVD), **hypovolemia,** or **dehydration.** In the strict sense, dehydration is not an ECF deficit but a water deficit only.

ECF deficit can occur because of an abrupt decrease in fluid intake or a marked increase in fluid output, i.e., an acute loss of secretions or excretions. The body's initial response to a fluid deficit is depletion of the intravascular compartment. Then fluid is drawn from the interstitial compartment into the intravascular compartment, depleting the interstitial compartment. To compensate for the decreased interstitial volume, the body then draws intracellular fluid out of the cells.

In clients with ECF deficit, the total volume of fluid and associated electrolytes is reduced; the proportions, however, usually remain normal. For the signs of ECF deficit, see the accompanying box. ECF deficits generally occur as a result of abnormal losses through the skin, gastrointestinal tract, or kidney; decreased intake of fluid; bleeding; or movement of fluid into **third-space.** Third-spacing is the movement of fluid into body spaces such as the interstitial spaces, and the pleural, peritoneal, pericardial, or joint cavities. It commonly occurs in clients with burns and other traumatic injuries but may occur after abdominal surgery; it can lead to hypovolemia, renal failure, and shock. Third-spacing occurs when tissue injury increases capillary membrane permeability. This allows not only fluid but also blood proteins (e.g., albumin) to move out of the capillary into the interstitial space. The movement of proteins decreases the plasma osmotic force and increases the interstitial osmotic force, pulling even more fluid from the plasma to the insterstitium.

Changes brought about by *hypovolemia* are (a) reduced extracellular fluid (ECF) volume and (b) hypertonicity or a hyperosmolar fluid imbalance. These changes occur because there is more solute in proportion to fluid. When the body is deprived of water, the extracellular fluid compartment, including interstitial fluid, is reduced. However, water passes into plasma immediately. The water gained passes by osmosis from the intracellular compartments through interstitial fluid to the plasma. This transfer of water tends to preserve the circulating blood plasma volume. If the kidneys are functioning normally, they will attempt to retain water and salt by reducing the excretion of sodium chloride and water to minimal amounts. As the fluid deficit progresses, the concentrations of the sodium ion (Na^+) and the chloride ion (Cl^-) in plasma rise, thus increasing blood concentration (increased serum osmolarity).

Clients go into **hypovolemic shock** when intravascular fluid compartments become greatly depleted. Shock indicates that the deficits are so great that the regulatory mechanisms of the body can no longer maintain the plasma volume. It is responsible for such manifestations as a rapid weak pulse, fall in blood pressure, and increased concentration of blood solutes. Since the kidneys rely on sufficient arterial blood pressure to produce urine, hypovolemia results in **oliguria** (decreased urine output). Oliguria can progress to **anuria** (absence of urine). As a consequence, met-

---

Clinical Signs of ECF Deficit

Observations:
- Postural hypotension
- Weight loss
- Dryness of mucous membranes
- Decreased tissue turgor
- Weak, rapid pulse
- Sunken eyeballs
- Oliguria—may be less than 30 ml/hr
- Skin pale

Laboratory findings:
- Increased specific gravity of urine
- Elevated hematocrit
- Decreased central venous pressure (CVP)

abolic wastes accumulate, the client quickly becomes disoriented and comatose, and death ensues due to the effects of the acid waste products on the cells.

Extracellular Fluid (ECF) Excess

An excess of extracellular fluid, also called *fluid volume excess* (FVE), can lead to (a) **hypervolemia** (increased blood volume or **circulatory overload**) and (b) **edema** (excess fluid in the interstitial compartment). **Overhydration** is another term sometimes used synonymously with ECF excess. However, overhydration is an increase only in the amount of water (not electrolytes) in the extracellular space. Normally, the interstitial fluid compartment is not bogged with water; rather, it is compact, elastic, and expandable, with just enough fluid to fill the crevices between tissues. This compact state facilitates diffusion of nutrients from the plasma to the intracellular fluid (ICF) and diffusion of the metabolic wastes from the cells to the plasma. When the interstitial spaces are filled with fluid and the extracellular osmotic pressure increases, fluid is pulled from within the cells, resulting in edema. Edema is most frequently observed around the eyes, and in the feet and hands. *Dependent edema* is found in the lowest body parts, e.g., in the feet and legs or in the sacrum of the sitting client. Edema can be localized or generalized in the body and can account for an increase in weight of at least 4.5 kg (10 lb) in an adult.

Edema can develop whenever there is increased formation of interstitial fluid or impaired removal of interstitial fluid. This commonly occurs when (a) the capillary permeability increases (e.g., burns, allergy), resulting in increased movement of fluid from the capillaries into the interstitial space or (b) the hydrostatic pressure in the capillaries increases (e.g., blood hypervolemia, venous blood circulation obstruction). As a result of the hypervolemia, more fluid is pushed out of the arterial capillary bed into the interstitial space. Venous obstruction results in an increased pressure in the venous capillaries, impeding the flow of fluid from the interstitial spaces into the venous capillaries. Edema can also occur when (c) removal of fluid from the interstitial space is decreased (e.g., lymphatic blockage).

Pitting edema is edema that leaves a small depression or pit after finger pressure is applied to the swollen area. The pit is caused by movement of fluid to adjacent tissue, away from the point of pressure. Within 10 to 30 seconds, the pit normally disappears. Pitting edema is never seen in clients with a pure water excess (Harvey et al. 1980, p. 56). See Chapter 19, page 370, for assessment of pitting edema. In *nonpitting edema,* the fluid in edematous tissues cannot be moved to adjacent spaces by finger pressure. Nonpitting edema is not a sign of ECF excess but often accompanies infections and traumas that cause fluid to collect and coagulate in tissue spaces. The coagulation prevents displacement of fluid to other areas by pressure.

Overloading of the vascular fluid compartment increases blood hydrostatic pressure, which forces fluid into the interstitial spaces. **Anasarca** (edema that is generalized throughout the body) is the result. Greatly increased hydrostatic pressure forces large amounts of fluid through the alveolar-capillary membrane into the alveoli of the lungs, causing pulmonary edema, a serious problem that can result in death by suffocation. Manifestations of pulmonary edema are frothy sputum, dyspnea, cough, and gurgling sounds on respiration. The most common cause of pulmonary edema is left-sided heart failure, with resulting increases in the pressure of the pulmonary blood capillaries and the interstitial spaces of the lung tissue.

Because there is no change in the tonicity of body fluids in ECF volume excess, fluid does not move into the ICF compartment. Thus, clients with ECF excess do not develop cerebral signs as do clients with isolated water excess. The serum sodium level and serum osmolarity also remain normal. The hematocrit may be normal or decreased. In persistent ECF excesses associated with heart failure or cirrhosis, the client's hematocrit is usually normal. In acute ECF excesses, however, the hematocrit decreases in proportion to the severity of the problem.

When fluid moves from the vascular compartment into the interstitial spaces, the blood volume drops. In response, the body releases antidiuretic hormone (ADH) and aldosterone, which stimulate the kidneys to retain fluid and sodium. This response adds to the existing problem because the retained fluid can also move into the interstitial spaces, thus augmenting the edema. Therefore, generalized edema is a self-perpetuating condition. See the accompanying box for clinical signs of ECF excess.

Clinical Signs of ECF Excess

Observations:

- Peripheral edema
- Weight gain
  - a. Mild: 2% in an adult
  - b. Moderate: 5% in an adult
  - c. Severe: 8% in an adult
- Distended neck veins
- Moist crackles in lungs
- Distended peripheral veins
- Ascites
- Bounding full pulse

Laboratory findings:

- Decreased hematocrit due to plasma dilution
- Decreased BUN due to plasma dilution

Sodium (Na$^+$)

Normal sodium concentrations in the extracellular fluid are regulated by ADH and aldosterone. Aldosterone, a hormone produced by the adrenal cortex, acts to maintain sodium concentrations, although its action can be overridden by ADH and the thirst mechanism described earlier. *ADH* regulates the amount of water absorbed into the blood from the renal tubules. *Aldosterone* regulates the amount of sodium reabsorbed into the blood. When aldosterone is secreted and the reabsorption of sodium is increased, the sodium concentration of the extracellular fluids rises. In a feedback mechanism, the increased extracellular sodium causes the adrenal cortex to decrease the secretion of aldosterone. If the body must conserve sodium for any reason, it can excrete sodium-free urine.

Sodium not only moves into and out of the body but also moves in careful balance among the three fluid compartments. It is found in most body secretions, e.g., saliva, gastric and intestinal secretions, bile, and pancreatic fluid. Therefore, continuous excretion of any of these fluids, e.g., via intestinal suction, can result in a sodium deficit.

Sodium functions largely in the control and regulation of the body fluids. When sodium is reabsorbed into the blood from the tubules of the glomeruli, chloride is reabsorbed with it. The combined reabsorption increases the fluid held in the body. Sodium also helps maintain blood volume and interstitial fluid volume through this mechanism. With potassium, sodium helps maintain the electrolyte balance of intracellular and extracellular fluids by means of the active transport mechanism, the sodium-potassium pump. Sodium is also involved in the transmission of nerve impulses. For additional information about sodium see Table 39–3, page 995.

Hyponatremia is a sodium deficit in the blood plasma. It is the result of:

1. *Net gain of water.* The intake of water exceeds the corresponding intake of sodium, e.g., drinking excessive quantities of water or administering excessive amounts of 5% dextrose in water (D5W) intravenously.

2. *Loss of sodium-rich fluids that are replaced only by water.* Excessive sodium loss can be the result of excessive sweating or the prolonged use of strong diuretics. Also, clients can lose abnormally large amounts of sodium through the gastrointestinal tract. The sodium content of pancreatic secretions and gastric mucus is especially high. Severe, prolonged diarrhea or a draining pancreatic fistula can result in abnormally high sodium loss. Gastric suction, which withdraws gastric mucus along with other gastric fluids, can also be the cause.

Hypernatremia is sodium excess in the blood plasma. Hypernatremia is the result of:

1. *Net loss of water.* Body water loss exceeds sodium loss in situations of water deprivation (dehydration). Also,

clients may lose more water than sodium through a draining intestinal wound or through untreated watery diarrhea. A client who is not treated for watery diarrhea may experience hypernatremia on about the fifth or sixth day after onset.

2. *Excessive sodium intake.* Sodium intake rarely exceeds water intake but may occur when a person, for example, mistakenly ingests a large number of sodium chloride tablets or is given a hypertonic saline solution intravenously.

The clinical signs of hyponatremia and hypernatremia are shown in the box above.

Chloride (Cl$^-$)

Chloride is the major anion of extracellular fluid. Chloride is found in blood, interstitial fluid, and lymph. A very small amount is found in intracellular fluid. It functions as sodium

---

Clinical Signs of Hyponatremia and Hypernatremia

Hyponatremia

Observations:
- Feelings of apprehension
- Lethargy
- Muscle cramps
- Anorexia, nausea, vomiting
- Postural hypotension
- Seizures, coma

Laboratory findings:
- Serum sodium below 135 mEq/L
- Serum osmolality below 285 mOsm/kg
- Urine sodium varies depending on cause

Hypernatremia

Observations:
- Extreme thirst
- Dry, sticky mucous membranes
- Tongue red, dry, swollen
- Elevated body temperature
- Severe hypernatremia
  a. Agitated behavior
  b. Fatigue
  c. Restlessness

Laboratory findings:
- Serum sodium above 145 mEq/L
- Serum osmolality above 295 mOsm/kg

does to maintain the osmotic pressure of the blood. Its reabsorption in the kidney is secondary to that of sodium; i.e., each sodium ion reabsorbed is accompanied by the chloride or bicarbonate ion. Because aldosterone controls the reabsorption of sodium, it controls the reabsorption of chloride indirectly. **Hypochloremia** (a deficit in serum chloride) and **hyperchloremia** (an excess serum chloride) usually develop along with sodium disturbances. The normal serum chloride of an adult is 95 to 108 mEq/liter.

Potassium (K⁺)

Potassium is the major cation of intracellular fluid. Potassium balance is regulated in the kidneys by two mechanisms: exchange with sodium ions in the kidney tubules and secretion of aldosterone. Aldosterone is extremely important in controlling potassium concentrations in extracellular fluids. The aldosterone-potassium feedback system works in three steps:

1. Increased potassium concentration in extracellular fluid causes an increase in the production of aldosterone.

2. The elevated aldosterone level increases the amount of potassium excreted by the kidneys.

3. As potassium excretion increases, the concentration of potassium in the extracellular fluid decreases. In turn, aldosterone production decreases.

Potassium affects the functions of most body systems, including the cardiovascular system, the gastrointestinal system, the neuromuscular system, and the respiratory system. Of particular importance is potassium's role in transmitting electrical impulses to the heart and other muscles, to lung tissues, and to intestinal tissues. Most of the body's potassium is found inside the cells. A small amount is found in the plasma and interstitial fluids. See Table 39–3, page 995, for additional information about potassium.

Potassium is usually excreted by the kidneys. However, the kidneys do not regulate potassium excretion as effectively as sodium excretion. Therefore, an acute potassium deficiency can develop rapidly. Of the body's secretions, the gastrointestinal secretions are high in potassium.

Like other electrolytes, potassium moves continually in and out of the cells. This movement from the interstitial fluid, which has less potassium, to the intracellular fluid, which has a greater concentration, is influenced by the adrenal steroids, testosterone, pH changes, glycogen formation, and hyponatremia. If tissues are damaged, the body can lose potassium quickly.

Hypokalemia is a potassium deficit in the blood plasma. Hypokalemia can develop quickly in people who are starving. The combined effects of inadequate potassium intake and potassium loss because of prolonged diarrhea can deplete potassium stores acutely. A leading cause of potassium deficit is the use of powerful diuretics. Surgical procedures, particularly those involving the digestive tract, often result in a potassium deficit unless supplemental potassium is supplied.

Hyperkalemia is a potassium excess in the blood plasma. Hyperkalemia is most often caused by a decreased urinary excretion of potassium, leakage of potassium from the body's cells, e.g., after severe burns, or by excessive ingestion of potassium, e.g., the intravenous administration of excessive amounts of potassium when kidney function is impaired. The clinical signs of hypokalemia and hyperkalemia are shown in the accompanying box.

Clinical Signs of Hypokalemia and Hyperkalemia

Hypokalemia

Observations:

- Muscle weakness, leg cramps
- Fatigue
- Anorexia, nausea, vomiting
- Decreased bowel sounds

Laboratory findings:

- Serum potassium below 3.5 mEq/L
- Arterial blood gases (ABGs) may show increased pH and HCO_3^-
- Electrocardiogram may show flattening of the T waves and depression of the ST segment

Hyperkalemia

Observations:

- Gastrointestinal hyperactivity, diarrhea
- Irritability, apathy, confusion
- Cardiac arrhythmia, bradycardia, cardiac arrest
- Muscle weakness, numbness, **areflexia** (absence of reflexes)

Laboratory findings:

- Serum potassium above 5.0 mEq/L

Calcium (Ca²⁺)

The richest sources of calcium are milk and milk products. Drinking water in some parts of the country also contains an absorbable calcium. See Table 39–3, page 995.

Calcium functions in bone formation and in the transmission of nerve impulses, muscle contraction, blood coagulation, and activation of certain enzymes, e.g., pancreatic lipase and phospholipase. Only 1% of the body's calcium is found in ECF.

Hypocalcemia is a calcium deficit in the blood plasma. Two causes of hypocalcemia are hypoparathyroidism and excessive loss of intestinal secretions, which contain a great deal of calcium. Mild hypocalcemia may be reflected as a tingling sensation in the fingers and around the mouth, and as abdominal and skeletal muscle cramps. Severe depletion can cause **tetany** (muscle spasms, sharp flexion of the wrists and ankles, cramps), which can lead to convulsions. Adults experience hypocalcemia when the serum calcium level falls below 4.3 mEq/liter.

Hypercalcemia is an excess of calcium in the blood plasma. It can be due to prolonged immobilization, hyperparathyroidism, or a tumor of the parathyroid glands. The clinical signs of hypocalcemia and hypercalcemia are given in the accompanying box.

Magnesium (Mg^{2+})

Magnesium, the fourth most abundant cation in the body, is important for maintaining neuromuscular activity within the body. Like calcium, magnesium is regulated by the parathyroid glands. It is absorbed from the intestinal tract. The magnesium content of the body is affected by the potassium concentration. If magnesium is deficient, the kidneys tend to excrete more potassium. Increased extracellular magnesium levels (**hypermagnesemia**) depress nervous system activity and skeletal muscle contractions. Low magnesium concentrations (**hypomagnesemia**), by contrast, cause increased irritability of the nervous system, peripheral vasodilation, and cardiac arrhythmias (Guyton 1986, p. 872). For clinical signs of hypomagnesemia (magnesium deficit) and hypermagnesemia (magnesium excess), see the box on page 1048.

Calcium is excreted in urine, feces, bile, digestive secretions, and sweat. The concentration of body calcium is controlled indirectly by the effect of parathyroid hormone on bone reabsorption. When calcium levels in extracellular fluid fall too low, the parathyroid glands are stimulated to increase parathyroid hormone (parathormone) secretion. This hormone acts directly on the bones to increase the release of calcium into the blood. When the bones run out of calcium, parathyroid hormone acts on both the kidney tubules and the intestinal mucosa to increase the reabsorption of calcium from the kidneys and the intestine.

Another hormone, *calcitonin,* has an effect nearly opposite that of the parathyroid hormone. Calcitonin reduces the concentration of calcium ions in the blood. Calcitonin, which is secreted by the thyroid gland, stimulates the deposition of calcium in bone and depresses the formation of osteoclasts in the bone. However, the effect of calcitonin on plasma concentration levels of adults is minimal (Guyton 1986, p. 947) because the parathyroid hormone counteracts the effect of calcitonin within hours.

Phosphate (PO_4^-)

The phosphate anion is found both in intracellular and extracellular fluid. Most of the phosphorus (P^+) in the body exists as PO_4^-. Together with calcium, phosphate is involved in bone and tooth formation. It is also involved in many chemical actions of the cells. Many of the B vitamins are effective only when combined with phosphate (Metheny and Snively 1983, p. 58). Phosphate is absorbed exceedingly well from the intestine, and it is excreted in the urine. Phosphate is a threshold substance because none is lost in urine when blood plasma concentrations fall below a critical level. When the concentration is above the critical level, however, it is excreted in proportion to the increase. Therefore, the kidneys regulate the concentration of phosphate in the extracellular fluid. In addition, phosphate excretion is regulated by the parathyroid hormone. See the box on page 1048 for clinical signs of **hypophosphatemia** (phosphate deficit) and **hyperphosphatemia** (phosphate excess). Table 40–6 summarizes data about body fluids and electrolytes.

Clinical Signs of Hypomagnesemia and Hypermagnesemia

Hypomagnesemia

Observations:

- Neuromuscular irritability with tremors
- Increased reflexes, tremors, convulsions
- Positive Chvostek's and Trousseau's signs (see Table 40–8)
- Tachycardia
- Disorientation and confusion

Laboratory findings:

- Serum magnesium below 1.5 mEq/L

Hypermagnesemia

Observations:

- Lethargy, drowsiness
- Coma
- Impaired respirations
- Nausea, vomiting
- Muscle weakness, paralysis
- Hypotension

Laboratory findings:

- Serum magnesium above 2.5 mEq/L
- Electrocardiogram shows prolonged QT interval and an atrioventricular (AV) block may occur

Clinical Signs of Hypophosphatemia and Hyperphosphatemia

Hypophosphatemia

Observations (Acute):

- Confusion, seizures, coma
- Muscle pain
- Decreased muscle strength

Observations (chronic):

- Memory loss
- Fatigue
- Bone pain and joint stiffness

Laboratory findings:

- Serum phosphate below 1.2 mEq/L
- Decreased cardiac function

Hyperphosphatemia

Observations:

- Anorexia, nausea, and vomiting
- Hyperreflexia, tetany
- Tachycardia

Laboratory findings:

- Serum phosphate level above 3.0 mEq/L
- Electrocardiogram shows shortened ST segment and QT interval

TABLE 40–6 *Fluid and Electrolyte Data*

Clinical Factor (Normal)	Food Sources	Predisposing Conditions	Nursing Intervention
Extracellular fluid (infant: 29% of body weight; adult: 15% of body weight)	Oral fluids, fruits, vegetables	*Deficit:* Nausea, vomiting, anorexia, diarrhea, insufficient fluid intake, third-spacing	*Deficit:* Give oral fluids as permitted. Administer and monitor IV fluids as ordered. Monitor fluid intake and output. Assess for signs of dehydration. Monitor vital signs.
		Excess: Excessive intake of fluids with NaCl, renal failure, congestive heart failure, diet high in sodium	*Excess:* Assist adherence to sodium-restricted diet as ordered. Monitor response to diuretics, weigh daily. Monitor intake, output, and vital signs. Restrict fluids as ordered.

Clinical Factor (Normal)	Food Sources	Predisposing Conditions	Nursing Intervention
Sodium (Na$^+$) (135–45 mEq/L [serum])	Table salt (NaCl), cheese, pork, salted meats, canned vegetables, potato chips	*Deficit:* Excessive perspiration, gastrointestinal loss, excessive administration of fluid without NaCl	*Deficit:* Monitor fluid intake and output. Assess for presence of symptoms such as anorexia, nausea, vomiting. Assist with intake of foods and fluids containing sodium.
		Excess: Excessive intake of sodium, deprivation of water, excessive loss of water, i.e. diarrhea	*Excess:* Monitor fluid intake and output. Monitor for presence of symptoms (see page 1045). Assist with fluid intake. Advise regarding low-sodium foods and fluids as ordered.
Potassium (K$^+$) (3.6–5.0 mEq/L [serum])	Bananas, broccoli, cantaloupe, citrus fruits, potatoes, nuts, fish	*Deficit:* Diarrhea, vomiting, certain kidney diseases, potassium-losing diuretic therapy, excessive stress	*Deficit:* Monitor cardiac changes (e.g., weak, irregular pulse). Administer potassium as ordered. Teach client about food sources high in potassium. Monitor for presence of symptoms. Monitor intake and output.
		Excess: Excessive potassium administration, renal disease	*Excess:* Monitor cardiac function for irregular pulse rate and bradycardia. Restrict potassium in diet. Monitor serum potassium.
Calcium (Ca^{2+}) (4.3–5.3 mEq/L [serum])	Milk, milk products, grains, cereals, fruits, nuts, greens	*Deficit:* Increased calcium loss, e.g., intestinal suction, hypoparathyroidism, chronic renal failure	*Deficit:* Administer calcium supplement as needed. Advise to increase or decrease regular dietary calcium. Initiate seizure precautions. Monitor serum calcium. Assess client for signs of hypocalcemia.
		Excess: Prolonged immobilization hyperparathyroidism, hypophosphatemia	*Excess:* Monitor serum calcium. Assess client for signs of hypercalcemia. Inspect urine for calculi.
Chloride (Cl$^-$) (98–108 mEq/L [serum])	Table salt, dairy products	*Deficit:* Increased HCO$_3^-$, loss through vomiting, excessive ECF loss through intestinal fistula	*Deficit:* Usually associated with hyponatremia (see sodium, above). Monitor serum sodium and chloride.
		Excess: Increased Na$^+$, excessive fluid loss through kidneys, severe dehydration	*Excess:* Usually associated with hypernatremia (see sodium, above).
Magnesium (Mg^{2+}) (1.5–2.5 mEq/L [serum])	Whole grains, green leafy vegetables	*Deficit:* Chronic alcoholism, acute pancreatitis, prolonged gastric suction, diarrhea, intestinal malabsorption syndrome	*Deficit:* Monitor breathing. Employ safety precautions if confusion or seizures are anticipated. Assist with magnesium replacement as ordered.
		Excess: Excessive use of magnesium-containing antacids, renal failure, Addison's disease	*Excess:* Monitor vital signs. Monitor level of consciousness.

TABLE 40-6 *Fluid and Electrolyte Data* (continued)

Clinical Factor (Normal)	Food Sources	Predisposing Conditions	Nursing Intervention
Phosphate (PO_4^-) (1.2–3.0 mEq/L [serum])	Milk, cheese, fish, poultry, milk products, whole grains	*Deficit:* Excessive use of phosphate-binding antacids, malabsorption syndrome	*Deficit:* Monitor serum phosphate levels. Assess neurologic signs and orientation. Administer IV phosphate as ordered. Teach client about food sources high in phosphorus.
		Excess: Renal insufficiency, hypoparathyroidism, Vitamin D intoxication, myelogenous leukemia, lymphoma	*Excess:* Administer magnesium or calcium or antacids as ordered. Assist with diet low in phosphorus.

ACID-BASE BALANCE

The body's cellular activity requires an alkaline medium. Alkalinity and its opposite, acidity, are measured in terms of hydrogen ion concentration, expressed on a scale called **pH.** Body fluids are normally maintained at a pH of about 7.4. Alterations of pH of even a few tenths can be incompatible with cellular activity. The normal pH range of extracellular fluid is 7.35 to 7.45. See Figure 40–1. This precise balance is maintained as long as the ratio of 1 carbonic acid molecule to 20 bicarbonate ions is maintained in the extracellular fluid. The ratio, rather than the specific amount of each, is important.

Opposing the body's alkalinity are cellular chemical processes that are constantly producing large amounts of acid as by-products of metabolism. Fortunately, precise control mechanisms maintain the pH of body fluids within a very narrow range. The pH is controlled by buffer systems in all body fluids and by respiratory and kidney regulatory systems.

Buffer Systems

A buffer system resists change in the pH of a fluid by chemically binding excess hydrogen ions to prevent an increase in pH or by releasing hydrogen ions to prevent a decrease in the pH. Buffers do not neutralize; acid-base buffers decrease the effect of strong acids and strong bases, so that the pH of a body fluid falls or rises only slightly.

There are three main buffer systems in the body: the bicarbonate buffer, the phosphate buffer, and the protein buffer.

Bicarbonate Buffer System The bicarbonate (HCO_3^-) buffer system is important in controlling the pH of *extracellular* fluids of the body. It consists of sodium bicarbonate ($NaHCO_3$) or potassium bicarbonate ($KHCO_3$) and carbonic acid (H_2CO_3) in the same solution.

If a strong acid, such as hydrochloric acid (HCl) is introduced into an unbuffered system, such as a glass of water, the pH of the fluid drops significantly to 1 or 2. However, if a bicarbonate buffer system is already present in the water, the HCl quickly combines with the buffer, producing a weaker acid (carbonic acid), and the pH drops only slightly. This is the reaction:

$$HCl + NaHCO_3 \rightarrow H_2CO_3 + NaCl$$

(hydrochloric acid)	(sodium bicarbonate)	(carbonic acid)	(sodium chloride)

A strong acid is a compound that completely dissociates its hydrogen ions; for example, HCl yields H^+ and Cl^-. A weak acid frees only some of its hydrogen ions; for example, H_2CO_3 yields H^+ and HCO_3^-. One hydrogen ion is free, the other is not.

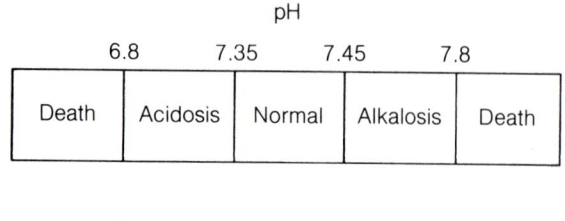

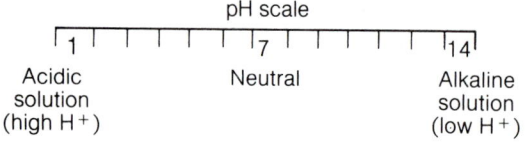

Figure 40–1 Body fluids are normally slightly alkaline, between a pH of 7.35 and 7.45.

Alkalis (bases) undergo a similar change. When a strong base such as sodium hydroxide is added to body fluids, it combines with carbonic acid to form a weaker base, sodium bicarbonate:

$$NaOH + H_2CO_3 \rightarrow NaHCO_3 + H_2O$$
(sodium hydroxide)   (carbonic acid)   (sodium bicarbonate)   (water)

Although the bicarbonate buffer system is not the strongest buffer system in the body (the most powerful and plentiful one consists of the proteins of plasma and cells), it is important, because the concentration of sodium bicarbonate is regulated by the kidneys and the concentration of carbonic acid by the respiratory system.

Phosphate Buffer System   The phosphate buffer system is an important *intracellular* buffer system. Phosphate ions (HPO_4^{2-}), like bicarbonate ions and ammonia ions, are present in the urine. The phosphate buffer system is composed of two elements, $H_2PO_4^-$ and HPO_4^{2-}. These elements exchange a hydrogen ion for a sodium ion mainly in the kidney tubules. For example, when hydrochloric acid (HCl, a strong acid) is added to these two elements, the HCl is removed and replaced by a weakly acidic compound (NaH_2PO_4):

$$HCl + Na_2HPO_4 \rightarrow NaH_2PO_4 + NaCl$$
(strong acid)   (buffer)   (weak acid)   (sodium chloride)

By contrast, when sodium hydroxide (NaOH, a strong base) is added to the buffer system, a very weak base (Na_2HPO_4) is formed:

$$NaOH + NaH_2PO_4 \rightarrow Na_2HPO_4 + H_2O$$
(strong base)   (buffer)   (weak base)   (water)

This phosphate buffer system is particularly important in buffering the fluids in the kidney tubules and the fluid inside the cells.

Protein Buffer System   The protein buffer system is the largest buffer system in the body. The buffers are the proteins of the cells and of the plasma. It has been shown that about three-fourths of all chemical buffering in the body takes place inside the cells and results from intracellular proteins (Guyton 1986, p. 442). Important protein buffers are hemoglobin in the red blood cells, and histone proteins and nucleic acids inside the cells.

Respiratory Regulation

Elimination of carbon dioxide by the lungs also regulates acid-base balance. The carbon dioxide that a person exhales comes from carbonic acid as follows:

$$H_2CO_3 \rightarrow CO_2 + H_2O$$

The more CO_2 exhaled, the more H_2CO_3 is removed from the blood, thus elevating the blood pH to a more alkaline level. Hyperventilation is an example of a mechanism by which respiratory regulation of acid-base balance is achieved. Increasing the ventilation rate raises the pH. By contrast, holding one's breath, or hypoventilating, causes the body to retain CO_2, which is then available to form carbonic acid, reducing the pH and acidifying body fluids. Respiratory alterations, therefore, change the pH of body fluids significantly and rapidly.

Renal Regulation

The kidney's role in maintaining acid-base balance is complex. A simplified account of the process follows. The kidneys excrete hydrogen ions and form bicarbonate ions in specific amounts as indicated by the pH of the blood. When the plasma pH drops (becomes more acidic), hydrogen ions (acid) are excreted, and bicarbonate ions (base) are formed and retained. Conversely, when the plasma pH rises (becomes more alkaline), hydrogen ions are retained in the body, and bicarbonate ions are excreted.

Primary Acid-Base Imbalances

Imbalances in pH can result in either acidosis or alkalosis. **Acidosis** (blood pH below 7.35) occurs with increases in blood carbonic acid or with decreases in blood bicarbonate. It is also referred to as **acidemia**. **Alkalosis** (blood pH above 7.45) occurs with increases in blood bicarbonate or decreases in blood carbonic acid. It is also referred to as **alkalemia.** A client will not become acidotic or alkalotic, however, unless the normal ratio of 1 carbonic acid molecule to 20 bicarbonate ions is altered.

The primary general cause or origin of a pH imbalance is indicated by the terms *metabolic* or *respiratory.* Metabolic acidosis and metabolic alkalosis are imbalances brought about by changes in bicarbonate levels as a result of metabolic alterations. Respiratory acidosis and respiratory alkalosis are imbalances brought about by changes in carbonic acid levels as a result of respiratory alterations.

In all acid-base imbalances, there is a corrective body response by both the kidneys and the lungs called **compensation.** Any given acid-base imbalance can be described as compensated until body reserves are used up. Then the condition is described as uncompensated. In compensated acidosis or alkalosis, the kidneys and lungs are able to restore the altered ratio of 1 carbonic acid molecule to 20 bicarbonate ions, thereby maintaining a normal pH. For example in (compensated) respiratory acidosis, the plasma pH is maintained at normal even though there is an increase in the carbonic acid because the kidneys retain bicarbonate.

Respiratory Acidosis (Carbonic Acid Excess)
Respiratory acidosis occurs when exhalation of carbon dioxide is inhibited, creating a carbonic acid excess in the

body. Hypoventilation is its general cause. Two major conditions that cause hypoventilation are central nervous system depression and obstructive lung disease. Morphine poisoning and anesthesia are examples of central nervous system depression, whereas asthma and emphysema are obstructive lung diseases. See the box above for the clinical signs of respiratory acidosis.

Respiratory Alkalosis (Carbonic Acid Deficit)

Respiratory alkalosis occurs when exhalation of carbon dioxide is excessive, resulting in a carbonic acid deficit. Its root cause is hyperventilation, which can be due to fever, anxiety, or pulmonary infections. A hyperventilating client blows off abundant carbon dioxide, resulting in lowered carbonic acid blood levels. The box below lists the clinical signs of respiratory alkalosis. These signs reflect the primary imbalance, renal compensation, and associated electrolyte imbalances.

Metabolic Acidosis (Base Bicarbonate Deficit)

Metabolic acidosis occurs when levels of base bicarbonate are low in relation to carbonic acid blood levels. The kidneys normally retain bicarbonate (HCO_3^-) or excrete hydrogen ions (H^+) in response to altered blood pH. Starvation, renal impairment, and diabetes mellitus are among the conditions that deluge the plasma with acid metabolites. With renal impairment, related electrolyte imbalances may develop. Prolonged diarrhea can decrease bicarbonate. See the box above for clinical signs of metabolic acidosis.

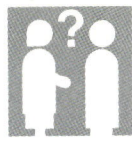

Metabolic Alkalosis (Bicarbonate Excess)

Metabolic alkalosis occurs when the level of base bicarbonate is high. Metabolic alkalosis may be due to excess intake of baking soda and other alkalis, prolonged vomiting, and other conditions that flood plasma with the bicarbonate anion. Prolonged vomiting causes the body to lose chloride (Cl^-) and hydrogen (H^+) ions. Loss of chloride ions causes a proportionate increase of bicarbonate in the blood. Related electrolyte imbalances account for some of the clinical signs. The clinical signs of metabolic alkalosis are summarized in the box on the opposite page.

ASSESSING

Assessment of clients with or at risk for developing fluid and electrolyte disturbances includes (a) taking a nursing history; (b) obtaining clinical measurements, e.g., daily weights, vital signs, and fluid intake and output; (c) per-

forming a physical examination; and (d) reviewing results of laboratory tests performed to evaluate fluid, electrolyte, and acid-base balance.

Nursing History

Fluid and electrolyte disturbances are characterized by numerous signs and symptoms that affect many areas of body function and are often interrelated. The nurse therefore needs to elicit specific data about many aspects of the client's needs and functional health patterns. Although each specific imbalance is manifested as a unique syndrome, the history must not be focused on any one specific problem from the start. Data must be obtained about the client's fluid and food intake; fluid output; recent fluid losses; signs of fluid deficit or excess; common signs of electrolyte and acid-base problems; long-term and recent disease processes, and medications and treatments that alter fluid and electrolyte balance. Examples of interview questions to elicit this information are shown in the box above.

Clinical Measurements

Three simple clinical measurements that the nurse can initiate without a physician's order are daily weights, vital signs, and fluid intake and output.

Daily Weights   Daily weight measurements can provide a relatively accurate assessment of a client's fluid status. Notable changes in weight are indicative of *acute* fluid changes. Each kilogram of weight gained or lost is equivalent to one liter of fluid gained or lost. Such fluid gains or losses indicate total body fluid volume changes in all of the fluid compartments rather than in any specific compartment, such as the intravascular compartment. Rapid losses or gains of 5% to 8% of total body weight indicate moderate to severe fluid volume deficits or excesses.

To obtain accurate weight measurements, the nurse should balance the scale before each use and weigh the client (a) at the same time each day (e.g., before breakfast and after the first morning void), (b) while wearing the same or similar clothing, and (c) on the same scale. The type of scale (i.e., standing, bed, chair) should be documented.

Vital Signs   Changes in the vital signs may indicate fluid, electrolyte, and acid-base imbalances or compensating mechanisms for maintaining balance. Table 40–7 shows possible implications of changes in vital signs.

Fluid Intake and Output (I & O)   The measurement and recording of all fluid intake and output during a 24-hour period provide important data about the client's fluid and electrolyte balance. Generally, intake and output are measured for at-risk clients (see the accompanying box).

The unit used to measure intake and output is the milli-

TABLE 40–7   *Changes in Vital Signs That May Indicate Fluid, Electrolyte, or Acid-Base Imbalances*

Vital Sign	Implications	Vital Sign	Implications
Body temperature Increased	May result from hypernatremic dehydration. May lead to diaphoresis and increased insensible fluid loss. Fever also causes (a) increased metabolism, producing more metabolic wastes and increased urine output, and (b) hyperpnea, resulting in increased insensible fluid loss through the lungs.	*Pulse (continued)* Irregular rhythm *Respirations* Increased rate and depth (hyperventilation)	May indicate potassium or magnesium deficit. Increases insensible fluid loss. May be result of fever, anxiety, or pulmonary infection. May cause carbonic acid deficit (respiratory alkalosis) or be compensatory mechanism for metabolic acidosis.
Decreased *Pulse* Increased	May result from hypovolemia. May occur with fluid volume deficit and hyponatremia as compensating mechanism to increase cardiac output. May also occur with potassium or magnesium deficits.	Shallow respirations or respiratory embarrassment (hypoventilation) Shortness of breath, crackles, or rhonchi	Decreases exhalation of carbon dioxide, creating a carbonic acid excess (respiratory acidosis). May be compensatory mechanism for metabolic alkalosis. May indicate fluid volume excess due to fluid accumulation in the lungs.
Decreased Weak, thready	May indicate potassium or magnesium excess. May indicate fluid volume deficit as a result of reduced intravascular volume (hypovolemia).	*Blood Pressure* Decreased systolic pressure from the lying to sitting or standing position (postural hypotension)	A postural decrease exceeding 10 mm Hg usually indicates a fluid volume deficit, specifically hypovolemia with reduction in stroke volume.
Bounding	May result from fluid volume excess, which can increase the volume of blood ejected by the left ventricle and the strength of left ventricular contraction.	Elevated systolic pressure	May indicate fluid volume excess and an increase in stroke volume.

ing fluids need to be recorded:

- *Oral fluids.* Water, milk, juice, soft drinks, coffee, tea, cream, soup, sherry, and wine. Include water taken with medications. To assess the amount of water taken from a water pitcher, measure what remains and subtract this amount from the volume of the full pitcher. Then refill the pitcher.

- *Ice chips.* Record these as fluids at approximately one-half their volume.

- *Foods that are or tend to become liquid at room temperature.* These include ice cream, sherbert, custard, and gelatin (Jello). Do *not* measure foods that are pureed, since purees are simply solid foods prepared in a different form.

- *Tube feedings.* Remember to include the 30- to 60-ml water rinse at the end of intermittent feedings or during continuous feedings.

- *Parenteral fluids.* The exact amount administered is to be recorded, since some fluid containers may be overfilled. Blood transfusions are included.

- *Intravenous medications.* IV medications that are prepared with sterile water and administered with an infusion, for example, must also be included (e.g., Tobramycin sulfate 80 mg in 50 ml of sterile water).

- *Catheter or tube irrigants.* Fluid used to irrigate urinary catheters, nasogastric tubes, and intestinal tubes must be measured and recorded.

liter (ml) or cubic centimeter (cc); these are equivalent metric units of measurement. In household measures, 30 ml is roughly equivalent to 1 fluid ounce, 500 ml is about 1 pint, and 1000 ml is about 1 quart. To measure fluid intake, nurses must convert household measures such as a glass, cup, or soup bowl to metric units. Most agencies provide conversion tables, since the sizes of dishes vary from agency to agency. A table is often provided on or with the bedside I & O record. Examples of equivalents are given in the accompanying box.

Most agencies have a form for recording I & O, usually a bedside record on which the nurse lists all items measured and their quantities per shift (see Figure 17–5 on page 305). Some agencies have another form for recording the specifics of intravenous fluids, such as the type of solution, additives, time started, amounts absorbed, and amounts remaining per shift.

Nurses must inform clients, family members, and all caregivers that accurate measurements of the client's fluid intake and output are required, explaining why and emphasizing the need to use a bedpan or urinal (unless a urinary drainage system is in place). Clients who wish to be involved in recording these measurements need to be taught how to compute the values and what foods are considered fluids.

To measure *fluid intake,* the nurse records on the I & O form each fluid item taken (if the client has not already done so), specifying the time and type of fluid. All of the follow-

To measure *fluid output,* the nurse must measure the following fluids:

 ■ *Urinary output.* Following each voiding, pour the urine into a measuring container, observe the amount, and record it and the time of voiding on the bedside I & O form. For clients with retention catheters, note and record the amount of urine at the end of the shift, and then empty the drainage bag. Drainage bags are usually calibrated to indicate the amount of urine. If there is any doubt about the amount in the drainage bag, empty it into an accurate measuring container. In critical care areas, the urine ideally is measured hourly.

If the client is incontinent of urine or is extremely diaphoretic, estimate and record these outputs. For example, of an incontinent client the nurse might record "Incontinent × 3" or "Drawsheet soaked in 12-in diameter." A more accurate estimate of the urine of incontinent clients may be obtained by first weighing diapers or incontinent pads that are dry, and then subtracting this weight from the weight of the soiled items.

 ■ *Vomitus and liquid feces.* The type of fluid and time need to be specified.

■ *Diaphoresis.* For a diaphoretic client, record "Perspiring profusely [or + + + +]. Gown and drawsheet changed × 2." Follow agency practices in this regard.

 ■ *Tube drainage,* e.g., gastric or intestinal drainage.

■ *Wound drainage* and *draining fistulas.* Wound drainage may be recorded by documenting the type and number of dressings or linen saturated with drainage or by measuring the exact amount of drainage collected in a vacuum drainage (e.g., Hemovac) or gravity drainage system. Note that excessive fluid transfers also occur with extensive burns.

■ *Rapid, deep respiratory rate.* Since hyperventilation can contribute to insensible fluid loss, the rate and depth of respirations in such clients should be recorded.

Fluid intake and output measurements are totaled at the end of the shift (every 8 or 12 hours), and the totals are transferred to the correct column on the client's permanent record. In some critical care areas, the nurse may need to record intake and output hourly.

To determine whether the fluid output is proportional to fluid intake or whether there are any changes in the client's fluid status, the nurse (a) compares the total fluid output measurement with the total fluid intake measurement and (b) compares both to previous measurements. Urinary output is normally equivalent to the amount of fluids ingested; the usual range is 1500 to 2000 ml in 24 hours, or 40 to 80 ml in 1 hour. Clients whose output substantially exceeds intake are at risk for fluid volume deficit. By contrast, clients whose intake substantially exceeds output are at risk for fluid volume excess. Inadequate intakes and outputs need to be reported to the nurse in charge. In adults, for example, a urine output of less than 500 ml in 24 hours or less than 30 ml per hour is considered inadequate.

Physical Examination

The client is examined for clinical signs of fluid, electrolyte, and acid-base imbalances. The nurse needs a knowledge of significant signs as well as the normal clinical picture presented by the client. Tables 40–6 and 40–9 (in this chapter) describe some common clinical signs of fluid, electrolyte, and acid-base imbalances.

The physical examination for assessing a client's fluid and electrolyte status is focused on the skin, the oral cavity, the eyes, the jugular veins, the veins of the hand, and the neurologic system. Data from this physical examination expand and verify information obtained during the nursing history. See Table 40–8 for significant findings and their implications.

Laboratory Tests

Many laboratory studies are conducted to determine the existence of fluid, electrolyte, and acid-base imbalances. Some of the more common tests are discussed here.

Serum Electrolytes Serum electrolyte levels are often routinely ordered for any client admitted to hospital as a screening test for electrolyte and acid-base imbalances. The most commonly ordered serum tests are for sodium, potassium, chloride, and bicarbonate ions. Normal values are shown in Table 40–6, earlier.

Anion Gap For optimum health, the body must maintain a state of electrical neutrality or electrolyte equilibrium between anion and cation groups in extracellular fluids. Because simultaneous measurement of all electrolytes is seldom performed, a calculaton of the **anion gap** (difference between the unmeasured serum anions and cations) can demonstrate the anion-cation balance. A simple formula using the values of the most frequently assessed electrolytes (sodium, potassium, chloride and bicarbonate) can yield the anion gap (Byrne, Saxton, Pelikan, and Nugent 1986, p. 272):

$$\text{Anion gap} = (\text{sodium} + \text{potassium}) - (\text{chloride} + \text{bicarbonate})$$

The anion gap value obtained from this calculation approximates the difference between unmeasured calcium and magnesium ions minus the sum of unmeasured protein, phosphate, organic acid, and sulfate ions. Note, however, that a normal anion-cation balance does not necessarily exclude the possibility of one or more abnormal values for individual ions. Compensations to preserve electrolyte equilibrium may have occurred.

TABLE 40–8 *Physical Assessment Findings Associated With Fluid and Electrolyte Imbalances*

Findings	Implications	Findings	Implications
Skin		**Veins (continued)**	
Dry skin	May indicate fluid volume deficit.		seconds, and lowering the hand will refill them in 3–5 seconds. An interval of longer than 3–5 seconds for emptying indicates fluid volume excess; for filling, a fluid volume deficit.
Warm, flushed skin	Due to peripheral vasodilation. May indicate metabolic acidosis.		
Pale, cool skin	Due to peripheral vasoconstriction. May indicate severe fluid volume deficit, i.e., compensatory mechanism for hypovolemia.	**Neurologic and Neuromuscular**	
		Change in level of consciousness	May occur with changes in serum sodium and acute acid-base imbalances.
Reduced skin turgor over forehead, sternum, scapula, forearm, dorsum of hand, or inner aspect of thighs	May be due only to decrease in skin elasticity in elderly clients or may indicate fluid volume deficit if pinched skin remains elevated or tented for several seconds.	Restlessness and confusion	May occur with fluid volume deficit or acid-base imbalance.
		Neuromuscular excitability (e.g., hyperactive deep-tendon reflexes)	Occurs with calcium and magnesium deficits, metabolic alkalosis, and sodium excess.
Dependent edema or pitting edema (over bony surface such as tibia or sacrum)	Indicates expanded interstitial fluid volume and retention of excess sodium and water (at least 3–5 kg).	Depressed neuromuscular function (e.g., diminished reflexes)	Occurs with calcium and magnesium excesses, sodium and potassium deficits, and acidosis.
Oral Cavity			
Dry mucous membrane between the cheek and gums	Indicates fluid volume deficit.	Positive Trousseau's sign (ischemia-induced carpal spasm) elicited by applying a blood pressure cuff to the upper arm and inflating it past the systolic BP for 2 minutes	Can occur with calcium and magnesium deficits.
Dry and sticky mucous membrane	May indicate sodium excess.		
Increased longitudinal furrowing of the tongue	Suggests fluid volume deficit.		
Red and swollen tongue	May indicate sodium excess.		
Absence of salivation	Indicates fluid volume deficit.	Positive Chvostek's sign (unilateral contraction of the facial and eyelid muscles) elicited when percussing the facial nerve about 2 cm anterior to the earlobe	As above.
Eyes			
Periorbital edema, blurred vision	Suggests significant fluid retention.		
Sunken, soft eyeballs with dry conjunctiva	Due to decreased intraocular pressure. Indicative of severe fluid volume deficit.		
Veins		Neuromuscular symptoms of tingling, paresthesias, weakness, and flaccid paralysis	May occur with potassium excess. Parethesias are common with metabolic alkalosis.
Jugular vein distention (See page 410 for method of assessment)	Values above 3 cm suggest fluid volume excess or decreased cardiac function.		
Delayed filling and emptying of veins of hands	Normally, elevating the hand will collapse the veins in 3–5	Tetany	Occurs with alkalosis (metabolic and respiratory).

The normal values for the anion gap are approximately 14 mEq/liter, or a range of 11 to 17 mEq/liter. A difference of less than 10 mEq/liter or more than 17 mEq/liter between these values indicates a serious illness. The anion gap is a helpful diagnostic tool in differentiating metabolic acidosis and alkalosis, and in monitoring therapy for excess anion accumulation.

Complete Blood Count (CBC)

The complete blood count, another basic screening test, includes information about the hematocrit and hemoglobin levels. The **hematocrit** measures the volume (percentage) of whole blood that is composed of red blood cells (RBCs). Since the hematocrit is a measure of the volume of cells in relation to plasma, it is affected by changes in plasma volume. Thus, the hematocrit increases with severe dehydration and hypovolemic shock and decreases with severe overhydration. Normal hematocrit values are 40% to 54% (males) and 37% to 47% (females).

An increase in hemoglobin levels may accompany an increase in hematocrit levels. Decreased levels of hemoglobin are found with severe hemorrhage. Normal adult values are 95% to 98% by electrophoresis.

Osmolality   **Osmolality** is an indicator of the concentration or number of particles dissolved in serum and urine. They are reported as milliosmoles of solute per kilogram of fluid (mOsm/kg). *Serum osmolality* is a measure of the solute concentration of the blood. The particles included are sodium ions, glucose, and urea (blood urea nitrogen, or BUN). Serum osmolality can be estimated by doubling the serum sodium, since sodium and its associated chloride ions are the major determinants of serum osmolality. More precise estimates of serum osmolality, however, take sodium, glucose, and urea into account, as the following formula shows:

$$\text{Serum osmolality} = 2Na^+ + \frac{\text{serum glucose}}{18} + \frac{\text{urea (BUN)}}{2.8}$$

Glucose and urea are measured by weight (mg/dl); these values must be converted to concentration or numbers of particles by dividing their weight per liter of solution by their molecular weight (18 and 2.8, respectively).

Serum osmolality levels are the major regulator of antidiuretic hormone (ADH) release, which, in turn, controls the rate of water reabsorption by the kidneys and therefore urine osmolality. An increased plasma osmolality level stimulates ADH secretion, which causes the reabsorption of water from the renal tubules and thus increases the concentration and osmolality of urine. Serum osmolality values are used primarily to measure the extent of dehydration, since they reflect the balance of osmotic pressure between tissue cells and body fluids. Normal values are 275 to 300 mOsm/kg. An increase in serum osmolality indicates a fluid volume deficit; a decrease reflects a fluid volume excess.

Urine osmolality is a measure of the solute concentration of urine. The particles included are nitrogenous wastes, such as creatinine, urea, and uric acid. Normal values are (Byrne, Saxton, Pelikan, and Nugent 1986, p. 276) as follows:

For healthy males:	390 to 1090 mOsm/kg 770 to 1630 mOsm in 24 hours
For healthy females:	300 to 1090 mOsm/kg 430 to 1150 mOsm in 24 hours
For infants:	213 mOsm/kg

An increased urine osmolality indicates a fluid volume deficit; a decreased urine osmolality reflects a fluid volume excess.

Osmolality determinations help to diagnose fluid and electrolyte imbalances. For example, during intravenous fluid therapy, increased osmolality values may indicate that the client is receiving too many electrolytes for the amount of fluid. Conversely, decreased osmolality values may indicate that the client is receiving too much water for the amount of electrolytes.

The ratio between urine and serum osmolality values is important in interpreting the significance of abnormal values. The normal ratio of urine osmolality to serum osmolality is 1.0 to 3.0, i.e.,

$$\frac{\text{Urine osmolality}}{\text{Serum osmolality}} = \frac{1.0}{3.0}$$

Values greater than 3.0 normally occur after an overnight fast, which causes concentrated urine. A ratio close to 1.0 (dilute urine) usually indicates loss of concentrating ability by the kidneys and advanced renal disease. A ratio below 1.0 (extremely dilute urine) commonly occurs after excessive water intake or excessive water loss in diabetes insipidus.

Urine pH   Measurement of urine pH may be obtained by laboratory analysis or by using a dipstick on a freshly voided specimen. See Chapter 43, page 1202. Since the kidneys play a critical role in regulating acid-base balance, assessment of urine pH can be useful in determining whether the kidneys are responding appropriately to metabolic acid-base imbalances. Normally, the pH of the urine is relatively acidic, averaging about 6.0, but a range of 4.6 to 8.0 is considered normal. In metabolic acidosis, urine pH should decrease, indicating that the kidneys are responding appropriately; in metabolic alkalosis, the pH should increase. Increases of the pH in metabolic acidosis or decreases of the pH in metabolic alkalosis are abnormal.

Urine Specific Gravity   Specific gravity is discussed in detail in Chapter 43, page 1201. Although it is a less reliable indicator of concentration than urine osmolality, the test can be performed quickly and easily by nursing personnel. Specific gravity is affected by both the number and weight of solutes. Therefore, the presence of a few large solutes such as protein or glucose can cause a deceptively high specific gravity. Other substances that may also give a falsely high specific gravity include dextran, radiographic contrast material, and some medications.

Arterial Blood Gases (ABGs)   Specimens of arterial blood are taken to determine the adequacy of alveolar gas exchange and evaluate the ability of the lungs and kidneys to maintain the acid-base balance of body fluids. ABGs routinely include pH, P_{CO_2} (carbonic acid concentration), bicarbonate (HCO_3^-), P_{O_2}, and O_2 saturation.

Normally, arterial blood has a pH of 7.35 to 7.45. Any variation from normal can reflect a problem in the bicarbonate and carbonic acid buffer system.

The P_{CO_2} is a measure of the pressure exerted by carbon dioxide gas dissolved in the blood. The P stands for partial arterial pressure—here, the pressure exerted by CO_2 in the arterial blood. This pressure is regulated by the lungs and reflects the amount of carbonic acid available to the bicarbonate and carbonic acid buffer system. A normal P_{CO_2} is 35 to 45 mm Hg.

Serum bicarbonate (HCO_3^-) is the major renal component of acid-base regulation. It is excreted or regenerated by the kidneys to maintain a normal acid-base environment. Normal values are 21 to 28 mEq/liter. Decreased HCO_3^- levels are indicative of metabolic acidosis (seen frequently as a compensatory mechanism for respiratory alkalosis). Increased HCO_3^- levels reflect metabolic alkalosis or may indicate compensatory alteration in response to respiratory acidosis.

Partial pressure of oxygen (P_{O_2}) is the pressure exerted by the small amount of oxygen dissolved in the plasma. This oxygen is separate from the oxygen carried by the hemoglobin of the erythrocytes. Normal values of P_{O_2} are 80 to 100 mm Hg in arterial blood. The P_{O_2} has no major role in acid-base regulation if it is within normal limits.

Oxygen saturation (O_2 Sat) is a measure of the degree to which hemoglobin is saturated with oxygen. Normal values are 95% to 98% in arterial blood and 60% and 85% in venous blood. Oxygen saturation provides some indication of the efficiency of the client's lung ventilation.

To interpret the blood gases, the nurse follows these steps (see also Table 40–9):

1. Determine the acidity or alkalinity of the blood from the pH value. Below 7.35 is acidotic; above 7.45 is alkalotic.
2. Identify the cause of the pH by checking the P_{CO_2} (carbonic acid) and HCO_3^- values. Abnormalities in the P_{CO_2} indicate respiratory acid-base imbalances; abnormalities in the HCO_3^- levels indicate metabolic acid-base imbalances. An increased P_{CO_2} signals *respiratory acidosis*; a decreased P_{CO_2}, *respiratory alkalosis*. Both of these values are in an inverse relationship with the pH; i.e., if the P_{CO_2} is increased, the pH is decreased; if the P_{CO_2} is decreased, the pH is increased.

If, however, the P_{CO_2} is normal but the HCO_3^- levels are abnormal, *metabolic acidosis* (reduced HCO_3^-) or *metabolic alkalosis* (increased HCO_3^-) is the cause. Note that in metabolic acid-base imbalances, the pH and HCO_3^- are in direct relationship—i.e., both are increased or decreased.

TABLE 40–9 Compensated and Uncompensated Acid-Base Imbalances

Acid-Base Imbalance	Findings		
	pH	P_{CO_2}	HCO_3^-
Respiratory acidosis	↓ pH (below 7.35)	↑ P_{CO_2} (above 45 mm Hg)	Normal HCO_3^-
Respiratory alkalosis	↑ pH (above 7.45)	↓ P_{CO_2} (below 35 mm Hg)	Normal HCO_3^-
Metabolic acidosis	↓ pH (below 7.35)	Normal P_{CO_2}	↓ HCO_3^- (below 21 mEq/L)
Metabolic alkalosis	↑ pH (above 7.45)	Normal P_{CO_2}	↑ HCO_3^- (above 28 mEq/L)
Compensated respiratory acidosis	↓ pH or near normal	↑ P_{CO_2}	↑ HCO_3^- (renal compensation by retention of HCO_3^- ions)
Compensated respiratory alkalosis	↑ pH or near normal	↓ P_{CO_2}	↓ HCO_3^- (renal compensation by excretion of HCO_3^- ions)
Compensated metabolic acidosis	↓ pH or near normal	↓ P_{CO_2} (hyperventilation; attempt to blow off more acid)	↓ HCO_3^-
Compensated metabolic alkalosis	↑ pH or near normal	↑ P_{CO_2} (compensation by depressed respiration)	↑ HCO_3^-

TABLE 40–10 *Examples of Assessment Data Clusters and Related Nursing Diagnosis*

Data Cluster	Nursing Diagnoses
Merlyn Chapman, a 27-year-old sales clerk, reported generalized weakness, malaise, and symptoms of flu for 3–4 days. She was unable to tolerate fluids even though thirsty because of nausea and vomiting and had liquid stools 2–4 times per day. Physical findings indicated dry oral mucosa, furrowed tongue, cracked lips, mild fever (38.6 C) and scanty concentrated urine output (specific gravity: 1.035).	**Fluid volume deficit** related to excessive fluid loss (vomiting, diarrhea)
Luella Fisher, a frail 93-year-old with congestive heart failure, uses a daily diuretic (furosemide). She has recently had a stroke that impairs her swallowing. A nasogastric tube and catheter are in place. Appetite is poor.	**Potential fluid volume deficit** related to inadequate fluid intake, loss of fluid through indwelling tubes, and diuretic therapy
Tom Bricker, a 67-year-old pensioner who has a history of heart disease, has experienced a weight gain of 4–5 kg over the past month. He states his rings are too tight to remove, his ankles are swollen, his heart pounds at times, he gets breathless with exertion, and feels bloated. Physical findings reveal jugular vein distention above 3 cm, delayed emptying of hand veins, bounding pulse (86), pitting edema in feet, ankles, and lower legs, and lung crackles.	**Fluid volume excess** related to **altered cardiac output: decreased**
Fred Boysniak was admitted to emergency after being found with an empty bottle of codeine tablets by his bed. He appears very lethargic and stuporous, pulse is 120, respirations 12 and very shallow. Blood gases reveal pH of 7.1, Pco_2 49 mm Hg, and HCO_3^- 29 mEq/liter.	**Impaired gas exchange** related to hypoventilation secondary to overdose of respiratory depressant drug.

3. Determine whether the body is compensating for the pH change. If both the Pco_2 and HCO_3^- are abnormal, the value that deviates the most from normal parameters points to the primary disturbance causing the altered pH. Compensating elements or a mixed respiratory and metabolic disturbance may be present. When the plasma pH becomes more acidic, the kidneys excrete more hydrogen ions and retain the bicarbonate ions as a buffer. Conversely, when the plasma pH becomes too alkaline, the kidneys retain hydrogen ions and excrete bicarbonate ions to produce more acidity.

4. Check the Po_2 and oxygen saturation to determine whether they are normal, decreased, or increased. A high Po_2 may indicate the need to decrease the concentration of oxygen being delivered. A decrease of both Po_2 and O_2 saturation can lead to lactic acidosis and may suggest the need for increased concentrations of oxygen.

DIAGNOSING

Nursing diagnoses that relate to fluid, electrolyte, and acid-base imbalances include the following:

- **Fluid volume deficit,** the state in which an individual experiences vascular, cellular, or intracellular dehydration related to:
  1. *Failure of regulatory mechanisms, or*
  2. *Active loss*
- **Potential fluid volume deficit,** the state in which an individual is *at risk of* experiencing vascular, cellular, or intracellular dehydration due to active or regulatory losses of body water in excess of needs.
- **Fluid volume excess,** the state in which an individual experiences increased *fluid retention* and *edema.*
- **Impaired gas exchange,** the state in which an individual experiences an imbalance between oxygen uptake and carbon dioxide elimination at the area of gas exchange—the alveolar-capillary membrane.

These diagnoses with possible contributing factors are shown below. Examples of assessment data clusters and related nursing diagnoses are shown in Table 40–10.

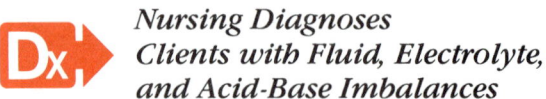

Nursing Diagnoses Clients with Fluid, Electrolyte, and Acid-Base Imbalances

Fluid volume deficit related to excessive fluid loss (e.g., vomiting, diarrhea, diaphoresis, hemorrhage, extensive burns)

Potential fluid volume deficit related to

- Inadequate fluid intake
- Increased fluid output
- Loss of fluid through abnormal routes (e.g., indwelling tubes)
- Loss of fluid through physiologic routes (e.g., vomiting, diarrhea)
- Knowledge deficit about required fluid volume
- Hypermetabolic state (e.g., fever)
- Deviation affecting absorption of fluids
- Medication (e.g., diuretic)

Fluid volume excess related to

- Excess sodium intake
- Excessive fluid intake (e.g., excessive intravenous infusion)
- Drug therapies (e.g., tolbutamide, chlorpropamide, vincristine sulfate)

Other relevant diagnoses for clients with fluid, electrolyte, or acid-base imbalances may include:

Altered oral mucous membrane related to fluid volume deficit

Impaired skin integrity related to dehydration and/or edema

Altered cardiac output: decreased related to hypovolemia

Altered tissue perfusion related to altered cardiac output: decreased secondary to fluid volume deficit

---

PLANNING

The overall goals for clients with actual or potential fluid, electrolyte, and acid-base imbalances are to regain or maintain adequate fluid, electrolyte, and/or acid-base balance and to prevent potential associated risks such as skin breakdown, loss of tissue integrity, and decreased cardiac output. Appropriate nursing interventions and outcome criteria that relate to these broad goals are then identified in accordance with the written diagnosis. The following are among the strategies the nurse should consider:

- Ensure an appropriate oral fluid intake in accordance with the client's needs, e.g., increased or decreased fluid intake.
- Measure fluid intake and output.
- Develop a dietary plan to resolve electrolyte imbalances.

- Monitor vital signs; weight; urine pH and specific gravity; serum electrolyte values; hemoglobin and hematocrit; breath sounds.
- Assess oral mucous membranes, skin turgor, abdominal girth, and ankle circumference as required.
- Prevent complications of fluid excess. For example, apply elastic stockings, encourage deep breathing and coughing, position the client in Fowler's position to facilitate ventilation and elevate the client's legs to minimize dependent edema and avoid skin breakdown.
- As ordered, administer medications (e.g., antiemetics, antidiarrheals) to prevent further fluid losses or diuretics to prevent fluid retention.
- Administer and monitor the flow rate of intravenous infusions, electrolytes, blood, blood products, and plasma expanders as ordered by the physician.
- Instruct the client and family about reasons for fluid and electrolyte deficits or excesses; reasons for treatments; dietary alterations; purposes, dosages, and side-effects of ordered medications; ways to prevent recurrences; and plans for follow-up care.

Examples of outcome criteria to evaluate the achievement of client goals and the effectiveness of nursing interventions are shown below.

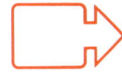 *Outcome Criteria*
Clients with Fluid, Electrolyte,
and Acid-Base Imbalances

The client with **Actual** or **Potential fluid volume deficit:**

- Has a balanced fluid intake and output (average of 2500 ml per day) for 3 days.
- Has good skin turgor.
- Has moist mucous membranes.
- Is free of thirst.
- Is free of vomiting and diarrhea.
- Has a normal urine specific gravity (1.010 to 1.025).
- Has normal vital signs for age, sex, and health status.
- Explains reasons for fluid/electrolyte imbalance.
- Explains purposes and side-effects of ordered medications.
- Identifies amounts and types of foods and fluids to consume to prevent recurrence.

The client with **Fluid volume excess** in addition:

- Is gradually free of edema, i.e., able to wear shoes again.

- Has intact skin.
- Is free of dyspnea and able to breathe in the supine position.
- Loses ____ kg body weight within 1 week and then maintains stable body weight.

The client with **Acid-base imbalance:**

- Resumes normal diaphragmatic breathing pattern.
- Experiences no mental disorientation or agitation.
- Has normal ABGs.

IMPLEMENTING

Providing Fluids and Electrolytes Orally

Fluids and electrolytes can be provided orally in the home and hospital if the client's health permits, i.e., the client is not vomiting, has not experienced an excessive fluid loss, and has an intact gastrointestinal tract. Some clients who are unable to ingest solid foods are often able to ingest fluids.

Fluids　*Increased* fluids (ordered as "push fluids") are often prescribed for clients with actual or potential fluid volume deficits arising, for example, from mild diarrhea or mild to moderate fevers. Clients recovering from anesthesia and certain types of surgery (e.g., bladder surgery) are also commonly given only clear liquids initially and then, if these are tolerated, are advanced to a regular diet. Guidelines for helping clients increase fluid intake are shown in the accompanying box.

Restricted fluids may be necessary for clients who have fluid retention (fluid volume excess) as a result of renal failure, congestive heart failure, syndrome of inappropriate antidiuretic hormone (SIADH), or other disease process. Fluid restrictions vary from "nothing by mouth" to a precise amount ordered by a physician. In addition, the client may be limited to only clear fluids (see Chapter 39, page 1014). The restriction of fluids can be difficult for some clients, particularly if they are experiencing thirst. Guidelines for helping clients restrict fluid intake are shown in the box on the opposite page.

Foods　Specific fluid and electrolyte imbalances may require simple dietary changes. For example, clients receiving potassium-depleting diuretics are commonly given potassium supplements. In addition, the client needs to be informed about foods with a high potassium content (e.g.,

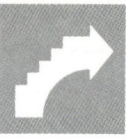

CLINICAL GUIDELINES
Facilitating Normal or Increased Fluid Intake

- Explain to the client the reason for the required intake and the specific amount needed. This gives the client a rationale for the requirement and promotes compliance.
- Establish a 24-hour plan for ingesting the fluids. Generally, half of the total volume is ingested during the day shift, and the other half is divided between the evening and night shifts, with the majority ingested during the evening shift. For example, if 2500 ml is to be ingested in 24 hours, the plan may specify 7–3 (1500 ml); 3–11 (700 ml); and 11–7 (300 ml). Try to avoid the ingestion of large amounts of fluid before bedtime to prevent the need to urinate during sleeping hours.
- Set short-term goals that the client can realistically meet. Examples include ingesting a glass of fluid every hour while awake or a pitcher of water by 12 noon.
- Identify fluids or fluidlike substances the client likes and make available a variety of those items, including fruit juices, tea, coffee, and milk (if allowed).
- Help clients to select foods that tend to become liquid at room temperature (e.g., gelatin, ice cream, sherbert, custard), if these are allowed.
- For clients who are confined to bed, supply appropriate cups, glasses, and straws to facilitate appropriate fluid intake and keep the fluids within easy reach.
- Make sure fluids are served at the appropriate temperature: hot fluids hot and cold fluids iced and cold.
- Encourage clients when possible to participate in maintaining the fluid intake record. This assists them to evaluate the achievement of preestablished goals.

bananas, oranges, and leafy greens). Some clients with fluid retention due to hypernatremia need to avoid foods high in sodium. Most healthy clients can benefit from foods high in calcium. Nurses can often help clients by giving them a list of foods and fluids high in the electrolytes they require or need to avoid. See Table 40–6 for foods high in specific electrolytes.

Administering Intravenous Therapy

Intravenous (IV) fluid therapy is a common practice today. It is an efficient and effective method of supplying fluids directly into the extracellular fluid compartment, specifically the venous system. Intravenous fluid therapy is ordered by the physician. The nurse is responsible for administering and maintaining the therapy.

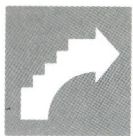

CLINICAL GUIDELINES
Helping Clients Restrict Fluid Intake

- Explain the reason for the restricted intake and how much and what types of fluids are permitted orally. Many clients need to be informed that ice chips, gelatin, and ice cream, for example, are considered fluid.

- Help the client decide the amount of fluid to be taken with each meal, between meals, before bedtime, and with medications. Generally, half of the total volume is scheduled during the day shift, when the client is most active, receives two meals, and often most oral medications. A large part of the remainder is scheduled for the evening shift to permit fluids with meals and evening visitors.

- Identify fluids or fluidlike substances the client likes and make sure that these are provided, unless contraindicated. A client who is allowed only 200 ml of fluid for breakfast, for example, should receive the type of fluid the client favors.

- Set short-term goals that make the fluid restriction more tolerable. For example, schedule a specified amount of fluid at one or two hourly intervals between meals. Some clients may prefer fluids between meals only since the food provided at mealtime may help relieve feelings of thirst.

- Provide the client with small fluid containers that make the container appear to contain more fluid than it actually does.

- Periodically offer the client ice chips as an alternative to water, since ice chips when melted are approximately one-half of the frozen volume.

- Help clients to rinse their mouths with water if they can do so without swallowing the fluid.

- Ensure meticulous oral care.

- Instruct the client to avoid ingesting or chewing salty or sweet foods (hard candy or gum), since these foods tend to produce thirst. Sugarless gum may be an alternative for some clients.

- Encourage the client when possible to participate in maintaining the fluid intake record.

Intravenous therapy can be prescribed for these reasons:

1. To supply fluid when clients are unable to take in an adequate volume of fluids by mouth

2. To provide salts needed to maintain electrolyte balance

3. To provide glucose (dextrose), the main fuel for metabolism.

4. To provide water-soluble vitamins and medications

5. To establish a lifeline for rapidly needed medications

Common Types of Solutions   Common solutions administered intravenously include nutrient solutions, electrolyte solutions, alkalizing and acidifying solutions, and blood volume expanders. *Nutrient solutions* contain some form of carbohydrate (e.g., dextrose, glucose, or levulose) and water. Water is supplied for fluid requirements and carbohydrate for calories and energy. For example, 1 liter of 5% dextrose provides 170 calories. Nutrient solutions are useful in preventing dehydration and ketosis but do not provide sufficient calories to promote wound healing, weight gain, or normal grown in children. Common nutrient solutions are 5% dextrose in water (D5W) and 5% dextrose in 0.45% sodium chloride (dextrose in half-strength saline).

Electrolyte solutions contain varying amounts of cations and anions. Commonly used solutions are normal saline (0.9% sodium chloride solution), Ringer's solution (which contains sodium, chloride, potassium, and calcium), and lactated Ringer's solution (which contains sodium, chloride, potassium, calcium, and lactate). Lactate is a salt of lactic acid that is metabolized in the liver to form bicarbonate (HCO_3^-). Saline solutions are frequently used as initial hydrating solutions. Multiple electrolyte solutions approximate the ionic profile of plasma and are used to prevent dehydration or to restore or correct fluid and electrolyte imbalances.

Alkalizing solutions are administered to counteract metabolic acidosis. One commonly used solution is lactated Ringer's solution. *Acidifying solutions,* in contrast, are administered to counteract metabolic alkalosis. Examples of acidifying solutions are 5% dextrose in 0.45% sodium chloride and 0.9% sodium chloride solution.

Blood volume expanders are used to increase the volume of blood following severe loss of blood (e.g., from hemorrhage) or plasma (e.g., from severe burns, which draw large amounts of plasma from the bloodstream to the burn site). Common blood volume expanders are dextran, plasma, and human serum albumin.

Peripheral Venipuncture Sites   The site chosen for venipuncture varies with the client's age, the infusion time, the type of solution used, and the condition of veins. For adults, veins in the arm are commonly used; for infants, veins in the scalp are used. The larger veins of the forearm are preferred to the metacarpal veins of the hand for infusions that need to be given rapidly and for solutions that are hypertonic, are highly acidic or alkaline, or contain irritating medications.

The most convenient veins for venipuncture in the *adult* are the basilic and median cubital veins in the crease of the elbow (antecubital space). See Figure 40–2. Laboratory technicians often withdraw blood for examination from these large superficial veins. Unfortunately, use of these veins for prolonged infusions limits arm mobility, because a splint is needed to stabilize the elbow joint. For prolonged therapy, veins on the back of the hand and on the forearm are preferred. The metacarpal, basilic, and cephalic veins are

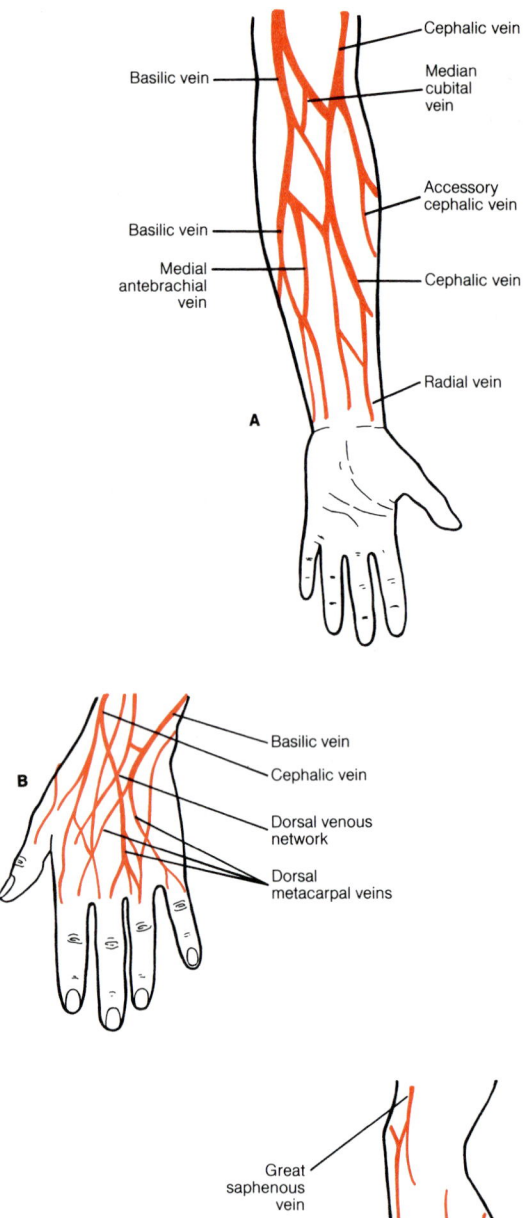

Figure 40–2 Commonly used venipuncture sites of the *A,* arm; *B,* hand; *C,* foot.

commonly used. The ulna and radius act as natural splints at these sites, and the client has greater freedom of arm movements for activities such as eating.

Because *infants* do not have large veins in the antecubital fossa, blood specimens for examination are usually taken from the external jugular vein and femoral veins. If an infusion is to be maintained for a long period, veins in the temporal region of the scalp, or sometimes the back of the hand or the dorsum of the foot, are used.

Central Venous Sites   Most clients receiving intravenous therapy have a peripheral line in place, but in some instances a central venous line is inserted. A **central venous line** is a catheter inserted into a large vein located centrally in the body. The tip of the catheter may terminate in the vein, e.g., the superior vena cava, or in the right atrium of the heart. See Figure 40–3. The catheters are radiopaque so that they will show up on fluoroscopy or x-ray films. Correct placement of the catheter is confirmed by x-ray film.

Central venous lines are usually inserted by physicians. They are inserted primarily for the following reasons: (a)

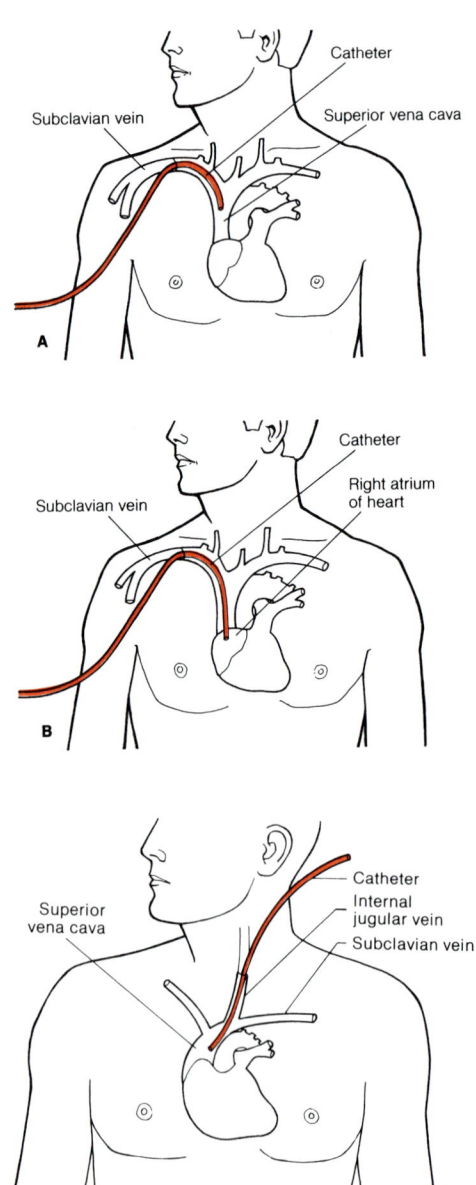

Figure 40–3   Central venous lines with *A,* the catheter tip in the superior vena cava; *B,* the catheter tip in the right atrium of the heart; and *C,* left jugular insertion and catheter tip placement in the superior vena cava.

to administer nutritional solutions that are highly irritating to smaller veins, (b) to administer irritating medications, (c) to monitor central venous pressure (CVP), and (d) to withdraw central venous blood samples.

Insertion of a central venous catheter may be a nonsurgical or surgical procedure. In the nonsurgical procedure, two approaches may be used:

1. The *infraclavicular approach* (below the clavicle), in which the catheter is inserted into the right or left subclavian vein. This site permits freedom of movement for ambulation.

2. The *supraclavicular approach* (above the clavicle), in which the catheter is inserted through the right or left jugular vein. This site hinders head and neck movement somewhat but provides a straight line to the subclavian vein (and superior vena cava).

The surgical insertion of a central venous catheter involves an incision into the tissues of the chest and the placement of an implantable venous access device (see page 1069). Many types of single- and multiple-lumen catheters are available for central venous infusions.

Equipment　Because equipment varies according to the manufacturer, the nurse must become familiar with the equipment used in each particular agency.

Solution containers are available in various sizes (50, 100, 250, 500, or 1000 ml); the smaller containers are often used to administer medications. Most solutions are currently dispensed in plastic bags. See Figure 40–4. However, glass bottles may need to be used if the administered medications are incompatible with plastic. Some glass solution bottles have a tube inside the bottle that serves as an air vent, so that air replaces the solution as it runs out of the bottle. See Figure 40–5. Containers without air vents require a vent on the administration set. See Figure 40–6. Air vents usually have filters to remove any contamination from the air that enters the container. Air vents are not required for plastic solution containers because plastic bags collapse under atmospheric pressure when the solution enters the client's vein.

Administration sets consist of an insertion spike, a drip chamber, a roller valve or screw clamp, tubing, and a protective cap over the needle adapter. See Figure 40–7. The insertion spike is kept sterile and inserted into the solution container when the equipment is set up and ready to start. The drip chamber permits a predictable amount of fluid to be delivered. A commonly used drip chamber is the macrodrip, which delivers 10 to 20 drops per milliliter of solution. This information is found on the package. There are also microdrip sets, which deliver 60 drops per milliliter of solution. The roller valve or screw clamp, which compresses the lumen of the tubing, controls the rate of the flow. The protective cap over the needle adapter maintains the sterility of the end of the tubing so that it can be attached to a sterile needle inserted in the client's vein.

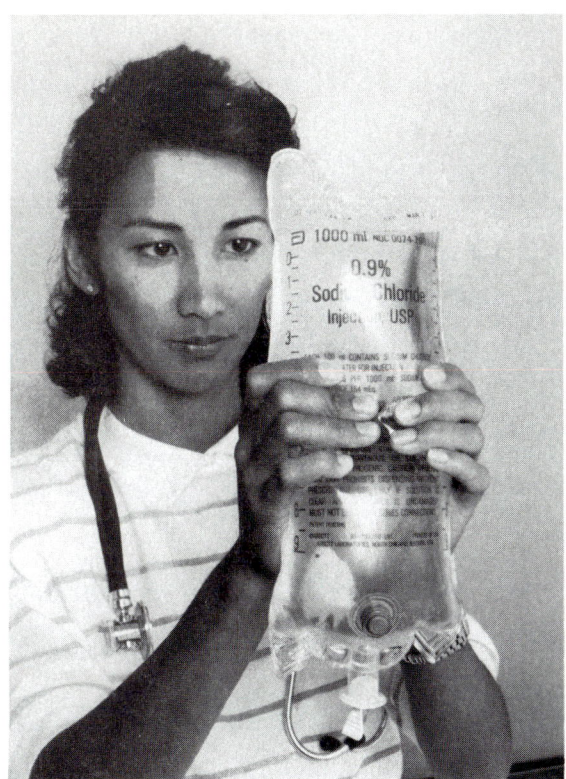

Figure 40–4　A plastic intravenous fluid container.

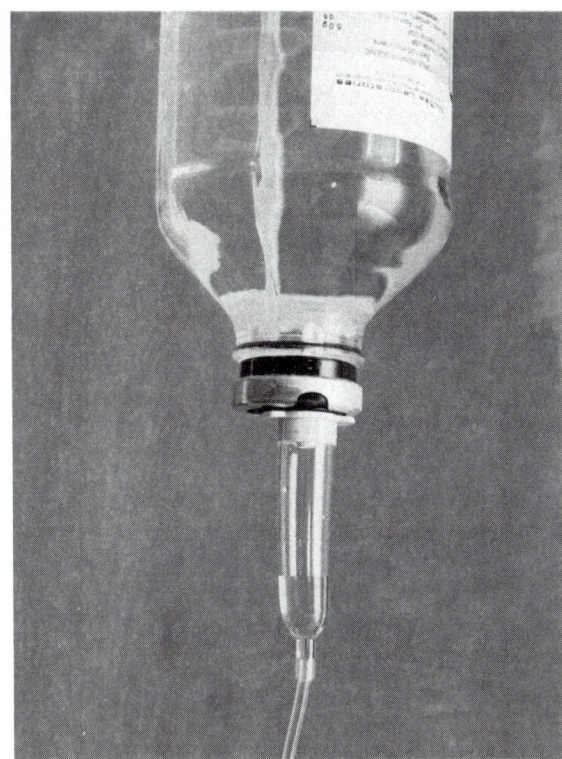

Figure 40–5　An intravenous container with an inside air vent.

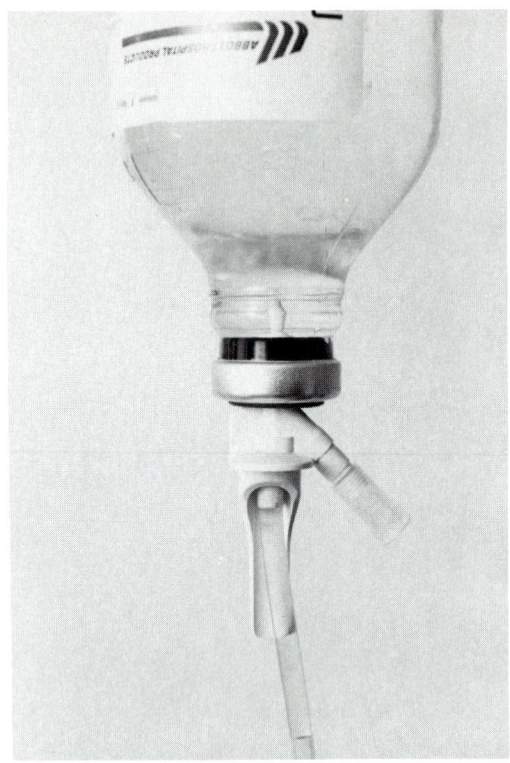

Figure 40–6 A nonvented intravenous container. Note the air vent on administration tubing.

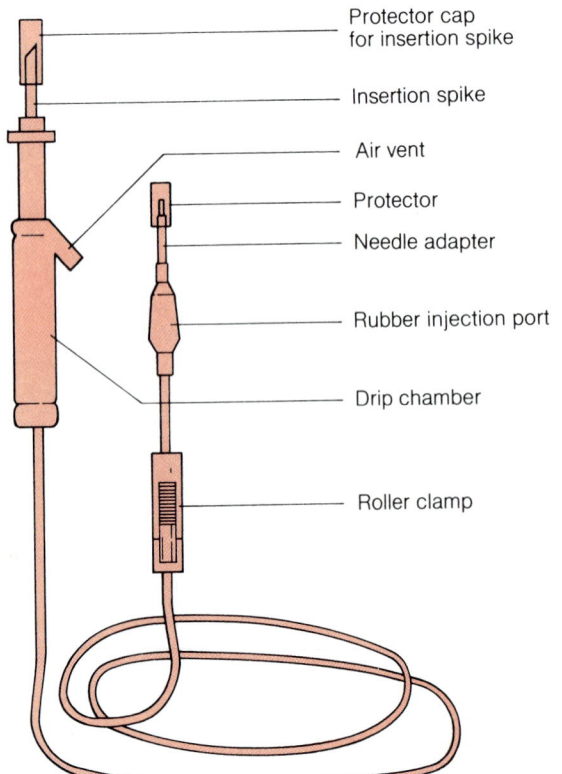

Protector cap
for insertion spike

Insertion spike

Air vent

Protector

Needle adapter

Rubber injection port

Drip chamber

Roller clamp

Figure 40–7 Schematic of a standard vented administration set.

IV poles (rods) are needed to hang the solution container. Some poles are attached to hospital beds; others stand on the floor or hang from the ceiling. Still others are floor models with casters that can be pushed along when a client is up and walking. The height of most poles is adjustable. The higher the solution container, the greater the force of the solution as it enters the client and the faster the rate of flow.

Many kinds of needles and catheters are commonly used for intravenous infusions. *Butterfly or wing-tipped needles* with plastic flaps attached to the shaft are shown in Figure 40–8. The flaps are held tightly together to hold the needle securely as it is inserted; after insertion, they are flattened against the skin and secured with tape. They vary in length from 1.5 to 3 cm (½ to 1¼ in), and from #25 to #17 gauge in diameter. The larger the gauge number, the smaller the diameter of the shaft. Needles of #20 to #22 gauge and short lengths are commonly used for adults. A *catheter* or *angiocatheter* is a plastic tube inserted into the vein. Some catheters fit over a needle during insertion, whereas others fit inside a needle. See Figure 40–9. An angiocatheter has a metal stylet (needle), which is used to pierce the skin and vein and is then withdrawn, leaving the catheter in place.

IV filters are increasingly being used to remove air, particulate matter, and microbes from intravenous infusions and to reduce the risk of contamination and complications (e.g., infusion-related phlebitis) associated with routine intravenous therapies. In addition, most agencies advise use of a filter if the infusion contains KCl or if the site is to be used for medication administration. Although all clients may benefit from the use of filters, the National Intravenous Therapy Association (NITA) recommends them for clients at risk (e.g., those receiving long-term infusion therapy, total parenteral nutrition (discussed later in this chapter), and intra-arterial infusion chemotherapy. Further research to prove the value of filters in preventing clinical infection is needed.

Most IV filters in current use consist of a membrane (pore size of 0.22 μm, although sizes vary). Ideally, the filter should be located within the intravenous line as close to the venipuncture site as possible (Crow 1987, p. 101). Some problems associated with filters include (a) clogging of the filter surface, which may stop or slow the flow rate when debris accumulates, and (b) drug binding of some drugs (e.g., insulin and amphotericin B) to the surface of the filter. When using filters, the nurse should remember that the filter should never be considered a substitute for quality care and meticulous aseptic technique.

Variations from the Standard Infusion When more than one solution needs to be infused at the same time, *secondary sets* are used. Two set-ups are used for this purpose: the tandem setup and the piggyback set up. In a *tandem setup,* a second container is attached to the line of the first container at the lower, secondary port. See Figure 40–10, *A.* It permits medications to be administered intermittently or simultaneously with the first solution.

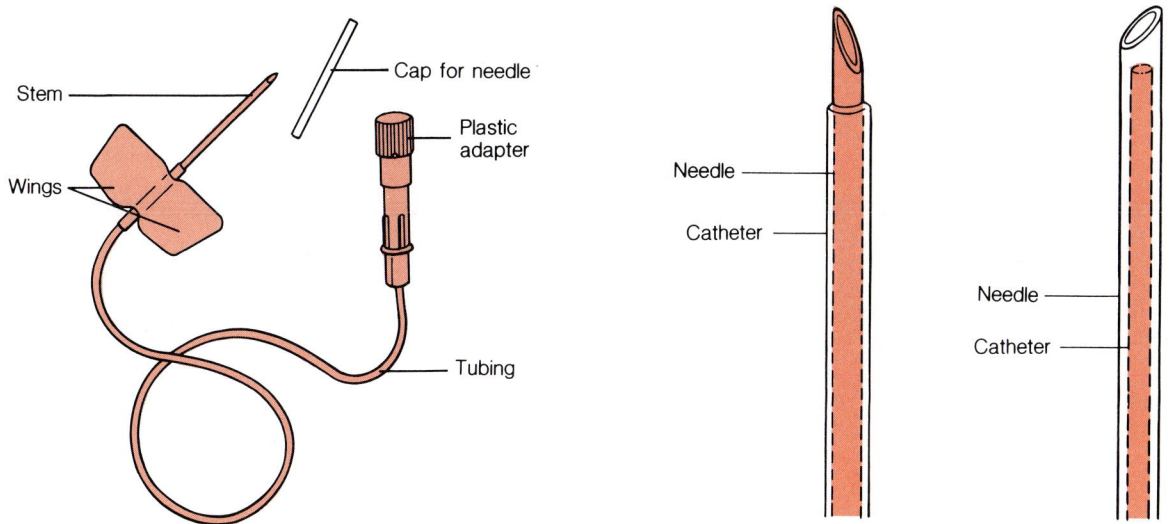

Figure 40–8 Schematic of a butterfly needle with adapter.

Figure 40–9 Schematic of an over-the-needle catheter and an inside-the-needle catheter.

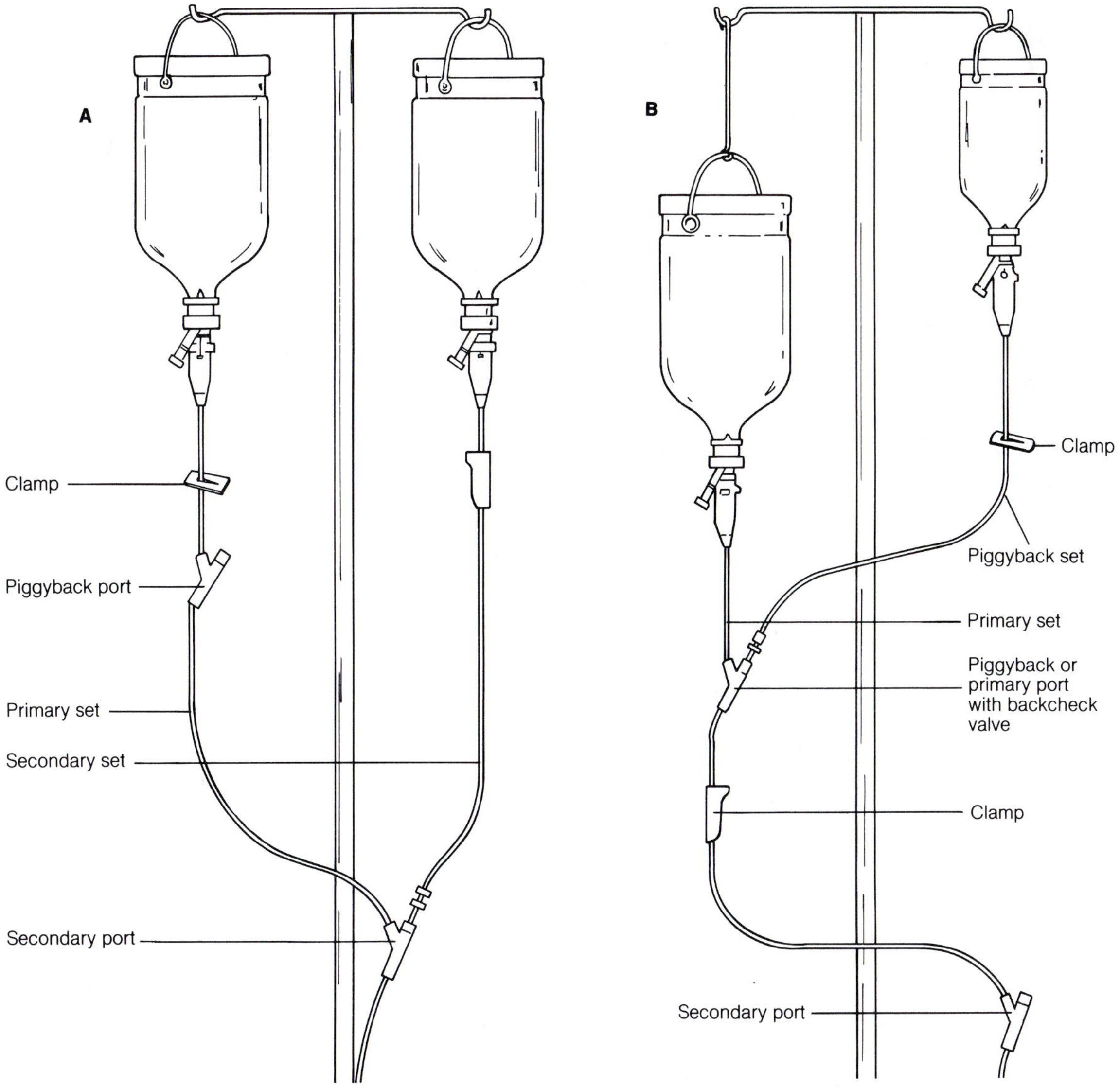

Figure 40–10 Secondary intravenous lines: *A*, a tandem intravenous alignment; and *B*, a piggyback intravenous alignment.

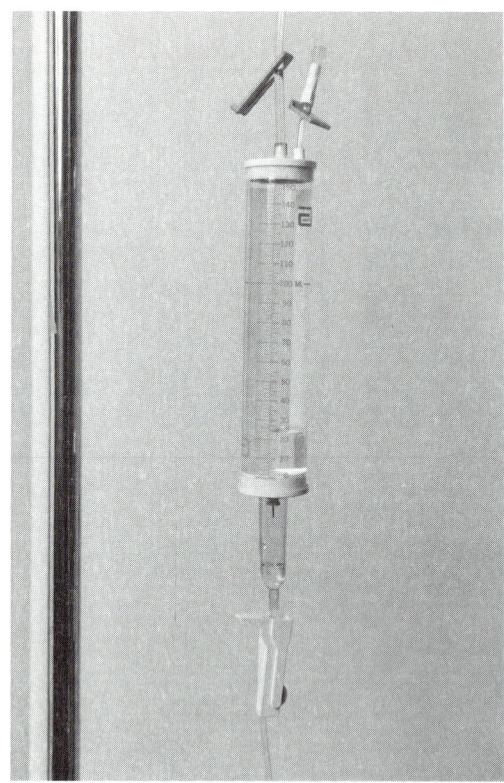

Figure 40–11 A volume-control set above the drip chamber of an intravenous infusion.

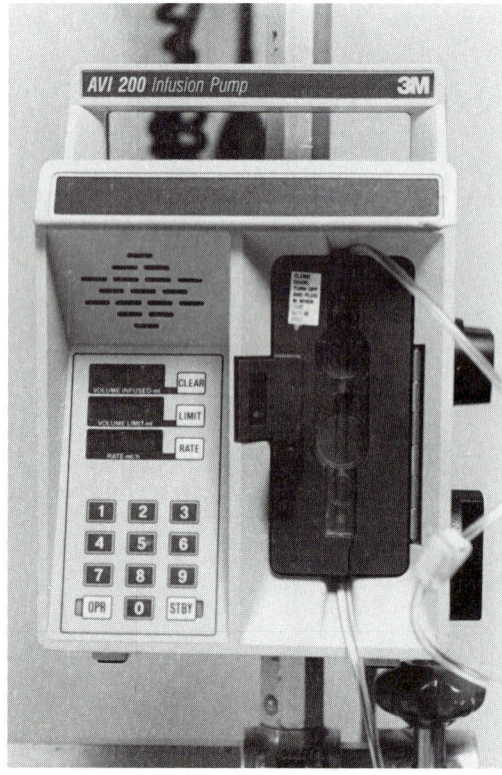

Figure 40–12 An intravenous infusion pump.

In the piggyback alignment, a second set connects the second container to the tubing of the first at the upper port. This setup is used solely for intermittent drug administration. See Figure 40–10, *B.* Various manufacturers describe these sets differently, so the nurse must check the manufacturer's labeling and directions carefully.

Another variation is a *volume-control set,* which is used if the volume of fluid administered is to be carefully controlled. The set is attached below the solution container, and the drip chamber is placed below the set. See Figure 40–11. Volume-control sets are frequently used in pediatric settings, where the volume administered is critical.

Pumps and Controllers   A number of kinds of electronic pumps and controllers are available to control intravenous flow rates more precisely than the standard IV system. A pump (see Figure 40–12) delivers fluids intravenously by exerting positive pressure on the tubing or on the fluid. In situations where the fluid flow is unrestricted, the pump pressure is comparable to that of gravity flow. However, if restrictions develop (increased venous resistance) the pump can maintain the fluid flow by increasing the pressure applied to the fluid. A controller, by contrast, operates solely by gravitational force. The delivery pressure depends on the height of the container in relation to the venipuncture site. The container must be at least 76 cm (30 in) above the venipuncture site for a controller to work. A controller does not have the ability to add pressure to the line and to overcome resistances to fluid flow.

Two types of delivery systems are provided: drops per minute and milliliters per hour. The drops-per-minute models, also referred to as rate consistent devices, are useful when fluid needs to be delivered at a constant and consistent rate to maintain a specific drug level in the client's blood or to achieve a desired client response. The milliliters-per-hour system, or volumetric device, is useful when a specific volume of fluid is to be delivered over a unit of time, e.g., 500 ml in 2 hours. Newborns, burn victims, and clients with renal or congestive heart failure usually require volumetric accuracy.

Some or all of the following special features may be included on pumps and controllers (Wittig and Semmler-Bertanzi 1983, p. 1023):

- *Alarms.* Both visible and audible alarms are usually available. In controllers, the alarm is triggered when the infusion flow cannot be maintained by gravity to the selected rate. In pumps, an occlusion alarm sounds when a restriction to flow cannot be overcome as the pump increases its pressure. When an alarm is activated, some devices automatically stop; others maintain a low flow rate (e.g., 1 to 4 ml/hour) to keep the vein open. Some devices may also be equipped to trigger a remote alarm at the nurse-call system. The nurse needs to explain and demonstrate the alarm to clients so that they will know what to expect when it comes on later.

- *Meters.* Some meters indicate the amount of fluid that has been delivered; others indicate the amount of fluid to be delivered.
- *Flow rate settings.* On most models, the flow rate setting is simply set to the desired rate, i.e., in either drops/minute or milliliters/hour.
- *Drop sensor.* The drop sensor is a photoelectric device placed on the drip chamber. It detects drops as they form and activates the alarm when no drops are formed (e.g., when the solution container is empty or when the tubing is occluded).
- *Air detector.* Some models activate an alarm when air is in the tubing.
- *Infiltration detector.* This flat rubber pad containing two temperature sensors is taped to the skin at the venipuncture site. The two temperature sensors compare skin temperature at separate points. When fluid that is relatively cool compared to skin temperature infiltrates the tissues, the detector activates an alarm.
- *Occlusion detector.* The pump sensor activates an alarm when back pressure becomes greater than the pump's preset limit (e.g., 10 or 15 psi). Most pumps have a psi rating that describes the maximum pressure at which the pump will trigger an occlusion alarm. This pressure rating differs from the actual pressure of fluid delivery. Excessive back pressure may be caused by kinked or pinched tubing, an unopened tubing clamp, or an obstructed in-line filter or bottle airway. Accurate functioning of the occlusion alarm can be ascertained by pinching or clamping the tubing once or twice each shift.
- *Battery.* To allow client mobility, most models are equipped with a rechargeable battery that operates the device from 1 to 4 hours.

Sterile Injection Cap (Heparin or Saline Lock)

This device may be attached to an existing intravenous catheter to keep the route of venous access available for the administration of intermittent or emergency medications. The device is commonly referred to as a *heparin or saline lock* because periodic injection with heparin or saline is used to keep blood from coagulating within the tubing. The lock consists of small plastic tubing with one self-sealing end into which medications can be injected (see Figure 45–51, on page 1292). The other end is inserted into the intravenous catheter.

Implantable Venous Access Devices
Recently developed implantable venous access devices or ports are used in the management of clients with chronic illness who require long-term intravenous therapy (e.g., intermittent medications, continuous infusions of fluid, blood, or parenteral nutrition fluids, and frequent blood samples). The device is designed to provide repeated access to the central

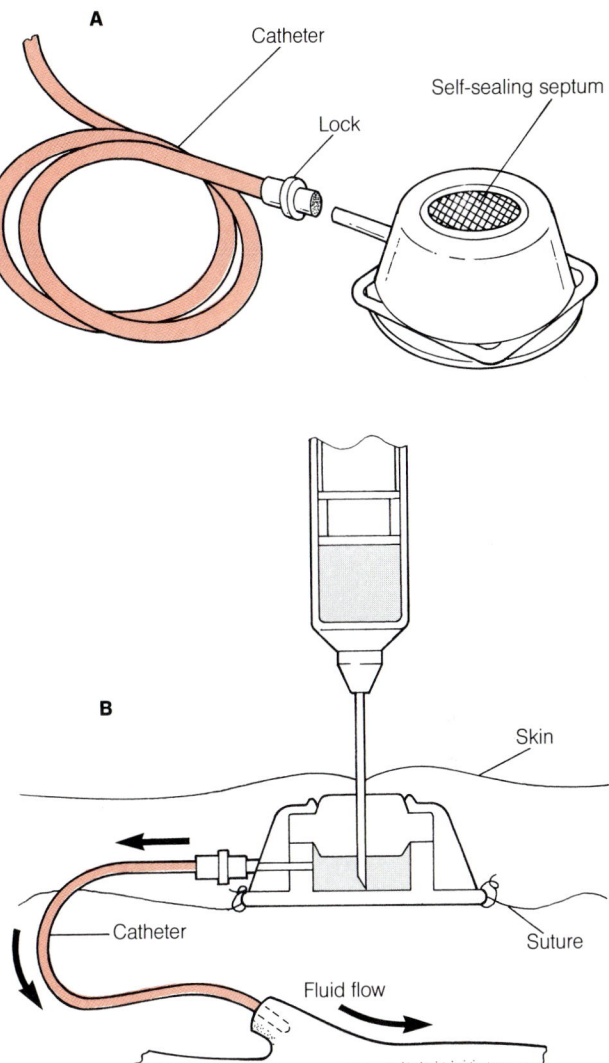

Figure 40–13 An implantable venous access device: *A,* components; *B,* the device in place.

venous system, hence avoiding the trauma and complications of multiple venipunctures.

The device consists of a radiopaque silicone catheter and a plastic or stainless steel injection portal with a self-sealing silicone-rubber septum. See Figure 40–13. Current brand names of the implantable ports are Port-a-Cath, Infuse-A-Port, Mediport, and Chemo-Port. Manufacturers guarantee the septum for a specific number of punctures (e.g., 1000 to 2000). Implantable ports are surgically placed into a small subcutaneous pocket, using local anaesthesia, usually over the third or fourth rib lateral to the sternum. The distal end of the catheter is inserted into the desired central venous blood vessel (see the discussion of central venous sites, earlier in this chapter); the proximal end is routed through a subcutaneous tunnel to the injection portal. These ports can be used immediately after placement. However, a special *Huber needle* must be used to access the port. The delivery opening of this needle is on the side rather than the tip. The needle is inserted at a 90° angle. The site of the port is located by palpation. Agency protocol must be followed when accessing these devices. Before use, aseptic skin preparation is required; after every use, the port must be flushed with heparinized saline to maintain catheter patency.

Setting Up an Intravenous Infusion

An intravenous infusion is set up before venipuncture so that the infusion can be quickly attached to the needle or catheter immediately after it is inserted. Before preparing the infusion, the nurse first verifies the physician's order indicating the type of solution, the amount to be administered, and the rate of flow of the infusion.

When selecting containers, the nurse should avoid using containers with greater volumes than ordered. For example, if 750 ml D5NS (750 ml of 5% dextrose in normal saline) has been ordered, obtain one 500-ml container and one 250-ml container, which total 750 ml. Do not obtain a 1000-ml container with the intention of stopping the solution after 750 ml has been administered. Too often, the incorrect amount can be instilled. If a 1000-ml solution container *must* be used, remove 250 ml before starting the infusion. Note that some agencies use abbreviations to describe commonly used solutions, e.g., DW (distilled water), NS (nor-

mal saline), D5W (5% dextrose in water), D5NS (5% dextrose in normal saline). The nurse should therefore become familiar with the abbreviations used by the agency.

It is essential that the solution be sterile and in good condition, i.e., clear. Cloudiness, evidence that the container has been opened previously, or leaks indicate possible contamination. The nurse should also check the expiration date on the label. A plastic solution bag can be squeezed and inspected for leaks or hairline cracks. The nurse must return any unsatisfactory container to the central supply or distributing department, indicating the reason for the return.

Selection of an appropriate administration set depends on several factors:

- *Vents.* Tubing appropriate for either the rigid or flexible container should be selected.

- *Drop size.* For accurate regulation, a *microdrip* set is usually required if the fluid is to be administered at a rate of 50 to 75 ml/hr or less; a *macrodrip* should be selected when large quantities of solution or fast rates are required.

- *IV ports.* Ports are required to administer secondary infusions and medications.

- *Volumetric chamber.* This will be required if small doses of medication or fluid are to be delivered over an extended period of time.

To set up the intravenous infusion, see Procedure 40–1.

PROCEDURE 40–1

SETTING UP AN INTRAVENOUS INFUSION

Equipment

Correct container(s) of sterile intravenous solution

Appropriate administration set

IV pole

Medication labels for the infusion container if required

Label for the IV tubing

IV filter according to agency policy

Infusion control pump (optional)

Intervention

1. **Open and prepare the administration set.**

- Remove tubing from the container, and straighten it out.
- Slide the tubing clamp along the tubing until it is just below the drip chamber to facilitate its access.
- Close the clamp.

- Leave the ends of the tubing covered with the plastic caps until the infusion is started. *This will maintain the sterility of the ends of the tubing.*

2. **Spike the solution container.**

For a bottle with a rubber stopper:

- Remove the metal disc while maintaining the sterility of the stopper.

If the stopper becomes contaminated while you are removing the metal disc, swab it with disinfectant.

- Remove the cap from the tubing, and insert the spike firmly through the rubber stopper into the port, maintaining sterile technique.

For a bottle with an indwelling vent:

- Remove the metal disc and the

rubber diaphragm, keeping the stopper sterile, and listen for a hissing sound as the air rushes into the bottle. If there is no hissing sound, discard the container, because it was probably not sealed.

- Insert the spike into the larger hole (the one without the vent).

For spiking a plastic bag:

- Remove the protective cover from the entry site and insert the spike. See Figure 40–14.

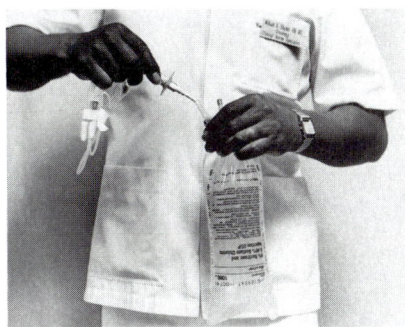

Figure 40–14   Inserting the spike.

3. Hang the solution container on the pole.

- Adjust the pole so that the container is suspended about 1 m (3 ft) above the client's head. *This height is needed to enable gravity to overcome venous pressure and facilitate flow of the solution into the vein.*

4. Partially fill the drip chamber with solution.

For a flexible drip chamber:

- Squeeze the chamber gently until it is half full of solution. See Figure 40–15.

For a firm drip chamber:

- The chamber will usually fill automatically. *The drip chamber is partly filled with solution to prevent air from moving down the tubing.*

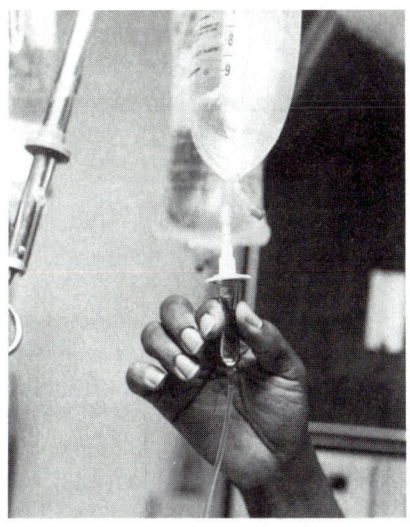

Figure 40–15   Squeezing the drip chamber.

5. Prime the tubing.

For protective caps without air vents:

- Remove the protective cap, and hold the tubing over a cup or basin. Maintain the sterility of the end of the tubing and the cap.

- Release the clamp, and let the fluid run through the tubing until all bubbles are removed. Tap the tubing if necessary with your fingers to help the bubbles move. *The tubing is primed to prevent the introduction of air into the client. Air bubbles in large amounts can act as emboli in the bloodstream.*

- Reclamp the tubing, and replace the tubing cap, maintaining sterile technique.

For caps with air vents:

- Do not remove the cap when priming this tubing. The flow of solution through the tubing will cease when the cap is moist with one drop of solution.

- If an infusion control pump or controller is being used, follow the manufacturer's directions for inserting the tubing and setting the infusion rate.

6. Apply a medication label to the solution container according to agency policy.

- In many agencies, medications and labels are applied in the pharmacy; if they are not, apply the label upside down on the container (see Figure 45–44 on page 1286). *The label is applied upside down so it can be read easily when the container is hanging up.*

7. Label the IV tubing.

- Label tubing with date, time of attachment, and initials (see Figure 40–16). This labeling may also be done at the time the infusion is started. *The tubing is labeled to ensure that it is changed at regular intervals* (i.e., every 24 to 72 hours according to agency policy).

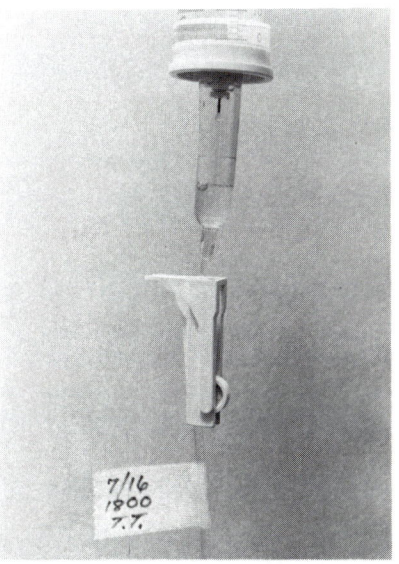

Figure 40–16   Tubing labeled with date, time of attachment, and nurse's initials.

8. Apply a timing label on the solution container.

- The timing label may be applied at the time the infusion is started. Follow agency practice. See discussion of regulating infusion flow rates on page 1075 and Figure 40–22 on page 1075.

Guidelines for Vein Selection

- Use distal veins of the arm first.
- Use the client's nondominant arm whenever possible.
- Use veins in the feet and legs only when arm veins are inaccessible, since they are more prone to thrombus formation and subsequent emoboli.
- Select a vein that:
  a. Is easily palpated and feels soft and full
  b. Is naturally splinted by bone
  c. Is large enough to allow adequate circulation around the catheter

Avoid using the following veins:

- Those in areas of flexion (e.g., the antecubital fossa)
- Those that are highly visible, since they tend to roll away from the needle
- Those damaged by previous use, phlebitis, infiltration, or sclerosis
- Those continually distended with blood or that have become knotted or tortuous
- Veins of a surgically compromised or injured extremity (e.g., following a mastectomy) because of possible impaired circulation and discomfort for the client.

Selecting a Venipuncture Site

As a general rule, distal veins of the hands and arms should be used when initiating intravenous therapy. Guidelines for vein selection are shown in the accompanying box. The extremity must be observed and palpated before a vein is chosen.

Starting an Intravenous Infusion

Agency practices vary about which nurses perform venipunctures and start intravenous infusions. In many settings, nurses must be supervised and certified before they are permitted to start infusions on their own. Some agencies have teams of specially prepared nurses who initiate all intravenous infusions. Before starting an infusion, the nurse must determine the following:

- The physician's exact orders.
- Whether the client has any allergies, e.g., to tape or povidone-iodine.
- The agency policy about shaving the area before a venipuncture. Some agencies advise against shaving because of the possibility of nicking the skin and subsequent infection.

To start an intravenous infusion, see Procedure 40–2.

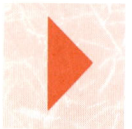

PROCEDURE 40–2

STARTING AN INTRAVENOUS INFUSION USING A BUTTERFLY NEEDLE OR AN ANGIOCATHETER

Equipment ☑

Sterile butterfly (wing-tipped) needle. A 2.5-cm (1-in) needle, #21 or #23 gauge, is used for most infusions; a #19 needle is used for whole blood
or
Angiocatheter of suitable size, e.g., #22 gauge for clear liquid infusions, #20 gauge for infusing drug boluses or peripheral fat solutions

Antiseptic swabs

Tourniquet

Receptacle for discarded fluid

Adhesive or nonallergenic tape

Skin preparation materials if the skin at the site will be shaved

Container of sterile parenteral solution

Intravenous administration set

Intravenous stand (pole)

Towel or pad

Arm splint, if required

Gauze squares or other appropriate dressings

Antiseptic ointment, e.g., povidone-iodine (Betadine)

Gloves to protect the nurse from contamination by the client's blood

Intervention

1. Prepare the client.

■ Explain the procedure to the client. A venipuncture can cause discomfort for a few seconds, but there should be no discomfort while the solution is flowing. Clients often want to know how long the process will last. The physician's order may specify the length of time of the infusion, e.g., 3000 ml over 24 hours.

■ Provide any scheduled care before establishing the infusion to minimize movement of the affected limb during the procedure. *Moving the limb after the infusion is established could dislodge the needle.*

■ Make sure that the client's gown can be removed over the IV apparatus if necessary. Some agencies provide special gowns that open over the shoulder and down the sleeve for easy removal.

■ Wash hands.

2. Set up the infusion equipment if not already prepared.

■ See Procedure 40–1 on page 1070.

■ Prepare strips of adhesive tape to stabilize the needle once it is inserted.

3. Select and prepare the venipuncture site.

■ Starting at the distal end of the vein, select a site by palpating accessible veins. Veins can become sclerotic from irritation by the infusion or the needle. Sclerosis may then interfere with venous flow. If so, more proximal parts of the veins can be used.

■ If necessary, shave the skin where adhesive tape will be applied (about a 2-inch area around the intended site). Check agency policy.

4. Dilate the vein.

■ Place the extremity in a dependent position (lower than the client's heart). *Gravity slows venous return and distends the veins. Distending the veins makes it easier to insert the needle properly.*

■ Apply a tourniquet firmly 15 to 20 cm (6 to 8 in) above the venipuncture site. The tourniquet must be tight enough to obstruct venous flow but not so tight that it occludes arterial flow. *Obstructing arterial flow inhibits venous filling.* If a radial pulse can be palpated, the arterial flow is not obstructed.

■ If the vein is not sufficiently dilated:
   a. Massage or stroke the vein distal to the site and in the direction of venous flow toward the heart. *This action helps fill the vein.*
   b. Encourage the client to clench and unclench the fist rapidly. *Contracting the muscles compresses the distal veins, forcing blood along the veins and distending them.*
   c. Lightly tap the vein with your fingertips. *Tapping may distend the vein.*

■ If the above steps fail to distend the vein so that it is palpable, remove the tourniquet and apply heat to the entire extremity for 10 to 15 minutes. *Heat dilates superficial blood vessels, causing them to fill.* Then repeat the steps above.

5. Don gloves and clean the venipuncture site.

■ Clean the skin at the site of entry with a topical antiseptic swab, e.g., alcohol, and then an anti-infective solution e.g., povidone-iodine (Betadine).

■ Use a circular motion, moving from the center outwards for several inches. *This motion carries micro-*

organisms away from the site of entry.

6. Insert the needle or angiocatheter and initiate the infusion.

■ Use one thumb to pull the skin taut below the entry site. *This stabilizes the vein and makes the skin taut for needle entry. It can also make initial tissue penetration less painful.*

For a butterfly needle:

■ Hold the needle, pointed in the direction of the blood flow, at a 30° angle, with the bevel up, and pierce the skin beside the vein about 1 cm (½ in) below the site planned for piercing the vein. See Figure 40–17.

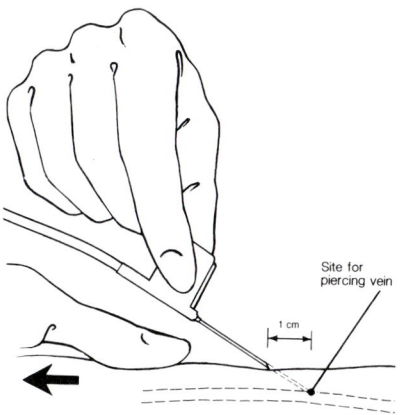

Site for piercing vein

1 cm

Figure 40–17 Inserting a butterfly needle.

■ Once the needle is through the skin, lower the needle so that it is almost parallel with the skin. *Lowering the needle reduces the chances of puncturing both sides of the vein.* Follow the course of the vein, and pierce one side of the vein.

■ When blood flows back into the needle tubing, insert the needle farther up the vein 2 to 2.5 cm (¾ to 1 in) or to the hub of the butterfly needle. Sudden lack of resistance can be felt as blood enters the needle.

- Release the tourniquet, attach the infusion, and initiate flow as quickly as possible. *Attaching the tubing quickly prevents blood from clotting and obstructing the needle.*

For an angiocatheter:

- Insert the catheter by the direct or indirect method. The direct method is preferred for large veins and the indirect method for smaller veins (Peck 1985, p. 40). For the *direct method,* hold the catheter with bevel up, at a 15° to 20° angle, and insert the catheter through the skin and into the vein in one thrust. For the *indirect method,* first pierce the skin, then reduce the angle and advance the catheter into the vein. Sudden lack of resistance is felt as the catheter enters the vein.

- Once blood appears in the catheter or you feel the lack of resistance, advance the catheter another 0.6 cm (¼ in). *The catheter is advanced to ensure that it, and not just the metal needle, is in the vein.*

- Release the tourniquet.

- Remove the protective cap from the distal end of the tubing, and hold it ready to attach to the catheter, maintaining the sterility of the end.

- Grasp the hub of the catheter with your thumb and index finger, and withdraw the needle. See Figure 40–18.

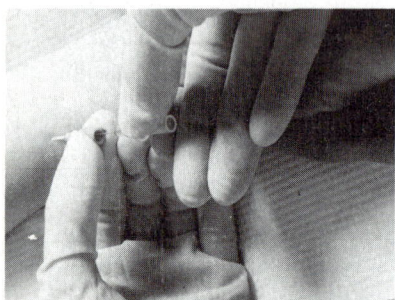

Figure 40–18 Withdrawing the needle from an angiocatheter.

- Advance the catheter up to the hub or until you feel resistance.

- Attach the end of the infusion tubing to the catheter hub. Initiate the infusion.

7. **Secure the needle or catheter with tape.**

- Tape the butterfly needle securely by the H method (see Figure 40–19) or crisscross (chevron) method (see Figure 40–20). Place a cotton ball or small gauze square under the needle, if required. *The gauze keeps the needle in position in the vein.*

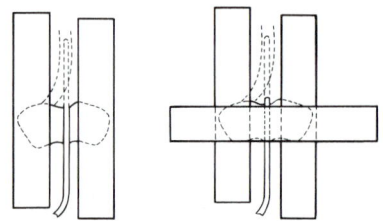

Figure 40–19 Taping the butterfly needle by the H method.

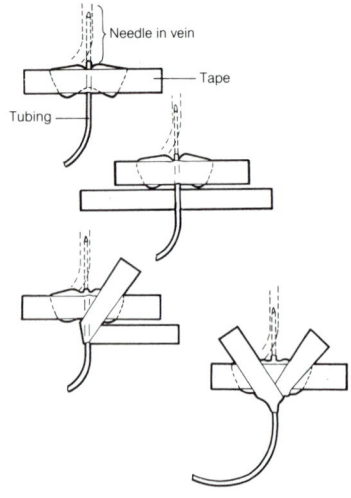

Figure 40–20 Taping the butterfly needle by the crisscross (chevron) method.

- Tape the catheter:
  a. Place the first tape, sticky side up, under the catheter hub, and fold the sticky sides down on the skin along each side of the catheter distal to the insertion point.
  b. Place the second strip, sticky side down, across the catheter hub.
  c. Place the third strip, sticky side up, under the catheter hub distal to the second strip, and fold each side diagonally across the catheter.

8. **Dress and label the venipuncture site according to agency policy.**

- In some agencies, the nurse puts a small amount of antiseptic ointment, e.g., povidone-iodine, over the venipuncture site, then a gauze square. In other agencies, a sterile transparent occlusive dressing is applied. This permits assessment of the site without disturbing the dressing. This type of dressing can be left on for 72 hours, unless there are complications (Peck 1985, p. 32).

- Loop the tubing, and secure it to the dressing with tape. *Looping and securing the tubing prevent the weight of the tubing or any movement from pulling on the needle or catheter.*

- Label a piece of tape with the date and time of insertion, type and gauge of needle or catheter used, and your initials. Apply the tape label over the venipuncture dressing. See Figure 40–21.

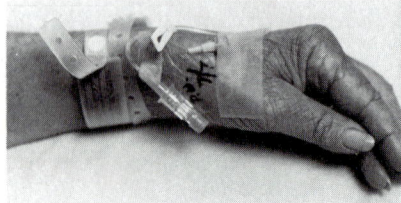

Figure 40–21 Properly labeled tape over venipuncture dressing.

Regulating Intravenous Flow Rates

An important nursing function is to regulate the flow rate of an intravenous infusion. The physician usually describes in the order how long an infusion should last, e.g., 3000 ml over 24 hours. It is then a nursing responsibility to calculate the correct flow rate and regulate the infusion. Problems that can result from incorrectly regulated infusions include hypervolemia and hypovolemia. Unless a regulating device (i.e., a controller, infusion pump, or in-line manual adjuster) is being used, the nurse administering the intravenous solution must regulate the drops per minute manually by using the roller clamp to ensure that the prescribed amount of solution will be infused in the correct time span.

There are a number of commercially prepared infusion sets, each with its own type of drip chamber; so, it is important to know the number of drops per milliliter of solution for a particular drip chamber before calculating a drip rate. This rate, called the **drop** or **drip factor**, is printed on most commercially prepared packages. Common drop factors are 10, 15, and 20 for macrodrips (regular infusion sets) and 60 for microdrips (mini-drip infusion sets).

To calculate flow rates, the nurse must know the volume of fluid to be infused and the specific time for the infusion. Two commonly used methods of indicating flow rates are designating the number of milliliters to be administered in 1 hour (ml/hr) and the number of drops to be given in 1 minute (gtt/min). Since 1 milliliter of fluid displaces 1 cubic centimeter of space, the volume to be infused in the first method may also be designated as cubic centimeters per hour (cc/hr).

Milliliters per hour Hourly rates of infusion can be calculated by dividing the total infusion volume by the total infusion time in hours. For example, if 3000 ml is infused in 24 hours, the number of milliliters per hour is

$$\frac{3000 \text{ ml (total infusion volume)}}{24 \text{ hr (total infusion time)}} = 125 \text{ ml/hr}$$

Nurses need to check infusions at least every hour to ensure that the indicated milliliters per hour have been infused. A strip of adhesive marking the exact time and/or amount to be infused may be taped to the solution bottle. Some agencies make premarked labels available. See Figure 40–22.

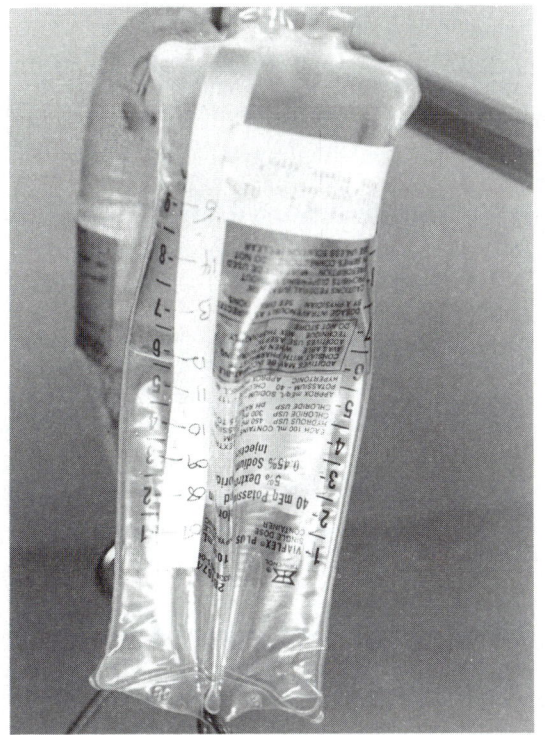

Figure 40–22 Timing label on an intravenous container.

---

9. Ensure appropriate infusion flow.

- Apply a padded arm board to splint the elbow or wrist joint if needed.
- Adjust the infusion rate of flow according to the order.

10. Document relevant data including assessments.

- Record the start of the infusion on the client's chart. Some agencies

provide a special form for this purpose. Include the date and time of the venipuncture; amount and type of solution used, including any additives (e.g., kind and amount of medications); absorption time; container number; drip rate; type and gauge of the needle or catheter; venipuncture site; and client's general response.

Sample Recording

Date 6/8/91	Time 1800

IV #1–1000 ml D5W started in the right basilic vein. BF needle #21G inserted. Drip rate 125 ml/hr. Completion time 0200 hours. IV running at prescribed rate's signs of infiltration. No discomfort voiced. — Dino C. Anastasio, NS

Drops per minute

The nurse who begins an infusion must regulate the drops per minute to ensure that the prescribed amount of solution will infuse. Drops per minute are calculated by the following formula:

$$\text{Drops per minute} = \frac{\text{Total infusion volume} \times \text{drops/ml (or drop factor)}}{\text{Total time of infusion in } \textit{minutes}}$$

If the requirements are 1000 ml in 8 hours (480 minutes) and the drip factor is 20 drops/ml, the drops per minute should be

$$\frac{1000 \text{ ml} \times 20 \text{ drops/ml}}{480 \text{ min}} = 41 \text{ drops/min}$$

Approximating this rate as 40 drops/min, the nurse must then regulate the drops per minute by tightening or releasing the intravenous tubing clamp and counting the drops the same way a pulse is counted. Devices such as battery-operated rate meters and infusion pumps with alarm systems facilitate a regulated flow.

Factors influencing flow rates

No matter how often flow rates are regulated, several factors can change the rate of flow of an intravenous solution. If an infusion is too fast or too slow, the nurse needs to consider several factors:

1. *The position of the forearm.* Sometimes a change in the position of the client's arm decreases flow. Slight pronation, supination, extension, or elevation of the forearm on a pillow can increase flow.

2. *The position and patency of the tubing.* Not infrequently, the tubing is obstructed by the client's weight, a kink, or a clamp closed too tightly. The flow rate also diminishes when part of the tubing dangles below the puncture site.

3. *The height of the infusion bottle.* Elevating the height of the infusion bottle a few inches can speed the flow by creating more pressure.

4. *Possible infiltration or fluid leakage.* Swelling, a feeling of coldness, and tenderness at the venipuncture site may indicate infiltration.

Monitoring and Maintaining an Intravenous Infusion

Intravenous infusions must be carefully monitored so that the correct solution is maintained at the correct rate and any problems (e.g., fluid infiltration, phlebitis, circulatory overload, and blockage of the infusion flow) are prevented. See Table 40–11 for an intravenous infusion checklist.

Compare the rate of flow regularly, e.g., every hour, against the schedule. If the rate is too fast, slow it so that the infusion will be completed at the planned time. If it is too slow, check agency practice. Some agencies permit nursing personnel to adjust a rate of flow of 3 ml/min or less. Adjustments above 3 ml/min may require a physician's order. If the rate of flow is 150 ml/hr or more, the rate of flow must be checked more frequently, e.g., every 15 to 30 minutes. Infusions that are off schedule can be harmful to a client. Solution that is administered too slowly can supply insufficient fluid, electrolytes, or medication for a client's needs. Solution administered too quickly may cause a significant increase in circulating blood volume (which is about 6 liters in an adult). Hypervolemia may result in pulmonary edema and cardiac failure. The clinical signs of cardiac failure are dyspnea, reduced urine output, edema, weak and rapid pulse, and shallow, rapid respirations. The clinical signs of pulmonary edema are dyspnea, coughing, frothy sputum, and rales on lung auscultation.

As part of the ongoing assessment of each client receiving intravenous therapy, the nurse should inspect the client's infusion site for fluid **infiltration**, i.e., the escape of intravenous fluid into the interstitial tissues, usually near the insertion site. Infiltration occurs when the needle or catheter has become dislodged from the client's vein, allowing the intravenous fluid to flow into the subcutaneous tissue. The clinical signs are swelling, coolness, pain, pallor at the site, and discomfort. To ascertain the presence of infiltration, the nurse:

1. Palpates the surrounding tissue for edema.
2. Feels the surrounding skin for changes in temperature.

If infiltration is not evident, the following measures can determine whether the needle is dislodged from the vein:

1. Gently pinch the IV tubing adjacent to the needle site. This will cause blood to flow (flash back) into the tubing if the needle is in the vein.
2. Use a sterile syringe of saline to withdraw fluid from the rubber at the end of the tubing near the venipuncture site. If blood does not return, discontinue the intravenous infusion.
3. Try to stop the flow by applying a tourniquet 10 to 15 cm (4 to 6 in) above the insertion site and opening the roller clamp wide. If the infusion continues to flow slowly, the needle is in subcutaneous tissue (it has infiltrated.) If the infusion has infiltrated, the nurse should immediately discontinue the infusion. See page 1079.

Inspecting for **phlebitis** (inflammation of a vein) is an essential part of the initial and ongoing assessment of a client receiving intravenous therapy. It is recommended that an infusion site be inspected and palpated every 8 hours (Lonsway 1987, p. 107). Phlebitis can occur as a result of injury to a vein, e.g., because of mechanical trauma or chemical irritation. Chemical injury to a vein can occur from intravenous electrolytes (especially potassium and magnesium) and medications. The clinical signs are redness, warmth, and swelling at the intravenous site. Should phlebitis develop, pain along the course of a vein may be detected.

the infusion should be discontinued, warm compresses applied to the venipuncture site, and the injured vein should not be used for further infusions.

Ongoing assessment should also include inspection for *bleeding* at the intravenous site. Oozing or bleeding into the surrounding tissues can occur while the infusion is freely flowing but is more likely to occur after the needle has been removed from the vein. The site of insertion should always be inspected for evidence of blood, particularly in clients who bleed readily, e.g., clients receiving anticoagulants.

Another nursing responsibility is to ensure that the *correct solution* is being infused. If the solution is incorrect, the nurse slows the rate of flow to a minimum to maintain the patency of the catheter. If the infusion is terminated, the client will have to have another venipuncture before the new solution is administered. The error is reported to the nurse in charge and the solution is changed to the correct one. Agencies have different policies about how and to whom to report an incident.

In addition to assessing the client, the nurse should also *inspect the system* to make sure that it is intact. If there is leakage, the nurse locates the source. If the leak is at the catheter connection, the tubing into the catheter is tightened. If the leak cannot be stopped, the nurse slows the infusion as much as possible without stopping it and replaces the tubing with a new sterile set, estimating the amount of solution lost if it was substantial. The system should be inspected for blockages. The flow of solution can be blocked or impeded for several reasons, and systematic assessment helps the nurse identify and correct problems rapidly. If blockage is suspected:

1. Inspect the tubing for any kinks. Arrange the tubing so that it is lightly coiled and under no pressure. Sometimes the tubing becomes caught under the client's arm, and the weight of the arm blocks the flow.

2. Determine whether the bevel of the catheter is blocked against the wall of the vein. If it is blocked, pull back gently, turn it slightly, or carefully raise or lower the angle of insertion slightly, using a sterile gauze pad underneath to protect the skin and change the position of the catheter bevel.

3. Examine the tubing clamp. If it is closed, adjust it to the open position.

4. Observe the position of the solution container. If it is less than 1 m (3 ft) above the IV site, readjust it to the correct height on the pole. If the container is too low, the solution may not flow into the vein because there is insufficient gravitational pressure to overcome the pressure of the blood within the vein.

5. Observe the position of the tubing. If it is dangling below the venipuncture, coil it carefully on the surface of the bed. The solution cannot flow upward into the vein against the force of gravity.

TABLE 40-11 Checklist for an Intravenous Infusion

Component	Data
Solution Container	
Name of solution	_____
Amount of solution	_____
Number of container	_____
Date and time	_____
Time of completion	_____
Next Solution	
Name of solution	_____
Amount of solution	_____
Number of container	_____
Date and time	_____
Time of completion	_____
Tubing	
Intact	_____
Coiled smoothly	_____
Unobstructed	_____
Drip Chamber	
Appropriately filled	_____
Dripping at correct rate	_____
Client	
Venipuncture site	_____
Dry or wet	_____
Bleeding	_____
Swelling	_____
Skin color	_____
Skin temperature	_____
Pain	_____
Respirations	_____
Pulse	_____
Urine output	_____
Edema	_____
Sputum and cough	_____
Psychologic concerns	_____

Changing Intravenous Containers and Tubing

Intravenous solution containers are changed when only a small amount of fluid remains in the neck of the container and fluid still remains in the drip chamber. The Centers for Disease Control (CDC) (1982) recommend that tubing be changed every 48 hours to decrease the incidence of phlebitis and infection. However, recent studies indicate that 72-hour intervals may be appropriate (Josephson et al. 1985, p. 367; Snydman et al. 1987, p. 116). Tubing is changed most easily when a new container is added. Procedure 40–3 provides guidelines for changing an intravenous container and tubing.

6. Observe the drip chamber. If it is less than half full, squeeze the chamber to allow the correct amount of fluid to flow in. See Figure 40–15.

   The nurse needs to teach clients when to call for assistance, e.g., if the solution stops dripping or the venipuncture site becomes swollen. To help the client maintain the intravenous infusion, instruct the client to.

   1. Avoid sudden twisting or turning movements of the arm with the needle or catheter.
   2. Avoid stretching or placing tension on the tubing.
   3. Try to keep the tubing from dangling below the level of the needle.
   4. Notify a nurse if:
      a. There is a sudden change in the flow rate.
      b. The solution container is nearly empty.
      c. There is blood in the IV tubing.
      d. He or she feels discomfort at the IV site.

PROCEDURE 40–3

CHANGING AN INTRAVENOUS CONTAINER AND TUBING

☑ Equipment

Container with the correct kind and amount of sterile solution

Administration set, including sterile tubing and drip chamber

Tape

Sterile gauze square for positioning the needle

Antiseptic solution and/or ointment for cleaning the site. Check agency practice.

Sterile swabs

Receptacle (e.g., a basin) for discarded fluid

Gloves to protect the nurse from contamination by the client's blood

Intervention

1. Obtain the correct solution container.
- Verify the physician's order.
- Compare the number on the new container against the number on the used container.
- Read the label of the new container.

2. Assess the client and the IV system.
- Assess the client for signs of infiltration, circulatory overload, and phlebitis. Evidence of such signs indicates the need to change the venipuncture site and possibly the volume of fluid.
- Inspect the IV system for blockages.

3. Set up the intravenous equipment with the new container and label them.
- See Procedure 40–1 earlier.
- Apply a timing label to the container.
- Prime the tubing.
- Label the tubing as shown in Figure 40–16, earlier in this chapter.

4. Remove the venipuncture dressing to expose the needle or catheter hub.
- Loosen the tape at the venipuncture site.
- Don gloves to prevent exposure to the client's secretions.

5. Disconnect the used tubing.
- Remove the tape and the dressing from around the needle or catheter, taking care not to dislodge the needle or catheter from the vein.
- Place a sterile swab under the hub of the catheter. *This absorbs any leakage that might occur when the tubing is disconnected.*
- Holding the hub of the needle with the nondominant hand, loosen the tubing with the dominant hand, using a twisting, pulling motion. *Holding the needle firmly but gently maintains its position in the vein.*
- Clamp and remove the used tubing.
- Place the end of the tubing in the kidney basin or other receptacle.

RESEARCH NOTE

How Often Should IV Tubing Be Changed?

The CDC recommends that the cannulae for intravenous therapy be removed and the infusion restarted in another site every 48 to 72 hours (CDC 1982). This recommendation was made because the incidence of infection tends to increase with the duration of cannulation. However, many hospitals began to change intravenous tubing routinely every 48 hours. These researchers, questioning the need to change the tubing more frequently than the cannula, examined the incidence of IV infection in tubing changed at 48-hour intervals compared to tubing changed only when the cannula site was changed.

During the course of the study, 219 courses of intravenous therapy were followed over an 11-month period. In one group, the tubing was changed every 48 hours; in the other, the tubing was changed when the cannula site was changed. The fluid contamination was found to be low in both groups: 0.87% in the 48-hour group, and 0.96% in the other.

Implications: Based on data, the researchers recommend that tubing be changed at a 3- or 4-day frequency. The 3-day (72-hour) frequency would serve clients whose IV site is changed every 72 hours.

A. Josephson, M. D. Gombert, M. F. Sierra, L. V. Karanfil, and G. F. Tansino. The relationship between fluid contamination and the frequency of tubing replacement, *Infection Control,* September 1985, 6:367–70.

Discontinuing an Intravenous Infusion

Discontinuing an intravenous infusion, which is indicated when the amount of solution ordered by the physician has been infused, is not uncomfortable for a client. Before removing a catheter or needle from the vein, the nurse must determine whether a sterile injection cap (heparin lock) should be attached to the catheter so that intravenous medications can be administered intermittently (see discussion on page 1069).

When discontinuing an infusion, obtain a sterile gauze (dry or soaked in antiseptic), an adhesive bandage strip or small sterile dressing and tape, and gloves for the nurse. First, clamp the infusion tubing, and then loosen the tape by pulling it toward the site so as not to dislodge the needle or catheter accidently. Apply gloves. Remove the dressing, and discard it in a moisture-proof container. After removing the dressing, hold a sterile gauze over the venipuncture site with the nondominant hand and apply slight pressure. With the dominant hand, withdraw the needle or catheter by pulling it steadily along the line of the vein. Pulling in this direction is less likely to injure the vein or break the needle or catheter. Immediately apply firm pressure for 2 to 3 minutes to prevent any bleeding. Clients who have received heparin or who have had a heparin lock require longer pressure because of the action of heparin on blood-clotting mechanisms. Inspect the needle or catheter carefully to make sure it is intact. Any broken device must be reported to the nurse in charge promptly because the piece in the vein could move centrally in the client's circulatory system. After making sure there is no bleeding, apply the adhesive bandage strip or sterile dressing to the site to prevent

---

▶ **PROCEDURE 40–3** *(continued)*

ing from the insertion point out-

7. Clean the venipuncture site, and apply a sterile dressing with label.

- Clean the venipuncture site, working from the insertion point outward in a circular manner. Iodine or ethyl alcohol is frequently used. Some agencies also place water-soluble iodine ointment, e.g., Beta-dine, at the site.
- Tape the needle in place. See Procedure 40–2.
- Apply a sterile dressing over the site.
- Remove gloves.
- Apply a labeled tape over the dressing. The label should include (a) the date and time the dressing is applied; (b) the original date and time of the venipuncture; (c) the size of the catheter or needle; and

6. Connect the new tubing, and reestablish the infusion.

- Continue to hold the needle, and grasp the new tubing with the dominant hand.
- Remove the protective tubing cap, and, maintaining sterility, insert the tubing end securely into the needle hub. Twist it to secure it.
- Open the clamp to start the solution flowing.

8. Regulate the rate of flow of the solution according to the order on the chart.

9. Document relevant information.

- Record the change of the solution container and/or tubing in the appropriate place on the client's chart. Also record the fluid intake according to agency practice. Record the number of the container if the containers are numbered at the agency. Also record your assessments.

(d) your initials, as the nurse who changed the dressing.

Administering Blood Transfusions

A **blood transfusion** is the introduction of whole blood or components of the blood (e.g., plasma or erythrocytes) into the venous circulation. See Table 40–12 for blood and blood products and indications for their use. Blood transfusions are given for the following reasons:

1. To restore blood volume after severe hemorrhage
2. To restore the capacity of the blood to carry oxygen
3. To provide plasma factors, e.g., antihemophilic factor (AHF) or factor VIII, or platelet concentrates, which prevent or treat bleeding

Blood Matching

Blood groups   Human blood is classified into four main groups (A, B, AB, and O) on the basis of polysaccharide antigens on the erythrocyte surface. These antigens, type A and type B, commonly cause antibody reactions and are called **agglutinogens.** In other words, group A blood contains type A agglutinogen, group B blood contains type B agglutinogen, group AB blood contains both A and B agglutinogen, and group O blood contains neither agglutinogen. In addition to agglutinogens on the erythrocytes, **agglutinins** (antibodies) are present in the blood plasma. No individual can have agglutinins and agglutinogens of the same type; that person's system would attack its own cells. Thus, group A blood does not contain agglutinin A but does contain agglutinin B. Group B blood does not contain agglutinin B but does contain agglutinin A. Group AB blood does not contain either agglutinin, and Group O contains both anti-A and anti-B agglutinins. Blood transfusions must be matched to the client's blood type in terms of compatible agglutinogens. Mismatched blood will cause a hemolytic reaction. See Table 40–13 for blood groups and compatibility.

Rhesus (Rh) and other factors   Rh antigens, also on the surface of erythrocytes, are present in about 85% of the population and can be a major cause of hemolytic reactions. Persons who possess the **Rh factor** are referred to as **Rh positive**; those who do not are referred to as **Rh negative**. Some other blood factors are the M, N, S, s, P, Kell, Lewis, Duffy, Kidd, Diego, and Lutheran factors (Guyton 1986, p. 73). These rarely cause major reactions because their antigenic properties are poor.

The Rh factor differs from the A and B agglutinogens in that it cannot cause a hemolytic reaction on the first exposure to mismatched blood. This is because the Rh antibody

microorganisms from entering the open area. The site should be kept dry for 24 hours to promote healing. Document on the client's record the date, time, discontinuation of the infusion, the appearance of the site and the intactness of the catheter or needle. Also, record the amount of fluid infused, the container number, type of solution, and additional assessments. The attachment of a heparin lock should also be documented.

TABLE 40–12   Blood and Blood Products

Product (Volume)	General Information
Citrated whole human blood (500 ml)	Contains RBCs and plasma and anti-coagulation preservative. Expands intravascular volume; increase in RBCs; increases tissue oxygenation. Has a hematocrit of 35–40%.
Red blood cells (packed cells) (250 ml)	Has a hematocrit of approximately 75%. Increases tissue oxygenation. Some are prepared with a preservative solution. Should raise hematocrit.
Platelet concentrates (30 ml)	Used to treat or prevent bleeding. Administer rapidly through a filter.
Granulocyte concentrates	Used to treat infections. Administer through a filter. Requires pretransfusion RBC compatibility testing.
Plasma (200 ml)	Provides coagulation factors. Can transmit infections. Transfuse with a filter.
Cryoprecipitate (10 – 20 ml)	Blood product containing high concentrations of fibrinogen and antihemophilic factor (factor VIII). May transmit infections. Transfuse with a filter.
Albumin (50 ml)	Expands blood volume rapidly. Increases plasma albumin level. Does not transmit infection.
Plasma protein fraction (Plasmanate)	Expands blood volume rapidly. Does not transmit infection.
Clotting factors (Fibrinogen) (10 ml)	Used to prevent or treat bleeding. Monitor blood volume.
Immune globulins, gamma-globulin, hepatitis B globulin	Used to treat exposure to Hepatitis A or B. Administer intramuscularly, intravenously.

TABLE 40 – 13 Blood Compatibility

Blood Group	Percentage of Population	Antibodies Present in Plasma	Compatible RBCs	Compatible Plasma
O	47	Anti-A, Anti-B	O	O, A, B, AB
A	41	Anti-B	A, O	A, AB
B	9	Anti-A	B, O	B, AB
AB	3	Neither Anti-A nor Anti-B	AB, A, B, O	AB

Rh Type	Percentage of Population	RBC Rh Type for Transfusion	Plasma Rh Type for Transfusion
Positive	85	Positive or negative	Positive or negative
Negative	15	Negative	Positive or negative

is *not* normally present in the plasma of persons who are Rh negative.

Transfusion Reactions Transfusion reactions can be categorized as hemolytic, febrile (bacterial), allergic, and hypervolemic. The assessments and nursing interventions for each type of reaction are outlined in Table 40–14. The *hemolytic reaction*, which can be a fatal response, occurs when agglutinins and agglutinogens of the same type come in contact; e.g., type A agglutinogen and anti-A agglutinin, or type B agglutinogen and anti-B agglutinin. **Agglutination** (clumping) and **hemolysis** (rupture) of the red cells

TABLE 40 – 14 Transfusion Reactions

Reaction	Assessment	Nursing Intervention
Hemolytic	Chills, fever, headache, backache, dyspnea, cyanosis, chest pain, tachycardia, hypotension	Discontinue transfusion immediately. Keep vein open with normal saline. Send remaining blood and sample of client's blood to laboratory for repeat cross-matching and typing. Notify physician immediately. Monitor vital signs. Monitor fluid intake and output. Administer medications as ordered.
Febrile (Bacterial)	Fever, chills, warm, flushed skin, headache, nausea, hematemesis, diarrhea	See above.
Allergic	*Mild:* Urticaria, bronchial wheezing, nasal congestion, mild edema. *Severe:* Dyspnea, circulatory collapse	*Mild:* Slow transfusion. Notify physician. Administer medications as ordered. *Severe:* Stop transfusion. Keep vein open with normal saline. Notify physician immediately. Monitor vital signs. Administer medications, oxygen as ordered.
Hypervolemia	Cough, dyspnea, hemoptysis, edema, distended peripheral veins, bounding, full pulse	Slow transfusion. Notify physician. Monitor vital signs. Administer medications as ordered.

PROCEDURE 40–4

STARTING, MAINTAINING, AND TERMINATING A BLOOD TRANSFUSION

☑ Equipment

Unit of whole blood

Blood administration set, either a straight line or a Y-set (the Y-set is preferred)

Venipuncture set containing a #18 needle or catheter (if one is not already in place) or, if blood is to be administered quickly, a #15 needle or a larger catheter (e.g., #14)

Container of 250 ml of normal saline solution

IV pole

Alcohol swabs

Tape

⬗ Gloves to protect the nurse from contamination by the client's blood

---

of the four blood types. Table 40–13 summarizes compatibility among blood groups.

Febrile reactions (bacterial reactions) are rare. They occur as a result of contaminated blood or sensitivity to the donor's white blood cells. *Allergic reactions* are relatively common and are thought to be due to allergenic substances or antibodies in the donor's plasma. *Hypervolemic reactions* are rare and tend to occur when a transfusion has been administered too quickly or when too much blood has been given.

Blood Administration   Blood is usually provided in plastic bags by the blood bank. One unit of whole blood is 500 ml of blood in a container. No more than one blood component or unit is obtained for the client at a time.

There are two types of blood administration sets: the straight line and the Y-set. The Y-set is preferred because the vein can be kept open with saline if any adverse effects arise from the transfusion. See Figure 40–23. In many instances, however, the tubing must also be changed. The infusion tubing has a filter inside the drip chamber. The tubing clamp should be just under the drip chamber. A Y-set can also be used when a saline solution is needed to run with the blood (e.g., when giving packed cells) or to flush the line before the blood enters the tubing (e.g., when running an intravenous infusion that is not saline). Some agencies recommend that saline be run through the tubing before and after a blood transfusion. Saline is used because it simulates plasma isotonicity.

Blood transfusions are administered through a #18 needle or catheter. When blood is to be administered quickly, a #15 needle or a larger catheter, e.g., #14, is often used. Large-gauge needles prevent damage to red blood cells (RBCs).

To start, maintain, and terminate a blood transfusion, see Procedure 40–4.

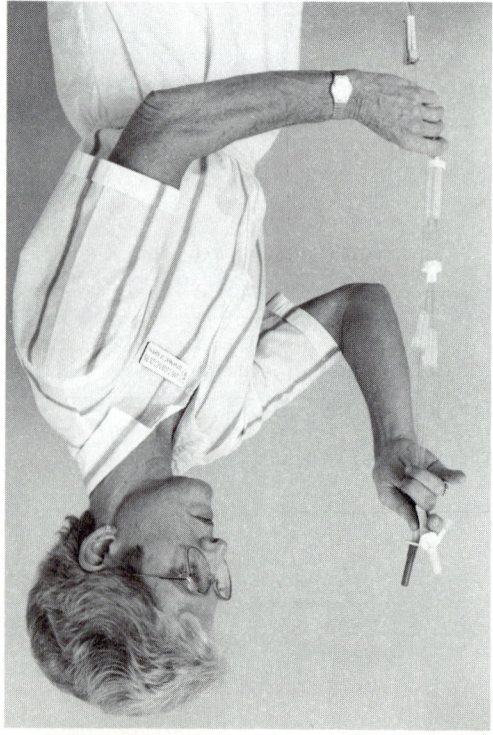

Figure 40–23   A Y-set for blood administration.

result from such contact. It is essential, therefore, to match the donor's blood type to the recipient's. Otherwise, the agglutinins present in the recipient's plasma will agglutinate the red cells donated. Because type O blood has neither A nor B agglutinogens, it can be donated to recipients with any of the four types of blood; a person with this type is called a **universal donor.** A person with type AB blood, because it has neither anti-A nor anti-B agglutinins in plasma, is referred to as a **universal recipient,** able to receive any

Intervention

1. **Obtain client consent and baseline data before the transfusion.**

- Obtain signed consent form if required.
- Assess vital signs for baseline data.
- Determine any known allergies or previous adverse reactions to blood.
- Note specific signs related to the client's pathology and reason for transfusion. For example, for an anemic client, note the hemoglobin level.

2. **Prepare the client.**

- Explain the procedure and its purpose to the client. Instruct the client to report promptly any sudden chills, nausea, itching, rash, dyspnea, or other unusual symptoms.
- If the client has an intravenous solution infusing, check whether the needle and solution are appropriate to administer blood. The needle should be #18 gauge or larger, and the solution must be saline. If the infusing solution is not compatible, remove it and dispose of it according to agency policy. Dextrose, which causes lysis of RBCs, Ringer's solution, medications and other additives, and hyperalimentation solutions are incompatible.
- If the client does not have an intravenous solution infusing, check agency policies. In some agencies an infusion must be infusing before the blood is obtained from the blood bank. In this case, you will need to perform a venipuncture on a suitable vein (see Procedure 40–2) and start an IV infusion of normal saline.

3. **Obtain the correct blood component for the client.**

- Check the physician's order with the requisition.
- Check the requisition form and the blood bag label with a laboratory technician or according to agency policy. Specifically check the client's name, identification number, blood type (A, B, AB, or O) and Rh group, the blood donor number, and the expiration date of the blood.
- With another nurse (the agency may require an RN), compare the laboratory blood type record with
  a. The client's name and identification number. Ask the client to state the full name as a double check.
  b. The number on the blood bag label.
  c. The ABO group and Rh type on the blood bag label.
- Sign the appropriate form with the other nurse according to agency policy.
- Make sure that the blood is left at room temperature for no more than 30 minutes before starting the transfusion. *RBCs deteriorate and lose their effectiveness after 2 hours at room temperature.* Agencies may designate different times at which the blood must be returned to the blood bank if it has not been started. *As blood components warm, the risk of bacterial growth also increases.*

4. **Verify the client's identity.**

- Ask the client's full name.
- Check the client's arm band. Do not administer blood to a client without an arm band.

5. **Set up the infusion equipment.**

- Ensure that the blood filter inside the drip chamber is suitable for whole blood or the blood components to be transfused. Blood filters have a surface area large enough to allow the blood components through easily but are designed also to trap clots.
- Close all the clamps on the Y-set: the main flow rate clamp and both Y-line clamps.
- Spike a container of 0.9% saline solution with the Y-set spike containing the vented tubing.
- Insert the remaining Y-set spike into the blood bag.
- Hang the saline solution and blood with the Y-set attached on an IV pole about 1 m (36 in) above the planned venipuncture site.

6. **Prime the tubing with saline solution.**

- Open the clamp on the normal saline tubing, and squeeze the drip chamber until it is one-third full.
- Remove the IV tubing needle adapter cover, open the main flow rate clamp, and prime the tubing. Close both clamps, and replace the needle adapter cover.

7. **Perform venipuncture if required.**

- See Procedure 40–2.

8. **Establish the saline infusion.**

- Connect the primed tubing to the IV needle.
- Tape the tubing to the IV needle securely.
- Open the saline solution clamp and the main roller clamp.
- Close the saline solution clamp and the main flow clamp.

9. **Establish the blood transfusion.**

- Invert the blood bag gently several times to mix the cells with the plasma. *Rough handling can damage the cells.*
- Expose the port on the blood bag by pulling back the tabs. See Figure 40–24.

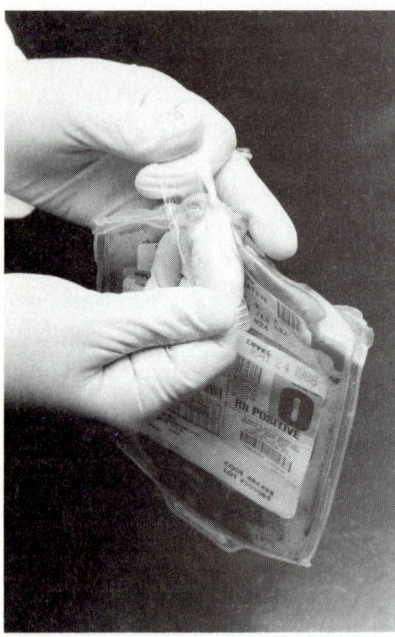

Figure 40–24 Exposing the port on the blood bag by pulling back the tabs.

- Open the blood line clamp.
- Squeeze the blood drip chamber until the filter is completely immersed in blood.
- Open the main flow rate clamp and regulate the blood's flow rate.

10. Observe the client closely for the first 5 to 10 minutes.

- Run the blood for the first 15 minutes at 20 drops per minute.
- Note adverse reactions such as chilling, nausea, vomiting, skin rash, or tachycardia. *The earlier a transfusion reaction occurs, the more severe it tends to be. Identifying such reactions promptly helps to minimize the consequences.*

- Remind the client to call you immediately if any unusual symptoms are felt during the transfusion.
- If any of these reactions occur, see Table 40–14, earlier in this chapter, for appropriate nursing action.

11. Document relevant data.

- Record starting the blood, including vital signs, type of blood, blood unit number, sequence number (e.g., #1 of three ordered units), site of the venipuncture, size of the needle, and drip rate.

12. Monitor the client.

- Fifteen minutes after initiating the transfusion, check the client's vital signs. If there are no signs of a reaction, establish the required flow rate. Most adults can tolerate receiving one unit of blood in 1½ to 2 hours.
- Assess the client every 30 minutes or more often, depending on the health status, including vital signs.

13. Terminate the transfusion.

- Don gloves.
- If no infusion is to follow, clamp the blood tubing and remove the needle.
- If the primary IV is to be continued, flush the line with saline solution, attach the primary IV container, and adjust the drip to the desired rate. *Often a normal saline or other solution is kept running in case of a delayed reaction to the blood.*

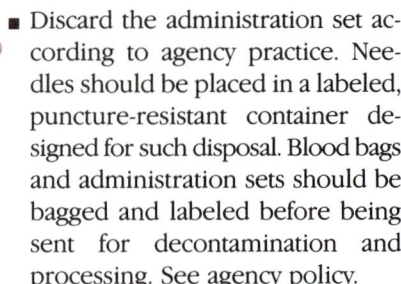

- Discard the administration set according to agency practice. Needles should be placed in a labeled, puncture-resistant container designed for such disposal. Blood bags and administration sets should be bagged and labeled before being sent for decontamination and processing. See agency policy.
- Remove gloves.
- Again monitor vital signs.

14. Follow agency protocol for appropriate disposition of the blood bag.

- On the requisition attached to the blood unit, fill in the time the transfusion was completed and the amount transfused.
- Attach one copy of the requisition to the client's record and another to the empty blood bag.
- Return the blood bag and requisition to the blood bank.

15. Document relevant data.

- Record completion of the transfusion, the amount of blood absorbed, the blood unit number, and the vital signs. If the primary intravenous infusion was continued, record connecting it.

Sample Recording

Date 12/12/91	Time: 1100

1 unit whole blood administered. No adverse reactions. BP stable at 120/70, TPR 37, 88, 14. 500 ml saline started at 10 gtt/min. ——————— Selina L. Ward, SN

Total Parenteral Nutrition

Total parenteral nutrition (TPN), also referred to as **intravenous hyperalimentation (IVH),** is the parenteral administration of solutions of dextrose, water, fat, proteins, electrolytes, vitamins, and trace elements; it is the provision of all needed calories. Because TPN solutions are *hypertonic* (highly concentrated in comparison to the solute concentration of blood), they are injected only into high-flow central veins, where they are diluted by the client's blood.

TPN is a means of achieving an anabolic state in clients who are unable to maintain a normal nitrogen balance. Such clients may include those with severe malnutrition, severe burns, bowel disease disorders (e.g., ulcerative colitis or enteric fistula), acute renal failure, hepatic failure, metastatic cancer, or major surgeries where nothing may be taken by mouth for more than 5 days.

 Infection control is of utmost importance during TPN therapy. The nurse must always observe surgical aseptic technique when changing solutions, tubing, dressings, and filters.

TPN solutions are a mixture of 10% to 50% dextrose in water, amino acids, and special additives such as vitamins (e.g., B complex, C, D, K), minerals (e.g., potassium, sodium, chloride, calcium, phosphate, magnesium), and trace elements (e.g., cobalt, zinc, manganese). Additives are adapted to each client's nutritional needs. Fat emulsions may be given to provide essential fatty acids to correct and/or prevent essential fatty acid deficiency or to supplement the calories for clients who, for example, have high calorie needs or cannot tolerate glucose as the only calorie source.

Because TPN solutions are high in glucose, infusions are started gradually to prevent hyperglycemia. The client needs to adapt to TPN therapy by increasing insulin output from the pancreas. For example, an adult client may be given 1 liter (40 ml/hr) of TPN solution the first day, if the infusion is tolerated; the amount may be increased to 2 liters (80 ml/hr) for 24 to 48 hours, and then to 3 liters (120 ml/hr) within 3 to 5 days. When TPN therapy is to be discontinued, the TPN infusion rates are decreased slowly to prevent hyper-insulinemia and hypoglycemia. Weaning a client from TPN may take up to 48 hours but can occur in 6 hours as long as the client receives adequate carbohydrates either orally or intravenously.

EVALUATING

To evaluate whether client goals have been achieved, the nurse collects data pertaining to the established outcome criteria at specified intervals. Evaluation activities may include the following:

- Measuring fluid intake and output
- Measuring vital signs
- Measuring body weight
- Assessing skin turgor, intactness, and appearance
- Obtaining current values of laboratory tests
- Measuring urine specific gravity and pH
- Observing the client for specific signs of fluid excess (edema, dyspnea) or fluid deficit (dry mucous membrane, concentrated urine)
- Asking the client about reasons for fluid/electrolyte therapy or about purposes and side-effects of medications

Examples of evaluative statements indicating goal achievement are "The client's fluid intake and output have been balanced for three days (specify range)," "The client has lost 2.6 kg in 2 days," and "The client's serum sodium is 142 mEq/ml."

ASSESSMENT DATA

Nursing Assessment

Mrs. Joan O'Brien is a 46-year-old waitress who underwent a cholecystectomy yesterday for treatment of acute cholecystitis/cholelithiasis. She has had an intolerance of fatty foods and indigestion for several months. For 2 days prior to surgery, she had experienced acute pain and tenderness in the upper right abdomen and severe nausea and vomiting. In addition, she has been anorexic for several days. Mrs. O'Brien returned from surgery with a nasogastric tube connected to low intermittent suction and a T-tube to gravity drainage. She is NPO and is receiving intravenous infusions at an 8-hour rate. Her skin and mucous membranes are dry. Her subcostal abdominal incision is painful, and as a result she is taking shallow, rapid respirations with splinting.

Physical Examination

Height: 160 cm (5'3")
Weight: 66.2 kg (146 lb)
Temperature: 38.1 C (100.6 F)
Pulse rate: 96 BPM
Respirations: 28 per minute
Blood pressure: 110/70 mm Hg
Skin turgor poor
Skin dry and mucous membranes dry and sticky
Dark amber urine

Diagnostic Data

Chest x-ray film: Negative
Serum sodium: 155 mEq/liter
Serum osmolarity: 298 mOsm/kg
Serum potassium: 3.2 mEq/liter
Serum bicarbonate: 33 mEq/liter
Plasma pH 7.48

CARE PLAN

Nursing Diagnosis	Client Goals and Outcome Criteria	Nursing Interventions and Rationales	Evaluation
Fluid volume deficit related to nausea, vomiting, nasogastric suctioning resulting in decreased skin turgor, dry skin and mucous membranes, decreased urinary output, increased serum sodium.	Client Goal: Normal hydration and electrolyte status. Outcome Criteria: Fluid and electrolyte balance will be evidenced by day 3. Skin and mucous membranes will be moist by day 2. Urinary output will be approximately 2000 ml per day.	Maintain accurate I & O. *Rationale:* Provides data about fluid balance. Assess client for dry skin, dry mucous membranes, and poor skin turgor. *Rationale:* Denotes dehydration. Irrigate nasogastric tube with normal saline. *Rationale:* Keeps tube patent and decreases chance of further electrolyte imbalance. Administer fluids and electrolytes intravenously as ordered. *Rationale:* Replaces fluids and electrolytes and maintains hydration and nutrition. Assess wound and T-tube drainage. *Rationale:* Excessive drainage may increase fluid imbalance and need for increase in fluid replacement.	On day 3, client's skin and mucous membranes are moist. Her nasogastric tube has been removed, and she is taking sips of water and ice chips. Her 24-hr IV intake has been 2000 ml, and her urinary output has been 1500 ml. Her lab values are Potassium: 3.8 mEq/liter Sodium: 137 mEq/liter Serum osmolarity: 287 mOsm/kg

Ineffective breathing pattern due to subcostal abdominal incision resulting in shallow respiration, ineffective coughing, splinted/guarded respirations.	Client Goal: Maintain effective breathing pattern and have no respiratory complications. Outcome Criteria: Coughs and deep breathes q1 hr within first 48 hrs. Absence of adventitious breath sounds by day 2. Splints abdomen when coughing or deep breathing by day 2.	Assess for shallow breathing and adventitious breath sounds. *Rationale:* Ineffective breathing may result in atelectasis or pneumonia. Encourage coughing, turning, and deep breathing q1–2 hrs. *Rationale:* Assists in mobilizing secretions and decreasing development of atelectasis and other complications. Instruct client to splint incision while coughing and deep breathing. *Rationale:* Splinting incision provides support and decreases pain. Assist client with use of incentive spirometer. *Rationale:* Use of incentive spirometer will improve the volume of inspiration.	On day 2, client splints her abdominal incision while coughing and deep breathing a minimum of every 2 hrs. Her breath sounds are clear; no adventitious breath sound are noted.

CHAPTER HIGHLIGHTS

▶ A balance of both fluids and electrolytes in the body is necessary for health and life.

▶ The body fluid is divided into two major reservoirs: the intracellular fluid (ICF) inside the cells and extracellular fluid (ECF) outside the cells.

▶ Extracellular fluid is subdivided into two compartments: intravascular (plasma) and interstitial. It constitutes about one-fourth to one-third of total body fluid.

▶ ECF is in constant motion throughout the body. It is the transport system that carries nutrients to and waste products from the cells.

▶ Secretions and excretions, also part of the body's total fluid volume, are part of the ECF.

▶ The percentage of total body fluids varies according to the individual's age, body fat, and sex. The younger the person, the higher the proportion of water in the body. The less body fat present, the greater the proportion of body fluid. Postadolescent females have a smaller percentage of fluid in relation to total body weight than do men.

▶ There are two types of body electrolytes (ions): positively charged ions (cations) and negatively charged ions (anions).

▶ The principal ions of ECF are sodium and chloride; the principal ions of ICF are potassium and phosphate.

▶ Fluids and electrolytes move among the body compartments by diffusion, osmosis, and active transport.

▶ The major fluid pressures exerted as part of the movement of fluid and electrolytes from one compartment to another are oncotic pressure and hydrostatic pressure.

▶ The three sources of body fluid are fluids taken orally, food ingested, and the oxidation of food. Fluid intake is regulated by the thirst mechanism.

▶ Fluid output occurs chiefly through excretion of urine, although body fluid is also lost through sweat, feces, and insensible vapor loss.

▶ In healthy adults, measurable fluid intake and output should balance (about 1500 ml per day). The output of urine normally approximates the oral intake of fluids. Water from food and oxidation is balanced by fluid loss through the skin, respiratory process, and feces.

▶ Fluid and electrolyte imbalances include
  a. Fluid volume deficit (FVD), also referred to as hypovolemia, dehydration, and extracellular fluid deficit. In a strict sense, dehydration is a water deficit only.
  b. Fluid volume excess (FVE), also referred to as hypervolemia, edema, overhydration, and extracellular fluid excess. Overhydration is a water excess only.

▶ The most common electrolyte imbalances are deficits or excesses in sodium, potassium, and calcium.

▶

CHAPTER HIGHLIGHTS *(continued)*

▸ Fluid and electrolyte imbalance is most accurately determined through laboratory examination of blood plasma.

▸ The acid-base balance (pH range) of body fluids is maintained within a precise range of 7.35 to 7.45. This pH is controlled by buffer systems in all body fluids (bicarbonate, phosphate, and protein) and by respiratory and kidney regulating systems.

▸ Acid-base imbalance occurs when the body fluids are higher or lower than the normal pH range. Imbalances may result in respiratory or metabolic disturbances; either can result in acidosis or alkalosis.

▸ Assessment relative to fluid, electrolyte, and acid-base balance includes (a) a nursing history; (b) measurement of body weight, vital signs, and fluid intake and output; (c) physical examination of the skin, oral cavity, eyes, jugular vein, veins of the hand, and the neurologic system; and (d) various diagnostic studies of blood and urine.

▸ A nursing history includes data about the client's fluid and food intake; fluid output; signs of fluid, electrolyte, and acid-base imbalances; and medications, therapies, or disease processes that may disrupt these balances.

▸ NANDA approved nursing diagnoses that relate specifically to fluid and electrolyte imbalances include **Fluid volume deficit, Potential fluid volume deficit,** and **Fluid volume excess.** Other diagnoses that may be relevant are **Altered oral mucous membrane, Impaired skin integrity, Altered cardiac output: decreased,** and **Altered tissue perfusion.**

▸ In many instances, fluids and electrolytes can be provided orally to clients who are experiencing or at risk of developing fluid deficits. The nurse needs to establish with the client a 24-hour plan for ingesting the necessary fluids and to respect the client's fluid preferences.

▸ For clients with fluid retention, fluids may need to be restricted; a schedule and short-term goals that make the fluid restriction more tolerable need to be developed.

▸ For clients experiencing excessive fluid losses, the administration of fluids and electrolytes intravenously is necessary. Meticulous aseptic technique is required when caring for clients with intravenous infusions.

▸ Preventing complications such as infiltration, phlebitis, hypervolemia (circulatory overload), and infection are an important aspect of intravenous therapy.

▸ The administration of blood transfusions involves accurately matching and identifying the blood for the individual, correctly identifying the recipient, and monitoring the client throughout the procedure for transfusion reactions.

▸ The hypertonic solutions used in total parenteral nutrition are infused in a central vein and are given to achieve a positive nitrogen balance and weight gain.

READINGS AND REFERENCES

SUGGESTED READINGS

Feldstein, A. January 1986. Detect phlebitis and infiltration before they harm your patient. *Nursing 86* 16:44–47.
  More than 70% of hospitalized clients receive IV therapy. Preventing phlebitis and infiltration necessitates selecting the right cannula and right vein. Feldstein explains these two problems, indicates the clinical signs, and explains what nurses should do in the event they identify any of the clinical signs.

Heitkemper, M. M., and Bond, E. January/February 1988. Fluid and electrolytes: Assessment and interventions. *Journal of Enterostomal Therapy* 15:18–23.
  The authors review normal fluid and electrolyte distribution in the body and discuss osmolality in reference to body water balance. A table lists the clinical findings and selected nursing management of water deficit and excess and saline deficit and excess. Heitkemper and Bond also describe fluid and electrolyte imbalances commonly seen in clinical settings.

McAdams, R. C., and McClure, K. December 1986. Hypovolemia: When to suspect it. *RN* 49:34–37; Hypovolemia: How to stop it. *RN* 49:38–42.
  The authors describe the therapy of a 71-year-old hypovolemic client and review the assessments and the problem of circulatory overload. They discuss colloid and crystalloid solutions and the hydrostatic and osmotic pressures concerned with body fluid movement. The authors also explain the nursing actions required to treat hypovolemia.

Mathewson, M. February 1989. Intravenous therapy. *Critical Care Nurse* 9:21–23, 26–28, 30–36.
  Mathewson discusses the clinical indications for IV therapy and describes isotonic, hypotonic, and hypertonic solutions, electrolyte imbalances, and fluid volume imbalances. Assessment, nursing diagnoses, planning, intervention, and evaluation for clients undergoing IV therapy conclude the article.

Young, M. E., and Flynn, K. T. August 1988. Third-spacing: When the body conceals fluid loss. *RN* 51:46–48. The authors explain third-spacing and the normal dynamics of fluid filtration and reabsorption. Two phases in surgical clients are described: (1) 24 to 48 hours postoperatively, when tissue injury permits fluid and proteins to leave the capillaries; and (2) 48 to 72 hours postoperatively, when reabsorption begins. The authors discuss assessment of a client during both phases and monitoring for fluid overload.

RELATED RESEARCH

DeMonaco, H. J.; Cronin, C. M.; Dempsey, M. J.; and Tulley, S. November/December 1986. Comparison of phlebitis rates with Buretrol and Harvard Mini-infuser for administration of I.V. piggyback medications. *Journal of the National Intravenous Therapy Association* 9:475–77.

Drew, D., and Schumann, D. November/December 1986. Homogeneity of potassium chloride in small volume intravenous containers. *Nursing Research* 35:325–29.

Josephson, A.; Gombert, M. E.; Sierra, M. F.; Karanfil, L. V.; and Tansino, G. F. September 1985. The relationship between intravenous fluid contamination and the frequency of tubing replacement. *Infection Control* 6:367–70.

Snydman, D. R.; Donnelly-Reidy, M.; Perry, L. K.; and Martin, W. J. March 1987. Intravenous tubing containing burettes can be safely changed at 72-hour intervals. *Infection Control* 8:113–16.

SELECTED REFERENCES

Boykoff, S. L; Boxwell, A. O.; and Boxwell, J. J. February 1988. Six ways to clear air from an IV line. *Nursing 88:* 46–48.

Bryan, C. S. June 1987. "CDC says . . .": The case of IV tubing replacement. *Infection Control* 8:255–56.

Byrne, C. J.; Saxton, D. F.; Pelikan, P. K.; and Nugent, P. M. 1986. *Laboratory tests: Implications for nursing care.* 2d ed. Menlo Park, Calif.: Addison-Wesley Publishing Co.

Carpenito, L. J. 1989. *Nursing diagnosis: Application to clinical practice.* 3d ed. Philadelphia: J. B. Lippincott Co.

Centers for Disease Control. 1982. Guidelines for prevention of intravascular infections. *Infection Control* 3:61–72.

Chenevey, B. December 1987. Overview of fluids and electrolytes. *Nursing Clinics of North America* 22:749–59.

Committee on Transfusion Practice, American Association of Blood Banks. October 1986. The latest protocols for blood transfusions. *Nursing 86* 16:34–41.

Crow, S. March/April 1987. Infection risks in IV therapy *Journal of the National Intravenous Therapy Association* 10:101–5.

Frawley, L. W. December 1985. Cost-effective application of the Centers for Disease Control guideline for prevention of intravascular infections. *American Journal of Infection Control* 13:275–77.

Gaspar, P. M. July/August 1988. What determines how much patients drink? *Geriatric Nursing* 9:221–24.

Goodinson, S. M. February 1990. The risks of I.V. therapy. *Professional Nurse* 5:235–36.

Guyton, A. C. 1986. *Textbook of medical physiology.* 7th ed. Philadelphia: W. B. Saunders Co.

Heitkemper, M. M., and Bond, E. January/February 1988. Fluid and electrolytes: Assessment and interventions. *Journal of Enterostomal Therapy* 15:18–23.

Holder, C., Alexander, J. February 1990. A new and improved guide to I.V. therapy . . . protocols for intravenous therapy. *American Journal of Nursing* 90:43–47.

Horne, M. M., and Swearingen, P. L., editors. 1989. *Pocket guide to fluids and electrolytes.* St. Louis: C. V. Mosby Co.

Janusek, L. W. July 1990. Metabolic acidosis: Pathophysiology, signs and symptoms. *Nursing 90* 20:52–53.

Josephson, A.; Gombert, M. E.; Sierra, M. F.; Karanfil, L. V.; and Tansino, G. F. September 1985. The relationship between intravenous fluid contamination and the frequency of tubing replacement. *Infection Control* 6:367–70.

Kim, M. J.; McFarland, G. K.; and McLane, A. M. 1989. *Pocket guide to nursing diagnoses.* 3d ed. St. Louis: C. V. Mosby Co.

Knox, L. S. January/February 1987. Implantable venous access devices. *Critical Care Nursing* 7:70–73.

Lancaster, L. E. December 1987. Renal and endocrine regulation of water and electrolyte balance. *Nursing Clinics of North America* 22:761–72.

Larkin, M. May/June 1987. Home I.V. therapy. *Journal of the National Intravenous Therapy Association* 10:171.

LaRocca, J. C., and Otto, S. E. 1989. *Pocket guide to intravenous therapy.* St. Louis: C. V. Mosby Co.

Lenox, A. C. March 1990. I.V. Therapy: Reducing the risk of infection. *Nursing 90* 20:60–61.

Lonsway, R. A. March/April 1987. Research, standards, and infection control: The impact of I.V. nursing. *Journal of the National Intravenous Therapy Association* 10:106–9.

McAdams, R. C., and McLure, K. December 1986a. Hypovolemia: How to stop it. *RN* 49:38–42.

———. December 1986b. Hypovolemia: When to suspect it. *RN* 49:34–37.

Mathewson, M. February 1989. Intravenous therapy. *Critical Care Nurse* 9:21–23, 26–28, 30–36.

Metheny, N. M. June 1990. Why worry about I.V. fluids? *American Journal of Nursing* 90:50–57.

Metheny, N. M., and Snively, W. D. 1983. *Nurses' handbook of fluid balance.* 4th ed. Philadelphia: J. B. Lippincott Co.

Millan, D. A. March 1988. Managing complications of IV therapy. *Nursing 88* 18:34–43.

NANDA approved nursing diagnostic categories for clinical use and testing. Summer 1988. *Nursing Diagnosis Newsletter* 15:1–3.

Peck, N. May, June, and July. Perfecting your IV therapy techniques. (3 parts.) *Nursing 85* 15:38–43; 48–51; 32–35.

Poyss, A. S. December 1987. Assessment and nursing diagnosis in fluid and electrolyte disorders. *Nursing Clinics of North America* 22:773–83.

Snydman, D. R.; Donnelly-Reidy, M.; Perry, L. K.; and Martin, W. J. March 1987. Intravenous tubing containing burettes can be safely changed at 72-hour intervals. *Infection Control* 8:113–16.

Townend, M. January/March 1990. The importance of developing and using standards of practice for I.V. therapy. *CINA Journal* 6:4.

Weinstein, S. May 1987. Intravenous filters. *Infection Control* 8:113–116.

Winskunas, C.A. March/April 1990. A creative approach to comprehensive I.V. therapy documentation. *Journal of Intravenous Nursing* 13:115–118.

Wiseman, M. April 1985. Setting standards for home IV therapy. *American Journal of Nursing* 85:421–23.

Wittig, P., and Semmler-Bertanzi, D. J. July 1983. Pumps and controllers: A nurse's assessment guide. *American Journal of Nursing* 83:1022–25.

Young, M. E., and Flynn, K. T. August 1988. Third-spacing: When the body conceals fluid loss. *RN* 51:46–48.

CHAPTER

41

Oxygenation

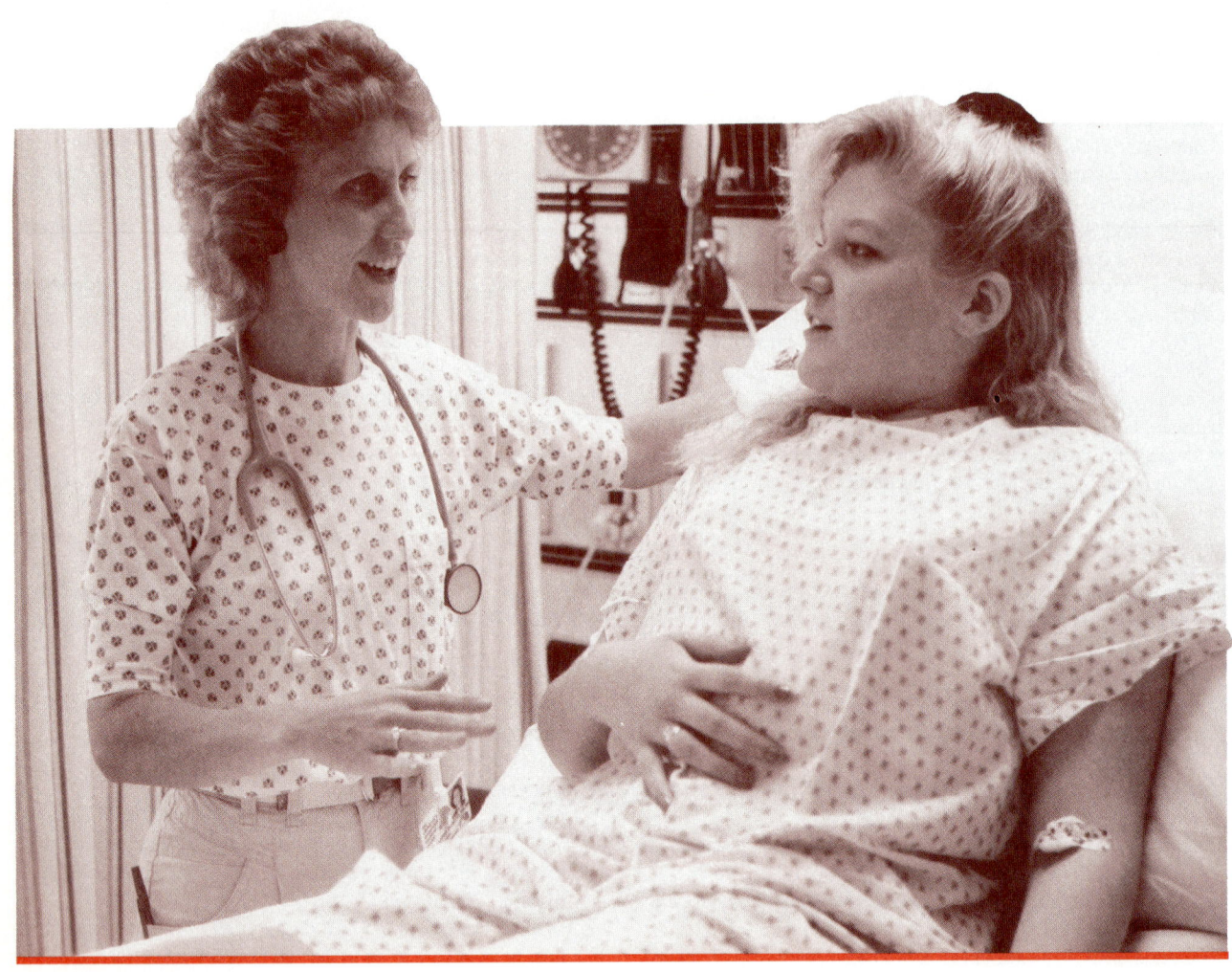

CONTENTS

CONTENTS (continued)

OBJECTIVES

▶ Explain the three phases of respiration.

▶ Describe the basic mechanics of breathing.

▶ Identify the requirements of adequate ventilation.

▶ Explain mechanisms regulating the respiratory process.

▶ Describe factors that influence the rate of diffusion of gases through the respiratory membrane.

▶ Explain how oxygen is transported to the tissues and how carbon dioxide is transported from the tissues.

▶ Identify factors influencing respiratory and circulatory function.

▶ Describe clinical signs of hypoxia.

▶ Describe common altered breathing patterns.

▶ List the signs of an obstructed airway.

▶ Identify common responses to alterations in respiratory and circulatory status.

▶ Describe positions that facilitate oxygenation.

▶ Explain the importance of hydration in promoting adequate oxygenation.

▶ Describe the use of selected inhalation therapy devices and practices.

▶ Explain oropharyngeal and nasopharyngeal suctioning.

▶ Describe various methods to administer oxygen.

▶ Compare administering oxygen therapy by nasal cannula and face mask.

▶ State outcome criteria for evaluating client responses to implemented measures to promote adequate oxygenation.

▶ Describe various types of chest drainage systems.

▶ Monitor clients with chest drainage effectively.

PHYSIOLOGY OF RESPIRATION

Respiration is the process of gaseous exchange between the individual and the environment. The process has three parts:

1. Pulmonary ventilation, or the inflow and outflow of air between the atmosphere and the alveoli of the lungs

2. Diffusion of gases (oxygen and carbon dioxide) between the alveoli and pulmonary capillaries

3. Transport of oxygen and carbon dioxide via the blood to and from the tissue cells

Pulmonary Ventilation

Ventilation of the lungs is accomplished through the act of breathing (inspiration and expiration). The degree of chest expansion during ventilation is minimal with normal breathing but can reach maximum capacities during strenuous activity. See Mechanics and Control of Breathing in Chapter 18, page 342.

Breathing during strenuous exercise or illness requires greater chest expansion and effort. The greater chest expansion of heavy breathing is accomplished by intercos-tal and other muscles that elevate or depress the rib cage. During inspiration, the rib cage is pulled upward by the action of the anterior neck muscles and contraction of the external intercostals. During expiration, the rib cage is pulled downward by the anterior abdominal muscles. Active use of these muscles and noticeable effort in breathing are seen in clients with obstructive respiratory disease.

Pulmonary Volumes   The volume to which the lungs expand during ventilation depends on whether breathing is normal and whether maximum inspiration and expiration occur. The normal volume of air inspired and expired is referred to as the **tidal volume.** See Figure 41–1. In young adults, the tidal volume is about 500 ml in males and 400 ml in females. Volumes may be smaller in small persons or greater in large or athletic persons. There are three other volumes: the **inspiratory reserve volume,** the **expiratory reserve volume,** and the **residual volume.** These three volumes added to the tidal volume yield the **total lung capacity,** which is the maximum volume to which the lungs can expand. See Table 41–1.

Pulmonary Capacities   Pulmonary volumes are often grouped in combinations of two or more. These com-

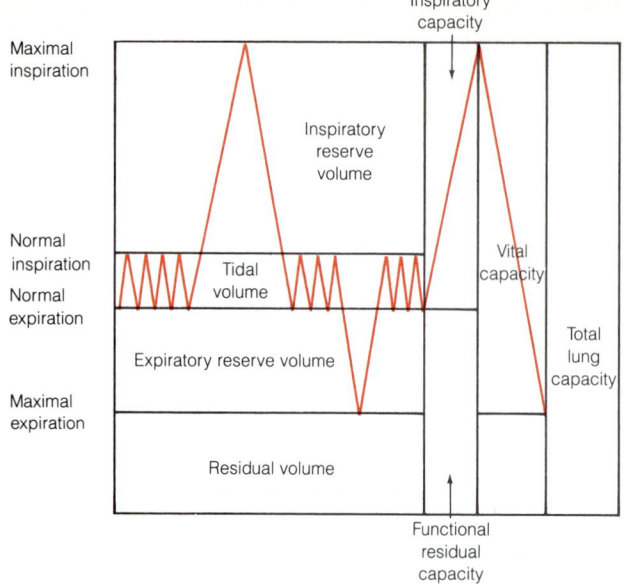

Figure 41–1   Pulmonary volumes and capacities.

bined volumes are referred to as the **pulmonary capacities** and include total lung capacity plus the **inspiratory capacity,** the **functional residual capacity,** and the **vital capacity.** See Table 41–1. The residual volume is normally about 20% of the total lung capacity.

Individual vital capacity varies with (a) anatomical build, (b) position, (c) strength of the respiratory muscles, (d) distensibility of the lungs and thorax, and (e) age. An adult's vital capacity is normally about 4500 to 5000 ml. A tall, thin person has a higher capacity than an obese person. Athletes may develop vital capacities up to 7000 ml. Standing increases vital capacity, whereas lying down reduces it. When a person is lying down, the abdominal organs tend to push against the diaphragm and the volume of pulmonary blood increases, both of which effects reduce pulmonary space and air. Weakness or paralysis of respiratory muscles, such as occurs in quadriplegics, can decrease the vital capacity to a point that is just adequate to sustain life (500 to 1000 ml). Diseases that impair lung distensibility, such as pulmonary edema and lung cancer, seriously reduce vital capacity.

Pulmonary Pressures   Breathing produces changes in **intrapulmonic pressure** (pressure within the lungs) and in **intrapleural pressure** (pressure outside or around the lungs). These pressure changes are related to the changes in the lung volumes in accordance with *Boyle's Law,* which states that the volume of a gas at constant temperature varies inversely with its pressure. On inspiration, the volume of the lungs increases, and thus the intrapulmonic pressure decreases. This decreased pressure allows atmospheric air to enter, since its pressure is greater. Conversely, on expiration the volume of the lungs decreases, and the intrapulmonic pressure increases. This allows the air to escape to

TABLE 41–1   *Summary of Respiratory Volumes and Capacities*

Measurement	Adult male Average Value*	Description
Respiratory Volumes		
Tidal volume (TV)	500 ml	Amount of air inhaled or exhaled with each breath under resting conditions
Inspiratory reserve volume (IRV)	3100 ml	Amount of air that can be forcefully inhaled after a normal tidal volume inhalation
Expiratory reserve volume (ERV)	1200 ml	Amount of air that can be forcefully exhaled after a normal tidal volume exhalation
Residual volume (RV)	1200 ml	Amount of air remaining in the lungs after a forced exhalation
Respiratory Capacities		
Total lung capacity (TLC)	6000 ml	Maximum amount of air contained in lungs after a maximum inspiratory effort: TLC = TV + IRV + ERV + RV
Vital capacity (VC)	4800 ml	Maximum amount of air that can be expired after a maximum inspiratory effort: VC = TV + IRV + ERV (should be 80% TLC)
Inspiratory capacity (IC)	3600 ml	Maximum amount of air that can be inspired after a normal expiration: IC = TV + IRV
Functional residual capacity (FRC)	2400 ml	Volume of air remaining in the lungs after a normal tidal volume expiration: FRC = ERV + RV

*Female values are 20% to 25% smaller.

Source: E. N. Marieb, *Human anatomy and physiology* (Redwood City, Calif.: Benjamin/Cummings, 1989), p. 727. Used with permission.

the atmosphere, where the pressure is lower than that in the lungs. At sea level, atmospheric pressure is about 760 mm Hg. Only very small pressure changes are required to move air in and out of the lungs. On inspiration, the intraalveolar pressure drops to less than 1 mm Hg below atmospheric pressure, whereas on expiration it rises to 1 mm Hg above atmospheric pressure. Although very little pressure is required to move air in and out of the lungs, pressures can increase substantially, as, for example, in certain lung diseases. In a healthy man, a maximum expiratory effort can raise the intraalveolar pressure to as high as 140 mm Hg; a maximum inspiratory effort can depress the intraalveolar pressure to as low as −100 mm Hg (Guyton 1986, p. 46).

Unless the chest cavity is damaged or opened, the intrapleural pressure is always negative. This negative pressure is essential because it creates the suction that holds the visceral pleura and the parietal pleura together as the chest cage expands and contracts. The recoil tendency of the lungs is a major factor responsible for this negative pressure. The fluid in the intrapleural space, however, provides even more negative pressure. Intrapleural fluid causes the pleura to adhere together, much as a film of water can cause two glass slides to adhere together.

Ventilation of the lungs depends on

1. adequate atmospheric oxygen
2. clear air passages
3. adequate pulmonary compliance and recoil
4. regulation of respiration

Regulation is discussed on page 1095.

The presence of atmospheric oxygen in adequate concentration is basic to adequate respirations. Concentrations of oxygen are lower at high altitudes than at sea level. In some instances people at very high altitudes need supplementary oxygen.

During inspiration, air passes through the nose, pharynx, larynx, trachea, bronchi, and bronchioles to the alveoli, and expiration reverses that course. The nose performs three important functions. It warms, moistens, and filters the air. Large particles in the air are filtered by the hairs at the entrance of the nares, and smaller particles are filtered by nasal turbulence. Each time air contacts the nasal turbinates or nasal septum it must change direction, and in the process small particles are trapped.

Air passages are cleared by the mucous membrane lining, which contains **cilia** (hairlike projections of the respiratory mucous membrane). Mucus entraps organisms or other small foreign material while the cilia move the trapped material. The cilia beat continually at a rate of 10 to 20 times per second, directed toward the pharynx. Thus the cilia in the lower respiratory passageways (e.g., the bronchi) beat upward, and the cilia in the nose beat downward. Material can be moved as much as 1 cm per minute along the trachea (Guyton 1986, p. 475).

The cough reflex and the sneeze reflex are also essential cleaning mechanisms. The *cough reflex* is triggered by irritants that send nerve impulses through the vagus nerve to the medulla. Any foreign matter in the larynx, trachea, or bronchi initiates the cough reflex. A particularly sensitive area is the **carina,** the ridge or junction where the main bronchi meet at the trachea. The cough reflex process is described in the accompanying box. The *sneeze reflex* is to the nasal passages as the cough is to lower respiratory passages. Sneezing is initiated when irritating impulses pass by way of the fifth cranial nerve to the medulla. Sneezing involves a series of reactions similar to the cough reflex; however, the uvula is depressed so that a large volume of air passes rapidly through the nose as well as the mouth, thus helping to clear the nasal passages (Guyton 1986, p. 475).

Lung compliance is lung expansibility or stretchability. It generally includes expansibility of both the lungs and the thorax but sometimes denotes compliance of the lungs alone. Compliance can be measured by noting the increase in lung volume produced by units of increased intraalveolar pressure.

Inadequate compliance can result from any condition that destroys lung tissue, such as edema or tumors, or any condition that inhibits thoracic expansion, such as paralysis or kyphosis.

In contrast to lung compliance is **lung recoil.** The lungs have a continual tendency to collapse away from the chest wall. Two factors are responsible for this recoil tendency: (a) elastic fibers present in lung tissue and (b) surface tension of the fluid lining the alveoli. The latter accounts for two-thirds of the recoil phenomenon. Counterbalancing this surface tension in the alveoli is a lipoprotein mixture called **surfactant.** When surfactant is absent, lung expansion is exceedingly difficult and the lungs collapse. Normally, the secretion of surfactant by the alveoli is stimulated several times each hour by yawning, sighing, or deep breaths. Surfactant stimulation is important for clients on automatic ventilation. The alveoli must be stretched several times every hour by a sigh mechanism on the respirator.

Diffusion of Gases

After the alveoli are ventilated, the second phase of the respiratory process—*the diffusion of oxygen from the alveoli and into the pulmonary blood vessels*—begins. **Diffusion** is the movement of gases or other particles from an area of greater pressure or concentration to an area of lower pressure or concentration. Because the alveolar walls are very thin and are surrounded by a closely intertwined network of blood capillaries, these membranes together are often referred to as the **respiratory membrane.**

Four factors influence the rate of diffusion of gases through the respiratory membrane (Guyton 1986, p. 488):

1. Thickness of the membrane
2. Surface area of the membrane
3. Diffusion coefficient of the gases
4. Pressure difference on each side of the membrane

The thickness of the respiratory membrane increases in clients with pulmonary edema or certain other pulmonary diseases. Any increase in the thickness of this membrane can seriously decrease gaseous diffusion. Similarly, any alteration of surface area of the membrane influences the rate of diffusion. Conditions such as **emphysema** (in which alveoli coalesce) or lobectomy (the surgical removal of a portion of the lung) impede gaseous exchange. In clients at rest, the loss of some surface area is not a serious deficit. However, a loss of more than 25% is serious. Also, when for some reason (e.g., exercise or certain diseases) there is increased pulmonary demand, a loss of less than 25% can be a serious deficit.

The diffusion coefficients of oxygen and carbon dioxide are also a significant factor. This **diffusion coefficient** depends on the molecular weight of the gas and its solubility in the membrane. Carbon dioxide diffuses about 20 times more rapidly than oxygen. Thus, in some situations an oxygen lack is seen without a carbon dioxide buildup.

Pressure differences in the gases on each side of the respiratory membrane obviously affect diffusion. When the pressure of oxygen is greater in the alveoli than in the blood,

oxygen diffuses into the blood. Normally the oxygen pressure gradient between the alveoli and the blood entering the pulmonary capillaries is about 40 mm Hg. The **partial pressure** (the pressure exerted by each individual gas in a mixture according to its concentration in the mixture) of oxygen (Po_2) in the alveoli is about 100 mm Hg, whereas the Po_2 in the entering venous blood of the pulmonary arteries is about 60 mm Hg. These pressures equalize very rapidly, however, so that the arterial pressure also reaches about 100 mm Hg. By contrast, carbon dioxide in the venous blood entering the pulmonary capillaries has a partial pressure of about 45 mm Hg, whereas that in the alveoli has a partial pressure of about 40 mm Hg. These partial pressures frequently are used diagnostically to assess deficiencies or excesses of oxygen and carbon dioxide in persons with pulmonary disease.

Transport of Oxygen and Carbon Dioxide

The third part of the respiratory process involves the transport of respiratory gases. Oxygen needs to be transported from the lungs to the tissues, and carbon dioxide must be transported from the tissues back to the lungs. Normally, most of the oxygen (97%) combines loosely with the **hemoglobin** (oxygen-carrying red pigment) in the red blood cells and is carried to the tissues as **oxyhemoglobin** (the compound of oxygen and hemoglobin). The remaining oxygen is dissolved and transported in the fluid of the plasma and cells.

The amount of oxygen that the blood will absorb before reaching saturation is about 20 ml per 100 ml of blood. This ratio is expressed as 20 vol%. After it has released oxygen to the tissues, hemoglobin is referred to as **reduced hemoglobin.** Normally, only about 25%—or 5 ml (¼ of 20 ml)—of oxygen per 100 ml of blood is diffused to the tissues (utilization coefficient). However, this rate of release can increase to 75% during periods of stress or increased exercise, since more oxygen is utilized by the cells. In situations of extreme oxygen lack in the tissues caused by a sluggish blood flow or a very high metabolic rate, the tissues can remove 100% of the oxygen from the blood (Guyton 1986, pp. 496–97). Several factors affect the rate of oxygen transport from the lungs to the tissues:

1. Cardiac output
2. Number of erythrocytes
3. Exercise
4. Blood hematocrit

Normal **cardiac output** (amount of blood pumped by the heart) is approximately 5 liters per minute. Any pathologic condition that decreases cardiac output (e.g., damage to the heart muscle, blood loss, or pooling of blood in the peripheral blood vessels) diminishes the amount of oxygen delivered to the tissues. Generally, the heart compensates for inadequate output by increasing its pumping rate. Normally, compensatory cardiac output can increase the oxygen transport fivefold; but when disease conditions exist, this is not possible.

The second factor influencing oxygen transport is the number of **erythrocytes** (red blood cells, or RBC). In men the number of circulating erythrocytes normally averages about 5 million per cubic milliliter of blood, and in women, about 4½ million per cubic milliliter. Reductions in these normal values can be brought about by anemia of any cause.

Exercise also has a direct influence on oxygen transport. In well-trained athletes, oxygen transport can be increased up to 20 times normal, due in part to an increased cardiac output and to increased utilization of oxygen by the cells (utilization coefficient).

The **hematocrit** is the percent of the blood that is erythrocytes. It is also referred to as the packed cell volume per 100 ml. Normally this ratio is about 40% to 54% in men and 37% to 47% in women. Excessive increases in the blood hematocrit increase the blood viscosity, reduce the cardiac output, and therefore reduce oxygen transport. Excessive reductions in the blood hematocrit, such as occur in anemia, also reduce oxygen transport. It is interesting to note that persons who develop elevated hematocrits when acclimatizing to high altitudes seldom have oxygen transport problems, probably because of an associated increase in the numbers and sizes of peripheral blood vessels.

A moderate amount of carbon dioxide (30%) is transported by reduced hemoglobin (which is able to combine with carbon dioxide to form **carbaminohemoglobin**). The largest amount (about 65%) is carried in the form of bicarbonate (HCO_3^-) inside the red blood cells. Smaller amounts (5%) are transported in solution in the plasma and as **carbonic acid** (the compound formed when CO_2 combines with water). In the normal resting person, about 4 ml of CO_2 in each 100 ml of blood is transported from the tissues to the lungs.

the distended lungs and chest. A second function of the dorsal group is the control of respiratory rhythm.

The *ventral respiratory group* is also located in the medulla. These neurons become active when there is a need for increased respiratory ventilation, stimulating increased respiratory inspiration and expiration. This group of neurons remains inactive during normal, quiet respiration. The *pneumotaxic center,* the third group, is located in the upper part of the pons. Impulses from this area function primarily to control the duration of inspiration. The main function of the pneumotaxic center is to limit inspiration.

A **chemosensitive** center in the medulla oblongata is highly responsive to increases in blood CO_2 or hydrogen ion concentration. By influencing other respiratory centers, this center can increase the activity of the inspiratory center, the rate of respirations, and the rate and depth of inspirations. In addition to direct chemical stimulation of the respiratory center in the brain, there are special receptors sensitive to decreases in O_2 concentration located outside the central nervous system, in the carotid bodies (just above the bifurcation or the common carotid arteries) and aortic bodies. Impulses from these **chemoreceptors** travel along Hering's nerves to the glossopharyngeal nerves and then to the dorsal respiratory area in the medulla. Decreases in arterial oxygen concentrations stimulate the chemoreceptors in the aortic and carotid bodies, and they, in turn, stimulate the respiratory center to increase ventilation. Of the three blood gases (hydrogen, oxygen, and carbon dioxide) that can trigger chemoreceptors, increased carbon dioxide concentration stimulates respiration most strongly.

In clients with certain lung ailments, such as emphysema, however, oxygen concentrations, *not carbon dioxide concentrations,* play a major role in regulating respiration. For such clients, decreased oxygen concentrations are the main stimuli for respiration. This is sometimes called the *hypoxic drive.* Increasing the concentration of oxygen depresses the respiratory rate. Thus, only low concentrations of supplemental oxygen are administered to these clients.

REGULATION OF RESPIRATION

Respiratory regulation of oxygen, carbon dioxide, and hydrogen ions in body fluids includes both neural and chemical controls. Respiratory control basically functions to maintain the correct concentrations. The nervous system of the body adjusts the rate of alveolar ventilations to meet the needs of the body so that Po_2 and Pco_2 remain relatively constant. The body's "respiratory center" is actually a number of groups of neurons located in the medulla oblongata and pons. There are three main groups: a dorsal respiratory group, a ventral respiratory group, and the pneumotaxic center. The *dorsal respiratory group* is located in the medulla. Stimulation of this group causes inspiration. Expiration, by contrast, is produced passively, by elastic recoil of

FACTORS AFFECTING OXYGENATION

Factors that influence oxygenation affect the cardiovascular system as well as the respiratory system. These factors include environment, exercise, emotions, life-style, health status, and narcotics.

Environment   Altitude, heat, cold, and air pollution affect oxygenation. The higher the *altitude,* the lower the partial pressure of the oxygen (Po_2) an individual breathes. As a result, the person at high altitudes has increased respiratory and cardiac rates and increased respiratory depth, which usually become most apparent when the individual exercises.

In response to *heat,* the peripheral blood vessels dilate; consequently, blood flows to the skin, increasing the amount of heat lost from the body surface. With vasodilation, the lumens of blood vessels enlarge, thus decreasing the resistance to the blood flow. In response, the heart increases output to maintain blood pressure. The increased cardiac output requires additional oxygen, which is acquired through increased rate and depth of breathing. In a *cold* environment, by contrast, the peripheral blood vessels constrict, raising the blood pressure, which decreases cardiac action, thereby reducing the need for oxygen.

Healthy people exposed to *air pollution,* e.g., smog, often experience stinging of the eyes, headache, dizziness, coughing, and choking. Persons who have a history or existing lung disease and altered respiratory function experience varying degrees of respiratory difficulty in a polluted environment. Some are unable to maintain self-care activities in such an environment.

Exercise   Physical exercise or activity increases the rate of respirations and the heart rate and hence the supply of oxygen in the body. The mechanism underlying this effect is not completely known; however, it is thought that a number of factors are involved, including chemical, neural, and temperature changes.

Emotions   An accelerated heart rate may also be a response to emotions such as fear, anxiety, and anger. It is thought that sympathetic nervous stimulation is responsible for this phenomenon.

Life-Style   The client's life-style is an important factor that may influence oxygenation status. Cigarette smoking and certain occupations predispose an individual to lung disease. For example, silicosis is seen more often in sandstone blasters and potters than in the rest of the population; asbestosis in asbestos workers; anthracosis in coal miners; and organic dust disease in farmers and agricultural employees who work with moldy hay. Activity patterns are also a factor. Sedentary persons lack the alveolar expansion and deep breathing patterns of persons who exercise on a routine basis and are therefore less able to respond effectively to respiratory stressors.

Health Status   In the healthy person, the cardiovascular and respiratory systems can provide sufficient oxygen to meet the body needs. However, diseases of the cardiovascular system often affect the delivery of oxygen to the cells of the body. In addition, diseases of the respiratory system can adversely affect the oxygenation of the blood. In both instances, **hypoxemia** (a condition characterized by low partial pressure of oxygen in arterial blood or a low saturation of oxyhemoglobin) can result.

One cardiovascular condition that affects oxygenation is **anemia.** There are many causes of anemia, including malnutrition, loss of blood, and the effect of chemicals. Because hemoglobin carries oxygen and carbon dioxide, as explained earlier, anemia can affect the delivery of these gases to and from the body cells.

Narcotics   Narcotics such as morphine and meperidine hydrochloride (Demerol) decrease the rate and depth of respirations by depressing the respiratory center in the medulla. When administering narcotic analgesics, the nurse must monitor respiratory rates and depths.

RESEARCH NOTE

What Are the Smoking Practices Among Nursing Students?

Studies of the smoking practices of nursing students are less prevalent than those of registered nurses. These authors compare and contrast the findings of two 1986 studies: one in Buffalo, New York by Haughey, Dittmar, O'Shea, and Brasure, and another in Portland, Maine by Casey. The mean age of the nurses studied was 24 years, although the ages ranged from 17 to 55 years. Both samples included only a few males (7%). Smoking rates were found to be similar to those of the female population in the U.S. and were not unlike the national estimates of 29% for registered nurses. In the Buffalo sample, 30% of the students were smokers compared to only 23% in the Portland sample. Both studies found that of the students who smoke, many (75% in Buffalo and 70% in Portland) began smoking while they were in nursing school. The reasons for beginning to smoke included the following: that it was "the thing to do," the pleasure it provided, peer pressure, the desire to be more relaxed in social situations, pressures at nursing school and at work, and the desire to lose weight. More than 90% of the students were aware of smoking's association with coronary artery disease, lung cancer, chronic bronchitis, oral cancer, pulmonary emphysema, laryngeal cancer, and low birth weight syndrome. Almost 30% of students in both samples, however, were unaware of the association with bladder cancer.

Implications: Because it is important for nurses to act as role models for clients and as positive influences on clients who smoke, the authors emphasize the challenging opportunity for nurse educators to study and implement strategies to prevent smoking initiation and encourage cessation among future nurses.

F. S. Casey, B. P. Haughey, S. S. Dittmar, R. M. O'Shea, and J. Brasure. Smoking practices among nursing students: A comparison of two studies. *Journal of Nursing Education,* November 1989. 28:397–401.

ALTERATIONS IN RESPIRATORY FUNCTION

Respiratory function can be altered by conditions that affect three areas of function:

1. The movement of air into or out of the lungs
2. The diffusion of oxygen and carbon dioxide between the alveoli and the pulmonary capillaries
3. The transport of oxygen and carbon dioxide via the blood to and from the tissue cells

Three major alterations in respiration are hypoxia, altered breathing pattern, and obstructed or partially obstructed airway.

Hypoxia

Hypoxia is a condition of insufficient oxygen anywhere in the body, from the inspired gas to the tissues. It can be related to any of the three parts of respiration: ventilation, diffusion of gases, or transport of gases by the blood, and can be caused by any condition that alters one or more parts of the process. At high altitudes the partial pressure of oxygen is low; therefore, the alveolar and the arterial oxygen partial pressures are low. This form of hypoxia is called *hypoxic hypoxia*.

Another cause of hypoxia is **hypoventilation,** i.e., inadequate alveolar ventilation due to decreased tidal volume. Whatever the reason for a decreased tidal volume (for example, diseases of the respiratory muscles, drugs, or anesthesia), carbon dioxide often also accumulates in the blood. This condition is called **hypercarbia (hypercapnia).** Additional terms relating to hypoxia are given in the accompanying box.

Hypoxia can also develop when the lungs' ability to diffuse oxygen into the arterial blood decreases, as with pulmonary edema, or can result from problems in the delivery of oxygen to the tissues (e.g., anemia, cardiac failure, and embolism). See Table 41–2 for the early and late clinical signs of hypoxia. **Cyanosis** (bluish discoloration of the skin, nail beds, and mucous membranes, due to reduced oxygen levels of hemoglobin) may be present; however, a client can be hypoxic without exhibiting cyanosis. Cyanosis of the skin and mucous membranes requires these two conditions: the blood must contain about 5 g or more of unoxygenated hemoglobin per 100 ml of blood, and the surface blood capillaries must be dilated. Any factors that interfere with either of these conditions (e.g., severe anemia or the administration of adrenaline) will eliminate cyanosis as a sign even if the client is experiencing hypoxia.

Other clinical signs of *acute* hypoxia are nausea, vomiting, oliguria, and possibly anuria. The client may also report headache, apathy, dizziness, irritability, and memory loss. Adequate oxygenation is essential for cerebral functioning. The cerebral cortex can tolerate hypoxia for only 3 to 5 minutes before permanent damage occurs. The face of the acutely hypoxic person usually appears anxious, tired, and drawn. The person usually assumes a sitting position, often leaning forward slightly to permit greater expansion of the thoracic cavity. The hypoxic client may or may not experience pain on breathing. Although lung tissue lacks pain receptors, pain can arise from the pleura, chest wall, or upper respiratory tract.

With *chronic* hypoxia, the client often appears fatigued and is lethargic. The body often adapts to the lack of oxygen in the following manner: (a) pulmonary ventilation increases, (b) the red blood cell count increases, and (c) the hemoglobin concentration increases. The client's fingers may be clubbed as a result of long-term lack of oxygen in the arterial blood supply to the fingers. With clubbing, the base of the nail becomes swollen and the ends of the fingers and toes increase in size. The angle between the nail and the base of the nail increases to more than 160°. See Figure 19–16, page 373.

Altered Breathing Patterns

Breathing patterns refer to the rate, volume, rhythm, and relative ease or effort of respiration. Normal respiration (**eupnea**) is quiet, rhythmic, and effortless. **Tachypnea**

TABLE 41–2 *Clinical Signs of Hypoxia*

Early Signs	Late Signs
Increased pulse rate	Decreased pulse rate
Increased rate and depth of respirations	Decreased systolic blood pressure
Slight increase in systolic blood pressure	Dyspnea
	Cough
	Hemoptysis

(rapid rate) is seen with fevers, metabolic acidosis, and pain and with hypercapnia (elevated blood CO_2) or anoxemia (decreased oxygen in the blood). Bradypnea is an abnormally slow respiratory rate, which may be seen in clients who have taken drugs such as morphine sulphate (a respiratory depressant), who have metabolic acidosis, or who have increased intracranial pressure (e.g., from brain injuries).

Hyperventilation is an excessive amount of air in the lungs. It is often called alveolar hyperventilation because the amount of air in the alveoli exceeds the body's metabolic requirements; that is, more CO_2 is eliminated than is produced. Hyperventilation usually results from an increase in the rate and depth of respirations. One particular type of hyperventilation that accompanies metabolic acidosis is Kussmaul breathing, by which the body attempts to compensate (give off excess body acids) by blowing off the carbon dioxide through deep and rapid breathing. Hyperventilation can also occur after the administration of amphetamines because of the increased metabolic rate such drugs induce.

Hypoventilation is inadequate alveolar ventilation, i.e., ventilation that does not meet the body's requirements. As a result, carbon dioxide is retained in the bloodstream. Hypoventilation can occur as a result of collapse of the alveoli, leaving too few functioning alveoli to meet the body's ventilation needs; or it may result from airway obstruction or the side effects of some drugs. Hypoventilation is indicated when the arterial P_{CO_2} is above 35 to 45 mm Hg. (Byrne et al. 1986, p. 285).

Abnormal respiratory *rhythms* create an irregular breathing pattern. Four abnormal respiratory rhythms are:

- **Cheyne-Stokes.** Marked rhythmic waxing and waning of respirations from very deep to very shallow breathing and temporary apnea (cessation of breathing); common causes include congestive heart failure, increased intracranial pressure, and drug overdose.
- **Kussmaul's** (or *hyperventilation*). Increased rate and depth, often exceeding 20 breaths per minute; seen in metabolic acidosis and renal failure.
- **Apneustic.** Prolonged gasping inspiration followed by a very short, usually inefficient, expiration; associated with central nervous system disorders.
- **Biot's.** Shallow breaths interrupted by apnea; may be seen in healthy people and in clients with central nervous system disorders.

Normal breathing is effortless, and respirations are evenly spaced and vary little in depth. Difficult or labored breathing is called dyspnea. The dyspneic person often appears anxious and may say, "I can't catch my breath." Often the nostrils are flared because of the increased effort of inspiration. The skin may appear dusky; heart rate is increased. Orthopnea is the inability to breathe except in an upright sitting or standing position.

Obstructed Airway

A complete or partially obstructed airway can occur anywhere along the upper or lower respiratory passageways. An upper airway obstruction—i.e., in the nose, pharynx, larynx, or trachea—can arise because of a foreign object, such as food; because the tongue falls back into the oropharynx when a person is unconscious; or when secretions collect in the passageways. In the latter instance, the respirations will sound gurgly or bubbly as the air attempts to pass through the secretions. Lower airway obstruction involves partial or complete occlusion of the passageways in the bronchi and lungs.

Maintaining an open (patent) airway is a frequent nursing intervention, one that often requires immediate action. Partial obstruction of the upper airway passages is indicated by a low-pitched snoring sound during inhalation. Complete obstruction is indicated by extreme inspiratory effort that produces no chest movement. Such a client, in an effort to obtain air, may also exhibit marked sternal and intercostal retractions. Lower airway obstruction is not always as easy to observe. The client may have altered arterial blood gas levels, restlessness, dyspnea, and **adventitious** (abnormal) **breath sounds.** See Table 19–15, page 403.

ASSESSING

Nursing assessment of oxygenation status includes a history, physical assessment, and review of relevant diagnostic data.

Nursing History

A comprehensive nursing history relevant to oxygenation status should include data about current and past respiratory and cardiovascular problems; life-style; presence of cough, sputum, pain, medications for heart, blood pressure, or breathing; and presence of risk factors for impaired oxygenation status. Examples of interview questions to elicit this information are shown in the accompanying box.

Physical Assessment

In assessing a client's oxygenation status the nurse uses all four physical assessment techniques: inspection, palpation, percussion, and auscultation. The nurse first observes the rate, depth, rhythm, and quality of respirations, noting the position the client assumes for breathing. Some clients with chronic respiratory problems prefer to bend forward at the waist to ease breathing or to sit leaning over a table because these positions permit greater lung expansion. Lying on the back or on either side restricts expansion of part of the thorax (the underlying portion). This relatively small increase in expansion may be important to a dyspneic client. Chapter 18 provides additional information on assessing respirations.

Current Respiratory Problems

- What recent changes have you experienced in your breathing pattern (e.g., shortness of breath, difficulty in breathing, need to be in upright position to breathe, or rapid and shallow breathing)? See below for cough, sputum, and pain.

- Which of your activities might cause the above symptom(s) to occur?

- Have you been exposed to any pollutants?

History of Respiratory Disease

- Have you had colds, allergies, croup, asthma, tuberculosis, bronchitis, pneumonia, or emphysema?

- How frequently have these occurred? How long did they last? And how were they treated?

Current or Past Cardiovascular Problems

- Do you have a history of cardiac or blood circulation problems (e.g. anemia, hypertension, heart disease)?

Life-Style

- Do you smoke? If so, how much?

- Does any member of your family smoke?

- Are there smokers or other pollutants (e.g., fumes, dust, coal, asbestos) in your workplace?

Presence of Cough

- How often and how much do you cough?

- Is it *productive,* i.e., accompanied by sputum, or *nonproductive,* i.e., dry?

- Does the cough occur during certain activity or at certain times of the day?

Description of Sputum

- When is the sputum produced?

- What is the amount, color, thickness, odor?

- Is it ever tinged with blood?

Presence of Chest Pain

- Do you experience any pain with breathing or activity?

- Where is the pain located?

- Describe the pain, i.e., how does it feel?

- Does it occur when you breathe in or out?

- How long does it last, and how does it affect your breathing?

- What activities precede your pain?

- What do you do to relieve the pain?

Presence of Risk Factors

- Do you have a family history of lung cancer, cardiovascular disease (including strokes), or tuberculosis?

- The nurse should also note the client's weight, activity pattern, and dietary assessment. In addition to smoking, risk factors include obesity, sedentary lifestyle, and diet high in saturated fats.

Medication History

- Have you taken or do you take any over-the-counter or prescription medications for heart, blood pressure, or breathing (e.g., bronchodilator, inhalant, narcotic)?

- Which ones? And what are the dosages, times taken, and results, including side-effects?

Variations in the shape of the thorax may indicate adaptation to chronic respiratory conditions. For example, clients with emphysema frequently develop a *barrel chest.* See Figure 19–59 on page 400 for an illustration of variations in the shape of the chest. The lungs and heart should be assessed very carefully. See Chapter 19. Terms commonly used in recording physical assessment findings related to respiratory function are shown in the boxes on the following pages.

Diagnostic Studies

The physician may order various diagnostic tests to assess respiratory status, function, and oxygenation. Included are sputum specimens, throat cultures, venous and arterial blood samples, visual inspection procedures, and thoracentesis.

Often it is the nurse who collects specimens to be sent to the laboratory for analysis.

Specimens Sputum is the mucous secretion from the lungs, bronchi, and trachea. It is important to differentiate it from *saliva,* the clear liquid secreted by the salivary glands in the mouth, sometimes referred to as "spit." Healthy individuals do not produce sputum. Clients need to cough to bring sputum up from the lungs, bronchi, and trachea into the mouth in order to expectorate it into a collecting container. Sputum specimens are usually collected for one or more of the following reasons:

- For *culture and sensitivity* to identify a specific microorganism and its drug sensitivities.

Breathing Patterns and Sounds

Breathing Patterns

Rate

- *Eupnea*—normal respiration that is quiet, rhythmic, and effortless

- *Tachypnea*—rapid respiration marked by quick, shallow breaths

- *Bradypnea*—abnormally slow breathing

- *Apnea*—cessation of breathing

Volume

- *Hyperventilation*—an increase in the amount of air in the lungs characterized by prolonged and deep breaths; may be associated with anxiety

- *Hypoventilation*—a reduction in the amount of air in the lungs; characterized by shallow respirations

Rhythm

- *Cheyne-Stokes breathing*—rhythmic waxing and waning of respirations, from very deep to very shallow breathing and temporary apnea; often associated with cardiac failure, increased intracranial pressure, or brain damage

Ease or effort

- *Dyspnea*—difficult and labored breathing during which the individual has a persistent, unsatisfied need for air and feels distressed

- *Orthopnea*—ability to breathe only in upright sitting or standing positions

Breath Sounds

Audible without amplification

- *Stridor*—a shrill, harsh sound heard during inspiration with laryngeal obstruction

- *Stertor*—snoring or sonorous respiration, usually due to a partial obstruction of the upper airway

- *Wheeze*—continuous, high-pitched musical squeak or whistling sound occurring on expiration and sometimes on inspiration when air moves through a narrowed or partially obstructed airway

- *Bubbling*—gurgling sounds heard as air passes through moist secretions in the respiratory tract

Audible by stethoscope

- *Crackles* (formerly called *rales*)—dry or wet crackling sounds simulated by rolling a lock of hair near the ear. Generally heard on inspiration as air moves through accumulated moist secretions. *Fine to medium* crackles occur when air passes through moisture in small air passages and alveoli. *Medium to coarse* crackles occur when air passes through moisture in brochioles, bronchi, and trachea.

- *Gurgles* (formerly called *rhonchi*)—coarse, dry, wheezy, or whistling sound more audible during expiration as the air moves through tenacious mucus or narrowed bronchi

- *Pleural friction rub*—coarse, leathery, or grating sound produced by the rubbing together of inflamed pleural

Chest Movements

- *Intercostal retraction*—indrawing between the ribs

- *Substernal retraction*—indrawing beneath the breast bone

- *Suprasternal retraction*—indrawing above the breast bone

- *Supraclavicular retraction*—indrawing above the clavicles

- *Tracheal tug*—indrawing and downward pull of the trachea during inspiration

- *Flail chest*—the ballooning out of the chest wall through injured rib spaces; results in *paradoxical breathing,* during which the chest wall balloons on expiration but is depressed or sucked inward on inspiration

Secretions and Coughing

- *Hemoptysis*—the presence of blood in the sputum

- *Productive cough*—a cough accompanied by expectorated secretions

- *Nonproductive cough*—a dry, harsh cough without secretions

---

- For *cytology* to identify the origin, structure, function, and pathology of cells. Specimens for cytology often require serial collection of three early morning specimens and are tested to identify cancer in the lung and its specific cell type.

- For *acid-fast bacillus* (AFB), which also require serial collection, often for 3 consecutive days, to identify the presence of tuberculosis (TB). Some agencies use a special glass container when the presence of AFB is suspected.

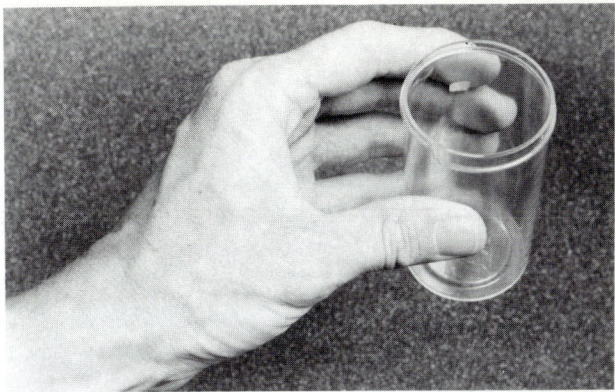

Figure 41–2   Sputum specimen container.

should include the amount, color, odor, consistency (thick, tenacious, watery, etc.), and the presence of hemoptysis. Normal sputum often contains the same kinds of microorganisms found in the upper respiratory passages. The normal flora found in sputum are listed in the box below.

A **throat culture** sample is collected from the mucosa of the oropharynx and tonsillar regions using a culture swab. The sample is then cultured and examined for the presence of disease-producing microorganisms. To obtain a throat culture specimen, the nurse inserts the swab into the oropharynx and runs the swab along the tonsils and areas on the pharynx that are reddened or contain exudate. The gag reflex, active in some clients, may be decreased by having the client sit upright if health permits, open the mouth,

- To assess the *effectiveness of therapy.* Sputum specimens are often collected in the morning. Upon awakening, the client can cough up the secretions that have accumulated during the night. Sometimes specimens are collected during postural drainage, when the client can usually produce sputum. When a client cannot cough, the nurse must sometimes use pharyngeal suctioning to obtain a specimen.

To collect a sputum specimen, the client should have mouth care first so that the specimen is not contaminated by microorganisms in the mouth. Then the client breathes deeply and coughs up 1 to 2 tablespoons of sputum (15 to 30 ml, or 4 to 8 fluid drams). The client then **expectorates** (spits out the sputum) into the specimen container, taking care that the sputum does not contact the outside of the container (see Figure 41–2). If the outside of the container should become contaminated, the nurse washes it with a disinfectant. The nurse's hands should be gloved to avoid direct contact with the client's sputum, particularly if **hemoptysis** (the presence of blood in the sputum) is suspected. The client might wish a mouth wash after producing the specimen, to remove any unpleasant taste. When recording the collection of the sputum specimen the nurse

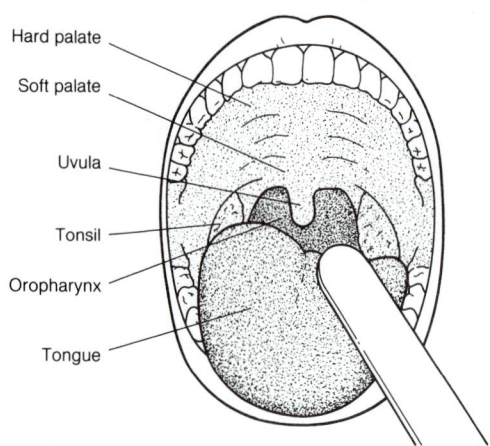

Hard palate

Soft palate

Uvula

Tonsil

Oropharynx

Tongue

Figure 41–3 Diagram of the mouth.

extend the tongue and say "ah," and by taking the specimen quickly. The sitting position and extension of the tongue help expose the pharynx; saying "ah" relaxes the throat muscles and helps minimize contraction of the constrictor muscle of the pharynx (the gag reflex). If the posterior pharynx cannot be seen, use a light, and depress the tongue with a tongue blade (see Figure 41–3).

Specimens of venous blood are taken for a *complete blood count* (CBC), which includes hemoglobin and hematocrit measurements, erythrocyte (RBC) count, leukocyte (WBC) count, and a differential red cell and white cell count.

The **hematocrit** is the packed cell volume. It denotes the percent of a given volume of whole blood occupied by erythrocytes (RBCs). Therefore, a hematocrit level of 25% indicates that erythrocytes make up 25% of the total volume of whole blood. Hematocrit levels are usually related to hemoglobin values.

Erythrocyte counts show the number of red blood cells in 1 μL or 1 mm^3 of whole blood. The level of red blood cells is regulated by their rate of formation in the bone marrow. The rate of red blood cell formation normally remains relatively constant; however, in clients with hypoxia, **erythropoiesis** (the formation of red blood cells) is stimulated.

A *white blood cell count* determines the number of circulating leukocytes (white blood cells) in 1 μL or 1 mm^3 of whole blood. Above-normal WBC counts indicate increased production of leukocytes by the bone marrow, often in response to the presence of bacterial pathogens in the body. Decreased WBC levels, by contrast, are due to decreased production of leukocytes, often because of the presence of viruses or toxic chemicals in the body.

Differential leukocyte and erythrocyte counts enumerate the different kinds of white and red blood cells in the blood specimen. A number of white blood cells are identified and classified according to their **morphology** (their form and structure). The percentage distribution of the different kinds

of white blood cells can assist in diagnosis because characteristic patterns of distribution are consistent with certain disorders. Red blood cells are examined for their size, shape, color, maturation, and content.

Measurement of *arterial blood gases* is another important diagnostic procedure. Specimens of arterial blood are normally taken by specialty nurses or medical technicians. Arterial blood is often tested for partial pressure of oxygen (Po$_2$), partial pressure of carbon dioxide (Pco$_2$), oxygen saturation (So$_2$ or O$_2$Sat), hydrogen ion concentration (pH), and the amount of bicarbonate (HCO$_3$ $^-$), and base excess (BE). Blood for these tests is taken from the radial, brachial, or femoral arteries. Because of the relatively great pressure of the blood in these arteries, it is important to prevent hemorrhaging by applying pressure to the puncture site for about 5 minutes after removing the needle.

Pulmonary function tests measure lung volume and capacity, discussed earlier in this chapter. Clients undergoing pulmonary function tests, which are usually carried out by a respiratory therapist, do not require an anesthetic. The client breathes into a machine. The tests are painless, but the client's cooperation is essential. Nurses need to explain the tests to people beforehand and help clients to get rest afterward, because the tests are often tiring. See Table 41–1 for a description of the measurements taken and the normal adult values.

A number of **visualization procedures** can be done to view parts of the respiratory tract. Roentgengraphy, fluroscopy, lung scan and endoscopy (bronchoscopy and laryngoscopy) are a few. See Chapter 48.

A *lung scan* records on a photographic plate the emissions of radioactive waves from a substance injected intravenously as it circulates through the lung. It usually involves a perfusion and ventilation scan. The *perfusion scan* (Q scan) measures the integrity of the blood vessels and evaluates blood flow abnormalities (e.g., emboli). The *ventilation scan* (V scan), performed after the perfusion scan, detects ventilation abnormalities, particularly in clients with emphysema. For this scan, the client inhales a radioactive gas through a mask and then exhales it into room air. The client needs to be informed that the radioactive isotopes disintegrate and are removed from the circulation within 8 hours.

DIAGNOSING

Five main categories of NANDA nursing diagnoses relate to oxygenation:

- **Ineffective airway clearance,** the state in which an individual is unable to clear secretions or obstructions from the respiratory tract to maintain airway patency.

- **Ineffective breathing pattern,** the state in which an individual's inhalation and/or exhalation pattern does not enable adequate ventilation.

- **Decreased cardiac output,** the state in which the blood pumped by an individual's heart is sufficiently reduced that it is inadequate to meet the needs of the body's tissues.

- **Impaired gas exchange,** the state in which an individual experiences an imbalance between oxygen uptake and carbon dioxide elimination at the alveolar capillary membrane gas exchange area.

- **Altered tissue perfusion** (cerebral, cardiopulmonary, gastrointestinal, peripheral, renal), the state in which an individual experiences a decrease in nutrition and oxygenation at the cellular level because of a deficit in capillary blood supply.

Other diagnoses that may result from the effects of insufficient oxygenation on the client's daily living patterns include **Activity intolerance, Anxiety, Ineffective individual coping, Fear, Powerlessness,** and **Sleep pattern disturbance.** These diagnoses with possible contributing factors are shown below. Examples of assessment data clusters and related nursing diagnoses are shown in Table 41–3.

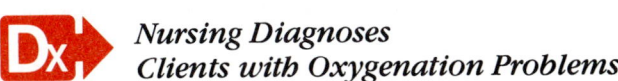

Nursing Diagnoses
Clients with Oxygenation Problems

Ineffective airway clearance related to:

- Tracheobronchial infection, obstruction, secretions
- Decreased energy and fatigue
- Trauma (e.g., inhalation injury)
- Dehydration

Ineffective breathing pattern related to:

- Neuromuscular/musculoskeletal impairment
- Pain
- Anxiety
- Decreased energy and Fatigue
- Inflammatory process
- Decreased lung expansion
- Tracheobronchial obstruction
- Alteration of normal O_2/CO_2 ratio (e.g., O_2 therapy in presence of chronic obstructive pulmonary disease, or COPD)

Decreased cardiac output related to:

- Structural alterations (e.g., valvular disease, ventricular aneurysm, ventricular-septal rupture)
- Electrical alterations in rate, rhythm, conduction
- Mechanical alteration in *preload* (e.g., altered myocardial contractility, decreased venous return), *afterload* (e.g., systemic vascular resistance), and *inotropic changes* in the heart.

Impaired gas exchange related to:

- Altered oxygen supply (e.g., altitude increase)
- Alveolar-capillary membrane changes
- Altered oxygen-carrying capacity of the blood (e.g., anemia, carbon monoxide poisoning)
- Altered blood flow

Altered tissue perfusion related to:

- Interrupted venous or arterial flow
- Hypovolemia
- Hypervolemia

Activity intolerance related to:

- Imbalance between oxygen supply and demand
- Sedentary life-style

Anxiety related to:

- Ineffective airway clearance
- Ineffective breathing pattern

Ineffective individual coping related to activity intolerance associated with impaired gas exchange

Fear related to feeling of suffocation associated with ineffective airway clearance

Powerlessness related to:

- Impaired verbal communication associated with endotracheal tube
- Self-care deficit and decreased cardiac output

Sleep pattern disturbance related to:

- Ineffective breathing pattern (orthopnea)
- Anxiety associated with ineffective airway clearance

PLANNING

Planning for a client's actual or potential oxygenation problems involves facilitating pulmonary ventilation, the diffusion of gases, and the transport of oxygen and carbon dioxide. *Facilitating pulmonary ventilation* may include ensuring a patent airway, positioning, encouraging deep breathing and coughing, and ensuring adequate hydration. Other nursing interventions helpful to ventilation are suctioning, lung inflation techniques, administration of analgesics before deep breathing and coughing, postural drainage, and percussion and vibration. Nursing strategies to *facilitate the diffusion of gases* through the alveolar membrane include encouraging coughing, deep breathing, and suitable activity. To *promote the transport of oxygen and carbon dioxide,* the nurse can optimize cardiac output by reducing stress,

TABLE 41–3 *Examples of Assessment Data Clusters and Related Nursing Diagnoses*

Data Cluster	Nursing Diagnosis
Barry Galloway reports recent flu with malaise, diaphoresis, headache, nausea, and vomiting. Now has fever and chills, chest pain, and painful nonproductive cough. Rhonchi auscultated anteriorly over bronchi.	**Ineffective airway clearance** related to inflammatory process and dehydration
Mr. Michael Parry has shortness of breath, moist cough, and fatigue. His lips and nailbeds are cyanotic. Respirations are 32 and shallow. Uses pursed-lip breathing and accessory muscles (intercostal and supraclavicular) to exhale. Blood gases indicate elevated Pco_2. Has history of COPD. Is most comfortable sitting in orthopneic position.	**Impaired gas exchange** related to alveolar-capillary membrane changes
Gloria Way, 32 years old, reports severe upper abdominal pain and abdominal distention on her first postoperative day following cholecystectomy. Is reluctant to perform deep breathing and coughing exercises. Respirations are 18 but shallow.	**Ineffective breathing pattern** related to upper abdominal incisional pain
Bessie Peacock, 78 years old, has history of cardiac failure. She reports marked fatigue and shortness of breath on exertion and has decreased pedal pulses. There is pitting edema of both ankles, and the overlying skin is cool, taut, and shiny.	**Altered peripheral tissue perfusion** related to altered circulation secondary to **Altered cardiac output: decreased**

reduce cardiac workload, and to maintain tissue perfusion and cellular oxygenation. Outcome criteria that relate to these broad goals are then identified. See examples below.

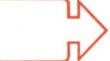

Outcome Criteria
Clients with Oxygenation Problems

The client with **Ineffective airway clearance:**

- Has a patent airway.
- Readily expectorates secretions.
- Has clear breath sounds bilaterally.
- Has normal respiratory rate, rhythm, and depth.
- Has skin, nails, lips, and earlobes of natural color.
- Identifies potential complications.
- Explains medications and treatments for home use and plans for follow-up care.

The client with **Ineffective breathing pattern** or **Impaired gas exchange:**

- Establishes a normal effective respiratory pattern of 12 to 20 per minute, effortless breathing (no use of accessory muscles), and symmetric chest expansion on inhalation.
- Is free of cyanosis.
- Has normal arterial blood gases.
- Performs activities of daily living without shortness of breath.
- Demonstrates appropriate life-style changes.
- Explains purposes and side-effects of medications (e.g., bronchodilator, expectorant, anti-infective, antihistamine, corticosteroid).
- Explains treatments for home care and plans for follow-up care.

The client with **Altered cardiac output: decreased:**

- Has normal heart rhythm and rate within 20 beats of normal.
- Has a maximum systolic blood pressure of 140 mm Hg and maximum diastolic blood pressure of 90 mm Hg.
- Has clear breath sounds bilaterally.
- Has appropriate peripheral pulses.
- Performs activities of daily living without fatigue *or* alters activities to reduce cardiac workload.
- Verbalizes knowledge of condition, risk factors, and treatment plan (e.g., exercise, stress management, medications such as diuretics and vasodilators).

The client with **Altered tissue perfusion:**

- Has all pulses palpable and strong.
- Has warm extremities of color normal for the individual.
- Has normal vital signs.

planning appropriate activities, and positioning the client for improved vascular blood flow. A client's nursing care plan should also include appropriate dependent nursing interventions such as oxygen therapy, tracheostomy care, and maintenance of a chest tube.

Overall client goals for individuals with oxygenation problems are to maintain airway patency, to maintain adequate ventilation, to maintain adequate cardiac output, to

- Has intact skin on extremities.
- Is free of edema.
- Has a balanced fluid intake and output.
- Identifies causative factors.
- Verbalizes knowledge of condition, therapy, medications (e.g., anticoagulants).
- Demonstrates life-style changes to improve circulation (e.g., cessation of smoking, exercise program).

IMPLEMENTING

Positioning

Normally, adequate ventilation is maintained by frequent changes of position, ambulation, and exercise. When persons become ill, however, their respiratory functions may be inhibited, for a variety of reasons. One common reason is immobility induced by surgery or medical therapy. Lying too long in one position compresses the thorax, limits chest expansion, and thus inhibits the movement of air through the lungs. Sitting in a slumped position also inhibits chest expansion, since the abdominal contents are pushed up against the diaphragm. Another frequent cause of limited chest expansion is abdominal pain or chest pain. The client often voluntarily limits chest movements to relieve the pain.

Shallow respirations inhibit both diaphragmatic excursion and lung distensibility. The result of inadequate chest expansion is stasis and pooling of respiratory secretions, which ultimately harbor microorganisms and promote infection. This situation is often compounded in the hospitalized client who receives narcotics for pain, because narcotics further depress the rate and depth of respiration.

Interventions by the nurse to maintain the normal respirations of clients include

- Positioning the client to allow for maximum chest expansion
- Encouraging or providing frequent changes in position
- Encouraging ambulation
- Implementing measures that promote comfort, such as giving pain medications

The semi-Fowler's or high-Fowler's position allows maximum chest expansion in bedfast clients, particularly dyspneic clients. The nurse encourages clients who cannot assume this position to turn from side to side frequently, so that alternate sides of the chest are permitted maximum expansion. In the hospital, dyspneic clients often sit in bed and lean over their overbed tables (which are raised to a suitable height), usually with a pillow for support. This *orthopneic position* is an adaptation of the high-Fowler's position. It has a further advantage in that, unlike in high-Fowler's, the abdominal organs are not pressing on the diaphragm.

CLIENT TEACHING
Deep Breathing and Coughing

Abdominal (Diaphragmatic and Pursed-Lip) Breathing

- Assume a comfortable semi-sitting position in bed or chair *or* a lying position in bed with one pillow.
- Flex your knees to relax the muscles of the abdomen.
- Place one or both hands on your abdomen, just below the ribs.
- Breathe in deeply through the nose, keeping the mouth closed.
- Concentrate on feeling your abdomen rise as far as possible; stay relaxed, and avoid arching your back. If you have difficulty raising your abdomen, take a quick, forceful breath through the nose.
- Then purse your lips as if about to whistle, and breathe out slowly and gently, making a slow "whooshing" sound without puffing out the cheeks. This *pursed-lip breathing* creates a resistance to air flowing out of the lungs, increases pressure within the bronchi (main air passages), and minimizes collapse of smaller airways, a common problem for people with chronic obstructive pulmonary disease.
- Concentrate on feeling the abdomen fall or sink and tighten (contract) the abdominal muscles while breathing out to enhance effective exhalation. Count to seven during exhalation.
- If indicated, cough two or more times during exhalation.
- Use this exercise whenever feeling short of breath, and increase gradually to 5 to 10 minutes four times a day. Regular practice will help you do this type of breathing without conscious effort. The exercise, once learned, can be performed when sitting upright, standing, and walking.

Also, a client in the orthopneic position can press the lower part of the chest against the table to help in exhaling.

Deep Breathing and Coughing

The nurse can facilitate respiratory functioning by encouraging *deep-breathing exercises and coughing* to remove secretions. Breathing exercises are frequently indicated for clients with restricted chest expansion, e.g., people with chronic obstructive pulmonary disease (COPD) or clients recovering from thoracic surgery. Commonly employed breathing exercises are abdominal (diaphragmatic) and pursed-lip breathing, apical expansion, and basal expansion exercises. *Abdominal (diaphragmatic) breathing* permits deep full breaths with little effort. See the box above for client instructions. *Apical or basal expansion exercises*

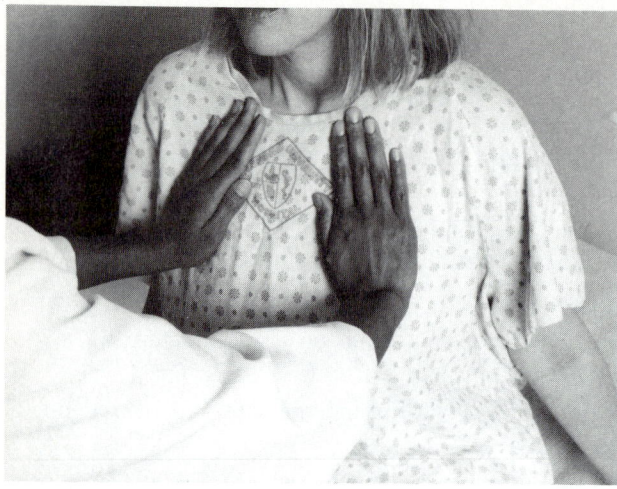

Figure 41–4 Assisting the client to carry out apical expansion exercises.

are often required for clients who restrict their upper or lower chest movement because of pain from a severe respiratory disease, chest surgery, or upper abdominal surgery.

To assist the client with *apical* expansion exercises, the nurse places the fingers below the client's clavicles and exerts moderate pressure; alternatively, clients place their own fingers over the same area. See Figure 41–4. This hand position facilitates evaluation of the depth of apical inhalation. The nurse instructs the client to concentrate on expanding the upper chest forward and upward while inhaling. This helps aerate the apical areas of the upper lung lobes. To promote aeration of the alveoli, the client holds the inhalation for a few seconds before slowly, qui-

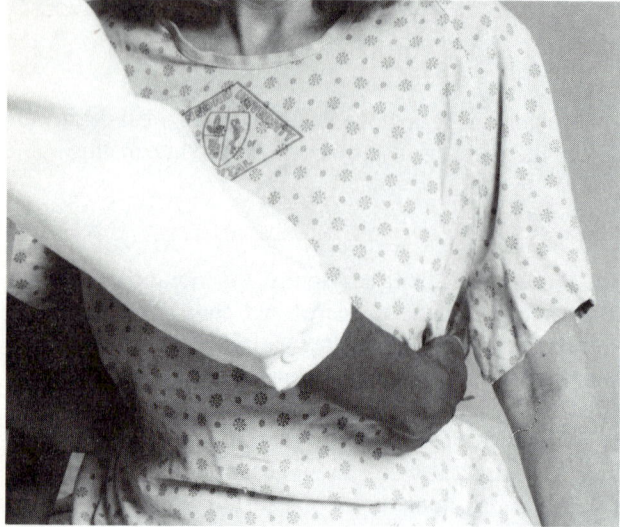

Figure 41–5 Assisting the client to carry out basal expansion exercises.

etly, and passively exhaling through the mouth or nose. Performing this exercise several times a day (e.g., five respirations four times a day) helps to reexpand lung tissue, move secretions to promote effective elimination, and minimize flattening of the upper chest wall from disuse.

To assist the client with *basal* expansion exercises, the nurse places the palms of the hands in the area of the lower ribs along the midaxillary lines and exerts moderate pressure; alternatively, clients place their own hands over the same area. See Figure 41–5. This hand position facilitates evaluation and comparison of the depth of bilateral basal inspiration. The nurse instructs the client to concentrate on moving the lower chest outward upon inhalation and then to exhale slowly, quietly, and passively. If the client appears to be having difficulty in exhaling or if the upper chest draws in upon exhalation, the nurse should have the client do pursed-lip exhalation. The nurse should have the client purse the lips as if about to whistle and to breathe out slowly and gently, tightening the abdominal muscles to exhale more effectively. Pursing the lips creates a resistance to air flowing out of the lungs.

Hydration

Adequate hydration maintains the moisture of the respiratory mucous membranes. Normally, respiratory tract secretions are thin and therefore moved readily by ciliary action. However, when the client is dehydrated or when the environment has a low humidity, the respiratory secretions can become thick and tenacious. The mucous membranes then become irritated and prone to infection. Nursing measures to increase and monitor fluid intake thus assume a high priority. Appropriate measures are discussed in Chapter 40.

Humidifiers are devices that add water vapor to inspired air. Their purposes are to prevent mucous membranes from drying and becoming irritated and to loosen secretions for easier expectoration. All humidifiers employ the simple method of passing the gas through sterile water so that water vapor is picked up before the gas reaches the client. The more bubbles are created during this process, the more water vapor is produced. Some humidifiers heat the water vapor, thus increasing the humidity provided. Three main types are the room humidifier (ordinarily for home use), the cascade humidifier, and the cold bubble diffuser (oxygen humidifier).

A *room humidifier* (see Figure 41–6) can provide either cool mist or steam. Some types can be used with gas lines, e.g., oxygen, to provide moistened air directly to the client. A *cascade humidifier* can deliver 100% humidity at body temperature. The temperature of the vapor can be controlled, and the machine can be used to provide humidified oxygen to clients on ventilators.

An *oxygen humidifier* (see Figure 41–7) is used with all oxygen equipment to moisten the oxygen before it is inhaled. This device provides 20% to 40% humidity. The oxygen passes through sterile distilled water and then along a line

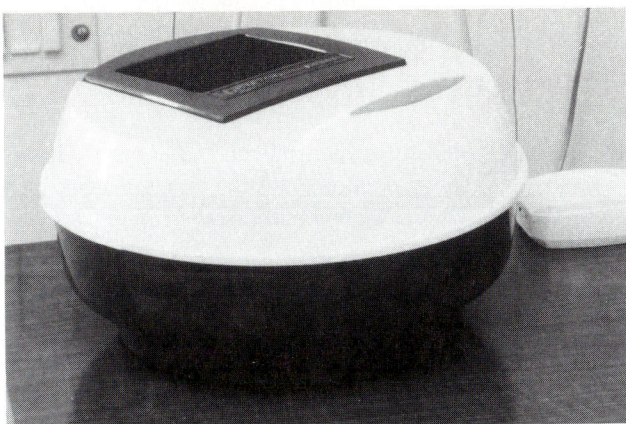

Figure 41–6   A room humidifier.

to the device through which the moistened oxygen is inhaled (e.g., a cannula, nasal catheter, or oxygen mask). See the discussion of oxygen therapy, later in this chapter.

A *nebulizer* is used to deliver a fine spray of medication or moisture to a client. **Nebulization** is the production of a fog or mist.

There are two kinds of neubulization: atomization and aerosolization. In *atomization,* a device called an *atomizer* produces rather large droplets for inhalation. When the droplets are suspended in a gas, such as oxygen, the process is **inhalation** (aerosol) **therapy.** The smaller the droplets, the further they can be inhaled into the respiratory tract. When a medication is intended for the nasal mucosa, it is inhaled through the nose; when it is intended for the trachea, bronchi, and/or lungs, it is inhaled through the mouth.

A *large-volume nebulizer* can provide a heated or cool mist. It is used for long-term therapy, such as that following a tracheostomy. These nebulizers have a 250-ml capacity and deliver oxygen or room air. The *ultrasonic nebulizer* (see Figure 41–8) provides 100% humidity and can provide particles small enough to be inhaled deeply into the respiratory tract. There are two types of ultrasonic nebulizers: one has a cup filled with sterile distilled water; the other requires a continuous supply of sterile distilled water from a bag connected by tubing to the nebulizer bottle.

The *hand nebulizer* (see Figure 41–9 on the next page) is a container of medication that can be compressed by hand to release the medication through a nosepiece or mouthpiece. The force with which the air moves through the nebulizer causes the large particles of medicated solution to break up into finer particles, forming a mist or fine spray. Aerosol inhalers must be used properly to ensure correct delivery of the prescribed medication. The *mini-nebulizer* is used with oxygen or a pressurized gas source, e.g., air. With this device, the client inhales and exhales independently. Medication is administered during inhalation. A *side-stream nebulizer* provides a medication to a client on a ventilator or receiving intermittent positive pres-

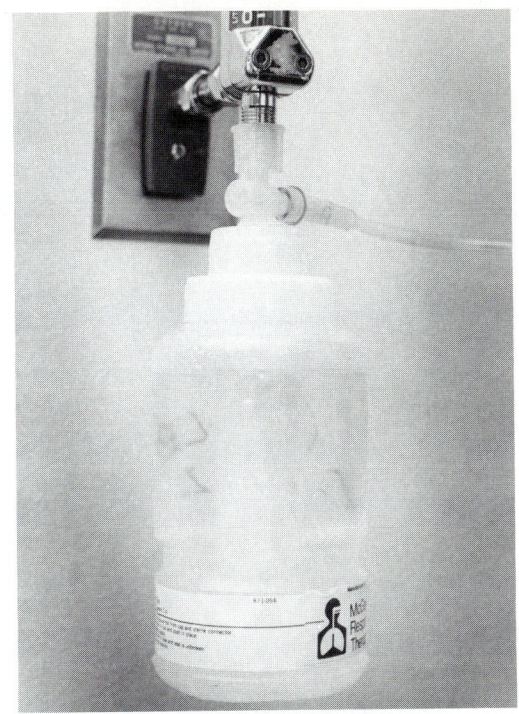

Figure 41–7   An oxygen humidifier.

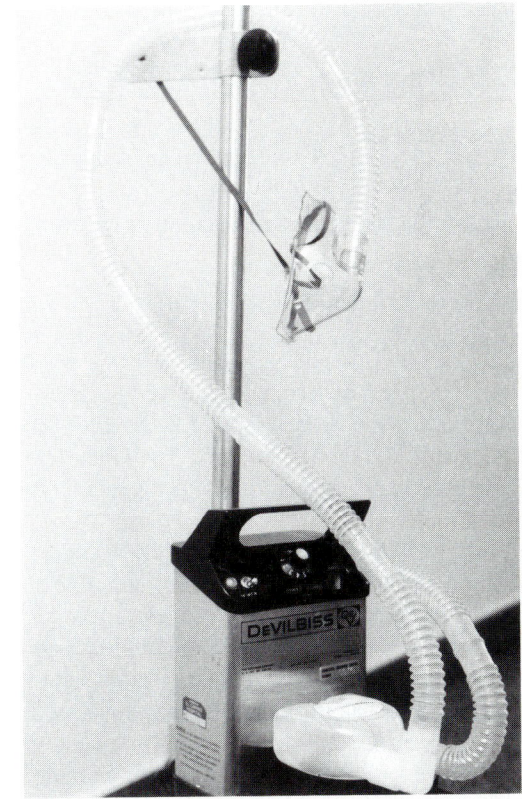

Figure 41–8   An ultrasonic nebulizer.

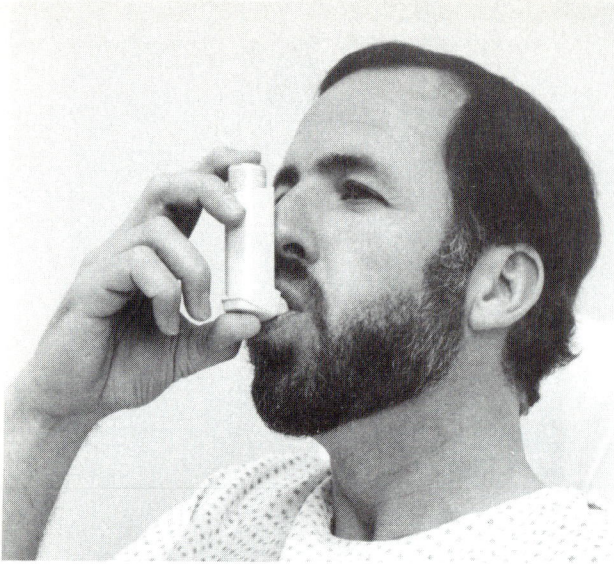

Figure 41–9 A hand nebulizer.

sure breathing (IPPB) therapy. The gas, e.g., oxygen, passes through a device containing the medicated solution and then into the ventilator and to the client. The accompanying box gives clients instructions on how to use a hand nebulizer.

Lung Inflation Devices

Lung inflation devices are used to

- Improve pulmonary ventilation
- Counteract the effects of anesthesia and/or hypoventilation
- Loosen respiratory secretions
- Facilitate respiratory gaseous exchange
- Expand collapsed alveoli

Incentive spirometers, also referred to as *sustained maximal inspiration devices* (SMIs), measure the flow of air inhaled through the mouthpiece. They therefore offer an incentive to improve *inhalation.* Two general types are the flow-oriented spirometer and the volume-oriented spirometer. The *flow-oriented SMI* consists of one or more clear plastic chambers containing freely movable colored balls or discs. The balls or discs are elevated as the client inhales. The client is asked to keep them elevated as long as possible with a maximal sustained inhalation. Figure 41–10 shows a Triflo II SMI. Flow-oriented SMIs are low-cost devices, are often disposable, and can be used independently by clients. They do not measure the specific volume of air inhaled, however.

Volume-oriented SMIs measure the inhalation volume maintained by the client. A plastic *disposable* device is shown in Figure 41–11. When the client inhales, the accordion-pleated cylinder rises from the bottom as the cylinder col-

CLIENT TEACHING
Using a Hand Nebulizer

- Make sure the canister is firmly and fully inserted into the outer shell or actuator. Press the canister firmly into the actuator with a twisting motion, and rotate back and forth several times.
- Remove the cap from the mouthpiece. Hold the inhaler in the hand and shake by inverting it several times.
- Breathe out slowly until no more air can be expelled from the lungs, then immediately *(for the next step there are two alternatives, depending on the technique preferred by the physician):*
- Place the mouthpiece over the tongue and well into the mouth. Close the lips tightly around the mouthpiece. Press the top of the canister firmly between forefinger and thumb, while inhaling deeply and slowly, *or*
- Place the inhaler directly in front of the mouth. Begin a slow inward breath through the wide open mouth, at the same time pressing the canister down firmly into the inhaler.
- Continue inhaling to carry the spray deep into the lungs. Hold the breath for as long as is comfortable.
- Release the pressure on the canister. Remove the inhaler away from mouth and breathe out gently.
- *Before the second puff,* wait for at least 30 seconds for the valve pressure to rebuild. Then rotate the canister back and forth, and again shake several times before reusing.

Common Problems in Using an Inhaler

- Not taking the medication as prescribed, but taking either too much or too little.
- Incorrect activation. This usually occurs through pressing the canister before taking a breath. Both should be done simultaneously so that the drug can be carried down to the lungs.
- Forgetting to shake the inhaler. Because the drug is in a suspension, particles may settle. If the inhaler is not shaken, it may not deliver the correct dose of the drug.
- Not waiting long enough (30 seconds) between puffs. The whole process should be repeated to take the second puff; otherwise, the dose may be incorrect, or the drug may not penetrate the lungs.

lapses. Markings on the side indicate the volume of inspiration achieved by the client. The goal is to make the cylinder collapse as much as possible.

More expensive *nondisposable volume-oriented SMIs*

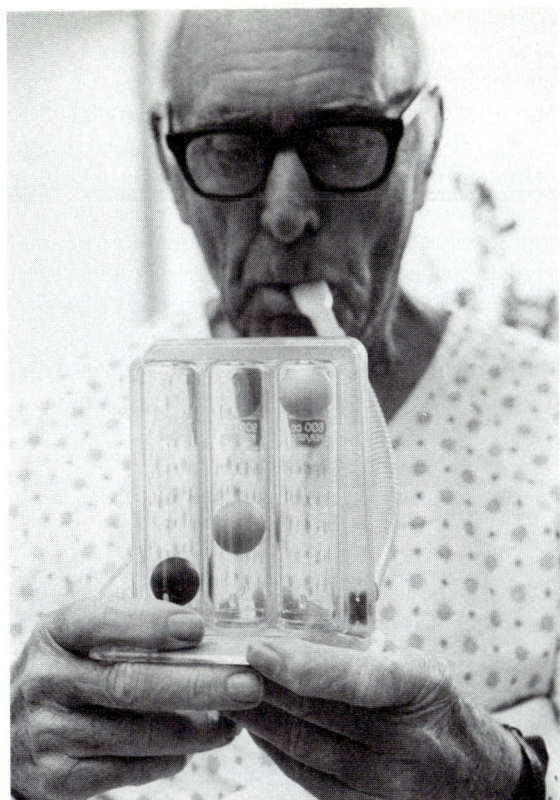

Figure 41–10 Sustained maximal inspiration device (SMI).

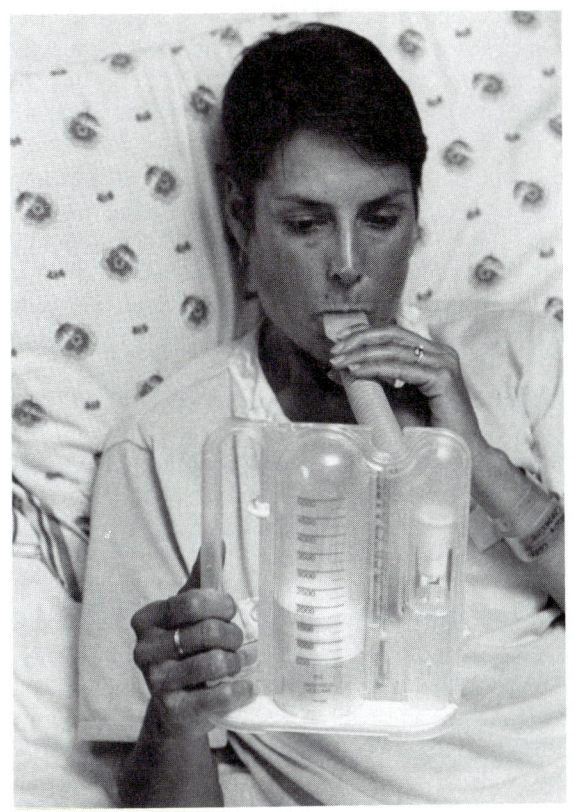

Figure 41–11 Plastic disposable volume-oriented SMI.

CLIENT TEACHING
Using an Incentive Spirometer

- Hold or place the spirometer in an upright position. A tilted *flow-oriented* device requires less effort to raise the balls or discs; a volume-oriented device will not function correctly unless upright.

- Exhale normally.

- Seal the lips tightly around the mouthpiece.

- Take in a *slow, deep breath* to elevate the balls or cylinder, and then hold the breath for 2 seconds initially, increasing to 6 seconds (optimum), to keep the balls or cylinder elevated if possible.

- For a flow-oriented device, avoid brisk, low-volume breaths that snap the balls to the top of the chamber. Greater lung expansion is achieved with a very slow inspiration than with a brisk, shallow breath, even though it may not elevate the balls or keep them elevated while you hold your breath. Sustained elevation of the balls or cylinder ensures adequate ventilation of the alveoli (lung air sacs).

- If you have difficulty breathing only through the mouth, a nose clip can be used.

- Remove the mouthpiece, and exhale normally.

- Cough after the incentive effort. Deep ventilation may loosen secretions, and coughing can facilitate their removal.

- Relax, and take several normal breaths before using the spirometer again.

- Repeat the procedure several times and then four or five times hourly. Practice increases inspiratory volume, maintains alveolar ventilation, and prevents atelectasis (collapse of the air sacs).

- Clean the mouthpiece with water and shake it dry. Change disposable mouthpieces every 24 hours.

measure the inhalation volume maintained by the client very precisely. These devices contain pistons or bellows that are raised by the client's inhalation to a predetermined volume. Some volume-oriented devices feature an achievement counter or light. The light will not turn on until the inspiration is held at the minimum predetermined volume for a specified time period.

Client preparation and instruction is essential for effective use of lung inflation devices. The client should be assisted preferably to an upright sitting position in bed or in a chair when using any of these devices. This position facilitates maximum ventilation. The accompanying box lists instructions for clients in the use of incentive spirometers.

If nondisposable devices are used in hospitals, the nurse will need to check the physician's or respiratory therapist's order and set the spirometer to the predetermined volume. Volume ranges vary from 0 to 5000 ml, depending on the type of spirometer. Battery-operated SMIs will also need to be checked for proper functioning. In all situations, the nurse should auscultate the client's lungs before and after the procedure and compare the findings. When recording the procedure, include the type of spirometer, number of breaths taken, volume or flow levels achieved, and results of ausculation. For a flow SMI, calculate the volume achieved by multiplying the setting by the length of time the client kept the balls elevated. For example, if the setting was 500 ml and the balls were kept suspended for 2 seconds, the volume is 500 × 2 = 1000 ml. For a volume SMI, take the volume directly from the spirometer, e.g., 1500 ml.

Intermittent positive pressure breathing (IPPB) is a lung inflation technique for delivering air or oxygen into the lungs at positive (above atmospheric) pressure during inspiration and automatic releasing of the pressure when the predetermined positive pressure level is reached in the air passages. Thus, expiration occurs passively. Some IPPB machines can exert pressure during expiration, and the abbreviations IPPB/I (inspiratory) and IPPB/E (expiratory) are sometimes used to differentiate the two methods. Generally, however, IPPB refers to positive pressure therapy administered during inspiration, a safer and more common practice.

Use of IPPB therapy has decreased since the advent of incentive spirometers. Advocates of IPPB therapy, however, believe that IPPB devices are more effective in expanding the lungs, moving secretions, promoting coughing, and

delivering aerosol medications into the deeper, smaller air passages. Because they require less effort by the client, they are prescribed for selected clients.

Various IPPB machines are marketed. Two commonly used types are the Bird respirator and the Bennett respirator. Assembly and maintenance of respirators is usually handled by respiratory therapists. The machine is connected to an oxygen supply and is equipped with an in-line humidifier, which must be filled with distilled water. The client breathes through a mouthpiece or a mask attached to the end of the respirator tubing. See Figure 41–12.

Usually, IPPB treatments are given by respiratory therapists. The nurse must observe the client's progress and response to such therapy.

Percussion, Vibration, and Postural Drainage (PVD)

Percussion, vibration, and postural drainage are dependent nursing functions performed according to a physician's order. **Percussion,** sometimes called *clapping,* is forceful striking of the skin with cupped hands. Mechanical percussion cups and vibrators are also available. When the hands are used, the fingers and thumb are held together and flexed slightly to form a cup, as one would to scoop up water. Percussion over congested lung areas can mechanically dislodge tenacious secretions from the bronchial walls. Cupped hands trap the air against the chest. The trapped air sets up vibrations through the chest wall to the secretions. Before percussion, ensure that the area to be percussed is covered, e.g., by a gown or towel, since percussing the unprotected skin can cause discomfort. Ask the client to breathe slowly and deeply to promote relaxation. To percuss, alternatively flex and extend the wrists rapidly to slap the chest. The hands must remain cupped so the air cushions the impact, to avoid injuring the client. See Figure 41–13. Percuss each affected lung segment for 1 to 2 minutes. When done correctly, the percussion action should produce a hollow, popping sound. Percussion is avoided over certain easily injured structures, such as the breasts, sternum, spinal column, and kidneys.

Vibration is a series of vigorous quiverings produced by hands that are placed flat against the client's chest wall. Vibration is used after percussion to increase the turbulence of the exhaled air and thus loosen thick secretions. It is often done alternately with percussion.

To vibrate, place your hands palms down, one hand over the other, with fingers together and extended, on the chest area to be drained. See Figure 41–14. Alternatively, the hands may be placed side by side. Ask the client to inhale deeply and exhale slowly through the nose or pursed lips. During the exhalation, tense all your hand and arm muscles, and, using mostly the heel of the hand, vibrate (shake) your hands, moving them downward. Stop the vibrating when the client inhales.

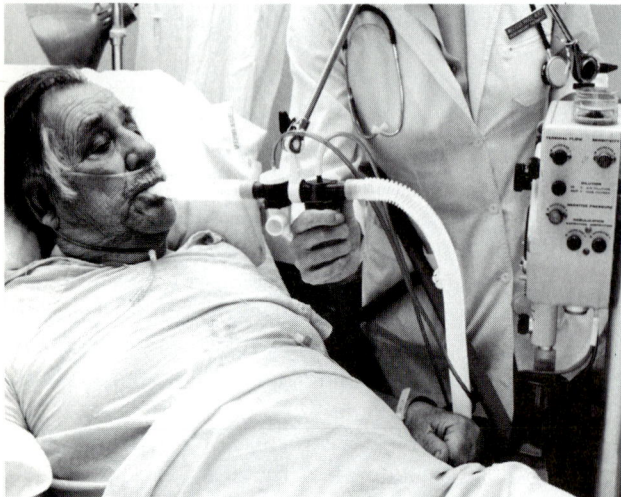

Figure 41–12 Intermittent positive pressure breathing (IPPB).

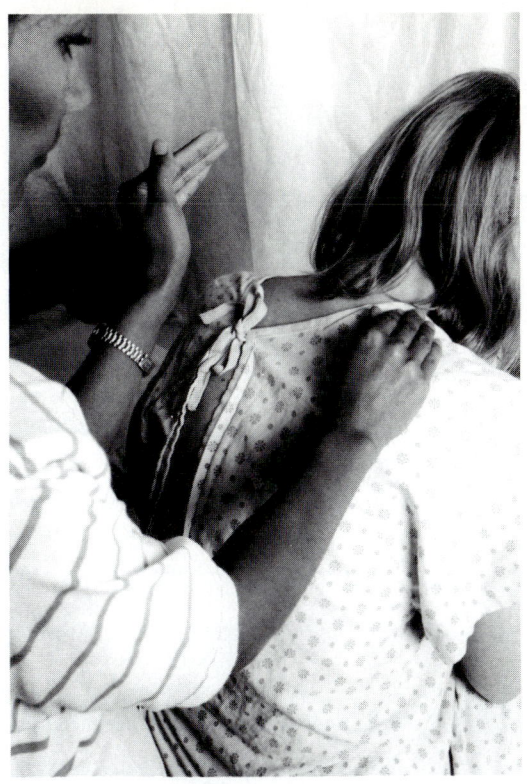

Figure 41–13 Percussing the upper posterior chest.

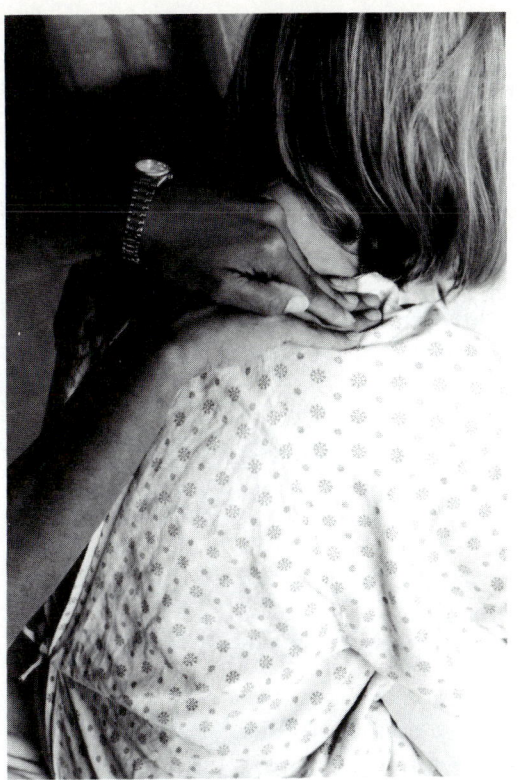

Figure 41–14 Vibrating the upper posterior chest.

Vibrate during five exhalations over one affected lung segment. After each vibration encourage the client to cough and expectorate secretions into the sputum container.

Postural drainage is the drainage, by gravity, of secretions from various lung segments. Secretions that remain in the lungs or respiratory airways promote bacterial growth and subsequent infection. They also can obstruct the smaller airways and cause atelectasis. Secretions in the major airways, such as the trachea and the right and left main bronchi, are usually coughed into the pharynx, where they can be expectorated, swallowed, or effectively removed by suctioning.

A wide variety of positions is necessary to drain all segments of the lungs, but not all positions are required for every client. Only those positions that drain specific affected areas are used. The lower lobes require drainage most frequently, since the upper lobes drain during normal daily activities. Prior to postural drainage, the client may be given a bronchodilator medication or nebulization therapy to loosen secretions. Frequently, postural drainage treatments are scheduled two or three times daily, depending on the degree of lung congestion. The best times include before breakfast, before lunch, in the late afternoon, and before bedtime. It is best to avoid hours shortly after meals because postural drainage at these times can be tiring and can induce vomiting.

The nurse needs to evaluate the client's tolerance of postural drainage by assessing the stability of the client's vital signs, particularly the pulse and respiratory rates, and by noting sings of intolerance, such as pallor, diaphoresis, dyspnea, and fatigue. Some clients do not react well to certain drainage positions, and the nurse must make appropriate adjustments. For example, some become dyspneic in Trendelenburg's position and require only a moderate tilt or a shorter time in those positions.

The sequence for PVD is usually as follows: positioning, percussion, vibration, and removal of secretions by coughing or suction. Each position is usually assumed for 10 to 15 minutes, although beginning treatments may start with shorter times and gradually increase. Usually, the entire treatment, including preparatory nebulization and deep breathing as well as all postures, takes 30 minutes. Postural drainage position and percussion areas for specific lung segments are shown in Table 41–4.

Following PVD, the nurse should auscultate the client's lungs, compare the findings to the baseline data, and document the amount, color, and character of expectorated secretions.

TABLE 41–4 *Postural Drainage for Adults*

Upper Lobes

Lung Segment
Apical segments

Client Position
Lies back at 30° angle

Percussion/Vibration Area
Between the clavicles and above the scapulae

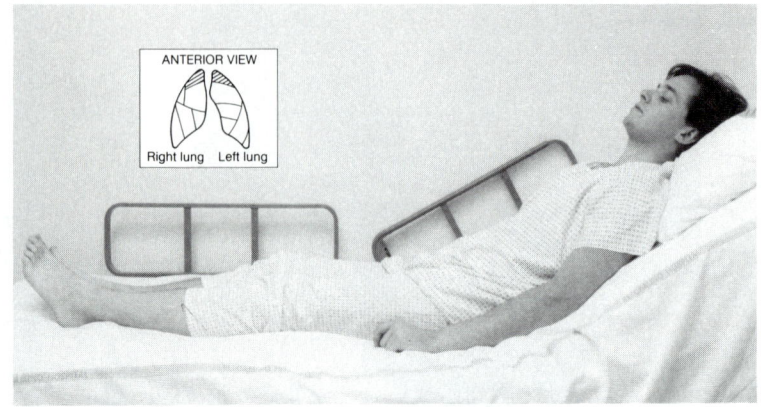

Lung Segment
Posterior segments

Client Position
Sits upright in a chair or in bed with head bent slightly forward

Percussion/Vibration Area
Between the clavicles and the scapulae

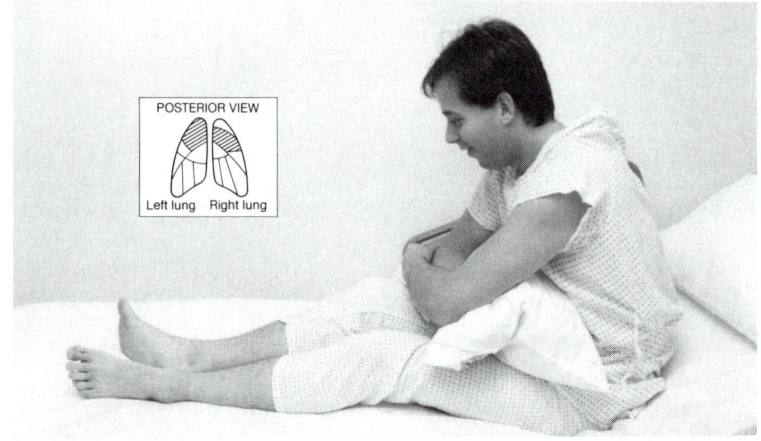

Lung Segment
Anterior segments

Client Position
Lies on a flat bed with pillows under the knees to flex them

Percussion/Vibration Area
Upper chest below the clavicles down to the nipple line, except for women

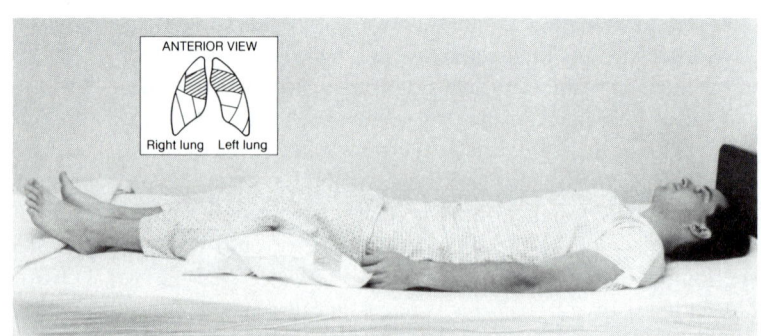

TABLE 41–4 *Postural Drainage for Adults*   (continued)

Right Middle Lobe

Lung Segment

Right lateral and medial segments

Client Position

Lies on the left side and leans back slightly (about a quarter turn) against pillows, extending at the back from the shoulder to the hip. Nurse elevates foot of bed about 15° or 40 cm (15 in).

Percussion/Vibration Area

For *male* client: Over the right side of the chest at the level of the nipple between the fourth and sixth ribs

For *female* client: Beneath the breast; position the heel of your hand toward her axilla with your cupped fingers extending forward beneath the breast

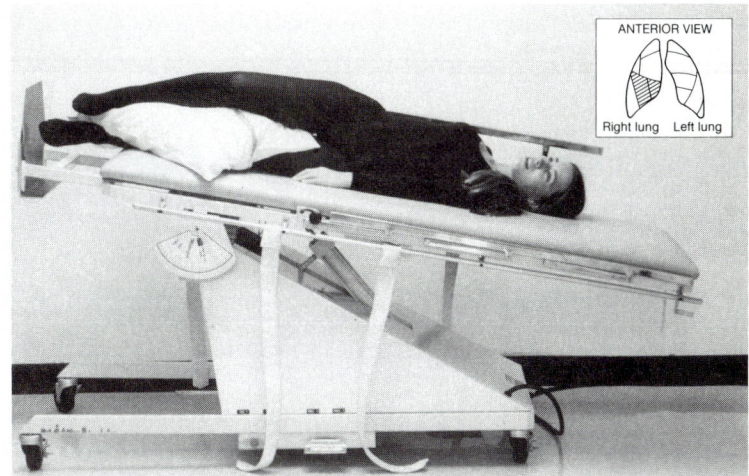

Lower Division of Left Upper Lobe (Lingula)

Lung Segment

Left lingular segments

Client Position

As above for right middle lobe, but on the *right* side

Percussion/Vibration Area

As above for right middle lobe, but on the *left* side

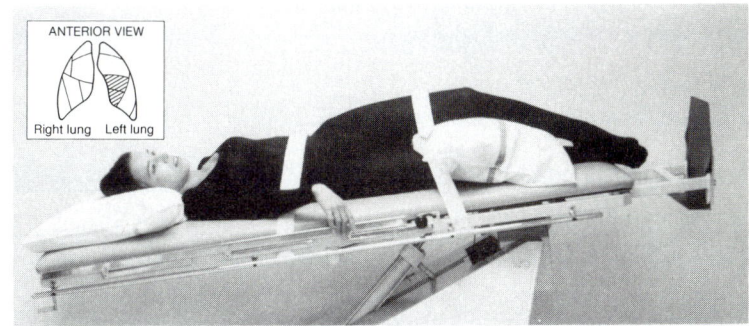

Lower Lobes

Lung Segment

Superior segments

Client Position

Lies on the abdomen on a flat bed, and nurse places two pillows under the hips

Percussion/Vibration Area

The middle area of the back (below the scapulae) on both sides of the spine

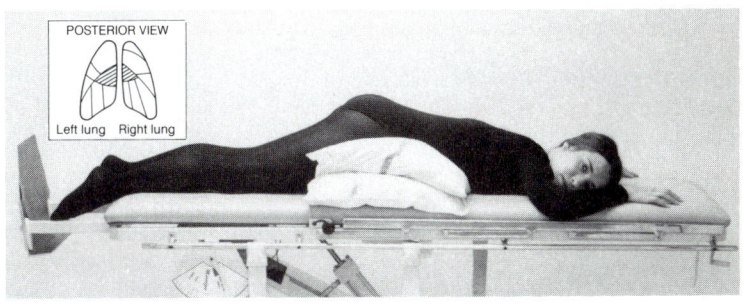

TABLE 41–4 *Postural Drainage for Adults* (continued)

Lower Lobes (continued)

Lung Segment
Anterior basal segments

Client Position
Lies on unaffected side with the upper arm over the head and pillow between knees. Nurse elevates the foot of the bed about 30° or 45 cm (18 in) or to height tolerated by the client. A pillow under the head is optional.

Percussion/Vibration Area
Over the lower ribs inferior to the axilla on the affected side of the chest

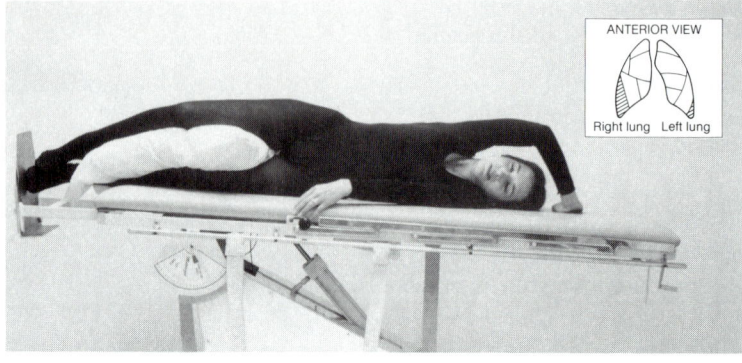

Lung Segment
Lateral basal segments

Client Position
Lies partly on unaffected side and partly on the abdomen. Nurse elevates the foot of the bed about 30° or 45 cm (18 in) or to height tolerated, or elevates client's hips with pillows.

Percussion/Vibration Area
The uppermost side of the lower ribs

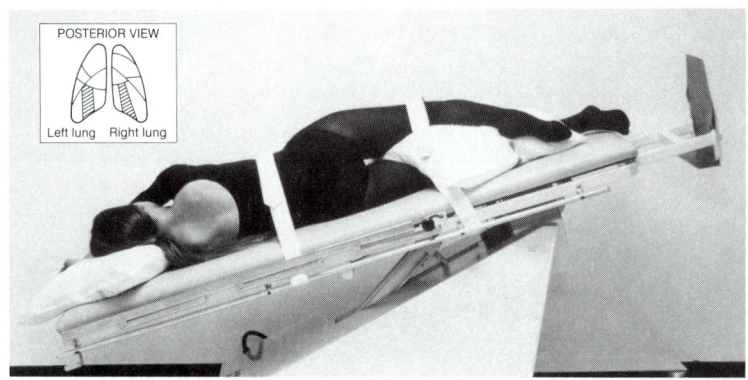

Lung Segment
Posterior basal segments

Client Position
Lies prone. Nurse elevates foot of bed about 45 cm (18 in), and elevates client's hips on two or three pillows to produce a jackknife position from the knees to the shoulders.

Percussion/Vibration Area
Over the lower ribs on both sides close to the spine, but not directly over the spine or kidneys

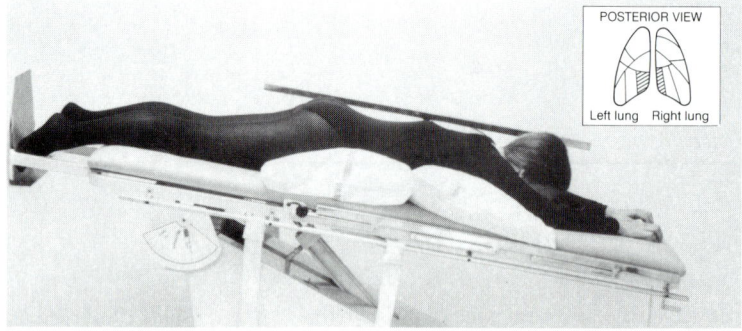

Suctioning Oropharyngeal and Nasopharyngeal Cavities

The nurse must sometimes apply suction to the oropharynx and nasal passages of clients who have difficulty swallowing or expectorating secretions. **Suctioning** is the aspiration of secretions, often through a rubber or polyethylene catheter connected to a suction machine or wall outlet. It is recommended that sterile technique be used for all suc-

tioning, so that microorganisms are not introduced into the pharynx, where they can multiply and move into the trachea and bronchi. This is particularly important for debilitated clients, who are more susceptible to infection.

The purposes of suctioning are

- To remove secretions that obstruct the airway
- To facilitate respiratory ventilation
- To obtain secretions for diagnostic purposes

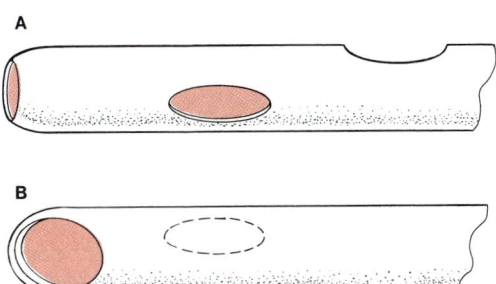

Figure 41–15 Types of pharyngeal suction catheters: *A,* open-tipped; *B,* whistle-tipped.

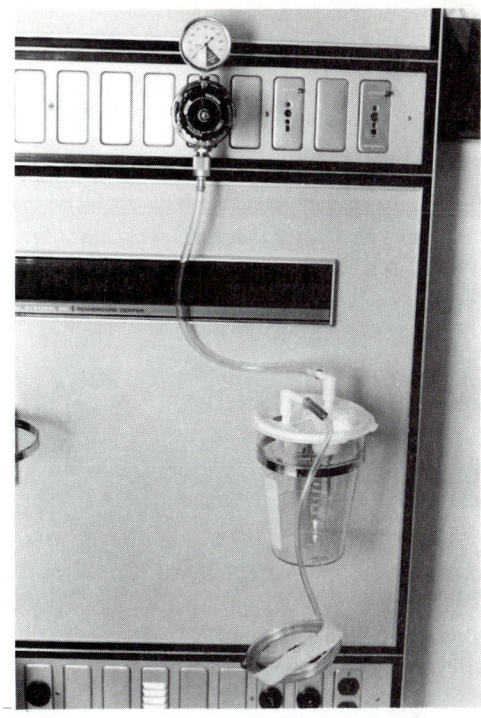

Figure 41–16 A wall suction unit.

■ To prevent infection that may result from accumulated secretions

Several types of catheters are available for suctioning. The open-tipped catheter has an opening at the end and several openings along the sides. See Figure 41–15, *A*. It is effective for thick mucus plugs, but it can irritate tissue. The whistle-tipped catheter has a slanted opening at the tip. See Figure 41–15, *B*. Most catheters have a thumb port on the side, which is used to control the suction. The tip of a suction catheter has several openings along the sides to distribute the negative pressure of the suction over a wide area, thus preventing excessive irritation of any one area of the respiratory mucous membrane.

The suction apparatus includes a collection bottle, a tubing system connected to the suction catheter, and a gauge that registers the degree of suction. These apparatus are either portable or wall mounted. See Figure 41–16.

Oropharyngeal or nasopharyngeal suctioning removes secretions from the upper respiratory tract. Deeper suctioning, called *endotracheal suctioning,* removes secretions from the trachea and the bronchi. Deep suctioning requires considerably more skill and is usually carried out by a critical-care nursing specialist or an experienced nurse.

Suctioning of the upper respiratory airways is indicated when the client is unable to cough or swallow and makes light bubbling or rattling breath sounds that signal the accumulation of secretions. Guidelines for oropharyngeal and nasopharyngeal suctioning are described in Procedure 41–1.

PROCEDURE 41–1

OROPHARYNGEAL AND NASOPHARYNGEAL SUCTIONING

Equipment

Portable or wall suction machine with tubing and collection receptacle
Sterile suction catheter
Sterile gloves

Sterile disposable container for sterile fluids
Water-soluble lubricant
Sterile normal saline or water
Y-connector

Sterile gauzes
Towel or pad
Moisture-resistant disposal bag
Sputum trap

Intervention

1. **Assess the need for suctioning.**

■ Suction *only* when necessary, i.e., when secretions are audible during respiration or when adventitious breath sounds are auscultated.

■ Establish baseline data by auscultating the chest, assessing the client's mental status, and briefly observing the rate and pattern of respirations and the pulse rate and rhythm.

2. **Prepare the client.**

■ Explain to the client that suctioning will relieve breathing difficulty and that the procedure is painless but may stimulate the cough, gag, or sneeze reflex. *Knowing that the procedure will relieve breathing problems is often reassuring and enlists cooperation.*

■ Position a *conscious* person who has a functional gag reflex in the semi-Fowler's position with the head turned to one side for oral suctioning or with the neck hyperextended for nasal suctioning. *These positions facilitate the insertion of the catheter and help prevent aspiration of secretions.*

■ Position an *unconscious* client in the lateral position, facing you. *This position allows the tongue to fall forward, so that it will not obstruct the catheter on insertion. Lateral position also facilitates drainage of secretions from the pharynx and prevents the possibility of aspiration.*

■ Place the towel over the pillow or under the chin.

3. **Prepare the equipment.**

■ Set the pressure on the suction gauge, and turn on the suction. Many suction devices are calibrated to three pressure ranges:

Wall unit
Adult: 100 to 120 mm Hg
Child: 95 to 110 mm Hg
Infant: 50 to 95 mm Hg
Portable unit
Adult: 10 to 15 mm Hg
Child: 5 to 10 mm Hg
Infant: 2 to 5 mm Hg

■ Open the sterile suction package.
  a. Set up the cup or container, touching only its outside.
  b. Pour sterile water or saline into the container.
  c. Don the sterile gloves or don a nonsterile glove on the nondominant hand and then a sterile glove on the dominant hand. *The sterile gloved hand maintains the sterility of the suction catheter and the unsterile glove prevents the transmission of the microorganisms to the nurse.*

■ With your sterile gloved hand, pick up the catheter, and attach it to the suction unit. See Figure 41–17.

■ Open the lubricant if performing nasopharyngeal suctioning.

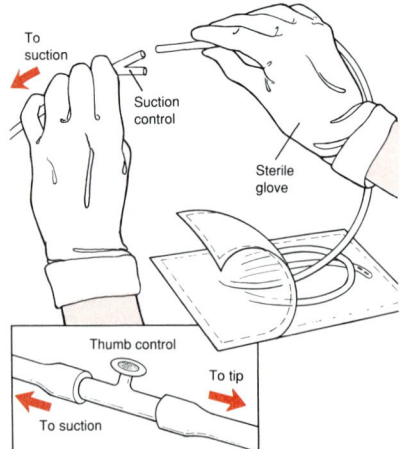

Figure 41–17 Attaching the catheter to the suction unit.

4. **Make an approximate measure of the depth for the insertion and test the equipment.**

■ Measure the distance between the tip of the client's nose and the earlobe, or about 13 cm (5 in) for an adult.

■ Mark the position on the tube with the fingers of the sterile gloved hand.

■ Test the pressure of the suction and the patency of the catheter by applying your sterile gloved finger or thumb to the port or open branch of the Y-connector (the suction control) to create suction.

5. **Lubricate and introduce the catheter.**

■ For nasopharyngeal suction, lubricate the catheter tip with water-soluble lubricant; for oropharyngeal suction, moisten the tip with sterile water or saline. *This reduces friction and eases insertion.*

For an oropharyngeal suction:

■ Pull the tongue forward, if necessary, using gauze.

■ Do not apply suction during insertion. *Doing so causes trauma to the mucous membrane.*

■ Advance the catheter about 4 to 6 in along one side of the mouth into the oropharynx. *Directing the catheter along the side prevents gagging.*

For a nasopharyngeal suction:

■ Without applying suction, insert the catheter into either naris and advance it along the floor of the nasal cavity. *This avoids the nasal turbinates.*

■ Never force the catheter against an obstruction. If one nostril is obstructed, try the other.

6. **Perform suctioning.**

■ Apply your finger to the suction control port to start suction, and gently rotate the catheter. *Gentle rotation of the catheter ensures that all surfaces are reached and prevents trauma to any one area of the respiratory mucosa due to prolonged suction.*

- Apply suction for 5 to 10 seconds, then remove your finger from the control, and remove the catheter.

- A suction attempt should last only 10 to 15 seconds. During this time, the catheter is inserted, the suction applied and discontinued, and the catheter removed.

- It may be necessary during oropharyngeal suctioning to apply suction to secretions that collect in the vestibule of the mouth and beneath the tongue.

7. Clean the catheter and repeat suctioning as above.

- Wipe off the catheter with sterile gauze if it is thickly coated with secretions.

- Flush the catheter with sterile water or saline.

- Relubricate the catheter, and repeat suctioning until the air passage is clear.

- Allow 20- to 30-second intervals between each suction, and limit suction to 2 minutes in total. *Applying suction for too long may cause secretions to increase or decrease the client's oxygen supply.*

- Alternate nares for repeat suctionings.

8. Encourage the client to breathe deeply and cough between suctions. *Coughing and deep breathing help carry secretions from the trachea and bronchi into the pharynx, where they can be reached with the suction catheter.*

9. Obtain specimen if required.
Use a sputum trap (see Figure 41–18) as follows:

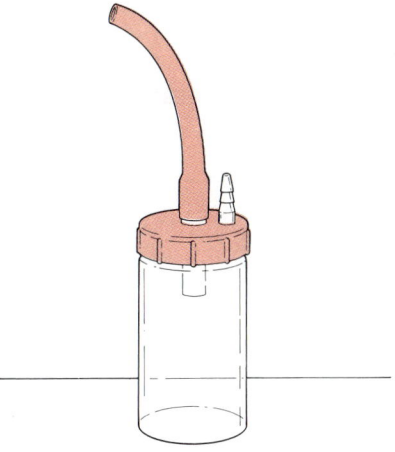

Figure 41–18   A sputum collection trap.

- Attach the suction catheter to the rubber tubing of the sputum trap.

- Attach the suction tubing to the sputum trap air vent.

- Suction the client's nasopharynx or oropharynx. The sputum trap will collect the mucus during suctioning.

- Remove the catheter from the client. Disconnect the sputum trap rubber tubing from the suction catheter. Remove the suction tubing from the trap air vent.

- Connect the rubber tubing of the sputum trap to the air vent. *This retains any microorganisms in the sputum trap.*

- Flush the catheter to remove secretions from the tubing.

10. Promote client comfort.

- Offer to assist the client with oral or nasal hygiene.

11. Dispose of equipment and ensure availability for next suction.

- Dispose of the catheter, gloves, water, and waste container. Wrap the catheter around your sterile

glove and roll it inside the glove for disposal.

- To ensure that equipment is available for the next suctioning, change suction collection bottles and tubing daily or more frequently as necessary.

12. Assess the effectiveness of suctioning.

- Auscultate the client's breathing sounds to ensure they are clear of secretions.

13. Document relevant data.

- Record the procedure: the amount, consistency, color, and odor of sputum, (e.g., foamy, white mucus; thick, green-tinged mucus; or blood-flecked mucus) and the client's breathing status before and after the procedure.

Sample Recording

Date: 5/12/91	Time: 0200

Oropharyngeal suctioning for 2 min. 35 ml thick, greenish sputum. Respirations 20/min, wet. Cyanotic. No response to painful stimuli. Positioned in left Sims'. -
———— Rozelle L. Schwartz, RN

- If the technique is carried out frequently e.g., q1h, it may be appropriate to record only once, at the end of the shift; however, the frequency of the suctioning must be recorded.

Sample Recording

Date: 5/12/91	Time: 0700

Nasopharyngeal suctioning q.1h. for 3 min. × 6. Nares alternated. 175 ml thick, greenish sputum obtained with 6 suctionings. Respirations remain dyspneic, 30–32/min. No response to verbal stimuli. Position changed q.1h. × 6. ————
———— Rozelle L. Schwartz, RN

Oxygen Therapy

Additional oxygen is indicated for numerous clients who have *hypoxemia,* for example, people who have reduced lung diffusion of oxygen through the respiratory membrane, heart failure leading to inadequate transport of oxygen, or substantial loss of lung tissue due to tumors or surgery. Oxygen therapy is prescribed by the physician, who specifies the specific concentration, method, and liter flow per minute. The concentration is of more importance than the liter flow per minute. When the administration of oxygen is an emergency measure, the nurse may initiate the therapy. The signs of hypoxemia generally include the following, in order of occurrence:

1. Increased rapid pulse
2. Rapid, shallow respirations and dyspnea
3. Increased restlessness or lightheadedness
4. Flaring of the nares
5. Substernal or intercostal retractions
6. Cyanosis

 Safety precautions are essential during oxygen therapy (see the accompanying box). Although oxygen by itself will

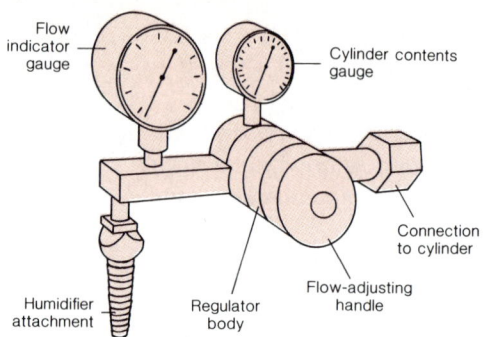

Figure 41–19 An oxygen regulator.

not burn or explode, it does facilitate combustion. For example, a bed sheet ordinarily burns slowly when ignited in the atmosphere; however, if saturated with free-flowing oxygen and ignited by a spark, it will burn rapidly and explosively. The greater the concentration of the oxygen, the more rapidly fires start and burn, and such fires are difficult to extinguish. Because oxygen is colorless, odorless, and tasteless, people are often unaware of its presence.

Oxygen is supplied in hospitals in two ways: by liquid portable systems (cylinders) and from wall outlets. Oxygen cylinders are made of steel. Large ones contain 244 cubic feet of oxygen stored at a pressure of 2200 pounds per square inch (psi). Smaller cylinders are available for emergency and ambulatory use. Piped-in oxygen is stored at much lower pressure, usually 50 to 60 psi.

Oxygen administered from a cylinder or wall-outlet system is dry. Dry gases dehydrate the respiratory mucous membranes. Humidifying devices are thus an essential adjunct of oxygen therapy, particularly for liter flows over 2 liters/minute.

Oxygen cylinders are generally encased in metal carriers equipped with wheels for transport and a broad flat base on which the cylinder stands at the bedside to prevent it from falling. A cap on the top protects the valves and outlets. Accidentally opened outlets can turn a stable tank into a dangerous projectile. A regulator and a humidifier must be attached before the cylinder is used. The purpose of the regulator is to release oxygen at a safe level and at a desirable rate. The regulator has two gauges: the *cylinder contents gauge* nearest the tank indicates the pressure or amount of oxygen in the tank; the *flow meter gauge* indicates the gas flow in liters per minute. To ensure that the regulator is firmly attached, the inlet nut is tightened with a wrench. See Figure 41–19. A humidifier bottle with distilled water is then attached below the flow meter gauge, and the specific oxygen tubing and equipment prescribed for the client, e.g., nasal cannula or mask, is attached to it.

Before the regulator is attached, any dust particles in the outlets must be removed to prevent them from being forced into the regulator. This task is accomplished by slightly opening the handwheel at the top of the cylinder counterclockwise and then quickly closing it. This procedure, referred to as "cracking the cylinder," releases a small amount

---

Oxygen Therapy Safety Precautions

- Place cautionary signs reading "No Smoking: Oxygen in Use" on the client's door, at the foot or head of the bed, and on the oxygen equipment.

- Instruct the client and visitors about the hazard of smoking with oxygen in use.

- Request other clients in the room and visitors to smoke in areas provided elsewhere in the hospital.

- Make sure that electrical equipment, such as razors, hearing aids, radios, televisions, and heating pads, is in good working order to prevent the occurrence of short-circuit sparks.

- Avoid materials that generate static electricity, such as woolen blankets and synthetic fabrics. Cotton blankets are used, and nurses are advised to wear cotton fabrics.

- Avoid the use of volatile, flammable materials, such as oils, greases, alcohol, and ether, near clients receiving oxygen. Avoid alcohol back rubs and take nail polish removers or the like away from the immediate vicinity.

- Ground electric monitoring equipment, suction machines, and portable diagnostic machines.

- Make known the location of fire extinguishers, and make sure personnel are trained in their use.

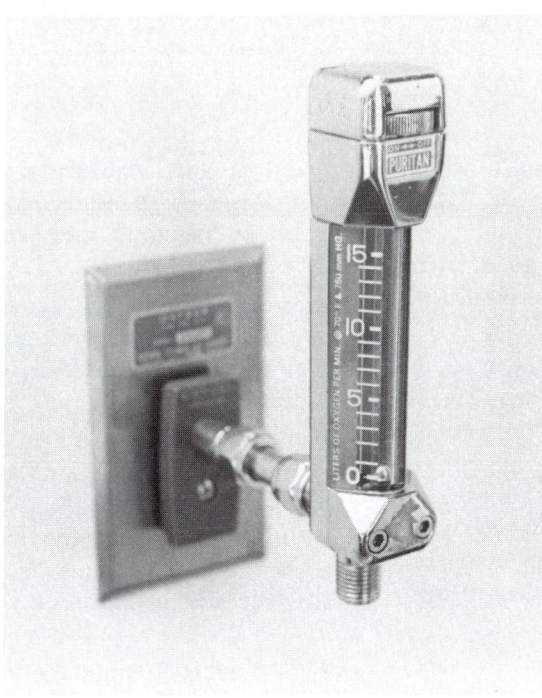

Figure 41-20 An oxygen flow meter attached to a wall outlet.

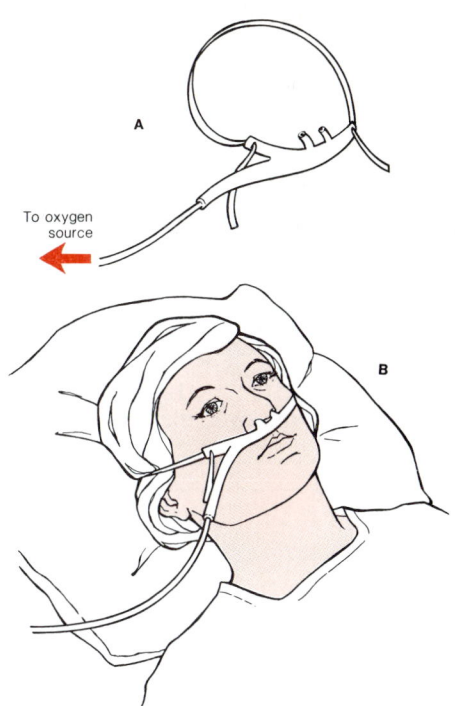

Figure 41-21 *A,* nasal cannula; *B,* the cannula in place.

of oxygen that flushes out the outlet. The force of this oxygen release causes a loud hissing noise that is startling and frightening to most people. Nurses should therefore forewarn clients and others or prime the tank away from the bedside. Oxygen cylinders need to be handled and stored with caution and strapped securely in wheeled transport devices or stands to prevent possible falls and outlet breakages. They should be placed away from traffic areas and heaters.

To use an oxygen wall outlet:

1. Attach the flow meter to the wall outlet, exerting firm pressure. The flow meter should be in the off position. See Figure 41-20.

2. Fill the humidifier bottle with distilled water. (This can be done before coming to the bedside.)

3. Attach the humidifier bottle to the base of the flow meter. See Figure 41-7 on page 1107.

4. Attach the prescribed oxygen tubing and delivery device to the humidifier.

5. Regulate the flow meter to the prescribed level.

Oxygen is administered by either low-flow or high-flow systems. The fraction of inspired oxygen (Fio_2) is variable, depending on the client's respiratory rate and volume and the oxygen liter flow. *Low-flow administration devices* include nasal cannula, simple face mask, partial rebreathing mask, nonrebreathing mask, Croupette, and oxygen tent. A low-flow system is contraindicated when a client requires a carefully monitored oxygen concentration.

A *high-flow oxygen system* delivers all the gas required. It provides a precise amount of oxygen, regardless of the client's respirations. The ratio of room air to oxygen is regulated and does not vary with the client's respirations. The Venturi mask is an example of a high-flow administration device. Some devices can be used for both low- and high-flow administration, e.g., the face tent, oxygen hood, and incubator (Isolette).

The **nasal cannula** (nasal prongs) is the most common low-flow device used to administer oxygen. It consists of a rubber or plastic tube that extends around the face, with 0.6- to 1.3-cm (¼ to ½-in) curved prongs that fit into the nostrils. One side of the tube connects to the oxygen tubing and oxygen supply. The cannula is often held in place by an elastic band that fits around the client's head or under the chin. See Figure 41-21. For clients who are confused or particularly active, it may be helpful to secure the cannula in place with small pieces of tape on each side of the face.

The nasal cannula is easy to apply and does not interfere with the client's ability to eat or talk. It also is relatively comfortable and permits some freedom of movement. It delivers a relatively low concentration of oxygen (24% to 45%) at flow rates of 2 to 6 liters per minute. Higher concentrations and flow rates can be administered; however, above 6 liters per minute there is a tendency for the client to swallow air and for the nasal and pharyngeal mucosa to become irritated.

Administering oxygen by cannula is detailed in Procedure 41-2.

ADMINISTERING OXYGEN BY CANNULA

Equipment ☑

Oxygen supply with a flow meter

Humidifier with sterile distilled water

Nasal cannula and tubing

Tape, if needed, to secure the cannula in place

Gauzes to pad the tubing over the cheekbones

Intervention

1. Determine the need for oxygen therapy and verify the physician's order.

■ Perform a respiratory assessment to determine the need for O_2 therapy.

■ Check the physician's order for the method of delivery and percentage of oxygen or liter flow.

2. Prepare the client and support persons.

■ Assist the client to a semi-Fowler's position if possible. *This position permits easier chest expansion and hence easier breathing.*

■ Explain that oxygen is not dangerous when safety precautions are observed and that it will ease the discomfort of dyspnea. Inform the client and support persons about the safety precautions connected with oxygen use.

3. Set up the oxygen equipment and the humidifier. See page 1118.

4. Turn on the oxygen at the prescribed rate and ensure proper functioning.

■ Check that the oxygen is flowing freely through the tubing. There should be no kinks in the tubing, and the connections should be airtight. There should be bubbles in the humidifier as the oxygen flows through the water. You should feel the oxygen at the outlets of the cannula.

■ Set the oxygen at the flow rate ordered, e.g., 2 to 6 liters per minute.

5. Apply the cannula.

■ Put the cannula over the client's face, with the outlet prongs fitting into the nares and the elastic band around the head. Some models have a strap to adjust under the chin.

■ If the cannula will not stay in place, tape it at the sides of the face.

■ Slip gauze pads under the tubing over the cheekbones to prevent skin irritation as necessary.

6. Assess the client regularly.

■ Assess the client's color and ease of respirations and provide support while adjusting to the cannula.

■ Assess the client in 15 to 30 minutes, depending on the client's condition, and regularly thereafter. Assess vital signs, color, breathing patterns, and chest movements.

■ Assess the client regularly for clinical signs of hypoxia: tachycardia, confusion, dyspnea, restlessness, and cyanosis.

■ Assess the client's nares for encrustations and irritation. Apply a water-soluble lubricant as required to soothe the mucous membranes.

7. Inspect the equipment regularly.

■ Check the liter flow and the level of water in the humidifier in 30 minutes and whenever providing care to the client.

■ Make sure that safety precautions are being followed.

8. Document relevant data.

■ Record initiation of the therapy and all nursing assessments.

Sample Recording

Date: 12-5-91	Time: 0730

P 96, R 24. Slightly cyanotic, dyspneic on exertion, and restless. O_2 by cannula at 3 L/min. applied. Susan de Camillis, SN

	Time: 0800

No cyanosis apparent. P 84, R 16. States "breathing is easier." Is less restless. ——
———————— Susan de Camillis, SN

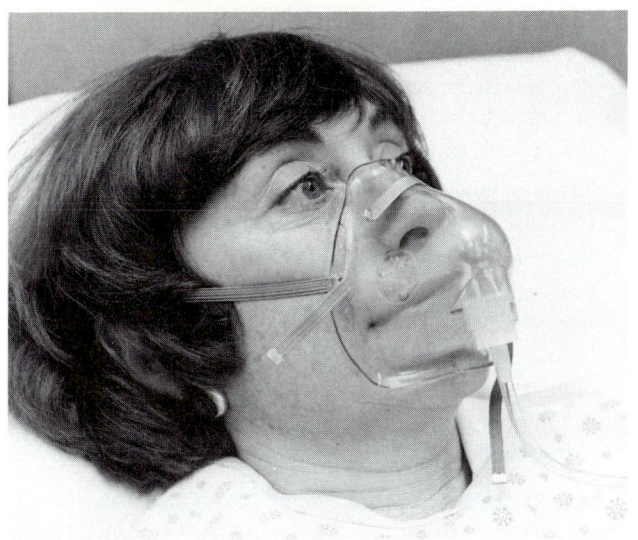

Figure 41–22   A simple face mask for a low-flow oxygen system.

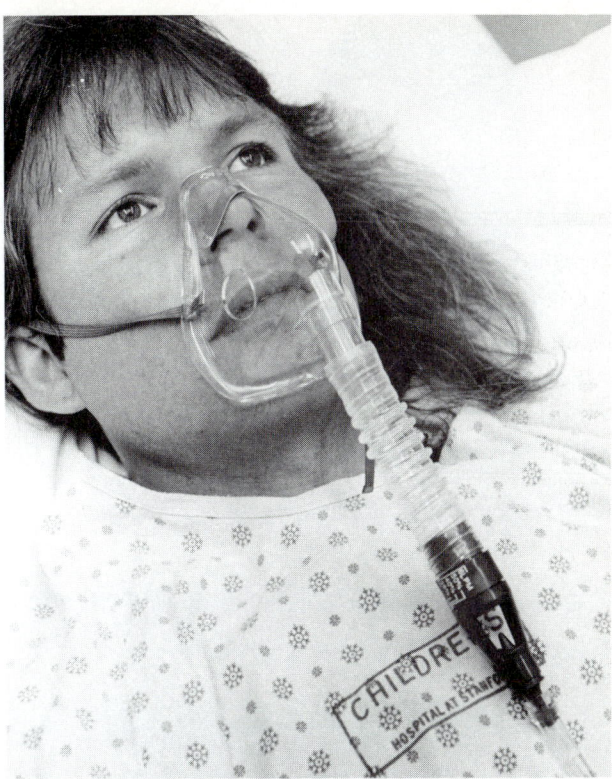

Figure 41–23   A Venturi mask for a high-flow oxygen system.

Face masks that cover the client's nose and mouth may be used for oxygen inhalation. Most masks are made of clear, pliable plastic or rubber that can be molded to fit the face. They are held to the client's head with elastic bands. Some have a metal clip that can be bent over the bridge of the nose for a snug fit. There are several holes in the sides of the mask (exhalation ports) to allow the escape of exhaled carbon dioxide.

Some masks have reservoir bags, which provide higher oxygen concentrations to the client. A portion of the client's expired air is directed into the bag. Because this air comes from the upper respiratory passages (e.g., the trachea and bronchi), where it does not take part in gaseous exchange, its oxygen concentration remains the same as that of inspired air.

A variety of oxygen masks are marketed:

- The *simple face mask* (low-flow system) delivers oxygen concentrations from 40% to 60% at liter flows of 5 to 8 liters per minute. See Figure 41–22.

- The *partial rebreather mask* (low-flow system) delivers oxygen concentrations of 60% to 90% at liter flows of 6 to 10 liters per minute. The oxygen reservoir bag that is attached allows the client to rebreathe about the first third of the exhaled air. The partial rebreather bag must not totally deflate during inspiration. If this problem occurs, increase the liter flow of oxygen.

- The *nonrebreather mask* (low-flow system) delivers the highest oxygen concentration possible by means other than intubation or mechanical ventilation, i.e., 95% to 100%, at liter flows of 6 to 15 liters per minute. Using a nonrebreather mask, the client breathes only the source gas from the bag. One-way valves on the mask and between

the reservoir bag and the mask prevent the room air and the client's exhaled air from entering the bag. The non-rebreather bag must not totally deflate during inspiration. If it does, this problem can be corrected by increasing the liter flow of oxygen.

- The *Venturi mask* (high-flow system) delivers oxygen concentrations precise to within 1% and is often used for clients with COPD. See Figure 44–23. Oxygen concentrations vary from 24% to 40% or 50%, depending on the brand, at liter flows of 4 to 8 liters per minute. The Venturi mask is designed with wide-bore tubing and various color-coded jet adapters. Each color code corresponds to a precise oxygen concentration and a specific liter flow. For example, a blue adapter delivers a 24% concentration of oxygen at 4 liters per minute, and a green adapter delivers a 35% concentration of oxygen at 8 liters per minute. Optional humidification adapters are also available for clients who require them, e.g., those receiving oxygen concentrations in excess of 30%.

Initiating oxygen by mask is much the same as initiating oxygen by cannula, except that the nurse must find a mask of appropriate size. Smaller sizes are available for children. When fitting a client with a face mask, the nurse needs to

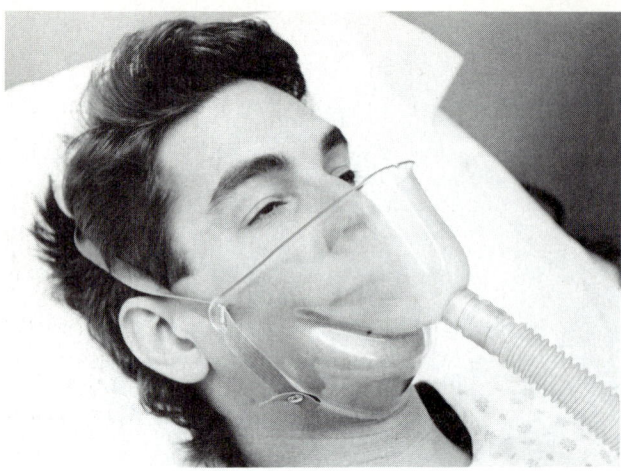

Figure 41–24   An oxygen face tent.

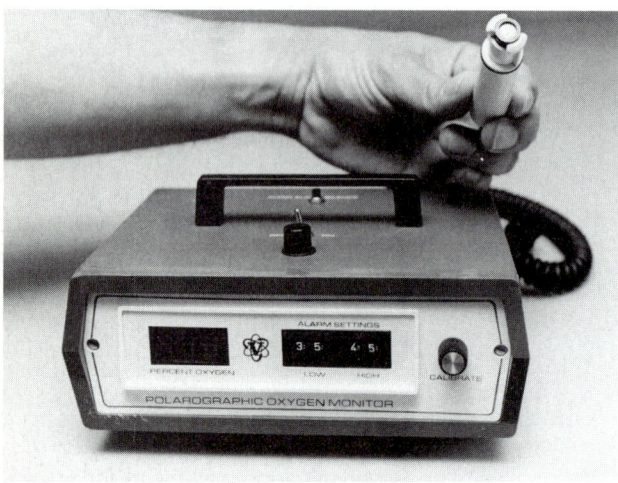

Figure 41–25   An oxygen analyzer.

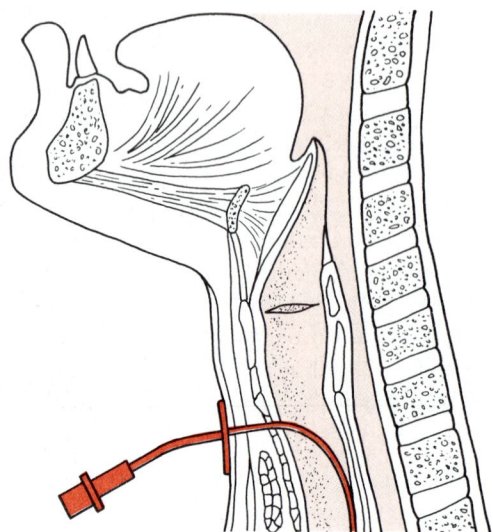

Figure 41–26   A transtracheal oxygen catheter in place.

1. Familiarize the client with the mask when possible. Allow the client to hold the mask, guide it toward the face, and get used to the sensation of the mask covering the nose and mouth. Instruct the client to put on the mask from the nose downward during expiration.

2. Turn on the oxygen to the prescribed rate of flow. When the mask has a reservoir bag, the nurse should first flush the mask with oxygen until it is partially inflated.

3. Gradually fit the mask to the contours of the face, and encourage the client to breathe normally. The mask should be molded to prevent oxygen escaping upward into the client's eyes or around the cheeks or chin. Pad the band behind the ears and over bony prominences to prevent skin irritation.

Face tents can replace oxygen masks when masks are poorly tolerated by clients (e.g., children). See Figure 41–24. When a face tent alone is used to supply oxygen, the concentration of oxygen varies; therefore, it is often used in conjunction with a Venturi system. Face tents provide varying concentrations of oxygen at 8 to 10 liters per minute. Frequently inspect the client's facial skin for dampness or chafing, and dry and treat as needed. As with face masks, the client's facial skin must be kept dry.

Oxygen analyzers (see Figure 41–25) measure the concentration of oxygen being received by the client. The analyzer is first used to measure the concentration of oxygen in the room. It should register 0.21 (21%). If it does not, the nurse adjusts the dial to this calibration. Then the sampling tube is placed next to the client's nose, and the reading on the analyzer is monitored. The nurse adjusts the oxygen flow rate to obtain the desired fraction of inspired oxygen (FiO_2).

Home delivery devices are now available to clients who require continuous oxygen therapy at home. *Transtracheal oxygen delivery* refers to oxygen given through a small narrow plastic cannula that is inserted through the skin at the base of the neck directly into the trachea. See Figure 41–26. A chain around the neck holds the catheter in place. With this delivery system, the client requires less oxygen because all of the flow delivered enters the lungs. Portable oxygen devices last much longer between refills, and therapy is thus obtained at a lower cost. Clients also report improved mobility, comfort, and appearance in comparison to the nasal cannula. To be considered for this type of delivery system, the client must have a PaO_2 below 55 mm Hg or an oxygen saturation below 85% while breathing room air at rest and when exercising. The catheter is kept patent by injecting 1.5 ml normal saline into it, moving a cleaning rod in and out of it and then injecting another 1.5 ml of saline solution. This is done two or three times a day.

A new device referred to as *Oxy-Frames* delivers oxygen through specially designed eyeglasses that provide the same liter flow as nasal cannulae. The oxygen tubing is camouflaged in grooves on the inside of the frames. It extends down the inside of the frames and around the perimeter of the lens and terminates in a small plastic cannula that enters the nares. The portion of the cannula entering the nares can be detached for maintenance or replaced.

Another option is the *Nocturnal Cannula,* oxygen tubing held in place with a headband. The plastic tubing extends from the headband around the forehead along the sides of the nose into the nares. This device is useful for clients whose nasal cannula tends to become dislodged during sleep. It can also be used during the day to relieve pressure points on the cheeks and ears obtained from the nasal cannula.

Reservoir cannulae or *Oxymizers* are nasal cannula devices with plastic reservoirs that store oxygen and deliver a 20-ml bolus of oxygen during the first part of the inspiratory cycle. The plastic reservoirs inflate with 20 ml of oxygen during expiration and deflate at the beginning of inspiration when delivering this 20-ml bolus, which goes directly to the alveoli. After the bolus is delivered, oxygen is received as usual through the nasal cannula. Some nasal breathing on both inspiration and expiration is needed to trigger the device. One type of oxymizer consists of a reservoir worn under the nose in the mustache area. Another, less visible, type is the oxymizer pendant, which consists of a large storage pendant and tubing larger than standard. Because of its weight, the pendant oximizer may cause soreness in the area where the device is anchored to the ears. Oxymizers are helpful for clients who require a liter flow greater than 4 liters/minute. The client can be away from home for longer periods, since the reservoir extends the time a portable unit lasts between refills.

Demand devices (Pulsair, Oxymatic) are battery-operated devices that deliver a bolus of oxygen *only* at the beginning of inhalation. They conserve oxygen, since oxygen delivery during exhalation and late inhalation is avoided. These devices are triggered to deliver oxygen when negative pressure at the tip of the nasal cannula is sensed.

Artificial Airways

Artificial airways are inserted to maintain a patent air passage for clients whose airway has become or may become obstructed. A patent airway is necessary so that air can flow to and from the lungs. Four of the more common types of intubation are oropharyngeal, nasopharyngeal, endotracheal, and tracheostomy.

Oropharyngeal intubation is done most frequently for clients who have had general anesthesia and for those who are semiconscious and are likely to obstruct their own airways with their tongues. An oropharyngeal tube is inserted in some instances for pharyngeal suctioning. It is not inserted in clients who are conscious, because it stimulates the gag reflex and thus can cause vomiting. Oropharyngeal tubes are somewhat S-shaped and usually made of plastic. Adult, child, and infant sizes are available. The tube is inserted through the mouth and terminates in the posterior pharynx. See Figure 41–27.

To insert an oropharyngeal airway, the nurse dons dis-

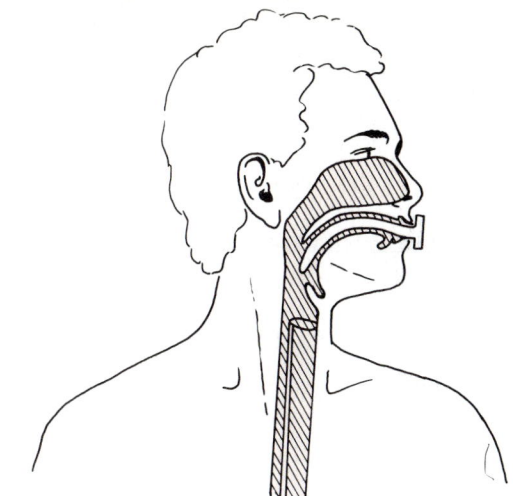

Figure 41–27   An oropharyngeal tube in place.

posable gloves, opens the client's mouth, and removes any dentures present. The client should be in a supine position, with the neck hyperextended or with a pillow placed under the shoulders so that the tongue cannot fall back to block the pharynx. This position may be contraindicated for clients with head, neck, or back injuries. The nurse then lubricates the airway with a water-soluble lubricant and advances the airway sideways along the roof of the mouth until the flange touches the mouth. The airway is rotated when introducing it over the tongue to the pharynx. If necessary, the nurse tapes the airway in position and suctions secretions as necessary.

Nursing interventions for intubated clients include the following:

- Maintain the client in a lateral or semiprone position so that blood, vomitus, and mucus will drain out of the mouth and not be aspirated.

- Remove the airway once the client has regained consciousness and has the swallow, gag, and cough reflexes.

Nasopharyngeal intubation is carried out if the oropharyngeal route is contraindicated, e.g., following oral surgery. A nasopharyngeal tube may also be inserted to protect the nasal and pharyngeal mucosa during nasopharyngeal or nasotracheal suctioning. The tube is inserted through a nostril and terminates in the pharynx, below the upper edge of the epiglottis. See Figure 41–28 on page 1124. Tubes vary in size for adults, children, and infants. They are usually made of latex rubber.

To insert a nasopharyngeal tube, the nurse lubricates the entire tube with a topical anesthetic (if ordered) to prevent irritation of the nasopharyngeal mucosa and undue discomfort. The nurse then holds the airway by the wide end and inserts the narrow end into the naris, applying gentle inward and downward pressure when advancing the airway to follow the natural course of the nasal structures. The nurse

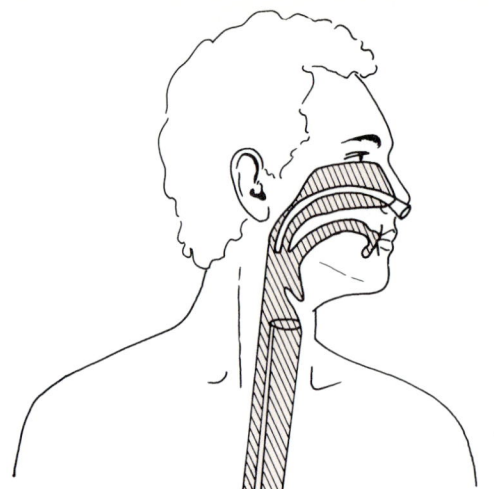

Figure 41–28 A nasopharyngeal tube in place.

removes excess lubricant from the client's face and nares before securing the tube in place with tape.

Nursing interventions for clients with nasopharyngeal tubes include the following:

- Remove the tube, and insert it in the other nostril at least every 8 hours, or as ordered by the physician, or more often to prevent irritation of the mucosa.

- Provide nasal hygiene every 4 hours or more often if needed.

- Monitor the client closely for stimulation of the vagus nerve if nasotracheal suctioning is carried out. Vagal stimulation can lead to cardiac arrest.

Endotracheal tubes are most commonly inserted for clients who have had general anesthetics or for those in emergency situations where mechanical ventilation is required. An endotracheal tube is a curved polyvinylchloride tube that is inserted through either the mouth or the nose and into the trachea with the guide of a laryngoscope. See Figure 41–29. It terminates just superior to the bifurcation of the trachea into the bronchi. Because an endotracheal tube passes through the epiglottis and splits it open, an inflated cuff is needed to close the system. Nursing interventions for clients with endotracheal tubes in place include the following:

- Maintain the client in a lateral or semiprone position so that blood, vomitus, or secretions can drain from the mouth and are not aspirated.

- Provide oral or nasal hygiene every 3 hours or as needed.

- For an oral insertion, provide a bite block so that the client cannot bite the tube and occlude the airway.

- Assess the condition of the nasal or oral mucosa for irritation and notify the physician should the need to change a nasal endotracheal tube arise; reposition an oral endotracheal tube from one side of the mouth to the other every 8 hours or as required.

- Closely monitor the air pressure in the endotracheal cuff. If it is greater than 20 mm Hg, necrosis of the tracheal tissues can result.

- Tape the airway in place to prevent accidental slippage or extubation.

- Change the tape daily, and position the tube on the opposite side of the mouth at each change.

- Provide continuous humidification or aerosol therapy to prevent undue drying and irritation of the mucous membranes, if the tube is left in for more than a short time (e.g., for days or weeks).

- Deflate and reinflate the cuff according to the manufacturer's directions.

- Communicate frequently with the client and provide a notepad or other means for the client to communicate. Most clients cannot speak with an inflated cuff since no air can pass over the vocal cords.

Tracheostomy tubes are inserted to provide and maintain a patent airway, to remove tracheobronchial secretions from clients unable to cough, to replace endotracheal tubes, to permit the use of positive pressure ventilation, and to prevent unconscious clients from aspirating secretions.

A tracheostomy tube is a curved tube that is inserted into a tracheostomy (a surgical incision in the trachea just below the first or second tracheal cartilage). See Figure 41–30. The tube extends through the tracheostomy stoma into the trachea. See Figure 41–31. Tracheostomy tubes come in different sizes and may be made of metal, plastic, or foam. Plastic tubes are increasingly popular, because they are lightweight, their parts are interchangeable, and crusting from the tissues rarely forms on plastic materials.

The main parts of a tracheostomy set are the outer tube, the inner tube or inner cannula, and the obturator. See

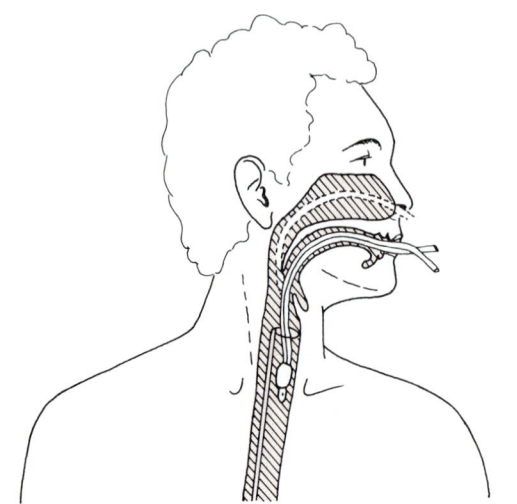

Figure 41–29 An endotracheal tube in place.

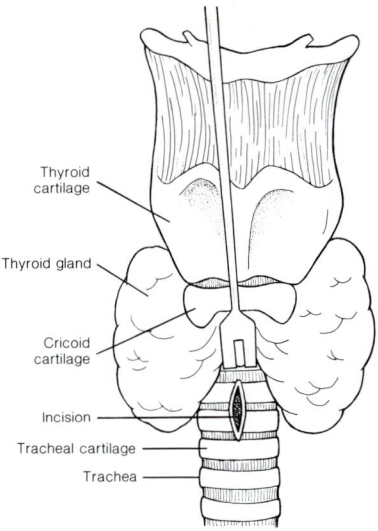

Figure 41-30   Site of a tracheostomy incision.

Thyroid
cartilage

Thyroid gland

Cricoid
cartilage

Incision

Tracheal cartilage

Trachea

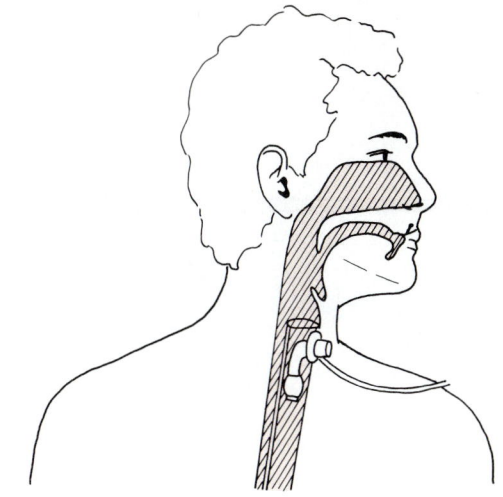

Figure 41-31   A tracheostomy tube in place.

Figure 41–32. The obturator is used only to insert the outer tube. It is removed once the outer tube is in place. The outer tube usually has ties to secure it around the client's neck, although many plastic tubes are cuffed with a soft balloon that can be inflated to hold the tube in place (see below). Fitted inside the outer tube is an inner cannula. (Some plastic sets do not have this, because it is unnecessary to change the tube. They are called *single-cannula tubes.*) In double-cannula sets, the inner cannula is inserted and locked in place after the obturator is removed; it acts as a removable liner for the more permanent, outer cannula. The inner tube is withdrawn for brief periods to be cleaned.

Cuffed tracheostomy tubes are surrounded by an inflatable cuff that produces an airtight seal between the tube and the trachea. This seal prevents aspiration of orophar-

yngeal secretions and air leakage between the tube and the trachea. Cuffed tubes are often used immediately after a tracheostomy in adults and infants and are essential when ventilating a tracheostomy client with a ventilator. Children do not require cuffed tubes, since their tracheas are resilient enough to seal the air space around the tube.

Some tubes have high-pressure cuffs, others have low-pressure cuffs. Some high-pressure tubes are double-cuffed; these can be inflated alternately to alter the pressure points on the trachea and prevent tracheal irritation and tissue damage. Alternate inflation also allows uninterrupted respirator function for people using ventilators. Commercially prepared cuffs are available for use on cuffless tracheostomy tubes.

Different cuffed tubes have different advantages and disadvantages. Cuffs that are bonded to the tracheostomy tube

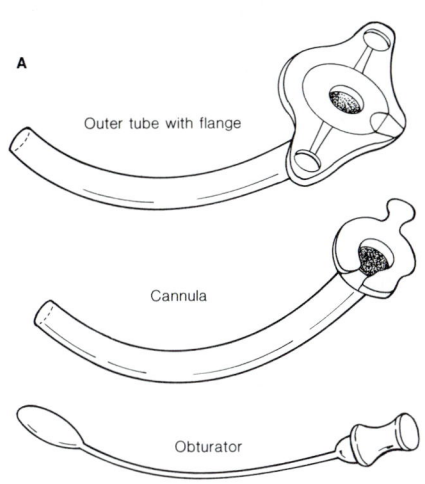

A

Outer tube with flange

Cannula

Obturator

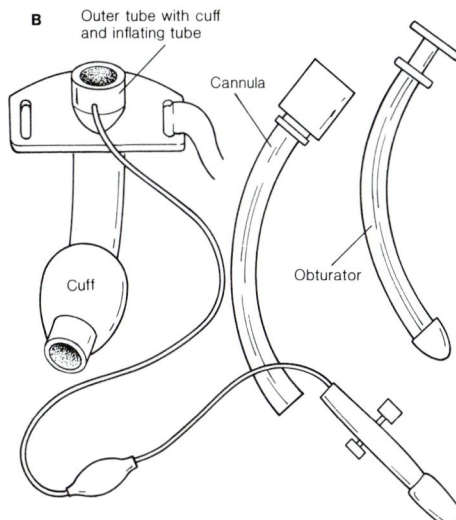

B   Outer tube with cuff
and inflating tube

Cannula

Cuff

Obturator

Figure 41-32   Two types of tracheostomy sets: *A,* noncuffed; *B,* cuffed.

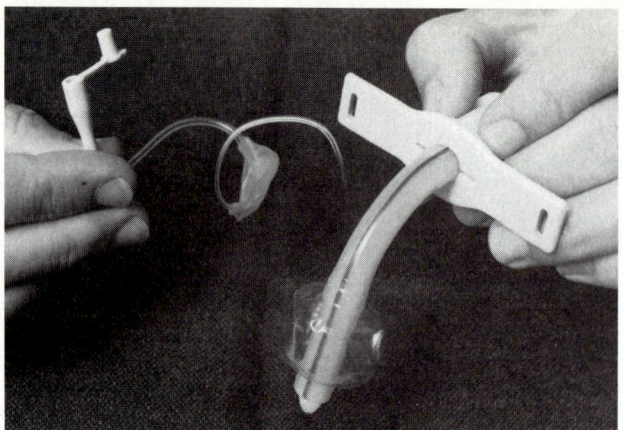

Figure 41–33 A tracheostomy tube with a foam cuff.

the risk of tissue necrosis with alternate inflation of cuffs but *only* if there is rigid adherence to the alternate inflation schedule. If tracheal damage does occur, a larger area of the trachea is involved with double-cuffed tubes.

A variation of the cuffed tube is the foam cuff. It does not require injected air; instead, when the port is opened, ambient air enters the balloon, which then conforms to the client's trachea. See Figure 41–33. The physician removes air from the cuff prior to insertion or removal of the tube.

For **tracheostomy and endotracheal suctioning and lavage,** the diameter of the suction catheter should be about half the inside diameter of the tracheostomy tube so that hypoxia can be prevented.

Sterile normal saline without a bacteriostatic preservative is often used for tracheal lavage. The amount used varies: 0.5 to 1 ml is generally used for infants, 2 ml for children, and 2 to 5 ml for adults. Suctioning a tracheostomy or endotracheal tube is discussed in detail in Procedure 41–3.

Double-cannula tracheostomy tubes are cleaned whenever necessary, but at least once per shift. See Procedure 41–4 on page 1128.

eliminate the risk of accidental detachment inside the trachea. Low-pressure cuffs, which are more costly than others, distribute a low, even pressure against the trachea, thus decreasing the risk of tracheal tissue necrosis. They do not need to be deflated periodically to reduce pressure on the tracheal wall. Double-cuffed high-pressure tubes may reduce

---

PROCEDURE 41–3

SUCTIONING A TRACHEOSTOMY OR ENDOTRACHEAL TUBE

Equipment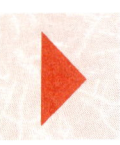

Equipment for suctioning the oropharyngeal cavity (see Procedure 41–1)

Sterile 2- to 10-ml syringe and sterile normal saline

Sterile towel

Resuscitation bag connected to 100% oxygen

Goggles and mask if necessary

Gown (if necessary)

Intervention

1. Prepare the client.

■ Inform the client that suctioning usually causes intermittent coughing and that this assists in removing the secretions.

■ If not contraindicated because of health, place the client in semi-Fowler's position to promote deep breathing, maximum lung expansion, and productive coughing. *Deep breathing oxygenates the lungs, counteracts the hypoxic effects of suctioning, and may induce coughing. Coughing helps to loosen and move secretions.*

2. Prepare the equipment.

■ Attach the resuscitation apparatus to the oxygen source. See Figure 41–34. Adjust the oxygen flow to "100% flush."

■ Open the sterile supplies in readiness for use.

■ Place the sterile towel, if used, across the client's chest, below the tracheostomy.

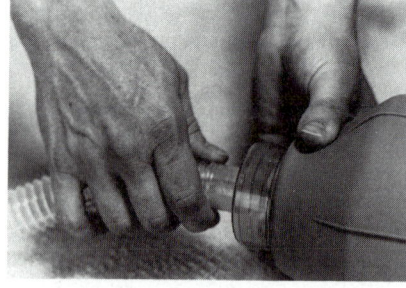

Figure 41–34 Attaching the resuscitation apparatus to the oxygen source.

■ Turn on the suction, and set the pressure in accordance with agency policy. For a wall unit, pressure of about 100 to 120 mm Hg is normally used for adults, 50 to 95 mm Hg for infants and children.

■ Put on goggles and mask (and gown if necessary).

■ Put on sterile gloves. Some agencies recommend putting a sterile glove on the dominant hand and an unsterile glove on the nondominant hand to protect the nurse.

■ Holding the catheter in the dominant hand and the connector in the nondominant hand, attach the catheter to the Y-connector or straight connector. See Figure 41–17, earlier.

3. Flush and lubricate the catheter.

■ Using the dominant hand, place the catheter tip in the sterile saline solution.

■ Using the thumb of the nondominant hand, occlude the thumb control, and suction a small amount of sterile solution through the catheter. *This determines that the suction equipment is working properly and lubricates the outside and the lumen of the catheter. Lubrication eases insertion and reduces tissue trauma during insertion.* Lubricating the lumen also helps prevent secretions from sticking to the inside of the catheter.

4. If the client does *not* have copious secretions, hyperventilate the lungs with a resuscitation bag before suctioning.

■ Summon an assistant, if one is available, for this step.

■ Using your nondominant hand, turn on the oxygen to 12 to 15 L/min.

■ If the client is receiving oxygen, disconnect the oxygen source from the tracheostomy tube using your nondominant hand.

■ Attach the resuscitator to the tracheostomy or endotracheal tube. See Figure 41–35.

■ Compress the Ambu bag five times as the client inhales. This is best done by a second person, who can use both hands to compress the

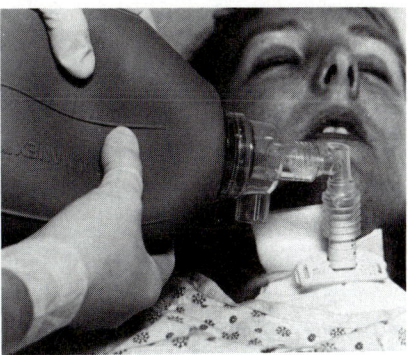

Figure 41–35 Attaching the resuscitator to the tracheostomy.

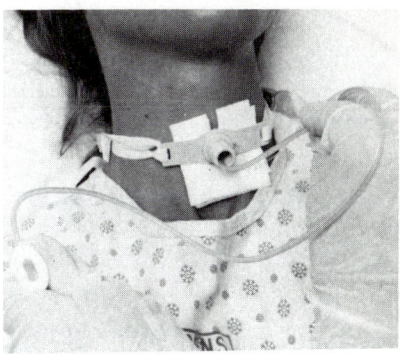

Figure 41–36 Inserting the catheter into the trachea through the tracheostomy tube.

bag, providing a greater inflation volume.

■ Observe the rise and fall of the client's chest to assess the adequacy of each ventilation.

■ Remove the resuscitation device and place it on the bed or the client's chest with the connector facing up.

5. If the client has copious secretions, do *not* hyperventilate with a resuscitator. Instead:

■ Keep the regular oxygen delivery device on, and increase the liter flow for a few minutes before suctioning. *Hyperventilating a client who has copious secretions can force the secretions deeper into the respiratory tract.*

6. Quickly, but gently, insert the catheter.

■ With your nondominant thumb off the suction port, quickly but gently insert the catheter into the trachea through the tracheostomy tube. See Figure 41–36. *To prevent tissue trauma and oxygen loss, suction is not applied during insertion of the catheter.*

■ Insert the catheter about 12.5 cm (6 in) or until the client coughs.

7. Perform suctioning.

■ Apply suction for 5 to 10 seconds by placing the nondominant thumb over the thumb port. *Suction time is restricted to 10 seconds or less to minimize oxygen loss.*

■ Rotate the catheter by rolling it between your thumb and forefinger while slowly withdrawing it. *This prevents tissue trauma by minimizing the suction time against any part of the trachea.*

■ Withdraw the catheter completely, and release the suction.

8. If secretions are thick, flush the catheter and perform tracheal lavage according to agency protocol.

■ Flush the catheter with sterile water or saline.

■ Insert 2 to 5 ml of sterile saline solution through the tracheostomy tube into the trachea. *This liquefies tenacious secretions so that they are more easily suctioned out.*

■ Then suction again.

9. Reassess the client's oxygenation status and repeat suctioning as above.

■ Observe the client's respirations and skin color. With your clean hand, check the client's pulse if necessary.

- Encourage the client to breathe deeply and to cough between suctions.

- Flush the catheter, and repeat suctioning until the air passage is clear and the breathing is relatively effortless and quiet.

- After each suction, pick up the resuscitation bag with your clean hand, and ventilate the client with five breaths.

10. Dispose of equipment and ensure availability for the next suction.

- Flush the catheter and suction tubing.

- Turn off the suction, and disconnect the catheter from the suction tubing.

- Wrap the catheter around your sterile hand, and peel the glove off, so that it turns inside out over the catheter.

- Discard the glove and the catheter in the moisture-resistant bag.

- Replenish the sterile fluid and supplies so that the suction is ready to be used again. *Clients who require suctioning often require it quickly, so it is essential to leave the equipment at the bedside ready for use.*

11. Provide for client comfort and safety.

- Assist the client to a comfortable, safe position that aids breathing. If the person is conscious, a semi-Fowler's position is frequently indicated. If the person is unconscious, Sim's position can assist the drainage of secretions from the mouth.

12. Document relevant data.

- Record the suctioning, including the amount and description of suction returns, the amount of sterile saline instilled, and any other relevant assessment (e.g., the client's respirations and breath sounds).

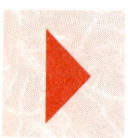

PROCEDURE 41–4

CLEANING A DOUBLE-CANNULA TRACHEOSTOMY TUBE

Equipment

Sterile bowls for the cleaning solutions

Hydrogen peroxide and sterile normal saline

Sterile nylon brush or pipe cleaners

Sterile gauze squares or sterile cotton-tipped applicator sticks

Sterile gloves (1 pair and 1 glove or 2 pairs)

Clean glove

Intervention

1. Don gloves, and suction the tracheostomy tube.

- Put on an unsterile glove on the nondominant hand and a sterile glove on your dominant hand.

- Suction the entire length of the inner cannula prior to its removal to remove secretions and ensure a patent airway. (See Procedure 41–3).

2. Remove and soak the inner cannula.

- With the nondominant hand, unlock the inner cannula by turning the lock about 90° counterclockwise. The nondominant hand is used to handle the flange of the cannula, which is not sterile.

- With the nondominant hand, remove the inner cannula by gently pulling it out toward you in line with its curvature.

- Soak the inner cannula in the hydrogen peroxide solution for several minutes. *This moistens and loosens dried secretions.*

3. Change gloves, and clean the cannula.

- Remove the gloves, and replace them with sterile gloves on both hands. Both hands are needed to clean the tube. *To maintain sterile technique, both hands must be gloved.*

- Remove the cannula from the soaking solution.

- Clean the lumen and entire inner cannula thoroughly, using the pipe cleaners or brush moistened with sterile saline.

■ Agitate the cannula for several seconds in the sterile saline. *This thoroughly rinses the cannula and provides a thin film of moisture to lubricate for insertion.*

■ Inspect the cannula for cleanliness by holding it at eye level and looking through it into the light. If encrustations are evident, repeat above steps.

■ After rinsing the cannula, gently tap it against the inside edge of the sterile solution bowl. *This removes excess liquid from the cannula and prevents possible aspiration of it by the client.*

4. Dry the *inside* of the cannula.

■ Use two or three pipe cleaners twisted together to dry the inside of the cannula. Do not dry the outer surface. *A thin film of moisture on the outer surface acts as a lubricant for insertion.*

5. Suction the outer cannula.
Secretions must be removed to prevent adherence of the two tubes when the inner cannula is inserted.

6. Clean the flange of the outer cannula if necessary.

■ Use clean cotton-tipped applicators or gauze squares moistened with sterile saline to clean the flange.

7. Insert the clean inner cannula, and secure it.

■ Grasp the outer flange of the inner cannula, and insert the cannula in the direction of its curvature.

■ Lock the inner cannula in place by turning the lock clockwise about 90° to an upright position.

■ Gently pull on the inner cannula to ensure that the position is secure.

8. Document relevant data.

■ On the client's chart record the removal, cleaning, and reinsertion of the cannula and all assessments.

A **minitracheostomy** (MT) is a technique in which a cannula with an internal diameter of 4 mm is inserted into the trachea, through the cricothyroid membrane. It is not recommended for children under age 12 years. MT is easily performed in the nursing unit under local anesthesia without sedation. Before the development of MT, the treatment of sputum retention depended on nasal/oropharyngeal suction and endotracheal intubation or tracheostomy. Because nasal or oral suction is very unpleasant for conscious clients and intubation interferes with talking and coughing abilities, MT offers distinct advantages for specific clients (Preston, Matthews, and Ready 1986, p. 496):

■ The client still breathes normally through the mouth and nose, thereby filtering and humidifying the air and reducing the risk of superadded infection.

■ No respiratory crises occur if the MT becomes blocked.

■ The client can talk and cough normally (when otherwise able).

■ The client can eat and drink normally.

■ The MT can remain in situ long-term if necessary.

■ The small stab incision heals very quickly after decannulation and is often airtight within one day.

Nursing interventions for a client who has a tracheostomy tube include the following:

■ Suctioning the tube to maintain its patency (see Procedure 41-3).

■ Cleaning the double cannula tube (See Procedure 41-4).

■ Deflating a cuffed tube at prescribed intervals to prevent prolonged pressure on the trachea.

■ Changing the tracheostomy dressing and tie tapes.

■ Plugging the tube for specified lengths of time before removal. A tracheostomy plug is usually inserted into a tracheostomy tube for specified lengths of time before the tube is removed. Suctioning of the client's nasopharynx and the tracheostomy is performed before the plug is inserted. While the tube is plugged, the client is carefully monitored for signs of respiratory distress. Often the length of time the tube is plugged is increased over a number of days if the person tolerates the procedure well.

Deflating and Inflating Cuffed Tracheostomy Tubes   The physician's orders must be checked to determine when a cuffed tracheostomy tube should be inflated. Cuffed tracheostomy tubes are generally inflated

■ During the first 12 hours after a tracheostomy

■ When the client is being ventilated or receiving IPPB therapy, to prevent air leakage

■ When the client is eating or receiving oral medications and for a prescribed period of time following meals or medications (e.g., 30 minutes), to prevent aspiration

■ When the client is comatose, to prevent aspiration of oropharyngeal secretions

At other times, the cuff is deflated. If double-cuffed tubes are used, deflation and inflation must be done at regular intervals according to the manufacturer's directions.

Before deflating a cuffed tube, the nurse assists the client to a semi-Fowler's position unless contraindicated. Clients receiving positive pressure ventilation should be placed in a supine position so that secretions above the cuff site are moved up into the mouth. The nurse then suctions the oropharyngeal cavity and discards the suction catheter. Suctioning prevents pooled oral secretions from descending into the trachea after the cuff is deflated. These secretions could cause irritation and infection. The catheter is discarded to avoid introducing microorganisms into the lower airway when it is suctioned later. If a hemostat is clamping the cuff inflation tube, it will need to be unclamped. Some tubes have one-way valves that replace the hemostat. To deflate the cuff, follow these steps:

1. Attach the 5- or 10-ml syringe to the distal end of the inflation tube, making sure the seal is tight.

2. While the client inhales, slowly withdraw the amount of air from the cuff indicated by the manufacturer, or as orders indicate, while providing a positive pressure breath with a manual resuscitator (Ambu bag). Removal of air on inhalation under positive pressure allows secretions to ascend from the bronchi.

3. Keep the syringe attached to the tubing. The syringe is left attached for reinflation of the cuff.

4. If the cough reflex is stimulated during cuff deflation, suction the lower airway with a sterile catheter. (Cuff deflation can stimulate the cough reflex, which may produce additional secretions.)

5. Assess the client's respirations, and suction the client as needed. If the client experiences breathing difficulties, reinflate the cuff immediately.

The cuff is reinflated to the *minimal occluding volume* (MOV) to prevent tracheal damage and is performed as follows:

1. Inflate the cuff on *inhalation* until you cannot hear a leak (a harsh, squeaking, or gurgling sound) when you listen with a stethoscope over the neck adjacent to the trachea.

2. The cuff is inflated sufficiently when
   a. You cannot hear the client's voice.
   b. You cannot feel any air movements from the client's mouth, nose, or tracheostomy site.
   c. You hear no leak from the positive pressure ventilation when auscultating the neck adjacent to the trachea during inspiration.

An alternative method is called the *minimal air-leak technique (MLT)*. The same steps are carried out, after which 0.1 ml is withdrawn to allow a small leak.

Following inflation, the cuff pressure is measured using a manometer specifically designed for this purpose. The cuff's pillow port is attached to the cuff pressure manometer tubing. The pressure should not exceed 15 to 20 mm Hg or 25 cm H_2O. Check physician's orders. Excessive cuff pressure causes tracheal edema, ulceration, and necrosis. Underinflation may cause inadequate ventilation and may allow aspiration of blood, food, or secretions. If the pressure is appropriate, the inflation tube is clamped with the hemostat, provided that the tube does not have a one-way valve. The syringe is then removed, and the exact amount of air used to inflate the cuff is determined. This helps prevent overinflation in subsequent cuff procedures.

A **tracheostomy dressing and the tie tapes** need to be changed whenever soiled. Soiled dressings harbor microorganisms and are a potential source of skin excoriation, breakdown, and infection. Usually, the dressing is changed after the cannula is cleaned, but a more frequent dressing change may be necessary. Dressing technique is described in Chapter 46. Sterile gloves should be worn. The incision site and flange of the tube are usually cleaned with sterile normal saline using gauze squares or applicator sticks. If encrustations are difficult to remove, a half-and-half solution of hydrogen peroxide and normal saline may be used. Because hydrogen peroxide can be irritating to the skin, the cleaned area must be thoroughly rinsed with normal saline and then dried. If agency protocol dictates, an antibiotic ointment may be applied around the incision site before the dressing is applied. Commercially prepared tracheostomy dressings of nonraveling material are available. If not available, a 4 × 4 square of *noncotton-filled gauze* may be opened and refolded as shown in Figure 41–37, *A–D*. Place the gauze as shown in Figure 41–37, *E* if drainage is heavy; if drainage is not heavy, the dressing is inserted from above. Use of cut and cotton-filled gauze squares is avoided because the client might aspirate cotton lint or frayed fibers which could subsequently cause a tracheal abscess. The tracheostomy tube must be securely supported when applying the dressing. Excessive movement of the tube is irritating to the trachea.

Tie tapes also often become soiled and require changing. It is best to have an assistant don a sterile glove and hold the tracheostomy tube in place while the nurse changes the ties. Holding the tube prevents accidental expulsion if the client coughs or moves. If an assistant is not available, the clean ties should be fastened *before removing the soiled ties*. The soiled ties will first have to be moved down to the bottom half of the slots of the tracheostomy plate.

Cotton twill tape is used to secure the tracheostomy tube. Two methods can be used: one uses two strips of twill tape, the other one strip.

For the two-strip method, cut the strips in different lengths (i.e., 25 cm [9 in] and 50 cm [20 in]) to enable fastening at the side of the neck for easy access; a knot at the back of the neck could create pressure, discomfort, and skin irritation. Cut slits into the end of each strip, first folding back the end of the tape onto itself and then cutting a slit in the middle of the tape from its folded edge. To make the tape easier to thread through the slots, cut the ends of the tape at an angle. After cutting or untying the soiled tapes, thread the slit end of one clean tape through the eye of the tracheostomy faceplate from the bottom side; then thread the other end of the tie through the slit of the tape, pulling it taut until it is securely fastened to the faceplate. Then tie the tapes together at the side of the client's neck using two square knots; these prevent slippage and possible tube dislodgement. When tying the tapes, ask the client to flex the neck, and have the assistant place one or two fingers under the tapes at the side of the client's neck. Flexion of the neck, like coughing, increases neck circumference. The assistant's finger placement also ensures that the tapes are not tied too tightly, causing choking or pressure on the jugular veins. Tape should be applied over the knot to avoid confusing the tracheostomy ties with the client's gown ties.

When using the one-strip method recommended by Dunleap (1987, p. 26), one long strip of twill tape is needed. To determine the length required, hold one end of the tape at the slot on one side of the tracheostomy plate, pull the tape around the back of the client's neck to the slot on the other side, and multiply this length by 2.5. To apply this tie, thread one end of the tape into the upper half of the slot on one side. Bring both ends of the tape together, and take them around behind the client's neck, keeping them flat and untwisted. Then thread the piece of tape closest to the client's neck from back to front through the other slot, and tie square knots with the loose tape. Implement the measures described above to ensure that the tape is not too tight and to avoid confusion with gown ties.

Cardiopulmonary Resuscitation for an Adult

A **cardiac arrest** is the cessation of cardiac function; the heart stops beating. Often a cardiac arrest is unexpected and sudden. When it occurs, the heart no longer pumps blood to any of the organs of the body. Breathing then stops, and the person becomes unconscious and limp. Within 20 to 40 seconds of a cardiac arrest, the victim is clinically dead. After 4 to 6 minutes, the lack of oxygen supply to the brain causes permanent and extensive damage. Causes of cardiac arrest are many and include electrocution, myocardial infarction (heart attack), respiratory failure, extensive hemorrhage, and brain injury.

The three cardinal signs of a cardiac arrest are apnea, absence of a carotid or femoral pulse, and dilated pupils. The person's skin appears pale or grayish and feels cool. Cyanosis is evident when respiratory function fails prior to heart failure.

A **respiratory** (pulmonary) **arrest** is the cessation of breathing. If often occurs as a result of a blocked airway, but it can occur following a cardiac arrest and for other reasons. A respiratory arrest is preceded by short, shallow breathing. The breathing becomes increasingly labored. Then the person becomes flushed and disoriented and experi-

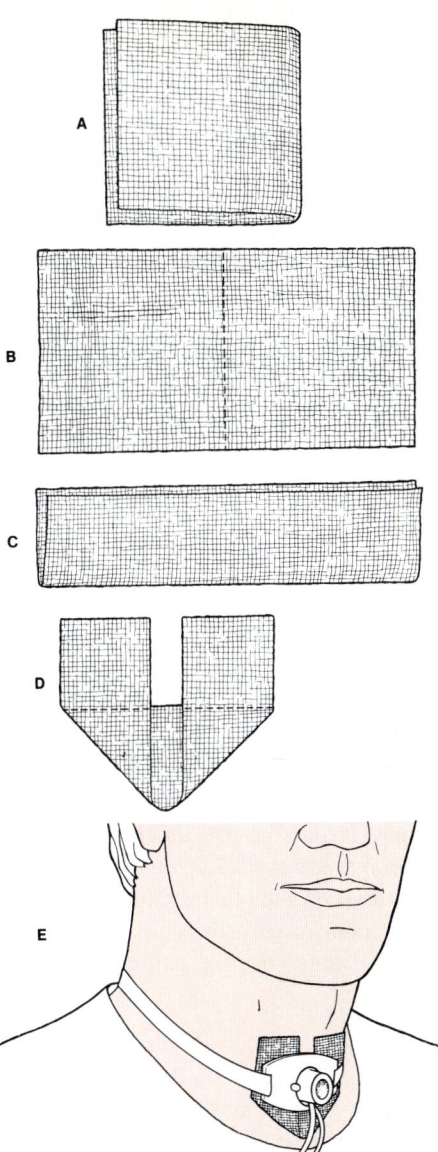

Figure 41–37 Applying the tracheostomy dressing.

ences feelings of suffocation. If the respiratory problem persists, the person becomes cyanotic, becomes comatose, and goes into cardiac arrest. Respiratory arrest leads to cardiac arrest because of the lack of oxygen to vital organs, especially the heart and the brain.

Resuscitation is restoration to consciousness or life; it includes all measures to revive individuals who have stopped breathing due to either respiratory or cardiac failure. **Artificial respiration** (e.g., oral resuscitation) is used when the victim's breathing has stopped while the heart continues to beat. **External cardiac massage** (or compression) is used when both the heartbeat and breathing have stopped; then both artificial respiration and external cardiac massage are applied at the same time. These combined measures are often called **cardiopulmonary resuscitation**

(CPR) or **basic life support (BLS).** Basic life support must be complemented by a rapid delivery of **advanced cardiac life support (ACLS).** ACLS includes the following:

1. Establishing an effective airway: endotracheal intubation is preferable
2. Establishing an intravenous line, preferably a central line
3. Defibrillation
4. Administering emergency cardiac drugs, such as nitroglycerine, verapamil, and amrinone. These are given intravenously, but some drugs may be given via the endotracheal tube (e.g., epinephrine (Adrenalin), lidocaine hydrochloride (Lidocaine), atropine sulfate (Atropine), naloxone hydrochloride (Narcan), and metaraminol bitartrate (Aramine).

The survival rate from cardiac arrest due to ventricular fibrillation clearly depends on the promptness of the initiation of CPR and ACLS. Studies show that there is a 43% survival rate if CPR is initiated within 4 minutes and ACLS within 8 minutes. Only 10% survive if ACLS is not initiated until 16 minutes have elapsed (McIntyre and Lewis 1983, p. 9). Recognizing the need for CPR and skill in performing it quickly and competently are essential functions of nurses. More and more laypersons are also being encouraged to learn CPR. Courses are available at national Red Cross and Heart Associations throughout the country. *Learning to perform these procedures correctly requires instruction from a certified instructor at these associations and supervised practice.*

CPR in a Hospital

Most health care agencies have established practices and policies governing CPR. Nurses need to learn immediately the following information:

- The agency procedure for external cardiac massage
- Where the emergency equipment is kept
- The agency's method of notification of a cardiac arrest
- The advised compression rates for adults, children, and infants.

Practices commonly include the following:

- The person who discovers a client who has had a cardiac arrest is responsible for obtaining assistance. The nurse may simply call out to others or may telephone to the hospital switchboard. The person then starts CPR immediately.
- Many hospitals have a special team (the crash team) that answers the call. The team usually consists of physicians and nurses who have had special education in CPR. The team will have a crash cart stocked with the special supplies and equipment required for CPR.
- Hospitals with a loudspeaker system to summon the special team usually use a code to notify the staff without

alarming visitors and clients. Some agencies use a number, such as "99," while others use a color, such as "Blue." The announcement may be "Code Blue West 8" or "Doctor 99 West 8" to tell the members of the team that the cardiac arrest is on the eighth floor of the west wing.

- When the special team arrives, it takes over the care of the client. The nursing staff may stay to assist or continue with other nursing responsibilities, depending on the situation.

- If external cardiac compression does not produce a heartbeat, the physician may decide to defibrillate the client. There are many types of defibrillators; most function by passing an electric current through the heart to establish normal cardiac rhythm. The two paddles of the defibrillator are lubricated and then placed on the person's chest: one to the right of the sternum, the other near the apex of the heart along the left axillary line. The axillary line extends inferiorly from the anterior axillary fold. Before the current is activated, all people stand away from the client so as not to receive the electric current. The effectiveness of the defibrillation can be determined by checking the carotid pulse, the movement of the pupils of the eyes, and the return of respirations or by referring to the cardiac monitor that may have been connected to the client.

ABCs of Cardiopulmonary Resuscitation

The ABCs of cardiopulmonary resuscitation (CPR) are

a. Clear the *airways.*
b. Initiate artificial *breathing* (oral resuscitation).
c. Initiate *cardiac compression* (artificial *circulation*).

This sequence is recommended because spontaneous breathing can occur after any one action, such as after the airway is opened or after a few artificial respirations are provided.

An *Emergpak,* containing a disposable CPR Microshield, adequately protects against biologic contact with the victim. The *CPR Microshield* is a patented one-way valve device that reduces rescuer/victim contact by providing a physical barrier during mouth-to-mouth resuscitation. This shield, intended for use by CPR-trained individuals only, delivers recommended volumes of air to the victim without affecting the basic resuscitation technique. A disposable ultrasoft barrier film that conforms to the victim's facial contours is attached to the mouthpiece. Some Emergpaks also contain gloves.

The assessment phases of BLS are of extreme importance. Each of the ABCs of CPR begins with an assessment phase:

a. *Airways:* Determine the person's air exchange and responsiveness.
b. *Breathing:* Determine the person's breathlessness.
c. *Circulation:* Determine the person's pulselessness.

Performing each assessment step ensures that the victim will not be subjected to any intrusive procedure (e.g., positioning, opening the airway, rescue breathing, external cardiac compression) until the need for it is determined.

Initial Steps
Initial steps when a rescuer arrives at the scene of the emergency include the following:

1. Assess consciousness. Grasp the shoulder of the person who appears unconscious; shake it, calling, "Are you all right?" If there is no response, the person is unconscious. If the person is conscious, determine the ability to speak or cough; pinch the earlobe or toes of an infant to determine if the child can cry in response to the pain.

2. Assess any injury. If injury to the head or neck is evident or suspected, avoid moving the victim inappropriately to prevent further injury and potential paralysis.

3. If the victim does not respond, call for help. When another rescuer arrives, have the person call an ambulance or the community emergency medical service (EMS).

4. Position the victim supine on a flat, firm surface, with the arms alongside the body. If the victim is lying face down, roll the body as a unit (head, shoulders, and trunk simultaneously) to prevent twisting and injury of the spine.

5. Kneel beside the victim's shoulders so you can perform rescue breathing and chest compression without moving your knees. If the victim is in bed, you may have to kneel on the bed.

Clearing an Obstructed Airway
Since there are several possible causes of airway obstruction, there are several different ways of clearing an obstructed airway. Causes include

- Aspirated food, mucus plug, or foreign bodies, such as partial dentures or small toys. Food is the most common cause of choking, particularly meat that has been ineffectively chewed.

- Unconsciousness or seizures, which cause the tongue to fall back and block the airway.

- Severe trauma to the nose, mouth, or neck that produce blood clots that obstruct the airway, especially in unconscious victims.

- Acute edema of the trachea, from smoke inhalation, facial and neck burns, or anaphylaxis. In these instances, a tracheostomy is often indicated.

Foreign bodies may cause either partial or complete airway obstruction.

When an airway is partially obstructed, the victim may either have good air exchange or poor air exchange. If sufficient air is obtained, even though there is frequent wheezing between coughs, do *not* interfere with the victim's attempts to expel the foreign object. If the partial obstruction remains, call the EMS. Partial obstructions with inadequate air exchange are dealt with in the same manner as complete obstructions.

The person with poor air exchange or complete airway obstruction clutches at the throat and is unable to speak; wheezes suddenly or has stridor (makes crowing sounds); becomes anxious, restless, and agitated; experiences a feeling of suffocation; has pale or cyanotic skin and/or mucous membranes; has exaggerated retractions (indrawing) of the chest wall on inhalation; has tachycardia; is unconscious.

The **Heimlich maneuver** (subdiaphragmatic abdominal thrusts) is recommended to relieve obstructions for persons over 1 year of age. By elevating the diaphragm, this maneuver forces air from the lungs to create an artificial cough to expel the obstruction. It may be necessary to perform this maneuver 6 to 10 times to clear the airway. The Heimlich maneuver can be performed when the victim is conscious and standing or sitting, and when the client is unconscious and lying flat. For infants under 1 year of age, a combination of back blows and chest thrusts is recommended. The Heimlich maneuver can cause intraabdominal injury in this age group.

Heimlich maneuver to a standing or sitting victim
To perform the Heimlich maneuver to a conscious person who is standing or sitting:

1. Stand behind the person, and wrap your arms around the person's waist.

2. Make a fist with one hand, tuck the thumb inside the fist, and place the flexed thumb against the person's epigastrium, i.e., below the xiphoid process. A protruding thumb could inflict injury.

3. With the other hand, grasp the fist (see Figure 41–38), and press it into the person's abdomen with a firm, quick upward thrust (see Figure 41–39). Avoid tightening the arms around the rib cage, and thrust in the direction of the chin. Deliver one quick thrust.

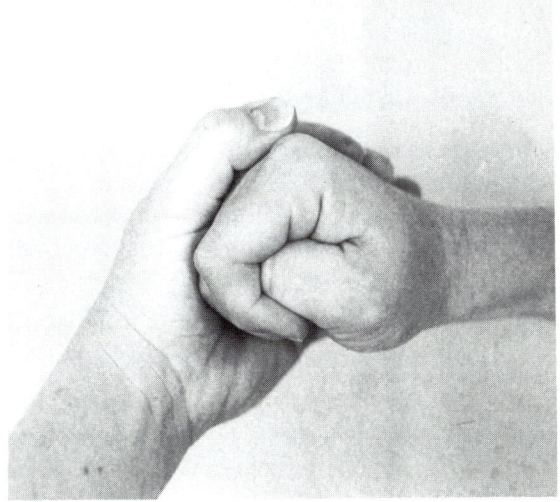

Figure 41–38 Making a fist for the Heimlich maneuver.

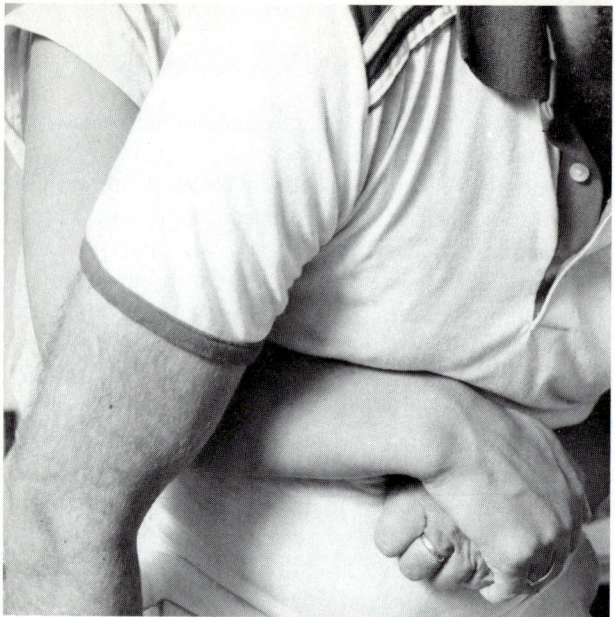

Figure 41–39   Arm position for the Heimlich maneuver.

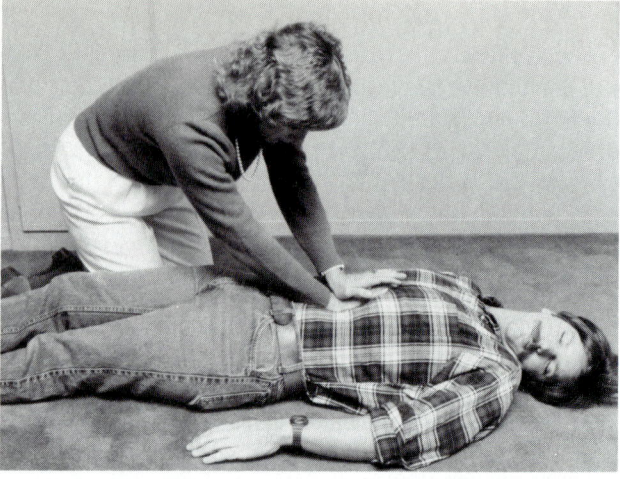

Figure 41–40   Position for the Heimlich maneuver when the victim is lying down.

4. Deliver successive thrusts as separate and complete movements.

Heimlich maneuver to a victim lying on the ground   To implement the Heimlich maneuver to an unconscious person who is lying on the ground:

1. Place the person supine and kneel preferably astride or to the side of the person's thighs.
2. Place the heel of one hand slightly above the person's navel and well below the tip of the xiphoid process, i.e., in the epigastric area.
3. Place the other hand directly on top of the first. Make sure the shoulders are over the person's abdomen and the elbows are straight.
4. Press the heel of the first hand into the abdomen with a quick upward thrust. See Figure 41–40. Be sure to direct the thrust in the midline of the abdomen and not to the left or to the right. The weight of your shoulders and trunk supplies power for the thrust.

Chest thrusts to standing or sitting victims   Chest thrusts are to be administered only to women in advanced stages of pregnancy and markedly obese persons who cannot receive the Heimlich maneuver. To administer chest thrusts:

1. Stand behind the person with your arms under the person's armpits and encircling the person's chest.
2. Place the thumb side of the fist on the *middle* of the breast bone, *not* on the xiphoid process.
3. Grab the fist with the other hand and deliver a quick backward thrust.
4. Repeat thrusts until the obstruction is relieved.

Chest thrust to a victim lying flat   Chest thrusts to unconscious persons lying on the ground are administered only to women in advanced stages of pregnancy or markedly obese persons. To administer this maneuver:

1. Position the person supine and kneel close to the side of the person's trunk.
2. Position the hands as for cardiac compression with the heel of the hand on the lower half of the sternum. (See Procedure 41–6, Step 2.)
3. Administer downward thrusts, each one slow and distinct.

Finger sweep   If foreign material is visible in the mouth, it must be expediently removed. The finger sweep maneuver *should be used only on unconscious persons and with extreme caution in infants and children* since the foreign material can be pushed back into the airway, causing increased obstruction. To digitally remove visible foreign material from the mouth:

1. Don disposable gloves if available.
2. Open the person's mouth by grasping the tongue and lower jaw between the thumb and fingers, and lifting the jaw upward. See Figure 41–41. This pulls the tongue away from the back of the throat.
3. To remove solid material, insert the index finger of your free hand along the inside of the person's cheek and deep into the throat. With your finger hooked, use a sweeping motion to try to dislodge and lift out the foreign object. If these measures fail, try more abdominal thrusts and back blows.
4. After removing the foreign object, clear our liquid material, such as mucus, blood, or emesis, with a scooping motion, using two fingers wrapped with a tissue or piece of cloth.
5. After the digital maneuver, assess air exchange. If it is ineffective, proceed with Procedures 41–5 and 41–6.

Oral Resuscitation　　Oral resuscitation is achieved in four ways: by mouth-to-mouth, mouth-to-nose, and mouth-to-mouth-and-nose resuscitation, or by the use of new face masks or a hand-compressible breathing bag (e.g., the Ambu bag). Many agencies provide rubberized breathing bags attached to face masks for respiratory resuscitation. The bags are compressed by hand to deliver air into the mask and rapidly self-inflate after compression. Exhaled air is released through an exhaust valve to prevent its entry back into the bag. Two significant advantages of the breathing bag are that supplemental oxygen can be attached to it and the nurse avoids direct contact with the person's mouth or nose.

Mouth-to-mouth resuscitation depends on the large amount of air that a normal person can inhale and therefore breathe into the victim's lungs. Although the oxygen content of expired air is slightly reduced, it is sufficient for revival. See Procedure 41–5.

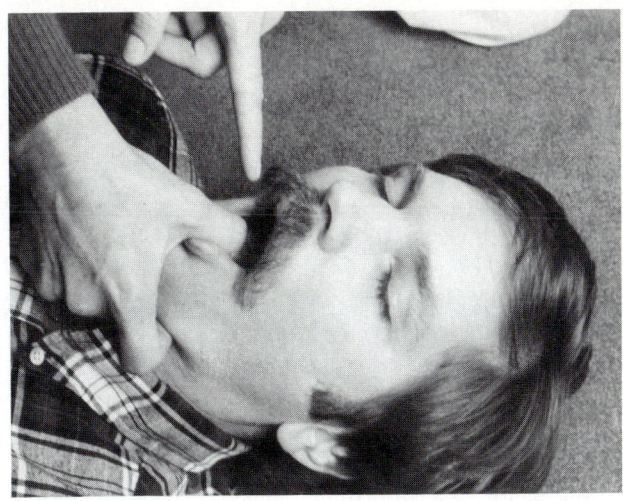

Figure 41–41　Finger sweep to remove an obstruction from the mouth or throat.

PROCEDURE 41–5

ADMINISTERING ORAL RESUSCITATION

Equipment ☑
Pocket face mask or mouth shields or hand-compressible breathing bag with mask, if available (see Figure 41–42)
Disposable gloves

Intervention

1. Clear the mouth and throat of obstructive material, and position the client appropriately.

- See "Finger Sweep" on page 1134. *A clear airway prior to resuscitation permits air to move freely in and out of the respiratory passages.*
- If the person is lying on one side or face down, turn the client onto the back, and kneel beside the head.

2. Open the airway.

- Use the head-tilt, chin-lift maneuver or the jaw-thrust maneuver. A modified jaw thrust is used for victims with suspected neck injury. In

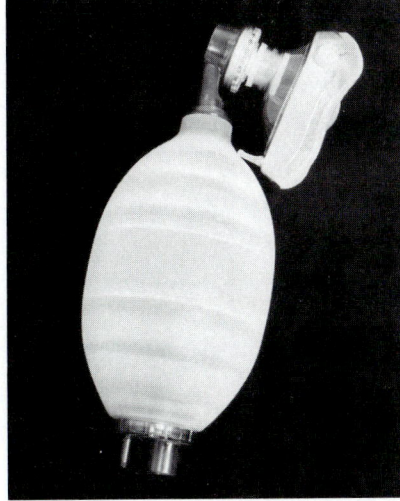

Figure 41–42　An Ambu bag with a face mask.

unconscious persons, the tongue lacks sufficient muscle tone, falls to the back of the throat, and obstructs the pharynx. *Because the tongue is attached to the lower jaw, moving*

the lower jaw forward and tilting the head backward lifts the tongue away from the pharynx and opens the airway. See Figure 41–43.

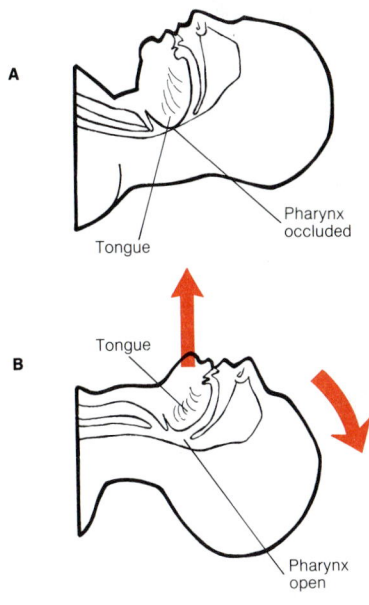

Figure 41–43　The position of an unconscious person's tongue: A, pharynx occluded; B, pharynx open.

Head-tilt, chin-lift maneuver:

■ Place one hand palm downward on the forehead.

■ Place the fingers of the other hand under the bony part of the lower jaw near the chin. The teeth should then be almost closed. The mouth should not be closed completely.

■ Simultaneously press down on the forehead with one hand, and lift the person's chin upward with the other. See Figure 41–44. Avoid pressing the fingers deeply into the soft tissues under the chin, since too much pressure can obstruct the airway.

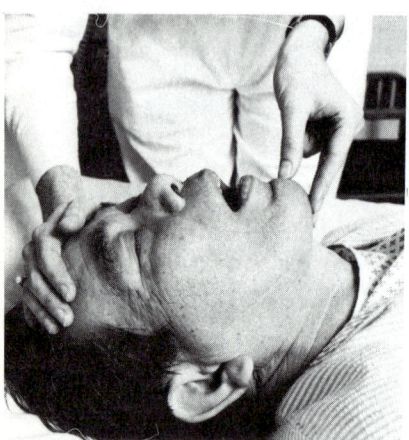

Figure 41–44 The head-tilt/chin-lift maneuver.

■ Open the person's mouth by pressing the lower lip downward with the thumb after tilting the head.

■ Remove dentures if they cannot be maintained in place. However, dentures that can be maintained in place make a mouth-to-mouth seal easier should rescue breathing be required.

Jaw-thrust maneuver:

■ Kneel at the *top* of the victim's head.

■ Grasp the angle of the mandible directly below the earlobe between your thumb and forefinger on each side of the person's head.

■ While tilting the head backward, lift the lower jaw until it juts forward and is higher than the upper jaw. See Figure 41–45.

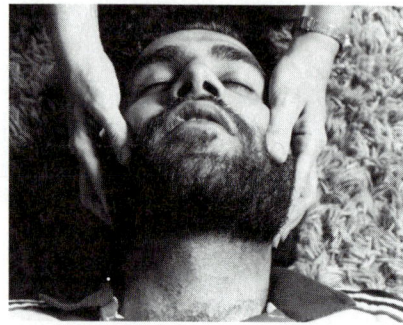

Figure 41–45 The jaw-thrust maneuver.

■ Rest your elbows on the surface on which the person is lying.

■ Retract the lower lip with the thumbs prior to giving artificial respiration.

■ If the victim is suspected of having a spinal neck injury, *do not hyperextend the neck.* Instead, *use the modified jaw thrust for a person with a spinal injury:*

Modified jaw-thrust maneuver:

■ Perform first two steps for jaw-thrust maneuver.

■ Do not tilt the head backward while lifting the lower jaw forward.

■ Support the head carefully without hyperextending it or moving it from side to side.

3. Determine the person's ability to breathe.

■ Place your ear and cheek close to the client's mouth and nose.

■ Look at the chest and abdomen for rising and falling movement.

■ Listen for air escaping during exhalation.

■ Feel for air escaping against your cheek.

4. If no breathing is evident, provide rescue breathing if required.

■ Use the mouth-to-mouth, mouth-to-nose method, pocket face mask method, or hand-compressible breathing bag method.

Mouth-to-mouth method:

■ Put on a mouth shield.

■ Maintain the open airway by using the head-tilt, chin-lift maneuver.

■ Pinch the person's nostrils with the index finger and thumb of the hand on the person's forehead. *Pinching closes the nostrils and prevents resuscitation air from escaping through them.*

■ Take a deep breath, and place the mouth, opened widely, around the victim's mouth. Ensure an airtight seal. See Figure 41–46.

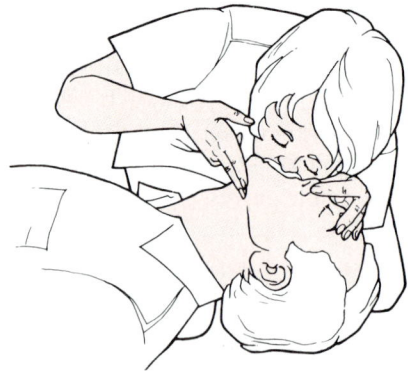

Figure 41–46 Mouth-to-mouth rescue breathing.

■ Exhale two full breaths (1 to 1½ seconds per breath). Pause and take a breath after the first ventilation. *The 1- to 1½-second time span closely matches the victim's inspiratory time, allows adequate time to provide good chest expansion, and decreases the possibility of gastric distention. Excessive air volumes and rapid inspiratory flow rates can cause pharyngeal pres-*

sures that are great enough to open the esophagus, thus allowing air to enter the stomach.

■ Ensure adequate ventilation by observing the person's chest rise and fall and by assessing the person's breathing as outlined in step 3. Adequate ventilation volumes for most adults are about 800 ml and do not need to exceed 1200 ml (American Heart Association 1986, p. 2917).

■ If the initial ventilation attempt is unsuccessful, reposition the person's head and repeat the rescue breathing as above. If the victim still cannot be ventilated, proceed to clear the airway of any foreign bodies using the finger sweep, Heimlich maneuver, or chest thrusts described earlier.

Mouth-to-nose method:

This method can be used when there is an injury to the mouth or jaw or when the client is edentulous (toothless), making it difficult to achieve a tight seal over the mouth.

■ Maintain the head tilt and chin lift.

■ Close the person's mouth by pressing the palm of your hand against the person's chin. The thumb of the same hand may be used to hold the bottom lip closed.

■ Put on a mouth shield

■ Take a deep breath, and seal your lips around the person's nose. Ensure a tight seal by making contact with the cheeks around the nose.

■ Deliver two full breaths of 1 to 1½ seconds each, and pause to inhale before delivering the second breath.

■ Remove your mouth from the nose, and allow the victim to exhale passively. It may be necessary to separate the victim's lips or to open the mouth for exhaling, since the

nasal passages may be obstructed during exhalation.

Pocket face mask method:

■ Remove the mask from its case and push out the dome.

■ Connect the one-way valve to the mask port.

■ Position yourself at the top of the person's head, and open the airway using the jaw-thrust maneuver.

■ Place the bottom rim of the mask between the person's lower lip and chin. Place the rest of the mask over the face using your thumbs on each side of the mask to hold it in place. *This keeps the mouth open under the mask.*

■ Perform the jaw-thrust maneuver to tilt the head backward. Use your index, middle, and ring fingers of both hands behind the angles of the jaw, and grasp the person's temples with the palms of your hands.

■ Maintain this head position while blowing intermittently into the mouthpiece.

Hand-compressible breathing bag method:

■ Stand at the person's head.

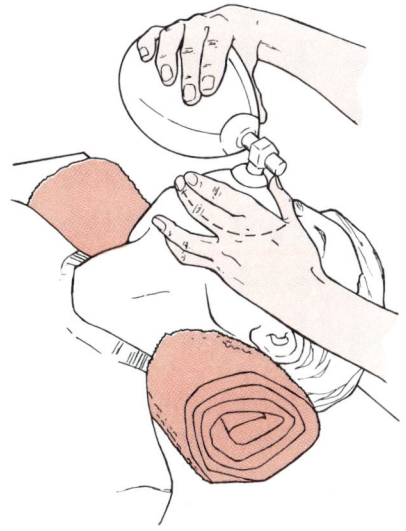

Figure 41–47 An Ambu bag in position.

■ Use one hand to secure the mask at the top and bottom and to hold the person's jaw forward. Use the other hand to squeeze and release the bag. See Figure 41–47.

■ Compress the bag until sufficient elevation of the person's chest is observed. Then release the bag.

5. Determine whether the person's breathing is restored. See step 3 above.

6. Determine the presence of a carotid pulse (see Figure 41–48).

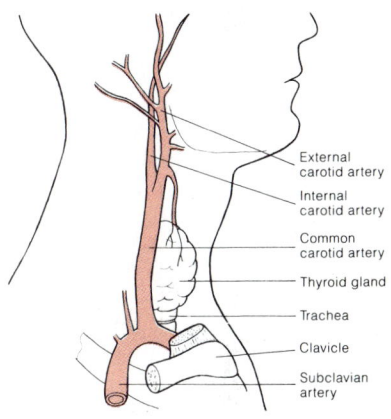

Figure 41–48 Location of the carotid artery.

■ Take about 5 to 10 seconds for this pulse check. *Adequate time is needed since the victim's pulse may be very weak and rapid, irregular, or slow.*

■ To palpate the carotid artery, first locate the larynx, then slide your fingers alongside it into the groove between the larynx and the neck muscles. Use gentle pressure. *This avoids compressing the artery. The carotid pulse site is used because the femoral pulse is difficult to locate on a fully clothed person and because a pulse can often be palpated there when more peripheral pulses, such as the radial, are imperceptible.*

- If you cannot feel a carotid pulse, check for a femoral pulse.

7. If the carotid pulse is palpable, but breathing is not restored, repeat rescue breathing.

- Inflate at the rate of 12 breaths per minute (1 breath every 5 seconds).
- Blow forcibly enough to make the person's chest rise.

- If chest expansion fails to occur, ensure that the head is hyperextended and the jaw lifted upward, or check again for the presence of obstructive material, fluid, or vomitus.

- After each inflation, move your mouth away from the person's mouth by turning your head toward the person's chest. *This movement allows the air to escape when the person exhales. It also gives the nurse time to inhale and to watch for chest expansion.*

8. Reassess the carotid pulse after every 12 inflations (after 1 minute).

- If you cannot locate the pulse, the person's heart has stopped, and cardiac compression also needs to be provided. See Procedure 41–6. **Accurate assessment of the person's pulse is essential** **because performing external chest compressions on victims who have a pulse can lead to serious medical complications.**

 A current problem facing resuscitators relates to the AIDS epidemic. Although there is no documented evidence to date that the human immunodeficiency virus (HIV) can be spread through saliva, manual resuscitation and pocket face masks are now available for mouth-to-mask resuscitation, eliminating mouth-to-mouth contact. In many agencies, pocket face masks are now kept at the bedside of every client, in the radiology department, and on CPR crash carts. The pocket face mask has these features (Juip and Harned 1988, p. 48):

- It is stored in a flat case and is designed with a push-out resuscitation dome.

- It has a one-way valve that eliminates direct contact with the victim's mouth and nose. This valve must be attached to the mask port when the mask is removed from the case.

- It provides an airtight seal over the face, even in many cases of severe facial trauma.

- It allows the provision of oxygen if needed.

- It is transparent, so that the rescuer can see the color of the victim's lips and the presence of vomitus.

- It has straps that can be used to attach the mask to the person's head if there is a need to perform both mouth-to-mask breathing and chest compressions. The rescuer can then work from the side of the person's head rather than the top.

External Cardiac Compression The external chest compression procedure consists of sequential, rhythmic applications of pressure over the lower half of the sternum. The pressure compresses the heart between the sternum and the vertebral column and squeezes blood out of the chambers of the heart. Circulation is thus provided to the lungs, heart, brain, and other essential organs.

External cardiac compression should never be practiced on a person with a functioning heart, because it could *interfere with the normal cardiac contractions.*

Performing external chest compression is described in detail in Procedure 41–6.

▶ **PROCEDURE 41–6**

ADMINISTERING EXTERNAL CARDIAC COMPRESSION

Intervention

1. Position the client appropriately if not already done.

- Place the person supine on a firm surface. *Blood flow to the brain will*

be inadequate during CPR if the victim's head is positioned higher than the thorax. A hard surface facilitates compression of the heart between the sternum and the hard surface.

- If the victim is in bed in a health care facility, place a cardiac board—preferably the full width of the bed—under the back. If necessary, place the victim on the floor.

▶

- If the person must be turned, turn the body as a unit while firmly supporting the head and neck so that the head does not roll, twist, or tilt backward or forward. *Turning the person as a unit prevents further injury (if present) to the neck or spine.*

- Elevate the lower extremities (optional). *This may promote venous return and augment circulation during external cardiac compressions* (American Heart Association 1986, p. 2919).

2. **Position the hands on the sternum.** Proper hand placement is essential for effective cardiac compression. Position the hands as follows:

- With the hand nearest the victim's legs, use your middle and index fingers to locate the lower margin of the rib cage.

- Move the fingers up the rib cage to the notch where the lower ribs meet the sternum. See Figure 41–49.

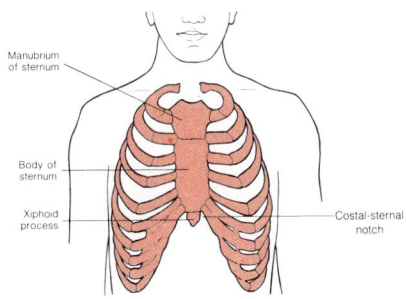

Figure 41–49 The sternum and ribs.

- Place the heel of the other hand (nearest the victim's head) along the lower half of the victim's sternum, close to the index finger that is next to the middle finger in the costal-sternal notch. *Proper positioning of the hands during cardiac compression prevents injury*

to underlying organs and the ribs. See Figure 41–50. *Compression directly over the xiphoid process can lacerate the person's liver.*

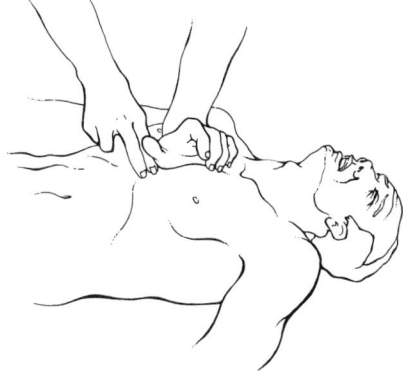

Figure 41–50 Proper positioning of hands during cardiac compression.

- Then place the first hand on top of the second hand so that both hands are parallel. The fingers may be extended or interlaced. *Compression occurs only on the sternum through the heels of the hands.*

3. **Administer cardiac compression according to American Heart Association guidelines** (1986, p. 2921).

- Lock your elbows into position, straighten your arms, and position your shoulders directly over your hands. See Figure 41–51.

- For each compression, thrust *straight down* on the sternum. For an adult of normal size, depress the sternum 3.8 to 5.0 cm (1.5 to 2 in). *The muscle force of both arms is needed for adequate cardiac compression of an adult. The weight of your shoulders and trunk supplies power for compression. Extension of the elbows ensures an adequate and even force throughout compression.*

- Completely release the compression pressure. However, do *not* lift your hands from the chest or

change their position. *Releasing the pressure allows the sternum to return to its normal position and allows the heart chambers to fill with blood. Leaving the hands on the chest prevents taking a malposition between compressions and possibly injuring the person.*

- Provide external cardiac compressions at the rate of 80 to 100 per minute. Maintain the rhythm by counting "One and, two and," and so on. *The specified compression rate and rhythm simulate normal heart contractions.*

- Administer 5 or 15 external compressions, depending on the number of rescuers, and coordinate them with rescue breathing. See CPR performed by one rescuer or by two rescuers, next.

Variation: CPR performed by one rescuer

- Assess responsiveness.

- Call for help and have another person call for EMS. In many

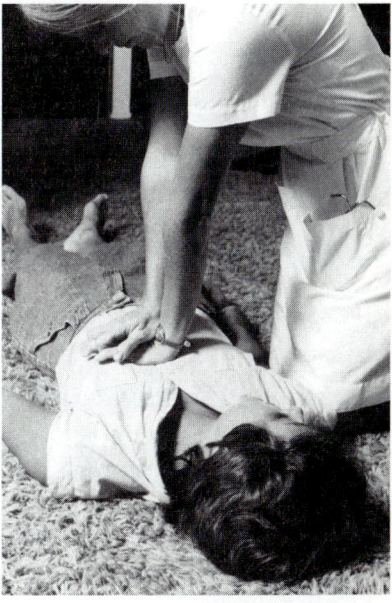

Figure 41–51 Arm and hand position for external cardiac massage.

communities the emergency telephone number is 911. The American Heart Association (1986, p. 2918) recommends that the person who calls the local EMS be able to impart all of the following information:

a. Location of the emergency
b. Telephone number from which the call is being made
c. What happened
d. Number of people needing assistance
e. Condition of the victim(s)
f. What aid is being given
g. Any other information that is requested

■ If no help comes and the rescuer is alone, CPR should be performed for 1 minute and then help summoned.

■ Position the client on the back on a flat, firm surface.

■ Kneel beside the person's chest. If the person is in bed, you may have to kneel on the bed.

Airway:

■ Clear the airway, if you suspect airway obstruction from food or some other foreign object.

■ Open the airway with the head-tilt, chin-lift maneuver or, if neck injury is suspected, the modified jaw thrust.

Breathing:

■ Assess breathing: *Look for* chest movement; *listen for* exhalation; and *feel for* air flow against the cheek.

■ Ventilate the person, if breathing is not restored. See Procedure 41–5 for detailed steps.

■ Deliver two full breaths into the person's mouth. Between the breaths, remove your mouth, turn your head to the side, and pause to take a breath.

■ If unable to give two breaths, repo-

sition the client's head, and attempt to ventilate again.

■ If still unsuccessful, remove foreign bodies from the victim's airway. See digital removal of material from the mouth, earlier.

Circulation:

■ Assess the carotid or femoral pulse for 5 seconds.

■ If pulse is present:
a. Continue rescue breathing at 12 times per minute while monitoring the pulse.
b. Call for EMS.

■ If pulse is absent:
a. Call for EMS.
b. Begin external chest compression.
c. Perform chest compression: 15 external chest compressions at the rate of 80 to 100 per minute. Count, "One and, two and, three and . . ." up to 15.
d. Open the airway, and give two rescue breaths.
e. Repeat 15 chest compressions.
f. Perform four complete cycles of 15 compressions and two ventilations.

■ Assess the client's carotid pulse after four sets of 15 compressions, each followed by two lung inflations. If there is no pulse, continue with CPR and check for return of pulse every few minutes. Do *not* interrupt CPR for more than 7 seconds.

Variation: CPR performed by two rescuers

When help arrives, one rescuer can provide external cardiac compression, and the other can provide pulmonary resuscitation, inflating the lungs once after every five compressions, a 5:1 ratio. The second rescuer follows these initial steps:

■ Tell the first rescuer, "Stop CPR after two ventilations."

■ Check the carotid or femoral pulse for 5 seconds.

■ If no pulse is felt, state, "No pulse."

■ The second rescuer then
a. Gives two breaths.
b. Provides compression.
c. Sets the pace, counting aloud, "One and, two and, three and, four and, five and, ventilate."

■ The first rescuer:
a. Provides one ventilation after every five chest compressions.
b. Observes each breath for effectiveness.
c. Assesses the carotid pulse frequently between breaths to assess the effectiveness of cardiac compression.
d. Observes for abdominal (gastric) distention, which can result from overinflation of the lungs. If distention occurs, the rescuer reduces the force of the ventilations, but ensures sufficient ventilation to elevate the ribs.
e. Assesses the person's pupils every 5 minutes (optional). Pupil changes are not the best indicator of restored circulation, however.

■ When the person compressing the chest becomes fatigued, positions should be changed. To initiate a change in positions, the person compressing states, "Change one and, two and, three and, four and, five and"; moves to the person's head; and counts the pulse for 5 seconds. CPR should never be interrupted for more than 7 seconds.

■ The person ventilating gives the breath and moves into position to provide compression.

■ If there is no pulse, the original person compressing states, "No pulse—start compression," gives one full breath, and CPR is again initiated.

When relieved from CPR

- Stand by to assist. Often a person is needed to take notes, document the actions taken, and record the drugs given by the cardiac arrest team.
- Provide support to the victim's support persons and others who may have witnessed the cardiac arrest. This is often a frightening experience for others because it is so sudden and so serious.
- Document the time CPR began, the time a physician arrived, the drugs and techniques employed, the time CPR was terminated, and all nursing assessments.

Terminating CPR

A rescuer terminates CPR only when one of the following events occurs:

- Another person takes over.
- The victim's heartbeat and breathing are reestablished.
- Adjunctive life-support measures are initiated.
- A physician states that the individual is dead and that CPR is to be discontinued.
- The rescuer becomes exhausted, and there is no one to take over.

Chest Tubes

Chest tubes are usually inserted through an intercostal space into the pleural cavity. They are used following chest surgery or trauma and for pneumothorax and/or hemothorax. A **pneumothorax** is a collection of air or other gas in the pleural space that causes the lung to collapse. A **hemothorax** is the accumulation of blood and fluid in the pleural cavity, usually as a result of trauma or surgery. Clinical signs of penumothorax include sharp pain on the affected side; weak, rapid pulse: pallor; vertigo; faintness; dyspnea; diaphoresis; excessive coughing; and blood-tinged sputum.

Chest tubes that are used to remove air are usually inserted superiorly (i.e., through the second intercostal space) and anteriorly, because air tends to rise in the pleural cavity. Tubes used to drain fluids are inserted more inferiorly, often in the eighth or ninth intercostal space, and more posteriorly. Sometimes a tube used to drain air is inserted inferiorly and threaded superiorly in the pleural space. When a client requires drainage of both fluid and air, two chest tubes may be inserted. These are sometimes joined externally by a Y-connector.

Drainage Systems

Because the pleural cavity normally has negative pressure, any drainage system connected to it must be sealed so that air or liquid cannot enter. Such a drainage system is called a water-sealed (underwater) drainage or a disposable pleural drainage system. In water-sealed drainage, fluid in the bottom of the container prevents air from entering the chest tube and thus entering the pleural cavity. The system must be kept below the level of the client's chest so that the fluid in the container is not drawn into the pleural cavity by gravity. it is also very important to maintain the patency of the tubing.

Drainage systems use three mechanisms to drain fluid and air from the pleural cavity; positive expiratory pressure, gravity, and suction. When the pleural cavity contains some air or fluid, a positive pressure develops during expiration. This positive pressure is abnormal, but it does help expel the air and to some extent fluid from the space. Gravity acts as an evacuation force when the tubing is placed so that it descends from the insertion site to the drainage receptacle. Suction is used in conjunction with the other two forces in some drainage systems.

There are several kinds of water-sealed drainage systems: one- and two-bottle gravity systems, two- and three-bottle suction systems, and disposable unit systems.

Bottle systems

In a **one-bottle system,** a single receptacle receives both the fluid and/or air from the client and seals the system. See Figure 41–52, *A.* The air or fluid enters through the collection inlet, which terminates under sterile water. The air then exits through the water and through the air vent; the fluid remains in the bottle. The fluid in this bottle then is a combination of fluid from the client and sterile water—it forms the water seal. The one-bottle system depends upon gravity and positive expiratory pressure for drainage.

A **two-bottle system** uses one bottle to receive the fluid or air from the client and the second bottle to create the water seal. See Figure 41–52, *B.* The air or fluid from the pleural cavity is received into bottle A. The air from bottle A is passed into bottle B. The air then passes through the sterile water and exits from bottle B through the air vent. The fluid from the pleural cavity remains in bottle A. This system uses gravity and positive expiratory pressure for drainage.

The **three-bottle system** has a collection bottle (A), a water-seal bottle (B), and a suction-control bottle (C). See Figure 41–52, *C.* Fluid from the pleural cavity collects in

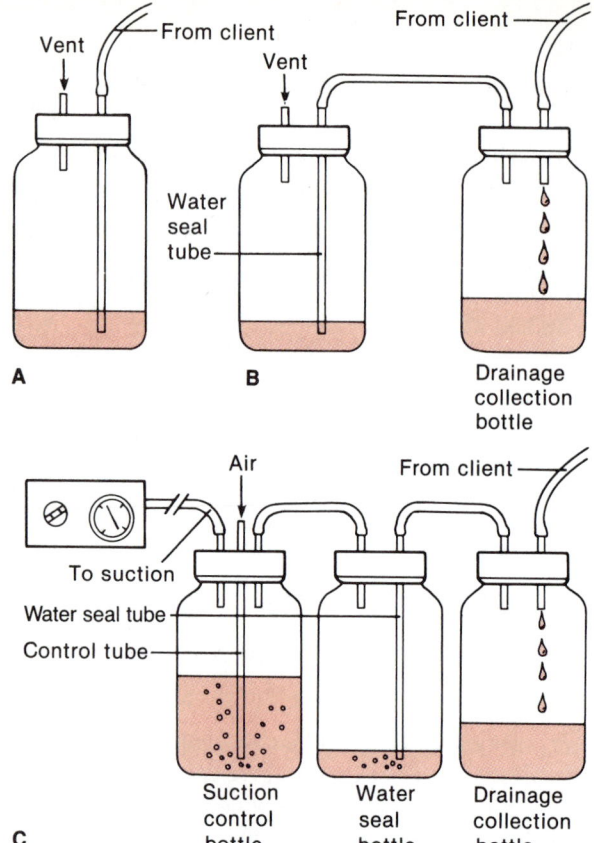

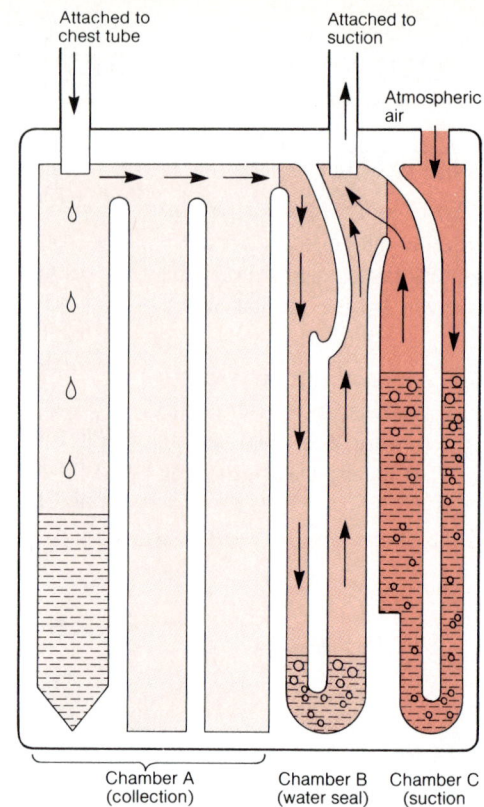

Figure 41–53 A Pleur-evac chest drainage system.

Figure 41–52 Drainage systems for chest tubes. *A*, one bottle-system; *B*, two-bottle system; *C*, three-bottle system. **Source:** C. Kneisl and S. Ames, *Adult health nursing* (Redwood City, Calif.: Addison-Wesley Publishing Co., 1986), p. 565. Used with permission.

bottle A, which is connected to a tube in bottle B that terminates below the fluid level. Bottle B is then connected to bottle C by a short tube. Bottle C also has a manometer tube submerged in sterile water. The depth to which this tube is submerged determines the amount of suction exerted in the pleural cavity. The suction-control bottle has another inlet, for suction. This sytem uses positive expiratory pressure, gravity, and suction for drainage.

Disposable unit systems Several types of disposable unit systems are available commercially. Two commonly seen are the Pleur-evac system and the Argyle system. A newer system is the Thora-Drain III system. The Pleur-evac system consists of three chambers. See Figure 41–53. Chamber A is the collection chamber. It receives fluid and/or air from the pleural cavity and is divided into three subchambers. The client's fluid remains in this chamber, while air from the client passes on to chamber B, the water-seal chamber. This chamber is U-shaped, and air from the pleural cavity passes through the water seal and exits at the suction outlet side of the U. Chamber C, the suction chamber, is also U-shaped. The height of the fluid in chamber C determines the amount of suction pressure exerted upon the client. Atmospheric air enters on the far left of this chamber, passes

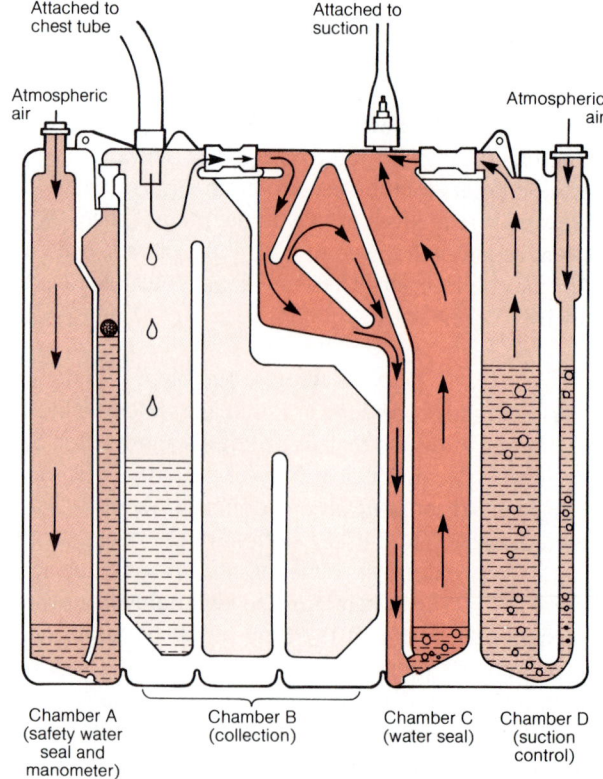

Figure 41–54 An Argyle chest drainage system.

through the suction-control water, and joins the air from the client. These then pass into the suction outlet.

The Argyle double-seal system consists of four chambers. See Figure 41–54. Chamber A is a water-seal chamber with a manometer. Chamber B is the collection chamber. Chamber C is another water seal. Chamber D is for suction control. Normally, the client's pleural air passes from chamber B into chamber C and to the suction source; however, if the suction becomes obstructed, the air can pass to chamber A and to the atmosphere. Chamber A thus serves as a safety vent.

The Thora-Drain III system consists of three chambers; a collection chamber, a water-seal chamber, and a suction-control chamber. The unique feature of this system is its replaceable collection chamber. When the collection chamber is filled with drainage it can be changed or replaced without interupting the entire system.

Assisting Clients with Chest Tubes Chest tubes are inserted and removed by the physician with the nurse assisting. Both procedures require sterile technique and must be done without introducing air or miocroorganisms into the pleural cavity. After the insertion, an x-ray film is taken to confirm the position of the tube. Procedure 41–7 provides guidelines for assisting with chest tube insertion.

The major objective of nursing care of clients with chest tubes is to facilitate drainage of fluid and air, thus promoting lung re-expansion. Essential aspects of care include maintaining the water seal, maintaining patency of the drainage system, and assessing the client's respiratory and cardiovascular status. Policies and procedures vary considerably from agency to agency in regard to chest drainage interventions. Certain interventions, such as milking a chest tube to maintain patency, may be prohibited. The nurse must therefore review agency policies before intervening. Procedure 41–8 on page 1145 provides guidelines for monitoring the client with a chest tube.

Chest tubes are generally removed within 5–7 days. Before removal, the tube is clamped with two large, rubber-tipped clamps for 1–2 days to assess for signs of respiratory distress and to determine whether air or fluid remains in the pleural space. An x-ray film of the chest is generally taken 2 hours after tube clamping to determine full lung expansion. If the client develops signs of respiratory distress or the film indicates pneumothorax, the tube clamps are removed, and chest drainage is maintained. If neither occurs, the tube is removed. Another x-ray film of the chest is often taken after removal to confirm full lung expansion. Procedure 41–9 on page 1148 provides guidelines for assisting with the removal of a chest tube.

PROCEDURE 41–7

ASSISTING WITH THE INSERTION OF A CHEST TUBE

Equipment ☑

Sterile chest tube tray, which includes

Drapes

10-ml syringe

Sponges

1-in #22 gauge needle

$\frac{5}{8}$-in #25 gauge needle

Scalpel

Forceps

Two rubber-tipped clamps for each tube inserted

Several 4 × 4 gauze squares

Split drain gauzes

Chest tube with a trocar

Suture materials (e.g., 2-0 silk with a needle)

Pleural drainage system with sterile drainage tubing and connectors

Y-connector, if two tubes will be inserted

Sterile gloves for the physician and the nurse

Vial of local anesthetic (e.g., 1% lidocaine) if required

Alcohol sponges to clean the top of the vial

Antiseptic (e.g., povidone-iodine)

Tape (nonallergenic is preferable)

Sterile petrolatum gauze (optional)

Intervention

1. Obtain baseline data.

■ Measure vital signs.

■ Auscultate lungs bilaterally for breath sounds. Diminished or ab-

sent breath sounds indicate inadequate lung expansion and recurrent pneumothorax after chest drainage is established.

■ Observe chest movements. A decrease in chest expansion on the

affected side can indicate pneumothorax.

■ Note presence of clinical signs indicative of pneumothorax (see page 1141).

2. **Prepare the client.**

- Explain placement and rationale for chest tube(s) to client and family.

- Assist the client to a lateral position with the area to receive the tube facing upward. Determine from the physician whether to have the bed in the supine position or semi-Fowler's position. *A supine position is generally preferred for tube insertion into the second or third intercostal space, a semi-Fowler's position for the sixth to eighth intercostal spaces.*

3. **Prepare the equipment.**

- Open the chest tube tray and the sterile gloves on the overbed table.

- Pour antiseptic solution onto the sponges.

- Be sure to maintain sterile technique.

4. **Support and monitor the client as required.**

5. **Provide an airtight dressing.**

After tube insertion

- Don sterile gloves. Wrap a piece of sterile petrolatum gauze around the chest tube. Place drain gauzes around the insertion site (one from the top and one from the bottom). Place several 4 × 4 gauze squares over these. *The gauze makes an airtight seal at the insertion site.*

- Remove your gloves and tape the dressings, covering them completely.

6. **Secure the chest tube appropriately.**

- Tape the chest tube to the client's skin away from the insertion site. *Taping prevents accidental dislocation of the tube.*

- Tape the connections of the chest tube to the drainage tube and to the drainage system. *Taping prevents inadvertent separation.*

- Coil the drainage tubing, and secure it to the bed linen, ensuring enough slack for the person to turn and move. *This prevents kinking of the tubing and impairment of the drainage system.*

7. **When all drainage connections are completed, ask the client to**

- Take a deep breath and hold it for a few seconds.

- Slowly exhale. *These actions facilitate drainage from the pleural space and lung reexpansion.*

8. **Ensure client safety.**

- Place rubber-tipped chest tube clamps at the bedside. *These are used to clamp the chest tube and prevent pneumothorax if the tube becomes disconnected from the drainage system or the system breaks or cracks.*

- Assess the client regularly for signs of pneumothorax and subcutaneous emphysema. *Subcutaneous emphysema can result from a poor seal at the chest tube insertion site.*

It is manifested by a "crackling" sound that is heard when the area around the insertion site is palpated.

- Assess the client's vital signs every 15 minutes for the first hour following tube insertion and then as ordered, e.g., every hour for 2 hours, then every 4 hours or as often as health indicates.

- Auscultate the lungs at least every 4 hours for breath sounds and the adequacy of ventilation in the affected lung.

9. **Document relevant information.**

- Document the date and time of chest tube insertion or removal and the name of the physician.

- Include the insertion site, drainage system used, presence of bubbling, characteristics of the drainage, vital signs, breath sounds by auscultation, and any other assessment findings.

Sample Recording

Date 12-6-91	Time: 2200

Sudden sharp pain in L chest, diaphoretic, pale, and dyspneic. —————
2300: BP 100/70, TPR 98.6, 105, 24. Diminished breath sounds in L lung and absence of chest movement. Two chest tubes inserted by Dr. Jung in L 2nd and 8th ICS. Connected by Y-connector and attached to Pleur-evac. Drainage system functioning. Drainage clear amber. —————
2305: BP 110/70, TPR 98.6, 100, 20. Breath sounds present in L lung. —————
————————— Karen P. Smith, RN

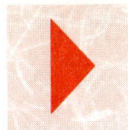

PROCEDURE 41–8

MONITORING A CLIENT WITH CHEST DRAINAGE

Equipment ☑

Two rubber-tipped Kelly clamps
Sterile gloves
Sterile petrolatum gauze
Sterile drainage system
Antiseptic swabs

Sterile 4 × 4 gauzes
Air-occlusive tape
Specimen supplies, if needed:
    Povidone-iodine swab
    Sterile #18 or #20 gauge needle

3- or 5-ml syringe
Needle protector
Label for the syringe
Laboratory requisition

Intervention

1. Assess the client.

■ Assess vital signs every 4 hours, or more often, as indicated.

■ Determine ease of respirations, breath sounds, respiratory rate and depth, and chest movements.

■ Monitor the client for signs of pneumothorax (see page 1141).

■ Inspect the dressing for excessive and abnormal drainage, such as bleeding or foul-smelling discharge. Palpate around the dressing site and listen for a crackling sound indicative of subcutaneous emphysema. Subcutaneous emphysema can result from a poor seal at the chest tube insertion site. It is manifested by a "crackling" sound that is heard when the area around the insertion site is palpated.

■ Assess level of discomfort. Analgesics often need to be administered before the client moves or does deep-breathing and coughing exercises.

2. Implement safety precautions.

■ Keep two 15- to 18-cm (6- to 7-in) rubber-tipped Kelly clamps within reach at the bedside, to clamp the chest tube in an emergency, e.g., if leakage occurs in the tubing.

■ Keep one sterile petrolatum gauze within reach at the bedside to use with an air-occlusive material if the chest tube becomes dislodged.

■ Keep an extra drainage system unit available in the client's room. In most agencies the physician is responsible for changing the drainage system except in emergency situations, such as malfunction or breakage. In these situations:

a. Clamp the chest tube close to the insertion site with two rubber-tipped clamps placed in opposite directions. See Figure 41–55.

b. Reestablish a water-sealed drainage system.

c. Remove the clamps, and notify the physician.

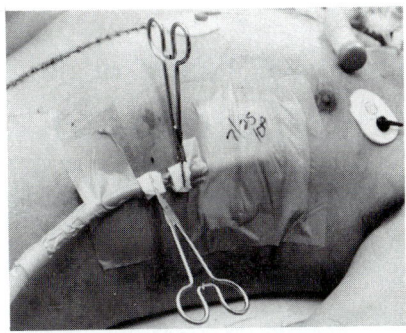

Figure 41–55 Clamping a chest tube.

■ Keep the drainage system below chest level and upright at all times, unless the chest tubes are clamped. *Keeping the unit below chest level prevents backflow of fluid from the drainage chamber into the pleural space. Keeping the unit upright maintains the glass tube below the water level, forming the water seal.*

3. Maintain patency of the drainage system.

■ Check that all connections are secured with tape to ensure that the system is airtight.

■ Inspect the drainage tubing for kinks or loops dangling below the entry level of the drainage system.

■ Inspect the air vent in the system periodically to make sure it is not occluded. A vent must be present to allow air to escape. *Obstruction of the air vent causes an increased pressure in the system that could result in pneumothorax.*

■ Milk or strip the chest tubing **as ordered and only in accordance with agency protocol.** Too vigorous milking can create excessive negative pressure that can harm the pleural membranes and/or *surrounding tissues.* Always verify the physician's orders before milking the tube; milking of only short segments of the tube may be specified (e.g., 10–20 cm or 4–8 in). To milk a chest tube, follow these steps:

a. Lubricate about 10–20 cm (4–8 in) of the drainage tubing with lubricating gel, soap, or hand lotion, or hold an alcohol sponge between your fingers and the tube. *Lubrication reduces friction and facilitates the milking process.*

b. With one hand, securely stabilize and pinch the tube at the insertion site.

c. Compress the tube with the thumb and forefinger of your other hand and milk it by sliding them down the tube, moving away from the insertion site. *Milking the tubing dislodges obstructions such as blood clots. Milking from the insertion site downward prevents movement of the obstructive material into the pleural space.*

d. If the entire tube is to be milked, reposition your hands farther along the tubing, and repeat steps a–c in progressive overlapping steps, until you reach the end of the tubing.

4. **Assess fluid level fluctuations and bubbling in the drainage system.**

- In gravity drainage systems, check for fluctuation (tidaling) of the fluid level in the water-seal glass tube of a bottle system or the water-seal chamber of a commercial system as the client breathes. Normally, fluctuations of 5–10 cm (2–4 in). occur until the lung has reexpanded. In suction drainage systems, the fluid line remains constant. *Fluctuations reflect the pressure changes in the pleural space during inhalation and exhalation. The fluid level rises when the client inhales and falls when the client exhales. The absence of fluctuations may indicate tubing obstruction from a kink, dependent loop, blood clot, or outside pressure (e.g., because the client is lying on the tubing), or may indicate that full lung reexpansion has occurred.*

- To check for fluctuation in suction systems, temporarily disconnect the system. Then observe the fluctuation.

- Check for intermittent bubbling in the water of the water-seal bottle or chamber. *Intermittent bubbling*

normally occurs when the system removes air from the pleural space, especially when the client takes a deep breath or coughs. Absence of bubbling indicates that the pleural space has healed and is sealed. Continuous bubbling or a sudden change from an established pattern can indicate a break in the system, i.e., an air leak, and should be reported immediately.

- Check for gentle bubbling in the suction-control bottle or chamber. *Gentle bubbling indicates proper suction pressure.*

5. **Assess the drainage.**

- Inspect the drainage in the collection container at least every 30 minutes during the first 2 hours after chest tube insertion and every 2 hours thereafter.

- Every 8 hours, mark the time, date, and drainage level on a piece of adhesive tape affixed to the container, or mark it directly on a disposable container (see Figure 41–56).

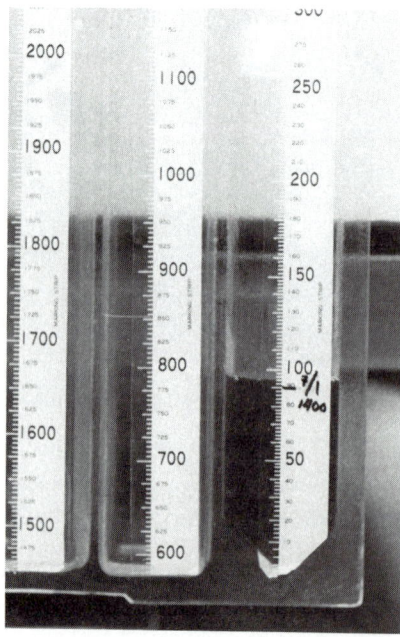

Figure 41–56 Marking the date, time, and drainage level.

- Note any sudden change in the amount or color of the drainage.

- If drainage exceeds 100 mL/hour or if a color change indicates hemorrhage, notify the physician immediately.

6. **Watch for dislodgement of the tubes and remedy the problem promptly.**

- If the chest tube becomes disconnected from the drainage system:
  a. Have the client exhale fully.
  b. Clamp the chest tube close to the insertion site with two rubber-tipped clamps placed in opposite directions.
  c. Quickly clean the ends of the tubing with an antiseptic, reconnect them, and tape them securely.
  d. Unclamp the tube as soon as possible.
  e. Assess the client closely for respiratory distress (dyspnea, pallor, diaphoresis, blood-tinged sputum, or chest pain). *Clamping the tube prevents external air from entering the pleural space. Two clamps ensure complete closure of the tube. Having the client exhale and clamping the tube for no longer than necessary prevents an air or fluid buildup in the pleural space, which can cause further lung collapse.*
  f. Check vital signs every 10 minutes.

- If the chest tube becomes dislodged from the insertion site:
  a. Remove the dressing, and immediately apply pressure with the petrolatum gauze, your hand, or a towel.
  b. Cover the site with sterile 4 × 4 gauze squares.
  c. Tape the dressings with air-occlusive tape.
  d. Notify the physician immediately.

e. Assess the client for respiratory distress every 10 to 15 minutes or as health indicates.

■ If the drainage system is accidentally tipped over:
  a. Immediately return it to the upright position.
  b. Ask the client to take several deep breaths. *Deep breaths help force air out of the pleural cavity that might have entered when the water seal was not intact.*
  c. Notify the nurse in charge and the physician.
  d. Assess the client for respiratory distress.

7. **If continuous bubbling persists in the water-seal collection chamber indicating an air leak, determine its source.** *Continuous bubbling in the water-seal collection chamber normally occurs for only a few minutes after a chest tube is attached to drainage, since fluid and air initially rush out from the intrapleural space under high pressure.*

■ To detect an air leak follow the next steps sequentially (Quinn, 1986 and Palau, 1986):
  a. Check the tubing connection sites. Tighten and retape any connection that seems loose. *The tubing connection sites are the most likely places for leaks to occur. Bubbling will stop if these are the source of the leak.*
  b. If bubbling continues, clamp the chest tube near the insertion site and see if the bubbling stops while the client takes several deep breaths. *Clamping the chest tube near the insertion site will help determine whether the leak is proximal or distal to the clamp. Chest tube clamping must be done only for a few seconds at a time. Clamping for long periods can aggravate an existing pneumothorax or lead to a recurrent pneumothorax.*

c. If bubbling stops, follow the next step. The source of the air leak is above the clamp, i.e., between the clamp and the client. It may be either at the insertion site or inside the client.
d. If bubbling continues, the source of the air leak is below the clamp, i.e., in the drainage system below the clamp. See *locating an air leak below the chest tube clamp.*

■ To determine whether the air leak is at the insertion site or inside the client:
  a. Unclamp the tube and palpate gently around the insertion site. If the bubbling stops, the leak is at the insertion site. To remedy this situation, apply a petrolatum gauze and a 4 × 4 gauze around the insertion site and secure these dressings with adhesive tape.
  b. If the leak is not at the insertion site, it is inside the client and may indicate a dislodged tube or a new pneumothorax, a new disruption of the pleural space. In this instance leave the tube unclamped, notify the physician, and monitor the client for signs of respiratory distress.

■ To locate an air leak below the chest tube clamp:
  a. Move the clamp a few inches farther down and keep moving it downward a few inches at a time. Each time the clamp is moved, check the water-seal collection chamber for bubbling. The bubbling will stop as soon as the clamp is placed between the air leak and the water-seal drainage.
  b. Seal the leak when you locate it by applying tape to that portion of the drainage tube.
  c. If bubbling continues after the entire length of the tube is clamped, the air leak is in the

drainage device. To remedy this situation the drainage system must be replaced and the physician notified.

8. **Take a specimen of the chest drainage as required.**

■ Specimens of chest drainage may be taken from a disposable chest drainage system, since these systems are equipped with self-sealing ports. If a specimen is required:
  a. Use a povidone-iodine swab to wipe the self-sealing diaphragm on the back of the drainage collection chamber. Allow it to dry.
  b. Attach a sterile #18 or #20 gauge needle to a 3- or 5-ml syringe, and insert the needle into the diaphragm.
  c. Aspirate the specimen, attach the needle protector, label the syringe, and send it to the laboratory with the appropriate requisition form.

9. **Ensure essential client care.**

■ Encourage deep-breathing and coughing exercises every 2 hours if indicated (this may be contraindicated in clients with a lobectomy). Have the client sit upright to perform the exercises, and splint the tube insertion site with a pillow or with a hand to minimize discomfort. *Deep breathing and coughing help to remove accumulations from the pleural space, facilitate drainage, and help the lung to reexpand.*

■ While the client takes deep breaths, palpate the chest for thoracic expansion. Place your hands together at the base of the sternum so that your thumbs meet. As the client inhales, your thumbs should separate at least 2.5–5 cm (1–2 in). Note whether chest expansion is symmetric.

■ Reposition the client every 2 hours. When the client is lying on the affected side, place rolled towels beside the tubing. *Frequent position changes promote drainage, prevent complications, and provide comfort. Rolled towels prevent occlusion of the chest tube by the client's weight.*

■ Assist the client with range-of-motion exercises of the affected shoulder three times per day to maintain joint mobility.

■ When transporting and ambulating the client:

a. Attach rubber-tipped forceps to the client's gown for emergency use.

b. Keep the water-seal unit below chest level and upright.

c. If it is necessary to clamp the tube, remove the clamp as soon as possible.

d. Disconnect the drainage system from the suction apparatus

before moving the client, and make sure the air vent is open.

10. **Document relevant information.**

■ Record patency of chest tubes; type, amount, and color of drainage; presence of fluctuations, appearance of insertion site; laboratory specimens, if taken; respiratory assessments; client's vital signs and level of comfort; and all other nursing care provided.

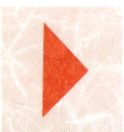

PROCEDURE 41–9

ASSISTING WITH THE REMOVAL OF A CHEST TUBE

Equipment ☑

Clean gloves to remove the dressing
Sterile gloves to remove the tube
Sterile suture removal set, with forceps and suture scissors

Sterile petrolatum gauze
Several 4 × 4 gauze squares
Air-occlusive tape, 2 or 3 in wide (nonallergenic is preferred)
Scissors

Absorbent linen-saver pad
Moistureproof bag
Sterile swabs or applicators in sterile containers to obtain a specimen (optional)

Intervention

1. **Prepare the client.**

■ Administer an analgesic, if ordered, 30 minutes before the tube is removed.

■ Ensure that the chest tube is securely clamped. *Clamping prevents air from entering the pleural space.*

■ Assist the client to a semi-Fowler's position or to a lateral position on the unaffected side.

■ Put the absorbent pad under the client beneath the chest tube. *The pad protects the bed linen from drainage and provides a place for the chest tube after removal.*

2. **Prepare sterile field and sterile air-tight gauze.**

■ Open the sterile packages, and prepare a sterile field.

■ Wearing sterile gloves, place the sterile petrolatum gauze on a 4 × 4 gauze square. *This will quickly provide an airtight dressing over the insertion site after the tube is removed.*

3. **Remove the soiled dressing.**

■ Be careful not to dislodge the tube when removing underlying gauzes.

■ Discard soiled dressings in the moisture-resistant bag.

4. **Prepare strips of air-occlusive tape.**

■ While the physician is removing the tube, remove gloves and prepare three 15-cm (6-in) strips of air-occlusive tape.

■ After the petrolatum gauze dressing is applied over the insertion site immediately after tube removal, completely cover it with the air-occlusive tape. *This makes the dressing as airtight as possible.*

5. **Obtain specimen as required.**

■ If a specimen is required for culture and sensitivity, use a swab to obtain drainage from inside the chest tube, while the physician holds the tube.

6. Assess the client.

■ Monitor the vital signs, and assess the quality of the respirations as health indicates, e.g., every 15 minutes for the first hour following tube removal and then less often.

■ Auscultate the client's lungs every hour for the first 4 hours to assess breath sounds and the adequacy of ventilation in the affected lung.

■ Assess the client regularly for signs of pneumothorax, subcutaneous emphysema, and infection.

7. Document relevant information.

■ Document the date and time of chest tube insertion or removal and the name of the physician.

■ Include the amount, color, and consistency of drainage, vital signs, and the specimen obtained for culture, if taken.

Sample Recording

Date 12-12-91	Time: 1000

Chest tubes removed by Dr. Jung. 100 mL clear pink drainage. BP 120/70, TPR 98.6, 76, 16. Specimen of chest tube drainage taken for culture and sensitivity and sent to lab. —————————Susan March, NS

EVALUATING

To evaluate whether client goals have been achieved, the nurse collects data pertaining to the established outcome criteria. Evaluation activities may include the following:

■ Observing the rate, depth, and character of respirations

■ Observing chest movements and symmetry of expansion

■ Observing ability to expectorate secretions

■ Auscultating breath sounds

■ Assessing pulse rate, volume, and rhythm

■ Assessing peripheral pulse volume

■ Inspecting color of skin, mucous membranes, lips, and earlobes

■ Observing the client demonstrating deep-breathing exercises as taught

■ Reviewing recent laboratory data, e.g., blood gas results

■ Asking the client about ability to perform activities of daily living without shortness of breath

■ Asking the client to describe purposes and side-effects of medications or to explain treatments prescribed for home care

Examples of evaluative statements indicating goal achievement are "The client's respirations are effortless, 16 per minute with symmetric chest expansion on inhalation," "Auscultated breath sounds are clear bilaterally," and "States can now perform hygienic care and toilet self without shortness of breath."

ASSESSMENT DATA

Nursing Assessment

Miss Ellen Martin is a 19-year-old secretary who was admitted to the hospital yesterday with an elevated temperature, a productive cough, and rapid, labored respirations. In taking a nursing history, Nurse Hayes finds that Miss Martin had a "bad cold" for several weeks that just wouldn't go away. She has been dieting for several months and skipping meals in order to decrease her caloric intake. Miss Martin mentions that in addition to her full-time job as a secretary, she is attending college classes 2 evenings a week and a dance class on Saturdays. Miss Martin, who is a smoker, states she has been unable to smoke for several days because of her cough and cold.

Physical Examination

Height: 167.6 cm (5'6")
Weight: 54.4 kg (120 lb)
Temperature: 39.4 C (103 F)
Pulse rate: 28 BPM
Blood pressure: 118/70 mm Hg
Skin pale, cheeks flushed, chills
Nasal flaring
Use of accessory muscles
Inspiratory rales with diminished breath sounds right base

Diagnostic Data

Chest x-ray film: R lobar infiltration
WBC: 14,000

CARE PLAN

Nursing Diagnosis	Client Goals and Outcome Criteria	Nursing Interventions and Rationales	Evaluation
Ineffective airway clearance related to thick sputum/pneumonia resulting in frequent productive cough, rapid respirations, nasal flaring, adventitious breath sounds, stabbing chest pain.	Client Goal: Normal breath sounds in right lung. Outcome Criteria: Coughs and deep breaths q1 hr within first 24 hrs. Ineffective coughing is eliminated by day 2. Expectorates secretions from airway whenever necessary. Increases fluid intake to 3000 ml to liquefy secretions by day 2. Lung sounds clear to auscultation by day 3.	Assess respirations and respiratory movements. *Rationale:* Aids in determining whether ventilation is adequate. Encourage coughing and deep breathing q1h. *Rationale:* Coughing in conjunction with deep breathing facilitates the movement and expectoration of respiratory tract secretions. Demonstrate effective coughing while splinting client's chest. *Rationale:* Ineffective coughing is tiring and will exhaust the client. Encourage fluid intake of 3000 ml/day. *Rationale:* Hydration will aid in liquefying thick, tenacious secretions and make them easier to expectorate as well as to replace fluid loss due to fever. Position client in semi-Fowler's or high Fowler's position. *Rationale:* Encourages maximum chest expansion. Assist with postural drainage 3 times daily. *Rationale:* Postural drainage will drain secretions from lung segments into tracheobronchial tree, from where they can be removed. Assist with IPPB and/or nebulizer treatments. *Rationale:* Facilitates the clearing of bronchial secretions by thinning secretions.	Client coughs and deep breaths purposefully q1–2 hrs during the day. While coughing, she splints her chest with her hands or a pillow. She coughs forcefully after taking a deep breath, using her abdominal and accessory respiratory muscles. Her fluid intake is approximately 3000 ml each day. Cough continues to be productive of moderately thick, rusty sputum. Inspiratory rales still present in right lung. Adventitious breath sounds still audible at base of right lung.

Impaired gas exchange related to accumulation of secretions in airways resulting in dyspnea, tachypnea, pallor, tachycardia, decreased activity tolerance, decreased P_{O_2}.	Client Goal: Increase O_2 and CO_2 exchange. Increase activity tolerance without experiencing dyspnea and chest pain. Outcome Criteria: Relief of symptoms of chest pain, tachypnea, dyspnea by day 5. Improved activity tolerance by day 5. Improved P_{O_2} by day 2.	Assess respiratory status and vital signs. *Rationale:* Vital signs and respiratory status will indicate adequacy of ventilation. Maintain oxygen 30% per nasal cannula at 5 liters. *Rationale:* Additional oxygen will reduce hypoxemia. Maintain bed rest and assist with ADLs. *Rationale:* Rest decreases metabolic rate and oxygen demand by tissues, thereby decreasing dyspnea. Monitor arterial blood gases. *Rationale:* Indicates adequacy of ventilation and perfusion.	On day 5, client is able to sit at the bedside 4× daily without chest pain and dyspnea. Her respirations are 22 per minute. She is assisting with her bed bath. Her P_{O_2} is 85 mm Hg.

CHAPTER HIGHLIGHTS

▶ Respiration, the process of gaseous exchange between the individual and the atmosphere, involves pulmonary ventilation, diffusion of gases, and transport of oxygen and carbon dioxide to and from the body's cells.

▶ Pulmonary ventilation, the inflow and outflow of air between the atmosphere and the alveoli of the lungs, is accomplished through the mechanical act of breathing (inspiration and expiration).

▶ The volume to which the lungs expand during ventilation depends on the pattern of breathing, the size and position of the individual, medical or surgical conditions affecting the thorax, and developmental variations in the shape of the chest.

▶ Ventilation depends upon adequate atmospheric oxygen, clear air passages, adequate pulmonary compliance and recoil, and neurochemical regulation of respiration.

▶ Diffusion of oxygen and carbon dioxide is the movement of the gases from areas of greater pressure or concentration to areas of lower pressure or concentration.

▶ The rate of diffusion of gases through the respiratory membrane is influenced by the thickness of the membrane, surface area of the membrane, diffusion coefficient of the gases, and pressure difference on either side of the membrane.

▶ Factors affecting the rate of oxygen transport include: cardiac output, the number of erythrocytes present in the blood, exercise, and blood hematocrit.

▶ In healthy individuals, decreased concentration of carbon dioxide in the blood stimulates respiration. Clients with respiratory disorders such as COPD have what is called a *hypoxic drive*, i.e., decreased levels of blood oxygen stimulate respiration.

▶ Factors that influence oxygenation of the body's tissues include altitude, air pollution, emotions, exercise, health, life-style, and narcotic analgesics.

▶ Respiratory function may be altered by any condition that affects the movement of air into or out of the lungs, changes in the diffusion rate of oxygen and carbon dioxide between the alveoli and the pulmonary capillaries, or alterations in the transport of oxygen and carbon dioxide via the blood to and from the tissue cells.

▶ Hypoxia is insufficient oxygenation of body tissues.

▶ Clinical signs of hypoxia may be early (increased heart and respiratory rates and slight rise in systolic blood pressure) or late (decreased pulse and systolic blood pressure, dyspnea, cough, and hemoptysis). Cyanosis is not a reliable sign.

▶ Normal respiration (eupnea) is quiet, rhythmic, and effortless. Common altered breathing patterns include: tachypnea, bradypnea, dyspnea, orthopnea, hyperventilation, and hypoventilation.

▶ The signs of airway obstruction include: labored noisy respirations, extreme inspiratory effort without chest movement, sternal or intercostal retractions, altered arterial blood gas values, restlessness, dyspnea, and abnormal or absent breath sounds.

READINGS AND REFERENCES

SUGGESTED READINGS

Eggland, E. T. January 1987. Teaching the ABCs of C.O.P.D. *Nursing 87* 17:60–64.

Because a COPD patient can never take breathing for granted, this home care nurse went "back to the basics" to help an elderly client breathe more easily. The ABCs include (A) airway pathophysiology, (B) better breathing techniques, and (C) controlled environment.

Hahn, K. April 1987. Slow-teaching the C.O.P.D. patient. *Nursing 87* 17:34–41.

This ANA/AACN approved continuing education article discusses essential information to teach a client experiencing chronic breathlessness. Included are ways to prevent exacerbations; three controlled-breathing techniques (floppy-lips breathing, abdominal breathing, and counted breathing); the three causes of COPD; common bronchial irritants; COPD medications; and proper use of inhalers.

Hoffman, L. A., and Wesmiller, S. W. April 1988. Home oxygen. Transtracheal and other options. *American Journal of Nursing* 88:464–69.

This article describes an array of new oxygen delivery systems for oxygen therapy clients at home. They include transtracheal insertion and maintenance, O_2 through eyeglass frames, two types of reservoir cannulae, and demand delivery devices. Using eight photographs and one table, the authors compare the systems in terms of advantages and disadvantages and oxygen conservation.

Mims, B. C. July 1987. The risks of oxygen therapy. Part 2. *RN* 50:20–26.

In this second article on respiratory problems, Mims discusses identifying patients who need oxygen, recognizing oxygen deficit, and low-flow and high-flow methods of oxygen delivery. Two case studies emphasize that giving more oxygen may not cure hypoxia and that oxygen is not always the best solution for clients with COPD.

RELATED RESEARCH

Balazs, I. B.; Walton, C. B.; Briggs, S.; and Goldstein, M. January 1987. A clinical evaluation of an oxygen insufflation/suction catheter. *Heart and Lung* 16:39–46.

Bostick, J., and Wendelgass, S. T. September 1987. Normal saline instillation as part of the suctioning procedure: Effects on Pao_2 and amount of secretions. *Heart and Lung* 16:532–37.

Casey, F. S.; Haughey, B. P.; Dittmar, S. S.; O'Shea, R. M.; and Brasure, J. November 1989. Smoking practices among nursing students: A comparison of two studies. *Journal of Nursing Education* 28:397–401.

Pierce, J. B., and Piazza, D. E. January 1987. Differences in postsuctioning arterial blood oxygen concentration values using two postoxygenation methods. *Heart and Lung* 16:34–38.

Winslow, E. H.; Lane, L. D.; and Gaffney, F. A. May/June 1985. Oxygen uptake and cardiovascular responses in control adults and acute myocardial infarction patients during bathing. *Nursing Research* 34:164–69.

SELECTED REFERENCES

Acee, S. July/August 1984. Helping patients breathe more easily. *Geriatric Nursing* 5:230–33.

Albanese, A. J., and Toplitz, A. D. April 1982. A hassle-free guide to suctioning a tracheostomy. *RN* 45:24–29.

American Heart Association. 1986. Standards and guidelines for cardiopulmonary resuscitation (CPR) and emergency cardiac care (ECC). *Journal of the American Medical Association* 255:2841–3044.

Birdsall, C., and Ruggio J. August 1987. Mouth-to-mouth resuscitation—is there a safe, effective alternative? . . . face mask with wide, flexible tubing. *American Journal of Nursing* 87:1019.

Byrne, C. J.; Saxton, D. F.; Pelikan, P. K.; and Nugent, P. M. 1986. *Laboratory tests: Implications for nursing care.* 2d ed. Menlo Park, Calif.: Addison-Wesley Publishing Co.

Carpenito, L. J. 1989. *Nursing diagnosis: Application to Clinical Practice.* 3d ed. Philadelphia: J. B. Lippincott Co.

Carroll, P. F. January 1985. Action stat! Dislodged trach tube. *Nursing 85* 15:46.

———. December 1986. The ins and outs of chest drainage systems. *Nursing 86* 16:26–34.

———. May 1988. Lowering the risks of endotracheal suctioning. *Nursing 88* 18:46–50.

Crocco, J. A.; Francis, P. B.; and Lefrak, S. S. May 15, 1987. When the patient needs oxygen—stat. *Patient Care* 21:83–86, 89.

Dennison, R. D. October 1987. Managing the patient with upper airway obstruction. *Nursing 87* 17:34–42.

Dunleap, E. August 1987. Safe and easy ways to secure breathing tubes. *RN* 50:26–27.

Fuchs, P. L. 1983a. Humidifiers. pp. 458–62. *The nurse's reference library: Procedures.* Nursing 83 Books, Springhouse, Pa.: Intermed Communications.

———. 1983b. Nebulizers. pp. 462–66. *The nurse's reference library: Procedures.* Nursing 83 Books, Springhouse, Pa.: Intermed Communications.

———. May 1984a. Streamlining your suctioning techniques. Part 1. Nasotracheal suctioning. *Nursing 84* 14:55–61.

———. July 1984b. Streamlining your suctioning techniques. Part 2. Tracheostomy suctioning. *Nursing 84* 14:39–43.

Green, E., and Sumner, S. November 1988. Does nursing need its own ACLS course? . . . advanced cardiac life support. *Nursing 88* 18:40–42.

Guyton, A. C. 1986. *Textbook of medical physiology.* 7th ed. Philadelphia: W. B Saunders Co.

Hoffman, L. A., and Maszkiewicz, R. C. January 1987. Airway management for the critically ill patient. *American Journal of Nursing* 87:39–53.

Hoffman, L. A., and Wesmiller, S. W. April 1988. Home oxygen: Transtracheal and other options. *American Journal of Nursing* 88:464–69.

Juip, M., and Harned, J. C. December 1988. Giving mouth-to-mouth ventilations? *Nursing 88* 18:48–49.

Kim, M. J. July 1984. Respiratory muscle training: Implications for patient care. *Heart and Lung* 13:333–40.

Kim, M. J.; McFarland, G. K.; and McLane, A. M. 1989. *Pocket guide to nursing diagnoses.* 3d ed. St. Louis: C. V. Mosby Co.

Knauss, P. J. December 1985. Chest tube stripping: Is it necessary? *Focus on Critical Care* 12:41–43.

Lederer, J. R.; Marculescu, G. L.; Mocnik, B.; and Seaby, N. 1990. *Care Planning Pocket Guide.* 3d ed. Redwood City, Calif.: Addison-Wesley Nursing.

Lockhart, J. S., and Griffin, C. April 1987. Action STAT! Occluded trach tube. *Nursing 87* 17:33.

Lynch, J., and Bennett, B. February 1986. A review of airway devices. *Emergency Care Quarterly* 1:51–61.

McIntyre, K. M., and Lewis, A. J., editors. 1983. *Textbook of advanced cardiac life support.* Dallas, Texas: American Heart Association.

Mapp, C. S. July 1988. Trach care: Are you aware of all the dangers? *Nursing 88* 18:34–43.

Miller, K. S. February 1987. Chest tubes: Indications, techniques, management and complications. *Chest* 91:258–64.

Mims, B. C. July 1987. The risks of oxygen therapy. Part 2. *RN* 50:20–26.

NANDA approved nursing diagnostic categories for clinical use and testing. Summer 1988. *Nursing Diagnosis Newsletter* 15:1–3.

Newbold, D. June 24–30, 1987. The physiology of cardiac massage. Part 1. *Nursing Times* 83: 59–60, 62.

Palau D., Jones, S. October 1986. Test your skill at trouble shooting chest tubes. *RN* 49:43–45.

Preston, I. M.; Matthews, H. R., and Ready, A. R. October 10, 1986. Minitracheostomy: A new technique for tracheal suction. *Physiotherapy* 72:494–97.

Quinn, A. September 1986. Thora-Drain III: Closed chest drainage made simpler and safer. *Nursing 86* 16:46–51.

Reed, J. Jr. November 1987. Orotracheal and nasotracheal intubation. *Emergency Care Quarterly 2* 3:1–6.

Scherer, P. December 1986. ACLS guidelines: What nurses are saying about the drug changes. *American Journal of Nursing* 86:1352–58.

Shekleton, M. E., and Nield, M. March 1987. Ineffective airway clearance related to artificial airway. *Nursing Clinics of North America* 22:167–78.

Spearing, C., and Cornell, D. J. September 1987. Incentive spirometry: Inspiring your patient to breath deeply. *Nursing 87* 17:50–51.

Stevens, S. A., and Becker, K. L. January 1988. How to perform picture-perfect respiratory assessment. *Nursing 88* 18:57–63.

Sumner, S. November 1988. Another point of view. *Nursing 88* 18:42.

Sumner, S. M., and Gran, P. E. July 1982. Emergency! First aid for choking. *Nursing 82* 12:40–49.

Transtracheal oxygen: The nose knows the difference. April 1987. *American Journal of Nursing* 87:421–22.

Weaver, T. E. May 1985. Chronic ineffective gas exchange: When your patient goes from bad to worse. *Nursing 85* 15:7.

———. February 1981. New life for lungs through incentive spirometers. *Nursing 81* 11:54–58.

Willens, J. S., and Copel, L. C. January 1989. Performing CPR on adults. *Nursing 89* 19:34–43.

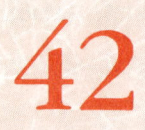
Fecal Elimination

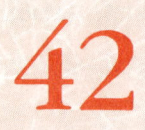

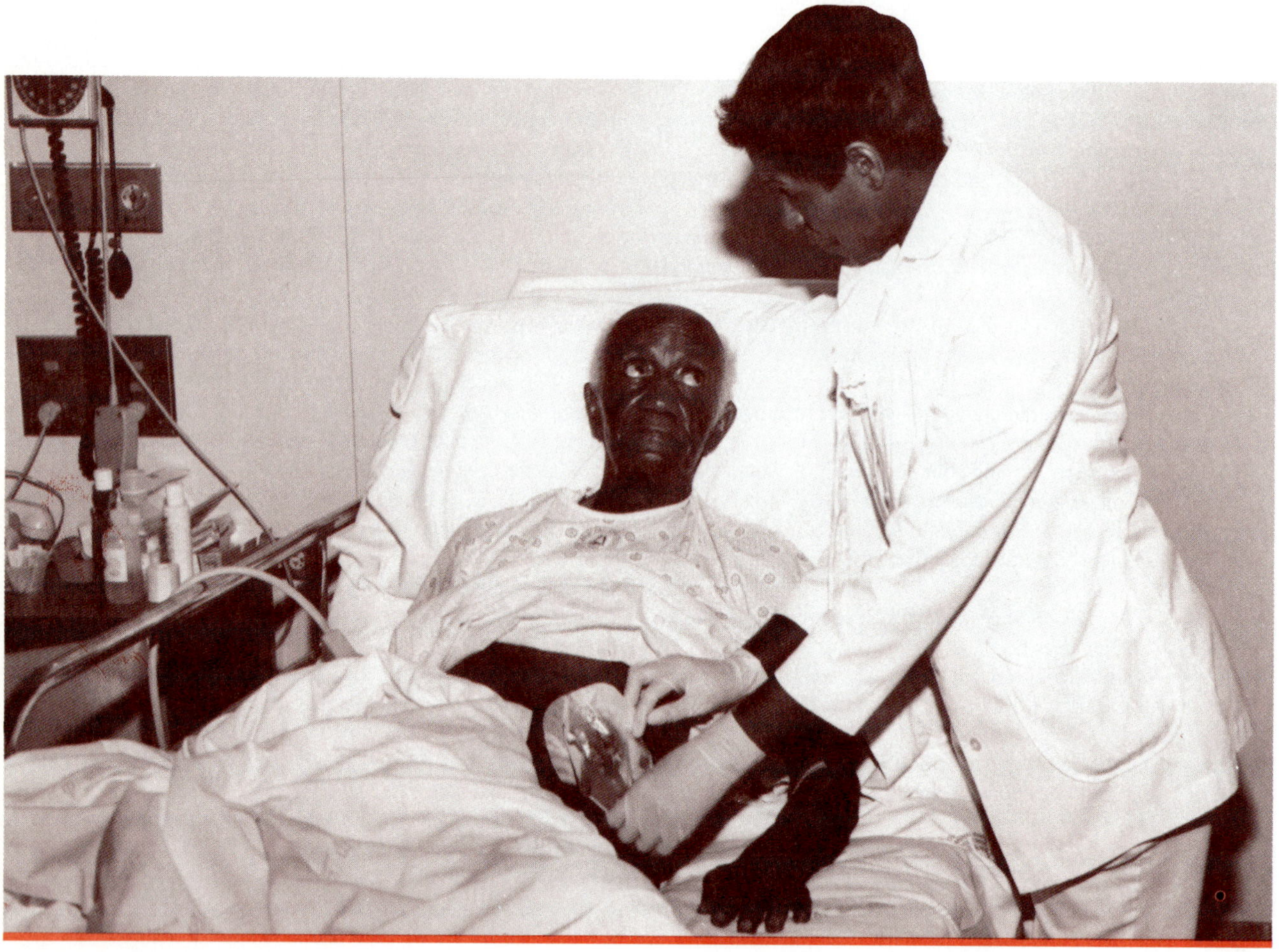

- Describe the functions of the lower intestinal tract.
- Identify factors that influence fecal elimination and patterns of defecation.
- Distinguish between normal and ab-

normal characteristics and constituents of feces.

- Describe methods used to assess the intestinal tract.
- Differentiate among specific common fecal elimination problems.
- Identify common causes and effects of selected fecal elimination problems.

- Identify measures that maintain normal fecal elimination patterns.
- Relate common interventions to specific fecal elimination problems.
- Give reasons for selected nursing interventions.
- Describe modifications for clients with ostomies.
- State outcome criteria essential for evaluating the client's progress.

PHYSIOLOGY OF DEFECATION

Elimination of the waste products of digestion from the body is essential to health. The excreted waste products are referred to as **feces** or **stool.**

Large Intestine

The large intestine extends from the ileocecal (ileocolic) valve, which lies between the small and large intestines, to the anus. The colon (large intestine) in the adult is generally about 125 to 150 cm (50 to 60 in) long. It has seven parts: the cecum; ascending, transverse, and descending colons; sigmoid colon; rectum; and anus or external orifice. See Figure 42–1.

The large intestine is a muscular tube lined with mucous membrane. See Figure 42–2. The muscle fibers are both circular and longitudinal, thus permitting the intestine to enlarge and contract in both width and length. The longitudinal muscles are shorter than the colon and therefore cause the large intestine to form pouches, or **haustra.**

The colon's main functions are the absorption of water and nutrients, the mucal protection of the intestinal wall, and fecal elimination. The contents of the colon normally represent foods ingested over the previous 4 days, although most of the waste products are excreted within 48 hours of **ingestion** (the act of taking food). The waste products leaving the stomach through the small intestine and then passing through the ileocecal valve are called **chyme.** The colon absorbs water and significant amounts of sodium and chloride as food passes along it. As much as 1500 ml of chyme passes into the large intestine daily, and all but about 100 ml is absorbed in the proximal half of the colon. The 100 ml of fluid is excreted in the feces (Guyton 1986, p. 796).

The colon also serves a protective function in that it secretes mucus. This mucus contains large amounts of bicarbonate ions. The mucus secretion is stimulated by excitation of parasympathetic nerves. Therefore, during extreme stimulation—e.g., as a result of emotions—large amounts of mucus are secreted, resulting in the passage of stringy mucus as often as every 30 minutes with little or no

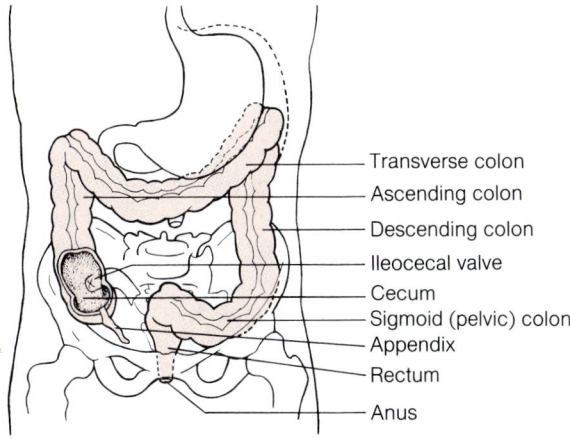

Figure 42–1 The large intestine and rectum.

Transverse colon
Ascending colon
Descending colon
Ileocecal valve
Cecum
Sigmoid (pelvic) colon
Appendix
Rectum
Anus

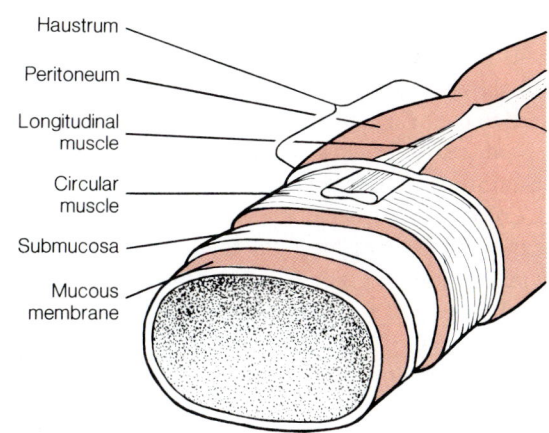

Figure 42–2 The layers of the wall of the large intestine.

Haustrum
Peritoneum
Longitudinal muscle
Circular muscle
Submucosa
Mucous membrane

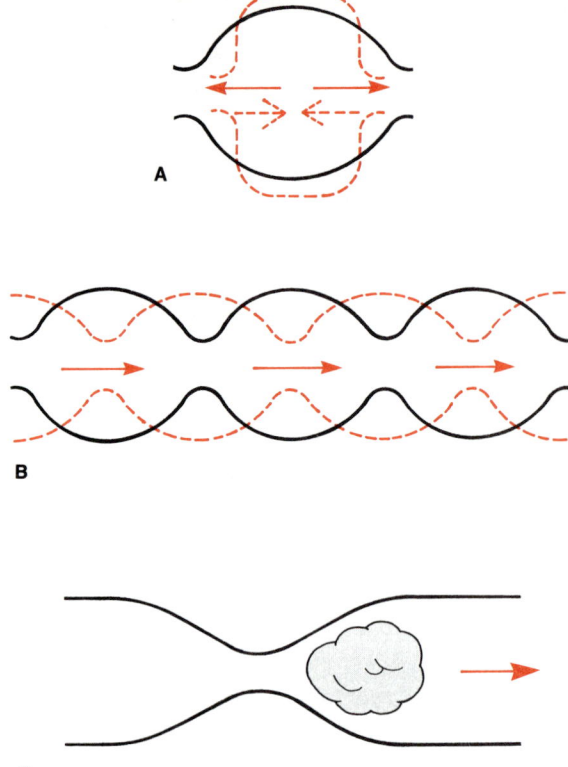

Figure 42–3 Three types of intestinal movements: *A,* haustral churning; *B,* peristalsis; *C,* mass peristalsis.

feces (Guyton 1986, p. 785). Mucus serves to protect the wall of the large intestine from trauma by the acids formed in the feces, and it serves as an adherent for holding the fecal material together. Mucus also protects the intestinal wall from bacterial activity.

The colon acts to transport along its lumen the products of digestion, which are eventually eliminated through the anal canal. These products are flatus and feces. Flatus is largely air and the by-products of the digestion of carbohydrates. Three types of movements occur in the large intestine: haustral churning, colon peristalsis, and mass peristalsis. See Figure 42–3. **Haustral churning** or **shuffling** involves movement of the chyme back and forth within the haustra. In addition to mixing the contents, this action aids in the absorption of water and moves the contents forward to the next haustra. **Peristalsis** is wavelike movement produced by the circular and longitudinal muscle fibers of the intestinal walls; it propels the intestinal contents forward. Colon peristalsis is very sluggish and is thought to move the chyme very little along the large intestine. **Mass peristalsis,** the third type of colonic movement, involves a wave of powerful muscular contraction that moves over large areas of the colon. Usually mass peristalsis occurs after eating, stimulated by the presence of food in the stomach and small intestine. In adults, mass peristaltic waves occur only a few times a day.

Rectum and Anal Canal

The rectum in the adult is usually 10 to 15 cm (4 to 6 in) long; the most distal portion, 2.5 to 5 cm (1 to 2 in) long, is the anal canal. In the rectum are three folds of tissue that extend across the rectum and several folds that extend vertically. Each of the vertical folds contains a vein and an artery. It is believed that these folds help retain feces within the rectum. When the veins become distended, as can occur with repeated pressure, a condition known as *hemorrhoids* occurs (see discussion later in the chapter).

The anal canal is bounded by an internal and an external sphincter muscle. See Figure 42–4. The *internal sphincter* is under involuntary control, and the external sphincter normally is voluntarily controlled. The *external sphincter*'s action is augmented by the levator ani muscles of the pelvic floor. The internal sphincter muscle is innervated by the autonomic nervous system; the external sphincter is innervated by the somatic nervous system.

Defecation

Defecation is the expulsion of feces from the anus and rectum. It is also called a bowel movement. The frequency of defecation is highly individual, varying from several times per day to two or three times per week. The amount defecated also varies from person to person. When peristaltic waves move the feces into the sigmoid colon and the rectum, the sensory nerves in the rectum are stimulated and the individual becomes aware of the need to defecate.

Defecation is normally initiated by two defecation reflexes. See Figure 42–5. When feces enter the rectum, distention of the rectal walls initiates a signal that spreads through the mesenteric plexus to initiate peristaltic waves in the descending and sigmoid colons and in the rectum. These waves force the feces toward the anus. As the peristaltic waves approach the anus, the internal anal sphincter becomes inhibited from closing and, if the external sphincter is relaxed, defecation occurs. This is called the *intrinsic defecation reflex.*

The second reflex, called the *parasympathetic defecation reflex,* is also actively involved in defecation. When nerve fibers in the rectum are stimulated, signals are transmitted to the spinal cord and then back to the descending and sigmoid colons and the rectum. These parasympathetic signals intensify the peristaltic waves, relax the internal anal sphincter, and intensify the intrinsic defecation reflex.

The *internal* anal sphincter relaxes, and feces move into the anal canal. After the individual is seated on a toilet or bedpan, the *external* anal sphincter is relaxed voluntarily. Expulsion of the feces is assisted by contraction of the abdominal muscles and the diaphragm, which increases abdominal pressure, and by contraction of the levator ani muscles of the pelvic floor, which moves the feces through the anal canal. Normal defecation is facilitated by (1) thigh flexion, which increases the pressure within the abdomen,

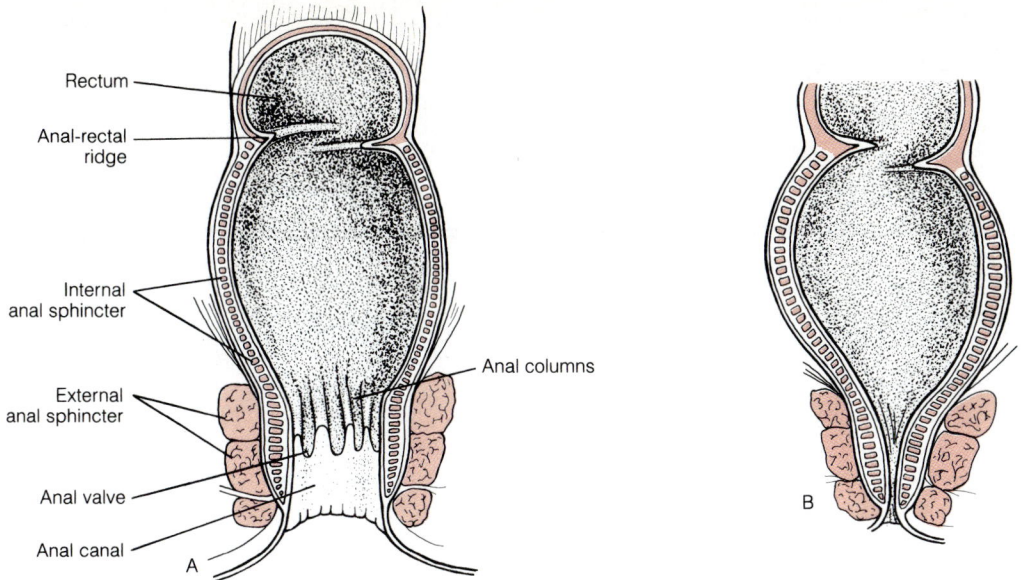

Figure 42–4 The rectum, anal canal, and anal sphincters: *A,* open; *B,* closed.

and (b) a sitting position, which increases the downward pressure on the rectum.

If the defecation reflex is ignored, or if defecation is consciously inhibited by contracting the external sphincter muscle, the urge to defecate normally disappears for a few hours before occurring again. Repeated inhibition of the urge to defecate can result in expansion of the rectum to accommodate accumulated feces and eventual loss of sensitivity to the need to defecate. Constipation can be the ultimate result.

FACTORS THAT AFFECT DEFECATION

Age and Development   Age affects not only the character of fecal elimination but also its control. The very young are unable to control elimination until the neuromuscular system is developed, usually between the ages of 2 and 3 years. The elderly also experience changes that can affect bowel evacuation. Two of these are **atony** (lack of normal muscle tone) of the smooth muscle of the colon, which can result in a slower peristalsis and thus hardened (drier) feces, and decreased tone of the abdominal muscles, which also decreases the pressure that can be exerted during bowel evacuation. Some elderly people also have decreased control of the anal sphincter muscles, which can result in an urgency to defecate.

Diet   Sufficient bulk (cellulose, fiber) in the diet is necessary to provide fecal volume. Certain foods are difficult or impossible for some people to digest. This inability results in digestive upsets and, in some instances, the passage of

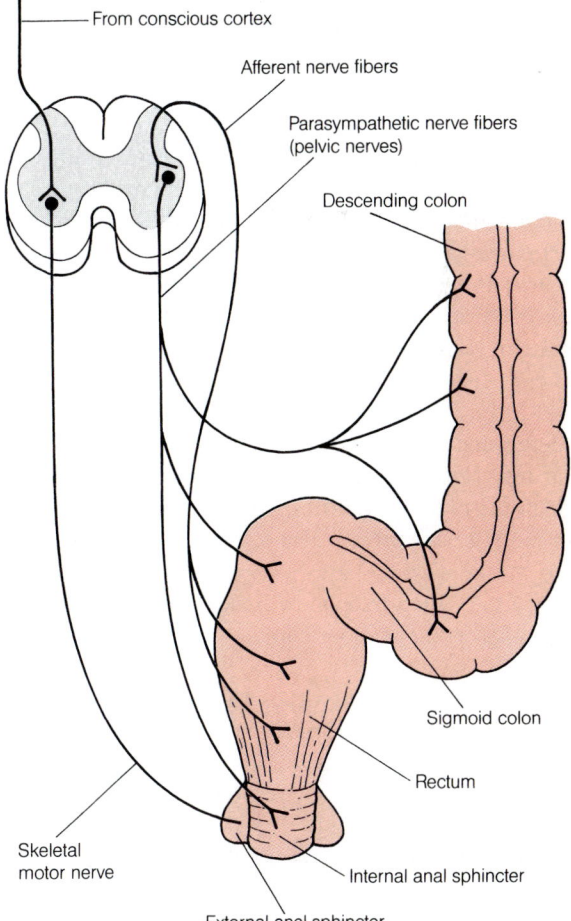

Figure 42–5 The afferent and efferent pathways of the parasympathetic nervous system for stimulating defecation.

watery stools. Irregular eating can also impair regular defecation. Individuals who eat at the same times every day have a regularly timed, physiologic response to the food intake and a regular pattern of peristaltic activity in the colon. Spicy foods can produce diarrhea and flatus in some individuals.

Fluid   When fluid intake is inadequate or output (urine or vomitus, for example) is excessive for some reason, the body continues to reabsorb fluid from the chyme as it passes along the colon. As a result the chyme becomes drier than normal, resulting in hard feces. In addition, reduced fluid intake slows the chyme's passage along the intestines, further increasing the reabsorption of fluid from the chyme. Healthy fecal elimination usually requires a daily fluid intake of 2000 to 3000 ml. If chyme moves abnormally quickly through the large intestine, however, there is less time for fluid to be absorbed into the blood; as a result, the feces are soft or even watery.

Activity   Activity also stimulates peristalsis, thus facilitating the movement of chyme along the colon. Weak abdominal and pelvic muscles are often ineffective in increasing the intraabdominal pressure during defecation or in controlling defecation. Weak muscles can result from lack of exercise, immobility, or impaired neurologic functioning.

Psychologic Factors   Certain diseases that involve severe diarrhea, such as ulcerative colitis, may have a psychologic component. It is also known that some people who are anxious or angry experience increased peristaltic activity and subsequent diarrhea. In addition, people who are depressed may experience slower intestinal motility, resulting in constipation.

Life-Style   Early bowel training may establish the habit of defecating at regular times, such as daily after breakfast, or it may lead to an irregular pattern of defecation. The availability of toilet facilities, embarrassment about odors, and the need for privacy also affect fecal elimination patterns. A client who shares a room in a hospital may be unwilling to use a bedpan because of the lack of privacy and embarrassment about odors.

Medications   Some drugs have side effects that can interfere with normal elimination. Some cause diarrhea; others, such as large doses of certain tranquilizers and repeated administration of morphine and codeine, cause constipation.

Some medications directly affect elimination. **Laxatives** are medications that stimulate bowel activity and so assist fecal elimination. There are medications that soften stool, facilitating defecation. Certain medications, such as dicyclomine hydrochloride (Bentyl), suppress peristaltic activity and sometimes are used to treat diarrhea.

Diagnostic Procedures   Before certain diagnostic procedures, such as visualization of the sigmoid colon (sigmoidoscopy), the client is allowed no food or fluid after midnight preceding the examination. Often the client is given a cleansing enema prior to the examination. In these instances the client will not usually defecate normally until eating has been resumed.

Barium (used in radiologic exams) presents a further problem. It hardens if allowed to remain in the colon, producing constipation and sometimes an impaction.

Anesthesia and Surgery   General anesthetics cause the normal colonic movements to cease or slow down by blocking parasympathetic stimulation to the muscles of the colon. Clients who have regional or spinal anesthesia are less likely to experience this problem.

Surgery that involves direct handling of the intestines can cause temporary cessation of intestinal movement. This is called *paralytic ileus,* a condition that usually lasts 24 to 48 hours. Listening for bowel sounds that reflect intestinal motility is an important nursing assessment following surgery. See Chapter 19 for assessment of bowel sounds.

Pathologic Conditions   Spinal cord injuries and head injuries, for example, can decrease the sensory stimulation for defecation. Impaired mobility may limit the client's ability to respond to the urge to defecate when the client is unable to reach a toilet or summon assistance. As a result, the client may experience constipation. Or a client may experience fecal incontinence because of poorly functioning anal sphincters (see discussion later in the chapter).

Irritants   Spicy foods, bacterial toxins, and poisons can irritate the intestinal tract and produce diarrhea and often large amounts of flatus.

Pain   Clients who experience discomfort when defecating, e.g., following hemorrhoid surgery, will often suppress the urge to defecate to avoid the pain. Such clients can experience constipation as a result.

COMMON FECAL ELIMINATION PROBLEMS

There are six common problems of fecal elimination: constipation, fecal impaction, diarrhea, fecal incontinence, flatulence, and hemorrhoids.

Constipation

Constipation refers to the passage of small, dry, hard stool or the passage of no stool for a period of time. It occurs when the movement of feces through the large intestine is slow, thus allowing time for additional reabsorption of fluid from the large intestine. Associated with constipation are difficult evacuation of stool and increased effort or straining of the voluntary muscles of defecation. It is important to define constipation in relation to the person's regular elimination pattern. Some people normally defecate only a few times a week and therefore are not necessarily constipated when they fail to defecate every day. Other people defecate more than once a day; to them, a movement only once a day can indicate constipation. Careful assessment of the person's habits is necessary before a diagnosis of constipation is made.

McShane and McLane (1988, pp. 31–32) describe three types of constipation: rectal, colonic, and perceived. In *rectal constipation,* the pattern of elimination is changed and characterized by fecal retention, normal fecal consistency, and delayed defecation as a result of biopsychosocial disruptions. *Colonic constipation* is manifested by the passage of hard, dry feces as a result of the delayed passage of food residue. *Perceived constipation* is a condition in which the person makes a self-diagnosis of constipation and ensures a daily bowel movement through overuse of laxatives, enemas, and suppositories. See the accompanying box for defining characteristics of constipation.

Many causes and factors contribute to constipation, among them:

- *Irregular defecation habits.* When the normal defecation reflexes are inhibited or ignored, these conditioned reflexes tend to be progressively weakened. When habitually ignored, the urge to defecate is ultimately lost. Children at play may ignore these reflexes; adults ignore them because of the pressures of time or work. Hospitalized clients may suppress the urge because of embarrassment about using a bedpan or because defecation is too uncomfortable.

- *Overuse of laxatives.* Overuse of laxatives has the same effect as ignoring the urge to defecate—natural defecation reflexes are inhibited. The habitual user of laxatives eventually requires larger or stronger doses, since they have a progressively reduced effect with continual use.

- *Increased psychologic stress.* Strong emotion is thought to cause constipation by inhibiting intestinal peristalsis through the action of epinephrine and the sympathetic nervous system. Stress can also cause a spastic bowel (spastic or hypertonic constipation or an irritable colon). Associated with this type of constipation are abdominal cramps, increased amounts of mucus, and alternating periods of constipation and diarrhea.

- *Inappropriate diet.* Bland diets and low-fiber diets are lacking in bulk and therefore create insufficient residue of waste products to stimulate the reflex for defecation. Low-residue foods such as rice, eggs, and lean meats move more slowly through the intestinal tract. Increasing fluid intake with such foods increases their rate of movement. A change in diet can also contribute to constipation.

Defining Characteristics of Constipation

- Decreased frequency of defecation
- Hard, dry stool
- Straining at stool
- Painful defecation
- Abdominal pain
- Abdominal distention
- Rectal pressure or fullness
- Palpable fecal mass (rectal constipation)
- Headache
- Impaired appetite
- Expected daily defecation (perceived constipation)
- Overuse of defecation aids (perceived constipation)

- *Insufficient fluid.* An insufficient fluid intake reduces the amount of fluid in the chyme, which enters the large intestine. This lack of fluid in turn results in drier, harder feces.

- *Medications.* Some drugs, such as morphine or codeine as well as adrenergic and anticholinergic drugs, slow the motility of the colon through their action on the central nervous system, thus causing constipation. Others, such as iron tablets, have an astringent effect and act more locally on the bowel mucosa to cause constipation. Iron also has an irritating effect and can cause diarrhea in some people.

- *Insufficient exercise.* In clients on prolonged bed rest, generalized muscle weakness extends to the muscles of the abdomen, diaphragm, and pelvic floor, which are used in defecation. Indirectly associated with lack of exercise is lack of appetite and possible subsequent lack of fiber.

- *Age.* The muscle weakness and poor sphincter tone that occur in some elderly people contribute to constipation. In addition, the decrease in mucus and intestinal secretions contributes to this problem.

- *Disease processes.* Several diseases produce constipation, such as bowel obstruction; paralysis, which inhibits the client's ability to bear down; and pelvic inflammatory conditions, which create paralysis or atony of the bowel.

Constipation can be hazardous to clients. Straining in order to defecate can place stress on abdominal or perineal sutures, rupturing them if the pressure is sufficiently great. In addition, straining often is accompanied by holding the breath. This Valsalva maneuver can present serious problems to people with heart disease, brain injuries, or respiratory disease. Holding the breath increases the intrathoracic and the intracranial pressures. To some degree this pressure can be reduced if the person exhales through the mouth while straining. However, avoiding any straining is the best precaution.

Fecal Impaction

Fecal impaction is a mass or collection of hardened, puttylike feces in the folds of the rectum. Impaction results from prolonged retention and accumulation of fecal material. In severe impactions the feces accumulate and extend well up into the sigmoid colon and beyond. Fecal impaction is recognized by the passage of liquid fecal seepage (diarrhea) and no normal stool. The liquid portion of the feces seeps out around the impacted mass. See Figure 42–6. Impaction can also be assessed by digital examination of the rectum, during which the hardened mass can often be palpated.

Along with fecal seepage and constipation, symptoms include frequent but nonproductive desire to defecate and rectal pain. A generalized feeling of illness results; the client becomes anorexic, the abdomen becomes distended, and nausea and vomiting may occur.

The causes of fecal impaction are usually poor defecation habits and constipation. Certain medications (see page 1158) also contribute to impactions. The barium used in radiologic examinations of the upper and lower gastrointestinal tracts can be a causative factor. Therefore, after these examinations, measures are usually taken to ensure removal of the barium. In the elderly, a combination of factors contribute to impactions: poor fluid intake, insufficient bulk in the diet, lack of activity, and weakened muscle tone. In some people, impactions tend to occur regardless of the measures taken to prevent them.

An impaction can sometimes be palpated through the client's abdomen. Digital examination of the impaction through the rectum should be done gently and carefully because stimulation of the vagus nerve in the rectal wall can slow the client's heart. Some nurses advise against digital rectal examination without a physician's order.

Diarrhea

Diarrhea refers to the passage of liquid feces and an increased frequency of defecation. It is the opposite of constipation and results from rapid movement of fecal contents through the large intestine. Rapid passage of chyme reduces the time available for the large intestine to reabsorb water and electrolytes. Some people pass stool with increased frequency, but diarrhea is not present unless the stool is relatively unformed and excessively liquid. The person with diarrhea finds it difficult or impossible to control the urge to defecate for very long. Diarrhea and the threat of incontinence are sources of concern and embarrassment. Often, spasmodic and piercing abdominal cramps are associated with diarrhea. Sometimes the client passes blood and excessive mucus; nausea and vomiting may also occur. With persistent diarrhea, irritation of the anal region extending to the perineum and buttocks generally results. The skin should be kept clean, washed with a mild soap, rinsed, and dried when soiled, and protective ointments such as zinc oxide or petrolatum applied to protect the skin. Fatigue, weakness, malaise, and emaciation are the results of prolonged diarrhea.

When the cause of diarrhea is irritants in the intestinal tract, diarrhea is thought to be a protective flushing mechanism. It can create serious fluid and electrolyte losses in the body, however, that can develop within frighteningly short periods of time, particularly in infants and small children. See Chapter 40 for further information concerning fluid and electrolyte losses in the body. Table 42–1 lists some of the major causes of diarrhea and the physiologic response of the body.

Fecal Incontinence

Fecal incontinence refers to loss of voluntary ability to control fecal and gaseous discharges through the anal sphincter. The incontinence may occur at specific times, such as after meals, or it may occur irregularly. Two types of fecal incontinence are described: partial and major. *Partial incontinence* is the inability to control flatus or to prevent minor soiling. *Major incontinence* is the inability to control feces of normal consistency (Hanauer 1988, p. 107).

Fecal incontinence is generally associated with impaired functioning of the anal sphincter or its nerve supply, such as in some neuromuscular diseases, spinal cord trauma, and tumors of the external anal sphincter muscle. It is estimated

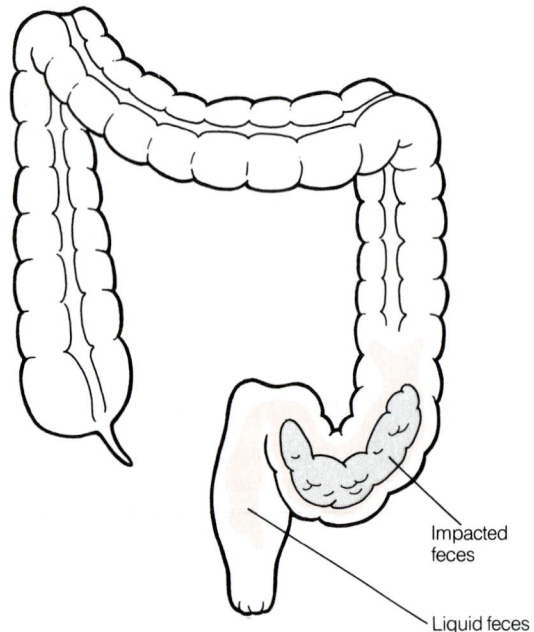

Impacted feces

Liquid feces

Figure 42–6 A fecal impaction with liquid feces passing around the impaction.

that 60% of the elderly may be affected by fecal incontinence at some time (Hanauer 1988, p. 105).

Fecal incontinence is an emotionally distressing problem that can ultimately lead to social isolation. Afflicted persons withdraw into their homes or, if in the hospital, the confines of their room to minimize the embarrassment associated with soiling. Such people may come to prefer easily washable night garments to street clothes. Incontinent feces are acidic and contain digestive enzymes that are highly irritating to skin. Therefore, the area around the anal region should be kept clean and dry and be protected with zinc oxide or other ointment.

More recently, a fecal collector has been used. This pouch is applied to the skin after the application of a protective barrier. The pouch, which is made of an odor-barrier film and has a drainage outlet, can be attached to a bedside receptacle when there is a high volume of loose feces (Mowlam et al. 1986, p. 59).

Flatulence

Air or gas in the gastrointestinal tract is called **flatus.** There are three primary causes of flatus: (a) action of bacteria on the chyme in the large intestine, (b) swallowed air, and (c) gas that diffuses from the bloodstream into the intestine. Normally all but 0.6 liters of this gas is absorbed into the intestinal capillaries (Guyton 1986, p. 805).

Flatulence is the presence of excessive flatus in the intestines and leads to stretching and inflation of the intestines (*intestinal distention*). This condition is also referred to as **tympanites.** Large amounts of air and other gases can accumulate in the stomach, resulting in gastric distention.

An adult usually forms 7 to 10 liters of flatus in the large intestine every 24 hours. The gases include carbon dioxide, methane, hydrogen, oxygen, and nitrogen. Some are swallowed with food and fluids taken by mouth, and others are formed through the action of bacteria on the chyme in the large intestine (Guyton 1986, p. 805).

Most gases that are swallowed are expelled through the mouth by **eructation** (belching). The gases formed in the large intestine are chiefly absorbed, through the intestinal capillaries, into the circulation. Flatulence can occur in the colon, however, from a variety of causes, such as abdominal surgery, anesthetics, or narcotics. If this gas cannot be expelled through the anus, it may be necessary to insert a rectal tube or provide a return flow enema to remove it.

Common causes of flatulence and distention are constipation; codeine, barbiturates, and other medications that decrease intestinal motility; and states of anxiety, during which large amounts of air are swallowed. Most people have experienced some flatulence and distention after eating such gas-forming foods as beans or cabbage. Postoperative distention after abdominal surgery is commonly seen in hospitals. This type of distention generally occurs on about the third postoperative day and is caused by the effects of anesthetics, narcotics, dietary changes, and reduction in activity.

TABLE 42–1 *Major Causes of Diarrhea*

Cause	Physiologic Response
Psychologic stress, e.g., anxiety	Increased intestinal motility and mucus secretion
Medications	
Antibiotics	Inflammation and infection of mucosa due to overgrowth of pathogenic intestinal microorganisms
Iron	Irritation of intestinal mucosa
Cathartics	Irritation of intestinal mucosa
Allergy to food, fluid/drugs	Incomplete digestion of food or fluid
Intolerance of food or fluid	Increased intestinal motility and mucus secretion
Diseases of the colon	
Malabsorption syndrome	Reduced absorption of fluids
Crohn disease	Inflammation of the mucosa often leading to ulcer formation
Others	
Surgical operations	
Imbalance of intestinal flora	Use of antibiotics destroys normal flora

Hemorrhoids

Hemorrhoids, also called *piles,* are distended veins in the anal area. They can be internal or external. Internal hemorrhoids occur in the anal canal, where they remain. External hemorrhoids prolapse through the anal opening and can be seen there. Hemorrhoids can occur as a result of increased pressure in the anal area, often secondary to chronic constipation, straining during defecation, pregnancy, or obesity.

Some hemorrhoids are asymptomatic; others cause pain, itching, and sometimes bleeding. Hemorrhoids are often treated conservatively with astringents (to shrink the tissues) and local anesthetics (to provide relief from the pain). Stool softeners may also be used, to decrease irritation during defecation. Sometimes the pain from hemorrhoids causes constipation.

ASSESSING

Assessment of fecal elimination includes taking a nursing history; performing a physical examination of the abdomen, rectum, and anus; and inspecting the feces. The nurse also should review any data obtained from relevant diagnostic tests.

ASSESSMENT INTERVIEW
Fecal Elimination

Defecation Pattern

- What is the frequency and time of day of defecation?
- Has this pattern changed recently?

Description of Feces and Any Changes

- How would you describe your stool in terms of color, texture (hard, soft, watery), shape, odor?
- Have you noticed any changes in your stool recently?

Fecal Elimination Problems

- What problems have you had or do you now have with your bowel movements (constipation? diarrhea? excessive flatulence? seepage or incontinence?)
- When and how often does it occur?
- What causes it (food, fluids, exercise, emotions, medications, disease, surgery)?
- What methods have you used to remedy the problem, and how effective were they?

Presence and Management of Ostomy

- What is your usual routine with your colostomy/ileostomy?
- What problems, if any, do you have with it?
- How can the nurses help you manage colostomy/ileostomy?

Factors Influencing Elimination

- *Use of elimination aids.* What routines do you follow to maintain your usual defecation pattern? Do you use natural aids such as specific foods or fluids (e.g., a glass of hot lemon juice before breakfast), laxatives, or enemas to maintain elimination?
- *Diet.* What foods do you believe affect defecation? What foods do you typically eat? What food do you always avoid? Do you take meals at regular times?
- *Fluid.* What amount and kind of fluid do you take each day (e.g., 6 glasses of water, 5 cups of coffee)?
- *Exercise.* What is your usual daily exercise pattern? (Obtain specifics about exercise rather than asking whether it is sufficient; ideas of what is sufficient vary among individuals.)
- *Medications.* Have you taken any medications that could affect the gastrointestinal tract (e.g., iron, antibiotics)?
- *Stress.* Are you experiencing any long-term or short-term stressors? If so, what are these? Do you think these affect your defecation pattern? How?

Nursing History

A nursing history for fecal elimination helps the nurse ascertain the client's normal pattern. The nurse elicits a description of usual feces and any recent changes and collects information about any past or current problems with elimination, the presence of an ostomy, and factors influencing the elimination pattern.

Examples of interview questions to elicit this information are shown in the accompanying box. The number of questions to ask is adapted to the individual client, according to the client's responses in the first three categories. For example, questions about factors influencing elimination are addressed perhaps only to clients who are experiencing problems.

When eliciting data about the client's defecation pattern, the nurse needs to understand that the time of defecation and the amount of feces expelled are as individual as the frequency of defecation. Some people normally defecate once a day; others defecate only three or four times a week. Some defecate after breakfast; others do so in the evening. Often, the patterns individuals follow depend largely on early training and on convenience. Most people develop the habit of defecating after breakfast, when the gastrocolic and duodenocolic reflexes cause mass movements in the large intestine.

Physical Examination

Physical examination of the abdomen, rectum, and anus is discussed in Chapter 19. Physical examination of the abdomen in relation to fecal elimination problems includes inspection, auscultation, percussion, and palpation with specific reference to the intestinal tract. Auscultation precedes palpation, since palpation can alter peristalsis. Examination of the rectum and anus includes inspection and palpation.

Characteristics of Feces

The client's stool is inspected for color, consistency, shape, amount, odor, and the presence of abnormal constituents. See Table 42–2 for a summary of normal and abnormal characteristics of stool and possible causes.

Diagnostic Studies

Diagnostic studies of the gastrointestinal tract include direct visualization techniques, indirect visualization techniques, and laboratory tests for abnormal constituents.

Visualization Studies *Direct visualization techniques* include **anoscopy,** the viewing of the anal canal; **proctoscopy,** the viewing of the rectum; **proctosigmoidoscopy,** the viewing of the rectum and sigmoid colon; and

TABLE 42-2 *Characteristics of Normal and Abnormal Feces*

Characteristic	Normal	Abnormal	Possible Cause
Color	Adult: brown Infant: yellow	Clay or white	Absence of bile pigment (bile obstruction); diagnostic study using barium
		Black or tarry	Drug (e.g., iron); bleeding from upper gastrointestinal tract (e.g., stomach, small intestine); diet high in red meat and dark green vegetables (e.g., spinach)
		Red	Bleeding from lower gastrointestinal tract (e.g., rectum); some foods (e.g., beets)
		Pale	Malabsorption of fats; diet high in milk and milk products and low in meat
		Orange or green	Intestinal infection
Consistency	Formed, soft, semisolid, moist	Hard, dry, constipated stool	Dehydration; decreased intestinal motility resulting from lack of fiber in diet, lack of exercise, emotional upset, laxative abuse
		Diarrhea	Increased intestinal motility (e.g., irritation of the colon by bacteria)
Shape	Cylindrical (contour of rectum) about 2.5 cm (1 in) in diameter in adults	Narrow, pencil-shaped, or stringlike stool	Obstructive condition of the rectum
Amount	Varies with diet (about 100 to 400 g per day)		
Odor	Aromatic: affected by ingested food and person's own bacterial flora	Pungent	Infection, blood
Constituents	Small amounts of undigested roughage; sloughed dead bacteria and epithelial cells; fat; protein; dried constituents of digestive juices (e.g., bile pigments); inorganic matter (calcium, phosphates)	Pus	Bacterial infection
		Mucus	Inflammatory condition
		Parasites	
		Blood	Gastrointestinal bleeding
		Large quantities of fat	Malabsorption
		Foreign objects	Accidental ingestion

colonoscopy, the viewing of the large intestine. *Indirect visualization* of the gastrointestinal tract is achieved by roentgenography. Roentgenography of the large intestine requires the introduction into the colon of barium, a radiopaque substance. Barium permits the viewing of the outline of the colon by either fluoroscopy or roentgenography.

Collecting Stool Specimens   The nurse is responsible for collecting stool specimens ordered for laboratory analysis. Before obtaining a specimen, the nurse needs to determine the reason for collecting the stool specimen and the correct method of obtaining and handling it (i.e., how much stool to obtain, whether a preservative needs to be added to the stool, and whether it needs to be sent immediately to the laboratory). It may be necessary to confirm this information by checking with the agency laboratory. In many situations, only a single specimen is required; in others,

timed specimens are necessary, and every stool passed is collected within a designated time period.

Nurses need to give clients the following instructions:

- Defecate in a clean or sterile bedpan or bedside commode.

- Do not contaminate the specimen, if possible, by urine or menstrual discharge. Void before the specimen collection.

- Do not place toilet tissue in the bedpan after defecation, since contents of the paper can affect the laboratory analysis.

- Notify the nurse as soon as possible after defecation, particularly for specimens that need to be sent to the laboratory immediately.

To secure a stool specimen from a baby or young child who is not toilet trained, the nurse obtains newly passed feces from the diaper.

When obtaining stool samples, i.e., when handling the client's bedpan, when transferring the stool sample to a specimen container, and when disposing of the bedpan contents, the nurse follows medical aseptic technique meticulously. The nurse wears disposable gloves to prevent hand contamination and takes care not to contaminate the outside of the specimen container. The nurse uses one or two clean tongue blades to transfer the specimen to the container and then wraps them in a paper towel before disposing of them in the waste container. This practice lessens the chance of contact with other articles and the spread of microorganisms. The amount of stool to be sent depends on the purpose for which the specimen is collected. Usually about 2.5 cm (1 in) of formed stool or 15 to 30 ml of liquid stool is adequate. For some timed specimens, however, the entire stool passed may need to be sent. Visible pus, mucus, or blood should be included in sample specimens. For a stool culture, the nurse dips a sterile swab into the specimen, preferably where purulent fecal matter is present, and, using sterile technique, places the swab in a sterile test tube.

Because fresh specimens provide the most accurate results, the nurse sends the specimen to the laboratory immediately. If this is not possible, the nurse follows the directions on the specimen container. In some instances refrigeration is indicated, since bacteriologic changes take place in stool specimens left at room temperature.

Testing Feces for Occult Blood
Several test products are available to test stool specimens for occult blood: the guaiac test, Hematest, and Hemoccult slide. Because results of occult blood tests may be positive if the client has eaten meat within 3 days, the client may need to refrain from eating red meat for 3 days before the test. Oral iron preparations may also be discontinued because, if partially undigested, they may mask the presence of occult blood in the stool. Before the test, the nurse should assess the client for hemorrhoids that may bleed. This is particularly important for clients who are constipated, since constipated stool can aggravate existing hemorrhoids. Any bleeding can affect test results.

 To perform the test, the nurse obtains a stool specimen, selects a test product, puts on gloves, and follows the manufacturer's directions:

- For a guaiac test, smear a thin layer of feces on a paper towel or filter paper with a tongue blade, and drop reagents onto the smear as directed.

- For a Hematest, smear a thin layer of feces on filter paper, place a tablet in the middle of the specimen, and add two drops of water as directed.

- For a Hemoccult slide, smear a thin layer of feces over the circle inside the envelope, and drop reagent solution onto the smear.

For all tests, a blue color indicates a positive result, i.e., the presence of occult blood.

DIAGNOSING

Common nursing diagnoses that relate to fecal elimination problems include **Constipation** (perceived and colonic), **Bowel incontinence,** and **Diarrhea.** Other diagnoses that may arise include **Potential fluid volume deficit** if diarrhea is severe or if there is abnormal fluid loss through an ostomy; **Body image disturbance** if, for example, the client has a bowel diversion ostomy; **Potential impaired skin integrity** if intestinal contents threaten skin integrity; and **Knowledge deficit** in clients requiring instruction in self-care skills to manage, for example, a new colostomy. These diagnoses and others, with possible contributing factors, are shown below. Examples of assessment data clusters and related nursing diagnoses are shown in Table 42–3.

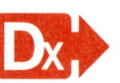 ***Nursing Diagnoses***
Clients With Fecal Elimination
Problems

Constipation related to:

- Inadequate fiber in diet
- Immobility or inadequate physical activity
- Inadequate fluid intake
- Pain on defecation
- Change in routine (e.g., diet intake)
- Abuse of laxatives
- Delaying defecation when urge is present
- Use of prescribed constipating medications (narcotic analgesic, iron, antacid, and anticholinergic)

Perceived constipation related to:

- Altered thought processes
- Family health beliefs
- Knowledge deficit about normal processes

Bowel incontinence related to:

- Diarrhea
- Fecal impaction
- Central nervous system disruption (e.g., stroke)
- Cognitive/perceptual impairment
- Demyelinating disease
- Extreme debilitation

Diarrhea related to:

- Dietary alteration
- Stress/anxiety
- Inflammation or irritation of bowel
- Drug side-effects
- Spoiled food

- Tube feeding
- Allergy

Potential fluid volume deficit related to:

- Diarrhea
- Abnormal fluid loss through ostomy

Potential impaired skin integrity related to:

- Prolonged diarrhea
- Bowel incontinence
- Bowel diversion ostomy

TABLE 42–3 *Examples of Assessment Data Clusters and Related Nursing Diagnoses*

Data Cluster	Nursing Diagnosis
Mrs. Amy Ballaster states she feels fullness in her rectum and wants to move her bowels but cannot, even with straining. Her last bowel movement was 3 days ago. She lives alone and tends to eat only tea, toast, and noodle soup. Because of arthritis, her activities (gardening and walking) have decreased. Bowel sounds are decreased.	**Constipation** related to inadequate physical activity and insufficient fiber in diet
Marvin Lombardi reports having loose, liquid, light brown stools for 2 days. Passage of stools is associated with cramping abdominal pain. Bowel sounds are increased. Temperature is 38 C (100.4 F). Has not taken any medications but reports feeling of general malaise. States he "ate at a fast-food restaurant 2 nights ago."	**Diarrhea** related to spoiled food
Mary Kuoko has had involuntary leakage of stool. States her clothing is soiled several times a day. Says she is too embarrassed to go out with her friends because of the fecal odor. Last bowel movement was more than 3 days ago. Digital examination reveals impaction.	**Bowel incontinence** related to fecal impaction.
Mr. John Deer had a bowel diversion ostomy 2 days ago. Effluent is continuous and liquid. Peristomal skin is intact. Disposable colostomy device applied.	**Potential impaired skin integrity** related to discharge from bowel diversion ostomy

PLANNING

The overall client goal for persons with fecal elimination problems is to maintain or restore a regular elimination pattern. For clients who have prolonged diarrhea, maintenance of fluid balance is also an essential goal.

Appropriate nursing interventions and outcome criteria that relate to these broad goals must be identified. Preventive and corrective interventions need to be included. Among the strategies the nurse should consider are the following:

- Implementing measures that promote normal defecation in hospitalized clients
- Implementing medically prescribed therapies, such as cathartics, antidiarrheal preparations, and enemas
- Checking for and digitally removing an impaction
- Teaching clients about appropriate life-style changes, such as increasing fluid intake, exercise, and intake of dietary fiber
- Providing special care for clients with bowel diversion ostomies and teaching them about ostomy management

Examples of outcome criteria to evaluate the achievement of client goals and the effectiveness of nursing interventions are shown below.

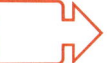 *Outcome Criteria: Clients With Fecal Elimination Problems*

The client with **Constipation:**

- Experiences regular soft brown bowel movements that are symmetric in contour.
- Resumes previously identified "normal" elimination schedule (e.g., every 1 to 3 days).
- Reports absence of distention, flatus, or feeling of rectal fullness before defecation.
- Reports absence of discomfort or straining during defecation.
- Establishes a regular time for defecation.
- Verbalizes satisfaction with present bowel habits.
- Consumes a well-balanced diet that includes fiber and 8 to 10 glasses of fluid daily.
- Names five foods high in fiber.
- Incorporates daily exercise (minimum of a 15-minute walk per day) into lifestyle.
- Attends to defecation urge when it arises.
- Takes oral laxative as prescribed and understands its desired effects.
- Takes over-the-counter laxatives rarely.

The client with **Diarrhea:**

- Has no more than two bowel movements per day.

- Defecates formed stool.
- Demonstrates signs of adequate hydration, e.g., well-hydrated skin and a urine output of 60 ml per hour.
- Is free of abdominal pain or discomfort, urgency, and perianal skin irritation.
- Alters contributing factors associated with diarrhea (e.g., avoids certain foods, implements stress-management techniques).
- States action and side-effects of prescribed medications.

The client with **Bowel incontinence:**

- Establishes a regular defecation pattern.
- Experiences fewer episodes of incontinence.
- Is free of perianal irritation and odor.
- Participates actively in bowel-training program.
- Resumes previous patterns of social interaction.

IMPLEMENTING

Promoting Regular Defecation

The nurse can help the client achieve regular defecation by attending to: (a) the provision of privacy, (b) timing, (c) nutrition and fluids, (d) exercise, and (e) positioning.

Privacy   Privacy during defecation is extremely important to many people. The nurse should therefore provide as much privacy as possible for such clients. Some clients also prefer to wipe, wash, and dry themselves after defecating. A nurse may need to provide water and a washcloth and towel for this purpose.

Timing   A client should be encouraged to defecate when the urge to defecate is recognized. To establish regular bowel elimination, the client and nurse can discuss when mass peristalsis normally occurs and provide time for defecation. Many people have well-established times and routines for defecation that should be part of the client's schedule. Other activities such as bathing and ambulating should not interfere with the defecation time. Also, clients should not be hurried but given adequate time to defecate.

Nutrition and Fluids   The diet a client needs for regular normal elimination varies, depending on the kind of feces the client currently has, the frequency of defecation, and the types of foods that the client finds assist normal defecation.

For the client who is constipated:

1. Increase daily fluid intake, and instruct the client to drink hot liquids and fruit juices, especially prune juice.

2. Include fiber in the diet, that is, foods such as prunes, raw fruit, bran products, and whole-grain cereals and bread.

For the client who has diarrhea, encourage oral intake of fluids and food. Because ingestion of foods and fluids stimulates the gastrocolic and duodenocolic reflexes, thus inducing more stool, the client may be reluctant to eat or drink. Eating small amounts of bland foods can be helpful, since they are more easily absorbed. Diarrhea can lead to great potassium losses, and the ingestion of food or fluids containing potassium should be encouraged. See the discussion of hypokalemia in Chapter 40. Excessively hot or cold fluids should be avoided, because they stimulate peristalsis. In addition, highly spiced foods and high-fiber foods can aggravate diarrhea.

For the client who has flatulence, limit carbonated beverages, the use of drinking straws, and chewing gum—all of which increase the ingestion of air. Gas-forming foods, such as cabbage, beans, onions, and cauliflower, should also be avoided.

Exercise   Regular exercise helps clients develop a regular defecation pattern and normal feces. Walking and swimming, for example, help stimulate normal motility of the intestines. Postsurgical clients often are encouraged to ambulate, with regaining normal intestinal motility as one of the reasons.

A client with weak abdominal and pelvic muscles (which impede normal defecation) may be able to strengthen them with the following isometric exercises.

- In a supine position, the client tightens the abdominal muscles as though pulling them inward, holding them for about 10 seconds and then relaxing them. This should be repeated five to ten times, four times a day, depending on the client's health.
- Again in a supine position, the client can contract the thigh muscles and hold them contracted for about 10 seconds, repeating the exercise five to ten times, four times a day. This helps the client confined to bed gain strength in the thigh muscles, thereby making it easier to use a bedpan.

Positioning   Clients who are confined to bed may need assistance to sit on a bedpan. There are two main types of bedpans, the regular high-back pan (see Figure 42–7, *A*) and the slipper or fracture pan (see Figure 42–7, *B*). The slipper pan has a low back and is used for clients unable to raise their buttocks because of physical problems or therapy that contraindicates such movement. Female clients use a bedpan for both urine and feces; male clients use a bedpan for feces and a urinal for urine (see Chapter 43).

A *commode* is sometimes used instead of a bedpan when the client can get out of bed but is unable to go to a bathroom. A commode is like an armchair with an open, toilet-

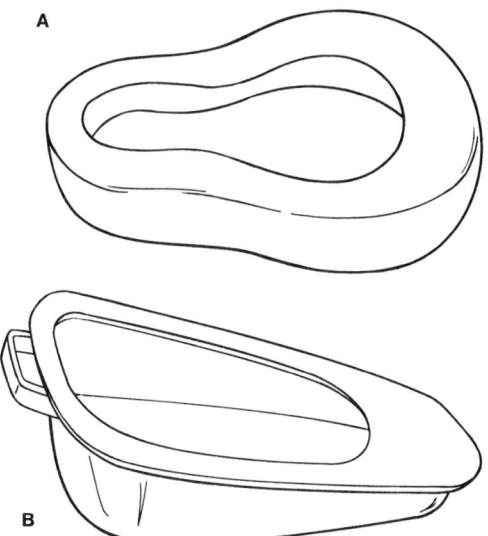

Figure 42–7 Two types of bedpans: *A,* the high-back, or regular pan; *B,* the slipper, or fracture pan.

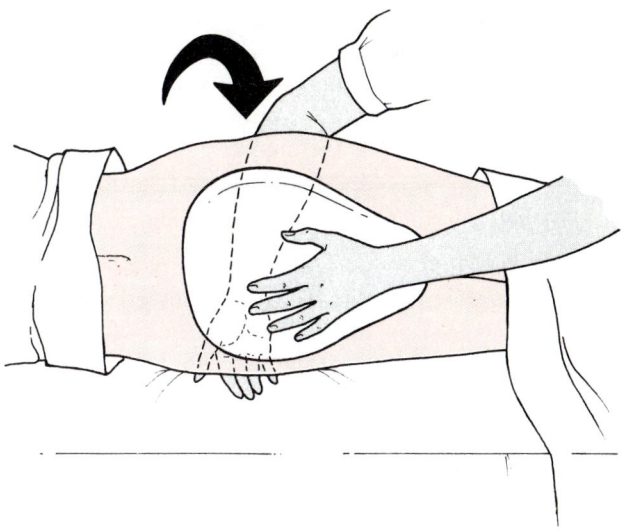

Figure 42–8 Placing a regular bedpan on the buttocks of an immobilized client.

like seat and a receptacle underneath for receiving the urine and feces. The receptacle may be specially fitted to the commode or simply a bedpan that fits under the toiletlike seat. A commode may or may not be on wheels and freely movable. Some commodes have an additional plain seat, thus doubling as a regular chair.

For clients who have difficulty in raising themselves from the toilet, an elevated toilet seat can be attached to a regular toilet. Clients then do not have to lower themselves as far onto the seat and do not have to lift as far off the seat.

A client confined to bed may require assistance getting on and off a bedpan. The nurse should bear in mind that clients using bedpans should not exert themselves unduly and therefore provide support while the client is seated on the bedpan to avoid muscle strain. For the client who can raise the buttocks, the nurse can place the bedpan under the client after the client has flexed the knees and raised the buttocks. A client can be assisted in this movement if the nurse places a hand, palm up, under the client's lower back, resting the elbow on the mattress and using the forearm as a lever. The nurse then can place a regular bedpan under the client's buttocks, with the narrow end toward the foot of the bed and the client's buttocks resting on the smooth, rounded rim. A slipper (fracture) pan should be placed with the flat end under the client's buttocks. For clients who cannot raise their buttocks on and off a bedpan:

1. Assist the client to a side-lying position, backside toward you.

2. Place the bedpan against the client's buttocks, with the open rim toward the foot of the bed.

3. Hold the far hip with one hand and the bedpan with the

other. Smoothly roll the client toward you and onto the back, with the bedpan in place (see Figure 42–8). Assume a wide stance, and shift weight from the front leg to the back leg when moving the client. The use of appropriate body mechanics prevents undue muscle exertion and strain. A bedpan should never be shoved under a client, because this can injure the client's skin.

4. Elevate the head of the bed to a semi-Fowler's position. This position relieves strain on the client's back and permits a more normal position for elimination.

5. Place a small pillow under the back for support if the client is unable to assume a semi-Fowler's position.

After placing tissues and the call light within easy reach, the nurse then leaves the client in privacy. The nurse should return to remove the bedpan when the client signals. If assistance cleaning the perineal area is required, the nurse should wrap toilet tissue several times around the hand and wipe the client from the pubic area to the anal area, using one stroke for each piece of tissue. (Cleaning from the less soiled to the more soiled area helps prevent the spread of microorganisms.) The nurse then turns the client on the side, spreads the buttocks, and cleans the anal area in the same manner. The anal area should be washed with soap and water, as indicated, and then thoroughly dried. Adequate washing and drying help prevent skin irritation and excessive accumulation of microorganisms.

To remove a bedpan from a client unable to assist:

1. Return the bed to flat position, if the client's health permits.

2. Fold the top bed linen down to the client's thighs.

3. Holding the bedpan securely with one hand, gently roll the client to a side-lying position. If unassisted, it is safer and easier to roll the client toward you rather than away from you. To prevent a fall while turning the client, raise the side rail or call another nurse.

4. Clean the anal area as described above. If the bed linens have become soiled, they should be changed.

Before the pan is emptied (either in the client's toilet or in a receptacle in the utility room), the contents should be observed and perhaps measured. Most hospitals have spray faucets to rinse the bedpan thoroughly.

Administering Prescribed Medications

Cathartics   **Cathartics,** frequently referred to as *laxatives,* are drugs that induce defecation. They vary in their degree and method of action. Cathartics can have a laxative effect or a purgative effect. A laxative effect is mild in comparison to a purgative effect, which produces frequent movements of the bowel, soft liquid stools, and sometimes abdominal cramps. Different cathartics have different effects, but even the same cathartic may have either a purgative or laxative effect depending on the dosage taken. A large dose of a cathartic may have a purgative effect, whereas a small dose of the same cathartic may have a laxative effect and produce a normal bowel movement. Table 42–4 describes the different types of cathartics.

The administration of cathartics is prescribed with caution by the physician. Constipation is not the only reason for prescribing cathartics. For example, cathartics are prescribed in preparation for radiologic examinations or surgery.

Laxative abuse is thought to be a common problem. The elderly, in particular, often use laxatives improperly. Research shows that the elderly spend millions of dollars on products to relieve constipation. Persistent self-administration of laxatives, however, can result in chronic constipation. There is a trend toward the "natural laxative" approach, that is, the use of increased dietary fiber such as that found in fruits

TABLE 42–4   *Types of Cathartics*

Type	Action	Examples	Pertinent Teaching Information
Bulk-forming	Increases the fluid, gaseous, or solid bulk in the intestines	Psyllium hydrophilic mucilloid (Metamucil)	May take 12 or more hours to act. Sufficient fluid must be taken.
Lubricant or emollient	Softens and delays the drying of the feces	Mineral oil, Haley's M-O	Refrigerated oil has less odor. Mixing with fruit juice decreases unpleasant taste. Prolonged use inhibits the absorption of some fat-soluble vitamins.
Wetting agents	Lower the surface tension of the feces, thus helping water to penetrate the feces	Docusate sodium (Colace, Disonate)	Slow-acting; may take several days.
Chemical (stimulant) irritant	Irritates the intestinal mucosa, causing rapid propulsion of the contents.	Castor oil, cascara sagrada, Bisacodyl	Fluid is passed with the feces. May cause cramps. Prolonged use may cause fluid and electrolyte imbalance.
Saline	Salts are not absorbed in the intestine; therefore, fluid bulk is increased because fluid absorption is decreased. Also, may lubricate the feces.	Epsom salts, magnesium hydroxide (Milk of Magnesia), magnesium citrate	May be rapid-acting. Can cause fluid and electrolyte imbalance, particularly in elderly people and children with cardiac and renal disease.

and vegetables to obtain a laxative effect. Unfortunately, the desired laxative effect may not persist (Osis 1987, p. 6). In the elderly, laxatives should always be used secondarily to dietary and life-style changes. Fluid intake should also be at least 1500 ml per day.

Cathartics are contraindicated in the client who has nausea, cramps, colic, vomiting, or undiagnosed abdominal pain (Fingl 1980, p. 1011). Clients at home should be aware of the dangers of laxative use. The first step is to eliminate laxative use and then to increase dietary fiber and regular exercise. In addition, the medication regimen should be examined, because it may adversely affect normal bowel activity. Sometimes medication can be changed to reduce undesirable side-effects such as constipation.

Suppositories

Suppositories   Some cathartics are given in the form of suppositories. These act in various ways: by softening the feces, by releasing gases such as carbon dioxide to distend the rectum, or by stimulating the nerve endings in the rectal mucosa. Suppositories need to be inserted beyond the internal anal sphincter. A disposable glove is worn by the nurse, and the suppository is well lubricated prior to insertion to prevent friction and tissue damage. For an adult, the suppository is inserted gently 7.5 to 10 cm (3 to 4 in), or the length of the nurse's index finger; less for a child or baby. The client is instructed to breathe through the mouth, because mouth breathing may relax the anal sphincter. To be effective, the suppository needs to be placed along the wall of the rectum rather than lodged in the feces. Immediately after inserting the suppository, the nurse can help dispel any urge the client has to expel the suppository by pressing the client's buttocks together for a few seconds. After the procedure, the nurse removes the glove (by turning it inside out) and discards it.

Generally, suppositories are effective within 30 minutes. The best results can be obtained by inserting the suppository 30 minutes before the client's usual defecation time or when the peristaltic action is greatest, such as after breakfast.

Antidiarrheal Medications

Antidiarrheal Medications   Clients who have diarrhea may require antidiarrhetics. Some of these mechanically coat the irritated bowel and act as protectives (**demulcents**). Others absorb gas or toxic substances from the bowel (**adsorbents**) or shrink swollen and inflamed tissues (**astringents**). In certain situations, sedatives and antispasmodics may also be required.

Administering Enemas

An **enema** is a solution introduced into the rectum and sigmoid colon. Its function is to remove feces and/or flatus. Enemas are classified into four groups, according to their action: cleansing, carminative, retention, or return flow. A *cleansing enema* stimulates peristalsis by irritating the colon and rectum and/or by distending the intestine with the volume of fluid introduced. Two kinds of cleansing enemas are the high enema and the low enema. The *high enema* is given to clean as much of the colon as possible. It is often used before diagnostic studies. Often about 1,000 ml (1 liter) of solution is administered to an adult. The client changes from the left lateral to the dorsal recumbent position and then to the right lateral position during the administration so that the fluid can follow the large intestine. See Figure 42–1, earlier. The fluid is administered at a higher pressure than for a low enema; that is, the container of solution is held higher. Cleansing enemas are most effective if held for 5 to 10 minutes. The *low enema* is used to clean the rectum and the sigmoid colon only. About 500 ml (0.5 liters) of solution is administered to an adult, and the client maintains the left sidelying position during its administration.

A **carminative** *enema* is given primarily to expel flatus. The solution instilled into the rectum releases gas, which in turn distends the rectum and the colon, thus stimulating peristalsis. For an adult, 60 to 180 ml of fluid is instilled.

A *retention enema* introduces oil into the rectum and sigmoid colon. The oil is retained for a relatively long period of time (e.g., 1 to 3 hours). It acts to soften the feces and to lubricate the rectum and anal canal, thus facilitating passage of the feces.

A *return flow enema,* sometimes referred to as the *Harris flush* or *colonic irrigation,* is used to expel flatus. Alternating flow of 100–200 ml of fluid into and out of the large intestine stimulates peristalsis and the expulsion of feces.

Various solutions are used for enemas. The specific solution may be ordered by the physician or dictated by agency practice. Table 42–5 lists some of these solutions, giving the quantity and proportions frequently used.

An enema is a relatively safe procedure for the client. The chief dangers are irritation of the rectal mucosa by too much

TABLE 42–5   *Types of Enemas Commonly Used for Adults*

Name	Constituents
Commercially prepared enema	90–120 ml of a hypertonic solution, such as sodium phosphate (see directions on the package)
Saline	9 ml of sodium chloride to 1,000 ml of water
Tap water	500–1,000 ml of tap water
Soap	20 ml of castile soap in 500–1000 ml of water
Oil, e.g., olive oil	90–120 ml of oil (commercially prepared): mineral, olive, or cottonseed

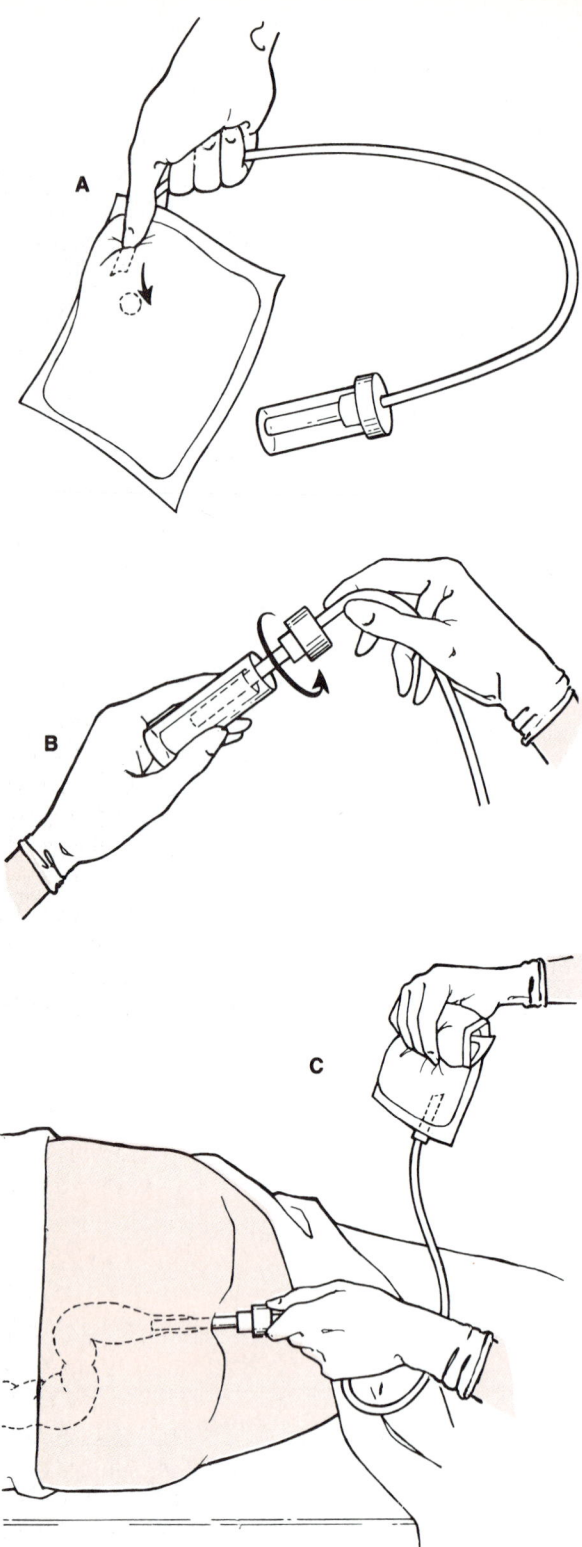

Figure 42–9 One type of commercially prepared disposable enema: *A,* the bead that seals the tube is expelled from the tube into the bag so that the solution can flow through the tubing; *B,* the protector cover of the insertion tip is rotated to distribute the lubricant on the tip before the cover is removed; *C,* after the tube has been inserted, the bag is inverted and compressed.

soap or an irritating soap and negative effects of a *hypertonic solution* (possessing a greater tonicity than blood) or *hypotonic solution* (possessing a lesser tonicity than blood) on the body fluid and electrolytes. A hypertonic solution, such as the phosphate solutions of some commercially prepared enemas, is slightly irritating to the mucous membrane and causes fluid to be drawn into the colon from the surrounding tissues. The process by which this happens is called *osmosis.* Because only a small amount of fluid is normally administered, the advantages of comfort, retention for only 5 to 7 minutes, and convenience generally outweigh these disadvantages.

The repeated administration of hypotonic solutions, such as tap water enemas, can result in absorption of the water from the colon into the bloodstream. This increases the blood volume and can produce water intoxication. For this reason, some health agencies limit to three the number of tap water enemas given consecutively. This is of particular concern when the order is "enemas until returns are clear"— for example, prior to a visual examination of the large intestine. Hypotonic solutions can also be unsafe for clients with decreased kidney function or acute heart failure.

Before administering an enema, determine if a physician's order is required. At some agencies, a physician must order the kind of enema and the time to give it, e.g., the evening before surgery or the morning of the examination. When the client has rectal pathology, the physician may also specify the size of the rectal tube to use. At other agencies, enemas are given at the nurses' discretion, i.e., as necessary on a prn order.

Some agencies use commercially prepared disposable enemas (see Figure 42–9). It is important that the nurse be aware that prepackaged enemas have their own instructions, which should be followed unless there are other instructions from the physician or the agency.

Enemas for adults are usually given at 40 to 43 C (105 to 110 F); those for children are given at 37.7 C (100 F), unless otherwise specified. Some oil retention enemas are given at 33 C (91 F). High temperatures can be injurious to the bowel mucosa; cold temperatures are uncomfortable for the client and may trigger a spasm of the sphincter muscles.

The amount of solution to be administered depends on the kind of enema, the age of the person, and the person's ability to retain the solution. The usual amount for an adult cleansing enema is 750 to 1000 ml. The nurse must select a rectal tube of the correct size. Adults usually require #22 to #30 Fr. Children require a smaller tube, such as #12 Fr. for an infant and #14 to #18 Fr. for the toddler or school-age child.

How long the client retains the enema solution depends on the purpose of the enema and the ability of the client to contract the external sphincter to retain the solution. Oil retention enemas are usually retained 2 to 3 hours. Other enemas are normally retained 5 to 10 minutes.

Procedure 42–1 explains how to administer an enema.

ADMINISTERING AN ENEMA

Equipment ☑

Disposable enema unit (see Figure 42–9, earlier)

Enema set with a container, tubing, clamp, rectal tube

Lubricant

Bath thermometer

Prescribed amount of solution at the correct temperature

Bath blanket

Waterproof absorbent pad

Paper towel

Bedpan or commode if the client is unable to reach the bathroom

Disposable gloves

Intervention

1. Prepare the client.

■ Explain the procedure to the client. Indicate that the client may experience a feeling of fullness while the solution is being administered.

■ Assist the client to a left lateral position, with the right leg acutely flexed. *This position facilitates the flow of solution by gravity into the sigmoid and descending colon, which are on the left side. Having the right leg acutely flexed provides for adequate exposure of the anus.* For infants and small children, the dorsal recumbent position is frequently used. Position them on a small padded bedpan with support for the back and head. Secure the legs by placing a diaper under the bedpan and then over and around the thighs.

■ Place the waterproof pad under the client's buttocks to protect the bed linen, and drape the client with the bath blanket.

2. Prepare the equipment.

■ Lubricate about 5 cm (2 in) of the rectal tube (some commercially prepared enema sets already have lubricated nozzles). *Lubrication facilitates insertion through the sphincters and minimizes trauma.*

■ Open the clamp, and run some solution through the connecting tubing and the rectal tube to expel any air in the tubing; then close the clamp. *Air instilled into the rectum, although not harmful, causes unnecessary distention.*

3. Don gloves, and insert the rectal tube.

■ Lift the upper buttock to ensure good visualization of the anus.

■ Insert the tube smoothly and slowly into the rectum, directing it toward the umbilicus (see Figure 42–10). *This angle follows the normal contour of the rectum. Slow insertion prevents spasm of the sphincter.*

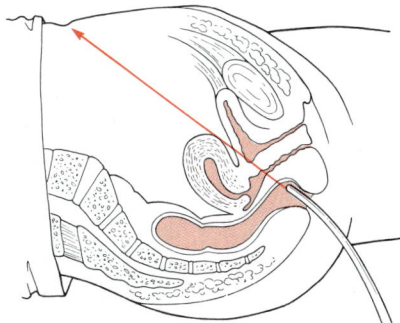

Figure 42–10   Inserting the rectal tube following the direction of the rectum.

■ Insert the tube 7 to 10 cm (3 to 4 in) in an adult (less for children). *Since the canal is about 2.5 to 5 cm (1 to 2 in) long, insertion to this point places the tip of the tube beyond the anal sphincter into the rectum.*

■ If resistance is encountered at the internal sphincter, ask the client to take a deep breath, then run a small amount of solution through the tube to relax the internal anal sphincter.

■ Never force tube entry. If resistance persists, withdraw the tube and report the resistance to the nurse in charge.

4. Slowly administer the enema solution.

■ Raise the solution container, and open the clamp to allow fluid flow. *or*
Compress a pliable container by hand.

■ During most adult enemas, hold the solution container no higher than 30 cm (12 in) above the rectum. *The higher the solution container is held above the rectum, the faster the flow and the greater the force (pressure) in the rectum. Damage to the mucosal lining may result if the container is held higher than 30 cm.* During a high enema, hold the solution container a little higher, e.g., 4 to 6 inches. *The fluid must be instilled farther to clean the entire bowel.* For children, lower the height of the solution container appropriately for the age of the child.

■ Administer the fluid slowly. If the client complains of fullness or pain, use the clamp to stop the flow for 30 seconds, and then restart the flow at a slower rate. *Administering the enema slowly and stopping the flow momentarily decrease the likelihood of intestinal spasm and premature ejection of the solution.*

■ If you are using a plastic commercial container, roll it up as the fluid is instilled. *This prevents subsequent suctioning of the solution.*

■ After all of the solution has been instilled or when the client cannot hold any more and wants to defecate (the urge to defecate usually indicates that sufficient fluid has been administered), close the clamp, and remove the rectal tube from the anus.

■ Place the rectal tube in a paper towel as you withdraw it.

5. Encourage the client to retain the enema.

■ Ask the client to remain lying down. *It is easier for the client to retain the enema when lying down than when sitting or standing because gravity promotes drainage and peristalsis.*

■ To assist an incontinent person in retaining the solution, apply firm pressure over the anus with tissue wipes, or press the buttocks together.

■ Ensure that the client retains the solution for the appropriate amount of time.

6. Assist the client to defecate.

■ Assist the client to a sitting position on the bedpan, commode, or toilet. *A sitting position facilitates the act of defecation.*

■ Ask the client who is using the toilet not to flush it. *The nurse needs to observe the feces.*

■ If a specimen of feces is required, ask the client to use a bedpan or commode.

7. Record and report relevant data.

■ Record administration of the enema; the amount, color, and consistency of returns; and the relief of flatus and abdominal distention.

Sample Recording

Date: 6/29/91	Time: 2100

1,000 ml saline enema given. Returned large amount of hard, white stool and large amount of flatus. Abdomen soft and less distended.P72.——Roxy-Ann B. Stanley, NS

Administering an Enema to an Incontinent Client   Occasionally a nurse needs to administer an enema to a client who is unable to control the external sphincter muscle and thus cannot retain the enema solution for even a few minutes. In that case the client assumes a supine position on a bedpan. The head of the bed can be elevated slightly, e.g., to 30° if necessary, and the client's head and back are supported by pillows. The nurse wears gloves to prevent direct contact with the solution and feces that are expelled over the hand into the bedpan during administration of the enema.

Administering a Return Flow Enema   Administering the return flow enema (the Harris flush, or colonic irrigation) is similar to administering and siphoning an enema. Initially, the solution (100 to 200 ml for an adult) is instilled into the client's rectum and sigmoid colon. Then the solution container is lowered so that the fluid flows back out through the rectal tube into the container. The inflow-outflow process is repeated five or six times (to stimulate peristalsis and the expulsion of flatus), and the solution is replaced several times during the procedure as it becomes thick with feces. A total of about 1000 ml of solution is usually used for an adult.

Siphoning an Enema   In some instances, a client may be unable to expel the solution after administration of an enema. The solution must then be siphoned off. In siphoning, the nurse uses the force of gravity to draw the fluid out of the rectum and colon.

The equipment required is a bedpan, a disposable large plastic volume enema container, rectal tube, lubricant, and a container of water at 40 C (105 F). During siphoning, the client assumes a *right* side-lying position so that the sigmoid colon is uppermost, thus facilitating drainage of the solution from the rectum and the colon. The client lies on the bed with hips close to the side of the bed. The nurse places a bedpan on a chair at the side of the bed near the client's hips. The chair must be lower than the bed. The rectal tube is lubricated and attached to the partially filled enema set. The tube is filled with solution, then pinched and gently inserted into the rectum as for an enema. The nurse holds the enema container about 10 cm (4 in) above the anus, releases the pinched rectal tube, and quickly lowers the enema container. This action should draw the fluid from the colon and rectum, permitting it to flow through the rectal tube into the solution container. The nurse then notes the amount of fluid siphoned off as well as the color, odor, and presence of any feces or abnormal constituents, such as blood or mucus.

Digital Removal of a Fecal Impaction

Digital removal of a fecal impaction is sometimes necessary. The nurse breaks up the fecal mass digitally and then removes portions of it. This procedure is distressing and uncomfortable, and clients may desire the presence of another nurse or family member for support. The nurse must take care to avoid injuring the bowel mucosa and thus to prevent bleeding. Also, rectal stimulation is contraindicated for some clients, since it may cause an excessive vagal response, resulting in cardiac arrhythmia. For these reasons, agency policies vary about who may break up impactions digitally. After disimpaction, follow-up measures to encourage normal defecation, such as administering enemas or suppositories, are implemented for a few days.

The procedure for digital removal of a fecal impaction is as follows.

1. The client assumes a side-lying position, with the knees flexed and the back toward you. Although some clients may prefer to stand by a toilet, the bed position is advised because disimpaction can be exhausting.

2. Place a waterproof bedpad under the client's buttocks and a bedpan nearby to receive stool.

3. Put on a pair of gloves, and liberally lubricate the index finger to be inserted.

4. Gently insert the index finger into the rectum, and move the finger toward the client's umbilicus, moving along the length of the rectum.

5. Loosen and dislodge stool by gently massaging around it. Break up stool by working the finger into the hardened mass. Take care to avoid injury to the mucosa of the rectum.

6. Carefully work stool downward to the end of the rectum and remove it in small pieces. Continue to remove as much fecal material as possible. Periodically assess the client for signs of fatigue, such as facial pallor, diaphoresis, or change in pulse rate. Manual stimulation should be minimal, since excessive vagal nerve stimulation could result in cardiac arrhythmia.

7. Following disimpaction, assist the client to clean the anal area and buttocks. Then assist the client onto a bedpan or commode for a short time, because digital stimulation of the rectum often induces the urge to defecate.

Decreasing Flatulence

There are several ways to reduce or prevent flatulence: not providing gas-producing foods, encouraging exercise, and repositioning clients are recommended. Encouraging ambulation is an effective means of reducing flatulence, since the motility stimulates reabsorption of gases in intestinal capillaries. A method of treating flatulence is to insert a rectal tube into the rectum and leave it there for varying lengths of time (generally no longer than 30 minutes, to prevent undue irritation to the rectal lining). The tube can then be reinserted, as needed, every 2 to 3 hours. Some nurses advocate connecting the open end of the rectal tube, via another tube, to a collecting receptacle. The passage of flatus is confirmed by noting bubbles in the water. The equipment required for relieving flatulence is shown in the accompanying box.

BOWEL DIVERSION OSTOMIES

Bowel diversion ostomies are often classified according to (a) whether they are permanent or temporary, (b) their anatomic location, and (c) the construction of the **stoma** (artificial opening in the abdominal wall). An *ileostomy* is an opening into the ileum (small bowel). A *colostomy* is an opening into the colon (large bowel). Figure 42–11 shows a colostomy stoma.

Permanence   Colostomies can be either temporary or permanent. Temporary colostomies are generally performed for traumatic injuries or inflammatory conditions of the bowel. They allow the distal diseased portion of the bowel to rest and heal. Permanent colostomies are performed to provide a means of elimination when the rectum or anus is nonfunctional as a result of disease or birth defect. They are commonly performed for diseases such as cancer of the bowel. The diseased portion may or may not be removed.

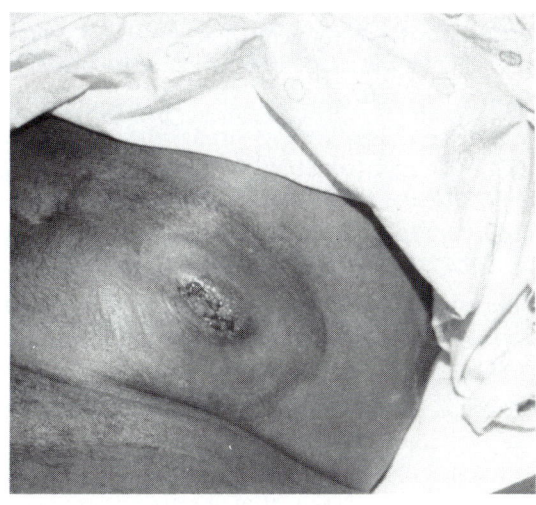

Figure 42–11   A colostomy stoma.

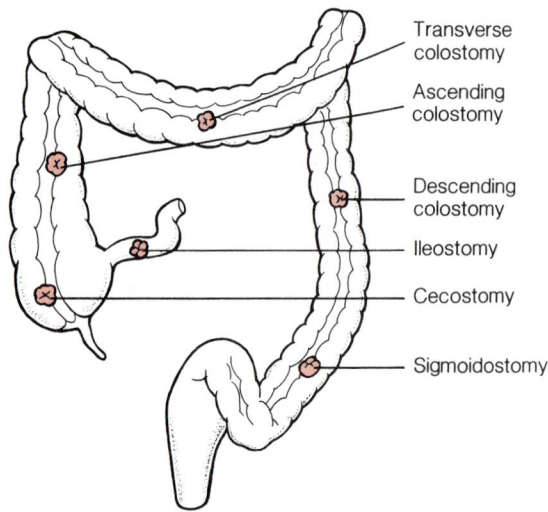

Figure 42–12 The locations of bowel diversion ostomies.

Transverse colostomy
Ascending colostomy
Descending colostomy
Ileostomy
Cecostomy
Sigmoidostomy

Anatomic Location

An ileostomy generally empties from the distal end of the small intestine. A cecostomy empties from the cecum (the first part of the ascending colon). An ascending colostomy empties from the ascending colon. A transverse colostomy empties from the transverse colon. A descending colostomy empties from the descending colon. A sigmoidostomy empties from the sigmoid colon. See Figure 42–12.

The location of the ostomy influences the character and management of the fecal drainage. The farther along the bowel, the more formed the stool, since the large bowel reabsorbs water from the fecal mass. In addition, more control over the frequency of stomal discharge can be established. For example:

1. An ileostomy produces liquid fecal drainage that drains continuously and cannot be regulated. Ileostomy drainage contains some digestive enzymes, which are damaging to the skin. Ileostomy clients must wear an appliance continuously and take special precautions to prevent skin breakdown. Odor is minimal, however, compared to colostomies, because fewer bacteria are present.

2. An ascending colostomy is similar to an ileostomy in that the drainage is liquid, passes through the ostomy several times a day, and cannot be regulated by the irrigation method. However, digestive enzymes are present, and odor is a problem requiring control (e.g., a deodorant inside the appliance).

3. A transverse colostomy produces a malodorous, mushy drainage because some of the liquid has been reabsorbed. There is usually no control.

4. A descending colostomy produces increasingly solid fecal drainage. Stools from a sigmoidostomy are of normal consistency, and the frequency of discharge can be regulated by irrigation. Clients with sigmoidostomies may

not have to wear an appliance at all times, and odors can usually be controlled.

The length of time an ostomy is in place also helps determine the consistency of the stool, particularly with transverse and descending colostomies. Over time, the stool becomes more formed because the remaining functioning portions of the colon tend to increase water reabsorption

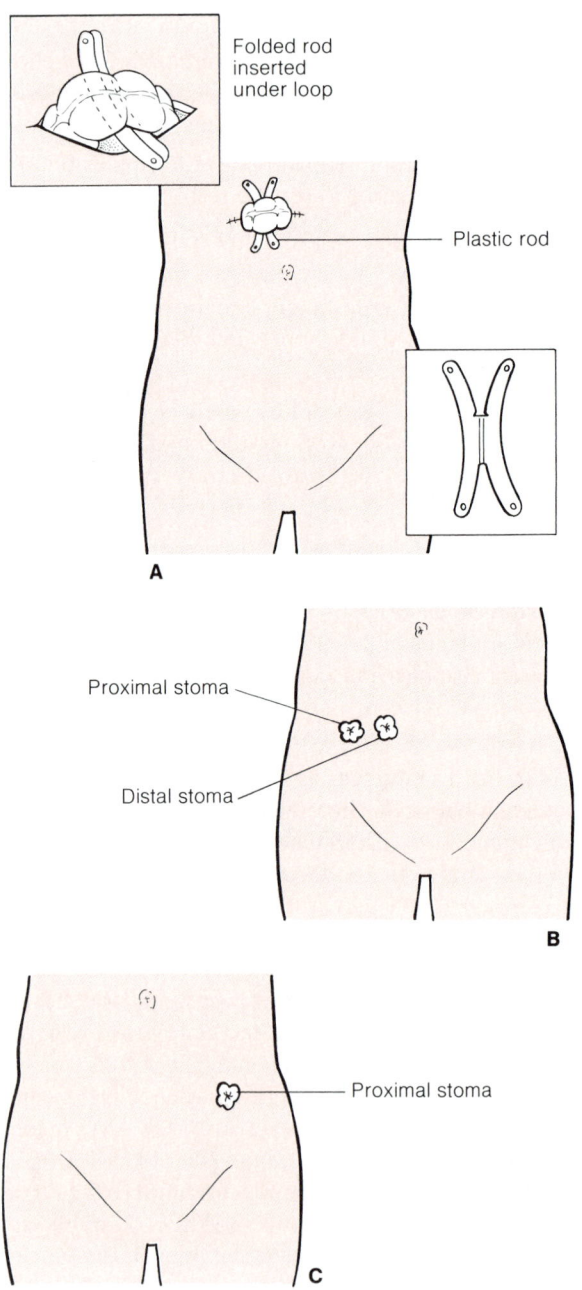

Folded rod inserted under loop
Plastic rod
A
Proximal stoma
Distal stoma
B
Proximal stoma
C

Figure 42–13 Three types of colostomies: *A,* the loop colostomy using a plastic rod; *B,* the double-barreled colostomy; *C,* the end colostomy. Note the plastic rod under the loop colostomy at the top.

in compensation. There are three major types of stoma constructions: the loop colostomy, the double-barreled colostomy, and the end colostomy. See Figure 42–13. See the accompanying box for stoma assessment.

Assessing prior to a bowel diversion should include:

- *Tape allergy.* The client may have a documented allergic reaction to the tape used to secure the ostomy appliance to the abdomen. A 24-hour tape-patch test, experimenting with at least three or four different types of tape (silk, paper, and foam) is best done *before* the client has surgery and on the nonoperative side. Cut strips of each type, label them with a marking pen, and place them on the client's abdomen. See Figure 42–14. The abdomen, rather than the inner arm, is used, since abdominal skin is more sensitive. Abdominal hair may first need to be removed (using scissors or an electric razor or clippers). During the next 24 hours, note complaints of itching or burning, and at the end of the period remove the tape and inspect the abdomen for redness and swelling. Document specific allergies, if present, on the client's chart, and provide the client with an allergic-alert arm band.

- *Learning needs* of the client and family members regarding the ostomy and self-care.

Assessing a Stoma

- *Stoma color.* The stoma should appear red, similar in color to the mucosal lining of the inner cheek. Very pale or darker-colored stomas with a bluish or purplish hue indicate impaired blood circulation to the area.

- *Stoma size and shape.* Most stomas protrude slightly from the abdomen. New stomas normally appear swollen, but swelling generally decreases in size over 2 or 3 weeks or for as long as 6 weeks. Lack of size decrease may indicate a problem, e.g., blockage.

- *Stomal bleeding.* Slight bleeding initially when the stoma is touched is normal, but other bleeding should be reported.

- *Status of peristomal skin.* Any redness and irritation of the peristomal skin (the 5 to 13 cm (2 to 5 in) of skin surrounding the stoma) should be noted. Transient redness after removal of adhesive is normal.

- *Amount and type of feces.* For ileal effluent and feces (colostomy effluent), assess the amount, color, odor, and consistency. Inspect for abnormalities, such as pus or blood.

- *Complaints.* Complaints of burning sensation under the faceplate may indicate skin breakdown. The presence of abdominal discomfort and/or distention also needs to be determined.

- *Emotional status* of the client.

A client who has a stoma usually requires nursing assistance in four major areas: psychosocial adjustment, diet, stoma and skin care, and odor control. Enterostomal therapy nurses are recognized specialists for such clients. A person who undergoes surgery resulting in a stoma is likely to have strong reactions to the operation. In some instances the ostomy is palliative treatment for an underlying disease, such as a malignancy of the rectum. Here the client faces not only adjustment to the stoma but also adjustment to a disease process that may not be cured. The client may feel that health is lost and that his or her life-style must change. Some clients and family members go through a process of grieving before accepting the ostomy and learning to deal with it.

A stoma means changes in both the method and pattern of defecation, which is a highly personal function. Most clients are very aware of other people's reactions to the stoma and particularly sensitive to any negative behavior that could be interpreted as meaning that he or she is offensive. It is important for nurses to communicate acceptance and understanding and to provide the same privacy during care that is normally provided for elimination.

In a client with an ileostomy, accumulated waste products can block the ileum, often at the point where it passes through the abdominal wall. Blockage is best prevented by teaching the client to chew potentially obstructing foods well and introducing them one at a time. In this way, the client learns to identify and avoid foods that cause blockage. Examples of potentially obstructing foods are corn, celery, and whole grains.

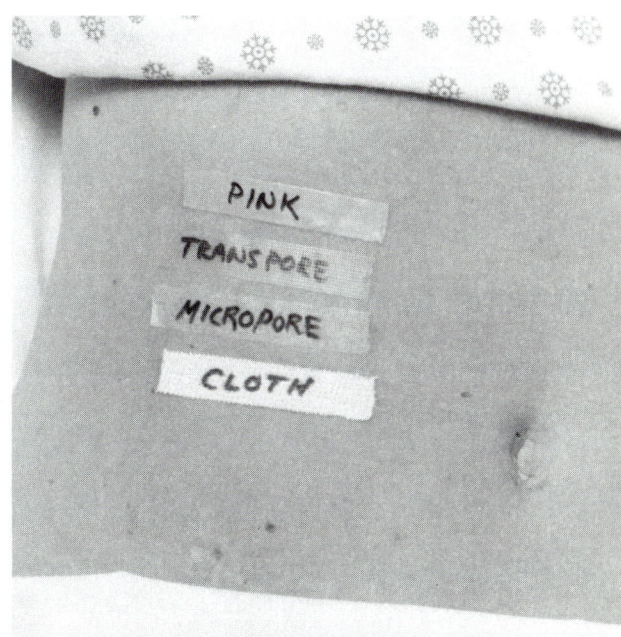

Figure 42–14   A 24-hour tape patch test.

RESEARCH NOTE

How Important is the ET Nurse to the Social Adjustment of Ostomy Clients?

The author's purpose was to determine the impact of the enterostomal nurse (ET nurse) on the social readjustment of ostomy clients. Forty clients, twenty of whom were hospitalized, participated in the study. Hedrick found that people who received an ET nurse's counseling during hospitalization had a better level of adjustment than people who did not receive counseling.

Implications: Counseling by an ET nurse will often assist a client's adjustment following ostomy surgery.

J. K. Hedrick. Effects of nursing interventions on adjustment following ostomy surgery, *Journal of Enterostomal Therapy*, November/December 1987, 14:229–39.

Fluid and electrolyte imbalance can occur because the client is without a functioning colon. The colon normally reabsorbs water and sodium through its wall into the blood circulation. Clients who have ileostomies tend to lose excessive amounts of sodium and fluid through the ileal effluent. Therefore, the diet should be high in fluids, sodium, and potassium, especially when the client has diarrhea or significant losses from other routes, e.g., high sodium loss due to excessive perspiration. Clients need to be taught to respond to thirst and the signs and symptoms of fluid electrolyte imbalance. Foods rich in potassium include bananas, chard, avocados, and fish.

Care of the stoma and skin is important for all clients who have ostomies. The fecal material from a colostomy or ileostomy is irritating to the peristomal skin. This is particularly true of ileal effluent, which contains digestive enzymes. It is important that the peristomal skin be assessed for irritation each time the appliance is changed. Any irritations or skin breakdown need to be treated immediately. The skin is kept clean by washing off any excretion and then dried thoroughly. A barrier such as karaya is applied over the skin around the stoma to prevent contact with any excretion. An appliance (bag) is then fitted to the stoma so that there is no leakage around it. It is exceedingly important to dry the skin before attaching the appliance. The pouch will not adhere to moist skin, causing effluent to leak onto the skin. Numerous pouch systems are commercially available. All appliances have three features in common: a pouch to collect the effluent, an outlet at the bottom for easy emptying, and a faceplate. Temporary, disposable pouches are made of transparent plastic and have a peel-off adhesive square into which a hole the size of the stoma is cut. Permanent pouches may be clear or opaque, rubber or vinyl and have a solid ring faceplate that fits around the stoma. See Figure 42–15.

Odor control is essential to clients' self-esteem. As soon as the client is out of bed, he or she can learn to work with the ostomy in the bathroom to avoid odors at the bedside. For odor control, it is necessary to use the appropriate kind of appliance. An intact appliance contains odors. The appliance should be rinsed thoroughly when it is emptied. Deodorizers can be placed in the pouch of the appliance, or

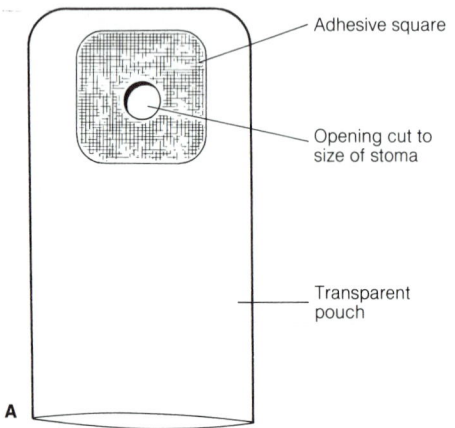

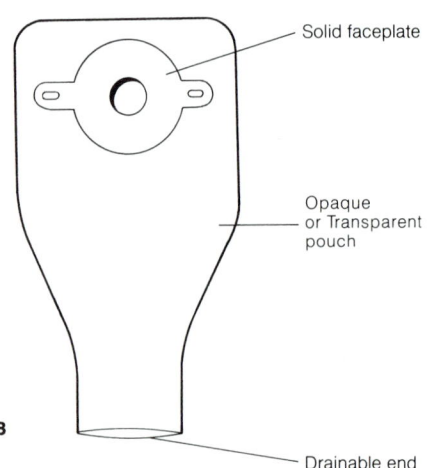

Figure 42–15 Ostomy appliances: *A,* temporary, disposable; *B,* permanent, reusable.

pouches with charcoal filter discs are available. Some recommend oral intake of charcoal or bismuth subcarbonate, which should be taken only with the physician's approval. See the accompanying box for criteria for ostomy appliances.

Disposable ostomy appliances can be applied for up to 7 days. They need to be changed whenever the effluent leaks onto the peristomal skin or when it cannot be rinsed completely away. Many people prefer to change them daily or whenever they become soiled, but this practice can be detrimental to the integrity of the peristomal skin and is expensive. Check agency practice in this regard. Erickson (1987, p. 314) recommends removing the pouch and skin barrier twice a week to clean and inspect the peristomal skin. If the peristomal skin is erythematous, Broadwell (1987, p. 331) recommends removing and changing the system every 48 to 72 hours; if the skin is eroded, denuded, or ulcerated, it should be changed every 24 to 48 hours to allow appropriate treatment of the skin. More frequent changes are recommended if the client complains of pain or discomfort. Procedure 42–2 explains how to change a bowel diversion ostomy appliance.

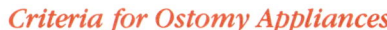

Criteria for Ostomy Appliances

The ostomy appliance should:

- Be odor-resistant
- Protect peristomal skin. The faceplate opening needs to fit closely around the stoma
- Stay secure for 3 to 5 days
- Be nonallergenic (bags with adhesive-backed discs)
- Be readily available, affordable, and appealing to the client
- Be invisible underneath clothing

Disposable postoperative pouches should be:

- Transparent, to allow assessment of the stoma
- Odorproof, to enhance client acceptability
- Drainable, so that the pouch can be emptied without removing it
- Adjustable, so that the size of the opening can be altered to accommodate changes in stoma shape and size as edema resolves

---

PROCEDURE 42–2

CHANGING A BOWEL DIVERSION OSTOMY APPLIANCE

Equipment ☑

Solvent (presaturated sponges or liquid)

Receptacle

Cleaning materials, including tissues, warm water, mild soap (optional), washcloth or cotton balls, towel

Tissue or gauze pad

Skin barrier (liquid protective covering or peristomal skin barrier)

Peristomal skin paste or powder

Measuring guide

Pen or pencil

Scissors

Tail closure or elastic band

Special adhesive and brush, if needed.

Stoma guidestrip

Deodorant (liquid or tablet) for a nonodorproof colostomy bag

Tape for securing a detachable faceplate as necessary

Disposable gloves

Intervention

1. Determine the need for appliance change.

- Assess the used appliance for leakage of effluent. *Effluent can irritate the peristomal skin.*
- Ask the client about any discomfort at or around the stoma. *A burning sensation may indicate breakdown beneath the faceplate of the pouch.*

- Assess the fullness of the pouch. Pouches need to be emptied when they are one-third to one-half full. *When the fluid level in the bag becomes too high, the weight of it may loosen the faceplate and separate it from the skin, causing the effluent to leak and irritate the peristomal skin.*
- If there is pouch leakage or discomfort at or around the stoma, change the appliance.

2. Select an appropriate time.

- Avoid times close to meal or visiting hours. *Ostomy odor and effluent may reduce appetite or be visibly distressing.*
- Avoid times immediately after the administration of any medications that may stimulate bowel evacuation. *Changing the pouch is facilitated when the ostomy is least likely to function.*

3. **Prepare the client and support persons.**

- Explain the procedure to the client and support persons. Changing an ostomy appliance should not cause discomfort, but it may be distasteful to the client. *Support persons are often more supportive if properly informed.*

- Communicate acceptance and support of the client. It is important to change the appliance competently and quickly and not to convey disgust.

- Provide privacy, preferably in the bathroom, where clients can learn to deal with the ostomy as they would at home.

- Assist the client to a comfortable sitting or lying position in bed or preferably a sitting or standing position in the bathroom. *Lying or standing positions may facilitate smoother pouch application, i.e., avoid wrinkles.*

- Don gloves, and unfasten the belt if one is being worn.

4. **Shave the peristomal skin of well-established ostomies as needed.**

- Use an electric or safety razor on a regular basis to remove excessive hair growth. *If the hair is allowed to grow and is regularly pulled out when the appliance and skin barrier are removed, hair follicles can become irritated or infected.*

5. **Empty and remove the appliance.**

- Empty the pouch contents through the bottom opening into a bedpan. *Emptying before pouch removal prevents spillage of effluent onto the client's skin.*

- Assess the consistency and amount of effluent.

- If needed, apply an adhesive solvent to remove the appliance. This is not needed in most cases and should be used only when absolutely necessary.

- Peel the bag off slowly while holding the client's skin taut. *Holding the skin taut minimizes client discomfort and prevents skin abrasion.*

- If the appliance is disposable, discard it in a moistureproof bag.

6. **Clean and dry the peristomal skin and stoma.**

- Use toilet tissue to remove excess stool.

- Use warm water, mild soap (optional), and cotton balls or a washcloth and towel to clean the skin and stoma. Check agency practice on the use of soap. *Soap is sometimes not advised because it can be irritating to the skin.*

- Use a special skin cleanser to remove dried, hard stool. *This emulsifies the stool, making removal less damaging to the skin.*

- Dry the area thoroughly by patting with a towel or cotton swabs. *Excess rubbing can abrade the skin.*

7. **Assess the stoma and peristomal skin.**

- Inspect the stoma for color, size, shape, and bleeding.

- Inspect the peristomal skin for any redness, ulceration, or irritation. Transient redness *after the removal of adhesive* is normal.

- Place a piece of tissue or gauze pad over the stoma, and change it as needed. *This absorbs any seepage from the stoma.*

8. **Apply paste-type skin barrier if needed.**

- Fill in abdominal creases or dimples with paste. *This establishes a smooth surface for application of the skin barrier and pouch.*

- Allow the paste to dry for 1 to 2 minutes or as recommended by the manufacturer.

9. **Prepare and apply the skin barrier (peristomal seal).**

For solid wafer or disc skin barrier:

- Use the guide to measure the size of the stoma. See Figure 42–16.

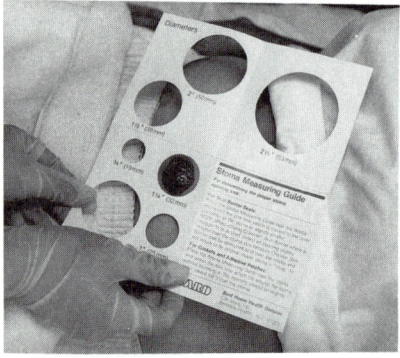

Figure 42—16   A guide for measuring the stoma.

- On the backing of the skin barrier, trace a circle the same size as the stomal opening.

- Make a template (mold) of the stoma pattern. *A template aids other nurses and the client with future appliance changes.* However, the template will need to be adjusted as the stoma size decreases.

- Cut out the traced stoma pattern to make an opening in the skin barrier.

- Remove the backing to expose the sticky adhesive side.

- Center the skin barrier over the stoma, and gently press it onto the client's skin, smoothing out any wrinkles or bubbles. See Figure 42–17.

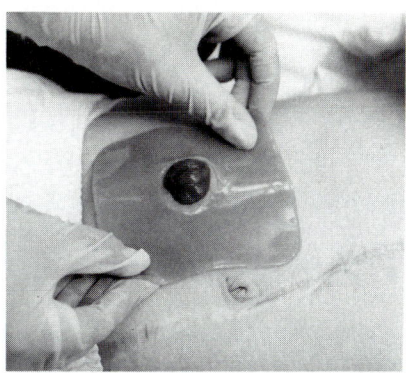

Figure 42-17 Centering the skin barrier over the stoma.

For liquid skin sealant:

- Cover the stoma with a gauze pad. *This prevents contact with the skin sealant.*

- Either wipe the product evenly around the peristomal skin, or use a brush to apply a thin layer of the liquid plastic coating to the same area.

- Allow the skin barrier to dry until it no longer feels tacky.

10. Fill in any exposed skin around an irregularly shaped stoma.

- Apply paste to any exposed skin areas. Use a nonalcohol-based product if the skin is excoriated. *Alcohol may cause stinging and burning.*
  or

- Sprinkle peristomal powder on the skin, wipe off the excess, and dab the powder with a slightly moist gauze or an applicator moistened with a liquid skin sealant. *This creates a barrier or seal.* Avoid using skin sealant. *Skin sealant burns if the area is excoriated.*

11. Prepare and apply the clean appliance.

- Remove the tissue over the stoma before applying the pouch.

For a disposable pouch with adhesive square:

- If the appliance does not have a precut opening, trace a circle ⅛ to ⅙ inch larger than the stoma size on the appliance's adhesive square. *The opening is made slightly larger than the stoma to prevent rubbing, cutting, or trauma to the stoma.*

- Cut out a circle in the adhesive. Take care not to cut any portion of the pouch.

- Peel off the backing from the adhesive seal.

- Center the opening of the pouch over the client's stoma, and apply it directly onto the skin barrier. See Figure 42-18.

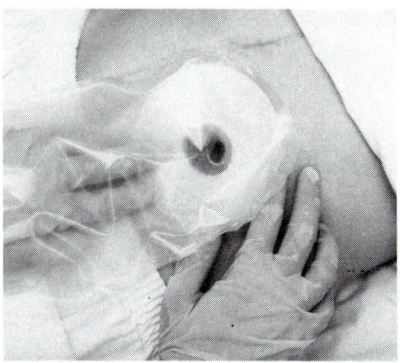

Figure 42-18 Applying the disposable pouch.

- Gently press the adhesive backing onto the skin and smooth out any wrinkles, working from the stoma outward. *Wrinkles allow seepage of effluent, which can irritate the skin or soil clothing.*

- Remove the air from the pouch. *Removing the air helps the pouch lie flat against the abdomen.*

- Place a deodorant in the pouch (optional).

- Close the pouch by turning up the bottom a few times, fanfolding its end lengthwise and securing it with a rubber band or tail closure clamp.

For a reusable pouch with faceplate attached:

- Apply either adhesive cement or a double-faced adhesive disc to the faceplate of the appliance, depending on the type of appliance being used. Follow the manufacturer's directions.

- Insert a coiled paper guidestrip (15-cm [6-in] strip of 1.3-cm [½-in] wide paper) into the faceplate opening. The strip should protrude slightly from the opening and expand to fit it. See Figure 42-19. *The guidestrip helps you center the appliance over the stoma and prevents pressure or irritation to the stoma by an ill-fitting appliance.*

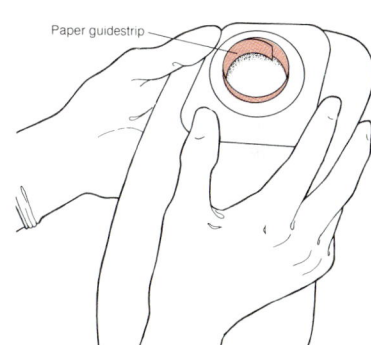

Paper guidestrip

Figure 42-19 The coiled paper guidestrip in the faceplate opening.

- Using the guidestrip, center the faceplate over the stoma.

- Firmly press the adhesive seal to the peristomal skin. The guidestrip will fall into the pouch; commercially prepared guidestrips will dissolve in the pouch.

- Place a deodorant in the bag if the bag is not odorproof. Most pouches are odorproof.

- Close the end of the pouch with the designated clamp.
- Attach the pouch belt, and fasten it around the client's waist (optional).

For a reusable pouch with detachable faceplate:

- Note allergies and results of tape patch test performed before surgery.
- Some nurses recommend applying a skin sealant (e.g., Skin Prep) to the faceplate before attaching the adhesive disc. *This makes it easier to remove the adhesive disc from the faceplate.*
- Remove the protective paper strip from one side of the double-faced adhesive disc.
- Apply the sticky side to the back of the faceplate.
- Remove the remaining protective paper strip from the other side of the adhesive disc.
- Center the faceplate over the stoma and skin barrier, then press and hold the faceplate against the client's skin for a few minutes to secure the seal.
- Press the adhesive around the circumference of the adhesive disc.
- Tape the faceplate to the client's abdomen using four or eight 7.5-cm (3-in) strips of hypoallergenic tape. Place the strips around the faceplate in a "picture-framing" manner, one strip down each side, one across the top, and one across the bottom. See Figure 42−20. The additional four strips can be placed diagonally over the other tapes to secure the seal.
- Stretch the opening on the back of the pouch, and position it over the base of the faceplate. Ease it over the faceplate flange.

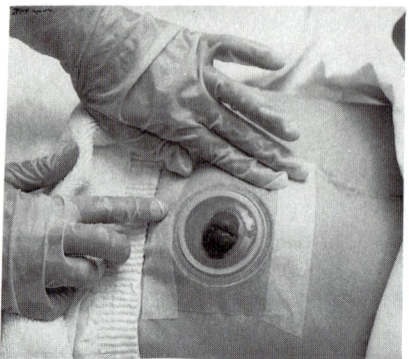

Figure 42−20   Taping the faceplate to the client's abdomen.

- Place the lock ring between the pouch and the faceplate flange (see Figure 42−21) to seal the pouch against the faceplate.
- Close the base of the pouch with the appropriate clamp.
- Attach the pouch belt, and fasten it around the client's waist (optional).

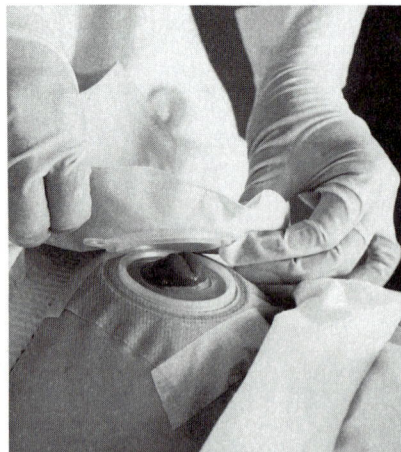

Figure 42−21   Sealing the pouch against the faceplate.

12. **Dispose of or clean reusable equipment.**

- Discard disposable bags in plastic bags before placing in the waste container.

- If feces is liquid, measure its volume before emptying the feces into a toilet or hopper.
- Wash reusable bags with cool water and mild soap, rinse, and dry.
- Wash a soiled belt with warm water and mild soap, rinse, and dry.
- Remove and discard gloves.

13. **Report and record pertinent assessments and interventions.**

- Report to the nurse in charge any increase in stoma size, change in color indicative of circulatory impairment, and presence of skin irritation or erosion.
- Record on the client's chart discoloration of the stoma; the appearance of the peristomal skin; the amount and type of drainage; the client's fatigue, discomfort, and significant behavior about the ostomy; and skills learned.
- Adjust the teaching plan and nursing care plan as needed. Include on the teaching plan the equipment and procedure used. *Learning to care for the ostomy is facilitated if procedures implemented by nurses are consistent.*

Sample Recording

Date: 10/5/91	Time: 1400

Colostomy appliance changed. 350 ml dark brown liquid feces. Stoma pink, 8 cm. Peristomal skin intact. No discomfort. Helped to clean the peristomal skin.——
————————Ramona L. de Santo, NS

Variation: applying the skin barrier and appliance as one unit.

If a disc- or wafer-type skin barrier is used, the skin barrier and appliance can be applied as one unit. Applying the skin barrier and the appliance together not only is quicker but also is thought by some to reduce the chance of wrinkles. It also is easier for the client to apply without help.

■ Prepare the skin barrier by measuring the size of the stoma, tracing a circle on the backing of the skin barrier, and cutting out the

traced stoma pattern to make an opening in the skin barrier.

■ Prepare the appliance by cutting an opening ⅛ to ⅙ inch larger than the stoma size (if not already present) and peeling off the backing from the adhesive seal.

■ Center the opening of the pouch over the skin barrier.

■ Remove the skin barrier backing to expose the sticky adhesive side.

■ Center the skin barrier and appliance over the stoma, and press it onto the client's skin.

Colostomy Irrigation

A colostomy irrigation, similar to an enema, is a form of stoma management used only for clients who have a sigmoid or descending colostomy. The purpose of irrigation is to distend the bowel sufficiently to stimulate peristalsis, which stimulates evacuation. When a regular evacuation pattern is achieved, the wearing of a colostomy pouch is unnecessary.

Routine daily irrigations for control of the time of elimination ultimately become the client's decision. Some clients prefer to control the time of elimination through rigid dietary regulation and not be bothered with irrigations, which can take up to an hour to complete. When regulation by irrigation is chosen, it should be done at the same time each day. Control by irrigations also necessitates some control of the diet. For example, laxative foods that might cause an unexpected evacuation need to be avoided.

For most clients, a relatively small amount of fluid (300 to 500 ml) stimulates evacuation. For others, up to 1000 ml may be needed, since a colostomy has no sphincter and the fluid tends to return as it is instilled. This problem is reduced by the use of a cone on the irrigating catheter. The cone helps to hold the fluid within the bowel during the irrigation.

Before starting an irrigation, assess the client's readiness to select and use the equipment. Because many types of irrigation sets are available, clients should begin with a "starter set" until they are familiar with the colostomy and the problems of irrigating it. Later, with the help of an enterostomal therapy nurse or a qualified person from a surgical supply house, the client can select the set most appropriate for the client's needs.

The equipment commonly used for a colostomy irrigation is shown in the accompanying box. Both commercially prepared equipment and standard equipment are available. See Figure 42–22 on page 1182.

Assist the client who must remain in bed to a side-lying position. Place a disposable bedpad on the bed in front of the client, and place the bedpan on top of the disposable pad, beneath the stoma. Assist an ambulatory client to sit on the toilet or on a commode in the bathroom. Ensure that the client's gown or pajamas are moved out of the way to prevent soiling, and cover the client appropriately with the bath blanket to prevent undue exposure. Throughout the technique, provide explanations, and encourage the client to participate as much as the client desires.

Equipment for a Colostomy Irrigation

■ A moisture-resistant bag

■ A clean colostomy appliance or dressings

■ Irrigation equipment

   a. A bag to hold the solution. With routine irrigations for regulation, the bag is usually filled with 500 ml of warm (body temperature) tap water, or other solution as ordered. For a bowel preparation, 1000 ml of solution is needed.

   b. Tubing attached to the bag

   c. A tubing clamp or flow regulator

   d. A #28 rubber colon catheter, calibrated in either centimeters or inches, with a stoma cone or seal

   e. A disposable stoma-irrigation drainage sleeve with belt to direct the fecal contents into the toilet or bedpan

■ Lubricant

■ Clean gloves to protect the nurse's hands from contamination, and one glove to dilate the stoma if ordered by the physician

■ A bath blanket

■ An IV pole

■ A disposable bedpad, bedpan, and cover, if the client is to remain in bed

---

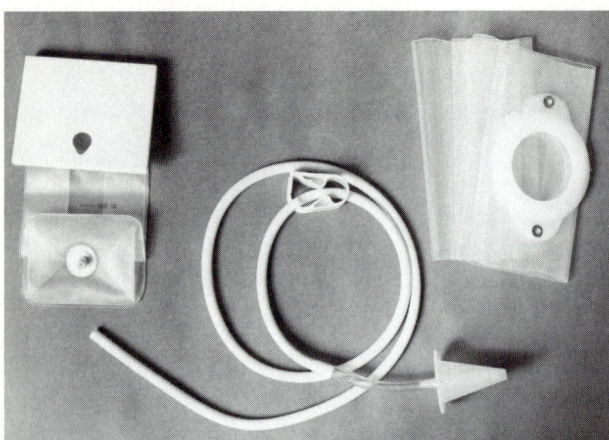

Figure 42–22 A commercially prepared colostomy irrigation set. The irrigation solution bag is on the left, and the collecting bag (irrigation drainage sleeve) on the right; the stoma cone is fitted to the catheter.

Hang the solution bag on an IV pole so that the bottom of the container is at the level of the client's shoulder, or 30 to 45 cm (12 to 18 in) above the stoma. This height provides a pressure gradient that allows fluid to flow into the colon. The rate of flow can be regulated with the tubing clamp. Attach the colon catheter securely to the tubing. Open the regulator clamp, and run fluid through the tubing to expel all air from it. Close the clamp until ready for the irrigation. Air should not be introduced into the bowel because it distends the bowel and can cause cramps. Remove the soiled colostomy bag, and place it in the moisture-resistant bag so that microorganisms are contained and odor is reduced. Center the irrigation drainage sleeve over the stoma, and attach it snugly to prevent seepage of the fluid onto the skin. Direct the lower open end of the drainage sleeve into the bedpan or between the client's legs into the toilet. If ordered by the physician, dilate the stoma:

1. Put on gloves.
2. Lubricate the tip of the little finger.
3. Gently insert the finger into the stoma, using a massaging motion. See Figure 42–23. A massaging motion relaxes the intestinal muscles.
4. Repeat steps 2 and 3 above, using progressively larger fingers until maximum dilation is achieved. Stoma dilation helps to stretch and relax the stomal opening and enables the nurse to assess the direction of the proximal colon prior to an irrigation.

Lubricate the tip of the stoma cone or colon catheter to ease its insertion and prevent injury to the stoma. Using a rotating motion, insert the catheter or stoma cone through the opening in the top of the irrigation drainage sleeve and gently through the stoma. See Figure 42–24. Insert a catheter only 7 cm (3 in); insert a stoma cone just until it fits snugly. Many practitioners prefer using a cone to avoid the risk of perforating the bowel. If you have difficulty inserting the catheter or cone, do not apply force. A rotating motion on insertion helps to open the stoma. Forcing the cone or catheter may traumatize or perforate the bowel. Open the tubing clamp, and allow the fluid to flow into the bowel. If

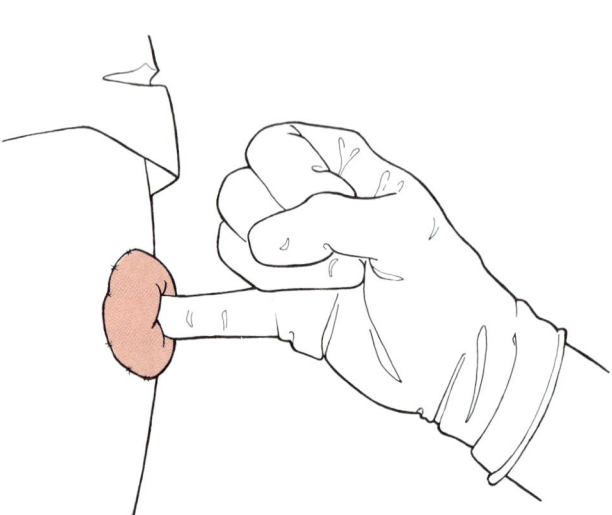

Figure 42–23 Dilating a colostomy stoma.

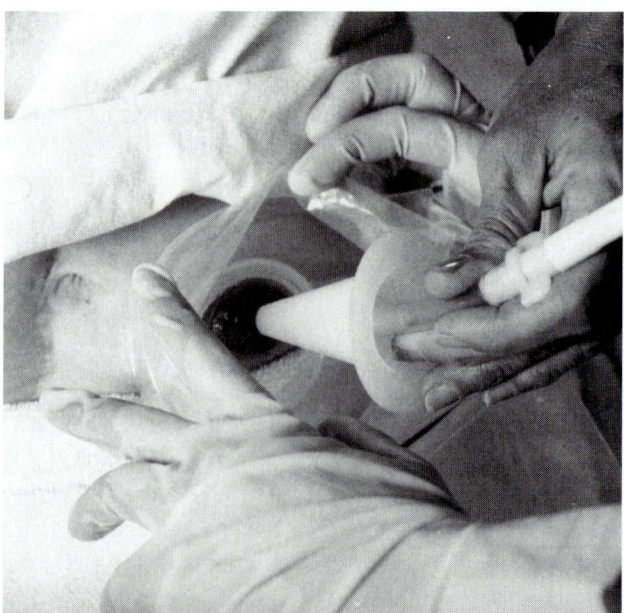

Figure 42–24 The client is participating in the colostomy irrigation by directing the cone.

cramping occurs, stop the flow until the cramps subside; then resume the flow. Fluid that is too cold or administered too quickly may cause cramps. If the fluid flows out as fast as you put it in, press the stoma cone or seal more firmly against the stoma to occlude it. If a stoma cone or seal is not available, press around the stoma with your fingers to close the stoma against the catheter. After all the fluid is instilled, remove the catheter or cone and allow the colon to empty. Although not always indicated, you may ask the client to gently massage the abdomen and sit quietly for 10 to 15 minutes until initial emptying has occurred. Massaging the abdomen encourages initial emptying. In some agencies the stoma cone is left in place for 10 to 15 minutes before it is removed.

Clean the base of the irrigation drainage sleeve, and seal the top and bottom off with a drainage clamp, following the manufacturer's instructions. Encourage an ambulatory client to move around for about 30 minutes, since complete emptying of the colon takes up to half an hour and moving around facilitates peristalsis. Empty the irrigation drainage sleeve, and remove it. Clean the area around the stoma, dry it thoroughly, and put a colostomy appliance on the client as needed.

Promptly report to the nurse in charge any problems, such as no fluid or stool returns, difficulties inserting the tube, peristomal skin redness or irritation, and stomal discoloration. Record the irrigation on the client's chart, the time of the irrigation, the type and amount of fluid instilled, the returns, and the client's response.

EVALUATING

To evaluate whether client goals have been achieved, the nurse collects data pertaining to the established outcome criteria at specified intervals. Evaluation activities may include the following:

- Observing the character of stool
- Recording the frequency of defecation
- Measuring the client's fluid intake and output
- Inspecting the anal, perianal, or peristomal skin
- Palpating the abdomen for distention
- Auscultating the abdomen for bowel sounds
- Asking the client about flatulence, feelings of rectal fullness, abdominal discomfort before or during defecation, straining at defecation, or urgency
- Observing the client demonstrate self-care skills for ostomy management
- Questioning the client about dietary intake, daily exercise, or other measures implemented to relieve or eliminate contributing factors

Examples of evaluative statements indicating goal achievement are "The client's perianal skin is intact"; "The client has established a regular defecation pattern (bowel movement three times a week) for 2 weeks"; or "The client was able to name five high-fiber foods."

NURSING CARE PLAN FOR EMMA BROWN

ASSESSMENT DATA

Nursing Assessment
Mrs. Emma Brown is a 78-year-old widow of 9 months. She lives alone in a low-income housing complex for the elderly. Her two children live with their families in a city approximately 150 miles away. She has always enjoyed cooking for her family in the past; however, now that she is alone, she does not enjoy cooking for herself. As a result, she has developed irregular eating patterns and tends to prepare soup-and-toast meals. She does not walk or exercise very much. She has bouts of insomnia since her husband's death. Lately, Mrs. Brown has been having a problem with constipation. She has a bowel movement approximately every 3 or 4 days, and her stools are hard and painful to excrete. When the housing complex sponsors a health fair, Mrs. Brown attends and seeks some assistance with her elimination problem from Laura Nakamura, the county public health nurse.

Physical Examination
Height: 162 cm (5'4")
Weight: 65 kg (143 lb)
Temperature: 36.2 C (97.2 F)
Pulse rate: 82 BPM
Respirations: 20 per minute at rest
Blood pressure: 128/74 mm Hg
Active bowel sounds
Abdomen slightly distended

Diagnostic Data
CBC: Hgb 10.8
Urine: Negative

Nursing Diagnosis	Client Goals and Outcome Criteria	Nursing Interventions and Rationales	Evaluation
Constipation related to low fiber intake and inactivity resulting in infrequent hard stools, painful defecation, abdominal distention.	Client Goal: Relief of constipation Outcome Criteria: Drinks 2000 to 3000 ml of fluid daily Eats bran flakes for breakfast 3 times per week. Eats 3 complete meals each day.	Encourage warm fluids, e.g., warm lemonade or coffee, early each morning. *Rationale:* Increased fluid intake decreases incidence of constipation and hot fluid stimulates peristalsis. Encourage foods such as bran, fresh fruits, and vegetables in daily diet. *Rationale:* High-fiber foods provide bulk that increases fecal volume. Discuss need to eat 3 or 4 regularly scheduled meals a day. *Rationale:* Eating at regular times promotes regular defecation. Increase physical activity through exercise, e.g., walking. *Rationale:* Exercise increases appetite and peristalsis.	Passes soft and formed stools daily. She drinks warm lemonade each morning before a breakfast that frequently includes bran flakes and prune juice. She now participates in the "Meals on Wheels" program and has joined the Seniors Exercise Club.
Altered nutrition: Less than body requirements, resulting in weight loss, inadequate intake of fiber, vitamins, and proteins.	Client Goal: Maintain normal body weight. Outcome Criteria: Identifies factors related to inadequate food intake. Gains weight at rate of 1 pound per month. Identifies two food sources high in fiber.	Instruct client to keep a diet log for 1 week. *Rationale:* A diary can identify types of foods eaten. Refer client to nutritionist regarding diet. *Rationale:* Proper food sources of protein and fiber can be identified and recommended. Discuss ways to modify eating behavior pattern. *Rationale:* Behavior modifications may assist in changing eating habits.	Client identifies two food sources high in fiber, protein, and vitamins after consulting with dietitian. She has gained 2 pounds in past month and feels less fatigued.

CHAPTER HIGHLIGHTS

▶ Primary functions of the large bowel are the excretion of digestive waste products and the maintenance of fluid balance.

▶ Patterns of fecal elimination vary greatly among people, but a regular pattern of fecal elimination with formed, soft stools is essential to health and a sense of well-being.

▶ A variety of factors affect defecation: age, diet, fluid intake, activity/exercise, psychologic stress, life-style, medications, diagnostic procedures, anesthesia, and pathologic conditions.

▶ Common fecal elimination problems include constipation, fecal impaction, diarrhea, fecal incontinence, flatulence. Each has specific defining characteristics and contributing causes that often relate to or are identical to the factors that affect defecation.

▶ Assessment relative to fecal elimination includes a nursing history; physical examination of the abdomen, rectum, and anus; and, in some situations, visualization studies and inspection and analysis of stool for abnormal constituents such as blood.

- A nursing history includes data about the client's defecating pattern, description of feces and any changes, problems associated with elimination, and data about possible factors altering bowel elimination.

- Physical examination of the abdomen includes methods of inspection, auscultation, percussion, and palpation. Physical examination of the rectum and anus includes inspection and palpation.

- When inspecting the client's stool, the nurse must observe its color, consistency, shape, amount, odor, and the presence of abnormal constituents.

- A major function of the nurse is to assist clients with endoscopic and radiographic studies of the large intestine. Client assistance for visualization involves diet and bowel preparation before the study and appropriate follow-up care after the study.

- Clients also often need assistance to obtain stool specimens for laboratory analysis. In many agencies, nurses test the stool for occult blood.

- NANDA approved nursing diagnoses that relate specifically to altered bowel elimination include **Constipation, Diarrhea,** and **Bowel incontinence.** However, because altered elimination patterns affect several areas of human functioning, diagnoses such as **Potential fluid volume deficit, Body image disturbance,** and **Potential impaired skin integrity** may also apply.

- Constipation can be categorized as rectal, colonic, or perceived. Clients with perceived constipation often require education because overuse of laxatives can itself cause constipation.

- Lack of exercise, irregular defecation habits, stress, and bland diets are all thought to contribute to constipation. Sufficient fluid and fiber intake are required to keep feces soft.

- An adverse effect of constipation is straining during defecation, during which the Valsalva maneuver may be used. Cardiac problems may ensue.

- An adverse effect of prolonged diarrhea is fluid and electrolyte imbalance.

- Digital removal of an impaction should be carried out gently because of vagal nerve stimulation and subsequent depressed cardiac rate. A physician's order is often necessary.

- Normal defecation is often facilitated in both well and ill clients by providing privacy, teaching clients to attend to defecation urges promptly, assisting clients whenever possible to normal sitting positions, encouraging appropriate food and fluid intake, and scheduling regular exercise.

- Additional nursing strategies include administering cathartics and antidiarrheals; administering cleansing, carminative, or retention enemas; removing an impaction digitally; inserting rectal tubes to decrease flatulence; applying protective skin agents; monitoring fluid and electrolyte balance; and instructing clients in ways to promote normal defecation.

- Clients who have bowel diversion ostomies require special care, with attention to psychologic adjustment, diet, and stoma and skin care. A variety of stomal management methods are available to these clients, depending on the type and position of the ostomy.

READINGS AND REFERENCES

SUGGESTED READINGS

Alterescu, V. November 1985. The ostomy. What do you teach the patient? *American Journal of Nursing* 85:1250–53.
    This article includes a discussion of some of the psychosocial implications of a colostomy. Preoperative and postoperative teaching is also included. Eleven do's and don'ts of ostomy-client teaching are provided as well as sample discharge instructions.
Cerrato, P. L. May 1989. Is American really constipated? *RN* 52:81–2, 84, 86.
    Americans spend almost $400 million a year on laxatives, reports the author. Cerrato offers two suppositions: constipation is a widespread problem, and advertising has made bowel function a nationwide obsession. It is thought that many people eat insufficient fiber; the average person consumes 20 grams of dietary fiber a day when the recommended intake is 40 grams. Other problems associated with constipation are inadequate fluids, prolonged bed rest and too little exercise, ignoring the urge to defecate, drugs and dietary supplements, and food intolerances. The author describes the various groups of laxatives but stresses that finding the right remedy to a client's constipation requires good nursing judgment.
Rolstad, B. S. June 1987. Innovative surgical procedures and stoma care in the future. *Nursing Clinics of North America* 22:341–56.
    The author describes the various types of urologic and enteric diversions and provides information about client selection and nursing management associated with these procedures. The author also discusses the educational needs of clients and their families.
Smith, D. B. November 1985. The ostomy, how is it managed? *American Journal of Nursing* 85:1246–49.
    This article describes how to assess a new colostomy and how to irrigate a colostomy. Ileostomy care is also covered. Includes a number of color photographs.

RELATED RESEARCH

Battle, E., and Hanna, C. September 1980. Evaluation of a dietary regimen for chronic constipation: Report of a pilot study. *Journal of Gerontological Nursing* 6:527–32.

Hedrick, J. K. November/December 1987. Effects of nursing interventions on adjustment following ostomy surgery. *Journal of Enterostomal Therapy* 14:229–39.

Willington, F. L.; Yarnell, J. W. G.; and Sweetman, P. M. March 1981. Cleansing incontinent patients: An evaluation of the use of nonionic detergents compared with soap. *Journal of Advanced Nursing* 6:107–9.

SELECTED REFERENCES

Alterescu, K. B. June 1987. Colostomy. *Nursing Clinics of North America.* 22:281–89.

Aman, R. A. September 1980. Treating the patient, not the constipation. *American Journal of Nursing* 80:1634–35.

Behm, R. M. July/August 1985. A special recipe to banish constipation. *Geriatric Nursing* 6:216–17.

Broadwell, D. C. June 1987. Peristomal skin integrity. *Nursing Clinics of North America* 22:321–32.

Ellickson, E. B. January 1988. Bowel management plan for the homebound elderly. *Journal of Gerontological Nursing* 14:16–19.

Erickson, P. J. June 1987. Ostomies: The art of pouching. *Nursing Clinics of North America* 22:311–20.

Fingl, E. 1980. In Goodman, L., and Gilman, A., editors. *Goodman and Gilman's The Pharmalogical Basis of Therapeutics.* 6th ed. New York: Macmillan Co.

Guyton, A. C. 1986. *Textbook of Medical Physiology.* 7th ed. Philadelphia: W. B. Saunders Co.

Hanauer, S. B. March 30, 1988. Fecal incontinence in the elderly. *Hospital Practice* 23:105–8.

Kim, M. J.; McFarland, G. K.; and McLane, A. M. 1987. *Pocket guide to nursing diagnoses.* 2d ed. St. Louis: C. V. Mosby Co.

Logio, T. February 1985. Suppository insertion—which end is first? *Nursing 85* 15:10.

McCann, J. A. S. March 1990. A guide to colostomies. *Nursing 90* 20:32.

McShane, R. E., and McLane, A. M. April 1988. Constipation: Impact of etiological factors. *Journal of Gerontological Nursing* 14:31–34.

Mager-O'Connor, E. May/June 1984. How to identify and remove fecal impactions. *Geriatric Nursing* 5:158–61.

Mowlam V.; North, K.; and Myers, C. November 26–December 2, 1986. Continence: Managing fecal incontinence. *Nursing Times* 82:55, 57, 59.

NANDA approved nursing diagnostic categories for clinical use and testing. Summer 1988. *Nursing Diagnosis Newsletter* 15:1–3.

Osis, M. Fall 1987. Laxatives: Are we making the best choice? *Gerontion* 2:5–7.

Resnick, B. July/August 1985. Constipation: Common but preventable. *Geriatric Nursing* 6:213–15.

Salter, M. May 2–8, 1990. Overcoming the stigma . . . irrigation and continent pouches. *Nursing Times* 86:67–9, 71.

Shipes, E. June 1987. Psychosocial issues: The person with an ostomy. *Nursing Clinics of North America* 22:291–302.

Smith, D. B. January/February 1983. Colostomy irrigations—so simple . . . Irrigation takes on complex variables and requires individualization in each situation. *Journal of Enterostomal Therapy* 10:22–23.

Urinary Elimination

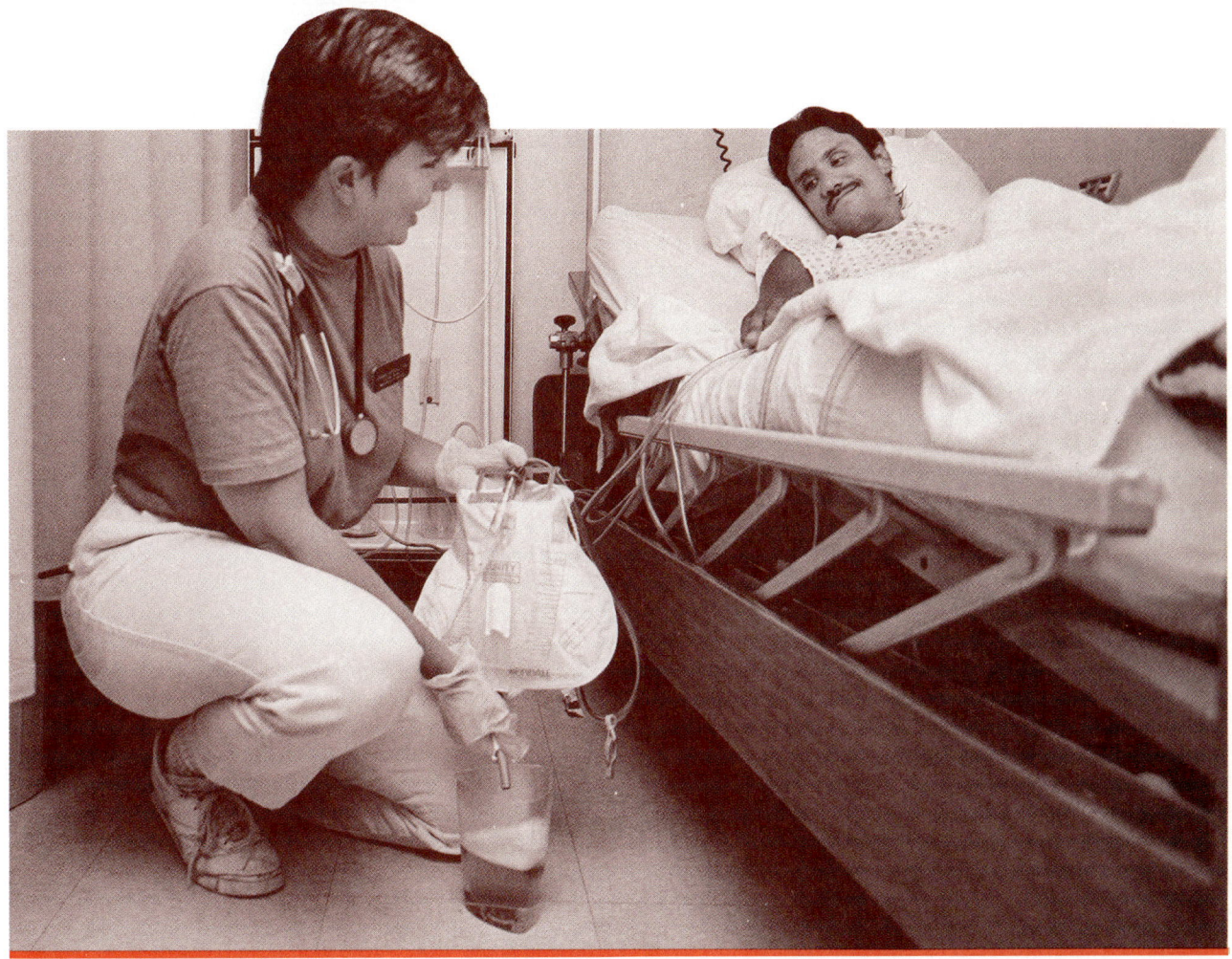

CONTENTS

CONTENTS (continued)

OBJECTIVES

▶ Describe the process of micturition.

▶ Identify factors that influence urinary elimination.

▶ Describe common alterations in urinary elimination.

▶ Identify common causes of selected urinary problems.

▶ Describe urinary diversion ostomies.

▶ Identify essential components of a urinary elimination nursing history.

▶ Describe physical examination methods used to identify urinary elimination problems.

▶ Identify normal and abnormal characteristics and constituents of urine.

▶ Describe diagnostic measures to assess kidney function and urinary tract abnormalities.

▶ Explain how to collect urine specimens and perform simple tests.

▶ Develop nursing diagnoses related to urinary elimination.

▶ Develop client goals and outcome criteria for clients with nursing diagnoses related to urinary elimination.

▶ Describe interventions to maintain normal urinary elimination and to assist clients with urinary incontinence and retention.

▶ Identify ways to prevent urinary infection.

▶ Identify interventions required for clients with retention catheters.

▶ Describe interventions to maintain normal urinary elimination and assist clients with urinary retention and incontinence.

PHYSIOLOGY OF URINARY ELIMINATION

Urinary elimination depends on effective functioning of four urinary tract organs: kidneys, ureters, bladder, and urethra.

Kidneys

The kidneys filter from the blood any products for which the body has no use. Each kidney has one *renal artery* that originates from the abdominal aorta and enters the kidney at the hilum. (See Figure 43–1). The renal vein exits through the hilum and joins the inferior vena cava. It is estimated that, in the average adult, 1200 ml of blood passes through the kidneys every minute. This figure represents about 21% of the cardiac output (5600 ml per minute). The body's total blood supply circulates through the kidneys approximately 12 times per hour (Richard 1986, p. 13).

From this blood, the **nephron** (the functional unit of the kidney—see Figure 43–2) forms a fluid called **glomerular filtrate** (about 180 liters daily, or 25 ml per minute). This volume-time ratio is referred to as the *glomerular filtration rate (GFR)*. The **glomerulus** is a tuft or cluster of blood vessels surrounded by Bowman's capsule. The pores of the glomerulus are large enough for water and some solutes to pass through but are too small for large molecules, such as protein and formed elements in the blood, to filter through. The glomerular filtrate is chemically almost the same as **plasma** but has only minute quantities of protein (0.03%) compared to the amount found in plasma (7%). **Protein-uria** (the presence of protein in the urine) is a sign of glomerular injury. Glomerular filtrate consists of water, electrolytes, creatinine, glucose, urea, amino acids, uric acid, bicarbonate, and other electrolytes.

After the filtrate enters Bowman's capsule, it passes into the tubular system, where about 99% of it is reabsorbed into the bloodstream. The remaining 1% forms the urine to be excreted from the body (Guyton 1986, p. 398). Thus, the function of the nephron is to return the majority of glomerular filtrate to the circulation. The kidneys are therefore the most important organs in regulating body fluid balance.

Ureters

Once the urine is formed in the kidneys, it enters the ureters via collecting ducts and then passes on to the bladder. See Figure 43–1. The ureters are from 25 to 30 cm (10 to

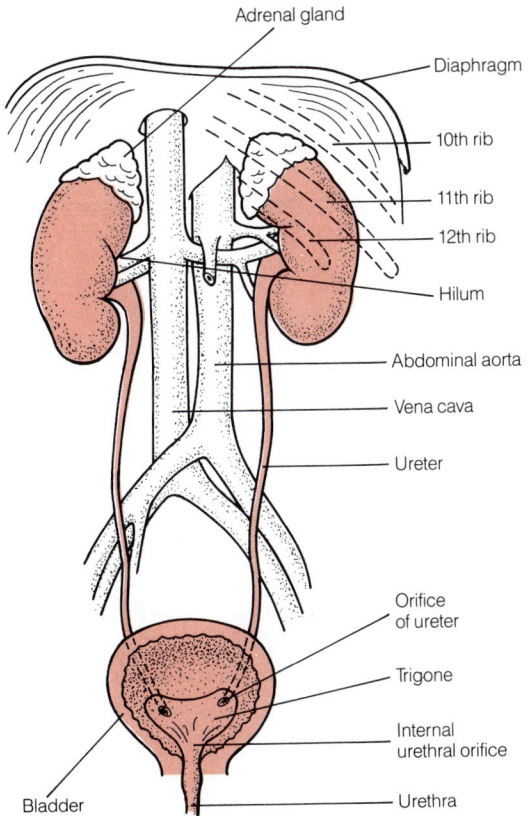

Figure 43–1 Anatomic structures of the urinary tract.

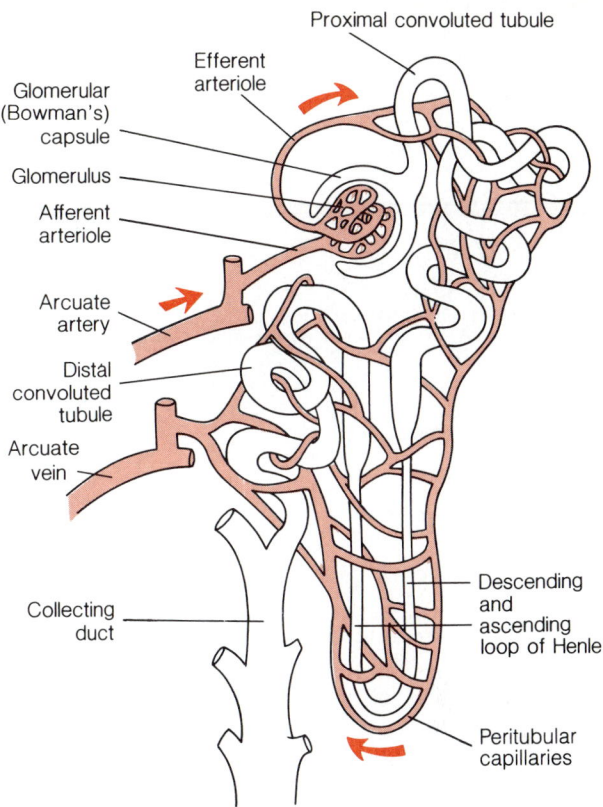

Figure 43–2 The nephrons of the kidney are composed of five parts: Bowman's capsule, proximal convoluted tubule, loop of Henle, distal convoluted tubule, and collecting duct.

12 in) long in the adult and about 1.25 cm (0.5 in) in diameter. The upper end of each ureter is funnel-shaped as it enters the kidney, forming what is referred to as the **renal pelvis**. The lower ends of the ureters enter the bladder at the posterior corners of the floor of the bladder. At this junction between the ureter and the bladder there is a flap-like fold of mucous membrane that acts as a valve to prevent **reflux** (backflow) of urine up the ureters to the kidneys.

Bladder

The urinary bladder is a hollow, muscular organ that serves as a reservoir for urine and as the organ of excretion. When empty, it lies behind the symphysis pubis. In the male, it lies in front of the rectum and above the prostate gland (see Figure 43–3); in the female, it lies in front of the uterus and vagina (see Figure 43–4). The wall of the bladder is made up of four layers: (a) an inner mucous layer that is continuous with that of the ureters and the urethra; (b) a submucous connective tissue layer; (c) a muscular layer consisting of three layers of smooth muscle fibers, some of which extend lengthwise, some obliquely, and some more or less circularly; and (d) an outer serous layer. The smooth muscle layers are collectively called the **detrusor muscle**.

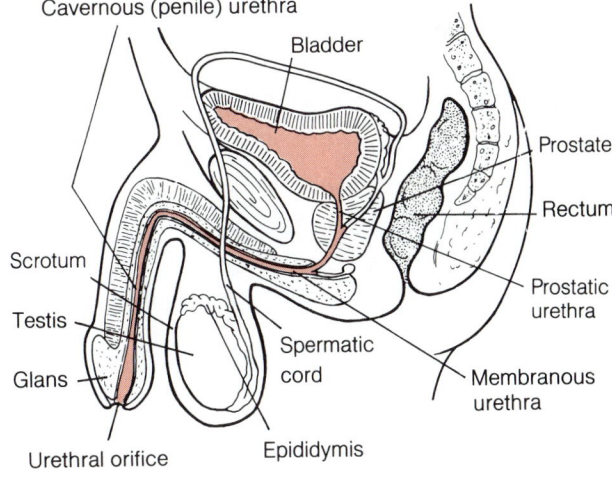

Figure 43–3 The male urogenital system.

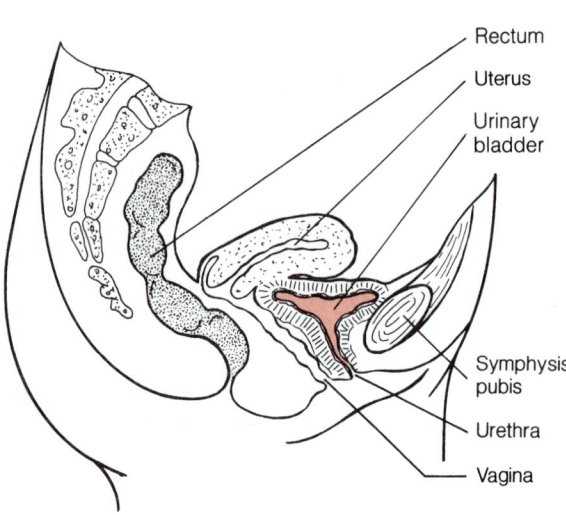

Figure 43-4 The female urogenital system.

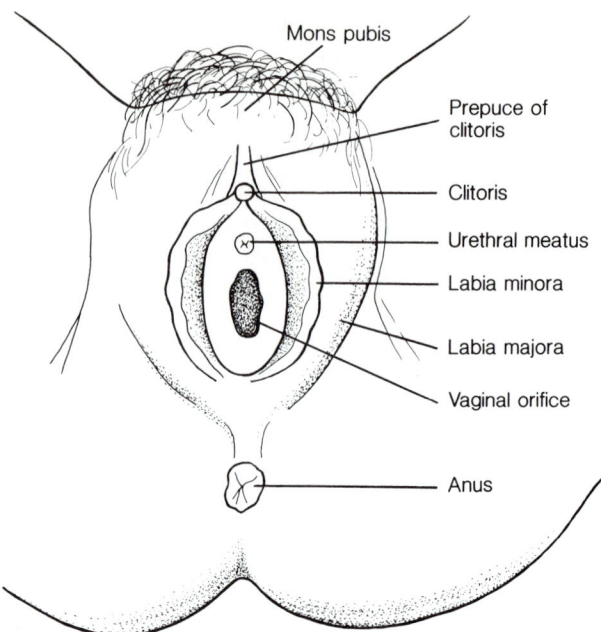

Figure 43–5 Location of the female urinary meatus in relation to surrounding structures.

The base of the bladder, called the **trigone**, is a triangular area marked by the ureter openings at the posterior corners forming the base and the opening of the urethra at the anterior inferior corner forming the apex. Urine exits from the bladder through the urethra.

The amount of urine normally stored in the bladder varies to some degree among individuals and with age. For an adult, the desire to void is normally experienced when the bladder contains between 250 and 450 ml of urine. Normal output of urine for an adult is about 1500 ml/day.

The bladder is capable of considerable distention because of *rugae* (folds) in the mucous membrane lining and because of the elasticity of its walls. When full, the dome of the bladder may extend above the symphysis pubis; in extreme situations it may extend as high as the umbilicus.

Urethra

The urethra extends from the bladder to the urinary **meatus** (opening, or passage) and is the exit passageway for the urine. It is lined with mucous membrane. In the adult male, the urethra—which functions as a passageway for reproductive fluid (semen) as well as urine—(see Figure 43–3).

In the adult female, the urethra lies directly behind the symphysis pubis, anterior to the vagina, and is about 3.7 cm (1.5 inches) in length. See Figure 43–4. It serves only as a passageway for the elimination of urine. The urinary meatus is located between the labia minora, in front of the vagina and below the clitoris (see Figure 43–5); in the male, it is located at the distal end of the penis.

In both the male and the female, the urethra has two **sphincter** muscles. The internal sphincter muscle is situated at the base of the urinary bladder and is involuntary. The second sphincter muscle is under voluntary control. In

the female it is situated at about the midpoint of the urethra; in the male it is distal to the prostatic portion of the urethra.

In both males and females, the urethra has a mucous membrane lining that is continuous with the bladder and the ureters. Thus, an infection of the urethra can readily extend through the urinary tract to the kidneys. Women are particularly prone to urinary tract infections because of the shortness of their urethras.

Urination

Micturition, voiding, and urination all refer to the process of emptying the urinary bladder. Urine collects in the bladder until pressure stimulates special sensory nerve endings in the bladder wall called *stretch receptors*. This occurs when the adult bladder contains between 250 and 450 ml of urine. In children, a considerably smaller volume, 50 to 200 ml, stimulates these nerves.

Once excited, the stretch receptors transmit impulses to the spinal cord, specifically to the voiding reflex center located at the level of the second to fourth sacral vertebrae. Some impulses continue up the spinal cord to the voiding control center in the cerebral cortex. If the time is appropriate to void, the brain then sends impulses through the spinal cord to the motor neurons in the sacral area, causing stimulation of the parasympathetic nerves. As a result, urine can be released from the bladder, but it is still impeded by the external urinary sphincter. If the time and place are appropriate for urination, the conscious portion of the brain relaxes the external urethral sphincter muscle, and urination takes place. If the time and place are inappropriate, the micturition reflex usually subsides until the bladder becomes more filled and the reflex is stimulated again. The sympathetic nervous system also innervates the bladder, causing it to relax.

Voluntary control of urination is possible only if the nerves supplying the bladder and urethra, the neural tracts of the cord and brain, and the motor area of the cerebrum are all intact. The individual must be able to sense that the bladder is full. Injury to any of these parts of the nervous system— by, for example, a cerebral hemorrhage or spinal cord injury above the level of the sacral region— results in intermittent involuntary emptying of the bladder. Elderly people whose cognition is impaired may not be aware of bladder fullness. Involuntary micturition is called **incontinence.** When there is damage to the spinal cord above the sacral vertebrae, the micturition reflex may remain intact and urination may occur reflexively. This situation is referred to as an *automatic bladder*.

Occasionally a person is unable to void even though the bladder contains an excessive amount of urine. This con-dition is known as **retention.** Catheterization (introduction of a tube—known as a **catheter**—through the urethra into the bladder to remove urine) relieves the discomfort that accompanies retention. A more serious complication, which is also characterized by the inability to void, is called **suppression.** In this situation the person cannot void because the kidneys are not secreting any urine; the bladder is empty.

FACTORS AFFECTING VOIDING

Numerous factors affect the volume of urine formed and the process of voiding.

Growth and Development

Voiding changes throughout the life cycle. See Table 43–1.

TABLE 43–1   *Changes in Urinary Elimination Through the Life Cycle*

Stage	Variations
Fetus	The fetal kidney begins to excrete urine between the 11th and 12th week of development.
	Fetal urine is hypotonic to plasma
	The placenta serves as a pseudo-kidney in regulating fetal fluid and electrolyte balance.
	The kidney does not function independently until after birth.
Infant	Ability to concentrate urine is minimal; therefore, urine appears light yellow.
	Voluntary urinary control is absent.
Children	Kidney function reaches maturity between the first and second year of life; urine is concentrated effectively and appears a normal amber color.
	Voluntary control of urine begins at 18 to 24 months of age, when the child starts to recognize bladder fullness, holds urine beyond the urge to void, and warns parents of the urge to void.
	Full urinary control is not gained until age 4 or 5 years; daytime control is usually achieved by age 2 years.
	Boys are slower than girls in gaining control.
	The kidneys grow in proportion to overall body growth.
Adults	The kidneys reach maximum size between 35 and 40 years of age.
	After age 50 the kidneys begin to diminish in size and function. Most shrinkage occurs in the cortex of the kidney, due primarily to the loss of glomeruli.
Elderly adults	There is an estimated 30% loss of glomeruli by age 80 (Richard 1986, p. 38).
	Renal blood flow decreases because of vascular changes and a decrease in cardiac output.
	Urine concentratability declines.
	Excessive urination at night and increased frequency of urination occur because of loss of concentratability and diminished bladder muscle tone.
	Residual urine may increase due to diminished bladder muscle tone and contractability, which increases the risk of bacterial growth and infection.
	Urinary incontinence may occur due to mobility problems or neurologic impairments.

Psychosocial Factors

Certain psychosocial factors may be associated with retention. Many people have developed a set of behaviors that help stimulate the micturition reflex. Examples are privacy, normal position, sufficient time, and, occasionally, running water. North Americans, in contrast to many Europeans, expect private toilet facilities; many Europeans more readily accept communal toilet facilities. The need for privacy also differs between the sexes. Women are used to enclosed cubicles in public facilities; men are used to sharing more open facilities. Circumstances that counter the client's usual set of behaviors may produce anxiety and muscle tension. In persons who are unable to relax abdominal and perineal muscles and the external urethral sphincter, voiding may be incomplete and result in urinary retention.

Fluid and Food Intake

The healthy body maintains a sensitive balance between the amount of fluid ingested and the amount of fluid eliminated. When the amount of fluid intake increases, therefore, the output normally increases. Certain fluids, such as alcohol, increase fluid output by inhibiting the production of antidiuretic hormone. Fluids that contain caffeine, e.g., coffee, tea, and cola drinks, also increase urine production. Foods that are high in fluid content, e.g., iceberg lettuce, milk, and cooked cereal, also increase fluid output. By contrast, food and fluids high in sodium can cause fluid retention.

Some foods and fluids can change the color of urine. For example, beets and blackberries can cause urine to appear red; foods containing carotene can cause the urine to appear yellower than usual.

Medications

Many medications interfere with the normal urination process and may cause retention:

- Anticholinergic-antispasmodic medications, such as atropine, belladonna, Donnatal, papaverine.
- Antidepressant-antipsychotic agents, such as phenothiazines and MAO inhibitors.
- Antiparkinsonism drugs, such as levodopa, trihexyphenidyl (Artane), and benztropine mesylate (Cogentin).
- Antihistamine preparations, such as Actifed and Sudafed.
- Beta-adrenergic blockers, such as a propranolol hydrochloride (Inderal).
- Antihypertensives, such as hydralazine hydrochloride (Apresoline) and methyldopa (Aldomet).

Diuretics (e.g., chlorothiazide, furosemide, and ethacrynic acid) increase urine formation by preventing the reabsorption of water and electrolytes from the tubules of the kidney into the blood stream. Diuretics are commonly taken for hypertension and cardiac disease.

Muscle Tone and Activity

People who exercise regularly will likely have good muscle tone, increased body metabolism, and good urine production. Poor muscle tone can lead to impaired bladder muscle contraction and poor control of the external urethral sphincter and thus poor urination control. The presence of an indwelling catheter can also lead to poor bladder muscle tone; the bladder does not fill and stretch, and the external sphincter does not completely close. When the catheter is removed, therefore, the client may have difficulty in regaining urinary control.

Pathologic Conditions

Specific pathologic conditions affect the formation and/or excretion of urine. Endocrine disorders such as diabetes insipidus increase urine formation. Diseases that impair blood flow to the kidneys, e.g., atherosclerosis, can decrease urine formation. Diseases of the kidneys themselves can reduce kidney function and perhaps eventually result in renal failure.

Any process that impairs the flow of the urine from the kidneys to the urethra can impair urine excretion. Hypertrophy of the prostate gland, which commonly occurs in older men, can interfere with the ability to empty the bladder. Febrile conditions can interfere with urine formation: Because the body loses excessive fluid through perspiration, less urine is formed in the kidneys to maintain the fluid and electrolyte balance. The urine formed under such circumstances is normally highly concentrated so that the waste products of metabolism are still excreted.

Surgical and Diagnostic Procedures

Some surgical and diagnostic procedures can affect the passage of urine and the urine itself. The urethra may swell following a cystoscopy, and surgical procedures on any part of the urinary tract may result in some postoperative bleeding; as a result, the urine may be red- or pink-tinged for a time.

Spinal anesthetics can also affect the passage of urine, because they decrease the client's awareness of the need to void. Other anesthetic agents can decrease blood pressure and glomerular filtration, thereby decreasing urine formation. Surgery on structures adjacent to the urinary tract (e.g., the uterus) can also affect voiding because of swelling in the lower abdomen and often necessitates the use of a retention catheter for a short time.

ALTERED URINE PRODUCTION

Although people's patterns of urination are highly individual, most people void about five or more time a day. People usually void when they first awaken in the morning, before they go to bed, and around mealtimes. Most people void about 70% of their daily urine during the waking hours and do not need to void during the night.

Polyuria

Polyuria, or **diuresis,** refers to the production of abnormally large amounts of urine by the kidneys, such as 2500 ml/day. Polyuria can be the result of (a) excessive fluid intake, (b) the ingestion of substances containing caffeine and alcohol, (c) diabetes mellitus, (d) hormone imbalances (e.g., deficiency of antidiuretic hormone, or ADH), or (e) chronic kidney disease. Other signs often associated with diuresis are **polydipsia** (intense thirst), dehydration, and weight loss.

Oliguria and Anuria

Oliguria refers to voiding scant amounts of urine, such as 100 to 500 ml/day. **Anuria** refers to voiding less than 100 ml/day. The terms *complete kidney shutdown, renal failure,* and *urinary suppression* have the same meaning. Oliguria may result from an extremely low fluid intake but may also follow disease. Both anuria and oliguria can result from kidney disease, severe heart failure, burns, and shock. These clinical signs can be fatal if some other means—such as an artificial kidney—is not used to remove body wastes. Oliguria may also normally accompany fever and heavy perspiration. Because of excessive fluid losses via the skin, urine production is decreased.

ALTERED URINARY ELIMINATION

Frequency and Nocturia

Frequency is generally considered voiding at frequent intervals, that is, more often than usual. Normally with an increased intake of fluid there is some increase in the frequency with which a person voids. Frequency without an increase in fluid intake may be the result of **cystitis** (an acutely inflamed bladder), stress, or pressure on the bladder (because of pregnancy, for example).

With frequency, the total amount of urine voided may be normal, since the amounts voided each time are small, such as 50 to 100 ml.

Nocturia, or *nycturia,* is increased frequency at night that is not a result of an increase in fluid intake. Like frequency, it is usually expressed in terms of the number of times the person gets out of bed to void, for example, "nocturia × 4."

Urgency

Urgency is the feeling that the person *must* void. There may or may not be a great deal of urine in the bladder, but the person feels a need to avoid immediately. Often the person hurries to the toilet with the fear of being incontinent. Urgency accompanies psychologic stress and irritation of the trigone and urethra. It is also common in young children who have poor external sphincter control.

Dysuria

Dysuria means voiding that is either painful or difficult. It can accompany a **stricture** (decrease in caliber) of the urethra, urinary infections, and injury to the bladder and/or urethra. Often clients will say they have to push to void or that burning accompanies or follows voiding. Burning during micturition is often due to an irritated urethra; burning following urination may be the result of a bladder infection when the irritated rugae (ridges) of the trigone rub together. The burning may be described as severe, like a hot poker, or more subdued, like a sunburn. Often, **hesitancy** (a delay and difficulty in initiating voiding) is associated.

Enuresis

Enuresis is defined as repeated involuntary urination in children beyond the age when voluntary bladder control is normally acquired, usually 4 or 5 years of age (Whaley and Wong 1989, p. 489).

Enuresis can also be described as *primary,* meaning there has never been a long, dry, symptom-free period, or *secondary (acquired),* meaning the enuresis occurs after a dry period of at least a year. It is also described as *nocturnal* (nighttime), *diurnal* (daytime), or both. The incidence is approximately 5% to 17% in otherwise normal children between 3 and 15 years of age, with a male predominance (Whaley and Wong 1978, p. 489). Diurnal enuresis without nocturnal enuresis is unusual. There are many reasons for enuresis; several causes or contributing factors may exist in each individual situation.

Urinary Incontinence

Incontinence is a symptom, not a disease. Figures range from 10% to 47% (Turner and Plymat 1988, p. 133). There are different types of incontinence, e.g., total, stress, urge, functional, and reflex incontinence.

Total incontinence is a continuous and unpredictable loss of urine. Common causes are injury to the external urinary sphincter in the male, injury to the perineal musculature or a fistula between the bladder and vagina in the female, and congenital or acquired neurogenic disease.

Stress incontinence is the leakage of less than 50 ml of urine as a result of a sudden increase in intra-abdominal pressure, e.g., when one coughs, sneezes, laughs, or otherwise exerts oneself physically. This type of incontinence occurs most frequently in females who suffer pelvic relaxation due to childbirth trauma, loss of tissue tone, or aging.

Urge incontinence follows a sudden strong desire to urinate and is due to involuntary detrusor contraction. It is also sometimes referred to as *unstable bladder,* because the detrusor contractions are unreliable and bladder emptying cannot be controlled. The client is unable to stop urine flow when it starts and often fails to get to the bathroom in time. This is the most common type of incontinence found in the elderly: It occurs in 40% to 70% of elderly people who are incontinent (Orzeck and Ouslander 1987, p. 21). Loss of urine occurs at any time—not just as a result of straining— a characteristic that distinguishes urge from stress incontinence. Urge incontinence occurs in women with cystitis and in both men and women with other bladder diseases, such as neurologic pathology, calculi, and tumors. Inhibitory impulses that normally calm the bladder may be too weak, or some other imbalance of voiding reflexes due to central nervous system pathology, such as cerebral arteriosclerosis, may exist. The individual is unable to suppress the urge to void.

Functional incontinence is the involuntary, unpredictable passage of urine. It can exacerbate other types of incontinence, although it is generally not caused by genitourinary pathology (Orzeck and Ouslander 1987, p. 23). Functional incontinence is also defined as incontinence that persists because of a physical or mental disorder or some environmental factor that prevents the client from reaching the bathroom.

Reflex incontinence is an involuntary loss of urine occurring at somewhat predictable intervals when a specific bladder volume is reached. The client has no awareness of bladder filling.

Urinary retention with overflow is a dribbling incontinence that results when the bladder is greatly distended with urine because of an obstruction, e.g., an enlarged prostate gland. The client voids small amounts of urine frequently, or dribbles urine, while the bladder remains distended. The term **neurogenic bladder** describes any voiding problem relating to neurologic impairment or dysfunction. A flaccid type of neurogenic bladder occurs following spinal injury or other pathology at the sacral level (below T_{12}). The client is unaware of bladder filling; the bladder walls become overstretched and atonic. Urine "overflows" or dribbles when the pressure increases in the bladder to a point where it surpasses the urethral sphincter's resistance to urine. This is also called reflex incontinence.

RESEARCH NOTE

Does Incontinence Affect Your Client's Self-Concept?

A study was conducted using a sample of 43 females over the age of 60 who lived in a community setting. It aimed to (a) identify urinary incontinence, (b) identify hidden urinary incontinence, and (c) identify the self-concept of these elderly females.

The hypothesis that a negative self-esteem would result in hiding the symptoms of being incontinent was not supported: There were no statistical differences between the self-esteem scores in the continent and incontinent groups. The hypothesis that individuals tend to hide incontinence, however, *was* supported: 11 subjects (50%) identified as being incontinent did not reveal the symptom to a health care provider. The study also revealed that elderly women perceive urinary incontinence as an inevitable consequence of aging. It was found, in addition, that physicians lack interest in the problem.

Implications: Elderly women need to be informed that incontinence is not normal.

J. Simons, Does incontinence affect your client's self-concept? *Journal of Gerontological Nursing,* June 1985, 11:37–40, 42.

Retention   Urinary retention is the accumulation of urine in the bladder with associated inability of the bladder to empty itself. Because urine production continues, retention distends the bladder. An adult urinary bladder normally holds 250 to 450 ml of urine when the micturition reflex is triggered. With urinary retention, some adult bladders may distend to hold 3000 ml of urine. Prolonged retention leads to **stasis** (a slowing of the flow of urine) and stagnation of urine, which increase the possibility of urinary tract infection. According to Lapides, Diokno, Silber, and Lowe (1972, p. 460), the most common cause of increased susceptibility to bacterial invasion is decreased blood flow to the tissues. Distention causes reduced blood flow to the bladder, making it less resistant to invading gram-negative organisms. This reduced blood flow, rather than residual urine or organisms supposedly ascending through the urethra, is considered the major causative factor of urinary tract infections.

Clinical signs of retention are summarized in the box on the opposite page. Retention is distinguished from oliguria or anuria by the bladder distention. Bladder distention can be assessed by palpation and percussion above the symphysis pubis. Percussion of the suprapubic area produces a "kettle-drum" or dull sound when the bladder is full. The most common type of retention is post-operative retention.

Postpartum retention is commonly due to swelling around the urinary meatus that results from perineal trauma associated with vaginal delivery. It is also caused by conditions that contribute to spasm of the perineal musculature. Many medications interfere with the normal urination process and may cause retention. Examples are listed in the box in the right-hand column.

Certain psychosocial factors may be associated with retention. Many people have developed a set of behaviors that help stimulate the micturition reflex; these are discussed earlier.

URINARY DIVERSIONS

A urinary diversion is the surgical rerouting of the urine formed in the kidneys to a site other than the bladder. These operations are often necessary when the urine flow is obstructed by, for example, a malignancy of the bladder. A *stoma* is an artificial opening in the abdominal wall through which waste products such as urine can be excreted. There are four main types of urinary diversions: cutaneous ureterostomy, ileal conduit, continent vesicostomy, and ureterosigmoidostomy or ureteroileosigmoidostomy.

Permanent urinary diversions are indicated for any condition that requires a total cystectomy, e.g., cancer of the bladder. Temporary urinary diversion stomas are indicated for any condition requiring partial cystectomy, trauma to the lower urinary tract, or severe chronic urinary tract infections.

Cutaneous Ureterostomy

In cutaneous **ureterostomy**, the ureters are diverted to the abdominal wall or flank, and a ureteral stoma is formed. Ureterostomies are small compared to colostomies (about 0.5 mm, or 1/4 in, in diameter) and drain continuously. They may involve the right or left ureter (*unilateral ureterostomy,* Figure 43–6, *A*) or both ureters (*bilateral ureterostomy,* Figure 43–6, *B*), in which case each one is covered by a separate appliance, unless they are placed close to each other.

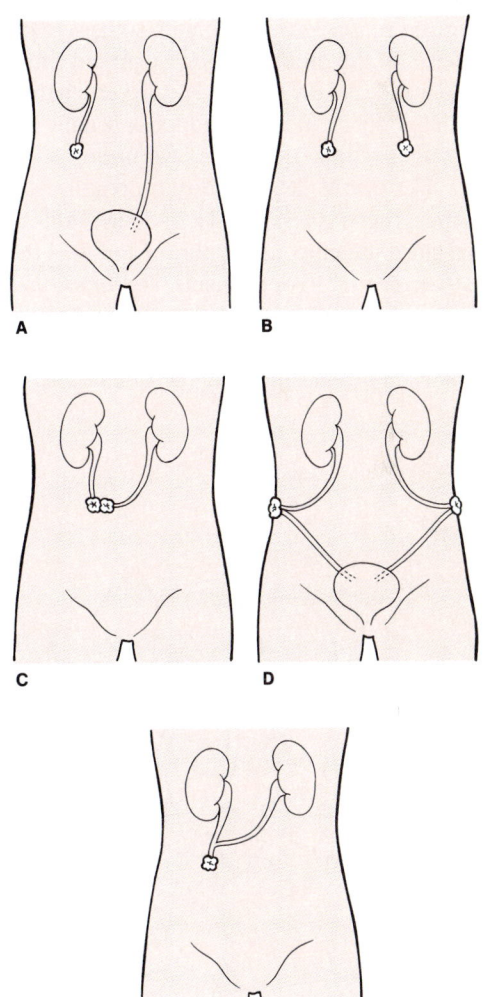

Figure 43–6 Five types of ureterostomies: *A,* right unilateral ureterostomy; *B,* bilateral ureterostomy; *C,* double-barreled ureterostomy; *D,* flank loop ureterostomy; *E,* transureteroureterostomy.

Variations of the bilateral ureterostomy include

1. The *double-barreled ureterostomy,* in which both ureters are brought to the skin surface to form side-by-side stomas. See Figure 43–6, *C.*

2. The *loop ureterostomy,* in which the ureters are looped out to the skin surface of each flank to form the stomas. See Figure 43–6, *D.*

3. The *transureteroureterostomy,* in which one ureter is first connected to the other, and then the receiving ureter is brought to the skin surface to form a stoma. See Figure 43–6, *E.*

Ileal Conduit

The ileal (ileo) conduit is also referred to as *ileal (ileo) loop, ileal (ileo) bladder, ureteroileostomy,* or *Bricker's loop.* See Figure 43–7. In this procedure, a segment of the ileum is removed and the intestinal ends are reattached. One end of the portion removed is closed with sutures to create an ileal pouch, and the other end is brought out through the abdominal wall to create a stoma. The ureters are implanted into the ileal pouch, and the bladder is usually removed. The advantages of this procedure over ureterostomies are that the ileal stoma is larger and more readily fitted with an appliance; there is less chance of an ascending kidney infection, since the mucous membrane lining of the ileum acts as a barrier to microorganisms; and the stoma is less likely to stenose, a major problem with ureterostomy stomas. For these reasons, the ileal conduit is one of the most commonly used urinary diversion procedures.

Continent Vesicostomy (Kock Pouch)

In vesicostomy, the anterior wall of the bladder is sutured to the abdominal wall, and a stoma is formed from the bladder wall. The urethral neck is sutured closed so that urine from the bladder empties directly through the stoma. To provide urinary control, a *continent vesicostomy* is usually performed. See Figure 43–8. In this procedure, a tube is formed from part of the bladder wall. A stoma is formed at one end of the tube. A nipplelike valve is created from the bladder wall at the internal end. Urine drains through this type of vesicostomy only after a catheter is inserted through the stoma into the bladder pouch.

Ureterosigmoidostomy

Ureterosigmoidostomy and ureteroileosigmoidostomy are two urinary diversion procedures that result in the excretion of urine through the rectum. In ureterosigmoidostomy, the more common procedure, the ureters are implanted into the sigmoid colon. See Figure 43–9, *A.* One major complication with this type of procedure is pyelonephritis (infection of the kidney pelvis) from reflux of fecal material and intestinal microorganisms into the ureters and kidney pelvis. In ureteroileosigmoidostomy, a segment of the ileum is reseated and connected to the sigmoid colon. The ureters are then implanted into this ileal pouch. See Figure 43–9, *B.* This procedure is thought to reduce the incidence of pyelonephritis. In both of these procedures, urine mixes with fecal material, resulting in very liquid stools and possible anal leakage of urine.

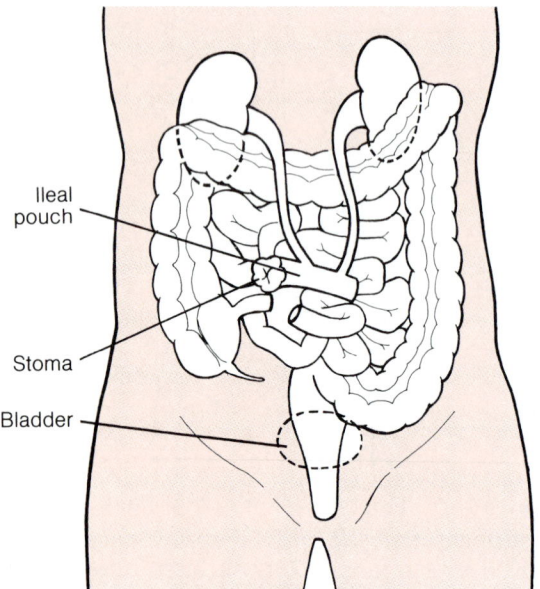

Figure 43–7   An ileal conduit.

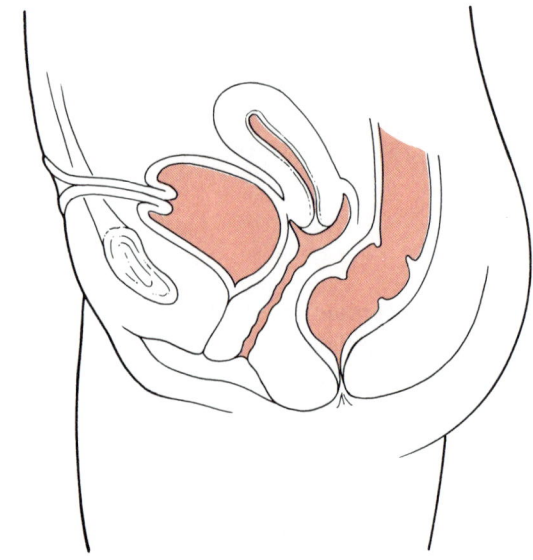

Figure 43–8   A continent vesicostomy (Kock pouch).

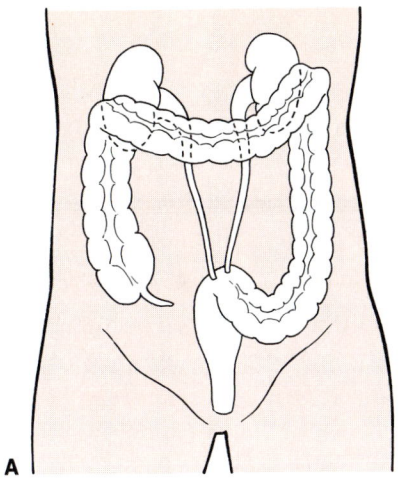
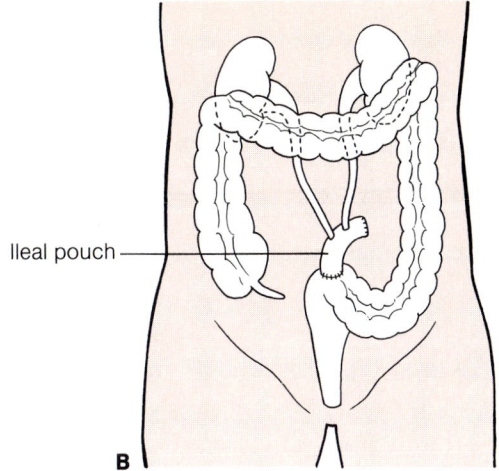

Figure 43–9 *A,* Ureterosigmoidostomy; *B,* Ureteroileosigmoidostomy.

Clients with urinary diversions usually are required to wear an external pouch to collect the urine. An exception is the person with a Kock pouch, who needs a small dressing over the stoma to protect the clothing from mucous drainage. The external appliances are made of either soft rubber or plastic and may be reusable or disposable. The appliance must be emptied several times a day before it becomes too heavy. Clients with urinary diversions may experience problems with their body image and may require assistance in coping with these changes and managing the stoma. People are usually able to resume their normal activities and life-style.

ASSESSING

Assessment of urinary elimination includes taking a nursing history; physical assessment of the kidneys, urinary bladder, urethral meatus, and skin; and measurement, inspection, and testing of the urine. The nurse also reviews any data from relevant diagnostic studies. Guidelines for assessment are summarized in the accompanying box.

In addition to assessing conditions that affect urinary function directly, the nurse needs to consider problems the client may have with mobility. Diseases such as rheumatoid arthritis or other degenerative musculoskeletal or neurologic disorders that impair the client's mobility may result in functional incontinence. Clients who have impaired hand coordination may have difficulty manipulating clothing fasteners. Assessment of these related conditions permits the nurse to identify relevant nursing diagnoses.

The client's medical history of elimination problems and urinary tract disease or surgery and other diseases may affect urinary elimination problems. Some of these conditions are:

1. Urinary tract infections of the kidney, bladder, or urethra
2. Urinary calculi
3. Urinary tract surgery, such as kidney surgery, bladder surgery, prostate removal, or other surgical procedures that alter urinary routes, e.g., ureterostomy
4. Cardiovascular disease such as hypertension or heart disease
5. Chronic diseases that alter urinary characteristics or impair urinary function, such as diabetes mellitus, neurologic disease (e.g., multiple sclerosis), and cancer.

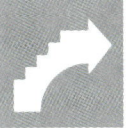

CLINICAL GUIDELINES
Assessing Urinary Elimination

Complete assessment includes:

- Developmental variables (see section earlier in this chapter)
- Usual patterns of urination
- Identification of any alterations in urinary elimination and influencing or associated factors
- Physical assessment (see the section to follow)
- Volume and characteristics of the client's urine
- Review of data obtained from diagnostic tests and examinations
- Past illnesses or surgery

Voiding Pattern

- How many times do you void during a 24-hour period?
- Has this pattern changed recently?
- Do you need to get out of bed to void at night? How often?

Description of Urine and Any Changes

- How would you describe your urine in terms of color, clarity (clear, transparent, or cloudy), and odor (faint or strong)?

Urinary Elimination Problems

What problems have you had or do you now have with passing your urine?

- Passage of large amounts of urine?
- Passage of small amounts of urine?
- Voiding at more frequent intervals?
- Trouble getting to the bathroom in time or feeling of urgency to void?
- Painful voiding?
- Difficulty starting urine stream?
- Frequent dribbling of urine or feeling of bladder fullness associated with voiding small amounts of urine?
- Reduced force of stream?
- Accidental leakage of urine? If so, when does this occur (e.g., when coughing, laughing, or sneezing; at night; during the day)?
- Past urinary tract illness such as urinary tract infection of the kidney, bladder, or urethra; urinary calculi; urinary tract surgery of kidney, ureters or bladder?

Presence and Management of Urinary Diversion Ostomy

- What is your usual routine with your ostomy?
- What problems, if any, do you have with it?
- How can the nurse help you manage it?

Factors Influencing Urinary Elimination

- *Medications.* Have you taken any medications that could increase urinary output (e.g., diuretic) or cause retention of urine (e.g., anticholinergic-antispasmodic, antidepressant-antipsychotic, anti-parkinsonism drugs, antihistamines, antihypertensives)? Note specific medication and dosage.
- *Fluid intake.* What amount and kind of fluid do you take each day (e.g., 6 glasses of water, 5 cups of coffee, 3 cola drinks with or without caffeine)?
- *Environmental factors.* Do you have any problems with toileting (mobility, dexterity with clothing, toilet seat too low, facility without grab bar)?
- *Presence of long-term catheter.* How do you care for your catheter? Do you have any discomfort with it or other problems? How can the nurse help you manage it?
- *Stress.* Are you experiencing any long-term or short-term stress? If so, what are the stressors? Do you think these affect your urinary pattern?
- *Disease.* Have you had or do you have any illnesses other than urinary tract disease that may affect urinary function, such as hypertension, heart disease, neurologic disease (e.g., multiple sclerosis), cancer, prostatic enlargement, diabetes mellitus, or diabetes insipidus?
- *Diagnostic procedures.* Have you recently had a cystoscopy or spinal anesthetic?

Nursing History

The nurse determines the client's normal voiding pattern and frequency, appearance of the urine and any recent changes, any past or current problems with urination, the presence of an ostomy, and factors influencing the elimination pattern.

Examples of interview questions to elicit this information are shown in the box above. The number of questions asked depends on the individual and the responses to the first three categories. Table 43–2 summarizes influencing and associated factors, related to altered urinary elimination patterns.

Physical Assessment

Complete physical assessment of the urinary tract is usually performed by a physician or nurse practitioner. It includes percussion of the kidneys to detect areas of tenderness and palpation for contour, size, tenderness, and lumps. Palpation and percussion of the bladder are performed also. See Chapter 19, pages 420–422. These aspects of physical

TABLE 43–2 *Selected Factors, Associated with Altered Urinary Elimination Patterns*

Altered Pattern	Selected Influencing and Associated Factors to be Determined	Altered Pattern	Selected Influencing and Associated Factors to be Determined
Polyuria	Increase in fluid intake and ingestion of fluids containing caffeine or alcohol	Dysuria	Presence of known urinary tract inflammation, infection, or injury
	Prescribed diuretic		Presence of other signs that may accompany dysuria, such as hesitancy, hematuria, pyuria, and frequency
	Presence of thirst, dehydration, and weight loss	Enuresis	Family history of enuresis
	Presence of or familial history of diabetes insipidus or kidney disease		Difficult access to toilet facilities
Oliguria, anuria	Decrease in fluid intake		Home stresses
	Signs of dehydration (see Chapter 40)		Strict bladder-training methods
	Presence of known kidney disease or familial history of kidney disease	Incontinence	Presence of known bladder inflammation or other disease
	Signs of renal failure, such as the presence of uremic frost (urea crystals) on the skin, an elevated BUN, and an aromatic odor to the skin; and signs of fluid and electrolyte imbalances (see Chapter 40)		Difficulties in independent toileting (mobility impairment)
			Leakage when coughing, laughing, sneezing
	Presence of febrile condition		Cognitive impairment
Frequency or nocturia	Pregnancy	Retention	Presence of distended bladder on palpation and percussion
	Increase in fluid intake		Associated signs, such as pubic discomfort, restlessness, frequency, and small urine volume
	Presence of known urinary tract inflammation or infection		Low fluid intake
	Any known contributing or initiating causes, such as stress		Recent anesthesia
Urgency	Presence of psychologic stress		Recent perineal surgery
	Presence of known urinary tract inflammation or infection		Presence of perineal swelling
			Medications prescribed
			Lack of privacy or other factors that initiate micturition

assessment are included in the ongoing assessment of the client as well and are routinely performed by the assigned nurse. The urethral meatus of both male and female clients is inspected during examination of the genitals (either during the physical examination or when bathing the client) for swelling, discharge, and inflammation.

Assessment of Urine

Normal urine consists of 96% water and 4% solutes. Organic solutes include urea, ammonia, creatinine, and uric acid. Urea is the chief organic solute. Inorganic solutes include sodium, chloride, potassium, sulfate, magnesium, and phosphorus. Sodium chloride is the most abundant inorganic salt. Assessment of urine involves measuring the volume of urine; comparing the output to the client's intake; inspecting the urine for color, clarity, and odor; testing urine

for specific gravity, glucose, ketone bodies, blood, and pH; and reviewing of data obtained from diagnostic tests. Characteristics of normal and abnormal urine are summarized in Table 43–3 on page 1200.

Urine volume depends on the amount of solutes to be excreted, loss of fluid in perspiration and exhaled air, the cardiac status and renal status of the client, hormonal influences, and the amount of fluid ingested. Normally, the kidneys produce urine continuously at the rate of 60 to 120 ml per hour (720 to 1440 ml per day) in the adult, but the rate may be as high as 2000 ml per day if fluid intake is high. Fluid balance and measurement of all fluid intake and output are discussed in Chapter 40. Urine outputs below 30 ml per hour may indicate kidney malfunction and must be reported. Urine production of more than 2000 ml per day or 55 ml per hr constitutes polyuria. In children, normal values for urine volumes are 300 to 1500 ml per day.

TABLE 43–3 *Characteristics of Normal and Abnormal Urine*

Characteristic	Normal	Abnormal	Possible Causes
Amount in 24 hours (adult)	1200–1500 ml	Under 1200 ml	Decreased fluid intake Kidney failure
		Over 1500 ml	Diabetes Diuretics Increased fluid intake
Color	Straw, amber	Dark amber	Insufficient fluid intake resulting in concentrated urine
	Transparent	Cloudy	Infectious process
		Dark orange	Drugs, e.g., phenazopyridine hydrochloride (Pyridium)
		Red or dark brown	Disease process causing blood in urine
Consistency	Clear liquid	Mucous plugs, viscid, thick	Infectious process
Odor	Faint aromatic	Offensive	Infectious process
Sterility	No microorganisms present	Microorganisms present	Infection of the urinary tract
pH	4.5 to 8	Under 4.5 Over 8	Urinary tract infections Uncontrolled diabetes Starvation Dehydration
Specific gravity	1.010 to 1.025	Under 1.010	Diabetes insipidus Kidney disease Overhydration
		Over 1.025	Diabetes mellitus Underhydration
Glucose	Not present	Present	Diabetes mellitus
Ketone bodies (acetone)	Not present	Present	Diabetic coma Starvation Prolonged vomiting
Blood	Not present	Occult Bright red	Kidney disease Hemorrhage

Normal urine is straw-colored or amber-colored. The latter is most likely early in the morning, when urine is most concentrated. Increased fluid intake throughout the day normally makes the urine less concentrated, and so it becomes paler in color. Abnormal urine colors can occur for a number of reasons. Table 43–4 summarizes some causes of urine discoloration.

Normal, freshly voided urine is clear or transparent. Urine may become cloudy due to the presence of mucus or pus, or because of a high protein concentration (e.g., with kidney disease). Urine that is left to stand for a while normally becomes cloudy. Similarly, normal, freshly voided urine has a characteristically faint aromatic odor but acquires a stronger odor the more concentrated it becomes. Bacterial decomposition may change the odor after urine stands for any length of time. Decomposition produces the characteristic pungent odor of ammonia. Additional odors may be due to a variety of causes (Byrne et al. 1986, p. 9), such as:

1. *A sweet or fruity smell.* Due to acetone and acetoacetic acid, which is associated with starvation, diabetes mellitus, or dehydration.

2. *An offensive odor.* Due to bacterial action on pus in heavily infected urine (**pyuria**).

3. *Certain ingested foods.* E.g., garlic or asparagus produce characteristic odors.

4. *Certain medications.* E.g., menthol, antibiotics, paraldehyde, and vitamins give characteristic odors.

Several simple urine tests are often done by nurses on the nursing units or are taught to clients, who perform them independently. Tests commonly performed on urine include

TABLE 43–4 *Selected Causes of Urine Discoloration*

Color	Cause	Color	Cause
Almost colorless (very pale greenish yellow)	Alcohol ingestion Chronic kidney disease Diabetes insipidus Diabetes mellitus Diuretic therapy Large fluid intake Nervousness Severe iron deficiency	Green or blue-green (often blue mixed with yellow urine)	Porphyrin Rifampin (Rifadin) Amitriptyline (Elavil hydrochloride) Azuresin (Diagnex Blue) Bilirubin-biliverdin Methocarbamol (Robaxin) Phenylsalicylate Vitamin B complex Yeast concentrate
Yellow	Acriflavine Cascara Nitrofurantoin (Furadantin) Phenacetin Quinacrine hydrochloride (Atabrine) Riboflavin (vitamin B_2)	Pale blue	Pyrenium
		Brown or black	Bilirubin-biliverdin Cascara (in acid urine) Chloroquine phosphate (Aralen) Furazolidone (Furoxone) Iron compounds (injectable) Levodopa (L-dopa) Melanin Nitrofurantoin Phenol Phenylhydrazine Porphyrin Sinemet
Orange	Azo Gantrisin Bilirubin Concentrated urine Multivitamins Nitrofurantoin Phenazopyridine hydrochloride (Pyridium) Restricted fluid intake Rhubarb, senna, santonin, cascara (in acid urine) Sulfonamides Thiamine hydrochloride Urobilin in excess	Cloudy	Bacteria Calculi "gravel" Clumps, pus, tissue Fecal contamination Leukocytes Mucin, mucous threads Phosphates, carbonates Prostatic fluid Red blood cells (smoky) X-ray contrast media
Pink, red, or reddish orange	Azo Gantrison Beets Cascara (in alkaline urine) Chlorpromazine hydrochloride (Thorazine) Dorbantyl Doxidan Ex-Lax Hemoglobin Phenothiazine Phenytoin (Dilantin)	Milky	Fat (lipuria, opalescent; chyluria, milky) Pyuria

Source: Adapted from C. J. Byrne, D. F. Saxton, P. K. Pelikan, and P. M. Nugent, *Laboratory tests implications for nursing care,* 2d ed. (Menlo Park, Calif.: Addison-Wesley Publishing Co., 1986), pp. 10–12. Used by permission.

those for specific gravity, pH, and presence of glucose and occult blood. **Specific gravity** is the weight or degree of concentration of a substance compared with that of an equal volume of another, such as distilled water, taken as a standard. The specific gravity of distilled water is 1.00 g/ml (in other words, 1 ml of water weighs 1 g).

The specific gravity of urine can be measured by a urinometer (**hydrometer**), calibrated in units of 0.001. The instrument is placed in a glass cylinder containing the urine.

See Figure 43–10. The scale on the urinometer progresses from 1.000 at the top to 1.060 at the bottom. The specific gravity of urine is normally about 1.010 to 1.025 g/ml. A low specific gravity is often the result of overhydration or a disease that affects the kidneys' ability to concentrate solutes in the urine. A high specific gravity may indicate dehydration or a disease that increases water reabsorption by the kidneys, causing concentrated urine. False positive results are caused by drugs such as dextran and radiopaque mate-

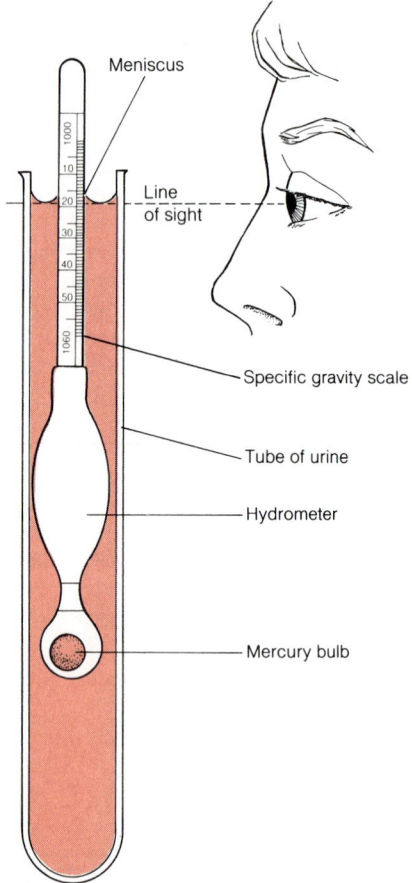

Meniscus

Line of sight

Specific gravity scale

Tube of urine

Hydrometer

Mercury bulb

Figure 43–10 A urinometer measurement of specific gravity is taken at the base of the meniscus.

rials used in x-ray examination of the urinary tract. To measure specific gravity with a urinometer, the nurse can do the following:

1. Pour at least 20 ml of a fresh urine sample in a glass cylinder, or fill the cylinder three-quarters full.

2. Place the urinometer into the cylinder and give it a gentle spin to prevent it from adhering to the sides of the cylinder.

3. Hold the urinometer at eye level, and read the measurement at the base of the meniscus at the surface of the urine. See Figure 43–10.

The concentration of the urine affects the degree to which the urinometer will float. The depth to which it sinks indicates the specific gravity.

Specific gravity can also be measured with a *spectrometer* or *refractometer*. In this instance the nurse places one or two drops of urine on a slide, turns on the instrument light, and looks into the instrument. The specific gravity appears on a scope. Manufacturer's directions are usually available for specific models.

Urinary pH is a measurement of the concentration of

hydrogen ions in the client's urine, which indicates its acidity or alkalinity. Discrete measurements of pH are made on a scale of 1 to 14, in which the value 7 is neutral, below 7 is acid, and above 7 is alkaline (base). Such quantitative measurements, however, are conducted in the agency laboratory, where specific reactive agents are used.

Urine becomes increasingly acidic when increasing amounts of sodium and excess acid are retained in the body. Ingestion of various foods also affects urinary pH. A diet rich in animal protein and cranberry juice decreases the pH and produces an acid urine. A diet high in citrus fruits, most vegetables, milk, and other dairy products increases the pH and produces an alkaline urine. Urine left at room temperature for several hours gradually becomes alkaline because of bacterial action.

Control of the urine pH is an important factor in certain medical therapies. For example, the formation of renal stones is partially dependent on the urinary pH; therefore, clients being treated for stones are often given diets or medications to alter the pH and prevent stone formation. Certain medications, such as streptomycin, neomycin, and kanamycin, are more effective for treating urinary tract infections if the urine is alkaline.

Measurement of pH involves dipping a strip of either red or blue litmus paper into the urine specimen, observing the color of the litmus paper, and comparing it to a standardized color chart on the bottle. The blue litmus paper, more commonly used, remains blue if the urine is alkaline and turns red if it is acidic. The red litmus paper remains red in the presence of acid urine and turns blue if the urine is alkaline. Whichever litmus strip is used, red always indicated acid urine; blue, alkaline urine.

Normal urine is free of blood and has negligible amounts of glucose and acetone. When blood is present, it may be clearly visible or not visible (occult). Commercial reagent strips and tablets are used to test the urine for these substances. The nurse dips the reagent strip into a sample of urine or applies a drop of urine to the tablet and compares the color change with a color chart.

Diagnostic Tests

Diagnostic tests and procedures to determine urinary tract disease or disorders of other body systems influencing the production of urine include laboratory analysis of urine (urinalysis), urine culture, radiographic examinations (KUB and IVP), cystoscopy, and blood tests. A routine screening urinalysis is usually performed on all clients when they are admitted to a health care agency. Routine urine examination is usually done on the first voided specimen in the morning, because it tends to have a higher, more uniform concentration and a more acid pH than specimens later in the day (Byrne et al. 1986, p. 5). In addition to the routine tests discussed previously (i.e., specific gravity, pH, presence of glucose, ketone bodies, and blood), the physical examination of the urine sample provides data about the presence of other abnormal constituents, such as protein, bilirubin, urobilinogen, and nitrite determinations. Microscopic examination provides information on urinary constituents such as red and white blood cells, epithelial cells, casts, crystals, bacteria, parasites, and yeast (Byrne et al. 1986, p. 37).

Urine culture and sensitivity tests are done to identify specific causative microorganisms of urinary tract infections and appropriate antimicrobial agents. The nurse's role in bacteriologic urine culture tests is to obtain a clean-catch specimen, also referred to as a clean voided midstream urine (CVMS). In the past, catheterization was the preferred method for acquiring uncontaminated culture specimens, particularly from females. Today, even though the clean-catch specimen may be somewhat contaminated by skin bacteria, it is considered better to have a contaminated specimen than to risk causing infection of the client's urinary tract by introducing a microorganism through catheterization. If a client has an indwelling catheter, the aspiration method is used.

Radiographic examinations involving the urinary tract include intravenous pyelography (IVP), x-ray films of the kidneys, ureters, and bladder (KUB), and renal scanning. These examinations provide data about the presence of tumors or other obstructions within the organs and distortions in the shapes or densities of the organs. Two **blood tests** commonly conducted to examine renal function are the blood urea nitrogen (BUN) clearance test and the creatinine clearance test. These measure how effectively the kidneys are excreting the respective substances.

Collecting Urine Specimens

The nurse is responsible for collecting urine specimens for a number of tests: clean voided specimens for routine urinalysis, *clean-catch* or *midstream urine specimens* for urine culture, and timed urine specimens for a variety of tests that depend on the client's specific health problem. Clients need varying degrees of instruction and assistance to provide clean voided specimens. Many clients are able to provide the specimen independently. Male clients generally have little difficulty voiding directly into the specimen container, but female clients usually need to stand over a toilet bowl and hold the container between their legs during the process of voiding. About 120 ml (4 oz) of urine is generally required. Clients who are seriously ill, physically incapacitated, or disoriented may need to use a bedpan or urinal in bed; others may require supervision and/or assistance in the bathroom. Whatever the situation, explicit directions are required.

The nurse should explain that all specimens must be free of fecal contamination, so voiding needs to occur at a different time from defecation. Instruct female clients to discard the toilet tissue in the toilet or in a waste bag rather than in the bedpan, since tissue in the specimen makes laboratory analysis more difficult. When the specimen is obtained, put the lid tightly on the container to prevent spillage of the urine and contamination of other objects. If the outside of the container has been contaminated by urine, clean it with a disinfectant. Make sure that the specimen label and the laboratory requisition carry the correct information, and attach them securely to the specimen. Inappropriate identification of the specimen can lead to errors of diagnosis or therapy for the client.

Clean-catch or mid-stream specimens must be as free as possible from external contamination by microorganisms near the urethral opening. Sterile specimen containers and lids are used for those specimens. Procedure 43–1 describes the steps involved in obtaining these specimens.

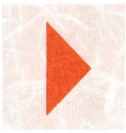

PROCEDURE 43–1

COLLECTING A URINE SPECIMEN FOR CULTURE AND SENSITIVITY BY CLEAN CATCH

Equipment ☑

Equipment used varies from agency to agency. Some agencies use commercially prepared disposable clean-catch kits. See Figure 43–11. Others are agency-prepared sterile trays. Both prepared trays and kits generally contain the following items:

Sterile cotton balls or 2- by 2-inch gauze pads

Antiseptic, such as povidone-iodine

Disposable gloves

Sterile specimen container

Specimen identification label

Completed laboratory requisition form

Bath blanket, if the client is not ambulatory

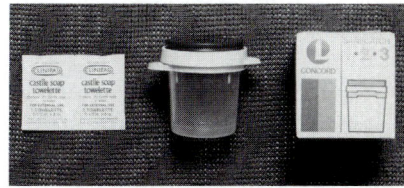

Figure 43–11 A commercially prepared disposable clean-catch kit.

Intervention

1. **Instruct and assist the client appropriately.**

- Inform the client that a urine specimen is required; give the reason, and explain the method to be used to collect it.

- Ask an *ambulatory* client to wash and dry the genitals and perineum thoroughly with soap and water. *A clean perineum is essential to reduce the number of skin bacteria and to minimize contamination of the specimen.*

- Assist the *ambulatory* client to the bathroom. The preferred method to collect specimens from ambulatory clients is to have them provide the specimen while standing over the toilet in the bathroom.

- Assist *nonambulatory* clients to an upright sitting position on a urine receptacle. Provide appropriate covers for the client: Drape the client in a bath blanket, exposing only the perineal area.

- Assist *female* clients to spread their legs enough to ensure that the urine does not touch the legs.

2. **Prepare the equipment, and implement body fluid precautions.**

- Open the sterile kit or tray, using sterile technique. *Sterile technique is essential to maintain the sterility of the specimen container.*

 - Put on the sterile gloves.

- Pour the antiseptic solution over the cotton balls.

3. **Clean the area at the external urinary meatus with the anti-**

septic. *The antiseptic reduces the number of bacteria near the urethral opening and minimizes contamination of the urine specimens.*

For female clients:

- Swab the labia minora from front to back, using one swab for each wipe. *Swabbing from front to back cleans from the area of least contamination to the area of greatest contamination.*

- Spread the labia minora well apart, using the thumb and another finger (e.g., the third finger) of one hand.

- Swab between the labia minora over the urethra from front to back. *The urethra is considered less contaminated than the vagina and anus.*

For male clients:

- Hold the penis with one hand, and clean the urinary meatus using a circular motion. First retract the foreskin of an uncircumcised male.

- Wash outward from the meatus in a circular motion, using one swab for each wipe and moving down the shaft of the penis a few inches. *This cleans from the area of least contamination to the area of greatest contamination.*

4. **Collect the specimen.**

- Ask the client to start voiding. *Initial voiding clears additional external contaminants at the urethral opening.*

- After the client has begun to void, place the specimen container under the stream of urine near to, but not touching, the meatus.

- Collect 30 to 60 ml of midstream urine.

- Handle only the outside of the container. *This protects the sterility of the inside.*

- Put the sterile cap tightly on the specimen container, touching only the outside of the cap. *Capping the container prevents spillage of urine and contamination of other objects. Touching only the outside of the cap retains the sterility of the inside of the cap.*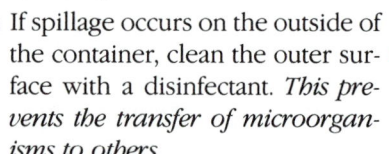

- If spillage occurs on the outside of the container, clean the outer surface with a disinfectant. *This prevents the transfer of microorganisms to others.*

- Remove your gloves, and wash hands.

5. **Label and transport the specimen.**

- Ensure that the specimen label and the laboratory requisition carry the correct information. Attach them securely to the specimen. *Inaccurate identification and/or information on the specimen container can lead to errors of diagnosis or therapy.*

- Arrange for the specimen to be sent to the laboratory immediately. *Bacterial cultures must be started immediately, before any contaminating organisms can grow, multiply, and produce false results.*

6. **Document pertinent data.**

- Record collection of the specimen, any pertinent observations of the urine in terms of color, odor, or consistency, and any difficulty in voiding that the client experienced.

Several urine tests require timed specimens. Urine specimens are collected at timed intervals, for short periods (1 to 2 hours) or long periods (12 to 24 hours). All timed urine specimens should be refrigerated to prevent bacterial growth and decomposition of the urine components, unless a special preservative has been added. Each voiding of urine is collected in a small, clean container and then emptied immediately into the large refrigerated bottle or carton. Some of the tests performed on timed urine specimens include:

1. **Quantitative albumin** (24 hours): Determines the daily amount of albumin lost in the urine in such conditions as kidney disease, hypertension, drug toxicity, or severe heart failure involving kidney damage.

2. **Amino acid** (24 hours): Determines acquired or congenital disease of the kidneys.

3. **Amylase** (2, 12, or 24 hours): Determine the amount of amylase, a pancreatic enzyme that may be excreted in the urine in certain diseases of the pancreas.

4. **Quantitative chlorides** (24 hours): Determines the total excretion of chloride; may be performed in the management of cardiac clients who are on low-salt diets.

5. **Concentration and dilution:** Determines disorders of the kidney tubules in concentrating and diluting urine. These specimens are collected over varying periods of time. Specimens are commonly collected at hourly intervals for 2 to 4 hours after the client has been given a specified amount of clear fluid to drink.

6. **Creatinine** or **creatinine clearance** (24 hours): Reflects the degree of kidney impairment. Creatinine is formed in the muscles from creatine in relatively constant daily amounts and is excreted in the urine. Elevated creatinine content indicates a disturbance in kidney function.

7. **Estriol determination** (24 hours): Measures the level of this hormone in the urine of high-risk pregnant women, e.g., those with toxemia or diabetes. Estriol is the major form in which estrogen is excreted in the urine. Low levels can indicate inadequate function of the placenta and possible fetal distress.

8. **Glucose tolerance** (24 hours): Determines disorders of glucose metabolism that may arise from malfunction of the liver or pancreas. Tests are performed on both the blood and the urine after the client is given a large amount of glucose orally or intravenously.

9. **17-hydroxycorticosteroid** (24 hours): Assesses the functioning of the adrenal cortex. Corticosteroids are hormones that are produced in the adrenal cortex, altered, and then excreted in the urine.

10. **Urobilinogen** (random times or 2 hours): Determines obstruction of the biliary tract, excessive destruction of red blood cells, or liver damage. These specimens need to be protected from light.

Appropriate specimen containers with or without preservative in accordance with the specific test are generally obtained from the laboratory and placed in the client's bathroom or in the utility room. Alert signs are placed in the client's unit to remind staff of the test in progress. Specimen identification labels need to indicate the date and time of each voiding in addition to the usual identification information. They may also be numbered sequentially, e.g., 1st specimen, 2nd specimen, 3rd specimen.

Clients need to be told explicitly why the test is being done and how they can assist. The nurse tells the client when the specimen collection will begin and end; e.g., a 24-hour urine test may begin at 0700 hours and ends at the same hour the next day. Instructions should include the following facts:

1. All urine must be saved and placed in the specimen containers once the test starts.

2. The urine must be free of fecal contamination and toilet tissue.

3. Each specimen must be given to the nursing staff immediately so that it can be placed in the appropriate specimen bottle.

The collection period is started by having the client void in the toilet or bedpan or urinal. This urine is usually discarded, but agency procedure needs to be checked. All subsequent urine specimens are collected, including the one at the end of the period.

The nurse needs to make sure that the client ingests a required amount of liquid for certain tests and instructs the client to void all subsequent urine into the bedpan or urinal and to notify the nursing staff for assistance and after each voiding. Some tests require that the client void at specified times. Each specimen must be placed in the appropriately labeled container. The nurse asks the client to provide the last specimen 5 to 10 minutes before the end of the collection period and informs the client that the test is completed. The starting time of the test and completion of the specimen collection are recorded on the client's chart. In addition, if indicated for the specific test, the time each urine specimen was collected is noted, as are the volume of each specimen, the appearance of the urine, and other relevant data such as fluid intake or restrictions.

DIAGNOSING

Nursing diagnoses that related to urinary elimination problems include **Incontinence, Altered patterns of urinary elimination,** and **Urinary retention.** The North American Nursing Diagnosis Association subcategorizes the diagnosis of **Incontinence** as follows:

- **Functional incontinence**
- **Reflex incontinence**
- **Stress incontinence**
- **Total incontinence**
- **Urge incontinence**

Definitions of these were discussed earlier on page 1193. Other diagnoses, depending on the data obtained, may arise:

- **Potential for infection** if the client has urinary retention or undergoes an invasive procedure such as catheterization or cystoscopic examination.

TABLE 43–5 *Examples of Assessment Data Clusters and Related Nursing Diagnoses*

Data Cluster	Nursing Diagnosis
Mrs. Amy Brown, 75 years old, reports accidental loss of urine before she is able to reach the toilet. She is aware of the urge to void but "because of my stroke I sometimes can't get there soon enough."	**Functional incontinence** related to mobility deficit
Anthony Cherry, a teenage victim of a spinal cord injury, has no awareness of bladder filling, the urge to void, or feelings of bladder fullness. He reports loss of urine at fairly regular intervals.	**Reflex incontinence** related to neurologic impairment (spinal cord lesion)
Tammy Tyndale reports dribbling whenever she laughs, coughs, or sneezes. She is 8 months pregnant.	**Stress incontinence** related to high intra-abdominal pressure associated with pregnancy
Mr. Gino Mingo is wheelchair-bound from the effects of multiple sclerosis. He has a constant flow of urine at unpredictable times, including nocturia. He is unaware of bladder filling and of incontinence.	**Total incontinence** related to neurologic impairment
Mrs. Gail Brady reports urinary urgency, difficulty in getting to the bathroom in time, frequency (more often than every 2 hours), and leakage of urine when unable to reach the toilet in time.	**Urge incontinence** to unknown etiology

- **Self-esteem disturbance** if the client is incontinent. Incontinence can be physically and emotionally distressing to clients because it is considered socially unacceptable. Often the client is embarrassed about dribbling or having an accident and may restrict normal activities for this reason.
- **Potential impaired skin integrity** if the client is incontinent. Bed linens and clothes saturated with urine irritate and excoriate the skin. Prolonged skin dampness leads to dermatitis (inflammation of the skin) and subsequent formation of decubitus ulcers.
- **Social isolation** if the client is incontinent (see also **Self-esteem disturbance**).
- **Self-care deficit: Toileting** if the client has functional incontinence.
- **Potential fluid volume deficit** or **Fluid volume excess** if the client has impaired urinary function associated with a disease process.
- **Body image disturbance** if the client has a urinary diversion ostomy.
- **Knowledge deficit** if the client requires self-care skills to manage, for example, a new urinary diversion ostomy.

These diagnoses with possible contributing factors are shown below. Examples of assessment data clusters and related nursing diagnoses are shown in Table 43–5.

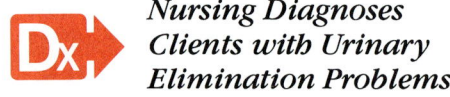

Nursing Diagnoses Clients with Urinary Elimination Problems

Functional incontinence related to:
- Altered environment (e.g., poor lighting or inability to locate toilet, reluctance to use call light or bedpan)
- Sensory or cognitive deficit (e.g., inattentiveness to voiding urge or use of sedation)
- Mobility deficit

Reflex incontinence related to neurologic impairment

Stress incontinence related to:
- Weak pelvic muscles and structural supports associated with age, surgery (cystocele, rectocele), or multiple deliveries
- High intra-abdominal pressure associated with obesity, pregnancy, or other factors

Total incontinence related to:
- Neurologic impairment
- Urinary diversion ostomy

Urge incontinence related to:

- Irritation of bladder stretch receptors, causing spasm (e.g., bladder infection; consumption of alcohol, caffeine, or increased fluids; or overdistention of bladder)
- Decreased bladder capacity (e.g., history of indwelling urinary catheter, surgery, pelvic inflammatory disease)
- Overdistention of bladder

Urinary retention related to:

- Urethral blockage
- Medication

Altered patterns of urinary elimination related to:

- Bladder infection
- Neurogenic disorder or injury
- Renal calculi
- Loss of perineal tissue tone
- Medication therapy (e.g., diuretic)

Potential for infection related to:

- Indwelling urethral catheter
- Urinary retention

Potential for impaired skin integrity related to:

- Incontinence
- Urinary diversion ostomy

PLANNING

The overall goals for clients with potential or actual urinary elimination problems are the maintenance or restoration of the client's normal urinary elimination pattern and the prevention of associated risks such as infection, skin breakdown, fluid and electrolyte imbalance, and lowered self-esteem.

Appropriate nursing interventions and outcome criteria that relate to these broad goals are then identified. Among the strategies the nurse should consider are the following:

- Implementing measures that promote normal urination for hospitalized clients.
- Implementing measures to control urinary incontinence, such as attending to environmental factors; modifying clothing; maintaining regular toileting schedules; teaching the client pelvic floor muscle exercises; establishing external urinary devices; and, as a last resort, inserting an indwelling catheter.
- Keeping the incontinent client's skin clean and dry.

- Encouraging appropriate fluid intake to prevent urinary infections.
- Teaching clients with bladder flaccidity Credé's maneuver (see page 1212).
- Providing special care for clients with urinary diversion ostomies.

Examples of outcome criteria to evaluate the achievement of client goals and the effectiveness of nursing interventions are shown below.

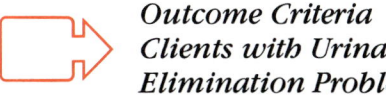

Outcome Criteria
Clients with Urinary
Elimination Problems

The client with **Incontinence:**

- Identifies interventions to prevent incontinence.
- Alters environment and clothing to accommodate needs.
- Attempts voiding every 2 hours and gradually increases to every 3 or 4 hours.
- Experiences a gradual decrease in episodes of incontinence to less than three times a week.
- Has intact skin around the urinary meatus and perineum (or under condom or urinary diversion stoma appliance).
- Establishes bladder conditioning regimen.
- Demonstrates techniques to strengthen pelvic floor muscles.
- Performs pelvic floor strengthening exercises three times a day for 4 months.
- Remains continent even with increased intra-abdominal pressure (stress incontinence).
- Manages incontinence sufficiently to maintain social functioning.
- Reports increased time interval between urge and involuntary loss of urine.
- Manages care of catheter or urinary diversion stoma appropriately.

The client with **Urinary retention:**

- Voids sufficient amounts with no palpable bladder distention.
- Has a postvoid residual urine of less than 50 ml.
- Is free of overflow dribbling.

The client with **Altered pattern of urinary elimination has:**

- Normal color, odor, and consistency of urine.
- A urinary output in balance with fluid intake.
- A negative urine culture.

- No dysuria or frequency.
- Urinary pH of less than 5.5.
- Urinary output of at least 1500 ml/day.
- Fluid intake of at least 2500 ml/day.

IMPLEMENTING

Maintaining Normal Urinary Elimination

Most interventions to maintain normal urinary elimination are independent nursing functions. These include maintaining an adequate fluid intake and promoting normal voiding habits.

Fluid Intake Increasing fluid intake increases urine production, which in turn stimulates the micturition reflex. A normal, average daily intake of 1200 to 1500 ml of measurable fluids is adequate for most clients. Additional amounts are required for clients whose fluid demands are great, e.g., those who have abnormal fluid losses from other routes, such as excessive perspiration, vomiting, or diarrhea.

Immobilized clients who are susceptible to calculi formation require daily intakes of 2000 to 3000 ml per day (unless medically contraindicated). Dilute urine helps prevent urinary tract stones and infection. Increased fluid intakes

are contraindicated in clients who require fluid restrictions, e.g., those with renal impairment or congestive heart failure. Fluid intake can also be increased by encouraging the client to eat plenty of raw fruits and vegetables, which have a high water content.

Voiding Habits Hospital routines and prescribed medical therapies can interfere with a client's normal voiding habits. Assisting clients to use bedpans is discussed in Chapter 42. Some female clients may prefer to use a female urinal. Figure 43–12, *B*, shows a female urinal; Figure 43–12, *A*, shows a male urinal.

Guidelines for helping clients maintain normal voiding habits are summarized in the accompanying Clinical Guidelines box.

Nursing Interventions for Clients with Urinary Incontinence

Independent nursing interventions for clients with urinary incontinence include a bladder-retraining program, meticulous skin care, and, for males, application of an external drainage device (condom). The physician may order urinary catheterization for clients unable to voluntarily control micturition. Nursing interventions for catheterized clients are discussed later in the chapter.

Bladder-Retraining Program A bladder-retraining program requires involvement of the nurse, the client, and support persons. Clients must be alert and physically able to follow a program. The goal of bladder retraining is to restore a normal pattern of voiding by inhibiting or stimulating voiding (Orzeck and Ouslander 1987, p. 20). Guidelines for bladder retraining are summarized in the accompanying box. A routine for voiding helps decrease the number of incontinent episodes.

Strengthening Pelvic Floor Muscles Pelvic floor exercises, referred to as perineal muscle tightening or *Kegel's exercises,* strengthen pubococcygeal muscles and can increase the incontinent female's ability to start and stop the stream of urine. The client can feel the perineal muscle group to be exercised by stopping urination midstream. The following technique is sometimes used to teach Kegel's exercises. Ask the client to think of her perineal muscles as an elevator. When the client relaxes, the elevator is on the first floor. To perform the exercise, contract the perineal muscles, bringing the elevator to the second, third, and fourth floors. Keep the elevator on the fourth floor for a few seconds, and then gradually relax the area. When the exercise is properly performed, contraction of the muscles of the buttocks and thighs is avoided.

Kegel's exercises can be performed anytime, anywhere, sitting or standing—even when voiding. Specific client

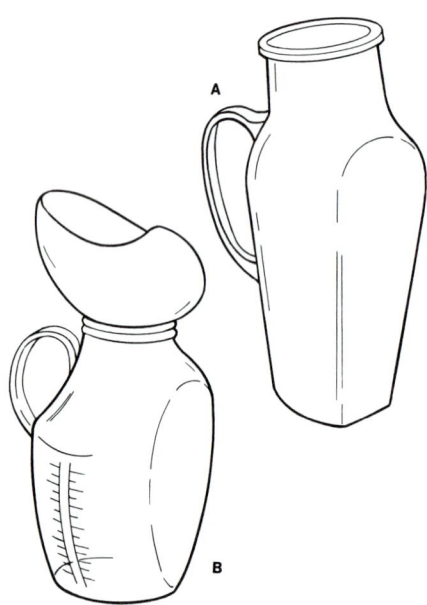

Figure 43–12 Two types of urinals: *A,* male urinal; *B,* female urinal.

CLINICAL GUIDELINES
Maintaining Normal Voiding Habits

Positioning

- Assist the client to a normal position for voiding: standing for males; for females, squatting or sitting. These positions enhance movement of urine through the tract by gravity.
- Use bedside commodes as necessary for females and urinals for males standing at the bedside.
- Encourage the client to push over the pubic area with the hands or to lean forward to increase intra-abdominal pressure and external pressure on the bladder.

Relaxation

- Provide privacy for the client.
- Allow the client sufficient time to void.
- Suggest the client read or listen to music.
- Provide sensory stimuli that may help the client relax. Pour warm water over the perineum of a female or have the client sit in a warm bath to promote muscle relaxation. Applying a hot-water bottle to the lower abdomen of both men and women may also foster muscle relaxation.
- Turn on running water within hearing distance of the client to mask the sound of voiding for persons who find this embarrassing.
- Relieve physical and emotional discomfort to decrease muscle tension and encourage the mental concentration that may be needed for micturition. Make sure to provide ordered analgesics and emotional support.

Timing

- Assist clients who have the urge to void immediately. Delays only increase the difficulty in starting to void, and the desire to void may pass.
- Offer toileting assistance to the client at usual times of voiding, e.g., on awakening, before or after meals, and at bedtime.

For Bed-Confined Clients

- Warm the bed pan. A cold bedpan may prompt contraction of the perineal muscles and inhibit voiding.
- Elevate the head of the client's bed to Fowler's position, place a small pillow or rolled towel at the small of the back to increase physical support and comfort, and have the client flex the hips and knees. This position simulates the normal voiding position as closely as possible.

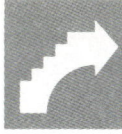

CLINICAL GUIDELINES
Bladder Retraining

- Determine the client's voiding pattern and encourage voiding at those times, or establish a regular voiding schedule and help the client to maintain it, whether the client feels the urge or not (e.g., upon awakening, every 1 or 2 hours during the day and evening, before retiring at night, every 4 hours at night). The stretching-relaxing sequence of such a schedule tends to increase bladder muscle tone and promote more voluntary control.
- When the client finds that voiding can be controlled, the intervals between voiding can be lengthened slightly without loss of continence.
- Regulate fluid intake, particularly before the client retires, to help reduce the need to void during the night.
- Encourage fluids about half an hour before the voiding time between the hours of 0600 and 1800, or allow 2 hours between the last fluid and bedtime. Large amounts of fruit juices and carbonated beverages should be avoided, since fruit juice alkalinizes the urine and soft drinks cause bladder irritation.
- Stimulants (e.g., tea, coffee, and alcoholic beverages) should be avoided at bedtime to decrease the possibility of nocturia.
- Schedule diuretics early in the morning.
- Explain to clients that adequate fluid intake is required to ensure adequate urine production to stimulate the micturition reflex. Clients who have fluid restrictions due to a medical condition may be maintained on 1500 ml per day.
- Apply protector pads to keep the bed linen dry, and provide specially made waterproof underwear to contain the urine and decrease the client's embarrassment. Avoid using diapers, which are demeaning and also suggest that incontinence is permissible.
- Assist the client with an exercise program to increase the tone of abdominal and pelvic muscles.
- Provide a system of positive and negative reinforcements to encourage continence. Such systems are commonly referred to as *behavior modification* and require the cooperation of all persons involved in the client's care.

CLIENT TEACHING
Routine for Kegel's Exercises

- First, sit or stand with the legs apart.
- Pull your rectum, urethra, and vagina up inside, and hold for a count of 5 seconds. The pull should be felt at the cleft of your buttocks.
- Initially perform each contraction 5 or 6 times. As the muscle group becomes stronger, increase the number to 25 or more each time. The goal is to perform 200 exercises daily but not all at once.
- Develop a schedule that will help remind you to do them, e.g., while driving to work or when working at the kitchen sink.
- Try to start and stop your stream of urine.
- To control episodes of stress incontinence, brace the muscles and use the Kegel maneuver when doing any activity that increases intra-abdominal pressure, such as coughing, laughing, sneezing, or lifting.

instructions for performing Kegel's exercises suggested by Kuhns-Hastings (1988, p. 82) are summarized in the box above.

 Maintaining Skin Integrity Skin that is continually moist becomes macerated. Over a period of time urine that accumulates on the skin is converted to ammonia, which is very irritating to the skin. Since both skin irritation and maceration predispose the client to skin breakdown and decubitus ulcers, the incontinent person requires meticulous skin care. To prevent alterations in skin integrity, the nurse washes the client's perineal area with soap and water after periods of incontinence, dries it thoroughly, and provides clean, dry clothing or bed linen. If the skin is irritated,

the nurse applies barrier creams such as zinc oxide ointment to protect it from contact with urine. If it is necessary to pad the client's clothes for protection, the nurse should use products that absorb wetness and leave a dry surface in contact with the skin.

Specially designed *incontinence drawsheets* that provide significant advantages over standard drawsheets for bedridden incontinent clients have been recently introduced in North America and Great Britain (Cefalu 1987; Pottle 1986). These sheets are like a drawsheet but are double layered, with a colored (e.g., yellow or pink) quilted upper nylon or polyester surface and an absorbent viscose rayon layer below. The rayon soaker layer generally has a waterproof backing on its underside. Fluid (i.e., urine) passes through the upper quilted layer and is absorbed and dispersed by the viscose rayon, leaving the quilted surface dry to the touch. This absorbent sheet helps maintain skin integrity; it does not stick to the skin when wet, decreases the risk of bedsores, and reduces odor.

Applying External Urinary Devices The application of a **condom,** also referred to as a *urinary sheath* or *external catheter,* and attachment of its base to a urinary drainage system are commonly prescribed for incontinent males. Use of a condom appliance is preferable to insertion of a retention catheter, because it avoids entrance into the urethra and bladder and minimizes the risk of urethral or bladder infection.

Methods of applying condoms vary according to the length of time the condom is to be worn. Condoms that are to be worn for short periods are generally applied with elastic tape only; if the condom is to be worn for longer periods (e.g., a few days), additional measures are required to protect the foreskin and to ensure secure attachment. The manufacturer's instructions need to be followed when applying a condom. Before applying the condom, the nurse determines when the client experiences incontinence. Some clients may require a condom appliance at night only, others continuously. Procedure 43–2 describes how to apply and remove a drainage condom.

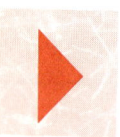

PROCEDURE 43–2

APPLYING AND REMOVING A DRAINAGE CONDOM

Equipment

Condom sheath

Elastic tape or velcro strap

Leg drainage bag with tubing or urinary drainage bag with tubing

Basin of warm water and soap

Washcloth and towel

Bath blanket

Disposable gloves

Intervention

1. Prepare the equipment.

- Assemble the leg drainage bag or urinary drainage bag for attachment to the condom sheath.

- Roll the condom outward onto itself to facilitate easier application. On some models an inner flap will be exposed. *This flap is applied around the urinary meatus to prevent the reflux of urine.* See Figure 43-13.

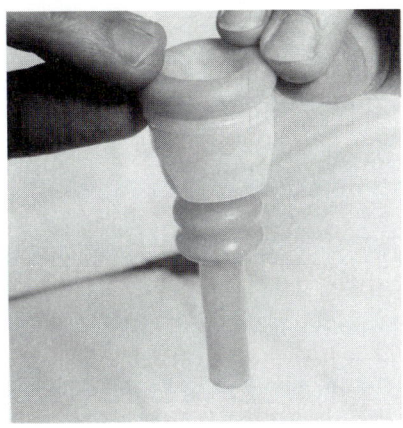

Figure 43-13 Before application, roll the condom outward onto itself.

2. Position and drape the client.

- Position the client in either a supine or a bed-sitting position.

- Drape the client appropriately, exposing only the penis.

3. Inspect and clean the penis.

- Don gloves.

- Inspect the penis for skin irritation (contact dermatitis), excoriation, swelling, or discoloration. *The nurse needs to obtain baseline data.*

- Clean the genital area, and dry it thoroughly. *This minimizes skin irritation and excoriation after the condom is applied.*

4. Apply and secure the condom.

- Roll the condom smoothly over the penis, leaving 2.5 cm (1 in) between the end of the penis and the rubber or plastic connecting tube. See Figure 43-14. *This space prevents irritation of the tip of the penis and provides for full drainage of urine.*

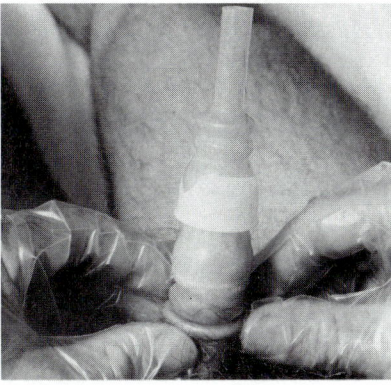

Figure 43-14 Rolling the condom over the penis.

- Secure the condom firmly, but not too tightly, to the penis by wrapping a strip of elastic tape or velcro around the base of the penis over the condom. Ordinary tape is contraindicated because it is not flexible and can stop bloodflow. The elastic or velcro strip should not come in contact with the skin and should hold the condom in place without impeding blood circulation to the penis.

5. Securely attach the urinary drainage system.

- Make sure that the tip of the penis is not touching the condom and that the condom is not twisted. *A twisted condom could obstruct the flow of urine.*

- Attach the urinary drainage system to the condom.

- Remove gloves.

- If the client is to remain in bed, attach the urinary drainage bag to the bed frame.

- If the client is ambulatory, attach the bag to the client's leg. See Fig-

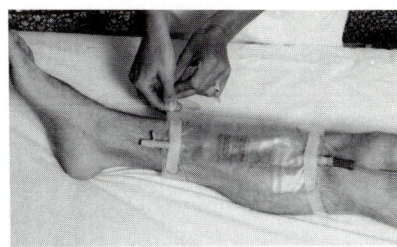

Figure 43-15 Attaching the urinary drainage bag to the leg.

ure 45-15. *Attaching the drainage bag to the leg helps control the movement of the tubing and prevents twisting of the thin material of the condom appliance at the tip of the penis.*

6. Teach the client about the drainage system.

- Instruct the client to keep the drainage bag below the level of the condom and to avoid loops or kinks in the tubing.

7. Document pertinent data.

- Record the application of the condom, the time, and pertinent observations, such as irritated areas on the penis.

8. Inspect the penis 30 minutes following the condom application, and check urine flow.

- Assess the penis for swelling and discoloration, which indicates that the condom is too tight.

- Assess urine flow. Normally, some urine is present in the tube if the flow is not obstructed.

9. Change the condom daily, and provide skin care.

- Remove the elastic or velcro strip, and roll off the condom.

- Wash the penis with soapy water, rinse, and dry it thoroughly.

- Assess the foreskin for signs of irritation, swelling, and discoloration.

Nursing Interventions for Clients with Urinary Retention

Interventions that assist the client to maintain a normal voiding pattern, discussed earlier, are applicable when dealing with urinary retention. If these actions are unsuccessful, the physician may order a cholinergic drug such as bethanecol chloride (Urecholine) to stimulate bladder contraction and facilitate voiding. For clients who have bladder **flaccidity** (weak, soft, and lax bladder muscles), manual exertion of pressure on the bladder may be necessary to force urine out. This is known as **Credé's maneuver** or *method*. It is not advised without a physician's order and is used only for clients who have lost and are not expected to regain voluntary bladder control. For clients who are expected to regain control, this maneuver does not promote increased bladder muscle tone and may cause damage to the urethral sphincters. When all measures fail to initiate voiding, urinary catheterization may be ordered.

Urinary Catheterization

Urinary catheterization involves the introduction of a catheter (latex or silicone tube) through the urethra into the urinary bladder. This is usually performed only when absolutely necessary, since certain hazards are incurred. Because the urinary structures are normally sterile except at the end of the urethra, the danger exists of introducing microorganisms into the bladder. This hazard is greatest for clients who have lowered resistance due to disease processes. Once an infection is introduced into the bladder, it can ascend the ureters and eventually involve the kidneys. Even after the catheter has been inserted and left in place for a time, the hazard of infection remains, since pathogens can be introduced through the catheter lumen. Thus, strict surgical aseptic technique is used for catheterizations.

Another hazard is trauma, particularly in the male client, whose urethra is longer and more tortuous. It is important to insert a catheter along the normal contour of the urethra. Damage to the urethra can occur if the catheter is forced through strictures or at an incorrect angle. For females, the urethra lies posteriorly, then takes a slightly anterior direction toward the bladder. See Figure 43–4. For males, the urethra is normally curved (see Figure 43–3), but it can be straightened by elevating the penis to a position perpendicular to the body.

Two categories of urinary catheters are straight catheters and retention catheters. The *straight* or *Robinson catheter* is a single-lumen tube with a small eye or opening about 1¼ cm (½ in) from the insertion tip. See Figure 43–16, *A*. It is used primarily for obtaining urine specimens and residual urine.

Residual urine (urine remaining in the bladder following the voiding) is normally not present in the bladder or consists of only a few milliliters. However, whenever there is a bladder outlet obstruction (e.g., enlargement of the

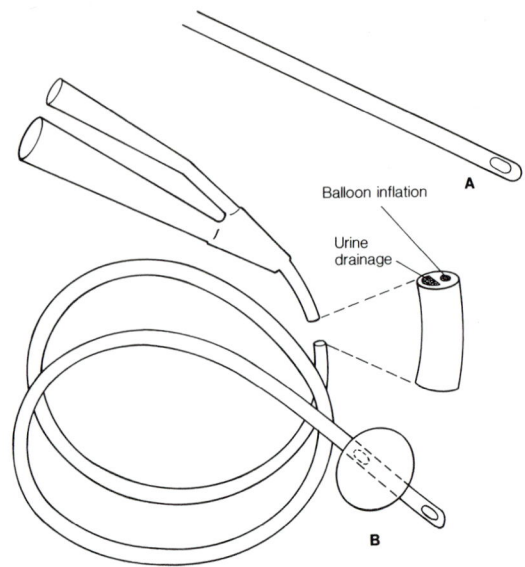

Figure 43–16 Two types of commonly used catheters: *A*, a straight (Robinson) catheter; *B*, a retention (Foley) catheter with the balloon inflated.

prostate gland) or loss of bladder muscle tone, there can be large amounts of residual urine. Incomplete emptying of the bladder may be suspected when the client experiences frequency and when only small amounts of urine are voided at a time (e.g., 100 ml in an adult). The consequence of incomplete emptying of the bladder is urinary stasis and, ultimately, infection. The purposes of measuring the residual urine are: (a) to determine the degree to which the bladder is emptying, and (b) to assess the need to establish therapy that will empty the bladder (e.g., insertion of a retention catheter).

To measure the residual urine, the nurse asks the client to void and then immediately catheterizes the client. Both the amount of urine voided and the amount of residual urine are measured and recorded. Generally, if the amount of residual urine exceeds 50 ml, an indwelling catheter is inserted.

The *retention* (*indwelling* or *Foley*) *catheter* contains a second, smaller tube throughout its length on the inside. This tube is connected to a balloon near the insertion tip. After catheter insertion, the balloon is inflated to hold the catheter in place within the bladder. The outside end of the retention catheter is bifurcated, that is, it has two openings, one to drain the urine, the other to inflate the balloon. See Figure 43–16, *B*.

There are several other types of retention catheters. One that is frequently used for a client requiring continual or periodic bladder irrigations is the *three-way Foley catheter.* It is similar to the two-way Foley catheter described above, except that it has a third channel through which sterile fluid can flow into the urinary bladder. See Figure 43–17.

All types of catheters are sized by the diameter of the

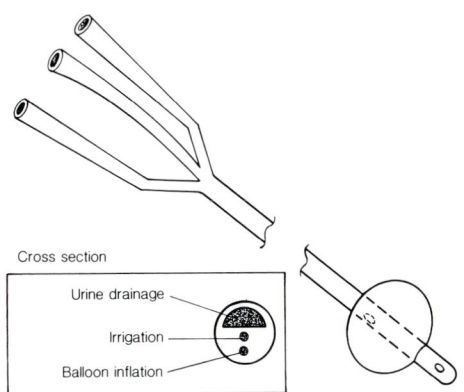

Cross section

Urine drainage

Irrigation

Balloon inflation

Figure 43–17 A three-way Foley catheter.

lumen and are categorized according to the French scale of numbers: the larger the number, the larger the lumen. Small sizes, such as #8 or #10, are used for children; #14, #16, and #18 are commonly used for adults. Men frequently require a larger size than women. The balloons of retention catheters are sized by the volume of fluid or air used to inflate them. The two commonly used sizes are 5-ml and 30-ml balloons. The size of the balloon is indicated on the catheter along with the diameter, e.g., "#18 Fr.—5 ml." The nurse uses as small a balloon as possible. A balloon

size of 5 to 10 ml will permit effective drainage, maintain the eyes of the catheter as low as possible in the bladder, and cause less discomfort in the majority of clients. Larger balloon sizes (e.g., 30 ml) may be required only for post-prostatectomy clients (Slade and Gillespie 1985).

There is controversy regarding the value of meatal cleansing using antiseptics before catheterization. Prospective trials have been unable to demonstrate any reduction in the rate of bacteriuria when various methods of meatal cleansing are used (Burke, Jacobsen, Garibaldi, Conti, and Alling 1983, p. 334; Conti and Eutropius 1987, p. 308).

The procedure for inserting a urinary retention catheter is similar to the basic catheterization procedure, with differences occurring primarily after the catheter is inserted. Prior to insertion of the catheter, the nurse tests the balloon of the retention catheter to see that it is intact and, following the insertion, inflates the balloon and attaches a urinary drainage system.

A simple urinary drainage system consists of a retention catheter, tubing, and a receptacle (collecting bag) for the urine. This is called a straight drainage system, and it depends on the force of gravity to move the urine from the urinary bladder to the collecting bag. When this system is not or cannot be opened anywhere along it from the catheter to the bag, it is referred to as a closed system. See Figure 43–18. Closed systems are being used increasingly because

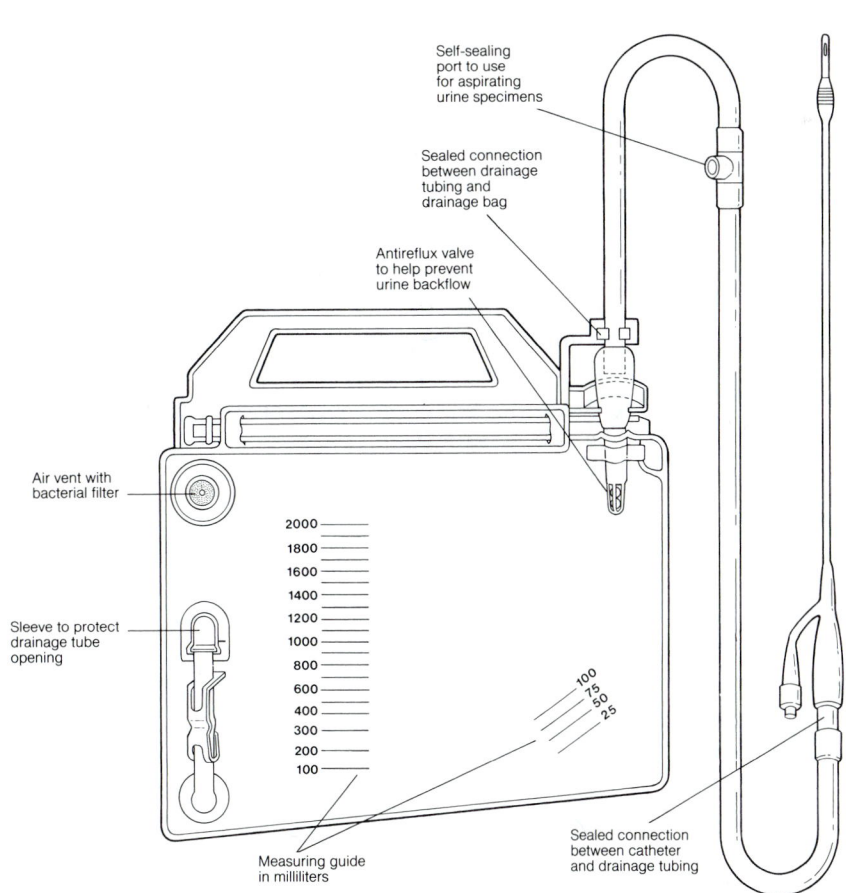

Self-sealing port to use for aspirating urine specimens

Sealed connection between drainage tubing and drainage bag

Antireflux valve to help prevent urine backflow

Air vent with bacterial filter

Sleeve to protect drainage tube opening

Measuring guide in milliliters

Sealed connection between catheter and drainage tubing

Figure 43–18 A closed urinary drainage system.

of the danger of microorganisms entering the urinary tract whenever the system is opened. The more traditional type of system is the open system, in which the tubing may be separated from the catheter.

Catheterization of females and males, using straight catheters, is described in Procedures 43–3 and 43–4, respectively. Procedure 43–5 outlines how to insert a retention catheter.

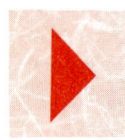

PROCEDURE 43–3

FEMALE URINARY CATHETERIZATION USING A STRAIGHT CATHETER

Equipment ☑

A sterile catheterization kit containing:
  Gloves
  Drapes
  Fenestrated drape (optional) to place over the perineum
  Antiseptic solution
  Cotton balls or gauze squares

Forceps
Water-soluble lubricant
Catheter of appropriate size (e.g., #14 or #16)
Receptacle for the urine
Specimen container if necessary

Bag or receptacle for disposal of the cotton balls

Flashlight or lamp
Mask, if required by agency policy
Bath blanket
Soap, a basin of warm water, a washcloth, and a towel
Disposable gloves

Intervention

1. **Percuss and palpate the bladder to assess for urinary retention.**

■ To percuss the bladder, place the middle finger of one hand against the skin, and strike it sharply with the middle finger of the other hand. When the bladder is full, the resulting sound will be duller than normal.

■ To palpate the bladder, indent the skin more than 1.3 cm (0.5 in) just above the symphysis pubis by pressing the fingers of one hand on the fingers of the other. See Figure 19–93. *This increases the pressure for palpation.*

2. **Prepare the client.**

■ Explain the catheterization to the client, and provide privacy. *Exposure of the genitals is embarrassing to most clients.* Some people fear that the procedure will be painful; explain that normally a catheterization is painless and that there may be a sensation of pressure. *Reliev-*

ing the client's tension can facilitate insertion of the catheter, because the urinary sphincters are more likely to be relaxed.

■ Assist the client to a supine position, with knees flexed and thighs externally rotated. Pillows can be used to support the knees and to elevate the buttocks. *Raising the client's pelvis gives the nurse a better view of the urinary meatus and reduces the risk of contaminating the catheter.*

■ Drape the client. *This maintains comfort and prevents unnecessary exposure.* Cover the client's chest and abdomen with a bath blanket. Pull the client's gown up over her hips. Cover her legs and feet with the bed sheet or another blanket. Place it diagonally on the client with a corner around each foot. See Figure 19–1 on page 362.

■ Wash the perineal-genital area with warm water and soap. Wear disposable gloves. *Cleaning reduces the number of microorganisms around the urinary meatus and*

the possibility of introducing microorganisms with the catheter.

■ Rinse and dry the area well. *Rinsing removes soap that could inhibit the action of the antiseptic later.*

■ Obtain assistance if the client requires help in maintaining the required position. *The client must remain still throughout the procedure to maintain a clear view of the urinary meatus and prevent contamination of the sterile field.*

3. **Prepare the equipment.**

■ Adjust the light to view the urinary meatus. It may be necessary to use a flashlight or to place a gooseneck lamp at the foot of the bed, so that it focuses on the perineal area.

■ Put on a mask, gown, and/or cap if required by agency policy (e.g., for reverse isolation).

4. **Create a sterile field.**

■ At the client's bedside, open a sterile kit and the catheter, if it is packaged separately, and put on the sterile gloves (see Procedure 20–3 on page 482).

- Drape the client with the sterile drapes, being careful to protect the sterility of the drapes and your gloves. Use the first drape as an underpad, and place it under the buttocks. Keep the underpad edges cuffed over your gloves. *This prevents contamination of the gloves against the client's buttocks.* If the other drape is fenestrated, place it over the perineal area, exposing only the labia. If a fenestrated drape is not available, place the two thigh drapes so that they overlap between the client's thighs. Place the thigh drapes from the side farthest to the side nearest you. *This prevents reaching across a sterile field and possible contamination of the new drape.*

- Place the sterile kit on the drape between the clients thighs. *This facilitates access to supplies.*

- Pour the antiseptic solution over the cotton balls, if they are not already prepared.

- Lubricate the insertion tip of the catheter liberally, and place it in the sterile container ready for use. *Water-soluble lubricant facilitates insertion of the catheter by reducing friction. Lubricate at this point, because you will subsequently have only one sterile hand available.*

- Open the urine specimen container, and keep the top sterile. *This prepares the container for specimen collection.*

5. Clean the meatus (if recommended by agency practice).

- With the non-dominant hand, separate the labia majora with the thumb and finger, and clean the labia minora on each side, using forceps and cotton balls soaked in antiseptic. Use a new swab for each

stroke. *This prevents the transfer of microorganisms.* Move downward from the pubic area to the anus. See Figure 43–19. *Cleaning from anterior to posterior cleans from the area of least contamination to the area of greatest contamination.*

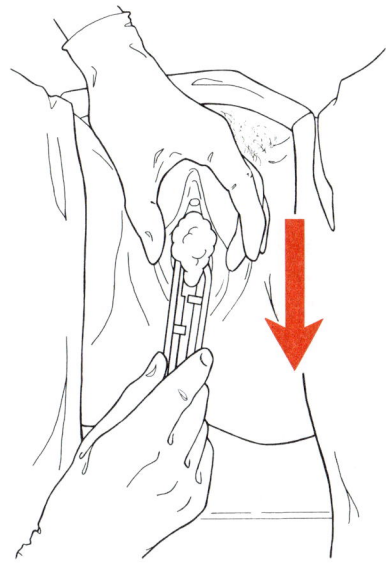

Figure 43–19   When cleaning the labia minora, move the swab downward.

- Then, separate the labia minora with two other fingers, still using the nondominant hand. See Figure 43–20.

- Expose the urinary meatus adequately by retracting the tissue of the labia minora in an upward (anterior) direction. See Figure 43–20. Clean first from the meatus downward and then on either side, using a new swab for each stroke. Once the meatus is cleaned, do not allow the labia to close over it. *Keeping the labia apart prevents the risk of contaminating the urinary meatus.*

Note: The hand that touches the client becomes unsterile. It remains in position exposing the urinary meatus, while the other hand

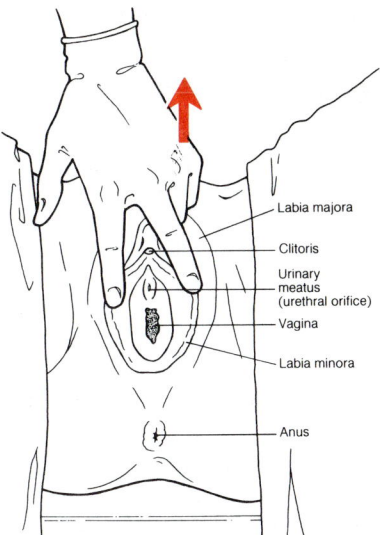

Figure 43–20   To expose the urinary meatus, separate the labia minora and retract the tissue upward.

remains sterile holding the sterile forceps.

6. Inspect the meatus.

- Assess any signs, such as excoriation of the tissues surrounding the urinary meatus, swelling of the urinary meatus, or the presence of discharge around the urinary meatus. *This assessment provides baseline data.* If discharge is present, refer to the nurse in charge for a culture order.

7. Insert the catheter until urine flows.

- Place the drainage end of the catheter in the urine receptacle. Pick up the insertion end of the catheter with your uncontaminated, sterile, gloved hand, holding it about 5 cm (2 in) from the insertion tip. *Because the adult female urethra is approximately 4 cm (1.5 in) long, the catheter is held far enough from the end to allow full insertion into the bladder and to maintain control of the tip of the catheter so it will not accidentally become contaminated.*

- Gently insert the catheter into the urinary meatus until urine flows. Insert the catheter in the direction of the urethra. If the catheter meets resistance during insertion, do not force it. *Forceful pressure exerted against the urethra can produce trauma.* Ask the client to take deep breaths. *This helps relax the external sphincter.* If this does not relieve the resistance, discontinue the procedure, and report the problem to the nurse in charge. Exercise caution to prevent the catheter tip from becoming contaminated. If it becomes contaminated, discard it.

- When the urine flows, transfer your hand from the labia to the catheter to hold it in place 2 cm from the meatus. *This prevents its expulsion by a possible bladder contraction.*

8. Collect a urine specimen.

- Pinch the catheter, and transfer the drainage end of it into the sterile specimen bottle. Usually, 30 ml of urine is sufficient for a specimen. Securely place the top on the spec-imen container, and set it aside for labeling later.

9. Empty or partially drain the bladder, and remove the catheter.

- For adults experiencing urinary retention, some orders limit the amount of urine drained to 700 to 1000 ml. Whether to limit the amount of urine drained has been a controversial issue. *Rapid removal of large amounts of urine is thought to induce engorgement of the pelvic blood vessels and hypovolemic shock. However, retained urine may serve as a reservoir for microorganisms to multiply.* Usually, agency policy or the physician indicates the amount to be removed and times at which the remaining urine is to be withdrawn. Recently, Bristol, Fadden, Fehring, Rohde, Prue, and Wohlitz (1989, p. 345) concluded from research that *complete* drainage of a distended bladder is likely to be more comfortable and certainly seems as safe as threshold clamping.

- Pinch the catheter. *This prevents leakage of urine.* Remove the catheter slowly.

10. Promote client comfort.

- Dry the client's perineum with a towel or drape. *Excess lubricant and solution in the area can irritate the skin.*

11. Assess the urine.

- Inspect the urine for color, clarity, odor, and the presence of any abnormal constituents, such as blood.

- Measure the amount of urine.

12. Document the catheterization.

- Include assessments before and after the procedure; type and size of catheter inserted; time; characteristics and amount of urine obtained; whether a specimen was sent to the laboratory; and client response to the procedure.

Sample Recording

Date 01-26-91	Time 1900

C/o pubic discomfort. Has not voided since surgery. Intake 2000 ml. Bladder palpable above symphysis pubis. Is restless. Catheterize with #14F catheter for 650 ml clear amber urine. States, "am more comfortable." Less restless. —————
————————— Sylvia F. Tompkins, RN

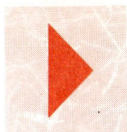

PROCEDURE 43–4

MALE URINARY CATHETERIZATION USING A STRAIGHT CATHETER

Equipment ☑

See Procedure 43–3. A #16 or #18 catheter is usually used for an adult male.

Intervention

1. Follow Procedure 43–3, step 1.

2. Prepare the client.

- Explain the catheterization, as in Procedure 43–3.

- Assist the client to a supine position, with the knees slightly flexed and the thighs slightly apart. *This allows greater relaxation of the abdominal and perineal muscles and permits easier insertion of the catheter.*

- Drape the client by folding the top bedclothes down so that the penis is exposed and the thighs are covered. Use a bath blanket to cover the client's chest and abdomen.

- Wash the perineal area, as in Procedure 43–3.

 3. Create a sterile field.

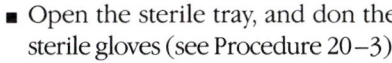

- Open the sterile tray, and don the sterile gloves (see Procedure 20–3).

- Place a drape under the penis and a second drape above the penis over the pubic area. If a fenestrated drape is available, place it over the penis and pubic area, exposing only the penis.

- Place the sterile kit on the sterile drape over the client's thighs or next to the thigh.

- Pour the antiseptic solution over the cotton balls, if they are not already prepared.

- Lubricate the insertion tip of the catheter liberally for about 5 to 7 cm (2 to 3 in). Place it in the sterile

container ready for insertion. *Water-soluble lubricant facilitates insertion of the catheter by reducing friction. Do this step before cleaning, since you will subsequently have only one sterile hand available.*

4. Clean the urinary meatus.

- Grasp the penis firmly behind the glans with the nondominant hand, and spread the meatus between the thumb and forefinger. Retract the foreskin of an uncircumcised male. The hand holding the penis is now considered contaminated. *Firmly grasp the penis to avoid stimulating an erection.*

- With the dominant hand, use sterile forceps to pick up a swab. Clean the meatus first, and then wipe the tissue surrounding the meatus in a circular motion. Discard each swab after only one wipe. *Using forceps maintains the sterility of your gloves.*

5. Insert the catheter.

- Place the drainage end of the catheter in the urine receptacle. Then, pick up the insertion end of the catheter with your uncontaminated, sterile, gloved hand, holding it about 8 to 10 cm (3 to 4 in) from the insertion tip for an adult or about 2.5 cm (1 in) for a baby or small boy. In some agencies, the catheter is picked up with forceps. *The male urethra is approximately 20 cm (8 in) long. Holding the catheter far enough from the end to maintain control of the tip of the catheter avoids accidental contamination.*

- Lift the penis to a position perpendicular to the body (90° angle), and exert slight traction (pulling or tension upward). Insert the catheter steadily about 20 cm (8 in) or

until urine begins to flow. *Lifting the penis perpendicular to the body straightens the downward curvature of the urethra.*

- To bypass slight resistance at the sphincters, twist the catheter, or wait until the sphincter relaxes. Ask the client to take deep breaths or try to void. If difficult resistance is met, discontinue the procedure, and report the problem to the nurse in charge. *Slight resistance is normally encountered at the external and internal urethral sphincters. Deep breathing can help to relax the external sphincter. Forceful pressure exerted against a major resistance can traumatize the urethra.*

- While the urine flows, lower the penis, and transfer your hand to hold the catheter in place at the meatus.

6. Drain the urine from the bladder.

- Collect a urine specimen (if required) after the urine has flowed for a few seconds. Pinch the catheter, and transfer the drainage end of the catheter into the sterile specimen bottle. Usually, 30 ml of urine is sufficient for a specimen.

- Empty the bladder, or drain the amount of urine specified in the order. See Procedure 43–3, step 9, for recent research.

7. Make the client comfortable.

- Dry the penis with a towel or drape.

- Replace the foreskin. *This prevents a mechanical phimosis (constriction), which may compromise circulation to the glans.*

8. Assess the client and the urine, as in Procedure 43–3, and document the procedure and the assessments.

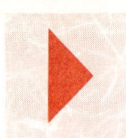

PROCEDURE 43–5

INSERTING A RETENTION CATHETER

Equipment ☑

In addition to the equipment used for a straight catheterization, the following equipment is needed:

Retention catheter, #14 or #16 for adults, #8 or #10 for children.

Prefilled syringe (sterile water is often used)

Nonallergenic tape

Safety pin or clip

Intervention

1. Prepare the client and the equipment.

- Explain to the client why the retention catheter is to be inserted, how long it will be in place, and how the urinary drainage equipment needs to be handled to maintain and facilitate the drainage of urine. Reassure the client that the procedure is painless. Some clients fear spillage of urine when they experience the urge to void during insertion of the catheter and for a short period of time after the catheter is in place. Reassure these clients that the catheter drains the urine and that the urge to void will disappear.

- Follow procedure as for straight catheterization up to and including draping the client.

2. Test the catheter balloon.

- Attach the prefilled syringe to the balloon valve, and inject the fluid. The balloon should inflate appropriately and not leak. Withdraw the fluid, and set aside the catheter with the syringe attached for later use. If the balloon leaks or does not inflate adequately, replace the catheter. In such a case, withdraw the fluid, and detach the syringe for later use. Ask another nurse to obtain a second catheter and open

the package for you, then test the new balloon.

or

Remove the equipment, and obtain another catheter. Then begin again with the new sterile equipment.

3. Follow steps as for straight catheterization.

- Lubricate the insertion tip of the catheter.

- Remove the sterile cap from the specimen container.

- Separate and clean the urinary meatus and surrounding tissues.

- Insert the catheter.

- Collect a urine specimen as required.

4. Move the catheter farther into the bladder, and inflate the balloon.

- Insert the catheter an additional 2.5 to 5 cm (1 to 2 in) beyond the point at which urine began to flow. The balloon of the catheter is located behind the opening at the insertion tip, and sufficient space needs to be provided to inflate the balloon. *This ensures that the balloon is inflated inside the bladder and not in the urethra, where it could produce trauma.*

- Inflate the balloon by injecting the contents of the prefilled syringe into the valve of the catheter. See Figure 43–21, *A*. Placement of the catheter and balloon in a male client is shown in Figure 43–21, *B*. If the client complains of discomfort or pain during the balloon inflation, withdraw the fluid, insert the catheter a little farther, and inflate the balloon again. Insert no more fluid than the balloon size indicates (e.g., 5 ml or 30 ml), and remove the syringe. A special valve prevents backflow of the fluid out of the catheter.

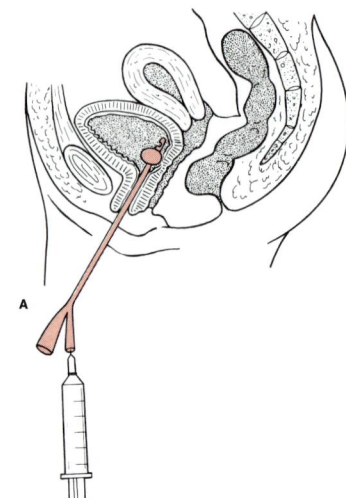

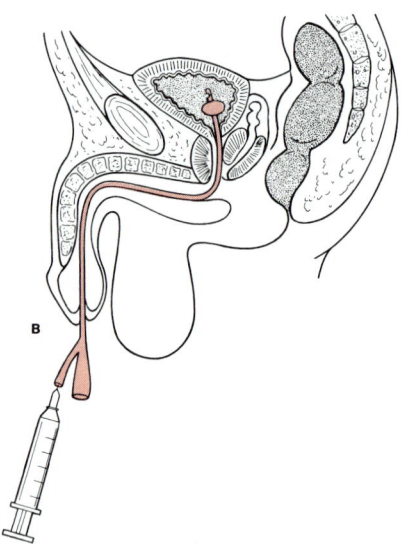

Figure 43–21 Placement of catheter and inflated balloon in *A,* female client; and *B,* male client.

- Follow agency policy when using a 30-ml balloon. Some agency policies state that only 15 ml of fluid is injected for inflation.

5. Ensure effective balloon inflation.

- When the balloon is safely inflated, apply slight tension on the catheter until you feel resistance. *Resis-*

tance indicates that the catheter balloon is inflated appropriately, and that the catheter is well anchored in the bladder.

■ Then, release the resistance on the catheter. This keeps the balloon from exerting undue pressure on the neck of the bladder.

6. **Anchor the catheter.**

■ Tape the catheter with nonallergenic tape to the inside of a female's thigh or to the thigh or abdomen of a male client. See Figures 43–22 and 43–23. Some nurses prefer taping the catheter to the abdomen whenever there is increased risk of penile scrotal excoriation. *Taping restricts the movement of the catheter, thus reducing friction and irritation in the urethra when the client moves. It also prevents skin excoriation at the penile-scrotal junction in the male.*

7. **Establish effective drainage.**

■ Ensure that the emptying base of the drainage bag is closed.

■ Secure the drainage bag to the bed frame, using the hook or strap provided. Suspend the bag off the floor, but keep it below the level of the client's bladder. See Figure 43–22. *Urine flows by gravity from the bladder to the drainage bag. The bag should be off the floor so that the emptying portion does not become grossly contaminated.*

■ Coil the drainage tubing loosely beside the client, so that the re-

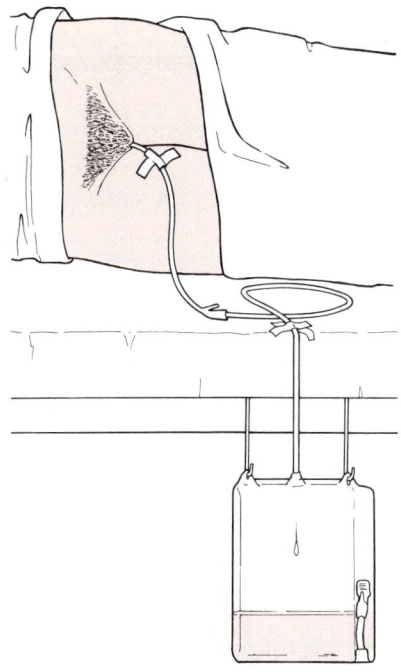

Figure 43–22 Tape the catheter to the inside of a female's thigh.

maining tubing runs in a straight line down to the drainage bag. Fasten the vertical tubing to the bedclothes with tape, a tubing clamp, or a safety pin and elastic band. See Figures 43–22 and 43–23. *The drainage tubing should not loop below its entry into the drainage bag, since this impedes the flow of urine by gravity.*

8. **Document pertinent data.**

■ Record the time and date of the catheterization; the reason; num-

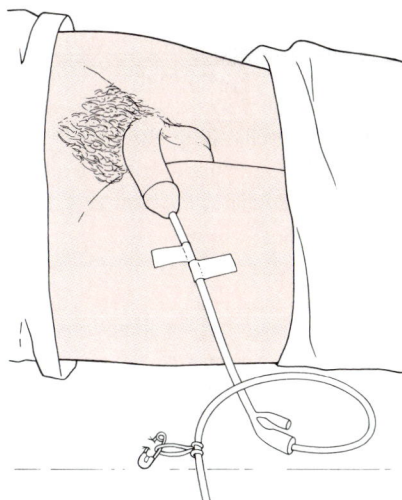

Figure 43–23 Tape the catheter to the thigh or abdomen of a male client.

ber of milliliters used to inflate the balloon; assessments before and after the procedure, including amount, color, and consistency of urine obtained; whether a specimen was taken and sent to the laboratory; whether all urine was emptied from the bladder; and the client's response.

Sample Recording

Date 07-12-91	Time 2000

#18 5-ml Foley catheter inserted and connected to drainage. 600 ml clear amber urine drained. Stated burning pain over pubic area relieved. Instructed about I & O. ————————— Ron J. Randall, SN

Nursing Interventions for Clients with Retention Catheters

Nursing care of the client with an indwelling catheter and continuous drainage is largely directed toward preventing infection of the urinary tract and encouraging urinary flow through the drainage system. It includes encouraging large amounts of fluid intake, accurate recording of the fluid intake and output, changing the retention catheter and tubing, maintaining the patency of the drainage system, preventing contamination of the drainage system, and teaching these measures to the client.

Fluids and Fluid Balance
An appropriate fluid balance is essential for the client with a retention catheter to minimize the risk of infection. The client should drink up to 3000 ml per day if permitted. Large amounts of fluid ensure a large urine output, which keeps the bladder flushed out and decreases the likelihood of urinary statis and subsequent infection. Large volumes of urine also minimize the risk of sediment or other particles obstructing the drainage tubing. Accurate recording of fluid intake and output is discussed in Chapter 40.

Dietary Measures
Many agencies implement prophylactic measures to acidify the client's urine to prevent urinary infection. By changing the composition of the diet, the urine can be made either acid or alkaline. Most vegetables and fruits yield an alkaline urine, whereas meat, fish, fowl, eggs, and cereals yield an acid urine. Alkalinization of the urine may be warranted to soothe an irritated bladder.

Perineal Care
Neither daily cleaning of the perineum with soap and water nor twice-daily cleaning with povidone-iodine solution has been shown to reduce the incidence of catheter-associated infections (Epstein 1985, p. 273). No special cleaning other than routine hygienic care is therefore officially recommended at this time. Nor is special meatal care recommended. Some studies have shown no improvement in catheter-associated infections and in fact a higher incidence of bacteriuria in groups of people receiving routine meatal care (Epstein 1985, p. 273). Agency practices regarding catheter care vary considerably. The nurse should check agency practice in this regard.

Changing the Catheter and Tubing
According to the CDC, "changing indwelling catheters at arbitrary fixed intervals" is not cost-effective and should not be performed (Epstein 1985, p. 274). Furthermore, the closed system should be maintained and the catheter and tubing not disconnected unless absolutely necessary. Clients should therefore be catheterized only when absolutely necessary and the retention catheter removed as soon as possible.

Agency policies may specify the frequency of catheter and tubing changes. Some agencies advocate that both be changed when sediment accumulates at the distal end. Sediment is present if sandy particles are felt when the end of the catheter is rolled between the thumb and fingers. The drainage bag and tubing are generally changed along with the catheter but need to be changed more frequently if sediment accumulates, if leakage occurs, or if a strong odor is evident. Recommendations for changes are made on the basis of reducing the incidence of infection and preventing unpleasant odors.

During tubing changes, strict surgical asepsis is essential to prevent contamination of the distal lumen of the catheter. The nurse acquires a new sterile drainage bag and tubing, a sterile towel or sterile gauzes, clamp, and antiseptic solution. After washing the hands well and setting up a sterile field, the nurse may don disposable gloves, then removes the protective cap from the drainage tube and places the open end of the tubing on the sterile field. The nurse then clamps the catheter above the tubing connector and cleans the catheter-tubing junction with an antiseptic solution. The nurse then disconnects the catheter from the old tubing, being careful not to contaminate the end of the catheter, and connects the catheter to the new tubing. She or he then unclamps the catheter, and establishes drainage by securing the tubing and drainage receptacle to the bed at an appropriate level. Applying waterproof tape around the connection site of the catheter and the tubing ensures a closed drainage system.

Ongoing assessment of clients with retention catheters is a high priority. The box below provides guidelines.

Ongoing Assessment of Clients with Retention Catheters

- Ensure that there are no obstructions in the drainage. Check that there are no kinks in the tubing, the client is not lying on the tubing, and the tubing is not clogged with mucus or blood.

- Check that there is no tension on the catheter or tubing, that the catheter is securely taped to the thigh or abdomen, and that the tubing is fastened appropriately to the bedclothes.

- Ensure that gravity drainage is maintained. Make sure there are no loops in the tubing below its entry to the drainage receptacle and that the drainage receptacle is below the level of the client's bladder.

- Ensure that the drainage system is well sealed or closed. Check that there are no leaks at the connection sites in open systems. Apply waterproof tape around the connection site of the catheter and tubing.

- Observe the flow of the urine every 2 or 3 hours, and note color, odor, and any abnormal constituents. If blood clots are present, check the catheter more frequently to ascertain whether it is plugged.

When emptying the drainage bag, the nurse must maintain surgical aseptic technique. The bag is emptied usually at the end of each shift of duty, and the tube at the bottom of the bag is used to drain the bag. The amount of drainage is noted in accordance with calibrations on the bag, or a graduated pitcher is brought to the bedside to assess the output. It is important for the nurse not to contaminate the end of the tubing and to reattach it appropriately when the bag is emptied.

Some agencies recommend instillation of hydrogen peroxide in the drainage bag of open systems to prevent the growth of microorganisms in the bag and to reduce odor. Agency policies vary, however. Guidelines to prevent catheter-associated urinary tract infections are given in the accompanying box.

Client Teaching   Usually nurses need to teach the client some principles about the gravity drainage system and the importance of maintaining a closed system. The client has to understand that the drainage tubing and drainage bag need to be kept lower than the bladder at all times. The client also needs to know how to prevent tension on the catheter tubing, to prevent loops or kinks in the drainage tubing, and to avoid lying on the tubing. Understanding how to manipulate the system when ambulating can give the client a sense of independence. Some clients also benefit from instruction about fluid intake measurement and perineal care. Clients who wish to be involved in recording fluid intake measurements need information about how to compute these values and which foods are considered fluids.

Removing Retention Catheters   Retention catheters are removed after their purpose has been achieved, usually on the order of the physician. A few days prior to removal the catheter may be clamped for specified periods of time (e.g., 2 to 4 hours) and then released. This causes some distention of the bladder and stimulation of the bladder musculature and may be ordered as "bladder training." In one research study, bladder reconditioning for as short a period as three cycles of 3 hours of clamping the catheter followed by 5 minutes of draining significantly helped women achieve regular voiding after being catheterized (Williamson 1982, p. 29). In most agencies, this must be ordered by a physician.

To remove a retention catheter, the nurse needs a receptacle for the catheter, e.g., a disposable basin; a clean, disposable towel; disposable gloves; and a sterile syringe to deflate the balloon. The syringe should be large enough to withdraw all the solution in the catheter balloon. The size of the balloon is indicated on the label at the end of the catheter.

Ask the client to assume a back-lying position as for a catheterization. Some agencies recommend that the nurse obtain a sterile specimen before removing the catheter. Remove the tape attaching the catheter to the client, and

Preventing Catheter-Associated Urinary Infections

- Have an established infection control program.
- Catheterize clients only when necessary, by using aseptic technique, sterile equipment, and trained personnel.
- Maintain a sterile closed-drainage system.
- Do not disconnect the catheter and drainage tubing unless absolutely necessary.
- Remove the catheter as soon as possible.
- Follow and reinforce good handwashing technique.
- Changing indwelling catheters at arbitrary, fixed intervals and regular bacteriologic monitoring of catheterized clients are not cost-effective practices and should not be performed.
- Avoid other measures until further data are available. New products that appear to be questionable or gimmicky probably should be avoided.
- Although instillation of H_2O_2 into the outlet tube of the drainage set or into the drainage bags has been associated with a reduction in bag contamination, studies indicate no difference in the rate of bag-source infection in clients with the suggested instillation of H_2O_2 into the drainage bag when compared with clients who had conventional closed-drainage systems (Epstein 1985).

then place the towel between the legs of the female client and over the thighs of the male. Insert the syringe into the balloon inflation tube of the catheter, and withdraw the fluid from the balloon. If not all the fluid can be removed, report this fact to the nurse in charge before proceeding. Do *not* pull the catheter while the balloon is inflated, since the urethra may be injured. Puncturing the balloon using sterile technique is a procedure usually performed by a physician. A sterile wire stylet is inserted up the lumen of the catheter, and the balloon is punctured. This will permit the fluid to flow out of the balloon (Mocsny 1980, p. 80).

After all the fluid is withdrawn from the balloon, gently withdraw the catheter, and place it in the waste receptacle. Dry the perineal area with the towel. Measure the urine in the drainage bag, and record the removal of the catheter. Include in the recording (a) the time the catheter was removed, (b) the amount, color, and clarity of the urine, and (c) the intactness of the catheter. Following removal of the catheter, determine the time of the first voiding and the amount voided over the first 8 hours. Compare this output to the client's intake. Clients who have had retention catheters for a prolonged period may lose some bladder muscle tone because the bladder remains relatively empty and thus is never stretched to its capacity. When a muscle is not stretched regularly, atrophy develops. When a catheter is removed, the client may have difficulty in regaining urinary control. Another potential problem is urine retention due to urethral swelling. Therefore, palpate the bladder for urinary retention following a retention catheter removal (see Chapter 19 for the technique).

Obtaining a Urine Specimen from a Retention Catheter
Sterile urine specimens can be acquired from closed drainage systems by inserting a sterile 1-in needle (#21 to #25 gauge), attached to a 3-ml syringe through a drainage port in the tubing. See Figure 43–24. Note that aspiration of urine from catheters can be done only with self-sealing rubber catheters, not plastic, silicone, or silastic catheters.

First, clean the entry point of the needle with a disinfectant swab. Then insert the needle at an angle to facilitate self-sealing of the rubber, at a place where it will not puncture the tube leading to the balloon. If the urine is not readily available, the drainage tubing is elevated slightly to return urine to the area, or the catheter is pinched or clamped about 5 to 7 cm (3 in) from its tip for a short period until urine appears.

After the urine is drawn into the syringe, transfer it to a *sterile* specimen container, cap the container, label it, and send it to the laboratory immediately for analysis or refrigeration.

Urinary Irrigations

An *irrigation* is a flushing or washing-out using a specified solution. A *bladder irrigation* is carried out on a physician's order, usually to wash out the bladder and/or apply an antiseptic solution to the bladder lining to treat a bladder infection. Sterile technique is used. *Catheter irrigations* are usually carried out to maintain or restore the patency of a catheter, e.g., to remove pus or blood clots that have formed in the bladder and are blocking the catheter. A physician's order may or may not be required, depending on agency policy.

There are three ways of irrigating a catheter or bladder: (1) maintaining the closed system and injecting the solution through an aspiration port, (2) irrigating through a three-way catheter (closed system), and (3) irrigating through a catheter after separating the catheter and tubing (open system). Although the open system may be used in some agencies, closed sterile drainage systems are recommended.

In the usual bladder irrigation, a two-way Foley catheter is usually in place. For a bladder irrigation, the frequency and the type, amount, and strength of solution to be used

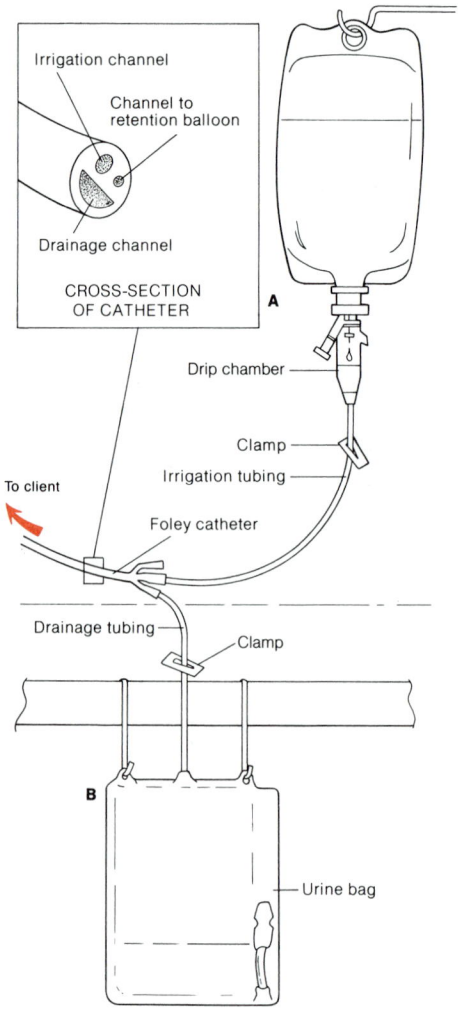

Figure 43–25 An intermittent bladder irrigation.

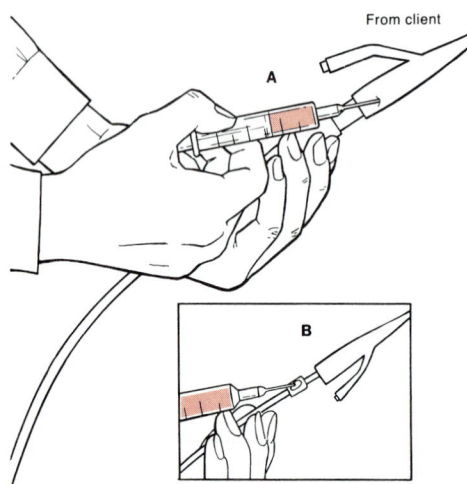

Figure 43–24 Obtaining a urine specimen from a retention catheter: *A*, from a specific area, sometimes designated by a patch, near the end of the catheter; *B*, from a drainage port in the tubing.

are ordered by the physician. If the physician has not specified these on the client's chart, check agency policies. Some agencies recommend the use of sterile normal saline at room temperature for both catheter and bladder irrigations. To irrigate an adult bladder, 1000 ml is commonly used; for a catheter irrigation, 200 ml is normally required.

Irrigations performed via straight gravity drainage are referred to as *plain irrigations.* A variation of the plain irrigation is the intermittent irrigation, in which one lumen of a three-way catheter is connected by tubing to a drip chamber and then to a container of sterile solution. The second lumen is attached to tubing and then to a urine receptacle. See Figure 43–25. There are clamps on both tubes. The clamp from the solution container (*A*) is released while the clamp to the urine bag (*B*) is closed. The fluid enters and remains in the bladder. The container tubing is then reclamped, and the urine receptacle tubing is unclamped, permitting the solution to flow out of the bladder. This process is carried out regularly. The same system can be used for continuous irrigations by carefully regulating the flow of fluid leaving the solution container and permitting it to flow freely out of the bladder into the urine bag.

There are several variations of this irrigation system. One requires a specific fluid pressure to build up in the urinary bladder before the irrigation system "trips," allowing the solution to flow out of the bladder into a receptacle. These systems are usually set up by a physician and monitored by nurses.

Procedure 43–6 outlines the steps in irrigating a catheter or bladder.

PROCEDURE 43–6

IRRIGATING A CATHETER OR BLADDER (CLOSED SYSTEM)

Equipment

Gloves

Sterile 30- or 50-ml syringe with a #19 to #23 needle

Sterile antiseptic swabs

Disposable, water-resistant towel

Sterile container of irrigating solution (generally at room temperature or warmed to body temperature).

Sterile receptacle

Intervention

1. **Determine that the catheter and tubing are indeed blocked.**

- Palpate the client's bladder to assess for urine retention.

- Compare the amount of urine in the bag with the drainage on the previous shift or with the client's fluid intake.

- If urine does not appear to be running freely, "milk" the catheter and tubing, working from the client toward the drainage bag. *This can dislodge an obstruction, avoiding the necessity of an irrigation to remove it. "Milk" away from the client so that the obstruction, e.g., a blood clot, is forced into the drainage bag and not into the urinary bladder.*

2. **Prepare the client.**

- Explain the procedure to the client. A bladder or catheter irrigation should not be painful, although solution that is not at body temperature may be uncomfortable to the client.

- Assist the client to a dorsal recumbent position. *This position facilitates the flow of the irrigating fluid into the bladder.*

- Fold back the top bedclothes to expose the retention catheter. Place a bath blanket across the client's chest and abdomen if they are exposed.

- Determine the amount of urine in the drainage bag. *This amount has to be deducted from subsequent measurements of the irrigating fluid returns.*

3. **Prepare the equipment.**

- Open the sterile set beside or between the client's thighs, using sterile technique.

- Don gloves.

- Place the sterile towel under the end of the catheter.

- For a bladder irrigation, clamp the drainage tubing distal to the irrigation port. *Clamping prevents the urine and solution from draining into the drainage bag.* For a catheter irrigation, leave the tubing unclamped.

- Remove the cap from the needle, and draw the irrigation solution into the syringe, maintaining the sterility of the syringe and the solution.

- Using the antiseptic swab, wipe the place on the catheter lumen or the port on the drainage tubing through which the solution is to be instilled. The correct place on the catheter lumen is usually marked.

4. Instill the fluid into the catheter.

■ Insert the needle into the port. See Figure 43–24, earlier.

■ Infuse the solution gently into the catheter. For each catheter infusion, instill about 30 to 40 ml of fluid for an adult; for each bladder infusion, instill about 100 to 200 ml. Use smaller amounts for children. *Gentle instillation avoids injury to the lining of the bladder and bladder spasms.*

■ Remove the needle from the port.

5. Drain the fluid.

■ For a catheter irrigation, immediately lower the catheter so that the fluid will run toward the distal end of the catheter into the drainage tubing.
  or

■ For a bladder irrigation, unclamp the drainage tubing so that the solution will run out of the bladder through the catheter and tubing.

■ Repeat the process outlined in step 4 until all of the solution has been used or until the purpose of the irrigation has been accomplished.

6. Calculate the amount of urine drained.

■ Empty the urine bag and subtract the amount of solution used from the volume of fluid in the bag.

7. Assess the client and drainage.

■ Note any change in discomfort.

■ Assess the drainage for color, clarity, and presence of abnormal constituents.

■ Assess the flow of urine in the catheter and tubing.

8. Document the irrigation.

■ Include assessments before and after the irrigation.

Sample Recording

Date 04-24-91	Time 1400

Bladder irrigated with 200 ml normal saline at room temperature. Returns slightly blood-tinged with some small blood clots. Catheter running freely. No discomfort. ——— Sandi R. Bailey, NS

Variation: Continuous irrigation using a three-way Foley catheter

1. Assemble the equipment.

■ Connect one port of the three-way catheter to the irrigation tubing which in turn is connected to the irrigation solution in a bag. Connect the second port of the catheter to the drainage tubing and bag, and the third port to the catheter balloon. See Figure 43–25, earlier.

2. Irrigate the bladder.

■ Open the flow clamp on the drainage tubing.

■ Adjust the flow rate, using the clamp on the irrigation tubing, as specified by the physician. If the order does not specify, the rate should be 40 to 60 drops per minute.

■ Inspect the fluid returns for amount, color, and clarity. The amount of returning fluid should correspond to the amount of fluid entering the bladder.

3. Document the assessments as above.

Variation: Irrigating a catheter or bladder using the open system.

■ After disinfecting the ends, separate the catheter from the drainage tubing, and place the tubing protector over the end of the tubing. Hold the catheter and the tubing at least 2.5 cm (1 in) from their ends. *This distance avoids contaminating the ends of the catheter and tubing.*

■ Draw the fluid into the syringe, then gently inject it into the catheter, maintaining the sterility of the end of the catheter, the syringe, and the solution. Remove the syringe, and allow the fluid to return through the catheter into the drainage receptacle. Repeat until the catheter is running freely or until the purpose of the irrigation has been accomplished.

■ Reattach the catheter to the tubing, maintaining the sterility of the ends of the tubing and the catheter.

■ Coil the drainage tubing carefully on the bed so that the urine can flow through it freely.

■ Make assessments as for irrigating using a closed system.

Suprapubic Catheter Care

A suprapubic catheter is inserted through the abdominal wall above the symphysis pubis into the urinary bladder. See Figure 43–26. The physician inserts the catheter using local anesthesia (in the client's bed unit) or using general anesthesia in conjunction with bladder or vaginal surgery (in the operating room). The catheter may be secured in place with sutures, with a commercial retention body seal, or with both sutures and a body seal. The catheter is then attached to a closed drainage system. When the catheter is removed, the muscle layers of the bladder contract over the insertion site to seal off the opening. Suprapubic catheters have several advantages over urethral catheters:

1. They are associated with a lower rate of urinary tract infections.
2. They are more comfortable for the client.
3. They allow the opportunity to evaluate the client's ability to void normally; the client can void normally when the suprapubic catheter is clamped. The urethral catheter, by contrast, must be removed before the client's ability to void normally can be assessed.
4. They facilitate evaluation of the client's residual urine.

Two commonly used suprapubic catheters are the *Cystocath* and the *Bonanno catheter.* See Figure 43–27. These are narrow-lumen catheters with a curl at the distal end that prevents the catheter from being expelled by the bladder through the urethra. The Cystocath has a disc that holds the catheter in place on the abdominal wall; the Bonanno catheter has wings for that purpose. Attachments of the catheter to the drainage system tubing also vary: The Cystocath is joined with a stopcock, the Bonanno with a Luer-Lok adapter.

The most common problem with the suprapubic catheter is blockage of drainage by sediment or clots or obstruction of the catheter or catheter tip by the bladder wall itself. Dislodgement of the catheter and hematuria following the use of a large-bore catheter are less common problems. Care of clients with suprapubic catheters includes regular assessments of the client's urine, fluid intake, and comfort; maintenance of a patent drainage system; skin care around the insertion site; periodic clamping of the catheter preparatory to removing it; and measurement of residual urine. The physician's order about management of the catheter is followed. Orders generally include leaving the catheter open to drainage for 48 to 72 hours, then clamping the catheter for 3- to 4-hour periods during the day until the client can void satisfactory amounts. Satisfactory voiding is determined by measuring the client's residual urine after voiding.

The client's urine needs to be assessed for color, consistency, clarity, and amount of urine drained, hourly for the first 24 hours and then at least three times daily. Fluid intake is carefully monitored to ensure it is adequate to maintain a satisfactory urine output. Bladder discomfort may occur because of bladder spasms. Bladder spasms may occur

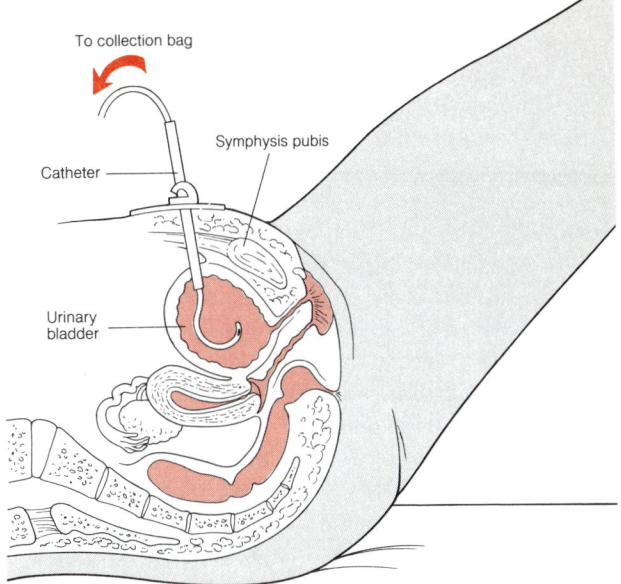

Figure 43–26 A suprapubic catheter in place.

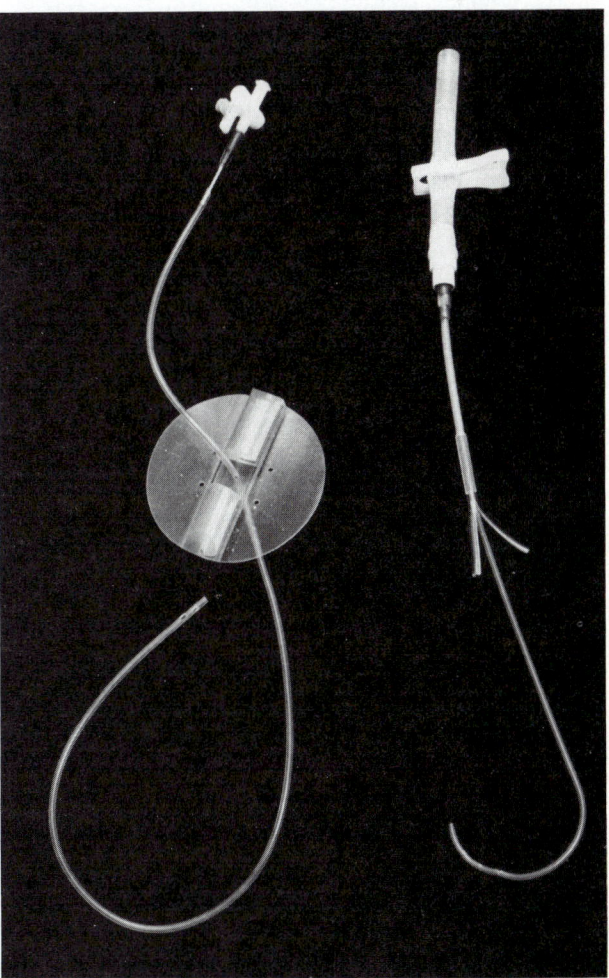

Figure 43–27 Two types of suprapubic catheters: a Cystocath (left) and a Bonanno (right).

during the first 24 to 48 hours. Spasms are identified by the presence of intermittent pain that does not affect the amount of urinary output.

Patency of the drainage system is maintained in the same manner as an indwelling catheter urinary drainage system. For example, the nurse makes sure that the catheter and drainage tubes are securely connected and taped, to avoid separation of the tubes, and ensures that the tubing is not kinked, that it runs straight up from the collection bag, and that excess tubing is coiled appropriately and taped to the client's abdomen or leg. Obstruction in the drainage system is identified by distention and tenderness of the bladder (assessed by palpation), feelings of fullness, pubic pain, and a reduction in urinary output.

Dressings around the suprapubic catheter are changed whenever they are soiled with drainage to prevent bacterial growth around the insertion site and reduce the potential for infection. A small amount of povidone-iodine ointment is applied around the insertion site and the site covered with gauze dressings. Procedures for cleaning wounds and changing dressings are discussed in Chapter 46. Any redness and discharge at the skin around the insertion site must be reported.

To ascertain the residual urine the suprapubic catheter is first closed with a clamp for 2 to 4 hours. The client then voids by the normal route, emptying the bladder as completely as possible. After this the residual urine is obtained by releasing the suprapubic catheter and allowing any remaining urine to drain into the drainage bag. Both the amount of urine voided and the amount of residual urine are measured. If the client can void a satisfactory amount (e.g., 150 to 350 ml) and the residual urine is less than 50 to 100 ml or volume specified by the physician, the catheter is often removed.

 To remove a suprapubic catheter, the nurse first dons gloves and then removes the dressing and any sutures holding the catheter in place. Suture removal is described in Chapter 46. The nurse then removes the catheter with a steady, continuous pull, applies pressure over the insertion site with gauze squares, cleans the site with antiseptic solu-tion or swabs, and applies povidone-iodine ointment and an Elastoplast bandage.

EVALUATING

To evaluate the achievement of client goals, the nurse collects data pertaining to the established outcome criteria at specified intervals. Evaluation activities may include the following:

- Observing the character of urine
- Recording the frequency of urination
- Measuring the client's fluid intake and output
- Inspecting the skin around the urinary meatus, perineum, and sacral area
- Percussing or palpating the bladder for distention
- Asking the client about dysuria, frequency, incontinence episodes (including overflow dribbling), time intervals between urge and involuntary loss of urine, methods used to prevent incontinence, and frequency of performing Kegel's exercises
- Observing the client demonstrate self-care skills for retention catheter, external urinary device, or urinary diversion stoma
- Measuring residual urine
- Measuring urine pH
- Determining results of urine cultures or other urinary function tests

Examples of evaluative statements indicating goal achievement are "The client experienced incontinence episodes only twice a week for 3 weeks"; "The client's perineal skin is intact"; "The client's residual urine is 45 ml"; "The client reported performing 15 Kegel exercises four times a day"; or "The client's fluid intake was 2000 ml/day and output in balance (i.e., from 1500 to 1800 ml/day) for 1 week."

NURSING CARE PLAN FOR JOHN BAKER

ASSESSMENT DATA

Nuring Assessment

Mr. John Baker is a 68-year-old shopkeeper who was admitted to the hospital early this morning because he has been unable to void since 7 o'clock last evening. Mrs. Fran Wittmer, the nurse, gathers the following information when taking a nursing history. He states he has noticed that for the past few weeks he has had to go to the bathroom more frequently during the day and that he doesn't always feel he has emptied his bladder after voiding. He has also noticed that he must get up a few times during the night to urinate. As of the past few days, he has noted some problems in starting urination and then dribbling urine afterward. He states that this is very embarrassing to him since he must deal with his customers during the day. Mr. Baker wonders what is causing his urinary problems.

Physical Examination

Height: 185.4 cm (6′1″)
Weight: 85.7 kg (189 lb)
Temperature: 37 C (98.6 F)
Pulse rate: 78 BPM
Respirations: 20 per minute
Blood pressure: 146/86 mm Hg
Retention catheter to closed drainage bag draining 800 ml amber urine

Diagnostic Data

CBC: Within normal range
Urine: Amber, clear, pH 7.5, specific gravity 1.025, negative for glucose, protein, ketone, RBC, and bacteria
IVP: evidence of enlarged prostate gland

CARE PLAN

Nursing Diagnosis	Client Goals and Outcome Criteria	Nursing Interventions and Rationales	Evaluation
Altered patterns of urinary elimination: Retention and incontinence related to bladder neck obstruction/ enlarged prostate gland resulting in urgency, dysuria, frequency, nocturia, dribbling, hesitancy, and bladder distention.	Client Goal: Establish normal urination pattern. Outcome Criteria: Experiences relief of urinary retention within 24 hrs. Output will balance intake by day 2. Experiences absence of dysuria by day 5. Verbalize increased self-esteem by day 5. Maintain negative urine culture by day 3.	Observe amount, color, and character of urinary output. *Rationale:* Determines adequacy of urinary tract function. Encourage fluid intake of approximately 3000 ml per day. *Rationale:* Increased fluids will increase urinary output and discourage bacterial growth. Encourage fluids, e.g., cranberry juice, that acidify urine. *Rationale:* Acidification of urine inhibits growth of bacteria. Maintain accurate I&O. *Rationale:* Serves as indicator of urinary tract and renal function and fluid balance. Maintain patency of retention catheter. *Rationale:* Prevents urinary stasis and bladder spasms. Provide perineal care. *Rationale:* Cleanliness of area will decrease chance of urinary infection. Tape retention catheter to lower abdomen. *Rationale:* Prevents erosion and pressure on penile-scrotal junction. Maintain drainage receptacle below level of client's bladder. *Rationale:* Prevents reflux flow to bladder.	Client's retention catheter remained patent, and his urinary output for the first 24 hrs was 2050 ml. For the past 48 hrs, his fluid intake has been 2000 to 3000 ml, and his urinary output has been 2500 ml. The results of his repeat urinalysis were negative. Client's retention catheter was removed on day 4, and he is voiding in the amounts of 200 to 300 ml q4–5 hrs. At times, he experiences some difficulty initiating a urinary stream, as well as some dribbling after voiding.

Nursing Diagnosis	Client Goals and Outcome Criteria	Nursing Interventions and Rationales	Evaluation
Knowledge deficit related to health problem (enlarged prostate gland and urinary retention) and its treatment resulting in anxious behavior, increased verbalization, inability to concentrate.	Client Goal: Understand prostatic hypertrophy and its treatment. Outcome Criteria: Describes function and anatomical location of gland by day 3. Describes 1 or 2 aspects of treatment for his condition by day 3. Experiences less anxiety as evidenced by use of coping mechanism by day 3.	Establish a good rapport with client by being supportive and empathetic. *Rationale:* Encourages client to ask questions and seek assistance. Encourage verbalization of concerns. *Rationale:* Assists client in working through his feelings and fears. Assess client's learning needs. *Rationale:* Will permit building upon client's present understanding of his condition. Adapt teaching to client's abilities. *Rationale:* Learning will be more meaningful to client. Reduce client's anxiety by explaining health problem. *Rationale:* Knowledge may decrease anxiety. Instruct client regarding dietary and activity restrictions. *Rationale:* Knowing what foods or activities to avoid will decrease symptoms of disease.	Client was able to relate his urinary problems to his enlarged prostate gland by day 3. He states he now knows to avoid spicy foods, alcohol, and coffee. He was able to verbalize his fears regarding his difficulty in voiding and the possibility of future surgery "to stop this dribbling."

CHAPTER HIGHLIGHTS

▶ Urinary elimination depends on normal functioning of the urinary, cardiovascular, and nervous systems.

▶ The normal process of micturition includes sufficient accumulation of urine in the bladder to stimulate the sensory stretch nerves in the bladder wall. Impulses from these stretch receptors then travel to the spinal cord, to the voiding reflex center and to the voiding control center in the cerebral cortex, where conscious control of micturition is regulated.

▶ In the adult, micturition generally occurs after 250 to 450 ml of urine has collected in the bladder.

▶ Many factors influence a person's urinary elimination including fluid intake, stress, activity, medications, and various diseases.

▶ Alterations in urinary elimination include polyuria, oliguria, anuria, frequency, nocturia, urgency, dysuria, enuresis, hematuria, incontinence, and retention. Each has various influencing and associated factors that need to be identified.

▶ A comprehensive assessment of a client's urinary function includes (a) a nursing history that identifies normal voiding patterns, usual urine and recent changes, past and current problems with urination, and factors influencing the elimination pattern; (b) a physical assessment of the kidneys, bladder, and urethral meatus; (c) inspection of the urine for amount, color, clarity, and odor, and, if indicated, (d) testing of urine for specific gravity, pH, and the presence of glucose, ketone bodies, and occult blood.

▶ Many NANDA approved nursing diagnoses may be applicable to clients with altered urinary elimination patterns, e.g., potential for infection.

▶ Incontinence can be physically and emotionally distressing to clients because it is considered socially unacceptable.

- Bladder-training programs can effectively reduce the incidence of incontinence episodes.

- Clients with urinary retention not only experience discomfort but also are at risk of urinary tract infection.

- The most common cause of urinary tract infection are invasive procedures such as catheterization and cystoscopic examination. Females in particular are prone to ascending urinary tract infections because of their short urethras.

- Nursing interventions related to urinary elimination are generally directed toward facilitating the normal functioning of the urinary system or toward assisting the client with particular problems.

- Interventions include (a) assisting the client to maintain an appropriate fluid intake, (b) assisting the client to maintain normal voiding patterns, (c) monitoring the client's daily fluid intake and output, and (d) maintaining cleanliness of the genital area.

- Urinary catheterization is frequently required for clients with urinary retention but is only performed when all other measures to facilitate voiding fail. Sterile technique is essential to prevent ascending urinary infections.

- Care of clients with indwelling catheters is directed toward preventing infection of the urinary tract and encouraging urinary flow through the drainage system.

READINGS AND REFERENCES

SUGGESTED READINGS

Cunha, B. A. July 1987. Nosocomial urinary tract infections. *Physician Assistant* 11:51–53, 56–57.

Urinary tract infections (UTIs) are the most common hospital-acquired infection in the United States. They can cause serious complications such as bacteremia and endocarditis, which significantly increase mortality and morbidity. Cunha discusses the major causes of UTI, its diagnosis, the difference between colonization and infection, and specific therapeutic approaches for catheter-related problems, bacteremia, and endocarditis in both normal and compromised hosts. Diligent hand washing between clients is emphasized as a major prevention and control measure.

McCormick, K. A.; Scheve, A. A. S.; and Leahy, E. March 1988. Nursing management of urinary incontinence in geriatric inpatients. *Nursing Clinics of North America* 23:231–264.

The authors describe the many management and treatment modalities for incontinence available to clients in long-term care facilities. Nursing implications for each modality are identified. The authors include staffing needed for an incontinence unit, management principles, assessing the client's ability to sense and communicate bladder fullness, manageable environmental factors, physical treatment regimens for urinary incontinence (drugs, devices, procedures, surgery), psychosocial treatment of incontinence, and behavioral interventions. Ten tables expand the above content.

Norton, C. March 1987. Continence and the older person. *Geriatric Nursing and Home Care* 7:9–13.

In this first article in her series on continence and the elderly, Norton outlines a knowledge base from which the nurse can work, discussing the aim of care, the prevalence of urinary incontinence, common causes of incontinence, essentials for maintaining continence, and possible side-effects of commonly prescribed drugs on bladder function (e.g., digoxin, chlorpromazine, and propantheline).

————. June 1987. Improving bladder function. *Geriatric Nursing and Home Care* 7:22–26.

In this fourth article in her series, Norton outlines the methods by which bladder function can be enhanced: bladder training; pelvic floor exercises; surgery for stress incontinence, outflow obstruction, and postprostatectomy incontinence; drugs to treat detrusor instability, stress incontinence, and incomplete bladder emptying; and clean intermittent catheterization for young persons with voiding difficulties (e.g., those with spinal injury or multiple sclerosis). A continence chart and two tables are included.

RELATED RESEARCH

Brink, C. A.; Wells, T. J.; and Diokno, A. C. June 1987. Urinary incontinence in women. *Public Health Nursing* 4:114–19.

Bristol, S. L.; Fadden, T.; Fehring, R. J.; Rohde, L.; Prue, K. S.; and Wohlitz, B. A. March 1989. The mythical danger of rapid urinary drainage. *American Journal of Nursing* 89:344–45.

Burgener, S. March 1987. Justification of closed intermittent urinary catheter irrigation/instillation: A review of current research and practice. *Journal of Advanced Nursing* 12:229–34.

Burke, J. P.; Jacobsen, J. A.; Garibaldi, R. A.; Conti, M.; and Alling, D. W. February 1983. Evaluation of daily meatal care with poly-antibiotic ointment in prevention of urinary catheter-associated bacteriuria. *Journal of Urology* 129:331–34.

Creason, N. S.; Grybowski, J. A.; Burgener, S.; Whippo, C.; Yeo, S.; and Richardson, B. February 1989. Prompted voiding therapy for urinary incontinence in aged female nursing home residents. *Journal of Advanced Nursing* 14:120–26.

Herzog, A. R.; Fultz, N. H.; Normolle, D. P.; Brock, B. M.; and Diokno, A. C. April 1989. Methods used to manage urinary incontinence by older adults in the community. *Journal of American Geriatric Society* 37:339–47.

SELECTED REFERENCES

Black, P. A. April 1990. Urinary incontinence: A many faceted problem. *Professional Nurse* 5:378, 380, 382+.

Blannin, J. February 1987. Incontinence: Men's problems. *Community Outlook:* 27,29.

Bristol, S. L.; Fadden, T.; Fehring, R. J.; Rohde, L.; Prue, K. S.; and Wohlitz, B. A. March 1989. The mythical danger of rapid urinary drainage. *American Journal of Nursing* 89:344–45.

Brogna, L., and Lakaszawski, M. L. February 1986. The continent urostomy . . . the Kock pouch. *American Journal of Nursing* 86:160–63.

Burke, J. P.; Jacobsen, J. A.; Garibaldi, R. A.; Conti, M.; and Alling, D. W. February 1983. Evaluation of daily meatal care with poly-antibiotic ointment in prevention of urinary catheter-associated bacteriuria. *Journal of Urology* 129:331–34.

Byrne, C. J.; Saxton, D. F.; Pelikan, P. K.; and Nugent, P. M. 1986. *Laboratory tests implications for nursing care.* 2d ed. Menlo Park, Calif.: Addison-Wesley Publishing Co.

Carpenito, L. J. 1989. *Nursing diagnosis: Application to clinical practice.* 3d ed. Philadelphia: J. B. Lippincott Co.

Cefalu, C. A. June 1987. Management of the bedridden patient with irreversible urinary incontinence. *Hospital Medicine* 23:183–87.

Conti, M. T., and Eutropius, L. March 1987. Preventing UTIs: What works? *American Journal of Nursing* 87:307–9.

Cunha, B. A. July 1987. Nosocomial urinary tract infections. *Physician Assistant* 11:51–53, 56–57.

Epstein, S. E. December 1985. Cost-effective application of the Centers for Disease Control Guidelines for prevention of catheter-associated urinary tract infections. *American Journal of Infection Control* 13:272–75.

Fader, M. January 1987. Assessing incontinence in the elderly. *Geriatric Nursing and Home Care* 7:10–12.

Frank, A., and Murray, S. M. June 1988. A no-guess guide for urinary color assessment. *RN* 51:46–47,49,51.

Gray, M., and Dougherty, M. C. July/August, 1987. Urinary incontinence: Pathophysiology and treatment. *Journal of Enterostomal Therapy* 14:152–62.

Greig, B. J. November/December 1986. Interventions of the ET nurse with the continent urinary Kock pouch patient. *Journal of Enterostomal Therapy* 13:226–31.

Gurevich, I. July 1985. Selection of closed urinary drainage systems: An update. *Infection Control* 6:289–90.

Guyton, A. C. 1986. *Textbook of medical physiology.* 7th ed. Philadelphia: W. B. Saunders Co.

Hahn, K. January 1988. Think twice about urinary incontinence. *Nursing 88* 18:65–67.

Hart, J. A. 1985. The urethral catheter: A review of its implication in urinary tract infection. *International Journal of Nursing Studies* 22(1):57–59.

Home Teaching Aid. July/August 1985a. Testing your urine for glucose and ketones. *Nursing Life* 5:32.

Home Teaching Aid. July/August 1985b. Urine self-testing: What your patient needs to know. *Nursing Life* 5:31.

Innes, B., and Bruga, M. Summer/Fall 1977. Postoperative voiding patterns and related contributing factors. *Washington State Journal of Nursing* 49:13–16.

Kim, M. J.; McFarland, G. K.; and McLane, A. M. 1989. *Pocket guide to nursing diagnoses.* 3d ed. St. Louis: C. V. Mosby Co.

Kirkpatrick, M. K., and Davies, C. July/August 1987. A bladder retraining program in a long-term-care facility. *Nursing Homes* 36:29–31.

Kuhns-Hastings, J. February 1988. Management of female incontinence with Kegel exercises. *American Association of Occupational Health Nurses Journal* 36:78–83.

Lapides, J.; Diokno, A. C.; Silber, S. J.; and Lowe, B. S. March 1972. Clean, intermittent self catheterization in the treatment of urinary tract disease. *Journal of Urology* 107:458–61.

Laycock, J. July 10, 1987. Graded exercises for the pelvic floor muscles in the treatment of urinary incontinence. *Physiotherapy* 73:371–73.

Lowthian, P. March 23–30, 1988. Steps to combat infection. *Nursing Times* 84:64–66.

McConnell, J. November/December 1984. Preventing urinary tract infections. *Geriatric Nursing* 5:361–62.

McConnell, E. A., and Zimmerman, M. I. 1983. *Care of patients with urologic problems.* Philadelphia: J. B. Lippincott Co.

McCormick, K. A. March 1988. Urinary incontinence in the elderly. *Nursing Clinics of North America* 23:135–37.

McCormick, K. A.; Scheve, A. A. S.; and Leahy, E. March 1988. Nursing management of urinary incontinence in geriatric inpatients. *Nursing Clinics of North America* 23:231–64.

Mocsny, N. March 1980. Puncturing catheter balloons. *Nursing 80* 10:88.

Mullhall, A.; Chapman, R.; and Crow, R. January 27–February 2, 1988a. Catheters: The acquisition of bacteriuria. *Nursing Times* 84:61–62.

———. January 27–February 2, 1988b. Catheters: Emptying urinary drainage bags. *Nursing Times* 84:64,66.

———. January 27–February 2, 1988c. Catheters: Meatal cleansing. *Nursing Times* 84:66,69.

NANDA approved nursing diagnostic categories for clinical use and testing. Summer 1988. *Nursing Diagnosis Newsletter* 15:1–3.

Newman, D. K., and Smith, D. A. May 1988. Rx: Homecare. Helping geriatric patients master self catheterization. *RN* 51:86.

———. March 1989. Incontinence: The problem patients won't talk about. *RN* 52:42–45.

Norton, C. March 1987a. Continence and the older person. *Geriatric Nursing and Home Care* 7:9–13.

———. April 1987b. Assessing incontinence. *Geriatric Nursing and Home Care* 7:24–26.

———. June 1987c. Improving bladder function. *Geriatric Nursing and Home Care* 7:22–26.

———. July 1987d. Maintaining continence. *Geriatric Nursing and Home Care* 7:25–27.

Orzeck, S., and Ouslander, J. G. January/February 1987. Urinary incontinence: An overview of causes and treatment. *Journal of Enterostomal Therapy* 14:20–27.

Palmer, M. H. March 1988. Incontinence: The magnitude of the problem. *Nursing Clinics of North America* 23:139–57.

Peterson, H. January 1985a. When the patient is incontinent. *Patient Care* 19:49–52,54,57.

———. March 1985b. Tips on using a urinary catheter. *Patient Care* 19:155–56, 158–60.

Petillo, M. H. June 1987. The patient with a urinary stoma: Nursing management and patient education. *Nursing Clinics of North America* 22:263–79.

Pottle, B. November 26–December 2, 1986. When the sheets were changed . . . absorbent sheets designed for incontinent patients. *Nursing Times* 82:64,66.

Ramphal, M. September/October 1987. Urinary incontinence among nursing home patients: Issues in research. *Geriatric Nursing* 8:249–54.

Rees-Williams, C.; Meyrick, M.; and Jones, M. October 5–11, 1988. Making sense of . . . urinary catheters. *Nursing Times* 84:46–47.

Richard C. J. 1986. *Comprehensive nephrology nursing.* Boston: Little, Brown & Co.

Roe, B. H. February 1990. Study of the effects of education on patient's knowledge of their indwelling urethral catheters. *Journal of Advanced Nursing* 15:223–31.

Rousseau, P. March/April 1990. Chronic urinary incontinence in the elderly. *Ostomy Wound Management* 27:24–8, 32–6.

Seth, C. February 1987. Male incontinence. *Community Outlook:* 20–21.

Sewell, C. M.; Koza, M. A.; Luchi, R. J. et al. April 1988. Risk factors associated with a cluster of urinary tract infections on a geriatric unit caused by *Klebsiella pneumoniae* resistant to multiple antibiotics. *American Journal of Infection Control* 16:66–71.

Slade, N., and Gillespie, W. A. 1985. *The Urinary tract and the catheter: Infection and other problems.* Chichester: John Wiley and Sons.

Smith, D. A. J. March 1988. Continence restoration in the homebound patient. *Nursing Clinics of North America* 23:207–19.

Stark, J. L. July 1988. A quick guide to urinary tract assessment. *Nursing 88* 18:56–58.

Tideiksaar, R. February 1987. Infections in the elderly. 1. Diagnosis and treatment. *Physician Assistant* 11:17–24,28,31.

Tulloch, G. J. January/February 1989. The incontinency taboo. *Geriatric Nursing* 10:19.

Tunink, P. M. April 1988. Focus: Nursing diagnosis. Alteration in urinary elimination. *Journal of Gerontological Nursing* 14:25–30.

Turner, S. L., and Plymat, K. R. May/June 1988. As women age: Perspectives on urinary incontinence. *Rehabilitation Nursing* 13:132–35.

Voith, A. M. May/June 1988. Alterations in urinary elimination: Concepts, research and practice. *Rehabilitation Nursing.* 13:122–31.

Voith, A. M., and Smith, D. A. December 1985. Validation of the nursing diagnosis of urinary retention. *Nursing Clinics of North America* 20:723–29.

Weigel, J. W. January/February 1988. Urinary incontinence. *Journal of Enterostomal Therapy* 15:24–29.

Wells, T. April 15–21, 1987. Diagnosing incontinence type. *Nursing Times* 83:89,91.

———. May/June 1990. Conquering incontinence. *Geriatric Nursing* 11:133–5. Whaley, L. F., and Wong, D. L. 1989. *Essentials of pediatric nursing.* 3d ed. St. Louis: C. V. Mosby Co.

Whitman, S., and Kursh, E. D. April 1987. Curbing incontinence. *Journal of Gerontological Nursing* 13:35–40.

Williamson, M. L. January/February 1982. Reducing post-catheterization bladder dysfunction by reconditioning. *Nursing Research* 31:28–30.

CHAPTER

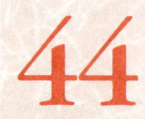

44

Sensory Perception and Cognition

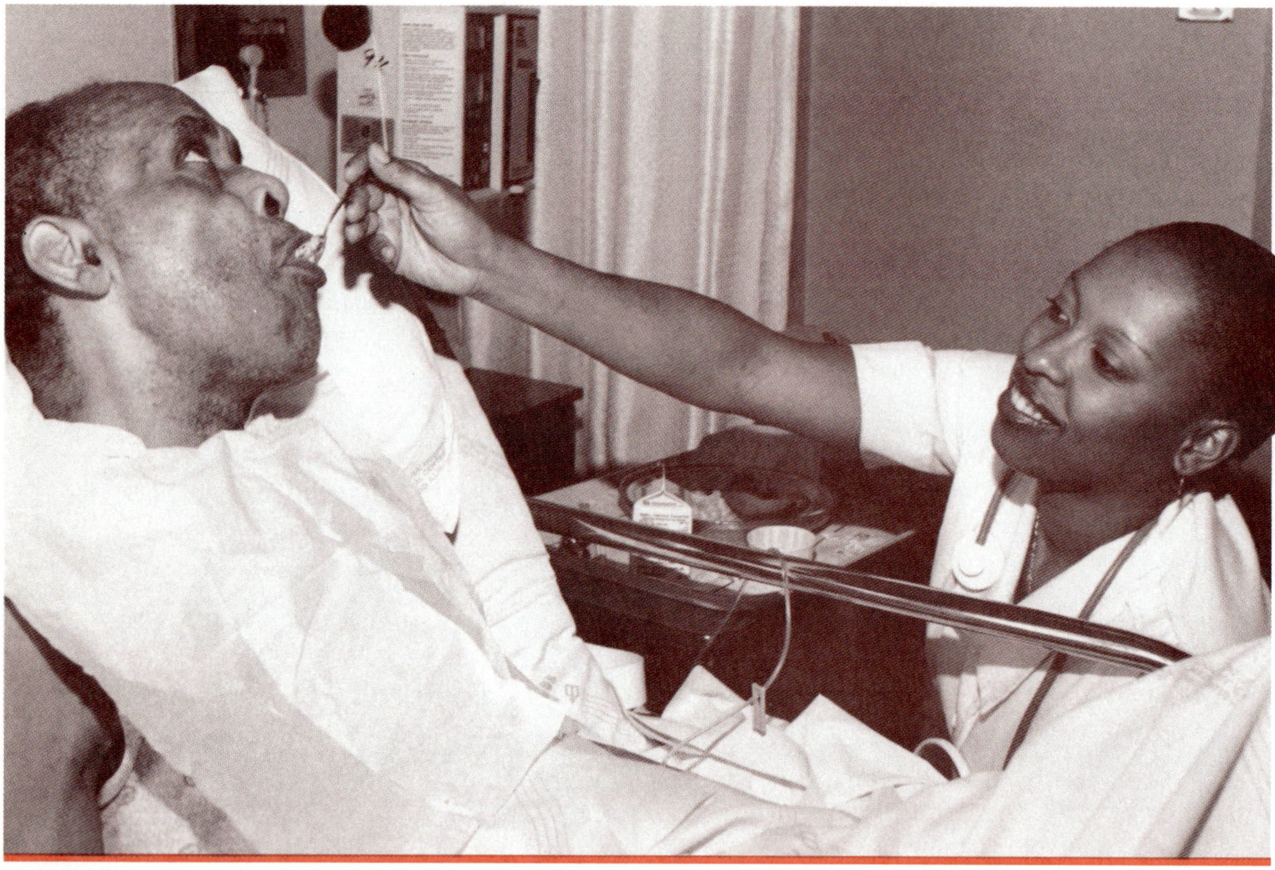

▶ Identify structural and physiologic elements of the sensory-perceptual process.

▶ Identify stages of awareness and consciousness.

▶ Identify causes and signs of three kinds of sensory disturbance.

▶ Identify factors influencing sensory function.

▶ Identify clients most at risk of sensory disturbances.

▶ Describe essential methods used to assess sensory/perceptual function and cognition.

▶ Identify clinical signs of sensory dysfunction.

▶ Develop nursing diagnoses for clients with impaired sensory and cognitive function.

▶ List outcome criteria to evaluate the effectiveness of goal achievement.

▶ Explain nursing interventions to promote and maintain sensory stimulation.

▶ Explain interventions that help the client adapt to altered sensory function and decrease further sensory loss.

THE SENSORY PROCESS

The sensory process involves two components: sensory reception and sensory perception. **Sensory reception** is the process of receiving stimuli or data. These stimuli are either external or internal to the body. External stimuli are **visual** (sight), **auditory** (hearing), **olfactory** (smell), **tactile** (touch), and **gustatory** (taste). Gustatory stimuli can be internal as well. Internal stimuli are kinesthetic or visceral. **Kinesthetic** refers to awareness of the position and movement of body parts. **Visceral** refers to any large organ in the body's interior. **Sensory perception** involves the organization and translation of the data or stimuli into meaningful information.

Sensory reception and perception are controlled by the nervous system. Once a stimulus triggers a sensory receptor, the stimulus travels along a neuron (sensory receptor I) to the central nervous system. From the spinal cord or brain stem, the impulses travel along sensory neuron II to the thalamus. These neurons synapse with sensory neurons III, which conduct the impulses from the thalamus to the somatosensory area of the postcentral gyrus of the parietal lobe of the brain, also called the primary sensory area. See Figure 44–1. In most instances, sensory pathways **decussate** (cross over) and register sensations from the opposite side of the body. Usually, decussation takes place at the level of sensory neuron II.

Sensory pathways carry information about heat, cold, touch, and pressure. **Stereognosis** (awareness of an object's size, shape, and texture), **kinesthesia** (ability to perceive muscle movement), vibratory sense, and two-point and weight discrimination are also sensory abilities that terminate in the primary sensory area. See Figure 44–2. Other special sensory areas are the visual, auditory, and olfactory association areas. The gustatory area is located in the parietal lobe deep in the lateral fissure.

After the reception and transmission of the stimuli, some data are integrated in the brain stem. It is this area that regulates many of the body's vital functions. The **reticular**

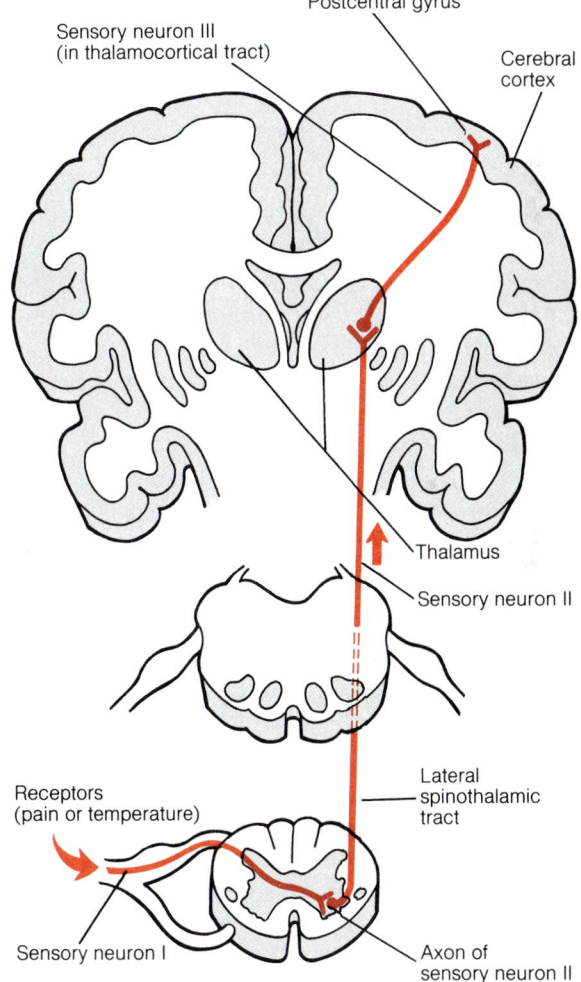

Figure 44–1 The lateral spinothalamic tract transmits impulses of crude touch, pain, and temperature up the spinal cord to the thalamus. The thalamocortical tract transmits impulses from the thalamus to the somatic sensory area of the cortex (postcentral gyrus).

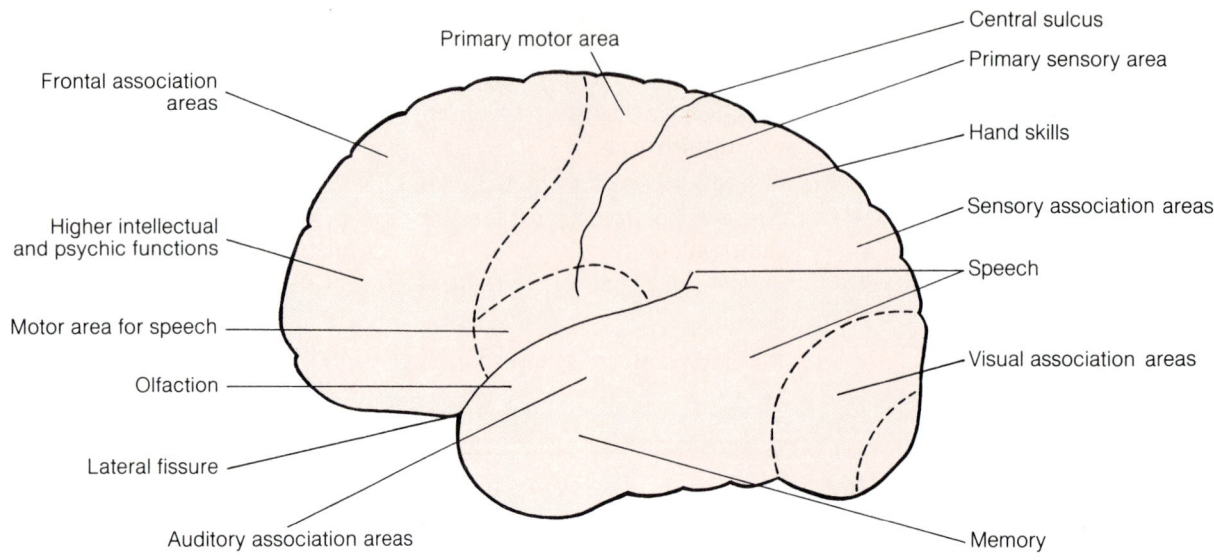

Figure 44–2 The lateral aspect of the functional areas of the left cerebral cortex.

formation, a diffuse network of neurons that extend throughout the brain stem, is situated here. See Figure 37–1, page 941. One part of the reticular formation, the **reticular activating system (RAS),** coordinates the input stimuli and regulates levels of awareness. The RAS, which extends from the lower level of the brain stem through the mesencephalon and thalamus to the cerebral cortex, activates the cerebral cortex and prepares it for incoming data. The role of the cortex is to process, interpret, use, and store the incoming data in an organized manner. For additional information on perception theory, see Chapter 4.

Cognition is cerebral functioning. It involves such processes as conscious thought, reality orientation, problem solving, judgment, and comprehension related to coping (personality, mental) disorders (Carpenito 1989, p. 726). The development of cognition is discussed in Chapter 24. **Awareness** is the ability to perceive environmental stimuli and body reactions and to respond appropriately through thought and action. The normal, alert person can assimilate many kinds of information at one time. The restaurant patron, for example, appreciates odors, tastes, conversation, and company at the same time. The normal person perceives reality accurately and acts on those perceptions.

FACTORS AFFECTING SENSORY STIMULATION

The need for sensory stimulation is called **sensoristasis.** Humans need constant and varied sensory stimuli. Insufficient stimuli cause sensory deprivation. Overstimulation at any one site causes **sensory adaptation,** a result of the ability of sensory receptors to adapt partially or completely to a repeated stimulus. At first, receptors respond at a very high impulse rate; with continued stimulation, the receptors respond less rapidly, and finally many do not respond at all. For this reason, the brain ceases to perceive the repeated stimulus. Extreme concentration produces a similar effect: The brain does not perceive extraneous stimuli. A number of factors affect sensory stimulation, including the person's development, culture, level of stress, medications, illness, and life-style.

Development   Perception of sensation is critical to the intellectual, social, and physical development of infants and children. As children grow, they learn that certain sensations provide cues for behavior already learned, e.g., stopping and looking both ways before crossing a street. Adults have many learned responses to sensory cues. Loss or impairment of any sense, therefore, has profound effects on both the child and young adult. The gradual diminishing of sensory perception that comes with age does not have as profound an effect.

Culture   An individual's culture often determines the amount of stimulation that person considers usual or "normal." For example, a child raised in a large, active Mexican-American family may be accustomed to more stimulation than one child raised in an Anglo-American family. In addition, the normal amount of stimulation associated with ethnic origin, religious affiliation, and income level, for example, also affects the amount of stimulation an individual desires and believes to be meaningful.

Stress During times of increased stress, people may find their senses already overloaded and thus seek to decrease sensory stimulation. For example, a client dealing with physical illness, pain, hospitalization, and diagnostic tests may wish to have only close support persons visit. In addition, the client may need the nurse's help to decrease unnecessary stimuli (e.g., noise) as much as possible.

Medications Certain medications can alter an individual's awareness of environmental stimuli. Narcotics and sedatives, for example, can decrease awareness of stimuli. Some antidepressants can alter perceptions of stimuli.

Illness Certain diseases, such as atherosclerosis, restrict blood flow to the receptor organ and the brain, thereby decreasing awareness and slowing responses. Uncontrolled diabetes mellitus can impair vision. Some central nervous system diseases cause varying degrees of paralysis and sensory loss.

Life-Style The amount of sensory stimulation varies according to a person's life-style. A nurse employed on a busy surgical unit of a hospital is accustomed to many diverse stimuli, whereas a nurse employed in a small long-term care unit is exposed to fewer, less diverse stimuli.

SENSORY ALTERATIONS

Alterations in sensory reception and sensory perception can lead to disorganized behavior.

Sensory Deprivation

Sensory deprivation, also called emotional-touch deprivation, results when the level of sensory input is too low for normal functioning. Sensory deprivation is situational. Ebersole and Hess (1985, p. 321) describe three reasons for sensory deprivation: (a) restricted environment, (b) reduced sensory input, and (c) decreased order and meaning from input.

When a person experiences sensory deprivation, the balance of the reticular activating system (RAS) is disturbed. The RAS is unable to maintain normal stimulation to the cerebral cortex. Because of this reduced stimulation, the person becomes more acutely aware of the remaining stimuli and perceives these in a distorted manner.

Elderly people are particularly susceptible to sensory deprivation, because of social isolation and a restricted environment. The elderly person can become socially isolated for a number of reasons, e.g., limited physical mobility, death of a spouse and/or friends, and changed living arrangements. The effects of sensory deprivation are cognitive, affective, and perceptual. See Table 44–1 for associated symptoms.

TABLE 44–1 *Symptoms of Sensory Deprivation*

Type	Symptoms
Cognitive	Reduced attention span; impaired memory and problem-solving ability; difficulty in concentrating
Affective	Inappropriate emotional response; depression; fear; anxiety; boredom; emotional lability
Perceptual	Inaccurate perception of stimuli; reduced motor coordination; disorientation

Sensory Overload

Sensory overload is more sensory stimulation in a given period than one can tolerate. Hospitalized clients, exposed to bright lights, noise, unfamiliar machinery, and too many visits from friends and health personnel, may suffer sensory overload. The person may appear fatigued, agitated, and confused. Two cognitive problems that may appear are hallucinations and illusions. **Hallucinations** are perceptions of external stimuli in the absence of such stimuli. **Illusions** are misinterpretations of external stimuli. For example, a person interprets a shadow as a person.

Sensory Deficits

A **sensory deficit** is impaired functioning of a sensory or perceptual process. Blindness and deafness are sensory deficits. When only one sense is affected, other senses may become more acute to compensate for the loss. However, sudden loss of eyesight can result in total disorientation.

When there is gradual loss of sensory function, individuals often develop behavioral alterations to compensate for the loss; sometimes, the behaviors are unconscious. For example, a person with gradual hearing loss in the right ear may unconsciously turn the left ear toward a speaker. When the loss is sudden, compensatory behavior often takes days or weeks to develop.

Some neurologic diseases cause changes in kinesthetic sense and tactile perceptions. Disease of the inner ear, for example, can cause loss of kinesthetic sense. Spinal cord injuries and cerebrovascular accidents cause paralysis and loss of tactile perception.

Vision Most people consider vision a critical sense. It can be affected by many disease conditions, e.g., uncontrolled diabetes mellitus, as well as age. Vision usually declines after age 45. Night vision, accommodation, and depth perception may be impaired, and sensitivity to glare may increase.

Hearing Hearing is often considered the second most important sense. Hearing impairment can lead to a decrease in self-esteem and to social isolation. Generally, elderly people experience loss of volume perception and pitch perception and impairment of hearing acuity (*presbycusis*). They often have difficulty in discriminating consonants, especially *s, f,* and *ch.*

Smell and Taste The sense of smell is often poorly developed. The receptors for smell are located in the mucous membrane. The sense of smell is an important safety factor aiding people to detect smoke and gas, and it also stimulates the appetite. Reduced sensitivity to odors is common in the elderly. The receptors for taste (gustation) are found in the mouth. There are four known tastes: salt, sweet, sour, and bitter. Both smell and taste are frequently diminished in chronic smokers.

Touch The receptors for the sense of touch (tactile sensation) are located in the skin. Receptors are sensitive to pressure, pain, temperature, and itching. Pain receptors protect the person from trauma; when pain is perceived, for example, the individual usually withdraws from the cause and seeks assistance. When the sense of touch is not functioning, a person can suffer injury and be unaware of it.

Alterations in Consciousness

Consciousness is awareness of environment, self, and others. It requires continuous stimulation of cortical neurons by impulses that pass through the reticular activating system. Illness and age can affect consciousness, as can hospitalization. Mildly confused hospitalized clients may momentarily forget they are not at home, wander from their rooms, misplace personal belongings, and so forth. Severely confused (disoriented) persons may not recognize family members or may think the nurse is a relative. Such persons may act atypically; severely confused people do not know where they are or what time of day or day of the week it is.

There are varying levels of consciousness. See Table 19–24 on page 429.

ASSESSING

When assessing the client for sensory/perceptual alterations, nurses should take a health history, examine the client for signs of sensory disturbance, perform required physical examinations, and identify clients at risk.

Nursing History

The nursing history focuses on sensory deficits. It includes not only the client's present sensory perceptions but also usual functioning and potential problems. In some instances,

significant others can provide data the person cannot. For example, a woman may detect her partner's hearing loss long before the partner is aware of it. Examples of interview questions to elicit data about the client's sensory/perceptual functioning are shown in the accompanying box.

Clinical Signs of Sensory/Perceptual Alterations

In addition to assessing the client for sensory deficits, the nurse observes clients for signs of sensory deprivation and sensory overload. Signs of both sensory deprivation and overload are similar and include the following:

- *Changes in attention span,* such as decreased concentration (inability to follow the flow of conversation), increased distractibility, restlessness, daydreaming. Persons who are daydreaming appear absorbed in their own thoughts and may talk and laugh to themselves. It may be difficult to engage such a person in conversation. These persons may confuse a daydream with reality and imagine a conversation that did not take place.
- *Changes in thought processes,* such as confusion about time, place, or person; disordered sequencing of time or events (e.g., the person may start a sentence on one subject and end it with an unrelated subject); difficulty in remembering what one was saying; difficulty in grasping ideas; slowness in communicating; indecision; bizarre thinking; illusions (e.g., interpreting a shadow as a man with a knife); and hallucinations.
- *Emotional lability,* such as rapid mood swings, irritability, exaggerated responses; apathy; ambivalence; emotional detachment; inappropriate reaction (e.g., laughing at bad news); anger; depression; anxiety, fear.
- *Changes in usual routines,* such as altered sleeping pattern (difficulty staying awake or difficulty sleeping) and altered eating pattern (e.g., loss of appetite). People tolerate the amount of environmental stimuli differently. For example, a mother of six active, noisy children may hardly notice the noise of her environment, whereas another person may find the noise bothersome. A child who has five brothers and sisters may be accustomed to a different level of sensory input than the only child. People whose developmental levels are characterized by short attention spans, a need for physical activity, and dependence on others for amusement are often more susceptible to sensory deprivation than people who are more self-reliant and contemplative. Likewise, persons who are stressed and anxious may have more difficulty in coping with sensory deprivation.

Physical Assessment

The nurse assesses vision, hearing, and olfactory, gustatory, tactile, and kinesthetic status. See Chapter 19 for additional information about these examinations. Physical assessment,

ASSESSMENT INTERVIEW
Sensory/Perceptual Functioning

Auditory

- Do you have any difficulty hearing, or have you had any recent changes in hearing?
- Do you wear a hearing aid? If so, when did you obtain it, and how well does it work for you?
- Can you locate the direction of sounds and distinguish various voices? (Persons with hearing aids often have difficulties in these areas.)
- Have you ever experienced a humming, ringing, buzzing, or crackling noise in the ears?

Visual

- Do you have any difficulty seeing near or far objects?
- Do you wear eyeglasses or contact lenses?
- Have you ever experienced any visual disturbances, such as blurred or double vision, rainbows or halos around lights or objects, blind spots, flashing lights, light sensitivity, troublesome spots or floaters?
- Have you or anyone in your family ever had glaucoma, cataracts, retinal detachment, or other eye problems?
- When did you last visit an ophthalmologist?

Gustatory

- Have you noticed any changes in your ability to taste (e.g., difficulty in differentiating sweet, sour, salty, and bitter tastes)?
- Do you find certain foods unpalatable? Which ones?

Olfactory

- Have you noticed any changes in your ability to smell (e.g., can you distinguish foods by their odors and tell when something is burning)?

Tactile

- Have you noticed any unusual sensations, such as "pins and needles" in your legs or arms?
- Have you ever had difficulty in perceiving heat, cold, or pain in your limbs? Have you had problems that alter your ability to do so?

Kinesthetic

- Have you ever noticed any difficulty in perceiving the position of parts of your body?

---

in particular, should reveal the client's specific visual and hearing abilities; perception of heat, cold, and pain in the limbs; and awareness of the position of the body parts.

Clients at Risk

Nurses need to be aware of those people who are particularly susceptible to sensory disturbances. By anticipating possible problems, the nurse can often implement measures to prevent them. The following circumstances may predispose the client to sensory disturbances.

- *Nonstimulating environments.* People who normally live alone and have little contact with others may experience sensory overload when they are hospitalized. This is particularly true of the elderly and of people who work at home alone. In their homes, these persons are at risk of sensory deprivation. People who live in institutions with unchanging social and perceptual stimuli are also at risk of sensory deprivation.
- *Therapeutic isolation.* Therapeutic isolation, either in the hospital or at home, can predispose the client to sensory

deprivation. Clients on protective asepsis are often confined to a room; gowned, masked personnel are their primary social contacts. Clients confined to bed, even if they are in rooms with other clients and allowed visitors, are also prone.

- *Medically intensive environments.* Clients in constantly staffed environments are often overloaded with stimuli. Clients in intensive care and coronary care units are never left alone. The noises, machines, and lights of such environments further the risk of sensory overload.
- *Known sensory deficits.* Clients with sensory deficits are at risk of both sensory deprivation and sensory overload. Persons with visual problems may be unable to read, watch television, or recognize nurses by sight. An unfamiliar environment can add to their confusion. The blind often have highly structured home environments, and the diversity and unfamiliarity of the hospital environment can create sensory overload. At the same time, impaired vision often means inability to move around readily or socialize with others. Deaf persons who cannot lip-read also may feel isolated.

See the box above for a summary of people at risk for sensory/perceptual alterations.

DIAGNOSING

The NANDA nursing diagnosis for clients with sensory perceptual problems is **Sensory/perceptual alteration** which must be specified as **visual, auditory, kinesthetic, gustatory, tactile,** or **olfactory.** It is defined as the state in which a person experiences or is at risk of experiencing a change in the amount or patterning of incoming stimuli. It is accompanied by a diminished, exaggerated, distorted, or impaired response to such stimuli. Because these specific deficits are often the result of a disease process or physiologic changes, the nurse may find that focusing on the client's responses to the deficit may be more appropriate (Carpenito 1989, p. 660). In this situation, the client's response becomes the diagnostic category, and the sensory/perceptual alteration becomes the etiology. For example, **Potential for injury** related to **Sensory/perceptual alteration: Visual** directs the nursing interventions more appropriately than **Sensory/perceptual alteration: Visual** related to the effects of cataracts. Many diagnostic categories discussed in detail throughout this book focus on *responses* to sensory/perceptual alterations, including **Impaired verbal communication, Impaired home maintenance management, Altered nutrition: Less than body requirements, Self-care deficit, Potential impaired skin integrity, Sleep pattern disturbance, Social isolation,** and **Altered thought processes** (a disruption in such mental activities as conscious thought, reality orientation, problem solving, judgment, and comprehension). Examples of these diagnoses and contributing factors are shown below. Examples of assessment data clusters and related nursing diagnoses are shown in Table 44–2.

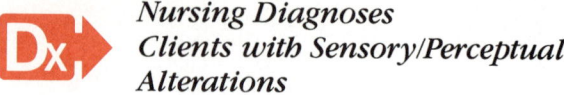

**Nursing Diagnoses
Clients with Sensory/Perceptual Alterations**

Potential for injury related to:

- Visual impairment (e.g., decreased depth perception)
- Reduced tactile sensation secondary to (specify—e.g., neurologic or circulatory alterations)
- Decreased sense of smell
- Decreased kinesthetic sense

Impaired verbal communication related to:

- Hearing impairment
- Sensory overload
- Sensory deprivation

Impaired home maintenance management related to declining visual abilities

Altered nutrition: Less than body requirements related to:

- Reduced sense of smell
- Sensory deprivation

Self-care deficit: Bathing/hygiene related to visual impairment

Potential impaired skin integrity related to reduced tactile sensation

Sleep pattern disturbance related to:

- Sensory deprivation
- Sensory overload

Social isolation related to:

- Impaired vision
- Impaired hearing

Altered thought processes related to:

- Sensory deprivation from imposed bed rest
- Sensory overload in intensive care unit

PLANNING

Overall client goals for persons with sensory/perceptual alterations include (a) maintaining or promoting the function of existing senses, (b) decreasing or eliminating signs of altered sensory function, (c) preventing injury, (d) maintaining nutrition, (e) maintaining or improving communication pattern, (f) maintaining or restoring ability to function in the environment safely, and (g) achieving self-care. Nursing interventions to achieve these goals may include adjusting environmental stimuli, providing a safe environment, encouraging as much independence as possible,

TABLE 44-2   Examples of Assessment Data Clusters and Related Nursing Diagnoses for Clients with Sensory Perceptual Alterations

Data Cluster	Nursing Diagnosis
Ralph Roberts, a 93-year-old widower, lives alone in his condominium. He can hear clearly spoken words close to left ear but cannot hear any sounds with right ear. He says he spends his time listening to the TV and radio (set at loud volumes). He tends to speak loudly and shout when talking with others, and nods and smiles when others speak. Daughter who visits says he refuses to wear a hearing aid (he says "it increases all the background sounds and doesn't help"). She has noticed recently that he has become withdrawn, appears absorbed in his own thoughts and talks and laughs to himself.	**Social isolation** related to declining auditory function associated with aging.
Flora Flower, an 86-year-old, has cataracts and wears bifocals. She reports difficulty with stairs (says "they all seem to blend together"), difficulty with bright lights and glare off shiny surfaces ("everything looks like a whitish blur"), and difficulty accommodating from a dark place to a sunny place or a brightly lit room to a dark room ("I don't seem to be able to adjust as I used to to light and dark"). Is able to read only large print with a magnifying glass and reports difficulty driving, especially at night.	**Potential for injury** related to declining vision secondary to aging and cataracts.
Tony Brown, a 52-year-old lawyer, has multiple sclerosis. Muscle strength in hands, arms, and legs has declined over past 2 years. He uses a three-wheeled motorized wheelchair to move about. Reports loss of sensation in lower limbs and inability to discern temperature differences. Wife assists with bathing/grooming hygienic care.	**Potential for injury** related to decreased tactile sensation secondary to neurologic impairment.

teaching clients ways to enhance existing sensory function, and informing clients how to prevent sensory loss. Examples of outcome criteria for clients with sensory/perceptual alterations follow.

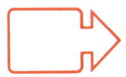

Outcome Criteria
Clients with Sensory/Perceptual Alterations

The client:

- Describes type, amount, and patterns of usual daily stimulation.
- Verbalizes presence of sensory overload or deprivation.
- Demonstrates decreased signs of sensory overload (or deprivation), as evidenced by, for example, communicating clearly with others, differentiating reality from fantasy, expressing fewer delusions, demonstrating fewer exaggerated emotional responses.
- Maintains orientation to time, place, and person.
- Demonstrates an increase in self-care activities.
- Remains free of injury.
- Demonstrates use of methods to alter environment.
- Sleeps at least 6 hours daily without awakening.
- Responds appropriately to questions and cues.
- Initiates interaction with others.

IMPLEMENTING

Nursing intervention can help reduce the effects of sensory overload and sensory deprivation and help clients with sensory deficits cope effectively.

Adjusting Environmental Stimuli

When a client is at risk of overstimulation or understimulation, nurses can adjust the environmental stimuli. A client who is understimulated needs to be provided with meaningful stimuli for all the senses. Clients who are overstimulated need a reduction in the number and type of stimuli. When a client is overstimulated, the nurse can counteract sensory overload by blocking stimuli and by helping the client organize the stimuli and alter responses to the stimuli.

Blocking Stimuli   Dark glasses can partially block light rays, and a sunscreen or a drape over a window can reduce visual stimulation. Ear plugs reduce auditory stimuli, as do soft background music and earphones. The odor from a draining wound can often be minimized by keeping the dressing dry and clean and applying a liquid deodorant on a gauze near the wound.

Another method of reducing sensory stimulation is to establish a nursing care plan that reduces novelty and surprise and provides rest intervals free of interruptions. Sometimes the number of visitors and the length of visits must be restricted. A nurse can organize care so that the client has long periods of little stimulation. If the nurse carries out several nursing measures together, the client can have a scheduled quiet period before the next activity.

Organizing Stimuli   If the nurse explains the sounds in the environment, the client can organize them mentally: A bell signals a change of shift; a buzzer, a change of IV. When clients understand their meaning, stimuli are frequently less confusing and more easily ignored.

Altering Responses   People can learn to alter their responses to stimuli. Clients can employ relaxation techniques to reduce anxiety and stress despite continual sensory stimulation. See Chapter 33 for additional information.

Promoting the Function of Existing Senses

Providing significant and meaningful stimuli can help the client use existing senses and prevent sensory alterations.

Vision   Because visual problems are commonly due to refractive errors, children and adults may need encouragement to have visual screening. To promote existing visual function, the nurse can teach the client to strengthen visual stimuli, use other senses to supplement sight, and establish a meaningful environment. See the accompanying box.

Hearing   The following measures can help maximize a person's residual hearing:

- Encouraging the client to have a hearing test
- Obtaining a telephone with an amplified ring and speaker
- Maintaining a hearing aid in good order
- Reducing background noise
- Keeping conversational groups small

The nurse communicates appropriately to the hearing-impaired client to convey respect, enhance the person's self-esteem, and ensure the exchange of correct information. The hearing-impaired person has to concentrate more than the unimpaired person and, therefore, tires more readily. Fatigue compounded by an illness can seriously alter the person's ability to hear.

The following guidelines can improve communication with the hearing-impaired person:

- Talk at a moderate rate and in a normal tone of voice. Shouting does not make your voice more distinct and, in some instances, makes understanding more difficult.
- Address the person directly. Do not turn away in the middle of a remark or story. Make sure the person can see your face easily and that it is well lighted.
- Avoid talking when you have something in your mouth, such as a pipe, cigar, cigarette, or chewing gum. Avoid covering your mouth with your hand.

Supporting Visual Function

Strengthening Visual Stimuli

- Arrange for suitable lighting, including night lights.
- Obtain reading material with large print.
- Obtain a magnifying glass and a phone dialer and wrist watch with large numbers.
- Use two side mirrors on a car to increase the visual field.
- Use contrasting colors to highlight material to be seen.
- Use colored rims on dishes.
- Color code dials on stoves, washer, and so on.

Increasing Use of Other Senses

- Provide materials that can be identified by other senses, i.e., materials of various textures and odors.
- Point out odors, shapes, and so on.
- Encourage handling of articles.
- Announce who you are when entering the room of a visually impaired person.

Establishing a Meaningful Environment

- Minimize glare by using soft, diffuse lighting.
- Use sunglasses and shades on windows.
- Keep furniture in its usual places.

- Keep your voice at about the same volume throughout each sentence, without dropping the voice at the end of each sentence.
- Always speak as clearly and accurately as possible. Articulate consonants in particular with care.
- Do not "overarticulate"; mouthing or overdoing articulation is just as troublesome as mumbling.
- Use longer phrases, which tend to be easier to understand than short ones. For example, "Will you get me a drink of water?" presents much less difficulty than "Will you get me a drink?" Word choice is important here: "Fifteen cents" and "fifty cents" may be confused, but "half a dollar" is clear.
- Pronounce every name with care. Make a reference to the name for easier understanding, e.g., "Joan, the girl from the office" or "the Bay, the big downtown store."
- Change to a new subject at a slower rate, making sure that the person follows the change to the new subject. A key word or two at the beginning of a new topic is a good indicator.

- When you are asked to repeat a sentence, find a different way of saying that same thing rather than repeating the original words over and over.
- Minimize background noise, such as traffic sounds, television, and a loud radio, which makes listening more difficult.

Taste   Maintaining good oral hygiene and hydration enhances the sense of taste. Foods need to be well seasoned, hot foods served hot, and cold foods served cold. Foods should also provide a variety of textures and be eaten separately.

Smell   Nurses can encourage clients to use the sense of smell. The aroma of fragrant flowers or cologne can make the environment more attractive. Nurses can eliminate unpleasant odors by ensuring adequate ventilation and by removing old dressings and equipment. Nurses and family can assist the client by refraining from wearing heavy perfumes.

 Touch   Clients with an impaired sense of touch must take protective measures to prevent injury. They may not be aware of hot temperatures, which can cause burns, or pressure on bony prominences, which can produce decubitus ulcers. Nurses can also provide the client with a variety of textures to enhance the remaining tactile sense.

Preventing Sensory Loss   Certain occupations or life-styles can produce or worsen sensory loss. For example, a person working in a noisy factory needs to wear protective ear covers to prevent hearing loss. People working where chemicals or solid materials are likely to fly into the eyes should wear goggles. Chemicals can burn the corneas, and small objects can penetrate the eyes, causing permanent injury.

Providing Meaningful Stimulation

Nurses should provide a variety of stimuli that appeal to different senses, e.g., newspapers, varied foods, and music. Clocks that differentiate night from day by color can help orient a client. Nurses can help by providing objects that are pleasant to touch. For example, many people obtain great joy from holding and stroking a pet.

Before planning interventions for the understimulated client, the nurse needs to determine the etiology of the sensory deprivation. Deprivation is usually due to inadequate stimuli, inability to receive stimuli, or inability to process stimuli.

Inadequate stimuli can mean insufficient stimuli. Stimuli are also inadequate when they are monotonous, infrequent, or too weak. A client who is confined to bed in a private room without television or radio and receives visitors only once a week is probably inadequately stimulated. After a

RESEARCH NOTE

What Foods Are Most Unpalatable to Cancer Clients Who Experience Changes in Taste Sensation?

Because a change in taste sensation is one cause of anorexia in cancer clients, Stubbs conducted a study to determine whether any particular foods were reported as tasting more unpleasant than others. A list of 25 foods and drinks representative of an average everyday diet was developed, and 218 clients with lung, cervical, and ovarian cancer participated. The clients were assessed after diagnosis, before receiving any treatment. Findings revealed that one in four clients experienced alterations in taste perception. Items clients found most unpalatable included protein-rich foods, such as meat, bacon, ham, and fried eggs; sweets and chocolates; and beverages such as tea, coffee, beer, wine, and spirits. Meat aversion was found to increase as the day progressed, and some clients found the taste of chilled or frozen foods more acceptable.

Implications: Dietary manipulations may be helpful for clients with cancer who experience changes in taste sensation. For example, a high-protein breakfast may benefit clients with meat aversion, which progresses throughout the day. Lentils, dried peas, beans, nuts, cheese, eggs, and fish may serve as alternatives for meat. The flavor of foods may be enhanced with herbs, spices, sugar, lemon, and tasty sauces.

L. Stubbs, Taste changes in cancer patients, *Nursing Times,* January 18–25, 1989, 85:49–50.

short time, e.g., several weeks, this client may experience sensory deprivation.

Providing Meaningful Communication

Aphasia   Clients with **aphasia** (impaired speech) may find it frustrating to be unable to express their thoughts coherently. Such persons can frequently think clearly even though their speech is impaired. Nurses can help aphasic clients communicate their needs and thoughts in writing or with a communication board. Some communication boards have pictures to which clients can point to express their needs. An important aspect of the aphasic client's care is teaching support persons how to enhance the client's independence. Sometimes people think it is kind to speak for the aphasic client, not realizing that the client should be encouraged to communicate by whatever means are available.

Altered Level of Consciousness   An altered level of consciousness can be frightening to both clients and their support persons. Often clients know that something is wrong and that they need help. The following interventions may help clients and support persons:

- Reorient the confused client to self, time, and place.
- Listen carefully to the client's and support person's concerns. Often they simply want to express them.
- Maintain the same schedule each day. Routine gives the client a sense of security and sometimes decreases confusion.
- Touch and stroke the unconscious client.
- Explain what is happening to the support persons, and encourage them to talk to and touch the unconscious client as though the client were conscious. This auditory and tactile stimulation supports the client and may restore some degree of consciousness.

If the client is unconscious, necessary nursing interventions include bathing, giving skin care, feeding, and meeting elimination needs. If the client is disoriented but conscious, the nurse may need to give instructions on how to perform these activities. Unless the person is totally incapacitated, it is preferable to foster independence and feelings of self-worth by helping the individual provide self-care than to give complete care to a passive client.

EVALUATING

Evaluative activities depend on the goals and the outcome criteria set in the planning phase. If the goal is to remain free of injury, the nurse simply asks or observes the client for verification of this. If the goal is to promote the function of existing senses (e.g., vision), the nurse needs to examine the client's visual function while using visual aids. If the goal is to maintain usual communication pattern, the nurse may need to determine whether the client responds to questions appropriately and initiates conversion with others.

NURSING CARE PLAN FOR JULIA HAGSTROM

ASSESSMENT DATA

Nursing Assessment

Mrs. Julia Hagstrom, an 80-year-old widow, has recently become a resident of an extended care facility. Just prior to her admission to the extended care facility, she underwent surgery for the removal of cataracts. She had also experienced increased difficulty in hearing. Her children, concerned about her physical safety and her lack of socialization, urged her to enter a nursing home. Up until the time Mrs. Hagstrom entered the extended care facility, she had lived alone in her home for 15 years and cared for herself independently. Three days after she was admitted to Valley View Home, her nurse, Marie Carter, finds Mrs. Hagstrom to be somewhat confused and disoriented to person, place, and time. She appears restless and withdrawn, and her syntax is sometimes confused. She states, "I'm afraid of all these strange creatures in this orphanage."

Physical Examination
Height: 160 cm (5'3")
Weight: 55.3 kg (122 lb)
Temperature: 37 C (98.6 F)
Pulse rate: 72 BPM
Respirations: 18 per minute
Blood pressure: 128/74 mm Hg
Rinne test: Negative

Diagnostic Data
Chest x-ray film: Negative
CBC: Negative
Urine: Negative

Nursing Diagnosis	Client Goals and Output Criteria	Nursing Interventions and Rationales	Evaluation
Altered thought processes related to change in environment and hearing loss, resulting in disorientation to time, place, and person; restlessness; fear; and altered behavior.	Client Goal: Demonstrate decreased symptoms and increased level of orientation to reality. Outcome Criteria: Is oriented to place, month, and year when questioned by day 3. Participates in self-care activities by day 3. Identifies 1 or 2 caregivers by name by day 4.	Assess for factors contributing to confusion. *Rationale:* Identification of contributing factors will assist in eliminating such factors. Establish daily routine. *Rationale:* Decreases novelty, surprise, and overstimulation. Provide for adequate rest periods. *Rationale:* Reduces overstimulation and fatigue. Attempt to assign same caregiver as often as possible. *Rationale:* Familiarity reduces confusion. Encourage caregivers to speak slowly and as one adult to another. *Rationale:* Enhances communication and client's dignity and self-esteem. Provide for meaningful sensory input. *Rationale:* Increases client's orientation to person, place, and time. Encourage client's participation in ADLs. *Rationale:* Increases client's self-esteem and sense of control.	Client identifies Miss Carter by sight and name. On December 3rd, during the course of the morning's conversation, she questions whether any shopping trips are planned for next week "since Christmas is only three weeks from now." She bathes herself each morning and makes her own bed.
Impaired verbal communication related to auditory impairment, resulting in decreased comprehension, inattention to voices/noises, and confusion.	Client Goal: Demonstrate improved ability to communicate. Outcome Criteria: Wears hearing aid during waking hours by day 2. Communicates effectively with care provider by day 5. Indicates feeling of well-being by day 5.	Assess ability to hear and speak. *Rationale:* Identifies client's specific problems of communication. Obtain client's attention before speaking. *Rationale:* Aids in establishing first step in communication. Lower sound on television or radio when communicating with client. *Rationale:* Extraneous environmental noises can interfere with communication for the hearing-impaired client. Speak slowly and distinctly while facing client. *Rationale:* Client will be better able to lip-read and comprehend speech. Assume a position for good eye contact. *Rationale:* Conveys interest and promotes better contact between client and caregiver. Establish therapeutic relationship. *Rationale:* Therapeutic relationship is necessary when dealing with communication problems.	Client's daughter has brought new batteries for client's hearing aid, and client now wears her hearing aid during the day. She recognizes Miss Carter by name and talks to her about her family and her former home. She states, "I guess at my age, it's best to have someone nearby at all times."

CHAPTER HIGHLIGHTS

- Awareness includes the ability to perceive environmental stimuli and respond appropriately.

- Sensoristasis is the need for sensory stimulation.

- Sensory stimuli can be visual, auditory, olfactory, tactile, gustatory, kinesthetic, and visceral.

- Sensory deprivation is a level of stimulation that is too low to permit normal functioning.

- Sensory overload is more sensory stimulation than a person can tolerate.

- Sensory deficit is an impairment in the sensory or perceptual process.

- The nurse needs to identify clients at most risk of developing sensory disturbances.

- A person who appears bored and sleeps excessively may be experiencing sensory deprivation.

- Sensory overload may be manifested as agitation and restlessness but can produce some of the same clinical signs that sensory deprivation produces.

READINGS AND REFERENCES

SUGGESTED READINGS

Chovaz, C. March 1989. Nursing the hearing impaired patient. *Canadian Nurse* 85:34–36.

This article presents a unique perspective on hearing loss. The client in this article is the nurse-author. She describes the meaning of her hearing loss, her reactions to this loss, and the problems she encountered. She also provides three suggestions to help allay the anxiety of the hearing-impaired person.

Hahn, K. February 1989. Think twice about sensory loss. *Nursing 89* 19:97–99.

The article describes the meaning of sensory impairment to an elderly female client with both impaired vision requiring cataract surgery and presbycusis. The article provides tips for the use of hearing aids and addresses the implications of taste impairment and touch deprivation.

RELATED RESEARCH

Fox, M. D. 1988. Elderly drivers' perception of their driving abilities compared to their functional visual perception skills and their actual driving performance. *Physical and Occupational Therapy in Geriatrics* 7:13–49.

Jones, D. A.; Vetter, N. J.; and Victor, C. R. August 1987. Visual disability and associated factors in the elderly *Health Visitor* 60:256–57.

Luckner, J. L. April/June 1989. Altering locus of control of individuals with hearing impairments by outdoor adventure courses. *Journal of Rehabilitation* 55:62–67.

Moss, J. R., and Craft, M. J. June 1989. Visual estimation accuracy. *Western Journal of Nursing Research* 11:352–60.

Stewart, N. J. Fall 1986. Perceptual and behavioral effects of immobility and social isolation in hospitalized orthopedic patients. *Nursing Papers* 18:59–74.

Stubbs, L. January 18–25, 1989. Taste changes in cancer patients. *Nursing Times* 85:49–50.

SELECTED REFERENCES

Alberti, P. W.; Ginsberg, I. A.; and Goode, R. L. February 15, 1988. Managing adult hearing loss. *Patient Care* 22:54–58, 63, 67.

Bentz, L. September 1987. Caring for and communicating with blind and visually impaired elderly persons. *Journal of Visual Impairment and Blindness* 81:326–27.

Brown, I. A. October 1985. The widespread influence of olfaction. *Journal of Neurological Nursing* 17:273–79.

Brown, J., and Hepler, R. April 1976. Stimulation: A corollary to physical care. *American Journal of Nursing* 76:578–81.

Callery, P. March 1990. Moral learning in nursing education: A discussion of the usefulness of cognitive–developmental and social learning theories. *Journal of Advanced Nursing* 15:324–8.

Carpenito, L. J. November 1985. Altered thoughts or altered perceptions? *American Journal of Nursing* 85:1283.

———. 1989. *Nursing diagnosis: Application to clinical practice.* 3d ed. Philadelphia: J. B. Lippincott Co.

Chodil, J., and Williams, B. September 1970. The concept of sensory deprivation. *Nursing Clinics of North America* 5(3):544–48.

Chovaz, C. March 1989. Nursing the hearing impaired patient. *Canadian Nurse* 85:34–36.

Christian, E.; Dluhy, N.; and O'Neill, R. November 1989. Sounds of silence: Coping with hearing loss and loneliness. *Journal of Gerontological Nursing* 15:4–9, 33–34.

Doenges, M. E., and Moorhouse, M. F. 1988. *Nurse's pocket guide: Nursing diagnoses with interventions.* 2d ed. Philadelphia: F. A. Davis Co.

Downs, F. S. March 1974. Bed rest and sensory disturbances. *American Journal of Nursing* 74:434–38.

Ebersole, P., and Hess, P. 1985. *Toward healthy aging: Human needs and nursing response.* 2d ed. St. Louis: C. V. Mosby Co.

Focus: Smell and taste disorders. October 1989. *American Association of Occupational Health Nurses* 35:463–64.

Foreman, M. D. May/June 1990. Complexities of acute confusion. *Geriatric Nursing* 11:136–9.

French, S. January 20–26, 1988. Understanding partial sight. *Nursing Times* 84:32–33.

Gioiella, E. C., and Bevil, C. W. 1985. *Nursing care of the aging client: Promoting healthy adaptation.* Norwalk, Conn.: Appleton-Century-Crofts.

Gould, D. February 1987. The biology of aging: The special senses. *Geriatric Nursing and Home Care* 7:15, 18–19.

Hahn, K. February 1989. Think twice about sensory loss. *Nursing 89* 19:97–99.

Kim, M. J.; McFarland, G. K.; and McLane, A. M. 1989. *Pocket guide to nursing diagnoses.* 3d ed. St. Louis: C. V. Mosby Co.

King, J. F. January/February 1988. Interacting with the deaf. *Nursing Homes* 37:20–21.

Kopac, C. A. June 1983. Sensory loss in the aged. The role of the nurse and the family. *Nursing Clinics of North America* 18:373–84.

Mahoney, D. F. September/October 1987. One simple solution to hearing impairment. *Geriatric Nursing* 8:242–45.

Maloney, C. C. Spring 1987. Identifying and treating the client with sensory loss. *Physical and Occupational Therapy in Geriatrics* 5:31–46.

Murphy, K. February 1987. Problems of impaired hearing. *Geriatric Nursing and Home Care* 7:9–11.

NANDA approved nursing diagnostic categories for clinical use and testing. Summer 1988. *Nursing Diagnosis Newsletter* 15:1–3.

Pace, K., Emerich, M. June 1990. Keeping track of confused patients. *Nursing 90* 20:64.

Perron, D. M. June 1974. Deprived of sound. *American Journal of Nursing* 74:1057–59.

Ravish, T. October 1985. Prevent social isolation before it starts. *Journal of Gerontological Nursing* 11:10–13.

Scura, K. W. October 1988. Audiological assessment program. *Journal of Gerontological Nursing* 14:19–25.

Suedfeld, P. 1985. Stressful levels of environmental stimuli. *Issues in Mental Health Nursing* 7:83–104.

Sullivan, N. April 1983. Vision in the elderly. Declining visual function in old age. Parts 1 and 2. *Journal of Gerontological Nursing* 9:228–35.

Walsh, C. October 1986. Commonsense nursing care for the patient with poor vision. *RN* 49:24–25.

Wyness, M. A. April 1985. Perceptual dysfunction: Nursing assessment and management. *Journal of Neurological Nursing* 17:105–10.

Zegeer, L. J. December 1986. The effects of sensory changes in older persons. *Journal of Neuroscience Nursing* 18:325–32.

IMPLEMENTING SPECIAL NURSING MEASURES

Medications

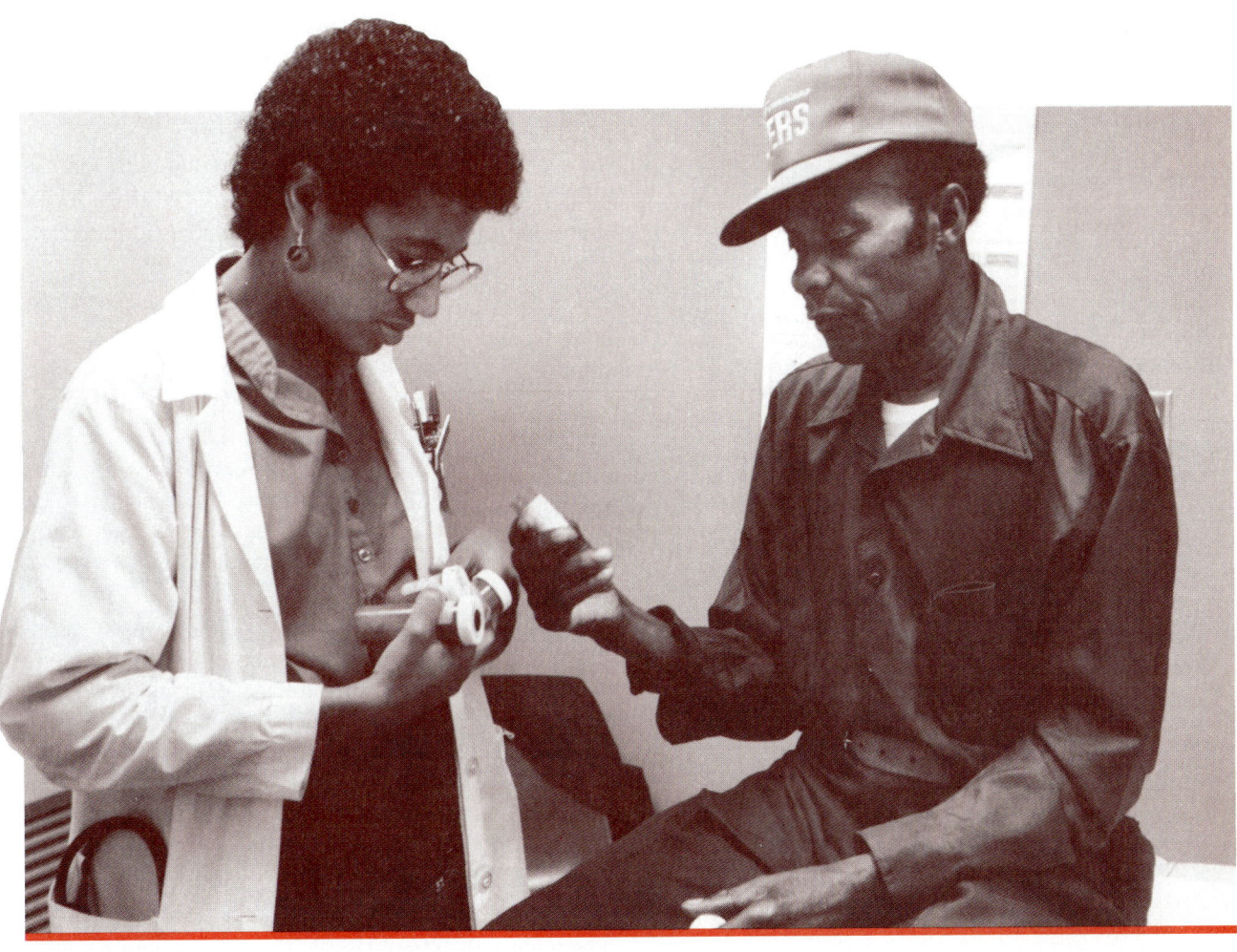

CONTENTS

▶

OBJECTIVES

▸ Define selected terms related to administration of medications.

▸ Describe legal aspects of administering drugs.

▸ Identify physiologic factors and individual variables affecting drug action.

▸ Describe various routes of drug administration.

▸ Identify essential parts of a drug order.

▸ Give examples of various types of medication orders.

▸ Recognize abbreviations commonly used in medication orders.

▸ List five essential steps to follow when administering drugs.

▸ Describe physiologic changes in elderly persons that alter drug administration and effectiveness.

▸ Outline steps required to administer oral medications safely.

▸ Identify equipment required for parenteral medications.

▸ Describe how to mix selected drugs from vials and ampules.

▸ Identify sites used for subcutaneous, intramuscular, and intradermal injections.

▸ Describe essential steps for safely administering parenteral medications by intradermal, subcutaneous, intramuscular, and intravenous routes.

▸ Describe essential steps in safely administering topical medications: dermatologic, ophthalmic, otic, nasal, vaginal, and rectal preparations.

NAMES AND TYPES OF MEDICATIONS

A **medication** is a substance administered for the diagnosis, cure, treatment, mitigation (relief), or prevention of disease. In the health care context, the words *medication* and *drug* are generally used interchangeably. The term **drug** also has the connotation of an illicitly obtained substance such as heroin, cocaine, or amphetamines. Medications have been known and used since antiquity. Crude drugs such as opium, castor oil, and vinegar were used in ancient times. Over the centuries the number of drugs available has increased greatly, and knowledge about these drugs has become correspondingly more accurate and detailed.

In the United States and Canada, medications are usually dispensed on the order of physicians and dentists. In some states in the United States, specially qualified nurse practitioners may also prescribe drugs. The written direction for the preparation and administration of a drug is called a **prescription.** One drug can have as many as four kinds of names: its generic name, official name, chemical name, and trademark or brand name. The **generic name** is given before a drug becomes official. The **official name** is the name under which it is listed in one of the official publications (e.g., the *United States Pharmacopeia*). The **chemical name** is the name by which a chemist knows it; this name describes the constituents of the drug precisely. The **trademark,** or **brand name,** is the name given by the drug manufacturer. Because one drug may be manufactured by several companies, it can have several trade names; for example, the drug hydrochlorothiazide (official name) is known by the trade names Esidrix and Hydro-Diuril. Medications are often available in a variety of forms. Common types of drug preparations are described in Table 45–1.

Pharmacology is the study of the effect of drugs on living organisms. Drugs are prepared by a **pharmacist,** a person licensed to prepare and dispense drugs and to make up prescriptions. A **clinical pharmacist** is a specialist

TABLE 45–1 *Types of Drug Preparations*

Type	Description	Type	Description
Aqueous solution	One or more drugs dissolved in water	Ointment	A semisolid preparation of one or more drugs used for application to the skin and mucous membrane
Aerosol spray or foam	A liquid, powder, or foam deposited in a thin layer on the skin by air pressure	Paste	A preparation like an ointment, but thicker and stiffer, that penetrates the skin less than an ointment
Aqueous suspension	One or more drugs finely divided in a liquid such as water	Pill	One or more drugs mixed with a cohesive material, in oval, round, or flattened shapes
Capsule	A gelatinous container to hold a drug in powder, liquid, or oil form	Powder	A finely ground drug or drugs; some are used internally, others externally
Cream	A nongreasy, semisolid preparation used on the skin	Spirit	A concentrated alcoholic solution of a volatile substance
Elixir	A sweetened and aromatic solution of alcohol used as a vehicle for medicinal agents	Suppository	One or several drugs mixed with a firm base such as gelatin and shaped for insertion into the body; the base dissolves gradually at body temperature, releasing the drug
Extract	A concentrated form of a drug made from vegetables or animals		
Fluid extract	An alcoholic solution of a drug from a vegetable source; the most concentrated of all fluid preparations	Syrup	An aqueous solution of sugar often used to disguise unpleasant-tasting drugs
Gel or jelly	A clear or translucent semisolid that liquefies when applied to the skin	Tablet	A powdered drug compressed into a hard small disc; some are readily broken along a scored line; others are enteric-coated to prevent them from dissolving in the stomach
Liniment	An oily liquid used on the skin		
Lotion	An emollient liquid that may be a clear solution, suspension, or emulsion used on the skin		
Lozenge (troche)	A flat, round, or oval preparation that dissolves and releases a drug when held in the mouth	Tincture	An alcoholic or water-and-alcohol solution prepared from drugs derived from plants

who often guides the physician in prescribing drugs. A **pharmacy assistant** is a member of the health team who in some states administers drugs to clients. **Pharmacy** is the art of preparing, compounding, and dispensing drugs. The word also refers to the place where drugs are prepared and dispensed.

DRUG STANDARDS

Drugs may have natural (e.g., plant, mineral, and animal) sources, or they may be synthesized in the laboratory. For example, digitalis and opium are plant derived, iron and sodium chloride are minerals, insulin and vaccines have animal or human sources, and the sulfonamides and propoxyphene hydrochloride (the analgesic Darvon) are the products of laboratory synthesis. Early drugs were derived from the three natural sources only. During the past 45

years, however, more and more drugs have been produced synthetically.

Drugs vary in strength and activity. Drugs derived from plants, for example, vary in strength according to the age of the plant, the variety, the place in which it is grown, and the method by which it is preserved. Drugs must be pure and of uniform strength if drug dosages are to be predictable in their effect. Drug standards have therefore been developed to ensure uniform quality. In the United States, official drugs are those so designated by the Federal Food, Drug, and Cosmetic Act. These drugs are officially listed in the *United States Pharmacopeia (USP)* and described according to their source, physical and chemical properties, tests for purity and identity, method of storage, assay, category, and normal dosages. In Canada, the *British Pharmacopoeia* is used for the same purpose, although some drugs used in Canada conform to the *USP* because they are obtained from the United States.

A **pharmacopoeia** is a book containing a list of products

used in medicine, with descriptions of the product, chemical tests for determining identity and purity, and formulas for certain mixtures. A **formulary** is a collection of formulas and prescriptions. The United States' *National Formulary* lists drugs and their therapeutic value and can include drugs that may still be used but not listed in the *USP.* The *Canadian Formulary* lists drugs used extensively in Canada but not necessarily listed in the *British Pharmacopoeia.*

Pharmacopoeias and formularies are invaluable reference sources for nurses and nursing students. Nurses not only administer thousands of medications but also are responsible for assessing their effectiveness and recognizing unfavorable reactions to drugs. Since it is impossible to commit to memory all pertinent information about a very large number of drugs, nurses must have a reliable reference readily available.

LEGAL ASPECTS OF DRUG ADMINISTRATION

The administration of drugs in both the United States and Canada is controlled by law. In the United States the major federal acts controlling drugs are the Food, Drug, and Cosmetic Act (1938), its amendments, and the Comprehensive Drug Abuse Prevention and Control Act (1970) (Controlled Substances Act). In Canada, three federal acts control drugs: The Food and Drugs Act (1953), the Proprietary or Patent Medicine Act (1908), and the Narcotics Control Act (1961).

See Table 45–2 for a summary of U.S. drug legislation. Table 45–3 provides a summary of Canadian drug legislation.

Nurses need to (a) know how nursing practice acts in their areas define and limit their functions and (b) be able to recognize the limits of their own knowledge and skill. To function beyond the limits of nursing practice acts or one's ability is to endanger clients' lives and leave oneself open to malpractice suits. Under the law, nurses are responsible for their own actions regardless of whether there is a written order. If a physician writes an incorrect order (e.g., Demerol 500 mg instead of Demerol 50 mg), a nurse who administers the written incorrect dosage is responsible for the error. Therefore, nurses should question any order that appears unreasonable and refuse to give the medication until the order is clarified.

Another aspect of nursing practice governed by law is the use of narcotics and barbiturates. In hospitals, narcotics are kept under double lock in a drawer or cupboard. Other medications, including barbiturates, are kept under single lock, although in some places barbiturates are kept with narcotics. Agencies have special forms for recording narcotics. The information required usually includes the name of the client, date and time of administration, name of the drug, dosage, and signature of the person who prepared and gave the narcotic. The name of the physician who ordered the narcotic may also be part of the record.

Included on the record are narcotics wasted during preparation. In most agencies, narcotic and barbiturate counts are taken at the end of each shift. The count total should tally with the total at the end of the last shift minus the number used. If the totals do not tally, the discrepancy must be reported immediately.

TABLE 45–2 *United States Drug Legislation*

Legislation	Content
Food, Drug, and Cosmetic Act (1938)	Implemented by Food and Drug Administration (FDA); requires that labels be accurate and that all drugs be tested for harmful effects
Durkham-Humphrey Amendment (1952)	Differentiates clearly between drugs that can be sold with and without a prescription
Kefauver-Harris Amendment (1962)	Requires proof of safety and efficacy of a drug for approval
Comprehensive Drug Abuse Prevention and Control Act (1970) (Controlled Substances Act)	Categorizes controlled substances and limits how often a prescription can be filled

TABLE 45–3 *Canadian Drug Legislation*

Legislation	Content
Proprietary or Patent Medicine Act (1908)	Protects the public against unsafe and ineffective over-the-counter drugs
Canada Food and Drugs Act (1953)	Prohibits advertising any food, drug, cosmetic, or device as a cure for certain specified diseases. Prohibits the sale of certain drugs unless approved by the federal government.
Canadian Narcotic Control Act (1961)	Allows only authorized people to possess narcotics. Specifies records about narcotics that must be kept

TABLE 45 – 4 *Therapeutic Actions of Drugs*

Drug Type	Description	Examples
Palliative	Relieves the symptoms of a disease but does not affect the disease itself	Morphine sulfate, aspirin for pain
Curative	Cures a disease or condition	Penicillin for infection
Supportive	Supports body functions until other treatment or the body's response can take over	Norepinephrine bitartrate for low blood pressure; aspirin for high body temperature
Substitutive	Replaces body fluids or substances	Thyroxine for hypothyroidism; insulin for diabetes mellitus
Chemotherapeutic	Destroys malignant cells	Busulfan for leukemia
Restorative	Returns the body to health	Vitamin, mineral supplements

EFFECTS OF DRUGS

The **therapeutic effect** of a drug, also referred to as the *desired effect,* is the primary effect intended, that is, the reason the drug is prescribed. For example, the therapeutic effect of morphine sulphate is analgesia, and the therapeutic effect of diazepam is relief of anxiety. See Table 45–4 for kinds of therapeutic actions.

A **side-effect,** or secondary effect, of a drug is one that is unintended. Side-effects are usually predictable and may be either harmless or potentially harmful. For example, digitalis increases the strength of myocardial contractions, but it can have the side-effect of inducing nausea and vomiting. Some side-effects are tolerated for the drug's therapeutic effect; hazardous side-effects justify the discontinuation of a drug.

Drug toxicity (deleterious effects of a drug on an organism or tissue) results from overdosage, ingestion of a drug intended for external use, and buildup of the drug in the blood because of impaired metabolism or excretion (cumulative effect). Some toxic effects are apparent immediately; some are not apparent for weeks or months. Fortunately, most drug toxicity is avoidable if careful attention is paid to dosage and monitoring for toxicity. An example of a toxic effect is respiratory depression due to the cumulative effect of morphine sulfate in the body.

A **drug allergy** is the immunologic reaction to a drug to which person has already been sensitized. When a client is first exposed to a foreign substance (antigen), the body may react by producing antibodies. A client can react to a drug as to an antigen and thus develop symptoms of an allergic reaction.

Allergic reactions can be either mild or severe. A mild reaction has a variety of symptoms, from skin rashes to diarrhea. See Table 45–5. It can occur anytime from a few hours to 2 weeks after the administration of the drug. A severe allergic reaction usually occurs immediately after the administration of the drug; it is called an **anaphylactic reaction.** This response can be fatal if the symptoms are not noticed immediately and treatment is not obtained promptly. The earliest symptoms are acute shortness of breath, acute hypotension, and tachycardia.

Drug tolerance exists in a person who has unusually low physiologic activity in response to a drug and who requires increases in the dosage to maintain a given ther-

TABLE 45 – 5 *Common Mild Allergic Responses*

Symptom	Description/Rationale
Skin rash	Either an intraepidermal vesicle rash or a rash typified by an urticarial wheal or macular eruption; rash is usually generalized over the body
Pruritus	Itching of the skin with or without a rash
Angioedema	Edema due to increased permeability of the blood capillaries
Rhinitis	Excessive watery discharge from the nose
Lacrimal tearing	Excessive tearing
Nausea, vomiting	Stimulation of these centers in the brain
Wheezing and dyspnea	Shortness of breath and wheezing upon inhalation and exhalation due to accumulated fluids and swelling of the respiratory tissues
Diarrhea	Irritation of the mucosa of the large intestine

apeutic effect. Drugs that commonly produce tolerance are opiates, barbiturates, ethyl alcohol, and tobacco. A **cumulative effect** is the increasing response to repeated doses of a drug that occurs when the rate of administration exceeds the rate of metabolism or excretion. As a result, the amount of the drug builds up in the client's body unless the dosage is adjusted. Toxic symptoms may occur. An **idiosyncratic effect** is unexpected and individual. Underresponse and overresponse to a drug may be idiosyncratic. Also, the drug may have a completely different effect from the normal one or cause unpredictable and unexplainable symptoms in a particular client.

A **drug interaction** occurs when administration of one drug before, at the same time as, or after another drug alters the effect of one or both drugs. The effect of one or both drugs may be either increased (*potentiating effect*) or decreased (*inhibiting effect*). Drug interactions may be beneficial or harmful. For example, Probenecid, which blocks the excretion of penicillin, is often given with penicillin to increase blood levels of the penicillin for longer periods (potentiating effect). Two analgesics, such as aspirin and codeine, are often given together because together they provide greater pain relief (additive effect).

Iatrogenic disease (disease caused unintentionally by medical therapy) can be due to drug therapy. Hepatic toxicity resulting in biliary obstruction, renal damage, and malformations of the fetus as a result of drugs taken during pregnancy are examples.

DRUG MISUSE

Drug misuse is the improper use of common medications in ways that lead to acute and chronic toxicity. Both over-the-counter drugs and prescription drugs may be misused. Laxatives, antacids, vitamins, headache remedies, and cough and cold medications are often self-prescribed and overused. Most people suffer no harmful effects from these drugs, but some people do. A persistent cough may go undiagnosed until the underlying problem is serious and advanced.

Drug abuse is inappropriate intake of a substance, either continually or periodically. By definition, drug use is abusive when society considers it abusive. For example, the intake of alcohol at work may be considered alcohol abuse, but intake at a social gathering may not. Drug abuse has two main facets, drug dependence and habituation. **Drug dependence** is a person's reliance on or need to take a drug or substance. The two types of dependence, physiologic and psychologic, may occur separately or together. **Physiologic dependence** is due to biochemical changes in body tissues, especially of the nervous system. These tissues come to require the substance for normal functioning. A dependent person who stops using the drug experiences withdrawal symptoms. **Psychologic dependence** is emotional reliance on a drug to maintain a sense of well-being, accompanied by feelings of need or cravings for that drug. There are varying degrees of psychologic dependence, ranging from mild desire to craving and compulsive use of the drug. In severe cases, the dependent person gives up other goals and satisfactions to satisfy the dependence. For example, a man highly dependent on tobacco may give up his job and increase a health problem rather than stop smoking.

Drug habituation denotes a mild form of psychologic dependence. The individual develops the habit of taking the substance and feels better after taking it. The habituated individual tends to continue the habit even though it may be injurious to health.

Illicit drugs, also called *street drugs,* are those sold illegally. Illicit drugs are of two types: (a) drugs unavailable for purchase under any circumstances, e.g., heroin (in the United States), and (b) drugs normally available with a prescription that are being obtained through illegal channels. Illicit drugs often are taken because of their mood-altering effect; i.e., they make the person feel happy or relaxed.

ACTIONS OF DRUGS ON THE BODY

The action of a drug in the body can be described in terms of its **half-life,** the time interval required for the body's elimination processes to reduce the concentration of the drug in the body by one-half. For example, if a drug's half-life is 8 hours, then the amount of drug in the body is as follows:

Initially: 100%

After 8 hours: 50%

After 16 hours: 25%

After 24 hours: 12.5%

After 32 hours: 6.25%

Since the purpose of most drug therapy is to maintain a constant drug level in the body, repeated doses are required to maintain that level. When an orally administered drug is absorbed from the gastrointestinal tract into the blood plasma, its concentration in the plasma increases until the elimination rate equals the rate of absorption. This point is known as the **peak plasma level.** See Figure 45–1. Unless the client receives another dose of the drug, the concentration steadily decreases. Key terms related to drug actions are listed and described in the box on the opposite page. The actions of drugs on the body can be described in terms of four general principles (Reiss and Melick 1984, pp. 14–15). These principles are summarized in the box on the opposite page.

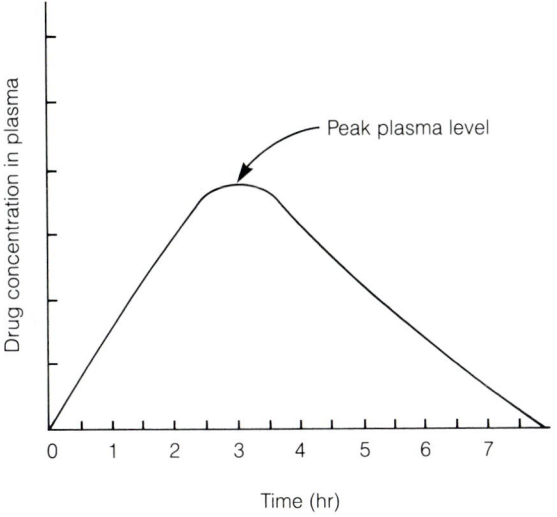

Figure 45–1 A graphic plot of drug concentration in the blood plasma following a single dose.

Key Terms Related to Drug Action

- *Onset of action:* The time after administration when the body initially responds to the drug
- *Peak plasma level:* The highest plasma level achieved by a single dose when the elimination rate of a drug equals the absorption rate
- *Drug half-life (elimination half-life):* The time required for the elimination process to reduce the concentration of the drug to one-half what it was at initial administration
- *Plateau:* A maintained concentration of a drug in the plasma during a series of scheduled doses

A drug that interacts with a receptor to produce a response is known as an **agonist.** Drugs that have no special pharmacologic action of their own but that inhibit or prevent the action of an agonist are called **specific antagonists.**

Pharmacokinetics

Pharmacokinetics is the study of the absorption, distribution, biotransformation, and excretion of drugs. **Absorption** is the process by which a drug passes into the bloodstream. Unless the drug is administered directly into the bloodstream, absorption is the first step in the movement of the drug through the body. For absorption to occur, the correct form of the drug must be given by the route intended.

The rate of absorption of a drug in the stomach is variable. Food, for example, can delay the dissolution and absorption of some drugs as well as their passage into the small intestine, where most drug absorption occurs. Food can also combine with molecules of certain drugs, thereby changing their molecular structure and subsequently inhibiting or preventing their absorption. Another factor that affects the absorption of some drugs is the acid medium in the stomach. Acidity can vary according to the time of day, foods ingested, and the age of the client. Some drugs do not dissolve or have limited ability to dissolve in the gastrointestinal fluids, decreasing their absorption into the bloodstream. Some drugs are absorbed by tissues before they reach the stomach. For example, nitroglycerin is administered under the tongue, where it is absorbed into the blood vessels that carry it directly to the heart, the intended site of action. If swallowed, this drug will be absorbed into the bloodstream and carried to the liver, where it will be destroyed.

General Principles Related to Drug Actions

- *Drugs act on existing cellular functions.* Drugs do not create new cellular function. For example, an antibiotic can slow microbial growth; laxatives can increase peristalsis.
- *Drugs act on the body in a number of ways.* Some drugs alter the chemical composition of a body fluid; e.g., an antacid decreases the acidity of the gastric contents. Other drugs accumulate in certain body tissues because of their attraction to that tissue; e.g., propylthiouracil (PTU) is an antithyroid drug with an affinity for the thyroid gland, which thereby prevents the formation of thyroid hormones in the gland. Still other drugs act by forming a chemical bond with a receptor in the body. This binding occurs only when the drug and the receptor are compatible.
- *Drugs that reach the same receptor can be expected to produce a similar drug response in a client.* For example, most penicillins, such as amoxillin and cyclacillin, have a similar action.

A drug administered directly into the bloodstream, i.e., intravenously, is immediately in the vascular system without having to be absorbed. This, then, is the route of choice for rapid action. Because subcutaneous tissue has a poorer blood supply than muscle tissue, absorption from subcutaneous tissue is slower. The rate of absorption of a drug can be accelerated by the application of heat, which increases blood flow to the area; conversely, absorption can be slowed by the application of cold. In addition, the injection of a vasoconstrictor drug such as epinephrine into the tissue can slow absorption of other drugs. Some drugs intended to be absorbed slowly are suspended in a low-solubility medium such as oil. The absorption of drugs from the rectum into the bloodstream tends to be unpredictable. Therefore, this route is used when other routes are unavailable or when the intended action is localized to the rectum or sigmoid colon (Reiss and Melick 1984, p. 16).

Distribution is the transportation of a drug from its site of absorption to its site of action. When a drug enters the bloodstream it is carried to the most vascular organs, i.e., liver, kidneys, and brain. Body areas with lower blood supply, i.e., skin and muscles, receive the drug later. The chemical and physical properties of a drug largely determine the area of the body to which the drug will be attracted. For example, fat-soluble drugs will accumulate in fatty tissue, whereas other drugs may bind with plasma proteins.

Biotransformation, also called **detoxification,** is a process by which a drug is converted to a less active form. Most biotransformation takes place in the liver, where many drug-metabolizing enzymes in the cells detoxify the drugs. The products of this process are called **metabolites.** There are two types of metabolites: active and inactive. An *active metabolite* has a pharmacologic action itself, whereas an *inactive metabolite* does not.

The biotransformation capability of a client's liver may be impaired. For example, an elderly client, just like a client with hepatic damage, may have a decreased ability to metabolize drugs. In these situations, nurses must be alert to the accumulation of the active drug in the client and to subsequent toxicity.

Excretion is the process by which metabolites and drugs are eliminated from the body. Most metabolites are eliminated by the kidneys in the urine; however, some are excreted in the feces, the breath, perspiration, saliva, and breast milk. Certain drugs, e.g., general anesthetic agents, are excreted in an unchanged form via the respiratory tract. In addition to metabolites, alcohol is eliminated, unchanged, through the lungs. The efficiency with which the kidneys excrete drugs and metabolites diminishes with age. Elderly people may require smaller doses of a drug because the drug and its metabolites may accumulate in the body. Also, kidney disease can impair excretion of drugs and metabolites.

Variables Influencing Drug Action

A number of factors influence the actions of drugs on the body. Among them are age, weight, sex, genetic and psychologic factors, illness and disease, time of administration, and environment. *Age* is a factor in that very young people and elderly people often are highly responsive to drugs and thus require lower doses. Immature liver and kidney function as well as diminished renal functioning due to aging can affect the action of a drug. *Body weight* also directly affects drug action; the greater the body weight, the greater the dosage required.

Sex-linked differences in the way men and women respond to drugs are chiefly due to two factors: differences in distribution of fat and water and hormonal differences. Because women usually weigh less than men, equal drug dosages are likely to affect women more than men. Women usually have more fatty pads than men, and men have more body fluid than women. Some drugs may be more soluble in fat, whereas others are more soluble in water. Thus, men absorb some drugs more readily than women, and vice versa.

Individuals may react differently to drugs as a result of *genetic factors*. A client may be abnormally sensitive to a drug or may metabolize a drug differently than most people because of genetic influences. Sometimes these reactions are mistaken for allergic reactions. *Psychologic factors* influence how one feels about a drug and what one believes it can do. A traditional example is the reaction of some people to a placebo, a substance (such as normal saline) often given to relieve pain. For some clients, the placebo has the same effect as an analgesic. See Chapter 38 for further information.

Illness and *disease* can also affect the action of drugs. For example, aspirin can reduce the body temperature of a feverish client but has no effect on the body temperature of a client without fever. Drug action is altered in clients with circulatory, liver, or kidney dysfunction. Diabetics need larger doses of insulin with fever or infection.

The *time of administration* of oral medications affects the relative speed with which they act. Orally administered medications are absorbed more quickly if the stomach is empty. Thus, oral medications taken 2 hours before meals act faster than those taken after meals. However, some medications, for example, iron preparations, irritate the gastrointestinal tract and need to be given after a meal, when they will be better tolerated. A client's sleep-wake rhythm may affect the action of a drug. Circadian variations in urine output and blood circulation, for example, may affect a client's response to a drug.

The client's *environment* can affect the action of drugs, particularly those used to alter behavior and mood. Therefore, nurses assessing the effects of a drug need to consider the drug itself as well as the client's personality and milieu. Environmental temperature may also affect drug activity. When environmental temperature is high, the peripheral blood vessels dilate, thus intensifying the action of vasodilators. In contrast, a cold environment and the consequent vasoconstriction inhibit the action of vasodilators but enhance the action of vasoconstrictors.

ROUTES OF ADMINISTRATION

Pharmaceutical preparations are generally designed for one or two specific routes of administration. See Table 45–6. The route of administration should be indicated when the

TABLE 45-6   *Routes of Administration*

Route	Advantages	Disadvantages
Oral	Most convenient Usually least expensive Safe, does not break skin barrier Administration usually does not cause stress	Inappropriate for clients nauseated or vomiting Drug may have unpleasant taste or odor Inappropriate when gastrointestinal tract has reduced motility Inappropriate when client cannot swallow or is unconscious Cannot be used before certain diagnostic tests or surgical procedures Drug may discolor teeth, harm tooth enamel Drug may irritate gastric mucosa Drug can be aspirated by seriously ill clients
Sublingual	Same as for oral, *plus*: Drug can be administered for local effect Drug is rapidly absorbed into the bloodstream Ensures greater potency because drug directly enters the blood and bypasses the liver	If swallowed, drug may be inactivated by gastric juice Drug must remain under tongue until dissolved and absorbed
Buccal	Same as for sublingual	Same as for sublingual
Rectal	Can be used when drug has objectionable taste or odor Drug released at slow, steady rate	Dose absorbed is unpredictable
Skin	Provides a local effect Few side-effects	May be messy and may soil clothes Drug can rapidly enter body through abrasions and cause systemic effects
Subcutaneous	Onset of drug action faster than oral	Must involve sterile technique because breaks skin barrier More expensive than oral Can administer only small volume Slower than intramuscular administration Some drugs can irritate tissues and cause pain Can be anxiety-producing
Intramuscular	Pain from irritating drugs is minimized Can administer larger volume than subcutaneous Drug is rapidly absorbed	Breaks skin barrier Can be anxiety-producing
Intradermal	Absorption is slow (this is an advantage when testing for allergies	Amount of drug administered must be small Breaks skin barrier
Intravenous	Rapid effect	Limited to highly soluble drugs Drug distribution may be inhibited by poor circulation
Inhalation	Introduces drug throughout the respiratory tract Rapid localized relief Drug can be administered when client is unconscious	Drug intended for localized effect can have systemic effect Only of use for the respiratory system

drug is ordered. When administering a drug, the nurse should ensure that the pharmaceutical preparation is appropriate for the route specified.

Oral   Oral administration is the most common, least expensive, and most convenient route for most clients. Since the skin is not broken as it is for an injection, oral administration is also a safe method.

The major disadvantages are possible unpleasant taste of the drugs, irritation of the gastric mucosa, irregular absorption from the gastrointestinal tract, slow absorption, and, in some cases, harm to the client's teeth. For example, hydrochloric acid can damage the enamel of teeth.

Sublingual   A drug may be placed under the tongue (**sublingual** administration), where it dissolves. See Figure 45–2. In a relatively short time, the drug is largely absorbed into the blood vessels on the underside of the tongue. The medication should not be swallowed. Drugs such as nitroglycerin are commonly given in this manner.

Buccal   **Buccal** means "pertaining to the cheek." In buccal administration, a medication (e.g., a tablet) is held in the mouth against the mucous membranes of the cheek until the drug dissolves. See Figure 45–3. The drug may act locally on the mucous membranes of the mouth or systemically when it is swallowed in the saliva.

Parenteral   **Parenteral** administration is administration other than through the alimentary tract, i.e., by needle.

Some of the more common routes for parenteral administration are

- **Subcutaneous (hypodermic)**—into the subcutaneous tissue, just below the skin
- **Intramuscular**—into a muscle
- **Intradermal**—under the epidermis (into the dermis)
- **Intravenous**—into a vein

Some of the less commonly used routes for parenteral administration are **intra-arterial** (into an artery), **intra-cardiac** (into the heart muscle), **intraosseous** (into a bone), and **intrathecal** or **intraspinal** (into the spinal canal). These less common injections are normally administered by physicians. Sterile equipment and sterile drug solution are essential for all parenteral therapy. The main advantage is fast absorption.

Topical   **Topical** applications are those applied to a circumscribed surface area of the body. They affect only the area to which they are applied. Topical applications include

- **Dermatologic preparations**—applied to the skin.
- **Instillations and irrigations**—applied into body cavities or orifices such as the urinary bladder, eyes, ears, nose, rectum, or vagina.
- **Inhalations**—administered into the respiratory tract by nebulizers or positive pressure breathing apparatuses. Air, oxygen, and vapor are generally used to carry the drug into the lungs. See Chapter 41.

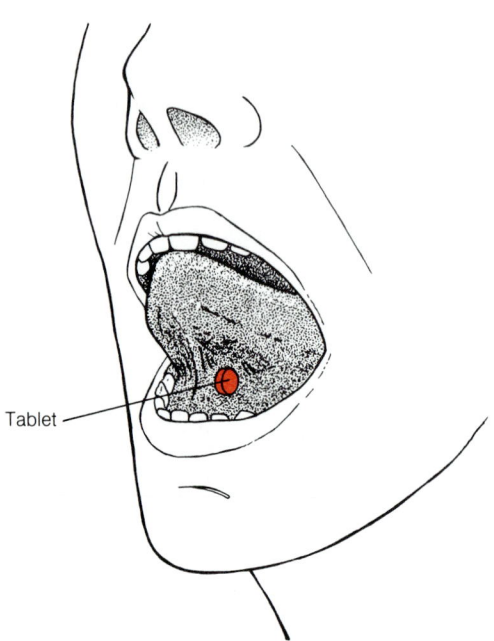

Figure 45–2   Sublingual administration of a tablet.

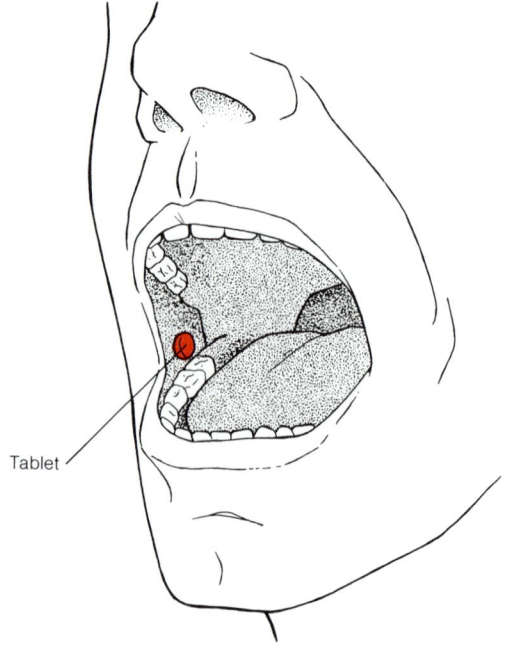

Figure 45–3   Buccal administration of a tablet.

MEDICATION ORDERS

A physician usually determines the clients' medications needs and orders medications, although in some settings nurse practitioners now order some drugs. Usually, the order is written, although telephone and verbal orders are acceptable in a number of agencies. Nursing students need to know the agency policies about medication orders. In some hospitals, for example, only licensed nurses are permitted to accept telephone and verbal orders.

Policies about physicians' orders vary considerably from agency to agency. For example, a client's orders are frequently automatically canceled after surgery or an examination involving an anesthetic agent. New orders must then be written. Most agencies also have lists of abbreviations officially accepted for use in the agency. Both nurses and physicians may need to refer to these lists if they have been working in a different agency. These abbreviations can be used on legal documents, such as clients' charts. See Table 45–7.

TABLE 45–7 *Common Abbreviations Used in Medication Orders*

Abbreviation	Explanation	Example of Administration Time	Abbreviation	Explanation	Example of Administration Time
ac	before meals	0700, 1100, and 1700 hrs	q$_{AM}$ (om)	every morning	1000 hours
			qh (q1h)	every hour	
ad lib	freely, as desired		q2h	every 2 hours	0800, 1000, 1200 hours, and so on
agit	shake, stir				
aq	water		q3h	every 3 hours	0900, 1200, 1500 hours, and so on
aq dest	distilled water				
bid	twice a day	0900 and 2100 hours	q4h	every 4 hours	1000, 1400, 1800 hours, and so on
c̄	with		q6h	every 6 hours	0600, 1200, 1800, 2400 hours
cap	capsule				
comp	compound		qhs	every night at bedtime	
dil	dissolve, dilute		qid	four times a day	1000, 1400, 1800, 2200 hours
elix	elixir				
h	an hour		qod	every other day	0900 hours on odd dates
hs	at bedtime				
IM	intramuscular		qs	sufficient quantity	
IV	intravenous		rept	may be repeated	
M or m	mix		Rx	take	
no.	number		s̄	without	
non rep	do not repeat		sc	subcutaneous	
OD	right eye		Sig or S	label	
OS or ol	left eye		sos	if it is needed	
OU	both eyes		ss or s̄s̄	one half	
pc	after meals	0900, 1300, and 1900 hours	stat	at once	
			sup or supp	suppository	
po	by mouth		susp	suspension	
prn	when needed		tid	three times a day	1000, 1400, and 1800 hours
q	every		Tr or tinct	tincture	

Types of Medication Orders

Four common medication orders are the stat order, the single order, the standing order, and the prn order:

1. A **stat order** indicates that the medication is to be given immediately and only once, e.g., Demerol 100 mg IM stat.

2. The **single order** is for a medication to be given once at a specified time, e.g., Seconal 100 mg hs before surgery.

3. The **standing order** may or may not have a termination date. A standing order may be carried out indefinitely (e.g., multiple vitamins daily) until an order is written to cancel it, or it may be carried out for a specified number of days (e.g., Demerol 100 mg IM q4h × 5 days). In some agencies, standing orders are automatically canceled after a specified number of days and must be reordered.

4. A **prn order** permits the nurse to give a medication when, in the nurse's judgment, the client requires it, e.g., Amphojel 15 ml prn. The nurse must use good judgment about when the medication is needed and when it can be safely administered.

Essential Parts of a Drug Order

The drug order has six essential parts, as listed in the box below. In addition, unless it is a standing order, it should state the number of doses or the number of days the drug is to be administered.

The *client's full name,* that is, the first and last names and middle initials or names, should always be used to avoid confusion between two clients who have the same last names. In some agencies the client's admission number is put on the order as further identification. Some hospitals imprint the client's name and hospital number on all forms. This imprinter is on the nursing unit; it is much like the credit card imprinters used in shops.

In addition to *the day, the month, and the year* the order was written, some agencies also require that the *time of day*

be written. Writing the time of day on the order can eliminate errors when nursing shifts change and makes clear when certain orders automatically terminate. For example, in some settings, narcotics can be ordered only for 48 hours after surgery. Therefore, a drug that is ordered at 1600 hours February 1, 1991 is automatically canceled at 1600 hours February 3, 1991. Many health agencies use the 24-hour clock, which eliminates confusion between morning and afternoon times. Time with the 24-hour clock starts at midnight, which is 0000 hours. See Chapter 17.

The *name of the drug* to be administered must be clearly written. In some settings, only generic names are permitted; however, trade names are widely used in hospitals and health agencies.

The *dosage of the drug* includes the amount, the times or frequency of administration, and in many instances the strength; for example, tetracycline *250 mg* (amount) *four times a day* (frequency); hydrochloric acid *10%* (strength) *5 ml* (amount) *three times a day with meals* (time and frequency). Dosages can be written in apothecaries' or metric systems.

Also included in the order is the *method of administering* the drug. This part of the order, like other parts, is frequently abbreviated. See Table 45–7 for abbreviations of routes of administration. It is not unusual for a drug to have several possible routes of administration; therefore, it is important that the route be included in the order.

The *signature* of the ordering physician or nurse makes the drug order a legal request. An unsigned order has no validity, and the ordering physician or nurse needs to be notified if the order is unsigned.

In agencies where telephone orders are taken, the nurse usually indicates the name of the person who phoned in the order. The nurse signs the order, but usually the person who ordered the drug must also sign at a later date. Some hospitals have policies that those who give orders by telephone must sign those orders within a certain time, for example, 48 hours after they have communicated the order.

When a physician writes a prescription for a client, the prescription also includes information for the pharmacist. Therefore, a prescription's content differs from that of a medication order in a hospital. Compare the parts of a prescription listed in the box next to Figure 45–4 with those shown in Figure 45–4.

Communicating a Medication Order

A drug order is written on the client's chart by a physician or by a nurse receiving a telephone or verbal order from a physician. Most agencies have a specified time frame (e.g., 24 or 48 hours) in which the physician issuing the telephone or verbal order must cosign the order written by the nurse. The medication order is then copied by a nurse or clerk to a Kardex and to a medication card or medication administration record (MAR). Increasingly, nurses are being provided with computer printouts of a client's medications

---

Drug Order: Essential Parts

- Full name of the client
- Date the order is written
- Name of the drug to be administered
- Dosage of the drug
- Method of administration
- Signature of the physician or nurse practitioner

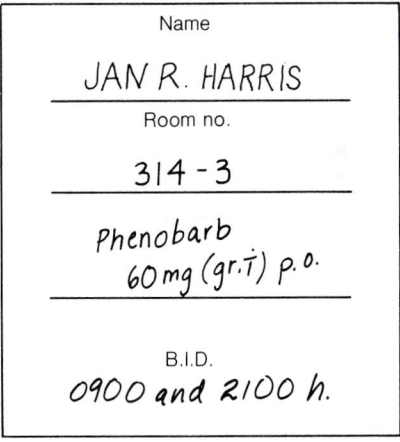

Name __Jane Smith_____ Age __36__

Address __3376 W. 141st St., Scottsdale__ Date __Dec. 3, 1991__

This prescription will be filled generically unless physician signs on line stating "Dispense as written."

R̸

Tetracycline   250 mgm
Disp.   #30
Sig.   1 qid

F. March

Dispense as Written   Substitution Permissable

Frederick March, M.D.   120 Madison Road   Scottsdale, NY
DEA #ER639524   Ph. No. __685-9533__

Figure 45–4 A prescription filled out by a physician.

instead of copying the physician's order. This method avoids errors of copying and saves nursing time.

Medication cards (see Figure 45–5) vary in form but include the client's name, room, and bed number; drug name and dose; and times and method of administration. In some agencies the date the order was prescribed and the date the order expires are also included, along with the signature of the person writing the order.

SYSTEMS OF MEASUREMENT

Three systems of measurement are used in North America: the metric system, the apothecaries' system, and the household system, which is similar to the apothecaries' system.

Metric System

The metric system, devised by the French in the latter part of the 18th century, is the system prescribed by law in most European countries and in Canada. The metric system is logically organized into units of ten; it is a decimal system. Basic units can be multiplied or divided by ten to form secondary units. Multiples are calculated by moving the decimal point to the right, and divisions by moving the decimal point to the left.

Basic units of measurement are the meter, the liter, and the gram. Prefixes derived from Latin designate subdivisions of the basic unit: deci (1/10 or 0.1), centi (1/100 or 0.01), and milli (1/1000 or 0.001). Multiples of the basic unit are designated by prefixes derived from Greek: deka (10), hecto (100), and kilo (1000). Only the measurements of volume (the liter) and of weight (the gram) are discussed

Name

JAN R. HARRIS

Room no.

314 - 3

Phenobarb
60 mg (gr. ī) p.o.

B.I.D.
0900 and 2100 h.

Figure 45–5 A sample medication card containing essential information.

in this chapter. These are the measures used in medication administration. See Figure 45–6. In nursing practice, the kilogram (kg) is the only multiple of the gram used, and the milligram (mg) and microgram (mcg or μg) are subdivisions. Fractional parts of the liter are usually expressed in milliliters (ml), for example, 600 ml; multiples of the liter are usually expressed as liters or milliliters, for example, 2.5 liters or 2500 ml.

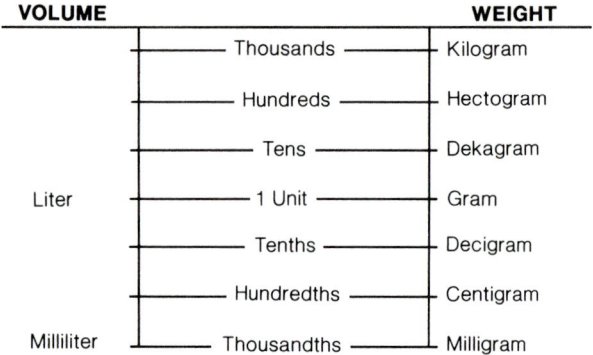

VOLUME		WEIGHT
	Thousands	Kilogram
	Hundreds	Hectogram
	Tens	Dekagram
Liter	1 Unit	Gram
	Tenths	Decigram
	Hundredths	Centigram
Milliliter	Thousandths	Milligram

Figure 45–6 Basic metric measurements of volume and weight.

Apothecaries' System

The apothecaries' system, older than the metric system, was brought to the United States from England during the colonial period. The basic unit of weight in the apothecaries' system is the grain, likened to a grain of wheat, and the basic unit of volume is the **minim,** a volume of water equal in weight to a grain of wheat. The word *minim* means "the least." In ascending order, the other units of weight are the scruple, the dram, the ounce, and the pound. Today, the scruple (scr) is seldom used. The units of volume are, in ascending order, the fluid dram, the fluid ounce, the pint, the quart, and the gallon.

Quantities in the apothecaries' system are often expressed by lowercase Roman numerals, particularly when the unit of measure is abbreviated. The Roman numeral follows rather than precedes the unit of measure. For example, a fluid ounce is abbreviated as f℥. Two fluid ounces are written as f℥ii, and 4 fluid ounces are written as f℥iv. One half fluid ounce is written as f℥ss, and 1½ fluid ounces as f℥iss. See Chapter 17, Table 17–2.

Household System

Household measures may be used when more accurate systems of measure are not required. Included in household measures are drops, teaspoons, tablespoons, cups, and glasses. Although pints and quarts are often found in the home, they are defined as apothecaries' measures. Equivalent units of the household system are in Appendix F.

Converting Units of Weight And Measure

Sometimes drugs are dispensed from the pharmacy in grams when the order specifies milligrams, or they are dispensed in milligrams though ordered in grains. The nurse prepar-

ing a medicated irrigation may find that the order calls for quarts and that the solution is dispensed in liter containers. In all situations, it is the nurse's responsibility to convert units of measure or weight, and thus nurses must be aware of approximate equivalents within each system of measurement and among systems.

Converting Weights within the Metric System

It is relatively simple to arrive at equivalent units of weight within the metric system, since the system is based on units of ten. Only three metric units of weight are used for drug dosages, the gram (g), milligram (mg), and microgram (mcg or μg): 1000 mg or 1,000,000 mcg equals 1 g. Equivalents are computed by dividing or multiplying; e.g., to change milligrams to grams, milligrams are divided by 1000. The simplest way to divide by 1000 is to move the decimal point three places to the left:

$$1000 \text{ mg} = 1 \text{ g}$$
$$500 \text{ mg} = 0.5 \text{ g}$$

Conversely, to convert grams to milligrams, the grams are multiplied by 1000, or the decimal point is moved three places to the right:

$$0.006 \text{ g} = 6 \text{ mg}$$

Converting Weights and Measures among Systems

When preparing client medications, a nurse may need to convert weights or volumes from one system to another. As an example, the pharmacy may dispense milligrams or grams of chloral hydrate, yet the nurse must administer an order that reads chloral hydrate grains viiss. To prepare the correct dose the nurse must convert from the apothecaries' to the metric system. To give clients a useful, realistic measure for home use, the nurse may have to convert from the apothecaries' or metric system to the household system. All conversions are approximate, that is, not totally precise.

Converting units of volume   Commonly used approximate equivalents are shown in Table 45–8.

By learning these equivalents, the nurse can make many conversions readily. For example, 15 minims = approximately 15 drops; therefore 1 minim is approximately 1 drop. Similarly, 1 quart approximates 1000 ml, and 1 gallon approximates 4000 ml; therefore 4 quarts is approximately 1 gallon.

The following are some situations in which nurses need to apply a knowledge of volume conversion.

1. Milliliter dosages may need to be fractionalized. The nurse can fractionalize milliliter dosages by remembering that 1 ml contains 15 drops or minims.

2. Fluid drams and ounces are commonly used in prescribing liquid medications, such as cough syrups, laxatives,

TABLE 45–8 Approximate Volume Equivalents: Metric, Apothecaries', and Household Systems

Metric		Apothecaries'		Household
1 ml	=	15 minims (min or m)	=	15 drops (gtt)
15 ml	=	4 fluid drams (f℥)	=	1 tablespoon (Tbsp)
30 ml	=	1 fluid ounce (f℥)	=	same
500 ml	=	1 pint (pt)	=	same
1000 ml	=	1 quart (qt)	=	same
4000 ml	=	1 gallon (gal)	=	same

TABLE 45–9 Approximate Weight Equivalents: Metric and Apothecaries' Systems

Metric		Apothecaries'
1 mg	=	1/60 grain
60 mg	=	1 grain
1 g	=	15 grains
4 g	=	1 dram
30 g	=	1 ounce
500 g	=	1.1 pound (lb)
1000 g (1 kg)	=	2.2 lb

antacids, and antibiotics for children. The fluid ounce is frequently converted to milliliters when measuring a client's fluid intake or output.

3. Liters and milliliters are the volumes commonly used in preparing solutions for enemas, irrigating solutions for douches, bladder irrigations, and solutions for cleaning open wounds. In some situations, the nurse needs to convert the volumes of such solutions.

Converting units of weight   The units of weight most commonly used in nursing practice are the gram, milligram, and kilogram and the grain and the pound. Household units of weight are generally not applicable.

Table 45–9 shows metric and apothecaries' approximate equivalents. Learning these equivalents helps the nurse make weight conversions readily, as, for example, in the following situations:

1. Converting a person's body weight from kilograms to pounds and vice versa

2. Converting grams and milligrams to grains and vice versa, for example, when preparing medications

When converting units of weight from the metric system to the apothecaries' system, the nurse should keep in mind that a milligram is smaller than a grain (1 mg = 1/60 grain and 1 grain = 60 mg). The result of converting a smaller unit (milligram) to a larger unit (grain) is a smaller number. Thus, the nurse must divide (by 60 if converting from milligrams to grains). Conversely, when converting from a larger unit to a smaller unit, the nurse multiplies (by 60 if converting from grains to milligrams), and the product is a larger number. In other words:

Small units (mg) to large units (grains)
= a smaller number
Large units (grains) to small units (mg)
= a larger number

$$\frac{3000\,mg}{60} = 50\ grains$$

$$50\ grains \times 60 = 3000\ mg$$

When converting pounds to kilograms, the nurse applies the same rule. The pound is a smaller unit than the kilogram, and the nurse converts by dividing or multiplying by 2.2:

$$\frac{110\,lb}{2.2} = 50\ kg$$

$$50\ kg \times 2.2 = 110\ lb$$

The conversion of milligrams to grams was previously discussed. The decimal point is moved three spaces to the left:

$$3000\ mg = 3\ g$$

Calculating Fractional Dosages

The need to calculate fractional dosages arises chiefly when small dosages must be administered to infants and children. Such calculation may also be necessary in preparing preoperative medications, injectable analgesics, and intravenous medications for adult clients.

Dosages for Children   Although dosage is stated in the medication order, nurses must understand something

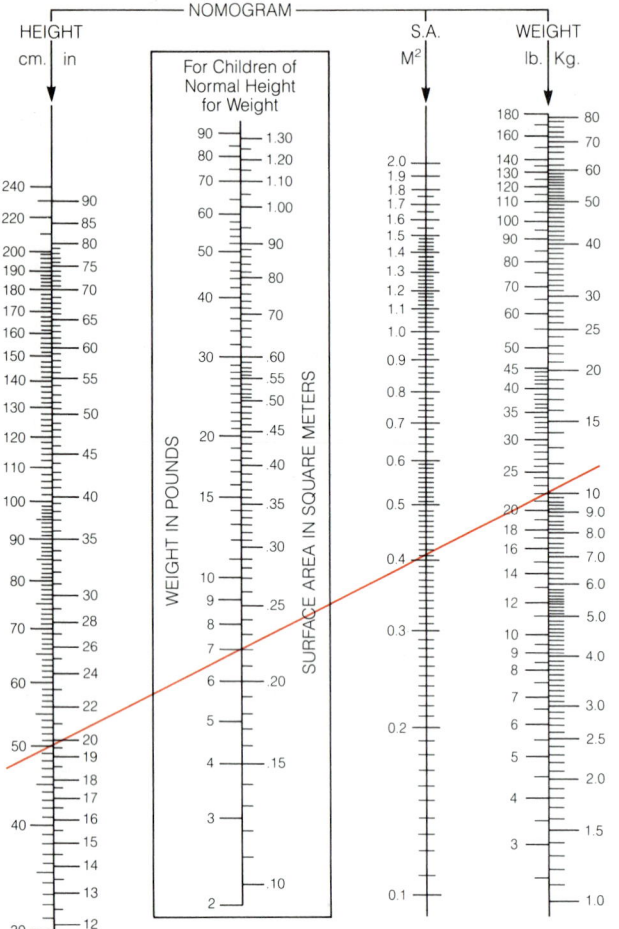

HEIGHT
cm. in

For Children of
Normal Height
for Weight

S.A.
M²

WEIGHT
lb. Kg.

WEIGHT IN POUNDS

SURFACE AREA IN SQUARE METERS

Figure 45-7 Nomogram with estimated body surface area. A straight line is drawn between the child's height (on the left) and the child's weight (on the right). The point at which the line intersects the surface area column is the estimated body surface area. *Source:* Courtesy of R. E. Behrman and V. C. Vaughan (editors), *Nelson textbook of pediatrics,* 13th ed. (Philadelphia: W. B. Saunders Co., 1987). Modified from data of E. Boyd by C. D. West.

about the safe dosage for children. Unlike adult dosages, children's dosages are not always standard. There are several formulas to determine pediatric dosages using body surface area and weight.

Body surface area   Body surface area is determined by using a nomogram and the child's height and weight. This is considered to be the most accurate method of calculating a child's dose. Standard nomograms give a child's body surface area according to weight and age. See Figure 45-7. The formula is the ratio of the child's body surface area to the surface area of an average adult (1.7 square

meters, or 1.7 m²), multiplied by the normal adult dose of the drug:

$$\text{Child's dose} = \frac{\text{Surface area of child (m}^2)}{1.7\,\text{m}^2} \times \begin{array}{l}\text{normal}\\\text{adult}\\\text{dose}\end{array}$$

For example, a child who weighs 10 kg and is 50 cm tall has a body surface area of 0.4 m². Therefore, the child's dose of tetracycline corresponding to an adult dose of 250 mg would be as follows:

$$\text{Child's dose} = \frac{0.4\,\text{m}^2}{1.7\,\text{m}^2} \times 250\,\text{mg}$$

$$= 0.23 \times 250 = 58.82\,\text{mg}$$

Clark's rule   Clark's rule, which applies to children of all ages, is less accurate than the above method for calculating pediatric dosages. It compares the child's body weight to the weight of a 150-pound (68-kilogram) adult and multiplies this ratio by the adult dose:

$$\text{Child's dose} = \frac{\text{Child's weight (lb)}}{150\,\text{lb}} \times \text{adult dose}$$

For example, for a child weighing 30 pounds and requiring Demerol, for which the adult dose is 100 mg:

$$\text{Child's dose} = \frac{30\,\text{lb}}{150\,\text{lb}} \times 100\,\text{mg}$$

$$= 0.2 \times 100 = 20\,\text{mg}$$

Fractional Dosages from Vials or Ampules

Many medications are already in liquid form and ready for use. Such medications are frequently packaged in vials and ampules. An **ampule** is a glass container usually designed to hold a single dose of a drug. It is made of clear glass and has a distinctive shape with a constricted neck. A **vial** is a small glass bottle with a sealed rubber cap. See Figure 45-17, later in this chapter. For example, meperidine hydrochloride (Demerol) is often distributed in large vials and prepared in dilutions of 50 mg per ml. Thus if the order calls for 100 mg, the nurse injects 2 ml, and if it calls for 75 mg, the nurse injects 1½ ml. To calculate the volume of solution that contains a certain milligram dosage, the nurse uses this formula:

$$\frac{D\,(\text{amount desired})}{H\,(\text{amount on hand})} = \text{Amount (volume) wanted}$$

$$\frac{40\,\text{mg}}{50\,\text{mg}} = \frac{4}{5}\,\text{ml}$$

The following is an example problem. Prepare 4 mg of a drug from a vial containing 20 mg in a 5-ml solution. Formula:

$$\frac{\text{Drug available}}{\text{Amount of solution}} = \frac{\text{Dose wanted}}{x\,\text{ml}}$$

$$\frac{20\,\text{mg}}{5\,\text{ml}} = \frac{4\,\text{mg}}{x\,\text{ml}}$$

Therefore

$$\frac{20}{5} = \frac{4}{x}$$

Cross multiply:

$$20x = 20$$

$$x = \frac{20}{20} = 1\,\text{ml}$$

ADMINISTERING MEDICATIONS SAFELY

The nurse should always assess a client's physical status prior to giving any medication. The extent of the assessment depends on the client's illness or current condition and the intended drug and route of administration. For example, the nurse assesses a dyspneic client's respirations carefully before administering any medication that might affect breathing. In general, the nurse assesses the client *prior* to administering any medication to obtain baseline data by which to evaluate the effectiveness of the medication. Clinical guidelines for administering medications are given in the accompanying box.

Process of Administering Medications

When administering any drug, regardless of the route of administration, the nurse must do the following.

1. *Identify the client.* Errors can and do occur, usually because one client gets a drug intended for another. In hospitals, most clients wear some sort of identification, such as a wristband with name and hospital identification number. Before giving the client any drug, the nurse should check the identification band with the medication card or medication administration record (MAR). As a double check, nurses also ask the client's name or ask another nurse to identify the client before administering any medication.

2. *Administer the drug.* Medication orders and cards or lists need to be read carefully and checked against the name on the medication envelope or on the drawer in which the client's medications are kept if a medication cart is used. The medication is then administered in the prescribed dosage, by the route ordered, at the correct time.

3. *Provide adjunctive interventions as indicated.* Clients may need help when receiving medications. They may

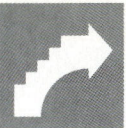

CLINICAL GUIDELINES
Administering Medications

- Nurses who administer medications are responsible for their own actions. Question any order that you consider incorrect.
- Be knowledgeable about the medications you administer.
- Federal laws govern the uses of narcotics and barbiturates. Keep these medications in a locked place.
- Use only medications that are in a clearly labeled container.
- Return liquid medications that are cloudy or have changed color to the pharmacy.
- Before administering a medication, identify the client correctly using the appropriate means of identification, e.g., identification bracelet and/or asking clients to state their names.
- Do not leave medication at the bedside, with certain exceptions, e.g., nitroglycerin, cough syrup. Determine agency policy.
- If a client vomits after taking an oral medication, report this to the nurse in charge.
- Take special precautions when administering certain medications; for example, have another nurse check the dosages of anticoagulants, insulin, and certain IV preparations.
- Most hospitals require new orders from the physician for the client's postsurgery care.
- When a medication is omitted for any reason, record the fact together with the reason.
- When a medication error is made, report it immediately to the nurse in charge.

require physical assistance, for instance, in assuming positions for intramuscular injections, or they may need explanations about the medications and guidance about measures to enhance drug effectiveness and prevent complications, e.g., drinking fluids. Some clients convey fear about their medications. The nurse can allay fears by listening carefully to clients' concerns and giving correct information.

4. *Record the drug administered.* The facts recorded in the chart, in ink or by computer printout, are name of the drug, dosage, method of administration, specific relevant data such as pulse rate (taken in most settings prior to the administration of digitalis), and any other pertinent information. The record should also include the

exact time of administration and the signature of the nurse providing the medication. Many medication records are designed so that the nurse signs once on the page and initials each medication administered. Often, medications that are given regularly are recorded on a special flow record, and prn or stat medications are recorded separately.

5. *Evaluate the client's response to the drug.* The kinds of behavior that reflect the action or lack of action of a drug and its untoward effects (both minor and major) are as variable as the purposes of the drugs themselves. The anxious client may show the desired effects of a tranquilizer by behavior that reflects a lowered stress level (e.g., slower speech or fewer random movements). The effectiveness of a sedative can often be measured by how well a client slept; the effectiveness of an antispasmodic, by how much pain the client feels. In all nursing activities, nurses need to be aware of the medications that a client is taking and record their effectiveness as assessed by the client and the nurse on the client's chart. The nurse may also report the client's response directly to the senior nurse and physician.

See the accompanying box for the five "rights" to accurate drug administration. In addition to adhering to these five "rights," the nurse should also be aware of clients' rights regarding medications. These are shown in the second box.

Developmental Considerations

Knowledge of growth and development is essential for the nurse administering medications to children. Oral medications for children are usually prepared in sweetened liquid form to make them more palatable. The parents may provide suggestions about what method is best for their child. Necessary foods such as milk or orange juice should not be used to mask the taste of medications, because the child may develop unpleasant associations and refuse that food in the future.

Children tend to fear any procedure in which a needle is used because they anticipate pain or because the procedure is unfamiliar and threatening. The nurse needs to acknowledge that the child will feel some pain; denying this fact only deepens the child's distrust. After the injection, the nurse (or the parent) can cuddle and speak softly to the infant and give the child a toy to dispel the child's association of the nurse only with pain.

The older person can present special problems, most of which are related to physiologic changes, to past experiences, and to established attitudes toward medications. The physiologic changes in elderly persons that may affect the administration and effectiveness of medications are included in the box on the opposite page.

Many of these changes enhance the possibility of cumulative effects and toxicity. For example, impaired circulation delays the action of medications given intramuscularly or subcutaneously. Digitalis, which is frequently taken by elderly people, can accumulate to toxic levels and be lethal. It is not uncommon for elderly clients to take several different medications daily. The possibility of error increases with the number of medications taken, whether self-administered at home or administered by nurses in a hospital. The greater number of medications also compounds the problem of drug interactions, because much is yet to be learned about the effects of drugs given in combinations. A general rule to follow is that elderly clients should take as few medications as possible.

Elderly persons usually require smaller dosages of drugs, especially sedatives and other central nervous system depressants. Reactions of the elderly to medications, particularly sedatives, are unpredictable and often bizarre. It is not uncommon to see irritability, confusion, disorientation, restlessness, and incontinence as a result of sedatives. Nurses therefore need to observe clients carefully for untoward reactions. The use of alcohol (e.g., brandy) as a bedtime relaxant and as an appetizer before meals is becoming more common. The moderate use of alcohol by people who are accustomed to it can contribute to a sense of well-being.

Attitudes of elderly people toward medical care and medications vary. Elderly people tend to believe in the wisdom of the physician more readily than younger people. Some older people are bewildered by the prescription of several medications and may passively accept their medications from nurses but not swallow them, spitting out tablets or capsules after the nurse leaves the room. For this reason, the nurse is advised to stay with clients until they have taken the medications. Others may be suspicious of medications and actively refuse them.

Elderly people are mature adults capable of reasoning. Therefore, the nurse needs to explain the reasons for and effects of medications. This education can prevent clients from taking a medication long after there is a need for it or discontinuing a drug too quickly. For example, clients should know that diuretics will cause them to urinate more frequently and may reduce ankle edema. Instructions about medications need to be given to all clients prior to discharge from a hospital. These instructions should include when to take the drugs, what effects to expect, and when to consult a physician.

Because some clients are required to take several medications daily and because visual acuity and memory may be impaired, the nurse needs to develop simple, realistic plans for clients to follow at home. For example, remembering to take drugs can be difficult for most persons, including the elderly. If medications are scheduled to be taken with meals or at bedtime, clients are not as likely to forget. Some clients may take their medications and then an hour later not remember whether they took them. One solution to forgetfulness is to use a special container or glass strictly for medications. An empty glass or container indicates that the person took the pills. Loss of visual acuity presents problems that can be overcome by writing out the plan in block letters large enough to be read. In some situations the help of a spouse, son, or daughter can be enlisted.

Medication History

The medication history includes information about the drugs the client is taken currently or has taken recently. This includes prescription drugs, over-the-counter drugs such as antacids, alcohol and tobacco, and nonsanctioned drugs such as marijuana. Sometimes one or more of these drugs may affect the choice of another, different medication, since they may be incompatible.

An important part of the history is clients' knowledge of their drug allergies. Some clients can tell a nurse, "I am allergic to penicillin, adhesive tape, and curry." Other clients may not be sure about allergic reactions. An illness occurring after a drug was taken may not be identified as an allergy, but the client may associate the drug with an illness or unusual reaction. The client's physician can often give information about allergies. During the history, the nurse tries to elicit information about drug dependencies. The frequency with which drugs are taken and the client's perceived need for them are measures of dependence.

Also included in the history are the client's normal eating habits. Sometimes the medication schedule needs to be coordinated with mealtimes or the ingestion of foods. Where a medication must be taken with food on a specified schedule, clients can often adjust their mealtime or have a snack, e.g., with a bedtime medication. In addition, certain foods are incompatible with certain medications; for example, milk is incompatible with tetracycline.

Any problems the client may have in self-administering a medication must also be identified. A client with poor eyesight, for example, may require special labels for the medication container; elderly clients with unsteady hands may not be able to hold a syringe or to inject themselves or another person.

ORAL MEDICATIONS

The oral route is the most common route by which medications are given. As long as a client can swallow and retain the drug in the stomach, this is the route of choice. See Procedure 45–1. Oral medications are contraindicated when a client is vomiting, has gastric or intestinal suction, or is unconscious and unable to swallow. Such clients in a hospital usually are on orders "nothing by mouth" (NPO).

PROCEDURE 45–1

ADMINISTERING ORAL MEDICATIONS

Equipment ☑

Medication tray or cart

Medication cards, medication administration record (MAR), or computer printout

Disposable medication cups: small paper or plastic cups for tablets and capsules, waxed or plastic calibrated medication cups for liquids

Pill crusher (optional)

Intervention

1. Organize the supplies.

- Assemble medication tray and cups in medicine room, or place medication cart outside the client's room.

- Plan to give medications first to clients who do not require assistance and last to those who do. Arrange the medication cards or records in this order.

- Assemble the medication cards or records for each client together so that medications can be prepared **S** for one client at a time. *Organization of supplies saves time and reduces the chance of error.*

2. Verify the client's ability to take medication orally.

- Determine whether the client can swallow, is on NPO, is nauseated or vomiting, or has gastric suction.

3. Verify the order for accuracy.

S
- Check the accuracy of the medication card, MAR, or printout with the physician's written order. It should contain the following: (a) client's name, (b) drug name and dosage, (c) time for administration, and (d) route of administration.

- Report any discrepancies in the order to the nurse in charge or the physician, as agency policy dictates.

4. Obtain the appropriate medication.

- Read the medication card or MAR, and take the appropriate medication from the shelf, drawer, or refrigerator. The medication may be dispensed in the bottle, box, or unit dose package.

S
- Compare the label of the medication container or unit dose package against the order on the medication card or MAR. If these are not identical, recheck the client's chart. If there is still a discrepancy, check with the nurse in charge.

5. Prepare the medication.

- Prepare the correct amount of medication for the required dose, without contaminating the medication. *Aseptic technique maintains drug cleanliness.*

S
- While preparing the medication, recheck each medication card or MAR with the prepared drug and container. *This second check reduces the chance of error.*

For tablets or capsules from a bottle:

- Pour the required number into the bottle cap, and then transfer the medication to the disposable cup without touching the tablets. See Figure 45–8. Usually all tablets or capsules to be given to the client are placed in the same cup.

- Keep medications that require specific assessments, e.g., pulse measurements, respiratory rate or depth, or blood pressure, separate from the others. *This enables the nurse to withhold the medication if indicated.*

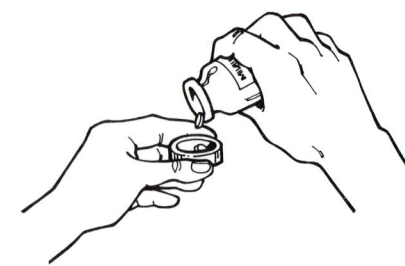

Figure 45–8 Pouring a tablet into the container lid.

- If the client has difficulty swallowing, crush the tablets to a fine powder in the mortar with the pestle or between two medication cups or spoons. Then, mix the powder with a small amount of soft food (e.g., custard, applesauce).

For liquid medication:

- Remove the cap, and place it upside down on the countertop to avoid contaminating it.

- Hold the bottle with the label next to your palm and pour the medication away from the label. See Figure 45–9. *This prevents the label from becoming soiled and illegible as a result of spilled liquids.*

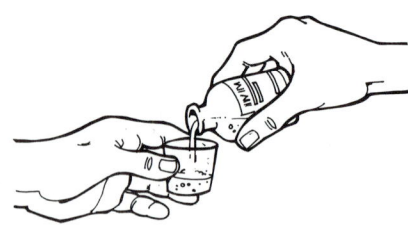

Figure 45–9 Pouring a liquid medication from a bottle.

- Hold the medication cup at eye level, and fill it to the desired level, using the bottom of the **meniscus** (crescent-shaped upper surface of a column of liquid) as the measurement guide. See Figure 45–10. *This method ensures accuracy of measurement.*

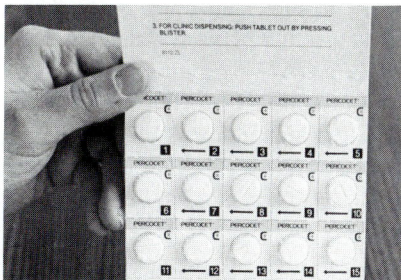

Figure 45–10 The bottom of the meniscus is the measuring guide.

- Before capping the bottle, wipe the lip with a paper towel. *This prevents the cap from sticking.*

For an oral narcotic:

- Check the narcotic record for the previous drug count and compare it with the supply available. Some narcotics are kept in specially designed plastic containers that are sectioned and numbered (see Figure 45–11).

Figure 45–11 Commercially packaged narcotics.

- Remove the next available tablet and drop it in the medicine cup.
- After removing a tablet, record the necessary information on the appropriate narcotic control record and sign it.

For a unit-dose medication:

- Place the *unwrapped* unit-dose medications directly into the medicine cup. *The wrapper keeps the medication clean and facilitates identification.*

For all medications:

- Place the prepared medication and medication card together on the tray or cart.
- Return the bottle, box, or envelope to its storage place, and recheck the label on the container. *This third check further reduces the risk of error.*
- Avoid leaving prepared medications unattended. *Accidental disarrangement of the medication could occur.*

6. Administer the medication at the correct time.

- Identify the client by comparing the name on the medication card or list with the name on the client's identification bracelet or by asking the client to tell you his or her name. *Accurate identification is essential to prevent error.*
- Explain the purpose of the medication and how it will help, using language that the client can understand. Include relevant information about effects, e.g., tell the client receiving a diuretic to expect an increase in urine. *Information facilitates acceptance of and compliance with the therapy.*
- Assist the client to a sitting position or, if not possible, to a lateral position. *These positions facilitate swallowing and prevent aspiration.*
- Take the required assessment measures, e.g., pulse and respiratory rates or blood pressure. The pulse rate is taken before administering digitalis preparations. Blood pressure is taken before giving hypotensive drugs. The respiratory rate is taken prior to administering narcotics, since narcotics depress the respiratory center. If the rate is below 12, consult the nurse in charge.
- Give the client sufficient water or juice to swallow the medication. *Fluids ease swallowing and facilitate absorption from the gastrointestinal tract.* Liquid medications are generally diluted with 15 ml (½ oz) of water to facilitate absorption.
- If the client is unable to hold the pill cup, use the pill cup to introduce the medication into the client's mouth, and give only one tablet or capsule at a time. *Putting the cup to the client's mouth maintains the cleanliness of the nurse's hands. Giving one medication at a time eases swallowing.*
- If the client has difficulty swallowing, ask the client to place the medication on the back of the tongue before taking the water. *Stimulation of the back of the tongue produces the swallowing reflex.*
- If the medication has an objectionable taste, ask the client to suck a few ice chips beforehand, or give the medication with juice, applesauce, or bread. *The cold will desensitize the taste buds, and juices or bread can mask the taste of the medication.*
- If the client says that the medication you are about to give is different from what the client has been receiving, do not give the medication without checking the original order. Most clients are familiar with the appearance of medications taken previously. *Unfamiliar drugs may signal a possible error.*
- Stay with the client until all medications have been swallowed. *The nurse must see the client swallow the medication before the drug administration can be recorded.* A physician's order or agency policy is required for medications left at the bedside.

7. Document each medication given.

- Record the medication given, dosage, time, any complaints or assessments of the client, and your signature.

- If medication was refused or omitted, record this fact on the appropriate record, and document the reason when possible.

8. Dispose of supplies appropriately.

- Return the medication cards or records to the appropriate file for the next administration time.

- Replenish stock, e.g., medication cups, and return cart to medicine room.

- Discard used disposable supplies.

9. Evaluate the effects of the medication.

- Return to the client when the medication is expected to take effect (usually 30 minutes) to evaluate the effects of the medication, e.g., relief of pain or any adverse effects.

PARENTERAL MEDICATIONS

Parenteral medications are given by nurses subcutaneously, intramuscularly, intradermally, or intravenously. Because parenteral medications are absorbed more quickly than oral medications and are irretrievable once injected, the nurse must prepare and administer them carefully and accurately. Administering parenteral drugs requires the same nursing knowledge as administering oral and topical drugs, plus considerable manual dexterity and the use of sterile technique.

Equipment

Syringes To administer parenteral medications, nurses use injectable equipment (i.e., syringes, needles, vials, and ampules). Syringes have three parts: the tip, which connects with the needle; the barrel, or outside part, on which the scales are printed; and the plunger, which fits inside the barrel. See Figure 45–12. Most syringes used today are made of plastic and are individually packaged for sterility in a paper wrapper or a rigid plastic container. Glass syringes are used when the medication is incompatible with plastic.

There are several kinds of syringes, differing in size, shape, and material. The three most commonly used types are the standard hypodermic syringe, the insulin syringe, and the tuberculin syringe. See Figure 45–13. *Hypodermic syringes* come in 2, 2.5, and 3 ml sizes. They usually have two scales marked on them: the minim and the milliliter. The milliliter scale is the one normally used; the minim scale is used for very small dosages.

Insulin syringes are similar to hypodermic syringes, but they have a scale specially designed for insulin: a 100-unit calibrated scale intended for use with U-100 insulin. Low-dose insulin syringes can hold a maximum of 50 units (½

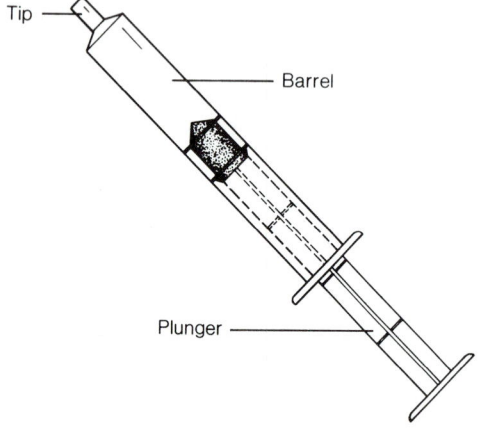

Figure 45–12 The three parts of a syringe.

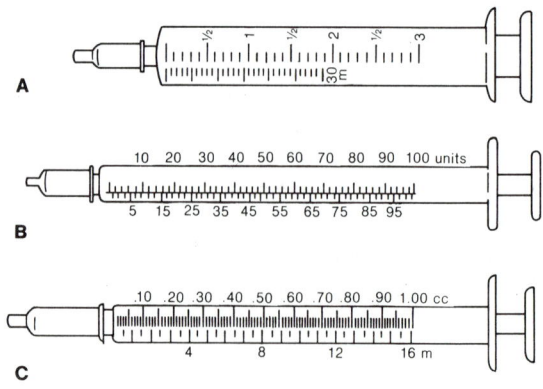

Figure 45–13 Three kinds of syringes: *A,* hypodermic; *B,* insulin; *C,* tuberculin.

ml) and frequently have a nonremovable needle. The *tuberculin syringe* was designed to administer tuberculin. It is a narrow syringe, calibrated in tenths and hundredths of a milliliter (up to 1 ml) on one scale and in sixteenths of a minim (up to 1 min) on the other scale. This type of syringe can also be useful in administering other drugs, particularly when small or precise measurement is indicated (e.g., pediatric dosages). Syringes are made in other sizes as well, for example, 5, 10, 20, and 50 milliliters. These are not generally used to administer drugs directly but can be useful for adding medications to intravenous solutions or for irrigating wounds.

The *disposable plastic syringe* is most frequently used today. The syringe is supplied with a needle, which may have a plastic cap over it. The syringe and needle may be packaged together or separately. See Figure 45–14.

Injectable medications are frequently supplied in *prefilled unit-dose syringes* with needles or cartridge-needle units. These prefilled syringes and cartridge-needle units are disposable. The cartridge-needle units, however, require special metal or plastic cartridge holders or syringes for administration. These syringes and cartridges come with manufacturer's directions for use.

Needles

Needles are made of stainless steel and most are disposable. Reusable needles (e.g., for special procedures) need to be sharpened periodically before resterilization, because the points become dull with use and are occasionally damaged or acquire burrs on the tips. A dull or damaged needle should *never* be used.

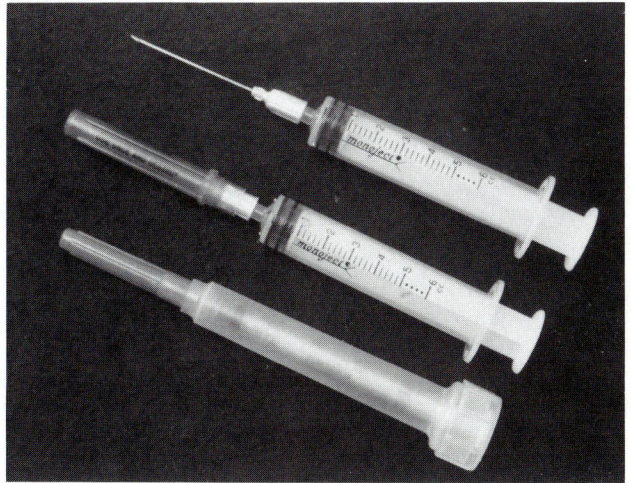

Figure 45–14 Disposable plastic syringes and needles: *top,* with syringe and needle exposed; *middle,* with plastic cup over the needle; *bottom,* with plastic case over the needle and syringe.

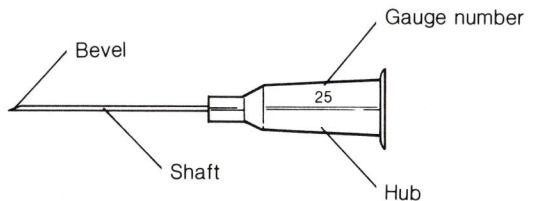

Figure 45–15 The parts of a needle.

A needle has three discernible parts: the hub, which fits onto the syringe; the cannula, or shaft, which is attached to the hub; and the bevel, which is the slanted part at the tip of the needle. See Figure 45–15. A disposable needle has a plastic hub. Needles used for injections have three variables:

1. *Slant or length of the bevel.* The bevel of the needle may be short or long. Longer bevels provide the sharpest needles and cause less discomfort and are commonly used for subcutaneous and intramuscular injections. Short bevels are used for intradermal and intravenous injections, because a long bevel can become occluded if it rests against the side of a blood vessel.

2. *Length of the shaft.* The shaft length of commonly used needles varies from ¼ to 5 in.

3. *Gauge (or diameter) of the shaft.* The gauge varies from #14 to #28. The larger the gauge number, the smaller the diameter of the shaft. Smaller gauges produce less tissue trauma, but larger gauges are necessary for viscous medications, such as penicillin.

For subcutaneous injections, it is usual to use a needle of #24 to #26 gauge and ⅜ to ⅝ in long. Obese clients may require a 1-in needle. For intramuscular injections, a longer needle, e.g., 1 to 1½ in, with a larger gauge, e.g., gauge #20 to #22, is used.

Needle Recappers

New devices, such as the On ● Gard Recapper™ (see Figure 45–16), allow the nurse to uncap and recap any needle safely and effectively, without changing current technique or needle brand. To use the On ● Gard Recapper, the nurse inserts the entire syringe in the center hole of the shield. The Recapper firmly grips the needle cap and holds it in place until it is ready to recap.

Ampules and Vials

Ampules and *vials* are frequently used to package sterile parenteral medications. See Figure 45–17. Most ampule necks have colored marks around them, indicating where they are prescored for easy opening. If the neck is not scored, it should be filed with a small file, then broken off at the neck. Vials come in different sizes, from single to multidose vials. They usually have a metal or plastic cap that protects the rubber seal.

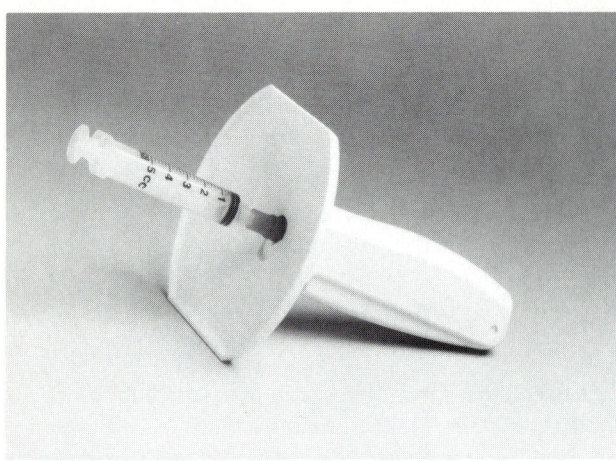

Figure 45–16 A device to prevent accidental needle sticks.

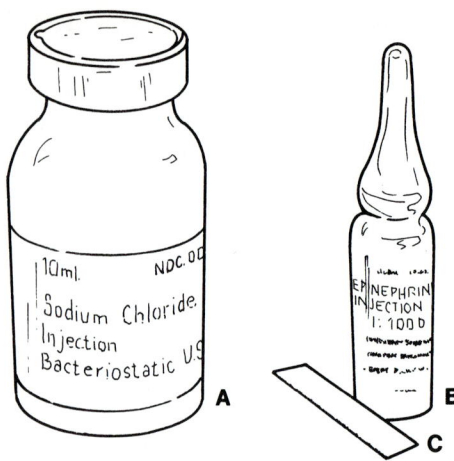

Figure 45–17 *A,* vial; *B,* ampule; *C,* ampule file.

Several drugs (e.g., penicillin) are dispensed as powders in vials. A liquid (solvent or diluent) must be added to a powdered medication before it can be injected. The technique of adding a solvent to a powdered drug to prepare it for administration is called **reconstitution.** Powdered drugs usually have printed instructions (enclosed with each packaged vial) that describe the amount and kind of solvent to be added. Commonly used solvents are sterile water or sterile normal saline. Some preparations are supplied in individual-dose vials; others come in multidose vials. The following are two examples of the preparation of powdered drugs:

1. *Single-dose vial:* Instructions for preparing a single-dose vial direct that 1.5 ml of sterile water be added to the sterile dry powder, thus providing a single dose of 2 ml. The volume of the drug powder was 0.5 ml. Therefore, the 1.5 ml of water plus the 0.5 ml of powder results in 2 ml of solution. In other instances, the addition of a solution does *not* increase the volume. Therefore it is important to follow the manufacturers' directions.

2. *Multidose vial:* A dose of 750 mg of a certain drug is ordered for a client. On hand is a 10-g multidose vial. The directions for preparation read: "Add 8.5 ml of sterile water, and each milliliter will contain 1.0 g or 1000 mg." Thus, after adding the solvent, the nurse will give $750/1000$ or $\frac{3}{4}$ ml (0.75 ml) of the medication.

Procedure 45–2 describes how to prepare medications from ampules and vials.

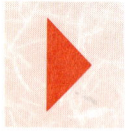

PROCEDURE 45–2

PREPARING MEDICATIONS FROM AMPULES AND VIALS

Equipment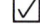

Vial or ampule of sterile medication
Alcohol swab
Needle and syringe

Special filter needle (optional) for withdrawing premixed liquid medications from multidose vials or from ampules to filter out glass slivers

Sterile water or normal saline, if necessary
File and small gauze square
Medication card, MAR, or computer printout

Intervention

1. **Ensure accuracy of the order and drug administration.**

■ Check the label on the ampule or vial carefully against the medica-

tion card, MAR, or client's chart to make sure that the correct medication is being prepared. See Procedure 45–1, Step 3.

■ Follow the three checks for admin-

istering medications. Read the label on the medication before it is taken off the shelf, before withdrawing the medication, and after placing it back on the shelf.

2. **Prepare the medication ampule or vial for drug withdrawal.**

Ampules:

■ Flick the upper stem of the ampule several times with a fingernail or, holding the upper stem of the ampule, make a large circle with the arm extended. *This will bring all the medication down to the main portion of the ampule.*

■ Partially file the neck of the ampule if necessary to start a clean break.

■ Place a piece of sterile gauze between your thumb and the ampule neck or around the ampule neck, and break off the top by bending it toward the gauze, i.e., away from you. See Figure 45–18. *The sterile gauze protects the fingers from the broken glass.*

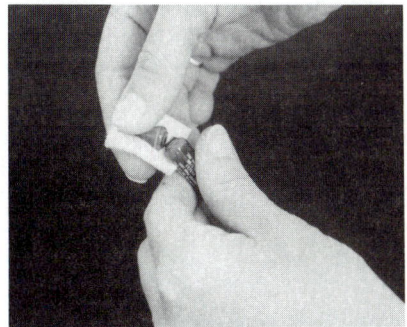

Figure 45–18 Breaking the neck of an ampule.

or

■ Place the antiseptic wipe packet over the top of the ampule before breaking off the top. *This method contains all the glass fragments in the packet and reduces the risk of cuts.*

Vials:

■ Mix the solution, if necessary, by rotating the vial between the palms of the hands, not by shaking. *Some vials contain aqueous suspen-*

sions, which settle when they stand. In some instances shaking is contraindicated because it may cause the mixture to foam.

■ Remove the protective metal cap, and clean the rubber cap with an antiseptic, such as 70% alcohol on a sterile gauze, by rubbing in a rotary motion. *The antiseptic cleans the cap so that the needle will remain sterile when it is inserted.*

3. **Withdraw the medication.**

Ampules:

■ Some nurses recommend using a needle with a filter to withdraw the medication in case there is any broken glass from the ampule in the medication. In this case, disconnect the regular needle, leaving its cap on, and attach the filter needle to the syringe.

■ Remove the cap from the needle, insert the needle in the ampule, and withdraw the amount of drug required for the dosage. See Figure 45–19.

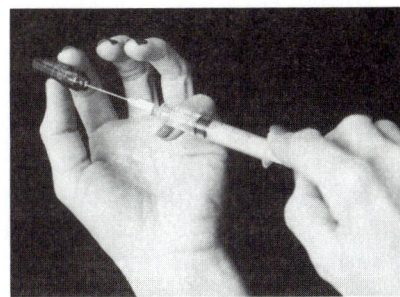

Figure 45–19 Withdrawing a medication from an ampule.

■ With a single-dose ampule, hold the ampule slightly on its side, if necessary, to obtain all the medication.

■ If a filter needle was used to withdraw the medication, replace it with a regular needle before injecting the client.

■ If a filter needle was not used, recap the needle. To recap a **sterile unused** needle safely (i.e., one that has *not* contacted body fluids or tissue of a person), hold the cap between two fingers, and brace the barrel against the palm. See Figure 45–20, *A.* Gently guide the tip of the needle into the opening of the cap, and release the fingers, allowing the cap to slide over the needle. See Figure 45–20, *B.* Tighten the cap.

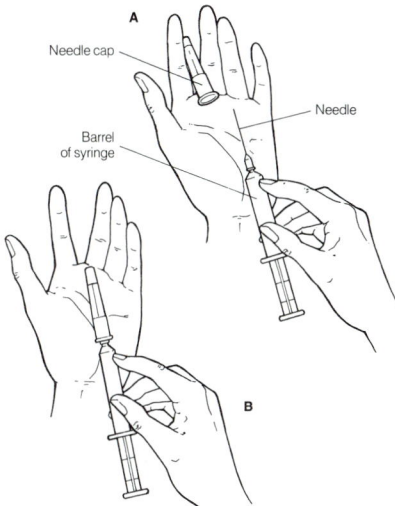

Needle cap

Needle

Barrel of syringe

Figure 45–20 Recapping a sterile unused needle.

Vials:

■ Attach a special filter needle as agency practice dictates to draw up premixed liquid medications from multidose vials. *The filter prevents any solid material from being drawn up through the needle.*

■ Remove the cap from the needle; then draw up into the syringe the amount of air equal to the volume of the medication to be withdrawn.

■ Carefully insert the needle into the vial through the center of the rubber cap, maintaining the sterility of the needle.

■ Inject the air into the vial, keeping the bevel of the needle above the surface of the medication. See Fig-

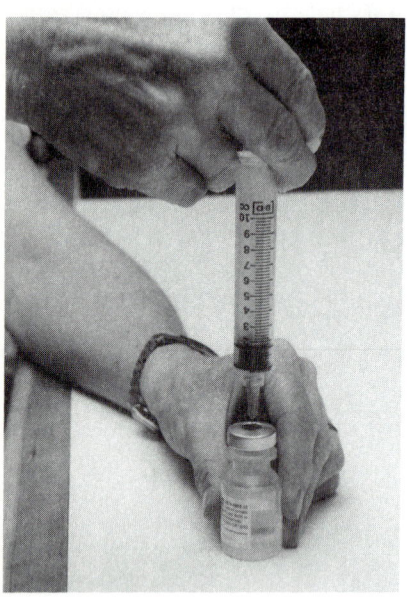

Figure 45–21 Injecting air into a vial.

ure 45–21. *The air will allow the medication to be drawn out easily, since negative pressure is not created inside the vial. The bevel is kept*

above the medication to avoid creating bubbles in the medication.

- Invert the vial, and hold it at eye level while withdrawing the correct dosage of the drug into the syringe. See Figure 45–22.
- Withdraw the needle from the vial, and replace the cap over the needle, thus maintaining its sterility.

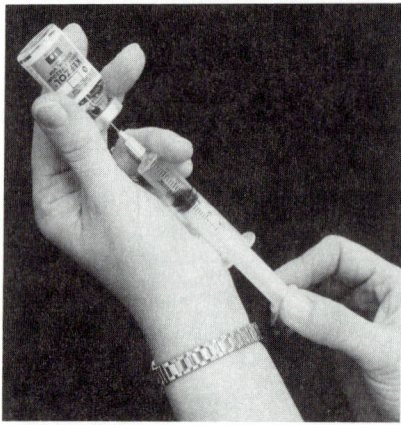

Figure 45–22 Withdrawing a medication from a vial.

or

Replace the filter needle with the regular needle.

___

Variation: preparing powdered drugs

- Read the manufacturer's directions.
- Withdraw an equivalent amount of air from the vial before adding the solvent, unless otherwise indicated by the directions.
- Add the amount of sterile water or saline indicated in the directions.
- If a multidose vial is reconstituted, label the vial with the date, time it was prepared, the amount of drug contained in each milliliter of solution, and your initials. Time is an important factor to consider in the expiration of these medications.
- Once reconstituted, store the medication in the vial in a refrigerator or as recommended by the manufacturer.

Mixing Medications

Frequently, clients need more than one drug injected at the same time. To spare the client the experience of being injected twice, two drugs (if compatible) are often mixed together in one syringe and given as one injection. It is common, for instance, to combine two types of insulin in this manner or to combine injectable preoperative medications such as morphine or meperidine (Demerol) with atropine or scopolamine. Drugs can also be mixed in intravenous solutions. When uncertain about drug compatibilities, the nurse should consult a pharmacist before mixing the drugs.

Mixing Medications from Two Vials   When withdrawing and mixing medications from two different vials, the nurse takes care not to contaminate the medication remaining in one vial with the other medication. To do this safely, the nurse inserts into vial A a needle attached to a syringe containing a volume of air equal to the volume of

medication to be withdrawn. The nurse then injects the air, making sure that the tip of the needle does not touch the solution. The nurse withdraws the needle and repeats the procedure with vial B; the nurse again injects a volume of air equal to the volume of medication to be withdrawn. The nurse then withdraws the required amount of medication from vial B. In this way, vial B is not contaminated by medication from vial A. When possible, the nurse then attaches a new, sterile needle to the syringe, inserts it into vial A, and withdraws the required amount of medication into the syringe. The syringe now contains a mixture of medications from vials A and B, and neither vial is contaminated by microorganisms or by medication from the other vial.

Often clients are given two types of insulin, short- and long-acting; these two types vary in content. Chemically, insulin is a protein that, when hydrolyzed in the body, yields a number of amino acids. Some insulin preparations contain an additional modifying protein, such as globulin or protamine, that slows absorption. This fact is particularly relevant when mixing two insulin preparations for injection, as many insulin syringes have needles that cannot be changed. A vial of insulin that does *not* have the added protein should never be contaminated with insulin that does have the added protein. For example, a vial of regular insulin (crystalline zinc insulin, CZ) should never be entered with a needle that had been previously used to withdraw protamine zinc, globin zinc, or isophane (NPH) insulins, all of which have added protein. See Figure 45–23.

The following is an example. At 0730 hours the nurse is to administer to a client 10 units of CZ and 30 units of NPH insulin, which contains protamine.

1. Inject 30 units of air into the NPH vial, and withdraw the needle. (There should be no insulin in the needle.) The needle should not touch the insulin.

2. Inject 10 units of air into the CZ vial, and immediately withdraw 10 units of CZ insulin.

3. Reinsert the needle into the NPH insulin vial, and withdraw 30 units of NPH insulin. (The air was previously injected into the vial.) See Figure 45–23.

By using this method, the nurse does not add NPH insulin to the CZ insulin.

Mixing Medications from One Vial and One Ampule

Because ampules do not require the addition of air prior to withdrawal of the drug, it is recommended that the nurse prepare the medication from the vial first,

RESEARCH NOTE

Should Diabetics Be Allowed to Administer Their Own Insulin in the Hospital?

Germain and Nemchik surveyed 73 persons concerning their beliefs about managing their diabetic care while in the hospital. A majority of persons (66%) stated that diabetics should manage their own care activities while hospitalized. Yet in most cases, care activities, such as administering insulin and testing blood glucose, were performed by the nurse more than 80% of the time. Diabetics who preferred to perform their own care activities felt that they "know more about their illness than anyone else." Those diabetics who preferred not to perform care activities stated it was nice to have a "vacation" from needles and counting food.

Implications: Every nurse should conduct a detailed interview with diabetics to identify what self-care activities they wish to perform while hospitalized. This information should be documented on the care plan to promote individualized patient care.

C. Germain and R. Nemchik, Diabetes self-management and hospitalization, *Image: Journal of Nursing Scholarship,* Summer 1988, 20:74–78.

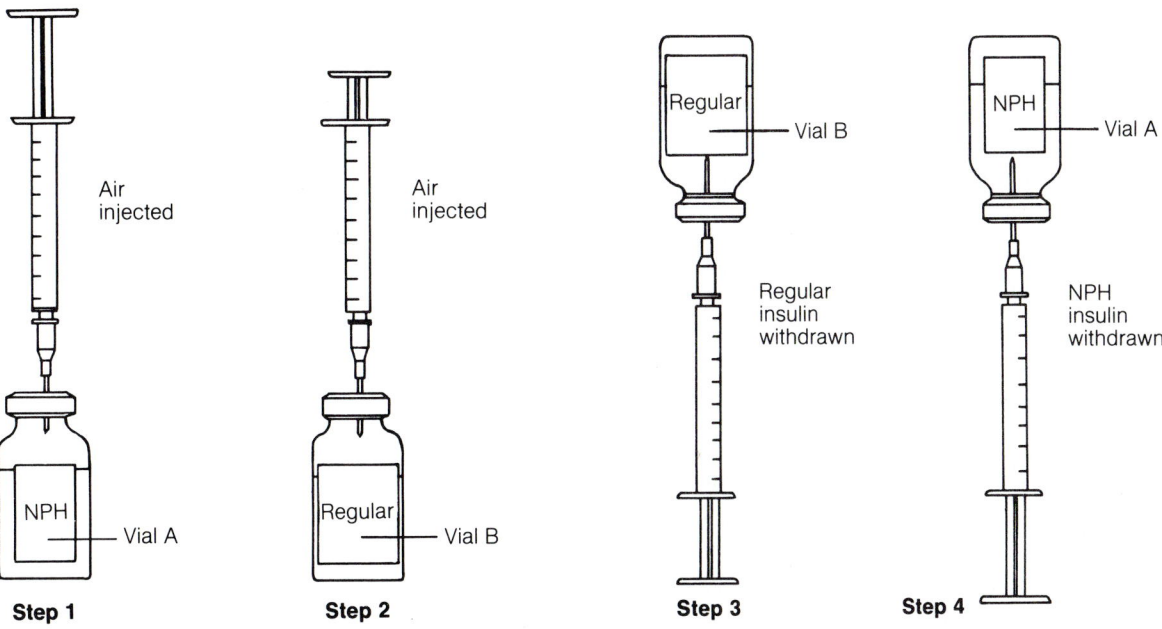

Figure 45–23 Mixing together two types of insulin.

then withdraw the medication from the ampule. To mix two medications from a cartridge and a vial or ampule, the nurse first ensures that the correct dose of the medication is in the cartridge. Any excess medication should be discarded. Then the nurse should draw up the required medication from a vial or ampule into the cartridge. If the total volume to be injected exceeds the capacity of the cartridge, a syringe with sufficient capacity should be used to withdraw the desired amount of medication from the vial/ampule, and the required amount from the cartridge should be transferred to the syringe.

Intradermal Injections

An intradermal injection is the administration of a drug into the dermal layer of the skin just beneath the epidermis. Usually only a small amount of liquid is used, for example, 0.1 ml. This method of administration is frequently indicated for allergy and tuberculin tests and for vaccinations. Common sites for intradermal injections are the inner lower arm, the upper chest, and the back beneath the scapulae. See Figure 45–24. Commonly the left arm is used for tuberculin tests and the right arm is used for all other tests.

The equipment normally used is a 1-ml syringe calibrated into hundredths of a milliliter. The needle is short and fine, frequently a #25, #26, or #27 gauge, ¼ in to ⅝ in long. After the site is cleaned, the skin is held tautly, and the syringe is held at about a 15° angle to the skin, with the bevel of the needle upward. The needle is then inserted through the epidermis into the dermis, and the fluid is injected. The drug produces a small bleb just under the skin. See Figure 45–25. The needle is then withdrawn quickly, and the site is very lightly wiped with an antiseptic swab. The area is not massaged because the medication may dis-

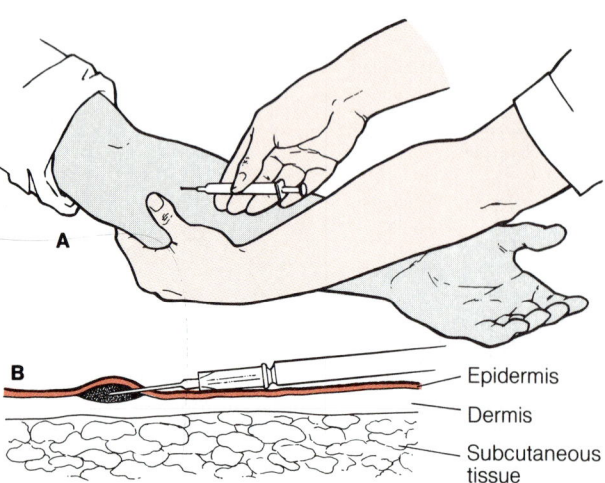

Figure 45–24 Body sites commonly used for intradermal injections.

Figure 45–25 For an intradermal injection: *A*, the needle enters the skin at a 15° angle; and *B*, the medication forms a bleb under the epidermis.

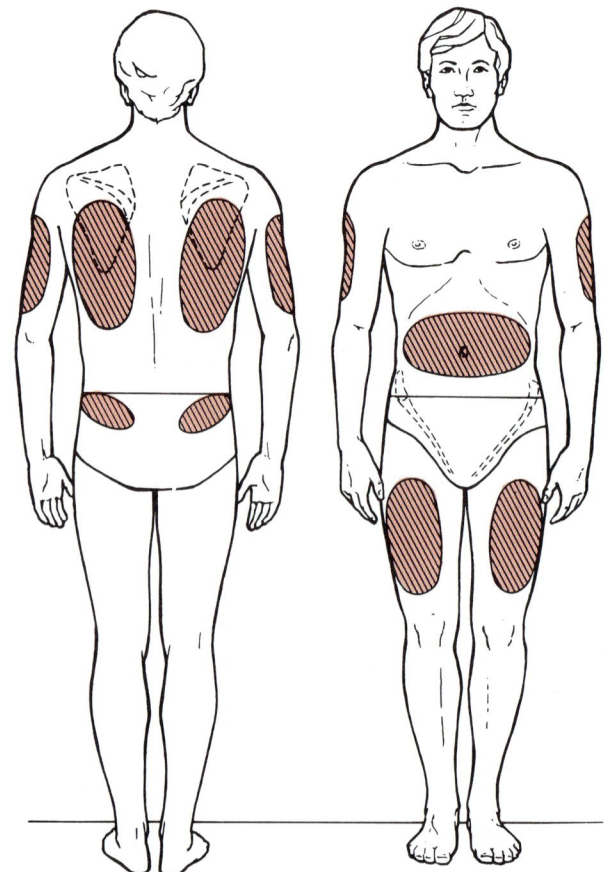

Epidermis
Dermis
Subcutaneous tissue

Figure 45–26 Body sites commonly used for subcutaneous injections.

perse into the tissue or out through the needle insertion site. Intradermal injections are absorbed slowly through blood capillaries in the area.

Subcutaneous Injections

Among the many kinds of drugs administered subcutaneously are vaccines, preoperative medications, narcotics, insulin, and heparin. Common sites for subcutaneous injec-

tions are the outer aspect of the upper arms and the anterior aspect of the thighs. These areas are convenient and normally have good blood circulation. Other areas that can be used are the abdomen, the scapular areas of the upper back, and the upper ventrogluteal and dorsogluteal areas. See Figure 45–26. Clients who administer their own injections, such as diabetics requiring insulin, usually use the abdomen and anterior thigh sites. Heparin, however, is given only in the abdomen (see Procedure 45–3).

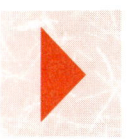

PROCEDURE 45–3

ADMINISTERING A SUBCUTANEOUS INJECTION

Equipment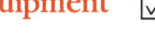

Client's medication card, MAR, or computer printout

Vial or ampule of the correct sterile medication

Sterile syringe and needle (e.g., 2-ml syringe, #25 gauge ⅝- or ½-in needle)

Sterile antiseptic-soaked swabs

Dry sterile gauze for opening an ampule (optional)

Gloves (according to agency protocol)

Intervention

1. Verify the medication order for accuracy.

■ See Procedure 45–1, Step 3.

2. Prepare the medication from the vial or ampule.

■ See Procedure 45–2, page 1272.

3. Identify the client, and assist the client to a comfortable position.

■ Check the client's arm band, and ask the client to tell you his or her name.

■ Assist the client to a position in which the arm, leg, or abdomen can be relaxed, depending on the

site to be used. *A relaxed muscle at the site minimizes discomfort.*

4. Select and clean the site.

■ Select a site free of tenderness, hardness, swelling, scarring, itching, burning, or localized inflammation. Select a site that has not been used frequently. *These conditions could hinder the absorption of the medication and also increase the likelihood of an infection at the injection site.*

■ As agency policy indicates, clean the site with an antiseptic swab. Start at the center of the site and clean in a widening circle to about 2″. Allow the area to dry thoroughly. *The mechanical action of swabbing removes skin secretions, which contain microorganisms.*

■ Place and hold the swab between the third and fourth fingers of the nondominant hand. *Doing so keeps the swab readily accessible when the needle is withdrawn.*

5. Prepare the syringe for injection.

■ Remove the needle cap while waiting for the antiseptic to dry. Pull the cap straight off to avoid contaminating the needle by the outside edge of the cap. *The needle will become contaminated if it*

touches anything but the inside of the cap, which is sterile.

■ Expel any air bubbles from the syringe by inverting the syringe and gently pushing on the plunger until a drop of solution can be seen in the needle bevel. If air bubbles still remain, flick the side of the syringe barrel.

6. Inject the medication.

■ Grasp the syringe in your dominant hand by holding it between your thumb and fingers with palm facing to the side or upward for a 45° angle insertion or with the palm downward for a 90° angle insertion. See Figure 45–27.

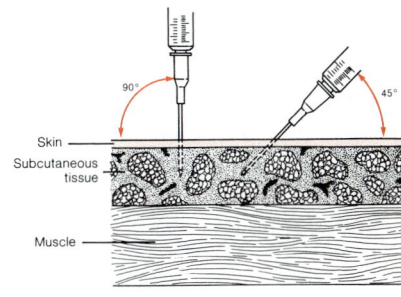

Figure 45–27 Inserting a needle into the subcutaneous tissue using 90° and 45° angles.

■ Using the nondominant hand, pinch or spread the skin at the site, and insert the needle, using the dominant hand and a firm steady push. See Figure 45–28. Recommendations vary about whether to pinch or spread the skin. *Pinching the skin is thought to desensitize the area somewhat and thus lessen the sensation of needle insertion. Spreading the skin can make it firmer and facilitate needle insertion.* Some recommend neither pinching nor spreading the skin (Pitel 1971, p. 79). The nurse needs to judge which method to use depending on the client's tissue firmness.

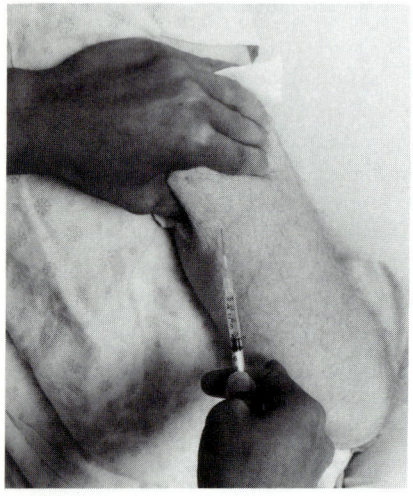

Figure 45–28 Administering a subcutaneous injection.

■ When the needle is inserted, move your nondominant hand to the end of the plunger. Some nurses find it easier to move the nondominant hand to the barrel of the syringe and the dominant hand to the end of the plunger.

■ Aspirate by pulling back on the plunger. If blood appears in the syringe, withdraw the needle, discard the syringe, and prepare a new injection. If blood does not appear, continue to administer the medication.

Aspiration determines whether the needle has entered a blood vessel. Subcutaneous medications may be dangerous if placed directly into the bloodstream; they are intended for the subcutaneous tissues, where the absorption time is greater.

■ Inject the medication by holding the syringe steady and depressing the plunger with a slow, even pressure. *Holding the syringe steady and injecting the medication at an even pressure minimizes discomfort for the client.*

7. Remove the needle, and massage the site.

■ Remove the needle quickly, pulling along the line of insertion while depressing the skin with your nondominant hand. *Depressing the skin places countertraction on it and minimizes the client's discomfort when the needle is withdrawn.*

■ Massage the site lightly with a sterile antiseptic-soaked swab, or apply slight pressure. *Massage is thought to disperse the medication in the tissues and facilitate its absorption. Massaging is omitted with heparin and insulin injections.*

■ If bleeding occurs, apply pressure to the site with a dry sterile gauze until it stops. Bleeding rarely occurs after subcutaneous injection.

8. Dispose of supplies appropriately.

■ Discard the uncapped needle and and attached syringe into designated receptacles. *Proper disposal protects the nurse and others from injury and contamination. The CDC does not recommend capping before disposal to reduce the risk of needle-prick injuries.*

9. Document relevant information.

■ Document the medication given,

dosage, time, route, assessments, and add your signature.

■ Many agencies prefer that medication administration be recorded on the medication record. The nurse's notes are used when prn medications are given or when there is a special problem.

10. Assess the effectiveness of the medication when it is expected to act.

Variation: Administering a heparin injection

The subcutaneous administration of heparin requires special precautions because of the drug's anticoagulant properties.

■ Select a site on the abdomen above the level of the iliac crests. *These areas are away from major muscles and are not involved in muscular activity, as the arms and legs are; thus, the possibility of hematoma is reduced.*

■ Use a ½-in #25 or #26 gauge needle, and insert it at a 90° angle. Draw 0.1 ml of air into the syringe when preparing the heparin, and inject it after the heparin. *This step fills the needle with air and prevents any leakage of heparin into the intradermal layers when the needle is inserted and when the needle is withdrawn, thus minimizing the possibility of a hematoma.*

■ Check agency practices regarding aspiration. *Some nurses recommend not to aspirate to determine needle placement because this can cause the needle to move, possibly damaging tissue and rupturing small blood vessels, causing bleeding and severe bruising.*

■ Do *not* massage the site after the injection. *Massaging could cause bleeding and ecchymoses.*

■ Alternate sites of subsequent injections.

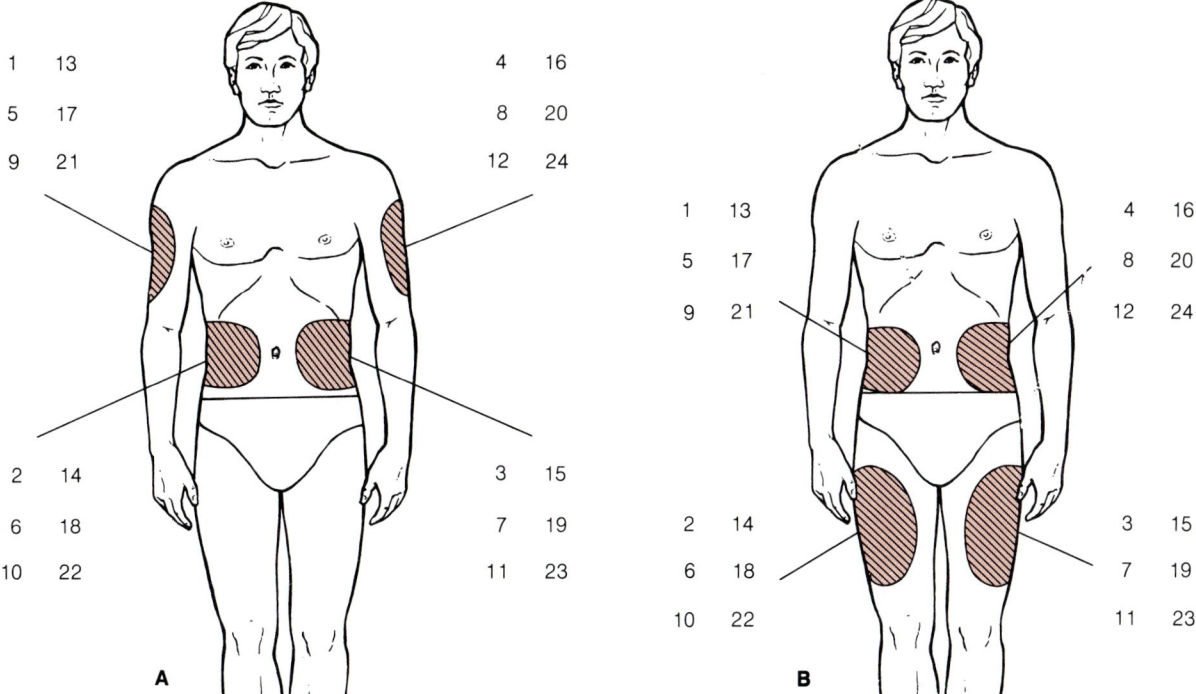

Figure 45–29 A commonly used system of rotating body injection sites for injecting insulin: *A,* sites used by the nurse; *B,* sites used by the client.

Subcutaneous injection sites need to be rotated in an orderly fashion to minimize tissue damage, aid absorption, and avoid discomfort. This is especially important for clients who must receive repeated injections, e.g., diabetics. The nurse or client can prepare a diagram indicating the sites to be used and after each injection mark its location on the diagram. See Figure 45–29.

Generally, a 2-ml syringe and a #25 gauge needle are used for subcutaneous injections. The length of the needle depends on the amount of adipose tissue at the site and the angle used to administer the injection. Generally, a ⅝-in needle is used for adults when the injection is administered at a 45° angle; a ½-in needle is used at a 90° angle. Shorter needles, e.g., ⅜ in, may be used for children, and longer ones, e.g., 1 in, may be necessary for very obese adults. To determine the appropriate length of the needle for a 90° angle injection, the nurse pinches a fold of skin between the thumb and forefinger at the injection site, then measures the width of the skinfold by placing a needle that will not be used for the injection against the skin surface. The appropriate needle length is one-half the width of the skinfold (Pitel 1971, p. 78). When this method of measuring is used, the needle is inserted without pinching the skin.

The steps for administering a subcutaneous injection are described in Procedure 45–3.

Intramuscular Injections

The intramuscular (IM) injection route is ordered for the following reasons:

- The speed of absorption is faster than by the subcutaneous route because of the greater blood supply to the body muscles.

- Muscles can usually take a larger volume of fluid without discomfort than subcutaneous tissues, although the amount varies among people, chiefly with muscle size and condition.

- Medications that irritate subcutaneous tissue may safely be given by intramuscular injection.

A number of body sites are used for intramuscular injections. Frequently used sites are the dorsogluteal, ventrogluteal, vastus lateralis, rectus femoris, and deltoid muscles. Only healthy muscles should be used for injections.

Dorsogluteal Site The dorsogluteal site is composed of the thick gluteal muscles of the buttocks. See Figure 45–30. The dorsogluteal site can be used for adults and for children with well-developed gluteal muscles. Because these muscles are developed by walking, it should not be used for infants under 3 years. The nurse must choose the injection site carefully to avoid striking the sciatic nerve, major blood vessels, or bone. The nurse palpates the posterior superior iliac spine, then draws an imaginary line to the greater trochanter of the femur. This line is lateral to and parallel to the sciatic nerve. The injection site is, then, lateral and superior to this line. See Figure 45–31. Palpating the ilium and the trochanter is important; visual calculations alone can result in an injection that is placed too low and injures other structures.

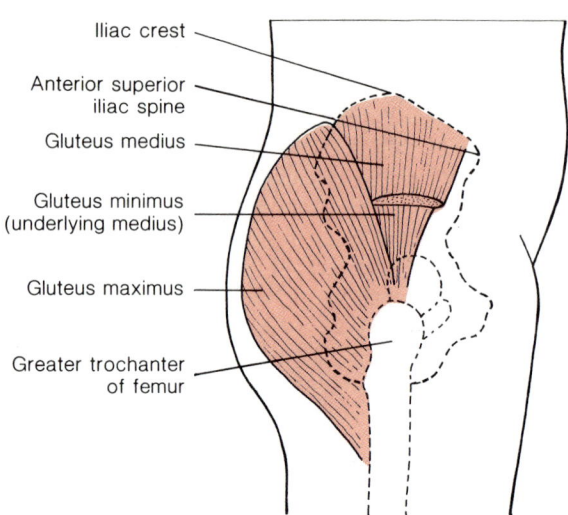

Figure 45–30 Lateral view of the right buttock showing the three gluteal muscles used for intramuscular injections.

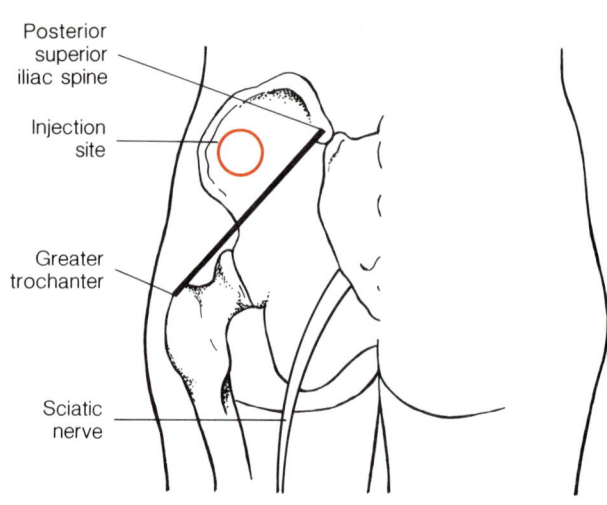

Figure 45–31 One method of establishing the dorsogluteal site for an intramuscular injection.

A second method for establishing the dorsogluteal site is to divide the buttock by imaginary lines as in Figure 45–32. The vertical line extends from the crest of the ilium to the gluteal fold. The horizontal line extends from the medial fold to the lateral aspect of the buttock. From these landmarks, the upper outer aspect of the upper outer quadrant is established. See Figure 45–32. The nurse palpates the crest of the ilium to ensure that the chosen site is high enough.

Usually, a 2- to 5-ml syringe is needed. Some medications,

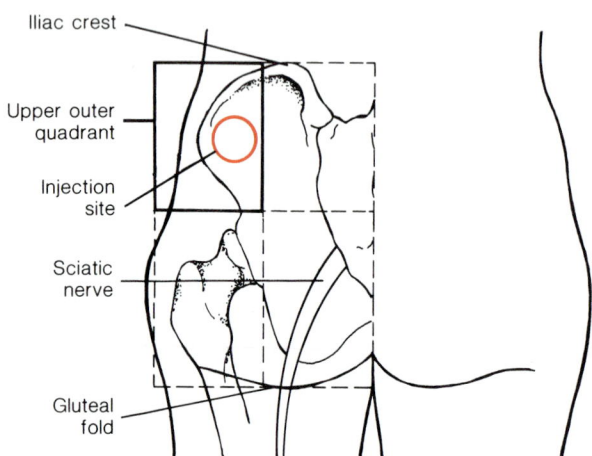

Figure 45–32 A second method of establishing the dorsogluteal site for an intramuscular injection.

medication interacts with plastic. The standard prepackaged intramuscular needle is 1½ inches and 21 or 22 gauge. However, the size and length of the needle should be determined by the muscle to be used, the type of solution, the amount of adipose tissue covering the muscle, and the age of the client. A large muscle, such as the gluteus medius, usually requires a #20 to #23 gauge needle, 1½ to 3 in long, whereas the deltoid muscle requires a smaller, #23 to #25 gauge needle, ⅝ to 1 in long. Oily solutions such as paraldehyde require a thicker needle, e.g., #21 gauge instead of #23 gauge. Also, the greater the amount of adipose tissue over the muscle, the longer the needle must be to reach the muscle. Therefore, 3-in needles may be needed for obese clients, whereas ½-in needles are used for thinner people. Infants and young children usually require smaller, shorter needles (#22 to #25 gauge, ⅝ to 1 in long).

To administer an injection into the dorsogluteal site, the nurse asks the client to assume a prone position with the toes pointing medially. A side-lying position can also be used, with the upper leg flexed at the thigh and the knee and placed in front of the lower leg. Both positions promote relaxation of the gluteal muscles. In the past, the dorsogluteal site was most commonly used for intramuscular injections. However, because of the problems caused by inaccurately locating the site, it is losing favor as the best intramuscular site.

Ventrogluteal Site The ventrogluteal site is the preferred site for intramuscular injections because there are no large nerves or blood vessels in the area and less fat than in the buttock area. It is also farther from the rectal area and tends to be less contaminated, which is a consid-

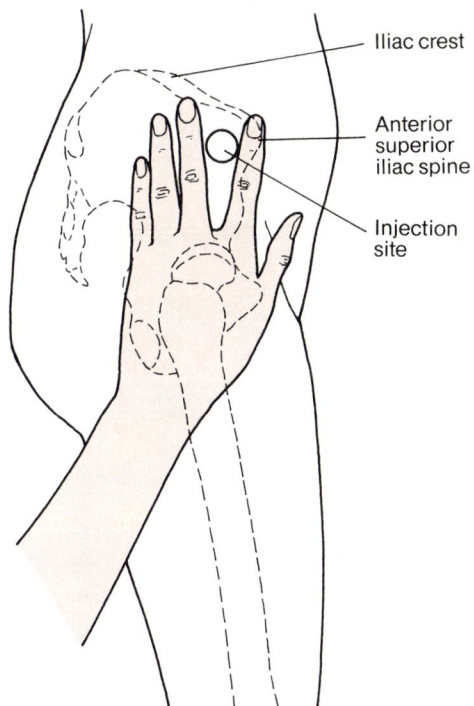

Figure 45–33   The ventrogluteal site for an intramuscular injection.

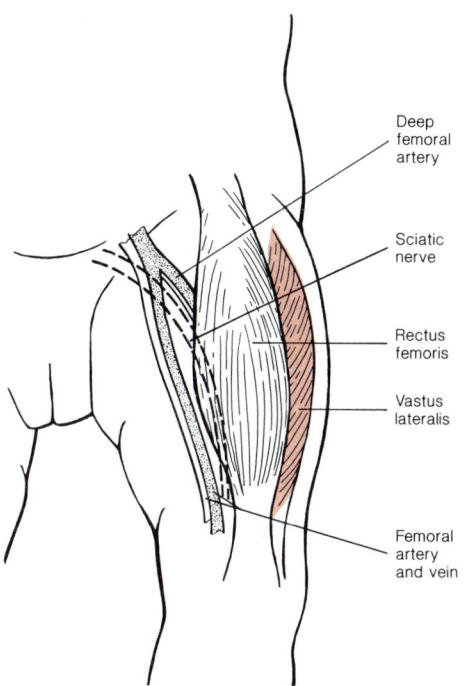

Figure 45–34   The vastus lateralis muscle of the upper thigh, used for intramuscular injections.

eration when giving injections to infants and incontinent adults. The ventrogluteal site, also known as von Hochstetter's site, is in the gluteus medius muscle, which lies over the gluteus minimus. See Figure 45–30. To establish the exact site, the nurse places the heel of the hand on the client's greater trochanter, with the fingers pointing toward the client's head. The right hand is used for the left hip, and the left hand for the right hip. With the index finger on the client's anterior superior iliac spine, the nurse stretches the middle finger dorsally, palpating the crest of the ilium and then pressing below it. The triangle formed by the index finger, the third finger, and the crest of the ilium is the injection site. See Figure 45–33. This site is suitable for infants, children, and adults. It is particularly suitable for immobilized clients whose dorsogluteal muscles may be atrophying. The client position for the injection can be a back- or side-lying position with the knee and hip flexed to relax the gluteal muscles.

Vastus Lateralis Site   The vastus lateralis muscle is usually thick and well developed in both adults and children. It is increasingly recommended as the site of choice for intramuscular injections for infants because there are no major blood vessels or nerves in the area. It is situated on the anterior lateral aspect of the thigh. See Figure 45–34. The middle third of the muscle is suggested as the site. It is established by dividing the area between the greater trochanter of the femur and the lateral femoral condyle into thirds and selecting the middle third. See Figure 45–35. The client can assume a back-lying or a sitting position for an injection into this site.

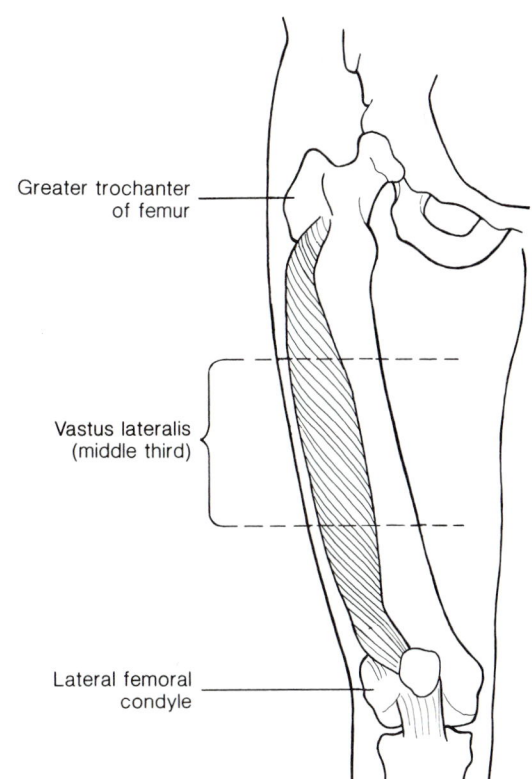

Figure 45–35   The vastus lateralis site for an intramuscular injection.

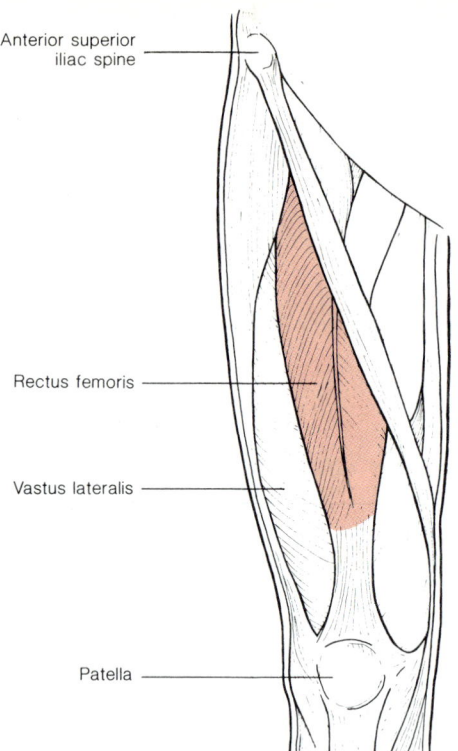

Figure 45-36 The rectus femoris muscle of the upper right thigh, used for intramuscular injections.

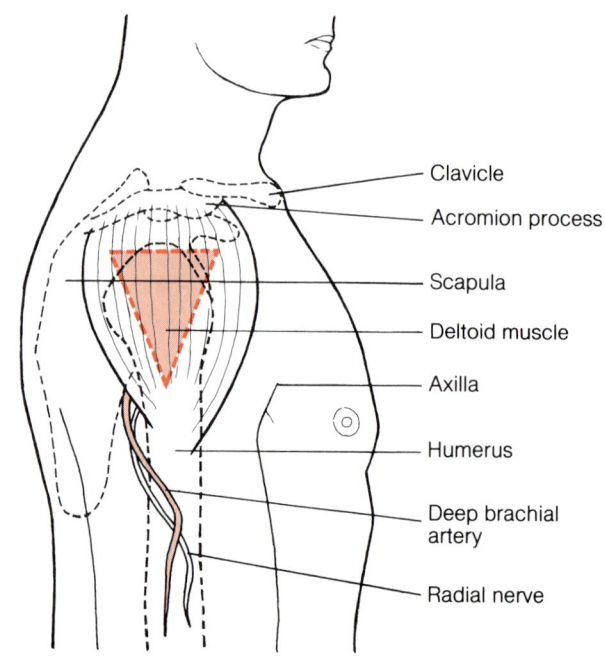

Figure 45-37 The deltoid muscle of the upper arm, used for intramuscular injections.

Rectus Femoris Site   The rectus femoris muscle, which belongs to the quadriceps muscle group, can also be used for intramuscular injections. It is situated on the anterior aspect of the thigh. See Figure 45–36. This site can be used for occasional injections for infants and children and for adults when other sites are contraindicated. Its chief advantage is that clients who administer their own injections can reach this site easily. Its main disadvantage is that an injection here may cause considerable discomfort for some people. The client assumes a sitting or back-lying position for an injection at this site.

Deltoid Site   The deltoid muscle is found on the lateral aspect of the upper arm. It is not used often for intramuscular injections because it is a relatively small muscle and is very close to the radial nerve and radial artery. To locate the densest part of the muscle, the nurse palpates the lower edge of the acromion and the midpoint on the lateral aspect of the arm that is in line with the axilla. A triangle within these boundaries indicates the deltoid muscle about 5 cm (2 in) below the acromion. See Figure 45–37. Another method of establishing the deltoid site is to place four fingers across the deltoid muscle, with the first finger on the acromion; i.e., the site is three finger breadths below the acromion. See Figure 45–38.

Procedure 45–4 describes how to administer an intramuscular injection.

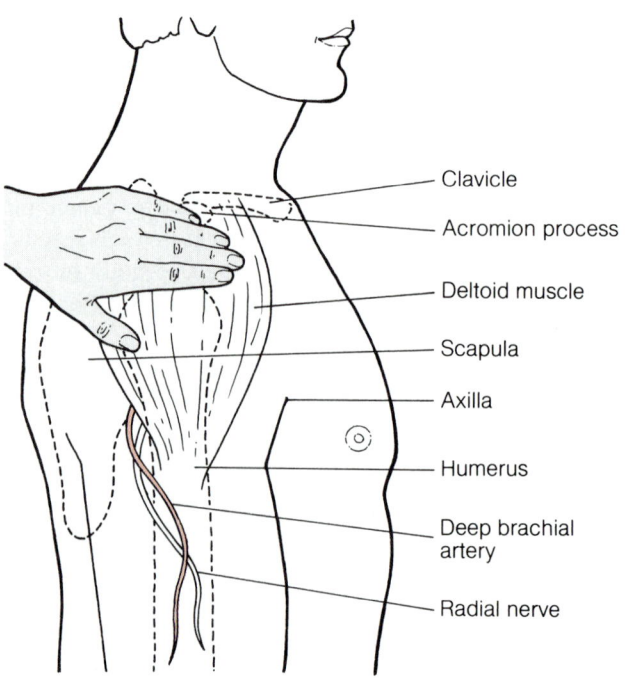

Figure 45-38 A method of establishing the deltoid muscle site for an intramuscular injection.

PROCEDURE 45–4

ADMINISTERING AN INTRAMUSCULAR INJECTION

Equipment ☑

Medication card, MAR, or computer printout

Sterile medication (usually provided in an ampule or vial)

Sterile syringe and needle of a size appropriate for the amount of solution to be administered

Swab saturated in an antiseptic solution

Dry sterile gauze or an unopened alcohol swab, if an ampule must be opened (optional)

Gloves (according to agency protocol)

Intervention

1. **Verify the medication order for accuracy.**

■ See Procedure 45–1, Step 3.

2. **Prepare the medication from the vial or ampule.**

■ See Procedure 45–2, page 1272.

■ If the medication is particularly irritating to subcutaneous tissue, change the needle on the syringe before the injection. *Because the outside of the new needle is free of medication, it does not irritate subcutaneous tissues as it passes into the muscle.*

3. **Identify the client, and assist the client to a comfortable position.**

■ Check the client's arm band, and ask the client to tell you his or her name.

■ Assist the client to a supine, lateral, prone, or sitting position, depending on the chosen site.

4. **Select, locate, and clean the site.**

■ Select a site free of skin lesions, tenderness, swelling, hardness, or localized inflammation and one that has not been used frequently.

■ If injections are to be frequent, alternate sites. If necessary, discuss an alternative method of providing the medication with the physician prescribing it.

■ Determine whether the size of the muscle is appropriate to the amount of medication to be injected. An average adult's deltoid muscle can usually absorb 0.5 ml of medication, although some authorities believe 2 ml can be absorbed by a well-developed deltoid muscle, and the gluteus medius muscle can absorb 1 to 5 ml (Newton and Newton 1979, p. 19), although 5 ml may be very painful.

■ Locate the exact site for the injection. See the discussion of sites earlier in this chapter.

■ Clean the site with an antiseptic swab. Using a circular motion, start at the center and move outward about 5 cm (2 in).

■ Transfer and hold the swab between the third and fourth fingers of your nondominant hand in readiness for needle withdrawal.

5. **Prepare the syringe for injection.**

■ Remove the needle cover without contaminating the needle.

■ Invert the syringe, and expel excess air, leaving only 0.2 ml of air. *This technique, referred to as the air-lock or air-bubble technique, prevents tracking of the medication through sensitive subcutaneous tissues in two ways: (a) it keeps the needle clean of medication on insertion, and (b) since the air bubble moves to the end of the plunger when the needle is pointed downward, the*

air bubble is injected behind the medication to clear the needle of medication again. See Figure 45–39.

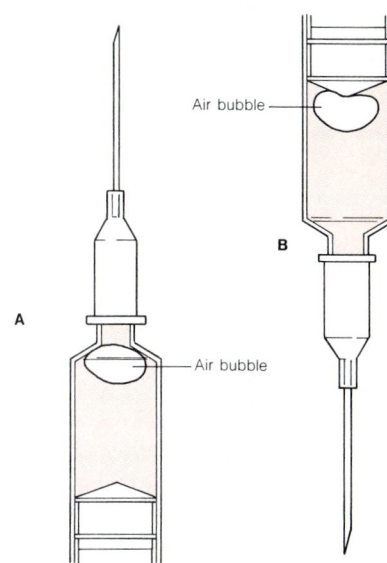

Figure 45–39 An air bubble in the medication in the syringe: *A,* needle pointed up; *B,* needle pointed down.

6. **Inject the medication.**

■ Use the nondominant hand to spread the skin at the site. *Spreading the skin makes it firmer and facilitates needle insertion.* Under some circumstances, e.g., for an emaciated client or an infant, the muscle may be pinched.

■ Holding the syringe between the thumb and forefinger, pierce the

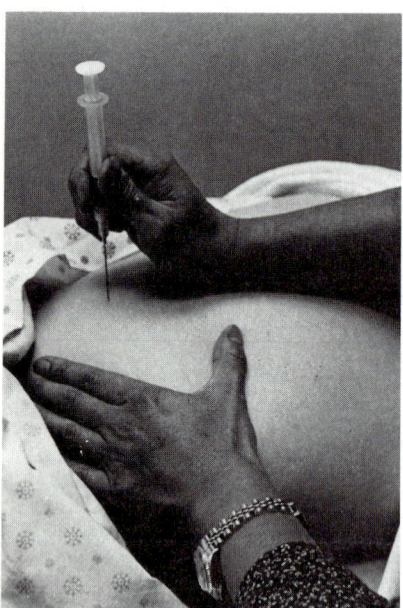

Figure 45–40 Administering an intramuscular injection.

skin quickly at a 90° angle (see Figure 45–40), and insert the needle into the muscle (see Figure 45–41). *Using a quick motion lessens the client's discomfort.*

- Aspirate by holding the barrel of the syringe steady with your nondominant hand and by pulling back on the plunger with your dominant hand. If blood appears in the syringe, withdraw the needle, discard the syringe, and prepare a new injection. *This step determines whether the needle is in a blood vessel.*

- If blood does not appear, inject the medication steadily and slowly, holding the syringe steady. *Injecting medication slowly permits it to disperse into the muscle tissue, thus decreasing the client's discomfort. Holding the syringe steady minimizes discomfort.*

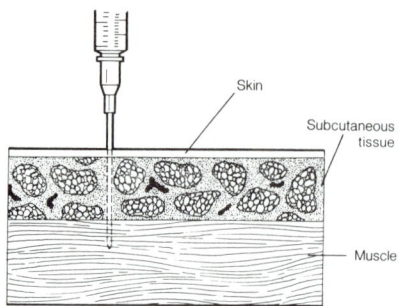

Figure 45–41 An intramuscular needle inserted into the muscle layer.

7. **Remove the needle, and massage the site.**

- See Procedure 45–3, step 7, for withdrawing the needle and massaging the site.

8. **Discard the uncapped needle and attached syringe into the proper receptacle.**

9. **Document relevant information.**

- Include time of administration, drug name, dose, route, and any complaints of the client.

Variation: Administering a Z-tract injection

This variation of the standard intramuscular technique is used to administer intramuscular medications that are highly irritating to subcutaneous and skin tissues.

- Follow steps 1 through 4.

- Attach a clean sterile needle to the syringe. *A new needle will not have* *any medication adhering to the outside that could be irritating to tissues.*

- Prepare an air lock (see step 5, above).

- With the nondominant hand, pull the skin and subcutaneous tissue about 2.5 to 3.5 cm (1 to 1¼ in) to one side at the injection site (see Figure 45–42).

- Insert the syringe and medication as in step 6. Withdraw the plunger with the dominant hand while holding the syringe to ascertain placement of the needle.

- Maintain the traction while removing the needle, and then permit the skin to return to its normal position.

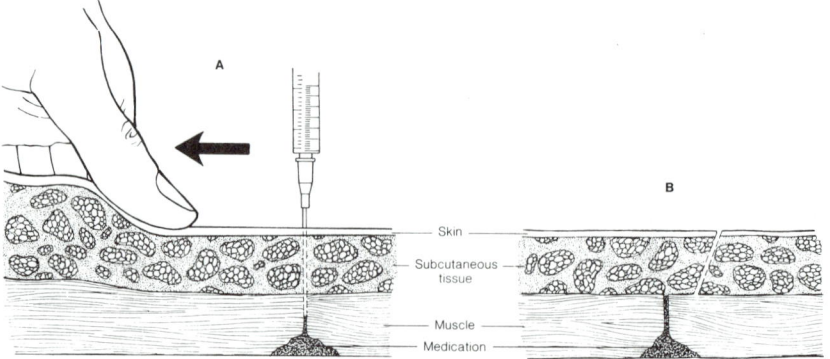

Figure 45–42 Inserting the needle using the Z-tract method: *A,* skin pulled to the side; *B,* skin released.

Intravenous Medications

Because intravenous (IV) medications enter the client's bloodstream directly, they are appropriate when a rapid effect is required (e.g., in a life-threatening situation such as cardiac arrest). This route is also appropriate when medications are too irritating to tissues to be given by other routes. When an intravenous line is already established, this route is desirable because it avoids the discomfort of other parenteral routes. Medications are administered intravenously via

1. Bottle or bag (continuous infusion)
2. Additional container (intermittent infusion by piggy-back [IVPB] or partial-fill [IVPF])
3. Volume-control administration set (often used for children)
4. Intravenous push (IVP or bolus)

There are, however, potential hazards in giving intravenous medications: infection and rapid, severe reactions to the medication. To prevent infection, the nurse uses sterile technique during all aspects of administering intravenous medication. To safeguard the client against severe reactions, the nurse must administer the drug slowly, following the manufacturer's recommendations. The nurse assesses the client closely during the administration, and discontinues the medication immediately if an untoward reaction occurs.

Continuous Infusions

For continuous infusions, medications can be added to a new fluid container prior to hanging it or to a fluid container that is already attached and running. Electrolytes (e.g., potassium chloride) and vitamins (e.g., Solu-B) are commonly administered by this method. Before administering any intravenous medication, the nurse (a) inspects and palpates the intravenous insertion site for signs of infection, infiltration, or a dislocated catheter; (b) inspects the surrounding skin for redness, pallor, or swelling; and (c) palpates the surrounding tissues for coldness and presence of edema, which could indicate leakage of the IV fluid into the tissues. The nurse then takes the vital signs for baseline data and makes sure that the drug and solutions are compatible. A nurse may need to consult a pharmacist for this information. An **incompatibility** is an undesired chemical or physical reaction between a drug and an infusion solution, between two or more drugs, or between a drug and the container or tubing (e.g., the incompatibility of some medications with plastic containers or syringes). See Procedure 45–5.

PROCEDURE 45–5

ADDING MEDICATIONS TO INTRAVENOUS FLUID CONTAINERS

Equipment ☑

Correct solution container, if a new one is to be attached

Medication card, MAR, or computer printout

Correct sterile medication

Diluent for medication in powdered form (see manufacturer's instructions)

Antiseptic swabs

Sterile syringe of appropriate size (e.g., 5 or 10 ml) and a 1- to 1½-in, #20 or #21 gauge sterile needle

Medication label

Intervention

 1. Verify the medication order for accuracy, and confirm compatibility of the drugs and solutions being mixed.

- Check the physician's orders carefully for the medication, dosage, and route. Verify which infusions are to be used with the medication. For example, the order may say to infuse the medication with 1000 ml of 5% dextrose and water rather than with normal saline.

- Consult a pharmacist, if required, to confirm compatibility of the drugs and solutions being mixed.

2. Prepare the medication from a vial or ampule.

- See Procedure 45–2, page 1272.

- Check the agency's practice about using a special filter needle to withdraw premixed liquid medications from multidose vials.

3. Confirm the sterility of the solution container (if a new one is to be attached), and locate and clean the injection port.

- Be sure that the solution container has no cracks or leaks, that the fluid is not discolored, and that the seal is undamaged.

■ If a glass container is vented, remove the metal cap and the rubber disc to locate the injection port. An injection port may be designated in several ways, e.g., by a triangle, cross, or circle. Do *not* inject medication through the port for the administration spike or through an air vent port if there is an injection port.

or

■ For a plastic container, locate the separate, self-sealing, soft rubber injection port.

■ Clean the injection port with an antiseptic swab. *This reduces the risk of introducing microorganisms into the container when the needle is inserted.*

4. Inject the medication into the container.

■ Remove the needle cover from the medication syringe, and inject the medication into the port. See Figure 45–43.

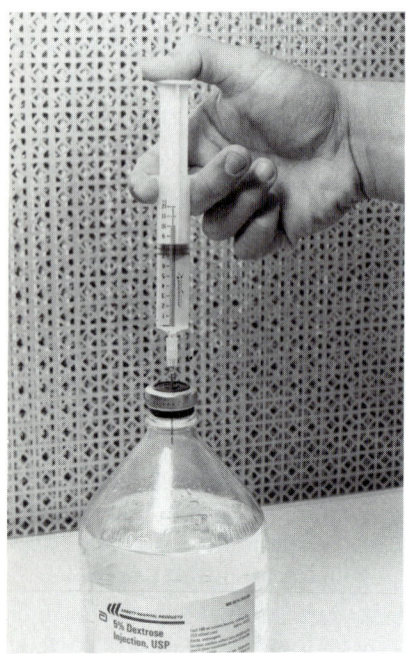

Figure 45–43 Inserting a medication into an intravenous bottle.

■ Remove the needle.

■ For a glass container, cover the top immediately either with (a) an antiseptic swab with the metal IV cap taped over it or (b) the special sterile cap provided by the manufacturer. *An open tubing port increases the risk of fluid contamination by microorganisms. Plastic containers have self-sealing ports.*

5. Attach a medication label.

■ Apply the medication label upside down to the fluid container. *This makes the label easy to read when the container is hanging.*

■ See Figure 45–44 for the information to be included on the medication label.

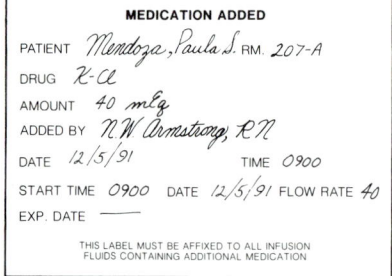

MEDICATION ADDED

PATIENT *Mendoza, Paula S.* RM. *207-A*
DRUG *K-Cl*
AMOUNT *40 mEq*
ADDED BY *N.W. Armstrong, RN*
DATE *12/5/91*   TIME *0900*
START TIME *0900*   DATE *12/5/91* FLOW RATE *40*
EXP. DATE ———

THIS LABEL MUST BE AFFIXED TO ALL INFUSION
FLUIDS CONTAINING ADDITIONAL MEDICATION

Figure 45–44 A medication label for an intravenous infusion.

6. Establish the infusion.

■ Spike and hang the container.

■ Regulate the flow rate according to the dosage required. *This prevents rapid infusion of the medication and fluid and subsequent complications.*

7. Document relevant information.

■ Record the type and amount of solution, medication and dose added, and times of starting and completing the infusion. Some

agencies have a special parenteral fluid form for this purpose.

■ Record fluid volume on the intake and output record.

8. Monitor the client and the infusion.

■ During the administration, observe the client for signs of an adverse reaction, such as noisy respirations, changes in pulse rate, chills, nausea, or headache. If any adverse sign occurs, follow agency policy (i.e., slow rate or stop flow), and notify the physician or nurse in charge. Also monitor the client for signs of the intended action of the medication.

■ Carefully monitor the infusion to maintain delivery of the medication and fluid at the specified rate.

Variations: Adding medications to an infusing container

For an IV container with a vented administration set (i.e., a nonvented container):

■ Make sure there is sufficient solution in the bottle to ensure proper dilution of the drug.

■ Close the IV flow clamp. *Closing the clamp is essential to prevent the medication from infusing to the client before it is properly diluted with the solution. Undiluted medication can produce a severe reaction.*

■ Detach the air vent cap, taking care not to contaminate the end.

■ Insert the tip of the medication syringe, *without the needle,* into the air vent port. See Figure 45–45.

■ Instill the medication.

■ Reattach the air vent.

For a vented IV bottle:

■ After ensuring that there is sufficient solution in the bottle, close the IV flow clamp.

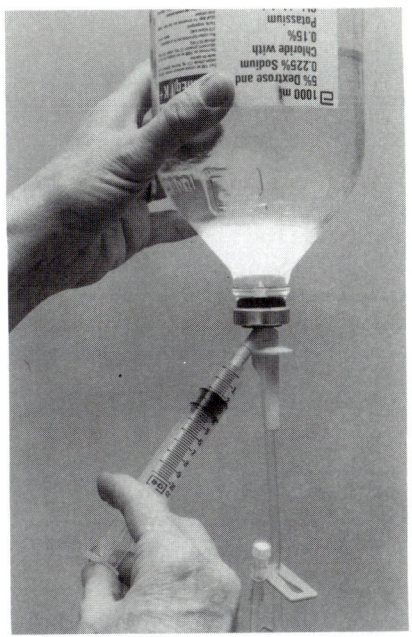

Figure 45–45 Instilling a medication into a hanging intravenous bottle.

■ Clean the medication port with an antiseptic swab.

■ Insert the syringe needle through the port and instill the medication. The medication port is usually marked (e.g., by a triangular imprint).

For a plastic IV bag:

■ After ensuring that there is sufficient solution in the bag, close the IV flow clamp.

■ Clean the medication port with an antiseptic swab.

■ While supporting and stabilizing the bag with your thumb and forefinger, carefully insert the syringe needle through the port and inject the medication. See Figure 45–46. *The bag is supported while injecting the medication to avoid punctures.*

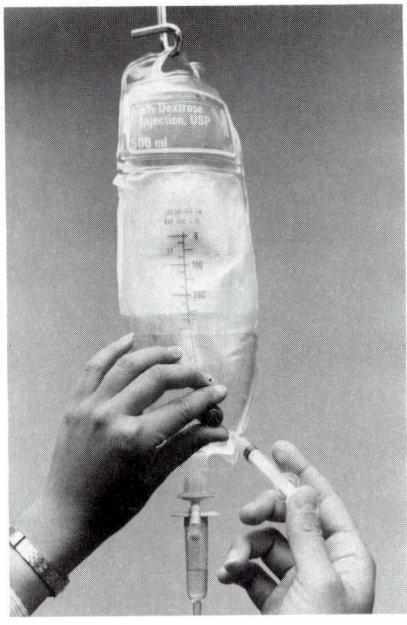

Figure 45–46 Instilling a medication into a hanging intravenous bag.

For all infusing methods:

■ Attach a medication label to the IV container.

■ Gently lift and rotate the container to mix the solution and medication.

■ Follow steps 6 through 8.

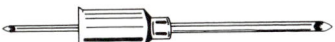

Figure 45–47 A transfer needle.

Variation: Using a transfer needle

A special transfer needle (see Figure 45–47) can be used to put medications in vials into a *plastic* IV container, provided the entire amount of medication is to be transferred to the IV container. After cleaning the top of the medication vial and the medication port on the IV bag with an antiseptic sponge, insert the small end of the transfer needle into the medication vial and the large end into the port of the IV container. To mix the medication and solution:

■ Invert the bag, so that the medication bottle is on top.

■ Gently squeeze the bag to transmit some air from the bag into the medication vial.

■ Release the pressure on the bag to allow medication to drain into the bag.

■ Repeat squeezing and releasing pressure until all the medication is transferred into the IV solution. The transfer needle may need to be pulled down so that all the medication is obtained from the vial.

■ Remove the needle, and gently rotate the bag to disperse the medication.

Intermittent Infusions   For intermittent infusions, additional fluid containers and secondary tubing sets are sometimes attached to a primary infusion to administer intravenous medications. These intermittent medications may be given simultaneously with the primary infusion (provided that the medications are compatible and the client is able to tolerate the additional fluid), or the primary line may be clamped while the intermittent medication is infusing. The medication is commonly injected into a small container of intravenous solution (usually 50 to 100 ml of D5W or NS). At some facilities, these containers are called intravenous partial-fills (IVPF) or additives (addits). When infusion pumps and controllers are used to administer inter-

mittent medications via secondary lines, the nurse should follow the manufacturer's instructions for setting up the intermittent infusion.

Depending on how the secondary infusion is set up, the intermittent infusion may be called an intravenous piggy-back (IVPB) or a tandem intravenous alignment (see Figure 40–10 on page 1067). The term *piggy-back* refers to the positioning of the additive container higher than the primary infusion container. Manufacturers provide the extension hook to lower the primary container. When the IVPB is connected to a port that has a backcheck valve, the valve automatically stops the flow of the primary infusion so that only the secondary infusion flows. See Figure 45–48. After the IVPB has infused and the level of solution in the tubing is below the level of the primary infusion drip chamber, the backcheck valve is released, and the primary infusion automatically starts running again. Thus, nurses need to leave the primary line unclamped when using this type of intermittent infusion setup.

When any intermittent medication is infusing, the nurse calculates the desired flow rate and estimated time of infusion. The nurse then adjusts the flow rate by counting the drops per minute in the secondary set drip chamber, manually setting a flow adjustment device attached to the secondary set or setting the rate on an infusion pump or controller. The nurse should assess the client at least every 15 minutes (or more frequently, e.g., when the client is receiving vasoactive drugs), to ensure that the medication is infusing satisfactorily. With some medications (e.g., potassium chloride), it may be necessary to dilute the medication in larger amounts of fluid (e.g., 250 ml) or infuse the medication at a slow rate with the primary line running at the usual rate to decrease irritation of the vein.

A *tandem intravenous alignment* may be set up by connecting the additive infusion to the primary line via a secondary port without a backcheck valve, more proximal to the client than the piggy-back port. This type of setup requires a longer secondary tubing set than does a piggy-back setup. Both the primary and the secondary infusions are positioned at the same height. Frequently, the primary infusion is temporarily clamped while the additive infuses, but this is required only when the two solutions are incompatible or when a more rapid infusion of the additive is desired. When the solutions are incompatible, the nurse must first clamp the primary line and flush the tubing between the secondary port and the client with a sterile solution (usually normal saline) before connecting and initiating the secondary infusion. The saline flush serves as a buffer between the two incompatible solutions. When the secondary infusion is complete, the nurse should again flush the line before restarting the primary infusion. Whenever the primary line is clamped, the nurse should carefully assess the client every 15 minutes (and more frequently when the secondary infusion is nearly complete), to maintain continuous patency. See Procedure 45–6.

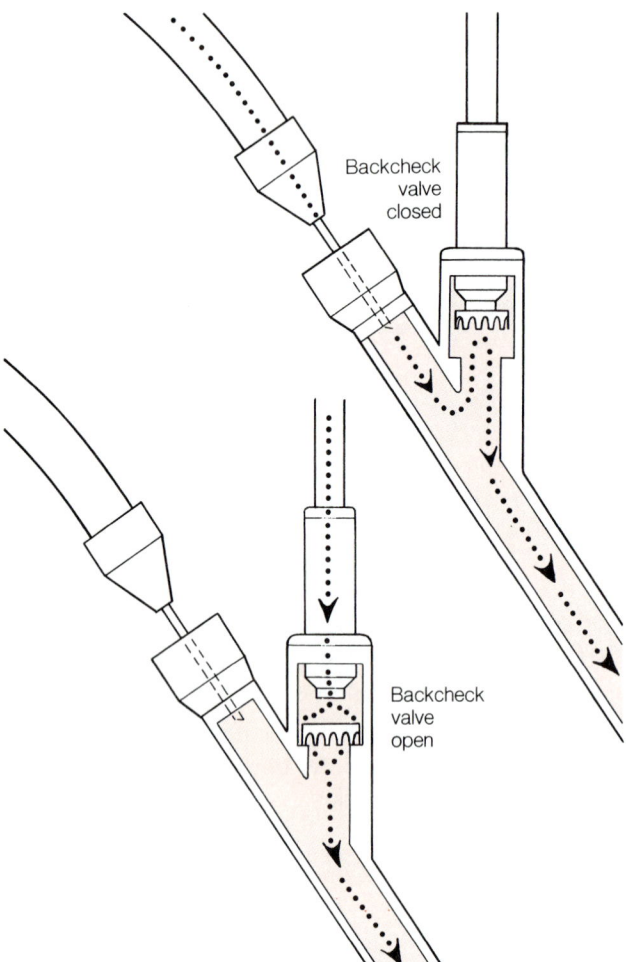

Backcheck valve closed

Backcheck valve open

Figure 45–48   Backcheck valve in a piggy-back set that stops the flow of the primary infusion.

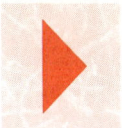

PROCEDURE 45–6

ADMINISTERING AN IV MEDICATION BY USING ADDITIVE SETS

Equipment ☑

Physician's order, medication card, or MAR

Medication label

Antiseptic swab

Adhesive tape

Sterile needle, syringe, and saline if medication is incompatible with the primary infusion

For piggy-back:

50- to 100-ml infusion bag with medication (most piggy-backs are prepared by the pharmacist)

Microdrip or macrodrip infusion set

Needle (1-in, #21 or #23 gauge)

Extension hook

For tandem setup:

Solution container with medication added

Long secondary tubing set

Intervention

1. Verify the medication order for accuracy, and confirm compatibility of the medication.

- See Procedure 45–5, step 1, page 1285.

2. Add the medication to the additive set if required.

- Prepare the medication from an ampule or vial. See Procedure 45–2, page 1272.
- Add the medication to the additional container. See Procedure 45–5, step 4, page 1286.
- Apply medication label.

3. Assemble the secondary infusion.

- Spike the secondary infusion container.
- Hang the secondary container at or above the level of the primary infusion. Use the extension hook to lower the primary infusion if a piggy-back setup is required.
- Attach the 1-in needle to the tubing, prime the tubing, and close the clamp.
- Replace the needle cover to keep the needle sterile before attaching it to the primary IV line.

4. Attach the secondary infusion to the primary infusion.

- Clean the Y-port on the primary IV line with an antiseptic swab. Clean the *primary port* (that furthest from the client) for a piggy-back alignment and the *secondary port* (that closest to the client) for a tandem setup.
- If the medication is *not* compatible with the primary infusion, flush the primary line with a sterile saline solution before attaching the secondary set. To flush the line, wipe the port with an antiseptic swab, clamp the primary line, and, using a sterile needle and syringe, instill a few milliliters of sterile saline through the port to wash any primary infusion fluid out of the infusion tubing.
- Insert the needle of the secondary line through the injection port of the primary line.
- Secure the needle with adhesive tape. *Tape prevents needle dislodgment.* Some agencies recommend that a needle guard be taped alongside the needle to support the needle placement and keep the needle guard handy for use when discontinuing the secondary attachment.

5. Administer the medication.

For piggy-back:

- Ensure that the primary line is unclamped if the port has a back-check valve. *The valve automatically stops the flow of the primary infusion while the additive set infuses and automatically starts it running after the piggy-back solution has been administered.*
- Open the clamp on the piggy-back line, and regulate it in accordance with the recommended rate for that medication. Usually, medications are administered in 30 to 60 minutes.

For tandem infusion:

- Open the clamp on the secondary line, and regulate its flow.
- For *continuous* infusion, set the secondary solution to the appropriate drip rate for the medication, and then adjust the primary solution to achieve the desired total infusion flow.
- For *intermittent* infusion, clamp the primary line and adjust the primary drip rate after the secondary solution is completed.

6. Document relevant data.

- Record date, time, medication, dose, route, and solution; assessments of IV site, if appropriate; and client response.
- Enter fluid intake according to agency protocol.

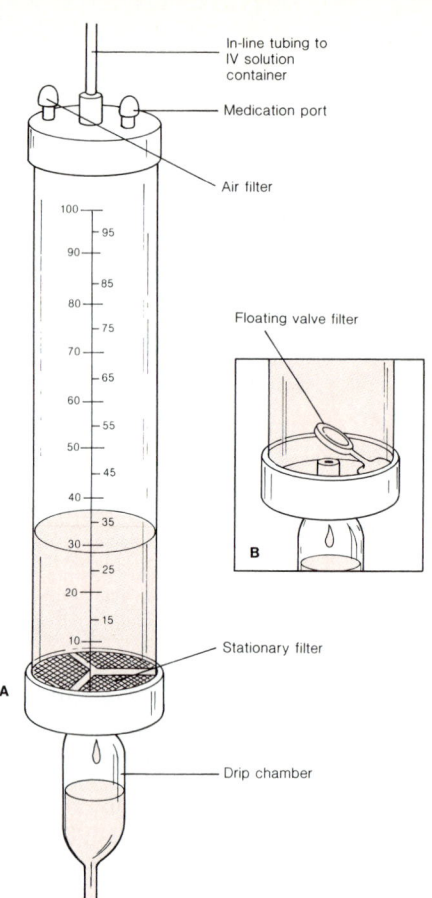

In-line tubing to IV solution container

Medication port

Air filter

Floating valve filter

B

Stationary filter

A

Drip chamber

Intermittent medications may also be administered by volume-control sets (e.g., Buretrol, Soluset, Volutrol, Pediatrol). They are small fluid containers (100 to 150 ml in size) attached below the primary infusion container. Volume-control sets are equipped with either a stationary membrane filter or a floating valve filter at the base of the container and are designed for fine control of the amount of infusing fluid. See Figure 45–49. Volume-control administration sets serve the following purposes:

- To administer intravenous medications (such as some antibiotics) that do not remain stable for the length of time it takes an entire solution container to infuse

- To administer medications intermittently

- To avoid mixing medications that are incompatible

- To dilute a drug so that it is less irritating to the veins than if given by direct intravenous push

- To deliver medications diluted in precise amounts of fluid

See Procedure 45–7.

◀ *Figure 45–49* A volume-control intravenous infusion set: *A,* with a stationary filter; *B,* with a floating valve filter.

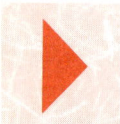

PROCEDURE 45–7

ADDING AN IV MEDICATION TO A VOLUME-CONTROL ADMINISTRATION SET

Equipment ☑

Correct solution container

Volume-control administration set

Physician's order, medication card, or MAR

Correct sterile medication

Antiseptic swabs

Sterile syringe of appropriate size (e.g., 5 or 10 ml)

1- to 1½-in, #20 or #21 gauge, sterile needle

Sterile filter needle if needed to withdraw the medication

Medication label for the volume-control set

Intervention

1. **Verify the medication order, and confirm compatibility of the medication.**

- See Procedure 45–5, step 1, page 1285.

2. **Prepare the medication from an ampule or vial.**

- See Procedure 45–2, page 1272.

3. **Attach the volume-control set to the infusion container.**

- Insert the spike of the volume-control set into the solution container and hang the container on the pole.

- Open the air vent clamp on the volume-control set.

- Position the lower clamp on the tubing below the drip chamber, and clamp it.

4. **Fill the volume-control device, and prime the tubing.**

For a set with a stationary membrane filter:

- Open the upper clamp, and allow the fluid chamber to fill with about 30 ml of solution, then close this clamp.

- Open the lower clamp, and flatten the drip chamber with two fingers and the thumb of your opposite hand. *The membrane filter can be damaged if the drip chamber is squeezed while the lower clamp is closed.*

- While keeping the drip chamber flattened, close the lower clamp. *These actions create a vacuum, so that solution from the fluid chamber will then flow into the drip chamber.*

- Release your pressure on the drip chamber, and reshape it until it becomes about half full.

- Repeat the above steps as necessary.

- Open the lower clamp, prime the tubing, and close the clamp.

For a set with a floating valve filter:

- Open the upper clamp, and squeeze the fluid chamber until it is filled with about 30 ml of solution.

- Close the clamp, and again gently squeeze the drip chamber until it is about half full.

- Open the lower clamp, prime the tubing, and close the clamp.

5. **Administer the medication.**

- Ensure that there is sufficient fluid in the volume-control fluid chamber to dilute the medication. Generally, 50 to 100 ml of fluid is used. Check the directions from the drug manufacturer.

- Close the inflow to the fluid chamber by adjusting the upper roller or slide clamp above the fluid chamber; also ensure that the clamp on the air vent of the chamber is open.

- Clean the medication port on the volume-control fluid chamber with an antiseptic swab.

- Insert the needle of the medication syringe into the port. See Figure 45–50.

- Inject the medication.

- Gently rotate the fluid chamber until the fluid is well mixed.

- Open the line's upper clamp, and regulate the flow by adjusting the lower roller or slide clamp below the fluid chamber.

6. **Attach a medication label to**

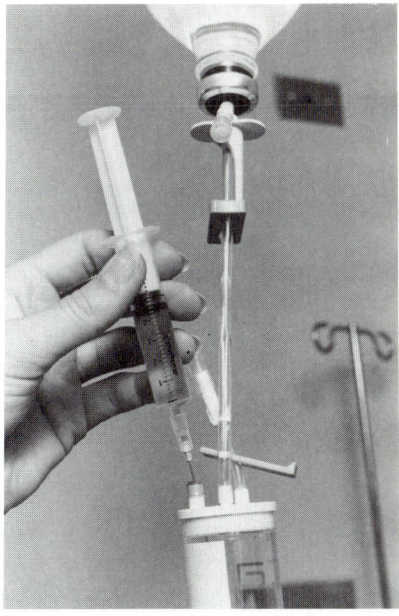

Figure 45–50 Adding medication to the port of a volume-control administration set.

the volume-control fluid chamber.

7. **Document relevant data, and monitor the client and the infusion.**

- See steps 7 and 8, Procedure 45–5, page 1286.

Intravenous Push   An **intravenous push** (**IVP** or **bolus**) is the intravenous administration of a medication that cannot be diluted or that is needed in an emergency. Also, certain drugs are administered this way to achieve maximum effect. It is important to remember that the rapid administration of an IVP could be dangerous for the client. An IVP can be administered directly into a vein through venipuncture, into an existing intravenous apparatus through an injection port (see Figure 45–51 in Procedure 45–8), or through an intermittent infusion set (heparin lock) when the client does not have an IV running but does have a heparin lock in place. The heparin lock (Figure 45–52 in Procedure 45–8), also called a male adapter plug (MAP), is used primarily for clients who require regular intermittent intravenous medications but not the fluid volume of an intravenous infusion. The set usually consists of an indwelling catheter attached to a plastic tube with a sealed injection tip. It is called a **heparin lock** because small amounts of heparin are injected into the catheter to maintain its patency. Some agencies now recommend that saline, rather than heparin, be used. After administering an IVP, the nurse discards the used syringe and needle in a designated container without recapping the needle, as for any other type of injection. See Procedure 45–8.

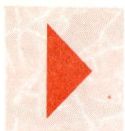

ADMINISTERING MEDICATION BY IV PUSH

Equipment ☑

Physician's order, medication card, or MAR

Correct sterile medication

Sterile syringe of the appropriate size for the volume of medication

Sterile 2.5-cm (1-in) #25 gauge needle to prevent large puncture holes in the injection port

Alcohol swabs

Gloves (optional)

In addition, for a beparin lock:

Sterile syringe and needle with a heparin flush solution (optional)

One or two syringes and needles, each with 2 ml (or amount prescribed by the agency) of normal saline

---

Intervention

1. Verify the medication order.

- Check the physician's order carefully for the medication, dosage, route, and rate of administration. *A medication that is injected too rapidly can create concentrations in the blood plasma that are toxic.*

2. Prepare the medication and heparin and/or saline as required.

- Prepare the medication according to Procedure 45–2. Label the syringe with the name of the medication and the dosage if other syringes for the heparin lock are needed.

- In a separate syringe, prepare the heparin solution according to agency practice, if needed. Many hospitals advocate the use of 100 units/ml of solution, and 0.5 ml is generally used. Label this syringe. A prepackaged heparin syringe may be used.

- In other syringes, prepare the saline solution if needed. Label these syringes.

3. Administer the medication.

To administer medication into an existing line:

- Inspect the injection site for any signs of infiltration, then identify an injection port nearest the client. Some ports have a circle indicating the site for the needle insertion. *An injection port must be used because it is self-sealing. Any puncture to the plastic tubing will leak.*

- Clean the port with an antiseptic swab.

- Stop the IV flow by closing the clamp or pinching the tubing above the injection port (see Figure 45–51).

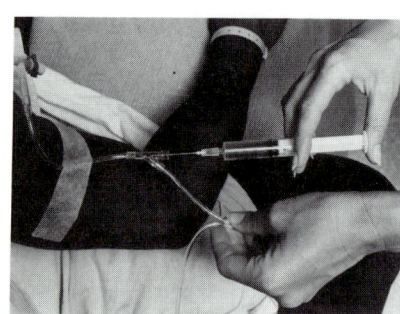

Figure 45–51 Administering medication through an injection port of an existing IV apparatus.

- While holding the port steady, insert the needle into the port.

- Draw back on the plunger to withdraw some blood into the IV tubing (not into the syringe). *This shows that the needle or catheter is in the vein.*

- Inject the medication at the ordered rate, withdraw the needle, reopen the clamp, and reestablish the intravenous infusion at the correct rate. If the medication is particularly irritating to the veins, run the IV rapidly for about a minute to dilute the medication, and then adjust the rate.

To administer medication into an intermittent infusion set:

- Swab the injection port with an antiseptic swab.

- Insert the needle attached to the normal saline syringe into the port, and aspirate for blood return. See Figure 45–52. *This ensures that the heparin lock catheter is in the vein. In some situations, blood will not return even though the heparin lock is patent.*

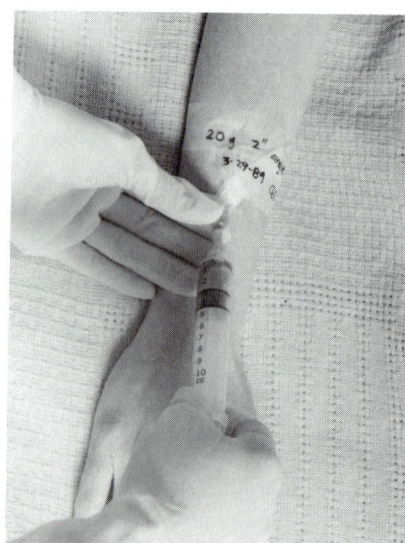

Figure 45–52 Administering medication through an intermittent infusion set.

■ Inject ½ to 2 ml of normal saline. This step is *optional.* Check agency practice. *This is done to flush the heparin from the catheter and to verify patency of the vein.* If the client experiences a burning or stinging sensation, this may be normal, or it may indicate that the needle or catheter is not in the vein and the fluid is infiltrating the tissue. In this case, withhold the medication until the heparin lock is replaced.

■ Remove the saline syringe.

■ Insert the needle attached to the medication syringe into the injection port.

■ Inject the medication slowly at the recommended rate of infusion. Observe the client closely for adverse reactions. Remove the needle and syringe when all medication is administered.

■ Attach the second saline syringe, and inject the recommended amount of saline. *The saline injec-tion flushes the medication through the catheter and prepares the lock for the heparin. Heparin is incompatible with many medications.*

■ If heparin is to be used, insert the heparin syringe, and inject the heparin slowly into the set. See Figure 45–53.

■ Check the patency of the heparin lock at least every 8 hours or according to agency practice.
  a. Aspirate for return blood flow.
  b. Flush the catheter with ½ to 2 ml of normal saline.
  c. Refill the heparin lock with new heparin solution (optional).

■ Check agency practice about recommended times for changing the heparin lock. Some agencies advocate a change every 48 to 72 hours.

4. Document relevant information.

■ Record the date, time, drug, dose, and route; client response; and assessments of infusion or heparin lock site if appropriate.

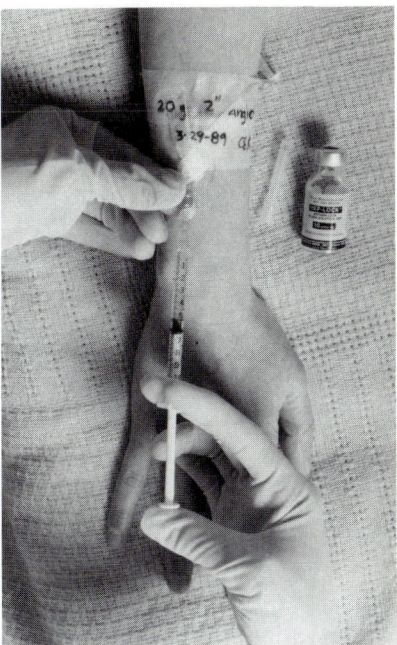

Figure 45–53 Injecting heparin into an intermittent infusion set.

TOPICAL MEDICATIONS

Topical medications include dermatologic medications and irrigations and instillations. Irrigations may or may not be medicated. *Dermatologic medications* are commonly applied for one of the following reasons:

■ To decrease itching (pruritus)

■ To lubricate and soften the skin

■ To cause local vasoconstriction or vasodilation

■ To increase or decrease secretions from the skin

■ To provide a protective coating to the skin

■ To apply an antibiotic or antiseptic to treat or prevent infection

In addition, some medications that are routinely administered by other routes may also be available for use trans-dermally by applying a "patch" to provide sustained action. Examples of these are nitroglycerin patches and anti–motion sickness preparations. Absorption is facilitated by washing the area well before the application. Dermatologic preparations include lotions, liniments, ointments, pastes, and powders. See Table 45–1, earlier in the chapter.

Unless contraindicated by a specific order, the nurse washes and carefully dries the area, using a patting motion, before applying a dermatologic preparation. Skin encrustations and discharges harbor microorganisms and cause local infections. They can also prevent the medication from coming in contact with the area to be treated. Nurses should always use surgical asepsis when an open wound is present. If a client has lesions, the nurse must wear gloves or use tongue depressors. In this way, the nurse's hand will not come in direct contact with microorganisms in and around the lesions. See Table 45–10 for general guidelines for applying topical medications.

TABLE 45–10 *Topical Applications*

Medication	Application
Lotion	Shake before use to distribute suspended particles.
	Pour onto sterile gauze, and pat onto affected area.
	To avoid aggravating affected area, do not rub.
Liniment	Pour onto hands, and rub into client's skin with long, smooth strokes.
Ointment and paste	Usually applied with a tongue blade or with gloves. Some must be applied thinly over the area, e.g., cortisone. Sterile dressing may be applied over ointment.
Powder	Sprinkle over the surface and cover with a dressing.

An **irrigation (lavage)** is the washing out of a body cavity by a stream of water or other fluid. An **instillation** is the insertion of a medication into a body cavity. Irrigation is performed for one or more of the following reasons:

- To clean the area; i.e., to remove a foreign object or discharge
- To apply heat or cold
- To apply a medication, such as an antiseptic
- To prepare an area for surgery, e.g., the eye

 Surgical asepsis is required when there is a break in the skin (e.g., in a wound irrigation), or whenever a sterile body cavity (e.g., the bladder) is entered. Some irrigations (e.g., an eye irrigation to remove foreign material; or a vaginal, rectal, or gastric irrigation) are safely conducted using medical asepsis.

A number of different kinds of syringes are used for irrigations. The most common are the Asepto, the rubber bulb, the Toomey, and the Pomeroy. The syringes are often calibrated, permitting the nurse to determine the amount of irrigant being delivered at any given time. The *Asepto syringe* is a plastic (or glass) syringe with a rubber bulb. See Figure 45–54, *A*. Squeezing the air out of the bulb produces negative pressure, and fluid can be sucked into the syringe. When the bulb is squeezed again, the fluid is ejected from the syringe. Asepto syringes come in several sizes, e.g., 30 ml (1 oz), 60 ml (2 oz), and 120 ml (4 oz).

The *rubber bulb syringe* is often used for irrigating the ears. See Figure 45–54, *B*. Like the Asepto syringe, it comes in a range of sizes. The *Toomey syringe,* which is made of plastic or glass, is also calibrated. See Figure 45–54, *C*. This syringe has a removable tip of metal or plastic that can fit into the end of tubing such as a catheter. Toomey syringes are used for deep-wound irrigations that require a catheter and for some types of bladder irrigations. The *Pomeroy syringe* is a metal syringe commonly used for ear irrigations. A shield near the tip prevents the solution from spraying outward (see Figure 45–54, *D*).

Ophthalmic Irrigations and Instillations

An eye irrigation is administered to wash out the conjunctival sac of the eye. In a hospital, sterile equipment is usually used. Medications for the eyes are instilled in the form of liquids or ointments. Eye drops are packaged in monodrip plastic containers that are used to administer the preparation. Ointments are usually supplied in small tubes. All containers must state that the medication is for ophthalmic use. Usually, sterile preparations are used, but sterile technique is not always indicated. Prescribed liquids are usually dilute, e.g., less than 1% strength. Procedure 45–9 illustrates how to administer irrigations and instillations.

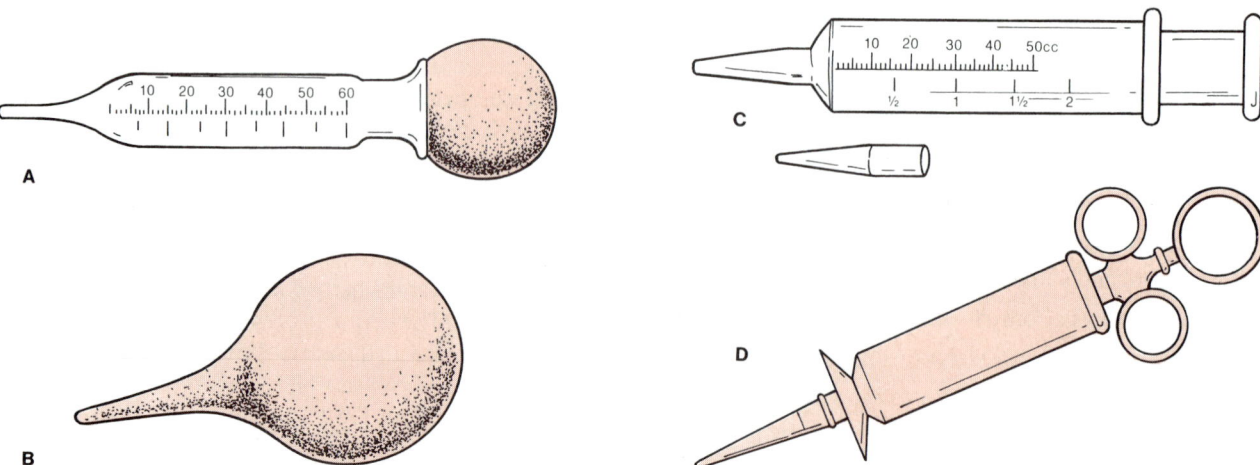

Figure 45–54 Four types of syringes commonly used for irrigations: *A,* Asepto; *B,* rubber bulb; *C,* Toomey with adapter tip to fit into tubing; *D,* Pomeroy.

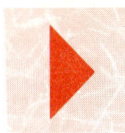

ADMINISTERING OPHTHALMIC IRRIGATIONS AND INSTILLATIONS

Equipment ☑

For an irrigation:

Sterile container for the irrigating solution

Irrigating solution (usually 60 to 240 ml (2 to 8 oz) of solution at 37 C (98.6 F) is appropriate)

Sterile eye syringe or eye irrigator (eyedropper can be used if only small amounts of solution are required)

Sterile kidney basin

Sterile cotton balls

Sterile normal saline (optional)

Moistureproof drape

Sterile gloves

For an instillation:

Medication

Dry sterile absorbent sponges

Sterile absorbent sponges soaked in sterile normal saline

Sterile eye dressing (pad) as needed and paper eye tape to secure it

Sterile gloves

Intervention

1. **Verify the medication or irrigation order.**

For an instillation:

- Check the physician's order for the preparation, strength, and number of drops. Also confirm the prescribed frequency of the instillation and which eye is to be treated. Abbreviations are frequently used to identify the eye: OD (right eye), OS (left eye), OU (both eyes).

For an irrigation:

- Check the type, amount, temperature, and strength of the solution and the frequency of the irrigation.

2. **Prepare the client.**

- Explain the technique to the client. The administration of an ophthalmic irrigating solution or medication is not usually painful. Ointments are often soothing to the eye, but some liquid preparations may sting initially.

- Assist the client to a comfortable position, either sitting or lying. Tilt the client's head toward the affected eye, and ensure that the light source does not shine into the person's eyes. *The head is tilted so that the solution will run from the eye to the basin at the side, not to the other eye. The light source is directed slightly away from the eye, particularly if the person is photophobic.*

- Place the drape to protect the client and the bedclothes, and position the basin against the cheek below the eye on the affected side.

3. **Assess the eye.**

- Assess the eye for redness, the location and nature of any discharge, lacrimation, and swelling of the eyelids or of the lacrimal gland.

- Note any complaints, e.g., itching, burning, pain, blurring of vision, and photophobia.

- Observe the client's behavior, e.g., squinting, blinking excessively, frowning, or rubbing the eyes.

4. **Clean the eyelid and eyelashes.**

- Use sterile cotton balls moistened with sterile irrigating solution or sterile normal saline, and wipe from the inner canthus to the outer canthus. *If not removed, material on the eyelid and lashes can be washed into the eye. Cleaning toward the outer canthus prevents contamination of the other eye and the lacrimal duct.*

5. **Administer the irrigation or eye medication.**

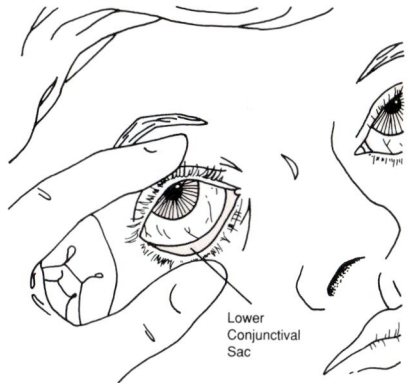

Figure 45–55 Exposing the lower conjunctival sac.

For an irrigation:

- Expose the lower conjunctival sac by separating the lids with the thumb and forefinger (see Figure 45–55). Or, to irrigate in stages, first hold the lower lid down, then hold the upper lid up. Exert pressure on the bony prominences of the cheekbone and beneath the eyebrow when holding the eyelids. *Separating the lids prevents reflex blinking. Exerting pressure on the bony prominences minimizes the possibility of pressing the eyeball and causing discomfort.*

- Fill and hold the eye irrigator about 2.5 cm (1 in) above the eye. *At this height the pressure of the solution will not damage the eye tissue, and the irrigator will not touch the eye.*

■ Irrigate the eye, directing the solution onto the lower conjunctival sac and from the inner canthus to the outer canthus. *Directing the solution in this way prevents possible injury to the cornea and prevents fluid and contaminants from flowing down the nasolacrimal duct.*

■ Irrigate until the solution leaving the eye is clear (no discharge is present) or until all the solution has been used.

■ Instruct the client to close and move the eye periodically. *Eye closure and movement help to move secretions from the upper to the lower conjunctival sac.*

■ Dry around the eye with cotton balls.

For an instillation:

■ Check the ophthalmic preparation as to name, strength, and number of drops if a liquid is used. Draw the correct number of drops into the shaft of the dropper if a dropper is used. If ointment is used, discard the first bead. *Checking medication data is essential to prevent a medication error. The first bead of ointment from a tube is considered to be contaminated.*

■ Instruct the client to look up to the ceiling. Give the client a piece of tissue. *The person is less likely to blink if looking up. While the client looks up, the cornea is partially protected by the top eyelid. A tissue is needed to press on the nasolacrimal duct after a liquid instillation or to wipe excess ointment from the eyelashes after an ointment is instilled.*

■ Expose the lower conjunctival sac by placing the thumb or fingers of your nondominant hand on the client's cheekbone just below the eye and gently drawing down the skin on the cheek. If the tissues are

edematous, handle the tissues carefully to avoid damaging them. *Placing the fingers on the cheekbone minimizes the possibility of touching the cornea, avoids putting any pressure on the eyeball, and prevents the person from blinking or squinting.*

■ Using a side approach, instill the correct number of drops onto the outer third of the lower conjunctival sac. Hold the dropper 1 to 2 cm (0.4 to 0.8 in) above the sac. See Figure 45–56. *The client is less likely to blink if a side approach is used. When instilled into the conjunctival sac, drops will not harm the cornea as they might if dropped directly on it. The dropper must not touch the sac or the cornea.*

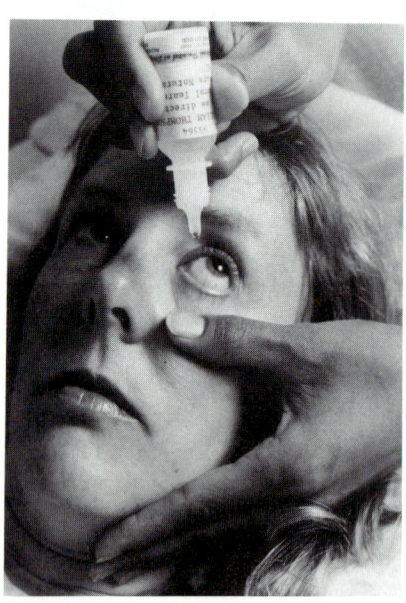

Figure 45–56   Instilling an eye drop into the lower conjunctival sac.

or

■ Holding the tube above the lower conjunctival sac, squeeze 3 cm (0.8 in) of ointment from the tube into the lower conjunctival sac from the inner canthus outward. See Figure 45–57.

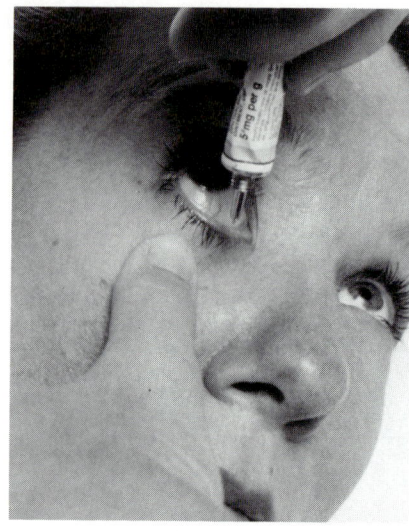

Figure 45–57   Instilling an eye ointment into the lower conjunctival sac.

■ Instruct the client to close the eyelids but not to squeeze them shut. *Closing the eye spreads the medication over the eyeball. Squeezing can injure the eye and push out the medication.*

■ For liquid medications, press firmly or have the client press firmly on the nasolacrimal duct for at least 30 seconds. See Figure 45–58.

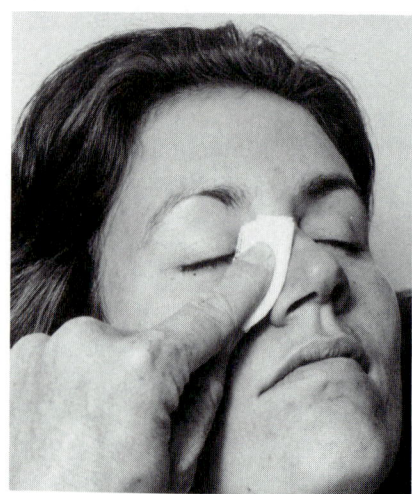

Figure 45–58   Pressing on the nasolacrimal duct.

Check agency practice. *Pressing on the nasolacrimal duct prevents the medication from running out of the eye and down the duct.*

6. **Clean the eyelids as needed.**

■ Wipe the eyelids gently from the inner to the outer canthus to collect excess medication.

7. **Apply an eye pad if needed, and secure it with paper eye tape.**

8. **Assess the client's response.**

■ Assess responses immediately after the instillation or irrigation and again after the medication should have acted.

9. **Document relevant information.**

■ Record nursing assessments and interventions relative to the instillation or irrigation. Include the name of the drug, the strength, the number of drops if a liquid, the time, and the response of the client.

Sample Recording

Date: 12/5/91	Time: 0900

C/o burning sensation OD. Moderate amount yellow purulent discharge at inner canthus and on eyelashes. Conjunctiva red. OD irrigated with 90 ml normal saline at 38 C. Returns cloudy. Stated "eye feels better" following irrigation. —————
—————————Deborah M. Mondeau, NS

Otic Irrigations and Instillations

Irrigations of the external auditory canal are generally carried out for cleaning purposes, although applications of heat and of antiseptic solutions are sometimes prescribed. Irrigations are usually performed in a hospital, using sterile supplies and equipment so that microorganisms will not be introduced into the ear. Normal saline at body temperature (37.0 C, or 98.6 F) is frequently used to irrigate the ear. The nurse uses a thermometer to ensure that the temperature of the solution is appropriate. Medical aseptic technique is used to instill medications to the ear unless the tympanic membrane is damaged, in which case sterile technique is used. The position of the external auditory canal varies with age. In the child under 3 years of age, it is directed upward. In the adult, the external auditory canal is an S-shaped structure about 2.5 cm (1 in) long. Procedure 45—10 explains how to administer otic irrigations and instillations.

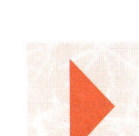

▶ *PROCEDURE 45—10*

ADMINISTERING OTIC IRRIGATIONS AND INSTILLATIONS

Equipment ☑

For an irrigation:

Container for the irrigating solution

Irrigating solution at the appropriate temperature, about 500 ml (16 oz) or as ordered

Syringe (rubber bulb or Asepto syringe is frequently used)

Basin, e.g., kidney basin

Moisture-resistant towel

Applicator swabs

Absorbent cotton balls

Gloves (optional)

For an instillation:

Correct medication bottle with a dropper

Cotton-tipped applicator

Flexible rubber tip (optional) for the end of the dropper, which prevents injury from sudden motion, e.g., by a child or disoriented client

Cotton fluff

Intervention

1. Verify the medication or irrigation order.

■ Check the physician's order for the kind of medication or irrigation; the time, amount, and dosage (if it is an instillation) or strength (if it is an irrigation); the temperature (if it is an irrigation); and which ear is to be treated.

2. Prepare the client.

For an irrigation:

■ Explain that the client may experience a feeling of fullness, warmth, and, occasionally, discomfort when the fluid comes in contact with the tympanic membrane.

■ Assist the client to a sitting or lying position with head turned toward the affected ear. *The solution can then flow from the ear canal to a basin.*

■ Place the moisture-resistant towel around the client's shoulder under the ear to be irrigated, and place the basin under the ear to be irrigated.

For an instillation:

■ Assist the client to a side-lying position with the ear being treated uppermost. See Figure 45–59.

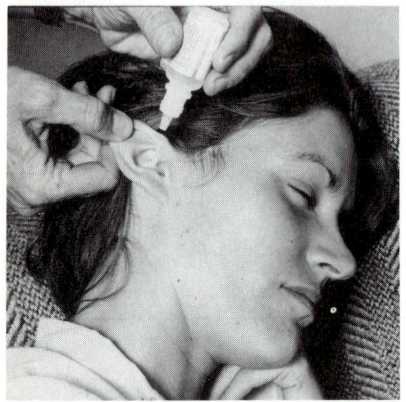

Figure 45–59 Instilling ear drops.

3. Assess the pinna of the ear and the meatus of the external auditory canal.

■ Inspect the ear and meatus for signs of redness and abrasions and the type and amount of any discharge.

■ Ask the client about complaints of discomfort.

■ If indicated, use an otoscope to assess (a) the external canal for any foreign bodies; (b) the external canal for swelling, redness, and discharge (the lining should be intact, pink, and without lesions); and (c) the intactness and appearance of the tympanic membrane. If the tympanic membrane is not intact or if foreign bodies are present in the external canal, do not proceed with the irrigation; report your findings to the nurse in charge.

4. Clean the pinna of the ear and the meatus of the ear canal.

■ Don gloves if indicated.

■ Use cotton-tipped applicators and solution to wipe the pinna and auditory meatus. *Any discharge is removed so that it will not be washed into the ear canal during an irrigation. It is cleaned before an instillation to remove any drainage.*

5. If doing an irrigation, prepare the equipment. (Omit this step for an instillation.)

■ Fill the syringe with solution.

or

■ Hang up the irrigating container, and run solution through the tubing and the nozzle. *Solution is run through to remove air from the tubing and nozzle.*

6. Administer the irrigation or ear medication.

For an irrigation:

■ Straighten the auditory canal. For an infant, gently pull the pinna downward. For an adult, pull the pinna upward and backward. See Figures 19–38 and 19–39, p. 386. *The auditory canal is straightened so that the solution can flow the entire length of the canal.*

■ Insert the tip of the syringe into the auditory meatus, and direct the solution gently upward against the top of the canal. *The solution will flow around the entire canal and out at the bottom. The solution is instilled gently because strong pressure from the fluid can cause discomfort and damage the tympanic membrane.*

■ Continue instilling the fluid until all the solution is used or until the canal is cleaned, depending on the purpose of the irrigation. Take care not to block the outward flow of the solution with the syringe.

■ Dry the outside of the ear with absorbent cotton balls. Place a cotton fluff in the auditory meatus to absorb the excess fluid.

■ Assist the client to a side-lying position on the affected side. *Lying with the affected side down helps drain the excess fluid by gravity.*

For an instillation:

■ Warm the medication container in your hand, or place it in warm water for a short time. *This promotes client comfort.*

■ Partially fill the ear dropper with medication.

■ Straighten the ear canal.

■ Instill the correct number of drops along the side of the ear canal.

■ Press gently but firmly a few times on the tragus of the ear. *Pressing on the tragus assists the flow of medication into the ear canal.*

■ Ask the client to remain in the side-lying position for about 5 minutes.

This prevents the drops from escaping and allows the medication to reach all sides of the canal cavity.

- Insert a small piece of cotton fluff loosely at the meatus of the auditory canal for 15 to 20 minutes. Do not press it into the canal. *The cotton helps retain the medication when the client is up. If pressed tightly into the canal, the cotton would interfere with the action of the drug and the outward movement of normal secretions.*

7. Assess the client's response.

- For an irrigation, assess the client for any discomfort and the appearance and odor of the fluid returns.

- For an instillation, assess the character and amount of discharge, appearance of the canal, discomfort, and so on, immediately after the instillation and again when the medication is expected to act. Inspect the cotton ball for any drainage.

8. Document relevant information.

- Document all nursing assessments and interventions relative to the procedure.

- For an irrigation include the type, concentration, amount, and temperature of the solution used; the appearance of the returns; and the presence of any discomfort.

- For an instillation, include the time, the dose, and any complaints of pain. Many agencies use flowsheets; others may require that a notation be made on the nurse's notes.

Sample Recordings

Date: 12/5/91	Time: 1100

Irrigated left ear with 60 ml normal saline at 40 C. Returns clear with several dark brown flecks. No complaints of discomfort. ———— Josephine A. deSanto, NS

Date: 12/5/91	Time: 0900

Auralgan instilled into left ear. States ear less painful. No discharge present.————————Margaret N. Kerr, NS

Nasal Instillations

Nasal instillations (nose drops) usually are instilled for their astringent effect (to shrink swollen mucous membranes) or to treat infections of the nasal cavity or sinuses. Prior to the instillation, the nurse should instruct the client to blow the nose to clear the nasal passages. Instilling nose drops requires that the client assume a back-lying position. A pillow is placed under the shoulders thus allowing the head to fall over the edge of the pillow.

To facilitate insertion of the drops, elevate the nares slightly by pressing the thumb against the tip of the nose. The dropper is held just above the nostril, and the drops are directed toward the midline of the superior concha of the ethmoid bone as the client breathes through the mouth. If the drops are directed toward the base of the nasal cavity, they will run down the eustachian tube. The mucous membranes of the nostrils should not be touched, to avoid injury to tissue and contamination of the dropper. The client remains in this position for 1 minute so that the solution will come into contact with all of the nasal surface. The nurse discards any medication remaining in the dropper before returning the dropper to the bottle. For administering medications by metered dose nebulizer, see Chapter 41, page 1108.

Vaginal Irrigations and Instillations

A vaginal irrigation (douche) is the washing of the vagina by a liquid at a low pressure. It is similar to the irrigation of the external auditory canal in that the fluid returns immediately after being inserted. Vaginal irrigations are not necessary for ordinary female hygiene but are used to prevent infection by applying an antimicrobial solution that discourages the growth of microorganisms, to remove an offensive or irritating discharge, and to reduce inflammation or prevent hemorrhage by the application of heat or cold. Commonly a betadine solution is prescribed.

In hospitals, sterile supplies and equipment are used; in a home, sterility is not usually necessary because people are accustomed to the microorganisms in their environments. Sterile technique is indicated if there is an open wound. Usually, 1000 to 2000 ml of irrigating solution at 40.5 C (105 F) is required. Check agency practice. Normal saline, tap water, sodium bicarbonate solution (8 ml of sodium bicarbonate to 1000 ml of water), and vinegar solution (8 ml of vinegar to 1000 ml of water) are commonly used. Before taking the equipment to the client, the nurse uses a thermometer to check the temperature of the solution.

Vaginal medications, or instillations, are inserted as creams, jellies, foams, or suppositories to relieve infection or to relieve vaginal discomfort, e.g., itching or pain. Medical aseptic technique is usually used. Vaginal creams, jellies, and foams are applied by using a tubular applicator with a plunger. Suppositories are inserted with the index finger of a gloved hand. Suppositories are designed to melt at body temperature, so they are generally stored in the refrigerator to keep them firm for insertion. See Procedure 45–11 for administering vaginal irrigations and instillations.

ADMINISTERING VAGINAL IRRIGATIONS AND INSTILLATIONS

Equipment ☑

For a vaginal irrigation:

Vaginal irrigation set (these are often disposable), containing a nozzle, tubing and a clamp, and a container for the solution

Moisture-resistant drape

Irrigating solution

Thermometer

Moistureproof pad

Bedpan

Tissues

Gloves

IV pole

For a vaginal instillation:

Correct vaginal suppository or cream

Disposable gloves

Lubricant for a suppository

Applicator for vaginal cream

Paper towel

Clean perineal pad and T-binder or sanitary belt

Intervention

1. Verify the medication or irrigation order.

■ Carefully check the physician's order for the specific medication or solution ordered, its dosage, and the time of administration.

2. Prepare the client.

■ Explain to the client that a vaginal irrigation or instillation is normally a painless procedure and, in fact, may bring relief from itching and burning if an infection is present. It usually takes about 10 minutes. Many people feel embarrassed about these procedures, and some may prefer to perform the procedure themselves if instruction is provided.

■ Provide privacy, and ask the client to void. *If the bladder is empty, the client will have less discomfort during the treatment, and the possibility of injuring the vaginal lining is decreased.*

3. Position and drape the client appropriately.

For an irrigation:

■ Assist the client to a back-lying position with the hips higher than the shoulders so that the solution will flow into the posterior fornix

of the vagina. Position the client on a bedpan, and provide comfortable support for the lumbar region of the back with a roll or pillow.

■ Place the waterproof drape under the bedpan to protect the bedding.

■ Provide a drape for the legs so that only the perineal area is exposed.

For an instillation:

■ Assist the client to a back-lying position with the knees flexed and the hips rotated laterally.

■ Drape the client appropriately so that only the perineal area is exposed.

4. Prepare the equipment.

For an irrigation:

■ Clamp the tubing. Hang the irrigating container on the IV pole so that the base is about 30 cm (12 in) above the vagina. *At this height, the pressure of the solution should not be great enough to injure the vaginal lining.*

■ Run fluid through the tubing and nozzle into the bedpan. *Fluid is run through the tubing to remove air and to moisten the nozzle.*

For an instillation:

■ Unwrap the suppository, and put it on the opened wrapper.

or

■ Fill the applicator with the prescribed cream, jelly, or foam. Directions are provided with the manufacturer's applicator.

5. Assess and clean the perineal area.

■ Don gloves. *Gloves prevent contamination of the nurse's hands from vaginal and perineal microorganisms.*

■ Inspect the vaginal orifice for inflammation

■ Note any odor or discharge from the vagina.

■ Ask about any vaginal discomfort.

■ Provide perineal care to remove microorganisms. *This decreases the chance of moving microorganisms into the vagina.*

6. Administer the irrigation or vaginal suppository, cream, foam, or jelly.

For an irrigation:

■ Run some fluid over the perineal area, then insert the nozzle carefully into the vagina. Direct the nozzle toward the sacrum, following the direction of the vagina.

■ Insert the nozzle about 7 to 10 cm (3 to 4 in), start the flow, and rotate the nozzle several times. *Rotating the nozzle irrigates all parts of the vagina.*

■ Use all the irrigating solution, permitting it to flow out freely into the bedpan. *Obstructing the flow of the returns could result in injury to the tissues from pressure.*

■ Remove the nozzle from the vagina.

■ Assist the client to a sitting position on the bedpan. *Sitting on the bedpan will help drain the remaining fluid by gravity.*

For a suppository:

■ Lubricate the rounded (smooth) end of the suppository, which is inserted first. *Lubrication facilitates insertion.*

■ Lubricate your gloved index finger.

■ Expose the vaginal orifice by separating the labia with your nondominant hand.

■ Insert the suppository about 8 to 10 cm (3 to 4 in) along the posterior wall of the vagina, or as far as it will go. See Figure 45–60. The posterior wall of the vagina is about 2.5 cm (1 in) longer than the anterior wall, since the cervix protrudes into the uppermost portion of the anterior wall. The anterior wall is usually about 6 to 7.5 cm (2½ to 3 in).

■ Withdraw the finger, and remove the gloves, turning them inside out and placing them on a paper towel. *Turning the gloves inside out prevents the spread of microorganisms.*

■ Ask the client to remain lying in the supine position for 5 to 10 minutes following insertion. The hips may also be elevated on a pillow. *This position allows the medication to flow into the posterior fornix after it has melted.*

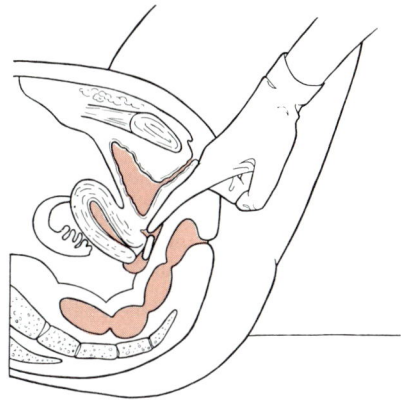

Figure 45–60 Instilling a vaginal suppository.

For a vaginal cream, jelly, or foam:

■ Gently insert the applicator about 5 cm (2 in).

■ Slowly push the plunger until the applicator is empty. See Figure 45–61.

■ Remove the applicator and place it on the paper towel. *The applicator*

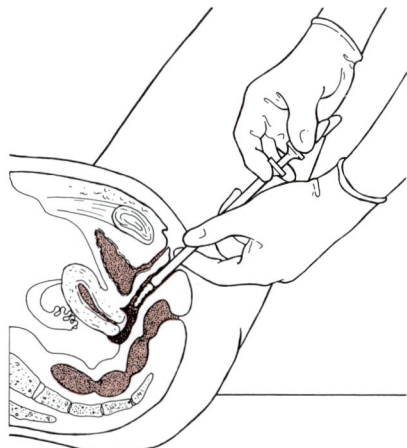

Figure 45–61 Using an applicator to instill a vaginal cream.

is put on a paper towel to prevent the spread of microorganisms.

■ Remove the gloves, turning them inside out, and place them on the paper towel.

■ Ask the client to remain in bed in the supine position for 5 to 10 minutes following the instillation.

7. Ensure client comfort.

■ Dry the perineum with tissues as required.

■ Remove the bedpan if used.

■ Remove the moisture-resistant pad and the drape.

■ Apply a clean perineal pad and a T-binder if there is excessive drainage.

8. Document relevant information.

■ To record the administration of the irrigation, note when it was administered; the amount, type, strength, and temperature of the irrigating solution; and all nursing assessments.

■ Record the instillation and assessments as you would other medications and instillations. See sample below.

9. Assess the client's response.

■ Assess the client's response to an instillation in terms of discharge, discomfort, and so forth when the medication is expected to act.

Sample Recording

Date: 3/15/91	Time: 1000

C/o pruritus around vaginal orifice. Thick, white, foul-smelling discharge apparent. Perineal care provided. Mycostatin suppository × i̇ inserted into vagina.——
——————————————Gloria Seng, NS

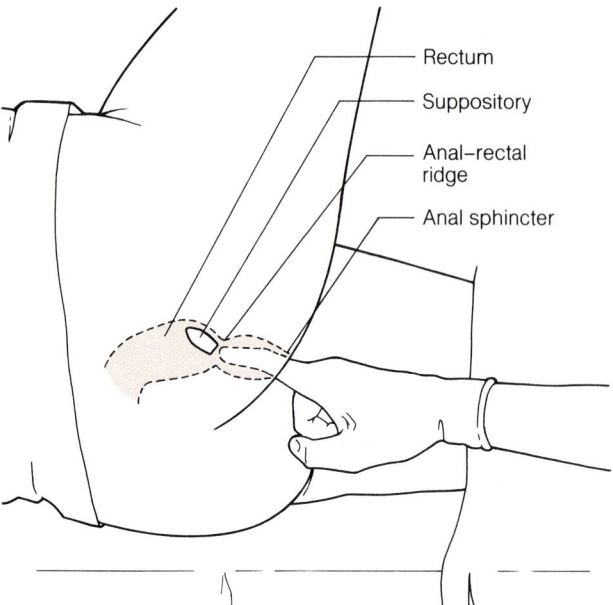

Rectum

Suppository

Anal–rectal ridge

Anal sphincter

Figure 45–62 A rectal suppository is inserted along the rectal wall beyond the internal anal sphincter.

Rectal Instillations

Rectal instillations (suppositories) are a convenient and safe method of giving certain medications. Rectal medications may have a local effect (e.g., a laxative suppository will soften feces and stimulate defecation) or a systemic effect (e.g., an aminophylline suppository will dilate the client's bronchi and ease breathing). The advantages of rectal instillation include the following:

- It avoids irritation of the upper gastrointestinal tract.
- Some medications are well absorbed across the mucosal surface of the rectum.
- Rectal suppositories are thought to provide higher bloodstream levels (titers) of medication, since the venous blood from the rectum is not transported through the liver (Hahn, Oestreich, and Barkin, 1986).

Prior to the insertion, the nurse helps the client to a lateral position, with the upper leg acutely flexed. Next, the nurse unwraps the suppository, puts it on the opened wrapper, and dons a glove on the hand that will insert the suppository. The glove prevents contamination of the nurse's hand by rectal microorganisms and feces. The nurse lubricates the smooth, rounded end of the suppository to prevent anal friction and tissue damage during insertion and lubricates the gloved index finger as well. To relax the client's anal sphincter, the nurse asks the client to breathe through the mouth. The suppository is inserted gently into the anus and along the wall of the rectum with the gloved index finger. In adults, suppositories are inserted to a depth of 10 cm (4 in); in children or infants, 5 cm (2 in) or less. See Figure 45–62. To be effective, the suppository needs to be placed along the wall of the rectum rather than embedded in feces. The nurse withdraws the finger, removes the glove by turning it inside out, and places it on a paper towel. Turning it inside out contains the rectal microorganisms and prevents their spread. To dispel the client's urge to expel the suppository, the nurse presses the client's buttocks together for a few seconds. If a laxative suppository has been given, the nurse asks the client to retain it for as long as possible (e.g., 15 to 20 minutes). The call signal should be within easy reach so that the client can summon assistance to use the bedpan or toilet.

CHAPTER HIGHLIGHTS

- ▶ Federal drug legislation in the United States and Canada regulates the production, prescription, distribution, and administration of drugs.

- ▶ Nursing practice acts define limits on the nurse's responsibilities regarding medications.

- ▶ Drugs are classified according to their overall action in the body.

- ▶ Primary actions of drugs in the body are stimulation and inhibition of tissue or organ functions.

- ▶ A drug may be incompatible with another drug or a particular food or an intravenous solution.

- ▶ Repeated doses of a drug will achieve a sustained level in the bloodstream.

- ▶ Obese clients require a larger dose of a drug than thin clients.

- ▶ Drugs given parenterally act more quickly than drugs given orally or topically.

- ▶ The five "rights" help ensure accurate administration of a drug.

- ▶ Parenteral administration of medications employs sterile technique.

- ▶ Clients receiving a series of injections should have the injection sites rotated.

READINGS AND REFERENCES

SUGGESTED READINGS

Birdsell, G., and Uretsky, S. October 1984. How do I administer medication by NG? *American Journal of Nursing* 84:1259–60, 1284.

The authors discuss which tablets can and cannot be crushed, how to deal with capsules, and how medications should be timed, with a description of the equipment used for administering the drugs.

Cohen, M. R. March 1990. Taking this test will help you avoid errors. *Nursing 90* 20:23–24.

Cohen provides an abbreviated version of a test given to nurses hired to work at Quakertown (Pennsylvania) Community Hospital. Nurses must attain a perfect score but may obtain the answers from textbooks, pharmacists, or other nurses.

Hayter, J. November/December 1981. Why response to medication changes with age. *Geriatric Nursing* 2:411–16, 441.

Hayter describes how absorption and distribution of a drug in an elderly person's body differs from that of other people, pointing out that the duration of action of a medication may be changed by decreased liver function. Hayter also discusses the toxic effects of drugs in older persons, their changing senses, and the implications of these changes on drug dosages.

Lenz, C. L. February 1983. Make your needle selection right to the point. *Nursing 83* 13:50–51.

The author describes how to select the correct needle length so that an intramuscular injection will be introduced into the center of the muscle. Lenz describes the pinch test, which can be used to calculate muscle size, considers the effect of the client's overall size, and points out that correct needle length prevents some of the complications of intramuscular injections.

Wiggins, M. S., and Sesin, P. April 1990. Guidelines for administering I.V. drugs. *Nursing 90* 20:145–52.

Wiggins and Sesin provide an easy-to-follow chart offering guidelines for administering common intravenous drugs by various methods: IV push, intermittent infusion, and continuous infusion. Developed by staff members at Boston's New England Deaconess Hospital, the chart also includes a column designating which intravenous solutions are compatible with the designated drug.

RELATED RESEARCH

Bayne, T., and Bindler, R. November/December 1988. Medication calculation skills of registered nurses. *Journal of Continuing Education in Nursing* 19:258–62.

Beecroft, P. C., and Redick, S. July/August 1989. Possible complications of intramuscular injections on the pediatric unit. *Pediatric Nursing* 15:333–36, 376.

Keen, M. F. Bomber, D., and Baer, C. 1989. *Using nursing research: Comparison of intramuscular injection techniques to reduce site discomfort and lesions* . . . The Z track technique. NLN Publication No. 15–2232. pp. 63–69, 70–73, 73–77. New York: National League for Nursing.

Wooldridge, J. B., and Jackson, J. G. September 1988. Evaluation of bruises and areas of induration after two techniques of subcutaneous heparin injection. *Heart and Lung* 17:476–82.

Worrell, P. J., and Hodson, E. March/April 1989. Posology: The battle against dosage calculation errors. *Nursing Educators Microworld* 14:27–31.

SELECTED REFERENCES

Burman, R., and Berkowitz, H. January/February 1986. I.V. bolus: Effective but potentially hazardous. *Critical Care Nurse* 6:22–28.

Chaplin, G.; Shull, H.; and Welk, P. C. September 1985. How safe is the air-bubble technique for I.M. injections? *Nursing 85* 15:59.

Clayton, M. June 1987. The right way to prevent medication errors. *RN* 50:30–31.

Cobb, M. D. March 1990. Dealing fairly with medication errors. *Nursing 90* 20:42–3.

Cohen, M. R. January 1990. Better way to transcribe orders. *Nursing 90* 20:9.

Cyganski, J. M.; Donahue, J. M.; and Heaton, J. S. June 1987. The case for the heparin flush. *American Journal of Nursing* 87:796–97.

Davis, N. M., and Cohen, M. R. March 1982. Learning from mistakes: 20 tips for avoiding medication errors. *Nursing 82* 12:65–72. Canadian ed. 12:23–30.

Gilman, A. G.; Goodman, L. S.; and Gilman, A. 1980. *The pharmacological basis of therapeutics.* 6th ed. New York: Macmillan Co.

Hahn, A. B.; Oestreich, S. J. K.; and Barkin, R. L. 1986. *Pharmacology in nursing.* 16th ed. St. Louis: C. V. Mosby Co.

Hahn, K. September 1989. Administering eye medications. *Nursing 89* 19:80.

Hayter, J. November/December 1981. Why response to medication changes with age. *Geriatric Nursing* 2:411–16.

Hudson, M. F. August 1984. Drugs and the older adult: Take special care. *Nursing 84* 14:47–54.

Keen, M. F. July/August 1986. Comparison of intramuscular injection techniques to reduce site discomfort and lesions. *Nursing Research* 35:207–10.

McConnell, E. A. February 1982. The subtle art of *really* good injections . . . IM, SC, and intradermal. *RN* 45:24–34.

———. March 1990. Giving intradermal injections. *Nursing 90* 20:70.

Monahan, F. D. March/April 1984. When swallowing pills is difficult. *Geriatric Nursing* 5:88–89.

Motz-Harding, E., and Good, F. February 1985. The right solution: Mixing I.V. drugs thoroughly. *Nursing 85* 15:62–64.

Newton, D. W., and Newton, M. July 1979. Route, site, and technique: Three key decisions in giving parenteral medication. *Nursing 79* 9:18–21, 23, 25.

Pitel, M. January 1971. The subcutaneous injection. *American Journal of Nursing* 71:76–79.

Reiss, B. S., and Melick, M. E. 1984. *Pharmacological aspects of nursing care.* Albany, New York: Delmar.

Scharf, L. June 1986. Safe needle disposal: A timely reminder. *RN* 49:42.

Thatcher, G. August 1985. Insulin injections: The case against random rotation. *American Journal of Nursing* 85:690–92.

Todd, B. January/February 1983. Drugs and the elderly: Using eye drops and ointments safely. *Geriatric Nursing* 4:53–56.

———. May/June 1983. Drugs and the elderly: Topical analgesics. *Geriatric Nursing* 4:152, 192, 196.

———. July/August 1985. Drugs and the elderly: Identifying drug toxicity. *Geriatric Nursing* 6:231, 234.

Winfrey, A. July 1985. Single-dose I.M. injections: How much is too much? *Nursing 85* 15:38–39.

Wong, D. L. August 1982. Significance of dead space in syringes. *American Journal of Nursing* 82:1237.

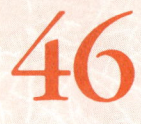

46

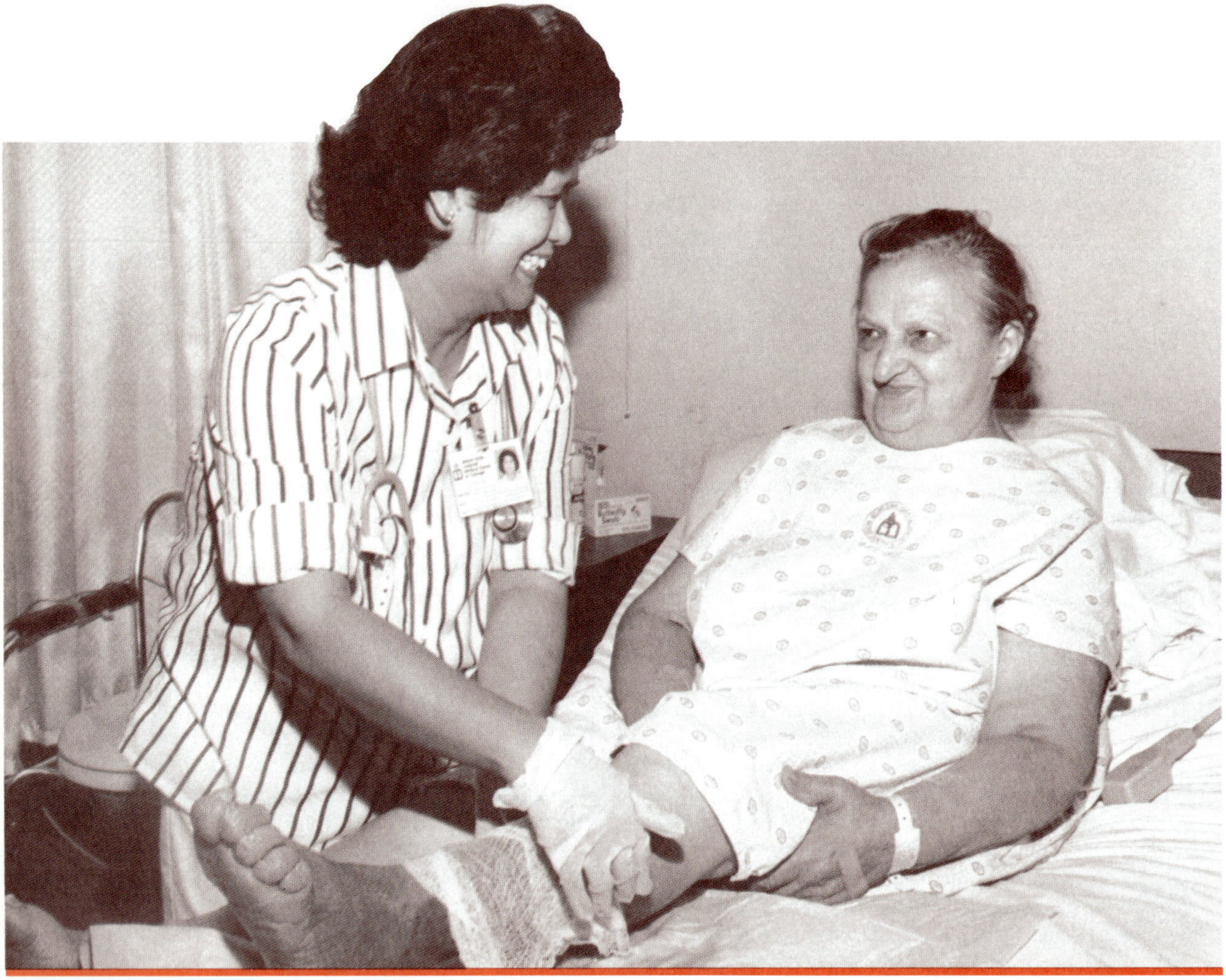

Wound Care

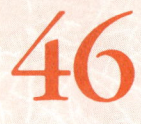

OBJECTIVES

▶ Define terms commonly used to describe wounds.

▶ State two basic ways in which wounds heal.

▶ Describe factors that affect wound healing.

▶ Identify the main complications of wound healing.

▶ Describe assessment criteria of a clean, healing wound.

▶ Identify nursing diagnoses for clients with various types of wounds.

▶ List suggested nursing strategies to promote wound healing and prevent complications of wound healing.

▶ Describe open and closed methods of wound care.

▶ Identify commonly used dressing materials and binders.

▶ Give reasons for selected steps of wound care procedures outlined in this chapter.

▶ Identify physiologic responses to heat and cold and purposes of heat and cold.

▶ Describe methods of applying dry and moist heat and cold.

▶ List outcome criteria by which to gauge whether wound healing has been achieved.

TYPES OF WOUNDS

The skin encloses the body structures and the body fluids, thereby protecting them from external assault. When this protective barrier is penetrated, the inflammatory process of the individual's immune response is enacted to eliminate the foreign material, if possible, and prepare the injured body area for healing. This injured body area, whether internal or external, is called a **wound.**

Body wounds are either intentional or unintentional. *Intentional* traumas occur during therapy. Examples are operations, venipunctures, or radiation burns. Although removing a tumor is therapeutic, the surgeon must cut into body tissues, thus traumatizing them. *Unintentional* wounds are accidental; e.g., a person may fracture an arm in an automobile collision. If the tissues are traumatized without a break in the skin, the wound is *closed.* The wound is *open* when the skin or mucous membrane surface is broken.

Wounds are frequently described according to how they are acquired: incised, contused, abraded, punctured, lacerated, or penetrating. An **incision** is made with a sharp instrument. It can be intentional, e.g., a cut made with a surgeon's scalpel, or accidental, e.g., a cut from a sharp knife. A **contusion** is a closed wound that is the result of a blow from a blunt instrument. The skin appears bruised (**ecchymotic**) because blood from the damaged blood vessels is released into the tissues. Contused wounds are usually unintentional, although they may result from surgical manipulation.

An **abrasion** is an open wound that results from friction, e.g., a scraped knee from a fall on a road surface. It involves the skin only. Abraded wounds can be intentional. In a dermal abrasion, for example, the superficial layers of the skin are removed, either by sandpapering or applying abrasion with a special machine, to obliterate scars and pockmarks. A **puncture wound** is an open wound made by a sharp instrument that penetrates the skin and underlying tissues. Puncture wounds can be accidental, e.g., a wound caused by stepping on a nail, or intentional, e.g., a wound made by a surgeon for the purpose of inserting a drain. Venipuncture and intramuscular injections are other common puncture wounds induced intentionally.

A **laceration** results when the tissues are torn apart, producing irregular edges. Lacerations are unintentional and often result from automobile or industrial accidents. A **penetrating wound** results when an instrument is inserted deeply into the tissues through the skin or mucous membrane. Usually, penetrating wounds are accidental, e.g., those from bullets or metal fragments. A bullet or other object making a penetrating wound may lodge in an internal organ.

Wounds can be further described according to the likelihood and degree of wound contamination (Garner 1986, p. 73).

■ *Clean wounds* are uninfected wounds in which no inflammation is encountered and the respiratory, alimentary, genital, and urinary tracts are not entered. Clean wounds are primarily closed wounds; or, if necessary, they are drained with closed drainage.

- *Clean-contaminated wounds* are surgical wounds in which the respiratory, alimentary, genital or urinary tract has been entered. Such wounds show no evidence of infection.
- *Contaminated wounds* include open, fresh, accidental wounds and surgical wounds involving a major break in sterile technique or a large amount of spillage from the gastrointestinal tract. Contaminated wounds show evidence of inflammation.
- *Dirty or infected wounds* include old, accidental wounds containing dead tissue and wounds with evidence of a clinical infection, e.g., purulent drainage.

WOUND HEALING

Following injury, the process of healing takes place. Only certain tissues of the body are capable of **regeneration** (renewal); those that are not form scars. Healing takes place by primary or secondary intention.

Primary Intention Healing

Primary intention healing occurs when the tissue surfaces are or have been **approximated** (closed) and there is minimal or no tissue loss; it is characterized by the formation of minimal granulation tissue and scarring. Also called *primary union* or *first intention healing,* primary intention healing has three stages: the defensive stage, the reconstructive stage, and the maturative stage.

Defensive Stage

The defensive stage begins at the time of injury and lasts 4 to 6 days. It has three major mechanisms: hemostasis, inflammation, and cell migration.

Hemostasis (the cessation of bleeding) results from vasoconstriction of the blood vessels in the affected area, retraction (drawing back) of injured blood vessels, and the deposition of fibrin and the formation of blood clots in the area. The blood clots, formed from blood platelets, provide a matrix of fibrin that becomes the framework for cell repair. A scab also forms on the surface of the wound. Consisting of clots and dead and dying tissue, this scab serves to aid hemostasis and inhibit contamination of the wound by microorganisms. Below the scab, epithelial cells migrate into the wound from the edges. This process of epithelization is slowed if the tissue becomes excessively dry (Pollack 1981, p. 16). The epithelial cells, which move from both sides of the wound and meet within 48 hours (Pollack 1981, p. 17), serve as a barrier between the body and the environment, preventing the entry of microorganisms.

Inflammation involves vascular and cellular responses intended to remove any foreign substances and dead and dying tissues. The blood supply to the wound is increased, bringing with it substances and nutrients needed in the healing process. The area appears reddened and edematous as a result.

During cell migration leukocytes move into the interstitial space (emigration), and erythrocytes pass through the blood vessel walls by a process known as *diapedesis*. Leukocytes (neutrophils) appear first and are replaced by monocytes. Leukocytes engulf bacteria and cellular debris by a process known as *phagocytosis*. Fibroblasts also migrate into the wound beginning about the second or third day as the inflammatory process subsides. New blood capillaries then form in the wound.

Reconstructive Stage

The reconstructive stage commences before the defensive processes are completed. The fibroblasts in the wound synthesize mucopolysaccharides, glycoproteins, and collagen. This process, called *fibroplasia,* requires 2 to 4 weeks, depending on the size and site of the wound. **Collagen** is a whitish protein substance that adds tensile strength to the wound. As the amount of collagen increases, so does the strength of the wound; thus, there is progressively less chance that the wound will open. During this time, the wound appears as a purplish, irregular, raised scar.

Maturative Stage

During the maturative stage, the scar changes in shape and size. This can take months or even years. The collagen fibers change to preinjury configuration. Although the wound gets progressively stronger, a healed wound usually does not attain the strength of preinjured tissue (Bruno 1979, p. 677). However, visceral wounds, e.g., to the stomach, regain strength sooner than skin wounds.

Secondary Intention Healing

A wound heals by secondary intention when it is extensive and there is considerable tissue loss. **Secondary intention healing** differs from primary intention healing in three ways: (a) the repair time is longer; (b) the scarring is greater; and (c) the susceptibility to infection is greater.

The healing process takes longer because dead tissue in the wound must be removed and because the wound must become filled with connective scar tissue to replace the previous tissue framework, which has been lost. As a result of this scarring, contracture and loss of function can occur. In addition, inflammation tends to be amplified during secondary healing. With inflammation, it is macrophages and lymphocytes (not neutrophils) that usually predominate. Fibroblasts and capillary buds move slowly toward the center of the wound. As the capillary network develops, the tissue becomes a translucent red color. This tissue, called **granulation tissue,** is fragile, bleeds easily, may protrude above the wound margins, and may have a mucin covering. When the granulation tissue matures, marginal epithelial cells migrate to it, proliferating over this connective tissue base to fill the wound. If the wound does not close by epithelialization, the area becomes covered with dried plasma proteins and dead cells. This is called **eschar.** Initially, wounds healing by secondary intention seep serosanguineous drainage. Later, if they are not covered by epithelial cells, they become covered with thick, gray, fibrinous tissue that is eventually converted into dense scar tissue.

Kinds of Wound Drainage

There are three major types of **exudate** (material, such as fluid and cells, that has escaped from blood vessels during the inflammatory process and is deposited in tissue or on tissue surfaces): serous, purulent, and sanguineous. A **serosanguineous** exudate is commonly seen in surgical incisions; it consists of serous and sanguineous drainage. Descriptions of these exudates are given in Chapter 20, page 455.

Factors That Affect Wound Healing

Both internal and external factors can affect wound healing, either positively or negatively. *Internal factors* include vasculature, immune status, nutrition, obesity, drugs, smoking, and stress. See the accompanying box. *External factors* include preoperative stay, preoperative preparation, and intraoperative elements (Flynn and Rovee 1982, p. 1550). The Centers for Disease Control recommend the following (Garner 1986, p. 77) to control some of the external factors that affect wound healing:

- Bacterial infections should be treated before surgery.
- The preoperative hospital stay should be as short as possible.
- Malnourished clients should receive enteral or parenteral nutrition preoperatively if the surgery is not urgent.
- Clients having elective surgery should bathe with an antimicrobial soap the night before surgery.
- Hair near the operative site should not be removed unless absolutely necessary.
- If hair must be removed, it should be clipped or removed with a depilatory, rather than shaved.

The preoperative use of antibiotics is recommended where there is a high risk of infection (Nichols 1982, p.34). The timing and dosage of the antibiotics are important factors in preventing postoperative infections in high-risk clients. Nichols recommends administering parenteral antibiotics within 1 hour of surgery and continuing for 24 to 72 hours. This practice allows time for drugs to reach therapeutic levels in the tissues but does not permit bacterial resistance to develop (Nichols 1982, p. 34).

Older adults are at greater risk for poor wound healing. The accompanying box summarizes particular factors that inhibit healing.

Wound Healing: Effects of Internal Factors

- *Vasculature:* Good blood supply promotes healing; delayed healing occurs when the blood supply is insufficient to provide nutrients for tissue repair.
- *Compromised host:* Client is at risk for an additional reason (e.g., infection, diabetes mellitus, receiving radiation therapy); secondary condition poses additional demands on body's healing responses.
- *Nutrition:* Wound healing places additional nutritional demands upon the body; delayed healing occurs in poorly nourished clients.
- *Obesity:* Adipose tissue has limited blood supply (decreasing nutritional source for tissue repair) and is difficult to suture (increasing likelihood of wound dehiscence—separating of the wound edges).
- *Medications:* Immunosuppressive agents may retard healing; antiinflammatory drugs may mask symptoms of superimposed infection.
- *Smoking:* Reduces functional hemoglobin with resultant decrease in circulating oxygenation of body's tissues; also may increase aggregation of platelets, contributing to hypercoagulability.
- *Stress:* Places additional demands on body responses and thus interferes with healing.

Factors Inhibiting Wound Healing in the Elderly

- Vascular changes associated with aging, such as atherosclerosis and atrophy of capillaries in the skin, can impair blood flow to the wound.
- Reduced liver function can impair the synthesis of needed blood clotting factors.
- Changes in the immune system may reduce the formation of antibodies and lymphocytes necessary to prevent infection.
- Nutrition deficiencies may reduce the numbers of red blood cells and leukocytes, thus impeding the delivery of oxygen and the inflammatory response essential for wound healing. Oxygen is needed for the synthesis of collagen and the formation of new epithelial cells.

Complications of Wound Healing

There are three main complications of wound healing:

1. *Hemorrhage.* Some escape of blood from a wound is normal intraoperatively and postoperatively. **Hemorrhage** (persistent bleeding), however, is abnormal. It may be caused by a dislodged clot, a slipped ligature, or erosion of a blood vessel, for example.

2. *Infection.* Infections of a surgical wound may become obvious 2 to 11 days postoperatively (Wright 1983, p. 143). Drainage from a suspected infected wound should be cultured (Garner 1986, p. 79).

3. *Dehiscence with possible evisceration.* **Dehiscence** is the partial or total rupturing of a wound. Dehiscence often refers specifically to the opening of an abdominal wound in which the layers below the skin also separate. **Evisceration** is the protrusion of the internal viscera through an incision. A number of factors, including obesity, poor nutrition, multiple trauma, failure of suturing, excessive coughing, vomiting, and dehydration, heighten a client's risk of wound dehiscence. Wound dehiscence is more likely to occur when no healing ridge has appeared within 4 to 5 days postoperatively. This ridge normally develops along the entire length of an incision and is a sign that fibroplasia has occurred.

Table 46–1 summarizes the clinical signs indicating the presence of the complications of wound healing. The nurse should notify the physician if the signs of hemorrhage or infection are present. If dehiscence occurs, the area should be covered with sterile towels soaked in sterile saline to maintain tissue moistness, and the physician should be notified immediately. Wound dehiscence is an emergency situation requiring surgical resuturing. A nurse should remain with the client and support the wound, with gloved hands if necessary, to prevent evisceration.

ASSESSING WOUNDS

Nurses commonly assess both untreated and treated wounds. *Untreated wounds* usually are seen shortly after an injury (e.g., at the scene of an accident or in an emergency center). Assessment for these wounds is shown in the box on the opposite page. Guidelines for care follow.

1. Control severe bleeding by (a) applying direct pressure over the wound and (b) elevating the involved extremity.

2. Prevent infection by (a) cleaning or flushing abrasions or lacerations with water and (b) covering the wound with a clean dressing (a sterile dressing is preferred). When applying a dressing, wrap the wound tightly enough to apply pressure and approximate the wound edges if

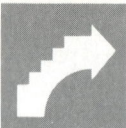

CLINICAL GUIDELINES
Assessing Untreated Wounds

- Assess client's condition. Determine the presence of a clear airway, adequacy of breathing, and presence of a carotid pulse.

- Assess the size and severity of the wound. If severe, have someone call an ambulance or, if in an emergency center, inform the physician.

- Inspect the wound for bleeding. The amount of bleeding varies according to the type of wound and location. Penetrating wounds may cause internal bleeding.

- Inspect the wound for foreign bodies (soil, broken glass, shreds of cloth, or other foreign substances).

- Assess associated injuries such as fractures, internal bleeding, spinal cord injuries, or head trauma.

- If the wound is contaminated with foreign material, determine when the client last had a tetanus toxoid injection. A tetanus antitoxin will be necessary if 5 years have elapsed.

possible. If the first layer of dressing becomes saturated with blood, apply a second layer. Do so without removing the first layer of dressing, because blood clots might be disturbed, resulting in more bleeding.

3. Control swelling and pain by applying ice over the wound and surrounding tissues.

4. If bleeding is severe or if internal bleeding is suspected, and if emergency equipment is available, assess vital signs.

Treated wounds, i.e., sutured wounds, are usually assessed during a dressing change unless a transparent dressing has been applied. If the wound itself cannot be directly inspected, the dressing is inspected and other data regarding the wound, e.g., the presence of pain, are determined. Many surgical wounds are covered with a transparent occlusive dressing that permits observation of the wound without exposing it to the air.

Clinical Assessment

Nurses assess wounds by visual inspection, palpation, and the sense of smell, noting the wound's appearance and any drainage, swelling, odor, dehiscence, and pain. The client is also assessed for any of the clinical signs of complications in Table 46–1.

As part of the ongoing assessment of each client with a wound, the nurse first checks the appearance of the wound itself for signs of healing and approximation of the wound edges. Taylor (1983, p. 44) and Bruno (1979, p. 670) outline the following *sequential* signs of primary wound healing:

TABLE 46–1 *Complications of Wound Healing*

Clinical Signs of Hemorrhage	Clinical Signs of Infection	Clinical Signs of Dehiscence
Increased pulse rate	Redness	Unexplained fever
Increased respiratory rate	Swelling	Unexplained tachycardia
Lowered blood pressure	Pain	Unusual wound pain
Restlessness	Induration (hardening of the tissues)	Prolonged paralytic ileus
Thirst	Fever	
Cold, clammy skin	Increased leukocyte count	

1. *Absence of bleeding and the appearance of a clot binding the wound edges.* The wound edges are well approximated and bound by fibrin in the clot within the first few hours after surgical closure.

2. *Inflammation (redness and swelling) at the wound edges for 1 to 3 days.*

3. *Reduction in inflammation when the clot diminishes,* as granulation tissue starts to bridge the area. The wound is bridged and closed within 7 to 10 days. Increased inflammation associated with fever and drainage is indicative of wound infection; the wound edges then appear brightly inflamed and swollen.

4. *Scar formation.* Collagen synthesis starts 4 days after injury and continues for 6 months or longer.

5. *Diminished scar size* over a period of months or years. An increase in scar size indicates keloid formation.

Additional assessment guidelines are presented in the box on the opposite page.

Laboratory Data

Laboratory data can often support the nurse's clinical assessment of the wound's progress in healing. A *decreased leukocyte count* can delay healing and increase the possibility of infection. *Blood coagulation studies* are also significant. Prolonged coagulation times can result in excessive blood loss and prolonged clot absorption. Hypercoagulability can lead to intravascular clotting. Intra-arterial clotting can result in **ischemia** (deficiency in blood supply) to the wound area. *Serum protein analysis* provides an indication of the body's nutritional reserves for rebuilding cells.

The most recently developed test for protein-calorie malnutrition is *thyroxine-binding prealbumin (TBP).* Because this test is more sensitive to small changes in protein status than serum albumin levels, it can identify malnutrition before it becomes severe. Readings between 10 and 15 mg/dl suggest a mild deficit; values of 5 to 10 mg/dl suggest a moderate deficit (Cerrato 1988, p. 74). This test must be done before surgery, because trauma can create false reduced

values. In agencies where TBP tests are not performed, the serum albumin test is performed; values below 3.5 g/dl suggest malnutrition. Other laboratory tests may be ordered as needed for individual clients.

Wound cultures can either confirm or rule out the presence of infection. Sensitivity studies are helpful in the selection of appropriate antibiotic therapy. Procedure 46–1 provides guidelines to obtain a wound culture.

CLINICAL GUIDELINES
Assessing Healing Wounds

Appearance

■ Inspect color of wound and surrounding area and approximation of wound edges. Note size and location of dehiscence, if present.

Drainage

■ Observe location, color, consistency, odor, and degree of saturation of dressings. Note number of gauzes saturated or diameter of drainage on gauze.

Swelling

■ Wearing sterile gloves, palpate wound edges for tension and tautness of tissues; minimal to moderate swelling is normal in early stages of wound healing.

Pain

■ Expect severe to moderate postoperative pain for 3 to 5 days; persistent severe pain or sudden onset of severe pain may indicate internal hemorrhaging or infection.

Drains or Tubes

■ Inspect drain security and placement, amount of character of drainage, and functioning of collecting apparatus, if present.

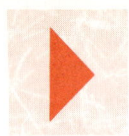

OBTAINING A SPECIMEN OF WOUND DRAINAGE

Equipment

Sterile dressing set, including dressings, cleaning solution, scissors, swabs, medications

Clean gloves

Sterile gloves (optional)

Moisture-resistant (plastic or waxed paper) disposal bag

Sterile culture tube or sterile syringe and needle (for an *aerobic culture,* use the standard culture tube with transport medium; for an *anaerobic culture,* use either a special culture tube containing carbon dioxide or nitrogen *or* a sterile 10-ml syringe and #21 gauge needle)

Completed labels for each container

Completed requisition to accompany the specimens to the laboratory

---

Intervention

1. Check agency practices about cleaning the wound before obtaining the specimen.

- In some agencies, the wound is cleaned with sterile water or normal saline to remove excessive exudate.

- In other agencies, only the area around the wound is cleaned with an alcohol or povidone-iodine sponge to minimize the risk of contaminating the specimen with skin bacteria.

2. Remove moist outer dressings.

- Put on clean gloves.

- Remove the outer dressing, and observe any drainage on it. Hold the dressing so that the client does not see the drainage. *The appearance of the drainage could upset the client.*

- Discard the dressing in the moistureproof bag. Handle it carefully so that the dressing does not touch the outside of the bag. *Touching the outside of the bag will contaminate it.*

- Remove your gloves, if used, and dispose of them properly.

3. Open the sterile dressing set using sterile technique.

- See Procedure 20–2 on page 479.

4. Assess the wound.

- Put on sterile gloves if you are not using sterile forceps.

- Assess the appearance of the tissues in and around the wound and the drainage. Infection can cause reddened tissues with a thick discharge, which may be foul smelling, whitish, or colored.

- Determine the amount of the drainage, e.g., one 2 × 2 gauze saturated with pale yellow drainage.

5. Obtain the culture.

For an aerobic culture:

- Open a specimen tube, and place the cap upside down on a firm, dry surface so that the inside will not become contaminated. Hold the tube in one hand, and pick up a swab in the other.

- Using the sterile swab, wipe the drainage at the designated point, i.e., at deep or active drainage areas of the wound. Absorb as much drainage as possible onto the swab. Wipe only once with one swab. *Only one wipe is taken with each swab to prevent contamination of other wound areas.*

- Insert the swab into the sterile container, taking care not to touch the top or the outside of the tube. *The outside of the container must remain free of pathogenic microorganisms to prevent their spread to others.*

- Close the container securely.

- If a specimen is required from another site, repeat the above steps. Specify the exact site (e.g., inferior drain site or lower aspect of incision) on the label of each container, if not labeled previously. Be sure to put each swab in the appropriately labeled tube.

For an anaerobic culture, using a special culture tube containing a swab:

- Remove the swab from the inner tube of the anaerobic culture tube without removing the rubber stopper of the larger tube. See Figure 46–1, *A.*

- Insert the sterile swab deeply into the draining body cavity.

- Rotate the swab gently.

- Remove the swab and quickly replace it into the inner tube.

- Depress the plunger of the inner tube to force it down into the larger tube. *Pushing the inner tube down into the larger tube exposes the specimen to the carbon dioxide or nitrogen environment.* See Figure 46–1, *B.*

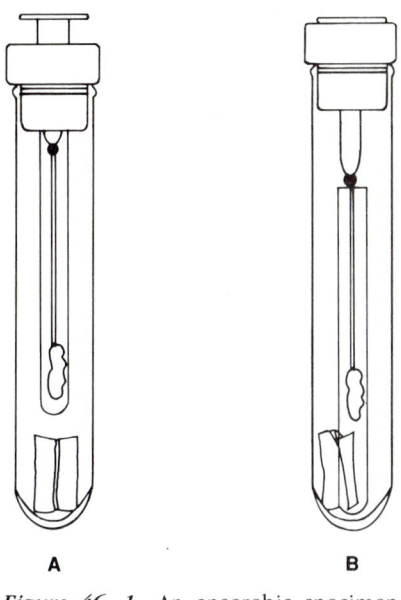

A   **B**

Figure 46–1 An anaerobic specimen culture tube with swab: *A,* before specimen collection; *B,* after specimen collection.

For an anaerobic culture, using a sterile syringe and needle:

- Insert a sterile 10-ml syringe (without needle) into the wound and aspirate 1 to 5 ml of drainage into the syringe.

- Attach the #21 gauge needle to the syringe, and expel all air from the syringe.

- Immediately inject the drainage into the anaerobic culture tube.

    or

- If a rubber stopper is available, insert the needle into the rubber stopper, and send the syringe of drainage to the laboratory immediately.

6. **Clean and dress the wound.**

- Clean the wound. See procedure 46–4 for appropriate method.

- Apply any ordered medication to the wound. Cover the wound with sterile dressings. See Procedure 46–4.

- Remove gloves, if worn, and dispose of them appropriately.

7. **Arrange for the specimen to be transported to the laboratory immediately. Be sure to include the completed requisition.**

8. **Document relevant information.**

- Record taking the specimen on the client's chart.

- Include the date and time; the appearance of the wound; the color, consistency, amount, and odor of any drainage; and any discomfort experienced by the client.

DIAGNOSING

Nursing diagnoses for clients with wounds or at risk of obtaining wounds largely reflect the need to prevent complications and to teach the client self-care. Depending on the assessment data obtained and the client's health status, some of the following NANDA diagnoses may be appropriate: **Potential for infection, Pain, Potential impaired skin integrity, Knowledge deficit, Altered tissue perfusion,** and **Body image disturbance.** Examples of these diagnoses with possible contributing factors are shown below. Defining characteristics are discussed elsewhere in this book.

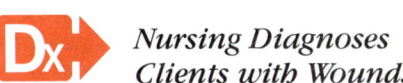 *Nursing Diagnoses Clients with Wounds*

Potential for infection related to:

- Impaired skin integrity (e.g., surgical incision, leg ulcer, Penrose drain)

Pain related to:

- Infected surgical incision
- Hematoma associated with hip injury
- Joint swelling secondary to knee injury

Altered tissue perfusion: Peripheral related to:

- Interrupted arterial blood flow
- Interrupted venous blood flow

Potential impaired skin integrity related to:

- Exposure to secretions (e.g., from draining fistula, ostomy, Penrose drain)
- Altered circulation
- Altered nutrition: Less than body requirements
- Impaired physical mobility

Body image disturbance related to:

- Altered body structure (e.g., loss of breast, extensive scarring associated with burns)
- Altered body function (e.g., ostomy)

Knowledge deficit (e.g., wound care, ostomy care, use of heating pad)

PLANNING TO AUGMENT HEALING

Just as there are many types of wounds, there are many ways of caring for wounds. In general, the care varies with the type of wound, its size, the amount of exudate present, its state (open or closed), the location, the personal preference of the physician, and the presence of complicating factors. Planning includes both independent and dependent nursing strategies to promote healing and prevent infection. Dependent strategies are those that stem largely from the wound care orders written by the physician.

Promoting wound healing is a goal for both the medical and nursing staff. The physician approximates the wound edges with sutures to ensure a good blood supply to provide essential nutrients. The nurse provides ongoing assessment of the healing wound and keeps the area free from body excretions. In addition, the nurse protects the surrounding tissues from skin excoriation when a wound is draining. This is accomplished by changing saturated dressings as required and by cleaning and drying wounds and surrounding skin areas. When drainage is excessive, as in some bowel (colostomy) or urinary surgery, the nurse may apply protective ointments or pastes to surrounding skin to prevent irritation and excoriation. The frequent removal of tape can also be irritating to the skin; thus, Montgomery straps (tie tapes) or newer tape products, which have minimal adhesive and are porous, are frequently used. These cause the least skin disruption.

The nurse can prevent infection from microorganisms entering a wound through the broken skin and mucous membranes by using surgical aseptic technique when caring for the wound, using antiseptic on the skin, and administering antibiotics as prescribed by the physician. Surgeons frequently place rubber or plastic tubes or drains into wounds or ducts to promote drainage. Some of these drains, commonly called **Penrose drains** (used primarily for infected wounds), are shortened progressively throughout the healing process. They ensure removal of inflammatory exudates and blood prior to closure of the overlying skin. Just as the drain serves as an outlet for waste from the wound, it is also an inlet for infectious organisms. Therefore, the nurse keeps the area around the drain outlet clean to decrease the risk of wound infection. Planning wound care also involves establishing outcome criteria by which to evaluate the client's progress. Examples of outcome criteria are shown below.

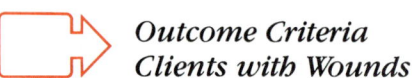

Outcome Criteria
Clients with Wounds

The client:
- Maintains normal or baseline vital signs.
- Achieves timely wound healing, as manifested by decreas-

ing inflammation and wound drainage and absence of purulent drainage.
- Accomplishes activities of daily living with minimal or no pain.
- Maintains adequate dietary intake for healing.
- Maintains intact skin around drainage site.
- Resumes normal activities within specified period.
- Demonstrates wound care as instructed.
- Reports understanding of discharge instructions.
- States signs of complications that require notification of the nurse or physician.

IMPLEMENTING

Caring for Open and Closed Wounds

In the *open method* of wound care, no dressings are used. The *closed method* involves applying a dressing. Dressings, which create an environment for optimum healing, have the following advantages:

- Absorbing drainage and debriding the wound when removed
- Protecting the wound from external microbial contamination
- Aiding in hemostasis when applied with elastic bandages
- Approximating wound edges
- Supporting and splinting the wound site, thus reducing mobility and trauma to the wound itself
- Covering unpleasant disfigurements

In some situations, the physician applies a protective covering such as collodion spray instead of a gauze dressing. This spray hardens like nail polish and can be either peeled from the skin when the wound is healed or removed with a special solution. A spray covering is often preferred to a dressing, because it eliminates friction and allows the wound to be seen through the translucent covering. Because the spray is moistureproof, the wound is protected from external contamination. For children, who are active and who heal quickly, spray is frequently used. However, it is not advised for draining wounds.

The *open method* avoids certain disadvantages of dressings. For example, dressings produce dark, warm, moist environments in which resident and nonresident microorganisms can multiply, and dressings can irritate wounds by friction. Exposing wounds to the air promotes drying and discourages the growth of microorganisms, which need moisture. The open method is frequently employed for burns.

Caring for wounds involves cleaning (both open and closed

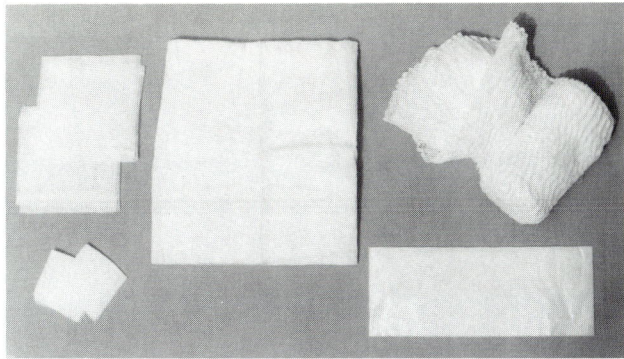

Figure 46–2 Some frequently used dressing materials (clockwise from bottom left): 2 × 2 gauze, 4 × 4 gauze, surgipad or abdominal pad, roller gauze, and nonadherent absorbent dressing.

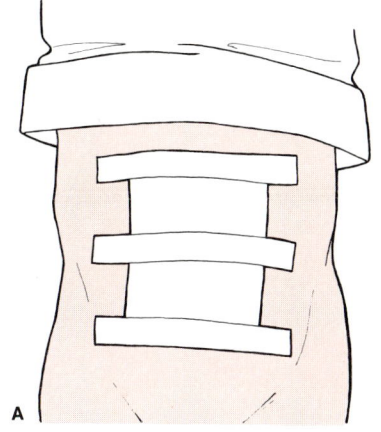

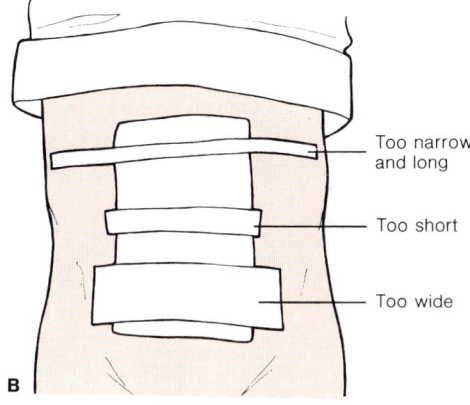

Figure 46–3 The strips of tape should be placed at the ends of the dressing and must be sufficiently long and wide to secure the dressing. *A,* correct taping; *B,* incorrect taping.

wounds) and covering the wound. Cleaning agents vary considerably. Examples include Betadine, 70% alcohol, and sterile normal saline. The choice depends on agency protocol and physician preference. Some nurses prefer cotton balls to clean wounds because of their absorbent qualities; others prefer gauze squares, claiming that threads of cotton balls can stick to sutures.

Several sizes of gauze are available to cover wounds. See Figure 46–2. The standard sizes are 10 × 10 cm (4 × 4 in) and 10 × 20 cm (4 × 8 in). The size and the number of pads used depend on the nature of the wound, the amount of exudate, and the location of the wound. These decisions are left to the nurse's judgment. Sometimes the gauze is precut halfway through one side to make it fit around a drain, or it is folded in a special way.

Telfa gauze is a special type. It has a shiny, nonadherent surface on one or both sides and is applied with the shiny surface on the wound. Exudate seeps through this surface and collects on the absorbent material on the other side or is sandwiched between the two nonadherent surfaces. Since the dressing does not adhere, it does not cause injury to the wound when removed. *Petrolatum* gauze, another nonadherent type, is impregnated with petroleum jelly. It is placed against the wound and usually covered with 4 × 4 gauze. Nonadherent dressings should not be used when wound **debridement** (removal of infected and necrotic material) is desired.

Larger and thicker gauze dressings, called *surgipads* or *abdominal pads,* are used to cover small gauzes. They not only hold the other gauzes in place but also absorb and collect excess drainage. Surgipads are more absorbent on one side, and this side is placed toward the wound; the less absorbent, more protective side is placed outward to protect the wound from external contamination. The outer side is often indicated with a blue stripe.

The nurse tapes the dressing over the wound ensuring that the dressing covers the entire wound and does not become dislodged. The correct type of tape must be selected for the purpose. Elastic tape can provide pressure; nonallergenic tape is used when a client is allergic to other tape. The nurse follows these steps:

1. Place the tape so that the dressing cannot be folded back to expose the wound. Place strips at the ends of the dressing, and space tapes evenly in the middle. See Figure 46–3.

2. Ensure that the tape is long and wide enough to adhere to the skin but not so long or wide that it loosens with activity. See Figure 46–3.

3. Place the tape in the opposite direction from the body action, e.g., across a body joint or crease, not lengthwise. See Figure 46–4.

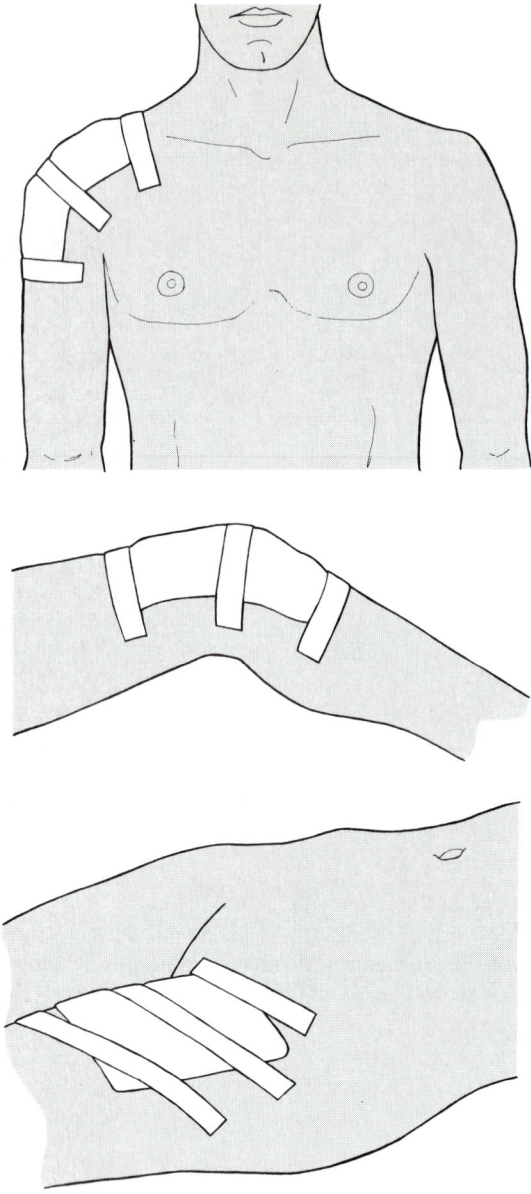

Figure 46–4 Dressings over moving parts must remain secure in spite of the movement.

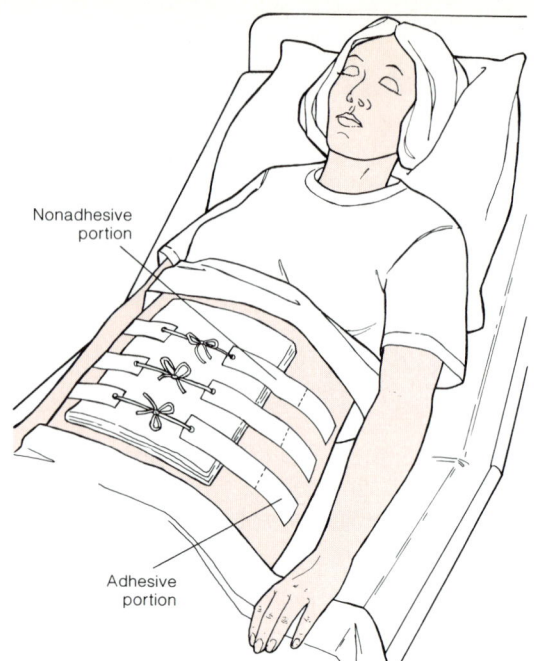

Figure 46–5 Montgomery straps, or tip tapes, are used to secure large dressings that require frequent changing.

After surgery, an elastic adhesive tape may be applied over wounds because of its ability to compress, thereby controlling hemorrhage. The original tape is removed during the initial dressing change, and a lighter dressing is applied. The nurse secures the dressing at both ends and across the middle and uses tape of a sufficient width for the dressing and the wound.

Montgomery straps (tie tapes) are commonly used for wounds requiring frequent dressing changes. See Figure 46–5. These straps prevent skin irritation and discomfort caused by removing the adhesive each time the dressing is changed. Nonallergenic tie tapes are available for people with sensitive skin. If these are not available, the nurse can protect the skin by applying tincture of benzoin to the site where the adhesive is to be placed.

Supporting and Immobilizing Wounds

Bandages   A **bandage** is a strip of cloth used to wrap some part of the body. Bandages are available in various widths, most commonly 1.5 to 7.5 cm (0.5 to 3 in), and are usually supplied in rolls for easy application to a body part. The purposes of bandages and binders are summarized in the box on the opposite page.

Many types of materials are used for bandages. Gauze is one of the most commonly used; it is light and porous and readily molds to the body. It is also relatively inexpensive, so it is generally discarded when soiled. Gauze is frequently used to retain dressings on wounds and to bandage the fingers, hands, toes, and feet. It supports dressings and at the same time permits air to circulate; it can also be impregnated with petroleum jelly or other medications for application to wounds.

Many kinds of elasticized bandages are applied to provide pressure to an area. They are commonly used as tensor bandages or as partial stockings to provide support and improve the venous circulation in the legs. Some elasticized bandages have an adhesive backing and can be secured to the skin; these are most frequently used to retain dressings and at the same time provide some support to a wound.

Plastic adhesive bandages are also used to retain dressings. They are waterproof and thus retain wound drainage or keep an area dry. They have some elastic properties and therefore provide some pressure.

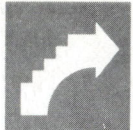

Purposes of Bandages and Binders

- Supporting a wound, e.g., a fractured bone
- Immobilizing a wound, e.g., a strained shoulder
- Applying pressure; e.g., elastic bandages apply pressure to the lower extremities to improve venous blood flow
- Securing a dressing, e.g., for an extensive abdominal surgical wound
- Retaining splints (this applies chiefly to bandages)
- Retaining warmth, e.g., a flannel bandage on a rheumatoid joint

The width of the bandage used depends on the size of the body part to be bandaged. For example, a 2.5-cm (1-in) bandage is used for a finger, a 5-cm (2-in) bandage for an arm, and a 7.5-cm or 10-cm (3-in or 4-in) bandage for a leg. The larger the circumference of the part, the wider the bandage. Padding (e.g., abdominal pads and gauze squares) are frequently used to cover bony prominences, such as the elbow, or to separate skin surfaces, such as the fingers.

Before applying a bandage, the nurse needs to know its purpose and the area requiring support. This area also should be assessed. See the upper right-hand box for assessment guidelines.

Applying bandages to various parts of the body involves one or more of five basic bandaging turns: circular, spiral, spiral reverse, recurrent, and figure-eight. *Circular* turns are used to anchor bandages and to terminate them. They are also used to bandage certain areas, such as the proximal aspect of a finger or a wrist. Circular turns usually are not applied directly over a wound because of the discomfort the bandage would cause.

Spiral turns are used to bandage parts of the body that are fairly uniform in circumference, e.g., the upper arm or upper leg. *Spiral reverse* turns are used to bandage cylindrical parts of the body that are not uniform in circumference, e.g., the lower leg or forearm. *Recurrent* turns are used to cover distal parts of the body, e.g., the end of a finger, the skull, or the stump of an amputation. *Figure-eight* turns are used to bandage an elbow, knee, or ankle, because they permit some movement after application. The *spica* bandage is a variation of the figure-eight bandage. It is commonly used to bandage the hip, groin, shoulder, breast, or thumb. A 2.5-cm (1-in) bandage is frequently used for a thumb spica, and a 7.5-cm (3-in) bandage for a hip or shoulder spica.

Some basic guidelines for bandaging are listed in the accompanying box. Procedure 46–2 illustrates how to apply basic bandages using the turns described above.

CLINICAL GUIDELINES
Assessing Before Applying Bandages or Binders

- Inspect and palpate the area for swelling.
- Inspect for the presence of and status of wounds (open wounds will require a dressing before a bandage or binder is applied).
- Note the presence of drainage (amount, color, odor, viscosity).
- Inspect and palpate for adequacy of circulation (skin temperature, color, and sensation). Pale or cyanotic skin, cool temperature, tingling, and numbness can indicate impaired circulation.
- Ask the client about any pain experienced (location, intensity, onset, quality).
- Assess the ability of the client to reapply the bandage or binder when needed.
- Assess the capabilities of the client regarding activities of daily living, e.g., to eat, dress, comb hair, bathe, and assess the assistance required during the convalescence period.

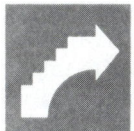

CLINICAL GUIDELINES
Bandaging

- Whenever possible, bandage the part in its normal position, with the joint slightly flexed to avoid putting strain on the ligaments and the muscles of the joint.
- Pad between skin surfaces and over bony prominences to prevent friction from the bandage and consequent abrasion of the skin.
- Always bandage body parts by working from the distal to the proximal end to aid the return flow of venous blood.
- Bandage with even pressure to prevent interference with blood circulation.
- Whenever possible, leave the end of the body part (e.g., the toe) exposed so that you will be able to determine the adequacy of the blood circulation to the extremity.
- Cover dressings with bandages at least 5 cm (2 in) beyond the edges of the dressing to prevent the dressing and wound from becoming contaminated.
- Face the client when applying a bandage to maintain uniform tension and the appropriate direction of the bandage.

BASIC BANDAGING

Equipment ☑

Clean bandage of the appropriate material and width

Padding such as ABD pads or gauze squares

Tape, special metal clips, or a safety pin

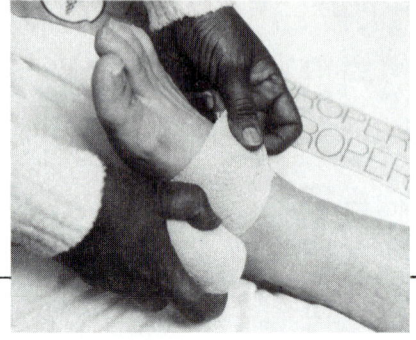

Figure 46-6 Starting a bandage with two circular turns.

Intervention

1. **Position and prepare the client appropriately.**

- Provide the client with a chair or bed, and arrange support for the area to be bandaged. For example, if a hand needs to be bandaged, ask the client to place the elbow on a table, so that the hand does not have to be held up unsupported. *Because bandaging takes a little time, holding up a body part without support can fatigue the client.*

- Make sure that the area to be bandaged is clean and dry. Wash and dry the area if necessary. *Washing and drying remove microorganisms, which flourish in dark, warm, moist areas.*

- Align the part to be bandaged with slight flexion of the joints, unless this is contraindicated. *Slight flexion places less strain on the ligaments and muscles of the joint.*

2. **Apply the bandage.**

Circular turns:

- Hold the bandage in your dominant hand, with the roll uppermost and unroll the bandage about 8 cm (3 in). *This length of unrolled bandage allows good control for placement and tension.*

- Apply the end of the bandage to the part of the body to be bandaged. Hold the end down with the thumb of the other hand. See Figure 46-6.

- Encircle the body part a few times or as often as needed, each turn directly covering the previous turn. *This provides even support to the area.*

- Secure the end of the bandage with tape, metal clips, or a safety pin over an uninjured area. *Clips and pins can be uncomfortable when situated over an injured area.*

Spiral turns:

- Make two circular turns. *Two circular turns anchor the bandage.*

- Continue spiral turns at about a 30° angle, each turn overlapping the preceding one by two-thirds the width of the bandage. See Figure 46-7.

- Terminate the bandage with two circular turns, and secure the end as described for circular turns.

Spiral reverse turns:

- Anchor the bandage with two circular turns, and bring the bandage upward at about a 30° angle.

- Place the thumb of your free hand on the upper edge of the bandage. See Figure 46-8, A. *The thumb will hold the bandage while it is folded upon itself.*

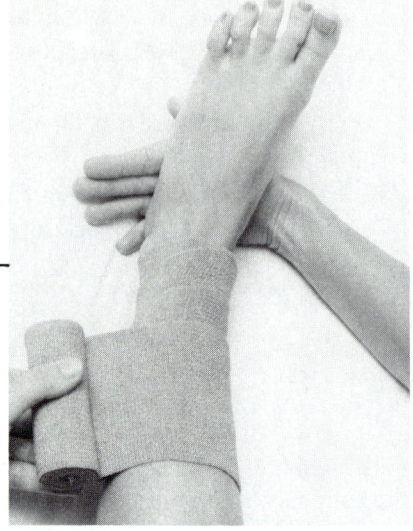

Figure 46-7 Applying spiral turns.

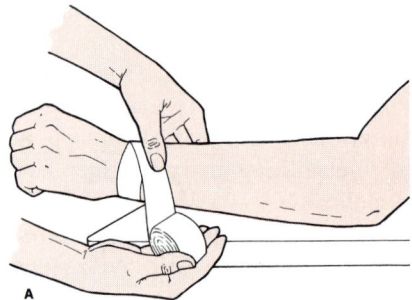

A

Circular turns / Bandage folded over to make spiral reverse turn

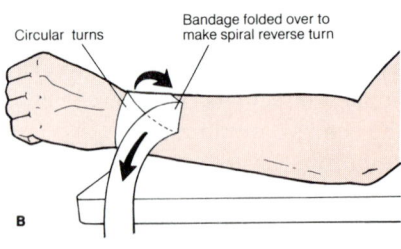

B

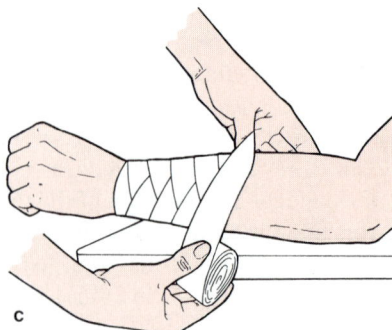

C

Figure 46-8 Applying spiral reverse turns.

- Unroll the bandage about 15 cm (6 in), then turn your hand so that the bandage falls over itself. See Figure 46–8, *B*.
- Continue the bandage around the limb, overlapping each previous turn by two-thirds the width of the bandage. Make each bandage turn at the same position on the limb so that the turns of the bandage will be aligned. See Figure 46–8, *C*.
- Terminate the bandage with two circular turns, and secure the end as described for circular turns.

Recurrent turns:

- Anchor the bandage with two circular turns.
- Fold it back on itself, and bring it centrally over the distal end to be bandaged. See Figure 46–9.

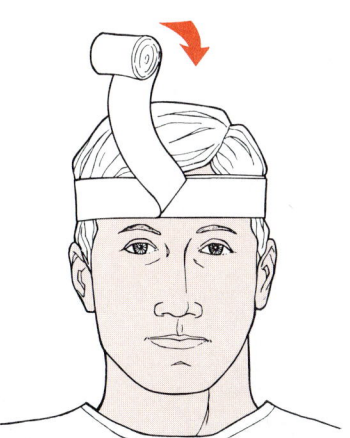

Figure 46–9 Starting a recurrent bandage with two circular turns.

- Holding it with the other hand, bring the bandage back over the end to the right of the center bandage but overlapping it by two-thirds the width of the bandage.
- Bring the bandage back on the left side, also overlapping the first turn by two-thirds the width of the bandage.

- Continue this pattern of alternating right and left until the area is covered. Overlap the preceding turn by two-thirds the bandage width each time.
- Terminate the bandage with two circular turns. See Figure 46–10. Secure the end appropriately.

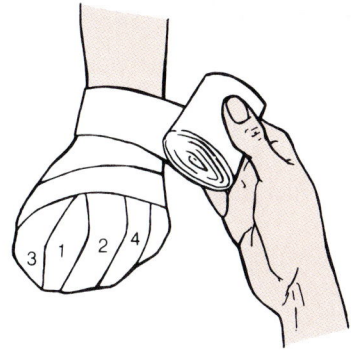

Figure 46–10 Completing a recurrent bandage with two circular turns.

Figure-eight turns:

- Anchor the bandage with two circular turns.
- Carry the bandage above the joint, around it, and then below it, making a figure eight. See Figure 46–11.

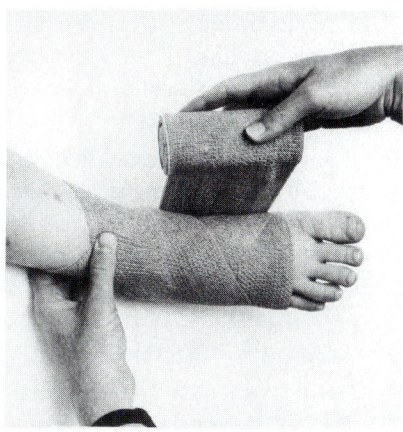

Figure 46–11 Applying a figure-eight bandage.

- Continue above and below the joint, overlapping the previous turn by two-thirds the width of the bandage.

- Terminate the bandage above the joint with two circular turns, and secure the end appropriately.

Thumb spica:

- Anchor the bandage with two circular turns around the wrist.
- Bring the bandage down to the distal aspect of the thumb, and encircle the thumb. Leave the tip of the thumb exposed if possible. *This enables the nurse to check blood circulation to the thumb.*
- Bring the bandage back up and around the wrist, then back down and around the thumb, overlapping the previous turn by two-thirds the width of the bandage.
- Repeat the above two steps, working up the thumb and hand until the thumb is covered. See Figure 46–12.
- Anchor the bandage with two circular turns around the wrist, and secure the end appropriately.

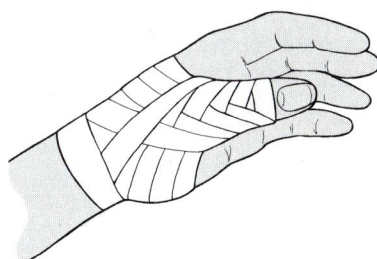

Figure 46–12 A thumb spica bandage.

3. Document relevant information

- Document the type of bandage applied, the area to which it is applied, and nursing assessments, including skin problems or neurovascular problems.

Sample Recording

Date: 4/7/91	Time: 0700

Elastic spiral bandage applied to right leg. Toes warm and pink. No numbness.———
——————— Laura R. Stenhouse, NS

Binders   A **binder** bandage is designed for a specific body part; for example, the triangular binder (sling) fits the arm. Binders are used to support large areas of the body, such as the abdomen, arm, or chest. Most binders are made of muslin (plain-woven cotton fabric), flannel, or synthetic material that may or may not be elasticized. Some abdominal binders are made of an elasticized netlike material that fits the body contours and allows air to circulate around the body part.

There are four commonly used types of binders:

1. *Triangular arm binder (sling):* Usually applied as a full triangle to support the arm, elbow, and forearm of the client or to reduce or prevent swelling of a hand.

2. *Breast binder:* To provide pressure on the breasts (e.g., when drying up the milk flow after childbirth) or to support the breasts (e.g., after surgery). Breast binders are pinned in the front and usually have shoulder straps to prevent the binder from slipping down.

3. *T-binder (single or double T):* To retain pads, dressings, or packs in the perineal area. Single T-binders are often used for females, and double T-binders for males to prevent undue pressure on the penis. The double T-binder can also provide greater support for large dressings on both males and females.

4. *Straight abdominal binder:* To provide support to the abdomen. This binder is a rectangular piece of material long enough to encircle the client's abdomen with some overlap. It can be made from any material, e.g., a towel.

Abdominal pads are used to protect bony prominences (e.g., the iliac crests for an abdominal binder) or to prevent skin surfaces from rubbing together and becoming exoriated (e.g., the skin beneath the breasts for a breast binder).

Procedure 46–3 describes how to apply the various binders.

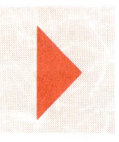

PROCEDURE 46–3

APPLYING BINDERS

Equipment ☑

Appropriate binder

Abdominal (ABD) pads as required for padding

Safety pins or tape

Intervention

1. **Prepare the client.**

■ If the binder is being placed directly against the skin and the area is soiled, wash and dry the area.

■ Assist the client to a comfortable lying or sitting position, supporting the area as appropriate.

2. **Apply the binder.**

Triangular arm sling:

■ Ask the client to flex the elbow to an 80° angle or less, depending on the purpose. The thumb should be facing upward or inward toward the body. *An 80° angle is sufficient to support the forearm, to prevent swelling of the hand, and to relieve pressure on the shoulder joint (e.g., to support the paralyzed arm of a stroke client whose shoulder might otherwise become dislocated). A more acute angle is preferred if there is swelling of the hand (see how to apply a sling for maximum hand elevation, below).*

■ Place one end of the unfolded triangular binder over the shoulder of the uninjured side so that the binder falls down the front of the chest of the client with the point of the triangle (apex) under the elbow of the injured side.

■ Take the upper corner, and carry it around the neck until it hangs over the shoulder on the injured side.

■ Bring the lower corner of the binder up over the arm to the shoulder of the injured side. Using a square knot, secure this corner to the upper corner at the side of the neck on the involved side. See Figure 46–13. *A square knot will not slip. Tying the knot at the side of the neck prevents pressure on the bony prominences of the vertebral column at the back of the neck.*

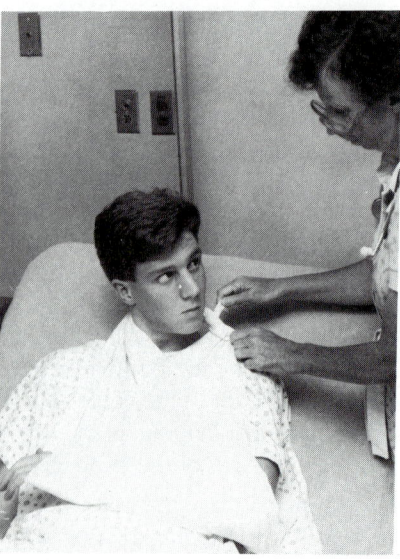

Figure 46–13   A large arm sling.

- Make sure the wrist is supported, to maintain alignment.

- Fold the sling neatly at the elbow, and secure it with safety pins or tape. It may be folded and fastened at the front.

- Remove the sling periodically to inspect the skin for indications of irritation, especially around the site of the knot.

Small arm sling (cravat binder):

- Make a cravat binder by folding the triangular binder in on itself, starting at the apex. See Figure 46–14, *A.*

- Apply the sling as in Figure 46–14, *B,* with the knot on the affected side.

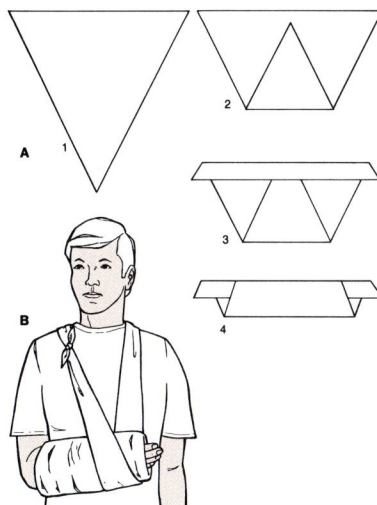

Figure 46–14 *A,* Making a cravat: (1) lay the triangular bandage on a flat surface; (2) fold the point up toward the base of the bandage; (3) fold the base over on itself to make a smooth edge; (4) fold the cravat from the other side to the desired width. *B,* The cravat applied as a small arm sling.

Triangular arm sling for maximum hand elevation:

- Flex the client's arm so that the hand rests on the clavicle of the unin-

jured side. *This position provides maximum elevation of the hand.*

- Place the binder over the shoulder of the uninjured side and *over the arm* (i.e., in front of the arm) so that the apex of the binder extends beyond the elbow of the injured side. See Figure 46–15, *A.*

- Tuck the base of the binder under the arm, bring the free end across the client's back, and—using a square knot—tie it to the other free end at the shoulder on the *uninjured* side. The knot should rest in the hollow of the clavicle to prevent pressure on the clavicle. See Figure 46–15, *B.*

- Bring the apex of the sling toward the back, tuck it in, and secure it with a safety pin or pins. See Figure 46–15, *C.*

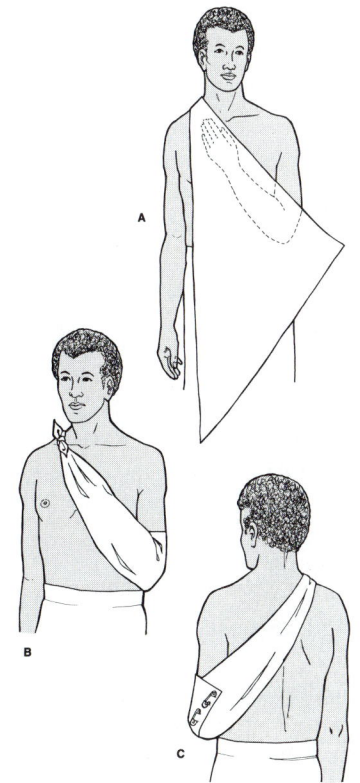

Figure 46–15 A triangular arm sling applied to provide hand elevation.

Hand or foot mitt:

- Apply the triangular bandage as a mitt to cover hand or foot dressings. See Figure 46–16.

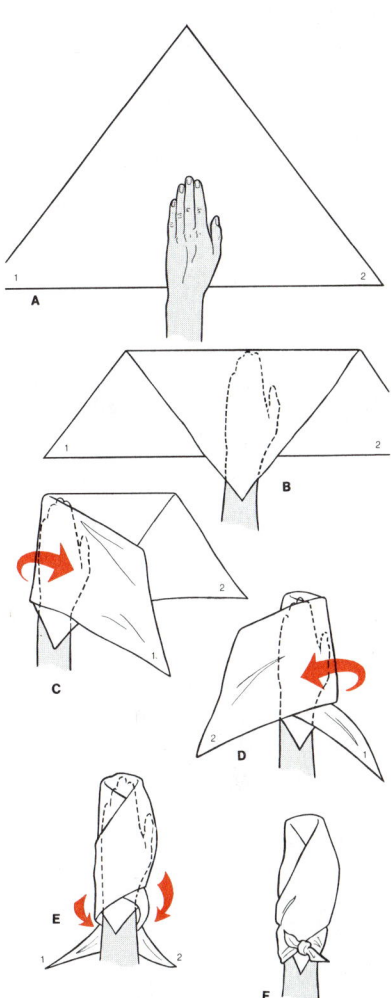

Figure 46–16 Wrapping a hand with a triangular bandage: *A,* lay the hand in the center of the triangular bandage; *B,* fold the apex over the wrist; *C, D,* wrap the corners (1 and 2) around the hand; *E,* bring the corners around the wrist; *F,* tie a square knot on the dorsum of the wrist.

Breast binder:

- Spread the binder on the bed, and ask the client to lie in a supine position on top of it. Center the binder, place the lower edge at the waistline, and allow adequate armhole space. *Adequate armhole space is needed to prevent the material from chafing the axillae.*

■ If the breasts are large, place padding under each breast. *This prevents skin excoriation caused by pressing the two skin surfaces tightly together.*

■ Pull the binder tightly across the breast tissue at the nipple line, and fasten it at the midline with a safety pin placed vertically. Ask the client to help by pressing the palms of her hands against the sides of the breasts.

■ While continuing to compress the breasts, pin the binder alternately above and below the first fastening. Place the pins vertically except for the lowest one, which is placed horizontally. See Figure 46–17.

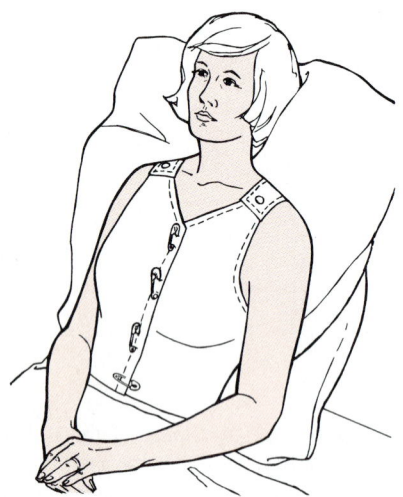

Figure 46–17 A breast binder.

Fastening the pins alternately above and below distributes pressure equally, thereby providing maximum support. Placing the lowest pin horizontally allows for more comfort when moving.

■ Fasten the shoulder straps, if required, with pins.

T-Binder:

■ Select the appropriate binder for the client, and place it smoothly under the person with the waistband at waist level and the tails running down the midline at the back. Double T-binders may be used for females if a dressing is large (e.g., after extensive surgery).

■ Bring the waist tails around the client, overlap them, and secure them with a pin placed horizontally. *The pins placed horizontally allow comfort when bending at the waist and moving.*

■ Bring the center tail up between the legs. See Figure 46–18, *A.* The two tails of the double T-binder are brought up on either side of the penis. See Figure 46–18, *B.* When dressings are in place, take care to touch only the outside of the dressings to prevent contamination of the wound or yourself.

■ Fasten the ties at the waist with a safety pin placed horizontally.

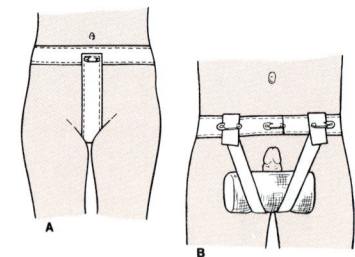

Figure 46–18 T-binders: *A,* single tail; *B,* two tails.

Straight abdominal binder:

■ With the client in a supine position, place the binder smoothly under the body, with the upper border of the binder at the waist and the lower border at the level of the gluteal fold. *A binder placed over the waist interferes with res-*

piration; one placed too low interferes with elimination and walking.

■ Apply padding over the iliac crests if the client is thin.

■ Bring the ends around the client, overlap them, and secure them with pins. See Figure 46–19. Place the top pin horizontally at the waist to allow for comfort when moving.

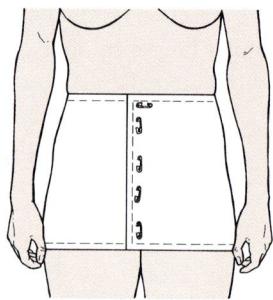

Figure 46–19 A straight abdominal binder.

3. Ensure client comfort.

■ Ensure that there are no wrinkles or creases against the body. *Wrinkles and creases cause pressure on the skin and subsequent excoriation.*

4. Document relevant information.

■ Determine the agency's policies about recording application of a binder. Binders are generally not recorded when applied to hold a dressing in place. However, an arm sling, breast binder, or abdominal binder may be recorded, together with the assessment data.

Sample Recording

Date: 8/17/91	Time: 1000

Breast binder applied. Breasts are enlarged, hard, engorged, and painful.——
——————— Page O. Mills, NS

Promoting Healing and Preventing Complications

Adequate nutrition is essential for wound healing. Proteins, vitamins, and trace metals play a major role in the healing process. Preventing stress on a wound, e.g., vomiting, abdominal distention, or strenuous coughing, is also important during the healing process. Vomiting is often prevented by withholding food and oral fluids until there is no nausea. Clients unable to eat a diet that provides sufficient calories and nutrients for wound healing may require a central line for total parenteral nutrition or an enteral feeding tube.

Abdominal distention often can be prevented by frequent position changes and early ambulation. Ambulation improves respiration and blood circulation, aiding the delivery of nutrients and oxygen to the wound area. Electrolyte imbalance also can contribute to abdominal distention and delayed wound healing (Cooper and Schumann 1979, p. 716). Specifically, imbalances due to hydrogen ion loss through gastric suctioning and excessive loss of potassium through the kidneys contribute to smooth muscle inactivity and abdominal distention. A distended urinary bladder can impair wound healing by displacing affected tissue and stretching an incision. Therefore, careful monitoring of fluid intake and output is important, as is prompt initiation of measures to promote urinary elimination when appropriate.

Preventing Infection

The Centers for Disease Control recommend the following wound care practices for preventing wound infection (Garner 1986, pp. 78–79).

1. Wash hands before and after caring for surgical wounds.
2. Touch an open or fresh surgical wound only when wearing sterile gloves or using sterile forceps. After the wound is sealed, sterile gloves are no longer required.
3. Remove or change dressings over open and closed wounds when they become wet.
4. Take a specimen of any drainage from the wound that is suspected of being infected. Send the specimen to the laboratory for culture and Gram stain.

To prevent transmission of human immunodeficiency virus (HIV), the causative agent of acquired immunodeficiency syndrome (AIDS), the CDC (1987) makes the following recommendations specific to wound care:

- Wear gloves when touching blood and body fluids, mucous membranes, or nonintact skin of all clients, and when handling items or surfaces soiled with blood or body fluids.
- Wash hands thoroughly after removing gloves, and if contaminated with blood or body fluids.
- Take precautions to prevent injuries by needles, sharp instruments, or sharp devices.
- Avoid direct client care if you have open or weeping lesions or dermatitis.
- Wear gloves, surgical masks, and protective eyewear as appropriate if procedures commonly cause droplets or splashing of blood or body fluids.

Changing Dressings

Dry Dressings   Sterile dry dressings are used for wounds that have minimal drainage and no tissue loss and heal by *primary intention* (e.g., surgical incisions). Most dressings have three layers:

1. A nonadhering contact dressing that covers the incision and part of the surrounding skin and that collects fibrin, blood products, and debris from the wound
2. An absorbent gauze dressing that acts as a reservoir for excess secretions
3. A thicker outer dressing that protects the wound from external contamination

A number of materials are used for dressings. See Table 46–2. Not all surgical dressings require changing. Sometimes surgeons apply a dressing in the operating room that remains in place until the sutures are removed, and no further dressings are required. In most situations, however, surgical dressings are changed regularly to prevent the growth of microorganisms.

In some instances, a client may have a Penrose drain inserted. The main surgical incision is considered cleaner than the surgical stab wound made for the drain insertion, because there usually is considerable drainage. The main incision is therefore cleaned first, and under no circumstances are materials used to clean the stab wound used subsequently to clean the main incision. In this way, the main incision is kept free of the microorganisms around the stab wound. Changing a dry sterile dressing is detailed in Procedure 46–4.

Wet-to-Dry Dressings   Sterile wet-to-dry dressings may be prescribed for debridement of wounds with extensive tissue loss that heal by *secondary intention*. Examples of such wounds are burns, varicose ulcers, or decubitus ulcers. These wounds are not amenable to suturing.

Wet-to-dry dressings consist of a moistened contact dressing layer that touches the wound surface. This layer is allowed to dry between dressing changes every 4 to 6 hours. The wet gauze traps necrotic material in its spaces as it dries. Dry dressings do not trap the debris as effectively. Wet dressings that do not dry out enough to trap debris promote bacterial growth in the damp environment and can cause tissue breakdown. Generally, 4 × 4 non-cotton-filled gauze dressings are used. Cotton fibers are contraindicated because they pull loose and remain in the wound, encouraging bacterial growth and contamination. See Table 46–2 for types of dressings.

TABLE 46-2 Types of Dressings

Dressing	Description	Purpose
Dry-to-dry	A layer of wide-mesh cotton gauze lies next to the wound surface. A second layer of dry absorbent cotton or Dacron is on top.	Necrotic debris and exudate are trapped in the interstices of the contact (gauze) layer. These are removed when the dressing is removed.
Wet-to-dry	Next to the wound surface is a layer of wide-mesh cotton gauze saturated with saline or an antimicrobial solution. This layer is covered by a moist absorbent material, i.e., moistened with the same solution.	Necrotic debris is softened by the solution and then adheres to the mesh gauze as it dries. It is removed when the dressing is removed. Also, moisture helps dilute viscous exudate.
Wet-to-damp	A variation of the wet-to-dry dressing, this dressing is removed before it has completely dried.	The wound is debrided when the gauze is removed.
Wet-to-wet	A layer of wide-mesh gauze saturated with antibacterial or physiologic solution lies next to the wound surface. Above is a second layer of absorbent material saturated with the same solution. The entire dressing is kept moist with wetting agent.	The wound surface is continually bathed. Moisture dilutes viscous exudate.
Synthetic dressings (e.g., Op-Site, Tegaderm)	One layer is placed on the wound, or the dressing is placed and changed according to manufacturer's instructions.	Necrotic material is liquefied.
Topical enzymes (e.g., Elase ointment)	The preparation is applied according to the manufacturer's instructions.	The preparation hastens separation of necrotic tissue.
Hydrophilic beads, gels, powders	The dressing is applied according to the manufacturer's instruction and washed off, e.g., with saline, when it becomes saturated.	Exudate is absorbed, and the wound is cleansed.

Source: Adapted from J. Z. Cuzzell, Wound care forum: Artful solutions to chronic problems, *American Journal of Nursing,* February 1985, 85:162–66.

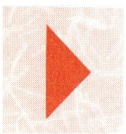

PROCEDURE 46-4

CHANGING A DRY STERILE DRESSING

Equipment ☑

Sterile dressing set; if none is available, gather the following sterile items from a central supply cart

Drape or towel

Cotton balls or gauze squares

Container for the cleaning solution

Antimicrobial solution

Two pairs of forceps (thumb or artery)

Gauze dressings and surgipads

Applicators or tongue blades to apply ointments

Additional supplies required for the particular dressing, e.g., extra gauze dressings and ointment or powder, if ordered

Disposable gloves

Sterile gloves (optional)

Mask (optional)

Moistureproof bag

Tape or tie tapes

Bath blanket (if necessary)

Acetone or another solution (if necessary to loosen adhesive)

Intervention

1. Prepare the client and assemble the equipment.

■ Acquire assistance for changing a dressing on a restless or confused adult. *The person might move and contaminate the sterile field or the wound.*

■ Assist the client to a comfortable position in which the wound can be readily exposed. Expose only the wound area, using a bath blanket to cover the client, if necessary. *Undue exposure is physically and psychologically distressing to most people.*

■ Make a cuff on the moistureproof bag for disposal of the soiled dressings, and place the bag within reach. It can be taped to the bedclothes or bedside table. *Making a cuff keeps the outside of the bag free from contamination by the soiled dressings and prevents subsequent contamination of the nurse's hands or of sterile instrument tips when discarding dressings or sponges. Placement of the bag within reach prevents the nurse from reaching across the sterile field and the wound and potentially contaminating these areas.*

■ Don a face mask if required. *Some agencies require that a mask be worn for surgical dressing changes to prevent contamination of the wound by droplet spray from the nurse's respiratory tract.*

2. Remove outer dressings.

■ Remove binders, if used, and place them aside. Untie tie tapes, if used.

■ If adhesive tape was used, remove it by holding down the skin and pulling the tape gently but firmly toward the wound. *Pressing down on the skin provides countertraction against the pulling motion. Tape is pulled toward the incision to prevent strain on the sutures or wound.*

■ Use a solvent to loosen tape, if required. *Moistening the tape with acetone or a similar solvent lessens the discomfort of removal, particularly from hairy surfaces.*

■ Don gloves, and remove the outer abdominal dressing or surgipad by hand if the dressing is dry, or using a disposable glove if the dressing is moist. *The outer surgipad is considered contaminated by the client's clothing and linen.*

■ Lift the dressing so that the underside is away from the client's face. *The appearance and odor of the drainage may be upsetting to the client.*

3. Dispose of soiled dressings appropriately.

■ Place the soiled dressing in the waterproof bag without touching the outside of the bag. *Contamination of the outside of the bag is avoided to prevent the spread of microorganisms to the nurse and subsequently to others.*

■ Remove glove(s), dispose of them in the waterproof bag, and wash your hands.

4. Remove inner dressings.

■ Open the sterile dressing set, using surgical aseptic technique.

■ Place the sterile drape beside the wound, and don sterile gloves (optional).

■ Remove the under dressings with tissue forceps or sterile gloves, taking care not to dislodge any drains. If the gauze sticks to the drain, use two pairs of forceps, one to remove the gauze and one to hold the drain, or secure the drain with one hand. *Forceps or gloves are used to prevent contamination of the wound by the nurse's hands and contamination of the nurse's hands by wound drainage.*

■ Assess the location, type (color, consistency), and odor of wound drainage, and the number of gauzes saturated or the diameter of drainage collected on the dressings.

■ Discard the soiled dressings in the bag. To avoid contaminating the forceps tips on the edge of the paper bag, hold the dressings 10 to 15 cm (4 to 6 in) above the bag, and drop the dressings into it.

■ After the dressings are removed, discard the forceps, or set them aside from the sterile field. *These forceps are now contaminated by the wound drainage.*

5. Clean the wound.

■ Clean the wound, using the second pair of artery or tissue forceps and gauze swabs moistened with antiseptic solution.

■ Keep the forceps tips lower than the handles at all times. *This prevents their contamination by fluid traveling up to the handle and back to the tips. The handle is contaminated by the nurse's bare hand.*

■ Clean with strokes from the top to the bottom, starting at the center and continuing to the outside. See Figure 46-20.

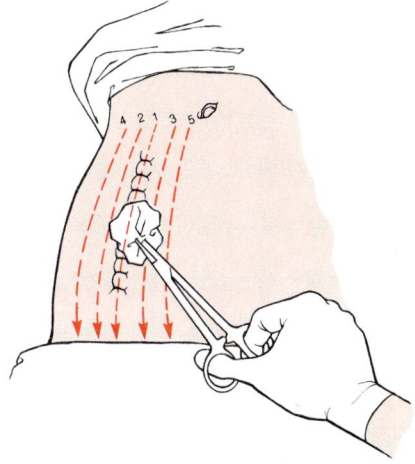

Figure 46-20 Cleaning a wound from top to bottom, starting at the center.

or

■ Clean with strokes outward from the incision on one side and then outward on the other side. See Figure 46-21. *The wound is cleaned from the least to the most contaminated area, e.g., from the top of the incision, which is drier, to the bottom of the incision, where any drainage will collect and which is considered more contaminated, or from the incision outward.*

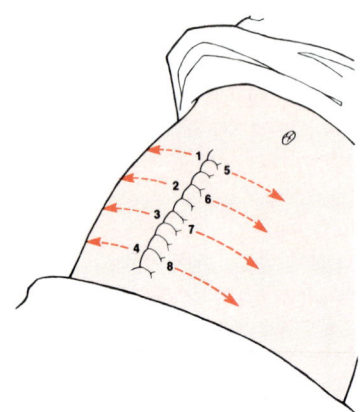

Figure 46–21 Cleaning a wound outward from the incision.

■ Use a separate swab for each stroke, and discard each swab after use. *This prevents the introduction of microorganisms to other wound areas.*

■ If a drain is present, clean it after the incision.

■ For irregular wounds, such as a decubitus ulcer, clean from the center of the wound outward, using circular strokes.

■ Repeat the cleaning process until all drainage is removed.

■ Dry the wound with dry gauze swabs as required, using the strokes described above.

6. **Assess the overall appearance of the wound.**

■ See the guidelines on page 1315.

7. **Apply ordered powder or ointment.**

■ Shake powders directly onto the wound. Antibiotic powders may be ordered by the physician.

■ Use sterile applicators or tongue blades to apply ointments. *Ointments can protect the skin from irritation if drainage is profuse.*

8. **Apply sterile dressings.**

■ Apply sterile dressings one at a time over the wound, using sterile forceps or sterile gloves. Start at the center of the wound and move progressively outward. The final surgipad can be picked up by hand, touching only the outside, which is often marked by a blue line down the center.

■ Remove and discard gloves, if worn.

■ Secure the dressing with tape, tie tapes, or a binder.

9. **Document the dressing change and all nursing assessments.**

Sample Recording

Date: 12/5/91	Time: 1500

Abdominal dressing changed. Incision cleaned with Alcohol 70%. Two 4 × 4 gauzes saturated with serous drainage at base of incision. Wound clean, edges closely approximated. No redness on incision line or surrounding tissue. 4 × 4 gauze and surgipads secured with tie tapes. No discomfort voiced.———————
————————————Evangeline R. Puritos, RN

The type of solution used for a wet dressing depends on the condition of the wound and the purpose of the dressings. Normal saline is often used to moisten necrotic tissue to help loosen and remove it. Betadine (10% solution) is often used for draining wounds infected with *Staphylococcus* or aerobic bacteria; it can cause burning and stinging, and some clients may be allergic to it. Acetic acid (0.25% solution) is often used for wounds infected with *Pseudomonas* or gram-positive and gram-negative organisms; it can be irritating to the skin surrounding the wound. Hydrogen peroxide (3% solution), not used as frequently today as in the past, is a debriding agent that facilitates removal of necrotic tissue. Sodium hypochlorite (Dakin's solution) is an antiseptic that dissolves necrotic tissue and retards *Pseudomonas* growth. Dakin's solution can cause skin breakdown, so it is used only on necrotic tissue. See Procedure 46–5 for applying wet-to-dry dressings.

Moist Transparent Wound Barriers Transparent wound barriers such as Op-Site, Tegaderm, and Bio-occlusive are often applied to ulcerated or burned skin areas. Advantages of these dressings include the following:

■ They are nonporous, self-adhesive dressings that do not require changing as other dressings do. They are often left in place until healing has occurred or as long as they remain intact.

■ Because they are transparent, the wound can be assessed through them.

■ Because they are occlusive, the wound remains moist and retains the serous exudate, which hastens healing and reduces the risk of infection.

■ Because they are elastic, they can be placed over a joint without disrupting the client's mobility.

■ They adhere only to the skin area around the wound and not to the wound itself, because the wound is kept moist.

■ They allow the client to shower or bathe without removing the dressing.

See Procedure 46–6 on page 1326 for applying a moist transparent wound barrier.

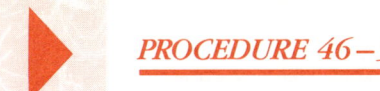

PROCEDURE 46–5

APPLYING WET-TO-DRY DRESSINGS

Equipment

Sterile dressing equipment (see Procedure 46–4)

Sterile thin, fine-mesh gauze

Sterile round or kidney-shaped container for the solution

Ordered solution

Clean disposable gloves

Sterile gloves

Mask (optional)

Moistureproof bag

Tape or tie tapes

Intervention

1. Ensure that the client's medication has been given before the procedure is begun.

- Check the physician's orders and the nursing progress notes. Clients are usually medicated before this procedure.

2. Assemble all equipment, prepare the client, and remove the outer dressings.

- See steps 1 to 3 in Procedure 46–4, pages 1322–1323.

3. Gradually free the wet-to-dry dressing as quickly as possible.

- Do not moisten the dressing. *Wet-to-dry dressings are intended to clean wounds by debridement of the exudate or necrotic tissue.*

- Dispose of soiled dressings appropriately in the moistureproof bag.

- Remove the disposable gloves, and discard them in the bag.

- Wash your hands.

4. Assess the wound.

- Assess the character and amount of drainage on the dressings and the appearance of the wound, i.e., the progress of healing by secondary intention.

- Observe the development and amount of granulation tissue.

5. Apply the wet-to-dry dressing.

- Open the packages of the sterile dressing set, fine-mesh gauze, and sterile solution container.

- Pour the ordered solution into the solution container.

- Don the sterile gloves.

- Place the fine-mesh gauze dressings into the solution container, and thoroughly saturate them with solution. *The entire gauze must be moistened to enhance its absorptive abilities.*

- If agency policy indicates, clean the wound gently, using a circular motion. Work outward from the center of the wound to its edge and beyond. Use a separate gauze swab for each cleaning stroke.

- Wring out excess moisture from the saturated fine mesh gauze dressings. *Dressings that are too wet will not dry out in 4 to 6 hours.*

- Pack the moistened dressings into all depressions and grooves of the wound, ensuring that all exposed surfaces are covered. If necessary, use forceps to feed the gauze gradually into deep depressed areas. *Necrotic tissue is usually more prevalent in depressed wound areas and needs to be covered with the wet-to-dry gauze.*

6. Cover the wet-to-dry dressing with dry dressings.

- Apply a dry 4 × 4 gauze over the wet dressings. *The dry gauze absorbs excess drainage.*

- Cover the dressings with a surgipad or abdominal pad. *The pad protects the wound from external contaminants.*

- Remove your gloves, and discard them.

- Secure the dressing at the edges only, with tape, tie tapes, bandage, or binder. Do *not* apply an airtight occlusive covering. *Occlusive dressings prevent air circulation and hinder drying of the fine-mesh gauze.*

7. Document the dressing change and nursing assessments.

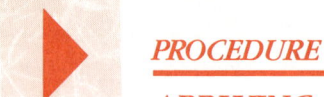

PROCEDURE 46–6

APPLYING A MOIST TRANSPARENT WOUND BARRIER

Equipment

Soap and water

Razor (optional) or clippers

Alcohol or acetone

Wound barrier

Sterile gauze and the wound-cleaning agents specified by the physician or agency (e.g., sterile saline, hydrogen peroxide, or Betadine)

Sterile gloves

Scissors

Paper tape

Sterile #26 gauze needle and syringe

Intervention

1. Obtain assistance as needed.

■ If the size of the wound necessitates it, acquire the assistance of a coworker to help apply the dressing.

2. Thoroughly clean the skin area around the wound.

■ Clean the skin with soap and water.

■ Clip the hair about 5 cm (2 in) around the wound area if indicated.

■ Rub the area with alcohol or acetone, and allow it to dry. *Alcohol or acetone defats the skin. Defatted and clean, dry skin ensures better adhesion of the dressing.*

3. Clean the wound if indicated.

 ■ Don sterile gloves.

■ Clean the wound with the prescribed solution.

4. Assess the wound.

■ See the guidelines on page 1315.

5. Apply the wound barrier.

■ Remove part of the paper backing on the dressing. If you have an assistant, remove all of the paper backing; the two of you should hold the colored tabs attached to the dressing.

■ Apply the dressing at one edge of the wound site, allowing at least 2.5-cm (1-in) coverage of the skin surrounding the wound.

■ Gently lay or press the barrier over the wound. Keep it free of wrinkles, but avoid stretching it too tightly. *A stretched dressing restricts mobility.*

■ Cut off the colored tabs after the wound is completely covered.

■ Remove and discard gloves.

6. Reinforce the dressing as needed.

■ Apply paper or other porous tape to the edges of the dressing.

7. Assess the wound at least daily.

■ Determine the extent of serous fluid accumulation under the dressing, wound healing, and the need to repair the dressing.

■ If excessive serum has accumulated, use a #26 gauge needle to aspirate the fluid. Then patch the needle hole.

■ If the dressing is leaking, remove it, and apply another dressing.

8. Document the procedure and all nursing assessments.

Monitoring Wound Drains and Suction

Surgical drains are inserted to permit the drainage of excessive serosanguineous fluid and purulent material and to promote healing of underlying tissues. These drains may be inserted and sutured through the incision line, but they are most commonly inserted through stab wounds a few centimeters away from the incision line so that the incision itself may be kept dry. Without a drain, some wounds would heal on the surface and trap the discharge inside. Then the tissues under the skin could not heal because of the discharge, and an abscess might form. These drains, e.g., the Penrose drain, have an open end that drains onto a dressing.

Drains vary in length and width. The length can be 25 to 35 cm (10 to 14 in), and the width 2.5 to 4 cm (0.5 to 1.5 in). To facilitate drainage and healing of tissues from the inside to the outside, or from the bottom to the top, the physician may order that the drain be pulled out or shortened 2 to 5 cm (1 to 2 in) each day. When a drain is completely removed, the remaining stab wound usually heals within a day or two. In some agencies, this shortening procedure is performed only by physicians; in others, it is ordered by the physician and performed by nurses. When changing a dressing or a draining wound, the nurse should be careful not to dislodge the drain. Shortening the drain is usually done when the dressing is changed. See Procedure 46–7.

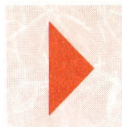

PROCEDURE 46–7

CLEANING A DRAIN SITE AND SHORTENING A PENROSE DRAIN

Equipment ☑

Sterile dressing equipment, including gauzes, container for the cleaning solution, towel or drape, surgipads and/or gauze dressings, antiseptic solution, and two pairs of forceps, including at least one hemostat

Sterile cotton-tipped applicators

Sterile dressing materials sufficient to cover the surgical incision and the drain site (at least two 4 × 4 gauzes are usually needed to dress the drain site, more if drainage is copious; a sterile precut gauze is needed to apply first around the drain site)

Sterile suture scissors (if the drain has *not* been shortened previously)

Sterile scissors

Sterile safety pin (add this to the sterile dressing set)

Disposable gloves (optional)

Sterile gloves

Moistureproof bag

Tape, tie tapes, or other binding supplies

Mask for the nurse and one for the client, if necessary

Intervention

1. Verify the physician's order.

■ Confirm that the drain is to be shortened by the nurse and the length it is to be shortened, e.g., 2.5 cm (1 in).

2. Prepare the client.

■ Inform the client that the drain is to be shortened and that this procedure should not be painful.

■ Explain that there may be a pulling sensation for a few seconds when the drain is being drawn out before it is shortened.

■ Position the client as for a dressing change.

3. Remove dressings, and clean the incision.

■ See Procedure 46–4, steps 2 to 5, page 1323. *The incision is cleaned first, since it is considered cleaner than the drain site. Moist drainage facilitates the growth of resident skin bacteria around the drain.*

4. Clean and assess the drain site.

■ Clean the skin around the drain site by swabbing in half or full circles from around the drain site outward, using separate swabs for each wipe. See Figure 46–22. You may

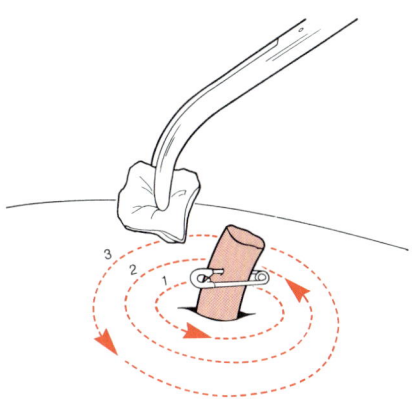

Figure 46–22 Cleaning the skin around a drain site.

hold forceps in the nondominant hand to hold the drain erect while cleaning around it. Clean as many times as necessary to remove the drainage.

■ Assess the amount and character of drainage, including odor, thickness, and color.

5. Shorten the drain.

■ If the drain has *not* been shortened before, cut and remove the suture. See Procedure 46–10. *The drain is sutured to the skin during surgery to keep it from slipping into the body cavity.*

■ With a hemostat, firmly grasp the drain by its full width at the level

of the skin, and pull the drain out the required length. *Grasping the full width of the drain ensures even traction.*

■ Wearing sterile gloves, insert the sterile safety pin through the base of the drain as close to the skin as possible by holding the drain tightly against the skin edge and inserting the pin above your fingers. See Figure 46–23. *The pin keeps the drain from falling back into the incision. Holding the drain securely in place at the skin level and inserting the pin above the fingers prevents the nurse from pulling the drain further out or pricking the client during this step.*

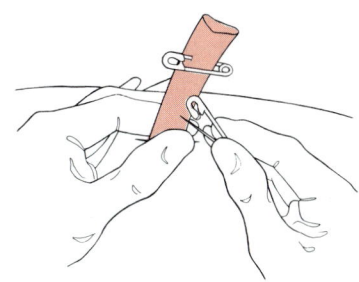

Figure 46–23 Pinning a drain.

■ Cut off the excess drain so that about 2.5 cm (1 in) remains above the skin. See Figure 46–24. Discard the excess in the waste bag.

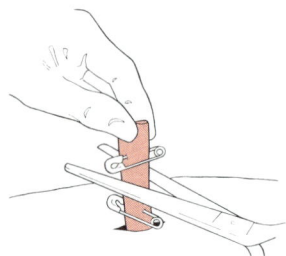

Figure 46−24   Shortening a drain.

the skin. *Using precut gauze or folding it as described, instead of cutting the gauze, prevents any threads from coming loose and getting into the wound, where they could cause inflammation and provide a site for infection.*

■ Apply the sterile dressings one at a time, using sterile gloved hands or sterile forceps. Take care that the dressings do not slide off and

become contaminated. Place the bulk of the dressings over the drain area and below the drain, depending on the client's usual position. *Layers of dressings are placed for best absorption of drainage, which flows by gravity.*

■ Apply the final surgipad by hand; remove gloves, and dispose of them; and secure the dressing with tape or ties.

6. **Apply dressings to the drain site and the incision.**

■ Place a precut 4 × 4 gauze snugly around the drain (see Figure 46−25), or open a 4 × 4 gauze to 4 × 8, fold it lengthwise to 2 × 8, and place the 2 × 8 around the drain so that the ends overlap. *This dressing absorbs the drainage and helps prevent it from excoriating*

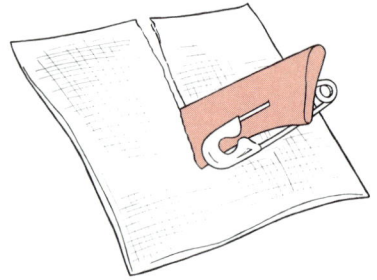

Figure 46−25   Precut gauze in place around a drain.

7. **Document the procedure and nursing assessments.**

Sample Recording

Date: 12/5/91	Time: 1025

Penrose drain shortened 2.5 cm. Three 4 × 4 gauzes saturated with brownish yellow drainage. Dry dressings × 4 applied. Skin intact; no redness or irritation.————
———————— Maria L. Antonio, RN

A *closed wound drainage system* consists of a drain connected to either an electric suction or a portable drainage suction, such as a Hemovac (see Figure 46−26) or Jackson-Pratt. The closed system eliminates the possible entry of microorganisms into the wound through the drain. The drainage tubes are sutured (stitched) in place and connected to a reservoir. For example, the Jackson-Pratt drainage tube is connected to a reservoir that maintains constant low suction. These portable wound suctions also provide for accurate measurement of the drainage.

The surgeon inserts the wound drainage tube during surgery. Generally, the suction is discontinued from 3 to 7 days postoperatively or when the wound is free from drainage. Nurses are responsible for maintaining the patency of the tube used for wound suction, which hastens the healing process by draining excess exudate that might otherwise interfere with the formation of granulation tissue. See Procedure 46−8 for establishing and maintaining a plastic bellows wound suction.

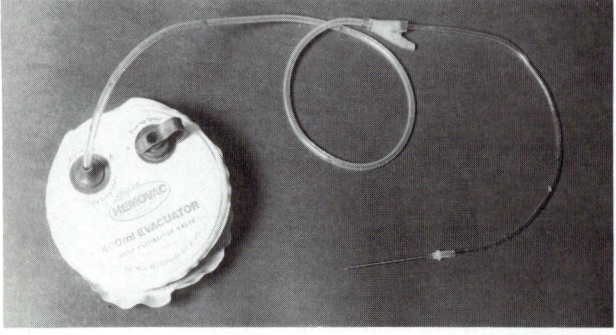

Figure 46−26   Closed wound drainage system (Hemovac).

Irrigating Wounds

An **irrigation (lavage)** is the washing or flushing out of an area. Sterile technique is required for a wound irrigation, because there is a break in the skin integrity. Wounds are usually irrigated to (a) clean the area, (b) apply heat and hasten the healing process, or (c) apply a medication, such as an antimicrobial solution.

Using piston syringes to irrigate a wound reduces the risk of aspirating drainage. For deep wounds with small openings, a sterile straight catheter may also be necessary. Frequently used irrigation solutions are sterile normal saline, Dakin's solution, hydrogen peroxide, and antibiotic solutions. See Procedure 46−9.

PROCEDURE 46–8

ESTABLISHING AND MAINTAINING A CLOSED WOUND DRAINAGE SYSTEM

Equipment ☑

Disposable gloves

Drainage receptacle, e.g., solution basin

Calibrated pitcher

Intervention

1. Establish suction if it was not already initiated.

■ Place the evacuator bag on a solid, flat surface.

■ Open the drainage plug on top of the bag, without contaminating it.

■ Compress the bag; while it is compressed, close the drainage plug to

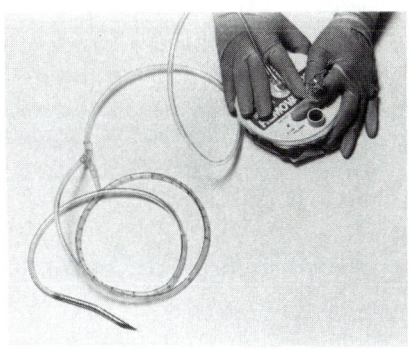

Figure 46–27 Compressing the Hemovac.

retain the vacuum. See Figure 46–27.

2. Empty the evacuator bag.

■ When the drainage fluid reaches

the line marked "Full," don disposable gloves, and open the drainage plug.

■ Invert the bag, and empty it into the collecting receptacle.

■ Reestablish suction as in step 1.

■ Measure the amount of drainage, and note its characteristics.

3. Document relevant information.

■ Record the emptying of the evacuator bag and nursing assessments on the nursing progress notes.

■ Record the amount and type of drainage on the intake and output record.

PROCEDURE 46–9

IRRIGATING A WOUND

Equipment ☑

Sterile dressing equipment and dressing materials (see Procedure 46–4)

Sterile irrigating syringe, (e.g., a 50-ml piston syringe)

Sterile basin for the irrigating solution

Sterile basin to receive the irrigation returns

Irrigating solution, usually 200 ml (6.5 oz) of solution at 32 to 35 C (90 to 95 F), according to the agency's or physician's choice

Sterile gloves

Moistureproof sterile drape

Sterile petroleum jelly

Sterile tongue blade

Intervention

1. Verify the physician's order.

■ Confirm the type and strength of the solution.

2. Prepare the client.

■ Assist the client to a position in which the irrigating solution will

flow by gravity from the upper end of the wound to the lower end and then into the basin.

■ Place the waterproof drape over the client and the bed, and position the sterile basin on it below the wound, to catch the irrigating solution.

■ Remove the old dressing, and clean the wound. See Procedure 46–4.

3. Protect the skin around the wound as required.

■ If an irrigating solution, such as Dakin's solution, is being used, apply sterile petroleum jelly to the skin around the wound, using the sterile tongue blade.

4. Irrigate the wound.

- Using the syringe, gently instill a steady stream of irrigating solution into the wound. Make sure all areas of the wound are irrigated.

- If you are using a catheter, insert the catheter into the wound until resistance is met. Do not force the catheter. *Forcing the catheter can cause tissue damage.*

- Continue irrigating until the solution becomes clear (no exudate is present) or until all the solution has been used. *The irrigation* *washes away tissue debris and drainage so that later returns are clearer.*

- Using dressing forceps or sterile gloves and sterile gauze, dry the area around the wound. *Moisture left on the skin promotes the growth of microorganisms and can cause skin irritation.*

5. Assess and dress the wound.

- Assess the appearance of the wound, noting in particular the type and amount of exudate and the presence and extent of granulation tissue. See the guidelines on page 1309.

- Apply a sterile dressing to the wound as described in Procedure 46–4.

6. Document relevant information.

- Document the irrigation, the solution used, the appearance of the irrigation returns, and nursing assessments. Note the presence of any exudate and sloughing tissue.

Assessing and Removing Sutures

Sutures are stitches used to sew body tissues together. *Suture* can also refer to the material used to sew the stitch. In some agencies, only physicians remove sutures; in others, registered nurses, licensed vocational nurses, and nursing students with appropriate supervision may do so. Various suture materials, e.g., silk, cotton, linen, wire, nylon, and Dacron (polyester fiber) threads are used. Silver wire clips are also available. The physician orders the removal of sutures. Usually, skin sutures are removed 7 to 10 days after surgery. Sterile technique and special suture scissors are used. The scissors have a short, curved cutting tip that readily slides under the suture. See Figure 46–28. Wire clips or staples are removed with a special instrument that squeezes the center of the clip to remove it from the skin. See Figure 46–29.

Retention sutures (stay sutures) are very large sutures used in addition to skin sutures for some incisions. See Figure 46–30. They attach underlying tissues of fat and muscle as well as skin and are used to support incisions in obese individuals or when healing may be prolonged. They are frequently left in place longer than skin sutures (14 to 21 days) but in some instances are removed at the same time as the skin sutures. To prevent these large sutures from irritating the incision, the surgeon may place rubber tubing over them or a roll of gauze under them extending down the incision line. Several forms of retention surfaces are

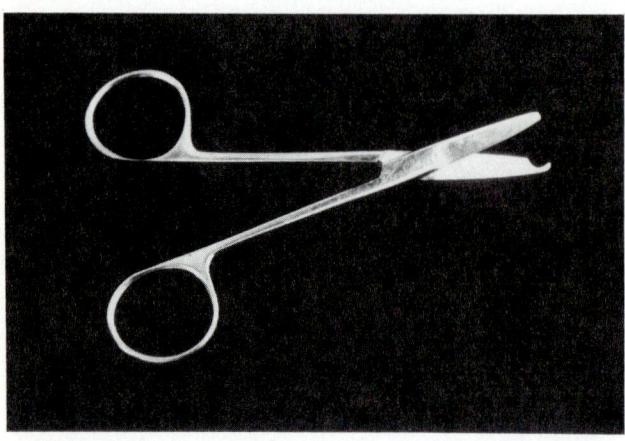

Figure 46–28 Suture scissors.

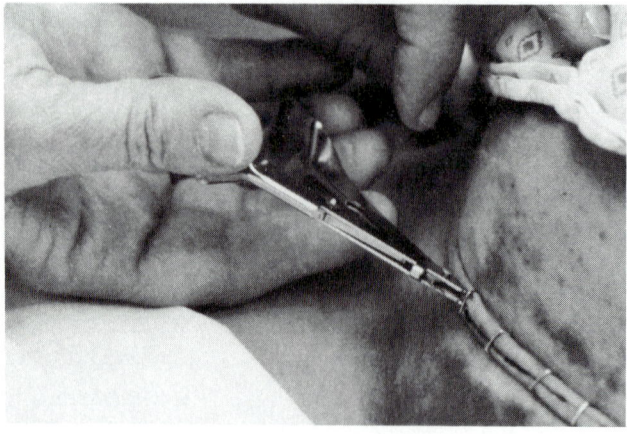

Figure 46–29 Removing surgical clips.

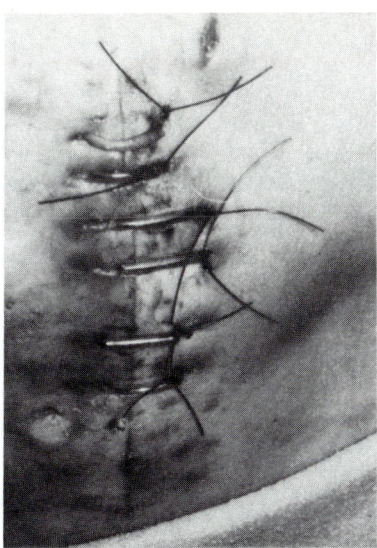

Figure 46–30 A surgical incision with retention sutures.

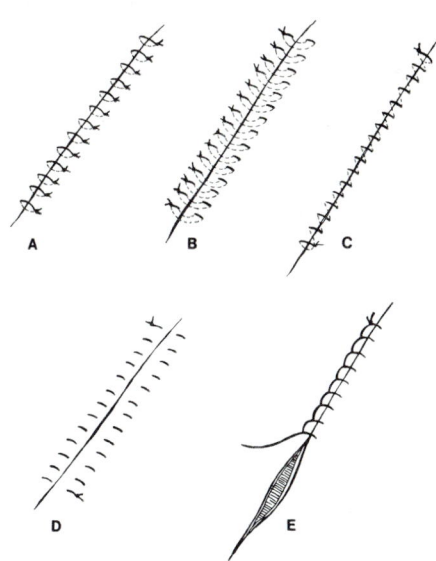

Figure 46–31 Common sutures: *A*, plain interrupted; *B*, mattress interrupted; *C*, plain continuous; *D*, mattress continuous; *E*, blanket continuous.

used, and agency policies about them may vary. The nurse should verify whether they are to be removed and who may remove them.

There are various methods of suturing. Skin sutures can be broadly categorized as either *interrupted* (each stitch is tied and knotted separately) or *continuous* (one thread runs in a series of stitches and is tied only at the beginning and at the end of the run). Common sutures are illustrated in Figure 46–31. The technique for removing skin sutures is described in Procedure 46–10.

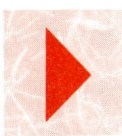

PROCEDURE 46–10

REMOVING SKIN SUTURES

Equipment ☑

Sterile dressing equipment (see Procedure 46–4)

Sterile suture scissors

Sterile butterfly tape (optional)

Moistureproof bag

Light sterile gauze pad and tape (if a dressing is to be applied)

Sterile gloves

Intervention

1. Verify the physician's order.

- Determine whether all or alternate sutures are to be removed. Many

times only *alternate* interrupted sutures are removed one day, and the remaining sutures are removed a day or two later.

2. Prepare the client.

- Inform the client that suture removal may produce slight discomfort, such as a pulling or stinging sensation, but should not be painful.

3. Remove dressings, and clean the incision.

- See Procedure 46–4, steps 2 through 5, page 1323.
- Don gloves.

- Clean the suture line with an antimicrobial solution before and after suture removal. *This is generally done as a prophylactic measure to prevent infection.*

4. Remove the sutures.

For plain interrupted sutures:

- Grasp the suture at the knot with a pair of forceps.

- Place the curved tip of the suture scissors under the suture as close to the skin as possible, either on the side opposite the knot (see Figure 46–32) or directly under the knot. Cut the suture. *Sutures are cut as close to the skin as possible* ▶

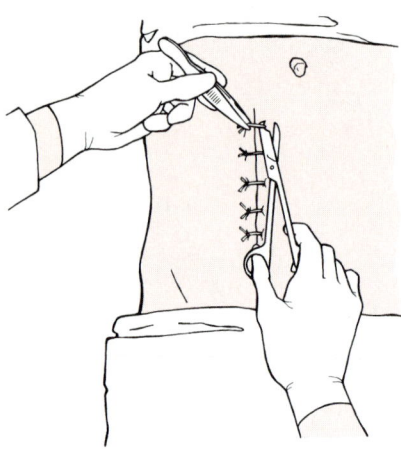

Figure 46–32 Removing a plain interrupted skin suture.

on one side of the visible part because the suture material that is visible to the eye is in contact with resident bacteria of the skin and must not be pulled beneath the skin during removal. Suture material that is beneath the skin is considered free from bacteria.

- With the forceps, pull the suture out in one piece. Inspect the suture carefully to make sure that all suture material is removed. *Suture material left beneath the skin acts as a foreign body and causes inflammation.*

- Discard the suture onto a piece of sterile gauze or into the moisture-proof bag, being careful not to contaminate the forceps tips. Sometimes the suture sticks to the forceps and needs to be removed by wiping the tips on a sterile gauze.

- Continue to remove *alternate sutures,* i.e., the third, fifth, seventh, and so forth. *Alternate sutures are removed first so that remaining sutures keep the skin edges in close approximation and prevent any dehiscence from becoming large.*

- If no dehiscence occurs, remove the remaining sutures. If dehis-

cence does occur, do not remove the remaining sutures, and report the dehiscence to the nurse in charge.

- If a little wound dehiscence occurs, apply a sterile butterfly tape over the gap:
  a. Attach the tape to one side of the incision.
  b. Press the wound edges together.
  c. Attach the tape to the other side of the incision. See Figure 46–33. *The butterfly tape holds the wound edges as close together as possible and promotes healing.*

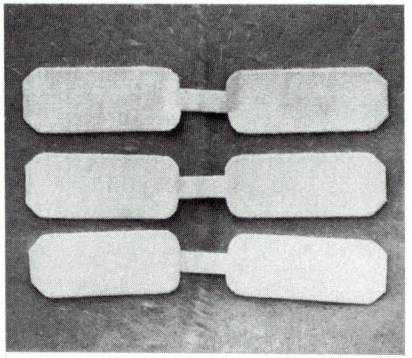

Figure 46–33 Butterfly tapes.

- If a large dehiscence occurs, cover the wound with sterile gauze, and report the problem immediately to the nurse in charge or physician.

For mattress interrupted sutures:

- When possible, cut the visible part of the suture close to the skin at *A* and *B* in Figure 46–34, opposite

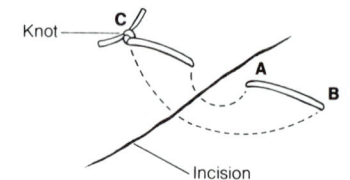

Figure 46–34 Mattress interrupted sutures.

the knot, and remove this small visible piece. Discard it as described above. In some sutures, the visible part opposite the knot may be so small that it can be cut only once.

- Grasp the knot (*C*) with forceps. Remove the remainder of the suture beneath the skin by pulling out in the direction of the knot.

For plain continuous sutures:

- Cut the thread of the first suture opposite the knot at *A* in Figure 46–35. Then cut the thread of the second suture on that same side at *B*.

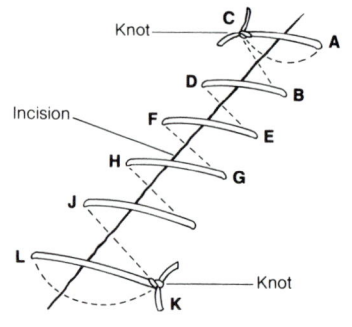

Figure 46–35 Plain continuous sutures.

- Grasp the knot (*C*) with the forceps, and pull. This removes the first stitch and the piece of thread beneath the skin, which is attached to the second stitch. Discard the suture.

- Cut off the visible part of the second suture at *D,* and discard it.

- Grasp the suture at *E,* and pull out the underlying loop between *D* and *E.*

- Cut the visible part at *F,* and remove it.

- Repeat the above two steps at *G* through *J,* until the last knot is reached. Note that after the first stitch is removed, each thread is cut down the same side, below the original knot.

■ Cut the last suture at *L,* and pull out the last suture at *K.*

For blanket continuous sutures:

■ Cut the threads that are opposite the looped blanket edge; i.e., cut at *A* through *F* in Figure 46–36.

■ Pull each stitch out at the looped edge.

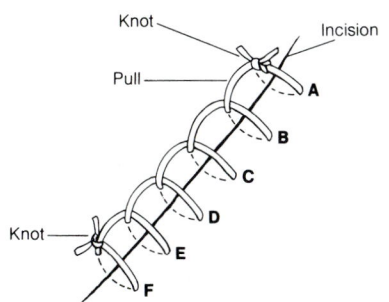

Figure 46–36   Blanket continuous sutures.

For mattress continuous sutures:

■ Cut the visible suture at both skin edges opposite the knot (at *A* and *B* in Figure 46–37) and the next suture opposite the knot (at *C* and *D*). Remove and discard the visible portions as described above.

■ Pull the first suture out by the knot at *E.*

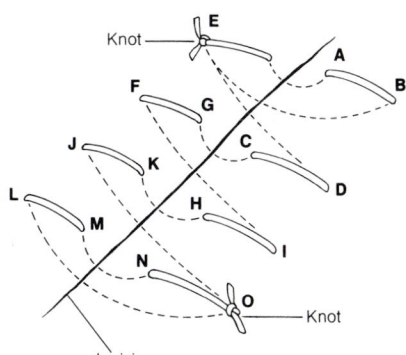

Figure 46–37   Mattress continuous sutures.

■ Lift the second suture between *F* and *G* to pull out the underlying suture between *G* and *C.* Cut off the visible part at *F* as close to the skin edge as possible.

■ Go to the opposite side between *H* and *I.* Lift out the suture between *F* and *I,* and cut off all the visible part close to the skin at *H.*

■ Lift the suture between *J* and *K* to pull out the suture between *H* and *K,* and cut the suture close to the skin at *J.*

■ Repeat the above 2 steps, working from side to side of the incision, until the last suture is reached.

■ Cut the visible suture opposite the knot at *L* and *M.* Pull out all remaining pieces of suture at *O.*

5. **Clean and cover the incision.**

■ Clean the incision again with antimicrobial solution.

■ Apply a small, light, sterile gauze dressing if any small dehiscence has occurred or if this is agency practice.

6. **Instruct the client about follow-up wound care.**

■ Generally, if a wound is dry and healing well, the person can take showers in a day or two.

■ Instruct the client to contact the physician if wound discharge appears.

7. **Document the suture removal and assessment data on the appropriate records.**

Sample Recording

Date: 12/5/91	Time: 1105

Abdominal sutures removed. Wound dry, edges approximated closely. No signs of inflammation. Gauze dressing applied.— ———————— Gwen E. Owens, NS

Applying Heat and Cold

Heat and cold are applied to the body to promote the repair and healing of tissues. The form of thermal applications generally depends on their purpose. Cold applied to a body part draws heat from the area; heat, of course, warms the area. The application of heat or cold produces physiologic changes in the temperature of the tissues, size of the blood vessels, capillary blood pressure, capillary surface area for exchange of fluids and electrolytes, and tissue metabolism. The duration of the application also affects the response. See Table 46–3 for a summary of the physiologic effects of heat and cold.

Heat is an old remedy for aches and pains; people often equate heat with comfort and relief. Heat causes **vasodi-**

lation (an increase in the inner diameter of blood vessels) and increases blood flow to the affected area, bringing oxygen, nutrients, antibodies, and leukocytes. Heat accelerates the inflammatory process by increasing both the action of phagocytic cells that ingest microorganisms and other foreign material and the removal of the waste products of infection and metabolic processes. Vasodilation produces skin redness and warmth that can be assessed by touch.

Application of heat promotes soft tissue healing and increases suppuration. The increase in blood flow also dissipates the heat, or draws it away from the affected area. A possible disadvantage of heat is that it increases capillary permeability, which allows extracellular fluid and substances such as plasma proteins to pass through the capillary walls and may result in edema (excessive amounts of

TABLE 46–3 *Physiologic Effects of Heat and Cold*

Body Part or Process	Effect of Heat	Effect of Cold
Local circulatory response	Vasodilation (reddened skin)	Vasoconstriction (pale, bluish skin)
Capillary permeability	Increased	Decreased
Cellular metabolism	Increased	Decreased
Inflammatory process	Increased	Decreased
Muscles	Relaxation	Decreased contractility
Nerves	Increased conduction rate	Decreased conduction rate
Synovial fluid	Increased viscosity	Decreased viscosity
Pain	Promotes comfort	Initial discomfort; later, numbness and paresthesia

fluid in the tissues) or an increase in preexisting edema. Heat is often used for clients with musculoskeletal problems such as joint stiffness from arthritis, contractures, and low back pain; and for those with open wounds needing debridement. See Table 46–4.

Heat can be applied to the body in both dry and moist forms. Dry heat is applied locally, for heat conduction, by means of a hot water bottle, electric pad, aquathermia pad,

or disposable heat pack. The heat lamp and bed cradle provide dry heat by radiation. Moist heat can be provided, through conduction, by compress, hot pack, soak, or sitz bath.

Cold therapy is more recent than heat therapy. Generally, its physiologic effects are opposite to the effects of heat. Cold lowers the temperature of the skin and underlying tissues and causes **vasoconstriction** (a decrease in the inner diameter of blood vessels). Vasoconstriction reduces blood flow to the affected area and thus reduces the supply of oxygen and metabolites, decreases the removal of wastes, and produces skin pallor, or a bluish discoloration, and coolness. Vasoconstriction and its consequent lowered blood flow to an area help control bleeding after injury. Prolonged exposure to cold results in impaired circulation, cell deprivation, and subsequent damage to the tissues from lack of oxygen and nourishment. The signs of tissue damage due to cold are a bluish-purple mottled appearance of the skin, numbness, stiffness, pallor, and sometimes blisters and pain. Cold is most often used for active young people with sports injuries (e.g., sprains, strains, fractures) to limit post-injury swelling and bleeding. It is increasingly being used for clients with rheumatoid arthritis, since it is thought to inhibit the activity of certain destructive enzymes that exacerbate joint problems (Lehmann and DeLateur 1982b). See Table 46–5.

Applications of cold may also be dry or moist. Dry cold is administered for local effect by the use of ice bags, ice collars, ice gloves, and disposable cold packs. Moist cold is applied for either local or systemic effects. Cold moist compresses are administered to body parts for a local effect; tepid sponge baths are given for a systemic cooling effect. Cold is often applied to the body to decrease bleeding by constricting blood vessels; to decrease inflammation by causing vasoconstriction; and to decrease pain by slowing nerve conduction rate, producing numbness, and acting as a counterirritant.

TABLE 46–4 *Selected Indications for Heat*

Indication	Effect of Heat
Muscle spasm	Relaxes muscles and increases their contractility
Inflammation	Increases blood flow, bringing more phagocytes (to facilitate exudate formation) and essential nutrients for healing; also enhances removal of wastes and debris formed in the inflammatory process. Moist heat softens exudates
Contracture	Reduces contractures and increases joint range of motion by allowing greater distention of muscles and connective tissue
Joint stiffness	Reduces joint stiffness by decreasing the viscosity of synovial fluid and increasing tissue distensibility
Pain	Relieves pain, possibly by promoting muscle relaxation, increasing circulation to ischemic areas, promoting psychologic relaxation and a feeling of comfort, and acting as a counterirritant

Source: P. S. Tepperman and M. Devlin, Therapeutic heat and cold. A practitioner's guide, *Postgraduate Medicine,* January 1983, 73:69.

TABLE 46–5 *Selected Indications for Cold*

Indication	Effect of Cold
Traumatic injury	Decreases bleeding by constricting blood vessels; decreases edema by reducing capillary permeability
Inflammation	Decreases inflammation by causing vasoconstriction, decreasing capillary permeability, decreasing blood flow, decreasing cellular metabolism, and slowing phagocytosis
Muscle spasm	Increases muscle relaxation by decreasing muscle contractility
Pain	Decreases pain by slowing nerve conduction rate and blocking nerve impulses, by producing numbness, by acting as a counterirritant, and by increasing the pain threshold

Source: P. S. Tepperman and M. Devlin, Therapeutic heat and cold. A practitioner's guide, *Postgraduate Medicine,* January 1983, 73:69.

Adaptation of Thermal Receptors   Thermal receptors adapt to temperature changes. When a cold receptor is subjected to an abrupt fall in temperature or when a warmth receptor is subjected to an abrupt rise in temperature, the receptor is strongly stimulated initially. This strong stimulation declines rapidly during the first few seconds and then more slowly during the next half hour or more as the receptor adapts to the new temperature (Guyton 1986, p. 604). This adaptive mechanism explains why people feel very cold at first when they go outdoors from a heated room on a cold day or feel very warm when they go from a cold environment to a heated room or from a warm room to a hot tub.

 Nurses need to understand this adaptive response when applying heat and cold. Clients may be tempted to change the temperature of a thermal application because of the change in thermal sensation following adaptation. Increasing the temperature of a hot application after adaptation has occurred can result in serious burns. Decreasing the temperature of a cold application can result in pain and

serious impairment of circulation to the body part. See Table 46–6 for recommended temperatures of hot and cold applications.

Rebound Phenomenon   The **rebound phenomenon** occurs at the time the maximum therapeutic effect of the hot or cold application is achieved and the opposite effect begins. For example, heat produces maximum vasodilation in 20 to 30 minutes; continuation of the application beyond 30 to 45 minutes brings tissue congestion, and the blood vessels then *constrict* for reasons unknown. If the heat application is continued further, the client is at risk for burns, since the constricted blood vessels are unable to dissipate the heat adequately via the blood circulation.

With cold applications, maximum vasoconstriction occurs when the involved skin reaches a temperature of 15 C (60 F). Below 15 C, vasodilation begins. This rebound phenomenon is thought to be the result of paralysis of the mechanism that contracts the vessel wall, or blockage of the nerve impulses to the vessels, or inactivation of the vasoconstric-

TABLE 46–6 *Recommended Temperatures for Hot and Cold Applications*

Description	Centigrade	Fahrenheit	Application
Very cold	Below 15	Below 59	Ice bags
Cold	15 to 18	59 to 65	Cold pack
Cool	18 to 27	65 to 80	Cold compress
Tepid	27 to 37	80 to 98	Alcohol and tepid sponges
Warm	37 to 40	98 to 105	Warm bath
Hot	40 to 46	105 to 115	Aquathermia, soaks, sitz baths, irrigations, moist sterile compresses, hot water bags for debilitated or young clients
Very hot	Above 46	Above 115	Hot water bags for adults, heat cradles

Variables Affecting Physiologic Tolerance to Heat and Cold

■ *Body part.* The back of the hand and foot are not very temperature-sensitive. In contrast, the inner aspect of the wrist and forearm, the neck, and the perineal area are temperature-sensitive.

■ *Size of the exposed body part.* The larger the area exposed to heat and cold, the lower the tolerance.

■ *Individual tolerance.* Tolerance to heat and cold is to some degree affected by age and condition of the skin, nervous system, and circulatory system. The very young and the very old generally have the lowest tolerance. Persons who have neurosensory impairments may have a high tolerance, but the risk of injury is greater.

■ *Length of exposure.* People feel hot and cold applications most while the skin temperature is changing. After a period of time, tolerance is increased.

■ *Intactness of skin.* Injured skin areas are more sensitive to temperature variations.

tor chemicals (Lehmann and DeLateur, 1982a). This mechanism is protective: It helps to prevent freezing of body tissues normally exposed to cold, such as the nose and ears. It also explains the ruddiness of the skin of a person who has been walking in cold weather.

An understanding of the rebound phenomenon is essential for the nurse. Thermal applications must be halted *before* the rebound phenomenon begins.

Systemic Effects

Heat applied to a localized body area, particularly a large body area, may increase cardiac output and pulmonary ventilation. These increases are a result of excessive peripheral vasodilation, which diverts large supplies of blood from the internal organs and produces a drop in blood pressure. A significant drop in blood pressure can cause fainting. Clients who have heart or pulmonary disease and who have circulatory disturbances such as arteriosclerosis are more prone to this effect than healthy persons.

With extensive cold applications and vasoconstriction, a client's blood pressure can increase, because blood is shunted from the cutaneous circulation to the internal blood vessels. This shunting of blood, a normal protective response to prolonged cold, is the body's attempt to maintain its core temperature. Shivering, another generalized effect of prolonged cold, is a normal response as the body attempts to warm itself.

Tolerance

Various parts of the body differ in tolerance to heat and cold. The physiologic tolerance of individuals also varies. See the accompanying box.

Specific conditions contraindicate the use of hot or cold applications. For example, heat increases bleeding and therefore is not used during the first 24 hours after traumatic injuries. See Table 46–7 for conditions that contraindicate the use of heat or cold. In addition, certain conditions call for precautions in administering heat and cold therapy:

■ *Neurosensory impairment.* Persons with sensory impairments are unable to perceive that heat is damaging the tissues and are at risk for burns or are unable to perceive discomfort from cold and prevent tissue injury.

■ *Impaired mental status.* People who are confused or have an altered level of consciousness need monitoring and supervision during applications to ensure safe therapy.

■ *Impaired circulation.* Persons with peripheral vascular disease, diabetes, or congestive heart failure lack the normal ability to dissipate heat via the blood circulation, which puts them at risk for tissue damage with heat applications. Note that cold applications are contraindicated for these people.

■ *Open wounds.* Tissues around an open wound are more sensitive to heat and cold.

Before applying heat or cold, the nurse assesses the area to be treated and the client's history and current health status to (a) determine the client's ability to tolerate the therapy and (b) identify conditions that contraindicate the therapy (see Table 46–7). The area to which the heat and cold will be applied also needs to be assessed. See the box below.

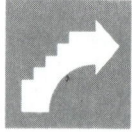

CLINICAL GUIDELINES
Assessing Body Areas Before Applying Heat or Cold

■ Observe alterations in skin integrity, such as the presence of edema, bruises, redness, open lesions, discharge, and bleeding.

■ Assess circulatory status (color, temperature, and sensation). Tissues that feel cold, have a pale or bluish hue, and lack sensation or feel numb indicate circulatory impairment.

■ Assess level of discomfort experienced by the client, and range of motion if muscle spasm or pain is being treated.

■ Determine pulse, respirations, and blood pressure. Assessing these factors is particularly important before hot or cold is applied to large body areas.

TABLE 46–7 *Conditions Contraindicating the Use of Heat and Cold*

Heat	Cold
During the first 24 hours after traumatic injury. Heat increases bleeding and swelling.	*Open wounds.* Cold can increase tissue damage by decreasing blood flow to an open wound.
Active hemorrhage. Heat causes vasodilation and increases bleeding.	*Impaired circulation.* Cold can further impair nourishment of the tissues and cause tissue damage. In clients with Raynaud's disease, cold increases arterial spasm.
Noninflammatory edema. Heat increases capillary permeability and edema.	*Allergy or hypersensitivity to cold.* Some clients have an allergy to cold that may be manifested by an inflammatory response, e.g., erythema, hives, swelling, joint pain, and occasional muscle spasm. Some react with a sudden increase in blood pressure, which can be hazardous if the person is hypersensitive.
Acute inflammation. Heat on such areas can increase edema; e.g., it can rupture an appendix.	
Localized malignant tumor. Because heat accelerates cell metabolism and cell growth and increases circulation, it may accelerate metastases (secondary tumors).	
Developing fetus. Heat to the abdomen of a pregnant woman can cause mutation in the fetal germinal cells and affect fetal growth.	
Skin disorder that causes redness or blisters. Heat can burn or cause further damage to the skin.	
Metallic implants such as a pacemaker or knee or hip replacements. Because metal is a good conductor of heat, medical diathermy—which uses electric current to heat deep tissues—can burn deep tissues.	

Applying Dry Heat   The *aquathermia* or *aquamatic pad* (also referred to as a *K-pad*) is a device commonly used in hospitals to provide heat to a body part. The pad is attached by tubing to an electrically powered control unit that has an opening for water and a temperature gauge. See Figure 46–38. Some aquathermia pads have an absorbent surface through which moist heat can be applied. The other surface of the pad is waterproof. These pads are disposable.

The reservoir of an aquathermia unit should be filled two-thirds full. The desired temperature is set, the pad is covered, placed on the body part, and maintained in place with roller gauze if needed. The nurse should check the manufacturer's instructions to regulate the temperature with a key if the temperature has not been preset. Normal temperature is 40.5 C (105 F), and treatment is usually continued for 10 to 15 minutes. If unusual redness or pain occurs, treatment is discontinued and the client's reaction reported and recorded.

Dry heat can be supplied by *commercially prepared disposable hot packs.* See Figure 46–39. *Directions* on the package tell how to initiate the heating process, e.g., by striking, squeezing, or kneading the pack. Hot packs provide a specified amount of heat for a specified time.

Lamps also provide dry heat to localized areas. A *heat lamp* is often a gooseneck lamp with either a special or an ordinary 40-watt or 60-watt bulb. An *infrared lamp* may also be used. Before a heat lamp is used, the affected area should be cleaned and dried to lessen the likelihood of burning. A heat lamp with a 40- or 60-watt bulb or a small infrared

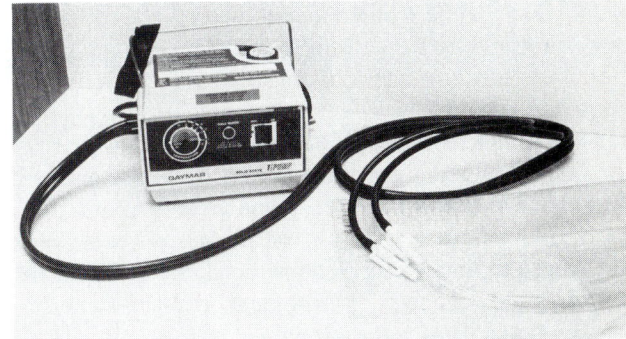

Figure 46–38   An aquathermia heating unit.

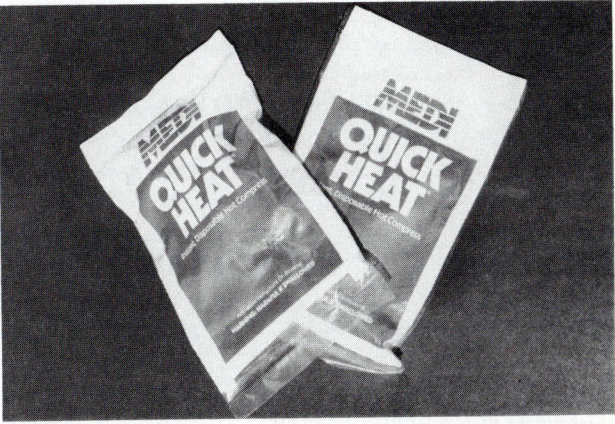

Figure 46–39   Commercially prepared disposable hot packs.

lamp is usually placed 45 to 60 cm (18 to 24 in) from the client. A large infrared lamp is placed 60 to 75 cm (24 to 30 in) away. The treatment usually lasts 15 to 20 minutes, provided that the client tolerates the heat. The client should be checked every 5 minutes for discomfort, burning, or any untoward reaction. The client is cautioned not to touch the infrared lamp, and the lamp should not be draped or placed under any bedclothes because of the risk of fire. At the first sign of skin redness or discomfort, the treatment should be discontinued and the reaction reported and recorded.

A *hot water bottle or bag* is a common source of dry heat used in the home. It is convenient and relatively inexpensive. However, because of the danger of burning from improper use, many agencies use other means.

The following temperatures of the water in the bag are considered safe in most situations and provide the desired effect: normal adult, 52 C (125 F); debilitated or unconscious adult, 40.5 to 46 C (105 to 115 F); child under 2 years, 40.5 to 46 C (105 to 115 F). Hot water bags usually are filled about two-thirds full. The remaining air is expelled and the top secured. The hot water bag can then be readily molded to a body part. Before application, the bag is dried and held upside down to test for leakage. If it is secure, it is then wrapped in a towel or cover and placed on the body site. A hot water bottle will usually stay hot for 45 minutes before needing to be replaced.

Electric pads provide a constant, even heat, are lightweight, and can be molded to a body part. Electric pads, however, can burn if the setting is too high. In some agencies, the controls on the pads are set to a specific temperature to prevent burning.

When using electric pads, the nurse needs to ensure that the body area is dry, since electricity in the presence of moisture can conduct a shock. Some models have waterproof covers for use when the pad is placed over a moist dressing. The nurse also cautions the client not to insert any sharp objects into the pad; doing so may cause an electric shock and damage the wiring.

A *heat cradle* is a metal frame with a row of 25-watt light bulbs used to provide less localized dry heat than a heat lamp. The cradle is placed over the client and usually covered with a bath blanket or sheet. The temperature inside the cradle normally should not exceed 51.6 C (125 F), and the treatment normally lasts 10 to 15 minutes. The heat source inside the cradle should be 45 to 60 cm (18 to 24 in) away from the client. The client should be checked every 10 minutes for discomfort or any untoward reaction.

Applying Moist Heat

Soaks and sitz baths may be ordered for these reasons:

- To hasten suppuration, soften exudates, and enhance healing

- To apply medications to a designated area

- To clean a wound in which there is sloughing tissue or an exudate

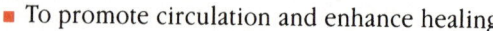

- To promote circulation and enhance healing

A *soak* refers to immersing a body part, e.g., an arm, in a solution or to wrapping a part in gauze dressings and then saturating the dressing with a solution. Sterile technique is generally indicated for open wounds, e.g., a burn or an unhealed surgical incision. Dry dressings are usually applied between the soaks.

A **sitz bath,** or hip bath, is used to soak a client's pelvic area. The client sits in a special tub or chair and is usually immersed from the midthighs to the iliac crests or umbilicus. Special tubs or chairs are preferred (see Figure 46–40); when the legs are also immersed, as in a regular bathtub, blood circulation to the perineum or pelvic area is decreased. Disposable sitz baths are also available; they are commonly used in homes but may be used in hospitals as well.

The temperature of the water should be from 40 to 43 C (105 to 110 F), unless otherwise ordered by the physician, or unless the client is unable to tolerate the heat. Some sitz tubs have temperature indicators attached to the water taps. The duration of the bath is generally 15 to 20 minutes, depending on the client's condition.

To prevent undue pressure on the sacrum or posterior aspects of the thighs, towels can be placed in or on the edges of a sitz tub. When a disposable sitz bath is used, a footstool can prevent pressure on the back of the thighs. Precautions also need to be taken to prevent chilling, burning, or fainting. Often, placing a bath blanket over the client's shoulders and eliminating drafts during the bath prevents chilling. Maintaining the temperature of the bath is important. The nurse tests the water temperature at least once during the bath and adjusts it as necessary.

Some clients, particularly those who have just had surgery, feel faint and dizzy during a sitz bath. Therefore, the nurse observes the client closely during the sitz bath for an

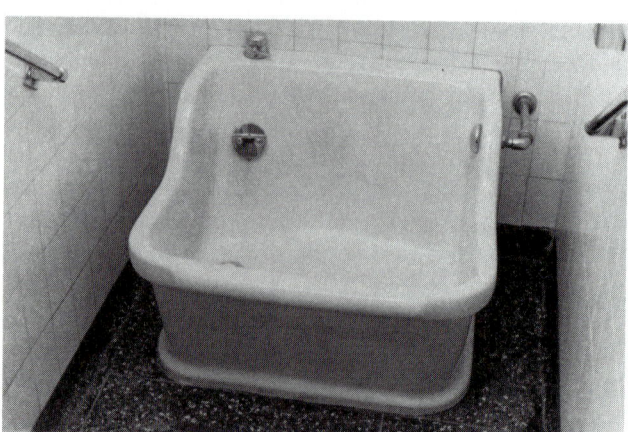

Figure 46–40   A sitz bath used in hospitals.

accelerated pulse or pallor. Clients need to be instructed beforehand to signal for the nurse if they feel weak so that they can be assisted promptly. Following the sitz bath, the nurse helps the client to dry the area and reapplies dressings (e.g., a perineal pad and T-binder) after reassessing the perineal area.

Applying Dry Cold

Applying cold to an affected area may be helpful in

- Relieving headaches caused by vasodilation
- Preventing swelling of tissues and pain immediately following an injury or surgery
- Preventing, decreasing, or terminating bleeding following an injury or surgery

The *ice bag,* commonly used in many homes and hospitals, is a moderate-sized rubber or plastic bag with a removable cap. Ice is placed inside the bag. Commercially prepared ice bags are available in some agencies. Such bags are filled with an alcohol-based solution and sealed; they are kept in freezing units in a central supply area. An *ice collar* is similar to an ice bag but is long and narrow (see Figure 46–41). It is designed for use around the neck, although it can be used on other body parts. An *ice glove* is simply a plastic glove filled with ice chips or a solution of alcohol and water and tied at the open end. It is applied to a small body area, such as the eye. Ice gloves can be stored in the freezer when not in use.

Disposable cold packs are similar to disposable hot packs. They come in a variety of sizes and shapes and provide a specific degree of coldness for a specified period of time, as indicated on the package. By striking, squeezing, or kneading the package, the nurse activates chemical reactions that release the cold. The manufacturer's instructions must be followed. Most commercially prepared cold packs have soft outer coverings so that they can be applied directly to the body part.

Administering a Cooling Sponge Bath

The purpose of a cooling sponge bath is to reduce a client's fever by promoting heat loss through conduction and vaporization. The cooling sponge bath consists of water or a combination of alcohol and water that is below body temperature. Alcohol evaporates at a low temperature and therefore removes body heat rapidly. However, alcohol-and-water sponge baths are less frequently used than in the past because alcohol has a drying effect on the skin. The temperatures for cooling sponge baths range from 18 to 32 C (65 to 90 F). A *tepid* sponge bath generally refers to one in which the water temperature is 32 C (90 F) throughout the bath. For a *cool* sponge bath, the water temperature is 32 C (90 F) at the beginning of the bath and is gradually lowered to 18 C (65 F) by adding ice chips during the bath. A fan is sometimes used to increase air movement around the

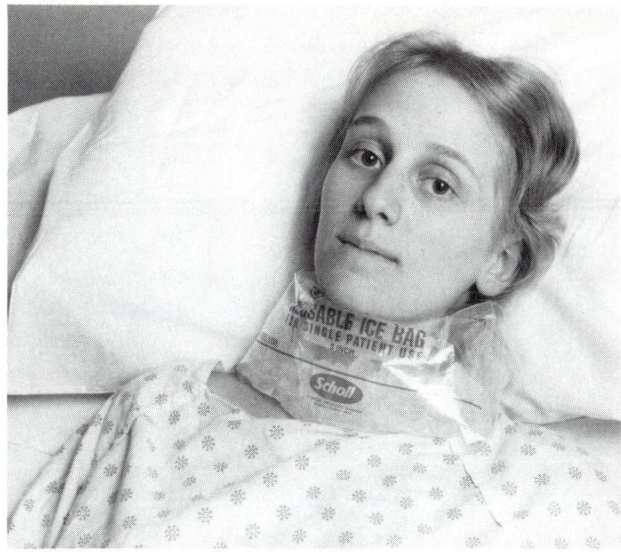

Figure 46–41   A disposable ice collar in place.

client, which lowers the body temperature through convection. In this case, drafts are not usually eliminated during the sponge bath. Cool sponge baths are used with extreme caution because of potential deleterious effects such as shock.

The decision to give a tepid sponge bath is generally made only after a marked fever is noted or a temperature increase of 1 to 2 C or 2 to 3 F. Some agencies require a physician's order; others permit a decision by the nurse in charge. Procedure 46–11 on page 1340 describes how to administer a cooling sponge bath.

Applying Compresses and Moist Packs

Compresses and moist packs can be either hot or cold. A **compress** is a moist gauze dressing applied frequently to an open wound. When hot compresses are ordered, the solution is heated to the temperature indicated by the physician, e.g., 40.5 C (105 F). When there is a break in the skin or when the body part (e.g., an eye) is vulnerable to microbial invasion, sterile technique is necessary; therefore, sterile gloves or sterile forceps are needed to apply the compress, and all materials (solution, container, thermometer, towels, gauze squares, and petroleum jelly) must be sterile. If a sterile thermometer is not available, the nurse pours a small amount of the solution into a clean basin, measures the temperature, and then discards the solution, since it is no longer sterile. The nurse adjusts the temperature of the solution according to the findings.

A hot or cold **pack** is a hot or cold moist cloth applied to an area of the body. Packs are usually unsterile; after application, they are covered with a water-resistant material (e.g., plastic wrap) to contain the moisture and prevent the transfer of airborne microorganisms to the area. For a

ADMINISTERING A COOLING SPONGE BATH

Equipment ☑

Basin for the solution

Bath thermometer

Solution at the correct temperature

(water or equal portions of 70% alcohol and water)

Ice chips (for a cool sponge bath)

Several washcloths and bath towels (fewer are needed if ice bags or cold packs are used)

Bath blanket

Thermometer to measure the client's temperature

Fan (optional)

Intervention

1. Obtain relevant baseline data.

■ If not already recorded prior to the sponge bath, measure the client's body temperature, pulse, and respirations to provide comparative baseline data.

■ Assess the client for other signs of fever: skin warmth, flushing, complaints of heat or chilling, diaphoresis, irritability, restlessness, general malaise, or delirium.

2. Prepare the client.

■ Explain that the face, arms, legs, back, and buttocks will be sponged (*not* the chest and abdomen) and that the procedure takes about 30 minutes.

■ Remove the gown, and assist the client to a comfortable supine position.

■ Place a bath blanket over the client.

■ If ice bags or cold packs are not used, place bath towels under each axilla and shoulder. *Bath towels protect the lower bed sheet from getting wet.*

3. Sponge the face.

■ Sponge the client's face with plain water only, and dry it.

■ Apply an ice bag or cold pack to the head for comfort.

4. Place cold applications in the axillae and groins.

■ Wet four washcloths; wring them out so that they are very damp but not dripping. *Washcloths need to be as moist as possible to be effective.*

■ Place washcloths in the axillae and groins.

   or

■ Place ice bags or cold packs in these areas. *The axillae and groins contain large superficial blood vessels, which aid the transfer of heat.*

■ Leave washcloths in place for about 5 minutes, or until they feel warm. Rewet and replace them as required during the bath. *Washcloths warm up relatively quickly in such vascular areas.*

5. Sponge the arms and legs.

■ Place a bath towel under one arm and sponge the arm *slowly* and *gently* for about 5 minutes or as tolerated by the client. *Slow, gentle motions are indicated because firm rubbing motions increase tissue metabolism and heat production. Cool sponges given rapidly or for a short period of time tend to increase the body's heat production mechanisms by causing shivering.*

   or

■ Place a saturated towel over the extremity, and rewet it as necessary. Give the client enough time to adjust to the initial reaction of chilliness and for the body to cool.

■ Dry the arm, using a patting motion rather than a rubbing motion.

■ Repeat the above steps for the other arm and the legs.

■ When sponging the extremities, hold the washcloth briefly over the wrists and ankles. *The blood circulation is close to the skin surface in the wrists and ankles.*

6. Reassess the client's vital signs after 15 minutes.

■ Compare findings with data taken before the bath. *The vital signs are checked to evaluate the effectiveness of the sponge bath.*

7. Sponge the back and buttocks.

■ Sponge the back and buttocks for 3 to 5 minutes.

■ Pat these areas dry.

8. Remove cold applications from the axillae and groins.

9. Reassess vital signs.

10. Document assessments, including the vital signs, as well as type of sponge bath given.

sterile moist pack, the container, solution, thermometer, and all materials must be sterile. In addition, sterile gloves or forceps are required to maintain the sterility of the pack when it is wrung out and applied.

Hot compresses usually are applied to hasten the suppurative process and healing. Cold compresses are applied either to decrease or prevent bleeding or to reduce inflammation. Hot packs are applied to relieve muscle spasm or pain, to reduce the pressure of accumulated fluid in a tissue or joint, and to reduce congestion in an underlying organ. Cold packs are used to prevent swelling due to tissue trauma and inflammation and to anesthetize tissues and temporarily reduce pain.

After a compress or a pack has been applied, it is advisable to apply external heat or cold, such as a hot water bottle, heating pad, or ice bag, to help maintain the temperature of the application. Application of compresses and moist packs is described in Procedure 46–12.

PROCEDURE 46–12

APPLYING COMPRESSES AND MOIST PACKS

Equipment

(Use sterile equipment and supplies for an open wound)

Compress:

Container for the solution

Solution at the strength and temperature specified by the physician or the agency

Thermometer

Petroleum jelly

Gauze squares

Insulating towel

Plastic

Hot water bottle or aquathermia pad (optional)

or

Ice bag (optional)

Ties, e.g., roller gauze or masking tape

Disposable gloves

Sterile gloves, forceps, and cotton applicator sticks (if compress must be sterile)

Moist pack:

Flannel pieces or towel packs

Hot-pack machine for heating the packs

or

Basin of water with some ice chips

Insulating material, e.g., flannel or towels

Plastic

Hot water bottle (optional)

or

Ice bag (optional)

Thermometer if a specific temperature is ordered for the pack

Petroleum jelly

Sterile gloves or forceps (if sterility must be maintained)

Intervention

1. **Prepare the client.**
- Assist the client to a comfortable position.
- Expose the area for the compress or pack.
- Provide support for the body part requiring the compress or pack.
- Don disposable gloves, and remove the wound dressing, if present. A dry, sterile dressing is often placed over open wounds between applications of moist heat or cold.

2. **Moisten the compress or pack.**
- Place the gauze in the solution.

   or
- Heat the flannel or towel in a steamer.

3. **Protect surrounding skin as indicated.**
- With a cotton swab or an applicator stick, apply petroleum jelly to the skin surrounding the wound, not on the wound or open areas of the skin. *Jelly protects the skin*

from possible burns, maceration, and irritating effects of some solutions.

4. **Apply the moist heat.**
- Wring out the gauze compress so that the solution does not drip from it. For a sterile compress, use sterile forceps or sterile gloves to wring out the gauze.
- Apply the gauze lightly and gradually to the designated area and, if tolerated by the client, mold the

compress close to the body. Pack the gauze snugly against all wound surfaces. *Air is a poor conductor of cold or heat, and molding excludes air.*

or

- Wring out the flannel (for a sterile pack, use sterile gloves).
- Apply the flannel to the body area, molding it closely to the body part.

5. Immediately insulate and secure the application.

- Cover the gauze or flannel quickly with a dry towel and a piece of plastic. *This step helps maintain the temperature of the application and thus its effectiveness.*
- Secure the compress or pack in place with gauze ties or tape.
- Optional: Apply a hot water bottle or aquathermia pad or ice bag over the plastic to maintain the heat or cold.

6. Monitor the client.

- Assess the client for discomfort at 5- to 10-minute intervals. If the client feels any discomfort, assess the area for erythema, numbness, maceration, or blistering.
- For applications to large areas of the body, note any change in the pulse, respirations, and blood pressure.
- In the event of unexpected reactions, terminate the treatment and report to the nurse in charge.

7. Remove the compress or pack at the specified time.

- Compresses and packs with external heat or cold usually retain their temperature anywhere from 15 to 30 minutes. Without external heat or cold, they need to be changed every 5 minutes.
- Apply a sterile dressing if one is required.

8. Document relevant information.

- Document the technique, the time, and the type and strength of the solution.
- Record assessments, including the appearance of the wound and surrounding skin area.

Sample Recording

Date: 5/12/91	Time: 0910

Sterile normal saline compress with K-Matic 37.7 °C applied to 2.5 cm sacral ulcer. Pink tissue surrounding ulcer. 1 cm diameter serosanguineous discharge on dressing. No discomfort voiced.————
———————— Olga R. Resnicoff, NS

Date: 5/12/91	Time: 0940

Compress removed. No further discharge. Ulcer packed with petrolatum gauze and sterile dry dressing applied.–
———————— Olga R. Resnicoff, NS

EVALUATING

To evaluate the effectiveness of nursing interventions and the achievement of client goals, the nurse obtains data relevant to the outcome criteria established in the planning phase. To elicit such data, the nurse may do the following:

- Assess the client's vital signs at specified intervals
- Inspect the wound and drainage site each time it is cleaned or dressed
- Observe the client's ability to perform self-care
- Ask the client about degree of pain experienced
- Monitor the client's food and fluid intake
- Watch the client demonstrate required home wound care
- Question the client about discharge instructions and symptoms or signs warranting notification of health personnel

Examples of evaluative statements follow. These need to be dated and signed.

"Wound edges are well approximated; incision line is dry; slight redness at wound edges."

"Skin is intact around drainage site."

"Client stated four out of five signs indicating problems with wound healing: increased pain, persistent bleeding, presence of pus, elevated temperature. Omitted wound gaping."

NURSING CARE PLAN FOR JOSÉ ALONZO

ASSESSMENT DATA

Nursing Assessment

José Alonzo is a 42-year-old construction worker who was injured at work when a wheelbarrow filled with cement rolled into him and pushed him off a four-foot ledge. He suffered several bruises and one 3.5-in (9-cm) laceration on the anterior aspect of the lower left leg. The laceration was covered with a sterile compression dressing at the scene by paramedics. Prior to irrigation and cleansing with normal saline and betadine, the wound contained particles of cement and dirt. Dr. James sutured the wound with silk suture and discharged Mr. Alonzo to home care. Mr. Alonzo is to return to the outpatient clinic for suture removal in 10 days. He asks the nurse whether he can use an aloe herbal ointment on the wound and drink a healing herbal tea that his wife makes.

Physical Examination

Height: 177.8 cm (5'10")
Weight: 72.7 kg (160 lb)
Temperature: 37 C (98.6 F)
Pulse: 88 BPM
Respiration: 24 per minute
Blood Pressure: 136/90

CARE PLAN

Nursing Diagnosis	Client Goals and Outcome Criteria	Nursing Interventions and Rationales	Evaluation
Potential for infection related to traumatic injury (contaminated by cement and dirt), as manifested by 3.5-in laceration on anterior aspect of left lower leg and multiple contusions on lower legs and right hip	Client Goal: Healed laceration and bruises without complications Outcome Criteria: Vital signs remain normal. No evidence of tissue inflammation in area of laceration. Laceration edges are closed and healing well on day 10 (suture removal appointment).	Establish rapport with client by being supportive and empathetic. *Rationale:* Encourages the client to ask questions and to seek assistance. Assess the client's knowledge about wound care. *Rationale:* Knowing the client's understanding of wound care enables the nurse to reinforce appropriate practices while discouraging potentially harmful practices. Instruct client to keep dressing clean and dry. *Rationale:* Wet and/or dirty dressings increase the potential for infection. Instruct client to change dressing and assess wound daily for signs of infection (redness, pain, warmth). *Rationale:* Early recognition of infection can enable the client to obtain prompt treatment. Instruct client about foods high in protein and/or vitamin C and encourage adequate intake. *Rationale:* Protein and vitamin C are essential for tissue repair. Allow client to use cultural remedies that will not interfere with healing (e.g., herbal tea). *Rationale:* Shows respect for client's cultural beliefs and encourages compliance with treatment plan.	Temperature, pulse, respiration and blood pressure normal at suture removal visit (day 10). No evidence of infection or inflammation in area of laceration on day 10. Wound is closed and healing well on day 10.

CHAPTER HIGHLIGHTS

- There are six types of wounds: incisions, contusions, abrasions, lacerations, punctures, and penetrating wounds.

- Wounds heal by either primary intention or secondary intention, depending on the extent of tissue loss.

- Internal factors affecting wound healing include vasculature, age, immune status, nutrition, obesity, smoking, stress, and medications.

- External factors affecting wound healing include preoperative stay, preoperative preparation, and intraoperative factors.

- The main complications of wound healing are hemorrhage, infection, dehiscence, and evisceration.

- Wound assessment is an ongoing process to evaluate healing; the nurse assesses wounds by visual inspection, palpation, and the sense of smell.

- Nursing diagnoses related to wound care include **Potential for infection, Pain, Potential impaired skin integrity, Knowledge deficit, Altered tissue perfusion,** and **Body image disturbance.**

- The care of wounds varies considerably in accordance with the type of wound, size and location, amount of exudate, presence of complicating factors, and sometimes the personal preference of the physician.

- Major nursing responsibilities related to wound care include preventing infection, preventing further tissue damage, preventing hemorrhage, promoting healing, cleaning wounds of foreign debris, and preventing skin excoriation around draining wounds.

- Open and closed methods of wound care have advantages and disadvantages that make them appropriate for different circumstances.

- Wound care may involve applying bandages and binders, changing dressings, maintaining drains, irrigation, and applying heat and cold.

- Five basic turns—spiral, circular, spiral reverse, recurrent, and figure-eight—are used in bandaging specific body parts.

- Before changing dressings, the nurse needs to ascertain the physician's orders, the presence of drains, the amount of wound drainage, and the cleaning solutions to be used.

- Each of five common types of sutures—plain interrupted, mattress interrupted, plain continuous, mattress continuous, and blanket continuous—is removed by a specific procedure.

- Heat and cold produce specific local physiologic responses that account for their therapeutic effects.

READINGS AND REFERENCES

SUGGESTED READINGS

Cuzzell, J. Z. February 1985. Wound care forum: Artful solutions to chronic problems. *American Journal of Nursing* 85:162–66.
According to Cuzzell, there are two general purposes to the care of chronic wounds: (1) cleaning a dirty, infected wound to prepare for surgical closure, and (2) protecting a clean wound until it can heal by the processes of contracture and epithelialization. Different types of dressings are described: dry-to-dry, wet-to-dry, wet-to-damp, and wet-to-wet, as well as synthetic dressings, topical enzyme preparations, and products that absorb exudates and cleanse a wound surface.

———. October 1988. The new RYB color code: Next time you assess an open wound, remember to protect red, cleanse yellow, and debride black. *American Journal of Nursing* 88:1342–46.
Cuzzell discusses the usefulness of the three-color concept of wound classification recently introduced by Marion Laboratories, Inc. It applies to any wound allowed to heal by secondary intention. Goals and details of wound management are included for each of the three colors.

Redheffer, G. July 1989 and August 1989. Treating wounds on the scene. Parts 1 and 2. *Nursing 89* 19:51–57; 47–51.
In Part 1 of this series, Redheffer discusses the management of abrasions, lacerations, punctures, sucking chest wounds, and wounds with embedded foreign objects. Part 2 includes emergency care for partial and complete amputations.

SELECTED REFERENCES

Bale, S., and Harding, K. G. February 1990. Using modern dressings to effect debridement. *Professional Nurse* 5:244, 246, 248.

Brozenec, S. April 1985. Caring for the postoperative patient with an abdominal drain. *Nursing 85* 15:55–57.

Bruno, P. December 1979. The nature of wound healing: Implications for nursing practice. *Nursing Clinics of North America* 14:667–82.

Bruno, P., and Craven, R. F. December 1982. Age challenges to wound healing. *Journal of Gerontological Nursing* 8:686–91.

Bukata, W. R.; Mathes, S. J.; and McCabe, J. B. May 30, 1988. Wound management. *Patient Care* 22:66–71, 73–78, 83.

Carpenito, L. J. 1989. *Nursing diagnosis: Application to clinical practice.* 3d ed. Philadelphia: J.B. Lipincott Company.

Centers for Disease Control: Recommendations for prevention of HIV transmission in health care settings. MMWR 1987:36:55.

Cerrato, P. L. June 1988. Nutritionist on call. What diet does for wound healing. *RN* 51:73–74, 76.

Changing the dressing: Proceed with care. June 1988. *Nursing 88* 18:34–37.

Cooper, D. M. March 1990. Wound healing. *Nursing Clinics of North America* 25:163–64.

———. March 1990. Optimizing wound healing: A practice within nursing's domain. *Nursing Clinics of North America* 25:165–80.

Cooper, D. M., and Schumann, D. December 1979. Postsurgical nursing intervention as an adjunct to wound healing. *Nursing Clinics of North America* 14:713–26.

Cuzzell, J. Z. February 1985. Wound care forum: Artful solutions to chronic problems. *American Journal of Nursing* 85:163–66.

Flynn, M. E., and Rovee, D. T. October 1982. Wound healing mechanisms. *American Journal of Nursing* 82:1544–50.

Garner, J. S. April 1986. CDC guidelines for the prevention and control of nosocomial infections: Guideline for prevention of surgical wound infections, 1985. *American Journal of Infection Control* 14:71–80.

Guyton, A. C. 1986. *Textbook of medical physiology.* 7th ed. Philadelphia: W. B. Saunders Co.

Kim, M. J., McFarland, G. K., and McLane, A. M. 1989. *Pocket guide to nursing diagnoses.* 3d ed. St. Louis: C. V. Mosby Company.

Lederer, J. R., Marculescu, G. L., Mocnik, B., and Seaby, N. 1990. *Care planning pocket guide.* 3d ed. Redwood City, Calif.: Addison-Wesley Nursing.

Lehmann, J. F., and DeLateur, B. J. 1982a. *Therapeutic heat and cold.* 3d ed. Baltimore: Williams and Wilkins Co.

———. 1982b. Diathermy and superficial heat and cold therapy. In Kottke, F. J.; Stillwell, G. K.; and Lehmann, J. F. *Krusen's handbook of physical medicine and rehabilitation.* 3d ed. Philadelphia: W. B. Saunders Co.

Lomas, C. September 21–27, 1988. From theory to practice . . . wound care. *Nursing Times* 84:63, 65–66.

McConnell, E. A. June 1990. How to tape a dressing. *Nursing 90* 20:23.

Meehan, P. A., and Mayz, E. J. June 1988. Nursing management of an open abdominal wound. *Critical Care Nurse* 8:29–30, 32–34.

Morison, M. J. February 1989. Wound cleansing—which solution? *Professional Nurse* 4:220–22, 224–25.

Neuberger, G. B., and Reckling, J. B. February 1985. A new look at wound care. *Nursing 85* 15:1 (Canadian ed., pp. 34–41).

Nichols, R. L., January/February 1982. Techniques known to prevent post-operative wound infection. *Infection Control* 3:34–37.

Piper, S. M. May 1989. Effective use of occlusive wound dressings. *Professional Nurse* 4:402–4.

Pollack, S. V. November/December 1981. Wound healing: A review: I. The biology of wound healing. *Journal of Enterostomal Therapy* 8:16–18, 19, 21, 39.

———. January/February 1982a. Wound healing: A review: II. Environmental factors affecting wound healing. *Journal of Enterostomal Therapy* 9:14–16, 35.

———. March/April 1982b. Wound healing: A review: III. Nutritional factors affecting wound healing. *Journal of Enterostomal Therapy* 9:28–29, 32–33.

Sieggreen, M. Y. June 1987. Healing of physical wounds. *Nursing Clinics of North America* 22:439–47.

Slahetka, F. May/June 1984. Dakin's solution for deep ulcers. *Geriatric Nursing* 5:168–69.

Sutton, J. September 20–26, 1989. Accurate wound assessment. *Nursing Times* 85:68, 71.

Taylor, D. L. May 1983. Wound healing: Physiology, signs and symptoms. *Nursing 83* 13:44–45.

Thomason, S. S. September/October 1989. Front-line antiseptics. *Geriatric Nursing* 10:235–36.

Westaby, S., editor. 1986. *Wound care.* St. Louis: C. V. Mosby Co.

Whitney, J. D. September 1989. Physiologic effects of tissue oxygenation on wound healing. *Heart and Lung* 18:466–76.

Wooding-Scott, M. December 1988. No wound is too big for resourceful nurses. *RN* 51:22–25.

Wright, N. E. July/August 1983. Abdominal wounds: Breakdown and dehiscence. *Journal of Enterostomal Therapy* 10:143–44.

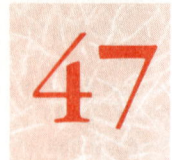
Perioperative Care

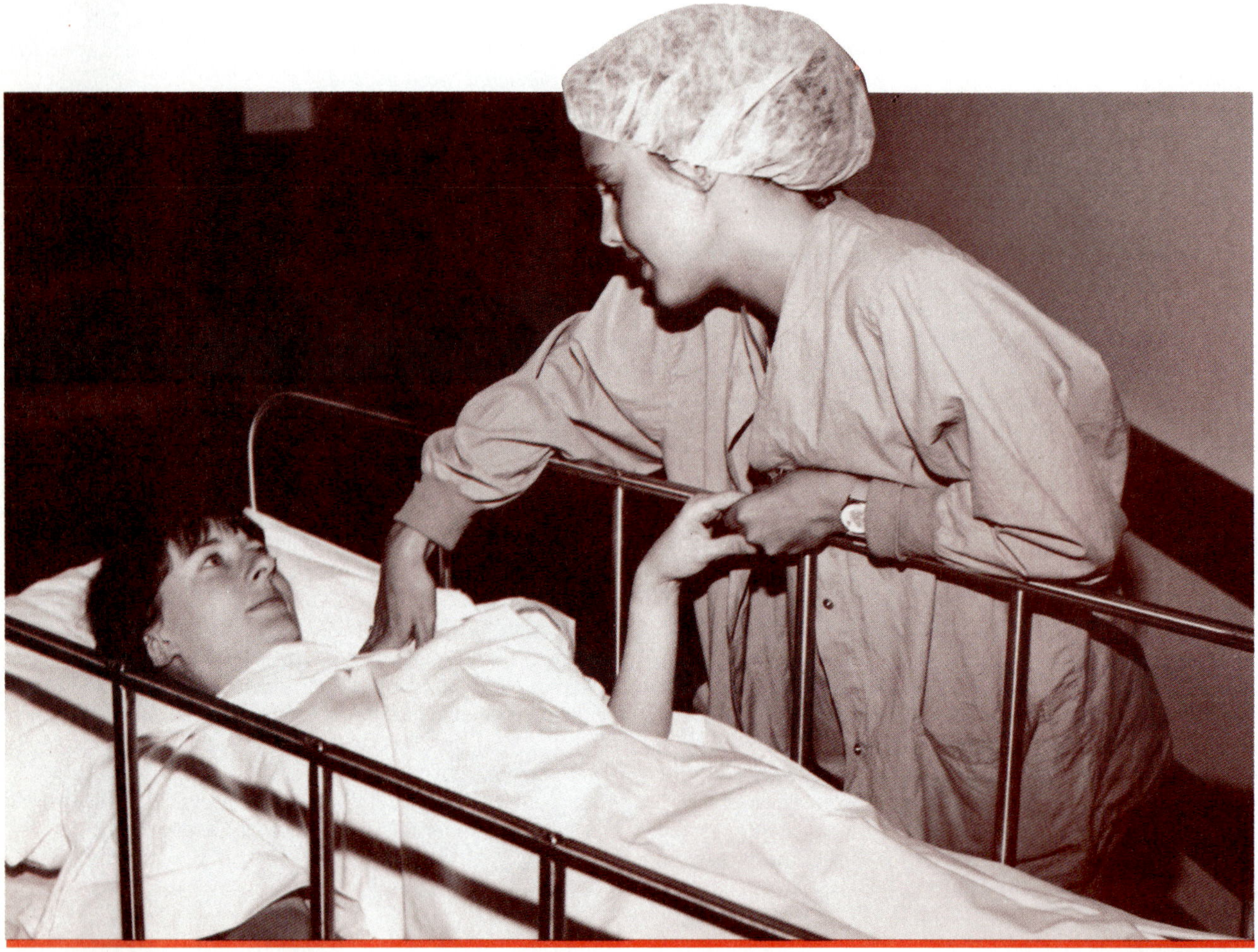

OBJECTIVES

▶ Describe the phases of the perioperative period.

▶ Discuss the legal aspects of surgery.

▶ Describe the elements of surgical risk.

▶ Outline the various aspects of preoperative assessment.

▶ Give examples of pertinent nursing diagnoses for surgical clients.

▶ Identify the essential nursing responsibilities included in planning perioperative nursing care.

▶ Describe how to teach clients to move, perform leg exercises, and perform coughing and deep breathing exercises.

▶ Identify the essentials of preoperative skin preparation.

▶ Explain why gastric intubation may be used for surgical clients.

▶ Describe some of the ways to protect a client from injury.

▶ Identify circumstances in which the nurse monitors a client.

▶ Discuss the importance of documentation with reference to preoperative, intraoperative, and postoperative recording.

▶ Identify potential postoperative complications and describe nursing interventions to prevent them.

▶ Identify outcome criteria by which to evaluate the effectiveness of perioperative nursing interventions.

THE PERIOPERATIVE PERIOD

Operations are traumatic for both clients and their support persons. Although increasing numbers of elective and minor surgical procedures are being performed in day-surgery centers, most operations still take place in hospitals, which many people associate with pain and death. Because many clients equate operations with disfigurement and pain, the nurse must be sensitive to the psychologic as well as physiologic needs of clients having operations.

The **perioperative** period is the time before, during, and after an operation; it encompasses three phases: preoperative, intraoperative, and postoperative. The **preoperative phase** begins when the decision for surgical intervention is made, and it ends when the client is transferred to the operating room bed. The preoperative client is prepared psychologically and physically for surgery. An important aspect of preoperative nursing is teaching clients what they need to know. The **intraoperative phase** begins when the client is transferred to the operating room bed, and it terminates when the client is admitted to the postanesthetic area. The main intraoperative nursing function is to maintain the client's safety.

The **postoperative phase** is the time following surgery. It begins with admission to the Post Anesthetic Care Unit (PACU), also referred to as the Recovery Room (RR), and ends when the client has completely recovered from the surgery. Major postoperative nursing functions are

- Helping the client recover from anesthesia
- Maintaining the client's body systems
- Preventing postoperative complications
- Preventing undue discomfort

Prior to any surgical procedure, clients must sign a surgical consent form. See Figure 47–1. This requirement protects clients from having any surgical procedure they do not want or do not know about. It also protects the hospital and the health personnel from a claim by client or family that permission was not granted. The consent form becomes a part of the client's record and goes to the operating room with the client.

Obtaining legal, informed consent to perform surgery is the responsibility of the surgeon. Informed consent is possible only when the client is told in advance of the character and importance of the surgery, its probable consequences, the chances for success, and alternative measures. Often a nurse is responsible for witnessing a consent. Nurses must be aware of their responsibilities regarding consents and of the particular hospital's policies. See Chapter 8, page 153, for information about informed consent.

Types of Surgery

Surgical procedures are commonly grouped into three general categories according to (a) urgency, (b) risk, and (c) purpose.

Degree of Urgency   In terms of urgency, surgery can be classified into three types: urgent, elective, and optional. **Urgent surgery** is performed for reasons of health, such as the removal of an inflamed appendix. Urgent surgery is always essential but not always an emergency. An emergency operation to control internal hemorrhaging is one kind of urgent surgery; another type is breast surgery for a malignancy. **Elective surgery** is performed for the client's well-being though not absolutely necessary for life, such as

EL CAMINO HOSPITAL DISTRICT
AUTHORIZATION AND CONSENT TO SURGERY, ANESTHESIA, DIAGNOSTIC OR THERAPEUTIC PROCEDURES

YOUR DOCTOR IS _____

THE OPERATION(S) OR PROCEDURE(S) TO BE PERFORMED IS/ARE:

_____
(MEDICAL TERMINOLOGY)

_____
(LAY TERMINOLOGY)

1. The hospital maintains personnel and facilities to assist your doctor in his performance of various surgical operations and other special diagnostic and therapeutic procedures. These operations and procedures may all involve risks of unsuccessful results, complications, injury, or even death, from both known and unforeseen causes, and no warranty or guarantee is made as to result or cure. You have the right to be informed of such risks as well as the nature and purpose of the operation(s) or procedure(s) and the available alternative methods of treatment and this form is not a substitute for such explanations which are provided by the above named physician. Except in cases of emergency, the operation(s) or procedure(s) is/are not performed until the patient has had the opportunity to receive such explanations. You may refuse any proposed operation or procedure anytime prior to its performance.

2. Your doctor has recommended the operation(s) or procedure(s) set forth above. Upon your authorization and consent, such operation(s) or procedure(s), together with any different or further procedure(s) which in the opinion of your doctor may be indicated due to any emergency, will be performed on you. The operation(s) or procedure(s) will be performed by the doctor named above together with associates and assistants, including anesthesiologists and radiologists from the medical staff of El Camino Hospital. Your attending physician, surgeon, assistant surgeon, anesthesiologist, and other physicians are not agents, servants or employees of the hospital or your doctor but are independent contractors, and therefore your agents.

3. Your signature below authorizes the hospital pathologist to use his or her discretion in disposition of any member, organ or other tissue removed from your person during the above-named procedure(s).

4. Your signature below constitutes your acknowledgement (1) that you have read and agree to the foregoing; (2) that the operation(s) or procedure(s) set forth above has/have been adequately explained to you by your doctor and that you have received all of the information you desire concerning such operation(s) or procedure(s); (3) that you authorize and consent to the performance of the operation(s) or procedure(s); (4) and that you acknowledge receipt of a copy of this authorization.

SIGNATURE:_____   _____
          PATIENT/PARENT/LEGAL GUARDIAN   DATE AND TIME

_____   _____
             RELATIONSHIP   WITNESS (NOT PATIENT'S DOCTOR)

_____
     REASON PATIENT UNABLE TO SIGN

Figure 47–1 A sample surgical consent form. **Source:** Courtesy of El Camino Hospital, Mountain View, California.

straightening a bent finger. It may be planned weeks or months ahead. **Optional surgery** is requested by the client though not necessary for physical health. Usually an operation such as facial plastic surgery is optional, being performed for psychologic reasons.

Degree of Risk   Surgery is classified as major or minor according to the degree of risk to the client. **Major surgery** involves a high degree of risk, for a variety of reasons: it may be complicated or prolonged; large losses of blood may occur; vital organs may be involved; or postoperative complications may be likely. Examples of major surgery are organ transplant, open heart surgery, and removal of a kidney. In contrast, **minor surgery** involves little risk, produces few complications, and may be performed in a "day surgery." Examples are breast biopsy, removal of tonsils, and removal of polyps from the nose.

Purpose   Surgical procedures are also categorized according to their purpose. **Diagnostic surgery** enables the surgeon to confirm a diagnosis. **Exploratory surgery** is frequently performed to determine the extent of a pathologic process and sometimes to confirm a diagnosis. For example, an exploratory laparotomy (opening into the abdomen) may be done to assess the extent of a cancerous growth. **Palliative surgery** is performed to relieve symptoms of a disease process without correcting the disease causing the symptoms. For example, if a client has an inoperable, obstructive malignant tumor of the bowel, an intestinal bypass operation (colostomy) may be done to relieve the discomfort caused by the obstruction. **Reconstructive surgery** refers to the repair of tissues or organs whose appearance or function has been damaged. Two examples are a vaginal repair and plastic surgery to repair a body part following extensive scarring from a burn. **Constructive surgery** is performed to correct a congenitally malformed organ or tissue, such as a harelip. **Ablative surgery** refers to the removal of a diseased organ such as the gallbladder or appendix. The term *ablate,* of Latin derivation, means "take away or cut off."

Types of Anesthesia

General anesthesia is the loss of all sensation and consciousness. A general anesthetic acts by blocking awareness centers in the brain so that amnesia (loss of memory), analgesia (insensibility to pain), hypnosis (artificial sleep), and relaxation (rendering a part of the body less tense) occur. General anesthetics are administered by intravenous infusion or by inhalation of gases or vapors delivered through a mask or through an endotracheal tube inserted into the trachea. Often, an intravenous drug such as thiopental sodium (Pentothal) is used to render the client unconscious and is then supplemented with other agents to produce surgical anesthesia.

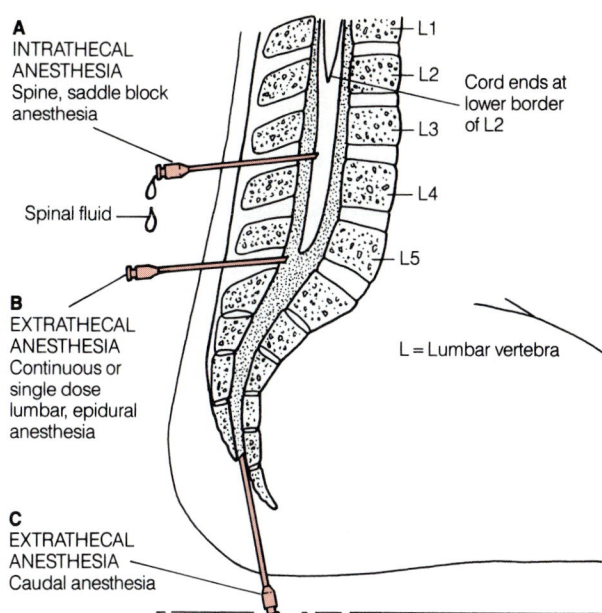

Figure 47–2   Anatomic sites for spinal anesthetics.

General anesthesia has certain advantages. Because the client is unconscious rather than awake and anxious, respiration and cardiac function are readily regulated. Also, the anesthesia can be adjusted to the length of the operation and the client's age and physical status. Its chief disadvantage is that it depresses the respiratory and circulatory systems. Some clients become more anxious about a general anesthetic than about the surgery itself. Often this is because they fear losing the capacity to control their own bodies.

Regional anesthesia is the loss of sensation in one area of the body due to the blockage of sensory impulses to the brain. The client remains conscious. A number of methods are employed, such as spinal anesthesia, nerve block, and epidural block. **Spinal anesthesia** requires a lumbar puncture. See Figure 47–2, *A.* The physician injects the anesthetic into the spinal canal (subarachnoid space). One type of spinal anesthesia is the saddle anesthesia, a "low spinal," which affects the lower lumbar nerves (L1–5) and sacral nerves (S1–4). Commonly used anesthetic agents are lidocaine hydrochloride (Xylocaine) and tetracaine hydrochloride (Pontocaine). A **nerve block** involves the injection of an anesthetic agent into a nerve plexus to anesthetize part of the body. For instance, injecting tetracaine into the brachial plexus interrupts the nerve impulses and anesthetizes the arm. For **lumbar epidural anesthesia,** the agent is injected through the lumbar interspace into the epidural space, i.e., outside the spinal canal. See Figure 47–2, *B.* The agent infiltrates the tissues and affects a band around the client's body at the level of the injection. In **caudal anesthesia,** the needle is inserted through the sacral hiatus into the caudal canal. See Figure 47–2, *C.* The client may assume a lateral or knee-chest position for the administration of a caudal anesthetic.

Local anesthesia is the loss of sensation in a small area of tissue. An anesthetic agent may be sprayed onto the skin or mucous membrane or injected into the tissue. For instance, proparacaine hydrochloride (Alcaine) commonly is used in a 0.5% solution to anesthetize the eye. Tetracaine, lidocaine (Xylocaine), and bupivacaine hydrochloride (Marcaine) are commonly used as injectable anesthetic agents. The chief advantage of this method is that the anesthetic acts quickly and has few side-effects.

PREOPERATIVE ASSESSING

Preoperative assessment includes clinical assessment of the client for identification of surgical risk factors and collection of a database used during postoperative evaluation.

The nurse also ensures that scheduled screening tests are completed, preparing the client beforehand and monitoring afterward when necessary.

Assessing Surgical Risk

The degree of risk involved in a surgical procedure is affected by the client's age, nutritional status, fluid and electrolyte status, general health, use of medications, and mental health and attitude.

Age   Very young and elderly clients are greater surgical risks than children and adults. A neonate's physiologic response to surgery is substantially different from an adult's. Factors that affect the risk are the neonate's circulation, which is largely central, and renal function, which is not fully developed until about 6 months of age. The neonate can respond to an additional need for oxygen only with an

TABLE 47–1   *Risk Factors for the Elderly Surgical Client*

Physiologic Change	Preoperative Nursing Interventions
Integumentary System	
Vulnerable skin due to venous stasis and poor venous return	Teach passive and active exercises.
	Measure the client for antiemboli stockings.
Cardiovascular System	
Reduced cardiac reserve due to changes in the myocardium	Determine usual pattern of ADLs and how quickly the client tires.
Tachycardia from anxiety, which is tolerated poorly in the elderly heart	Teach about and support anxiety reduction.
Decreased compliance of blood vessels due to atherosclerosis	Teach leg exercises and turning.
	Obtain baseline data re vital signs.
	Monitor blood pressure closely for hypertension.
Respiratory System	
Reduced vital capacity due to lowered expansibility of the rib cage	Teach deep breathing and coughing.
	Obtain baseline data re respirations.
Urinary System	
Reduced blood flow to the kidneys.	Obtain baseline urine output for 24 hours.
Reduced ability to excrete toxins due to reduced glomerular filtration	Initiate fluid intake and output recordings.
Fluids and Electrolytes	
Dehydration from repeated enemas.	Assess hydration status for baseline data.
Hypokalemia due to diarrhea	Monitor fluid intake and output.
Neurologic System	
Reduced sensory acuity	Orient client to surroundings.
Decreased reaction time	Allow time for client to proceed at own pace.

increased respiratory rate, and limited blood volume results in a limited fluid reserve.

Elderly persons are frequently at additional risk from surgery because of impaired circulation due to arteriosclerosis and limited cardiac function. Energy reserves are often limited, and hydration and nutritional status may be poor. In addition, the older person may be highly sensitive to medications such as morphine sulfate and barbiturates, frequently used preoperatively and postoperatively. See Table 47–1 for risk factors for the elderly surgical client.

Nutritional Status

Two nutritional problems that can increase surgical risk are obesity and malnutrition due to protein, iron, and vitamin deficiencies. Surgery for obese clients is often deferred, except in emergencies. The obese often have overtaxed hearts and elevated blood pressures. In addition, incisions in overly fatty tissue are difficult to suture and prone to infection.

Nutritional deficiencies are particularly common among elderly clients and chronically ill clients. Protein and vitamins are needed for wound healing; vitamin K is essential for blood clotting.

Fluid and Electrolyte Status

Dehydration and hypovolemia predispose a client to problems during surgery. Electrolyte imbalances often accompany fluid imbalances. Imbalances in calcium, magnesium, potassium, and hydrogen ions are of particular concern during surgery. See Chapter 40.

General Health

Surgery is least risky when the client's general health is good. Any infection or pathophysiology increases the risk. Of particular concern are upper respiratory tract infections, which together with a general anesthetic can adversely affect respiratory function. Common health problems that increase surgical risk and may lead to the decision to postpone or cancel surgery are listed in the accompanying box.

Medications

The regular use of certain medications can increase surgical risk.

- *Anticoagulants.* Increase blood coagulation time.
- *Tranquilizers.* May cause hypotension and thus contribute to shock.
- *Heroin and other depressants.* Decrease central nervous system responses.
- *Antibiotics.* May be incompatible with anesthetic agents, resulting in untoward reactions.
- *Diuretics.* May precipitate electrolyte (especially potassium) imbalances.

 Since some medications interact adversely with other medications and with anesthetic agents, preoperative assessment should include careful collection of a medica-

---

Health Problems that Increase Surgical Risk

- *Cardiac conditions* such as angina pectoris, recent myocardial infarction, severe hypertension, and severe congestive heart failure. Well-controlled cardiac problems generally pose minimal operative risk.
- *Blood coagulation disorders* that may lead to severe bleeding, hemorrhage, and subsequent shock.
- *Upper respiratory tract infections* or *chronic obstructive lung diseases,* such as emphysema. These conditions, especially when exacerbated by the effects of general anesthesia, adversely affect pulmonary function. They also predispose the client to postoperative lung infections.
- *Renal disease* that impairs the regulation of the body's fluids and electrolytes, e.g., renal insufficiency.
- *Diabetes mellitus,* which predisposes the client to wound infection and delayed healing.
- *Liver disease,* e.g., cirrhosis, which impairs the liver's abilities to detoxify medications used during surgery, produce the prothrombin necessary for blood clotting, and metabolize nutrients essential for healing.
- *Uncontrolled neurologic disease,* such as epilepsy.

---

tion history. Clients may be unaware of the potential adverse interactions of medications and may fail to report the use of medications used for conditions unrelated to the indication for surgery. The astute nurse interviewer may question the client and family about the use of commonly prescribed medications (and over-the-counter preparations) for specific conditions mentioned during the nursing history.

Mental Health and Attitude

Extreme anxiety can increase surgical risk. The level of anxiety does not always correspond to the seriousness of the surgical procedure. The surgeon needs to know if a person fears death during surgery. In some instances, professional counseling and a delay in the surgery are indicated.

Clients who have shown poor psychologic adjustment for some time may not be able to cope with the additional stress of surgery. People who cope only minimally in a stable, familiar environment can develop emotional problems postoperatively.

Nursing History

The nursing history obtained before surgery provides client data that help the nurse to plan preoperative and postoperative care. Although forms vary considerably among

Preoperative Nursing History

- *Physical condition.* General appearance (i.e., skin coloring, weight, hydration status, and energy level)
- *Mental attitude.* Mild anxiety is a normal response to surgery; severe anxiety can increase surgical risk.
- *Understanding of surgical procedure.* A well-informed client knows what to expect and in general accepts and copes more effectively with surgery and convalescence.
- *Previous experience.* May influence the physical and psychologic responses to the planned surgery.
- *Expected outcomes.* May alter a client's body image and life-style to varying degrees.
- *Medications.* List all current medications. Certain medications, such as anticonvulsants and insulin, must be continued throughout the operative period to prevent adverse effects. A physician's order to this effect is required, however.
- *Smoking.* Smokers' lung tissue may be chronically irritated, and a general anesthetic agent irritates it further.
- *Alcohol.* Heavy, consistent use can lead to problems during anesthesia, surgery, and recovery.
- *Coping resources.* Employing previously effective coping mechanisms or developing new strategies (e.g., diversional activities such as reading and relaxation exercises) may be helpful.
- *Self-concept.* A healthy, positive self-concept predisposes clients to approach a surgical experience with confidence that they can handle it successfully.
- *Body image.* Possible disfigurement or change in physical identity may be a concern prior to surgery. Providing accurate information often allays fears based on misconceptions.

agencies, essential preoperative information that should be included is summarized in the box above.

Screening Tests

The physician orders preoperative radiologic and laboratory tests and examinations. Abnormalities may warrant treatment prior to surgery. The nurse's responsibility is to check the orders carefully, to see that they are carried out, and to ensure that the results are obtained prior to surgery. See Table 47–2 for routine preoperative screening tests. In addition to these routine tests, diagnostic tests directly related to the client's disease are usually appropriate (e.g., stomach roentgenography to clarify the pathologic condition before gastric surgery).

PREOPERATIVE DIAGNOSING

Examples of nursing diagnoses for the preoperative client are shown below.

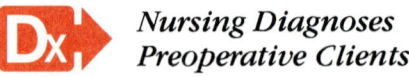 **Nursing Diagnoses**
Preoperative Clients

Fear related to:
- Effects of surgery on ability to function in usual roles
- Outcome of exploratory surgery for malignancy
- Risk of death
- Loss of control during anesthesia or waking up during anesthesia
- Perceived inadequate postoperative analgesia

Knowledge deficit (preoperative routines and postoperative exercises and activities)

Sleep pattern disturbance related to:
- Hospital routines
- Psychologic stress

Anticipatory grieving related to:
- Perceived loss of body part associated with planned surgery

Ineffective individual coping related to:
- Conflicting values (e.g., need for blood transfusion versus the religious values of a Jehovah's Witness)
- Lack of clear outcomes of surgery
- Unresolved past negative experience with surgery

PREOPERATIVE PLANNING

The duration of the preoperative period often affects preoperative care and planning. When the preoperative period lasts several days, nurses can draw up a nursing care plan and a teaching plan. When the preoperative period is just an hour, only the essentials can be carried out. In this case, the learning needs of the client must be met prior to admission to the clinical agency during the postoperative period.

Planning for the preoperative period should involve the client and support persons. The following are essential nursing responsibilities.

- Identify and meet the learning needs of clients and support persons
- Promote the client's peace of mind
- Meet fluid and nutritional needs

TABLE 47–2 *Routine Preoperative Screening Tests*

Test	Rationale
Urinalysis	To detect urinary tract infections and glucose in the urine.
Chest roentgenography	To identify lung pathology and heart size and location.
Electrocardiography (usual for clients who have cardiac pathology)	To determine cardiac pathology
Complete blood count (CBC)	To determine Hgb, Hct, RBC (i.e., the blood's ability to carry oxygen), and WBC, which signals infection when elevated
Blood grouping and cross-matching	To establish blood type for possible blood transfusion
Serum electrolytes (Na^+, K^+, Mg^{2+}, Ca^{2+}, H^+)	To determine electrolyte imbalances
Fasting blood sugar	To detect presence of glucose in the blood, which may indicate metabolic disorders, e.g., diabetes mellitus
Blood urea nitrogen (BUN) or creatinine	To assess urinary excretion

■ Promote rest

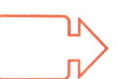

■ Ensure appropriate physical preparation to prevent aspiration, injury, infection, and other complications associated with anesthesia

■ Protect the client's personal property during the intraoperative period

The overall goal in the preoperative period should reflect that the client is physically and psychologically prepared for surgery. Examples of outcome criteria to evaluate achievement of these goals and the effectiveness of nursing interventions follow.

Outcome Criteria Preoperative Clients

The client:

■ Describes in general terms the proposed surgical procedure, reason for it, subsequent therapy, and expected length of stay in hospital.

■ Verbalizes understanding of events (e.g., transfer to post-anesthesia room or intensive care unit) and therapeutic devices (e.g., monitoring equipment, infusions) in all perioperative phases.

■ States reasons for preoperative and postoperative procedures (e.g., skin prep, bowel prep) and practices (e.g., deep breathing, coughing, turning, leg exercises).

■ Demonstrates deep breathing, coughing, splinting, leg exercises, and moving techniques as taught.

■ Verbalizes expectations and understanding of usual postoperative pain control and activity.

■ Expresses feelings about the surgery and its expected outcomes.

■ Expresses feelings of achieving adequate rest and sleep.

■ Demonstrates balanced fluid intake and output.

■ Remains free from infection, as manifested by baseline temperature and pulse rate.

PREOPERATIVE IMPLEMENTING

Preoperative Teaching

An explanation of perioperative care informs the client and the support persons about the perioperative period. Usually, people are anxious at this time, and many have misconceptions about surgery and surgical care. Clients often

RESEARCH NOTE

Does Relaxation Training Affect Postoperative Pain?

Nurses play a role in the prevention, observation, and treatment of postoperative pain. In this study, postoperative distress was compared for cholecystectomy and hysterectomy clients. Only hysterectomy clients who reported lower pain levels were found to benefit from relaxation training. Earlier studies also have supported the idea that relaxing becomes more difficult as pain sensations increase in intensity. Thus, the value of relaxation training appears to be only in relieving the distress caused by painful sensations, not in ameliorating their intensity.

Implications: This study emphasizes the demonstrated value of relaxation training and suggests preliminary definition of those clients who will benefit most from such a program.

J. Morgan, N. Wells, and E. Robertson, 1985. Effects of preoperative teaching on postoperative pain: A replication and expansion, *International Journal of Nursing Studies,* 22(3):267–80.

ask nurses about the operation after the surgeon has gained informed consent and left the client's room. The surgeon should be notified if the client is anxious about the procedure or has questions about the surgery that the nurse cannot answer.

Clients and their support persons need to know the time and type of surgery. The surgeon usually arranges the date and may specify it in the orders. The exact time may not be known until the surgical schedule for the hospital is distributed. If a nurse does not know the exact time of surgery, the nurse should say so and inform the client and support persons as soon as the time is decided.

The nurse needs to listen attentively and carefully to help the client identify specific concerns or fears and talk them through. Typical questions are: What will happen during surgery? How will I feel after the operation? What will the surgeon find? How long will the hospital stay be? Some clients may worry about finances. Those whose surgery involves disfigurement may have problems with their self-image.

This is also the time to clarify any misconceptions the client may have. Providing accurate information and acting supportively will help the client deal with identified concerns. The nurse should not dismiss the client's concerns by saying, "Everything will be all right." Unknowns or misconceptions can produce unrealistic fears and anxiety.

The client also may have specific learning needs regarding postoperative care. For example, learning to attend to a colostomy requires preparation *before* surgery. Pain is common postoperatively; learning *beforehand* how to min-

---

Preoperative Instructions

Preoperative regimen:

- Explain the need for preoperative tests (e.g., laboratory, x-ray, ECG).
- Discuss bowel preparation, if required.
- Discuss skin preparation, including operative area and preoperative bath or shower with antimicrobial agents.
- Discuss preoperative medications.
- Explain individual therapies ordered by the physician, such as intravenous therapy, the insertion of a urinary catheter or nasogastric tube, use of a spirometer or intermittent positive pressure breathing (IPPB) machine, or antiemboli stockings.
- Discuss the visit by anesthetist.
- Explain the need to restrict food and oral fluids at least 8 hours before surgery.
- Provide a general timetable for perioperative events.
- Discuss the need for the removal of jewelry, makeup, and all prostheses (e.g., eyeglasses, hearing aids, complete or partial dentures, wig) immediately before surgery.
- Confirm time of surgery.
- Inform client about the preoperative holding area, and give the location of the waiting room for support persons.

Postoperative regimen:

- Discuss postanesthesia recovery room routines and emergency equipment.
- Review type and frequency of assessment activities.

- Teach deep-breathing and coughing exercises, leg exercises, ways to turn and move, and splinting techniques.
- Discuss pain management.
- Explain usual activity restrictions and precautions used to help clients get up for the first time postoperatively.
- Describe usual dietary alterations.
- Discuss postoperative dressings and drains.
- Provide an explanation and tour of intensive care unit if client is to be transferred there postoperatively.

Day-surgery clients:

- Confirm place and time of surgery, including when to arrive (e.g., 1 to 1½ hours before scheduled surgery) and where to register (e.g., reception desk).
- Discuss what to wear (e.g., clients having hand surgery should wear a garment with large sleeve openings to fit over a bulky dressing; all clients need to leave valuables at home).
- Explain the need for someone to accompany the client home, and arrange a place for pickup.
- Review available medical and insurance forms.
- Review with the client any tests ordered and need for a urine specimen the morning of surgery.
- Communicate, by telephone, the evening before surgery to confirm time of surgery and arrival time, and call again the evening after surgery to assess progress.

---

imize it (e.g., by holding a pillow against the abdomen when moving after abdominal surgery) reassures the client. It also is important that clients know they will receive analgesics postoperatively to minimize discomfort.

When children are involved, the nurse should provide explanations in a language they can understand and at a rate that keeps their attention and does not overwhelm them. It will also help to show the child the anesthetic equipment and the postanesthesia room ("wake-up room") before surgery, explaining all postoperative care and dis-comfort clearly and simply, for example, "You will have a sore tummy." Confirm when the parents will visit, because this is the most essential piece of information the nurse can give the child.

A summary of preoperative instructions is shown in the box on the opposite page. Clients need to be informed about what activities to expect, when to expect them, and why they are being done. Procedure 47–1 provides guidelines for teaching moving, leg exercises, deep-breathing exercises, and coughing.

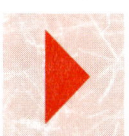

PROCEDURE 47–1

TEACHING MOVING, LEG EXERCISES, DEEP-BREATHING EXERCISES, AND COUGHING

Intervention

1. Show the client ways to turn in bed and to get out of bed.

■ Instruct a client who will have a right abdominal incision or a right-sided chest incision to turn to the left side of the bed and sit up as follows:

  a. Flex the knees.

  b. Hold the left arm and hand or a small pillow against the incision to splint the wound.

  c. Turn to the left while pushing with the right foot and grasping a partial side rail on the left side of the bed with the right hand.

  d. Come to a sitting position on the side of the bed by using the right arm and hand to push down against the mattress.

■ Ask a client with a left abdominal or left-sided chest incision to perform the same procedure but splint with the right arm and turn to the right.

■ For clients with orthopedic surgery (e.g., hip surgery), use special aids, such as a trapeze, to assist with movement.

2. Teach the client the following three leg exercises.

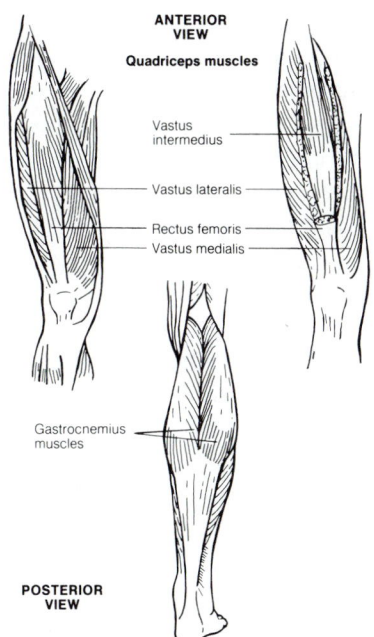

Figure 47–3 Leg muscles: anterior and posterior views.

■ Alternate dorsiflexion and plantar flexion of the feet. *This exercise is sometimes referred to as calf pumping, since it alternately contracts and relaxes the calf muscles, including the gastrocnemius muscles. See Figure 47–3.*

■ Flex and extend the knees, and press the backs of the knees into the bed while dorsiflexing the feet. See Figure 47–4. Instruct clients who cannot raise their legs to do isometric exercises that contract and relax the muscles.

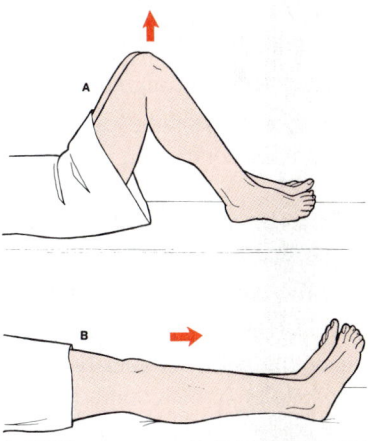

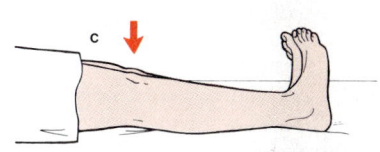

Figure 47–4 Flexing and extending the knees.

■ Raise and lower the legs alternately from the surface of the bed. Extend the knee of the moving leg. See Figure 47–5. *This exercise contracts and relaxes the quadriceps muscles.*

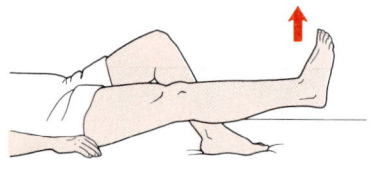

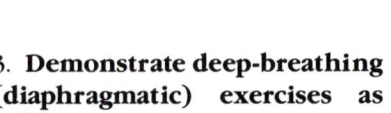

Figure 47–5   Raising and lowering the legs.

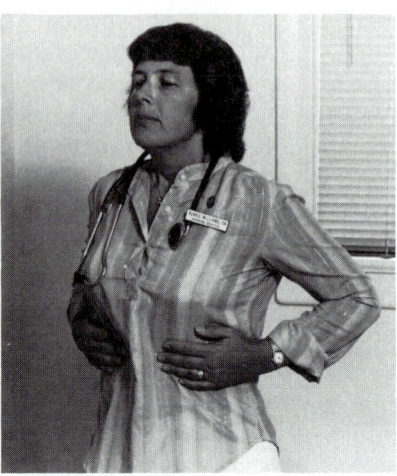

Figure 47–6 Demonstrating deep breathing.

3. Demonstrate deep-breathing (diaphragmatic) exercises as follows.

■ Place your hands palms down on the border of your rib cage, and inhale slowly and evenly through the nose until the greatest chest expansion is achieved. See Figure 47–6.

■ Hold your breath for 2 to 3 seconds.

■ Exhale slowly through the mouth.

■ Continue exhalation until maximum chest contraction is achieved.

4. Help the client perform deep-breathing exercises.

■ Ask the client to assume a sitting position.

■ Place the palms of your hands on the border of the client's rib cage to assess respiratory depth.

■ Ask the client to perform deep breathing, as described in step 3.

5. Instruct the client to cough voluntarily after a few deep inhalations.

■ Ask the client to inhale deeply, hold the breath for a few seconds, and then cough once or twice.

■ Ensure that the client coughs deeply and does not just clear the throat.

6. Demonstrate ways to splint the abdomen when coughing, if the incision will be painful when the client coughs.

■ Show the client how the nurse can support the incision by placing the palms of the hands on either side of the incision or directly over the incision, holding the palm of one hand over the other. *Coughing uses the abdominal and other accessory respiratory muscles. Splinting the incision may reduce pain while coughing if the incision is near any of these muscles.*

■ Show the client how to splint the abdomen with clasped hands and a firmly rolled pillow held against the abdomen. See Figure 47–7.

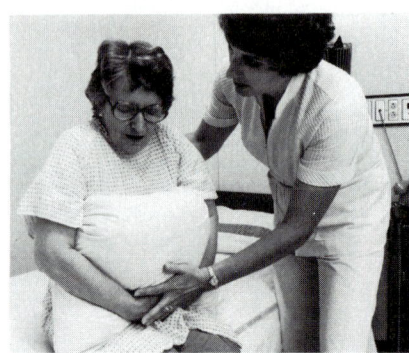

Figure 47–7   Splinting an incision with a pillow.

7. Inform the client about the expected frequency of these exercises.

■ Instruct the client to start the exercises as soon after surgery as possible.

■ Encourage clients with abdominal or chest surgery to carry out deep breathing and coughing at least three or four times daily and at each session to take a minimum of five breaths. Note, however, that the number of breaths and frequency of deep breathing varies with the client's health. People who are susceptible to pulmonary problems may need deep-breathing exercises every hour. People with chronic respiratory disease may need special breathing exercises, e.g., pursed-lip breathing, abdominal breathing, exercises using blow bottles and various kinds of incentive spirometers. See Chapter 41.

Physical Preparation

Preoperative preparation includes the following areas: nutrition and fluids, elimination, hygiene, rest, medications, care of valuables and prostheses, special orders, and surgical skin preparation. In many agencies on the day of surgery, a preoperative checklist is used. See Figure 47–8. The nurse checks the agency's forms and follows appropriate recording procedures. It is essential (a) that all pertinent records (laboratory records, x-ray films, consents) be assembled and completed so that operating and recovery room personnel can refer to them and (b) that all physical preparation is completed to ensure client safety.

Nutrition and Fluids   Adequate hydration and nutrition promote healing. Nurses need to record any sign of malnutrition. A perioperative record of the client's weight is one way to determine one aspect of nutritional status. If the client is on intravenous fluids or on measured fluid intake, nurses must ensure that the fluids are carefully measured.

Because anesthetics depress gastrointestinal functioning and because there is a danger the client may vomit and aspirate vomitus during administration of a general anesthetic, the client usually fasts at least 6 to 8 hours before surgery. The surgical client and support persons need to understand the necessity of fasting. Usually, the nurse

---

Form NS-68

ST. PAUL'S HOSPITAL
Vancouver, B.C.

PRE-OPERATIVE PREPARATION

EVENING PRIOR TO SURGERY—CHECK	Yes	Not Applicable
1. History—completed with signature		
2. Consultation (when necessary) on chart		
3. Treatment and operative consents—signed and witnessed		
4. Telephone no. of next of kin or friend:		
5. Identaband on wrist		
6. Allergy sign on chart and wristband		
7. Operative area prepared		
8. Pre-op bath or shower		
9. Pre-op teaching: a. Attended "Operation Tomorrow"		
b. Demonstrated deep breathing, coughing, and leg exercises		
c. Stated approximate time to OR and return to ward		
d. Stated expectations: • surgery planned		
• incision and dressing area		
• activity progression		
• pain and effect of analgesic		
• NPO, intravenous, diet progression		
• pre-op urine specimen		
e. Verbalized probable discharge plans		
10. H.S. sedation administered or refused—charted on anesthetic record		
11. Fasting sign posted		

DATE _____   SIGNATURE _____

IMMEDIATELY PRIOR TO SURGERY	Yes	Not Applicable
1. Pre-operative urine specimen sent		
2. Reports attached to chart—Lab, X-ray, ECG		
3. Old chart		
4. Addressograph plate attached		
5. Contact lens, wig, jewelry, make-up removed, prosthesis off		
6. Dentures and partial plates removed		
7. Voided _____ Catheterized—time _____ amount _____		
8. Patient in hospital gown		
9. Blood pressure, pulse and respirations taken at least an hour prior to pre-op medication—charted on clinical record		
10. Pre-medication administered and charted on the anesthetic record		
11. Notation made in nurses notes of time to surgery		

DATE _____   SIGNATURE _____

OPERATING ROOM	Yes	Not Applicable
1. Patient identified by circulating nurse		
2. Site of surgery checked by circulating nurse a. Left side _____ Right side _____		
b. Slate _____ Surgeon _____ History _____ Consent _____		

SIGNATURE _____

Figure 47–8   A sample preoperative checklist.
Source: Courtesy of St. Paul's Hospital, Nursing Department, Vancouver, British Columbia.

removes food and fluids from the bedside and places a fasting sign at the bed the evening before surgery. The client can use a mouthwash if the mouth feels dry but must not swallow any. If the client ingests food or fluids during the fasting period, the nurse must notify the surgeon.

Elimination   The nurse should ascertain whether the client has emptied the bowels and bladder the day of surgery. If an enema is ordered, the order will specify whether it should be given the evening prior to or the day of surgery. If it is ordered for the day of surgery, it should be administered soon enough on that day to allow the client time to expel it. A series of enemas may be needed if surgery on the bowel is planned. Sometimes, a rectal suppository is ordered instead of an enema. An enema or suppository is given because anesthesia and abdominal surgery decrease bowel activity for a few days postoperatively.

A retention catheter, if ordered, is usually inserted the day of surgery. The purpose of the catheter is to ensure that the bladder remains empty to prevent inadvertent injury to the bladder, particularly during pelvic surgery.

Hygiene   In some settings, clients are asked to bathe or shower using an antimicrobial agent the evening or morning of surgery (or both). The bath includes a shampoo whenever possible. Immediately before surgery, the client's nails should be trimmed and free of polish and all cosmetics removed so that the nail beds, skin, and lips are visible when circulation is assessed during and following surgery.

Surgical caps may be donned the day of surgery by clients in some hospitals. The surgical caps contain the client's hair and any microorganisms on the hair and scalp.

On the day of surgery, the nurse removes, or asks the client to remove, all hair pins and clips; these may cause pressure or accidental damage to the scalp when the client is unconscious. Long hair can be braided and fastened with elastic bands to keep it in place.

Rest   Nurses should do everything to help the client sleep the night before surgery. Often a sedative is ordered. Adequate rest helps the client manage the stress of surgery.

Medications   Preoperative medications also may be ordered for the day of surgery. Usually a narcotic (e.g., morphine) and a medication to dry the secretions of the mouth and respiratory tract (e.g., atropine) are given by injection. Sometimes, the surgeon orders oral sedatives (e.g., secobarbital) or tranquilizers to be administered before the injectable medications are given. A narcotic, sedative, or tranquilizer calms the client before general anesthesia and enhances a smooth anesthesia induction. Atropine or a similar drying drug minimizes the danger of aspirating secretions into the lungs. A newer trend is to give *no* preoperative medications, but if these are ordered, nurses need to administer them exactly at the time specified. Giving preoperative medications on time is essential because of their desired effect in combination with the anesthetic.

After giving the preoperative medications, the nurse informs the client that the medication will cause drowsiness and instructs the client to remain quietly in bed. The nurse raises the side rails and lowers the bed for safety, placing the call light within reach. Also, the nurse explains that scopolamine or atropine may cause thirst and that although a mouth wash may be used, no fluids should be swallowed.

Valuables and Prostheses   Valuables such as jewelry and money should be labeled and placed in safekeeping if support persons cannot take them home. In most hospitals, valuables can be kept in special envelopes and locked in a storage area on the unit. If a client wishes not to remove a wedding band, the nurse can tape it in place. Wedding bands must be removed, however, if there is danger of the fingers swelling after surgery. Situations warranting removal of a wedding band include surgery of or cast application to an arm and a mastectomy that involves removal of the lymph nodes. (Mastectomies may cause edema of the arm and hand.)

All prostheses (artificial body parts, such as partial or complete dentures, contact lenses, artificial eyes, and artificial limbs), as well as eyeglasses, wigs, false eyelashes, and hearing aids, must be removed before surgery. The nurse also checks for the presence of chewing gum or loose teeth, a common problem with 5- or 6-year-olds undergoing tonsillectomy. In some hospitals, dentures are placed in a locked storage area; in others they are placed in labeled containers and kept at the client's bedside. Partial dentures can become dislodged and obstruct an unconscious client's breathing. Loose teeth can become dislodged and be aspirated during anesthesia. Other prostheses may become damaged.

Special Orders   The nurse checks the surgeon's orders for special requirements, e.g., the insertion of a nasogastric tube prior to surgery; the administration of medications, such as insulin; or the application of antiemboli stockings. For the technique of inserting and removing a nasogastric tube, see Procedure 39–1, p. 1023.

Surgical Skin Preparation   The surgeon usually indicates the type of surgery in the preoperative orders on the client's chart. From this information, the nurse determines the kind and extent of skin preparation required (if not already specified on the order). Agencies often have protocols to follow regarding skin preparation areas; for example, the area should be larger than the incision area. In many hospitals skin preparation is done by operating room personnel.

The purpose of a surgical skin preparation is to reduce the risk of postoperative wound infection. This is done by

- Removing soil and transient microbes from the skin
- Reducing the resident microbial count to subpathogenic

amounts in a short period of time and with the least amount of tissue irritation

■ Inhibiting rapid rebound growth of microbes

Prior to any skin preparation, the nurse carefully inspects the prospective surgical area for growths, moles, rashes, pustules, irritations, exudate, abrasions, bruises or any broken or ischemic areas. These should be recorded and reported to the surgeon. In addition, the nurse must determine whether the client is allergic to any of the solutions used in the skin preparation, e.g., a depilatory.

The Association of Operating Room Nurses states that cleansing can be accomplished before surgery by having the client shower, by washing the operative site in the client unit, and/or by washing the operative site immediately before applying the antimicrobial agent in the operating room. (AORN 1988, p. 950).

Hair removal of an operative site is not recommended unless the hair interferes with the surgical procedure, e.g., craniotomy. If hair removal is required at the operative site, it should be performed in a client care area that provides privacy and good lighting. There are three methods:

1. Applying a **depilatory** (cream hair remover), which can be used before the client's arrival in the surgical suite (a skin sensitivity test should be done before application)

2. Using an electric clipper with a disposable or removable head that can be sterilized between clients

3. Shaving with a sharp, well-designed disposable or terminally sterilized razor.

Hair should be shaved only when other methods of hair removal are not available or when time does not permit their use. Shaving should be done as close to the time of the operative procedure as possible. The wet method of shaving is preferred. Persons performing the shave prep should wear protective gloves (AORN 1988, p. 951). Surgical skin preparation is detailed in Procedure 47–2.

Antiemboli Stockings   Antiemboli (elastic) stockings are indicated for clients who have problems with circulation to their feet and legs. The elastic material compresses the veins of the legs and thereby facilitates the return of venous blood to the heart. These stockings are frequently applied preoperatively as well as postoperatively.

There are several types of stockings. One type extends from the foot to the knee and another from the foot to midthigh. These stockings usually have a partial foot that exposes either the heel or toes so that extremity circulation can be assessed. See Figure 47–9. Elastic stockings usually come in small, medium, and large sizes. The accompanying box summarizes the assessments the nurse should make before applying antiemboli stockings.

Procedure 47–3 describes how to measure and apply antiemboli stockings. Many agencies use a measuring guide supplied by the stocking manufacturer.

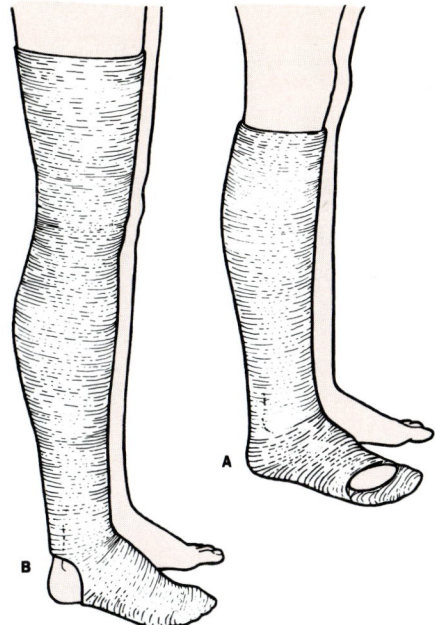

Figure 47–9 Two types of antiemboli stockings: *A,* extending to the knee, with an opening above the toes; *B,* extending to mid-thigh, with the heel exposed.

Criteria for Antiemboli Stockings

■ *Inadequate arterial blood circulation:* cool skin temperature in a warm environment; pallor; shiny, taut skin; mild edema.

■ *Insufficient venous blood return:* thickening of the skin; increased pigmentation around the ankles; pitting edema (edema in which firm finger pressure on the skin produces an indentation, or pit, that remains for several seconds); peripheral cyanosis.

■ *Altered posterior tibial* and *dorsalis pedis pulses:* Rates, volumes, and rhythms.

■ *Pain in the calf of the leg.* The nurse dorsiflexes the client's foot abruptly and firmly while the client's knee is straight or slightly flexed to assess pain in the calf (Homans' sign). The presence of pain is a positive Homans' sign.

■ *Distended superficial veins in the legs:* Normally veins may appear distended in a dependent position but collapse when the limb is elevated.

Equipment ☑

Adequate lighting for clear visibility of the hair on the skin

Bath blanket

Depilatory:

Cream hair remover with or without applicator

Washcloth

Gauze squares

Lukewarm water

Clipping:

Electric clippers with sharp heads and unbroken teeth

Scissors for long hair, if needed

Antimicrobial solution and applicators, if needed

Wet shave:

Skin preparation set containing a disposable razor, compartmentalized basin for solutions, moistureproof drape, soap solution, sponges, and cotton-tipped applicators

Warm water

Disposable gloves

Intervention

1. Drape the client appropriately.

■ Expose only the area to be prepared. If using clippers or a razor, expose only small areas at a time. You will clip or shave about 15 cm (6 in) at a time.

2. If a depilatory is to be used, test the client's reaction to it. *Some people may experience irritation or an allergic reaction, even after prior use without an adverse effect.*

■ Apply a small amount of the depilatory on a small part of the area where hair is to be removed. Use an area at the periphery of the skin prep area or area advised by the agency policy.

■ Apply the cream to the test area smoothly and thickly. Do not rub it in.

■ Leave the cream on for the specified time.

■ Remove the depilatory by rinsing the area thoroughly with lukewarm water and a washcloth. Do not use soap.

■ Pat, rather than rub, the area dry with gauze squares.

■ Wait for 24 hours, and assess the client's skin for redness or other responses.

3. Remove hair.

Depilatory:

■ If the client's skin appears normal after the skin test, apply the depilatory.

  a. Apply the depilatory as described above, and leave it in place for the *minimum* time specified by the manufacturer.

  b. Check a small area. If hair does not wipe off easily, wait a few minutes and check again, but do not leave the cream on longer than the *maximum* time recommended by the manufacturer.

  c. Remove all the depilatory as described in step 2, and pat the area dry.

Clipping:

■ Make sure the area is dry.

■ Remove hair with clippers; do not apply pressure. *Pressure can cause abrasions, particularly over bony prominences.*

■ Move the drape, and repeat the above steps until the entire area to be prepared is clipped.

■ If applying antimicrobial solution, follow Step 4.

Wet shave:

■ Place the moistureproof towel under the area to be prepared.

■ Lather the skin well with the soap solution. *Lathering makes the hair easier and softer to remove.*

■ Stretch the skin taut, and hold the razor at about a 45° angle to the skin.

■ Shave in the direction in which the hair grows. Use short strokes, and rinse the razor frequently. *Rinsing removes hairs and lather that can obstruct the blade.*

■ Wipe excess hair off the skin with the sponges.

■ Move the drape and repeat the above steps until the entire area to be prepared is shaved.

4. Clean and disinfect the surgical area according to agency practice.

■ This may be done in the operating room.

■ Clean any body crevices, such as the umbilicus, nails, and ear canals, with applicators and solutions. Dry with swabs.

■ If an antimicrobial solution is used, apply to the area immediately after it is clipped. Leave it for the designated time, then dry the area with clean swabs. Agency policy will guide you on whether to use an antimicrobial solution and, if so, which to use and how long to leave it on.

5. Inspect the skin after hair removal.

- Closely observe the skin for reddened or broken areas.
- Report to the nurse in charge any skin lesions.

6. Dispose of used equipment appropriately.

⚠ - Dispose of razor blade, if used, according to agency policy to prevent injury to others.
- Discard disposable supplies.

7. Document relevant information.

- Record the procedure, area prepared, and status of skin in the skin preparation area.

Sample Recording

Date: 12/5/91	Time: 0830

Area clipped on left lower extremity. Skin intact. Appeared tense. Stated: "I hope the scar won't show much." ————
————————Eunice L. Lentz, NS

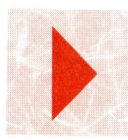

PROCEDURE 47–3

MEASURING AND APPLYING ANTIEMBOLI STOCKINGS

Equipment ☑

Measuring tape
Size chart
Correct size of elastic stockings

Intervention

1. Select an appropriate time to apply the stockings.

- Apply stockings in the morning, if possible, before the client arises. *In sitting and standing positions, the veins can become distended and edema occurs; the stockings should be applied before this happens.*
- Assist the client who has been ambulating to lie down and elevate the legs for 15 to 30 minutes before applying the stockings. *This facilitates venous return and reduces swelling.*

2. Obtain measurements to ascertain stocking size.

For knee-length stockings:

- Measure the circumference of the calf at the widest point, i.e., 15 cm (6 in) below the inferior aspect of the patella. See Figure 47–10.

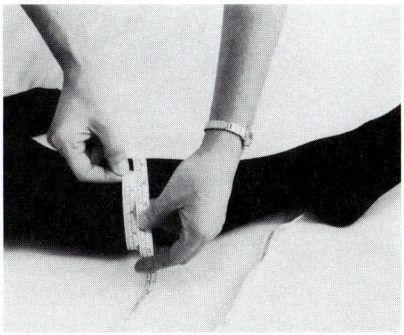

Figure 47–10 Measuring the calf circumference.

- Measure the length of the leg from the heel to the popliteal space. See Figure 47–11.

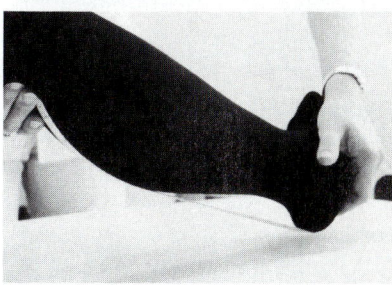

Figure 47–11 Measuring from the heel to the popliteal space.

For thigh-length stockings:

- Measure the circumference of the calf as above.

- Measure the circumference of the thigh at the widest point, i.e., 15 cm (6 in) above the superior aspect of the patella. See Figure 47–12.

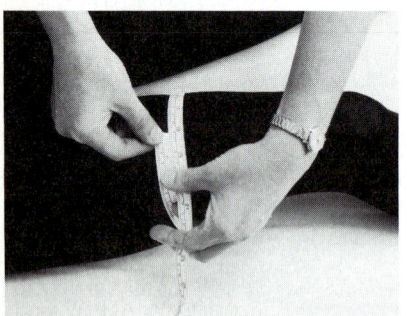

Figure 47–12 Measuring the thigh circumference.

- Measure the length of the leg from the heel to the gluteal fold. See Figure 47–13.

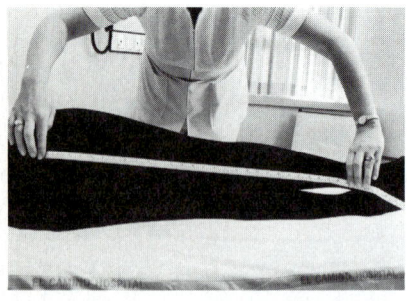

Figure 47–13 Measuring from the heel to the gluteal fold.

For waist-length stockings:

- Measure the circumference of the calf as above.

- Measure the circumference of the thigh as above.

- Measure the leg length from the bottom of the heel to the waist along the side of the body.

For all types of stockings:

- Compare the measurements to the size chart to obtain stockings of correct size.

3. **Apply the elastic stocking to the foot.**

- Assist the client to a lying position in bed.

- Dust the ankle with talcum powder, and ask the client to point the toes. *These measures ease application.*

- Turn the stocking inside out by inserting your hand into the stocking from the top and grabbing the heel pocket from the inside. The foot portion should now be inside the stocking leg.

- Remove your hand, and, with the heel pocket downward, hook your index and middle fingers of both hands into the foot section.

- Face the client, and slip the foot portion of the stocking over the client's foot, toes, and heel. See Figure 47–14. As you move up the foot, stretch the stocking sideways.

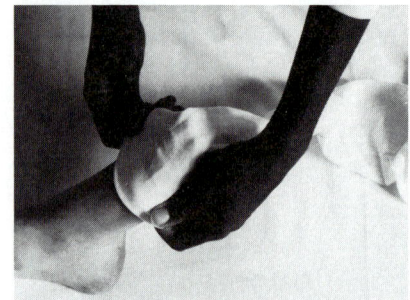

Figure 47–14 Applying the inverted stocking over client's toes.

- Support the client's ankle with one hand while using the other hand to pull the heel pocket under the heel.

- Center the heel in the pocket.

4. **Apply the remaining inverted portion of the stocking.**

- Gather the remaining portion of the stocking up to the toes, and pull only this part over the heel. With the foot already covered, the remainder of the stocking should slide easily over it.

- At the ankle, grasp the gathered portion between index and middle fingers, and pull the stocking up the leg to the knee. You may need to support the ankle with one hand and use the other hand to stretch the stocking and distribute it evenly.

- For *thigh- or waist-length stockings,* ask the client to straighten the leg while stretching the rest of the stocking over the knee.

- Ask the client to flex the knee while pulling the stocking over the thigh. Stretch the stocking from the top (front and back) to distribute it evenly over the thigh. The top should rest 2.5 to 7.5 cm (1 to 3 in) below the gluteal fold.

- For a *waist-length stocking,* ask the client to stand and continue extending the stocking up to the top of the gluteal fold.

- Apply the adjustable belt that accompanies thigh- and waist-length stockings, making sure that it does not interfere with any incision or external device (e.g., drainage tube or catheter).

- Adjust the foot section by tugging on the toe section to ensure toe comfort and stocking smoothness. Make sure a toe window is properly positioned.

PREOPERATIVE EVALUATING

To evaluate the achievement of the preoperative client's goals, the nurse collects data in relation to the outcome criteria. Evaluative activities may include

- Asking the client (a) to describe the proposed surgery, the reason for it, and expected length of stay; (b) to describe events that will occur in intraoperative and postoperative periods; and (c) to give reasons for specific preoperative and postoperative procedures.
- Listening attentively while encouraging the client to verbalize feelings about (a) the surgery and expected outcomes and (b) obtaining sufficient rest and sleep.
- Asking the client to demonstrate deep breathing, coughing, splinting, leg exercises, and moving techniques.
- Measuring vital signs and fluid intake and output.

The following are examples of evaluative statements: "Client stated, 'I'm really worried that this breast biopsy will reveal cancer and that I'll have to have more surgery' "; "Client stated, 'I had a good sleep last night since you told me what to expect after the surgery' "; "Client is able to relate reasons for deep breathing, coughing, and leg exercises but not for turning and movement"; and "Vital signs same as baseline findings 7/10/xx."

INTRAOPERATIVE PHASE

Clients undergo a wide variety of surgical procedures. Some have *day surgery,* arriving at the hospital on the day of the operation and leaving that same day. Others have a longer hospital stay, from a few days to several weeks. The prefixes and suffixes of the names of surgical procedures help the student understand the nature of the operation. See Appendix D.

During the intraoperative phase, nurses in the operating room protect the client from injury and infection, monitor the client, and maintain appropriate documentation.

 Protecting the Client Clients who have had an anesthetic are vulnerable to injury because they are unaware of the surroundings and cannot protect themselves. Nurses observe the following measures when positioning clients for surgery:

- Protecting the client's skin from injury while moving and positioning.
- Maintaining the client's position within the limits of the involved joint's range of motion.
- Using appropriate safety devices, e.g., side rails of a gurney and safety straps.

Monitoring the Client Monitoring the client's physiologic responses is the responsibility of an anesthetist or anesthesiologist. However, nurses monitor clients receiving local anesthetic. "Each client should be monitored for reaction to drugs and for behavioral and physiological changes" (Association of Operating Room Nurses 1986, p. 111:16–1).

Maintaining Documentation The intraoperative record focuses on nursing interventions, including notes about sponges; instrument and needle counts; grounding location for the electrosurgical unit; monitors used; tourniquet location, times, and pressure set; implant and lot numbers; dressings; drains; specimens and cultures; medications; client position on the operating room table; and types of safety devices, e.g., hand restraints (Kneedler and Dodge 1983, p. 463).

Nursing Roles During Surgery

Two types of nurses, the scrub nurse and the circulating nurse, assist during surgery. The scrub nurse is attired in a sterile gown, cap, mask, and gloves and has these responsibilities:

- Handing the surgeon sterile instruments and supplies from the sterile tray. Because many instruments are required during certain operations, a scrub nurse must have an extensive knowledge of all instruments and how they are used.
- Counting sponges, needles, and instruments. Counting is done before the surgeon closes the incision so that none are left inside the client.
- Disposing of used instruments.

The circulating nurse's responsibilities include

- Helping to position the client on the operating room table.
- Helping to drape the client and assisting the surgeon and scrub nurse to don sterile gowns and gloves.
- Opening packages so that the scrub nurse can remove the sterile supplies.
- Arranging for transfer of biopsy specimens to the laboratory.
- Adjusting operating room lights.
- Obtaining additional supplies and equipment.

Preparing for the Postoperative Client

While the client is in the operating room, the client's bed and room are prepared for the postoperative phase. In some agencies, the client is brought back to the unit on a stretcher and transferred to the bed in the room. In other agencies, the client's bed is brought to the recovery room (RR), and the client is transferred there. In the latter situation, the surgical bed needs to be made as soon as the client goes to the operating room so that it can be taken to the RR at any time. In addition, the nurse must obtain and set up special equipment as needed, such as an intravenous pole, suction, oxygen equipment, and orthopedic appliances (e.g., traction). If these are not requested on the client's record, the nurse should consult with the nurse in charge.

The surgical bed is also referred to as the *recovery bed, anesthetic bed,* or *postoperative bed.* It may be used not only for clients who have undergone surgical procedures but also for clients who have been given anesthetics for certain examinations.

There are four reasons for making a surgical bed:

1. To arrange the top bed linen so the client can be readily transferred to the bed

2. To provide as clean an environment as possible for the client

3. To provide a bed foundation that can be changed quickly and easily if it becomes soiled

4. In some instances, to provide extra warmth through the use of flannelette sheets

Procedure 47–4 provides instructions for making a surgical bed.

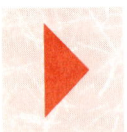

PROCEDURE 47–4

MAKING A SURGICAL BED

Equipment

Two clean sheets

Clean cotton drawsheet

Clean flannelette sheet

Clean bedspread

Disposable incontinence or drainage pad (optional)

Intervention

1. Strip the bed.

- See Procedure 22–7, step 3, on page 554.

- Place and leave the pillows on the bedside chair. *Pillows are left on a chair to facilitate transferring the client into the bed.*

2. Make the foundation of the bed.

- See Procedure 22–7, steps 4 and 5.

- Place the flannelette sheet on the foundation of the bed, if this is agency practice. *A flannelette sheet provides additional warmth.*

- Place a disposable pad for the client's head (optional).

3. Apply and fanfold the top bedding.

- Spread the top covers on the bed. Do not tuck them in, miter the corners, or make a toe pleat.

- Fold the hanging edges of the top covers up over the top of the bed so that the folds are at the mattress edge (fold the sides first, then the top and bottom). Then fanfold the covers in either of the following ways:

a. Fanfold them lengthwise at one side of the bed. See Figure 47–15.

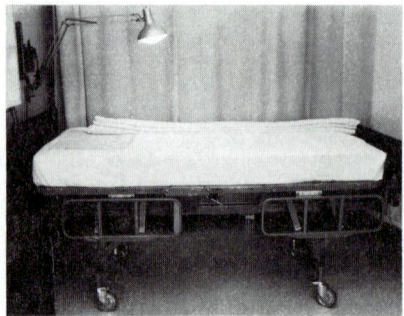

Figure 47–15 Surgical bed with top covers folded to the side.

b. Fanfold them crosswise at the bottom of the bed. See Figure 47–16. *The covers are fanfolded for ease in transferring the client into bed.*

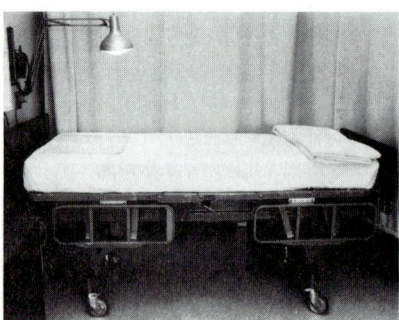

Figure 47–16 Surgical bed with top covers folded to the bottom.

4. Arrange the furniture and equipment appropriately.

- Arrange the furniture and equipment so that there is room near the bed for a stretcher or room to move the bed out of the room if the bed is to be transported to the operating room.

- Make sure any additional equipment, e.g., suction, is in readiness for use when the client returns from surgery.

5. Stabilize and raise the bed.

■ Lock the wheels of the bed if the bed is not to be moved. *Locking the wheels keeps the bed from roll-* *ing when the client is transferred from the stretcher to the bed.*

■ Leave the bed in the high position to meet the level of the stretcher. *The high position facilitates the transfer of the client.*

6. Notify appropriate people that the surgical bed is ready.

■ In some hospitals, a porter service or the like takes the bed to the recovery room.

POSTOPERATIVE PHASE

Nursing during the postoperative phase is especially important for the client's recovery. Anesthesia impairs the ability of clients to respond to environmental stimuli and to help themselves, although the degree of consciousness of clients will vary. Moreover, surgery itself traumatizes the body by decreasing its energy and resistance. Nursing interventions include monitoring the client's cardiovascular status, fluid balance, and neurologic status; providing comfort and safety; encouraging mobility; and preventing complications.

Immediate postanesthetic care is usually provided in a postanesthetic room (PAR) or recovery room (RR). Recovery room nurses have specialized skills to care for clients recovering from anesthesia and surgery. Once the health status has stabilized, the client is returned to the nursing unit or, in the case of a day-surgery client, to the day-surgery area before discharge. Recovery room assessment is summarized in the accompanying box.

 During the immediate postanesthetic stage, an unconscious client is positioned on the side, with the face slightly down. A pillow is not placed under the head. In this position, gravity keeps the tongue forward, preventing occlusion of the pharynx and allowing drainage of mucus or vomitus out of the mouth rather than down the respiratory tree.

The nurse ensures maximum chest expansion by elevating the client's upper arm on a pillow. The upper arm is supported because the pressure of an arm against the chest reduces chest expansion potential. Once the reflexes return, the client can usually assume a back-lying position. An artificial airway is maintained in place, and suction is supplied until reflexes for controlling coughing and swallowing return. Generally, the client spits out an oropharyngeal airway when coughing returns. Endotracheal tubes are not removed until clients are awake and able to maintain their own airways. Before any artificial airway is removed, suction is applied to the airway and the pharynx. The client is then helped to turn, cough, and take deep breaths, provided that vital signs are stable. See Chapter 41 for information about artificial airways.

After general anesthesia, clients usually awaken in the following sequence:

1. Responsive to stimuli (e.g., to loud noises or to their name spoken loudly)

2. Drowsy

3. Awake but not oriented

4. Alert and oriented (McConnell 1977a, p. 34)

The return of the client's reflexes, such as swallowing and gagging, indicates that anesthesia is ending. Time of recovery from anesthesia varies with the kind of anesthetic agent used, its dosage, and the individual's response to it. Nurses should arouse clients by calling them by name, and in a normal tone of voice repeatedly telling them that the surgery is over and that they are in the RR.

Once the health status has stabilized, the client is returned to the nursing unit or, in the case of a day-surgery client, to the day-surgery area, for *continuing postoperative care.*

Postoperative Assessing

As soon as the client returns to the nursing unit, the nurse conducts an initial assessment. See Figure 47–17 for a postoperative checklist. The sequence of these activities varies

---

Recovery Room Assessment

■ Respiratory function

■ Cardiovascular function (circulation)

■ Fluid and electrolyte balance

■ Dressings, tubes, and drains

■ Neurologic status

■ Pain

■ Safety

POSTOPERATIVE INITIAL ASSESSMENT CHECKLIST

1. **Time of arrival** ______
2. **Vital signs**
   Pulse ____ Respirations ____ Blood pressure ____
3. **Skin**
   Color ______
   Condition ______
4. **Level of consciousness**
   Conscious ___ Semiconscious ___ Unconscious ___
5. **Dressing**
   Dry ______ Drainage present ______
   Blood ______ Intact ______
6. **Intravenous**
   Type of solution ______
   Amount in bottle ______ Drip rate ______
   Venipuncture site ______
7. **Drainage tubes**
   Type ______
   Attached to suction or drainage container ______
   Appearance and amount of drainage ______
   ______
8. **Patient position** ______
9. **Side rails** ______
10. **Pain**
    Type of analgesic ______
    Time last given ______
11. **Other discomforts** ______
    ______
    ______

Figure 47–17 A sample postoperative checklist.

Postoperative Risk Factors in Elderly Adults

- Vulnerable skin due to venous stasis and poor venous return
- Reduced cardiac reserve due to changes in the myocardium
- Tachycardia from anxiety, which is tolerated poorly in the elderly heart
- Decreased compliance of blood vessels due to atherosclerosis
- Reduced vital capacity due to lowered expansibility of the rib cage
- Reduced blood flow to the kidneys
- Reduced ability to excrete toxins due to reduced glomerular filtration

with the situation. For example, the nurse may need to check the physician's stat orders before conducting the initial assessment; in such a case, nursing interventions to implement the orders can be carried out at the same time as assessment.

The nurse records the client's condition, including the assessment, on the chart. Many hospitals have postoperative protocols for regular assessment of clients. In some agencies, assessments are made every 15 minutes until vital signs stabilize, every hour thereafter the same day, and every 4 hours for the next 2 days. It is very important that the assessments be made as often as the client's condition requires. The nurse assesses the client's level of consciousness. At this point, most postoperative clients are conscious but drowsy. A fully conscious person responds verbally, is alert, and is aware of time, place, and person. A semiconscious person has fluctuating states of awareness. An unconscious person does not respond verbally, has variable responses to stimuli such as noise or pain, and may be incontinent of urine or feces. The nurse notifies the support persons that the client has returned from surgery. It may be necessary to caution them about the client's drowsiness and about not staying too long. Special assessments should be made with older adults. See the box in the left column for postoperative risk factors.

The client's *vital signs* need to be taken at least every 4 hours, or more frequently if they are abnormal. See Table 47–3 for assistance in analyzing the meaning of altered vital signs. The client's *skin color and temperature,* particularly that of the lips and nail beds, should be assessed, because the color of the lips and nail beds are indicators of **tissue perfusion** (passage of blood through the vessels). Pale, cyanotic, cool, and moist skin may be a sign of circulatory problems. In addition, the client should be assessed for signs of common circulatory problems: hemorrhage and shock, cardiac arrest, and postoperative hypotension. Disruption of sutures and insecure ligation of blood vessels can cause hemorrhage. Shock occurs as a result of massive hemorrhage or cardiac insufficiency. Signs of shock are summarized in the box below.

Clinical Signs of Shock

- Increased pulse and respiratory rates
- Restlessness
- Lowered blood pressure
- Cold, clammy skin
- Thirst
- Pallor

TABLE 47–3 *Potential Postoperative Problems*

Problem	Description	Cause	Clinical Signs	Preventive Interventions
Respiratory				
Pneumonia	Inflammation of the alveoli	Commonly *Diplococus pneumoniae,* a resident bacteria in the respiratory tract	Elevated temperature, cough, expectoration of blood-tinged or purulent sputum, dyspnea, chest pain	Deep-breathing and coughing exercises, moving in bed, early ambulation
Lobar pneumonia	Involves one or more lobes			
Bronchopneumonia	Originates in bronchi and involves patches of lung tissue	Poor lung expansion and circulation, resulting in stagnation of secretions		
Hypostatic pneumonia	Poor or stagnant circulation causing inflammation of lung tissue			
Atelectasis	Collapse of the alveoli, with retained secretions	Mucous plugs blocking bronchial passageways, inadequate lung expansion, analgesics, immobility	Marked dyspnea, cyanosis, pleural pain, prostration, tachycardia, increased respiratory rate, fever, productive cough, auscultatory crackling sounds	Deep-breathing and coughing exercises, turning, early ambulation, adequate fluid intake
Pulmonary embolism	Blood clot that has moved to the lungs and obstructs a pulmonary artery, thus inhibiting blood flow to one or more lung lobes	Stasis of venous blood from immobility, venous injury from fractures or during surgery, use of oral contraceptives high in estrogen, preexisting coagulation or circulatory disorder	Sudden chest pain, shortness of breath, cyanosis, shock (tachycardia, low blood pressure)	Deep-breathing and coughing exercises, turning, ambulation, antiemboli stockings
Circulatory				
Hemorrhage	Bleeding internally or externally	Disruption of sutures, insecure ligation of blood vessels	Rapid weak pulse, increasing respiratory rate, restlessness, lowered blood pressure, cold clammy skin, thirst, pallor, reduced urine output	Early recognition of signs
Hypovolemic shock	Markedly reduced volume of circulating blood resulting in inadequate tissue perfusion	Hemorrhage	Same as Hemorrhage	Early recognition of signs
Thrombophlebitis	Inflammation of the veins, usually of the legs and associated with a blood clot	Slowed venous blood flow due to immobility or prolonged sitting; trauma to vein, resulting in inflammation and increased blood coagulability	Aching, cramping pain; affected area is swollen, red, and hot to touch; vein feels hard; discomfort in calf when foot is dorsiflexed or when client walks (Homans' sign)	Early ambulation, leg exercises, antiemboli stockings, adequate fluid intake

TABLE 47–3 *Potential Postoperative Problems (continued)*

Problem	Description	Cause	Clinical Signs	Preventive Interventions
Circulatory (continued)				
Thrombus	Blood clot attached to wall of vein or artery most commonly the leg veins	Venous stasis; vein injury resulting from surgery of legs, pelvis, abdomen; factors causing increased blood coagulability, e.g., use of estrogen	Same as for Pulmonary Embolism; if lodged in heart or brain, cardiac or neurologic signs	Same as for Thrombophlebitis
Embolus	Clot that has moved from its site of formation to another area of the body, e.g., the lungs, heart, or brain	Same as for Thrombus	Same as for Thrombus	Same as for Thrombophlebitis
Urinary				
Urinary retention	Accumulation of urine in the bladder and inability of the bladder to empty itself	Depressed bladder muscle tone from narcotics and anesthetics; handling of tissues during surgery on adjacent organs (rectum, vagina)	Fluid intake larger than output; inability to void or frequent voiding of small amounts, bladder distention, suprapubic discomfort, restlessness	Monitoring of fluid intake and output, interventions to facilitate voiding
Urinary infection	Inflammation of bladder	Immobilization and limited fluid intake	Burning sensation when voiding, urgency, cloudy urine, lower abdominal pain	Adequate fluid intake, early ambulation, good perineal hygiene
Gastrointestinal				
Constipation	Infrequent or no stool passage for abnormal length of time, e.g., within 48 hours after solid diet started	Lack of dietary roughage, analgesics (decreased intestinal motility)	Absence of stool elimination, abdominal distention and discomfort	Adequate fluid intake, high-fiber diet, early ambulation
Singultus	Intermittent spasms of the diaphragm	Irritation of the phrenic nerve—for a variety of reasons, e.g., abdominal distention	Hiccups	Prevent the cause
Tympanites	Retention of gases within the intestines	Slowed motility of the intestines due to handling of the bowel during surgery and the effects of anesthesia	Obvious abdominal distention, abdominal discomfort (gas pains), absence of bowel sounds	Early ambulation, IV fluid progressing to clear fluids, full fluids and regular diet when peristalsis returns

▶

TABLE 47—3 *(continued)*

Problem	Description	Cause	Clinical Signs	Preventive Interventions
Gastrointestinal (continued)				
Nausea and vomiting		Pain, abdominal distention, ingesting food or fluids before return of peristalsis, certain medications, anxiety	Complaints of feeling sick to the stomach, retching or gagging	IV fluids until peristalsis returns; then clear fluids, full fluids, and regular diet; antiemetic drugs if ordered; analgesics for pain
Wound				
Wound infection	Inflammation and infection of incision or drain site	Poor aseptic technique; laboratory analysis of wound swab identifies causative microorganism	Purulent exudate, redness, tenderness, elevated body temperature, wound odor	Keeping wound clean and dry, surgical aseptic technique when changing dressings
Wound dehiscence	Separation of a suture line before the incision heals	Malnutrition (emaciation, obesity), poor circulation, excessive strain on suture line	Increased incision drainage, tissues underlying skin become visible along parts of the incision	Adequate nutrition, appropriate incisional support and avoidance of strain
Wound evisceration	Extrusion of internal organs and tissues through the incision	Same as for Wound Dehiscence	Opening of incision and visible protrusion of organs	Same as for Wound Dehiscence
Psychologic				
Postoperative depression	See Clinical Signs	News of malignancy, severely altered body image	Anorexia, tearfulness, loss of ambition, withdrawal, rejection of others, feelings of dejection, sleep disturbances (insomnia, excessive sleeping)	Adequate rest, physical activity, opportunity to express anger and other negative feelings

The nurse must inspect the client's dressings and the bedclothes underneath the client. Excessive bloody drainage on dressings or on bedclothes, often appearing underneath the client, can indicate hemorrhage. The amount of *drainage* on dressings is recorded by describing the diameter of stains. It is extremely important for the nurse to ensure that replacement of fluids lost during surgery is sufficient to maintain blood pressure. Nurses also must determine the color, consistency, and amount of drainage from all tubes and suction apparatuses. All tubes should be patent, and tubes and suction equipment should be functioning properly.

The client's *fluid intake and output* are monitored. In addition to watching for shock, the nurse assesses the client for signs of circulatory overload. See Chapter 40. During surgery, aldosterone production increases, and, as a result, the body conserves sodium and fluid. Therefore, care must be taken not to overload the body with fluid. In addition, the client is assessed for signs of fluid or electrolyte imbalance.

The surgeon may prescribe intravenous fluids or blood components to be administered in the surgical nursing unit. See Chapter 40.

Postoperative Diagnosing

Because surgery can involve many body systems both directly and indirectly and is a complex experience for the client, the nursing diagnoses focus on a wide variety of actual and potential problems. Certain diagnoses are more likely to apply during the intraoperative phase of the perioperative period. Examples are shown below.

Dx **Nursing Diagnoses Postoperative Clients**

Potential ineffective airway clearance related to:

- Effects of anesthesia (e.g., diminished cough reflex, retained secretions)
- History of smoking

Potential ineffective breathing pattern related to:

- Pain in high abdominal incision
- Effects of analgesic on ventilation

Potential for injury related to:

- Inability to adapt to environmental hazards secondary to anesthetized status
- Impaired physical mobility secondary to incisional pain and imposed restrictions to movement (e.g., intravenous line, cast)

Potential for infection related to:

- Impaired skin integrity (surgical incision)
- Knowledge deficit (wound or drainage tube care)

Knowledge deficit (wound care and activity restrictions after discharge)

Pain related to:

- Activity and surgical incision

Potential fluid volume deficit related to:

- Excessive wound drainage
- Inadequate fluid intake

Self-care deficit: Bathing/hygiene, dressing/grooming, toileting related to:

- Imposed activity restrictions
- Restrictive devices to movement

Potential urinary retention related to:

- Effects of anesthesia
- Swelling of urethra associated with bladder surgery

Postoperative Planning

Most people recover from surgery without incident. Complications or problems are relatively rare, yet nurses must be aware of such possibilities and their clinical signs. See Table 47–3. Many sources of data are relevant to the planning of a client's postoperative nursing needs (e.g., the preoperative nursing history, postoperative orders, the recovery room report, and the client). See the box above for significant data in the recovery room record. The nurse consults the surgeon's postoperative orders to learn the following:

- Food and fluids permitted by mouth
- Intravenous solutions and intravenous medications
- Position in bed
- Medications ordered, e.g., analgesics, antibiotics
- Laboratory tests
- Intake and output, which in some agencies are monitored for all postoperative clients
- Activity permitted, including ambulation

    Client goals during the postoperative period include

- Being free of surgical complications
- Experiencing minimal discomfort
- Achieving adequate rest
- Being free of injury
- Maintaining a healthy attitude toward self
- Resuming the highest possible level of wellness

Nursing interventions to achieve these goals are discussed below. Examples of outcome criteria to evaluate the achievement of goals and the effectiveness of nursing interventions follow.

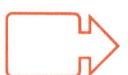 **Outcome Criteria Postoperative Clients**

The client:

- Maintains normal baseline vital signs.
- Performs deep-breathing exercises and voluntary coughing every 2 hours when awake, as instructed.

- Has adequate respiratory excursion (depth).
- Has clear lung sounds on auscultation.
- Performs specified leg exercises at least every 4 hours when awake, as instructed.
- Has negative Homans' sign.
- Has balanced fluid intake and output.
- Has good tissue turgor of the skin.
- Has clear amber urine.
- Experiences no burning sensation or urgency when voiding.
- Has active bowel sounds within 48 hours.
- Resumes normal defecation within 3 days.
- Is free of purulent wound drainage.
- Ambulates, performs self-care activities, and rests with minimal or no pain.
- Reports satisfactory sleep pattern each night.
- Reports feelings of increasing wellness each day.

Postoperative Implementing

Positioning   Position the client as ordered. Clients who have had spinal anesthetics usually lie flat for 8 to 12 hours. Agencies often have protocols regarding this practice. An unconscious or semiconscious client is placed on a side, if possible, or in a position that allows fluids to drain from the mouth. Otherwise, the nurse follows the client's preference. Most people prefer a back-lying position.

Deep-Breathing and Coughing Exercises   Deep-breathing exercises help remove mucus, which can form and remain in the lungs due to the effects of a general anesthetic and analgesics. These drugs depress the action of both the cilia of the mucous membranes lining the respiratory tract and the respiratory center in the brain. By increasing lung expansion and preventing the accumulation of secretions, deep breathing helps prevent pneumonia, which may result from stagnation of fluid in the lungs. See Table 47–3. Deep breathing frequently initiates the coughing reflex. Voluntary coughing in conjunction with deep breathing facilitates the movement and expectoration of respiratory tract secretions.

The nurse encourages the client to do deep-breathing and coughing exercises hourly, or at least every 2 hours, during waking hours for the first few days. The nurse should assist the client to a sitting position in bed or on the side of the bed. The client can splint the incision with a pillow when coughing, or the nurse can splint the incision for the client to reduce discomfort. To assist clients who have difficulty with deep-breathing and coughing exercises, the nurse should check about the use of incentive spirometers (see Chapter 41). Clients unable to cough up secretions may require suction (see Chapter 41).

Leg Exercises   The client should be encouraged to do leg exercises every hour, or at least every 2 hours, during waking hours. Muscle contractions compress the veins, preventing the stasis of blood in the veins, a cause of **thrombus** formation and subsequent **thrombophlebitis** and **emboli.** See Table 47–3. Contractions also promote arterial blood flow.

Moving and Ambulation   The client must be turned from side to side every 2 hours. Turning allows alternating maximum expansion of the uppermost lung. The nurse avoids placing pillows or rolls under the client's knees because pressure on the popliteal blood vessels can slow the blood circulation to and from the lower extremities. Clients who before surgery had practiced turning usually find it easier to do. The client should ambulate as soon as possible after surgery in accordance with the surgeon's orders. Generally, clients begin ambulation the evening of the day of surgery or the first day after surgery, unless the surgeon orders otherwise. Early ambulation prevents respiratory, circulatory, urinary, and gastrointestinal complications. It also prevents general muscle weakness. See Table 47–3. Ambulation should be scheduled for periods after the client has taken an analgesic or when the client is comfortable. And it should be gradual, starting with the client sitting on the bed and dangling the feet over the side. A client who cannot ambulate should be periodically assisted to a sitting position in bed, if allowed, and turned frequently. The sitting position permits the greatest lung expansion.

Hydration   The nurse should maintain intravenous infusions as ordered. Intravenous infusions are given to balance loss of body fluids during surgery (e.g., blood loss, perspiration, vomiting, and fasting). Only small sips of water should be offered to clients who can have fluids by mouth, until they establish tolerance. Large amounts of water can induce vomiting, since anesthetics and narcotic analgesics temporarily inhibit the motility of the stomach. Ice chips, if permitted, may be offered. The client who cannot take fluids by mouth *may* be allowed to suck ice chips; the surgeon's orders should be checked. Mouth care should be provided, and a mouthwash should be placed at the client's bedside. Postoperative clients often complain of thirst and a dry, sticky mouth. These discomforts are a result of the preoperative fasting period, preoperative medications (such as atropine or scopolamine), and loss of body fluid.

The client's fluid intake and output should be measured for at least 2 days or until fluid balance is stable without an intravenous infusion. Ensuring adequate fluid balance is important. Sufficient fluids keep the respiratory mucous membranes and secretions moist, thus facilitating the expectoration of mucus during coughing. Also, an adequate fluid balance will prevent dehydration and the resulting concentration of the blood that, along with venous stasis, is conducive to thrombus formation.

Diet   The surgeon orders the client's postoperative diet. Depending on the extent of surgery and the organs involved, some clients may be given intravenous fluids and nothing by mouth for a few days, whereas others may progress from a diet of clear liquids to full fluids, to a light diet, and then to a regular diet within a few days, provided that gastrointestinal functioning is normal. The return of peristalsis can be assessed by auscultating the abdomen. Gurgling and rumbling sounds indicate peristalsis (see Chapter 19). Anesthetic agents, narcotics, handling of the intestines during abdominal surgery, changes in fluid and food intake, and inactivity all inhibit peristalsis. Therefore, bowel sounds should be carefully assessed every 4 to 6 hours. Oral fluids and food are usually started after the return of peristalsis. The nurse may need to assist the very weak client to eat. In addition, the nurse observes the client's tolerance of the food and fluids ingested.

Urinary Elimination   The nurse may provide measures that promote urinary elimination. For example, the nurse helps male clients stand at the bedside, ensures that clients are free from pain, ensures that fluid intake is adequate, and helps clients walk. The nurse determines whether the client has any difficulties voiding and assesses the client for bladder distention (see Chapter 19, Figure 19–93). The nurse reports to the surgeon if a client does not void within 8 hours following surgery, unless another time frame is specified.

Anesthetic agents temporarily depress urinary bladder tone, which usually returns within 6 to 8 hours after surgery. Surgery in the pubic area, vagina, or rectum, during which the surgeon may manipulate the bladder, often causes urinary retention. If all measures to promote voiding fail, the physician usually orders urinary catheterization. See Chapter 43. The nurse measures the liquid intake and output of all clients with urinary catheters or other drainage devices. I & O records are kept for at least 2 days and until the client reestablishes fluid balance without a catheter in place.

Pain   Pain is usually greatest 12 to 36 hours after surgery, decreasing on the second or third day. Analgesics are usually administered every 3 or 4 hours the first day; by the third day most clients require only oral analgesics. Analgesics are also administered in infusions. Some may refuse to take analgesics on a regular schedule because they are not in severe pain. In this situation, the nurse assesses the need for analgesics (see Chapter 38) and, if indicated, informs the client that analgesics are most effective if given *before* pain becomes severe. The nurse also provides comfort measures to relax the client, e.g., back rubs, position changes, rest periods, and diverting activities, since tension increases pain perception and responses. Analgesics are given as ordered and as required. The accompanying box provides guidelines for ongoing postoperative assessment.

Closed Wound Suction   Closed wound drainage, e.g., the *Hemovac,* is used to apply suction to wounds. See Chapter 46.

Suction   The manner in which suction is applied to drainage tubes depends on the type of equipment available in the agency and the amount of suction required. The following are the most commonly used:

1. *Portable electric motor suction.* Portable electric units are plugged into electric wall outlets. The units have an on-off switch, a motor that generates the negative pressure, and a drainage bottle. The bottle needs to be monitored regularly to prevent overflow of drainage into the motor, which can cause irreparable damage to the apparatus.

2. *Gomco thermotic pump.* The Gomco pump is electrically operated but consists of a pump rather than a motor. It provides intermittent suction by alternating the air pressure, i.e., expanding and contracting the air. As the pressure alternates, red and green lights flash on and off. The amount of suction is regulated by a "high" or "low"

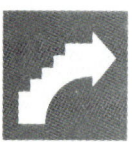

CLINICAL GUIDELINES
Ongoing Postoperative Care

■ Watch for signs indicating acute pain: pallor, perspiration, tension, and reluctance to perform deep-breathing and coughing exercises or to move or ambulate.

■ Give analgesics *before* activities (e.g., ambulation or meals) or rest periods (e.g., at bedtime) and assess the effectiveness of the analgesics.

■ Do not assume that the pain is caused by the incision (other causes include tight dressings, irritation from drainage tubes, or muscle strains resulting from positioning on the operating table).

■ Assess the abdominal area. Note and report the passage of flatus or abdominal distention.

■ Inspect dressings regularly to ensure that they are clean, dry, and intact. Excessive drainage can indicate hemorrhage, infection, or dehiscence. See Table 47–3. Change dressings, using sterile technique as required, when they are soiled with drainage or in accordance with the surgeon's or nursing orders. (See Chapter 46).

■ Report wound separations promptly to the nurse in charge and the surgeon. If a large dehiscence or evisceration occurs, cover the wound with sterile, moist saline towels or dressings.

pressure button. The pump is commonly used to suction gastrointestinal tubes.

3. *Wall suction.* In some agencies, wall suction units with piped-in negative pressure are available. These units consist of a suction pressure regulator and a drainage receptacle, which needs to be checked regularly to prevent overflow.

Gastrointestinal tubes   Some clients return from surgery with a gastric or intestinal tube in place and orders to connect the tube to suction. For more information about gastrointestinal tubes, see Chapter 39. The suction ordered can be continuous or intermittent. Intermittent suctioning is less likely to harm the mucous membrane lining near the tip of the suction tube.

Nasogastric tubes are generally irrigated (a) before and after the installation of medications, (b) before and after tube feedings, and (c) as ordered to prevent clogging. Check agency policies and practices. Nasogastric irrigation may require a physician's order. Excessive irrigation can lead to metabolic alkalosis.

Procedures 47–5 through 47–7 give details about gastrointestinal suction.

Postoperative Evaluating

To evaluate goal achievement and the effectiveness of nursing interventions, the nurse collects data related to the outcome criteria. Data collection for the postoperative client may include the following:

- Measurement of vital signs and fluid intake and output
- Auscultation of the lungs for breath sounds and the abdomen for bowel sounds
- Inspection of the client's wound and urine
- Observing the client when performing deep-breathing, coughing, and leg exercises
- Asking the client about problems with pain, voiding, defecation, or sleep
- Observing how well the client performs activities
- Performing other specific assessments, such as testing tissue turgor or testing for the presence of Homans' sign.

The following examples of evaluative statements: "Bilateral lung sounds are clear"; "Wound is dry, with only slight inflammation around suture line"; "Client states, 'I can get out of bed more easily today—my stomach isn't as sore.'"

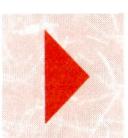

PROCEDURE 47–5

INITIATING GASTROINTESTINAL SUCTION

Equipment ☑

Gastrointestinal tube in place in the client. This may have been inserted prior to or following surgery (or prior to establishing the suction on a nonsurgical client).

Suction device for either continuous or intermittent suction

50-mL syringe with an adapter

Basin

Connector and connecting tubing

Stethoscope

Gloves (optional)

Intervention

1. Assess the client.

- Palpate the abdomen for distention and discomfort.
- Ausculate the abdomen for bowel sounds and gastrointestinal function.
- Inspect the nostrils for irritation by the tube.

2. Position the client appropriately.

- Assist the client to semi-Fowler's position if it is not contraindicated because of health. *In semi-Fowler's position the tube is not as likely to lie against the wall of the stomach and will therefore suction most efficiently. Semi-Fowler's position also prevents reflux of gastric contents, which could lead to aspiration.*

3. Confirm that the tube is in the stomach.

- Aspirate stomach contents and check their acidity.

- Insert air into the tube with the syringe and listen with a stethoscope over the stomach (just below the xiphoid process) for a swish of air.
- Use other methods in accordance with agency protocol. See Chapter 39, pages 1017–1018.

4. Set and check the suction.

- Adjust the suction machine for the recommended suction pressure, in accordance with agency policy or the physician's order. Some suctions are preset and cannot be adjusted. If using a Gomco thermotic pump, the suction is usually set on intermittent "low" suction for a single-lumen nasogastric tube or on "high" suction for a double-lumen nasogastric tube (e.g., Salem sump tube).

■ Turn on the suction machine, and check that the suction is working. The Gomco thermotic drainage pump has a red indicator light in the middle of the front panel; it blinks continuously when the machine is functioning. When using other suction machines, test for proper suctioning by holding the open end of the suction tube to the nurse's ear. Suctioning is confirmed by a sucking noise.

5. Establish gastric suction.

■ Connect the gastrointestinal tube to the tubing from the suction by using the connector.

■ If a Salem sump tube is in place, connect the larger lumen to the suction equipment. This double-lumen tube has a smaller tube running inside the primary suction tube. *The smaller tube provides a continuous flow of atmospheric air through the drainage tube at its distal end and prevents excessive suction force on the gastric mucosa at the drainage outlets. Damage to the gastric mucosa is thus avoided.*

■ Always keep the air vent tube of a Salem sump tube open when suction is applied. *Closing the vent would stop the sump action and cause mucosal damage.*

■ After suction is applied, watch the tubing for a few minutes until the gastric contents appear to be running through the tubing into the receptacle. A Salem sump tube makes a soft, hissing sound when it is functioning correctly.

■ If the suction is not working properly, check that the rubber stopper in the collection bottle and all tubing connections are tightly sealed and that the tubing is not kinked.

■ Coil and pin the tubing on the bed so that it does not loop below the suction bottle. *If the tubing falls below the suction bottle, the suction may be obstructed because of the pressure required to push the fluid against gravity.*

6. Assess the drainage.

■ Observe the amount, color, odor, and consistency of the drainage. Normal gastric drainage has a mucoid consistency and is either colorless or yellow-green because of the presence of bile. A coffee-grounds color and consistency may indicate bleeding.

■ Test the gastric drainage for pH and blood (by using Hematest) when indicated. A person who has had gastrointestinal surgery can be expected to have some blood in the drainage.

7. Document relevant information.

■ Document initiating the suction and the time. Also record the pressure established, the color and consistency of the drainage, and nursing assessments.

Sample Recordings

Date: 9/18/91	Time 1400

Suction initiated 100 mm Hg. Returns watery, bright red. Abdomen firm and slightly distended. Bowel sounds irregular and high pitched.————————
———————————— Molly Jones, RN

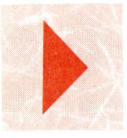

PROCEDURE 47–6

MAINTAINING GASTROINTESTINAL SUCTION

Equipment ☑

Cotton-tipped applicators

Ointment or lubricant

Graduated container as required to measure gastric drainage

Gloves

Intervention

1. Assess the client and the suction system regularly.

■ Assess the client regularly, e.g., every 30 minutes until the system is running effectively and then every 2 hours, or as the client's health indicates, to ensure that the suction is functioning properly. If the client complains of fullness, nausea, or epigastric pain or if the flow of gastric secretions is absent in the tubing or the collection bottle, ineffective suctioning or blockage of the nasogastric tube is likely.

■ Inspect the suction system for patency of the system, e.g., kinks or blockages in the tubing, and tightness of the connections. *Loose connections can permit air to enter and thus decrease the effectiveness of the suction by decreasing the negative pressure.*

2. Relieve blockages if present.

■ Milk the suction tubing.

■ Check the suction equipment. To do this, disconnect the nasogastric tube from the suction over a collecting basin (to collect gastric drainage), and then, with the suction on, place the end of the suction tubing in a basin of water. If water is drawn into the drainage bottle, the suction equipment is functioning properly, but the nasogastric tube is either blocked or positioned incorrectly.

■ Reposition the client, e.g., to the other side, if permitted. This may facilitate drainage.

■ Rotate the nasogastric tube and reposition it. This step is contraindicated for clients with gastric surgery because moving the tube may interfere with gastric sutures.

■ Irrigate the nasogastric tube as agency protocol states or on the order of the physician. See Procedure 47−7.

3. Prevent reflux into the vent lumen of a Salem sump tube.

Reflux of gastric contents into the vent lumen may occur when stomach pressure exceeds atmospheric pressure. In this situation gastric contents follow the path of least resistance and flow out the vent lumen rather than the drainage lumen. To prevent reflux:

■ Place the vent tubing above the client's midline. *A vent lumen placed below the midline acts as a siphon and allows gastric contents to flow through the air vent lumen.*

■ Always keep the drainage receptacle below the client's midline. *A drainage receptacle placed above midline and the fluid level in the client's stomach will cause reflux of gastric contents through the air vent lumen.* To avoid reflux when wall suction units are used, place the drainage container on the side of the bed or on the floor and attach a connecting tube from the drainage container to the wall outlet.

■ Keep the drainage lumen free of particulate matter that may obstruct the lumen. See irrigating a nasogastric tube in Procedure 47−7.

4. Ensure client comfort.

■ Clean the client's nostrils every 3 hours or as needed, using the cotton-tipped applicators and water. Apply a water-soluble lubricant or ointment.

■ Provide mouth care every 3 hours or as needed. Some postoperative clients are permitted to suck ice chips or a moist cloth to maintain the moisture of the oral mucous membranes.

5. Empty the drainage receptacle every 8 hours, or whenever it becomes three-quarters full.

■ Clamp the nasogastric tube and turn off the suction. Don gloves.

■ If the receptacle is graduated, determine the amount of drainage.

■ Disconnect the receptacle.

■ If not already measured, empty the contents into a graduated container and measure.

■ Inspect the drainage carefully for color, consistency, and presence of substances, e.g., blood clots.

■ Rinse the receptacle with warm water.

■ Reattach the receptacle to the suction.

■ Turn on the suction and unclamp the nasogastric tube.

■ Observe the system for several minutes to make sure function is reestablished.

6. Document relevant information.

■ Record assessments, supportive nursing measures, and data about the suction system.

Sample Recordings

Date: 10/7/91	Time: 0800

250 ml light brown thick drainage. No complaints of pain. Bowel sounds hyperactive, increased pitch. Abdomen soft upon palpation. No irritation in nostrils. Nostrils cleaned with water and lubricant applied. Vital signs q2h. BP 140/80, P 90, R 18 and stable. ———— R. Woo, SN

IRRIGATING A GASTROINTESTINAL TUBE

Nasogastric tubes are generally irrigated (a) before and after the instillation of medications, (b) before and after tube feedings, and (c) as ordered to prevent clogging. Check agency policies and practices. Nasogastric irrigation may require a physician's order. Excessive irrigation can lead to metabolic alkalosis.

Equipment ☑

Disposable irrigating set containing:
 Sterile 50-ml syringe
 Moisture-resistant pad

Basin

Graduated container

Sterile normal saline (500 ml) or the ordered solution

Stethoscope

Gloves

Intervention

1. Prepare the client and equipment.

- Place the moisture-resistant pad under the end of the gastrointestinal tube.

- Turn off the suction.

- Don gloves.

- Disconnect the gastrointestinal tube from the connector.

- Determine that the tube is in the stomach. See Procedure 47–5, step 3. *This ensures that the irrigating solution enters the stomach.*

2. Irrigate the tube.

- Draw up the ordered volume of irrigating solution in the syringe; 30 ml of solution per instillation is isual, but up to 60 ml may be given per instillation if ordered.

- Attach the syringe to the nasogastric tube and slowly inject the solution.

- Gently aspirate the solution. *Forceful withdrawal could damage the gastric mucosa.*

- If the nurse encounters difficulty in withdrawing the solution, inject 20 ml of air and aspirate again, and/or reposition the client or the nasogastric tube. *Air and repositioning may move the end of the tube away from the stomach wall.* If aspirating difficulty continues, reattach the tube to intermittent low suction and notify the nurse in charge or physician.

- Repeat above steps, until the ordered amount of solution is used.

- Note: A Salem sump tube can also be irrigated through the vent lumen without interrupting suction. However, only small amounts of irrigant can be injected via this lumen compared to the drainage lumen.

- After irrigating a Salem sump tube, inject 10 to 20 ml of air into the vent lumen while applying suction to the drainage lumen. *This tests the patency of the vent and ensures sump functioning.*

3. Reestablish suction.

- Reconnect the nasogastric tube to suction.

- If a Salem sump tube is used, inject the air vent lumen with 10 ml of air after reconnecting the tube to suction.

- Observe the system for several minutes to make sure it is functioning.

4. Document relevant information.

- Record verification of tube placement; the time of the irrigation; the amount and type of irrigating solution used; the amount, color, and consistency of the returns; the patency of the system following the irrigation; and nursing assessments.

Sample Recordings

Date: 9/19/91	Time 1600

Tube placement confirmed by injecting 10 ml air. Tube irrigated with 30 ml normal saline × 2. 30 ml × 2 returns cloudy, pink with small clots. Suction running with drainage noted. Abdomen soft, no discomfort, vital signs stable.— R. Woo, SN

NURSING CARE PLAN FOR GEORGE HANSEN

ASSESSMENT DATA

Nursing Assessment

George Hansen is a 22-year-old college student who was admitted to the surgical unit with a diagnosis of appendicitis. He was in good health until about 3 days ago, when he started experiencing nausea, anorexia, and vague abdominal discomfort. He was brought to the emergency department by his roommate today with pain in the right lower quadrant. He has been scheduled for an appendectomy later today. He has been medicated with meperidine 75 mg IM for pain. His abdomen has been shaved and prepped for surgery. Mr. Hansen has never been hospitalized and expresses concern about the operation. He asks the nurse if he will be asleep during the procedure and if there will be much pain afterward. He is drowsy but startles easily and appears anxious. He asks the nurse to stay with him.

Physical Examination

Height: 188 cm (6′2″)
Weight: 68.2 kg (150 lb)
Temperature: 37.2 C (99.6 F)
Pulse: 92 BPM
Respirations: 26 per minute
Blood pressure: 122/84
Hemoglobin (Hgb): 16 g/dl
Hematocrit (Hct): 48%
White Blood Count (WBC): 18,000/μl
Urinalysis: normal

CARE PLAN

Nursing Diagnosis	Client Goals and Outcome Criteria	Nursing Interventions and Rationales	Evaluation
Anxiety related to surgery (appendectomy) and **Fear** of the unknown as manifested by client's wish not to be alone, concern about pain, and slightly elevated pulse and respirations.	Client Goal: Anxiety will be decreased. Outcome Criteria: Client acknowledges fears. Verbalizes decreased anxiety. Appears relaxed and resting. Vital signs within normal limits and consistent with relaxed client.	Encourage client to verbalize feelings about surgery. *Rationale:* Identification of fears enables client and nurse to deal with them realistically. Provide information about the operative experience. *Rationale:* Assists client with a realistic understanding of the experience and dispels any misconceptions he might have. Minimize external stimuli (e.g., noise, movement). *Rationale:* Extraneous noises and movement may increase anxiety. Monitor vital signs (pulse, respirations, and blood pressure). *Rationale:* Changes in vital signs may be indicative of changes in level of anxiety. Administer medications (pain relief, sedatives) as indicated. *Rationale:* Will promote rest and reduce anxiety. Teach client about postoperative care. *Rationale:* Knowing what to expect and how he can assist with care will decrease anxiety.	Client verbalizes fears upon admission to unit. Client discusses the operative experience openly. Vital signs: pulse 74, respirations 18, blood pressure 118/84 two hours after admission to unit. Client resting quietly 2 hours after admission to unit.

Nursing Diagnosis	Client Goals and Outcome Criteria	Nursing Interventions and Rationales	Evaluation
Potential for injury related to altered sensory perception caused by sedation.	Client Goal: Client will be free of injury related to sedated state (e.g., falls, burns) Outcome Criteria: Identifies hazards related to drowsiness caused by sedation. Understands the need for side rails on bed. States will use call bell to obtain staff assistance for personal needs. Refrains from smoking in bed.	Give simple and brief directions to client. *Rationale:* Sedation may impair cognitive thinking and make it difficult for the client to understand involved instructions. Have client void prior to sedation. *Rationale:* Anticipating the client's need to void minimizes the possibility of the client trying to get out of bed to void when sedated. Place call bell within easy reach of client. *Rationale:* If the call bell is conveniently placed, client is more likely to use it. Appropriate placement negates the need to lean over side rails or attempt to get out of bed. Instruct client in the use of the call bell. *Rationale:* If the client understands how the call bell works, he is more likely to use it. Ensure that identification bracelet is securely fastened. *Rationale:* Prevents errors in identification of the sedated client. Instruct client not to smoke in bed while sedated. *Rationale:* A sedated client may fall asleep and set the bed linens on fire. Place side rails up and bed in low position when leaving client unattended in his room. *Rationale:* Side rails serve as a reminder to the client to not get out of bed. Bed in low position decreases the risk of injury should the client attempt to get out of bed. Encourage client to call for assistance. *Rationale:* The client may feel that he is bothering the staff by calling for assistance. Frequent reinforcement of staff availability will encourage the client to call for assistance.	Client is free of any injury prior to transport to the operating room. Client does not smoke while sedated.

CHAPTER HIGHLIGHTS

▶ The perioperative period includes three phases: preoperative, intraoperative, and postoperative.

▶ Nurses should assess the risk factors prior to a client's surgery whenever possible.

▶ Nursing history data are an important source for planning preoperative and postoperative care.

▶ The surgical excision of a part of the body may affect a client's self-image.

▶ Preoperative teaching should include moving, leg exercises, and coughing and deep-breathing exercises.

▶ Many aspects of preoperative teaching are intended to prevent postoperative complications.

▶ A surgical skin preparation should be carried out as close to the time of surgery as possible.

▶ Antiemboli stockings are intended to facilitate venous blood return.

▶ A preoperative checklist provides a guide and documentation of a client's preparation before surgery.

▶ A postoperative initial assessment checklist provides the nurse with a concise guide.

▶ Nurses may need to establish and monitor gastric suctions postoperatively.

READINGS AND REFERENCES

SUGGESTED READINGS

Blackwood, S. January 1986. Back to basics: The preop exam. *American Journal of Nursing* 86:39–44.
    Blackwood describes the preoperative examination, including essential methods, e.g., palpation, percussion, and auscultation. Included are illustrations of late clubbing, the location of the jugular veins, and measuring the legs for edema. A table summarizes the assessment techniques and normal and abnormal data.
Jackson, M. F. January 1988. High risk surgical patients. *Journal of Gerontological Nursing* 14:8–15.
    Jackson opens the article by pointing out that the mortality and morbidity rates for clients aged 90 to 95 who undergo elective surgery is double that of clients aged 70 to 75. Cardiovascular and pulmonary complications are major risks. The author then summarizes other factors, such as respiration, nutrition, and psychologic state, that should be assessed prior to surgery. Complications that can occur during the postoperative period are also discussed.
Montanari, J. August 1985. Documenting your postop assessment findings. *Nursing 85* 15:31–35.
    Montanari describes the transfer of a postoperative client from the RR to the nursing unit. The article includes a detailed description of postoperative assessment, including a two-page postoperative assessment form.

RELATED RESEARCH

Biley, F. C. July 1989. Nurses' perceptions of stress in preoperative surgical patients. *Journal of Advanced Nursing* 14:575–81.
Takahashi, J. J., and Bever, S. C. November 1989. Preoperative nursing assessment: A research study. *AORN Journal* 50:1022, 1024–29, 1031–32.
Yount, S. T.; Edgell, Sr. J.; and Jakovec, V. February 1990. Preoperative teaching: A study of nurses' perceptions. *AORN Journal* 51:572, 574–75, 577–79.

SELECTED REFERENCES

Association of Operating Room Nurses. 1986. *AORN standards and recommended practices for perioperative nursing.* Denver: Association of Operating Room Nurses, Inc.
———. November 1988. Recommended practices: Preoperative skin preparation. *AORN Journal* 48:950–51, 953–55, 958.
Croushore, J. M. April 1979. Postoperative assessment: The key to avoiding the most common nursing mistakes. *Nursing 79* 9:46–50.
Drain, C. B. August 1984. Managing postoperative pain . . . It's a matter of sighs. *Nursing 84* 14:52–55.
Erickson, R. July 1982. Tube talk principles of fluid flow in tubes. *Nursing 82* 12:54–61.
Garner, J. S. April 1986. CDC guidelines for the prevention and control of nosocomial infections: Guideline for prevention of surgical wound infections, 1985. *American Journal of Infection Control* 14:71–80.
Jackson, M. F. October 1989. Implications of surgery in very elderly patients. *AORN Journal* 50:859, 862–64, 866.
Kam, B. W., Werner, P. W. May 1990. Self-care theory: Application to Perioperative nursing. *AORN Journal* 51:1365–67.
Kneedler, J. A. and Dodge, G. H. 1983. *Perioperative patient care.* Boston: Blackwell Scientific Publications, Inc.
LeMaitre, G. D., and Finnegan, J. A. 1980. *The patient in surgery: A guide for nurses.* 4th ed. Philadelphia: W. B. Saunders Co.
Lierman, J. February 1988. Preoperative assessment: Can we afford to do without them? *AORN Journal* 47:586, 588, 590.
Luciano, K. November 1974. The who, when, where, what and how of preparing children for surgery. *Nursing 74* 4:64–65.
McConnell, E. A. September 1975. All about gastrointestinal intubation. *Nursing 75* 5:30–37.
———. March 1977. After surgery. *Nursing 77* 7:32–39.
———. September 1977. Ensuring safer stomach suctioning with a Salem sump tube. *Nursing 77* 7:54–57.
———. April 1979. Ten problems with nasogastric tubes . . . and how to solve them. *Nursing 79* 9:78–81.

Northrop, C. E. 1988. Legal aspects of nursing. In McCann Flynn, J. B., and Heffron, P. B. *Nursing: From concept to practice.* 2d ed. Norwalk, Conn.: Appleton & Lange.

Page, S. M., and Beresford, L. A. February 1988. Planning and documentation: Addressing patient needs in a day surgery setting. *AORN Journal* 47:526, 528, 530, 532–35, 537.

Reeder, J. M. December 1989. Ethical dilemmas in perioperative nursing practice. *Nursing Clinics of North America* 24:999–1007.

Ryan, R. October 1976. Thrombophlebitis: Assessment and prevention. *American Journal of Nursing* 76:1634–36.

Wiseman, S. J. March 1990. Patient advocacy: The essence of perioperative nursing in ambulatory care surgery. *AORN Journal* 51:754, 756, 758–591 + .

Special Studies

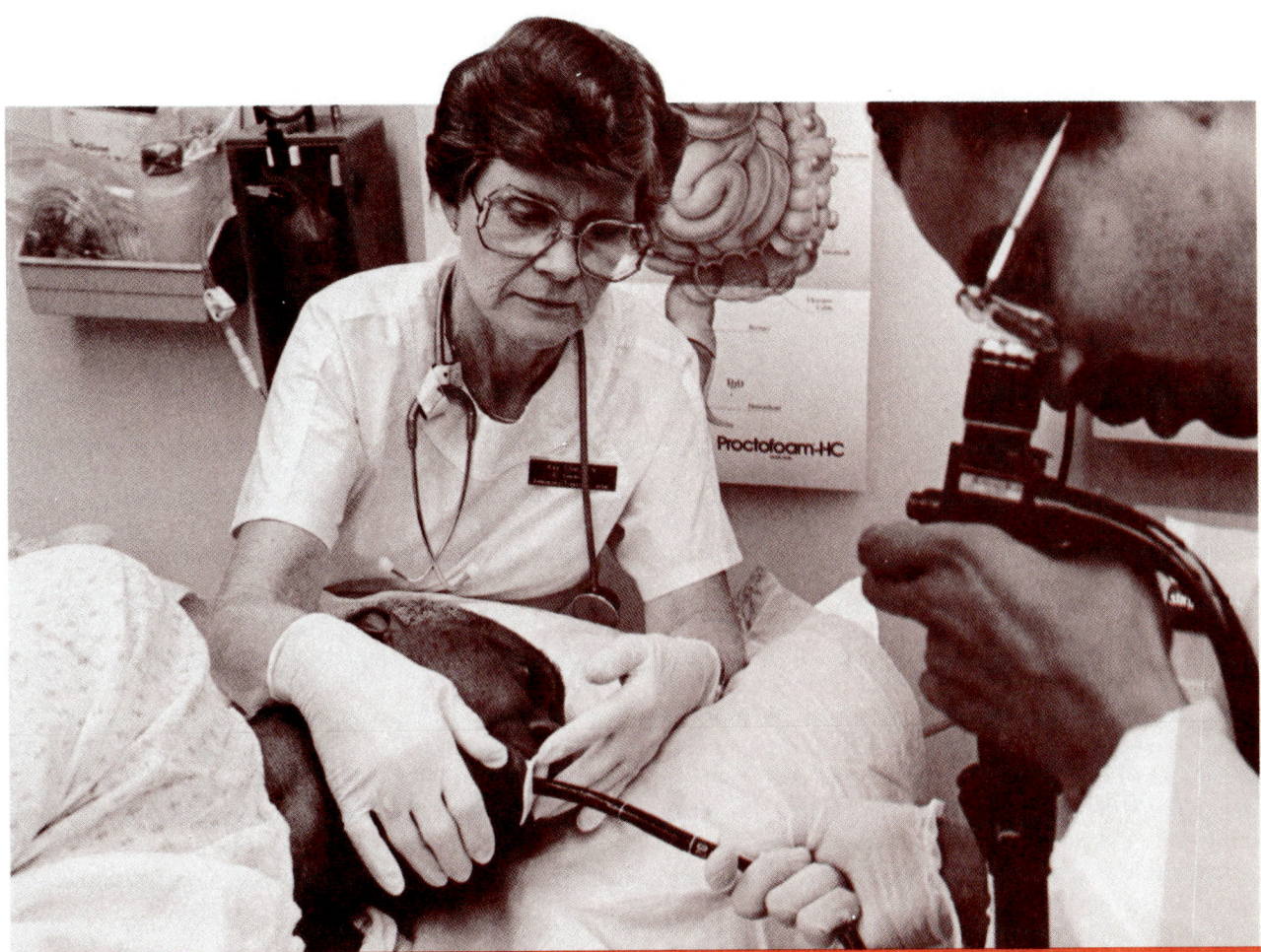

CONTENTS

▶ Define terms related to selected special procedures used in diagnosing and treating clients.

▶ Describe the purposes and sequencing of selected procedures.

▶ Identify assessment data required for specific procedures.

▶ Identify education needs of clients about to have certain tests and treatments.

▶ Outline measures to prepare the client physically for specific procedures.

▶ Identify the nursing responsibilities during selected procedures.

▶ Describe guidelines for evaluating and recording client responses after special procedures.

GENERAL NURSING GUIDELINES

In this technological society, health care practitioners frequently use highly specialized procedures and diagnostic equipment to better assess the health status of clients. This chapter focuses on providing information about some of the more commonly used special procedures to enable the nurse to better prepare clients for these procedures, skillfully care for clients during these procedures, and competently assess clients after these procedures.

Tests and treatments are frightening to many people. People may fear pain, the results of tests, or their reactions to either the pain or the findings of a test. Fear of the unknown increases these misgivings. Nurses need to be aware of the needs of clients and their support persons and to help them meet these needs by preparing them psychologically as well as physically.

The client and, very often, the support persons need to know why a test or treatment is necessary and what it will entail. The explanation should be adjusted to the client's needs; a small child requires an explanation different from that required by a curious adult. Some persons want to know every detail, but others need only a general explanation. The nurse must be honest with the client; if the client will feel sharp pain during the test, it is better to say so than not to mention it.

Often clients want to know where the test will take place, who will do it, how long it will last, and when the results will be available. The last question is often associated with fear. The nurse can base answers on knowledge of the test and on experience. An honest answer (e.g., "I don't know, but I'll try to find that out for you") is more psychologically supportive than an ambiguous answer (e.g., "Well, we'll see about that") or a condescending one ("Now, don't you worry about that at all").

The client needs to sign a consent form before any procedure. Obtaining the client's informed consent is the responsibility of a physician. To give truly informed consent, the client must understand what the procedure entails, what the risks are, and what the alternatives are. Before invasive procedures, e.g., lumbar puncture, the client must often sign a special consent form in addition to the general consent signed upon admission to a health agency. See Chapter 8 for more information about informed consent.

It is usually the nurse's responsibility to assemble the equipment for tests and treatments carried out at a hospitalized client's bedside or in an adjacent treatment room. Maintaining the sterility of sterile equipment is also a nursing responsibility. When a client goes to another area for the procedure, that department assumes responsibility for assembling the equipment.

Before any procedure, nurses should obtain information that can be used as baseline data for assessment during and following the procedure. Before a lumbar puncture, for example, the nurse records the client's vital signs (temperature, pulse, blood pressure) as well as any client complaints of headache or neurologic signs, e.g., tingling in the feet or legs. These clinical signs will be assessed after the lumbar puncture. In addition, signs that the client's life is threatened (e.g., falling blood pressure; irregular, weak pulse; or dyspnea) must be reported to the physician before the procedure.

If a client appears unduly anxious about the procedure, the nurse should intervene and attempt to relieve the anxiety. Often, repeated explanations of what the physician has said to the client, clarification of certain aspects of the procedure, or validation of the client's feelings may reduce anxiety. Unrelieved anxiety must be reported to the physician, who may give additional information and reassurance and in some instances order a tranquilizer or other medication.

During the treatment or test, the nurse continues to assess the client and provide emotional support. The nurse should be sensitive to signs of distress, such as pallor, profuse sweating, accelerated pulse, or signs of nausea or acute pain. Any distress needs to be reported immediately to the physician conducting the procedure. The nurse can support the client by providing information, for instance: "It will be about only 2 minutes more," "The needle is all the way in now," or "You won't feel any additional discomfort." Sometimes, the nurse can distract the client by asking questions; however, some clients do not respond well to this tactic.

Specimens obtained during a procedure should be appropriately labeled. Hospital specimens usually are marked with the client's name, identification number, and date. Some specimens require special care if not sent directly to the laboratory. Some urine specimens are refrigerated, and some fecal specimens are kept warm to keep microorganisms alive.

The nurse also assesses the client after any test or treatment. The interval between assessments depends on the client's condition and the procedure performed. Even if there are no adverse reactions, in many instances clients should be assessed immediately after the procedure and 30 minutes thereafter. Data obtained during the assessments are compared with the baseline data to evaluate any changes in the client's health status. After a procedure, the nurse assists the client to a prescribed or comfortable position. After a lumbar puncture, the client usually assumes a dorsal recumbent position.

Preprocedure assessments and nursing interventions are recorded before the procedure starts. After the procedure, the nurse records what treatment or test was performed, when it was done, who carried it out, and whether a specimen was taken. The nurse also records specific information, such as spinal fluid pressures, and any assessments and nursing interventions carried out during and after the procedure.

Support persons need to be told when a procedure is completed and when they can see the client or take the ambulatory client home. It is usually best to remove equipment before support persons enter the treatment room, because many people find long needles and similar equipment disquieting. The ambulatory client who is returning home after the procedure should receive written directions for any follow-up measures. People are often anxious and preoccupied at these times and find it difficult to remember verbal directions.

EXAMINATIONS INVOLVING ELECTRIC IMPULSES

A number of machines measure and record electric impulses. The **electrocardiograph** receives impulses from the heart; the **electroencephalograph,** from the brain; and the **electromyograph** from muscles. These machines have electrodes that are sensitive to electric activity, which is recorded graphically. The graphic reading can also be shown on an oscilloscope screen.

Electrocardiography

An **electrocardiogram** (**ECG** or **EKG**) is a graph of electric impulses from the heart. The heart muscle is **polarized,** or charged, when it is at rest. When the muscle cells of the ventricles and the atria contract, they **depolarize,** or lose their charge. During a resting stage, they regain their electric charge, or **repolarize.** Cardiac depolarization and repolarization are recorded on an EKG. Figure 48–1 shows a normal EKG and indicates the intervals of depolarization and repolarization. The *P wave* arises when the impulse from the **sinoatrial (SA) node** causes the atria to contract or depolarize. The *QRS complex* occurs

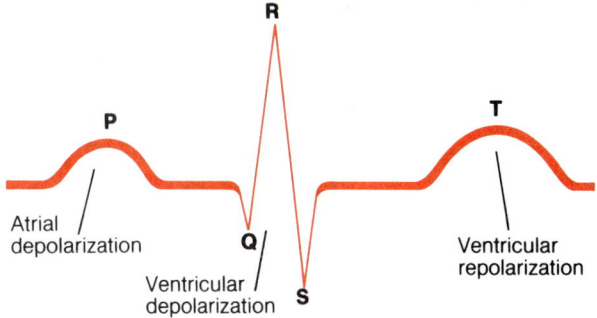

Figure 48–1 Schematic of a normal electrocardiogram.

with contraction and depolarization of the ventricles. The *T wave* represents the resting or repolarization of the ventricles.

Repolarization of the atria occurs during the QRS segment of the graph; it is normally not seen on an EKG. The EKG is produced on finely lined paper. The horizontal lines represent the voltage of the electric impulse, and the vertical lines represent time. See Figure 48–2. The graph waves can be abnormal in size, position, and form when cardiac disease exists.

Electrocardiography is painless and usually takes about 10 minutes, although newer computerized electrocardiograph machines are much quicker. Some physicians order an EKG as part of routine physical examinations of clients over age 40. No special preparation is required before the test unless the physician so specifies, e.g., "exercise strenuously for 5 minutes just prior to EKG." If the client is critically ill, the heart may be monitored continually. For such clients, a **cardiac monitor** is used. This machine shows cardiac waves on an oscilloscope.

Before the EKG is taken, the nurse assesses the client's vital signs (body temperature, pulse, respirations, and blood pressure) for baseline data, if not already available. The

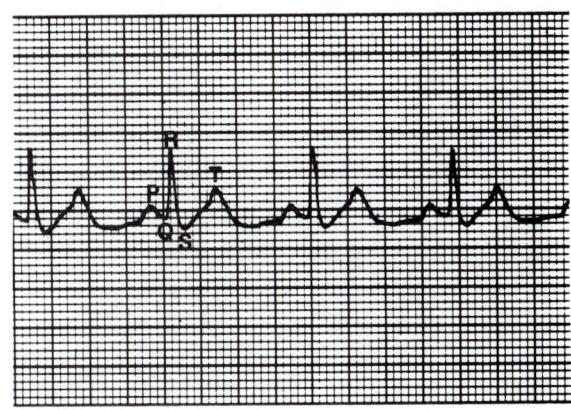

Figure 48–2 A normal electrocardiogram.

nurse also determines whether the client has had an EKG before and explains the procedure, as the client requires. The client may be anxious, not about the test, which is painless, but about the results, which might indicate a problem with the heart.

For an electrocardiogram, electrodes are attached by leads to the electrocardiograph. The electrodes are attached to the client's body with paste, suction cups, or tape. One electrode is attached to the lower part of each limb, and a fifth electrode is moved to six different positions on the chest. The first position is on the right sternal border; subsequent positions follow the general outline of the heart around to the left sternal border and laterally as far as the midaxillary line. The heart's electric impulses register on a graph that the machine produces during the procedure.

Following the procedure, the nurse assesses any reported discomfort, pulse, respirations, and blood pressure. The nurse also records the time the EKG was carried out, the person who performed it, and all assessments. If the client is particularly anxious about the test, the nurse notifies the physician so that the results can be explained as soon as possible.

Electroencephalography

Electroencephalograms (EEGs) are recordings of electric activity in the brain. Electroencephalographs have leads to electrodes that attach to the client's scalp with paste or small needles. The client lies in a dorsal recumbent position in a darkened room. The client may be asked to hyperventilate, and readings may also be taken while the client sleeps. If performed on a sleeping client, the test may take 2 hours; otherwise it lasts no more than 1 hour. The test is normally painless, although the client may feel occasional pinpricks if needle electrodes are used in the scalp.

Preparation for an EEG varies. Some agencies advise that on the day of the test the client not take stimulants, such as coffee, or depressants, such as alcohol. Usually, the client takes no medications prior to the test, and the client's hair is shampooed; it should be free of hair spray, hair creams, and the like.

In some instances, serial EEGs are ordered by the physician. These are taken at 12- or 24-hour intervals to detect possible changes in brain activity in brain-injured clients. Hospital policy and/or legal requirements may influence the number and sequencing of serial EEGs being performed prior to discontinuing life-support systems.

Electromyography

An **electromyogram (EMG)** is a record of the electric potential created by the contraction of a muscle. Two electrodes are attached with paste or small needles to the skin over the muscle. This test is used to discern muscle abnormalities such as **fasciculation** (abnormal contraction involving the whole motor unit). No special preparation is necessary for this procedure. The client may experience some discomfort when the needle electrodes are inserted and some residual discomfort if many muscles are tested.

EXAMINATIONS INVOLVING VISUAL INSPECTION

Visual inspection or direct visualization techniques involve the use of special instruments called **endoscopes,** through which interior parts of the body can be seen. Originally, endoscopes were straight, rigid, metal tubes. Today, most endoscopes are fiberoptic; i.e., they are flexible, easily maneuvered, brightly lighted tubes. These fiberoptic endoscopes or fiberscopes make examination easier to perform and more comfortable for the client. Some endoscopes are equipped with a camera that takes color photographs, which can be studied following the examination; others allow the attachment of a second eyepiece (see Figure 48–3) so that another diagnostician or student can observe the procedure simultaneously.

Endoscopes and the examinations performed with them assume their names from the body part to be examined. For example, a *bronchoscope* is used to visualize the bronchi of the lungs, and the examination is called a *bronchoscopy.* Endoscopic examinations are usually performed in surgery or special treatment rooms. They generally take about 30 to 60 minutes to complete. See Table 48–1 for nursing responsibilities before, during, and after each type of endoscopic examination.

Laryngoscopy and **bronchoscopy** are sterile procedures using a laryngoscope and bronchoscope, respectively. A general or local anesthetic may be given before the examination. If a general anesthetic is given, routine preoperative care is given. See Chapter 47. A local anesthetic,

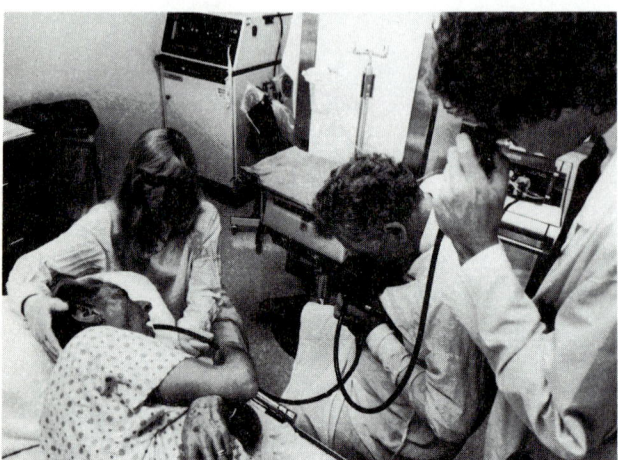

Figure 48–3   An endoscopic procedure in progress.

TABLE 48–1   *Nursing Interventions for Endoscopic Examinations*

Examination	Preprocedure	During Procedure	Postprocedure
Laryngoscopy or bronchoscopy	Explain the procedure and clarify concerns of the client. Explain that a local spray or gargle will be given or that some medications will be injected through a needle in the vein, that the client will rest the teeth against a small plastic mouthpiece, that the procedure is painless but some pressure may be felt. Explain that the test will take about 30 to 60 minutes. Assess vital signs, sputum, and character of respirations for baseline data. Remove dentures, necklaces, earrings, hairpins, and combs. Ensure good oral hygiene. Ensure nothing by mouth 6 to 8 hours beforehand. Confirm that the client is not allergic to any medications that will be given. Administer analgesic, sedative, antianxiety agent, and medication to dry secretions, if ordered.	Assist the physician as required, e.g., to hold the head piece or to move the client's head. Monitor the client's pulse and respirations. Support the client using touch and verbal communication.	1. Monitor vital signs every 30 minutes or as needed during the recovery period, and compare results to baseline data. 2. Withhold fluids until the gag reflex is restored and the client is conscious. 3. Position the client as ordered or indicated. Place the unconscious client in the lateral position so that secretions are not aspirated. 4. Inspect the client's sputum for blood caused by tissue damage. 5. Observe the client for signs of dyspnea, stridor, and shortness of breath, which may result from laryngeal edema or laryngospasm. 6. Provide ice chips and warm saline gargles or throat lozenges and administer ordered analgesics as required for throat discomfort. 7. Advise the client to contact the physician if there is difficulty with breathing, blood in sputum, fever, or pain.
Esophagoscopy, gastroscopy, and duodenoscopy	As above for bronchoscopy, with the exception of assessing sputum. Explain that the client may feel pressure in the stomach as the tube is moved about and fullness or bloating, like that after eating a large meal.	As above for bronchoscopy. Administer oral simethicone (Mylicon) before test if ordered; it decreases air bubbles in the stomach. If atropine is given intravenously to reduce gastrointestinal spasm, carefully monitor the client's pulse rate. Atropine increases the heart rate.	1. Follow steps 1 to 3 and 6, as for bronchoscopy. 2. Inspect emesis for blood and test it for occult blood if agency practice indicates. 3. Advise the client to contact the physician if client has persistent difficulty swallowing, pain, fever, blood in vomitus, or black stools.
Cystoscopy	Assess vital signs, frequency of urination, dysuria, amount and consistency of urine for baseline data. Administer enema if ordered. A clear bowel is necessary if x-ray films are planned. Ensure nothing by mouth for 6 to 8 hours or only IV fluids if general anesthetic is being given.	Support the client emotionally. Monitor vital signs. Label specimens, if taken, appropriately. Assist the physician as requested.	1. Monitor vital signs, urination, and urine, and compare with baseline data. 2. Position the unconscious client appropriately (as above for bronchoscopy). 3. Inspect the client's urine for blood and report bright red bleeding.

▶

Examination	Preprocedure	During Procedure	Postprocedure
Cystoscopy (continued)	Ensure appropriate fluid intake, if ordered, for the client having a local anesthetic to ensure an adequate flow of urine for the collection of specimens. Administer sedative and medication to dry secretions, if ordered.		4. Report inability to urinate by 8 hours. 5. Encourage increased fluid intake to decrease irritation of urinary tissue. 6. If dyes were used in the procedure, warn the client that the urine may be an unusual color. 7. Administer analgesics, as ordered, for pain. 8. If the client is discharged, advise the client to report persistent difficulty passing urine, bright blood in urine, pain, or fever.
Anoscopy, proctoscopy, sigmoidoscopy, and colonoscopy	Assess vital signs and consistency of feces for baseline data. Ensure appropriate preexamination diet and fluid intake. Some agencies provide a light evening meal the day before and only fluid the day of the examination. Administer laxative, if ordered, the evening before. Administer enemas until returns are clear or suppository as ordered the morning of the examination. Ensure that the client voids before the examination. The pressure during the procedure may injure a full bladder. Administer sedative beforehand, if ordered. Just before the endoscope is inserted explain (a) that the client will experience the sensation of having to move the bowels due to the pressure of the instrument, and (b) that the client may experience some abdominal cramping when air is introduced to distend the bowel.	Support the client physically in the knee-chest position, as needed. Monitor pulse and respiratory rates. Label specimens, if taken, appropriately. Support the client emotionally. Acknowledge feelings the client experiences, e.g., cramps, and assure the client that they are not unusual.	1. Monitor vital signs and compare with baseline data. 2. Inspect the next few stools for blood. 3. Allow the client to rest. This procedure may be physically and emotionally tiring. 4. Provide fluids and food.

if given, is sprayed on the client's pharynx to prevent gagging; alternatively, the client gargles with an anesthetic to anesthetize the throat. The bronchoscope is then inserted to visualize the larynx or bronchi. In some cases, a section of tissue is taken for biopsy. For this procedure, the client usually lies supine on the examining table. See Table 48–1 for nursing interventions before, during, and after the examination.

Esophagoscopy (visual examination of the esophagus), **gastroscopy** (visual examination of the stomach), and **duodenoscopy** (visual examination of the duodenum) are performed with a gastroscope. This is a clean rather than a sterile procedure. The preparation and care of the client are the same as for laryngoscopy and bronchoscopy. During these procedures, a tissue sample may be taken for biopsy, and samples of secretions may be taken for study of digestive enzymes. See Table 48–1 for nursing interventions.

Cystoscopy is the visualization of the interior of the urinary bladder; this examination requires insertion of a cystoscope into the bladder via the urethra. It is a sterile procedure. A general or local anesthetic is given, and the preparation is similar to that for bronchoscopy. During cystoscopy, catheters may be inserted up the ureters into each kidney. Contrast medium is then injected into the kidneys, and x-ray photographs are taken. This procedure is known as **retrograde pyelography.** The x-ray film shows the kidney calyces, the kidney pelvis, the ureters, and the urinary bladder. When a pyelogram is to be taken, the client is given laxatives and enemas to free the intestines of feces and gas. **Intravenous pyelography (IVP)** or **urography (IVU)** is roentgenography of the kidneys after the injection of dye into the arterial system. An intravenous pyelogram shows the same structures as a retrograde pyelogram. This examination does not require an anesthetic and normally lasts about 1 hour. See Table 48–1 for nursing interventions.

Anoscopy, proctoscopy, sigmoidoscopy, and **colonoscopy** are endoscopic procedures of the mucosa of the anus, rectum, sigmoid colon, and colon, respectively. A proctoscope or sigmoidoscope is used to examine the anus, rectum, and sigmoid colon. A colonoscope is used to examine the large bowel.

Preparation generally includes the administration of laxatives or enemas begun the evening before to clear the bowel of feces. General anesthesia is not usually necessary, although the client may experience some discomfort. The client assumes a knee-chest position on a special examining table during the examination.

EXAMINATIONS INVOLVING REMOVAL OF BODY FLUIDS AND TISSUES

Certain body fluids and tissues can help physicians diagnose disease. Table 48–2 lists some common procedures for removing body fluids and tissues. The procedures are normally performed by a physician at the bedside, in an examining room, or sometimes in the emergency department of a hospital. All the procedures described here involve inserting an instrument, often a needle, through the skin and withdrawing some fluid or tissue. The fluid or tissue is usually placed in a special container and sent to the laboratory for examination. During each procedure, the nurse's responsibility is to assist the physician as requested (maintaining sterile technique), to observe the client and to support the client verbally, describing the steps of the procedure if the physician does not do so.

Lumbar Puncture

A **lumbar puncture (LP, spinal tap)** is the insertion of a needle into the subarachnoid space of the spinal canal to withdraw cerebrospinal fluid (CSF). An adult normally has

TABLE 48–2 *Common Aspiration Studies*

Name	Type of Specimen	Source	Key Postprocedure Assessments
Lumbar puncture	Spinal fluid	Subarachnoid space of the spinal canal	Vital signs, neurologic signs, headache
Abdominal paracentesis	Ascitic fluid	Peritoneal cavity	Blood pressure, pulse, skin color, weight, abdominal girth
Thoracocentesis	Pleural fluid	Pleural cavity	Pulse, respirations, skin color
Pericardial aspiration	Pericardial fluid	Pericardial sac	As for thoracocentesis
Bone marrow biopsy	Bone marrow	Iliac crest, posterior superior iliac spine, or sternum	Leakage at site, pain
Liver biopsy	Liver tissue	Liver	Blood pressure, pulse, respirations, bleeding at site

about 150 ml of CSF (Guyton 1986, p. 374). The major function of the spinal fluid is to cushion the brain within the skull. Lumbar punctures are carried out for a number of diagnostic and therapeutic reasons, e.g., to analyze the constituents of the CSF. The site of the lumbar puncture is usually between the third and fourth or the fourth and fifth lumbar vertebrae. Inserted at this level, the needle does not damage the spinal cord and major nerve roots. See Figure 48–4. The fourth lumbar interspace is the most common lumbar puncture site for adults, but the site is usually lower for the infant or small child, whose spinal cord extends almost into the sacral region.

A lumbar puncture requires sterile technique. Many hospitals have disposable lumbar puncture kits. The equipment required includes: sterile sponges; antiseptic solution; local anesthetic and #21 and #24 gauge needles and syringes for injection; lumbar puncture needle 5 to 12.5 cm (2 to 5 in) long, depending on the age and size of the client (infants require a 5 cm needle); specimen containers; manometer to measure spinal fluid pressure; three-way stopcock; small dressing to put over the puncture site; sterile gloves for the physician and the nurse; and masks (optional).

Medical Technique

The physician applies an antiseptic to the area, injects local anesthetic, and inserts the needle into the intravertebral space. When the flow of CSF is established, the stopcock and manometer are attached to obtain an initial CSF pressure reading. Normal opening pressures are 60 to 180 mm of water. Pressures above 200 mm are considered abnormal.

A Queckenstedt-Stookey test may also be done while the manometer is attached. Someone (often the nurse) exerts digital pressure on one or both of the client's internal jugular veins. Normally digital pressure temporarily increases the manometer reading. If there is a blockage in the spinal canal, digital pressure affects CSF pressure minimally or not at all.

The physician usually takes specimens of CSF and hands the specimen tubes to the nurse, who numbers them in the sequence taken. Specimens of CSF are often tested in the laboratory for sugar, bacteria, and cell count. Normal CSF is a clear, colorless fluid. Blood may give the fluid a reddish cast, and infection may make the fluid cloudy.

Nursing Intervention

Preprocedure Assess the client's vital signs, pertinent health status, e.g., level of consciousness and neurologic status, to obtain baseline data. Determine drug allergies, particularly to local anesthetics and skin antiseptics.

Explain the following to the client, even if the client appears stuporous or confused:

- That the physician will be taking a small sample of spinal fluid from the lower spine

- That a local anesthetic will be given so that the client will feel no pain

- When and where the procedure will occur, e.g., at the bedside or in the treatment room

- Who will be present, i.e., the physician and the nurse

- How long the procedure will take, e.g., about 15 minutes

In addition, tell the client what to expect during the procedure. The client may feel slight discomfort (like a pinprick) when the local anesthetic is injected and a sensation

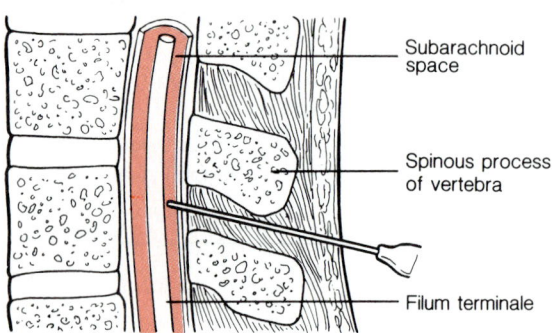

Figure 48–4 A diagram of the vertebral column, indicating the site for a lumbar puncture.

of pressure when the spinal needle is being inserted. Remind the client that it is important to remain still and in one position throughout the procedure. A restless client or a child will need to be held to prevent movement.

Have the client empty the bladder and bowels prior to the procedure to prevent unnecessary discomfort.

Position the client laterally with the head bent toward the chest, the knees flexed onto the abdomen, and the back at the edge of the bed or examining table. See Figure 48–5. Place a very small pillow under the client's head to maintain the horizontal alignment of the spine. In this position, the back is arched, increasing the spaces between the vertebrae so that the spinal needle can be inserted readily. Drape the client to expose only the lumbar spine.

Open the lumbar puncture set, and supply the physician with the sterile gloves and antiseptic in a container or poured onto sterile gauze squares, if necessary.

During the procedure Stand in front of the client, and support the back of the client's neck and knees if the client needs help remaining in this position without moving. See Figure 48–5. Reassure the client throughout the procedure by explaining what is happening. Encourage the client to breathe normally and relax as much as possible; excessive muscle tension, coughing, or changes in breathing can increase CSF pressure, resulting in a false reading.

If the Queckenstedt-Stookey test is being done, place digital pressure on the client's jugular veins. See Figure 48–6. Label the specimen tubes in sequence if they are not already labeled. While handling the tubes, wear gloves because the CSF may contain virulent microorganisms, e.g., those that cause meningitis. Place a small sterile dressing over the site of the puncture to help prevent infection after the needle is removed.

Postprocedure Assist the client to a dorsal recumbent position with only one pillow under the head. The client should not sit up for 8 to 24 hours, until the CSF is replenished (primarily by the choroid plexus in each ventricle of the brain). Determine the recommended time this position should be maintained according to physician's order or agency protocol. Some clients experience a headache after a lumbar puncture, and the dorsal recumbent position tends to prevent or alleviate it. Often analgesics are ordered and can be given for headaches.

Assess the client's pallor, changes in pulse rate and other vital signs, changes in neurologic status, swelling or bleeding at the puncture site, and complaints of faintness or headache. Be alert for complaints of numbness, tingling, or pain radiating down the legs, which may be due to nerve irritation. Observe the puncture site for leakage of CSF.

Ensure that the CSF specimens are correctly labeled and send them immediately to the laboratory, with the completed requisition.

Record the procedure on the client's chart, including the date and time it was performed; the name of the physician;

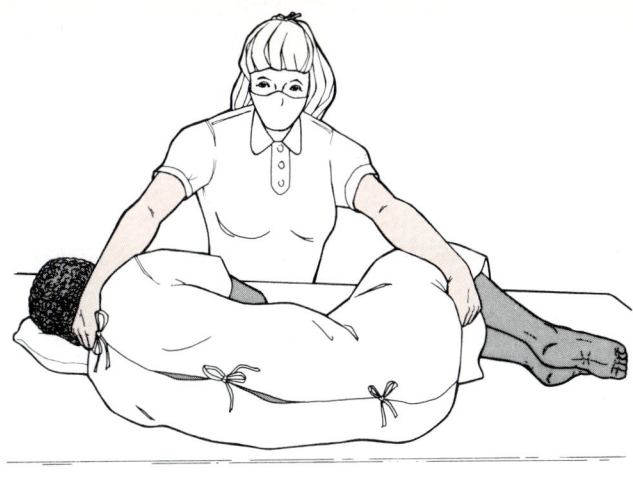

Figure 48–5 Positioning a client for a lumbar puncture.

the color, character (clear, cloudy), and amount of CSF obtained; the pressure readings; the number of specimens obtained; and the assessments of the client.

Abdominal Paracentesis

Abdominal paracentesis is the removal of fluid from the peritoneal cavity. Normally the peritoneum creates just enough fluid to lubricate the surface of the peritoneum and reduce friction between the peritoneum and the tissues with which it comes in contact. This fluid is absorbed into the lymph circulation through lymph vessels in the peritoneum. However, in some disease processes, such as cirrhosis of the liver, large amounts of fluid collect in the cavity;

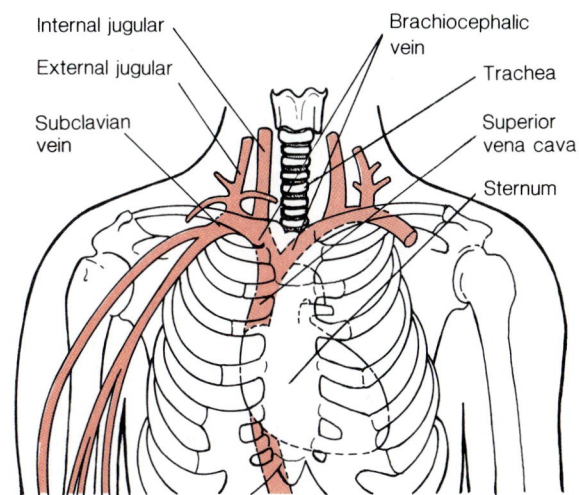

Figure 48–6 Location of the internal jugular vein, where digital pressure is applied during the Queckenstedt-Stookey test.

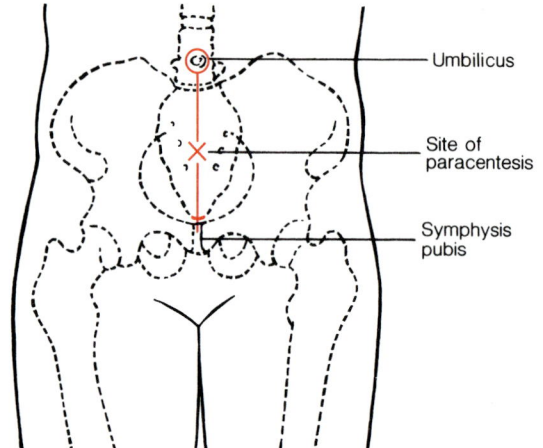

Figure 48–7 A common site for an abdominal paracentesis.

this condition is called **ascites.** Normal ascitic fluid is serous (clear and light yellow). An abdominal paracentesis is carried out to obtain a fluid specimen for laboratory study and to relieve pressure on the abdominal organs due to excess fluid. A common site for an abdominal paracentesis is midway between the umbilicus and the symphysis pubis in the midline. See Figure 48–7.

Abdominal paracentesis requires sterile technique. Paracentesis sets are usually available. These contain antiseptic; sponges; local anesthetic; syringe and #24 and #22 gauge needles to administer the anesthetic; fenestrated drape; small scalpel to make an incision in the abdomen; a needle holder and sutures to sew the incision; specimen containers; dressings; and an aspirating set. The aspirating set generally includes a receptacle for the fluid, tubing, and a trocar and cannula. A **trocar** is a sharp, pointed instrument that fits inside the cannula and pierces, in this case, the peritoneal cavity. A **cannula** is a tube through which plastic tubing can be threaded to drain fluid. The trocar and cannula (and the scalpel, sutures, and needle holder) are needed only if the purpose of paracentesis is to drain fluid. If the purpose is to obtain a specimen, an incision is not made. A long aspirating needle attached to a syringe is used in place of a trocar and cannula. Masks are optional. Also needed are sterile gloves for the physician and the nurse.

Medical Technique The physician applies an antiseptic to the site of the incision, drapes the area with sterile drapes, and administers a local anesthetic. After the area is numbed, the physician makes a small incision with a scalpel, inserts the trocar and cannula (the trocar inside the cannula), and then withdraws the trocar. Tubing is attached to the cannula, and the fluid flows through the tubing into a receptacle. Normally about 1500 ml is the maximum amount of fluid drained at one time, to avoid hypovolemic shock.

The fluid is drained very slowly for the same reason. Some fluid is placed in the specimen container before the cannula is withdrawn. The small incision may or may not be sutured; in either case, it is covered with a small sterile bandage.

Nursing Intervention

Preprocedure Assess the client's vital signs to obtain baseline data. Weigh the client, and measure the client's abdominal girth at the level of the umbilicus to obtain an indication of the amount of ascites. (See Chapter 19, Figure 19–82.) Determine any allergies, in particular to local anesthetics and antiseptics. Record your findings.

Explain the procedure to the client. Normally an abdominal paracentesis is not painful; when a client has considerable ascites, moreover, the procedure can relieve discomfort caused by the fluid. The procedure to remove ascitic fluid usually takes 30 to 60 minutes. Obtaining a specimen usually takes about 15 minutes. Emphasize that the client must remain still during the procedure. Explain when and where the procedure will occur and who will be present.

Ask the client to void just before the paracentesis to lessen the possibility of puncturing the urinary bladder. Notify the physician if the client cannot void prior to the procedure.

Help the client assume a sitting position in bed so that the fluid will accumulate in the lower abdominal cavity and so that gravity and the pressure of the abdominal organs will help the flow of the fluid from the cavity. Some clients may be able to sit on the edge of the bed with pillows to support the back. Cover the client to expose only the necessary area.

During the procedure Support the client verbally, and describe the steps of the procedure if the physician does not do so. Observe the client closely for signs of distress. A major concern is hypovolemic shock induced by the loss of fluid.

Place a small sterile dressing over the site of the incision after the cannula is withdrawn.

Postprocedure Assess the client's pulse rate, skin color, and blood pressure. Hypovolemic shock can occur when the fluid in the circulatory system is redirected to the abdominal area as a result of reduced pressure from the removal of the ascitic fluid. Shock is evidenced by pallor, dyspnea, diaphoresis (profuse perspiration), and a drop in blood pressure. Measure the abdominal girth with a tape measure in the same place as before the procedure, and weigh the client to establish fluid loss.

Arrange for the specimen with the completed requisition and label to be transported to the laboratory. Record the procedure on the client's chart, including the date and time; name of the physician; abdominal girth before and after the procedure; color, clarity, and amount of drained fluid; and nursing assessments.

Thoracocentesis (Thoracentesis)

Thoracocentesis (thoracentesis) is the withdrawal of fluid or air from the pleural cavity. Normally there is only enough fluid to lubricate the pleura so that they can move freely. However, excessive fluid or air can accumulate in the pleural cavity as a result of injury or disease. Pleural fluid is removed for both diagnostic and therapeutic purposes. Aspiration of air or fluid may be indicated to relieve pain, dyspnea, and other symptoms of pleural pressure. A thoracocentesis is also performed to introduce chemotherapeutic drugs intrapleurally.

A sterile thoracocentesis set usually contains these items:

- Sterile sponges or gauze squares with an antiseptic solution to apply to the site of the thoracocentesis.
- A drape or drapes to place over the client's chest. The drape is often fenestrated, and the opening is placed at the site of the thoracocentesis.
- A 2-ml syringe and #24 and #22 gauge needles to administer the anesthetic.
- A receptacle for the fluid. This may be a syringe (50 ml) and #16 gauge needle or an airtight container with negative pressure created by a pump or a suction machine. The negative pressure in the container must be greater than that of the pleural space. Negative pressure also prevents air from entering the pleural space and causing a pneumothorax (air in the pleural cavity).
- A three-way stopcock to prevent air from entering the pleural space.
- A two-way stopcock with connecting tubing to maintain the negative pressure in the receptacle and to direct the flow of pleural fluid into the container.
- A thoracocentesis needle, usually a #15 gauge needle about 5 to 7.5 cm (2 to 3 in) long.
- A specimen container.
- A local anesthetic. The anesthetic is usually packaged in an ampule.

 Sterile gloves for the physician and nurse are required. Masks for the nurse and the physician are optional. A completed laboratory requisition and label for the specimen are needed.

Medical Technique   The physician dons sterile gloves, cleans the site with an antiseptic solution, and administers a local anesthetic. The physician attaches a syringe and/or stopcock to the aspirating needle. The stopcock must be in the closed position so that no air will enter the pleural space. The physician inserts the needle through the intercostal space into the pleural cavity. In some instances, a small plastic tube is threaded through the needle and the needle is then withdrawn. (The tubing is less likely to punc-

ture the pleura.) If a syringe is used, the plunger is pulled out to draw out the pleural fluid as the stopcock is opened. If a large container is used to receive the fluid, the tubing is attached from the stopcock to the adapter on the receiving bottle. When the adapter and stopcock are opened, negative pressure in the container draws the fluid from the pleural cavity. After the fluid has been withdrawn, the physician removes the needle or plastic tubing.

Nursing Intervention

Preprocedure   Assess (a) vital signs (body temperature, pulse, respirations, and blood pressure) to obtain baseline data, if these are not already available; (b) respiratory depth and the movement of both sides of the chest during inspiration, to note differences between the two sides; (c) complaints of chest pain; (d) breath sounds; (e) dyspnea; (f) type and frequency of cough, if present; and (g) character and amount of sputum.

Also determine if the client has drug allergies, particularly allergies to the medications contained in local anesthetics and skin antiseptics. Administer any ordered cough medicine 30 minutes before the thoracocentesis to suppress coughing during the procedure.

Explain the procedure to the client. Normally a thoracocentesis is not painful, although the client may experience a feeling of pressure when the needle is inserted. The client may experience considerable relief if breathing has been difficult. The procedure takes only a few minutes, depending primarily on the time it takes the fluid to drain from the pleural cavity. It is important for the client not to cough while the needle is inserted, to avoid puncturing the lungs. Explain when and where the procedure will occur and who will be present.

Help the client assume a comfortable position. This is usually a sitting position with the arms above the head, which spreads the ribs and enlarges the intercostal space. Usually, the client either keeps the arm elevated and stretched forward (see Figure 48–8, A) or leans forward over pillows (see Figure 48–8, B). To make sure that the needle is inserted below the fluid level when fluid is to be removed (or above any fluid if air is to be removed), the physician palpates the chest and selects the exact site for insertion of the needle. A site on the lower posterior chest is often used to remove fluid, and a site on the upper anterior chest is used to remove air.

During the procedure   Support the client verbally, and describe the steps of the procedure if the physician does not do so. Observe the client closely for signs of distress, such as dyspnea, pallor, and coughing. If the client becomes distressed or has to cough, the procedure is halted briefly. The physician may withdraw the needle slightly to avoid puncturing the pleura.

Following the removal of the needle, place a small sterile dressing over the puncture site.

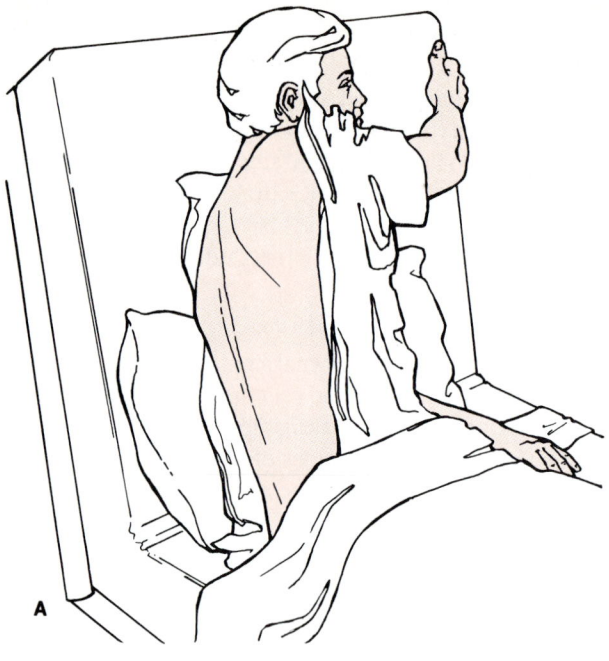

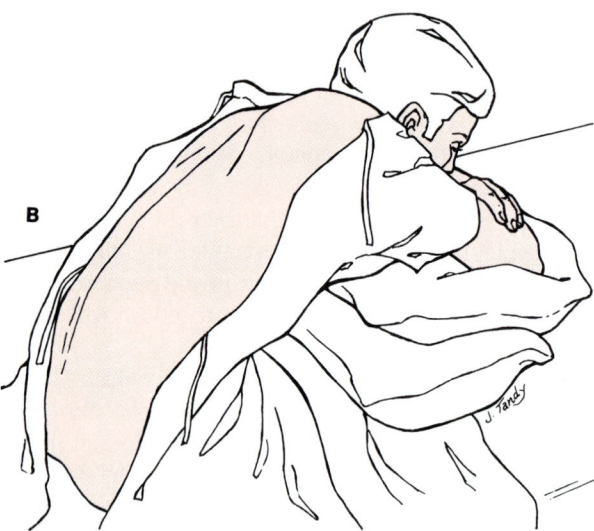

Figure 48–8 Two positions commonly used for a thoracocentesis: *A,* sitting on one side with the arm held to the front and up; *B,* sitting and leaning forward over pillows.

Postprocedure Assess the client's blood pressure, pulse, respiration rate, and skin color, because a shift in the mediastinum (heart and large blood vessels) can occur with removal of large amounts of fluid. Also observe any changes in the client's cough, sputum, respiration depth, breath sounds, and chest pain.

Arrange for the specimen and the completed requisition to be transported to the laboratory. Record the procedure on the client's chart, including the date and time; the name of the physician; the amount, color, and clarity of fluid drained; and any other significant assessments, such as the client's respiration rate.

Bone Marrow Biopsy

A bone marrow biopsy is the removal of a specimen of bone marrow for study in a laboratory. The biopsy makes it possible to study a bone marrow specimen for abnormal blood cell development and thus to detect anemia, leukemia, and other diseases of the blood. The sternum and the posterior superior iliac crests are common sites for biopsies. See Figure 48–9.

Bone marrow biopsy sets usually contain these items:

- A drape or drapes. One drape is often fenestrated, and the opening is placed over the aspiration site.
- Antiseptic to clean the skin.
- A local anesthetic.
- A 2-ml syringe and #25 gauge needle to administer the local anesthetic.
- A 10-ml syringe to withdraw the bone marrow.
- A bone marrow needle with stylet.
- Sterile gauze squares to apply the antiseptic and cover the wound.
- Test tubes and/or glass slides for the specimen.

Also needed are masks for the nurse and physician (optional), sterile gloves, and a completed laboratory requisition and labels for the specimen.

Medical Technique The physician administers a local anesthetic into the skin and the periosteum of the bone, then introduces a bone marrow needle with stylet through the skin and bone into the red marrow of the spongy bone. Once the needle is in the marrow space, the physician removes the stylet, attaches a 10-ml syringe to the needle, and draws the plunger back until 1 or 2 ml of marrow has been withdrawn. The physician replaces the stylet in the needle, withdraws the needle, and places the specimen in test tubes and/or on glass slides.

Nursing Intervention

Preprocedure Assess the client's vital signs for baseline data. Determine any client allergies, in particular to local anesthetics and skin antiseptics.

Explain the procedure to the client. The client may experience pain when the marrow is aspirated. There may be a crunching sound when the needle is pushed through the cortex of the bone. The entire procedure usually takes 15 to 30 minutes. Explain when and where the procedure will occur and who will be present.

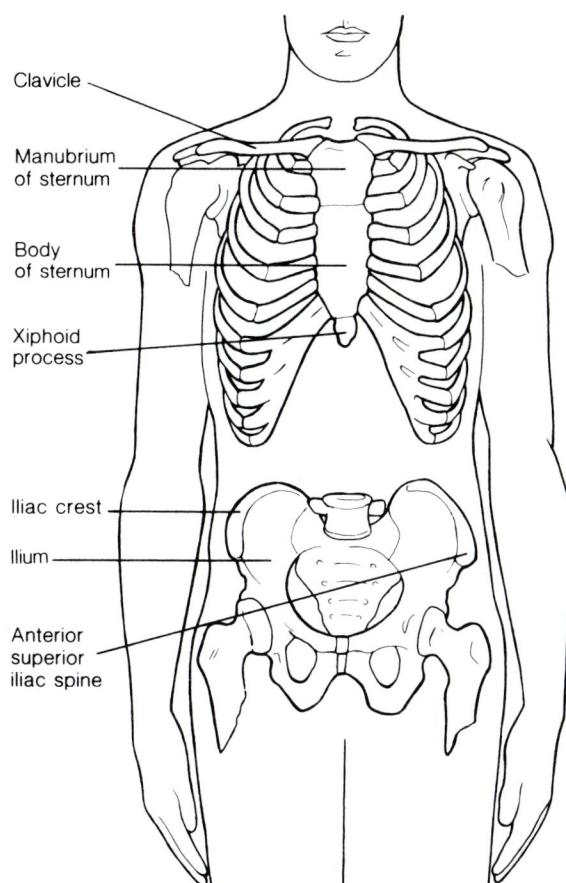

Figure 48–9   The sternum and iliac crests are common sites for bone marrow biopsies.

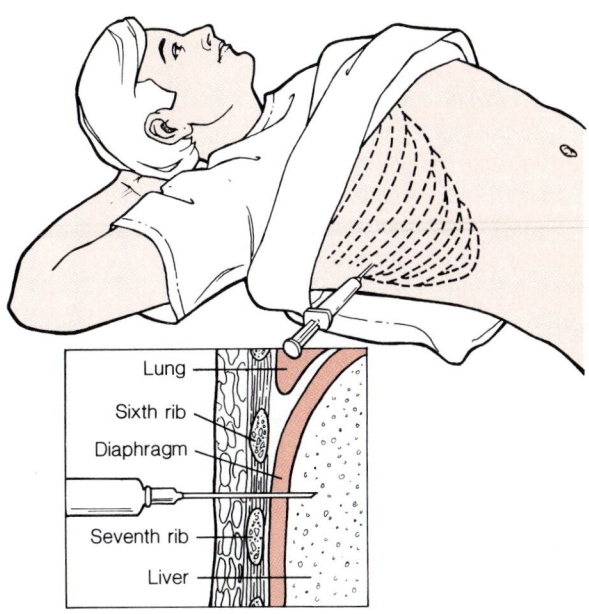

Figure 48–10   The site for a liver biopsy.

Help the client assume a supine position (with one pillow if desired) for a biopsy of the sternum (sternal puncture) or a prone position for a biopsy of either iliac crest. Fold the bedclothes back to expose the area.

During the procedure   Describe the steps of the procedure to the client, and provide verbal support. Observe the client for pallor, diaphoresis, and faintness. Place a small dressing over the site of the puncture after the needle is withdrawn.

Postprocedure   Assess the client's discomfort and any bleeding from the site. The client may experience some tenderness in the area. Bleeding and hematoma formation need to be assessed for several days. Provide an analgesic if required by the client and ordered by the physician.

Arrange for the specimen with the completed requisition and label to be transported to the laboratory. Record the procedure on the client's chart, including the data and time of the procedure, the name of the physician, and the assessments of the client.

Liver Biopsy

A liver biopsy is a short procedure, generally performed at the client's bedside. The physician inserts a needle into the liver to aspirate a sample of liver tissue. The site of insertion is either between two of the right lower ribs (see Figure 48–10) or through the abdomen below the right rib cage (subcostally). Liver biopsies are usually conducted to facilitate diagnosis of liver disease and to gain information about changes in liver tissue.

A liver biopsy requires sterile technique. Preassembled sterile sets are usually available containing sterile sponges or gauze squares with an antiseptic solution to apply to the skin site; a 2-ml syringe and #22 and #25 gauge needles (¾ in) to inject the local anesthetic; a large biopsy syringe and needle; drapes; a local anesthetic; sterile normal saline to clean the biopsy needle after insertion; and a specimen container with formalin to preserve the liver tissue. Also needed are face masks for the physician and the nurse (optional), sterile gloves, and a laboratory requisition and a specimen label.

Medical Technique   The physician puts on sterile gloves, applies an antiseptic to the biopsy site, drapes the area with sterile drapes, and injects the local anesthetic. When the area feels numb, the client holds the breath, and the physician inserts the biopsy needle, injects a small amount of sterile normal saline to clear the needle of blood or particles of tissue picked up during insertion, and aspirates liver tissue by drawing back on the plunger of the syringe. After the needle is withdrawn, the nurse applies pressure to the site to prevent bleeding.

Nursing Intervention

Preprocedure Assess the client's vital signs (body temperature, pulse, respirations, and blood pressure) for baseline data. Determine any drug allergies, particularly allergies to medications contained in the local anesthetics and skin antiseptics. Also assess the client's ability to hold the breath for up to 10 seconds. It is vitally important that the client do so and remain still while the biopsy needle is inserted.

Also determine the prothrombin time and platelet count from the client's record. Ensure that these are normal. Because many clients with liver disease have blood-clotting defects and are prone to bleeding, prothrombin time and platelet count are normally determined well in advance of the test. If the test results are abnormal, the biopsy may be contraindicated. Also determine if any preprocedural medications are required. Ensure that ordered medications have been given. Several days before the test, vitamin K may be administered intramuscularly to reduce the risk of hemorrhage. Vitamin K may be lacking in some clients with liver disease. It is essential for the production of prothrombin, which is a requisite for blood clotting.

Explain the procedure to the client, including what the physician will do, i.e., take a small sample of liver tissue by putting a needle into the client's side or abdomen; what will be done to prevent pain, i.e., a sedative and local anesthetic will be given; when and where the procedure will occur; who will be present; how long the procedure will last; and what to expect as the procedure is performed, i.e., the client may experience mild discomfort when the local anesthetic is injected and slight pressure when the biopsy needle is inserted.

Ensure that the client fasts for at least two hours before the procedure. Administer the appropriate sedative about 30 minutes beforehand or at the specified time. Help the

client assume a supine position, with the upper right quadrant of the abdomen exposed. Cover the client with the bedclothes so that only the abdominal area is exposed.

During the procedure Support the client in a supine position. Instruct the client to take a few deep inhalations and exhalations and to hold the breath after the final exhalation for up to 10 seconds as the needle is inserted, the biopsy obtained, and the needle withdrawn. Holding the breath after exhalation immobilizes the chest wall and liver and keeps the diaphragm in its highest position, avoiding injury to the diaphragm and laceration of the liver. Instruct the client to resume breathing when the needle is withdrawn. Apply pressure to the site of the puncture. Pressure will help stop any bleeding. Apply a small dressing to the puncture site.

Postprocedure Assist the client to a right side-lying position with a small pillow or folded towel under the biopsy site. See Figure 48–11. Instruct the client to remain in this position for several hours. The right lateral position compresses the biopsy site of the liver against the chest wall and minimizes the escape of blood or bile through the puncture site. Send the labeled specimen immediately to the laboratory along with the completed requisition.

Assess the client's pulse, respirations, and blood pressure every 15 minutes for the first hour following the test or until they are stable. Complications of a liver biopsy are rare, but hemorrhage from a perforated blood vessel can occur. Determine whether the client is experiencing abdominal pain. Severe abdominal pain may indicate bile peritonitis (an inflammation of the peritoneal lining of the abdomen caused by bile leaking from a bile duct). Observe the biopsy site for localized bleeding. Pressure dressings may be required if bleeding occurs. Record the procedure, including the date and time it was performed, the name of the physician, and nursing assessments.

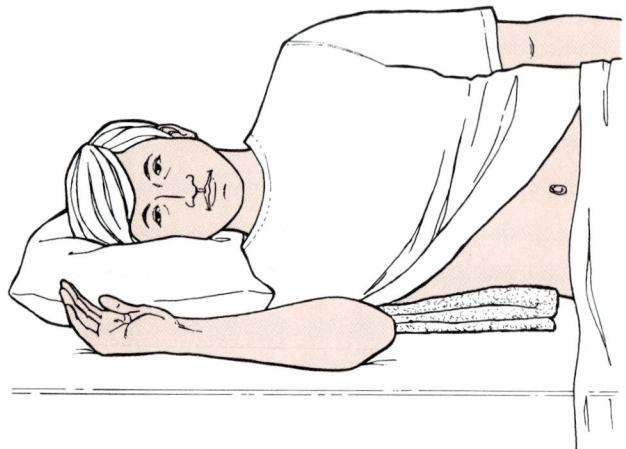

Figure 48–11 The position to provide pressure on a liver biopsy site.

HIGH-TECH STUDIES

With the technological advances of the twentieth century and those anticipated in the twenty-first century, more and more health assessment can be performed with relatively minimal discomfort to clients. This section highlights some of the more commonly performed technological procedures.

Roentgenography

Roentgen rays (x rays) are part of the spectrum of electromagnetic radiation. They travel at the speed of light and have considerably shorter wavelengths than light or radio waves. This distinctive property enables radiation to penetrate organs and tissues according to their thickness and density. High-voltage x rays have shorter wavelengths and produce a more penetrating (harder) radiation; low-voltage x rays have longer wavelengths and produce a more easily absorbable (softer) radiation. X rays that are not absorbed pass through the tissue to form an image on the photographic film (a plain, or static, radiograph) or on a fluorescent screen (fluoroscopy).

It is the differential absorption of x rays by the various tissues that makes roentgenography diagnostically useful. *Bones,* which are dense, permit fewer x rays to pass through to the film, so they appear as light areas. The *soft tissues* surrounding bone are less dense, so they appear darker on the film. Natural contrasts in density also occur between blood-filled cardiovascular structures and air-filled lung areas. Such natural contrasts, however, do not occur in the abdomen or between the soft tissue structures of the extremities. Thus, *contrast agents* must be introduced for certain body parts, e.g., the digestive tract and blood vessels, to show on the film.

Contrast materials (solids, liquids, or gaseous substances) must absorb either more or fewer x rays than the surrounding tissues. Commonly used contrast agents are compounds of iodine, barium, air, and carbon dioxide. Iodine and barium absorb more x rays than soft tissues; air and carbon dioxide absorb fewer. Contrast materials are introduced into the body in four ways to view specific organs:

1. Orally or rectally for the digestive tract (esophagus, stomach, intestines) and gallbladder. See Figure 48–12.

2. Intravenously for the blood vessels, bile ducts, and kidneys.

3. Into the subarachnoid space for the spine and the ventricles of the brain.

4. Through a nasotracheal tube or bronchoscope for the bronchial tree. (This method has been used infrequently since the advent of fiberoptic bronchoscopy, which has increased the area available to direct visual examination.)

Radiography of the gastrointestinal tract often involves fluoroscopy as well as a radiographic examination. **Fluoro-**

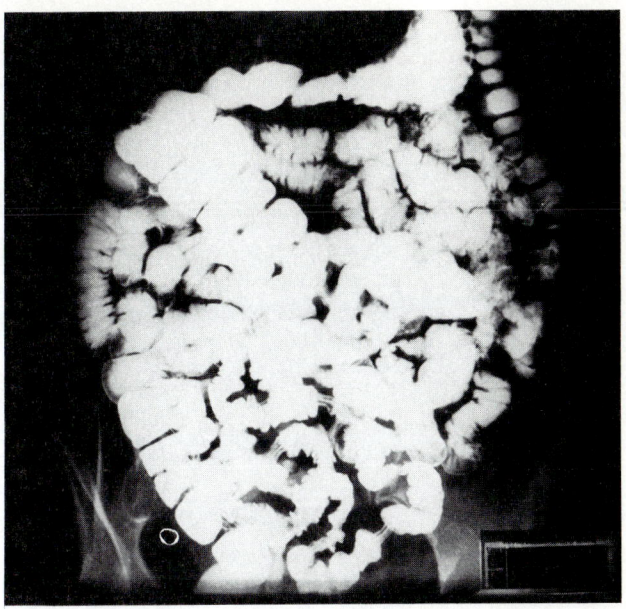

Figure 48–12 An x-ray film of the small and large intestines filled with a contrast medium.

scopy is an examination during which x rays are used to visualize body structures on a screen. A fluoroscope is a machine for examining internal structures by viewing the shadows they cast on the fluorescent screen after x rays travel through the structures. For example, a physician uses fluoroscopy to view the esophagus on a screen as barium passes through it. The following radiographic studies are frequently carried out:

■ Gastrointestinal tract: pharynx and esophagus, upper gastrointestinal tract (**barium swallow**), and lower gastrointestinal tract (**barium enema**). See Table 48–3.

TABLE 48–3 *Studies of the Gastrointestinal Tract*

| Name | Description | Nursing Intervention | |
		Preprocedure Teaching	Postprocedure
Barium swallow (usually part of an upper GI series)	The client swallows barium, and the pharynx and esophagus are outlined.	Procedure lasts 30 minutes. Client will be given a chalky substance (liquid barium) to drink.	Encourage fluids and activity to prevent constipation. Observe stool for whitish color, indicating client has passed barium in stool. Notify physician if barium not passed in 2 to 3 days (a laxative may be required).

TABLE 48–3 *Studies of the Gastrointestinal Tract (continued)*

Name	Description	Nursing Intervention	
		Preprocedure Teaching	**Postprocedure**
Upper gastroin-testinal (GI) series	The client swallows barium, and x-ray films are taken of its course through the esophagus, stomach, and duodenum.	Client must fast 4 to 6 hours before the examination. The client will be given a chalky sub-stance (liquid barium) to drink. Procedure lasts from 30 minutes to 1 hour. Client may experience a feeling of fullness. Client may need to assume several positions on the x-ray table.	Encourage fluids and activity to pre-vent constipation. Observe stool for whitish color, indi-cating client has passed barium in stool. Client may require a laxative or enema if client is constipated or does not pass barium in 2 to 3 days.
Lower gastroin-testinal series (barium enema)	A barium enema is given, and x-ray films are taken of the large intestine.	A laxative may be given the night before the test. Liquids are restricted after midnight before the test. Enemas or suppositories are given on the morning of the test to clean the bowel. The barium enema creates a feeling of fullness, and the client will feel the urge to defecate. Test usually lasts 30 to 45 minutes. There may be some cramping. Special tubes with balloons are often used to help the client retain the barium. The client will be asked to assume various positions, e.g., lying on the left side, then moving to the right side. Client will probably pass the barium at the x-ray department.	Provide a rest period afterward because procedure is fatiguing. Encourage fluids to prevent constipation. Observe stool for passage of barium, and assess regularity of movements. Notify physician if barium not passed in 2 to 3 days. An enema may be required if client does not pass all the barium.

- Gallbladder (**cholecystography**) and bile ducts (**chol-angiography**). See Table 48–4.
- Urinary tract (IVP or IVU). See Table 48–5.
- Central nervous system (**myelography**). See Table 48–5.
- Musculoskeletal system.
- Vascular system (**angiography**). See Table 48–5.

Mammography is radiologic examination of breast tis-sue. See Figure 48–13. It may be done with or without injec-tion of a contrast agent and is performed as a screening test or to study suspicious areas before a mass is distinguish-able. **Soft-tissue mammography** is done without a con-trast medium; the procedure is the same as a standard x-ray examination. Side and top-to-bottom views are taken of each breast. In **contrast (ductal injection) mammog-raphy,** a small-gauge needle is inserted successively into each mammary duct to be examined, and a radiopaque dye is injected before the x-ray films are taken. This test is usu-ally performed to detect an intraductal mass if there is nip-ple discharge. During this procedure, the client experi-ences moderate discomfort when the needle is inserted and when the dye that dilates the ducts is injected.

Xerography or **xeromammography** is mammography using a xerographic plate instead of film. The advantages of xerography are that smaller doses of radiation are used

TABLE 48–4   *Studies of the Gallbladder and Bile Ducts*

Name	Description	Nursing Interventions	
		Preprocedure	Postprocedure
Cholecystography (oral cholecystography)	X-ray films are taken of the gallbladder after a contrast dye has been given orally.	A fat-free supper is given the evening before. Check for allergy to the contrast dye, which contains iodine. A laxative may be given the evening before, or an enema the morning of the test. Six or more contrast pills (e.g., Telepaque) are given at 5-minute intervals the evening before the test, each with 4 to 6 oz water. The client fasts from midnight the evening before but may drink water. Explain that: • A fatty drink may be given during the test. • No discomfort is usually felt. • The procedure lasts about 30 to 45 minutes.	Provide a rest period. The client resumes a regular diet. A snack can be provided if the client is hungry. Assess allergy to the contrast dye.
Intravenous cholangiography	X-ray films are taken of the bile ducts after dye has been administered intravenously.	The client fasts from midnight the evening before the test but may drink water. The bowel is cleaned with a laxative the evening before or with an enema the morning of the test. Check for allergy to iodine contained in the dye. Explain that: • Iodine dye is given intravenously in the x-ray department. A test for allergy is given in the arm before the test. Study lasts 3 to 4 hours.	Assess for allergy to the dye. Observe IV site for bleeding, tenderness.
Percutaneous transhepatic cholangiography	A needle is inserted through the abdominal wall into the biliary radicle, and a contrast agent is injected. Test distinguishes between obstructive and nonobstructive jaundice.	See *Intravenous cholangiography* for preparation. Explain that procedure lasts about 30 minutes.	Monitor vital signs q15 minutes for 1 hour, q30 minutes for 4 hours, and then q4 hours until client is stable. Encourage bed rest. Position client on right side to place pressure on the puncture site to prevent bleeding. Monitor puncture site for bleeding.
Postoperative cholangiography	Dye is injected through the T-tube, and x-ray films are taken and fluoroscopy is done to determine if common bile duct is unobstructed.	See *Intravenous cholangiography.*	If T-tube is in place, clamp or attach to drainage as ordered. If T-tube is removed, apply sterile dressing.

TABLE 48–5 *Radiographic Studies: Intravenous Pyelography, Angiography, Myelography*

Name	Description	Nursing Interventions Preprocedure	Nursing Interventions Postprocedure
Intravenous pyleography or urography (IVP, IVU)	An intravenous injection of radiopaque material is given to examine the kidneys and ureters.	A strong laxative (e.g., castor oil) is given the afternoon before the test to clear the bowel of fecal material, which can obstruct the view of the urinary structures. The client fasts from midnight prior to the test. Check for allergy to iodine. Explain that: • An intravenous injection will be administered in the x-ray department. • The procedure lasts about 1 hour.	Encourage fluid intake. The client resumes a regular diet. Provide for rest, since the laxative and fasting can cause weakness. Observe for reactions to the radiopaque dye.
Angiography, e.g., cerebral angiography (vascular system of the brain), coronary arteriography (coronary arteries of the heart), renal angiography (vascular system of the kidneys), pulmonary angiography (vascular system of the lungs).	A radiopaque material is injected into an artery or vein to examine portions of the vascular system.	For some of these procedures, a catheter may be inserted into an artery or vein prior to the injection of radiopaque material. Before some procedures, the client is given a sedative. The client fasts from midnight prior to the test. A strong laxative may be given the evening before certain tests (e.g., renal arteriography). Client will be tested for allergy to iodine. The time needed for these procedures varies. Some may take up to 3 hours.	Bed rest is generally maintained for up to 12 hours. Monitor the client's radial pulse, respirations, and blood pressure every 15 to 30 minutes until they stabilize. Monitor peripheral pulses distal to the injection site. Observe the injection site for bleeding and swelling. Cold pack may prevent swelling. Determine any discomfort experienced by the client.
Myelography	A contrast material is injected into the subarachnoid space, and x-ray films are taken of the spinal cord, nerve roots, and vertebrae.	Fasting may be required from midnight prior to the test. The client may be given a sedative prior to the procedure. Explain that: • A radiopaque oil dye is injected via a lumbar puncture in the x-ray department. • The client will assume various positions, e.g., on the side for a lumbar puncture, then prone, and then tilted on x-ray table equipped with shoulder and foot supports. • Some pain may be felt when the oil is removed, due to irritation of the nerve roots. The procedure may last about 2 hours.	The client is generally positioned flat in bed for 24 hours to minimize headache and/or nausea, but may be positioned with the head elevated above the level of the spine if the dye has not been completely removed. This prevents the dye from moving to the head and causing an inflammation of the meninges (meningitis). Monitor vital signs and neurologic status, e.g., complaints of numbness, pain, or tingling in the extremities; muscle weakness. Monitor urinary output.

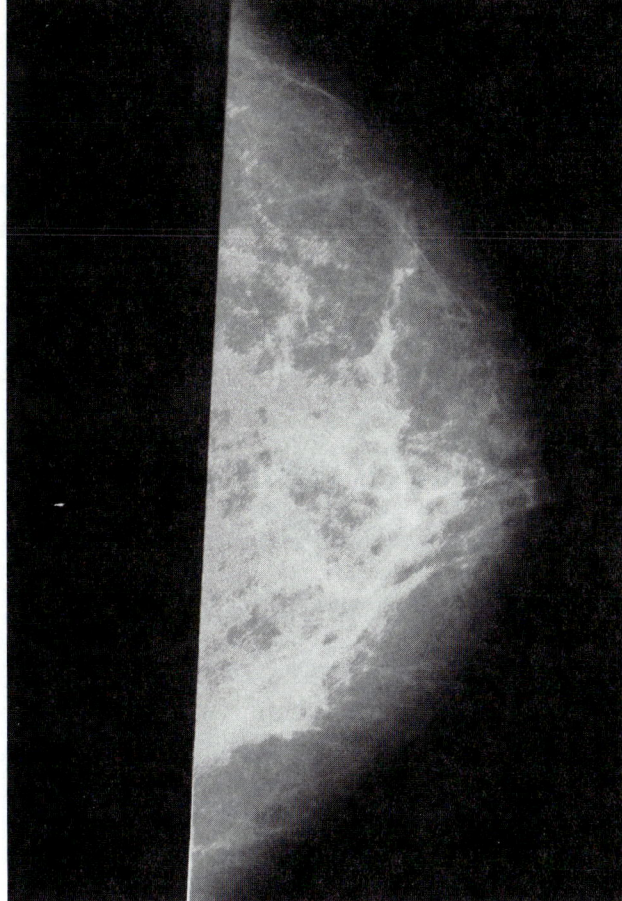

Figure 48–13　A normal mammogram of the breast.

and that the images of blood vessel patterns and tissue densities are more distinct. **Thermography** is a noninvasive screening procedure usually done before mammography. It measures and records the temperature distribution, especially areas of heat, of breast tissue. For this examination, the temperature of the breast skin must be as close as possible to room temperature. The woman usually must sit with her breasts exposed 5 to 10 minutes before the test.

Mammography is the chief method of detecting breast lesions. Extremely small, nonpalpable breast lesions that would otherwise not be detected can show up in this examination.

The nurse's role in assisting with an x-ray procedure is largely one of preparing the client (or teaching the client how to prepare) for the examination and providing follow-up care (or teaching the client to provide follow-up care).

Nuclear Medicine (Radioisotopes)

The instruments and **radioisotopes** (radioactive tracers) used in nuclear medicine are constantly changing, but the fundamental principles remain the same. A basic principle is that body constituents are dynamic, not static. Isotopes

enter into the same chemical reactions and metabolic processes as stable elements.

In nuclear medicine techniques, radioactive substances that have an affinity for specific body tissues are introduced orally or intravenously. For example, radioactive iodine may be given to measure the function of the thyroid gland. The thyroid gland normally picks up and uses iodine to produce the hormone thyroxine. When radioactive iodine is introduced, how much iodine the thyroid picks up and how it is distributed can be detected by a scanning device, allowing the examiner to detect any deficiencies in thyroid function. The scanning device may be a **scintillation counter** or a **scintillation camera.** The scintillation scanner has a probe that is passed back and forth over the body area being studied; the scintillation camera produces many images in rapid sequence, showing the transit of the isotope through blood vessels.

Radioisotopes are administered in extremely small doses, e.g., one billionth of a gram. For this reason, the body absorbs minimal amounts of radiation, and normal body cells are not damaged. The procedure is painless and has three steps:

1. Oral or intravenous intake of the radioisotope
2. A waiting period from 1 to 48 hours, during which the isotope is assimilated by the organ being studied
3. The scanning procedure, during which the client must remain still

Scintillation scanning (scintiscans) can be used to assess the function of an organ or detect a tumor. Organs commonly studied by nuclear medicine procedures include the thyroid, heart, brain, lungs, liver, spleen, bone marrow, bones, and kidneys. Radioisotopes are also used to measure blood volume, blood circulation rate, red blood cell turnover, cardiac output, and lung blood flow.

Computed Tomography (CT Scan)

Computed tomography is a painless, noninvasive x-ray procedure with the unique capability of distinguishing minor differences in the radiodensity of soft tissues. See Figure 48–14. For example, CT scans can be used to distinguish liver tissue from tumor or brain tissue from hematoma. Dense substances appear white; low-density substances appear dark. The organ to be studied gives the scan its name, e.g., brain scan, liver scan, lung scan.

In this technique, a planar slice of the body is subjected to sequential sweeps or **scans** of a narrow x-ray beam. The unabsorbed beam emerging through the tissues is measured by a radiation detector. Data obtained are stored in a computer, which produces an image, called a **tomogram,** on a viewing apparatus or printout machine. Photographs of the image can be reproduced.

The CT scan provides a three-dimensional view of the area under study. The scanner rotates 1° at a time through a 180° arc in about 5 minutes. At least five consecutive scans or "cuts" are taken of sequential parts of the organ. Follow-

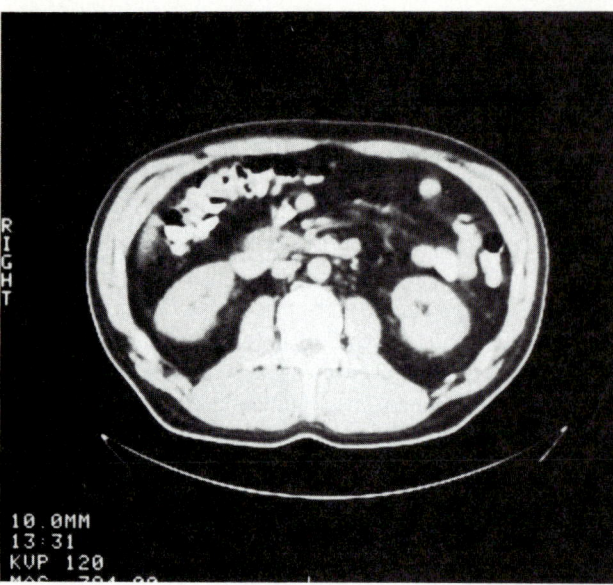

Figure 48–14 A CT scan showing a midabdomen cross section. The spine is at the base; the kidneys are to the right and left of the spine.

ing this initial scan, the client is usually given an intravenous injection of an iodine-containing contrast material, and the entire scan is repeated. This second scan is referred to as a "contrast enhancement" scan. The entire scanning procedure takes about 1 hour. The client must remain still throughout the scan to prevent false computer results.

The only risk involved with a CT scan is the possibility of allergic reaction to iodine; thus the client must always be asked about any known allergy to iodine before the test. Usually no special preparation is required. In some agencies, no food or fluids may be given 4 to 6 hours beforehand because the iodine-containing contrast medium may cause nausea. For other preprocedure nursing responsibilities, see the accompanying box.

There are usually no side-effects or limitations on client activity after the procedure. Additional scans may be performed at subsequent intervals, e.g., 2 hours, 24 hours, 48 hours, and 72 hours. The nurse observes for allergic reactions to the blocking agent.

Ultrasonography (Ultrasound)

Ultrasonography, another noninvasive technique, uses high-frequency sound waves well above the upper limit of human hearing. During this procedure, which has no known harmful effects, acoustic densities of tissues are measured. In contrast to usual radiography, ultrasound reveals the depth of a structure below the skin and the anteroposterior dimension of masses. Sound waves travel at different speeds, depending on the density of the structures through which they pass. Because sound is poorly conducted by gases and is well reflected by bone, structures containing air (such as

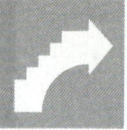

CLINICAL GUIDELINES
CT Scans

- Restless clients, e.g., children, may be given a sedative prior to the procedure so that they will lie still during the procedure.

- The nurse assures the client that there is no need to fear exposure to radiation; a CT scan exposes the client to less radiation than the usual x-ray procedure. A radioactive substance is given orally or intravenously.

- Depending on the substance used, a blocking agent may also be given to prevent uptake of the radioactive substance by organs other than the one being studied and to ensure that the substance goes into the organ being studied. Check for allergies to the blocking agents.
  a. Lugol's solution (iodine) may be given to block uptake by the thyroid (given orally with juice, since its taste is unpleasant), or a potassium compound may be given to clients allergic to iodine.
  b. Mercaptomerin sodium is given intramuscularly to block uptake by the kidneys.

- The nurse explains that
  a. The scan is performed in the nuclear medicine department.
  b. There will be a waiting period while the radioactive substance is taken up by the body.
  c. There is no discomfort.
  d. The client will be asked to assume various positions and must remain still while the scans are taken.

the lung) or surrounded by bone (such as the pelvis) are difficult to examine with ultrasound.

In this technique, a transducer or probe is used as both an emitter and a receiver. The probe is moved over the structure being examined, and an ultrasound beam is directed into the body. Echoes (sounds reflected back to the probe) are translated into a display unit for observation and photographic recording. The test usually takes 20 to 45 minutes. Ultrasound can

- Reveal the size, shape, and consistency of internal structures
- Show masses, fluid inflammation, and stones
- Differentiate cystic from solid masses
- Outline the boundaries of lesions and displacement of surrounding tissues
- Depict motion

Before many ultrasound examinations, the client requires no physical preparation. Food and fluids are withheld 8 to 10 hours before examination of the abdominal organs, and some physicians may order an enema or other agent to decrease the amount of intestinal gas, which impedes the sound reflection. For examinations of the pelvic organs, the client must have some urine in the bladder to enable better visualization. Inform the client to void 4 hours before the procedure and then not to void until after the procedure. If this is difficult for the client, 2 hours without voiding may be acceptable if the client drinks several glasses of fluid before the examination. The client also needs to know the following:

- Mineral oil or water-soluble jelly will be spread over the

skin. The oil prevents air from becoming trapped between the probe and the skin and facilitates acoustic contact.

- The procedure is painless. The client will merely feel the probe moving over the skin.
- The client will be asked to change positions on the table to allow visualization of the organ from different angles.
- During a scan of upper abdominal organs, the client may be asked periodically to inhale deeply and hold the breath for a few seconds. Inspiration displaces upper abdominal organs downward.

CHAPTER HIGHLIGHTS

▶ Tests and treatments are frightening for many people; they may fear pain, the findings of the tests, or their reactions to either the pain or the findings.

▶ The nurse must identify the concerns of the client and provide information and support to alleviate concern.

▶ Baseline assessment data are collected before the test and compared with the client's responses during and after the test.

▶ During the procedure, the nurse, if present, is usually the client's primary support person.

▶ The nurse is responsible for ensuring that specimens taken during the procedure are appropriately labeled, handled, and transported to the laboratory for study.

▶ Knowledge of the procedure and complications that may arise helps the nurse provide necessary interventions following the procedure to ensure the recovery and safety of the client.

READINGS AND REFERENCES

SUGGESTED READINGS

Davenport, D. O'G. June 1987. Computerized monitoring systems. *Nursing Clinics of North America* 22:495–501.

Computerized monitoring systems have proliferated in the last two decades. In this article, types of computer monitoring systems and their advantages and disadvantages are discussed. Although the most frequently computer-monitored element is the electrocardiogram, other parameters include arterial blood pressure, temperature, respirations, pulmonary artery pressure, central venous pressure, intracranial pressure, fluid intake and output, arterial blood gases, and several others.

Monroe, D. September 1989. Patient teaching for x-ray and other diagnostics. *RN* 52:50–56.

In this first in a new series of patient guides to x-ray examinations, Monroe discusses computerized tomography (CT scan) of the head, myelography, and cerebral arteriography. For each examination, she provides information about the test itself, why it is done, what the client needs to do to get ready for it, what happens during the test, how long it takes, what the potential risks are, and what the client can expect following the test.

RELATED RESEARCH

Hartfield, M. T.; Cason, C. L.; and Cason, G. J. July/August 1982. Effects of information about a threatening procedure on patient's expectations and emotional distress. *Nursing Research* 31:202–5.

SELECTED REFERENCES

Byrne, C. J.; Saxton, D. F.; Pelikan, P. K.; and Nugent, P. M. 1986. *Laboratory tests: Implications for nursing care.* 2d ed. Menlo Park, Calif.: Addison-Wesley Publishing Co.

Contrast radiography fact sheet: Update your knowledge of these contrast radiography studies. August 1984. *Nursing 84* 14:22–23.

Davenport, D. O'G. June 1987. Computerized monitoring systems. *Nursing Clinics of North America* 22:495–501.

Diagnostic scanning procedures and ultrasonography: Test yourself. November 1980. *American Journal of Nursing* 80:2005.

Guyton, A. C. 1986. *Textbook of medical physiology.* 7th ed. Philadelphia: W. B. Saunders Co.

Haughey, C. April 1981. Understanding ultrasonography. *Nursing 81* 11:36–40.

Markus, S. April 1981. Taking the fear out of bone marrow examinations. *Nursing 81* 11:64–67.

The Nurses' Reference Library. 1986. *Diagnostics.* 2d ed. Springhouse, Pa.: Intermed Communications.

Questions and answers about the CT scan exam: Patient education aid. April 15, 1985. *Patient Care* 19:185.

Rudolphi, D. M. April 1990. Duplex scanning. *American Journal of Nursing* 90:123–24.

Thrasher, S. B. September 1989. "What I didn't know really hurt me." . . . Preparing patients for diagnostic tests. *RN* 52:49–50.

APPENDIXES

CONTENTS

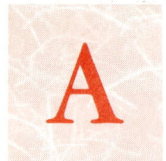

Significant Events in Nursing History

1–500 (circa) Care (mostly hygienic and comfort measures) for the destitute, homeless, and sick provided mainly by early Christians, working as committed individuals or in association with an organized church.

500–1500 (circa) Male and female religious, military, and secular orders with the primary purpose of caring for the sick came into being. Conspicuous among them were the Knights Hospitalers of St. John; the Alexian Brotherhood, organized in 1431; and the Augustinian sisters, the first purely nursing order.

1633 Sisters of Charity founded by St. Vincent de Paul in France. It was the first of many such orders with the same name (sometimes Daughters of Charity) organized under various Roman Catholic church auspices and largely devoted to caring for the sick.

1639 Augustinian sisters came to Canada, eventually establishing the Hotel Dieu in Quebec City.

1644 Jeanne Mance, known as the Florence Nightingale of Canada, founded the Hotel Dieu in Montreal.

——Mother Elizabeth Seton established the first American order of Sisters of Charity of St. Joseph, in Maryland.

1738 Mother d'Youville organized a noncloistered group of women to care for the sick in both hospitals and homes. These women became the Soeurs Grises or Grey Nuns.

1836 Theodor Fliedner reinstituted the Order of Deaconesses from earlier days, opening a small hospital and training school in Kaiserswerth, Germany. This was where Florence Nightingale received her "training" in nursing. The deaconess movement spread to four continents, the first motherhouse being established in Pittsburgh, Pennsylvania, in 1849.

1854–56 Florence Nightingale, long concerned with care of the sick, was named Superintendent of the Female Nursing Establishment of the English General Hospitals in Turkey, in charge of the nursing care of the soldiers during the Crimean War.

1859 Publication of *Notes on nursing: What it is and what it is not,* by Nightingale, in London. It was intended for the ordinary woman, not as a text for nurses.

1860 With a fund of 45,000 pounds (over $220,000 at that time) contributed by the grateful British public and soldiers, Nightingale established the first "modern" school of nursing at St. Thomas's Hospital in London. This date is considered the beginning of nursing as an organized profession. Nightingale believed not only in nursing the sick but also in promoting health.

1861–65 Dorothea Lynde Dix, better known for her earlier work in improving conditions of care for the mentally ill, was appointed superintendent of the first nurse corps of the United States Army during the Civil War.

1864 Jean Henri Dunant of Switzerland established the international conference that founded the Red Cross, for the relief of the suffering in war, in the Geneva Convention signed by 14 nations (the United States not among them).

1872 Woman's Hospital, Philadelphia, opened a training school for nurses.

——New England Hospital for Women and Children, Boston, opened a training school for nurses. Linda Richards, who graduated from the school in 1873, became known as America's first trained nurse.

——American Public Health Association established. Its primary concern at that time was with sanitary and environmental conditions. Later nurses became a significant part of its membership.

1873 First three schools of nursing patterned after (but not strictly according to) Nightingale principles were established at Bellevue Hospital, New York; Massachusetts General Hospital, Boston; and New Haven Hospital, Connecticut.

1874 First hospital training school (Mack Training School) for nurses formed in Canada at St. Catharines, Ontario.

1879 Mary Eliza Mahoney, first trained black nurse, graduated from the nursing school of New England Hospital for Women and Children.

1882 American National Red Cross organized by Clara Barton and linked with the international organization when the United States Congress ratified the Geneva Convention.

1885 Publication of *Textbook of nursing for the use of training schools, families and private students,* the first textbook written by an American Nurse (Clara Weeks Shaw) for nurses.

1893 Henry Street Settlement, New York, established by Lilian D. Wald and Mary Brewster to care for the sick and poor in their homes.

——American Society of Superintendents of Training Schools for Nurses (renamed the National League of Nursing Education [NLNE] in 1912) became the first organized nursing group in the United States and Canada.

1897 Nurses' Associated Alumnae of United States and Canada organized. Renamed the American Nurses' Association (ANA) in 1911.

——Victorian Order of Nurses established in Canada by Lady Aberdeen. It conducted practically all public health nursing.

1899 International Council of Nurses (ICN) established by Mrs. Bedford Fenwick of Great Britain, United States and Canadian nurses were among its founders, and their national associations were among the first admitted to membership.

1900 *American Journal of Nursing,* first nursing journal in the United States to be owned, operated, and published by nurses, launched. Its publisher, incorporated in 1902, now also publishes *Nursing Research,* established in 1952; *Nursing Outlook,*

1953; *International Nursing Index,* 1966; *MCN: American Journal of Maternal–Child Nursing,* 1976; and *Geriatric Nursing: American Journal of Care for the Aging,* 1980.

1901   United States Army Nurse Corps formally established by act of Congress.

1903   First nurse practice acts passed in North Carolina, New Jersey, Virginia, and New York.

1905   *Canadian Nurse* journal inaugurated. By 1959 it was published in both English and French.

1908   Canadian National Association of Trained Nurses (CNATN) established. It later became the Canadian Nurses' Association (CNA).

——National Association of Colored Graduate Nurses (NACGN) established.

——United States Navy Nurse Corps formed.

1912   National Organization for Public Health Nursing (NOPHN) established.

——United States Children's Bureau created by Congress as part of the Department of Commerce and Labor.

1916   Criteria for a profession, set forth by Abraham Flexner in "Is social work a profession?" (published in *School and society,* volume 1), became yardsticks for nursing and continue to serve this function.

1917   NLNE published its first *Standard curriculum for schools of nursing;* revised editions, under slightly different titles, appeared in 1927 and 1937.

1919   Ethyl Johns established the first baccalaureate degree program in nursing in the British Empire at the University of British Columbia, Vancouver.

1922   Sigma Theta Tau, national honor society of nursing in the United States, founded by six nursing students at Indiana Training School for Nurses.

1923   Publication of *Nursing and nursing education in the United States,* better known as the Goldmark (or Winslow-Goldmark) Report. Originally intended to study education for public health nursing, the study committee extended its work to include all of nursing education, criticizing the low standards, inadequate financing, and lack of separation of education from service.

——Yale University (New Haven, Connecticut) and Western Reserve University (Cleveland, Ohio), each with the aid of endowments, established independent schools of nursing. In 1934, both started requiring a baccalaureate degree for admission to the schools and granted masters of nursing degrees.

1928   Publication of *Nurses, patients, and pocketbooks,* first report of the Committee on Grading of Nursing Schools appointed two years earlier. The report indicated that there was an oversupply of nurses in general but an undersupply of adequately prepared ones.

1929   American Association of Nurse-Midwives formed. It merged in 1969 with the American College of Nurse-Midwifery to become the American College of Nurse-Midwives.

1931   Weir Report in Canada recommended integration of nursing education into the provincial education system.

1932   Association of Collegiate Schools of Nursing (ACSN) established to promote nursing education on a professional and collegiate level and to encourage research.

1933   ANA launched campaign for hospitals to employ graduate nurses instead of relying heavily on nursing students for patient care.

1934   Publication of *Nursing schools today and tomorrow,* final report of the Grading Committee (which never did grade schools

publicly). It confirmed the weaknesses in nursing education pointed out in the Goldmark Report, recommended graduate instead of student nursing staffs, and called for public support of nursing education.

1939   Graduate School of Midwifery created by the Frontier Nursing Service, Hyden, Kentucky.

1940   Formation of the Nursing Council on National Defense (retitled the National Nursing Council for War Service [NNCWS] in 1941), with representation from major nursing organizations and nursing service agencies, to unify all nursing activities directly or indirectly related to war.

1942   Committee appointed to develop what became the State Board Test Pool Examination (SBTPE). By 1950 all states were using the SBTPE.

——American Association of Industrial Nurses (now the American Association of Occupational Health Nurses) formed.

1943   United States Cadet Nurse Corps established. Through this corps, the federal government subsidized the cost of nursing education, in accelerated programs, for all students agreeing to serve after graduation in civilian or military nursing services for the duration of the war. It was discontinued in 1945.

1946   ANA adopted its economic security (now economic and general welfare) program legitimizing collective bargaining for nurses through their state nurses' associations.

1947   Passage of the Taft-Hartley Act, exempting nonprofit hospitals and other charitable institutions from the obligation to bargain collectively with their employees.

1948   Publication of *Nursing for the future,* report of a far-reaching study of "who would organize, administer, and finance *professional* schools of nursing." Commissioned by the National Nursing Council for War Services and carried out by anthropologist Esther Lucile Brown, the report recommended, among other things, that education for nursing belonged in colleges and universities, not in hospitals.

——NLNE formally established the National Nursing Accrediting Service for nursing educational programs.

——Nationwide movement toward "team nursing" started at Hartford Hospital, Connecticut.

——Metropolitan Demonstration School of Nursing in Windsor, Ontario, operated a 2-year nursing education program (from 1948 to 1952). The Lord Report in 1952 concluded that nurses could be trained at least as satisfactorily in 2 years as in 3 years.

1949   United States Air Force Nurse Corps created.

1950–53   United States nurses served in the Korean war, in Mobile Army Surgical Hospitals (M.A.S.H.).

1951   National Association of Colored Graduate Nurses dissolved itself, to be absorbed into the ANA.

1952   After years of study, the nursing profession in the United States was restructured into two national organizations: the ANA, which remained the membership organization, and the newly formed National League for Nursing (NLN), merging the former NLNE, NOPHN, and ACSN.

——Associate degree education for nursing begun in an experimental project at Teachers College, Columbia University, New York.

——*Nursing Research* launched due to the efforts of the ACSN.

1953   National Student Nurses' Association (NSNA) founded.

——United States Department of Health, Education, and Welfare (HEW) created. It became the Department of Health and Human Services (HHS) in 1980.

1954   Association of Operating Room Nurses formed.

1955 American Nurses' Foundation established by the ANA for research purposes.

1956 Federal nurse traineeship program established to aid registered nurses in advanced study.

1960 Publication of *Spotlight on nursing education* by Helen K. Mussallem, report of a pilot project for the evaluation of schools of nursing in Canada.

1963 Publication of *Toward quality in nursing,* report of the Surgeon General's Consultant Group in Nursing, another study of nursing and nursing education that projected the need for more and better prepared nurses.

1964 Ryerson Polytechnical Institute, Toronto, started the first diploma nursing program in Canada within a college institution.

——First Nurse Training Act allocated federal aid for nursing education in the United States.

1965 ANA issued its first (and famous) "Position paper on nursing education," calling for all nursing education to take place in institutions of higher education and stipulating the baccalaureate as minimum preparation for professional nursing practice, the associate degree for technical nursing practice.

1967 Pediatric nurse practitioner program initiated at University of Colorado, Boulder; a program at the University of California, San Francisco, gave nurses increased responsibility in ambulatory care. These marked the beginning of the "nurse practitioner" or "expanded role of the nurse" movement.

1969 Nurses' Association of the American College of Obstetricians and Gynecologists formed.

——American Association of Cardiovascular Nurses formed. It was broadened in 1972 to become the Association of Critical-Care Nurses.

——American Association of Colleges of Nursing (AACN) formed after two years of informal meetings.

1970 Canadian Nurses' Association established a national Testing Service (CNATS) to prepare examinations for graduate nurses seeking provincial registration.

——Publication of *An abstract for action,* report of the national Commission on Nursing and Nursing Education, and often referred to as the Lysaught report, after the study director. The report categorized nursing into episodic (illness) and distributive (preventive and health maintenance) care.

——Publication of *Extending the scope of nursing practice,* by HEW, endorsing extension of the nurse's traditional functions and responsibilities.

——Introduction of primary nursing as an alternative to team nursing.

——National Association of School Nurses formed.

1971 National Black Nurses' Association created.

——Lucille Kinlein became the first nurse to hang out her shingle as an independent practitioner. Today many nurses are in independent practice singly or in groups.

——Emergency Department Nurses' Association established.

1972 New York State amended its Nurse Practice Act to define professional nursing practice as diagnosing and treating human responses to actual or potential health problems.

——Nurses for Political Action, now Nurses' Coalition for Action in Politics (N-CAP), established to promote legislation in behalf of nursing; associated with the ANA.

1973 Federation of nursing specialty organizations and the ANA was created, after 2 years of preliminary meetings.

——ANA started certification program for nurses in specialty practice.

——American Academy of Nursing established, with appointment of 36 charter fellows. It was associated with the ANA.

——"External" associate degree program in nursing launched in New York. It permitted a degree to be awarded on the basis of independent study validated by examination. This was extended to the bachelor's degree in nursing in 1976.

——National Association of Pediatric Nurses formed.

——First national conference on nursing diagnoses held in St. Louis, Missouri.

1974 Amendments to the Taft-Hartley Act removed exemption of nonprofit institutions from the obligation to engage in collective bargaining.

——Association of Rehabilitation Nurses formed.

1975 Oncology Nursing Society started.

1976 Robert Wood Johnson Foundation launched a program of faculty fellowships in primary care.

1978 ANA House of Delegates resolved that "by 1985" minimum preparation for "entry into professional practice" would be the baccalaureate in nursing.

——Council of State Boards of Nursing separated from the ANA to form an autonomous body, the National Council of State Boards of Nursing.

1979 Committee on Credentialing in Nursing called for establishment of a free-standing national credentialing center, not endorsed by the ANA.

——Case Western Reserve University, Cleveland, initiated the first professional education program in nursing awarding the ND (Doctor of Nursing) degree.

1982 NLN endorsed the baccalaureate in nursing as minimum preparation for professional practice.

——ANA converted to a federation of constituent nurses' associations rather than an association of individual nurse members.

——National Association of Orthopedic Nurses established.

——North American Nursing Diagnosis Association (NANDA) established.

1983 Congress passed legislation changing Medicare reimbursement to hospitals to a system of prospective payment based on Diagnosis Related Groups (DRGs).

——Institute of Medicine report called for federally funded entity to place nursing research in the mainstream of scientific investigation.

——Center for Research for Nursing created by the American Nurses' Association.

1985 ANA House of Delegates voted to recommend titles for two levels of professional nursing practice: "registered nurse" for the baccalaureate-prepared nurse, and "associate nurse" for the associate degree (technical) nurse.

——National Institute of Nursing established.

1986 N-CAP (Nurses' Coalition for Action in Politics) renamed ANA-PAC.

——National Center for Nursing Research (within the National Institutes of Health in Bethesda, Maryland) established.

1988 The Secretary's Commission on Nursing, DHHS, issued its final report, which included 16 recommendations to improve recruitment and retention of an adequate supply of registered nurses.

1990 NCNIP (National Commission on Nursing Implementation Project) and the Advertising Council of America launched a multimillion dollar national advertising campaign to provide a more accurate image of nurses and nursing that would attract new recruits to the profession.

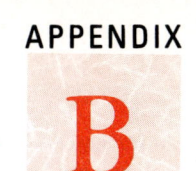
Nursing Organizations and Publications

INTERNATIONAL

Organization	Publications
International Council of Nurses (ICN) 3, rue Ancien-Port 1201 Geneva, Switzerland	
International Committee of Catholic Nurses Square Vergota 43, B1040 Brussels, Belgium	
North American Nursing Diagnosis Association (NANDA) St. Louis University Department of Nursing 3525 Caroline St. St. Louis, MO 63104	*Nursing Diagnosis*
Sigma Theta Tau International Honor Society of Nursing 1200 Waterway Blvd. Indianapolis, IN 46202	*Image: Journal of Nursing Scholarship, Reflections*
World Health Organization (WHO) Avenue Appia 1211 Geneva 27, Switzerland	

NATIONAL *(United States)*

Related to Scholarship

Organization	Publications
American Academy of Nurses (AAN) c/o American Nurses' Association 2420 Pershing Rd. Kansas City, MO 64108	*Nursing Outlook*
Sigma Theta Tau (see above)	
Alpha Tau Delta 14631 N. 2nd Dr. Phoenix, AZ 85023	*Captions of Alpha Tau Delta*

Related to Ethnic Origin

Organization	Publications
American Indian Nurses Association (AINA) P.O. Box 1588 Norman, OK 73071	*Newsletter of the AINA*
National Association of Hispanic Nurses 6905 Alamo Downs Pkwy. San Antonio, TX 78238	*Newsletter*
National Black Nurses Association P.O. Box 1835B Boston, MA 02118	*Journal of National Black Nurses Association*

General

Organization	Publications
American Nurses' Association (ANA) 2420 Pershing Road Kansas City, MO 64108	*American Journal of Nursing, The American Nurse*
Committee on Nursing of the Catholic Hospital Association 1438 S. Grand Blvd. St. Louis, MO 63104	
National Center for Nursing Ethics P.O. Box 2237 Cincinnati, OH 45201	
National Student Nurse Association (NSNA) 55 West 57th St. New York, NY 10019	*Imprint*
National League for Nursing (NLN) 10 Columbus Circle New York, NY 10019	*Nursing and Health Care*

Related to Occupation or Speciality

Organization	Publications
American Association for the History of Nursing P.O. Box 90803 Washington, DC 20003	*The Bulletin*

Organization	Publications	Organization	Publications
American Association of Critical Care Nurses (AACN) One Civic Plaza Newport Beach, CA 92660	*Heart and Lung*	**American Society of Ophthalmic Registered Nurses (ASORN)** P.O. Box 3030 San Francisco, CA 94119	*Insight*
American Nephrology Nurses' Association (ANNA) North Woodbury Road Box 56 Pitman, NJ 08071		**American Society of Plastic and Reconstructive Surgical Nurses** North Woodbury Road, Box 56 Pitman, NJ 08071	*Journal of Plastic and Reconstructive Surgical Nursing*
American Association of Neuroscience Nurses (AANN) 218 N. Jefferson St. Suite 204 Chicago, IL 60606	*Journal of Neuroscience Nursing*	**American Society of Post-Anesthesia Nurses (ASPAN)** P.O. Box 11083 Richmond, VA 23230	*Breathline, Journal of Post-Anesthesia Nursing*
American Association of Nurse Anesthetists (AANA) 216 Higgins Road Park Ridge, IL 60068-5790	*American Association of Nurse Anesthetists Journal*	**American Urological Association Allied** 6845 Lake Shore Dr. P.O. Box 9397 Raytown, MO 64133	*Urologic Nursing*
American Association of Occupational Health Nurses 50 Lenox Pointe Atlanta, GA 30324	*AAOHN Journal* *AAOH News*	**Association of Operating Room Nurses, Inc. (AORN)** 10170 East Mississippi Ave. Denver, CO 80231	*AORN Journal*
American Burn Association Burn Treatment Center Crozier-Chester Medical Center 15th and Upland Ave. Chester, PA 19013		**Association for Practitioners in Infection Control** 505 E. Hawley St. Mundelein, IL 60060	
American College of Nurse-Midwives (ACNM) 1522 K St. Suite 1120 Washington, DC 20005	*Journal of Nurse Midwifery*	**Association of Pediatric Oncology Nurses (APON)** Pacific Medical Center P.O. Box 7999 San Francisco, CA 94120	*APON Newsletter*
American Geriatric Society Room 1470 10 Columbus Circle New York, NY 10019		**Association of Rehabilitation Nurses** 2506 Gross Point Rd. Evanston, IL 60201	*Rehabilitation Nursing*
American Holistic Nurses Association 205 St. Louis St. Suite 506 Springfield, MO 65806	*Journal of Holistic Nursing, Beginnings*	**Dermatology Nurses' Association** North Woodbury Rd. Box 56 Pitman, NJ 08071	*DNA Focus*
American Public Health Association Public Health Nursing Section 1015 15th Street NW Washington, DC 20005	*American Journal of Public Health, The Nation's Health*	**Drug and Alcohol Nursing Association** P.O. Box 6126 Annapolis, MD 21401	*DANA Newsletter*
American Radiological Nurses Association c/o E. Deutsch 502 Forest Court Carrboro, NC 27510	*ARNA Images*	**Emergency Nurses Association (ENA)** Suite 1131 666 N. Lakeshore Dr. Chicago, IL 60611	

Organization	Publications	Organization	Publications

Flight Nurse Section
Aerospace Medical
  Association
Washington National Airport
Washington, D.C. 20001

International Association
  for Enterostomal
  Therapy
1701 Lake Avenue
Glenview, IL 60025

Journal of Enterostomal Therapy

National Association of
  Neonatal Nurses

Neonatal Network: The Journal of Neonatal Nursing

National Association of
  Orthopedic Nurses
North Woodbury Road
Box 56
Pitman, NJ 08071

Orthopedic Nursing

National Association of
  Pediatric Nurse
  Associates and
  Practitioners (NAPNAP)
1000 Maplewood Dr.
Suite 104
Maple Shade, NJ 08052

The Pediatric Nurse Practitioner

National Association of
  School Nurses, Inc.
Lamplighter Lane
P.O. Box 1300
Scarborough, ME 04074

School Nurse Journal

National Flight Nurses'
  Association
P.O. Box 68395
Virginia Beach, VA 23455

Aeromedical Journal

National Intravenous
  Therapy Association
87 Blanchard Rd.
Cambridge, MA 02138

NITA Journal, NITA Update

National Organization for
  the Advancement of
  Associate Degree
  Nursing
Amarillo College,
P.O. Box 447
Amarillo, TX 79178

Nurses Association of the
  American College of
  Obstetricians and
  Gynecologists
409 12th Street, SW
Washington, DC 20024-2191

Oncology Nursing Society
701 Washington Rd.
Pittsburgh, PA 15228

Oncology Nursing Forum

Society for Peripheral
  Vascular Nursing
P.O. Box 11356
Baltimore, MD 21239

SPVN Journal

Transcultural Nursing
  Society
College of Nursing
University of Utah
25 S. Medical Drive
Salt Lake City, Utah 84112

Biannual Newsletter

World Federation of
  Neurosurgical Nurses
Avenue Appia
1211 Geneva 27
Switzerland

Miscellaneous

Gay Nurses Alliance
P.O. Box 530
Back Bay Annex
Boston, MA 02117

National Male Nurses'
  Association
2308 State St.
Saginaw, MI 48602

National Nurses for Life
1998 Menold
Allison Park, PA 15104

Nurses Christian
  Fellowship
233 Langdon St.
Madison, WI 53703

Journal of Christian Nursing

Nurses' Environmental
  Health Watch, Inc.
33 Columbus Ave.
Somerville, MA 02143

Nurses House, Inc.
10 Columbus Circle
New York, NY 10019

CANADIAN

Canadian Association of
  Critical Care Nurses
P.O. Box 61
Welland, Ontario L3B 5N9

Canadian Critical Care Journal

Canadian Association of
  Enterostomal Therapy
4389 Prospect Rd.
North Vancouver, BC V7N 3L8

Canadian Association of
  Neurological and
  Neurosurgical Nurses
96 Palace Rd.
Kingston, Ontario K7L 4T3

Canadian Council of
  Cardiovascular Nurses
1200-1 Nicholas Street
Ottawa, Ontario K2P 1E2

Canadian Bulletin of Cardiovascular Nursing

Organization	Publications	Organization	Publications
Canadian Gerontological Nursing Association	*Perspectives*	**Canadian University Nursing Students Association**	
Continuing Nursing Education University of Saskatchewan Saskatoon, Saskatchewan S7W 0W0		School of Nursing Université de Montréal C.P. 6128 Montreal, Quebec H3T 1J4	
Canadian Intravenous Nurses Association	*Canadian Intravenous Nurses Association Journal*	**Dynamics of Critical Care Association of Canada**	
200-4433 Sheppard Ave. E. Agincourt, Ontario M1S 1V3		CNSC 200-4433 Sheppard Ave. E. Agincourt, Ontario M1S 1V3	
Canadian Nurses Association	*The Canadian Nurse*	**Operating Room Nurses Association of Canada**	*Canadian Operating Room Nurse Journal*
50 The Driveway Ottawa, Ontario K2P 1E2		213-52377 Range Rd. Sherwood Park, Alberta T8G 1B9	
Canadian Nurses Foundation		**Psychiatric Nurses Association of Canada**	*Canadian Journal of Psychiatric Nursing*
50 The Driveway Ottawa, Ontario K2P 1E2		1854 Portage Avenue Winnipeg, Manitoba R3J 0G9	
Canadian Nurses Respiratory Society Nurses Section		**Registered Nurses of Canadian Indian Ancestry**	
Canadian Lung Association 908-75 Albert Street Ottawa, Ontario K1P 5E7		500-275 Portage Ave. Winnipeg, Manitoba R3B 2B3	
Canadian Orthopedic Nurses Association		**TPN Nurses Association of Canada**	
43 Wellesley St. E. Toronto, Ontario M4Y 1H1		P.O. Box 62 Station K Toronto, Ontario M4P 2G1	
Canadian Society of Dialysis Perfusionists			
Dialysis Unit Health Sciences Centre 700 William Ave. Winnipeg, Manitoba R3E 0Z3			

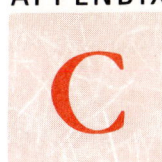
NANDA Taxonomy I (Revised 1990)

This list represents the NANDA approved nursing diagnostic categories for clinical use and testing (1990).

Pattern 1: Exchanging

Altered Nutrition: More than body requirements
Altered Nutrition: Less than body requirements
Altered Nutrition: Potential for more than body requirements
Potential for Infection
Potential Altered Body Temperature
Hypothermia
Hyperthermia
Ineffective Thermoregulation
Dysreflexia
Constipation
Perceived Constipation
Colonic Constipation
Diarrhea
Bowel Incontinence
Altered Patterns of Urinary Elimination
Stress Incontinence
Reflex Incontinence
Urge Incontinence
Functional Incontinence
Total Incontinence
Urinary Retention
Altered (Specify Type) Tissue Perfusion (Renal, cerebral, cardiopulmonary, gastrointestinal, peripheral)
Fluid Volume Excess
Fluid Volume Deficit (1)
Fluid Volume Deficit (2)
Potential Fluid Volume Deficit
Decreased Cardiac Output
Impaired Gas Exchange
Ineffective Airway Clearance
Ineffective Breathing Pattern
Potential for Injury
Potential for Suffocation
Potential for Poisoning
Potential for Trauma
Potential for Aspiration
Potential for Disuse Syndrome
Impaired Tissue Integrity
Altered Oral Mucous Membrane
Impaired Skin Integrity
Potential Impaired Skin Integrity
Altered Protection

Pattern 2: Communicating

Impaired Verbal Communication

Pattern 3: Relating

Impaired Social Interaction
Social Isolation
Altered Role Performance
Altered Parenting
Potential Altered Parenting
Sexual Dysfunction
Altered Family Processes
Parental Role Conflict
Altered Sexuality Patterns

Pattern 4: Valuing

Spiritual Distress (distress of the human spirit)

Pattern 5: Choosing

Ineffective Individual Coping
Impaired Adjustment
Defensive Coping
Ineffective Denial
Ineffective Family Coping: Disabling
Ineffective Family Coping: Compromised
Family Coping: Potential for Growth
Noncompliance (Specify)
Decisional Conflict (Specify)
Health Seeking Behaviors (Specify)

Pattern 6: Moving

Impaired Physical Mobility
Activity Intolerance
Fatigue
Potential Activity Intolerance
Sleep Pattern Disturbance
Diversional Activity Deficit
Impaired Home Maintenance Management
Altered Health Maintenance
Feeding Self Care Deficit
Impaired Swallowing
Effective Breastfeeding
Ineffective Breastfeeding
Bathing/Hygiene Self Care Deficit
Dressing/Grooming Self Care Deficit

Toileting Self Care Deficit
Altered Growth and Development

Pattern 7: Perceiving

Body Image Disturbance
Self Esteem Disturbance
Chronic Low Self-Esteem
Situational Low Self-Esteem
Personal Identity Disturbance
Sensory/Perceptual Alterations (Specify)(Visual, auditory,
    kinesthetic, gustatory, tactile, olfactory)
Unilateral Neglect
Hopelessness
Powerlessness

Pattern 8: Knowing

Knowledge Deficit (Specify)
Altered Thought Processes

Pattern 9: Feeling

Pain
Chronic Pain
Dysfunctional Grieving
Anticipatory Grieving
Potential for Violence: Self-directed or directed at others
Post-Trauma Response
Rape-Trauma Syndrome
Rape-Trauma Syndrome: Compound Reaction
Rape-Trauma Syndrome: Silent Reaction
Anxiety
Fear

Source: North American Nursing Diagnosis Association, 1990.

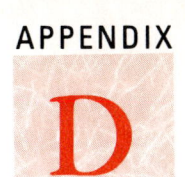

Root Words, Prefixes, and Suffixes

Word element	Meaning
ROOT WORDS	
Circulatory System	
cardio	heart
angio, vaso	vessel
hem, hema, hemato	blood
vena, phlebo	vein
arteria	artery
lympho	lymph
thrombo	clot (of blood)
embolus	moving clot
Digestive System	
bucca	cheek
os, stomato	mouth
gingiva	gum
glossa	tongue
pharyngo	pharynx
esophago	esophagus
gastro	stomach
hepato	liver
cholecyst	gallbladder
pancreas	pancreas
entero	intestines
duodeno	duodenum
jejuno	jejunum
ileo	ileum
caeco	cecum
appendeco	appendix
colo	colon
recto	rectum
ano, procto	anus
Skeletal System	
skeleto	skeleton
Respiratory System	
naso, rhino	nose
tonsillo	tonsil
laryngo	larynx
tracheo	trachea
bronchus, broncho	bronchus (pl. bronchi)
pulmo, pneuma, pneum	lung (sac with air)
Nervous System	
neuro	nerve

Word element	Meaning
cerebrum	brain
oculo, ophthalmo	eye
oto	ear
psych, psycho	mind
Urinary System	
urethro	urethra
cysto	bladder
uretero	ureter
reni, reno, nephro	kidney
pyelo	pelvis of kidney
uro	urine
Female Reproductive System	
vulvo	vulva
perineo	perineum
labio	labium (pl. labia)
vagino, colpo	vagina
cervico	cervix
utero	womb; uterus
tubo, salpingo	fallopian tube
ovario, oophoro	ovary
Male Reproductive System	
orchido	testes
Regions of the Body	
crani, cephalo	head
cervico, tracheo	neck
thoraco	chest
abdomino	abdomen
dorsum	back
Tissues	
cutis, dermato	skin
lipo	fat
musculo, myo	muscle
osteo	bone
myelo	marrow
chondro	cartilage
Miscellaneous	
cyto	cell
genetic	formation, origin
gram	tracing or mark

▶

Word element	Meaning	Word element	Meaning
graph	writing, description	hepa, hepato	liver
kinesis	motion	histo	tissue
meter	measure	homo	same
oligo	small, few	hydro	water
phobia	fear	hygro	moisture
photo	light	hyper	too much, high
pyo	pus	hypo	under, decreased
scope	instrument for visual examination	hyster	uterus
		ileo	ileum
roentgen	x-ray	in	in, within, into
lapar	flank; through the abdominal wall	inter	between
		intra	within
		intro	in, within, into
		juxta	near, close to

PREFIXES

Word element	Meaning	Word element	Meaning
		laryngo	larynx
a, an, ar	without or not	latero	side
ab	away from	lapar	abdomen
acro	extremities	leuk	white
ad	toward, to	macro	large, big
adeno	glandular	mal	bad, poor
aero	air	mast	breast
ambi	around, on both sides	medio	middle
amyl	starch	mega, megalo	large, great
ante	before, forward	meno	menses
anti	against, counteracting	mono	single
bi	double	multi	many
bili	bile	myelo	bone marrow, spinal cord
bio	life		
bis	two	myo	muscle
brachio	arm	neo	new
brady	slow	nephro	kidney
broncho	bronchus (pl. bronchi)	neuro	nerve
cardio	heart	nitro	nitrogen
cervico	neck	noct	night
chole	gall or bile	non	not
cholecysto	gallbladder	ob	against, in front of
circum	around	oculo	eye
co	together	odonto	tooth
contra	against, opposite	ophthalmo	eye
costo	ribs	ortho	straight, normal
cyto	cell	os	mouth, bone
cysto	bladder	osteo	bone
demi	half	oto	ear
derma	skin	pan	all
dis	from	para	beside, accessory to
dorso	back	path	disease
dys	abnormal, difficult	ped	child, foot
electro	electric	per	by, through
en	into, in, within	peri	around
encephal	brain	pharyngo	pharynx
entero	intestine	phlebo	vein
equi	equal	photo	light
eryth	red	phren	diaphragm, mind
ex	out, out of, away from	pneumo	air, lungs
extra	outside of, in addition to	pod	foot
ferro	iron	poly	many, much
fibro	fiber	post	after
fore	before, in front of	pre	before
gastro	stomach	proct	rectum
glosso	tongue	pseudo	false
glyco	sugar	psych	mind
hemi	half	pyel	pelvis of the kidney
hemo	blood	pyo	pus

▶

Word element	Meaning	Word element	Meaning
pyro	fever, heat	emia	blood
quadri	four	esis	action
radio	radiation	form	shaped like
re	back, again	genesis, genetic	formation, origin
reno	kidney	gram	tracing, mark
retro	backward	graph	writing
rhin	nose	ism	condition
sacro	sacrum	itis	inflammation
salpingo	fallopian tube	ize	to treat
sarco	flesh	lith	stone, calculus
sclero	hard, hardening	lithiasis	presence of stones
semi	half	lysis	disintegration
sex	six	megaly	enlargement
skeleto	skeleton	meter	instrument that
steno	narrowing, constriction		measures
sub	under	oid	likeness, resemblance
super	above, excess	oma	tumor
supra	above	opathy	disease of
syn	together	orrhaphy	surgical repair
tachy	fast	osis	disease, condition of
thyro	thyroid, gland	ostomy	to form an opening or
trache	trachea		outlet
trans	across, over	otomy	to incise
tri	three	pexy	fixation
ultra	beyond	phage	ingesting
un	not, back, reversal	phobia	fear
uni	one	plasty	plastic surgery
uretero	ureter	plegia	paralysis
urethro	urethra	rhage	to burst forth
uro	urine, urinary organs	rhea	excessive discharge
vaso	vessel	rhexis	rupture
		scope	lighted instrument for
SUFFIXES			visual examination
		scopy	to examine visually
able	able to	stomy	to form an opening
algia	pain	tomy	incision into
cele	tumor, swelling	uria	urine
centesis	surgical puncture to		
	remove fluid		
cide	killing, destructive		
cule	little		
cyte	cell		
ectasia	dilating, stretching		
ectomy	excision, surgical		
	removal of		

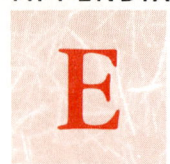

Canada's Food Guide (1985)

Variety   Choose different kinds of foods from within each group in appropriate numbers of servings and portion sizes.

Energy balance   Needs vary with age, sex, and activity. Balance energy intake from foods with energy output from physical activity to control weight. Foods selected according to the Guide can supply 1000–1400 kilo-calories. For additional energy, increase the number and size of servings from the various foods groups and/or add other foods.

Moderation   Select and prepare foods with limited amounts of fat, sugar and salt. If alcohol is consumed, use limited amounts.

Food group	Recommended number of servings (adults)	Some examples of one serving
Milk and milk products	2[a]	1 cup milk; ¾ cup yogurt; 1½ oz cheddar or process cheese
Meat, fish, poultry, and alternates	2	2–3 oz cooked lean meat, fish, poultry, or liver; 4 T peanut butter; 1 cup cooked dried peas, beans, or lentils; ½ cup nuts or seeds; 2 oz cheddar cheese; ½ cup cottage cheese; 2 eggs
Breads and cereals[b]	3–5	1 slice bread; ½ cup cooked cereal; ¾ cup ready-to-eat cereal; 1 roll or muffin; ½–¾ cup cooked rice, macaroni, spaghetti or noodles; ½ hamburger or wiener bun
Fruits and vegetables	4–5[c]	½ cup vegetables or fruits—fresh, frozen, or canned; ½ cup juice—fresh, frozen, or canned; 1 medium-sized potato, carrot, tomato, peach, apple, orange, or banana

[a]For children up to 11 years, 2–3 servings; adolescents, 3–4 servings; pregnant and nursing women, 3–4 servings.
[b]Whole grain or enriched. Whole grain products are recommended.
[c]Include at least two vegetables. Choose a variety of both vegetables and fruits—cooked, raw, or their juices. Include yellow, green, or green leafy vegetables.
Source: Minister of National Health and Welfare, Ottawa. Minister of Supply and Services Canada.

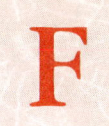
Weight and Volume Equivalents

Metric Equivalents

Weights

1 picogram	=	10^{-12} gram
1 nanogram	=	10^{-9} gram
1 microgram	=	10^{-3} milligram = 10^{-6} gram
1 milligram	=	1000 micrograms = 10^{-6} gram
1 centigram	=	10 milligrams = 10^{-1} decigram = 10^{-2} gram
1 decigram	=	100 milligrams = 10 centigrams = 10^{-1} gram
1 gram	=	1000 milligrams = 100 centigrams = 10 decigrams
1 kilogram	=	1000 grams

Volume

1 milliliter	=	1 gram
1 liter	=	1 kilogram = 1000 grams (milliliters)

Approximate Weight Equivalents: Metric and Apothecaries' Systems

Metric	Apothecaries'	Metric	Apothecaries'
0.1 mg	1/600 grain	30 mg	1/2 grain
1.12 mg	1/500 grain	40 mg	2/3 grain
0.15 mg	1/400 grain	50 mg	3/4 grain
0.2 mg	1/300 grain	60 mg	1 grain
0.25 mg	1/250 grain	100 mg (0.1 gm)	1-1/2 grains
0.3 mg	1/200 grain	150 mg (0.15 gm)	2-1/2 grains
0.4 mg	1/150 grain	200 mg (0.2 gm)	3 grains
0.5 mg	1/120 grain	300 mg (0.3 gm)	5 grains
0.6 mg	1/100 grain	400 mg (0.4 gm)	6 grains
0.8 mg	1/80 grain	500 mg (0.5 gm)	7-1/2 grains
1 mg	1/60 grain	600 mg (0.6 gm)	10 grains
1.2 mg	1/50 grain	1 gram	15 grains
1.5 mg	1/40 grain	1.5 gm	22 grains
2 mg	1/30 grain	2 gm	30 grains
3 mg	1/20 grain	3 gm	45 grains
4 mg	1/15 grain	4 gm	60 grains (1 dram)
5 mg	1/12 grain	5 gm	75 grains
6 mg	1/10 grain	6 gm	90 grains
8 mg	1/8 grain	7.5 gm	120 grains (2 drams)
10 mg	1/6 grain	10 gm	2-1/2 drams
12 mg	1/5 grain	30 gm	1 ounce (8 drams)
15 mg	1/4 grain	500 gm	1.1 pounds
20 mg	1/3 grain	1000 gm	2.2 pounds (1 kilogram)
25 mg	3/8 grain		

Approximate Volume Equivalents: Metric, Apothecaries', and Household Systems

Metric	Apothecaries'	Household
0.06 ml	1 minim (m)	1 drop (gt)
0.3 ml	5 minims	
0.6 ml	10 minims	
1 ml	15 minims	15 drops (gtt)
2 ml	30 minims	
3 ml	45 minims	
4 ml	60 minims (1 fluid dram [f℥])	60 drops (1 teaspoon [tsp])
8 ml	2 fluid drams	2 teaspoons
15 ml	4 fluid drams	4 teaspoons (1 tablespoon [Tbsp])
30 ml	8 fluid drams (1 fluid ounce [f℥])	2 tablespoons
60 ml	2 fluid ounces	
90 ml	3 fluid ounces	
200 ml	6 fluid ounces	1 teacup
250 ml	8 fluid ounces	1 large glass
500 ml	16 fluid ounces (1 pint)	1 pint
750 ml	1½ pints	
1000 ml (1 liter)	2 pints (1 quart)	1 quart
4000 ml	4 quarts	1 gallon

GLOSSARY

abdominal paracentesis removal of fluid from the peritoneal cavity

abduction movement of a bone away from the midline of the body

ablative surgery surgery to remove a diseased organ

abrasion wearing away of a structure, such as the skin or teeth

abscess a localized collection of pus and disintegrating body tissues

absorption (of drug) the process by which a drug passes into the blood stream

acapnia a decreased level of carbon dioxide in the blood

accommodation (Piaget) the process of change in which a person's cognitive processes are sufficiently matured so that he or she can solve problems that could not be solved previously

accountability being responsible for one's actions involving clients and/or colleagues and accepting the consequences for one's behavior

accreditation a process by which an agency appraises institutions or programs to determine whether they meet established standards for service or training

acculturation a process by which members of a society learn its culture and norms

acetylcholine an acetic acid ester of choline, which has an important function in the transmission of nerve impulses at the myoneural junction

acholic clay colored and free from bile

acidosis (acidemia) a condition that occurs with increases in blood carbonic acid or with decreases in blood bicarbonate; blood pH below 7.35

acne an inflammatory condition of the sebaceous glands

acromion (acromial process) the lateral projection of the scapula extending over the shoulder joint

active assistive exercise exercise carried out by the client with some assistance by the nurse

active exercise exercise carried out by the client, who supplies the energy to move the body parts

active immunity a resistance of the body to infection in which the host produces its own antibodies in response to natural or artificial antigens

active transport movement of substances across cell membranes against the concentration gradient

activities of daily living (ADLs) the tasks of daily life, such as eating and bathing

actual health problem a health problem that currently exists

actual loss a loss identifiable by others

acupuncture a Chinese practice of piercing specific superficial nerves with needles, often to treat pain

acute sharp or severe; describing a severe condition with a sudden onset and short course (as opposed to *chronic*)

adaptation the process of modifying to meet new, changing, or different conditions

adaptation (Piaget) the coping behavior of a person who has the ability to handle the demands of the environment

adaptive behavior the responses by which the whole person copes with internal and external environmental stimuli

adaptive mechanisms learned behaviors that assist an individual to adjust to the environment

adduction movement of a bone toward the midline of the body

adenosine triphosphate (ATP) a compound that stores energy from glucose oxidation

adherent sticking together, clinging

adhesion a fibrous band or structure by which parts are abnormally held together

adipose fat; of a fatty nature

adolescence a period of life beginning with the appearance of secondary sex characteristics and terminating with somatic growth, usually between ages 11 and 19

adrenocortical arising from the cortex of the adrenal gland

adrenocorticotrophic hormone (ACTH) a hormone produced by the pituitary gland that stimulates the adrenal cortex to produce hormones

adsorbent an agent that attracts other materials or particles to its surface, e.g., charcoal in the stomach and intestines

adventitious breath sounds abnormal breath sounds

advocate one who pleads the cause of another or argues or pleads for a cause or proposal

aerobe an organism that requires oxygen to live

aerobic requiring oxygen

aerobic exercise any activity during which the body takes in more or an equal amount of oxygen than it expends

affect feelings, emotions

agglutination the process of clumping together

agglutinin a specific antibody formed in the blood

agglutinogen a substance that acts as an antigen and stimulates the production of agglutinin

aggression an unprovoked attack or hostile, injurious, or destructive behavior or outlook

agnostic one who believes that the existence of God has not been proved or who doubts the existence of God

agonist a drug that interacts with a receptor to produce a response

albinism lack of melanin in the skin, hair, and eyes

albuminuria the presence of albumin in the urine

aldosterone a hormone produced by the adrenal cortex that regulates the level of sodium in the body

algor mortis the gradual decrease in body temperature after death

alkalosis (alkalemia) a condition that occurs with increases in blood bicarbonate or decreases in blood carbonic acid; blood pH above 7.45

alopecia abnormal loss of hair

alveolus saclike dilation or cavity in the body (plural: alveoli)

amblyopia reduced visual acuity in one eye

ambulation the act of walking

amino acid one of a group of organic acids containing nitrogen that are considered the components of protein

ampule a small, sealed glass flask, usually designed to hold a single dose of a medication

anabolism a process in which simple substances are converted by the body cells into more complex substances, e.g., building tissue; positive nitrogen balance

anaerobe an organism that does not require oxygen to live

analgesic a medication used to alter the perception and interpretation of pain

analyzing (or analysis) breaking down a whole into component parts

anaphylaxis (anaphylactic shock, anaphylactic reaction) a severe allergic reaction

anasarca generalized edema throughout the body

androgen any substance producing male characteristics

androgogy the art and science of helping adults learn

andropause (climacteric) the period of change in men when sexual activity decreases

androsperm sperm being a Y chromosome

anemia a condition in which the blood is deficient in red blood cells or hemoglobin

aneroid containing no liquid

anesthesia loss of sensation or feeling; induced loss of the sense of pain

aneurysm dilation of the wall of an artery, a vein, or the heart

anger an emotional state or a subjective feeling of animosity or strong displeasure

angiography a diagnostic procedure enabling x-ray visualization of the vascular system after injection of a radiopaque dye

anilingus anal stimulation provided orally

anion an ion carrying a negative charge

anion gap the difference between the unmeasured serum anions and cations

anisocoria unequal pupils

ankylosis permanent fixation of a joint; stiffening of a joint

anodyne a medication that relieves pain

anorexia lack of appetite

anorexia nervosa a psychologic condition in which the person eats little or nothing, leading to emaciation

anoscopy visual examination of the anal canal using a lighted instrument called an anoscope

anoxemia a condition in which the level of oxygen in the blood is below normal

anoxia systemic absence or reduction of oxygen in the body tissues below physiologic levels

answer (legal) a written response to a complaint

antecubital space the area in front of the elbow

anterior of, toward, or at the front

anthropometric measurement measurement of the size and composition of the body, e.g., height, weight, and skin folds

antibiotic a substance produced by microorganisms that has the capacity to inhibit the growth of or kill other microorganisms

antibody (immunoglobulin) a protective substance produced in the body to counteract antigens

anticipatory loss a loss experienced before it actually occurs

anticipatory socialization the process of preparing for roles to which one aspires

antidiuretic hormone (ADH) a hormone that is stored and released by the posterior pituitary gland and that controls water reabsorption from the kidney tubules; also referred to as *vasopressin*

antigen a substance capable of inducing the formation of antibodies

antipyretic a substance that is effective in relieving fever

antiseptic an agent that inhibits the growth of some microorganisms

anuria the failure of the kidneys to produce urine, resulting in total lack of urination or output of less than 100 ml per day in an adult

anxiety a state of mental uneasiness, apprehension, or dread producing an increased level of arousal due to an impending or anticipated threat to self or significant relationships

apathy lack of interest or feeling

Apgar score a system of numerically rating the condition of a newborn infant

aphasia the inability to communicate by speech, signs, or writing, resulting from an injury or disease

apical pulse the central pulse located at the apex of the heart

apical-radial pulse measurement of the apical beat and the radial pulse

APIE one format used to record the client's progress; it has four components: Assessment, Plan, Implementation, and Evaluation

apnea cessation of breathing

apneustic breathing prolonged, gasping inspiration followed by a very short, usually inefficient expiration

apocrine gland a large sweat gland whose duct usually opens into a hair follicle; sweat is released usually in response to emotional stimuli

approximate to bring close together (referring to wound or incision edges)

areflexia absence of reflexes

areola the circular area of different color around a central point, such as the circular pigmented area surrounding the nipple of the breast

arrhythmia an irregular pulse rhythm

arteriosclerosis a condition in which the walls of the arteries become hardened, thickened, and less compliant

artificial respiration forceful movement of air into and out of the lungs by means external to the person

ascites the accumulation of fluid in the abdominal cavity

asepsis freedom from infection or infectious material

asphyxia a condition resulting from a lack of oxygen in the inspired air

asphyxiation (suffocation) lack of oxygen due to interrupted breathing

aspirate to remove gases or fluids from a cavity by using suction

assault an attempt or threat to touch another person unjustifiably

assertiveness expression of oneself openly and directly without hurting others

assessing collecting, verifying, and organizing data about a client's health status; a continuous process carried out during all phases of the nursing process

assimilation (of a group) the blending of attitudes and beliefs of the members; process by which members of a foreign culture learn the values and behaviors of the culture into which they have immigrated

assimilation (Piaget) the process whereby humans are able to encounter and react to new situations by using the mechanisms they already possess

associative play play that occurs with other children

associative thinking a type of thinking that has little direction and often involves random thoughts (e.g., daydreaming)

assumptions statements of fact or suppositions that people accept as the underlying theoretical foundation for conceptualizations about a professional field

astigmatism a refractive error of the eye due to an uneven curvature of the cornea

astringent an agent that causes contraction or shrinkage of tissue; usually applied topically

ataxia failure of muscle coordination

atelectasis collapse of lung tissue

atheist one who denies the existence of God

athlete's foot (tinea pedis) a fungal infection of the foot; ringworm

atony lack of normal muscle tone

at-risk aggregate subgroup of a population who are at greater risk of illness or poor recovery

atrophic vaginitis vaginal atrophy characterized by thinning and drying of the vaginal wall, loss of elasticity, and decreased lubrication

atrophy a wasting away or decrease in size of a cell, tissue, body organ, or muscle

attitude a feeling tone directed toward a person, object, or idea

audit an examination or review of records

auditory related to or experienced through hearing

auricle a chamber of the ear or the heart

auscultation the practice of examining the body by listening to body sounds

authority the official or legitimized right to act and command

autoantigen an antigen that originates in the person's own body

autogenous (infection) originating from the client's own microbial flora

autonomy the state of being independent and self-directed without outside control

autopsy (postmortem examination) the examination of a body after death; performed by a physician

autoscope a lighted instrument used to examine the external ear canal

awareness the ability to perceive environmental stimuli and body reactions and to respond appropriately through thought and action

axilla the armpit (plural: axillae)

axillary line an imaginary line extending vertically from the anterior fold of the axilla

babbling prelinguistic repetitive sounds produced by infants

Babinski (plantar) reflex in infants up to 1 year, the normal fanning out of toes and dorsiflexion of the big toe elicited by stroking the sole of the foot (positive Babinski); after 1 year the normal curling of the toes at this stroking (negative Babinski)

bacteriocide an agent capable of destroying some microorganisms

bacteriocin substance produced by certain bacteria that kills other strains of bacteria

bacteriostatic agent an agent that prevents the growth and reproduction of some microorganisms

bacteriuria bacteria in the urine

balance stability; steadiness; a state of equipoise in which opposing forces counteract each other

bandage a material used to wrap a body part

barium a metallic element commonly used in solution as a contrast medium for x-ray filming of the gastrointestinal tract

barium enema x-ray filming of the large intestine using a contrast medium; also called a *lower gastrointestinal series*

barium swallow x-ray filming of the esophagus, stomach, and duodenum; also referred to as an *upper gastrointestinal series*

barrel chest a chest shape in which the ratio of the anteroposterior diameter to the lateral diameter is 1 to 1

basal metabolic rate (BMR) the rate of energy utilization in the body required to maintain body functions at rest

base of support the area on which an object rests

basophil granular leukocyte with two lobes

battery willful or negligent touching of a person or a person's clothes, which may or may not cause harm

Beau's line a deep line visible across a nail after its growth has been halted and then renewed

behavioral contract a written commitment by a client to follow through with selected actions

Being values (metaneeds) growth needs

belief something accepted as true by a judgment of probability rather than actuality

beneficence the doing or producing of good, such as performing an act of kindness

bereavement a subjective response of a person who has experienced the loss of a significant other through death

bevel a slanting edge

bilateral affecting two sides

bilirubin orange pigment in the bile

binder a type of bandage applied to large body areas, e.g., the abdomen or chest

biofeedback conscious control of physiologic responses under the control of the autonomic nervous system, such as heart rate and blood pressure

bioethics ethics concerning life

biologic sex sexual gender genetically determined at conception from the XX or XY chromosomal combination

biopsy the removal and examination of tissue from the living body

biorhythm an inner rhythm that appears to control a variety of biologic processes

Biot's respiration shallow breaths interrupted by apnea

biotransformation process by which a drug is converted to a less active form; also called detoxification

bleb (wheal) a small, smooth, slightly raised area on the skin, usually filled with fluid

blended family family composed of two previously existing family units; also called *reconstituted family*

blood pressure (arterial) the pressure of the blood as it pulsates through the arteries

body image an individual's perception of his or her own physical attributes, body functioning, sexuality, appearance, and state of wellness

body mechanics the efficient and coordinated use of the body to produce motion and maintain balance during activity

body temperature the balance between the heat produced by the body and the heat lost from the body

borborygmi abnormally intense and frequent bowel sounds

bottle mouth syndrome decay of teeth caused by constant contact with the sweet liquid from a bottle of formula

boundary (of a system) a real or imaginary line that differentiates one system from another system or a system from its environment

brachial pulse a pulse located on the inner side of the biceps muscle just below the axilla; usually palpated medially in the antecubital space

bradycardia an abnormally slow heart rate, below 60 beats per minute in an adult

bradykinin an amino acid chain that causes powerful vasodilation, increased capillary permeability, smooth muscle contraction, and stimulation of pain receptors

bradypnea abnormally slow respirations; usually fewer than 10 respirations per minute

brainstorming technique to generate ideas in which one person's idea elicits an idea from another person and so on

bromhidrosis foul smelling perspiration

bronchial sounds normal loud, harsh, hollow blowing sounds heard by auscultation over the trachea and major bronchi

bronchodilator an agent that dilates the bronchi of the lungs

bronchogram an x-ray film of the bronchial tree taken after injection of an iodized oil dye, used as a contrast medium

bronchophony an increase in vocal resonance; an abnormal voice sound heard on auscultation of the chest wall

bronchopneumonia an infection that originates in the bronchi and involves patches of lung tissue

bronchoscope a lighted instrument used to visualize the bronchi of the lungs

bronchoscopy visual examination of the bronchi using a bronchoscope

bronchovesicular sounds combination of bronchial and vesicular sounds heard by auscultation over parts of the chest where a bronchus is near lung tissue

bronchus a large air passageway of the lungs (plural: bronchi)

bruit abnormal blowing, swishing, or rippling sounds heard during auscultation

bruxism grinding of the teeth during sleep

bubbling gurgling sounds produced as air passes through moist secretions in the respiratory tract

buccal pertaining to the cheek

buffer an agent or system that tends to maintain constancy or that prevents changes in the chemical concentration of a substance

bulimia an uncontrollable compulsion to consume enormous amounts of food and then expel the food by self-induced vomiting or by taking laxatives

burden of proof (legal) evidence of the defendant's wrongdoing presented by the plaintiff

burning pain pain like the pain of burning skin

cachexia a state of weakness, emaciation, and malnutrition often seen in wasting diseases and terminal malignancies

calcitonin a hormone secreted by the thyroid gland that regulates blood calcium levels

calculus a stone composed of minerals that is formed in the body, e.g., a renal calculus formed in the kidney

calipers an instrument used to measure the thickness of folds of skin

callus hyperplasia or thickening of the horny layer of the epidermis, usually due to pressure

caloric density the number of kilocalories per unit weight of food

caloric value the amount of energy that nutrients or foods supply to the body

Calorie (large calorie, kilocalorie, C.) the amount of heat required to raise the temperature of 1 kilogram of water 1 degree centigrade

calorie (small calorie) the unit of heat required to raise the temperature of 1 gram of water 1 degree centigrade

calyx (calix) a cup-shaped organ or cavity

cannula a tube with a lumen (channel), which is inserted into a cavity or duct and is often fitted with a trocar during insertion

canthus the angle formed by the upper and lower eyelids; each eye has an inner and an outer canthus

capillary action the movement of fluid in a tube, caused by the adhesion of the fluid to the wall of the tube

capsule a soft, soluble container for a medication; an anatomic structure enclosing an organ or part of the body; (of a cell) a well-defined, gelatinous layer surrounding a bacterial cell

carbaminohemoglobin the chemical combination of carbon dioxide and hemoglobin

carbohydrate a nutrient composed of carbon, hydrogen, and oxygen, e.g., starches and sugars

carbonic acid the compound formed when carbon dioxide combines with water

cardiac arrest the cessation of heart function

cardiac output the amount of blood ejected from the heart per minute by ventricular contraction; it is the stroke volume times the heart rate per minute

cardiopulmonary resuscitation (CPR) artificial stimulation of the heart and lungs; also referred to as basic life support (BLS)

caries decay of a tooth or bone

carina the ridge or junction where the main bronchi meet the trachea

caring concern about persons, events, projects and things

carminative an agent that promotes the passage of flatus from the colon

carotid arteries major arteries lying on either side of the trachea and larynx

carotid receptors nerve endings that are found in the carotid bodies and carotid sinuses and that are sensitive to blood pH, changes in blood pressure, and excessive blood CO_2

carrier a person who harbors pathogens but is not ill

case management a system of delivering nursing care in which a nurse is responsible for nursing care throughout the client's stay in hospital

catabolism a destructive process in which complex substances are broken down into simpler substances, e.g., breakdown of tissue

cataplexy partial or complete muscle paralysis that can occur during narcolepsy

cataract opacity of the lens of the eye or its capsule

catarrh inflammation of the mucous membrane accompanied by a discharge

cathartic (laxative) a drug that induces evacuation of feces from the large intestine

catheter a tube of plastic, rubber, metal, or other material used to remove or inject fluids into a cavity such as the bladder

cation a positively charged ion

cauda a tail or taillike appendage

caudal anesthetic an anesthetic injected into the caudal canal, below the spinal cord

cavity a hollow space within the body or one of its organs

cellular fluid *see* intracellular fluid

cellulitis inflammation of cellular tissue

Celsius *see* centigrade

cementum a bonelike connective tissue surrounding the root of a tooth

center of gravity the point at which the mass (weight) of the body is centered

centigrade (Celsius) a thermometer scale used to measure heat; the freezing point of water is 0 C and the boiling point is 100 C

central venous pressure (CVP) a measurement of the pressure of the blood, in millimeters of water, within the vena cava or the right atrium of the heart

cephalocaudal proceeding in the direction from head to toe

cerebral death death that occurs when the cerebral cortex is irreversibly destroyed

cerebrospinal fluid fluid contained within the four ventricles of the brain, the subarachnoid space, and the central canal of the spinal cord

certification the practice of determining minimum standards of competence in specialty areas

cerumen waxlike material that protects the auditory canal

chancre a papular lesion (sore) occurring at the entry of infection in some diseases; the primary sore of syphilis

change process that leads to modifications in individual or institutional patterns of behavior

change agent an individual, such as a nurse, or group who operates to change the status quo in another individual or in a system

chaplain a member of the clergy who serves an institution

chart (medical record) a written account of a client's health history, current health status, treatment, and progress

charting (recording) the process of making written entries about a client on the medical record

cheilosis cracks or scaling at the corners of the lips

chemical name (of drug) the name by which a chemist knows a drug

chemical thermogenesis the production of heat by chemical means, e.g., production and circulation of ephinephrine

chemoreceptor a receptor that is sensitive to chemical substances

chemosensitive pain receptors pain receptors stimulated by chemicals

chemotaxis the movement of a cell or an organism in response to a chemical gradient

Cheyne-Stokes respirations rhythmic waxing and waning of respirations from very deep breathing to very shallow breathing with periods of temporary apnea, often associated with cardiac failure, increased intracranial pressure, or brain damage

chill shivering and shaking of the body with involuntary contractions of the voluntary muscles

cholangiogram an x-ray film of the biliary tract taken after the injection of a dye

cholecystogram an x-ray film of the gallbladder after the ingestion of a contrast dye; also called *oral cholecystography*

cholesterol a lipid that does not contain fatty acid but possesses many of the chemical and physical properties of other lipids

chordotomy *see* cordotomy

choroid plexus projections of the pia mater into the ventricles of the brain that secrete cerebrospinal fluid

chromosome a structure in the nucleus of a cell that contains DNA and transmits genetic information

chronic persisting over a long time

chyme semifluid material produced by gastric digestion of food in the stomach; it is found in the small and large intestines

cicatrical tissue *see* scar tissue

cicatrix scar

cicatrization formation of a scar

cilia hairlike projections from cells, e.g., of the mucous membrane of the respiratory tract

circadian rhythm rhythmic repetition of certain phenomena each 24 hours

circa dies about a day

circulatory overload a state in which the intravascular fluid compartment contains more fluid than normal

circumcision surgical removal of part or all of the foreskin of the penis; usually performed during infancy

circumduction movement of the distal part of a bone in a circle, with the proximal end remaining fixed

circumference the outer measurement or perimeter, e.g., the distance around the chest

cisterna an enclosed space that serves as a reservoir for body fluid

citric acid cycle (Krebs cycle) a complex series of chemical reactions by which the acetyl portion of acetyl coenzyme A is broken down into carbon dioxide and hydrogen

civil action a legal action between two or more individuals

civil (private) law rules that regulate or control relationships between people rather than between persons and governments

clean free of potentially infectious agents

clean technique a technique that maintains an area or articles free from infectious agents

clergy priests, rabbis, ministers, church elders, deacons, and any other spiritual advisers

client a person who engages the services of another who is qualified to provide this service

client contract a written agreement between a client and a nurse regarding a behavior change

client goal statement about the expected or desired change in a client's status after he or she receives nursing interventions

climacteric the point in development when reproduction capacity in the female terminates (menopause) and the sexual activity of the male decreases (andropause)

clinical pharmacist a person who specializes in drugs that are used for treatment, prevention, and diagnosis of disease

clitoris a small round mass of erectile tissue, blood vessels, and nerves located behind the junction of the labia minora; homologous to the penis

closed questions restrictive questions requiring only a short answer

closed system a system that does not exchange energy or matter with its environment

closed wound a wound in which there is no break in the skin

clubbing (of nails) an elevation of the proximal aspect of the nail and softening of the nail bed

coagulate to clot

cochlea a tubular structure in the inner ear that contains the organ for hearing

code of ethics formal guidelines for professional action

coercive power power derived from the perception of one's ability to threaten, harm, or punish others

cognition the process of knowing, including judgment and awareness

cognitive referring to intellectual processes such as remembering, thinking, perceiving, abstracting, and generalizing

cognitive appraisal (transactional stress theory) an evaluative process that determines why and to what extent a particular transaction or series of transactions between a person and the environment are stressful

cognitive development development of the faculties of remembering, thinking, perceiving, abstracting, and generalizing

cohabiting (communal) family family unit formed by unrelated individuals or families cohabiting or living under one roof

cohesive sticking together

cohesiveness (of a group) the degree of group unity or oneness

coitus sexual intercourse; from Latin, meaning "a coming together"

coitus interruptus a method of contraception during which the penis is withdrawn prior to ejaculation

colic paroxysmal intestinal cramplike pain

collaborative nursing action activity performed jointly with another member of the health care team or as a result of a joint decision by the nurse and another member of the health care team

collagen a protein found in connective tissue; a whitish protein substance that adds tensile strength to a wound

colloid substances, such as large plasma protein molecules, that do not readily dissolve in true solutions

colonization process by which strains of bacteria become resident flora

colonoscope a lighted instrument used to visualize the interior of the colon

colonoscopy visual examination of the interior of the colon with a colonoscope

colostomy an artificial abdominal opening into the colon (large bowel)

colostrum a yellow, milky fluid secreted by the mother's mammary glands a few days before or after childbirth

comatose a state of unconsciousness in which the person shows no response to maximum painful stimuli, absence of reflexes, and absence of muscle tone in the extremities

combustible able to burn; flammable

comedo a mass on the skin consisting of keratin, lipids, fatty acids, and bacteria; whiteheads and blackheads

commitment (of a group) an agreement, pledge, or obligation to do something or follow a course of action

commode a portable, chairlike structure used as a toilet

common law body of principles that evolves from court decisions (decisional law)

communicable disease (infectious disease) a disease that can spread from one person to another

communication exchange of thoughts, ideas, or feelings between two or more people

compensation defense mechanism in which a person substitutes an activity for one that he or she would prefer doing or cannot do

complaint (legal) a document filed by the plaintiff claiming that his or her legal rights have been infringed

compliance in learning, an individual's desire to learn and act on the learning; in drug therapy, the act of carefully following the prescription; of the arteries, distensibility or the ability to contract and expand

complier a person who follows a therapeutic regimen

compress a moist gauze dressing that is applied frequently to an open wound; it sometimes is medicated

concave hollowed or rounded inward

concept an abstract idea or mental image of phenomena or reality generalized from particular instances

conceptual framework set of concepts and statements that integrate the concepts into a meaningful configuration

conceptual model a basic structure in which a complex of ideas is united to portray a large general idea

concurrent audit an audit to review present practices

concurrent disinfection measures taken while a client is infectious to control the spread of the microorganisms

conditioning learning in which a response previously associated with one stimulus becomes associated with another stimulus

condom a sheath or cover, usually made of rubber or plastic, worn over the penis during coitus to prevent conception or infection; it may also be used to catch urine

conduction the transfer of heat from one molecule or object to another by contact

confer to consult another person or persons for advice, information, ideas, or instructions

confidentiality the right of a client or research subject that any information revealed by that individual will not be made public or available to others

conformity actions in accordance with specified standards

confusion a mental state in which a person appears bewildered and may make inappropriate statements and answers to questions

congenital existing at, and often before, birth

congestion excessive accumulation of blood in a part of the body

congruence (communication) a state in which one's verbal and non-verbal communications convey the same message

conjunctiva the delicate membrane that covers the eyeball and lines the eyelids

conjunctivitis inflammation of the conjunctiva

consciousness a person's normal state of awareness of the environment, self, and others

consensual reaction (eyes) a reaction in which one pupil constricts quickly in response to a bright light and the other pupil constricts also, but more slowly

consent permission given voluntarily by a person in his or her right mind; *informed consent* implies that the individual is knowledgeable about the consent and understands it

constant data information that is unchanging

constant fever minimal variance but constant elevation of body temperature

constipation passage of small, dry, hard stool or passage of no stool for an abnormally long time

constitutional law law stated in federal, state, or provincial constitutions

constructive surgery surgery to repair a congenitally malformed organ or tissue

consultation deliberation by two or more people

consumer an individual, group, or community that uses a service or a product

contaminated possessing disease-producing microorganisms

continuum a grid or graduated scale

contraception the prevention of fertilization of the ovum by any method

contract a written or verbal agreement between two or more people to do or not do some lawful act

contract law enforcement of agreements among private individuals

contraction the normal active shortening or tensing of a muscle

contractual obligation a duty to render service established by a formal or informal contract

contracture permanent shortening of a muscle and subsequent shortening of tendons and ligaments

contusion a closed wound that occurs as a result of a blow from a blunt instrument; a bruise

convection transfer of heat by movement of a liquid or gas, e.g., air currents

conversion a defense mechanism in which a mental conflict is converted into a physical symptom

convex curved or rounded like the external surface of a sphere

coping the process through which the individual manages the demands of the person-environment relationship that are stressful

coping behavior behavior learned in response to stress; immediate response to a threatening situation

coping mechanisms physical or emotional adaptive or defensive abilities

coping strategy an innate or acquired way of responding to a changing environment or specific problem or situation

copulation the act of coitus; from Latin, meaning "coupling or joining"

coraje a Hispanic term meaning rage in response to a particular situation

cordotomy (chordotomy) surgical severing of the spinothalamic portion of the anterolateral tract of the spinal cord, usually for the purpose of relieving pain

core-gender identity *see* sexual identity

core temperature temperature of the deep tissues of the body

corium *see* dermis

corn a hardening and thickening of the skin forming a conical mass pointing downward into the corium

cornea the transparent covering of the anterior eye that connects with the sclera

corneal reflex irritation of the cornea resulting in a reflex closing of the eyelids

cornification hardening

coroner a public official who is responsible for investigating any deaths that appear to be unnatural

cortical bone compact bone

corticoid a term applied to hormones of the adrenal cortex or substances with similar activity

cortisol the most abundant glucocorticoid; also called hydrocortisone

cortisone a hormone produced by the adrenal cortex that has antiinflammatory properties and is involved in the metabolism of glycogen to glucose

costal angle the angle formed between the ribs and the sternum

costal (thoracic) breathing breathing using chiefly the intercostal muscles

costovertebral angle the angle formed by a rib and the spine

counseling the process of helping a client to recognize and cope with stressful psychologic or social problems, to develop improved interpersonal relationships, and to promote personal growth

counterirritant an agent that produces an irritation with the intent of relieving some other problem

countershock phase part of the initial stage of the general adaptation syndrome during which the body changes produced in response to a stressor are reversed

covert data *see* subjective data

CPR *see* cardiopulmonary resuscitation

crackles (rales) rattling or bubbling breath sounds generally heard on inspiration

creatinine a nitrogenous waste that is excreted in the urine

creative thinking a pattern of thinking involving establishing new relationships and new concepts and solving problems innovatively

Credé's maneuver manual exertion of pressure on the bladder to force urine out

credentialing (nursing) the process of determining and maintaining competence in nursing practice

creed a set of guiding principles or beliefs

cremaster the inner layer of striated muscle and connective tissue in the scrotum

crepitus a grating sound caused by bone fragments rubbing together

creps (crepitation) a dry, crackling sound like that of crumpled cellophane, produced by air in the subcutaneous tissue or by air moving through fluid in the alveoli of the lungs

crime an act committed in violation of societal law

criminal action a legal action dealing with disputes between an individual and society as a whole

criminal law law that deals with actions against the safety and welfare of the public

crisis in psychosocial terms, a rapid change or event that disturbs a person's psychologic homeostasis; in fever, the sudden reduction of an elevated body temperature accompanied by flushed skin

criteria (of nursing care) indicators of the quality of nursing care or measures by which the nursing care is judged

criterion a standard or model that can be used in judging

critical thinking cognitive processes during which data are reviewed and explanations considered before an opinion is formed; a pattern of thinking based on knowledge, experience, and the abilities to conceptualize and analyse relationships

crown (of a tooth) the exposed part of the tooth outside the gum, covered by enamel

crutch palsy weakness of the hand, wrist, and forearm induced by prolonged pressure of a crutch on the axillary nerves

cryptorchidism failure of the testes to descend from the abdominal cavity to the scrotal sacs

crystalloid salts that dissolve readily in true solutions

cue a piece of information or data that influences decisions

cultural heritage values and beliefs unique to a particular culture that influence the family's structure, methods of interaction, health care practices, and coping mechanisms

cultural specifics practices, values, beliefs, and behavior patterns unique to a given culture

cultural universals attributes that are similar among different cultures

culture in microbiology, the cultivation of microorganisms or cells in a special growth medium; in sociology, the beliefs and practices that are shared by people and passed down from generation to generation

culture shock the shock that can occur when an individual changes quickly from one social setting to another where former patterns of behavior are often ineffective

cumulative effect the effect of a drug when the level builds up in the blood

cunnilingus oral stimulation of the clitoris and labia by a partner

cupula a gelatinous dome-shaped structure of the inner ear that contains sensory hair cells

curandero (female: curandera) a healer within the Hispanic community

curet a spoon-shaped instrument used for removing material from a body cavity

cyanosis bluish discoloration of the skin, nail beds, and mucous membranes, due to reduced oxygen in the blood

cyst an enclosed cavity or sac lined by epithelium and containing liquid or semisolid material

cystitis inflammation of the urinary bladder

cystocele protrusion of the urinary bladder through the vaginal wall

cystoscope a lighted instrument used to visualize the interior of the urinary bladder

cystoscopy visual examination of the urinary bladder with a cystoscope

cytology the study of the origin, structure, function, and pathology of cells

dacrocystitis inflammation of the lacrimal sac

Dakin's solution a buffered aqueous solution of sodium hypochlorite used as a bactericide

dandruff a dry or greasy, scaly material shed from the scalp

data information

data collection the process of gathering information about a client's health status

database (baseline data) all information known about a client; it includes the physician's history and physical examination, the nurse's assessment and history, and material contributed by other members of the health team

deamination the removal of the amino (NH_2) groups by hydrolysis from amino acids

debilitated having lost strength

debride to remove foreign and dying tissue from a wound so that healthy tissue is exposed

deceased dead; a person who is dead

decibel a unit used to measure or describe sound

deciduous teeth temporary teeth that are shed

decision (legal) the outcome of a trial, rendered by a judge

decisional law laws determined by the courts in ruling on cases, rather than by statutes

decoding the process of receiving a communication and sorting out the meaning of a message

decubitus ulcer an ulcer of the skin and underlying tissues produced by prolonged pressure

decussate to cross over

deductive reasoning making specific observations from a generalization

deductive theory a theory formulated by a process in which the idea is developed first, followed by observation of relevant supportive phenomena

deep breathing inhaling the maximum amount of air possible, then exhaling

defamation a communication that is injurious to a person

defecation expulsion of feces from the rectum and anus

defendant (legal) a person who is alleged to have infringed on the rights of another

defense mechanism unconscious psychologic processes that protect the person from anxiety

dehiscence a splitting open or rupture

dehydration insufficient fluid in the body

delegate to authorize another as one's representative or to entrust authority to another

delegation assigning to another an aspect of client care; sharing of responsibility and authority with others and holding them accountable for performance

delirious experiencing mental confusion, restlessness, and incoherence

demand feeding feeding the child when he or she is hungry

dementia decline in memory and other cognitive abilities

demineralization excessive loss of minerals or inorganic salts

demography the statistical study of population with reference to a distribution by age, place of residence, mortality, morbidity, and similar vital statistics

demulcent a drug that coats the intestine, thus protecting the lining

denial a defense mechanism in which painful or anxiety-producing aspects of reality are blocked out of consciousness

dental caries tooth decay

dental crown the exposed part of the tooth outside the gum, covered by enamel

dental plaque deposits on the teeth that serve as a medium for bacterial growth

dental pulp cavity a space in the center of the tooth containing blood vessels and nerves

dental root the part of the tooth that is imbedded in the jaw

dentifrice a paste or powder used to clean or polish the teeth

dentin the internal part of the tooth crown below the enamel

dentures a natural or artificial set of teeth; usually the term designates artificial replacements for natural teeth

deontology the theory or study of moral obligation

deoxyribonucleic acid (DNA) a nucleic acid found in all living cells; it is the carrier of genetic information

dependent edema edema that collects in the lower parts of the body, where hydrostatic pressure is greatest

dependent nursing action, intervention, or function activity by a nurse that is a result of a physician's order

depilatory an agent that removes body hair

depolarize to reduce a nonpolarized state; to cause loss of charge

depression feelings of sadness and dejection, often accompanied by physiologic change; a decrease of functional activity, as in depression of sensorium

dermatitis inflammation of the skin

dermatologic preparation a medication applied to the skin

dermis (corium) true skin, containing blood vessels, nerves, hair follicles, and glands

detrusor muscle the three layers of smooth muscle that make up the urinary bladder

detumescence the process of returning to a flaccid state, e.g., referring to the penis following ejaculation

development an individual's increasing capacity and skill in functioning, related to growth

developmental crisis a crisis that occurs as a result of stressors impeding development

developmental tasks skills and behavior patterns learned during development

dextrose a sugar; also called *glucose*

diagnosis a statement or conclusion concerning the nature of some phenomenon

diagnosing a process that results in a diagnostic statement or nursing diagnosis

diagnostic related group (DRG) a predetermined category of illnesses, injuries, surgical procedures, and/or other conditions requiring hospitalization for which the cost of care is established prior to a client's hospitalization

diagnostic surgery surgery performed to confirm a diagnosis

dialyzing membrane a membrane that permits water molecules and crystalloids in true solution to move through it but not particles in a colloid dispersion

diapedesis the movement of blood corpuscles through a blood vessel wall

diaphoresis profuse sweating

diaphragmatic (abdominal) breathing breathing that chiefly involves movement of the diaphragm and the abdomen

diarrhea defecation of liquid feces and increased frequency of defecation

diastole the period when the ventricles of the heart are relaxed

diastolic pressure the pressure of the blood against the arterial walls when the ventricles of the heart are at rest

dietitian a person who is skilled in the use of diets in health and disease

diffusion movement of gases or other particles from an area of greater pressure to an area of lower pressure or concentration; the continual intermingling of molecules in liquids, gases, or solids brought about by the random movement of the molecules

diffusion coefficient the rate of solubility of gases in the respiratory membrane

digital performed with the finger

dildo an artificial penis

dilemma a situation involving a choice between equally satisfactory or unsatisfactory alternatives or a difficult problem that seems to have no satisfactory solution

diploid number the original number of chromosomes in all cells of the body (23 pairs in humans)

diplopia double vision

direct interview highly structured questioning that elicits specific information

directed thinking a pattern of thinking that is purposeful and is used for forming judgments, problem-solving, and decision-making

disaccharide a sugar consisting of double molecules

discharge planning the process of anticipating and planning for client's needs after discharge from a hospital or other facility

discovery (legal) pretrial activities designed to gain all the facts of a situation

disease a morbid (unhealthful) process having definite symptoms

disengagement a mutual withdrawal between an older person and others

disequilibrium a disturbed state of equilibrium, either mental or physical; an unbalanced condition

disinfectant an agent that destroys pathogens other than spores

disinfection the process by which an article is rendered free of pathogens

disorientation a state of mental confusion; loss of bearings, time, and place

displacement a defense mechanism in which an emotional reaction is transferred from one object to another less threatening object

distal farthest from the point of reference

distention (abdominal) *see* tympanites

distraction a mechanism for relieving pain in which the person's attention is drawn away from the pain

distribution (of drug) the transportation of a drug from its site of absorption to its site of action

diuresis *see* polyuria

diuretic an agent that increases the production of urine

dorsal of, toward, or at the back

dorsal column stimulator an electrode attached to the dorsal column of the spinal cord for the purpose of relieving pain

dorsal flexion movement of the ankle so that the toes are pointing up

dorsalis pedis pulse a pulse located on the instep of the foot

dorsal recumbent position a back-lying position with the head and shoulders slightly elevated

drainage a discharge from a wound or cavity

dressing a material used to cover and protect a wound

drug (medication) a chemical compound taken for disease prevention, diagnosis, cure, or relief or to affect the structure or function of the body

drug abuse excessive intake of a substance either continually or periodically

drug allergy a hypersensitivity to a drug; the immunologic reaction to a drug

drug dependence inability to keep the intake of a drug or substance under control

drug habituation a mild form of psychologic dependence on a drug

drug interaction the beneficial or harmful interaction of one drug with another drug

drug misuse improper use of common medications in ways that can lead to acute and chronic toxicity

drug tolerance a condition in which successive increases in the dosage of a drug are required to maintain a given therapeutic effect

drug toxicity the quality of a drug that exerts a deleterious effect on an organism or tissue

DT diphtheria and tetanus toxoid

DTP diphtheria toxoid, tetanus toxoid, and pertussis vaccine

due process a constitutional clause that states fair procedures must be followed when rules are enforced

dullness (in percussion) decreased resonance or percussion sound that occurs over dense tissue or large amounts of fluid

duodenocolic reflex a mass peristaltic movement of the colon stimulated by the presence of chyme in the duodenum

duration (of sound) the length of the sound (long or short)

dyad a two-person group

dynamic equilibrium tendency of the body to maintain a state of balance or equilibrium while continually changing

dysmenorrhea painful menstruation

dyspareunia pain experienced by a woman during intercourse

dyspepsia indigestion

dysphagia difficulty or inability to swallow

dysphasia difficulty speaking

dysphoria disquiet, restlessness

dyspnea difficult and labored breathing in which the client has a persistent unsatisfied need for air and feels distressed

dysrhythmia an irregular pulse rhythm

dysuria painful or difficult urination

ecchymosis a blotchy area of discoloration of the skin; a bruise

ecchymotic appearing like a bruise

eccrine gland a sweat gland that secretes outward via a duct

echolalia the repetition by a person of words addressed to him or her

ecology the study of the relationship of humans and the environment

ectropion a rolling out of the eyelid

edema excess interstitial fluid

edentulous without teeth

effector organ a muscle or gland that responds to nerve impulses

efferent conveying away from the center

effluent urine or feces discharged through a stoma

ego (Freud) the part of the psyche that maintains its identity; the conscious sense of self

egocentricity concern about oneself

egocentric speech self-centered, noncommunicative speech

ego integrity feeling satisfied with one's life-style and accepting the inevitability of one's life cycle

egophony a type of bronchophony in which the voice has a nasal, bleating quality

ejaculation expulsion of semen from the penis

elective surgery surgery performed for a person's well-being but not absolutely necessary for life

Electra complex (Freud) the female child's attraction to her father; compare with *Oedipus complex*

electrocardiogram (ECG, EKG) a graph of the electric activity of the heart

electroencephalogram (EEG) a graph of the electric activity of the brain

electrolyte a chemical substance that develops an electric charge and is able to conduct an electric current when placed in water; an ion

electromyogram (EMG) a record of the electric potential created by the contraction of a muscle

electromyograph a machine that measures and records impulses from the muscles on an electromyogram

electron a negatively charged electric particle

emaciation excessive thinness

embalming a process of preserving a body chemically

embolus a blood clot (or a substance, such as air) that has moved from its place of origin and is obstructing the circulation in a blood vessel (plural: emboli)

emmetropia the normal refraction of the eye, which focuses objects on the retina

emollient an agent that soothes and softens skin or mucous membrane; often an oily substance

empacho a Hispanic term for a disease seen primarily in children that includes a swollen abdomen as a result of intestinal blockage

empathy seeing or feeling a situation the way another person sees or feels it

emphysema a chronic obstructive lung disorder in which the terminal bronchioles become distended and plugged with mucus

empirical by observation or experience

empirical data information collected from the observable world

emulsification a process by which lipids are broken up and evenly dispersed in an aqueous medium

emulsion a preparation in which one liquid is distributed throughout another

enamel (of a tooth) the hard, inorganic substance that covers the crown of a tooth

enanthema rash of the mucous membrane

encoding the selection of specific signs and symbols to transmit a message

endemic present in a community all the time

endogenous developing from within

endogenous opioid chemical regulators in the body that may modify pain

endorphin a polypeptide found throughout the body that is thought to relieve pain

endoscope a lighted instrument used to visualize the interior of a hollow organ

endothelium the layer of endothelial cells lining the blood vessels, cavities of the heart, and serous cavities

endotracheal tube tube inserted through either the mouth or the nose under the guidance of a laryngoscope

enema a solution injected into the rectum and the sigmoid colon

engorgement excessive fullness of an organ or passage

enkephalin a pentapeptide naturally occurring in the brain that has opiatelike effects

enteric referring to the intestines

enteric-coated surrounded with a special coating used for tablets and capsules that prevents release of the drug until it is in the intestines

enteric feeding a feeding administered directly into the small intestine through a tube

enteritis inflammation of the small intestine

enterocele any hernia of the intestine through the vaginal mucosa

enterostomal therapist a person who specializes in ostomy care

enterostomy an opening through the abdominal wall into the intestines

entropion an inturned eyelid

enuresis involuntary passing of urine in children after bladder control is achieved

environment all the conditions, circumstances, and influences surrounding and affecting the development of an organism or person

enzyme a biologic catalyst that speeds up chemical reactions

eosinophil a granular leukocyte with two lobes; readily stained with eosin

epidemic the occurrence of a disease in many people at the same time or in rapid succession in an area

epidemiology study of the occurrence and distribution of disease

epidermis the outermost, nonvascular layer of skin

epispadias opening of the urethra on the upper side of the penis

epistaxis nosebleed

equal protection (legal) a constitutional clause stating that like persons must be dealt with in like fashion

equilibrium a state of balance

equipoise a state of equilibrium

erection (penile) lengthening, widening, and hardening of the penis as it becomes congested with blood during sexual arousal

erogenous sexually sensitive

erotic stimuli sensations that cause sexual arousal

eructation ejection of gas from the stomach (belching)

erythema redness that is associated with a variety of rashes

erythematous of the nature of erythema

erythrocyte red blood cell

erythropoiesis the formation of red blood cells

eschar a slough of dried plasma proteins and dead cells; often produced by a burn, corrosive application, or gangrene

esophagoscopy visual examination of the interior of the esophagus with a lighted instrument

espanto a Hispanic term for a disease in which the individual is frightened by seeing supernatural spirits or events

ester a compound of alcohol and acid

ethics the rules or principles that govern right conduct

ethnic relating to races or to large groups of people with common traits and customs

ethnic group a set of individuals who share a unique cultural and social heritage passed on from one generation to another

ethnicity the condition of belonging to a specific ethnic group

ethnocentrism the belief that one's own culture is superior to all others

ethnoscience systematic study of the way of life of a designated cultural group to obtain accurate data regarding behavior, perceptions, and interpretations of the universe

etiology cause

Eucharist see Holy Communion

eupnea normal respiration that is quiet, rhythmic, and effortless

euthanasia the act or practice of killing for reasons of mercy

evacuator an instrument for removing fluid or small particles from a body cavity

evaluate to judge or appraise; to identify whether or to what degree a client's goals of care have been met

evaluating assessing the client's response to nursing intervention and then comparing the response to predetermined standards

evaporation conversion of liquid into a vapor

eversion turning outward

evisceration extrusion of the internal organs

exanthema skin rash

excise to cut off or out

excoriation loss of the superficial layers of the skin

excretion elimination of a waste product produced by the body cells from the body

exhalation (expiration) the act of breathing out; the outflow of air from the lungs to the atmosphere

exogenous developing from without

exophthalmos protruding eyeballs

exotoxin a toxic substance formed by bacteria and found outside the bacterial cell

expanded role increased responsibility assumed by a person by virtue of education and experience

expectorate to cough and spit up mucus or other materials

expert power power derived from one's expertise, talents, and skills

expert witness one who by education or experience possesses knowledge that the ordinary layperson does not have

expiration (exhalation) the outflow of air from the lungs to the atmosphere

expiratory reserve volume the maximum amount of air exhaled after a normal exhalation

expired dead

exploratory surgery surgery performed to confirm the extent of a pathologic process and sometimes to confirm a diagnosis

expressive language skill ability to use or to speak words

extended family the nuclear family plus other relatives such as uncles, aunts, and grandparents

extension increasing the angle of a joint (between two bones); the act of straightening

external cardiac massage rhythmic massage of the heart muscle over the sternum

external respiration interchange of oxygen and carbon dioxide between the alveoli of the lungs and the pulmonary blood

extinction (Skinner) a process in which a conditioned behavior is unlearned

extracellular outside the cells

extracellular fluid (ECF) fluid found outside the body cells

extrapolating inferring facts or data from known facts or data

extrathecal outside the sheath, e.g., outside the spinal canal

extravasation the escape of blood from a vessel into the body tissues

extreme unction the sacrament of anointing the sick

exudate material, e.g., fluid and cells, that has escaped from blood vessels and is deposited in tissues or on tissue surfaces during the inflammatory process

fad a practice followed by a time with exaggerated zeal

Fahrenheit a thermometer scale used to measure heat; the freezing point of water is 32 F, and the boiling point is 212 F

failure-to-thrive syndrome delayed development of infants without any physical cause

faith (Fowler) a relational phenomenon in which people invest love, commitment, belief, risk, and hope

family-centered nursing nursing that considers the health of the family as a unit in addition to the health of the individual family members

fantasy an adaptive mechanism in which wishes and desires are imagined as fulfilled

fasciculation abnormal contraction of a muscle involving the whole motor unit of the muscle

fasting abstinence from eating

fat an organic substance that is greasy and insoluble in water; adipose tissue, a whitish-yellow tissue that forms soft pads between various body organs and serves as an energy reserve; an ester of glycerol with fatty acids

fatty acid the basic structural unit of fat

fear an emotional response to an actual, present danger

febrile pertaining to a fever; feverish

fecal impaction a mass of hardened feces in the folds of the rectum

fecal incontinence inability to control the passage of feces through the anus

feces (stool) body wastes and undigested food eliminated from the rectum

feedback a process that enables a system to regulate itself; the response to some of a system's output, which acts as input for the purpose of exerting influence over a process; in communication, it is the response; in learning, it is the process of relating a person's performance to the desired goal

fellatio the oral stimulation of the male genitals by licking, blowing, or sucking

felony a crime of a serious nature punishable by imprisonment

femoral pulse the pulse found in the groin at the midpoint of the inguinal ligament

fenestrated perforated to provide a window or opening

fetus the unborn offspring in the postembryonic stage of development

fever elevated body temperature

fiber an indigestible carbohydrate derived from plants

fibrillation involuntary contractions of a muscle; cardiac arrhythmia characterized by extremely rapid, irregular, and ineffective contractions of the atria or ventricles

fibrin an insoluble protein formed from fibrinogen during the clotting of blood

fibrinogen plasma protein converted to fibrin when it is released into the tissues

fibrinous exudate exudate containing large amounts of fibrin

fibroplasia the formation of fibrous tissue

fibrous tissue common connective tissue composed of elastic and collagen fibers

first intention healing primary healing of a wound, which occurs when the tissue surfaces have been approximated

fissure a groove or deep fold such as that which separates the lobes of the lung

fistula an abnormal communication or passage usually between two organs or between an organ and the body surface

fixation (Freud) the inability of the personality to proceed to the next developmental stage

flaccid weak or lax

flaccid paralysis impaired muscle function with loss of muscle tone

flail chest the ballooning out of the chest wall through rib spaces during exhalation

flatness (in percussion) absence of resonance; extreme dullness

flatulence the presence of excessive amounts of gas in the stomach or intestines

flatus gas or air normally present in the stomach or intestines

flexion decreasing the angle of a joint (between two bones); the act of bending

flora collective vegetation in a given area

flowsheet a record used to chart the progress of specific or specialized data, such as vital signs, fluid balance, or routine medications

fluoroscope a device for examining internal structures using roentgen rays

fluoroscopy an examination using a fluoroscope

flushing (of the skin) transient redness of the skin, often of the face and neck; it may be generalized or restricted to a particular area

follicle (hair) a pouchlike depression in the skin in which a hair is enclosed

follicle stimulating hormone (FSH) a hormone produced by the anterior pituitary gland (adenohypophysis) that stimulates the development of the ovarian follicle

foment *see* hot pack

fomite an inanimate object other than food that can harbor disease-producing microorganisms and transmit an infection

fontanelle an unossified membranous gap in the bone structure of the skull

foot drop plantar flexion of the foot with permanent contracture of the gastrocnemius (calf) muscle and tendon

forceps an instrument with two blades and a handle used to grasp sterile supplies and to compress or grasp tissues

forensic medicine the application of medical knowledge to the law

foreplay physical stimulation to increase sexual arousal prior to intercourse; also called *precoital stimulation*

foreskin a covering fold of skin over the glans of the penis; also called the *prepuce*

formal operations stage (Piaget) the fourth cognitive developmental stage during ages 11 to 15 or 16 years

formulary a collection or list of prescriptions and formulas

Fowler's position a bed sitting position with the head of the bed raised to 45°

fracture a break in the continuity of bone

fracture board a support placed under the mattress of a bed to add rigidity

framework a basic structure supporting anything

fraud false presentation of some fact or facts with the intention that the information will be acted on by another person

frenulum a fold of mucous membrane that attaches the tongue to the floor of the mouth; a fold on the lower surface of the glans penis that connects it with the prepuce

fremitus vibration perceptible on palpation

frequency (of urination) voiding at more frequent intervals than usual

friction rubbing; the force that opposes motion

friction rub *see* pleural rub

frigidity a low or nondetectable sex drive, usually applied to females

frustration increased emotional tension due to inability to meet goals

fulcrum the fixed point of a lever

full disclosure provision of complete and truthful information to a client participating in a research study

functional residual capacity volume of air remaining in the lungs after a normal expiration

funnel chest (pectus excavatum) a congenital defect in which the sternum is depressed and the anteroposterior diameter of the chest is narrowed

gait the way a person walks

gastric pertaining to the stomach

gastrocolic reflex increased peristalsis of the colon after food has entered the stomach

gastroenteritis inflammation of the stomach and the intestines

gastroscope a lighted instrument used to visualize the interior of the stomach

gastroscopy visual examination of the stomach with a gastroscope

gastrostomy a surgical opening that leads through the abdomen directly into the stomach

gauge (of a needle) the diameter of the shaft of a needle

gavage administration of nourishment to the stomach through a nasogastric or orogastric tube; tube feeding

gay and lesbian families families in which the adult couple are homosexual partners

gelatinous like jelly

gender behavior behavior with masculine or feminine connotations

gender identity a person's sense of being masculine or feminine as distinct from being male or female

gender role (sexual role) all that a person says or does to indicate whether the person is male or female

gene the biologic unit of heredity, located on a chromosome

general adaptation syndrome (GAS) (Selye) a general arousal response of the body to a stressor that is characterized by certain physiologic events and that is dominated by the sympathetic nervous system

general inhibition syndrome (possum response) a response to a stressor that is characterized by inhibition of physiologic functioning and that is dominated by the parasympathetic nervous system

generativity (Erikson) concern for establishing and guiding the next generation

generic name (of drug) a drug name not protected by trademark and usually describing the chemical structure of the drug

genital stage (Freud) the final stage of maturity of an adult

genupectoral position a position in which the weight is borne by the knees and chest and the body is at a 90° angle to the hips

genu valgum a condition in which the medial aspects of the knees touch in the standing position while the feet remain apart; knock-knees

genu varum a condition in which, when the feet are held together, the knees remain apart; bowlegs

geriatrics the branch of medicine pertaining to elderly people

germicidal possessing the ability to kill microorganisms

gerontology the study of all aspects of aging

gingiva the gum tissue

gingivitis inflammation of the gums

glans penis the cap-shaped, expansive structure at the end of the penis

glaucoma an eye disease characterized by an increase in intraocular pressure that produces changes in the optic disc and the field of vision

global self the aggregate beliefs and images one holds about oneself

glomerular filtrate fluid formed in the nephron of the kidney that is similar to plasma in composition; the precursor of urine

glomerulus cluster of blood vessels surrounded by Bowman's capsule

glossitis inflammation of the tongue

glottis the vocal apparatus of the larynx

glucagon a hormone produced by the alpha cells of the islands of Langerhans in the pancreas; it stimulates the breakdown of liver glycogen

glucocorticoid a hormone produced by the adrenal glands that influences the metabolism of glucose, protein, and fat

gluconeogenesis the process by which the liver converts proteins and fats into glucose

glucose a monosaccharide occurring in food

glycerol the alcohol components of fats

glycogen the chief carbohydrate stored in the body, particularly in the liver and muscles

glycogenesis formation of glycogen

glycogenolysis the breakdown of glycogen to reform glucose

glycolysis the release of energy through the breakdown of glucose

glycosuria the presence of glucose in the urine; glucosuria

goal the desired outcome of nursing interventions

gonorrhea a sexually transmitted disease due to *Neisseria gonorrhoeae*

Good Samaritan act a law that protects physicians and sometimes nurses when rendering aid to a person in an emergency

goniometer a device that measures the angle of a joint in degrees

gout a condition characterized by excessive uric acid in the blood

governance the establishment and maintenance of social, political, and economic arrangements by which practitioners control their practice, self-discipline, working conditions, and professional affairs

granulation tissue young connective tissue with new capillaries formed in the wound healing process

granulosa cells a single layer of cells that surrounds the ovum

graphesthesia ability to recognize a figure traced on the skin with the tip of a finger, blunt pencil, or similar object

gravity the force that pulls objects toward the center of the earth

grief emotional suffering often caused by bereavement

grievance any disagreement arising out of the terms and conditions of employment

grounded theory a highly evolved and explicitly codified method for developing categories of theories and propositions about their relationships from qualitative data

grounding process of making an electrical connection between a conductor and the earth or a large body of zero potential

group two or more persons who have shared needs or goals

group dynamics (process) forces that determine the behavior of the group and its members

growth an increase in weight and height; an increase in physical size; the proliferation of cells

guilt the painful emotion associated with transgression of moral-ethical beliefs

gurgles see rhonchi

gustatory referring to the sense of taste

gynecology the branch of medicine that deals with processes of the female reproductive tract

gynosperm sperm bearing an X chromosome

habitus physique; body build or type

hair follicle a pouchlike depression in the skin enclosing the root of a hair

hair shaft the visible part of the hair

half-life (of drug) the time interval required for the body's elimination processes to reduce the concentration of the drug in the body by one half

halitosis bad breath

hallucinate to perceive through the senses something unreal; such as hearing voices or seeing things that do not exist

hallucinogens drugs that cause distortion of the sensory perception

hallux valgus bunion or lateral deviation of the big toe

haustrum a saclike formation of a part of the colon, produced by contraction of both the longitudinal and the circular muscles (plural: haustra)

health a state of being physically fit, mentally stable, and socially comfortable; it encompasses more than the state of being free of disease

health appraisal (family) assessment of the physical and psychosocial health of the family unit and its members

health behavior the action a person takes to understand his or her health state, maintain an optimal state of health, prevent illness and injury, and reach his or her maximum physical and mental potential

health beliefs concepts about health that an individual believes are true

health care system the totality of services offered by all health care disciplines

health-illness continuum a continuum (continuous process) with high-level wellness at one end and death at the other

health maintenance organization (HMO) an organization that provides a wide range of health services on a fixed contract basis, usually geared to preventive medicine

health practice an activity that a person carries out as a result of his or her health beliefs and definition of health

health practitioner a person who provides a health care service

health problem any condition or situation in which a person requires help to promote, maintain, or regain a state of health or to achieve a peaceful death

health promotion health care aimed at enhancing the wellness of individuals through education and encouragement of behavior changes or changes in the environment

health risk appraisal (HRA) tool that indicates a client's risk of diseases or injury over time by comparing the client with a large national sample with similar demographic data

health status the health of a person at a given time

health team a group of individuals with varying skills whose cooperative efforts are designed to assist people with their health

hectic fever *see* septic fever

height a vertical measurement extending from the highest point on the head to the surface on which the individual is standing, normally measured in centimeters or inches

Heimlich maneuver subdiaphragmatic abdominal thrusts used to clear an obstructed airway

hemangioma a large, persistent, bright red or dark purple vascular area of the skin

hematemesis the vomiting of blood

hematocrit the percentage of red blood cell mass in proportion to whole blood

hematoma a collection of blood in a tissue, organ, or body space due to a break in the wall of a blood vessel

hematuria the presence of blood in the urine

hemiplegia the loss of movement on one side of the body

hemoglobin the red pigment in red blood cells that carries oxygen

hemoglobinuria the presence of hemoglobin in the urine

hemolysis rupture of red blood cells

hemopneumothorax a collection of blood and air or gas in the pleural cavity

hemoptysis the presence of blood in the sputum

hemorrhage bleeding; the escape of blood from the blood vessels

hemorrhoids distended veins in the rectum

hemosiderosis deposition of iron in the skin, liver, spleen, and other organs

hemostat (artery forceps) a small pair of forceps used to constrict blood vessels

hemostasis cessation of bleeding

hemothorax a collection of blood in the pleural cavity

heparin a substance that prevents coagulation of blood

heparin lock an indwelling intravenous catheter attached to a plastic tube with a sealed injection tip

herb a leafy plant that does not have a wood stem and is valued for its medicinal, savory, or aromatic qualities

herbalist an herb doctor; one who prescribes herbs for treating people

hereditary factors risk factors related to genetically transmitted conditions or genetic predispositions to various conditions

Hering-Breuer reflex a reflex that inhibits inspiration

hernia protrusion of an organ or tissue through an abdominal opening

hesitancy (of urination) delay and difficulty initiating voiding

heterosexual a person whose primary sex orientation is to a member of the opposite sex

hex a jinx; a spell imposed by witchcraft

high Fowler's position a bed-sitting position in which the head of the bed is elevated 90°

hirsutism abnormal hairiness, particularly in women

histology the study of the structure and function of tissues

holism the view that a person is more than the sum of many parts

holistic health a model of health based on the belief that the whole is more than the sum of its parts

holophrasitic speech a type of speech in which one word expresses a whole sentence

Holy Communion a memorial sacrament practiced by Christians based on the mandate of Jesus Christ at the Last Supper; it is also called the *Eucharist* or the *Lord's Supper*

Homans' sign calf pain produced by dorsiflexion of the foot

homeodynamics the continual exchange of energy between humans and the external environment

homeostasis tendency of the body to maintain a state of balance or equilibrium while continually changing

homogeneity a high degree of likeness of attitudes and beliefs among members of a group

homosexual a person whose primary sexual orientation is to a member of the same sex

hordeolum inflammation of a hair follicle of the eyelid; a sty

hormone a chemical substance that is produced by the body and secreted into the bloodstream and that regulates the activity of certain body organs

hospice a health care facility for the dying

hostility overt antagonism; behavior in which the individual tends to be harmful or destructive

hot pack (foment) hot, moist cloth applied to an area of the body

humanism concern for human attributes

humidifier a device that adds water vapor to inspired air

humidity the amount of moisture in the air, expressed as a percentage

hyaluronidase an enzyme found in tissues; it catalyzes hydrolysis of hyaluronic acid, the cement substance of tissues

hydration the act of combining or being combined with water

hydraulics the branch of physics that deals with the physical actions of liquids

hydrocephalus a disease process resulting in excessive cerebrospinal fluid within the skull

hydrocortisone an adrenocortical steroid produced by the adrenal glands or produced synthetically; also called *cortisol*

hydrolysates hydrolyzed proteins or amino acids

hydrolysis the process of splitting a molecule in the presence of digestive enzymes with the addition of water

hydrometer an instrument used to determine the specific gravity of a fluid

hydrostatic pressure the pressure a liquid exerts on the sides of the container that holds it; also called *filtration force*

hygiene the science of health and its maintenance

hymen a thin fold of mucous membrane separating the vagina from the vestibule

hyperalgesia extreme sensitivity to pain

hyperalimentation *see* total parenteral nutrition

hypercalcemia excessive calcium in the blood plasma

hypercalciuria excessive calcium in the urine

hypercarbia (hypercapnia) accumulation of carbon dioxide in the blood

hyperchloremia an excess of serum chloride

hyperemia increased blood flow to an area

hyperesthesia greater than normal sensation

hyperextension further extension between two bones or stretching out of a joint

hyperglycemia an increased concentration of glucose in the blood

hyperhydrosis excessive perspiration

hyperkalemia excessive potassium in the blood

hyperlipidemia elevated concentration of lipids in the plasma

hypermagnesemia excessive magnesium in the blood plasma

hypernatremia an elevated level of sodium in the blood plasma

hyperopia farsightedness

hyperphosphatemia increased phosphorus levels in the blood plasma

hyperplasia an abnormal increase in the number of cells in a tissue or an organ

hyperpnea an abnormal increase in the rate and depth of respirations

hyperpyrexia an extremely elevated body temperature

hyperreflexia an exaggeration of the reflexes

hyperresonance a lower-pitched sound than resonance; booming sound

hypersensitivity an exaggerated response of the body to a foreign substance

hypersomnia excessive sleep

hypertension an abnormally high blood pressure

hyperthermia an abnormally high body temperature, sometimes induced as a therapeutic measure

hypertonicity excessive muscle tone or activity

hypertonic solution a fluid possessing a greater concentration of solutes than plasma

hypertrophy an increase in size of a cell, tissue, or body organ such as a muscle

hyperventilation an increase in the amount of air entering the lungs, characterized by deep, rapid breaths

hypervolemia an abnormal increase in the body's blood volume; circulatory overload

hypnosis an abnormally induced passive state in which an individual responds to suggestions that do not conflict with the person's conscious or unconscious desires

hypnotic (drug) a drug that induces sleep

hypoalbuminemia reduction in the level of albumin in the blood

hypocalcemia decreased calcium in the blood plasma

hypocarbia (hypocapnia) depressed level of carbon dioxide in the blood

hypochloremia a reduced concentration of chlorides in the blood plasma

hypodermic *see* subcutaneous

hypodermis (subcutaneous tissue) connective tissues beneath the skin

hypodermoclysis the introduction of fluid in the subcutaneous tissues

hypoesthesia less than normal sensation

hypofibrinogenemia an abnormally low level of fibrinogen in the blood

hypoglycemia a reduced amount of glucose in the blood

hypokalemia potassium deficit in the blood plasma

hypomagnesemia low magnesium in the blood plasma

hyponatremia an abnormally low amount of sodium in the blood plasma

hypophosphatemia phosphorus deficiency in the blood

hypophysis pituitary gland

hypopnea low rate of alveolar ventilation

hypoproteinemia small amounts of protein in the blood plasma

hypospadias opening of the urethra on the underside of the penis

hypostatic pneumonia an infection of lung tissue resulting from poor circulation or stagnation of secretions

hypotension an abnormally low blood pressure

hypothalamic integrator the center in the hypothalamus that controls the core body temperature

hypothalamus the part of the brain beneath the thalamus that forms the floor and part of the wall of the third ventricle

hypothermia an abnormally low body temperature

hypothesis a statement of the relationship between two or more concepts or variables; an assumption made to test its logical or empirical consequences

hypothesizing technique of predicting which actions will solve a problem or meet a goal

hypotonicity decreased muscle tone

hypotonic solution a fluid possessing a lesser concentration of solutes than plasma has

hypoventilation a reduction in the amount of air entering the lungs, characterized by shallow respirations

hypovolemia reduction in blood volume

hypovolemic shock a state of shock due to a reduction in the volume of circulating blood

hypoxemia low partial pressure of oxygen or low saturation of oxyhemoglobin in the arterial blood

hypoxia insufficient oxygen anywhere in the body

iatrogenic caused by the physician or medical therapy

id (Freud) the unconscious part of the personality that contains primitive desires and urges and is ruled by the pleasure principle

ideational forming images or objects in the mind

identification an adaptive or defense mechanism in which one assumes the attitudes, ideas, and behavior patterns of another person or persons

idiosyncratic effect a different, unexpected, or individual effect from the normal one usually expected from a medication; the occurrence of unpredictable and unexplainable symptoms

ileal conduit most commonly used urinary diversion procedure

ileostomy an artificial abdominal opening into the ileum (small bowel)

illicit drug a drug that is sold illegally; a street drug

illness sickness or deviation from a healthy state or the normal functioning of the total person

illness behavior the course of action a person takes to define the state of his or her health and pursue a remedy

illusion a false interpretation of some stimulus

imagination creation by the mind; forming a mental image of something not present to stimulate the senses

imitation copying the behaviors and attitudes of another person

immobility prescribed or unavoidable restriction of movement in any area of a person's life

immunity a specific resistance of the body to infection; it may be natural, endowed resistance or resistance developed after exposure to a disease agent

immunization the process of becoming immune or rendering someone immune

immunoglobulin a part of the body's plasma proteins; also called *immune bodies* or *antibodies*

immunologic reaction production of antibodies in response to an antigen; an allergic reaction

impaction a condition of being firmly wedged or lodged; in reference to feces, a collection of hardened puttylike feces in the folds of the rectum

imperforate abnormally closed; used to describe an opening, such as the anus or the hymen, that is not open

implementing putting the nursing strategies listed in the nursing care plan into action; intervening

impotence inability to achieve or to maintain an erection sufficiently to perform intercourse

incentive spirometer (sustained maximal inspiration device, SMI) a device that measures the flow of air through a mouthpiece

incision a cut or wound that is intentionally made, e.g., during surgery

incoherent engaging in actions or speech that lacks cohesion, orderly continuity, relevance, or consistency

incompatibility (of drug) undesired chemical or physical reaction between a drug and an infusion solution, between two or more drugs, or between a drug and the container or tubing

incontinence inability to control the elimination of urine (enuresis) or feces (fecal incontinence)

incorporation a process by which people or objects are internalized and become a part of one's understanding

incubation period the time between entrance of microorganism into the body and the onset of symptoms of the infection

incurvated (ingrown) nail a nail that has grown so that it impinges into surrounding soft tissues

independent nurse practitioner a nurse who practices independently in the health care system

independent nursing action (intervention or function) an activity initiated by a nurse as a result of her or his own knowledge and skills and without the physician's direct order

independent variable (IV) existing conditions or causes or those variables that a researcher manipulates to affect the dependent variable

indirect interview interview in which the nurse allows the client to control the purpose, subject matter, and pacing; also called *nondirect interview*

indirect services measures taken to provide or facilitate direct home care services

individual-client supply system (of drugs) medications supplied separately for each client in specified doses and quantities for a specified period of time

inductive reasoning making generalizations from specific data

inductive theory a theory formulated by a process in which certain phenomena are observed followed by the development of the idea relating the phenomena

induration hardening

inertia inactivity; inability to move spontaneously

infarct a localized area of necrosis (dead cells) usually owing to obstructed arterial blood flow to the part

infection the disease process produced by microorganisms

inference the interpretation of data from knowledge and past experience

inferential reasoning solving problems by means of inference; judgment or interpretation of cues

inferential statistics statistics that are inferred by generalization from other statistics

inferior situated below

infestation invasion of the body by insects, mites, and/or ticks

infiltration the diffusion or deposition into tissue of substances that are not normal to it

inflammation local and nonspecific defensive tissue response to injury or destruction of cells

influence (in a group) the result of the proper use of power

information power power derived from the perception that one controls key information

information processing the step-by-step mental operation used to solve problems

informed consent *see* consent

infradian rhythm a biorhythm that cycles monthly, such as the human menstrual cycle

infrared heat a radiant type of heat capable of penetrating body tissues to a depth of 10 mm; sources of infrared rays include heat lamps and incandescent light bulbs

infusion the introduction of fluid into a vein or part of the body

ingestion the act of taking in food or medication

ingrown toenail penetration of the edges of the toenail plate into the surrounding tissues

inhalation (inspiration) the act of breathing in; the intake of air or other substances into the lungs

inhalation therapist a respiratory technologist skilled in therapies for individuals with respiratory problems

inhalation (aerosol) therapy deliverance of droplets of medication or moisture suspended in a gas, such as oxygen, by inhalation through the nose or mouth

inner canthus the corner of the upper and lower eyelids near the nose

inorganic having no organs; not of organic origin; in chemistry, acids or compounds that do not contain carbon

input information, material, or energy that enters a system

inquest a legal inquiry into the cause or manner of a death

insensible heat loss heat loss that occurs from evaporation (vaporization) of moisture from the respiratory tract, mucosa of the mouth, and the skin

insensible perspiration unnoticeable sweating that evaporates immediately once it reaches the surface of the skin

insertion (of a muscle) the more movable point of attachment of a muscle

insomnia inability to obtain a sufficient quality or quantity of sleep

inspection visual examination to detect features perceptible to the eye

inspiration (inhalation) the act of drawing air into the lungs

inspiratory capacity the maximum amount of air that can be inhaled after a normal exhalation

inspiratory reserve volume the maximum amount of air inhaled after a normal inspiration

instillation application of a medication into a body cavity or orifice

insufflator an instrument used to blow air into a part of the body, e.g., the rectum

insulator a substance or material that inhibits conduction, e.g., of heat or electricity

insulin a hormone secreted by the beta cells of the islands of Langerhans in the pancreas; also a preparation for administration

integument the skin or covering of the body

integumentary system the skin, hair, and nails

intensity the loudness or softness of a sound

intensive services level of home care services in which clients require medical and professional nursing care as an alternative to hospitalization of skilled nursing home care

intercostal between the ribs

intercostal retractions indrawing between the ribs

interdependence a balance between dependence and independence

interdigital between the digits (toes and fingers)

intermediate services level of home care services in which clients require professional nursing supervision, direct care, physical or speech therapy, regular and periodic medical supervision, or some combination of these

intermittent (quotidian) fever a body temperature that alternates at regular intervals between periods of fever and periods of normal temperature

intermittent positive pressure breathing (IPPB) delivery of oxygen into the lungs at positive pressure and release of the pressure passively during expiration

intern a graduate of a basic health program who is taking planned practice experience, such as nursing or medicine, usually to obtain a license to practice

internal feedback positive or negative responses from oneself about a communication one has given either in writing or verbally

internal respiration the interchange of oxygen and carbon dioxide between the circulating blood and body cells

internal rotation a turning toward the midline, e.g., rotation of the hip joint

interpersonal skills verbal and nonverbal activities that people use when communicating directly with one another

interstitial between the cells of the body's tissues

interstitial cells of Leydig clusters of cells, located between the seminiferous tubules, that secrete male hormones

interstitial fluid fluid surrounding the body cells

intervention activities performed by the nurse and the client to change the effect of a problem

interview a structured consultation used to obtain information or to evaluate the progress of a person

intestinal distention (tympanites) stretching and inflation of the intestines due to the presence of air or gas

intraarterial within or inside an artery

intracardiac within or into the heart muscle

intracellular within a cell or cells

intracellular fluid (cellular fluid, ICF) fluid found within the body cells

intractable pain pain that is resistant to cure or relief

intradermal (intracutaneous) within the skin

intrafamily communication the pattern of verbal and nonverbally transmitted messages among family members

intramuscular within or inside muscle tissue

intraoperative period the time during surgery

intraosseous within or into the bone

intrapleural within the pleural cavity

intrapleural pressure pressure within the pleural cavity

intrapulmonic pressure pressure within the lungs

intraspinal *see* intravertebral

intrathecal within or into the spinal canal

intrauterine inside the uterus

intravascular within a blood vessel

intravascular fluid plasma

intravenous within a vein

intravenous cholangiogram an x-ray film of the bile ducts after a contrast dye has been administered intravenously

intravenous push (IVP, or bolus) administration of intravenous medications directly into a vein

intravenous pyelogram an x-ray film of the kidneys taken after intravenous injection of a radiopaque dye

intravenous pyelography (IVP) x-ray filming of the kidney and ureters after injection of a radiopaque material intravenously; also called *intravenous urography*

intravenous urography (IVU) *see* intravenous pyelography

intravertebral (intraspinal) within the vertebrae

introjection unconscious acceptance and incorporation of the patterns, attitudes, and ideals of another person as one's own

introversion direction of one's energy and interest toward oneself

intubation insertion of a tube

intuitionism the notion that people inherently know what is right or wrong

inunction application of a topical drug to the skin or mucous membrane for absorption

inversion a turning inward

involution a rolling or turning inward of a particular organ or the entire body, e.g., the uterus after the fetus is expelled

ion an atom or group of atoms that carry a positive or negative electric charge; an electrolyte

iritis inflammation of the iris

iron-deficiency anemia form of anemia caused by an inadequate supply of iron for the synthesis of hemoglobin

irradiation exposure to penetrating rays, such as x-rays, gamma rays, infrared rays, or ultraviolet rays

irrational confused as to time, place, and/or person

irrigation (lavage) the washing of a body cavity or a wound

irritant a substance that stimulates unpleasant responses, that is, irritates

ischemia lack of blood supply to a body part

isolation practice that prevents the spread of infection and communicable diseases

isometric having the same measure or length

isometric muscle contraction tensing of a muscle against an immovable outer resistance, which does not change muscle length or produce joint motion

isometric static exercise exercise in which a person consciously increases the tension of the muscle without moving the joint

isotonic having the same tonicity as the body fluids; the term is used to compare solutions of the same strength or concentration

isotonic exercise active exercise involving muscle contractions in which there is a marked shortening of muscle length

isotonic muscle contraction shortening of a muscle in the process of doing work that produces joint motion (e.g., range-of-motion exercises or weight lifting)

isthmus a narrow passage connecting two larger parts of an organ

jargon the technical or idiomatic terminology characteristic of a particular group

jaundice a yellowish tinge to the skin and mucous membrane

jejunum the portion of the small intestine that extends from the duodenum to the ileum

Kardex a portable card index file that organizes data about clients in a concise way and often contains nursing care plans

Kegel's exercises pelvic floor or perineal muscle tightening exercises

Kelly forceps a type of hemostat

keratin the protein found in epidermis, hair, and nails

keratinized cells dead cells that have been converted to protein

keratotic spots horny growths, such as warts or calluses

ketogenesis the process in which deaminated amino acids are converted into fatty acids, producing ketone bodies (acetone)

ketone any compound containing the carbonyl group, CO, and having hydrocarbon groups attached to the carbonyl group

ketosis a condition in which excessive ketones are formed in the body

kilocalorie (Calorie) the amount of heat required to raise the temperature of 1 kilogram of water 1 degree centigrade

kilogram a unit of weight equal to 1000 grams or approximately 2.2 pounds

kinesiology the study of the motion of the human body

kinesthesia the sense of the position and the movement of the body parts

kinesthetic referring to awareness of body position and movement

knee-chest position *see* genupectoral position

koilonychia an upward curvature of the nail from the nail bed

Korotkoff's sounds sounds of blood produced within the artery with each ventricular contraction

kosher sanctioned by Jewish law

Kussmaul breathing (Kussmaul-Kien respiration) deep rapid breathing; a dyspnea occurring in paroxysms often preceding diabetic coma: air hunger

kwashiorkor a condition occurring in children after weaning as a result of protein and calorie malnutrition; evidenced by growth failure, potbelly, edema, and mental apathy

kyphosis an exaggerated convexity in the thoracic region of the vertebral column, resulting in a stooped posture

labia majora the two longitudinal folds or lips of skin extending downward and backward from the mons pubis that protect the vaginal and urethral orifices

labia minor small folds of skin lying between the labia majora and the vaginal opening

labored breathing difficult or dyspneic breathing

labyrinth a system of interconnecting canals or cavities

lacerate to tear, rather than cut, a body tissue

lacrimal fluid tears produced by the lacrimal glands that lubricate the eye

lacrimal glands organs that are situated in a depression in the frontal bone at the upper, outer angle of the eye orbit, and that secrete tears

lacrimal sac the opening connecting the tear ducts in the inner canthus of the eye to the nasolacrimal duct, which empties into the nasal cavity

lacrimation the secretion and discharge of tears

lactase an enzyme that acts as a catalyst to convert lactose into glucose and galactose

lactate salt of lactic acid that is metabolized in the liver to form bicarbonate

lactation the secretion of milk; the period of milk secretion

lactiferous conveying or producing milk

lactoferrin iron-binding protein that inhibits the growth of invading microorganisms by making iron unavailable to them

lactose a carbohydrate found in milk

lalling repetitive sounds infants make based on what they hear

lanugo fine, wooly hair or down on the shoulders, back, sacrum, and earlobes of the unborn child; it may remain for a few weeks after birth

laryngeal mirror an instrument like a dental mirror used to view the pharynx, larynx, or structure of the mouth

laryngeal stridor a harsh, crowing sound heard during expiration when there is a laryngeal obstruction

laryngoscope a lighted instrument used to visualize the larynx

laryngoscopy visual examination of the larynx with a laryngoscope

laryngospasm spasmodic closure of the larynx

latch-key children working parents' school-age children who must care for themselves after school

latency period (Freud) the school-age years (6 to 12 years)

lateral to the side, away from the midline

lateral position a side-lying position

lavage an irrigation or washing of a body organ, such as the stomach

law system of principles and processes by which people attempt to control human conduct

laxative a medication that stimulates bowel activity

leading question question that directs the client's answer

learning a permanent change in behavior

learning need a need to change behavior or obtain information necessary to perform a function or care for self

learning principle an assumption thought to facilitate and maximize learning

legitimate power power derived from one's formal position or title in an organization

legume the fruit or pod of a leguminous plant, such as a pea or bean

lens a transparent, convex body that is the focusing device of the eye

lentigo senilis brown "age" spots as a result of clustered melanocytes

lesion the traumatic or pathologic interruption of a tissue or the loss of function of a body part

lethargy drowsiness; sleeping much of the time when not stimulated

leukocyte a white blood cell

leukocytosis an increase in the number of white blood cells

lever a rigid bar that moves on a fixed axis called a fulcrum

leverage force applied with the use of a lever

Levin tube a single-lumen nasogastric tube

liability the quality or state of being liable

liable legally responsible for one's obligations and actions and obliged to make financial restitution for wrongful acts

libel defamation by means of print, writing, or pictures

libido (Freud) the urge or desire for sexual activity; the energy form or life instinct; also called *sex drive* and *sexual motivation*

license a legal document authorizing an individual to offer knowledge and skills to the public

life expectancy the age to which a person is expected to live

life-style the values and behaviors adopted by a person in daily life

life-style assessment appraisal of the personal life-style and habits of the client as they affect health

ligament a broad, fibrous band that holds two or more bones together

line of gravity an imaginary vertical line running through the center of gravity

lingula (of the lung) the superior and inferior segments at the lower half of the long upper lobe of the left lung

liniment a topical liquid applied to the skin frequently to stimulate circulation or to relieve pain

lipid *see* fat

lithotomy position a back-lying position in which the feet are supported in stirrups

living will a statement of a person's wish not to be kept alive by artificial means or "heroic measures"

livor mortis discoloration of the tissues of the body after death

lobar pneumonia an infectious disease of one or more lobes of the lung

lobe a well-defined portion of an organ, e.g., of the lung or brain

local adaptation syndrome (LAS) the reaction of one organ or body part to stress

locus of control a concept about whether clients believe their health status is under their own or other's control

lordosis an exaggerated concavity in the lumbar region of the vertebral column

loss an actual or potential situation in which a valued ability, object, person, etc., is inaccessible or changed so that it is perceived as no longer valuable

lotion a liquid that often carries an insoluble powder

louse a parasitic insect that infests mammals (plural: lice)

lumbar puncture (LP, spinal tap) the insertion of a needle into the subarachnoid space at the lumbar region

lumen a channel within a tube, such as the channel of an artery in which blood flows

lung compliance expansibility of the lung

lung recoil the tendency of lungs to collapse away from the chest wall

lymph a transparent, slightly yellow fluid found within the lymphatic vessels

lymphadenitis inflammation of the lymph nodes

lymphangitis the inflammation of a lymphatic vessel or vessels

lymphatic referring to lymph or lymph vessels

lymphocyte mononuclear leukocyte formed chiefly by lymphoid tissue

lysis (of a fever) the gradual reduction of an elevated body temperature to normal

lysosome a minute body found in many types of cells; it is involved in intracellular digestion

lysozyme an enzyme in saliva and tears that functions as an antibacterial agent

maceration the wasting away or softening of a solid as if by the action of soaking; often used to describe degenerative changes and eventual disintegration

macrocephaly an abnormally large size of the head

macromineral minerals that people require daily in amounts over 100 mg

macrophage a large phagocytic cell that destroys microorganisms or harmful cells

malaise a general feeling of being unwell or indisposed

mal de ojo among Hispanics, the belief that disease can result from admiring a part of another person's body, e.g., the hair

malevolent transformation (Sullivan) the feeling that one lives among enemies

malignancy abnormal tissue with a tendency to grow and invade other tissues

malingering the willful feigning of the symptoms of illness to avoid facing something unpleasant

malleolus a rounded prominence on the distal end of the tibia or fibula

malnutrition a disorder of nutrition; insufficient nourishment of the body cells

malpractice professional misconduct or unreasonable lack of professional skill

mammography x-ray study of breast tissues

management the use of delegated authority to organize, direct, or control responsible subordinates to attain a goal

mandatory licensure laws that require all persons practicing in a field, such as nursing, to be licensed

manometer an instrument used to measure the pressure of fluids or gases

manslaughter an unlawful killing without previous intent; it is a felony

marasmus a condition of children under 1 year as a result of protein and calorie malnutrition; it is evidenced by wasting, wrinkled skin, thinness, eyes appearing large

margination the aggregating or lining up of substances along a surface or edge, e.g., the lining up of white blood cells against the wall of a blood vessel during the inflammatory process

marijuana an intoxicating agent from the leaves and flowers of the plant *Cannabis sativa;* commonly used in cigarettes

mastectomy surgical removal of the breast

masticate to chew, e.g., food

mastication chewing

masturbation self-stimulation of the genitals or other body parts to derive erotic pleasure

material culture objects, such as eating utensils, and the ways these are used by a society

matriarchy a system of social organization in which the mother is the head of the house or family

matrilineal relating to descent through the female line

maturation the process of becoming mature or fully developed; development of inherited traits

maturity state of maximal function and integration; state of being fully developed

meatus an opening, passage, or channel

mechanosensitive pain receptors pain receptors stimulated by mechanical stimuli

meconium black, tarry, odorless mucilaginous material found in the intestines of the newborn

medial toward the middle or midline

medical asepsis practices that limit the number, growth, and spread of microorganisms; clean technique

medical examiner a physician who investigates deaths that appear unnatural and who has advanced education in pathology and forensic medicine

medical record (chart) an account of the client's health history, current health status, treatment, and progress

medication (medicine, drug) a chemical or biologic compound administered to humans or animals for disease prevention, cure, or relief, or to affect the structure or function of the body

meditation mental exercise that directs the mind to think inwardly by closing the sense organs to external stimulation

melanin the dark pigment of the skin

melanocyte pigment-producing cell

menarche the first menstrual period, occurring sometime between the ages of 9 and 17

meniscus the crescent-shaped structure of the surface of a column of liquid; the crescent-shaped cartilage in the knee joint

menopause cessation of menstruation in the human female, usually occurring between ages 45 and 50

menses menstrual flow

mental (defense) mechanism *see* defense mechanism

mental well-being a state of contentment, peace of mind, and satisfaction with living and life

metabolism the sum of all the physical and chemical processes by which living substance is formed and maintained and by which energy is made available for use by the organism

metacarpal referring to the part of the hand between the wrist and the fingers

metaparadigm of nursing the concepts that influence nursing most significantly and determine its practice: the person, environment, health, and nursing actions

metatarsus adductus adduction of the anterior part of the foot with no deformity of the posterior part of the foot

microcephaly an abnormally small size of the head

microglia a type of nerve tissue with migratory cells that act as phagocytes to the waste products of nerve tissues

micromineral minerals that people require daily in amounts less than 100 mg

micronutrient nutrients, such as vitamins and minerals, required in small quantities by the body

microorganism minute living body visible under a microscope

micturate (urinate, void) to pass urine from the body

micturition (urination, voiding) the voluntary expulsion of urine

midclavicular line an imaginary line that runs inferiorly and vertically from the center of the clavicle

midsternal line an imaginary line that runs vertically through the middle of the sternum

milia (whiteheads) small, white nodules usually found over the nose and face of newborns

miliaria rubra a prickly heat rash of the face, neck, trunk, or perineal area of infants

milliequivalent (mEq) one-thousandth of an equivalent, which is the chemical combining power of a substance

milliliter (ml) a unit of volume in the metric system approximating 1 cubic centimeter

millimol one-thousandth of a mol

mineralocorticoid a steroid hormone of the adrenal cortex that acts to retain sodium in the body and to excrete potassium

minicomputer medium-sized computer system

minim the least; the basic unit of volume in the apothecaries' system, equal to 0.0616 ml

miosis constriction of the pupil

misdemeanor a crime less serious than a felony and punishable by a fine or short-term imprisonment or both

mitering a method of folding the bedclothes at the bed corners to maintain them securely

mitosis the process of cell division; the process by which the body replaces cells and grows

MMR combined measles, mumps, and rubella vaccine

mobility ability to move about freely

model (paradigm) an abstract outline or a theoretical depiction of a complex phenomenon

modeling observing the behavior of people who have successfully achieved a goal that one has set for oneself and, through observing, acquiring ideas for behavior and coping strategies

mol a molar solution of a substance

mongolian spots blue or black spots of varying size found largely in the sacral area of Oriental and black infants

monocyte mononuclear leukocyte formed in the bone marrow

monologue a long speech that occurs when there is no listener or responder

monosaccharide a sugar consisting of single molecules

monotheism belief in the existence of one God

mons pubis a pillow of adipose tissue situated over the symphysis pubis and covered by coarse hair; also called the *mons veneris*

Montgomery straps tie tapes used to hold dressings in place

morality a doctrine or system denoting what is right and wrong in conduct, character, or attitude

moralizing method of inculcating values in another

morbidity incidence of disease

mores values of members in a group

morgue a place where dead bodies are temporarily kept before release to a mortician

Moro's reflex the startle reflex of infants, in which the arms and legs are extended outward and retracted in response to a sudden stimulus such as a loud noise

morphology form and structure

mortality death; the death rate

mortician a person trained in the care of the dead; also called an *undertaker*

motivation desire

mourning the process through which grief is eventually resolved or altered

mucin the chief constituent of mucus

mucolytic destroying or dissolving mucus

mucous membrane epithelial tissue that forms mucus, concentrates bile, and secretes or excretes enzymes

mucus the lubricating, free slime of the mucous membranes

murmur (cardiac) harsh, rumbling sounds resulting from turbulent blood flow during systole and diastole

mydriasis enlargement of pupil(s)

mydriatic a medication that dilates the pupils of the eyes

myelogram an x-ray film of the spinal cord, nerve roots, and vertebrae after injection of a contrast media into the subarachnoid space

myocardial infarction cardiac tissue necrosis resulting from obstruction of the blood flow to the heart

myocardium the heart muscle; the middle layer of the heart tissue

myometrium the middle, thick, smooth muscle layer of the uterus

myopia nearsightedness

myotonia increased muscle tension

narcolepsy a condition in which an individual experiences an uncontrollable desire for sleep or attacks of sleep during the day

narcotic a strong analgesic

narcotic agonist-antagonist a drug with properties that simulate a narcotic and with properties that act against the effects of a narcotic

narrative charting a chronologic description (narration) of information

narrative notes records of a client's day-to-day progress which may be keyed to the SOAP format in the POMR or keyed chronologically in traditional client-records

nasogastric tube a plastic or rubber tube inserted through the nose into the stomach

nasopharynx the upper part of the pharynx adjoining the nasal passage

natriuresis increased excretion of sodium in the urine

naturopath a nonmedical practitioner who uses such things as light, heat, and water in therapy, but not drugs

nausea the urge to vomit

nebulization production of a fog or mist

nebulizer an atomizer or sprayer

necessary cause the one factor that must be present for a specific disease to occur

necrosis nonliving cells or tissue in contact with living cells

necrotic dying

need the lack of something requisite, desirable, or useful

negative feedback (homeostasis) a mechanism in which deviations from normal are sensed and counteracted

negative nitrogen balance a nitrogen output that exceeds nitrogen intake

negative reinforcement punishment for undesirable behavioral responses

negligence the omission of something a reasonable person would do or the doing of something a reasonable person would not do; an unintentional tort

neonatal mortality infant death within 28 days of birth

neoplasm any growth that is new and abnormal

nephritis inflammation of a kidney

nephron the functional unit of the kidney

nephrosis a disease of the kidney in which there is malfunctioning kidney tissue without inflammation; also called *nephrotic syndrome*

nerve block chemical interruption of a nerve pathway effected by injecting a local anesthetic

neurectomy interruption of the peripheral or cranial nerves, often to relieve localized pain

neurogenous arising in the nervous system

neurohypophysis the posterior part of the pituitary gland

neurologic pertaining to the nervous system

neuron a nerve cell and its processes; the functional unit of the nervous system

neutral question question seeking information without direction or pressure from the interviewer

neutrophil granular leukocyte with three to five lobes

night terrors (pavor nocturnus) nightmares that the person is unable to recall the next morning

nitrogen balance the state of protein nutrition

nociceptor a pain receptor

nocturia (nycturia) increased frequency of urination at night not as the result of increased fluid intake

nocturnal emission orgasm and emission of semen during sleep

nocturnal enuresis involuntary urination at night

nocturnal myoclonus frequent leg-kicking movements during sleep

noncompliance (drug use) failure to follow a prescription

noncomplier a person who does not follow a therapeutic regimen

nondirect interview rapport-building interview in which the nurse permits the client to control the purpose, subject matter, and pacing

nonmaleficence the duty to do no harm

nonmaterial culture the beliefs, customs, languages, and social institutions of a society

nonpathogen a microorganism that does not produce disease under normal conditions

nonproductive cough a dry, harsh cough without secretions

non-rapid-eye-movement sleep *see* NREM sleep

nonverbal communication (body language) communication other than words, including gestures, posture and facial expressions

norm an ideal or fixed standard; an expected standard of behavior of group members

normal saline an isotonic concentration of salt (NaCl) solution

normocephaly normal head circumference

nosocomial referring to or originating in a hospital or similar institution, e.g., a nosocomial infection

NREM sleep (non-rapid-eye-movement sleep) a deep restful sleep state; also called *slow wave sleep*

nuclear family the family unit composed of parents and children

null hypothesis statement that no relationship other than chance exists between a study's variables

nurse clinician a nurse who provides direct care in a specialized field

nurse theorist a person who seeks to define the basis and principles of nursing practice systematically

nursing assessment (nursing history) data collected during an interview between the nurse and client

nursing audit the review of clients' charts to evaluate nursing competence or performance

nursing care conference a meeting of a group of nurses to discuss possible solutions to certain problems of a client

nursing care plan written guide that organizes information about a client's health, focusing on the actions nurses must take to address identified nursing diagnoses and to meet the stated goals

nursing care rounds procedure in which a group of nurses visits all or selected clients at each client's bedside

nursing diagnosis a statement describing a combination of signs or symptoms indicative of an actual or potential health problem that nurses are able, licensed, and accountable to treat

nursing gerontology scientific study of the nursing care of the elderly

nursing goals goals stated in terms that guide the actions of the nurse

nursing health history systematic or structured method of collecting desired data about a client

nursing order specific action that a nurse takes to help a client meet established health care goals

nursing process a five-step systematic process used to plan and provide nursing care

nursing research research into human responses to actual or potential health problems and to the effects of nursing actions on such human responses

nursing standards optimum levels of nursing care against which actual performance of a nurse is compared

nursing strategy nursing action designed to achieve established client goals

nutrient an organic or inorganic substance found in food; nutrients are digested and absorbed in the gastrointestinal tract and then used in the body's metabolic processes

nutrition what a person eats and how the body uses it

nutritionist a specialist in food and nutrition

nutritive value the nutrient content of a specified amount of food

nystagmus involuntary rapid movement of the eyeball

obesity weight that is 20% greater than the ideal for height and frame

objective the aim of a maneuver or operation; without bias

objective data client information that can be determined by observation or measurement by laboratory or other means and that can be tested against an accepted standard

objective symptom a sign; evidence of a disease or body dysfunction that can be observed and described by others

obligatory heat the heat produced by the body as a result of the metabolism of food

obligatory loss the essential fluid loss required to maintain body functioning

observation the act or power of observing; gathering of information by noting facts or occurrences

observe to gather data using the five senses

obstetrics the branch of medicine dealing with the birth process and related events that precede and follow it

obtunded difficult to arouse from sleep; requiring shaking or a painful stimulus to awaken

obturator a disc or instrument that closes an opening; the obturator of a tracheostomy set fits inside and closes off the end of the outer tube

occult hidden

occupation an activity in which one engages

occupational therapist an individual who helps a client following illness or injury to develop skills necessary for the activities of daily living

Oedipus complex (Freud) the male child's attraction for his mother and accompanying hostile attitudes toward his father; compare with *Electra complex*

official name (of drug) the name under which a drug is listed in one of the official publications, such as, the *United States Pharmacopeia*

ointment a semisolid preparation applied externally to the body

olfactory referring to the sense of smell

oliguria production of abnormally small amounts of urine by the kidneys

oncotic pressure pulling force exerted by colloids that help maintain the water content of blood

opaque not admitting the passage of light

open-ended question broad question inviting a long answer

open system a system that exchanges matter, energy, and information with the environment

operative (intraoperative) period the time during surgery

ophthalmoscope an instrument used to examine the interior of the eye

opportunistic pathogen microorganism that causes disease only in a susceptible person

optional surgery surgery requested by the client but not necessary for health

oral referring to the mouth

oral stage (Freud) the stage of development during the 1st year of life, when the mouth is the principal area of activity

organic referring to an organ or organs; in chemistry, referring to compounds containing carbon; arising from an organism

orgasm the climax of sexual excitement, during which physiologic and psychologic release occurs; orgasm is characterized by rhythmic spasmodic contractions of the genitals

orgasmic dysfunction the inability of females to achieve orgasm

orientation awareness of time, place, and person

orifice an external opening of a body cavity; e.g., the anus is the orifice of the large intestine

oropharynx the part of the pharynx that lies between the upper aspect of the epiglottis and the soft palate

orthopnea the ability to breathe only in the upright position, i.e., sitting or standing

orthopneic position a sitting position in which the client leans over and is supported by an overbed table across the lap

orthostatic hypotension low blood pressure in a standing position

osmol the number of particles in 1 gram molecular weight of a disassociated solute

osmolarity (osmolality) the concentration of solutes in solution; the osmolar concentration of a solution expressed in osmols per liter of solution

osmosis passage of a solvent though a semipermeable membrane from an area of lesser solute concentration to one of greater solute concentration

osmotic pressure pressure exerted by the number of nondiffusable particles in a solution; the amount of pressure needed to stop the flow of water across a membrane

ossification the formation of bone or a bony substance

osteoarthritis noninflammatory degenerative joint disease

osteomalacia the softening of the bones; decalcification of bones in adults

osteoporosis decrease in bone density; demineralization of bone

-ostomy a suffix denoting the formation of an opening or outlet

otoscope an instrument used to inspect the eardrum and external ear canal

outcome (evaluative) criteria statements that describe specific, measurable, and observable responses of a client to nursing interventions; expected alterations in the health status of a client; standards for measuring success

output the energy, matter, or information released by a system as a result of its processes

outward rotation a turning away from the midline

overhydration *see* edema

overnutrition the oversupply of calories

overt data *see* objective data

overweight weight that is 10% greater than the ideal for height and frame

ovulation the discharge of a mature ovum from the Graafian follicle of the ovary

ovum (egg) the female reproductive cell, which becomes the embryo after fertilization

oxygen analyzer device that measures the amount of oxygen in room air and that being delivered during oxygen therapy

oxyhemoglobin the compound of oxygen and hemoglobin

pace the distance covered in a step when one walks or the number of steps taken per minute

packing filling an open wound or cavity with a material such as gauze

Paco$_2$ partial pressure of carbon dioxide (arterial blood)

pain a basically unpleasant sensation, localized or general, mild or intense, that represents the suffering induced by stimulation of specialized nerve endings; pain may be threatened or fantasied and may be induced by disease, injury, or mental derangement caused by disease or injury

pain reaction the autonomic nervous system and behavioral responses to pain

pain sensation *see* pain threshold

pain threshold the amount of stimulation required by a person to feel pain

pain tolerance the maximum amount and duration of pain that an individual is willing to endure

palate the roof of the mouth

palliative affording relief but not cure

palliative surgery surgery to relieve the symptoms of a disease process

pallor absence of normal skin color; a whitish-grayish tinge

palmar grasp reflex a reflex, normally present in newborns, that causes the fingers to curl around a small object placed in the palm of the hand

palpation the act of feeling with the hands, usually the fingers

pandemic an epidemic disease that is widespread

panic severe anxiety

Pao₂ partial pressure of oxygen (arterial blood)

Papanicolaou (Pap) smear a method of taking sample cervical cells for microscopic examination to detect malignancy

papule a small, superficial, round elevation of the skin

paracentesis the insertion of a needle into a cavity (usually the abdominal cavity) to remove fluid

paradigm *see* model

paradoxical breathing the ballooning out of the chest wall during expiration and depression or sucking inward of the chest wall during inspiration

parallel play play in which the child sits with other children but does not interact with them

paralysis the impairment or loss of motor function of a body part

paramedical having some connection with the practice of medicine

paraphrasing restating a person's message (thoughts and/or feelings) using similar words

paraplegia paralysis of the lower part of the body (including the legs) affecting both motor function and sensation

parasites plants or animals that live on or within another living organism

parasomnia a cluster of waking behaviors that occur during sleep and interfere with sleep

parenchyma the functional or essential elements of an organ

parenteral accomplished by a needle; occurring outside the alimentary tract; injected into the body through some route other than the alimentary canal, e.g., intravenously

paresis paralysis

paresthesia an abnormal sensation of burning or prickling

paronychia inflammation of the tissue surrounding the nail

parotitis (parotiditis) inflammation of the parotid salivary gland

paroxysm a sudden attack or sharp recurrence; a spasm

partial pressure the pressure exerted by each individual gas in a mixture according to its percentage concentration in the mixture

passive euthanasia allowing a person to die by withholding or withdrawing measures to maintain life

passive exercise exercise during which the muscles do not contract and the nurse, therapist, or client supplies the energy to move the client's body part

passive immunity a resistance of the body to infection in which the host receives natural or artificial antibodies produced by another source

passivity lethargy; receptivity to outside influence; lack of energy or will

paste a semisolid dermatologic preparation that tends to penetrate the skin less than an ointment

pastoral care an interpersonal relationship that focuses on the spiritual component of another person's life during distress

patent open, unobstructed, not closed

pathogen a microorganism capable of producing disease

pathogenic capable of producing disease

patient advocate a person who speaks on behalf of a client and can intercede on the client's behalf

patient (client) care standards *see* nursing standards

patient (client) goals goals stated as anticipated client outcomes, not as nursing activities

patriarchy a social system in which the father is the head of the household or family

patrilineal relating to descent through the male line

pavor nocturnus *see* night terrors

Pco₂ partial pressure of carbon dioxide (venous blood)

peak plasma level (of drug) the concentration of a drug in the blood plasma that occurs when the elimination rate equals the rate of absorption

pectoriloquy exaggerated bronchophony

pediculosis infestation with lice

pediculosis capitus infestation with head lice

peer a person of equal status

peer review the appraisal of a nurse's practice, education, or research by coworkers of equal status

penetrating wound a wound created by an instrument that penetrated the skin or mucous membranes deeply into the tissues

Penrose drain a flexible rubber drain

perceived loss loss experienced by a person that cannot be verified by others

perception the process of selecting, organizing and interpreting sensory stimuli into a meaningful framework; a person's awareness and identification of a person, thing, or situation

perception checking (consensual validation) verifying the accuracy of listening skills by giving and receiving feedback about what was communicated

percussion an assessment method in which the body surface is tapped or struck to elicit sound or vibrations from body structures below the struck area

percutaneous electric stimulation stimulation of major peripheral nerves by electricity

perfusion passage of fluid through the vessels of an organ or tissue

perineum the area between the anus and the posterior aspect of the genitals

periodontal disease inflammation of the tissues that surround and support the teeth

perioperative period the time before, during, and after an operation

periorbital around the eye socket

periosteum the connective tissue covering all bones

periostitis inflammation of the periosteum

peripheral at the edge or outward boundary

peripheral nerve implant an electrode implanted in a major sensory nerve for the purpose of relieving pain

peripheral pulse a pulse located in the periphery of the body

peristalsis wavelike movements produced by circular and longitudinal muscle fibers of the intestinal walls; it propels the intestinal contents onward

peristomal referring to the skin area that surrounds a stoma

peritoneal cavity the area between the layers of peritoneum in the abdomen; a potential space

peritoneum the membrane lining the abdominal walls

peritonitis inflammation of the peritoneum

permissive licensure the policy by which practitioners do not have to be licensed to practice but are not protected by the licensing body

perseveration the pattern of repeating the same response to different questions

personal space the physical distance people prefer to maintain in their interactions with others

personality the outward expression of the inner self

perspiration the fluid secreted by the sweat glands for excreting waste products and cooling the body

PES format the three essential components of a nursing diagnosis: problem (P), etiology (E), and signs and symptoms (S)

petechiae pinpoint red spots on the skin

pH a measure of the relative alkalinity or acidity of a solution; a measure of the concentration of hydrogen ions

phagocyte a cell, e.g., a white blood cell, that ingests microorganisms, other cells, and foreign particles

phagocytosis the process by which cells engulf microorganisms, other cells, or foreign particles

phalanx any bone of the fingers or toes (plural: phalanges)

phallic stage (Freud) the stage of development during the 4th and 5th years when sexual and aggressive feelings associated with the genital organs come into focus

phantom pain pain that remains after the perceived location has been removed, such as pain perceived in a foot after the leg has been amputated

phantom sensation a feeling that a missing body part is still present

pharmacist an individual licensed to prepare and dispense drugs and to make up prescriptions

pharmacokinetics the study of the absorption, distribution, biotransformation, and excretion of drugs

pharmacology the scientific study of the actions of drugs on living animals and humans

pharmacopoeia a book containing a list of drug products used in medicine, including their descriptions and formulas

pharmacy the skill of preparing, compounding, and dispensing medicines; the place where medicines are prepared and dispensed

pharmacy assistant a member of the health team who in some situations administers drugs to clients

phenomenal field the individual's frame of reference

phimosis an extremely narrowed opening of the foreskin of the penis

phlebitis inflammation of a vein

phlebothrombosis intravascular clotting with marked inflammation of a vein

phlebotomy opening a vein to remove blood

photophobia intolerance to light

photosensitive sensitive to light

phrenic referring to the diaphragm

physician a person licensed to practice medicine

physician's assistant a person educated to perform certain tasks under the direction of the physician

physiologic dependence biochemical changes occurring in the body as a result of excessive use of a drug

physiology the science concerned with the functioning of living organisms and their parts

physiotherapist (physical therapist) a member of the health team who provides assistance to clients with musculoskeletal problems

pica a craving for unnatural foods, often during pregnancy, some psychologic conditions, or extreme malnutrition

pigeon chest (pectus carinatum) a chest deformity in which there is a narrow transverse diameter, an increased anteroposterior diameter, and a protruding sternum

pinna the external part of the ear

pitch the number of vibrations per second or the frequency of vibrations

pitting edema edema in which firm finger pressure on the skin produces an indentation (pit) that remains for several seconds

placebo any form of treatment, e.g., medication, that produces an effect in the client because of its intent rather than its chemical or physical properties

placing reflex a reflex of infants demonstrated when the infant is placed vertically with one foot touching the edge of a table; the infant flexes the knee and hip of the same leg and tries to place the foot on the surface of the table

plaintiff the person who files a legal complaint claiming his or her rights have been infringed

planned change deliberate and collaborative process including a change agent and an individual or group

planning establishing a series of steps or designing or arranging the parts of something to achieve an end or goal; process of designing nursing strategies or interventions directed toward resolving health problems

plantar flexion movement of the ankle so that the toes point downward

plantar reflex *see* Babinski reflex

plantar wart a wart on the sole of the foot that is sensitive to pressure and caused by the virus *Papovavirus hominis*

plaque a film of mucus, bacteria, saliva, epithelial cells, and leukocytes that forms on the teeth

plasma the fluid portion of the blood in which the blood cells are suspended

pleural rub (friction rub) a coarse, leathery, or grating sound produced by the rubbing together of the pleura

pleximeter the nondominant hand used in percussion

plexor the dominant hand used in percussion

plexus a network, e.g., of nerves or veins

plumbism lead poisoning

pneumonia inflammation of the lung tissue

pneumothorax accumulation of air or gas in the pleural cavity

Po$_2$ partial pressure of oxygen (venous blood)

poison any substance that injures or kills through its chemical action

polarity the presence of two opposite poles

polarization (of a group) movement by members of a group toward a goal

polarized (cardiac) electrically charged

politics the process of influencing the allocation of scarce resources in the spheres of government, workplace, organizations, and community

polydipsia excessive thirst

polyneuritis inflammation of many nerves

polypnea an abnormal increase in the respiratory rate

polysaccharide a carbohydrate consisting of dozens of molecules of glucose

polysomnography an electroencephalogram, electromyogram, and electro-oculogram recorded simultaneously during sleep

polyuria (diuresis) the production of abnormally large amounts of urine by the kidneys

POMR (POR) *see* problem-oriented medical record

popliteal referring to the posterior aspect of the knee

port an opening or entrance

portal an entrance

positive reinforcement giving rewards such as praise for a learner's achievements

positive nitrogen balance nitrogen input exceeding nitrogen output

posterior of, toward, or at the back

posterior fornix a vaultlike space at the posterior aspect of the vagina

post-formal operations thinker a person who understands the temporary or relative nature of knowledge

postmortem examination *see* autopsy

postoperative (postsurgical) period the time following surgery

possible nursing diagnosis used when evidence about response is unclear or when related factors are unknown

postural drainage drainage of secretions from various lung segments by the use of specific positions and gravity

postural tonus sustained contraction of the muscles supporting an upright position

posture the bearing and position of the body; the relative arrangements of the various parts of the body

potency power; the ability of the male to engage in sexual intercourse

potential health problem the presence of risk factors that predispose persons and families to health problems

potential nursing diagnosis used when a client's responses can be predicted or when health promotion can contribute to well-being

power capacity to influence another person in some way or to produce change

powerlessness perceived lack of control over events

precedent a prior judicial decision used to justify or confirm a court ruling

precoital stimulation *see* foreplay

precordium the area of the chest over the heart or stomach

preferred provider organization (PPO) a group of physicians or a hospital that provides companies with health services at a discounted rate

preinteraction phase the planning stage before an interview or first face-to-face meeting

prelinguistic pertaining to sounds made by an infant that are not related to language

premature closure the acceptance of assumptions as fact

premature ejaculation the inability to control ejaculation prior to satisfaction of the partner or before 30 to 60 seconds after penetration

preoperational stage (Piaget) the phase of cognitive development that occurs during ages 3 to 7

preoperative period the time before an operation

prepuberty the period preceding puberty

prepubic urethra the part of the male urethra that is inferior to the pubis

prepuce *see* foreskin

presbycusis loss of hearing due to aging

presbyopia inability of the lens of the eye to accommodate initially to near objects and then to far objects as a result of the aging process

prescription the written direction for the preparation and administration of a remedy

pressoreceptor (baroreceptor) a receptor that is sensitive to changes in pressure, e.g., in the carotid sinus and the arch of the aorta

pricking pain pain like the pain of a knife piercing the skin

primary care the point of entry into the health care system at which initial health care is given

primary group a small, intimate group in which relations among the members are personal

primary intention healing wound healing that involves minimal or no tissue loss and in which there is minimal granulation tissue and scarring; also referred to as primary union or first intention healing

primary memory short-term memory

primary nursing a system of nursing in which the client is assigned on admission to one nurse, who has primary responsibility for nursing care 24 hours a day

primary prevention activities directed toward the protection from or avoidance of potential health risks

primary sexual characteristics characteristics that relate to the organs necessary for reproduction

primary socialization early socialization occurring from birth to adolescence

principle a fundamental law or doctrine; assumption

principled reasoning judgments made according to one's own principles in the face of conflicting societal rules or laws

priority setting process of establishing a preferential order for nursing strategies

privacy a deserved degree of social retreat that provides a comfortable feeling; the right of an individual participating in a research study to behave and think without the possibility of the behavior or thoughts being used to embarrass that person later

privileged communication information given to a professional such as a physician, who is not required to disclose it in a court of law

probate proceedings civil actions relating to wills and estates of deceased persons

probing asking for information chiefly out of curiosity

problem-oriented medical record (POMR, POR) a client's chart organized according to the client's problems and recording the reports of several health workers on each problem

process a series of actions directed toward a particular result; in anatomy, a prominence or projection, e.g., of a bone

process recording a word-for-word account of a conversation, including all verbal and nonverbal interactions

proctoscope a lighted instrument used to visualize the interior of the rectum

proctoscopy visualization of the interior of the rectum with a proctoscope

proctosigmoidoscope a lighted instrument used to visualize the rectum and sigmoid colon

proctosigmoidoscopy visual examination of the rectum and sigmoid colon with a proctosigmoidoscope

prodromal period the time from the onset of nonspecific symptoms to the appearance of specific symptoms

profession a calling that requires special knowledge, skill, and preparation

professional a person who practices a learned profession

professional socialization the process in which the knowledge, skills, and attitudes characteristic of a profession are acquired

prognosis the medical opinion about the outcome of a disease

projection a defense mechanism by which a person attributes his or her own undesired characteristics to another

proliferation rapid reproduction of parts or cells

pronation turning the palm downward; moving the bones of the forearm so that the palm of the hand turns from anterior to posterior in the anatomic position; also, flat feet

prone (prone position) lying on the abdomen with the face turned to one side

prophylaxis preventive treatment; prevention of disease

proposition statement that expresses the relationship between concepts

proprioceptor a sensory receptor that is sensitive to movement and the position of the body

prospective payment system (PPS) federal plan that establishes Medicare reimbursement rates in advance of hospitalization and according to diagnostic related groups

prostatectomy the removal of the prostate gland

prosthesis an artificial part, e.g., a glass eye, an artificial leg, or dentures

prostration extreme exhaustion

protein an organic substance that is composed of carbon, hydrogen, oxygen, and nitrogen and that yields amino acids upon hydrolysis

proteinuria the presence of protein in the urine

protocol written plan specifying the procedures to be followed in a particular situation

protraction moving a part of the body forward in a plane parallel to the ground

proxemics the study of physical distance between people in their interactions

proximal closest to the point of attachment

prudent diet a diet that is likely to benefit the individual even though it may not prevent disease

pruritus intense itching

psychogenic (functional) pain pain caused by psychologic factors

psychologic dependence (on a drug) a state of emotional reliance on a drug to maintain one's well-being; a feeling of need or craving for a drug

psychologic homeostasis emotional or psychologic balance or a state of mental well-being

psychomotor referring to motor actions; involving the hands

psychosomatic concerning the mind and the body; emotional disturbances manifested by physiologic symptoms

ptosis an eyelid that lies at or below the pupil margin; drooping eyelid

ptyalism excessive secretion of saliva

puberty the age during which the reproductive organs become active and secondary sex characteristics develop

public law rules regulating relationships between individuals and government

pudendum *see* vulva

pulmonary capacities the combinations of two or more pulmonary volumes

pulmonary embolus a blood clot that has moved to the lungs

pulse the wave of blood within an artery that is created by contraction of the left ventricle of the heart

pulse deficit a difference between the apical and the radial pulses

pulse pressure the difference between the systolic and the diastolic pressures

pulse rate the number of pulse beats per minute

pulse rhythm the pattern of pulse beats and of intervals between beats

pulse tension the elasticity of the arteries

pulse volume the force of the blood with each beat produced by contraction of the left ventricle; pulse strength

pulsus regularis equal lapses of time between beats of a normal pulse

puncture (stab) wound a wound made by a sharp instrument penetrating the skin and underlying tissues

purulent containing pus

purulent exudate an exudate consisting of leukocytes, liquefied dead tissue debris, and dead and living bacteria

pus a thick liquid associated with inflammation and composed of cells, liquid, microorganisms, and tissue debris

pustule a small elevation of the skin or mucous membrane or a clogged pore or follicle containing pus

putrid rotten

pyelogram an x-ray film of the kidney and ureter, showing the pelvis of the kidney

pyogenic pus-producing

pyorrhea purulent periodontal disease

pyrexia elevated body temperature; fever

pyrogen a substance that produces a fever

pyuria the presence of pus in the urine

quality (of sound) subjective description of a sound (e.g., whistling, gurgling, or snapping)

quality assessment examination of nursing services

quality assurance the evaluation of nursing services provided and the results achieved against an established standard and the efforts aimed at ensuring quality nursing care

rabbi a Jew ordained for professional religious leadership

race classification of humans into subgroups according to specific physical and structural characteristics

racism assumption of inherent racial superiority or inferiority and the consequent discrimination against certain races

radial pulse the pulse point located where the radial artery passes over the radius of the arm

radiating pain pain perceived at the source and in surrounding or nearby tissues

radiation the transfer of heat from a warm object to a cooler object by means of electromagnetic waves, without contact between the two objects; electromagnetic waves used in diagnostic tests and some kinds of therapy

radiopaque able to block the passage of radiant energy, such as x rays

rales *see* crackles

range of motion (ROM) the degree of movement possible for each joint

rapport an understanding between two or more people

rationale the scientific reason for selecting a specific nursing action

rationalization a defense mechanism in which good reasons, acceptable to the conscious mind, are given for behavior or circumstances instead of the real reason

reaction formation a defense mechanism in which one behaves exactly opposite to the way one is feeling

readiness the state of being ready; it is used to describe the developmental maturation and growth necessary before one can perform some activities, e.g., walking; in learning it is the behavior that reflects motivation at a specific time

rebound phenomenon (thermal) the time when the maximum therapeutic effect of a hot or cold application is achieved and the opposite effect begins

receptive language skill the ability to understand words

receptor (sensor) the terminal of a sensory nerve that is sensitive to specific stimuli

reconstituted family *see* blended family

reconstitution the technique of adding a solvent to a powdered drug to prepare it for injection

reconstructive surgery surgery to repair tissues whose function or appearance is damaged

record a collection of related data items about one file member

recording (charting) the process of making entries on clients' records

recovery index the sum of three 30-second pulse rates taken after increasing intervals of activity

rectocele (proctocele) a protrusion of part of the rectum into the vagina

recumbent length the distance from the soles of the feet to the vertex of the head of a person lying on the back

reduced hemoglobin hemoglobin that has released its oxygen

reduction (of bone) realignment of fractured bone fragments to their normal position

reexamining (reevaluating) the process of reassessing and replanning

referred pain pain perceived to be in one area but whose source is another area

referent power power derived from an individual's own vision and sense of self, and his or her ability to communicate these so that others are motivated to follow

referring the transfer of a client's care to another person

reflex an involuntary activity in response to a stimulus

reflexive vocalization nondescriptive sounds infants make in response to various stimuli and environmental conditions

reflexogenic erection an erection of the penis that occurs without apparent sexual stimuli

reflux backward flow

refractory period (sexual) the period immediately following orgasm when males cannot respond to sexual stimuli

regeneration the replacement of destroyed tissue cells by cells that are identical or similar in structure and function

regimen a regulated pattern of activity

registration the recording or entering of certain information about individuals

regression a defense mechanism in which one adapts behavior that was comforting earlier in life to overcome the discomfort and insecurity of the present situation

regurgitation the spitting up or backward flow of undigested food

rehabilitation the restoration of a person who is ill or injured to the highest possible capacity

rehabilitative services *see* intermediate services

relapsing fever a fever characterized by periods of normal temperature, lasting 1 or more days, between periods of fever

reliable criterion a criterion that produces consistent results on repeated use

reliability the degree to which an instrument produces consistent results on repeated use

religion an organized system of worship

remittent fever a fever characterized by a wide range of temperatures, all above normal, over a 24-hour period

REM sleep sleep during which the person experiences rapid eye movements; also called *paradoxical sleep*

renal relating to the kidney

renal dialysis a process in which blood flows from an artery through an artificial membrane that removes impurities; the blood then returns to the client through a vein

renal pelvis the funnel-shaped upper end of each ureter

renin a substance secreted by the kidneys when blood sodium levels are low; it controls aldosterone secretion

repolarized (cardiac) requiring an electric charge

repression a defense mechanism in which painful events are excluded from consciousness

research in nursing study of the nursing profession, including historic, ethical, and political areas

research process a series or steps of phases that are dynamic, flexible, and expandable, aimed toward generating useful knowledge

reservoir a source of microorganisms

resident flora microorganisms that normally reside on the skin, mucous membranes, and inside the respiratory and gastrointestinal tracts

residual urine the amount of urine remaining in the bladder after a person voids

residual volume (air) the amount of air remaining in the lungs after a person exhales both tidal and expiratory reserve volumes

resistive behaviors behaviors that inhibit involvement, cooperation, or change

resistive exercise exercise in which the client contracts a muscle against an opposing force, e.g., a weight

resonance a low-pitched, hollow sound produced over normal lung tissue when the chest is percussed

respiration the act of breathing; transport of oxygen from the atmosphere to the body cells and transport of carbon dioxide from the cells to the atmosphere

respiratory acidosis (hypercapnia) a state of excess carbon dioxide in the body

respiratory alkalosis a state of excessive loss of carbon dioxide from the body

respiratory arrest the sudden cessation of breathing

respiratory membrane the alveolar walls and the surrounding blood capillaries

respiratory technologist a therapist who provides diagnostic and therapeutic measures for clients with respiratory problems

responsibility reliability and trustworthiness; obligations associated with rights

rest calmness or relaxation without emotional stress

restitution an adaptive mechanism in which one performs restorative acts to relieve guilt

resuscitate to restore life; to revive

resuscitation the application of measures to reestablish breathing

retching the involuntary attempt to vomit without producing emesis

retention (urinary) the accumulation of urine in the bladder and the inability of the bladder to empty itself

retention (stay) suture a large plain suture that attaches to underlying tissues of fat and muscle in addition to the skin; retention sutures are used to support incisions

reticular activating system a portion of the reticular formation that coordinates input stimuli and regulates levels of awareness

reticular formation a diffuse network of neurons that extends throughout the brain stem

retraction moving a part of the body backward in a plane parallel to the ground; the act of drawing back

retrograde pyelogram an x-ray film taken after a contrast medium is injected through ureteral catheters into the kidneys

retroperitoneal behind the peritoneum

retrospective audit an audit of past events

reverse isolation (barrier technique) measures used to prevent certain clients, e.g., those with severe burns, from coming in contact with microorganisms

reverse Trendelenburg's position a position with the head of the bed raised and the foot lowered, while the bed foundation remains unbroken

reward power power derived from the perception of one's ability to bestow rewards or favors on others

Rh factor antigens present on the surface of some people's erythrocytes; persons who possess this factor are referred to as *Rh positive,* while those who do not are referred to as *Rh negative*

rhinitis inflammation of the mucous membrane of the nose

rhizotomy interruption of the anterior or posterior nerve root between the ganglion and the spinal cord, often for the purpose of relieving pain

rhonchi coarse, dry, wheezy, or whistling sounds, more audible during exhalation, as the air moves through tenacious mucus or a constricted bronchus

rickets a bone disorder resulting from a deficiency of vitamin D and calcium; decalcification of bone

rights privileges that individuals possess unless revoked by law or given up voluntarily

rights of human subjects the just claims of individuals who participate in research studies for full disclosure, self-determination, privacy, confidentiality, and freedom from harm

rigidity stiffness or inflexibility of a muscle

rigor mortis the stiffening of the muscles after death

Rinne test a hearing test that compares bone and air conduction of sound

risk factor a phenomenon that increases a person's chance of acquiring a specific disease or health problem

risk reduction planning and implementing nursing interventions to reduce health risks when possible or to optimize an individual's current health status when risks cannot be reduced

ritualistic behavior (ritualism) a series of repetitive acts performed compulsively, often to relieve anxiety

roentgen the unit of measurement of gamma rays (γ) or x-radiation

roentgenogram a film produced by photography with x rays

role the pattern of behavior expected of an individual in a situation or particular group

role conflict a clash between the beliefs, behaviors, etc., imposed by two or more roles fulfilled by one person

role performance the way a person performs a specific role

Romberg's sign inability to maintain balance while standing with the feet together

rooting reflex a reflex that causes newborns to turn their heads toward the side of a stimulated cheek or lip

rotation turning a bone around its central axis either toward the midline of the body *(internal rotation)* or away from midline of the body *(external rotation)*

rubefacient reddening the skin; a substance that reddens the skin

ruga a ridge or fold in the lining of an organ such as the vagina or the stomach (plural: rugae)

sacrament of the sick annointing the sick; a ritual of Roman Catholicism

Salem sump tube a double-lumen nasogastric tube

sanction punishment or a measure used to enforce normative behavior of group members

sanguineous bloody

sanguineous exudate an exudate containing large amounts of red blood cells

saphenous vein either of two superficial veins of the legs; the greater one extends from the foot to the inguinal region, while the lesser one extends from the foot up the back of the leg to the knee joint

sarcoidosis a disease in which affected tissues develop epithelioid cell tubercles; commonly affected organs are the lymph nodes, liver, spleen, lungs, skin, eyes, and small bones in the feet and hands

satiety a feeling of fullness as a result of satisfying the desire for food

saturated fat a fat whose molecular structure is saturated with hydrogen, such as fats in meat, butter, and eggs

scab the crust over a superficial wound

scald a burn from a hot liquid or vapor

scan a specialized type of x-ray procedure involving the use of a scanning device (probe), a computer, a printout machine, and a viewing apparatus

scar (cicatrical) tissue dense fibrous tissue derived from granulation tissue

Schwabach test hearing test that compares the client's and examiner's bone conduction of sound

scientific inquiry process in which observable, verifiable data are systematically collected to describe, explain, and/or predict events and phenomena

scientific method a logical, systematic approach to solving problems

sclerosis a process of hardening that occurs from inflammation and disease of the interstitial substance; the term is used to describe hardening of nervous tissues and arterioles

scoliosis a lateral curvature of a part of the vertebral column

scored marked with a line or groove

screening examination a brief review of essential functioning of various body parts or systems

scultetus binder an abdominal binder applied in strips that overlap each other

scurvy a condition resulting from vitamin C deficiency

sebaceous gland a gland of the dermis that secretes sebum

seborrheic dermatitis a chronic disease of the skin, characterized by scaling and crusted patches on various body areas, e.g., the scalp

sebum the oily, lubricating secretion of sebaceous glands in the skin

secondary care health care focusing on preventing complications of disease conditions

secondary group a group that is generally larger and more impersonal than a primary group

secondary intention healing wound healing that involves the formation of extensive granulation tissue and in which the repair time is lengthy and scarring is extensive; also referred to as *secondary union*

secondary memory long-term memory

secondary prevention activities designed for early diagnosis and treatment of disease or illness

secondary sexual characteristics characteristics that differentiate males and females but that do not relate directly to reproduction

secondary socialization the ongoing process of learning to adjust to new situations

secondary union (second intention) healing that requires the formation of considerable granulation tissue

secretion the product of a gland, e.g., saliva is the secretion of the salivary glands

sedative an agent that tends to calm or tranquilize

segmentation contractions contractions of segments of the intestine in contrast to contractions of large areas of the intestine

self-actualization (Maslow) the highest level of personality development in which people reach their full potential

self-care activities performed by individuals in their own behalf to maintain health and well-being

self-concept the combination of beliefs and feelings one holds about oneself at a given time

self-consistency the aspect of self that strives to maintain a stable self-image

self-determination the right of clients to feel free from undue influence

self-esteem self-acceptance; self-worth

self-expectancy what a person wants to become; the power a person perceives he or she has to meet self-expectations

self-ideal *see* self-expectancy

self-identity the conscious sense of individuality and uniqueness that continually evolves throughout life

self-image a person's perception of self at a specific time or over a period of time

self-terminating order on a client's record, an order whose termination time is implicit

semantics the study of the meaning of words

semen seminal plasma combined with sperm

semi-Fowler's position a bed sitting position in which the head of the bed is elevated at least 30°, with or without knee flexion; also referred to low Fowler's position

senescence the process of growing old

senility feebleness or loss of mental, emotional, or physical control that occurs in old age

sensitivity quick response, often referring to the response of microorganisms to an antibiotic

sensorimotor stage (Piaget) the initial phase of cognitive development between birth and 2 years

sensoristasis the need for sensory stimulation

sensorium a sensory nerve center

sensory adaptation ability of sensory receptors to adapt partially or completely to a repeated stimulus

sensory deficit partial or complete impairment of any sensory organ

sensory deprivation (input deficit) insufficient sensory stimulation for a person to function

sensory memory momentary perception of stimuli by the senses

sensory overload an overabundance of sensory stimulation

sensory perception the organization and translation of stimuli into meaningful information

sensory reception process of receiving environmental stimuli

separation anxiety anxious behavior when a child is separated from the parents

septic produced by putrefaction or decomposition

serosanguineous composed of serum and blood

serous of or like serum

serous exudate a watery exudate composed mainly of serum

serum (blood) blood plasma from which the fibrinogen has been separated during clotting

sex maleness or femaleness; sexual intercourse

sex behavior the behavior associated with sexual intercourse, including physiologic responses and sexual dysfunctions

sex drive *see* libido

sex-typed behavior the action that typically elicits different rewards for one sex or the other

sexual differentiation biologic sex determination of the fetus, during which male genitals or female genitals develop

sexual dimorphism the average differences between males and females in any given species

sexual dysfunction a perceived problem in achieving desired satisfaction of sexuality

sexual identity (core-gender identity) a person's inner feeling or sense of being male or female; more commonly indicates a person's sexual orientation

sexuality what constitutes male and female; the constitution of an individual in relation to sexual attitudes or activities

sexually transmitted (venereal) disease a disease that can be passed on through intercourse with an infected person

sexual motivation *see* libido

sexual role behavior sexual behavior and gender behavior

shiatsu form of massage in which firm, gentle pressure is applied to the acupuncture points of the body; also referred to as *acupressure*

shock acute circulatory failure

shock phase initial stage of the general adaptation syndrome during which the stressor may be perceived consciously or unconsciously and large amounts of epinephrine and cortisone are released in the body

shroud a large rectangular or square piece of material used to enclose a body after death

sickness a status or social entity usually associated with disease or illness

sick role behavior actions directed at getting well taken by the person who considers himself or herself ill

sickle cell anemia a genetic defect of hemoglobin synthesis that accounts for abnormally crescent-shaped erythrocytes; common to Afro-Americans

side effect (of a drug) an outcome that is not intended, such as an unintended action or complication of a drug

sigmoid colon the lower portion of the descending colon of the large intestine; it is shaped like the letter S

sigmoidoscope a lighted instrument used to examine the sigmoid colon

sigmoidoscopy examination of the interior of the sigmoid colon with a sigmoidoscope

sign *see* objective data

Sims' position semiprone position

sings healing ceremonies or rituals carried out by some Native Americans

singultus hiccups

sitz bath (hip bath) used to soak a client's pelvic or perineal area

slander defamation by spoken words

sleep a state of unconsciousness from which a person can be aroused by appropriate sensory or other stimuli

sleep apnea periodic cessation of breathing during sleep

slipper pan a bedpan with a flattened end to ease placement under the client; also called a *fracture pan*

smear material spread across a glass slide in preparation for microscopic study

smegma a thick, white, cheeselike secretion that collects between the labia and under the foreskin

SOAP the format used in the POR to record the client's progress; it has four components: Subjective data, Objective data, Assessment, and Planning

social communication unplanned communication

socialization the process by which individuals learn the knowledge, skills, and dispositions of their social group or society

socialized speech the exchange of thoughts between individuals, including questions, answers, commands, and criticisms of others

social support network others outside the immediate family unit who provide strength, encouragement, and assistance to the family, especially during a crisis

social worker an individual who assists persons and families with social problems

sociogram a diagram of the flow of verbal communication within a group during a specified period

sociopath a person who is unable to follow society's moral and ethical standards; one who has an antisocial personality

sodium cotransport theory a hypothesis about the mechanism for glucose transport in the presence of sodium

soixante-neuf (69) simultaneous oral-genital stimulation between two persons

solute a substance dissolved in a solution

solvent the component of a solution that can dissolve a solute

somatic referring to the physical body

somatogenic (organic) pain pain of physical origin

somatotype body type and personal tendencies of people

somnambulism sleepwalking

sordes the accumulation of foul matter (food, microorganisms, and epithelial elements) on the teeth and gums

souffle a blowing sound heard by auscultation

source-oriented medical record a traditional client's chart, organized according to the source of records (i.e., the person or department reporting); it includes separate records for the doctor, the nurse, the social worker, etc.

spasm involuntary contraction of a muscle or muscle group

spastic describing the sudden, prolonged involuntary muscle contractions of clients with damage to the central nervous system

specialty (in nursing) a defined area of clinical practice that has a narrow in-depth focus

specific gravity the weight or degree of concentration of a substance compared with the weight of an equal amount of another substance used as a standard (e.g., water used as a standard has a specific gravity of 1, while urine in comparison has a specific gravity of 1.010 to 1.025)

speculum a funnel-shaped instrument used to widen and examine canals of the body, e.g., the vagina or nasal canal

sperm the male germ cell (reproductive cell)

spermatogenesis production of sperm

spermicide foam, jelly, or cream inserted in the vagina before intercourse to destroy the sperm chemically

sphincter a ringlike muscle that opens or closes a natural orifice, such as the urethra, when it relaxes or contracts

sphygmomanometer an instrument used to measure the pressure of the blood in the arteries

spiritual belief a belief in a higher power, creative force, divine being, or infinite source of energy; the belief may or may not be associated with an organized religion

spiritual health (Ellison) a feeling of being generally alive, purposeful, and fulfilled; *spiritual well-being*

spiritual need what a client needs to maintain, increase, or restore his or her beliefs and faith and to fulfill religious obligations

spirometry the measurement of pulmonary volumes and capacities using a spirometer

splint a rigid bar or appliance used to stabilize a body part

spore a round or oval structure highly resistant to destruction that is formed in some bacterial cells

sprain injury of the ligaments and associated structure of a joint by wrenching or twisting; associated structures include tendons, muscles, nerves, and blood vessels

sputum the mucous secretion from the lungs, bronchi, and trachea that is ejected through the mouth

stability (of a group) the degree of permanence of a group

stab wound *see* puncture wound

stamina staying power or endurance

stammer involuntary repetitions and stops in vocal utterances

stance the manner in which a person stands

standard (norm) a measure of quantity, quality, weight, extent, or value that is set up as a rule

standards (in nursing) optimum levels of care against which actual performance is compared

standing order written document about policies, rules, regulations, or orders regarding client care that gives the nurse authority to carry out specific actions under certain circumstances, often when a physician is not available

stasis stagnation or stoppage of flow of body fluids, such as intestinal fluids, urine, or blood

static electricity stationary electric charges

station stance; the way a person stands

stature the height of a standing person

statutory law a law passed by a legislature (state, provincial, or federal)

stenosis constriction or narrowing of a body canal or opening

stepping reflex (walking, dancing reflex) a reflex of infants characterized by an up-and-down walking motion of the legs when the infant is held upright with the feet touching a flat surface

stereognosis ability to recognize objects by touching them

stereotype something that conforms to a fixed pattern; an oversimplified judgment or attitude about a person or group

sterile free from microorganisms, including spores

sterile field a specified area that is considered free from microorganisms

sterile technique *see* surgical asepsis

sterilization a process that destroys all microorganisms, including spores

stertor snoring or sonorous respiration, usually due to a partial obstruction of the upper airway

stethoscope an instrument used to listen to various sounds inside the body, such as the heartbeats

stimulus anything that arouses or incites action from a receptor

stock supply (of drugs) medications stocked in relatively large quantities in a nursing unit; individual doses are taken from the large supply

stoma an artificial opening in the abdominal wall; it may be permanent or temporary

stomatitis inflammation of the entire mouth

stool (feces) waste products excreted from the large intestine

stopcock a valve that controls the flow of fluid or air through a tube

strabismus squinting or crossing of the eyes; uncoordinated eye movements

strain (of a muscle) overexertion or overstetching of a muscle or part of a muscle

stress (as a stimulus) an event or set of circumstances causing a disrupted response; the disruption caused by a noxious stimulus or stressor

stressor (Selye) any factor that produces stress or alters the body's equilibrium

stress syndrome *see* general adaptation syndrome (GAS)

stretch receptors nerve receptors sensitive to changes in pressure, i.e., in the aorta and carotid sinus; also called *pressoreceptors or baroreceptors*

stricture a narrowing of a passageway or canal

stridor a shrill, harsh, crowing sound made on inhalation due to constriction of the upper airway or laryngeal obstruction

stroke volume the amount of blood ejected from the heart with each ventricular contraction

stroma tissue that forms the framework or structure of an organ

structural-functional theory a framework for studying the family unit that focuses on family membership and relationships among family members as well as the functions of the family

structured communication communication that has a definite planned content

stupor a condition of partial or nearly complete unconsciousness; stuporous clients are never fully awakened even when painfully stimulated

stuttering a speech problem evidenced by the repetition of letters or words and prolonged pauses

stylet a metal or plastic probe inserted into a needle or cannula to render it stiff and to prevent occlusion of the lumen by particles of tissue

subcostal below the ribs

subcutaneous (hypodermic) beneath the layers of the skin

subcutaneous tissue *see* hypodermis

subjective data client information that only the person personally can give, such as thoughts or feelings

sublimation the channeling of sexual and aggressive desires into socially acceptable forms of behavior

sublingual under the tongue

suborbital beneath the cavity or orbit

subscapular below the scapula

substance P a neurotransmitter in the dorsal horn of the spinal cord that enhances transmission of pain impulses

substernal retractions indrawing beneath the breastbone

substitution replacing one thing with another; an adaptive mechanism in which unattainable or unacceptable goals are replaced with ones that are attainable or acceptable

subsystem the low-level components of a system

sucking reflex a reflex sucking action in newborns, initiated by touching their lips

suctioning aspiration of secretions by a catheter connected to a suction machine or outlet

sudden infant death syndrom (SIDS) a condition of some children during the first year, resulting in death during sleep; crib death

sudoriferous gland a gland of the dermis that secretes sweat

suicide the taking of one's own life

sulcular technique a dental hygiene technique for removing plaque and cleaning under the gingival margins

superego (Freud) an unconscious part of the psyche that monitors the id and the ego; concerned primarily with ethics, conscience, and social standards

supination turning the palm upward; moving the bones of the forearm so that the palm of the hand turns from posterior to anterior in the anatomic position

supine (supine position) lying on the back with the face upward without support for the head and shoulders; also called *dorsal position*

support system the people and activities that can assist a person at a time of stress

suppository a solid, cone-shaped, medicated substance inserted into the rectum, vagina, or urethra

suppression the willful exclusion of a thought or feeling from consciousness; the sudden stoppage of a secretion or an excretion, e.g., urine

suppuration the formation of pus

supraclavicular retractions indrawing above the clavicles

supraoptic above the eye

suprapubic above the pubic arch

suprasternal retractions indrawing above the breastbone

suprasystem the highest level of interrelated subsystems

surfactant a lipoprotein mixture secreted in the alveoli that reduces surface tension of the fluid lining the alveoli

surgical asepsis measures that render and maintain objects free of all microorganisms including spores (sterile)

susto among Hispanics, a disease of emotional origin; fright caused by natural phenomena such as lightning or loud noises

suture in surgery, a surgical stitch used to close accidental or surgical wounds; in anatomy, a junction line of the skull bones

symbolization an adaptive mechanism by which objects are used to represent ideas or emotions too painful for a person to express; the creation of a mental image to stand for something

sympathectomy the severing of pathways of the sympathetic nervous system, often to relieve pain of a vascular origin

symptom (covert data) *see* subjective data

synapse the junction between two neurons, where nerve impulses are transmitted from one neuron to another

syncope fainting or temporary loss of consciousness

syndrome a group of signs and symptoms resulting from a single cause and constituting a typical clinical picture, such as the shock syndrome

synergist an agent that enhances the action of another so that their combined effect is greater than the effect of either

synovial joint a freely movable joint surrounded by a capsule enclosing a cavity that contains a transparent, viscid fluid

synthesis the process of putting together; assembling the parts of a whole

syphilis a sexually transmitted disease caused by the microorganism *Treponema pallidum*

syringe an instrument used to inject or withdraw liquids

system a set of identifiable parts or components

systemic pertaining to the body (or other system) as a whole

systems theory a framework applied to studying the family unit in which the family is viewed as a system whose members are interdependent, so that a change in one member influences the family unit as a whole

systole the period when the ventricles of the heart are contracted

systolic pressure the pressure of the blood against the arterial walls when the ventricles of the heart contract

tablet a medication in solid form that is often compressed and molded

tachycardia an excessively rapid pulse or heart rate, over 100 beats per minute in an adult

tachypnea abnormally fast respirations, usually more than 24 per minute, marked by quick, shallow breaths

tactile pertaining to the sense of touch

tactile (vocal) fremitus vibrations, palpable with the palms of the hands originating in the larynx and transmitted to the chest wall during speech

talipes equinovarus (clubfoot) a foot is malpositioned in plantar flexion at the ankle, with inversion and adduction of the heel and forefoot

Talmud the authoritative written body of Jewish tradition

Taoism Chinese mystical philosophy

tartar the film on teeth, often formed from plaque; dental calculus

taxonomy a classification system or set of categories, such as nursing diagnoses, arranged on the basis of a single principle or consistent set of principles

T-binder a cloth in the shape of a T often used to retain dressings in the genital region

Td combined tetanus and diphtheria toxoid used for people over 6 years of age; it has less diphtheria toxoid than DT

teaching an interactive process between a teacher and one or more learners in which specific learning objectives or desired behavior changes are achieved

team nursing the delivery of individualized nursing care to clients by a nursing team led by a professional nurse

technical assault and battery assault and battery without the intent to injure, e.g., when giving a hypodermic injection

technical skills "hands-on" skills such as skills required to manipulate equipment

teleology a doctrine that explains phenomena by results

temporal pulse a pulse point where the temporal artery passes over the temporal bone of the skull

tenacious sticky, adhesive

tenesmus straining; painful, ineffective straining during defecation or urination

territoriality the pattern of behavior arising from an individual's feeling that certain spaces and objects belong to him or her

tertiary care rehabilitation or long-term care

tertiary prevention activities designed to restore disabled individuals to their optimal level of functioning

testosterone a testicular hormone that stimulates the growth of the genitals and the development of male secondary sexual characteristics

tetany a syndrome manifested by muscle twitching, cramps, convulsions, and sharp flexion of the wrist and ankle joints

theism the belief in the existence of a god or gods

theory a scientifically acceptable general principle that governs practice or is proposed to explain observed facts

therapeutic healing; supportive of health

therapeutic communication communication that helps clients overcome temporary stress and get along with others

therapeutic effect (of a drug) the primary effect desired, or the reason the drug is prescribed

therapeutic touch a healing process by which energy is transmitted from one person to another via energy fields

therapy remedial treatment

thermography the use of an infrared camera to photograph the surface of the body, thus indicating surface temperatures

thermosensitive pain receptors pain receptors sensitive to heat and cold

thoracocentesis insertion of a needle into the pleural cavity for diagnostic or therapeutic purposes

thorax the chest cavity

thought disorganization a mental condition evidenced by difficulty remembering what one is saying, confusion about time, inappropriate verbal responses, and sensory distortions

thrill (cardiac) vibrating sensation indicating turbulent blood flow

thrombocytopenia an abnormal reduction in the number of platelets in the blood

thrombophlebitis inflammation of a vein followed by formation of a blood clot

thrombosis the development of a blood clot

thrombus a solid mass of blood constituents in the circulatory system; a clot (plural: thrombi)

throughput the process of transforming input so that it is useful to the system

thyroxine a hormone produced by the thyroid gland

tic a repetitive twitching of the muscles, often of the face or upper trunk

tick a small parasite that bites into tissue and sucks blood

tidal volume the volume of air that is normally inhaled and exhaled

tinea pedis *see* athlete's foot

tinnitus a ringing or buzzing sensation in the ears that is purely subjective

tissue perfusion passage of fluid, e.g., blood, through a specific organ or body part

tolerance the ability to endure without ill effects the term is often used with reference to taking medications

tomography a scanning procedure during which several x-ray beams pass through the body part from different angles

tonicity the normal condition of tension or tone, e.g., of a muscle

tonic neck reflex a reflex of the newborn, also called the *fencing reflex,* in which, when the head is forcibly turned to one side, the arm and leg on that side are extended while the opposite limbs are flexed

tonometer an instrument used to assess the pressure inside the eye

tonus the slight, continual contraction of muscles

topical applied externally, e.g., to the skin or mucous membranes

TOPV trivalent oral polio vaccine

torsion twisting

tort a civil wrong committed by a person against another person or the other person's property

torticollis limited range of motion of the neck, with lateral inclination and rotation of the head away from the midline of the body

tortuous twisted

total lung capacity the maximum volume to which the lungs can be expanded

total parenteral nutrition (TPN) or intravenous hyperalimentation (IVH) administration of a hypertonic solution of carbohydrates, amino acids, and lipids by an indwelling intravenous catheter placed into the superior vena cava via the jugular or subclavian vein

tourniquet a device, e.g., a rubber strip, that is wrapped around a body area to compress the blood vessels

toxemia a generalized intoxication due to the absorption of toxins in the body

toxic shock syndrome (TSS) serious, sometimes fatal illness, associated with tampon use

toxin a poison produced by some microorganisms, animals, and plants

toxoid a modified exotoxin that is no longer toxic but still has the ability to stimulate the production of antibodies

tracheal tug an indrawing and downward pulling of the trachea during inhalation

tracheostomy a procedure by which an opening is made in the anterior portion of the trachea and a cannula is introduced into the opening

traction the exertion of a pulling force

trademark (brand name) (of drug) name of drug given by the drug manufacturer

traditional family family unit in which both parents reside in the home with their children—the mother playing the nurturing role and the father providing necessary economic support

traditional health care mode of health care in which activities are aimed toward identifying and correcting a health problem that already exists

transcutaneous electrical stimulation the placement of electrodes on the surface of the skin over a peripheral nerve pathway for the purpose of relieving pain

transfusion (blood) the introduction of whole blood or its components, e.g., serum, erythrocytes, or platelets, into the venous circulation

transient flora microorganisms that are present episodically

transudation the passage of serum or other body fluids through a membrane or tissue

trapeze bar a triangular handgrip suspended from an overbed frame

trauma injury

tremor an involuntary muscle contraction, e.g., quivering, twitching, or convulsions

trend prevailing tendency or approach

Trendelenburg's position a bed position with the head of the bed lowered and the foot raised, while the bed foundation remains unbroken; in some agencies, the position involves elevation of the knees, with the feet lowered and the head lowered

triage picking, choosing, sorting, and selecting

trial legal proceedings during which all relevant facts are presented to a jury or judge

triglyceride a simple lipid or neutral fat consisting of three fatty acids for each glycerol base

trigone the triangular area at the base of the urinary bladder marked by the ureter openings at the posterior corners and the urethra at the anterior inferior corner

trimester a period of 3 months

trocar a sharp, pointed instrument that fits inside a cannula and is used to pierce body cavities

trochanter either of two processes below the neck of the femur

trochanter roll a rolled towel support placed against the hips to prevent external rotation of the legs

troche a lozenge

tubal ligation a surgical tying of the fallopian tubes, rendering the female sterile

tubercle a rounded eminence of bone

tumor an uncontrolled and progressive growth of cells

tunica dartos the middle layer of smooth muscle and tough connective tissue in the scrotum

tuning fork an instrument shaped like a two-pronged fork and made of metal; the prongs vibrate when struck

turgor normal fullness and elasticity

tympanites (distention) swelling of the abdomen due to the presence of excessive flatus in the intestines or peritoneal cavity

tympany a musical drumming sound produced on percussion over organs that contain gas or air

ulcer a localized sloughing of skin tissue or mucous membrane commonly associated with varicosities or hyperactivity of the gastrointestinal tract

ultradian rhythm a biologic cycle completed in minutes or hours

ultrasound high-frequency, mechanical, radiant energy

ultraviolet referring to radiation having wavelengths shorter than violet rays and longer than x rays; ultraviolet radiation has powerful chemical properties

unconscious incapable of responding to sensory stimuli; insensible

unconscious mind (Freud) the mental life of which a person is unaware

undernutrition inadequate caloric intake or nourishment

unilateral affecting one side

unit dose system (of drugs) prepackaged and labeled individual doses of medication for each client; the amount of medication the client is to receive at a prescribed hour

universal donor a person with type O blood

universal recipient a person with type AB blood

unpalatable distasteful, unpleasant to the taste

unsterile containing microorganisms; unsterile material may be clean or contaminated

untoward adverse

urban relating to or constituting a city

urea a substance found in urine, blood, and lymph; the main nitrogenous substance in blood

urea frost the appearance of the skin when the salt crystals remain after the evaporation of the sweat in urhidrosis

uremia the retention in the blood of excessive amounts of the byproducts of protein metabolism

ureteroileosigmoidostomy an artificial opening into the ureters in which a segment of the ileum is resected and connected to the sigmoid colon and the ureters are implanted into this ileal pouch

ureterosigmoidostomy an artificial opening into the ureters in which the ureters are implanted into the sigmoid colon

ureterostomy an artificial opening into the ureter

urethritis inflammation of the urethra

urgency (urinary) a feeling that one must urinate

urgent surgery surgery necessary for the client's health

urhidrosis a condition in which urinous materials, e.g., uric acid and urea, are present in the sweat

urinal a receptacle used to collect urine

urinalysis laboratory analysis of the urine

urinary diversion *see* urostomy

urine the fluid of water and waste products excreted by the kidneys

urobilin the oxidized form of urobilinogen, a compound formed from bilirubin, that is found in feces and occasionally in urine

urobilinogen a colorless compound found in the intestines from the reduction of bilirubin

urostomy (ureterostomy, urinary diversion) an opening through the abdominal wall into the urinary tract that permits the drainage of urine

urticaria an allergic reaction marked by smooth, reddened, slightly elevated patches of skin and intense itching

uvula a small fleshy mass projecting from the soft palate above the base of the tongue

vaccine a suspension of killed, attenuated, or living microorganisms administered to prevent or treat an infectious disease

vaginal diaphragm a round rubber cup inserted over the cervix of the uterus for contraception

vaginal orifice the external opening of the vagina

vaginal smear vaginal cells placed on a glass slide for laboratory analysis

vaginal sponge a contraceptive device that is saturated with spermicide and inserted into the upper vagina over the cervix

vaginismus painful, irregular, and involuntary contraction of the muscles around the outer third of the vagina during coitus

valid criterion a criterion that measures what it is intended to measure

validation the justification of a conclusion or diagnosis by the data

validity the degree to which an instrument measures what it is intended to measure

Valsalva maneuver forceful exhalation against a closed glottis, which increases intrathoracic pressure and thus interferes with venous return to the heart

value something of worth; a belief held dearly by a person

value conflict situation in which two or more values are incongruent

values clarification a process by which individuals define their own values

value system the organization of a person's values along a continuum of relative importance

vaporization evaporation; conversion of a solid or liquid into a gas (vapor)

varicosity the state of having swollen, distended, and knotted veins, especially in the legs

vasectomy ligation and cutting of the vas deferens, rendering the male sterile

vasoconstriction a decrease in the caliber (lumen) of blood vessels

vasodilation an increase in the caliber (lumen) of blood vessels

vasopressor an agent that causes the blood pressure to rise

vasospasm spasm or constriction of the blood vessels

vector an insect or other animal that transfers microorganisms from a reservoir to a host

vehicle a transporting agent or medium

vellus fine, nonpigmented body hair

ventilation the movement of air; the act of breathing

ventral of, toward, or at the front; anterior

ventricle a small cavity, such as those located in the brain or the heart

ventriculogram an x-ray film of the ventricles of the brain taken after the introduction of an opaque medium

ventriculography radiologic examination of the ventricles of the brain following the insertion of air or a radiopaque medium

verbal communication communication by the spoken or written word

verdict (legal) the outcome of a trial rendered by a jury

vermin external animal parasites, e.g., ticks, lice, and fleas

vernix caseosa the white, cheesy, greasy, protective material found on the skin of newborns

vertex the top of the head

vertigo dizziness

vesicostomy an artificial opening into the bladder in which the anterior wall of the bladder is sutured to the abdominal wall and a stoma is formed from the bladder wall

vesicular sounds normal, quiet, rustling or swishing respiratory sounds heard over the terminal bronchioles and alveoli during auscultation

vestibule a space or cavity at the entrance to a canal; the cleft between the labia containing the vaginal and urethral orifices, hymen, and openings of several ducts

viable fetus a fetus capable of extrauterine life

vial a glass medication container with a sealed rubber cap, for single or multiple doses

vibration (postural drainage) a technique of rapid agitation of the hands while pressing on a body area

violence exertion of physical force to injure or abuse

virulence ability to produce disease

virus minute infectious agents smaller than bacteria

viscera large interior organs in body cavities, e.g., the liver and stomach (singular: viscus)

visceral referring to viscera

visceral pain pain originating in the viscera

viscosity the quality of being viscous

viscous thick, sticky

vital capacity maximum amount of air that can be exhaled following a maximum inhalation

vital (cardinal) signs measurements of physiologic functioning, specifically temperature, pulse, respirations, and blood pressure

vitamins organic chemical substances found in food and essential for normal metabolism and life

vitiligo patches of hypopigmented skin

vocal resonance vibrations of the larynx transmitted during speech through the respiratory system to the chest wall

vocation the work that a person regularly performs and that especially suits a person

void urinate, micturate

volatile evaporating readily

vomitus material vomited; emesis

voodoo the practice of witchcraft or magic

vulnerable subjects individuals who because of diminished physical or mental capacity may be unable to give free and informed consent

vulva the external female genitals that surround the vaginal orifice and the urethra; also called the *pudendum*

walker a metal, rectangular frame used as an aid to ambulation

Weber's test a test that assesses bone conduction of sound

well-being a subjective perception of balance, harmony, and vitality

wellness active process of becoming aware and making choices toward a higher level of well-being

wheal *see* bleb

wheeze a whistling sound on exhalation that usually indicates narrowing of the bronchial air passages

will a declaration of how a person wishes to distribute his or her property after death

xiphoid process the lower portion of the sternum

x rays electromagnetic radiations with extremely short wavelengths

yang in Chinese folk medicine, a positive force that regulates health; it represents the male, warmth, light, and fullness

yin in Chinese folk medicine, a negative force that regulates health; it represents the female, coldness, darkness, and emptiness

yoga an Indian science that involves various physical postures and stationary exercises as well as psychologic measures to improve one's mental, social, and spiritual states

PHOTOGRAPHIC CREDITS

Chapter 1 Opener: Special Collections, The Library, University of California, San Francisco.

Chapter 2 Opener: Tom Ferentz.

Chapter 3 Opener: Suzanne Arms Wimberley.

Chapter 4 Opener: Sharon Beals.

Chapter 5 Opener: Judy Braginsky.

Chapter 6 Opener: Tom Ferentz.

Chapter 7 Opener: Suzanne Arms Wimberley.

Chapter 8 Opener: Tom Ferentz.

Chapters 9–14 Openers: Suzanne Arms Wimberley.

Chapter 15 Opener: Sharon Beals. Figures 15–1, 15–3, 15–5: Tom Thompson. Figure 15–4: © Robert Foothorap/Jeroboam, Inc.

Chapter 16 Opener: Judy Braginsky. Figure 16–1: Karen Stafford Rantzman.

Chapter 17 Opener: Judy Braginsky. Figure 17–2: © Lou De Matteis/ Jeroboam, Inc.

Chapter 18 Opener, 18–10, 18–14 B, C: Tom Ferentz.

Chapter 19 Opener: Tom Ferentz. Figures 19–7, 19–8, 19–84, 19–87: George B. Fry III. Figure 19–10: University of California, Los Angeles, School of Nursing. Figure 19–12: Karen Stafford Rantzman. Figures 19–22, 19–23, 19–24, 19–25, 19–26, 19–40, 19–42, 19–43, 19–44, 19–49, 19–50, 19–51, 19–67, 19–86, 19–92, 19–93, 19–95, 19–96, 19–97, 19–98, 19–99, 19–101, 19–102, 19–104, 19–105, 19–106: Tom Thompson. Figures 19–60, 19–64, 19–88, 19–89, 19–90, 19–100, 19–103: Tom Ferentz.

Chapter 20 Opener: Suzanne Arms Wimberley. Figures 20–3, 20–6, 20–7, 20–19, 20–20, 20–23, 20–29, 20–30, 20–31, 20–32, 20–33: Tom Thompson. Figures 20–21, 20–22: Tom Ferentz.

Chapter 21 Opener: Judy Braginsky. Figures 21–1, 21–3: Tom Ferentz. Figure 21–10: Karen Stafford Rantzman.

Chapter 22 Opener: © Emilio Mercado/Jeroboam, Inc. Figures 22–17, 22–18, 22–31, 22–42: Tom Ferentz. Figures 22–19, 22–32, 22–41: George B. Fry III. Figure 22–24: Tom Thompson.

Chapter 23 Opener: © Billy Barnes/Jeroboam, Inc.

Chapter 24 Opener: Kim Raftery.

Chapter 25 Opener, Figure 25–1: Judy Braginsky. Figures 25–2, 25–8: Karen Stafford Rantzman. Figure 25–6: Carol Stepanchuk.

Chaper 26 Opener: Suzanne Arms Wimberley. Figure 26–1, Karen Stafford Rantzman. Figure 26–2: © John Schoenwalter/ Jeroboam, Inc. Figure 26–4: © Emilio Mercado/Jeroboam, Inc.

Chapter 27 Opener: © Frank Siteman/Jeroboam, Inc. Figure 27–1, clockwise from top left: © Laima Druskis/Jeroboam, Inc.; Steve Malone, Jeroboam, Inc.; Shmuel Thaler/Jeroboam, Inc.; Bill Aron/Jeroboam, Inc. Figure 27–2, © Bob Clay/Jeroboam, Inc. Figure 27–3: Karen Stafford Rantzman.

Chapter 28 Opener: Suzanne Arms Wimberley.

Chapter 29 Opener: Suzanne Arms Wimberley.

Chapter 30 Opener: Sandra Weiner, The Image Works.

Chapter 31 Opener: Suzanne Arms Wimberley. Figure 31–2: Karen Stafford Rantzman. Figure 31–3: Judy Braginsky.

Chapter 32 Opener: Karen Stafford Rantzman.

Chapter 33 Opener: Judy Braginsky.

Chapter 34 Opener: Karen Stafford Rantzman.

Chapter 35 Opener: © Kathy Sloane/Jeroboam, Inc. Figure 35–5: Karen Stafford Rantzman. Figures 35–9 through 35–38: Tom Ferentz.

Chapter 36 Opener: © Frank Smith/Jeroboam, Inc. Figures 36–19, 36–25, 36–26, 36–30, 36–38, 36–50: Tom Thompson. Figures 36–32, 36–34, 36–37, 36–39: George B Fry III. Figure 36–33: Karen Stafford Rantzman. Figures 36–36, 36–51, 36–52: Tom Ferentz.

Chapter 37 Opener: Judy Braginsky.

Chapter 38 Opener: Judy Braginsky.

Chapter 39 Opener: Figures 39–9, 39–10: Karen Stafford Rantzman. Figures 39–2, 39–3, 39–4: Tom Ferentz. Figure 39–6: Judy Braginsky. Figure 39–11: George B. Fry III. Figures 39–12, 39–15, 39–17: Tom Thompson.

Chapter 40 Opener: Judy Braginsky. Figures 40–4, 40–11, 40–16, 40–18, 40–23, 40–24: Tom Thompson. Figures 40–12, 40–14, 40–15, 40-21, 40–22: Tom Ferentz.

Chapter 41 Opener: Judy Braginsky. Figures 41–2, 41–4, 41–5, 41–7, 41–10, 41–13, 41–14, 41–16, 41–20, 41–22, 41–23, 41–24, 41–25, 41–33, 41–36, 41–39, 41–45, 41–51, 41–55, 41–56: Tom Thompson. Figures 41-9, 41–40, 41–41, 41–42, Figures in Table 41–4: George B. Fry III. Figures 41–11, 41–34, 41–35, 41–38: Tom Ferentz. Figure 41–44: Karen Stafford Rantzman.

Chapter 42 Opener, Figure 42–11: Judy Braginsky. Figures 42–14, 42–16, 42–17, 42–18, 42–20, 42–21, 42–22, 42–24: Tom Thompson.

Chapter 43 Opener: Tom Ferentz. Figures 43–11, 43–13, 43–14, 43–15: Tom Thompson. Figure 43–27: George B. Fry III.

Chapter 44 Opener: Judy Braginsky.

Chapter 45 Opener: Suzanne Arms Wimberley. Figures 45–11, 45–40: Tom Ferentz. Figures 45–14, 45–18, 45–19, 45–21, 45–22: George B. Fry III. Figure 45–16: On•Gard Systems. Figures 45–28, 45–43, 45–45, 45–50, 45–51, 45–52, 45–53, 45–56, 45–57, 45–58, 45–59: Tom Thompson.

Chapter 46 Opener: Judy Braginsky. Figures 46–7, 46–11, 46–13, 46–39, 46–40, 46–41: Tom Thompson. Figures 46–27, 46–38: Tom Ferentz. Figures 46–28, 46–29, 46–30: George B. Fry III.

Chapter 47 Opener: Judy Braginsky. Figures 47–6, 47–7, 47–14: Tom Thompson. Figures 47–10, 47–11, 47–12, 47–13: George B. Fry III.

Chapter 48 Opener: © Kathy Sloane/Jeroboam, Inc.

INDEX

Colostomy irrigation, 1181–1183
Colostrum, 412
Coma, assessment of with Glasgow Coma Scale, 429t
Comedones, 638
Comfort, 957–984. See also Pain
Comfort measures, sleep and, 952, 953
Commandments, in nursing code of ethics, 132
COMMES, 48
Commitment, in group dynamics, 270
Commode, 1166–1167
Common advice, as nontherapeutic response, 262
Common law, 144
Communal family, 687
Communicable disease, 452
Communication
  ability of communicator affecting, 252
  assessing, 256–257
  attitudes affecting, 253–254
  client record as means of, 298
  cultural and ethnic background affecting, 746–747
  environment affecting, 253
  evaluating, 263, 263–265t
  family, 690–691
  importance of among health team members, 298
  meaningful, for clients with sensory/perceptual alteration, 1241–1242
  message in, 251
  modes of, 247–250
  and nontherapeutic responses, 261–263
  nonverbal, 247, 249–250
    assessing, 256–257
  in nursing, 247
  perceptions affecting, 252
  personal space affecting, 252–253
  planning for, 257–258
  privileged, 146
  problems in
    diagnosing, 257
    outcome criteria and, 258
  process of, 250–254
    factors affecting, 252–254
  receiver in, 251
  relationships affecting, 253
  response in, 252
  risk of injury affected by ability in, 490
  roles affecting, 253
  sender in, 251
  social, 247
  structured, 247
  style of
    assessing, 257
    in self-esteem development, 703
  territoriality affecting, 253
  therapeutic, 247
    techniques for, 258–261
  time affecting, 253
  verbal, 247, 247–249

impaired. See Impaired verbal communication
Communicator, ability of, communication affected by, 252
Communicator/helper, nurse as, 28
Community
  as base for political action, 53
  health promotion programs in, 565
  nutritional services of, 1017
Community health nurses, in occupational setting, 109
Compensation (compensatory mechanisms)
  in acid-base imbalance, 1051
  as defense mechanism, 803t
  in homeostasis, 792
Competence, personal, and self-esteem in children and adolescents, 714
Complaint, legal, 145
Complementary proteins, 990
Complete blood count, 1058, 1102
Complete proteins, 990
Completeness, in recording, 313–314
Compliance
  client, 93–94, 278
  lung, 1093
  vascular, 334
    blood pressure and, 346
Compound proteins, 990
Compresses, application of, 1339–1342
Compromised host, 461
  isolation precautions and, 475
  wound healing and, 1307
Computed tomography, 1399–1400
Computers
  and client records, 302–303
  nursing care plans written with, 48, 49f, 303
  and trends in nursing, 48–50
Concepts, and critical thinking, 227
Conceptual frameworks
  components of, 59–61
  definition of, 58–59
  for nursing, 58–80
  one versus several, 61
  relationship to nursing process, 61
  relationship to research, 66
  summary of major units from, 62–65t
Concreteness, in helping relationship, 245
Concurrent audit, 235, 238
Condescension, communication affected by, 253–254
Conditioning, behavioral, 589
Condoms, 727, 736, 737f
  for urinary drainage, 1210–1211
Conduction, heat loss by, 323–324
Conduction hearing loss, 387
Condyloid joint, 841t
Condyloma acuminatum, clinical signs of, 645t
Conference, nursing care, 316–317
Conferring, 316–317
Confidentiality

ethical responsibility of nurses and, 135–136
  right to in research project, 47
Conflict
  to implement change, 38
  role, 701–702
Confrontation, in helping relationship, 245
Congruence, communication affected by, 254
Conjunctiva
  assessment of, 376
  in elderly, 383
Conjunctivitis, 375
Connection power, 51
Conscience clauses, 134–135
Consciousness, 1236
  alterations in, 1236
    and providing meaningful communication, 1242
  level of, assessment of, 429
    in general survey, 368
    Glasgow Coma Scale for, 429t
  and risk of injury, 490
Consensual validation, in therapeutic communication, 260
Consensus decisions, in group dynamics, 270
Consent
  informed, 153–154
  surgical, 1347, 1348f
Consequences, in nursing models, 61
Constant data, 175
Constipation, 1158–1160, 1164, 1165t
  in dying client, 829t
  in elderly, 669, 676–677
  immobility and, 847, 864
  nutrition and, 1012
  outcome criteria and, 1165
  postoperative, 1368t
  tube feedings and, 1022t
Constitution of Canada, 143
Constitution of the United States, 143
Constitutional law, 145t
Constructive surgery, 1349
Consultant, computer as, 48
Consulting, 218–219
Consumer
  definition of, 9
  health care services affected by demands of, 104–105
  nursing practice affected by demands of, 40–41
Contact isolation, 470–471t
Contact lenses
  care of, 541
    teaching clients about, 542
  inserting, 541–543
  removing, 543–544
Contact transmission, in infection, 459
Continent vesicostomy, 1196
Continuing education, 16
Continuity theory of aging, 669
Continuous infusions, 1285

Continuous sutures, 1331
    removing, 1332–1333
Continuum, health-illness, 89, 90*f*
Contour position, for hospital bed, 551,
    552*f*
Contraception, 736–738
    chemical, 737
    surgical, 737–738
Contract law, 144, 145*t*, 148
Contracting, client, 292
Contracts, behavioral, in planning health
    promotion, 574
Contractual obligations, 149
Contractual relationships, 149
Contractures
    immobility and, 843
    and positioning clients in bed, 903
Contrast, definition of, 148
Contrast mammography, 1396
Control, perceived, health behavior
    affected by, 93
Controlled substances, and legal aspects
    of nursing practice, 154
Controller, intravenous infusion, 1068–
    1069
Contusion, 1305
    around eyes, 375
Convalescent period, 462
Convection, heat loss by, 324
Convenience groups, 266
Conversion, as defense mechanism, 804*t*
Converting units of weight and mea-
    sure, 1262–1263, 1417
Cooling sponge baths, 1339, 1340–1341
Cooperation, to implement change, 38–
    39
Coordination, in elderly, 437
Coping behavior, 176, 798. *See also*
    Coping/stress-tolerance pattern
    assessment of, 706
        in nursing health history, 360
    effective, 798
    family, 691
    ineffective, 798
        family. *See* Ineffective family coping
        individual. *See* Ineffective individ-
            ual coping
    in self-esteem development, 703
Coping mechanisms (coping strategies),
    798–799. *See also* Coping/stress-
    tolerance pattern
    family, 691
    pain and, 968, 969*t*
    in preschoolers, 623
Coping/stress-tolerance pattern, 186. *See
    also* Coping behavior; Coping
    mechanisms
    data obtained by, comparison of with
        body systems framework, 359*t*
Copper, 996*t*
Copulation, 727
Cordotomy, 979
Core self-concept, 701

Core temperature, 322. *See also* Body
    temperature
Corn, 522
Cornea
    assessment of, 377
        in elderly, 383
Corneal light reflex test, 380
Corneal sensitivity (reflex) test, 377
Cornstarch bath, 514*t*
Coroner, 157
Corticosteroids, urinary, 1205
Cortisol, in homeostasis, 794
Costal angle, 404
Costal breathing, 342
Cough
    nonproductive, 1100
    productive, 1100
Cough reflex, 1093
Coughing exercises, 873, 1105–1106
    postoperative, 1371
    preoperative teaching, 1356
Counseling, and changing behavior for
    health promotion, 575
Counselor
    in helping relationship, 243
    nurse as, 28–29
Countershock phase, of alarm reaction,
    796
Counting fingers, vision tested by, 379
Cover-uncover patch test, 380
Covert change, 279
Covert data, 175
CPR. *See* Cardiopulmonary resuscitation
Crab lice, 537
Crackles (rales), 403*t*, 1100
Cradle carry, 494
Cramps (menstrual), in adolescents, 644
Cranial nerves, 430*t*. *See also specific
    type*
    assessment of, 429
Craniosacral division of autonomic ner-
    vous system, in homeostasis, 792–
    793
Cravat binder, application of, 1319
Cream, 1251*t*
    vaginal, 1301
Creatinine, urinary, 1205
Creatinine clearance test, 1205
Creatinine excretion, 1008
Creative thinking, in implementing
    nursing care, 227
Credentialing, 146–148
    nursing practice affected by, 42
    principles of, 147*t*
Credé's maneuver/method, in urinary
    retention, 1212
Credibility, in verbal communication,
    249
Creed, in nursing code of ethics, 132
Creighton On-Line Multiple Modular
    Expert Systems, 48
Crepitations, 403, 1100
"Crib death", 615
Crib net, 499

Crimes (criminal actions), 145
    and liability in nursing, 151–152
    reporting, 153
Criminal law, 144, 145*t*
Crisis
    developmental, behaviors associated
        with, 703–704*t*
    family experiencing, 694–695
    of fever, 327
    loss as, 816–817
Crisis centers, 109
Criteria
    in measuring quality care, 238
    outcome. *See* Outcome criteria
    reliable, 238
    testing, 238
    valid, 238
Critical thinking
    in diagnostic process, 192
    in implementing, 227
Crown, 528
Crown-to-rump length, 601
Crust, 371*t*
Crutch stance, 929–930
Crutches, 926–933
    exercises for walking with, 928, 929*f*,
        929*t*
    gaits for walking with, 928–933
    and getting into chair, 932
    and getting out of chair, 932
    going down stairs with, 933
    going up stairs with, 932–933
    measuring clients for, 927–928
    muscles used in walking with, 929*t*
    teaching about use of, 928
Crying
    infants and, 614
    as response to stress, 802
Cryoprecipitate, 1080*t*
Crystalloids, 1039
CT scan. *See* Computed tomography
Cues, and comparing data against stan-
    dards or norms, 193–194
Cultural assimilation, 744–745
Culture. *See also* Ethnic group (ethnic
    affiliation); Race
    application of nursing process and,
        764–772
    assessment and, 765–770
    characteristics of, 745
    and clinical guidelines for client
        interaction, 772
    definition of, 744
    disease susceptibility and, 748
    diversity of North American society
        and, 745–748
    evaluating care and, 771–772
    family and, 688, 747
    folk healing and, 748–749
    food and nutritional practices and,
        747–748, 1002, 1003
    health care services affected by, 106
    health related factors and, 750–753*t*
    health status affected by, 91

Ethnoscience, 745
Ethyl alcohol. *See* Alcohol
Etiologic agent
  in chain of infection, 458
  and nursing interventions to break
    chain of infection, 460*t*
Etiology, definition of, 452–453
Eudaemonistic model of health, 85
Eupnea, 342, 1097, 1100
Eustachian tube, 383
Euthanasia, and legal aspects of nursing
    practice, 155
Evaluating, 169, 230–240. *See also specific subject and* Self-evaluation
  abilities needed for, 168*t*
  accountabilities related to, 171
  activities of, 167*t*
  collecting data for, 231
  communication, 263, 263–265*t*
  definition of, 231
  groups, 272, 273*t*
  identifying outcome criteria and, 231
  judging goal achievement and, 231,
    232–233*t*
  knowledge needed for, 168*t*
  learning, 293–294
  and modifying care plan, 234–235,
    236–237*t*
  process of, 231–235
  purpose of, 167*t*
  quality of nursing care, 235–239
    approaches to, 235–238
    historical perspective of, 235
    tools and methods for, 238–239
  and reexamining care plan, 234
  and relating nursing actions to client
    outcomes, 234
  SOAP format and, 311
  teaching, 293–294
Eversion, 842*t*
  foot, 857*t*
Evisceration, wound
  healing complicated by, 1308
  postoperative, 1369*t*
Examining. *See also* Physical assessment
  for data collection, 181–186
Exanthema, 462
Exception, charting by, 311
Excitement phase of sexual response
    cycle, 728
  physiologic changes associated with,
    728*t*
Excoriation, 371*t*
  at pressure area, 861
Excretion, drug, 1256
Excretions, 1037
  electrolyte composition of, 1039*t*
Exercise. *See also* Activity; Activity-exercise pattern
  in adolescents, 643
  aerobic, 653
  benefits of, 653*t*
  blood pressure affected by, 346
  body temperature affected by, 324

and cardiovascular problems of
    immobility, 872
  coughing, 873, 1105–1106
    postoperative, 1371
    preoperative teaching, 1356
  for crutch walking, 928, 929*f*, 929*t*
  deep breathing, 873, 1105–1106
    postoperative, 1371
    preoperative teaching, 1356
  diaphragmatic-abdominal, 873
  in elderly, 677–678
  fecal elimination affected by, 1158,
    1166
    immobility and, 874
  isometric, 866
  isotonic, 866
  leg
    postoperative, 1371
    preoperative teaching, 1355–1356
  and metabolic/nutritional problems
    of immobility, 873
  for middle-aged adults, 660–661
  and neurosensory problems of
    immobility, 874
  oxygenation affected by, 1096
  preambulatory, 924
  preparations for, 654*t*
  pulse rate affected by, 335
  range of motion
    active, 866
    active-assistive, 867–872
    passive, 866–867, 868–872*f*
  resistive, 872
  and respiratory problems of immobility, 873
  in school-age children, 632
  and urinary/endocrine problems of
    immobility, 873–874
  in young adults, 653–654
Exhalation, 342, 343*f*
Exhaustion stage, in stress adaptation,
    796
Expanded role, 13–14. *See also specific
    type*
Expectoration, for sputum collection,
    1101
Experimentation, in problem solving, 76
Expert power, 51
Expert witness, nurse as, 146
Expiration, 342, 343*f*. *See also*
    Respiration
Expiratory reserve volume, 1091, 1092*f*,
    1092*t*
Exploratory surgery, 1349
Exploring, in helping relationship, 245
Expression, facial, in nonverbal communication, 250
Expressive aphasia, 428
Expressive language skill, in toddlers,
    617
Extended family, 684
Extension, 842*t*
  of ankle, 856*t*
  of elbow, 854*t*

of fingers, 854*t*
  of hip, 855*t*
  of knee, 856*t*
  of neck, 852*t*
  of shoulder, 852*t*, 853*t*
  of thumb, 855*t*
  of toes, 857*t*
  of trunk, 857*t*
  of wrist, 854*t*
Extensor reflexes, 886
External cardiac compression, 1131,
    1138–1141
External ear canal, 382, 383*f*
  assessment of, 384–387
    findings in, 387*t*
    procedure for, 385–386
External limitations, outcome criteria
    and, 211
External respiration, 342
Extinction
  assessment of, 437
  and behavioral conditioning, 589
Extracellular fluid, 1036–1037, 1048*t*
  deficit of, 1043–1044, 1048*t*. *See also*
    Fluid volume deficit
  excess of, 1044, 1048*t*. *See also* Fluid
    volume excess
Extract, 1251*t*
Extraocular muscles, 379*f*
  testing, 379–380
Extrapolating, in generating nursing
    strategies, 212
Extremities
  lower, fine motor tests for, 433–435
    findings in, 434*t*
  upper, fine motor tests for, 433, 435*f*
    findings in, 434*t*
Extrinsic value, 125
Exudates, 455, 1307
  fluid loss and, 1043
  in inflammation, 455
  purulent, 455
  sanguineous (hemorrhagic), 455
  serosanguineous, 1307
  serous, 455
Eye(s), 539–545. *See also under Visual
    and* Vision
  artificial, 544
  assessment of, 374–381, 382*t*, 539,
    540
  "black", 375
  care of
    evaluating, 545
    general, 544–545
    implementing, 540–545
    planning, 540
  in elderly, 383, 668
  external structures of, 375*f*
    assessment of, 376–378
    in elderly, 383
  and infection protection, 453
  internal structures of, 375*f*
    assessment of, 380–381, 382*t*
    in elderly, 383

Hypotonic solution, 1039
  enema with, 1170
Hypoventilation, 342, 1097, 1098, 1100
Hypovolemia, 1043
Hypovolemic shock, 1043–1044
  postoperative, 1367t
Hypoxemia, 1096, 1101
  oxygen therapy in, 1118
Hypoxia, 1097, 1101
Hypoxic drive, 1095
Hypoxic hypoxia, 1097

I & O. See Intake and output record
    (twenty-four hour fluid balance
    record)
Iatrogenic disease, medications and,
    1254
Iatrogenic factors, infection and, 463
IC. See Inspiratory capacity
ICD. See International Classification of
    Diseases
Ice bag, 1339
ICN. See International Council of Nurses
ICT. See Intracellular fluid
Id, 586
Ideal self, 702
Identification
  as defense mechanism, 803t
  in preschoolers, 623
Identity
  gender, 720–721
  in self-concept, 702
    stressors affecting, 707
  and self-esteem in children and ado-
    lescents, 713
  sexual, 721
Idiosyncratic drug effect, 1254
IgA, 457t
  secretory, in defense against microor-
    ganisms, 453
IgD, 457t
IgE, 457t
IgG, 457t
IgM, 457t
Ileal (ileo) conduit/loop/bladder, 1196
Ileostomy, 1173
  anatomic location of, 1174
Illicit drugs, 1254
Illness, 94–98
  behaviors, 94–98
  in children, 98
  definition of, 86, 88f
  drug action affected by, 1256
  in elderly, 98
  family members affected by, 97–98,
    694
  fluid and electrolyte balance affected
    by, 1043
  health continuum and, 89, 90f
  of parents, 98
  present, in nursing health history,
    356–357
  prevention of, 563. See also Health,
    promotion of

sensory stimulation affected by, 1235
sexual motivation affected by, 731
sleep patterns affected by, 945–946
Illness period, of infection, 462
Imagery, guided, in pain control, 974,
    975
Imagination, in preschoolers, 623
Imitation, 590
Immediate postanesthetic care, 1365
Immediate recall, assessment of, 428
Immobility, 839–881. See also Impaired
    physical mobility; Mobility
  assessment of, 851–863
  cardiovascular system affected by,
    843–844, 858t, 872–873
  degrees of, 842
  endocrine system affected by, 846–
    847, 859t, 873–874
  evaluating care and, 878
  fecal elimination affected by, 847,
    859t, 874
  implementing care and, 865–878
  integumentary system affected by,
    510, 847, 860t, 875–878. See also
    Pressure sores
  metabolism affected by, 845–846,
    859t, 873
  musculoskeletal system affected by,
    843, 858t, 865–872
  neurosensory system affected by,
    847–848, 860t, 874
  nursing diagnoses related to, 863–
    864, 900, 900–901, 901t
  nutrition affected by, 845–846, 859t,
    873
  physiological responses to, 843–848
  planning care and, 864–865
  problems of
    assessing, 858, 858–860t
    preventing, 865–875
  psychosocial responses to, 848, 860t,
    874–875
  reasons for, 841
  respiratory system affected by, 844–
    845, 858–859t, 873
  skin affected by, 510, 847, 860t, 875–
    878. See also Pressure sores
  urinary system affected by, 846–847,
    859t, 873–874
Immoral act, 595
Immune globulins, for transfusion,
    1080t
Immune response. See also Immunity
  primary, 457
  secondary (booster), 457
Immunity, 456–458
  active, 456
  cellular, 457–458
  humoral (circulating), 456–457
  passive, 456
  types of, 456t
Immunizations, 465
  for adolescents, 641
  for elderly, 674

for infants, 610–611
for preschoolers, 625
schedule for, 610t, 611t
for school-age children, 630–631
for toddlers, 618
for young adults, 649–651
Immunoglobulins, 456. See also specific
    type under Ig
Impaired adjustment, 823, 824
Impaired gas exchange, 1060, 1103,
    1104t
  immobility and, 863
  outcome criteria for, 1104
Impaired home maintenance manage-
    ment, 692, 693
  mobility status and, 900, 901t
  sensory/perceptual alteration and,
    1238
Impaired physical mobility, 900, 901t
  in dying client, 829t
  foot care and, 524
  pain and, 972
Impaired skin integrity, 511
  fecal elimination and, 1165
  foot care and, 524, 525t
  hair and scalp problems and, 537
  immobility and, 864
  nutrition and, 1012
  sensory/perceptual alteration and,
    1238
  urinary elimination problems and,
    1206, 1207
  wounds and, 1311
Impaired tissue integrity, 511
  nose problems and, 549
  oral hygiene and mouth problems
    and, 531
Impaired verbal communication, 257,
    770
  sensory/perceptual alteration and,
    1238
Imperforate hymen, 731
Implantable venous access device,
    1069–1070
Implementing, 169, 223–229. See also
    specific subject
  abilities needed for, 168t
  accountabilities related to, 171
  activities of, 167t, 228
  definition of, 224
  and determining the need for assis-
    tance, 226
  knowledge needed for, 168t
  nursing actions in, 224–225
    communicating, 227
  of nursing strategies, 226–227
    guidelines for, 228
  process of, 225–227
  protocols and, 224–225
  purpose of, 167t
  and reassessing the client, 226
  skills for, 227–228
  SOAP format and, 311
  standing orders and, 224–225

Laboratory and diagnostic tests (special studies), 1381–1401. *See also specific type*
  in infection, 464
  infection risk affected by, 462
  as source of data, 176–177
Labyrinthine sense, 885
Laceration, 1305
Lack of interest, communication affected by, 254
Lacrimal apparatus, 375*f*
  assessment of, 377
Lacrimal gland, palpation of, 377*f*
Lacrimal sac, palpation of, 377*f*
Lacrimal tearing, drugs causing, 1253*t*
Lactase, 988*t*
Lacto-ovo-vegetarians, 999*t*
  dietary recommendations for, 1001
Lacto-vegetarians, 999*t*
  dietary recommendations for, 1001
Lactoferrin, in defense against microorganisms, 453
Ladder programs in nursing, 16
Laissez-faire, values transmission and, 127
Laissez-faire leadership, 31
Langerhans, islands of, 794
Language
  assessment of, 427
  changing patterns of, 712
  cultural and ethnic background affecting, 746–747
    assessment and, 769
  development of, 254–256
    assessing, 256
    bilingualism affecting, 255
    factors affecting, 255–256
    intelligence affecting, 255
    parental stimulation and, 256
    phases of, 254–255
    sex affecting, 255
    socioeconomic components of, 256
    and status as single child or twin, 255
    stimulating in children, 256
  in preschoolers, 623, 627
  in toddlers, 617
Large intestine, 1155–1156
  common bacteria in, 454*t*
Large-volume nebulizer, 1107
Laryngoscopy, 1384–1387
  nursing interventions for, 1385*t*
Larynx, infection of, common signs and symptoms of, 464*t*
LAS. *See* Local adaptation syndrome
Latchkey children, 686
Late adulthood, 665–682. *See also* Elderly persons
Lateral position, 909–910
  body pressure areas in, 850*f*
  procedure for supporting client in, 910
  turning client to, 914, 915–916
Laughing, as response to stress, 802

Lavage. *See also* Irrigations
  wound, 1328, 1329–1330
Law. *See also under Legal* and Legislation
  civil, 144, 145–146
  common, 144
  contract, 144, 145*t*, 148
  definition of, 143
  functions of in nursing, 143
  principles of, 144–145
  to protect nurses, 157–158
  source of, 143
  statutory, 143
  types of, 144, 145*t*
Lawsuit, 145–146
Laxatives, 1158
  administering, 1168–1169
  nutrition affected by, 1005*t*
  overuse of, 1159
    by elderly, 677
  types of, 1168*t*
Lazarus's model of stress, 796–798
Lead poisoning, 618–619
Leader, nurse as, 30–32
Leadership, 30. *See also* Management
  effective, 32
  styles of, 31
    in group dynamics, 270
Leading questions, for interviewing, 178
Leads, general, in therapeutic communication, 261
Learning. *See also* Teaching
  affective domain of, 283
  barriers to, 291*t*
  change and, 278–280
    acceptance of, 280, 281
    resistance to, 280–281
  cognitive domain of, 283
  domains of, 283
  evaluating, 293–294
  facilitating, 278–281, 281–282
  factors affecting
    facilitation, 281–282
    inhibition, 282–283
  observational, 590
  principles of, 281–283
  psychomotor domain of, 283
  Skinner's theory of, 589
  styles of, assessment of, 285
  theories of, 278
Learning needs, 278
  identifying, 284
  setting priorities for, 286
Leg blood pressure, 348. *See also* Blood pressure
Leg exercises
  postoperative, 1371
  preoperative teaching, 1355–1356
Leg positioning, protective, 872–873
Legal actions, kinds of, 145
Legal concepts. *See also* Law; Legislation
  general, 143–146
Legal document, client record as, 154, 298

Legal responsibilities, 145
  of nurses, 150*t*, 158–159
  of student nurses, 160
Legal rights, 145
  of nurse, 150*t*
Legislation, 143–144, 145*t*. *See also under Legal* and Law
  changes in, nursing practice affected by, 41–42
  nursing regulated by, 146–148
Legitimate power, 51
Leininger, Madeleine
  care and caring defined by, 71–72*t*
  nursing theory of, 4*t*
Length, at birth, 601
Lentigines, senile, 372
Lentigo senilis, 666
Lesbian family, 687–688
"Let the master answer", 149
Leukocyte count, differential, 1102
Leukocytes, in inflammation, 455
Leukocytosis, in inflammation, 455
Level of consciousness. *See also* Consciousness, alterations in
  assessment of, 429
    in general survey, 368
    Glasgow Coma Scale for, 429*t*
Lever, 886*t*
  in lifting, 888, 889*f*
Levin tube, 1017
Levine, Myra, nursing theory of, 4*t*
  summary of major units of, 62–63*t*
  and views of health, 83*t*
Lewin, Kurt, change theory of, 279–280, 280*t*
Liability, legal, 148
  insurance and, 158
  potential areas of in nursing, 151–153
Libel, 151
Libido, 586
  changes in, 731–732
Lice (pediculosis), 536–537
Licensed practical nurse (vocational nurse)
  education for, 14
  licensing and, 43
Licensure, 146–147
  titling and, 43
Lidocaine
  for local anesthesia, 1350
  for spinal anesthesia, 1349
Lids. *See* Eyelids
Life-stress review, 572
Life-style
  assessment of, 568
  body mechanics and ambulation affected by, 892
  changes in
    and health promotion, 565, 575
    providing and facilitating support for, 575
  defecation affected by, 1158
  diet affected by, 1003

sources of, 459*t*

transmission of, 459–461, 459*t*
  and nursing interventions to break
    chain of infection, 460*t*
  prevention of, 451–487

Micturition, 1190–1191. *See also* Urinary
    elimination; Voiding

Mid-upper-arm circumference, 1006,
    1007*f*

Midaxillary line, 397

Midclavicular lines, 397

Middle-aged adults, 655–662. *See also*
    Adults
  assessment of, 659–662
    guidelines for, 659
  cognitive development in, 658
  concept of death in, 817*t*, 818
  divorce in, 662
  exercise in, 660–661
  growth and development stages and,
    583*t*
  Havighurst's developmental tasks of,
    585*t*
  health maintenance visits for, 659–
    660
  health promotion and protection for,
    659–662
  loss experience in, 818
  male climacteric in, 656, 661
  menopause in, 661
  moral development in, 658–659
  nutrition in, 660
  physical development in, 656
  psychosocial development in, 657–
    658
  safety in, 660
  self-concept in, 661–662
  sexuality in, 724–725
  sleep patterns in, 945*t*
  spiritual development in, 659, 779*t*
  substance abuse in, 662
  teaching, 293

Midlife crisis, 658

Midsternal line, 397

Midstream urine specimen, collecting,
    1203–1204

MIF. *See* Migration inhibition factor

Migration inhibition factor, 458*t*

Miliaria rubra, 613

Milliequivalent system, 1038

Mind-body relationship, health status
    affected by, 91

Mineral supplements, immobility and,
    873

Mineralocorticoids, in homeostasis, 794

Minerals, 995, 995–996*t*

Mini-nebulizer, 1107

Minim, 1262

Minimal air-leak technique, for inflating
    tracheal tube cuff, 1130

Minimal occluding volume, inflating
    tracheostomy tube cuff to, 1130

Minimizing, and low self-esteem, 707

Minitracheostomy, 1129

Minor surgery, 1349

Minority decisions, in group dynamics,
    270

Minority group, 744

Miosis (constricted pupils), 378

Misdemeanor, 151

Mitered corners, making, 552, 553*f*

Mitosis, 722

Mitt restraint, 497, 498*f*

Mixed hearing loss, 387

Mixing medications, 1274–1276

MLT. *See* Minimal air-leak technique

Mobility, 839–881. *See also* Immobility;
    Impaired physical mobility
  assessment of, 851–863, 894–900
  career, 13
  factors affecting, 840–842
  implementing care and, 902–933
  joint, 840
  limited, and risk of injury, 490
  nursing diagnoses related to, 900–901
  planning care and, 901–902
  pressure sores and, 851

Modeling, 590
  health promotion and, 577
  by preschoolers, 623
  and self-evaluation, 712
  values transmission and, 127

Models, 58. *See also* Conceptual
    frameworks

Moist heat, application of, 1338–1339

Moist transparent wound barriers, 1324
  application of, 1326

Moisture
  pressure sores and, 851
  of skin, 371

Molybdenum, 996*t*

Monocytes, in infection, 464

Monosaccharides, 987

Monotheism, 779

Mons pubis (mons veneris), and erotic
    stimulation, 727

Montgomery straps, 1314

Montgomery's tubercles, 413

Mood. *See also* Affect
  assessment of in general survey, 367
  assessment of in nursing health his-
    tory, 360

Moon face, 374

Moral behavior, 125, 592, 593

Moral development, 126*t*, 592
  in adolescents, 640
  in elderly, 673
  in infants, 604
  in middle-aged adults, 658–659
  in preschoolers, 623
  in school-age children, 629
  theories of, 592–596
  in toddlers, 617
  in young adults, 648

Moral emotion, 593

Moral judgment, 593

Moral life, facets of, 594–595

Moral reasoning, 125

Morality, 592
  definition of, 125

Moralizing, values transmission and, 127

Morbidity, changes in rates of, 100

Mormon church (Church of Jesus Christ
    of Latter-Day Saints)
  basic beliefs of, 782
  death-related beliefs and practices of,
    830*t*

Morning care, 507

Moro reflex, 603

Morphine, continuous infusion of, in
    intractable pain, 978

Mortality, changes in rates of, 99–100

Mortician, 832

Moslem/Muslim (Islam)
  basic beliefs of, 782
  death-related beliefs and practices of,
    830*t*

Motivation, learning affected by, 281–
    282
  assessment and, 284–285

Motor aphasia, 428

Motor development, in infants, 605*t*

Motor function
  assessment of, 432–435
    findings in, 434*t*
  in infant, 603–604
  in preschoolers, 622
  in school-age children, 628
  in toddlers, 617

Mourning, 817

Mouth (oral cavity), 528–536. *See also*
    specific structure
  anatomic structures of, 392*f*
  assessment of, 389–393, 528–530
  common bacteria in, 454*t*
  common problems of, 530
    clients at risk for, 530
  in defense against microorganisms,
    453
  developmental variations of, 528
  in elderly, 392
  evaluating care of, 536
  floor of
    assessment of, 391–392
    lymph nodes of, 393*f*, 394*t*
  implementing care and, 532–535
  nursing diagnoses related to, 530–531
  planning care and, 531
  special care of, 534
    procedure for, 534–535

Mouth-to-mouth rescue breathing,
    1136–1137

Mouth-to-nose rescue breathing, 1137

MOV. *See* Minimal occluding volume

Movement. *See also* Activity
  capabilities and limitations for, assess-
    ment of, 897–898

Moving clients, 914–924. *See also* Posi-
    tioning clients
  in bed, 912–914, 915–919
  between bed and stretcher, 923

(continued)

Moving clients *(continued)*
  between bed and wheelchair, 920,
    921–922
  with mechanical lifter, 923–924
  postoperative, 1371
MT. *See* Minitracheostomy
MUAC. *See* Mid-upper-arm
    circumference
Mucous membranes (mucosa)
  as defense against microorganisms,
    453
  inner lip, assessment of, 389, 391*f*
    findings in, 390*t*
  oral, altered. *See* Altered oral mucous
    membrane
Multidimensional Health Locus of Con-
    trol, 570
Mummy restraint, 499
Murmurs (heart), 405
Muscle activity. *See also* Activity;
    Movement
  body temperature affected by, 323
  metabolism affected by, 987
  voluntary, 886
Muscle strength
  assessment of, 567
  grading, 427*t*
  tests of, 426*t*
Muscle tone, 426
  loss of in impending death, 825
  voiding affected by, 1192
Musculoskeletal system
  assessment of, 426–427
  changes in
    in elderly, 427, 667
    in middle-aged adult, 656*t*
  disorders of, body mechanics and
    ambulation affected by, 892–893
  immobility affecting, 843, 858*t*, 865–
    872
Muslim/Moslem (Islam)
  basic beliefs of, 782
  death-related beliefs and practices of,
    830*t*
Mustache care, 539
Mutual masturbation, 727
Mutual supplementation, 1000
Mydriasis, 378
Myelography, 1396, 1398*t*
Myoclonus, nocturnal, 950
Myopia, 620
  in preschoolers, 622

Na⁺. *See* Sodium
Nails, 526–528
  assessment of, 373–374, 526, 527
  clubbing of, 373
  in elderly, 374, 666
  ingrown, on toe, 522
  parts of, 373*f*
  spoon-shaped, 373
  trimming, 528
NANDA. *See* North American Nursing
    Diagnosis Association

Narcolepsy, 947
Narcotic agonist-antagonist, 976
Narcotics
  administration of, 976
    oral, 1269
  oxygenation affected by, 1096
Narrative charting, 306, 310*f*
Nasal cannula (nasal prongs), for oxy-
    gen administration, 1119–1120
Nasal cavities, assessment of, 388–389
Nasal instillations, 1299
Nasal passages
  common bacteria in, 454*t*
  in defense against microorganisms,
    453
Nasal speculum, 388
Nasogastric tube
  insertion of, 1023–1025
  irrigating, 1373, 1376
  removing, 1028
Nasogastric/nasointestinal feedings,
    1017–1028
  administering, 1025–1027
  clinical guidelines for, 1021
  formulas for, 1018–1020*t*
  inserting tube for, 1023–1025
  problems of, 1021–1023
  removing tube for, 1028
Nasolacrimal duct, palpation of, 377*f*
Nasopharyngeal suctioning, 1114–1117
Nasopharyngeal tubes, 1123–1124
National League for Nursing, 18, 1407
National Student Nurses Association, 18,
    1407
Native Americans (American Indians),
    749–755
  death-related beliefs and practices of,
    830*t*
  health-related factors and, 750*t*
  nursing implications for care of, 755
Natriuresis, immobility and, 846
Nausea
  drugs causing, 1253*t*
  postoperative, 1368*t*
Near vision, testing, 378
Nearsightedness, 375
Nebulization, 1107
Nebulizers, 1107–1108
Neck
  assessment of, 393–396, 852*t*
    in elderly, 396
  lymph nodes of, 393*f*, 394*t*
    assessment of, 394–395
  muscles of, 393*f*
    assessment of, 393–394
  range of motion of, 852*t*
  structures of, 393*f*
Needle recappers, 1271, 1272*f*
Needles, 1271
Needs
  human, 67–71. *See also* Human needs
  learning, 278
    identifying, 284
    setting priorities for, 286

physiologic, of dying client, 828, 829*t*
Negative feedback, in homeostasis, 792
Negative reinforcement, and learning
    motivation, 285
Negligence, 152
Neighborhood environment, assessment
    of in nursing health history, 360
Neonate. *See* Newborn
Neospinothalamic tract, in pain trans-
    mission, 961–962
Nephron, 1188, 1189*f*
Nerve block, 1349
  in pain control, 978
Nerve fibers, in pain transmission, 961
Nervous system. *See* Neurologic system
Neuman, Betty, nursing theory of, 4*t*
  summary of major units of, 62–63*t*
  and views of health, 83–84*t*
Neurectomy, 979
Neuritic plaque, 672
Neurofibrillary tangle, 672
Neurogenic bladder, 1194
Neurologic system
  assessment of, 427–437
  changes in in elderly, 437, 667
  disorders of, body mechanics and
    ambulation affected by, 892–893
  immobility affecting, 847–848, 860*t*,
    874
Neutral questions, for interviewing, 178
Neutrophils, in infection, 464
Newborn (neonate). *See also* Infant
  body alignment in, 897*t*
  fluid percentage of body weight in,
    1037*t*
  growth and development stages and,
    582*t*
  language development in, 254*t*
  sleep patterns in, 945*t*
  vital signs in, 325*t*
Niacin, 993*t*
Nicotine, use of in adolescents, 645–646
Nicotinic acid, 993*t*
Night terrors, 948
Nightingale, Florence, 3, 5
  views of health of, 84*t*
Nipples, assessment of, 413–424
Nitrogen balance, 991, 1007–1008
NLN. *See* National League for Nursing
No code order, 155–156
"No heroics" order, 156
Nociceptor, 959
Nocturia, 1193, 1199*t*
Nocturnal Cannula, for oxygen adminis-
    tration, 1123
Nocturnal emissions, in adolescents,
    643, 948
Nocturnal enuresis, 948
  in school-age children, 632
Nocturnal erections, in adolescents, 948
Nocturnal frequency, in elderly, 669
Nocturnal myoclonus, 950
Nodule, 371*t*
Noise, excessive, as health hazard, 502

Nursing diagnoses (continued)
  historical perspective of, 165, 199–200
  learning needs and, 285–286
  medical diagnoses differentiated from, 191
  possible, 198
  potential, 198
  taxonomy of, 200–202, 1411–1412
  writing, 197–198, 199t
Nursing gerontology, 666
Nursing health history, 186, 356–360. See also specific subject
  preoperative, 1351–1352
Nursing leadership, 30
Nursing models. See Conceptual frameworks
Nursing orders, 214–215
  with rationale, 216–217t
Nursing organizations. See Professional nursing organizations
Nursing practice, 9–14. See also Nursing
  change and, 38–40
  education and, 42–44
  factors influencing, 40–42
  legal facets of, 153–157
  legal responsibilities in, 158–159
  research and, 44–47
  standards of, 11–12, 148
    American Nurses' Association, 12t
    Canadian Nurses' Association, 12t
  unsafe, reporting, 153
Nursing process, 164–173. See also specific step
  abilities needed for, 168t
  activities of, 167t
  benefits of, 170–171
  characteristics of, 171
  components of, 166–170
  decision-making process compared with, 77t
  evolution of, 165–166t
  historical perspective of, 165
  and interrelationship with client and nurse, 167f
  introduction to, 164–173
  knowledge needed for, 168t
  medical process compared with, 170t
  problem-solving process compared with, 76t
  purposes of, 167t
  scientific method compared with, 76t
  teaching process compared with, 283t
Nursing research, 44–47
  on adults' definition of health, 85
  on career plans, 13
  on children's attitudes about alcohol, 633
  client records as source of data for, 298
  on clients likely to fall, 497
  on client's understanding of medical terminology, 284
  on client's vocabulary, 248

computers as tools in, 48–49
on culturally different client, 772
on effect of motherhood on development, 647
on effect of walking on fatigue in elderly, 678
on enterostomal nurse's impact, 1176
examples of studies, 44t
on hand decontamination practices, 468
on health promotion in family, 693
on health promotion practices of nursing students, 576
on homosexual clients, 724
on incident reports, 154
on insulin mixing by patient, 1275
on intershift reports, 316
on intravenous tubing changes, 1079
on intuition in nursing, 75
and investigative functions of nurses, 33–34t
on lifting methods, 889
on nurse's personal pain experience, 969
on nurses response to moral dilemmas, 136
on nursing behaviors affecting client satisfaction, 238
on nursing diagnosis use, 200
on nursing strategies, 213
on Opsite for decubitus ulcers, 877
on patient-controlled analgesia, 978
priorities for, 8
and protecting rights of human subjects, 45–47
on relaxation training in pain perception, 1353
on roles of faculty versus students, 27
on self-esteem in elderly, 714
on sleep patterns in elderly, 946
on smoking among nursing students, 1096
on spiritual care, 786
steps in, 45t
on stress and burnout, 795
on taste sensation changes in cancer, 1241
Nursing shortage, nursing practice affected by, 40
Nursing strategies, 211–214
  alternative, generating, 212, 213t
  choosing, 213–214
  consequences of, 213
  implementing, 226–227
    guidelines for, 228
  planning, 211–214
Nutrient solutions, in intravenous fluid therapy, 1063
Nutrient-drug interactions, 1005t
Nutrients, 987–995, 995–996t. See also specific type
  definition of, 986
Nutrition, 985–1034. See also Diet; Feeding; Food

for adolescents, 643
altered. See Altered nutrition
assessment of status of, 567, 1005–1010
body mechanics and ambulation affected by, 891
clinical signs indicating status of, 1008
community services and, 1017
counseling about, 1013
cultural and ethnic background affecting customs associated with, 747–748
  assessment of, 770
definition of, 986
for elderly, 675–676
enteral, 873. See also Tube feedings
evaluating care and, 1030
health status and, 1004
immobility affecting, 845–846, 859t, 873
implementing care and, 1012–1030
for infants, 613–614
infection risk affected by, 462
metabolism and, 986–987
for middle-aged adults, 660
nursing diagnoses related to, 1010–1011, 1011–1012
for older adults, 1000, 1001
parenteral, 873
planning care and, 1012
preoperative, 1357–1358
for preschoolers, 625
pressure sores and, 851
risk for problems with, 1010
for school-age children, 631–632
skin affected by, 510
and supporting body defenses, 465
surgical risk affected by, 1351
for toddlers, 620
total parenteral, 1085
wound healing and, 1307
for young adults, 652–653
Nutritional assessment, 567, 1005–1010
Nutritional history, 1008–1010
  in nursing health history, 357–358
Nutritional-metabolic pattern, 186
  data obtained by, comparison of with body systems framework, 359t
Nutritionist, as member of health care team, 112
Nutritive value, 986
Nutting, Mary Adelaide, 5
Nycturia, 1193
Nystagmus, 379

O₂ Sat. See Oxygen saturation
Oatmeal bath, 514t
Obesity, 1011
  in adolescents, 643
  blood pressure affected by, 345t, 346
  wound healing and, 1307
Objective data, 175, 306
Objectives, learning, 286
Obligatory fluid loss, 1041

Positive affect, in humanizing health care, 120
Positive feedback, in homeostasis, 792
Positive reinforcement, and learning motivation, 285
Positivism, in verbal communication, 249
Possum response, 798
Post-formal operations thinkers, 648
Postanesthetic care, immediate, 1365
Postanesthetic room, 1365
Postauricular lymph nodes (mastoid lymph nodes), 393*f*, 394*t*
Posterior axillary line, 397
Posterior tibial pulse
    location of, 335*f*, 336
    reasons for using, 336*t*
Postmortem examination, 157, 832
Postoperative bed (surgical bed), 1364
    making, 556, 1364–1365
Postoperative check list, 1366*f*
Postoperative cholangiography, 1397*t*
Postoperative phase, 1347, 1365–1376
    assessment during, 1365–1369
    depression during, 1369*t*
    evaluating care and, 1373
    implementing care and, 1371–1373, 1373–1376
    nursing diagnoses related to, 1370
    planning care and, 1370–1371
    potential problems during, 1367–1369*t*
    preparing for, 1363–1364
Postural drainage, 1111, 1112–1114*t*
    immobility and, 873
Postural hypotension (orthostatic hypotension), immobility and, 843–844
Postural reflexes, 885–886
Postural tonus, 885
Posture, 883. *See also* Body alignment
    assessment of in general survey, 367
    in nonverbal communication, 250
    problems of, 902–903
    in school-age children, 627
Potassium, 995*t*, 1046, 1049*t*
    in excretions/secretions/plasma, 1039*t*
    nutrition affected by, 1005*t*
Potassium permanganate bath, 514*t*
Poverty. *See also* Economic status
    culture of, 762–763
        health-related factors and, 752*t*
    and families at risk for health problems, 692
    health care services affected by, 107
Powder, 1251*t*
    application of, 1294*t*
    in skin care, 513*t*
    for wound dressing, 1322*t*
Powdered drugs in vials, 1272
    preparing, 1274
Power
    in group dynamics, 272
    professional change through, 51

Power-coercive strategies, to implement change, 38
Powerlessness, 709, 770
    dying client and, 826, 827
    immobility and, 864
    oxygenation and, 1103
PPO. *See* Preferred provider organization
PPS. *See* Prospective payment system
Practical nurse (vocational nurse)
    education for, 14
    licensing and, 43
Practical nursing programs, 14
Practice Acts. *See* Nurse Practice Acts
Praise, and positive self-evaluation, 712
Prayer
    Native American, 754
    as response to stress, 802
Preambulatory exercises, 924
Preauricular lymph nodes, 393*f*, 394*t*
Precoital stimulation, 726
Precordium
    anatomic sites of, 406*f*
    inspection and palpation of, 406
Preferred provider organization, 109
Pregnancy
    adolescent, 644
    breast changes during, 412
    sexual motivation affected by, 731–732
Prehelping phase (introductory phase) of helping relationship, 243–244
    tasks and skills for, 244*t*
Preinteraction phase of helping relationship, 243
    tasks and skills for, 244*t*
Prelinguistic phase of language development, 255
Premature closure, 175
Premature ejaculation, 732
Preoperative checklist, 1357*f*
Preoperative instructions, 1354
Preoperative medications, 1358
Preoperative phase, 1347
    assessment during, 1350–1351
    evaluating care and, 1363
    implementing care and, 1353–1363
    nursing diagnoses related to, 1352
    physical preparation in, 1357–1362
    planning care and, 1352–1353
Preoperative screening tests, 1351, 1352*t*
Preoperative teaching, 1353–1356
Prepuberty, 628
Presbycusis, 668
Presbyopia, 375, 668
Preschoolers, 622–627. *See also* Children
    assessment of, 624–627
        guidelines for, 624
    body alignment in, 897*t*
    cognitive development in, 623
    cognitive stimulation for, 627
    concept of death in, 817*t*
    dental health in, 625

elimination in, 625
goals for, 625*t*
growth and development stages and, 583*t*
health maintenance visits for, 625
health promotion and protection for, 624–627
immunizations in, 625
language development in, 254*t*, 627
moral development in, 623
nursing diagnoses for, 625*t*
nutrition in, 625
physical development in, 622
psychosocial development in, 622–623
rest/sleep in, 625–626
safety and, 625, 626*t*
sense of self in, 626–627
sleep patterns in, 945*t*
social interaction and, 627
spiritual development in, 623–624, 778*t*
and stimulation through play, 627
teaching, 293
Prescription, 1250. *See also* Medication order
    parts of, 1261
Present illness, in nursing health history, 356–357
Pressure areas, 850*f*
    assessment of, 860–861
    breakdown of, risk assessment form for, 861*t*
Pressure gradient, blood pressure and, 345
Pressure sores (pressure ulcers), 848–851
    and body pressure areas, 850*f*
    categories of, 849–851
    causes of, 848–849
    clients at risk for, 860–861, 862*t*
    factors affecting formation of, 851
    prevention of, 875–877
        mechanical devices for, 876
    stages of, 849–851
    treatment of, 877–878
Pressures
    partial. *See* Partial pressures
    pulmonary, 1092–1094
Prevention
    of injury. *See* Safety
    levels of, 563
Preventive health services, 564
Prickly heat, 613
Primary care, agencies providing, 108–109
Primary groups, 265–266
Primary intention healing, 1306
Primary nursing, as model for delivery of nursing care, 11
Primary prevention, 563
Primary sexual characteristics, development of during puberty, 638–639
Principled reasoning, 648

(continued)

acidification of, and urinary/endocrine problems of immobility, 874
altered production of, 1193
assessment of, 1199–1202
characteristics of, 1199–1202
  normal and abnormal, 1200*t*
collecting specimen of, 1203–1205
  clean catch, 1203–1204
  from retention catheter, 1222
culture and sensitivity tests of, 1203
discoloration of, selected causes of, 1201*t*
fluid loss and, 1041–1042
osmolality of, 1058
output of, 1199, 1200*t*
  in infants, 614
pH of, 1058, 1200*t*, 1202
specific gravity of, 1058, 1200*t*, 1201–1202
timed specimen of, 1205
Urine urea nitrogen, 1007–1008
Urinometer (hydrometer), 1201, 1202*f*
Urobilinogen, urinary, 1205
Urogenital tract. *See* Genitourinary system
Urography, intravenous, 1387, 1398*t*
Utilitarianism, 137
Uvula, 392*f*
  assessment of, 390*t*, 392

V scan, 1102
Vaccines, for immunization, 610
Vagina
  assessment of, 441
  common bacteria in, 454*t*
  in defense against microorganisms, 453
  in elderly, 442, 669
  microbial colonization of, 453
Vaginal diaphragm, for contraception, 736–737, 738*f*
Vaginal irrigations and instillations, 1299–1301
Vaginal speculum examination, 440–441
Vaginal sponge, for contraception, 737
Vaginismus, 733
Vaginitis, atrophic, in menopause, 661
Vagus nerve (tenth cranial nerve), function and assessment methods of, 430*t*
Validation, consensual, in therapeutic communication, 260
Valsalva maneuver
  and bedfast clients, 843, 872
  and straining in order to defecate, 1159–1160
Valuables, care of during surgery, 1358
Value conflicts, 132
Value set, 126
Value system
  definition of, 125
  in nursing models, 59–60
Value-belief pattern, 186

Values, 126–132
  acquisition of, 126–127
  being, 68
  body mechanics and ambulation affected by, 892
  client
    identifying, 130–132
    priority setting and, 208
  and clinical nursing practice, 128
  definition of, 125
  personal, 127–128
    identifying, 129–130
  professional, 127–128
  of professional nursing, 24–25
  societal, 128
  transmission of, 127–128
  unclear, behaviors indicating, 131
Values clarification, 128–129
  strategy for, 130
Vaporization, heat loss by, 324
Variable data, 175
Varicosities, of tongue, in elderly, 392
Vascular sounds, abdominal, auscultating for, 418–419
Vascular system
  peripheral
    assessment of, 408–411
    in elderly, 411
  wound healing and, 1307
Vasectomy, 737–738
Vasoconstriction
  cold causing, in wound care, 1334
  peripheral, stimulating, 872
Vasodilation, heat causing, in wound care, 1333, 1334*t*
Vasopressor, in homeostasis, 793
Vastus lateralis site, for intramuscular injection, 1281
VC. *See* Vital capacity
Vector, in transmission of microorganisms, 459–461
Vegans, 999*t*
Vegetarian diets, 999–1000, 1001
Vehicle transmission, in infection, 459
Venipuncture sites for intravenous fluid therapy
  central, 1064–1065
  peripheral, 1063–1064
  selecting, 1072
Venous access devices, implantable, 1069–1070
Venous circulation, altered, skin affected by, 510
Venous pressure, jugular, assessment of, 410
Venous valves, incompetent, immobility and, 844
Ventilation, 342, 1091. *See also* Breathing
Ventilation scan, 1102
Ventral respiratory group, 1095
Ventrogluteal site, for intramuscular injection, 1280–1281

Venturi mask, for oxygen administration, 1121
Verbal abuse, as response to stress, 802
Verbal communication, 247–249
  adaptability in, 249
  clarity in, 248
  credibility in, 249
  impaired. *See* Impaired verbal communication
  relevance in, 248–249
  simplicity in, 247–248
  timing in, 248–249
Verbal orders, and legal responsibility, 159
Verdict, in lawsuit, 145
Verifying, in therapeutic communication, 259–260
Vernix caseosa, 508
Vertebra prominens, 398
Vertebral line, 397
Vertical toe pleat, 555
Vesicle, 371*t*
Vesicostomy, continent, 1196
Vesicular breath sounds, 403*t*
Vestibule, of ear, 383
Vials, 1264, 1271–1272
  fractional dosages from, 1264–1265
  mixing drugs from, 1274–1276
  preparing medications from, 1272–1273
Vibration, for chest physiotherapy, 1110–1111
Vibratory sense, assessing, 436–437
Vicarious reinforcement, 590
Vietnamese Americans, 759
Virchow's triad, immobility and, 844
Virtues
  Erikson's, 593*t*
  hierarchy of, 595
Virulence of microorganisms, 452
Visceral pain, 959. *See also* Pain
Viscosity, blood pressure affected by, 346
Vision. *See also* Visual acuity
  assessment of, 374–381, 382*t*, 1237
  changes in, in elderly, 383, 668
  deficits in, 1235
  distance, testing, 378–379
  near, testing, 378
  in newborn, 602–603
  in preschoolers, 622
  in school-age children, 627–628
  supporting, 1240
  in toddlers, 619–620
Visual acuity. *See also* Vision
  assessment of, 378–379
  in elderly, 383, 668
  in toddlers, 616
Visual aphasia, 428
Visual fields, testing, 379
Visual reflexes, 885
Visual stimuli, 1233
Visualization, and self-evaluation, 712–713

nursing diagnoses related to, 1311
open method of care for, 1312–1314
penetrating, 1305
planning to augment healing of, 1312
postoperative infection of, 1369t
postoperative problems related to,
 1369t
preventing infection of, 1321
puncture, 1305
supporting, 1314–1320
types of, 1305–1306
Wrist, range of motion of, 854t

X rays, 1394. *See also* Roentgenography
Xerography, 1396–1399
Xeromammography, 1396–1399
Xylocaine. *See* Lidocaine

Y-set, for blood transfusion, 1082
Yin and yang, 758

Young adults, 646–655. *See also* Adolescents; Adults
 assessment of, 649–655
  guidelines for, 649
 battered or abused women and, 655
 cognitive development in, 648
 concept of death in, 817t, 818
 divorce and separation and, 655
 Erikson's developmental stages in,
  588t, 646
 exercise for, 653–654
 goals for, 649t
 growth and development stages in,
  583t
 Havighurst's developmental tasks of,
  585t
 health maintenance visits for, 649–
  651
 health promotion and protection for,
  649–655
 immunizations in, 649–651
 loss experience in, 818
 moral development in, 648
 nursing diagnoses for, 649t
 nutrition for, 652–653
 physical development in, 646
 psychosocial development in, 646–
  648
 safety and, 651–652
 sexual concerns of, 654–655
 sexuality in, 724–725
 sleep patterns in, 945t
 spiritual development in, 649, 779t
 substance abuse and, 655
 suicide in, 655
 teaching, 293
 work and career stress in, 654–655

Zinc, 996t